D1326193

Muir's textbook of

PATHOLOGY

Muir's textbook of PATHOLOGY

Thirteenth edition

EDITED BY

Roderick N M MacSween
BSc, MD, FRCPath, FRCP(Glasg & Edin), FRS(E), FIBiol
Professor of Pathology, University of Glasgow

and

Keith Whaley
MD, PhD, FRCP(Lond), FRCPath
Professor of Immunology, University of Leicester; formerly Titular Professor of Immunopathology, University of Glasgow

Edward Arnold
A member of the Hodder Headline Group
LONDON BOSTON MELBOURNE AUCKLAND

First published in Great Britain 1992
Reprinted with corrections, 1993

Distributed in the Americas by Little, Brown and Company
34 Beacon Street, Boston, MA 02108

British Library Cataloguing in Publication Data

MacSween, R. N. M.
Muir's textbook of pathology. – 13th ed.
I. Title II. Whaley, K.
616.07

ISBN 0-340-55145-3

Typeset in Century Old Style by Rowland Phototypesetting Limited, Bury St Edmunds, Suffolk. Printed and bound in Great Britain for Edward Arnold, a division of Hodder Headline PLC, Mill Road, Dunton Green, Sevenoaks, Kent TN13 2YA by Butler & Tanner Limited, Frome and London.

Preface

In his preface in 1924 to the first edition of the textbook with which he has been eponymously linked, Sir Robert Muir wrote:

> The subject of Pathology has now become so extensive that in a book of this size selection of subjects is essential for any satisfactory treatment, and in considering their relative importance I have been guided by two considerations. I have endeavoured, in the first place, to give due weight to the scientific aspect of the general pathological processes and, in the second, to describe those pathological changes in the various organs, which are of special importance in relation to Clinical Medicine and Surgery. The subject-matter thus falls into two main portions corresponding roughly with General and Special Pathology, though these terms are not used, as it seems inadvisable, in a book of this nature, to draw any sharp distinctions.

These remarks remain, in part, apposite some 68 years later as we introduce this thirteenth edition of his textbook. The division into general and systematic sections which Muir reluctantly introduced was accepted in subsequent editions and we have continued with this pattern. The text is divided into a general section comprising 11 chapters, a systematic section comprising 13 chapters; a final chapter deals with parasitic diseases.

In embarking on the daunting task of preparing this new edition we were aware that pathology, the study of disease by scientific methods, had, in the past decade, extended its frontiers to encompass advances in molecular biology which had first been made in the basic sciences as distinct from the more applied medical sciences. These advances are of particular relevance to the teaching of general pathology but will become increasingly important also in helping our understanding of system and organ diseases. The section on general pathology, therefore, has been restructured and almost completely rewritten, emphasizing the impact of cellular and molecular biology on our understanding of disease. We have deliberately sought to have dual or multi-authorship of most chapters. Thus, in the general section, in order to broaden our scope we have had contributions from colleagues in cell biology, clinical chemistry, immunology, immunopathology, medical genetics, microbiology and pharmacology. In addition, clinical colleagues have not only been consulted but have also contributed to this section and to some of the systematic chapters, thus increasing the clinical emphasis.

Chapter 1 deals with the structure and function of normal cells and extracellular matrix and explains how abnormalities may lead to disease. This is followed by a chapter on the genetic basis of inherited disease and the application of recombinant DNA technology to the detection and characterization of these diseases. Haemostasis and its disorders are transferred from the haematology section to the chapter on disturbances of body fluids and blood flow since it is relevant to the discussion of haemorrhage and thrombosis. Inflammation, healing and repair are incorporated into one chapter to emphasize that healing and repair are two of the possible outcomes of the inflammatory response. More attention has also been given to the chemical mediators of inflammation and the role of cytokines in these processes as these are potential areas for therapeutic intervention. Whereas, originally, we intended to have a single chapter covering basic immunology and immunopathology we were unable to condense the massively expanded body of immunological knowledge into a single comprehensive chapter. Thus, as in the twelfth edition, we still have two chapters dealing with these topics. A new chapter on metabolic disorders draws together a miscellaneous group of conditions which, in previous editions, were dealt with in various parts of the systematic pathology section. The chapter on microbial infections describes the host–parasite relationship and the pathology of common microbial infections. As these disorders often affect multiple organ systems and provide valuable examples of disease processes, this format is more appropriate. A full chapter is devoted to nutritional disorders; these, unfortunately, are probably still the commonest diseases of underdeveloped countries. The chapter dealing with growth and neoplasia describes and discusses the pathogenesis of tumours and their clinical behaviour. The last chapter in the general section deals with tissue injury produced by drugs and radiation; these diseases are often iatrogenic in origin. In contrast, drug abuse is usually a self-inflicted disease and the pathological mechanisms and consequences of this are briefly reviewed. The general section is extensively illustrated with some 200 line drawings.

In the systematic section we include diseases of the blood vessels and lymphatics in the chapter on the cardiovascular system. Emphasis is placed on the aetiology of the various diseases, their effects on structure and function and their clinicopathological correlations. Each chapter has been extensively revised and many recent advances have been included. The amount of systematic pathology covered is greater than most medical students require to assimilate during the undergraduate course in pathology, and students will therefore require guidance from their teachers. However, this book should continue to be of value throughout the 'clinical' years of the curriculum and indeed during vocational postgraduate training, not only in histopathology but in many disciplines. In some chapters, in order to provide comprehensive coverage, concise information has been provided in the form of extended tables. In every chapter a brief and limited list of further reading is included.

Glasgow
January 1992

R. N. M. MacSween
K. Whaley

Acknowledgements

We are deeply grateful to our fellow authors for their contributions. It is with much sadness that we record the death of Professor David Flenley; his contribution to Chapter 13 was virtually complete at the time of his death and has been incorporated with minor modifications. We thank all our authors for their tolerant acceptance of our editing of their manuscripts and for keeping to increasingly tight deadlines in order to meet the demand to publish by a specified date. The published text is our final responsibility; we earnestly hope we have achieved the correct balance in terms of content and that we have not introduced errors of fact or judgement.

In addition to named contributors we have received helpful advice from many of our colleagues in this department who have read chapters and commented on the balance of the content. They provided stimulating discussions on a number of topics, advised on lay-out and design and, most painstakingly of all, undertook proof reading duties. They include Dr M. E. Catto, Dr I. Gibson, Dr M. P. MacSween, Dr A. McPhaden and Dr E. A. Mallon. We gratefully acknowledge the contribution of Professor J. R. Anderson, co-editor or editor of the previous four editions. He encouraged us in our task and not only gave us a free hand with text material, but allowed us unrestricted use of many illustrations for this edition. Illustrations provided by colleagues from other departments are acknowledged in the legends. Dr A. J. Krajewski and Dr C. M. Steel kindly advised on some of the illustrations in Chapter 15.

We wish to thank Mr Peter Kerrigan and Mr David McComb who contributed considerably to the preparation of new photographic material. In particular we wish to record our debt to Mr I. Ramsden (University Department of Medical Illustration) for his skilful production of the numerous line diagrams which are a feature of this edition.

We are grateful to Mrs Maureen Ralston, senior academic secretary to the Department, who not only undertook the enormous additional organizational work stemming from revision of such a large multi-author text, but also typed a great deal of the text. In this she was most ably supported by Miss Sandra Howat. To them we owe a very great debt for their tolerance and forbearance in dealing with our editing and frequent re-editing, their intuitive ability to decipher our corrections and, literally, read between the lines, and for their willingness to work extended hours, at all times giving us cheerful encouragement.

It is a pleasure to thank the staff of our publishers Edward Arnold for their enthusiastic co-operation and Mrs Kathy Bayly who did excellent work as copy-editor.

Finally, we wish to thank our families for their support and encouragement over the prolonged period in which we were pre-occupied with 'Muir' and this to the exclusion of normal family life.

Glasgow
January 1992

R. N. M. MacSween
K. Whaley

Contents

Contributors

J. H. Adams DSc, MD, PhD, FRCP(Glasg), FRCPath, FRS(E)
Titular Professor of Neuropathology, The University of Glasgow

A. Barrett MD, FRCR, FRCP
Professor of Radiation Oncology, The University of Glasgow and Director, The Beatson Oncology Centre, Western Infirmary, Glasgow

W. M. H. Behan MD, FRCPath
Senior Lecturer in Pathology, The University of Glasgow

C. C. Bird MB, ChB, PhD, FRCPath, FRCP-(Edin)
Professor of Pathology, The University of Edinburgh

J. D. Briggs MB, ChB, FRCP
Consultant Nephrologist, Western Infirmary, Glasgow and Honorary Clinical Senior Lecturer, The University of Glasgow

R. A. Burnett MB, ChB, FRCPath
Consultant Pathologist, Western Infirmary, Glasgow and Honorary Clinical Senior Lecturer, The University of Glasgow

A. D. Burt BSc, MD, MRCPath
Senior Lecturer in Pathology, The University of Newcastle upon Tyne

J. M. Connor BSc, MD, FRCP(Edin & Glasg)
Professor of Medical Genetics (Burton Chair), The University of Glasgow

W. J. K. Cumming BSc, MD, FRCPI, FRCP
Consultant Neurologist, Alexandra Hospital, Cheadle, Cheshire

H. J. Dargie MB, ChB, FRCP
Consultant Cardiologist, Western Infirmary, Glasgow and Honorary Clinical Senior Lecturer, The University of Glasgow

C. W. Elston MD(Lond), FRCPath
Consultant Histopathologist, City Hospital, Nottingham and Clinical Teacher, University Medical School, Nottingham

D. C. Flenley (deceased) MB, ChB, FRCP(Edin), FRCP(Lond)
Formerly Professor of Respiratory Medicine, The University of Edinburgh

H. Fox MD, FRCPath
Professor of Reproductive Pathology, The University of Manchester

A. K. Foulis BSc, MD, MRCPath
Consultant Pathologist, Royal Infirmary, Glasgow and Honorary Clinical Senior Lecturer, The University of Glasgow

D. I. Graham MB, ChB, PhD, MRCP, FRCPath
Titular Professor of Neuropathology, The University of Glasgow

D. Heath DSc, MD, PhD, FRCP(Lond & Edin), FRCPath
Professor of Pathology, The University of Liverpool

J. M. Kay MD, FRCPC, FRCPath
Professor of Pathology, McMaster University, Hamilton, Ontario, Canada

J. M. Lackie MA, PhD
Director, Yamanouchi Research Institute, Oxford; formerly Senior Lecturer in Cell Biology, The University of Glasgow

F. D. Lee MD, MRCP(Glasg), FRCPath
Consultant Pathologist, Royal Infirmary, Glasgow and Honorary Clinical Professor, The University of Glasgow

W. R. Lee MD, FRCPath
Titular Professor of Ophthalmic Pathology, The University of Glasgow

K. R. Lees BSc, MD, MRCP(UK)
Lecturer in Medicine, Department of Medicine & Therapeutics, The University of Glasgow

G. B. M. Lindop BSc, MB, ChB, MRCPath
Senior Lecturer in Pathology, The University of Glasgow

S. B. Lucas MA, BM, BCh, MRCP, FRCPath
Senior Lecturer in Histopathology, University College Hospital and the London School of Hygiene and Tropical Medicine, the University of London

D. G. MacDonald RD, BDS, PhD, FRCPath, FDSRCPS(Glasg)
Titular Professor of Oral Medicine & Pathology, The University of Glasgow

D. R. McLellan MD, MRCPath
Consultant Pathologist, Victoria Infirmary, Glasgow and Honorary Clinical Senior Lecturer, The University of Glasgow

A. M. McNicol BSc, MD, MRCP(UK), FRCP(Glasg), MRCPath
Reader in Pathology, The University of Glasgow

R. N. M. MacSween BSc, MD, FRCP(Glasg & Edin), FRCPath, FRS(E), FIBiol
Professor of Pathology, The University of Glasgow

I. A. R. More BSc, MD, PhD, MRCPath
Senior Lecturer in Pathology, The University of Glasgow

A. McI. Mowat BSc, MB, ChB, PhD, MRCPath
Senior Lecturer in Immunology, The University of Glasgow

A. Mowat BSc, MB, ChB, MRCPath
Senior Registrar, Department of Pathology, Western Infirmary, Glasgow

T. H. Pennington MB, BS, PhD, FRCPath
Professor of Bacteriology, The University of Aberdeen

I. W. Percy-Robb MB, ChB, PhD, FRCP(Edin), FRCPath
Titular Professor of Pathological Biochemistry, The University of Glasgow

D. Pollock MSc, PhD
Senior Lecturer in Pharmacology, The University of Glasgow

J. L. Reid MA, DM, FRCP(Glasg & Lond)
Regius Professor of Medicine & Therapeutics, The University of Glasgow

R. P. Reid BSc, MB, ChB, MRCPath
Senior Lecturer in Osteoarticular Pathology, The University of Glasgow

R. M. Rowan MB, ChB, FRCP(Glasg & Edin)
Senior Lecturer in Haematology, The University of Glasgow

M. M. Seywright MB, ChB, MRCPath
Consultant Pathologist, Western Infirmary, Glasgow and Honorary Clinical Senior Lecturer, The University of Glasgow

A. Shenkin BSc, MB, ChB, PhD, FRCP(Glasg), FRCPath
Professor of Clinical Chemistry, The University of Liverpool

J. D. Sleigh MB, ChB, FRCPath, FRCP(Glasg)
Professor of Bacteriology, The University of Glasgow

I. D. Walker MD, FRCP(Edin), FRCPath
Consultant Haematologist, Royal Infirmary, Glasgow and Honorary Clinical Senior Lecturer, The University of Glasgow

K. Whaley MD, PhD, MRCPath, FRCP
Professor of Immunology, The University of Leicester; formerly Titular Professor of Immunopathology, The University of Glasgow

A. H. Wyllie PhD, MRCP, FRCPath, FRS(E)
Reader in Pathology, The University of Edinburgh

Introduction

What is Pathology?

Pathology is the study of disease by scientific methods. Disease may, in turn, be defined as an abnormal variation in the structure or function of any part of the body. There must be an explanation of such variations from the normal – in other words, diseases have causes – and pathology includes not only observation of the structural and functional changes throughout the course of a disease, but also elucidation of the factors which cause it. It is only by establishing the cause (aetiology) of a disease that logical methods can be sought and developed for its prevention or cure. Pathology may thus be described as the scientific study of the causes and effects of disease.

Pathology as defined in this way embraces a number of scientific specialties including: (a) histology and cytology in which the structural changes in diseased tissue are examined by naked eye inspection (macroscopic features) or by light and electron microscopy of tissue sections or smears (microscopic features); (b) clinical chemistry, in which the metabolic disturbances of disease are investigated by assay of various normal and abnormal compounds in the blood, urine, etc.; (c) microbiology, in which body fluids, mucosal surfaces, excised tissues, etc. are examined by microscopical, cultural and serological techniques to detect and identify the micro-organisms responsible for many diseases; (d) haematology – investigation of abnormalities of the cells of the blood and their precursors in haemopoietic tissue and of the haemostatic, including the clotting, mechanism; and (e) clinical genetics, in which inherited chromosomal abnormalities in the germ cells or acquired chromosomal abnormalities in somatic cells are investigated using the techniques of molecular biology.

These divisions of pathology have resulted from increasing specialization in techniques and from expanding knowledge within each discipline. They are each, however, of importance in the scientific study of disease. Even a cursory look at any of the systematic chapters in this book will immediately make the student appreciate how closely interlinked the disciplines are and how each variously contributes to our understanding of disease processes. Furthermore, it has to be emphasized that the pathologist, while sometimes removed from immediate patient contact, is nevertheless a clinical specialist who is frequently the first to establish a clinical diagnosis and whose experience is vitally important in clinical management and treatment. There is a compelling need therefore to learn pathology, irrespective of the branch of medicine the student intends to pursue. The pathological sciences are, and will continue to be, among subjects constituting the core course in medical curricula.

Pathological Processes

It was first pointed out by Virchow that all disturbances of function and structure in disease are due to cellular abnormalities and that the phenomena of a particular disease are brought about by a series of cellular changes. Pathological processes are of a dual nature, consisting first of the injurious effects of the causal agent and secondly, of reactive changes which are often closely similar to physiological processes. If death is rapid, as for example in cyanide poisoning, there may be little or no structural changes of either type. Cyanide inhibits the cytochrome-oxidase systems and thus halts cellular respiration before histological changes can become prominent. Similarly, blockage of a coronary artery cuts off the blood supply to part of the myocardium and death may result immediately from cardiac arrest or ventricular fibrillation. When this happens, no structural changes are observed. If, however, the patient survives for some days or more, the affected myocardium shows reactive changes which occur subsequent to cell death and the lesion becomes readily visible both macroscopically (p. 490) and microscopically (p. 493). Reactive changes may also, however, be closely similar to physiological processes. The increase in skeletal muscle size (i.e. hypertrophy) which is readily recognized as a normal adaptive response in the athlete is a similar process to the cardiac enlargement which occurs in the patient with high blood pressure and which, if the blood pressure is not controlled, may lead to cardiac failure. During the normal menstrual cycle the endometrium undergoes considerable increase in bulk by a process of hyperplasia, i.e. increase in cell numbers, but this ceases and the endometrium is shed during menstruation, the whole cycle being under hormonal control. If, however, there is hormonal imbalance then the hyperplasia may become an abnormal reactive response and the endometrium shows microscopic abnormalities.

The changes which are adaptive, as distinct from changes due to injury or those which are due to reaction, are often not as well defined as in the examples given above. Furthermore, the processes involved are often much more complex and this textbook sets out to provide an account of the mechanisms which are involved. In order to help in the understanding of these processes it is of value to introduce here a broad classification of causal factors in disease, citing a few examples.

The Causes of Disease

Causal factors in disease may be genetic or acquired. Genetically-determined disease is due to some abnormality of base sequence in the DNA of the fertilized ovum and the cells derived from it, or to reduplication, loss or misplacement of a whole or part of a chromosome. Such abnormalities are often inherited from one or both parents. Acquired disease is due to the effects of some environmental factor, e.g. malnutrition or micro-organisms. Most diseases are acquired but, very often, there is more than one causal factor and there may be many. Genetic variations may influence the susceptibility of an individual to environmental factors. Even in the case of infections, there is considerable individual variation in the severity of the disease. Of the adults who become infected with hepatitis B virus, most develop immunity without becoming ill, some have a mild illness and a few (less than 10%) develop chronic liver disease which progresses to cirrhosis. This illustrates the importance of host factors as well as causal agents. Spread of tuberculosis is favoured by poor personal and domestic hygiene, by overcrowding, malnutrition and by various other diseases. Accordingly, disease results not only from exposure to the major causal agent but also from the existence of predisposing or contributory factors.

Congenital Disease

Diseases may also be classified into those which develop during fetal life (congenital) and those which arise at any time thereafter during postnatal life. Genetically-determined diseases are commonly congenital, although some present many years after birth, a good example being adenomatous polyposis coli, which is due to an abnormal gene and consists of multiple tumours of the colonic mucosa, appearing in adolescence or adult life. Congenital diseases may also be acquired, an important example being provided by transmission of the virus of rubella (German measles) from mother to fetus during the first trimester of pregnancy. Depending on the stage of fetal development at which infection occurs, it can result in fetal death, or involvement of various tissues leading to mental deficiency, blindness, deafness or structural abnormalities of the heart. The mother can also transmit to the fetus various other infections, including syphilis and toxoplasmosis, with consequent congenital disease. Ingestion of various chemicals by the mother, as in the thalidomide disaster, may induce severe disorders of fetal development and growth. Another cause of acquired congenital disease is maternal–fetal incompatibility. Fetal red cells exhibiting surface antigens inherited from the father can enter the maternal circulation and stimulate antibody production: the maternal antibody may pass across the placenta and react with the fetal red cells, causing a haemolytic anaemia.

Acquired Disease

The major causal factors may be classified as follows:

(1) Deficiency diseases (p. 338). Inadequate diet still accounts for poor health in many parts of the world. It may take the form of deficiency either of major classes of food, usually high-grade protein, or of vitamins or elements essential for specific metabolic processes, e.g. iron for haemoglobin production. Often the deficiencies are multiple and complex. Disturbances of nutrition are by no means restricted to deficiencies, for in the more affluent countries obesity, due to overeating, has become increasingly common, with its attendant dangers of high blood pressure and heart disease.

(2) Physical agents. These include trauma, heat, cold, electricity, irradiation and rapid changes in environmental pressure. In all instances, injury is caused by a high rate of transmission of particular forms of energy (kinetic, radiant, etc.) to or from the body. Important examples in this country are mechanical injury, particularly in road accidents, and burns. Exposure to ionizing radiations cannot be regarded as entirely safe in any dosage (p. 430).

(3) Chemicals. With the use of an ever increasing number of chemical agents as drugs, in industrial processes, in agriculture and in the home, chemically-induced injury has become very common. The effects vary. At one extreme are those substances which have a general effect on cells such as cyanide (see above) which causes death almost instantaneously, with little or no structural changes. Many other chemicals, such as strong acids and alkalis, cause local injury accompanied by an inflammatory reaction in the tissues exposed to them. A third large group of substances produces a more or less selective injury to a particular organ or cell type. Hepatocytes play a major role in absorbing and metabolizing many toxic chemicals. They are therefore liable to injury by such substances, including paracetamol and alcohol in high dosage (p. 413). Many toxic chemicals or their metabolites are excreted by the kidneys and because of their concentrating function the renal tubular epithelial cells are exposed to high levels of such substances. Accordingly, toxic hepatic and renal tubular cell death are common. Fortunately both types of cell have a high regenerative capacity.

(4) Infective micro-organisms (p. 279). These include bacteria, protozoa, small metazoa, lower fungi and viruses. In spite of advances in immunization procedures and the extensive use now made of antibiotics, many important diseases still result from infection by micro-organisms, and the danger of widespread epidemics, e.g. of influenza and cholera, has been enhanced by air travel. The disease-producing capacity of micro-organisms depends on their ability to invade and multiply within the host, and on the possibility of their transmission to other hosts. The features of the disease produced by infection depend on the specific properties of the causal organism. Bacteria bring about harmful effects mainly by the production of chemical compounds termed toxins, and the biological effects of these, together with the response of the host, determine the features of the disease. Viruses multiply in host cells, usually with a direct cytopathic effect: features of virus disease depend largely on which cells are invaded and on the response of the host. Some viruses also become integrated, i.e. viral genes are inserted into the genome of the host cell, and this is probably a contributory cause in some forms of cancer (p. 391). Of the protozoa, the malaria parasite is of enormous importance as a cause of chronic ill health in whole populations.

(5) Metazoan parasites (p. 1142) are also an important cause of disease in many parts of the world. Hookworm infection of the intestine and schistosomiasis are causes of ill-health prevalent in many tropical countries.

(6) Immunological factors. The development of immunity is essential for protection against micro-organisms and parasites. Harmful effects, both local and more widespread, can, however, result from the reaction of antibodies and lymphocytes with parasites, microbes and their toxic products. Also, the immune system does not distinguish between harmful and harmless foreign antigenic materials and injury may result from immune reactions to either. Such hypersensitivity reactions (p. 204) are numerous and complex. Local examples include hay fever, asthma and some forms of dermatitis, while hypersensitivity to many foreign materials, including penicillin and other drugs, can cause generalized, sometimes fatal, reactions. Hypersensitivity reactions may also result from the development of autoimmunity in which antibodies and lymphocytes react with and injure normal cells and tissues; examples include chronic thyroiditis, commonly progressing to hypothyroidism, and the excessive destruction of red cells in autoimmune haemolytic anaemia.

In another group of disorders there is immune deficiency and the patient lacks defence against micro-organisms. This may result from abnormalities of fetal development, as an effect of various acquired diseases, most notably in infection by the human immunodeficiency virus (HIV) with the development of the acquired immunodeficiency syndrome (AIDS), or it may be induced by immunosuppressive therapy.

(7) Psychogenic factors. The mental stresses imposed by conditions of life, particularly in technologically advanced communities, are probably contributory factors in three important and overlapping groups of diseases. First, acquired mental disease such as depression, for which no specific structural or biochemical basis has yet been found. Second, diseases of addiction, particularly to alcohol, various drugs and tobacco. The heterogeneous third group, sometimes referred to as the psychosomatic disorders, includes peptic ulcer (p. 699), hypertension (p. 451) and coronary artery disease (p. 488); in these three conditions, anxiety, overwork and frustration (all of which are experienced by editors of textbooks) may be causal factors, although their modes of action are obscure.

1

Cells and Tissues in Health and Disease

Pathology is the study of disease by scientific methods; it involves the study of abnormality, of the failure of normal systems to operate, or their collapse following insult. Problems can arise either internally, through defects in the organism, or from external causes, such as infection or trauma. Not only is the study of pathology essential in understanding disease, it often provides valuable clues as to the functioning of normal systems. Equally, the pathologist must draw upon a range of disciplines to understand malfunction.

The human body is a clone of about 10^{13} cells together with the extracellular matrix they have made; complicated control mechanisms are required to keep it working in a co-ordinated fashion. Abnormalities may arise because of faulty genomic information or because of incorrect or untimely interpretations of the primary code. Obviously an inaccurate plan is likely to give rise to an abnormal system (Chapter 2) but it is less easy to see how the inappropriate expression of normal cellular information will cause abnormality. Thus, 'normal' behaviour in an abnormal site can cause serious problems.

One way of reducing the impact of malfunction is to have a repair and maintenance system, yet it is in these that we often see defects. This conundrum becomes understandable if we consider that if a primary system collapses then there is no body (or cell) to exhibit pathological features whilst a defective repair system leads to slow degenerative changes after a period of apparent normality. Thus, total failure of DNA replication would leave just a zygote whereas deficiency in the DNA repair system (e.g. in xeroderma pigmentosum – p. 390) leads to a high incidence of skin tumours. It is important to realize that biological structures at both cellular and tissue level are labile. Not only must the correct organization arise during embryonic development, it must be constantly maintained and renewed.

In this chapter, we will first discuss the structure and function of normal cells and tissues, concentrating on systems which cause problems if disturbed and draw attention to those areas of cell biology which help in understanding pathological mechanisms. Thereafter, we will examine some of the effects which result from tissue damage.

Normal Cell Structure and Function

A high level of complexity occurs in unicellular eukaryotic organisms (e.g. amoeba): here intracellular compartmentalization occurs with the development of intracytoplasmic organelles each with specific function (Fig. 1.1). There is a cost in terms of the informational energy required to establish and maintain compartments but this is offset by the ability to concentrate reactants and increase reaction rates. A multicellular mode of existence allows even more specialization, this time at the cellular level but more sophisticated control mechanisms are required to co-ordinate the functions of each cell type and the interaction between cell types.

Ultrastructural study of mammalian cells provides a fixed 'snapshot' of the cell at a particular time. The recent introduction of enhanced-contrast video microscopy has revealed dramatic movement within the cytoplasm, and has shown that even cytoskeletal elements may have half-lives of only minutes or seconds (Table 1.1).

Nucleus

The nucleus is the largest single compartment of the cell and is its central data store. Control arises through the interaction of nucleus and cytoplasm and neither one is autonomous as a controller. It is enclosed by the double membrane of the nuclear envelope which is perforated by nuclear pores, allowing passage of molecules including proteins and nucleic acids between nucleus and cytoplasm. The nuclear shape is stabilized by a group of polypeptides (**lamins**) which show some homology with intermediate filaments (see Table 1.3). The lamins bind to proteins of the inner membrane and form an electron dense layer on its nuclear aspect, the **nuclear lamina**.

Within the human nucleus are 46 chromosomes. Each consists of a single molecule of DNA approximately 5 cm long packed in a complex fashion (Fig. 1.2) with positively charged structural proteins (**histones**) to form a string of particles known as **nucleosomes**. Closely packed nucleosomes form electron dense **heterochromatin**, which is thought to be transcriptionally inactive, and is often concentrated at the periphery of the nucleus. In contrast, most RNA synthesis occurs in the more loosely arranged and thus electron lucent **euchromatin**. The arrangement of chromosomes within the nucleus appears to be non-random. For example, several chromosomes contain repeated genes for ribosomal RNA synthesis and these are clustered together to form nucleoli.

While the haploid set of chromosomes of each cell carries all the information needed for the entire organism, this information will only be correctly interpreted if the nucleus is in the cytoplasmic environment. The nucleus and cytoplasm are interdependent in the control of gene expression. An unusual feature of the nuclear compartment is that it is transient; at every cell division the nuclear membrane is broken down and then reformed. It is likely that nuclear structure and function are highly conserved since any major loss of content or alteration in function would be fatal to the organism. Minor alterations in the genetic code which

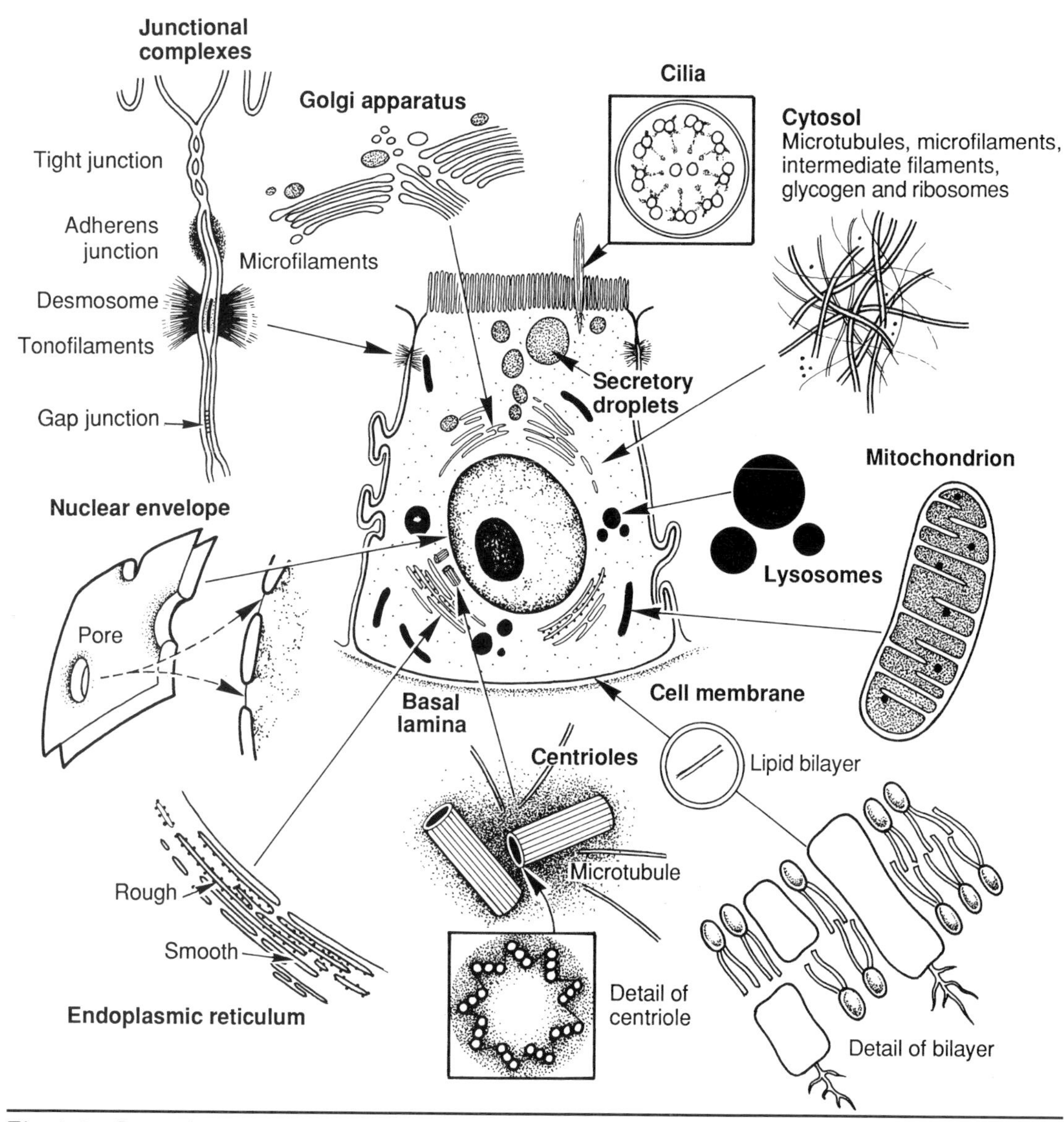

Fig. 1.1 Composite diagram of a secreting epithelial cell.

may be deleterious or advantageous are subject to natural selection.

Plasma Membrane

The plasma membrane (plasmalemma) is the boundary between the intracellular and extracellular spaces across which the passage of molecules occurs, regulated by pumps and channels. The plasma membrane interacts with adjacent cells, it may be electrically excitable, and is the location for many receptors, particularly those for hydrophilic signal molecules.

Like all cellular membranes, the plasma membrane comprises a bilayer of lipid molecules, in which are embedded membrane proteins (Fig. 1.3). In some regions the proteins are packed in a well ordered array, while in others they are more dispersed. The phospholipid bilayer is flexible, and

Table 1.1 Time-scale of various processes

Conformational changes	Microseconds?
Opening of ion channels	Microseconds?
Diffusion of soluble molecules	Seconds
Microfilament polymerization following stimulus	30 seconds
Change in shape of cells	Minutes
Half-life of microtubules	5 minutes
Recycling time of plasma membrane	10 minutes
Mitosis	1–2 hours
New expression of a gene	2–4 hours
DNA replication	4 hours
Cell cycle in rapidly proliferating cells	24 hours
Turnover of epithelium	4 days
Average lifespan of protein	4 days
Production cycle for leucocytes	12–14 days
Induction of immune responses	8 days
Repair of connective tissue	Weeks–months
Turnover of connective tissue	Months–years
Incubation period of slow viruses	Years
Senescence of organism	Lifetime
Senescence of cell population	60 doublings
Change in penetrance of a new allele	Generations

will conform to whatever shape is adopted by the moving cell, and is fluid, so that proteins can redistribute and interact within the plane of the membrane. The central hydrophobic region makes it fairly impermeable to hydrophilic molecules. The properties of membrane proteins are largely responsible for the properties of the membrane and distinguish the plasma membrane of one type of cell from another. Membrane proteins are diverse in their location, structure and function. Intrinsic proteins are embedded in the bilayer, either spanning it completely (**transmembrane proteins**) or protruding from it on only one face of the membrane. **Peripheral membrane proteins** are more loosely associated and are held in place

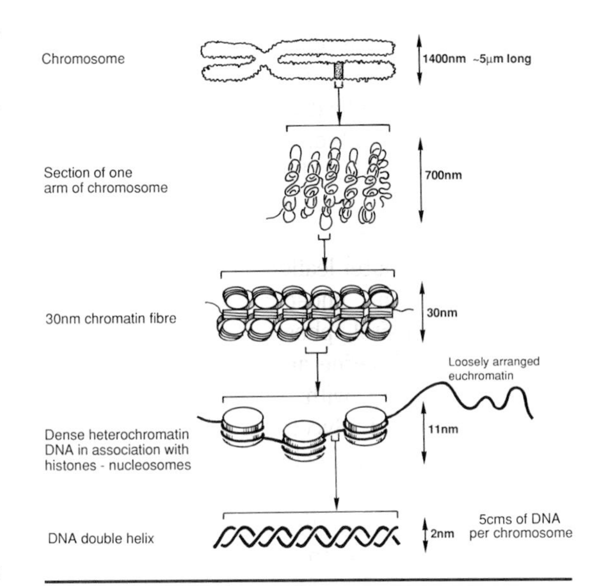

Fig. 1.2 Schematic representation of chromatin structure.

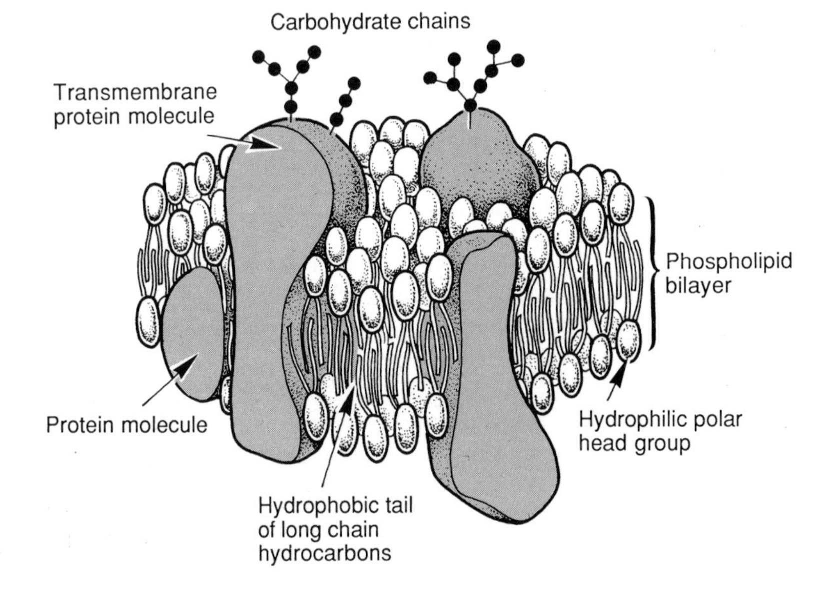

Fig. 1.3 Schematic representation of plasma membrane; outside uppermost.

by interactions with intrinsic proteins or are covalently bound to hydrophobic groups on molecules such as glycolipids. Many membrane proteins are glycosylated, particularly on their extracellular domains. The carbohydrate groups are different on different cells but their functions are not always clear.

The inner and outer leaflets of the plasma membrane differ in phospholipid composition; phosphatidyl inositol, phosphatidyl ethanolamine and phosphatidyl serine are largely restricted to the inner leaflet, with phosphatidyl choline, sphingomyelin and glycolipids the major components of the outer leaflet. In addition to their structural role, phospholipids, particularly phosphatidyl inositol, are also involved in signal–response transduction (p. 20).

The fluid properties of the membrane influence the mobility and sometimes the normal function of integral membrane proteins, for example by restricting conformational changes. Altering the activity of an ion pump may alter the transmembrane ion distribution needed for neural transmission; many anaesthetics probably act by modifying the lipid environment around particular proteins. Cholesterol regulates membrane fluidity, particularly in making cells less sensitive to temperature changes, so that the membrane maintains fluidity even at low temperatures.

Major defects in the structure of the plasma membrane are inconsistent with cell survival and damage to the cell membrane is often the cause of cell death. Acquired damage to the lipid bilayer by bacterial enzymes (e.g. lecithinase produced by *Clostridium welchii*) (p. 289), detergent, complement activation (p. 142), or attack by cytotoxic T cells (p. 196) allows small molecules to leak out and water to enter; therefore, the cell swells and dies (Fig. 1.4).

Few genetic defects affecting the cell membrane are known. In the so-called **transport diseases** specific small molecule transport proteins are absent. In Hartnup disease (p. 271) there is a defect in the transport of amino acids across the intestinal and renal tubular epithelium, leading to decreased intestinal absorption, particularly of tryptophan, and to abnormal amino-acid excretion in the urine. A defect in a membrane associated protein, dystrophin, has been identified in patients with Duchenne muscular dystrophy (p. 874) an X-linked recessive condition. Affected boys usually die of progressive muscle wasting and respiratory failure in their teens.

Cytoskeleton

Much of the mechanical strength of the cell is due to the array of microfilaments, microtubules and intermediate filaments, which are known as the cytoskeleton (Table 1.2). Microfilaments and microtubules are involved in motor activity of different kinds and also act as structural elements. Intermediate filaments act simply to resist tension. The cytoskeletal proteins are linked to integral membrane proteins by various subplasmalemmal proteins such as vinculin, ankyrin and spectrin. Details of the subplasmalemmal or membrane cytoskeleton were first worked out for the erythrocyte, which suffers enormous deformation as it traverses the microvasculature. Alterations in the erythrocyte cytoskeleton are responsible for disorders such as hereditary spherocytosis (Chapter 14) in which the red cell shape is abnormal due to lack of spectrin. Furthermore, the abnormal red cells cannot undergo deformation within the spleen, they stagnate in the cords of the red pulp, their survival is decreased and anaemia results. Similar membrane skeleton proteins are also present in other cell types including endothelium.

Microfilaments

Microfilaments are composed of filamentous (F) actin, a linear polymer of globular (G) actin. Their assembly is illustrated in Fig. 1.5a. They are very similar to the actin filaments of striated muscle, though they are not associated with troponin and only sometimes with tropomyosin. Striated muscle myosin will bind to microfilaments in an arrowhead fashion, revealing the intrinsic polarity of the polymer which is essential for movement.

Microfilaments are arranged in two ways: (1) as a meshwork underlying and anchored to the plasma membrane and which is responsible for

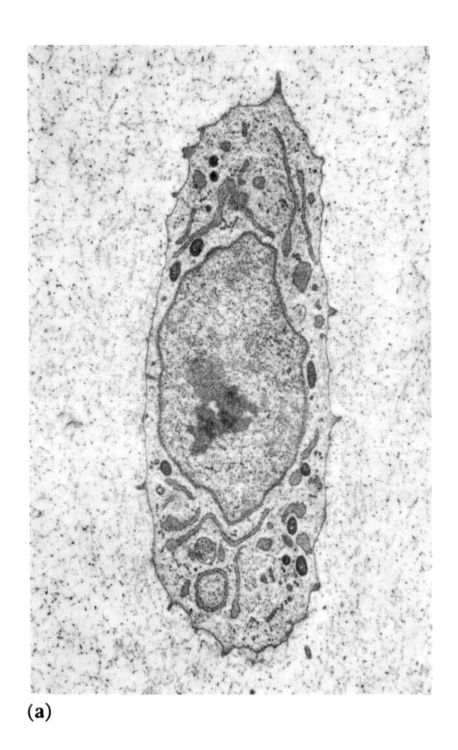
(a)

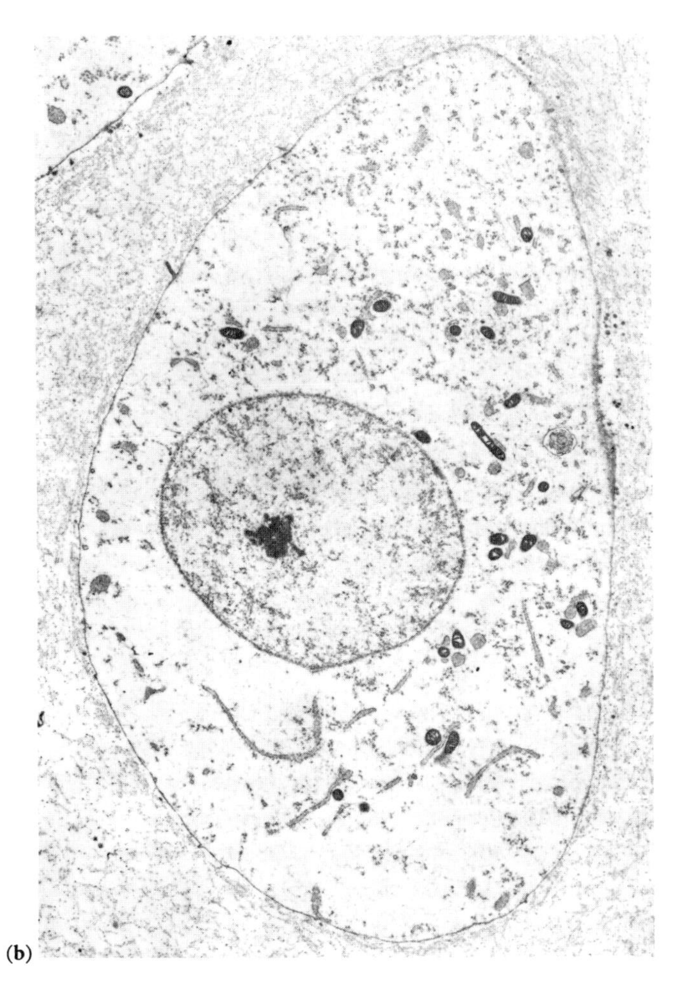
(b)

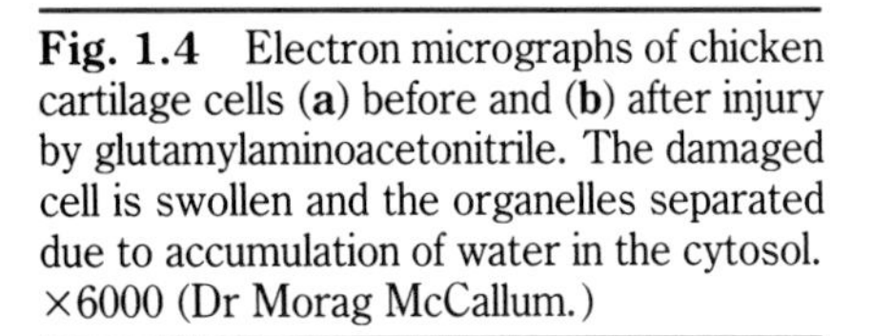
Fig. 1.4 Electron micrographs of chicken cartilage cells (**a**) before and (**b**) after injury by glutamylaminoacetonitrile. The damaged cell is swollen and the organelles separated due to accumulation of water in the cytosol. ×6000 (Dr Morag McCallum.)

many of the mechanical properties of the cell surface; and (2) as bundles attached to the plasma membrane at one end, and which are capable of linear contraction by the sliding of antiparallel filaments. Bundles of parallel actin filaments support the microvilli of intestinal epithelium. Actin is one of the most abundant cellular proteins (8–14% of total protein) and is very highly conserved, presumably because it interacts with so many other proteins. There are no known defects of actin.

Microtubules

Microtubules are also linear polymers, built up of tubulin heterodimers (Fig. 1.5b). Three classes, cytoplasmic, spindle and axonemal, are usually distinguished.

(1) **Cytoplasmic microtubules** arise from the microtubule organizing centre (MTOC) of the cell which is located in the pericentriolar region. Like microfilaments, microtubules have inherent polarity. Recently, microtubule-associated motor systems have been identified which are important in stabilizing the organization of cellular organelles. Two different motor molecules are involved, kinesin which transports organelles towards the peripheral ('plus') ends of microtubules, and cytoplasmic dynein which brings them back to the microtubule organizing centre. Disruption of the microtubule system with colchicine leads to dispersal of the Golgi apparatus, collapse of the endoplasmic reticulum network, and active redistribution of intermediate filaments to the perinuclear region, a process involving actin.

Table 1.2 Linear elements of the cytoskeleton

	Size (nm)	Subunit	Stability	Motor involvement	Inhibitors	Role
Microfilaments	5–7	Actin	Low	Myosin	Cytochalasins, phalloidin	Motor + skeletal
Microtubules	25	Tubulin	Low	Kinesin + dynein	Colchicine, taxol	Motor + skeletal
Intermediate filaments	10	Various	High	Nil	Unknown	Tension resistance

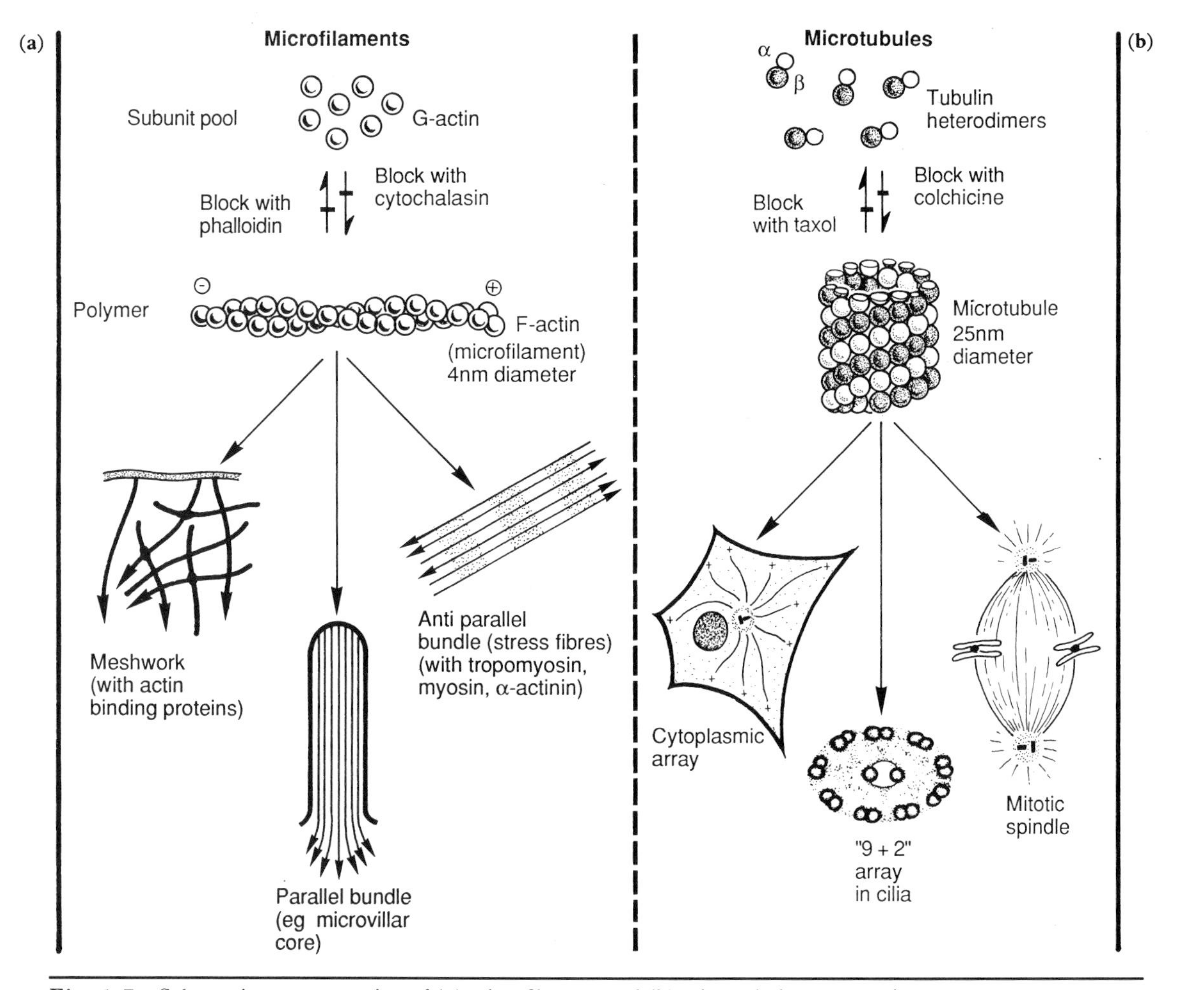

Fig. 1.5 Schematic representation of (**a**) microfilament and (**b**) microtubular aggregation.

Table 1.3 Intermediate filament proteins and proteins related by sequence homology

	Homology group		Mol. wt (kDa)	Cell type
Cytokeratins	I	(acidic)	40–60	Epithelia
	II	(neutral/basic)	50–70	
Vimentin	III		53	Many but predominantly mesenchymal
Desmin	III		52	Muscle
Glial fibrillary acidic protein	III		51	Glial cells, astrocytes
Neurofilament polypeptides	IV		57–150	Neurons
Nuclear lamins	V		60–70	All eukaryotes

Similar mechanisms are involved in transporting material to and from the main body of the neuron along axons (axoplasmic flow). Thus, normal cytoplasmic organization depends on the continued activity of these motor systems.

(2) **Spindle microtubules** are essential for mitosis and meiosis. Disruption of the spindle by colchicine leads to cessation of cell division at metaphase, so-called metaphase arrest.

(3) **Axonemal microtubules** are stabilized by interaction with other proteins and are an essential part of the ciliary motor system. A defect in axonemal dynein is responsible for the immobile cilia syndrome (Kartagener's syndrome), which leads to male infertility due to immobile spermatozoa and respiratory infection due to immobile respiratory mucosal cilia (p. 535).

Intermediate Filaments

Intermediate filaments are a group of fibrous proteins which have a structural or tension bearing role in the cell. Although there are several different groups of intermediate filaments of varying molecular weight and amino-acid sequence (Table 1.3), all have homologous regions and form 8–10 nm diameter filaments intermediate in size between microfilaments and thick (myosin) filaments. They are inserted into the cell membrane at the site of desmosomes (p. 14). The cells of different types of tissues contain different intermediate filaments which can be demonstrated by immunohistochemical techniques; this may be of value to histopathologists in determining the histogenesis of a poorly differentiated tumour. Malignant epithelial tumours (carcinomas) contain cytokeratin molecules, while malignant connective tissue tumours (sarcomas) contain vimentin. However, aberrant expression of inappropriate intermediate filaments by malignant tumours is sometimes seen. Thus, occasional sarcomas contain cytokeratin and carcinomas frequently express vimentin.

Damage to intermediate filaments may be seen in disease. In alcoholic liver disease intermediate filaments form discrete intracytoplasmic inclusions, Mallory bodies, in swollen hepatocytes (p. 763). The damage to the cytoskeleton may be a factor in the swelling or ballooning of the affected cells. Crooke's hyaline change in the pituitary (p. 1082) and the neurofibrillary tangle of Alzheimer's disease and Down's syndrome (p. 843) are also thought to be due to damage to the cytoskeleton.

Cell Locomotion

Movement of the whole cell, or movements which cause the cell to change shape, e.g. cell spreading or engulfment of particles, depend on microfilaments and, in some cases, myosin. Cell movement is important in morphogenesis, inflammation, wound healing, immune surveillance, tumour invasion and the ingrowth of new blood vessels (angiogenesis). Two different kinds of movement are involved in locomotion; first, the protrusion of a portion of the cell, and then contraction of the cell to bring the cell body forward. Of the two, protrusive activity is least well understood, but seems to depend almost completely upon actin filaments cross-linked with actin binding proteins. To achieve movement the formation of transient attachments to the substratum is required. It is important that the attachment is transient, as irreversible adhesion will trap a cell in place. Furthermore, when attachment is inadequate, movement will not occur.

Fibroblasts form discrete contacts with the substratum and can exert very substantial local forces on it. In wound healing, the myofibroblast acts like a winch, drawing its contacts together and causing wound contraction. Although this diminishes the size of a wound, there are potentially adverse effects, such as contractures following burns (p. 160) and the contraction of the vitreous of the eye which causes retinal detachment (p. 885). Most invasive cells do not exert substantial local stress upon the substratum or matrix, and have diffuse rather than focal adhesions. Diffuse adhesions allow a cell to move over substrata of low rigidity such as the surface of another cell. If a cell cannot crawl over surrounding cells it is locked in place – **contact inhibition**. Loss of contact inhibition of locomotion may allow the cell to lose positional control and become invasive. Not all invasive cells are of course malignant; for example, neutrophil polymorphs invade tissues during an inflammatory response (p. 117) and epithelial cells spread over territory occupied by fibroblasts during wound healing (p. 150).

Few defects in the basic motor systems of cells are known, reflecting the importance of the system. The major problems are in the control systems which regulate behaviour, particularly the social interactions with other cells. These basic cytoskeletal and motor systems are essential in so many cellular functions, including mitosis and cell movement, that any serious malfunction would be incompatible with development. Thus, in general, if defects do exist they are likely to be relatively subtle and to occur in control systems rather than in cytoskeletal structures. An example is the change seen in cultured fibroblasts transformed by a temperature sensitive Rous sarcoma virus. Within 20 minutes of shifting the cells to the permissive temperature (which allows viral transformation to be expressed) the organization of the microfilament system is completely changed and the cells behave in a manner characteristic of malignant cells. Alteration of the motor behaviour of malignant cells may allow invasion and metastasis (p. 385) although the basic mechanisms are not understood.

Membrane-bound Intracellular Compartments

The cytoplasm contains a series of membrane bound compartments, which are now recognized to be part of an interlinked system including the endoplasmic reticulum, the Golgi system and lysosomes. The interior of each of these organelles forms a separate compartment unconnected with the cytosol and topologically equivalent to the outside of the cell (Fig. 1.6). These membranous compartments are dynamic with constant interchange of membrane from one compartment to another by an energy-consuming system. This interchange leads to the recycling of membrane proteins through internal vesicles where they are inaccessible to the exterior. In this way membrane receptors can be internalized and material can be shuttled from the outside into cytoplasmic vesicles, or vesicle contents can be released to the exterior.

The possession of a particular set of membrane proteins determines the functional capacity of a membrane. Proteins must be targeted to the right membranes despite the chemical similarity of phospholipid bilayers. The protein must be inserted in the correct orientation, and the targeting must be constantly repeated as membrane components are renewed or recycled. Continual energy

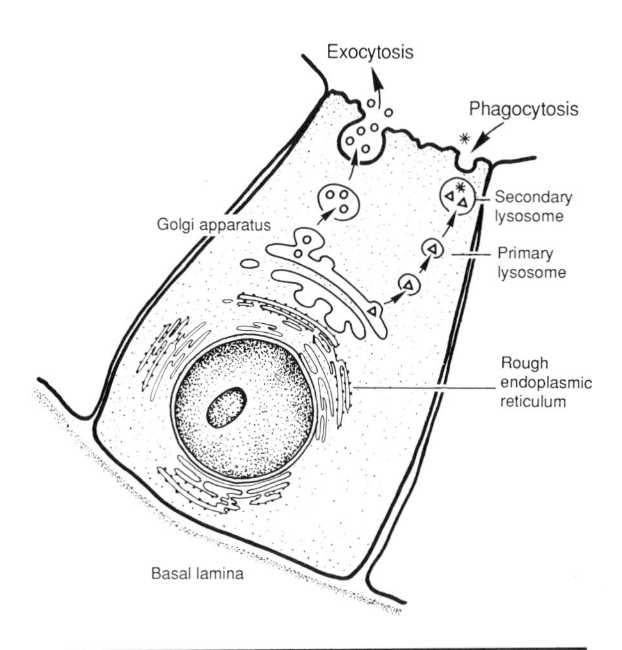

Fig. 1.6 Illustration of the various routes taken by membrane-bound vesicles within the cell. Proteins tagged with mannose-6-phosphate (△) are targeted to the lysosomal system whereas proteins lacking this marker (O) are directed to storage or secretory vesicles. Phagosomes containing ingested material (*) fuse with primary lysosomes to form secondary lysosomes.

input is required to maintain the asymmetry of structure.

Proteins destined for export are, in most cases, synthesized on mRNA–ribosome complexes bound to rough endoplasmic reticulum, and the protein is transferred into the cisternal space of the rough endoplasmic reticulum (RER) as it is synthesized. There are some rare exceptions, however, in which the secretory pathway of the protein is not known. The specific association with RER is determined by a recognition mechanism based upon the early amino-acid residues of the protein. This signal sequence is removed once the chain reaches the lumen of the endoplasmic reticulum. Partial transfer of a protein into the cisternal space will leave the protein as an integral membrane protein. Following transfer into the cisternal space the protein is partially glycosylated, moved to the Golgi where glycosylation is completed and then directed to various possible sites. If the protein is tagged with mannose-6-phosphate it binds to a receptor in the Golgi membrane. It is then transferred to a sorting compartment where the protein is released from the receptor and the phosphate removed, thus preventing return of the protein to the Golgi. The protein is then transferred to lysosomes and the receptor returns to the Golgi to be re-used as a shuttle. Proteins without the mannose-6-phosphate tag are directed to other vesicles either for storage or for immediate secretion from the cell.

A defect in this targeting mechanism is responsible for a very rare disorder, mucolipidosis-II or I-cell disease (p. 264). Patients homozygous for this recessive disorder have high levels of lysosomal enzymes in the extracellular fluids but are deficient in, or have none in their lysosomes. This is due to the lack of the enzyme which adds the mannose-6-phosphate recognition marker to hydrolases. The hydrolases therefore are not packaged into lysosomes but instead find their way into the secretory vesicles. It is probable that similar 'tagging devices' operate in other compartments. Mutations in secretory proteins are responsible for what are now recognized as endoplasmic reticulum storage diseases. Included in this group is the α_1-antitrypsin (α_1-AT) deficiency syndrome (p. 772) in which single amino-acid substitutions in the molecule are responsible for accumulation of α_1-AT in the RER of hepatocytes. The accumulation is morphologically identified as PAS positive/diastase resistant globules in hepatocytes (Fig. 1.7).

Membrane-bound vesicles are also selectively targeted to particular regions of the plasma membrane. In secretory epithelial cells, secretory products (such as mucin or digestive enzymes) are released on to the apical (luminal) surface, while basement membrane components (such as laminin and type IV collagen) are deposited on the basal surface. Thus, two distinct membrane domains are formed, the apical and the basolateral, with different functions and different integral proteins. Diffusion of membrane proteins between these domains is limited by tight junctions.

Many secretory products are stockpiled against sudden demand. For example, on receipt of an

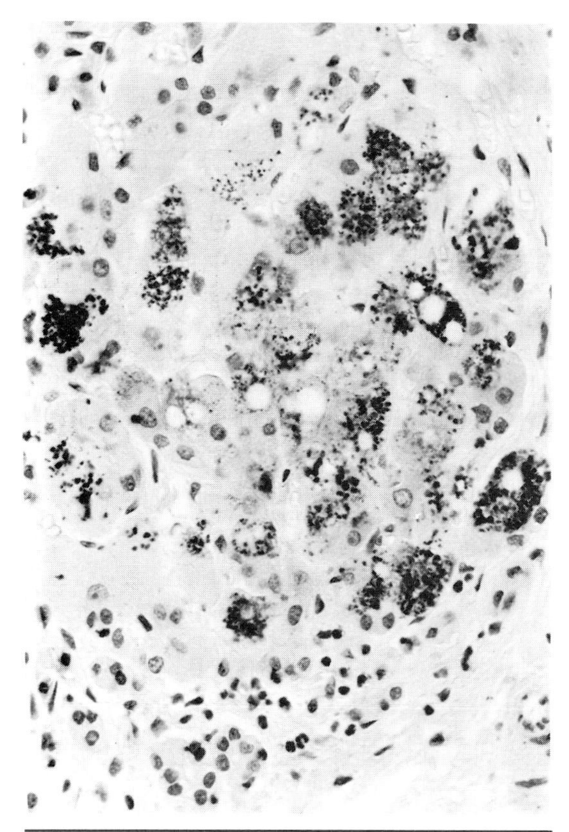

Fig. 1.7 The liver in α_1-antitrypsin deficiency. The hepatocytes have synthesized an abnormal form of protein which they cannot secrete. It is seen as numerous dark cytoplasmic globules which have been specifically stained with peroxidase-labelled antibody. ×570.

appropriate hormonal signal, pancreatic acinar cells release digestive enzymes, which are stored as inactive precursors in storage vesicles (zymogen granules). Fusion of the vesicle membrane with that of the apical plasma membrane releases the contents into the luminal space where enzymatic cleavage converts the inactive precursor to the active form. Active processes are involved in transferring the vesicles to the apical region of the cell; control of release involves regulation of intracellular calcium levels.

Receptor mediated endocytosis is a process where specific substances bind to cell surface receptors and are internalized, thus allowing efficient uptake of specific macromolecules. The molecules which bind to the receptors are known as **ligands**. An electron dense coat is found on the inner aspect of the cytoplasmic membrane at sites of internalization. This coat is rich in several proteins including clathrin. When binding of the appropriate ligand to receptors occurs, these **clathrin-coated pits** are rapidly internalized as **coated vesicles.**

One of the best studied examples, and one in which pathological alterations occur, is the low density lipoprotein (LDL) receptor system, the gene for which is located on chromosome 19. The uptake of LDL, which is cholesterol rich, is mediated by binding to a specific receptor. The receptor–ligand complexes are internalized in vesicles which fuse with each other to form larger vesicles called endosomes. These in turn fuse with primary lysosomes to form secondary lysosomes in which the cholesterol esters are hydrolysed. This makes cholesterol available for new membrane synthesis while the LDL receptors are recycled to the cell surface (Fig. 1.8). In familial hypercholesterolaemia there is failure of this uptake system leading to elevated blood cholesterol levels and the development of atheroma at an early age (p. 45). Various defects have been identified including partial or total absence of the LDL receptor, inefficient ligand binding and failure of the receptor–ligand complex to internalize.

Lysosomes

Lysosomes are bounded by a single membrane and contain a broad range of hydrolytic enzymes which, as has already been described, are directed to this compartment by a mannose-6-phosphate label. The majority of lysosomal enzymes are most active at acid pH. They are inactive unless the lysosome swells or fuses with a primary phagosome which may contain ingested particulate material or cytoplasmic components. In the latter case, this may arise through cell injury or programmed cell death – apoptosis. Fusion of lysosome and phagosome produces the secondary lysosome (phagolysosome) and leads to activation of acid hydrolases (see Fig. 1.6).

Lysosomes can be abnormal in several ways.

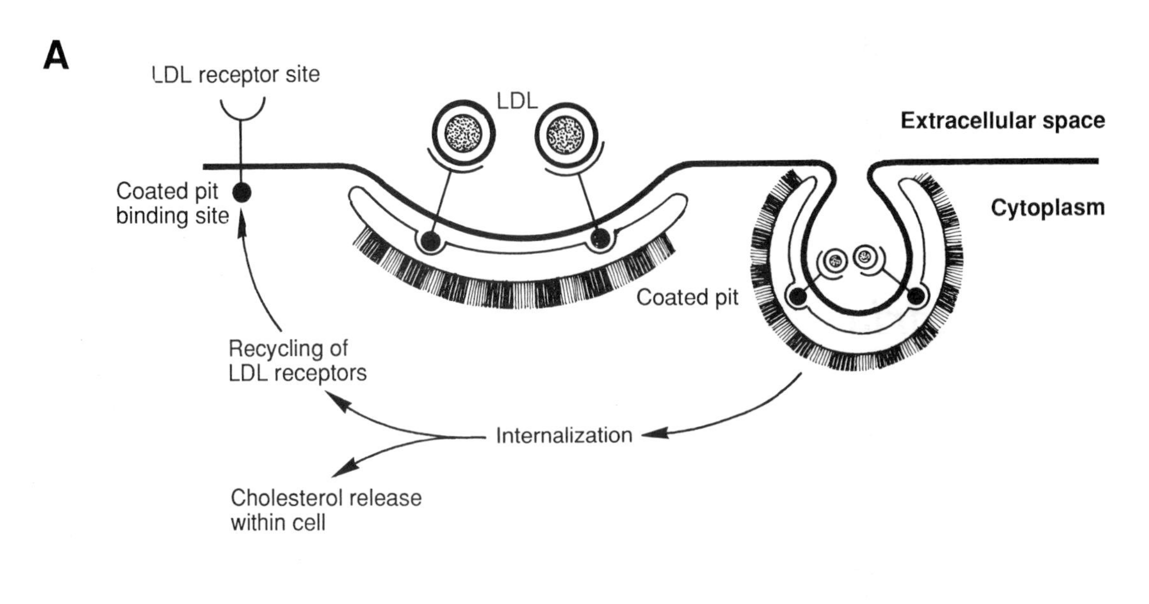

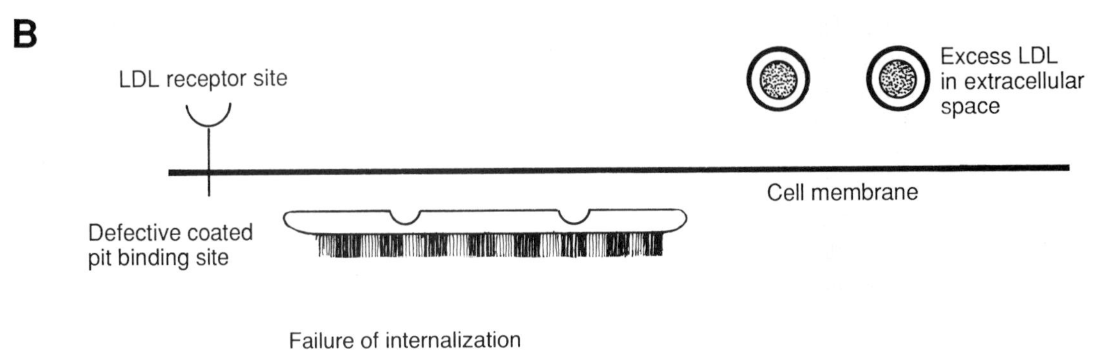

Fig. 1.8 Schematic representation of receptor mediated endocytosis: **A** with respect to low density lipoproteins (LDL); **B**: in familial hypercholesterolaemia.

Their permeability may be altered by bacterial toxins (e.g. streptococcal) or by surfactants (e.g. in hypervitaminosis A – p. 354). Inhaled silica is ingested by macrophages and partly converted to silicic acid which damages the phospholipids of the lysosomal membrane. This leads to pulmonary fibrosis and the condition known as silicosis (p. 569). Particles which are too large to be completely engulfed may nevertheless induce release of lysosomal enzymes directly into the extracellular space. Thus, in gout long, needle-shaped crystals of sodium urate are present in synovial fluid. These are engulfed by neutrophil polymorphs which release lysosomal enzymes, resulting in a severely inflamed joint (p. 996). In porphyria, ingested porphyrins in secondary lysosomes absorb light and cause chemical damage to lysosomal membranes (p. 276). Obviously, the release of degradative enzymes into the cytoplasm as a result of lysosomal damage is undesirable.

If cells are incapable of degrading a particular class of material, these will accumulate in secondary lysosomes, with the formation of residual bodies. Some common examples of these **lysosomal storage disorders**, in which specific lysosomal enzymes are deficient, are discussed in Chapter 7. Co-cultures of fibroblasts from patients with storage diseases with normal fibroblasts leads to restoration of full lysosomal function in the patient's cells. Theoretically, tissue transplantation might allow the specific enzyme to appear in the recipient's tissue. Liver transplantation has been carried out for the correction of enzyme defects primarily involving hepatocytes (e.g. glycogen storage disease types I and IV and type IV hyperlipidaemia).

Mitochondria

Mitochondria are the major site of adenosine triphosphate (ATP) production. The enzymes responsible for fatty acid and pyruvate degradation and for the citric acid cycle are found in the matrix while the enzyme systems involved in oxidative phosphorylation are arranged as arrays on the inner mitochondrial membrane. ATP generation requires the production of a proton gradient across the mitochondrial membrane, thus their existence as a closed compartment is essential to their function. Although usually shown as cylinders 0.5–1 μm long, mitochondria vary considerably in shape and may form an interconnected network.

Mitochondria are semi-autonomous in that they arise by growth and division of pre-existing mitochondria and have their own DNA and ribosomes. Many cell biologists accept the **symbiont hypothesis** which proposes that early in their evolution, eukaryotic cells became colonized by bacteria with the establishment of a symbiotic relationship. Thus, the bacterium/mitochondrion supplies the energy requirement of the host cell, while many mitochondrial proteins are encoded by nuclear DNA and are synthesized in the cytoplasm. Once these proteins have been selectively transported across mitochondrial membranes they undergo a conformational change which prevents them re-crossing mitochondrial membranes. Although mitochondrial replication is independent of cell division, it is not totally unregulated. The number of mitochondria is indicative of the energy requirements of the cell, and their location often indicates the major site of ATP consumption. In general, active mitochondria have more cristae, providing a larger surface on which to arrange the respiratory complexes.

Abnormalities of mammalian mitochondrial function are extremely rare; in mitochondrial myopathies (p. 876) there are defects in the respiratory chain which either result in the production of toxins which inhibit mitochondrial function, or in a shortage of oxygen needed for oxidative phosphorylation. Thus, the cell's stock of ATP is rapidly depleted and energy dependent systems cease to function. Chief among these are ion pumps such as the Na^+/K^+-ATPase of the plasma membrane which is responsible for the maintenance of the correct osmotic balance in the cell. Cell swelling is therefore a common sign of cell injury.

Cytosol

Once all the identifiable organelles have been considered, what remains? One view is that the remainder of the cytoplasm is just a protein-rich solution which is free to flow between the more highly ordered polymeric elements; an alternative view is that even this solution has structure, and that the proteins are arranged as a microtrabecular network. Since the cytoplasm does flow and since organelles and other large particles can move relatively freely within it, this arrangement, if it is not an artefact, must be very labile.

Cell–Cell and Cell–Matrix Interaction

In a multicellular organism interaction between cells is clearly of major importance. Cells must remain in contact with one another or with the extracellular matrix. Not only must there be mechanical linkage but there must also be communication between cells. Functional specialization leads to many different types of tissue which can, however, be broadly classified as epithelium and connective tissue. These differ principally in the relationship between cells and extracellular matrix. Neural tissues are a special case which will not be considered here.

Epithelium

Epithelial tissues consist of cohesive sheets of cells which rest upon and are firmly attached to a basement membrane (basal lamina). The cells adhere to one another by specialized junctions of several types (see Fig. 1.1).

Tight (occludens) junctions seal cells together to prevent even small molecules passing from one side of the sheet to the other, e.g. from the lumen of a gland to the basal aspect. They also act as barriers to the diffusion of proteins within the plasma membrane, maintaining separate apical and basolateral membrane domains.

Adherens junctions and ***desmosomes*** mechanically attach adjacent cells. Actin microfilaments are attached to adherens junctions and intermediate filaments (cytokeratins in epithelia) to desmosomes. Thus, both the cell membranes and their cytoskeletons are connected, giving mechanical strength to the epithelium. These adhesions can be disturbed in pathological states. Autoantibodies directed against desmosomal glycoproteins can be detected in the serum of patients with the skin disorder pemphigus (p. 1117). These antibodies bind to and disrupt desmosomes, causing loss of adhesion between cells with the formation of large intraepidermal blisters (bullae).

Gap junctions allow passage of small molecules and thus chemical or electrical messages can be transmitted between adjacent cells.

The many different functions of epithelia are reflected in the diversity of epithelial structure. Thus, in secretory epithelia, such as pancreatic acini, the cells are cuboidal, contain well developed RER and are arranged around ducts. Epithelia, such as skin where mechanical resistance is important, are stratified, contain abundant intermediate filaments and are joined by many desmosomes.

Basal Lamina

Epithelial cells produce the components of the basal lamina, which consists of a meshwork of type IV collagen, the glycoproteins laminin and entactin and proteoglycans, principally heparan sulphate. Cells are firmly bound to the basal lamina by **hemidesmosomes** into which are inserted cytoplasmic intermediate filaments. Adhesion between the cell and the collagen meshwork is made possible by laminin which binds both to cell surface receptors and to collagen. In bullous pemphigoid (p. 1119) autoantibodies reactive with the basement membrane of squamous epithelium are present in the serum and may be in part responsible for the subepidermal blisters (bullae) which occur.

Contact with basal lamina seems to be important for the maintenance of the differentiated characteristics of epithelia. In addition, the basal lamina forms a scaffolding along which cells may migrate during regeneration. Malignant epithelial cells have the capacity to digest and penetrate the basal lamina and thus invade surrounding tissues. Distant spread via the bloodstream requires that the vascular basal lamina must also be penetrated. The production of collagenases and other proteolytic enzymes is at least partly responsible for this.

Connective Tissue

Unlike epithelium the cells of connective tissue are dispersed more or less individually within an extracellular matrix (ECM) which may be solid (bone), or flexible (fibrous tissue). Indeed, blood may be regarded as a connective tissue in which the ECM is fluid (plasma) and the cells unusually mobile. Although largely separate, connective tissue cells are also capable of cell-to-cell interactions, junctions often being found between such cells. Contraction of smooth and cardiac muscle of course requires that adjacent cells are firmly attached.

The diversity of connective tissues depends on the different cell types present (e.g. fibroblasts, osteoblasts, chondrocytes), the chemical composition of the extracellular matrix which they produce, and the structural organization of the matrix components. These fall into three categories: (1) linear tension resisting elements (e.g. collagen); (2) space filling, compression resisting molecules (e.g. proteoglycans); and (3) link proteins (e.g. fibronectin) (Table 1.4). These individual components may also be organized in varying ways, e.g. collagen fibres may be arranged in parallel arrays (tendons), in orthogonal sheets (e.g. cornea) or a loose meshwork (vitreous humour).

Although turnover of ECM is relatively slow compared with cellular material, several disorders are known in which the inability to degrade ECM components leads to problems. For example, in osteopetrosis (p. 960) osteoclasts are unable to resorb the cartilage model of developing bones. The marrow space does not develop and severe anaemia results. There are also a number of defects of collagen biosynthesis with important clinical effects. In osteogenesis imperfecta (p. 961) abnormalities of the type I collagen gene lead to abnormally fragile bones which repeatedly fracture. In scurvy (p. 349) lack of vitamin C prevents hydroxylation of proline residues in collagen with consequent lack of cross-linking of collagen fibres. Increased cross-linking of collagen and elastin is responsible for many of the ageing changes in skin. Abnormalities of proteoglycans are found in cartilage in the degenerative joint disease, osteoarthritis.

Table 1.4 Constituents of connective tissue

Function of molecule	Major examples
Tension resistance	Collagen types I–III, V–XIII. Elastin
Space-filling/ incompressible	Hyaluronic acid Glycosaminoglycans Collagen IV? Hydroxyapatite Water
Link proteins	Fibronectin (and isoforms) Laminin

Cell Adhesion Molecules

As well as the specialized junctions described above, more transient interactions between cells and between cell and matrix are important. These include the interactions of leucocytes and platelets with vascular endothelium in the inflammatory response, the interactions between the various cell types in the immune response, the adhesion of leucocytes with bacteria which is required for phagocytosis, and the temporary adhesions between cell and matrix used in cell locomotion, and which are therefore important in invasion and wound healing. In addition there are interactions between like-cells in specialized tissue, e.g. epithelia and neural tissue.

There are two major theories of cell adhesion. The physicochemical theory proposes that the electrostatic repulsion forces between negatively charged cells are counterbalanced by electrodynamic attractive forces (London – van der Waals dispersion forces) acting between the phospholipids of the cell membranes. All cells carry net negative surface charge due to the carboxyl group of terminal sialic acid residues on membrane glycoproteins. The theoretical distances between cells predicted by this theory coincide well with those seen in the tissues. The non-specific nature of this mechanism does not matter provided there are quantitative differences in adhesion; if adhesion between similar cells is stronger than between dissimilar cells, then a mixture of cells will sort out into territories composed of similar cells.

The second theory is that receptor–ligand interactions are involved in cell adhesion, these interactions conferring specificity and also allowing for a diversity of functions. The molecules are referred to as cell adhesion molecules (CAMs), a term which is inaccurate in that they may also subserve other functions such as transmembrane signalling. Several groups of CAMs are recognized (Table 1.5). The table, however, is by no means complete and new molecules and additional functions are being increasingly recognized. The **selectins** are expressed on leucocytes and endothelial cells and are important in the acute inflammatory response and coagulation, facilitating the adhesion of leucocytes or platelets, respectively, to endothelial cells. The **integrins** comprise some 14 α/β heterodimeric transmembrane glycoproteins. There are a number of subfamilies based on differences in their β chains. The function of each integrin is determined by its unique α chain. The β_1 or very late activation (VLA) group react with extracellular matrix proteins and are important in cell movement during embryogenesis and wound healing;

Table 1.5 Examples of cell adhesion molecules (CAMs)

Family	Biochemical features	Examples and functions	
Selectins	Transmembrane glycoproteins, carbohydrate ligands	Endothelial cell adhesion molecule-1 (ELAM-1)	Neutrophil-endothelial attachment
		Leucocyte adhesion molecule (LAM-1)	Lymphocyte homing
		Platelet-activation-dependent granule external membrane proteins (PADGEM) or granule membrane proteins-140 (GMP 140)	Leucocyte-endothelial attachment
Integrins	α/β heterodimers; various ligands which include RGD (argenine-aspartate-glycine) LDV (leucine-aspartate-valine) sequences; Calcium dependent adhesion	β_1 family: very late activation (VLA 1–6) molecules	Six molecules whose ligands include collagen, fibronectin and laminin
		β_2 family: leucocyte function associated molecule-1 (LFA-1)	Reacts with intercellular adhesion molecules (ICAM)-1 and -2 expressed by endothelial cells and accessory cells
		MAC-1, p150, 95	Complement (C3bi) receptors
		β_3 family: VNR; group IIb/IIIa platelet glycoprotein	Vitronectin receptor; Platelet attachment factor
		β_4 family	Cell adhesion component of hemidesmosomes
Cadherins	Transmembrane glycoproteins; calcium dependent adhesion; usually homophilic binding	E-cadherin, N-cadherin, P-cadherin	*E*pithelial, *n*eural cell and *p*lacental cell adhesion
		Desmocollin	Desmosomal component
Immunoglobulin gene superfamily	Glycoproteins with immunoglobulin-like domains; calcium independent adhesion; may be homophilic or heterophilic binding	N-CAM	Neural cell adhesion molecule
		ICAM-1	Leucocyte-endothelial interaction with LFA-1
		VCAM-1	Leucocyte-endothelial interaction with β_1 integrin (VLA-4)

the β_2 or leucocyte integrins are involved in immune adherence and the expression of one of their ligands, ICAM-1, is up-regulated in some acute and chronic inflammatory conditions including viral infections and in renal and hepatic allograft rejection; the β_3 and β_4 families are similar to the β_1 group and include receptors for vitronectin and laminin. The **cadherins**, of which there are many families, are calcium-dependent molecules which are important in actions between 'like-cells' and there are many families of these. The **immunoglobin gene superfamily** includes receptors that react with antigens (T-cell receptor/CD3) and ligands which react with lymphocyte receptors.

Adhesion molecules undergo quantitative and qualitative alteration in expression in response to a variety of stimuli. Furthermore, the development of similar synthetic molecules using DNA technology (Chapter 2) or the use of specific monoclonal antibodies to these molecules may be of clinical value in modulating inflammatory and immunologically mediated tissue injury.

These adhesion molecules will only interact with a surface bearing the appropriate ligand. For a phagocyte, which must interact with previously unknown foreign surfaces, the problems are overcome, in some cases, by coating the surfaces with antibody or complement components, opsonization (p. 121), thereby allowing recognition and binding. A different strategy is to recognize some general property of alien surfaces. A correlation exists between the surface hydrophobicity of a particle and the ease with which it will be phagocytosed; pathogenic bacteria tend to have rather hydrophilic surfaces.

Information Processing

Intercellular communication demands that a variety of signals must be exchanged and messages must traverse the plasma membrane. Various chemical signalling mechanisms are seen. In classical **endocrine** action, the chemical is secreted into the bloodstream to affect target cells at a distant site. In **paracrine** signalling, messengers are released which act only in the immediate environment of the producing cell; this mode of action is widespread in the diffuse endocrine system. Finally, cells may secrete chemicals which bind to receptors on their surface and affect their own function, **autocrine** stimulation. Many systems (e.g. the endocrine, the central nervous system and the immune system) utilize not only similar mechanisms of signalling, but also the same chemical messengers. Thus, the same molecule may act as a hormone, a neurotransmitter, a cytokine or as a growth factor, depending on where it is released and what target cell is exposed to it.

Signal Transduction Mechanisms

Most signals are water soluble and few will easily cross the hydrophobic centre of the plasma membrane. Instead signals react with receptors on the cell surface. Receptors for such signal molecules are integral membrane proteins. The signal molecule, therefore, often does not itself enter the cytoplasm but stimulates the production of a second messenger. A number of problems must be solved in such a system: (1) the detector must be sufficiently sensitive to pick up the signal; (2) as the concentration of ligand is likely to be small, some form of amplification is necessary; (3) it may be necessary to integrate the input from several receptors and use the combined signal to activate different effectors; (4) the signal must be transient if it is to be used repeatedly; and finally (5) adaptation may be necessary to allow the system to operate over a range of signal intensities.

Signals cross the plasma membrane in one of the following ways (Fig. 1.9):

(1) by direct transfer of the signal molecule, e.g. steroid and thyroid hormones;
(2) by altering ion channels, e.g. neuromuscular junctions;
(3) by binding of the signal molecule to specific receptors, inducing a conformational change and triggering a series of events which activate intracellular proteins, e.g. many growth factors.

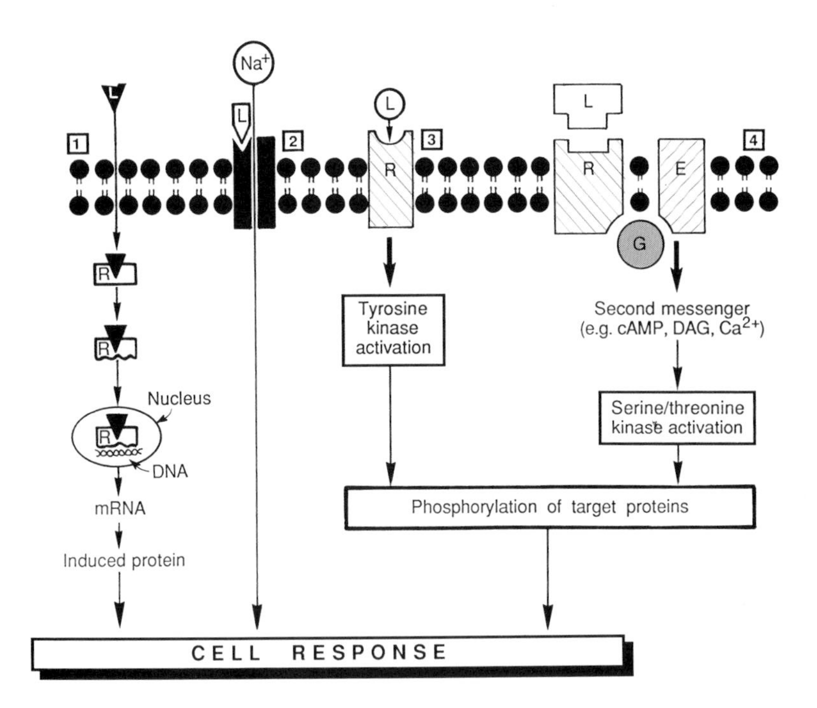

Fig. 1.9 Schematic representation of four common signal transduction mechanisms. L, ligand; R, receptor; G, G protein; E, effector enzyme.

Signalling Via Intracellular Receptors

Intracellular receptors (Fig. 1.9 [1]) are members of a nuclear receptor superfamily and include steroid, thyroid hormone, vitamin D and retinoic acid receptors. The receptors are polypeptides of around 800 amino acids and have three functional domains: the carboxyl-terminal hormone-binding domain, an internal domain which binds to DNA and an amino-terminal domain which activates (or inhibits) gene transcription. In the inactive state, the DNA binding domain is thought to be bound to an inhibitor protein. Some receptors are cytosolic when inactive, while others are nuclear. Binding of the hormone causes the receptor to dissociate from the inhibitory protein. Cytosolic receptors then move to the nucleus. Binding to specific sites within the DNA allows the receptor protein to interact with other regulatory proteins to alter the level of transcription of a small number of genes in any particular cell.

Channel-linked Receptors

Binding of the ligand results in the opening or closing of a specific ion channel (Fig. 1.9, [2]), thus altering the permeability of the cell membrane to that ion.

Tyrosine-kinase Activation

Phosphorylation is a common mechanism for altering the activity of a protein. There are two distinct types of protein kinases, one of which phosphorylates tyrosine residues and the other serine or threonine residues. Many catalytic receptors have been shown to be ligand activated tyrosine kinases. These include receptors for epidermal growth factor and platelet derived growth factor, implying that a tyrosine-kinase controlled step is important in cell proliferation, a suggestion supported by the finding that several oncogene products (p. 391) are also tyrosine kinases. Amplification of the signal is due to activation of tyrosine kinase (Fig. 1.9, [3])which may phosphorylate many different proteins, forming an enzyme cascade. Phosphatases which remove the phosphate group from the protein, thus diminishing its activity, are responsible for the transient effect of the signal. The modes of action of the phosphatases are as yet little understood, although they are clearly of major importance.

G-Protein Linked Receptors

These modulate the activity of the cell membrane associated enzymes via an intermediate GTP-binding (G) protein (Fig. 1.9, [4]). This may activate (or inactivate) a membrane bound enzyme or an ion channel. The levels of intracellular signalling molecules (or second messengers) such as cyclic AMP (cAMP) or Ca^{2+} can thus be changed, altering the activity of other cellular proteins. Two major G-protein linked signalling pathways are recognized.

Cyclic AMP pathway (Fig. 1.10). Cyclic AMP is generated from ATP by the enzyme adenylate cyclase which is located in the cell membrane. Increased levels of cAMP result in activation of cAMP-dependent protein kinase which triggers a series of phosphorylation reactions. Receptors which activate this pathway do so via a stimulatory G protein (G_s). Like all heterotrimeric G proteins, this comprises α, β and γ subunits. The α subunit contains the guanyl-nucleotide binding site which, in the inactive stage, binds GDP. The β and γ subunits form a complex which anchors the protein to the cell membrane. Receptor activation results in exchange of bound GDP for GTP by the α subunit, which then separates from the β and γ subunits and binds to adenylate cyclase, thus activating the enzyme.

In order to respond quickly to the body's changing requirements the levels of cAMP must be capable of rapid change. There are three processes which achieve this objective: (1) production of cAMP can continue only so long as messenger–receptor complexes persist at the cell surface, and such complexes are rapidly removed by endocytosis or by dissociation; (2) activated G_s protein is inactivated by the conversion of GTP to GDP by the endogenous GTPase activity of the α subunit. The subunit then reassociates with the β and γ subunits to form the inactive heterotrimer;

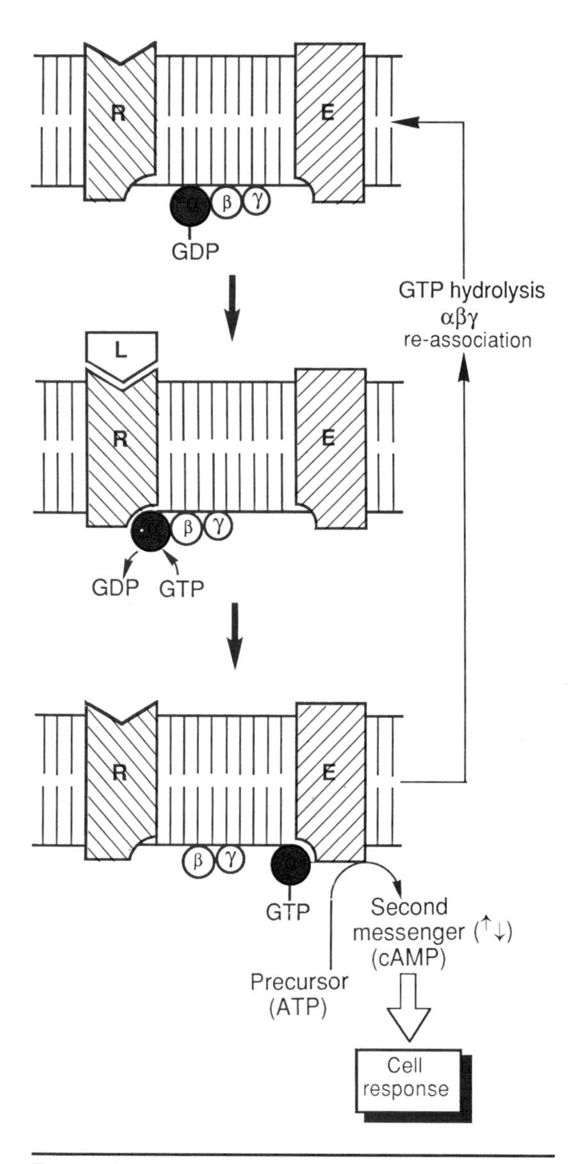

Fig. 1.10 Schematic representation of the G-protein-mediated activation of adenylate cyclase. Abbreviations are as in Fig. 1.9, and E represents the enzyme adenylate cyclase.

(3) cAMP is hydrolysed rapidly by phosphodiesterases.

In cholera, the enterotoxin of the bacterium *Vibrio cholera*, by preventing hydrolysis of GTP, produces persistent activation of the G_s protein in the intestinal epithelial cells. The persistent increase in the level of cAMP is responsible for the excessive secretion of water and electrolytes into the gut lumen and accounts for the intractable diarrhoea.

Some receptor–ligand interactions inhibit the activity of adenylate cyclase, via an inhibitory G protein (G_i) which has a different α chain, but the same β and γ subunits. It is activated in the same way as G_s. One of the toxins from *Bordetella pertussis*, which causes whooping cough, activates an inhibitory G protein and in so doing suppresses the normal immune response, improving survival for the bacterium but laying the host open to secondary infections which then constitute a major problem with this ailment.

Calcium and the phosphatidylinositol (PI) pathway (Fig. 1.11). The intracellular and extracellular concentrations of calcium are approximately equal. Most of the intracellular calcium is not in ionic form and is sequestered in various organelles or incorporated into calcium phosphate or bound by calcium binding proteins. The steep concentration of Ca^{2+} ions across the plasma membrane is maintained by energy derived from hydrolysis of ATP to pump Ca^{2+} against the gradient, both out of the cells and into the organelles.

The second messenger system activated by Ca^{2+}-mobilizing receptors is the phosphatidylinostol (PI) cycle (Fig. 1.11). Occupation of the receptor results in the activation of a polyphospho-inositide specific phosphodiesterase (PDE) via the action of a heterotrimeric G protein (Gp). PDE hydrolyses phosphatidylinositol 4,5-bisphosphate (PIP_2) to form two second messengers, diacylglycerol (DAG) and inositol 1,4,5-trisphosphate (IP_3). Diacylglycerol activates a calcium-dependent protein kinase (protein kinase C) which then phosphorylates specific proteins on serine or threonine residues. Phorbol esters act as analogues of diacylglycerol, but cause permanent activation of kinase C and this may explain their potent tumour promoting activity. Several oncogene products also act on this pathway, suggesting it is important in the development of malignancy (p. 391).

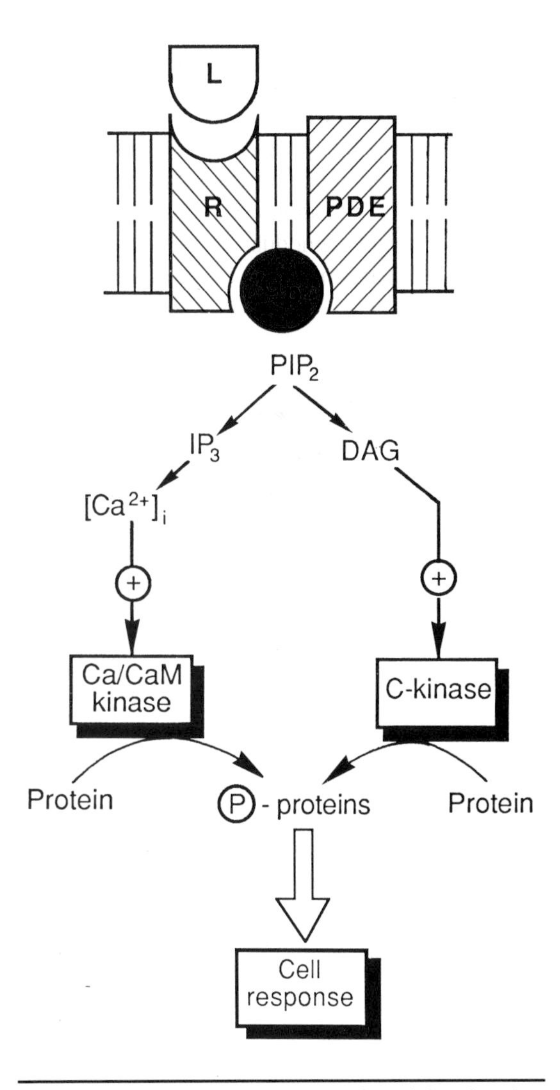

Fig. 1.11 Schematic representation of the phosphoinositide hydrolysis signalling system. Abbreviations as in Fig. 1.9.

IP_3 increases the level of intracellular Ca^{2+} by stimulating its release from stores in the endoplasmic reticulum. Like cAMP, the level of cytosolic Ca^{2+} can change rapidly. The rapid influx of extracellular Ca^{2+} or release of Ca^{2+} from intracellular stores is counterbalanced by efficient pumping of Ca^{2+} from the cytosol into organelles or into the extracellular fluid. Ca^{2+} activates a variety of intracellular enzymes, either directly or indirectly by binding to and activating the Ca^{2+} binding protein calmodulin (CaM). One of the important actions of calmodulin is the activation of a calmodulin-dependent protein kinase (Ca/CaM kinase).

Cell Proliferation

The control of cell proliferation is important in development and in tissue maintenance and repair. Tissues differ markedly in the extent to which their cell populations turn over. They can be regarded as **labile**, where continuing turnover occurs (e.g. skin, bone marrow), **stable** where little proliferation occurs in health, but where the ability to proliferate rapidly following damage is retained (e.g. liver), or **permanent**, where the ability to divide is lost (e.g. adult neurons). The size of a cell population is determined by the frequency of cell division, the proportion of the cells in the growth cycle and by the lifespan of cells. If the environment is unsuitable then the synthesis of new components will not proceed and growth will be stunted. The final size of a cell population or an individual is not determined purely by the available resources – a further level of control is needed, and this may be susceptible to pathological changes. For example, regulated secretion of somatotrophin (growth hormone) is required for normal growth and metabolism of tissues.

Excessive secretion of growth hormone results, in adults, in acromegaly (p. 1081) with bone enlargement and generalized organ and tissue hypertrophy. In childhood or adolescence excess growth hormone stimulates the immature skeleton producing gigantism, whereas its absence results in dwarfism (p. 1083).

Three patterns of cell proliferation occur. The two daughter cells may be identical (**binary division**) or they may have different fates (**dichotomous differentiation**), e.g. the fertilized ovum and many embryonic cells. In the **stem cell** pattern, one cell retains the primitive character, while the other follows a differentiating pathway, e.g. haemopoietic tissues and many epithelia. Although the full mechanism of control of proliferation is not understood, substantial progress has been made by the identification and characterization of molecules (cyclins) which control the progression of cells through the cell cycle. Excessive and inappropriate proliferation is a feature of neoplasia. These topics are discussed in detail in Chapter 10.

Homeostasis

Homeostasis can be considered at two levels, that of the cell itself, and that of the tissue. In the simplest of terms, there is a constant need to replace molecules which have gone past their 'sell-by' date, but there is also a need for turnover in order that novel transcriptional products can be expressed.

Intracellular proteins have very different half-lives, some being degraded within an hour of synthesis, others having half-lives of days or weeks. Much of this turnover occurs by the process of autophagy whereby molecules or organelles are enclosed by membrane vesicles which then fuse with lysosomes, but some occurs within the cytosol. In particular, some regulatory proteins have rapid turnover rates within the cytoplasm, and these short-lived proteins seem to have sequences rich in proline, glutamic acid, serine and threonine (PEST sequences). The formation of a complex between lysine amino groups of the protein and ubiquitin marks them for destruction by an ATP-dependent protease, releasing the ubiquitin for re-use. Ubiquitin is an abundant, highly conserved cytoplasmic protein, the free form of which is markedly diminished in concentration in the heat-shock response. Ubiquitin is associated with neurofibrillary tangles and senile plaques in Alzheimer's disease (p. 843) and other pathological inclusions.

Heat-shock proteins (stress proteins) are produced by a wide variety of cells in response to environmental insults, of which heat is only one. Several of these proteins seem to play a role in the assembly of membranes by stabilizing temporarily-folded proteins destined for membrane insertion. Increased production of these stabilizing proteins and reduced free ubiquitin levels may help the cell withstand further stress.

At a tissue level homeostasis involves the maintenance of the correct balance between cells and extracellular matrix, and the replacement of cells which have been damaged in some way. Extracellular matrix turnover is substantially slower than that of cytoplasmic proteins, but nevertheless still takes place. The correct balance between matrix degradation and replacement and between cell death and proliferation is undoubtedly altered in many pathological situations, an example of the importance of time relations.

Cell Injury and Death

Cells may be damaged as a result of some congenital defect, by some acquired insult, or as a consequence of programmed obsolescence. The acquired conditions include the effects of defective nutrition, hypoxia, physical damage, chemicals and drugs, infections and immunological reactions. Many of these entities will be dealt with in the appropriate chapters later in the book. Repair mechanisms exist within cells and thus injury, which is of short duration or minimal in extent, may cause damage which is capable of complete resolution. It is only if the cell's capacity for repair is exceeded that cell injury becomes manifest. In the extreme case this will result in cell death but lesser degrees may allow the cell time to adapt (e.g. by hypertrophy or metaplasia) so that it is able to withstand the injury.

Reversible Cell Injury

One of the commonest types of cell injury is due to ischaemia. The resultant hypoxia causes a reduction of available ATP and the cell switches over to anaerobic glycolysis in an attempt to maintain energy supply. Cellular stocks of glycogen diminish, there is a build-up in the concentration of lactic acid, a byproduct of anaerobic glycolysis, with a fall in the intracellular pH. Lack of ATP results in failure of the sodium pump mechanism and the resultant in-flow of sodium is accompanied by appropriate amounts of water to ensure isotonicity. The breakdown of cell constituents secondary to injury also causes an increase in the number of small molecules within the cytoplasm with a similar osmotically driven increase of intracellular water.

Direct injury to the plasma membrane can give an increase in permeability with similar effects. Acute cellular swelling is an early phenomenon in most varieties of reversible injury. The extra fluid within the cell may be seen by the light microscope as an increase in rather pale cytoplasm – hydropic change – whilst by the electron microscope there is dilatation of the endoplasmic reticulum with degranulation and dissociation of polyribosomes into single ribosomes. If water continues to accumulate it may produce clear vacuoles which can be seen in the light microscope – hence the term vacuolar degeneration.

Changes are also observed at the cell surface; microvilli are lost and surface blebs are seen. This may be due to changes in the cytoskeleton. Degenerative changes in lipid membranes produces myelin figures, stacks of lipid fragments which may roll up into closed vesicular structures. Nuclear changes are not striking in reversible injury although there may be mild clumping of chromatin and some separation of the nucleolus into its fibrillar and granular components.

Irreversible Cell Injury

It is not possible to establish reliable ultrastructural criteria by which irreversible cellular injury can be identified. There is a continuum from the reversibly injured cell through to the obviously necrotic and the point at which necrosis becomes inevitable cannot be discerned. Vacuolation within the cell becomes more severe, and woolly or flocculent densities may be found within mitochondria; mitochondrial damage is probably one of the most reliable early manifestations of irreversible cell injury. Damage to plasma membranes becomes obvious and is associated with loss of cell constituents into the extracellular space. Cytoskeletal changes involve the breakage of microfilaments and intermediate filaments. Perturbation of the membrane cytoskeleton may cause the formation of blebs on the surface. The drop in pH in injury to membranes is associated with the leakage of lysosomal enzymes (proteases, nucleases, glucosidases, phosphatidases and peroxidases) into the cytosol and to their activation. These acid hydrolases cause extensive digestion of both cytoplasmic and nuclear components, **autolysis**. The dead cell is finally represented by a mass of mainly membranous structures which can be phagocytosed by neighbouring cells or by macrophages.

Final Common Pathway in Irreversible Cell Injury

The cell may show a similar pattern of response in many types of injury. It may be that, although the initiating injury and the site of injury varies, in the irreversibly damaged cell there is a final common pathway which results in cellular demise. Cellular complexity and the close interaction and dependence of various aspects of cellular metabolism, one with the other, mean that injury to one part of a cell rapidly has repercussions elsewhere: in many instances it is therefore not possible to separate cause from effect in an injured cell.

The integrity of the compartmentalization within cells is central to their well-being. If the cell processes which produce and maintain these compartments are destroyed then the imbalance which exists between the inner and external environment of the cell is destroyed and the cell dies. These differences can be profound. Thus, in the case of calcium ions the external concentration is some 10^4 times that of the internal concentration, and the integrity of the plasma membrane in maintaining this difference seems to be all important.

Mechanism of Disruption of the Plasma Membrane

In ischaemic cellular injury reduction in blood supply leads to a diminution in the availability of ATP. If the duration of the ischaemia is short then the cell may recover on reinstatement of the blood supply. If the ischaemic period is more prolonged then reinstatement of the blood supply leads, not to recovery, but to further cell damage with loss of membrane permeability. This so-called **reperfusion injury** is secondary to the generation of toxic free radicals, mainly derived from oxygen, which are produced during the period of restored blood flow. Free radicals are chemical species which have a single unpaired electron in an outer orbital shell. They are highly reactive, markedly unstable, and are capable of stimulating autocatalytic reactions with the further generation of toxic species.

Oxygen Free Radicals

During the production of ATP, oxygen is reduced to water with the removal of four electrons. There are therefore three other oxygen species in which the reduction is partial, involving the loss of one, two or three electrons and generating superoxide (O_2^-), hydrogen peroxide (H_2O_2) and the hydroxyl radical ($OH^\bullet$) respectively. These species are not produced from the cytochrome oxidase chain but by other means.

Superoxide is generated utilizing xanthine oxidase or cytochrome P_{450}:

$$O_2 \xrightarrow[\text{oxidase}]{} O_2^-$$

Hydrogen peroxide is produced, either as a reaction product of the other free radicals or directly by various oxidases present in the peroxisomes.

Hydroxyl radicals are produced by the action of ionizing radiation on water and free radicals may also be produced by the reaction of hydrogen peroxide with transition metals as in the Fenton reaction:

$$H_2O_2 + Fe^{2+} \longrightarrow OH^- + OH^\bullet + Fe^{3+}$$

or by the Haber–Weiss reaction which involves superoxide:

$$O_2^- + H_2O_2 \longrightarrow O_2 + OH^- + OH^\bullet$$

These free radicals are highly unstable and may spontaneously decay. They may also be removed by a variety of antioxidants such as vitamin E, glutathione and D-penicillamine whose sulphydryl groups block the initiation of free radical formation. Enzymes such as superoxide dismutase convert superoxide to hydrogen peroxide and oxygen,

$$O_2^- + O_2^- + 2H^+ \longrightarrow H_2O_2 + O_2$$

catalase breaks hydrogen peroxide to water and oxygen and glutathione peroxidase converts hydroxyl radicals (and also hydrogen peroxide) to water.

Effects of free radicals. Free radicals react with the double bonds of unsaturated fatty acids and with sulphydryl groups in proteins. Hydroxyl radical is primarily involved in lipid damage. It reacts with the unsaturated bonds to produce a lipid free radical, which in turn reacts with oxygen to form a lipid peroxide. Lipid peroxide also acts as a free radical and reacts with a further unsaturated bond of a fatty acid to establish an autocatalytic chain reaction. The resultant damage to phospholipids causes changes in membrane permeability with the consequences which have been described. The reaction of free radicals with sulphydryl groups forms disulphide bonds with cross-linking of proteins. This may disrupt the functioning of enzymes or produce focal increases in membrane permeability.

Generation of Free Radicals in Pathological Processes

Free radicals have now been implicated in a number of pathological processes. In ischaemia they are involved in reperfusion injury. Bacterial killing by phagocytic cells is associated with a burst of oxygen consumption and some of the tissue damage associated with the process of inflammation is secondary to the production of toxic oxygen metabolites. Failure of phagocytic cells to produce free radicals leads to inefficient bacterial killing with serious consequences for the host, including the development of chronic granulomatous disease (p. 595).

Direct oxygen toxicity develops in patients exposed to high concentrations of the gas or for long periods of time. Exposure to ozone causes similar effects. Exposure to radiotherapy in the treatment of tumours (p. 433) owes its effects, at least in part, to the production of hydroxyl radicals secondary to the radiolysis of water. One of the theories of ageing postulates lipid peroxidation as a mechanism. In some chemical injuries there are also examples of free radical mediated damage: the toxic effects of carbon tetrachloride on liver cells is attributable to its metabolism in the smooth endoplasmic reticulum by the cytochrome P450 system with the production of the highly reactive trichloromethyl radical ($CCl_3^\bullet$). This moiety reacts with the double bonds of the unsaturated fatty acids in the membrane of the smooth endoplasmic reticulum, producing chloroform and a lipid radical. The latter then reacts with oxygen to initiate the autocatalytic reaction which will destroy the membrane system of the endoplasmic reticulum.

Necrosis

Necrosis is the death of cells or groups of cells which are still part of the living organism. The process may be rapid or gradual and the causes are many and varied. Tissue necrosis as a result of reduced blood supply and anoxia is termed **infarction** and the dead tissue is called an **infarct** (p. 103). Toxins and many bacterial toxins are directly membranolytic, as are some snake venoms. Membrane damage may be a consequence of the insertion of the membrane attack complex of complement (p. 142) or perforins from cytotoxic lymphocytes (p. 196). Virus infection of cells can cause their death and the result may be extremely serious as in poliomyelitis or hepatitis, or relatively trivial as in the case of cold sores caused by herpes simplex. Chemical poisons may affect cells non-selectively by causing protein denaturation or by disrupting the phospholipids of the plasma membrane, or may act on more restricted targets (e.g. cyanide inhibits the cytochrome oxidase system). Even though the primary target may be restricted the consequences can, however, be widespread. Thus, inhibition of ATP production by mitochondrial poisons removes the energy source for ion pumping, without which the plasma membrane resting potential is lost, and without electrically active membrane systems neuronal and muscular systems cease to work.

Physical damage and heat are obvious potential causes of death, the latter causing its effects by protein denaturation. Physical damage is also the cause of cell death in freezing where ice crystal formation ruptures cell membranes. Rapid freezing techniques and the use of cryoprotectants minimizes ice crystal formation and enable living cells to be stored in liquid nitrogen. Irradiation is a potent cause of cell damage though this is turned to advantage in the treatment of tumours.

Recognition of Necrosis

The gross changes brought about by the liberation of lytic enzymes from lysosomes (autolysis) take time to occur. Some of the early ultrastructural changes are described above but it is only after a few hours that changes can be seen in the light microscope. In a conventional haemotoxylin and eosin stained section there is cytoplasmic eosinophilia. This is due to loss of RNA with consequent loss of the normal cytoplasmic basophilia, plus increased binding of eosin to denatured cytoplasmic proteins. Some nuclei show decreased staining as they undergo dissolution – **karyolysis** (Fig. 1.12), other nuclei break up to give discrete fragments – **karyorrhexis** (Fig. 1.13) and some nuclei shrink and appear as densely staining masses (**pyknosis**).

The gross appearance of necrosis varies considerably and is, to some extent, dependent on the balance which is struck between the processes of denaturation and the autolytic changes which proceed concurrently. In **coagulative necrosis** the dead tissue becomes swollen and firm due to the deposition of thromboplastins and takes on a dull

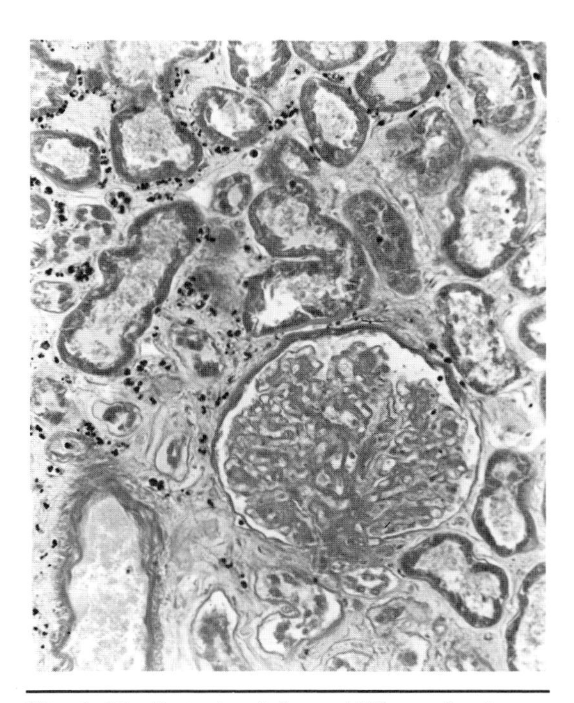

Fig. 1.12 Part of an infarct of kidney, showing coagulative necrosis. A glomerulus and tubules are seen, but the nuclei have disappeared and the structural details are lost. ×172.

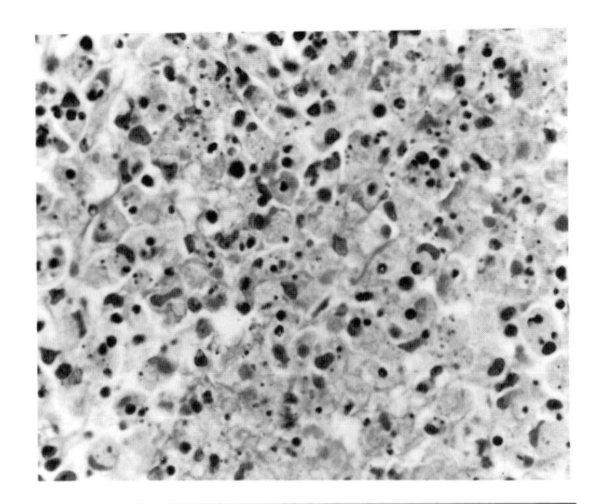

Fig. 1.13 Spreading necrosis with karyorrhexis in lymph node in typhoid fever. Note destruction of nuclei and numerous deeply stained granules of chromatin. ×312.

yellow colour (see Figs 10.28 and 10.29). In the light microscope ghost outlines of cells may still be visible and the dead area is brightly eosinophilic. These changes take place characteristically in heart, kidney and spleen, and generally in tissues damaged by heat denaturation of proteins in which enzyme (i.e. autolytic) activity is prevented. Tissues with a higher water content, such as brain, tend to show **colliquative necrosis**, a complete loss of tissue architecture with eventual cyst formation (p. 818). In such tissues the processes of autolysis predominate over the coagulative changes and hence tissue breakdown is extreme (see Fig. 21.18).

A similar effect is found in some bacterial infections when the chemotaxin induced accumulation of neutrophil polymorphonuclear leucocytes (p. 293) is associated with the release of their lysosomal contents and the consequent liquefaction of the tissues locally – an **abscess**. Other tissues lose their architecture and become amorphous, granular and eosinophilic with variable amounts of fat and an appearance reminiscent of cottage cheese, hence the term **caseation** (see Fig. 8.13). This pattern is commonly associated with tuberculosis but may also be found occasionally in some infarcts, in necrotic tumours and in inspissated pus.

Necrotic tissue may become secondarily infected by bacteria, particularly if the necrotic tissue is in contact with the skin or other mucosal surface. The combination of necrosis with bacterial invasion is referred to as **gangrene** (Fig. 1.14). In tissues in which the coagulative changes predominate the phenomenon is referred to as dry gangrene; if colliquative changes are present then the appearances are those of wet gangrene. The tissues so affected often become discoloured due to the deposition of sulphides derived from haemoglobin. A variety of anaerobic bacteria may be involved, in particular the clostridia group, which are commensals in the gastrointestinal tract. In gas gangrene, which is associated with penetrating injuries which may be contaminated by soil, *Clostridium welchii* produce hydrogen sulphide.

Finally, **fat necrosis** is a pattern of cell death found in fatty tissue. It is most commonly found in acute pancreatitis, where lipases liberated from damaged pancreatic acini act, not only on the local cells but also on fat cells throughout the peritoneal cavity. The lipases liberate free fatty acids from the triglycerides in the fat cells and, in the presence of calcium salts, calcium 'soaps' are precipitated. These appear as whitish chalky areas scattered throughout otherwise normal adipose tissue. Fat necrosis in breast tissue is associated with trauma.

Effects of Necrosis

The effects of tissue necrosis vary with the organ involved, the extent of the necrosis, the functional reserve of the tissue and the capacity of the surviving cells to proliferate and replace those which have been lost. Thus, the loss of a small amount of cardiac muscle may be fatal, whereas a comparable loss from a large skeletal muscle would be inconsequential; liver cells are rapidly replaced while neurons are not.

The necrotic area may eventually be completely restored to normal, the process of **resolution** (p. 130), although this is unusual. More commonly, there is an inflammatory reaction followed by the

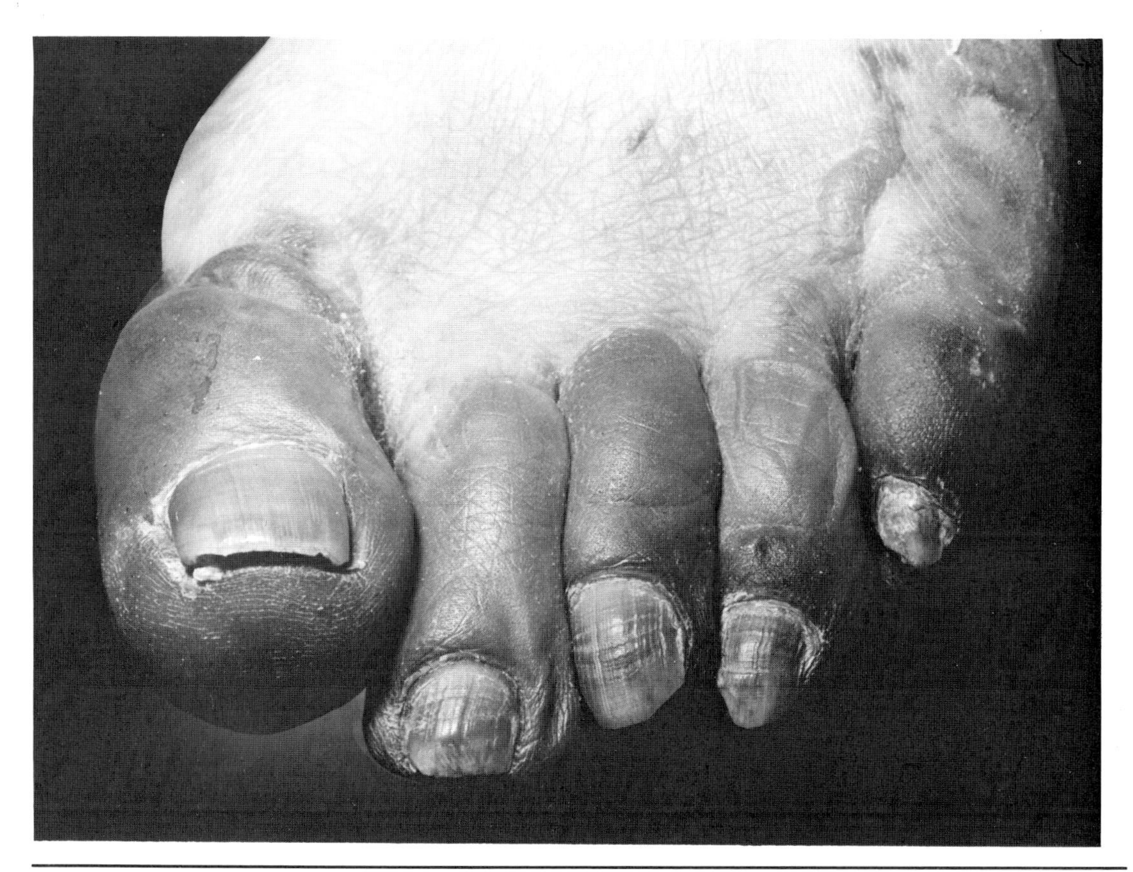

Fig. 1.14 Gangrene of toes.

process of **organization**. The dead tissue is removed by normal clearance mechanisms (largely phagocytic activity) and replaced by fibrous tissue. In very large areas the central portion of the necrotic tissue may be remote from the inflammatory process and may therefore persist for months to years. A variety of intracellular molecules are released following breakdown of the plasma membrane and elevated serum levels may act as diagnostic markers, e.g. the hepatic aminotransferases (p. 744). The released enzymes may cause non-specific effects such as a raised erythrocyte sedimentation rate and fever.

Necrotic tissue is a common site for **dystrophic calcification** – a process in which calcium salts are deposited in the tissues although the levels of calcium and phosphate are within the normal range. Calcification may be found in old infarcts, in areas of fat necrosis (p. 793), in the remains of dead parasites and in foci of inspissated pus: the previous sites of tuberculous caseation may be easily detected by X-ray examination. Although often associated with necrotic tissue, dystrophic calcification may also be found in the dense connective tissue of tendons, scarred heart valves, in some tumours (Fig. 1.15) and in the media of aged arteries where the Ca^{2+} may convert the vessel into a rigid tube which can be easily palpated and visualized by X-ray. Dystrophic calcification is contrasted with **metastatic calcification** in which there is the widespread deposition of calcium in otherwise normal tissues (Fig. 1.16) due to the raised levels of circulating or tissue calcium, e.g. secondary to hypervitaminosis

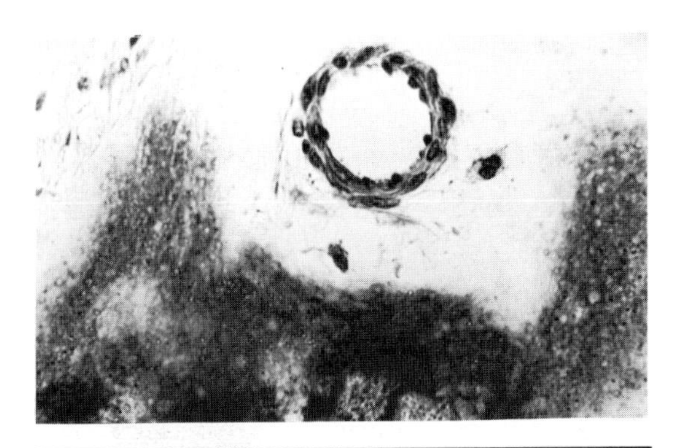

Fig. 1.15 Dystrophic calcification of hyaline connective tissue adjacent to a small blood vessel in a fibroma. The calcified tissue is stained by haematoxylin (even after decalcification), and presents a dark granular appearance. ×500.

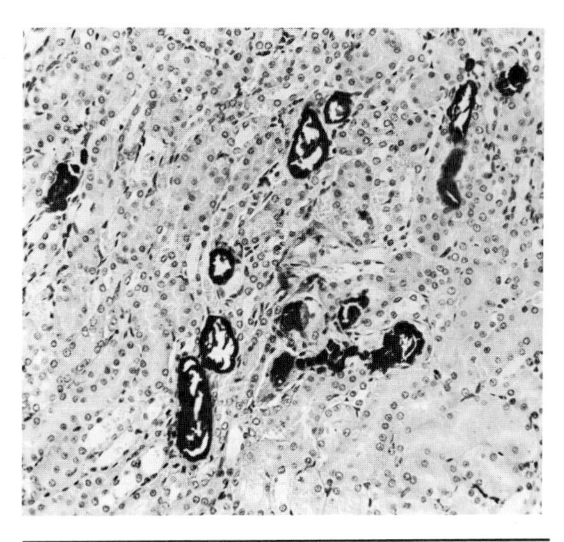

Fig. 1.16 Rat kidney in hypervitaminosis D. Note calcified small vessels and renal tubules. ×120.

D (p. 354), hyperparathyroidism (p. 1104), the milk-alkali syndrome, sarcoidosis (p. 313) and excess mobilization of calcium from the bones as in prolonged immobilization, the presence of secondary tumour or multiple myeloma (p. 948).

Programmed Cell Death

In many organs cells are shed as they come to the end of their lifespan. This programmed obsolescence involves cell death by the process of **apoptosis*** (Figs 1.17 and 1.18). Unlike necrosis, where groups of cells are killed, apoptosis tends to affect single cells surrounded by viable neighbours. It has a unique morphology characterized by chromatin condensation and shrinkage of cell volume. Apoptosis is an energy dependent process, unlike the passive autolysis which follows cell death induced by injury. The chromatin is broken down in a regular fashion by endonucleases, which are activated during the process.

*Note the second p is silent and the correct pronunciation is *apotosis*.

In addition, transglutaminases are activated, cross-link cytosolic proteins and help to convert the cell to a rigid, shrunken shell which shows intense eosinophilic staining. The dead cell breaks into fragments, some of which may be shed from free surfaces: others are phagocytosed by adjacent cells or by macrophages to form **apoptopic bodies**, secondary lysosomes containing cellular debris. New surface molecules appear on apoptotic cells which permit their recognition and phagocytosis. Unlike necrosis, apoptosis does not elicit an inflammatory response and underlines the physiological nature of programmed cell death.

Apoptosis is also prominent during embryological development, for example in the separation of digits in limb development. The initiation of apoptosis is regulated by growth factors, some turning it on whilst others delay or prevent it. Thus, falling progesterone and oestrogen levels trigger synchronous apoptosis and rapid endometrial cell loss at the time of menstruation. Apoptosis can also be a pathological process: it is found in tissues undergoing atrophy, in tissues which have been irradiated and in tissues injured by cytotoxic T lymphocytes. It is an important feature of tumours in which it may affect the rate of tumour growth (p. 362).

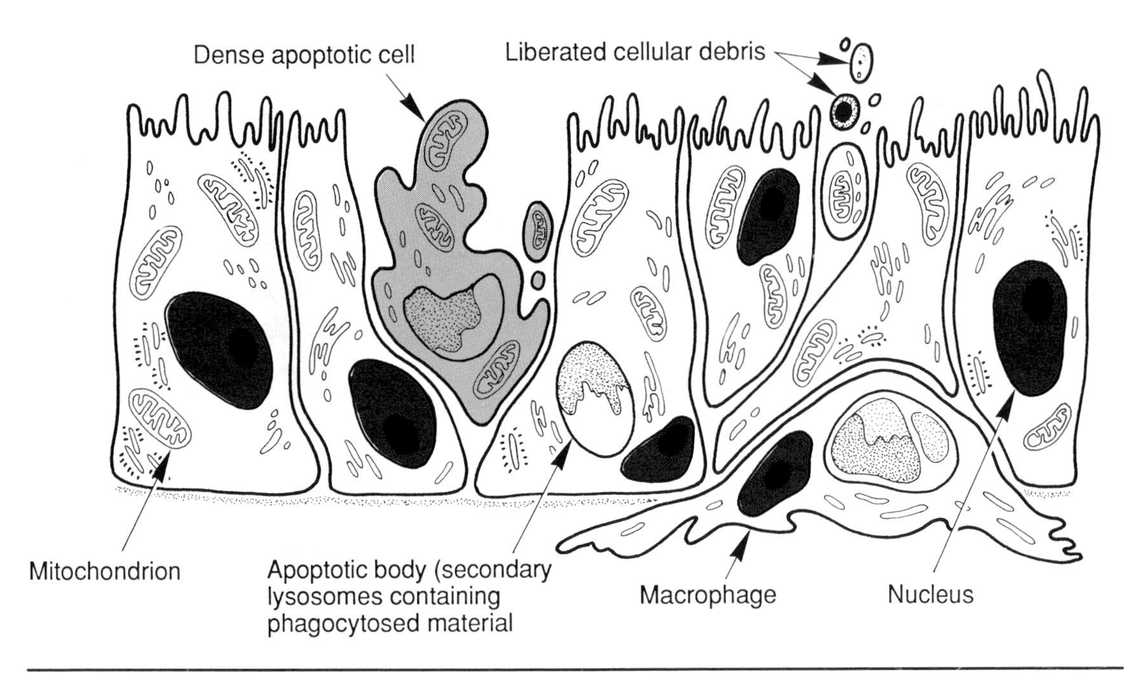

Fig. 1.17 Scheme of events in apoptosis. (By courtesy of Dr A. H. Wyllie.)

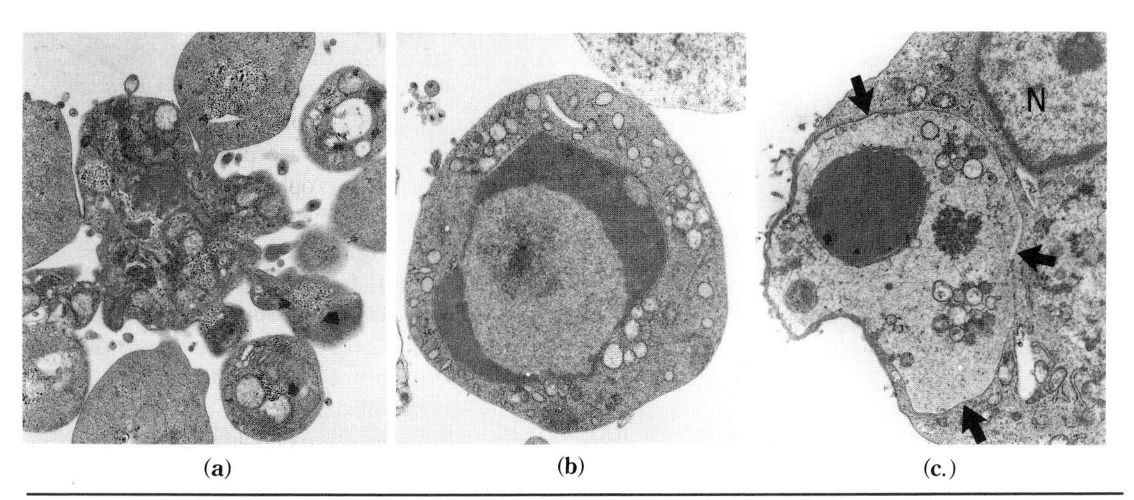

Fig. 1.18 Apoptosis in a rodent sarcoma cell. The electromicrographs show the traumatic shrinkage and blebbing (**a**), the characteristic nuclear chromatin condensation (**b**), and phagocytosis within a neighbouring cell whose own nucleus (N) is normal (**c.**) The boundaries of the phagosome are arrowed. (By courtesy of Dr A. H. Wyllie.)

Cellular Adaptation Mechanisms

The above text considers the two extremes with regard to a cell's ability to withstand insult, either complete recovery or death. Between these two extremes there lie a range of cellular reactions where the cell attempts to adapt to the insult. These reactions include atrophy, hypoplasia, hypertrophy, hyperplasia, metaplasia and the accumulation within the cell of a variety of materials which may be endogenous or exogenous in origin.

Hypoplasia and Atrophy

In hypoplasia and atrophy there is a decrease in the size of cells, or of the tissues as a result of decreased cell size or number. Hypoplasia is a failure of the tissue to reach normal size during development, whereas atrophy is a decrease in size at a later stage. Hypoplasia, which is the opposite of hyperplasia, may be due to reduced proliferation or a mismatch between replacement and death of cells. The atrophic cells tend to have diminished functional ability and this is reflected in a reduced number of cell organelles. It may be that the delicate balance between cellular synthetic and degradative processes is tipped in favour of the latter; as a consequence the cell decreases in volume and there is some loss of more specialized functions.

Hypoplasia can have various causes; in achondroplasia impaired growth of the cartilaginous skeleton is the result of a mutational event, whereas in some types of dwarfism the cause may be a reduced level of growth hormone as in pituitary hypofunction or a lack of growth hormone receptors as in Laron-type dwarfism. Other mechanisms include cell loss because of infection or poisoning. Rubella infection in early pregnancy may damage the fetal heart and lead to incomplete development of the cardiac septa, producing a number of congenital abnormalities.

Physiological atrophy. Atrophy is a normal aspect of ageing in many tissues, for example the loss of thymocytes and the shrinkage of the thymus after puberty, the reduction in endometrial cellularity after the menopause and of osteocytes in the ageing skeleton. Sexual glands decrease in size and the brain commonly atrophies in old age. Atrophy is quite commonly accompanied by the intracellular accumulation of lipofuscin, a yellowish-brown 'wear and tear' pigment.

Nutritional atrophy. This may be produced locally by arterial disease interfering with the blood supply to a part when the reduction is not sufficiently severe to cause necrosis. General atrophy occurs in starvation. Emaciation depends chiefly on utilization of the fat of the adipose tissues, but there is also wasting of the tissues, the liver and muscles being particularly affected. The term **cachexia** is often applied to the combination of wasting, anaemia and weakness, and is seen mainly in severely ill patients in whom loss of appetite and other gastrointestinal disturbances lead to diminished food intake. In most cases there are usually additional contributory factors such as the increased catabolism of fever. In patients dying of malignant disease the weight loss is a consequence of the action of the cytokine, tumour necrosis factor or cachectin (p. 145), produced by macrophages and possibly other cells in a response presumably designed to destroy the tumour.

Disuse atrophy. In general, diminished functional activity is associated with reduced catabolism, which in turn has a negative feedback on anabolism and leads to decrease in size of cells. A good example of this is the decrease in muscle bulk following prolonged immobilization or weightlessness in the case of astronauts. This leads to wasting, not only of muscle but also of bone from which calcium is lost. In paralysed limbs the bones become atrophic (Fig. 1.19). Unless such atrophy has become extreme, it is reversible and full functional activity may be restored.

Neuropathic atrophy develops when there is any destruction of lower motor neurons or their axons. After nerve section, the denervated muscles may lose half their mass. For at least a few weeks anabolic processes continue at a normal rate but catabolism is greatly accelerated. The affected muscles give abnormal electromyographic responses and complete return to normal is not possible.

Endocrine atrophy. Atrophy of thyroid, adrenals and gonads are seen when damage to the pituitary results in diminution of the appropriate trophic hormones. In turn marked atrophy of target organs may occur in endocrine hypofunction, e.g. the skin, hair follicles and sebaceous glands in hypothyroidism.

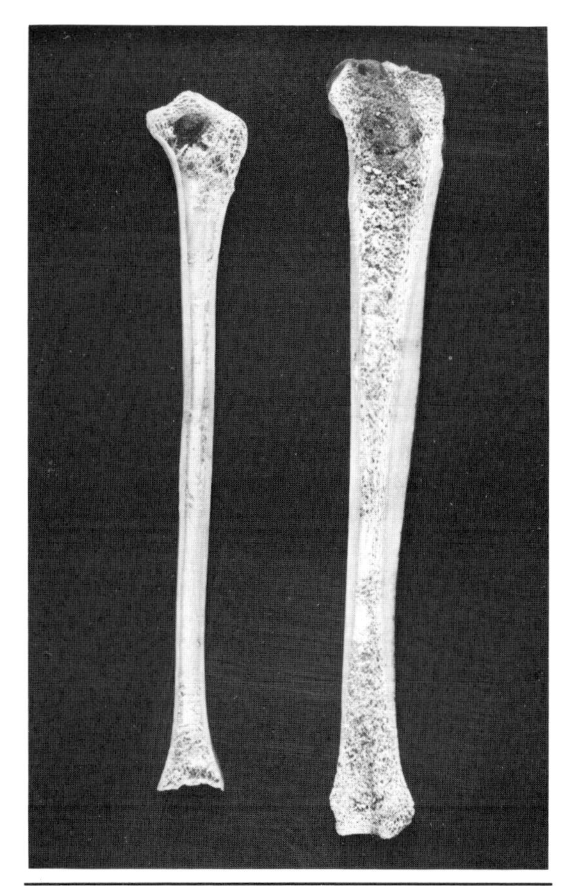

Fig. 1.19 Tibia from long-standing case of poliomyelitis, showing marked atrophy (left). Normal tibia for comparison (right). ×0.3.

Other types of atrophy. Increased catabolism in fever or following severe trauma may cause skeletal muscle atrophy. Pressure atrophy of an organ may result from benign tumours or cysts which interfere with the blood supply or function of the tissue. Post-irradiation atrophy is due to chromosomal damage which interferes with mitosis.

Hypertrophy and Hyperplasia

Stimulation of the parenchymal cells of an organ, usually by increased functional demand or by hormones, results in an increase in the total mass of the parenchymal cells. This may be brought about by enlargement of the cells – **hypertrophy** – or by an increase in their number – **hyperplasia**. The relative importance of the two processes varies in different organs. In some (e.g. skeletal muscle), the enlargement is purely by hypertrophy, but in most organs both hypertrophy and hyperplasia contribute.

The Response to Increased Functional Demand

This is illustrated by the hypertrophied muscles of manual labourers and athletes; the individual muscle fibres increase in thickness but not in number. A similar phenomenon can be seen in cardiac muscle in response to an increased workload, e.g. the left ventricle in hypertension (Fig. 1.20). Smooth muscle may also undergo hypertrophy, for example in the wall of the stomach in a patient with pyloric stenosis, or in the bladder obstructed by an enlarged prostate. Striking hypertrophy of smooth muscle is seen in the pregnant uterus in response to a combination of increased functional demand and hormonal stimuli, resulting in enlargement of fibres to more than a hundred times their original volume. In early pregnancy there is both hypertrophy and hyperplasia of muscle fibres. Compensatory hypertrophy may occur in the survivor of a pair of organs when one is removed. This is well exemplified in live kidney donors where the donor kidney nearly doubles in size through both hypertrophy and hyperplasia.

Hyperplasia without hypertrophy is unusual and one of the few common examples affects red blood cells. Residence at high altitude, where the O_2 content of the atmosphere is relatively low, leads to compensatory hyperplasia of red cell precursors in the bone marrow and an increased number of circulating red blood cells. Return to sea level causes a drop in the red blood cell numbers to normal values. An example of physiological hyperplasia is the enlargement of the breasts in preg-

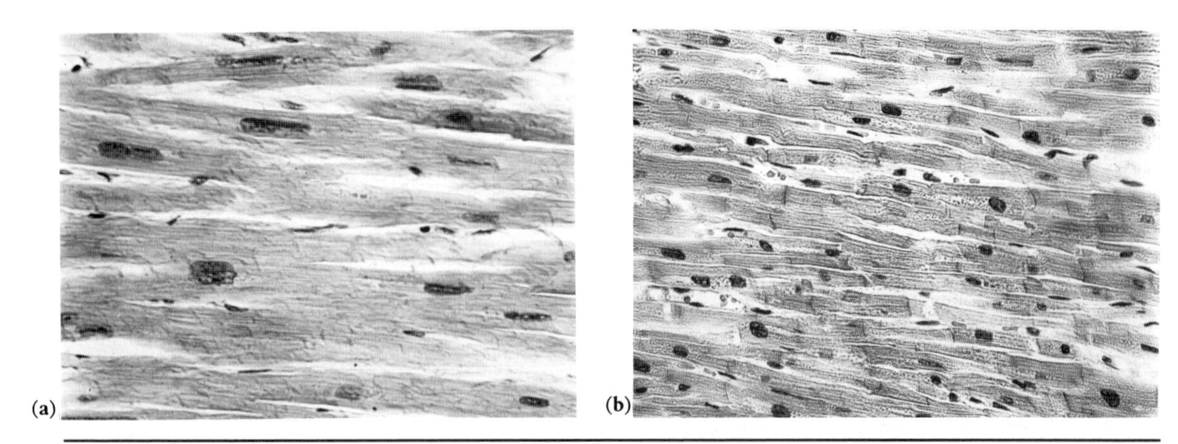

Fig. 1.20 (**a**) Hypertrophied muscle fibres of heart in a case of arteriosclerosis with high blood pressure. ×250. (**b**) Slightly atrophied heart muscle; to compare with **a**. ×250.

nancy (Fig. 1.21) when the mammary gland acini are stimulated by prolactin and oestrogens produced from the corpus luteum or placenta.

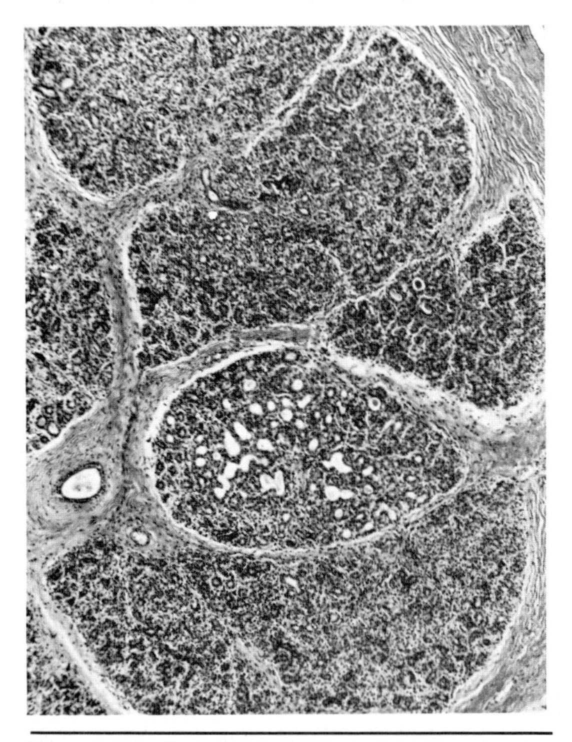

Fig. 1.21 Breast lobule in pregnancy showing marked hyperplasia. ×50.

Metaplasia

Metaplasia means the transformation of one type of differentiated tissue into another. An example is provided by the surface epithelium of the bronchi which commonly changes from the normal ciliated pseudostratified columnar epithelium to stratified squamous (Fig. 1.22). In this example it appears that chronic irritation or injury, often due to cigarette smoke, results in adaptive changes in the surface epithelium to a type more likely to be resistant to the cause of the irritation. Similarly, stratified squamous epithelium may form as a result of chronic irritation in the mucous membrane of the nose, salivary ducts, gall-bladder, renal pelvis and urinary bladder. In vitamin A deficiency, stratified squamous epithelium may replace the transitional and columnar epithelia of the nose, bronchi and urinary tract, and the specialized secretory epithelia of the lacrimal and salivary glands. In autoimmune chronic gastritis (p. 693), in which there is an immunological attack on the mucosa of the fundus of the patient's own stomach, there may be metaplasia to an intestinal type of mucosa with goblet cells and Paneth cells.

In connective tissues metaplasia occurs between fibrous tissue, bone and cartilage. Bone formation occasionally follows the deposition of calcium in such tissues as arterial walls (Fig. 1.23),

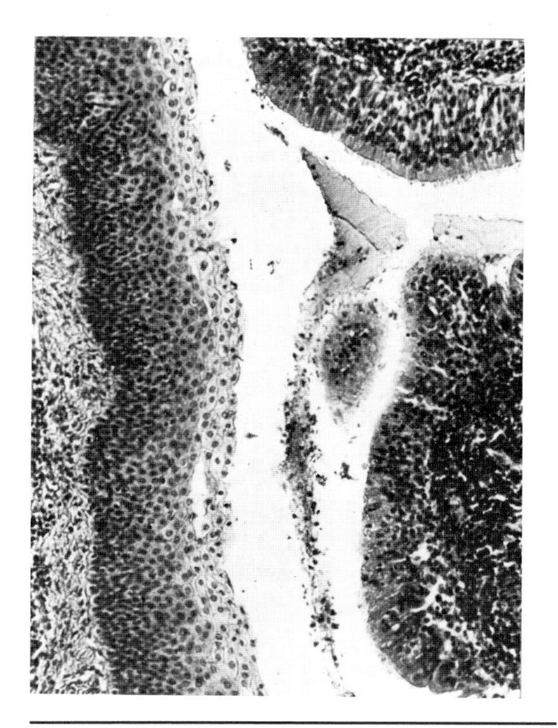

Fig. 1.22 Metaplasia of bronchial epithelium to stratified squamous type is seen on the left side, persistence of columnar ciliated epithelium on the right. ×200.

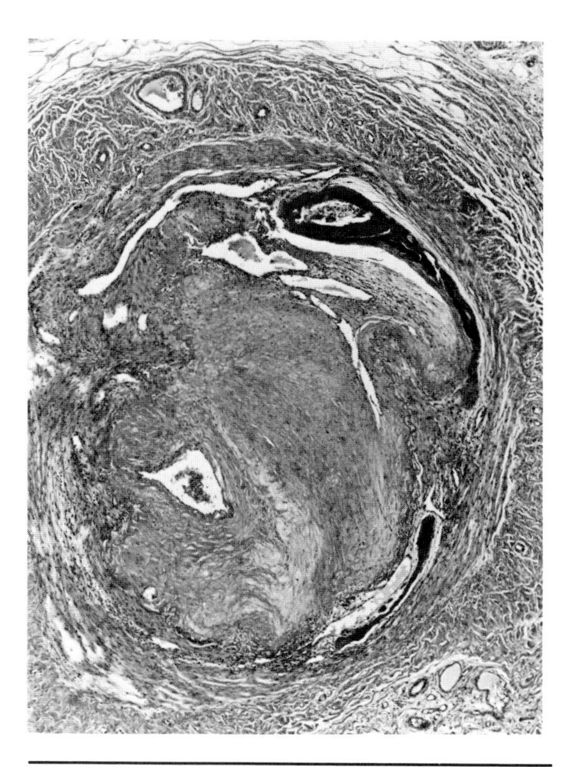

Fig. 1.23 Metaplastic bone formation in the wall of a largely obliterated artery. ×50.

bronchial cartilage and the uveal tract of the eye. In healing fractures cartilaginous metaplasia may occur, especially when there is undue mobility.

The examples of metaplasia described above are presumed to be due to gene activation and/or repression due to environmental signals. Alternatively it may be that the original cells are lost and a new population takes over. Many stimuli which give rise to metaplasia can induce neoplasia and metaplastic cells may give rise to tumours which exhibit the same type of metaplasia, e.g. squamous carcinoma of the bronchus.

There are other types of abnormal differentiation. In **heterotopia**, which arises during embryonic development, groups of cells differentiate in a manner which is inappropriate for their anatomical position in the body. An example is the presence of small clusters of pancreatic acini (sometimes with islets) in the wall of the stomach. The pathogenesis is unknown but focal errors in intercellular communication in the developing fetus seems likely. **Dedifferentiation** is a process whereby cells lose some of their specialized characteristics when they become atrophic.

Intracellular Storage

Variation in the supply of nutrients is offset by the normal process of intracellular storage. Excess storage can arise in a number of circumstances. It may be found when normal metabolism is upset by some toxin or drug, the result being the accumulation of a normal substance whose catabolism is now defective, e.g. fatty change. Alternatively, there may be a genetic defect resulting in the absence of some catabolic enzyme whose substrate therefore accumulates (see Chapter 7). Lastly, material which is incapable of further digestion or of transfer to other sites may accumulate. These compounds may be endogenous (lipofuscin, melanin, iron and bile pigments), or exogenous (carbon and tattoo pigments). In many instances the cell can tolerate the accumulation of large amounts of the appropriate product and appear unharmed, but in others the accumulated material causes cell injury.

Fatty Change

Fatty change is found most commonly in the liver which has a central role in fat metabolism; it is also described in heart and kidney. In normal conditions lipids are transferred to the liver from the gastro-intestinal tract and from adipose tissue and enter the hepatocytes as free fatty acids. They are there esterified to triglycerides which require the presence of a specific apoprotein molecule before they can be secreted from the cell. Triglycerides may therefore accumulate in the liver cells when excessive fatty acids are delivered to the liver for processing; this occurs in obesity, diabetes mellitus and, paradoxically, in starvation and in some chronic wasting illnesses, where there is mobilization of the fat stores (see Fig. 20.9). Starvation will also reduce protein synthesis, and in particular the formation of apoproteins, essential for normal lipid transformation (p. 339). Various toxins can also cause fatty change by interrupting the metabolism of lipid in the liver cell; the commonest of these is alcohol (p. 760).

Lipofuscin

Lipofuscin is a yellow-brown finely granular pigment which accumulates in the cytoplasm of cells. Associated with age and with apoptosis it is often referred to as a 'wear and tear' pigment but may also be found with increased frequency in malnourished patients, in those with wasting illnesses (e.g. cancer), in patients receiving radiotherapy and in atrophic cells or tissues. Whilst lipofuscin can be found in any cell it is particularly associated with liver and heart – 'brown atrophy' of the heart.

Ultrastructurally the pigment takes the form of autophagocytic vacuoles, often in a perinuclear position, containing mainly lipid residues of variable density. They are thought to be the indigestible end results of lipid peroxidation and to consist of polymers of lipid and phospholipid which are complexed with protein.

Melanin

Melanin is a black pigment produced by the dendritic melanocytes of the skin. Excess production is associated with exposure to sunlight. Addison's disease, failure of the adrenal cortex (p. 1102), is associated with a generalized increase in pigmentation due to increased synthesis of melanocyte stimulating hormone by the pituitary, whilst in chloasma the increased melanin is associated, in a minority of women, with the hormones of pregnancy.

Exogenous Pigment

Exogenous pigments may enter the body by inhalation, by ingestion or by injection. Atmospheric pollutants, in particular carbon particles, are taken up by alveolar macrophages and deposited as black particles in the draining lymph nodes. In workers in the mining industries the inhaled carbon can give the whole lung a black appearance and causes one form of inhalational dust disease – the pneumoconioses (p. 567). Tattooing, in which various dyes are introduced by needling into the skin, is self-explanatory. Drug abusers who 'mainline', i.e. inject drugs directly into the venous system, often introduce a variety of foreign materials into their circulation at the same time. Talc, chalk, starch and many other substances may be found in tissue macrophages.

Ageing

As individuals age they become susceptible to a variety of diseases, but the contribution of medical science to longevity has been to increase the number of people reaching old age rather than increasing the total lifespan. The degenerative changes associated with increasing age may be detected as early as the third decade when a progressive decline becomes apparent in cellular function in many tissues. Muscle power decreases, neural conduction time increases and there are decreased reserves of pulmonary, cardiac and renal function. With increasing age the skin loses its elasticity, connective tissue fibres become more cross-linked and less soluble (thereby affecting their turnover and ease of replacement), body fat increases and muscle bulk diminishes. The 'physiological' atrophy of old age becomes apparent.

The cause of the changes in ageing are essentially unknown although theories abound. At a cellular level there is a clear phenomenon of senescence and two main hypotheses have been advanced. In the **cumulative error hypothesis**, the suggestion is that random damage to genes for essential proteins eventually makes cellular homeostasis impossible. Insoluble protein debris and lipofuscin accumulate and swamp the system with useless molecules. Reduced output of essential hormones leads to metabolic disturbance, and developing insufficiency of the immune system makes the organism susceptible to infection or incapable of recognizing and responding to faulty cells – i.e. tumours can develop more easily.

An alternative hypothesis is that cells reach the end of a predetermined span, and undergo **programmed cell death**. For 'normal' cells in culture (*cell strains*) there seems to be a finite doubling potential of about 60 divisions, although cells can occasionally escape this limit and become immortal (*cell lines*). Such behaviour is difficult to accommodate in the cumulative error model. Despite the clear indication of a limit to proliferation in culture, it is also known that fibroblasts, even from very old individuals, have substantial doubling potential, though less than those from young donors. Undoubtedly there would be a selective advantage in having substantial capacity for repair, even though the limit might only be approached in injury prone areas. It could be that the doubling potential of a critical cell population might actually account for mortality of the organism as a whole, even though the less essential systems retain proliferative reserves. Certainly, similar lifespans are found in genetically similar individuals and there are inherited diseases such as *Down's syndrome* and *progeria* in which lifespan is characteristically shortened.

Further Reading

Alberts, B., Bray, D., Lewis, J., Raff, M., Roberts, K. and Watson, J. D. (1989). *Molecular Biology of the Cell*, 2nd edn. Garland, New York & London.

Fawcett, D. W. (1981). *The Cell*, 2nd edn. W. B. Saunders, Philadelphia.

Ghadially, R. N. (1988). *Ultrastructural Pathology of the Cell and Matrix*, 3rd edn, 2 volumes. Butterworth, London.

Lackie, J. M. and Dow, J. A. T., eds (1989). *Dictionary of Cell Biology*. Academic Press, London.

Toner, P. G. and Carr, K. E. (1982). *Cell Structure: an Introduction to Biomedical Electron Microscopy*, 3rd edn. Churchill Livingstone, Edinburgh.

2

Genetics and Disease

Physical Basis of Heredity

Heredity is in essence the transmission of information required to construct multiple proteins. These proteins have diverse roles and different subsets, are utilized by different cell types but all are encoded in the cell's DNA which is organized into discrete structures called chromosomes.

Chromosomes

Every cell nucleus contains a set of chromosomes (Greek: *chromos* = coloured; *soma* = body) which are named from their ability to take up certain stains. Each chromosome consists of a single molecule of **DNA** (deoxyribonucleic acid) together with associated acidic and basic proteins. Between cell divisions (interphase) the chromosomes are fully extended and are not individually distinguishable within the nucleus. During cell division each DNA molecule becomes coiled and condensed and the individual chromosomes can then be visualized with the light microscope.

Most human cells contain 46 chromosomes (**the diploid number**) with 22 pairs of autosomes which are alike in males and females and a pair of sex chromosomes: XX in a female and XY in a male (Fig. 2.1). Each chromosome has a narrow waist called the centromere which has a constant position for a given chromosome. According to the position of the centromere three subgroups of human chromosomes are identified: acrocentric, submetacentric and metacentric (Fig. 2.2).

The centromere divides each chromosome into short and long arms which are labelled p (from the French petit) and q respectively and the tip of each arm is called the telomere. Chromosomes 1, 3, 16, 19 and 20 are metacentric or nearly so. Chromo-

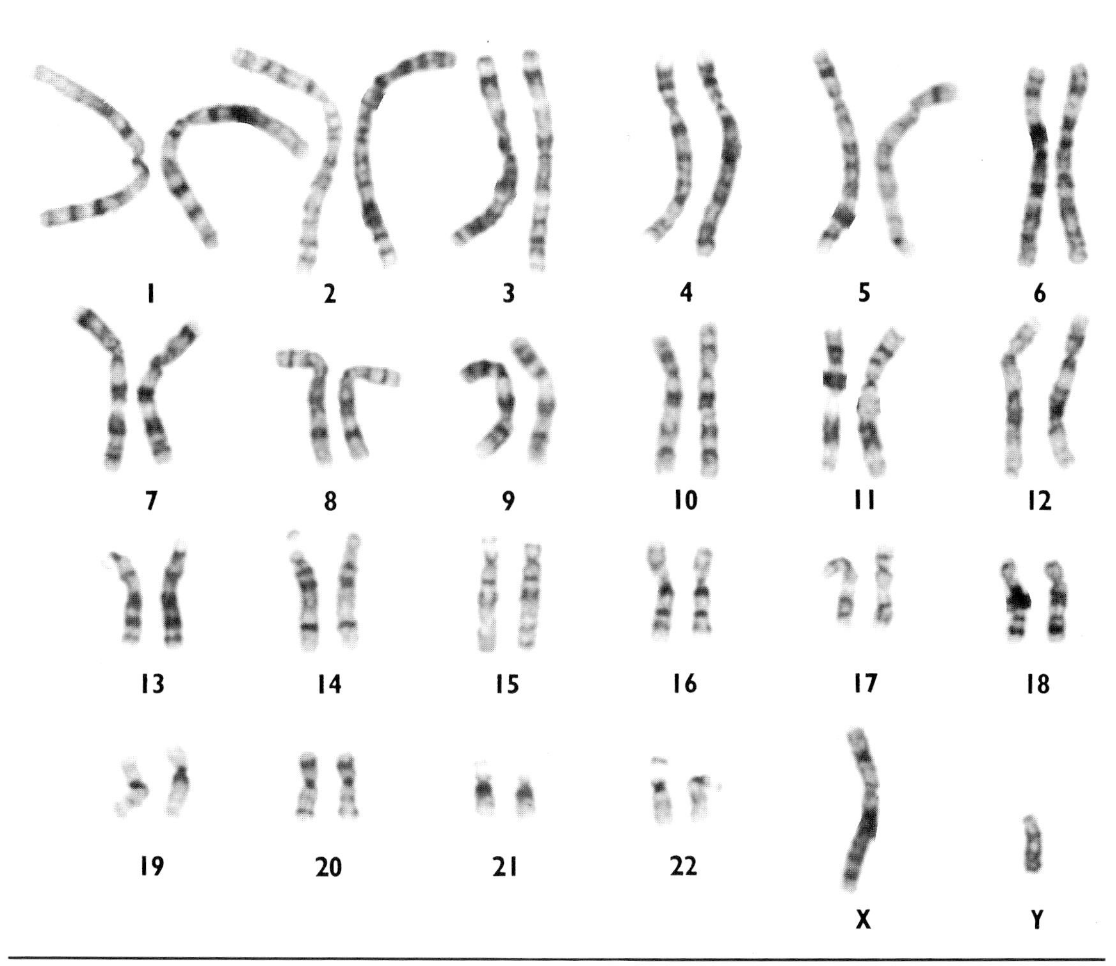

Fig. 2.1 Normal human male karyotype (Giemsa banded) with 22 pairs of autosomes and the sex chromosomes X and Y.

somes 13, 14, 15, 21, 22 and the Y are acrocentric and the remainder are submetacentric. The acrocentric chromosomes 13–15, 21 and 22 all have ribosomal genes located in their short arms and during cell division these areas often show a lack of condensation due to their involvement in the organization of nucleoli. Thus, the ends of their short arms appear as 'satellites' separated from the rest of the chromosome arm by narrow stalks known as secondary constrictions.

At **mitosis** each chromosome replicates to form a pair of sister chromatids which are held together at the centromere. Although exchanges of genetic material can occur by crossing over (sister chromatid exchanges, SCEs) during mitosis, as each sister chromatid is identical, clinical consequences do not arise. Thus, at the end of cell division each daughter cell has an identical set of 46 chromosomes (Fig. 2.3a).

In contrast, reduction cell division or **meiosis** results in cells with a half set (**haploid number**) of 23 chromosomes. Meiosis, which is confined to gonadal cells involved in gametogenesis, consists of two successive divisions in which the DNA replicates only once before the first division (Fig. 2.3b). Each mature egg thus normally contains one of each pair of autosomes and one X and each mature sperm has one of each pair of autosomes and the X or Y chromosome. At fertilization the diploid number is restored and in consequence half

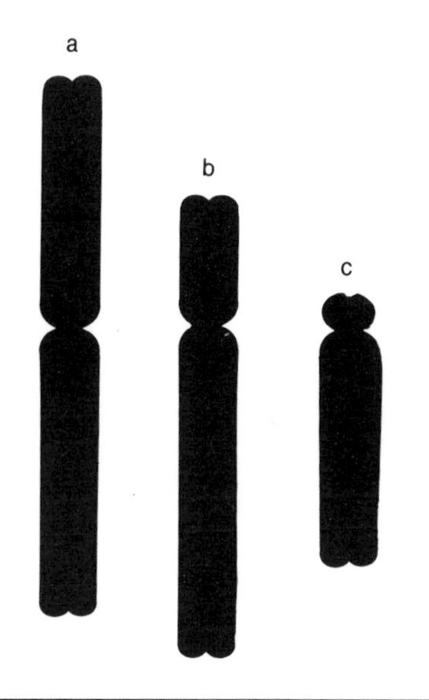

Fig. 2.2 Diagram of different types of human chromosomes: **a** metacentric; **b** submetacentric; **c** acrocentric.

of each individual's autosomes are derived from each parent and a female has an X from each parent whereas a male has a maternal X and a paternal Y sex chromosome.

DNA

Each molecule of DNA is composed of two nucleotide chains which are coiled clockwise around one another to form a double helix. Each component nucleotide consists of a nitrogenous base, a molecule of deoxyribose (in RNA ribose is used) and a phosphate molecule (Fig. 2.4).

The nitrogenous bases are of two types, purines and pyrimidines. In DNA there are two purine bases, adenine (A) and guanine (G), and two pyrimidine bases, thymine (T) and cytosine (C). The two nucleotide chains run in opposite direc-

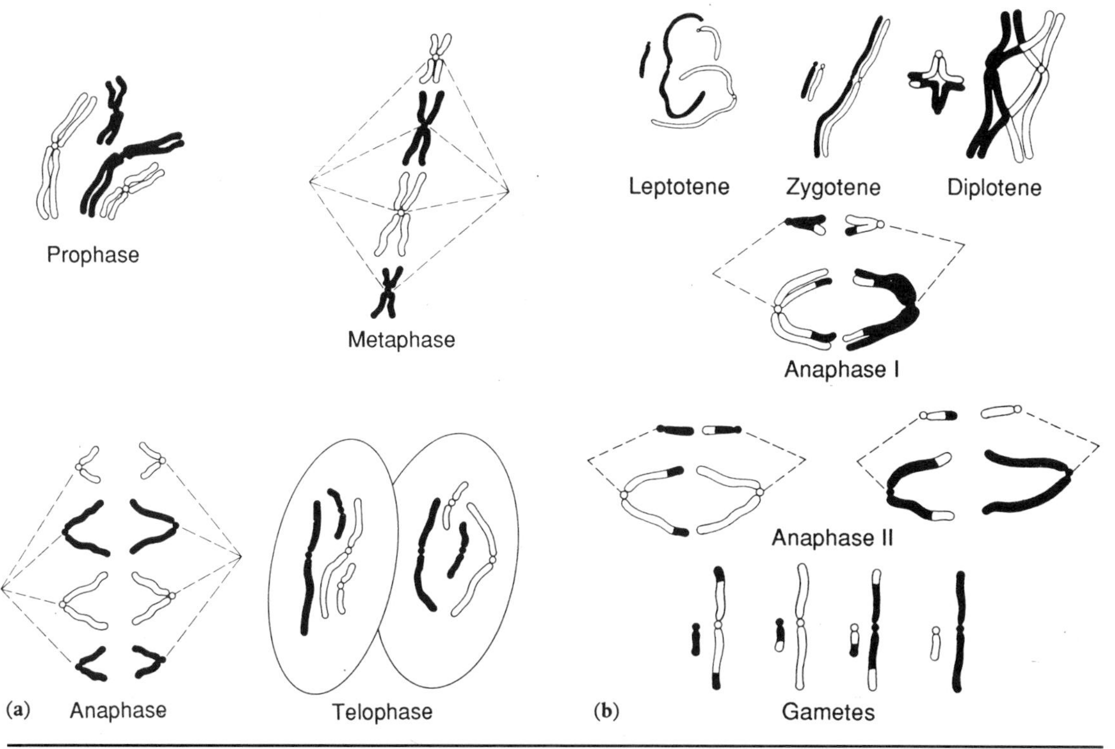

Fig. 2.3 **a** Diagram of mitosis. Only two chromosome pairs are shown; the chromosomes from one parent are in outline, those from the other are in black. **b** Diagram of meiosis. Only two chromosome pairs are shown; the chromosomes from one parent are in outline, those from the other are in black. Note exchange of chromosomal material as a result of recombination.

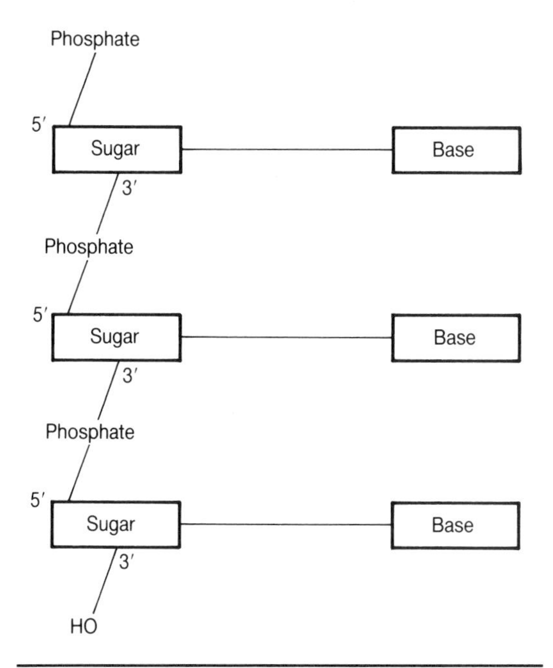

Fig. 2.4 Diagram of nucleic acid structure. The 5′ phosphate end is at the top and the 3′ hydroxyl group is at the bottom of this molecule.

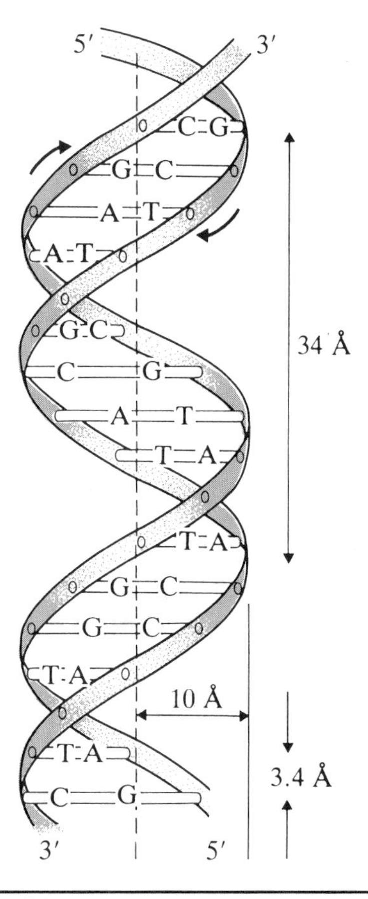

Fig. 2.5 Diagram of DNA double helix. The two phosphate-sugar chains are represented by ribbons and the pairs of bases holding the chains together are shown as horizontal rods.

tions and are held together by hydrogen bonds between A and T or between G and C. Since A:T and G:C pairing is obligatory the parallel strands must be complementary to one another. Thus, if one strand reads AATTGC the complementary strand must read TTAACG (Fig. 2.5).

The unit of length of DNA is the base pair (bp) with one thousand base pairs in a kilobase (kb) and one million base pairs in a megabase (Mb). The total length of DNA in the set of human chromosomes is 3000 million base pairs (or 3 million kb). An estimated 50 000 structural genes are encoded in the DNA, and as most of these have only one copy in the haploid genome, and if the average gene is perhaps 20 kb, they account for only one-third of the total DNA. Much of the remaining DNA consists of repetitive DNA, which may be moderately repetitive with several hundred copies or highly repetitive with many thousands of copies and may be dispersed or occur in clusters. The moderately repetitive DNA includes some functional genes which occur as multiple copies, including ribosomal RNA (300–400 copies) and the histone genes. In contrast, the highly repetitive DNA has no known function.

Proteins, whether structural components, enzymes, carrier molecules, hormones or receptors, are all composed of a series of amino acids. Twenty amino acids are known, and the order of these determines the form and function of the resulting protein. All proteins are encoded in DNA and, by definition, the unit of DNA which codes for a protein is its **gene**. The first stage in protein synthesis is **transcription**. The two strands of DNA separate in the area to be transcribed and one strand (the antisense strand) functions as a template, and messenger RNA (mRNA) is formed with a complementary nucleotide sequence under the influence of the enzyme RNA polymerase (Fig. 2.6).

Each set of three (a triplet or **codon**) DNA base pairs encodes an amino acid and as each base in the triplet may be any of four types of nucleotide (A, G, C, T), there are 64 possible combinations or codons (Table 2.1). By convention the codons for each amino acid are shown in terms of the messenger RNA so the corresponding DNA template codon will be complementary. All amino acids

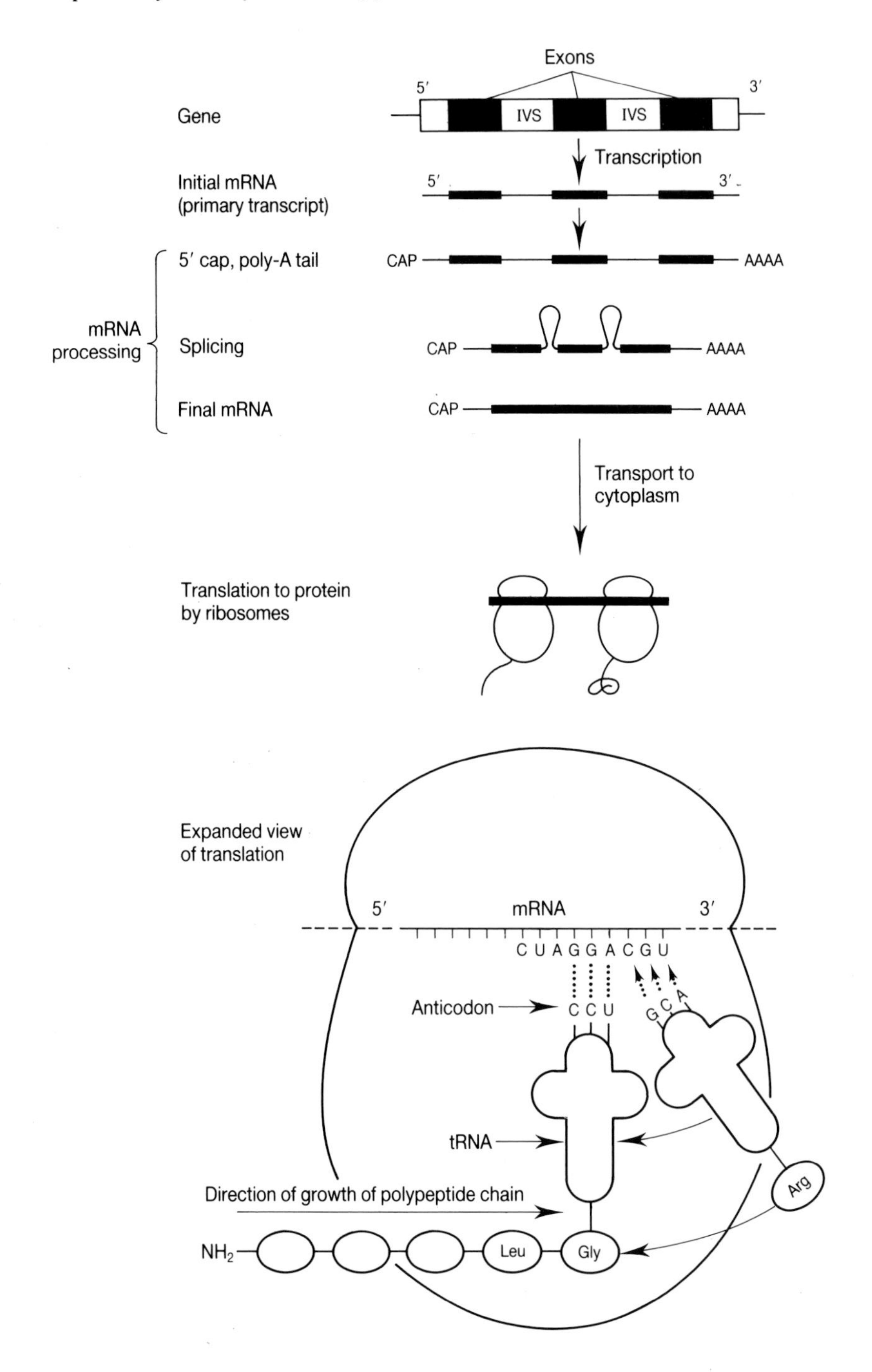

Fig. 2.6 Diagram of transcription, mRNA processing and translation. By convention the 5′ end of the mRNA molecule is placed to the left. IVS is the intervening sequence (intron) which is not translated.

Table 2.1 The genetic code with codons shown as messenger RNA. The corresponding DNA codons are complementary

First base	Second base: U		C		A		G		Third base
U	UUU	Phe	UCU	Ser	UAU	Tyr	UGU	Cys	U
	UUC	Phe	UCC	Ser	UAC	Tyr	UGC	Cys	C
	UUA	Leu	UCA	Ser	UAA	STOP	UGA	STOP	A
	UUG	Leu	UCG	Ser	UAG	STOP	UGG	Trp	G
C	CUU	Leu	CCU	Pro	CAU	His	CGU	Arg	U
	CUC	Leu	CCC	Pro	CAC	His	CGC	Arg	C
	CUA	Leu	CCA	Pro	CAA	Gln	CGA	Arg	A
	CUG	Leu	CCG	Pro	CAG	Gln	CGG	Arg	G
A	AUU	Ile	ACU	Thr	AAU	Asn	AGU	Ser	U
	AUC	Ile	ACC	Thr	AAC	Asn	AGC	Ser	C
	AUA	Ile	ACA	Thr	AAA	Lys	AGA	Arg	A
	*AUG	Met	ACG	Thr	AAG	Lys	AGG	Arg	G
G	GUU	Val	GCU	Ala	GAU	Asp	GGU	Gly	U
	GUC	Val	GCC	Ala	GAC	Asp	GGC	Gly	C
	GUA	Val	GCA	Ala	GAA	Glu	GGA	Gly	A
	GUG	Val	GCG	Ala	GAG	Glu	GGG	Gly	G

Abbreviations for amino acids (short code):

Ala	Alanine (A)	Leu	Leucine (L)
Arg	Arginine (R)	Lys	Lysine (K)
Asn	Asparagine (N)	Met	Methionine (M)
Asp	Aspartic acid (D)	Phe	Phenylalanine (F)
Cys	Cysteine (C)	Pro	Proline (P)
Gln	Glutamine (Q)	Ser	Serine (S)
Glu	Glutamic acid (E)	Thr	Threonine (T)
Gly	Glycine (G)	Trp	Tryptophan (W)
His	Histidine (H)	Tyr	Tyrosine (Y)
Ile	Isoleucine (I)	Val	Valine (V)

Other abbreviation:
STOP chain terminators
*Start codon for protein synthesis.

except methionine and tryptophan are encoded by more than one codon; three (UAA, UGA, UAG) designate termination of a message and one (AUG) acts as a start signal for protein synthesis. Transcription proceeds in a 5′ to 3′ direction until a chain termination codon is reached.

The vast majority of genes consist of alternating protein coding segments (**exons**) and non-protein coding segments of 10–10 000 bp called intervening sequences (**introns**) whose function is unknown. The initial mRNA is a complete transcript of the gene (including exons, introns and flanking sequences) but prior to its entry into the cytoplasm the segments corresponding to the introns are removed by splicing. Thus, the initial mRNA may be many times the length of the definitive message. The sequences around the exon/intron junctions serve as recognition sites for splicing enzymes and characteristically an intron begins GT (the 5′ or donor site) and ends AG (the 3′ or acceptor site). If splicing is defective then an abnormal protein or no protein will result. Histones, actins and some interferon genes do not contain introns but these are so far the only known human exceptions. The mRNA 5′ end is blocked or capped with 7-methylguanosine and a 3′ poly-A tail (with 100–200 adenine residues) is usually added to aid transport into the cytoplasm for ribosomal translation.

Translation occurs in the cytoplasm. Each mRNA molecule becomes attached to one or more ribosomes and as the ribosome moves along the mRNA from the 5′ to the 3′ end each codon is recognized by a matching transfer RNA (tRNA) which contributes its amino acid to the end of the growing protein chain. Many proteins are not in their final form after ribosomal translation and require post-translational processing before they assume their biologically active three-dimensional shape.

Gene Map

The first autosomal gene assignment was made in 1967 and by 1989, 1617 structural genes had been firmly localized to particular chromosomes. Figure 2.7 indicates some of the clinically more important of these localizations.

This represents under 4% of the estimated total of 50 000 structural genes but already certain observations are possible. Genes of related function are often clustered (e.g. β-globin cluster) and this undoubtedly represents ancestral gene duplication with subsequent divergence of function. In contrast, the genes for enzymes for different steps in the same metabolic pathway are scattered, rather than clustered as are the genes for lysosomal enzymes and for the mitochondrial and soluble forms of the same enzyme. Similarly, genes for subunits of complex proteins may be on different chromosomes. The map is similar in man and chimpanzee and the X chromosomal gene map appears similar in all mammals, but other homologies diverge in proportion to the timing of separation during evolution of the species.

Regulation of Gene Expression

All nucleated cells of an individual have an identical set of genes, yet the relative pattern of gene expression needs to vary widely not only for the differentiation of cells and tissues, but also to meet fluctuating demands for the synthesis of different proteins in each cell. In addition to the start and chain termination codons, areas of each gene and of the neighbouring DNA seem to play an important role in regulating transcription and hence, synthesis of each protein. Messenger RNA is transcribed from 5′ to 3′ and thus the beginning of a gene lies to the 3′ end of the DNA template strand (Fig. 2.8).

Upstream of the gene is the **promoter** which is involved in the attachment of RNA polymerase to the DNA sense strand. Promoters vary in their sequences and several promoter-specific transcription factors have now been identified which bind to specific promoters and activate transcription. The activity of many promoters is modulated by an **enhancer**, which is a separate regulatory element. The enhancer must be on the same molecule of DNA but can be 1000 bp or more from

Fig. 2.7 Some of the clinically more important assignments to the human gene map.

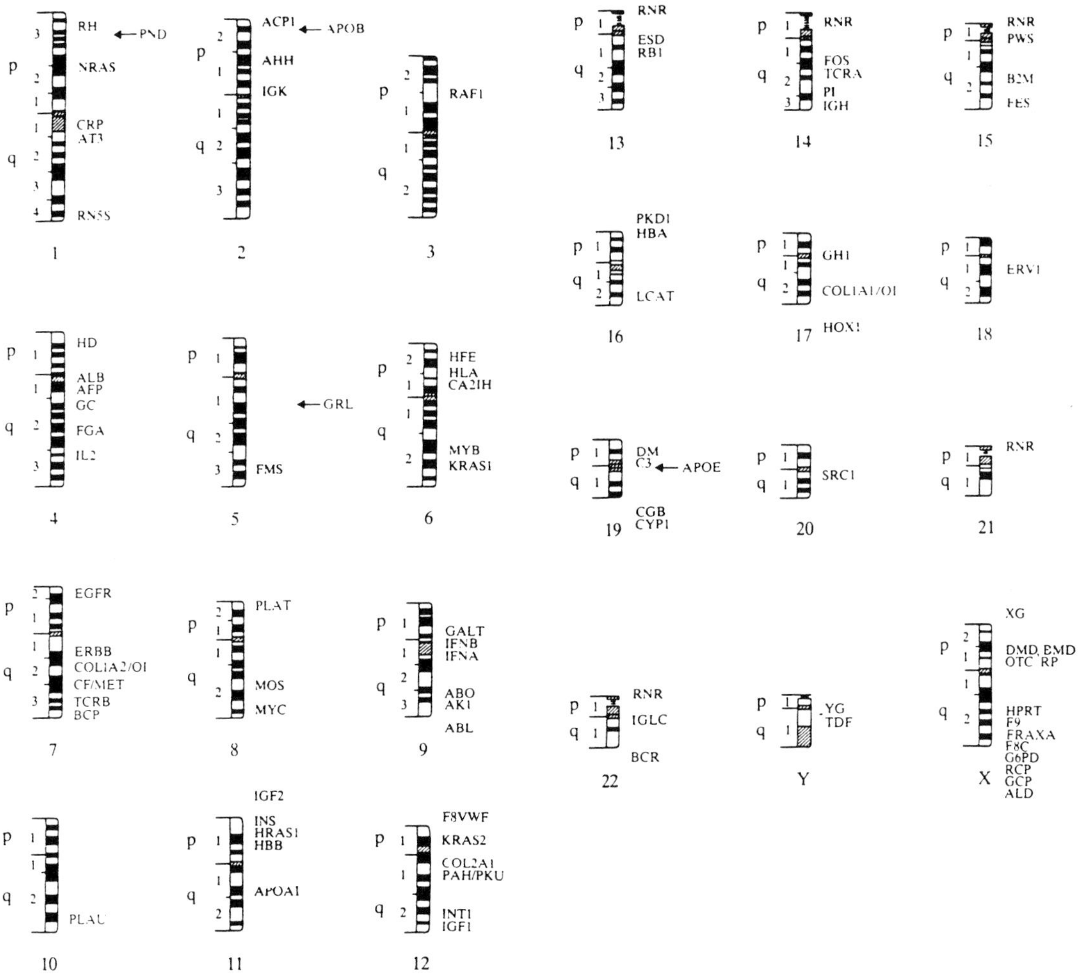

Chromosome 1	AT3	Antithrombin III
	CRP	C-reactive protein
	PND	Pronatriodilantin
	NRAS	Neuroblastoma v-*ras* oncogene homologue
	RH	Rhesus blood group
	RN5S	5S RNA gene(s)
Chromosome 2	ACP1	Acid phosphatase-1
	AHH	Aryl hydrocarbon hydroxylase
	APOB	Apolipoprotein-B
	IGK	Gene (cluster) for kappa light chain
Chromosome 3	RAF1	Murine leukaemia v-*raf*-1 oncogene homologue
Chromosome 4	AFP	Alpha-fetoprotein
	ALB	Albumin
	FGA	Fibrinogen, alpha chain
	GC	Group-specific component
	HD	Huntington disease
	IL2	Interleukin 2

Chromosome 5	FMS	McDonough feline sarcoma v-*fms* oncogene homologue
	GRL	Glucocorticoid receptor
Chromosome 6	CA2IH	Congenital adrenal hyperplasia
	HFE	Haemochromatosis
	HLA	Human leucocyte antigens
	KRAS1	Kirsten rat sarcoma v-Ki-*ras*-1 oncogene homologue
	MYB	Avian myeloblastosis v-*myb* oncogene homologue
Chromosome 7	BCP	Blue cone pigment
	CF	Cystic fibrosis
	COL1A2/OI	Collagen type I, alpha-2 chain/osteogenesis imperfecta
	EGFR	Epidermal growth factor receptor
	MET	*MET* proto-oncogene
	TCRB	T-cell receptor beta chain
Chromosome 8	MOS	Moloney murine sarcoma v-*mos* oncogene homologue
	MYC	Avian myelocytomatosis v-*myc* oncogene homologue
	PLAT	Tissue plasminogen activator
Chromosome 9	ABL	Abelson murine leukaemia v-*abl* oncogene homologue
	ABO	ABO blood group
	AK1	Adenylate kinase-1 (soluble)
	GALT	Galactose-1-phosphate uridyltransferase
	IFNA	Interferon, leucocyte
	IFNB	Interferon, fibroblast
Chromosome 10	PLAU	Urokinase plasminogen activator
Chromosome 11	APOAI	Apolipoprotein A-I
	HBB	Haemoglobin beta chain
	HRAS	Harvey rat sarcoma v-Ha-*ras* oncogene homologue
	IGF2	Insulin-like growth factor 2
	INS	Insulin
Chromosome 12	COL2A1	Collagen type II, alpha-1 chain
	F8VWF	Von Willebrand factor/disease
	IGF1	Insulin-like growth factor 1
	INT1	Murine mammary tumour virus integration site (v-*int*-1) oncogene homologue
	KRAS2	Kirsten rat sarcoma v-Ki-*ras*-2 oncogene homologue
	PAH/PKU	Phenylalanine hydroxylase/phenylketonuria
Chromosome 13	ESD	Esterase D
	RB1	Retinoblastoma
	RNR	Ribosomal RNA
Chromosome 14	FOS	Murine FBJ osteosarcoma v-*fos* oncogene homologue
	IGH	Immunoglobulin heavy chain gene cluster
	PI	Alpha-1-antitrypsin
	RNR	Ribosomal RNA
	TCRA	T-cell receptor alpha polypeptide
Chromosome 15	B2M	Beta-2 microglobulin
	FES	Feline sarcoma v-*fes* oncogene homologue
	PWS	Prader–Willi syndrome
	RNR	Ribosomal RNA
Chromosome 16	HBA	Haemoglobin alpha chain
	LCAT	Lecithin-cholesterol actyltransferase
	PKD1	Adult polycystic kidney disease
Chromosome 17	TP53	Tumour protein p 53
	COL1A1/OI	Collagen type I, alpha-1 chain/osteogenesis imperfecta
	GH1	Growth hormone
	HOX1	Homeo box region 1
Chromosome 18	ERV1	Endogenous retroviral sequence 1
Chromosome 19	APOE	Apolipoprotein E
	C3	Complement component 3
	CGB	Chorionic gonadotrophin, beta chain

	CYP1	Phenobarbitone-inducible P450
	DM	Myotonic dystrophy
Chromosome 20	SRC	Avian sarcoma v-*src* oncogene homologue
Chromosome 21	RNR	Ribosomal RNA
Chromosome 22	BCR	Breakpoint cluster region
	IGLC	Gene (cluster) for lambda light chain
	RNR	Ribosomal RNA
Chromosome X	ALD	Adrenoleucodystrophy
	BMD	Becker muscular dystrophy
	DMD	Duchenne muscular dystrophy
	F8C	Clotting factor VIII
	F9	Clotting factor IX
	FRAXA	Fragile X syndrome
	GCP	Green cone pigment (deutan colourblindness)
	G6PD	Glucose-6-phosphate dehydrogenase
	HPRT	Hypoxanthine-guanine phosphoribosyltransferase
	OTC	Ornithine transcarbamylase
	RCP	Red cone pigment (protan colourblindness)
	RP	X-linked retinitis pigmentosa
	XG	Xg blood group
Chromosome Y	TDF	Testis determining factor
	YG	Y homologue of Xg

the promoter and can be upstream or downstream. Some enhancers are tissue-specific whereas others mediate transcriptional responses of several genes in a non-tissue-specific manner, e.g. to steroid hormones.

The initial nucleotide of the mRNA non-coding leader is usually a purine and the first amino acid in the polypeptide chain is usually methionine, although this may be removed in later processing. At the end of the gene, the sequence AATAAA appears to be the signal for the addition of the poly-A tail (which aids transport to the cytoplasm), and the terminator codon signals RNA polymerase dissociation. Processing of the mRNA also appears to be regulated. For example, the calcitonin gene encodes calcitonin precursor, but by alternative splicing a different calcitonin gene-related neuropeptide is produced. The control of alternative splicing is obscure as is the role of DNA methylation. A lack of methylation of cytosine bases on the 5′ side of guanine residues of DNA is correlated with active gene expression and vice versa, but it is unclear if such methylation is responsible for regulation or is a secondary feature.

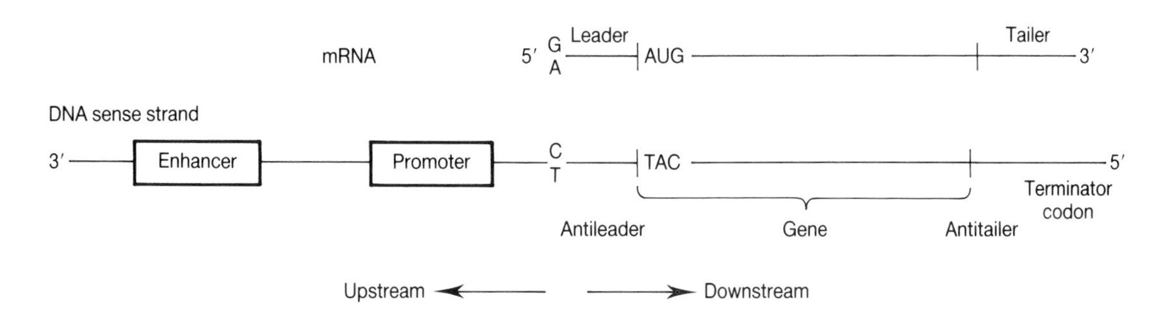

Fig. 2.8 Diagram of the sequences involved in the regulation of transcription.

Classification of Genetic Diseases

There are five main types of genetic disorder (Table 2.2). In chromosomal disorders there is a microscopically visible alteration in one or more chromosomes whereas the lesion in the other types may only be demonstrated by DNA analysis or inferred from family and pedigree analysis. Single gene disorders show characteristic patterns of inheritance and result from mutations in one member or both members of a pair of genes. In multifactorial disorders, an individual is rendered unduly susceptible to an environmental agent by virtue of the action of one or more genes. Mitochondria have their own chromosomes which are virtually all derived from the ovum and hence show maternal inheritance. Somatic cell genetic disorders arise after conception and are thus not inherited although they produce their effects via the DNA.

Although many genetic conditions are rare, there are many known disorders and collectively they represent a common problem. This is enhanced by the relative decline in importance of most infectious agents and by the realization of the genetic component in common multifactorial disorders, such as hypertension, and in common somatic cell genetic disorders such as cancer.

Pedigrees and Modes of Inheritance

Defining the distribution of a disorder in a particular family usually allows the pattern of inheritance to be determined. The family trees are drawn using standardized symbols to designate affected members, carriers and family relationships (Fig. 2.9).

Mitochondrial and single gene disorders often show diagnostic pedigree patterns. Mitochondrial disorders arise from mutations in the mitochondrial DNA which is inherited in the ovum and so all offspring of an affected mother receive the mutation, whereas offspring of an affected man are not at risk (Fig. 2.10).

The single gene disorders are subdivided according to whether the mutation is on an autosome or the X chromosome and according to whether a person with one mutant and one normal gene in a pair (**a heterozygote**) is affected. In autosomal dominant disorders the mutant gene is on an autosome and the heterozygote is affected. As indicated in Fig. 2.11, these autosomal dominant traits show a vertical type of pedigree pattern with approximately equal numbers of males and females affected. The affected person hands on either the normal gene or the mutant gene and thus, on average, 50% of the offspring will be affected.

So far 3047 autosomal dominant traits are known in man. Some of the commoner and more clinically important of these are shown in Table 2.3. In general they tend to be less severe than recessive traits and, whereas recessive traits usually result in defective enzymes, dominant traits often alter structural, carrier or receptor proteins.

Table 2.2 Types of genetic disease

Type	Number of subtypes	Combined frequency
Chromosomal disorders	>600 described	6/1000 live births
Single gene disorders	4937 (by March 1990)	> 12/1000 live births
Multifactorial disorders	>100	>150/1000 live births
Mitochondrial genetic disorders	8	Rare
Somatic cell genetic disorders	>100	>100/1000 live births

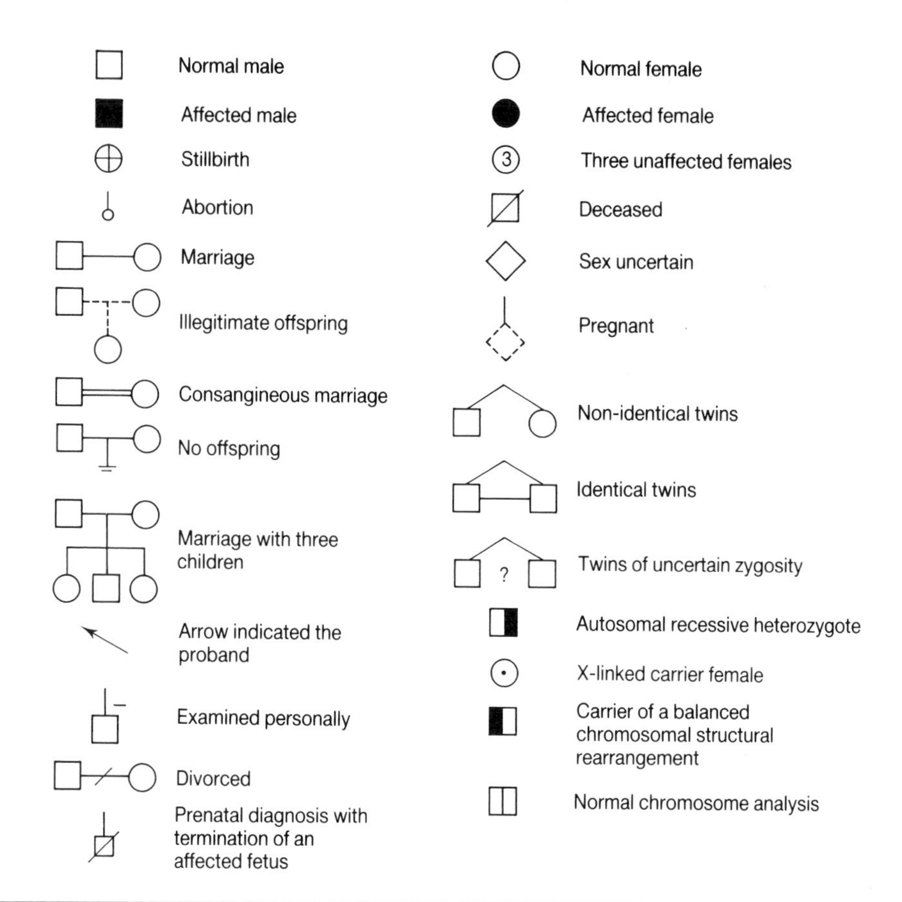

Fig. 2.9 Symbols used in pedigree construction.

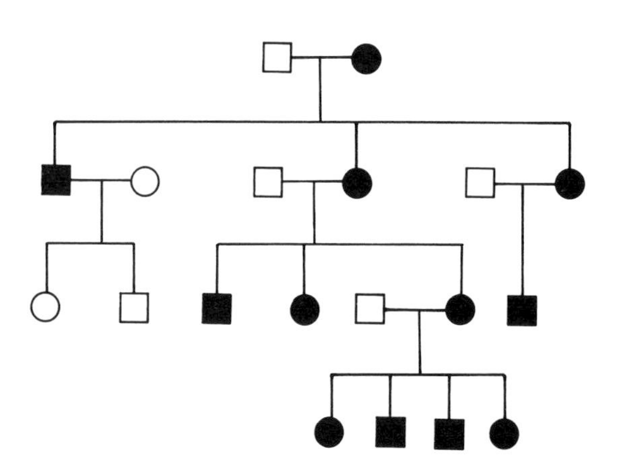

Fig. 2.10 Pedigree showing maternal inheritance of a mitochondrial DNA disorder.

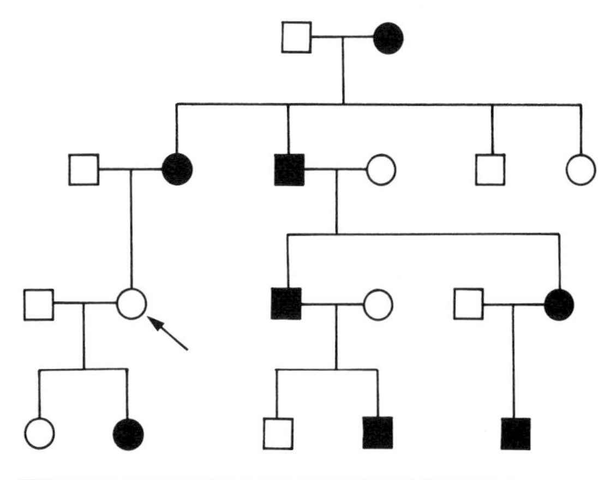

Fig. 2.11 Pedigree showing autosomal dominant inheritance and an example of non-penetrance (arrowed).

Table 2.3 Autosomal dominant diseases

Disease	Frequency/1000 births
Dominant otosclerosis	3
Familial hypercholesterolaemia	2
Adult polycystic kidney disease	1.0
Multiple exostoses	0.5
Huntington disease	0.5
Neurofibromatosis	0.4
Myotonic dystrophy	0.2
Congenital spherocytosis	0.2
Polyposis coli	0.1
Dominant blindness	0.1
Dominant congenital deafness	0.1
Others	1.9
Total	10/1000

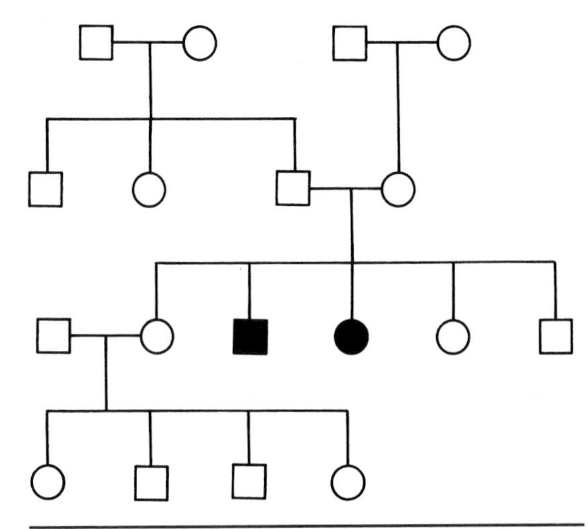

Fig. 2.12 Pedigree showing autosomal recessive inheritance. The parents of the affected children must be heterozygotes.

Many dominant traits show **variable expression**, which implies that the severity of the disorder varies in affected individuals in the same family (and with the same mutant gene). The basis for this is not understood, nor is the occasional occurrence of **non-penetrance** in some outwardly normal individuals who have inherited and transmitted the mutant gene (e.g. Fig. 2.11). Variable expression and non-penetrance are important considerations when counselling family members at risk. Another pitfall for the geneticist is **gonadal mosaicism** where the mutation is confined to the gonad of one parent. In this situation the parents of an affected child are clinically normal but, whereas a new mutation in the child would carry a very low recurrence risk for brothers and sisters, the recurrence risk for gonadal mosaicism may be as high as 50%.

Affected individuals with **autosomal recessive disorders** have mutations in both members of a gene pair (**homozygotes**). Usually the parents are unaffected clinically, yet each has one mutant gene and is thus a carrier or heterozygote. For two carrier parents the chance of further affected children is on average 1 in 4. The risk to other family members is relatively low and thus the pedigree is horizontal with brothers and sisters affected but usually no other family history (Fig. 2.12).

Many autosomal recessive traits affect enzyme proteins which have a large safety margin so that a reduction from the normal 100% activity to 50% in the heterozygote does not result in disease. Homozygotes with no normal gene product have little or no enzyme and within a family the disease tends to breed true. The chance of having a child with an autosomal recessive trait is increased if the parents are blood relatives (consanguineous) and, although not a prerequisite, consanguinity is an important clue that a disease is due to an autosomal recessive trait.

So far 1554 autosomal recessive traits are known in man. Some of the commoner and clinically more important of these are shown in Table 2.4. For many of these traits multiple different mutations may occur (**multiple allelism**) and an individual with two different mutant alleles at a locus is termed a genetic compound.

The uneven distribution of sex chromosomes results in a characteristic pattern of inheritance for **X-linked recessive disorders**. Males have only a single X chromosome (**hemizygous**) and thus are affected if any X-linked genes are mutant. Females have two X chromosomes and thus can compensate for a mutant gene on one X chromosome (carriers, heterozygotes). A carrier mother hands on the mutant X-linked gene on average to

Table 2.4 Autosomal recessive diseases

Disease	Frequency/1000 births
Cystic fibrosis	0.5
Recessive mental retardation	0.5
Congenital deafness	0.2
Phenylketonuria	0.1
Spinal muscular atrophy	0.1
Recessive blindness	0.1
Adrenogenital syndrome	0.1
Mucopolysaccharidoses	0.1
Others	0.3
Total	2/1000

one-half of her sons and to one-half of her daughters. If an affected male can reproduce then he transmits his X chromosome and hence the mutant gene to all of his daughters who will be carriers. His sons will receive his Y chromosome and are thus unaffected (Fig. 2.13).

X-linked recessive disorders tend to show consistent male severity within a family. Female carriers are usually clinically normal but may occasionally be mildly affected because of non-random inactivation of one of their X chromosomes (**Lyon hypothesis or Lyonization**). All early female embryos inactivate either the paternal or the maternal X chromosome in each cell at the sixteenth day after fertilization and all descendants of these cells retain the original active X. Occasionally this inactivation is non-random and if the X with the mutant gene is kept active in many cells of the target tissue then mild disease can result. So far 336 X-linked recessive disorders are known in man. Some of the commoner and more clinically important of these are listed in Table 2.5.

In contrast to the number of X-linked recessive disorders so far few human **X-linked dominant**

Table 2.5 Human X-linked disorders

Trait	UK frequency/ 10 000 males
Red–green colourblindness	800
Fragile X-associated mental retardation	5
Non-specific X-linked mental retardation	5
Duchenne muscular dystrophy	3
Becker muscular dystrophy	0.5
Haemophilia A (factor VIII deficiency)	2
Haemophilia B (factor IX deficiency)	0.3
X-linked ichthyosis	2
X-linked agammaglobulinaemia	0.1

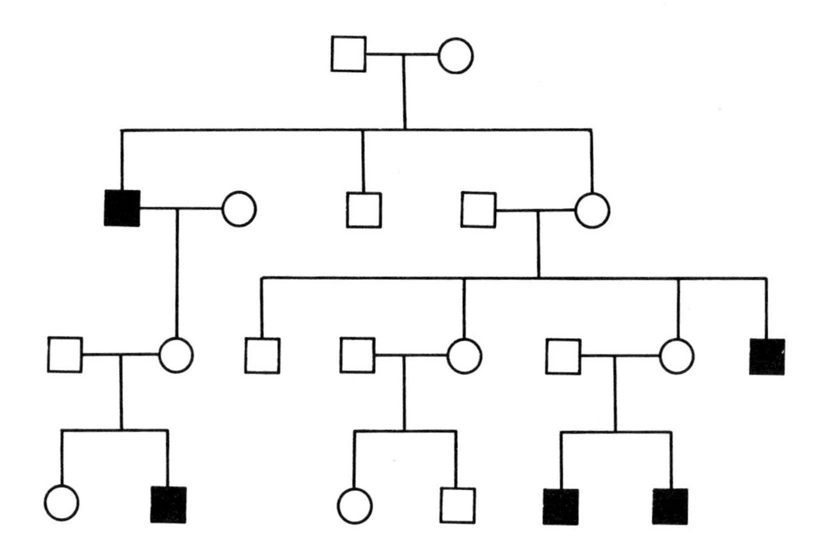

Fig. 2.13 Pedigree showing X-linked recessive inheritance. All the mothers of affected boys are carriers.

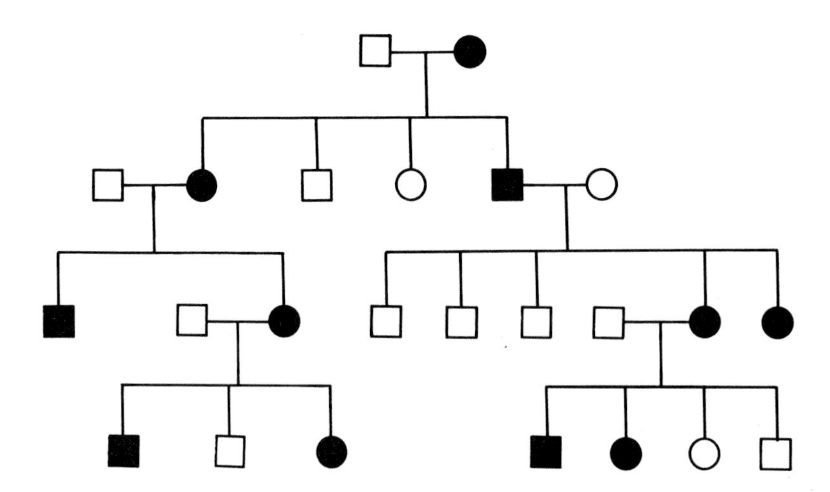

Fig. 2.14 Pedigree showing X-linked dominant inheritance.

disorders have been described (e.g. vitamin D resistant rickets) and most of these are very rare. Males and females are affected, with a uniformly severe disease in males but a more variable picture in heterozygous females, because of variable X-inactivation. Superficially, the family tree resembles that of an autosomal dominant trait but key differences are the lack of male-to-male transmission and the transmission from a male to all of his daughters (Fig. 2.14).

Apart from the genetic counselling difficulties mentioned earlier, many conditions which were believed to be single genetic entities are now known to be **genetically heterogeneous** (i.e. to have two or more different genetic causes). This is exemplified by albinism. In addition to the common type due to a lack of the enzyme tyrosinase, other variants are known with different (and not yet delineated) enzyme defects. These genetic mimics have different basic defects and thus different diagnostic tests and may have different modes of inheritance.

Laboratory Investigation of Genetic Disorders

Chromosomal Analysis

Chromosomes are conveniently studied in peripheral blood lymphocytes, but almost any growing tissue including bone marrow, cultivated skin fibroblasts or cells from amniotic fluid or chorionic villi can also be used. At autopsy, samples of *fascia lata* can be taken into culture medium and fibroblast culture from such samples may be possible even 3–4 days after death.

Routine Chromosomal Analysis

Five to ten millilitres of heparinized venous blood are required. The heparin prevents coagulation which would interfere with later separation of the lymphocytes. Samples must be delivered without delay but a **karyotype** can usually be obtained on a blood sample delivered by first class post. In the laboratory, the mitogen phytohaemagglutinin is added to the cultures set up from each sample and this stimulates T-lymphocytes to transform and divide. After 48–72 hours of incubation, cell division is arrested at metaphase by the addition of colchicine (which interferes with production of spindle microtubules) and a hypotonic solution is added to swell the cells and separate the individual chromosomes before fixation. Single drops of the fixed cell suspension are placed on to microscope slides and air-dried to spread the chromosomes out in one optical plane.

For routine karyotyping, **G (Giemsa) banding** is usually preferred. This produces 300–400 alternating light and dark bands which are characteristic for each chromosome pair and which reflect differential chromosomal condensation. Modern banding techniques allow precise identification of each chromosome, and missing or additional material of 4000 kb or greater can be visualized on routine chromosomal analysis. A standardized numbering system is used for the bands seen with G-banding and this permits accurate descriptions of structural chromosomal abnormalities (Fig. 2.15). The bands are numbered from centromere to telomere. Thus, for the term 1q23, 1q carries the band to the longer arm of chromosome one, while the 23 shows that it is the third band in the second group.

Karyotypes may be described using a shorthand system of symbols and in general this has the order: total number of chromosomes, sex chromosome constitution, and description of the abnormality. Thus a normal female karyotype is 46,XX and a normal male is 46,XY. Table 2.6 lists the other commonly used symbols.

Table 2.6 Symbols used for karyotype description

Symbol	Meaning
p	Short arm
q	Long arm
pter	Tip of short arm
qter	Tip of long arm
cen	Centromere
h	Heteromorphism
del	Deletion
der	Derivative of a chromosome rearrangement
dic	Dicentric
dup	Duplication
i	Isochromosome
ins	Insertion
inv	Inversion
mat	Maternal origin
pat	Paternal origin
r	Ring chromosome
t	Translocation
/	Mosaicism
+/−	Before a chromosome number indicates gain or loss of that whole chromosome
+/−	After a chromosome number indicates gain or loss of part of that chromosome

Specialized Techniques for Chromosomal Analysis

Constrictions at sites other than the centromeres are sometimes seen and these secondary constrictions may be particularly liable to chromatid breaks. Most of these are of no clinical consequence but a fragile site close to the end of the long arm of the X chromosome (Xq27) is associated with a common form of X-linked mental handicap (fragile X-syndrome). Demonstration of this fragile site requires culture of the lymphocytes in a special medium (deficient in folate or with thymidine excess) and this condition needs to be excluded in boys with otherwise unexplained mental handicap.

As indicated earlier, using routine chromosomal analysis the smallest visible gain or loss from a chromosome is 4000 kb, yet smaller deletions (microdeletions) are still clinically significant. In patients where microdeletions are suspected yet the routine analysis is apparently normal, two further types of analysis can be undertaken. **Prometaphase banding** is essentially the same as routine analysis except that the chromosomal condensation is arrested earlier at prometaphase (rather than at metaphase). With this approach over 1000 bands can be visualized.

A newer approach to the detection of sub-

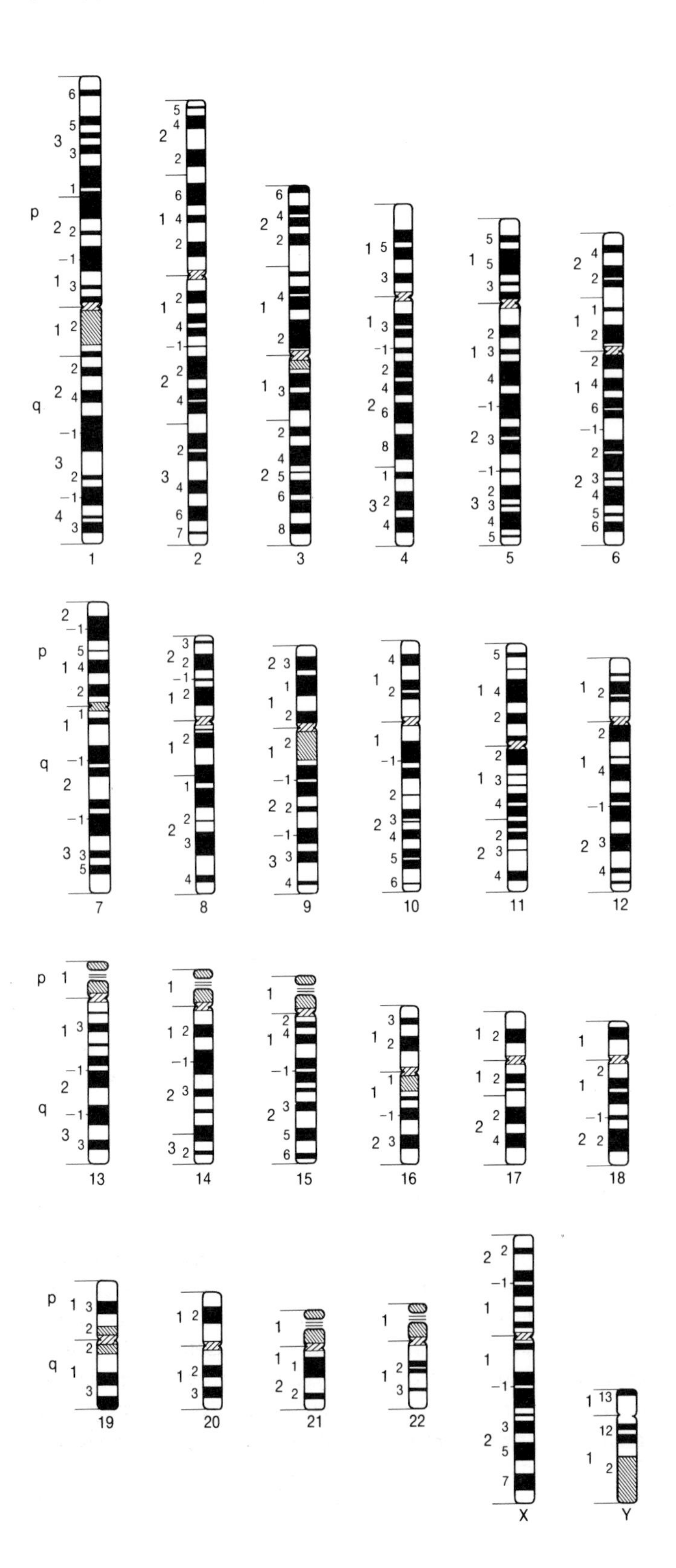

Fig. 2.15 Diagram of banding pattern of human chromosomes (Giemsa banding).

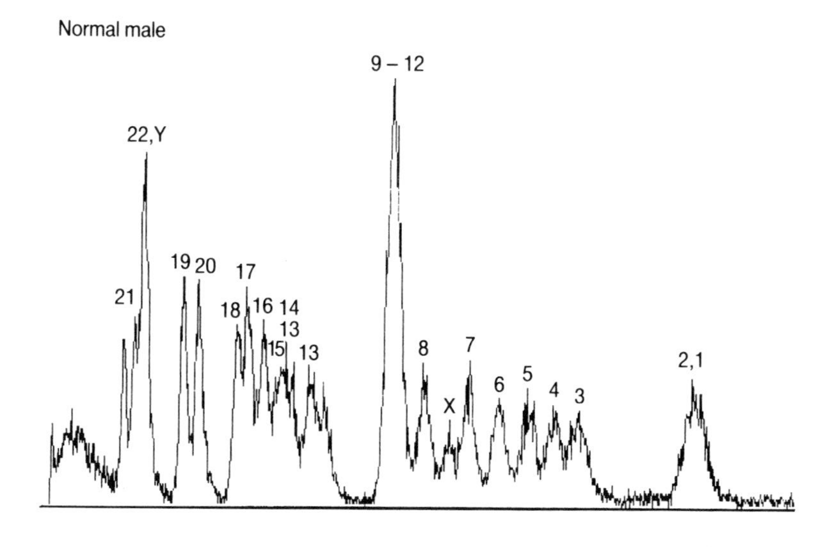

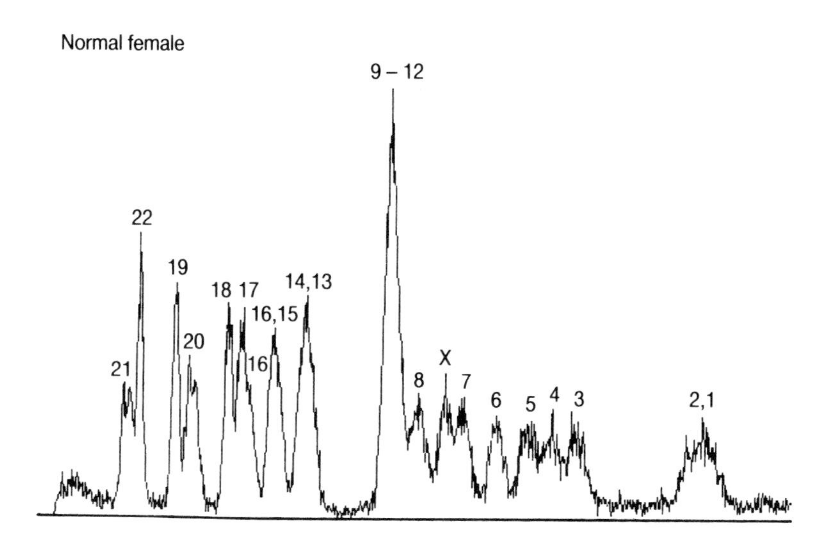

Fig. 2.16 Flow karyotype of a normal male and a normal female. The peaks correspond to individual chromosome pairs or groups of chromosomes as indicated.

microscopic abnormalities is **flow karyotyping.** In this technique a suspension of chromosomes is stained with a fluorescent dye (usually ethidium bromide) and this is passed through the laser beam of a fluorescence-activated cell sorter (FACS) at a speed of 2000 chromosomes per second. The fluorescence generated by the laser beam in each chromosome is collected in a photomultiplier and stored in a computer. After several minutes sufficient individual measurements have been collected to generate a histogram or flow karyotype which groups the chromosome measurements according to increasing DNA content (Fig. 2.16).

Many chromosomes form separate peaks and the median of each peak provides an accurate and reproducible measure of the relative DNA content of a particular pair of chromosomes. The area under each peak represents the relative number of chromosomes in each group. As shown in Fig. 2.16, male and female flow karyotypes are clearly distinguished by the size of the X chromosome peak, females having twice the size of the male peak. Using this technique chromosomes with small deletions will be shifted to the left in comparison with the normal homologue, and microdeletions as small as 2000 kb can be identified. Even smaller deletions can be identified by DNA analysis.

DNA Analysis

The ability to manipulate DNA *in vitro*, or genetic engineering, has a relatively brief but spectacular history. In 1972 the first recombinant DNA molecules were generated; in 1977 the first human gene (chorionic somatomammotrophin) was cloned; and in 1978 the first clinical diagnosis was made by DNA analysis (prenatal diagnosis of sickle cell disease). By the end of 1987 a complete linkage map of the human chromosomes had been developed and DNA diagnosis had become the mainstay for genetic counselling in over 20 important single gene disorders, including cystic fibrosis and Duchenne muscular dystrophy. These developments have all relied upon the specificity of base pairing or complementarity of DNA, and the discovery of special enzymes in bacteria (restriction enzymes) which cleave DNA molecules in a predictable manner.

Genomic DNA can be extracted from any nucleated tissue and the lymphocytes of a 20 ml venous blood sample yield 800–1000 μg which is sufficient for multiple DNA analyses. At autopsy, fresh spleen or liver should be taken into a dry sterile tube or snap-frozen in liquid nitrogen and stored at −20°C pending analyis.

DNA Probes

DNA probes are radioactively labelled fragments of DNA from tens of base pairs to several kilobases in size which are used to identify complementary base sequences. The probe is rendered single stranded (denatured) by heating and the target DNA sample is also rendered single stranded (often by exposure to a strong alkali). Upon identification of its complementary sequence(s) the single stranded proble and target DNA hybridize to form a radioactive double-stranded molecule which can be identified by autoradiography (Fig. 2.17).

Figure 2.18 illustrates the use of such a probe to identify its complementary sequence in serial dilutions of two DNA samples which are held on a DNA binding membrane (spot-blots). The radioactive signal is revealed by autoradiography and its intensity is proportional to the amount of target DNA present.

The same approach can be used to identify the site of production of single-stranded messenger RNA within a tissue (tissue RNA hybridization). Probes can also be used in a similar fashion to identify bacterial or viral DNA or RNA in tissue samples, and if a genomic probe is hybridized to a metaphase chromosome spread (rather than to extracted DNA or the whole tissue) then the site of hybridization on a chromosome will localize the point of origin of the probe (*in situ* hybridization, Fig. 2.19).

Restriction Fragment Length Polymorphisms (RFLPS)

Genomic probes can also be used to identify differences in the DNA sequence between a pair of chromosomes. Such differences appear to occur frequently (every 200–500 base pairs) throughout the chromosomes and the majority have no clinical significance. Each can, however, be of clinical value as a marker for that point of the DNA molecule. Identification of each of these differences requires a specific probe and restriction enzyme combination. **Restriction enzymes (restriction endonucleases)** are widespread in bacteria where they function as a defence mechanism against the incorporation of foreign DNA. More than 400 different restriction enzymes have

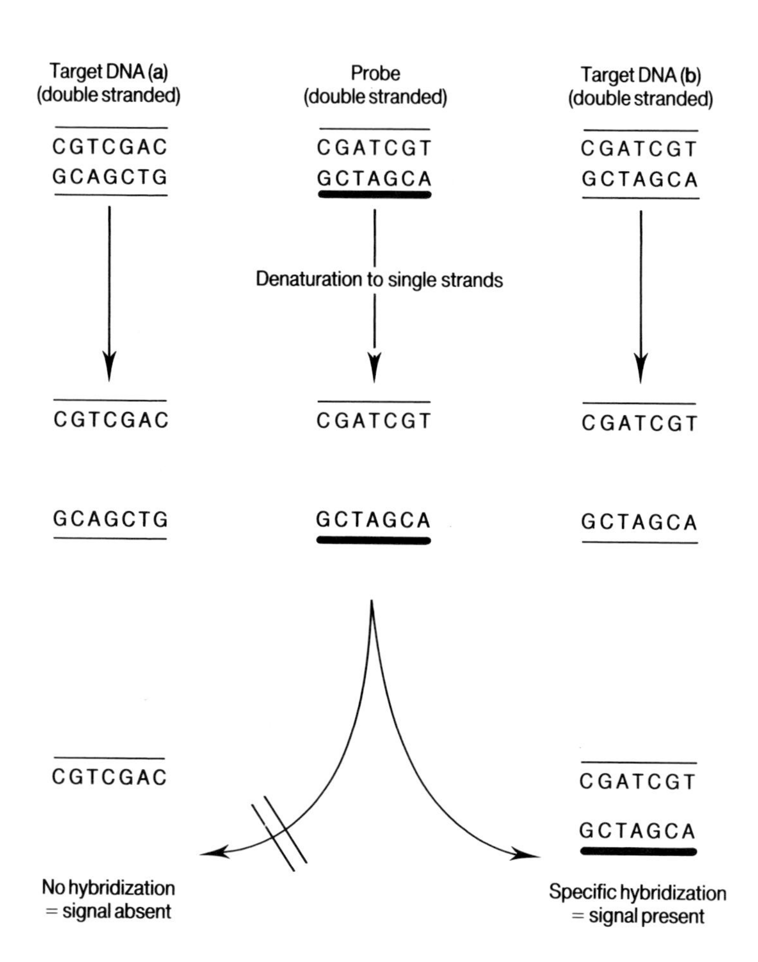

Fig. 2.17 Nucleic acid hybridization of complementary sequences.

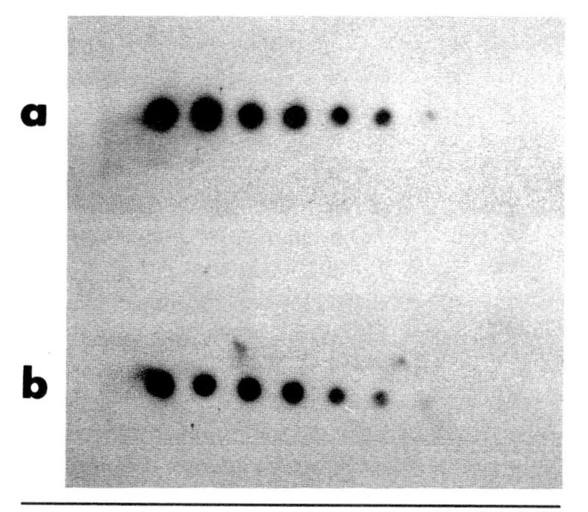

Fig. 2.18 Hybridization of a radiolabelled probe to its target sequence in serial dilutions of two DNA samples (**a** and **b**).

been described and over 100 are commercially available. Each is named after the organism from which it was first isolated, and each will only cleave at a specific DNA sequence, **the recognition site**, which is commonly 4 or 6 base pairs in length, to produce products with **flush (blunt)** or **staggered (sticky)** ends (Fig. 2.20). Thus, the enzyme *Taq*I will cut DNA at each point where the sequence TCGA occurs. Human DNA contains about one million *Taq*I recognition sites and so cleavage (digestion) with this enzyme yields about one million fragments of DNA. These fragments would be of variable length but each would have the same base order at their staggered ends. As these fragments differ in length they can be separated by electrophoresis and, following this, the fragments are transferred by the passage of a salt solution through the gel to a DNA binding mem-

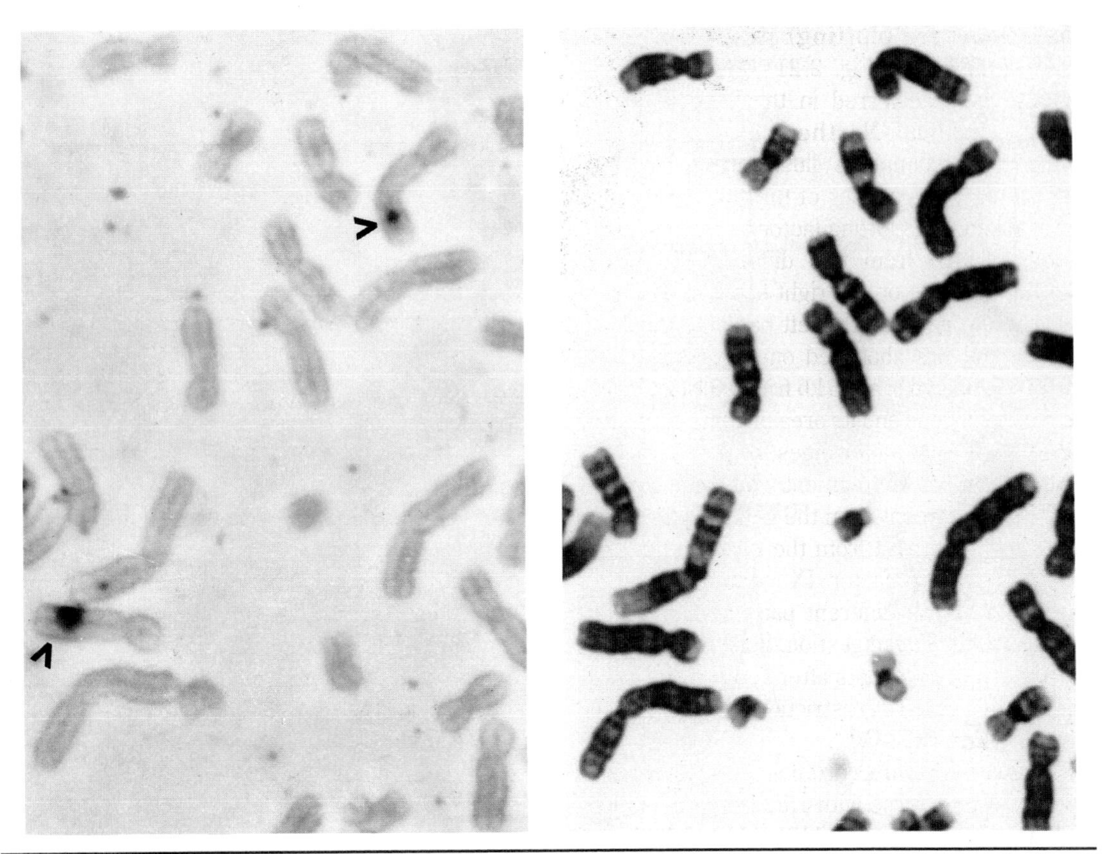

Fig. 2.19 Left: Specific *in situ* hybridization of a probe to copies of chromosome 4 (arrowed). Right: Same field with chromosome banding pattern shown.

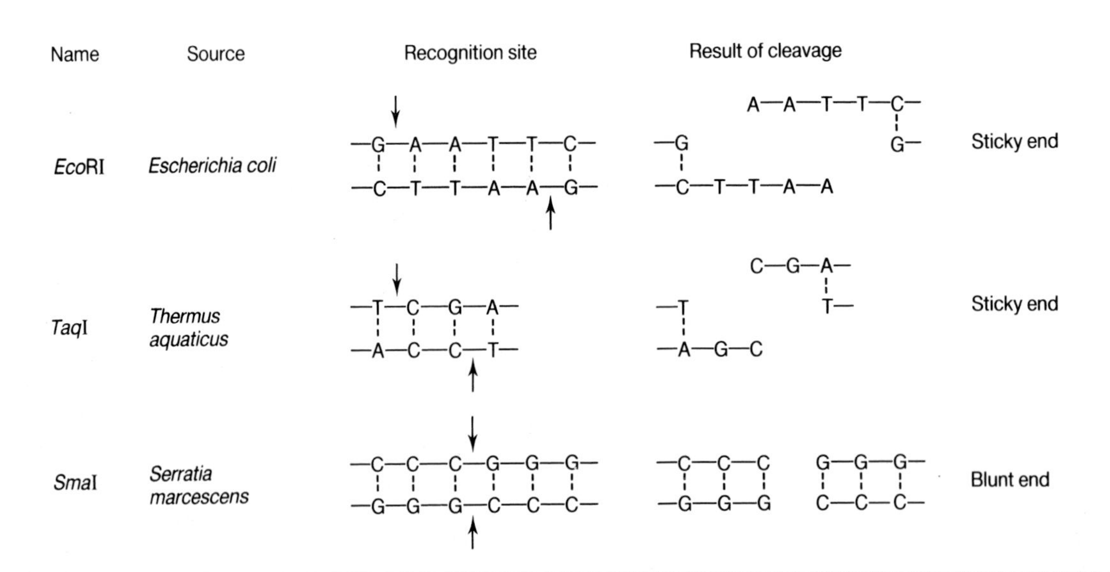

Fig. 2.20 Examples of restriction enzymes and their recognition sites.

brane (**Southern blotting**) and then hybridized to a specific probe (Fig. 2.21). Messenger RNA can also be transferred in this way to a DNA binding membrane (**Northern blotting**).

A specific example is illustrated in Fig. 2.22. This shows two portions of the clotting factor IX gene (absence of clotting factor IX is the cause of haemophilia B) from two different X chromosomes. The gene on the right has four *Taq*I sites whereas the gene on the left has only three as a base variant has abolished one recognition site. The probe shown is a 2.5 kb fragment from within the factor IX gene and its area of complementarity is indicated. Thus, after digestion it will hybridize to a constant 5.3 kb fragment from each gene and to a 1.8 kb fragment from the gene on the left and to a 1.3 kb fragment from the gene on the right. Thus, these two factor IX genes can be distinguished by the different pattern of fragments produced after *Taq*I digestion. Such a difference in the pattern of fragments after restriction enzyme digestion is called a restriction fragment length polymorphism (RFLP).

A female with two X chromosomes will generate one of three patterns with 1.8 kb fragments from each X chromosome (1.8 kb/1.8 kb), 1.3 kb fragments from each X chromosome (1.3 kb/1.3 kb) or

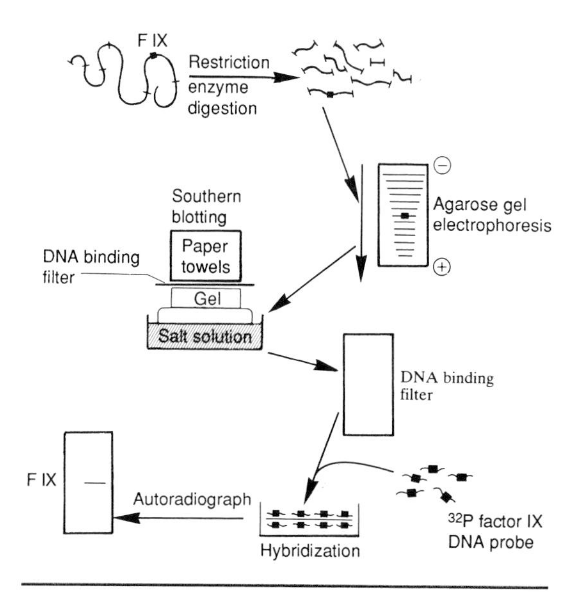

Fig. 2.21 Diagram of the steps involved in the identification of a restriction fragment length polymorphism.

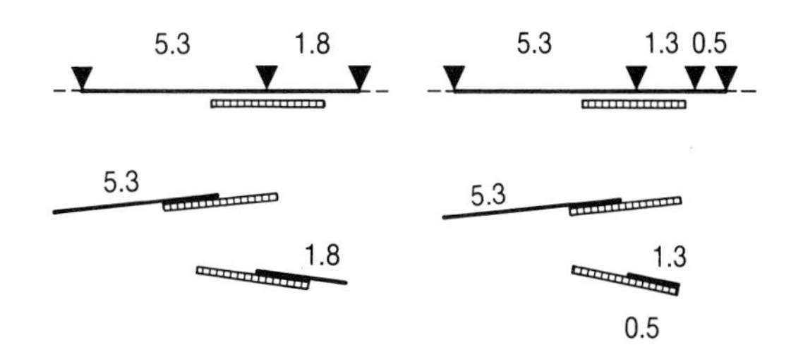

Fig. 2.22 Diagram of a coagulation factor IX intragenic restriction fragment length polymorphism in two X chromosomes. Arrows indicate restriction enzyme (*Taq*I) recognition sites and the hatched segment represents the DNA probe. Fragment sizes are in kilobases.

a 1.8 kb from one X chromosome and a 1.3 kb fragment from the other (1.8 kb/1.3 kb). Males with only a single X chromosome will generate only 1.8 kb or 1.3 kb fragments. Figure 2.23 shows this RFLP in a normal family. The mother is heterozygous for this RFLP (1.8/1.3) and she has inherited the 1.8 kb fragment from her father and handed it to one son. The other son must have received the grandmaternal factor IX gene, indicated by the 1.3 kb band.

Gene Tracking

Restriction fragment length polymorphisms (RFLPs) can be used to follow the inheritance of a part of a chromosome through a family. The family in Fig. 2.23 is normal but the same technique can be used to follow mutant genes through a family. Figure 2.24 illustrates a family with haemophilia B due to a deficiency of clotting factor IX.

The RFLP result for the factor IX RFLP of Figs 2.24 and 2.23 is shown for each family member. The affected son has inherited the 1.8 kb fragment from his heterozygous mother whereas the unaffected son has inherited the 1.3 kb fragment. The daughter at risk is homozygous for the 1.3 kb fragment and thus has inherited the normal factor IX gene from her mother and so is not a carrier for haemophilia B. This approach can also be used to test samples taken during a pregnancy for prenatal diagnosis in a fetus at risk.

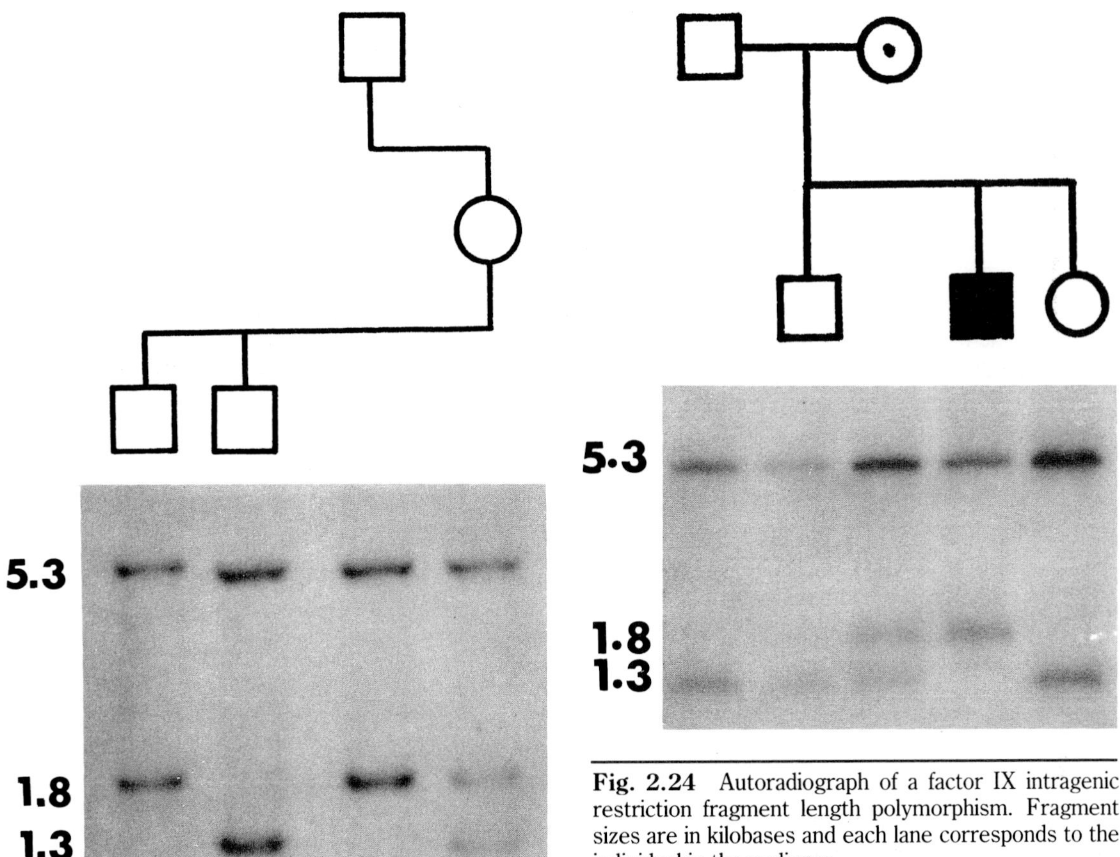

Fig. 2.23 Autoradiograph of a factor IX intragenic restriction fragment length polymorphism. Fragment sizes are in kilobases and each lane corresponds to the individual in the pedigree.

Fig. 2.24 Autoradiograph of a factor IX intragenic restriction fragment length polymorphism. Fragment sizes are in kilobases and each lane corresponds to the individual in the pedigree.

Gene tracking can use RFLPs from within the gene (intragenic RFLPs) or in neighbouring non-coding DNA (extragenic RFLPs). Intragenic RFLPs are to be preferred, as extragenic markers, especially if some distance from the gene of interest, carry error rates due to the possibility of recombination between the chromosomes. By 1989, 945 human structural genes had been cloned in addition to over 3400 intergenic DNA segments, and just under one-half of these genes or intergenic DNA segments detect RFLPs. Markers now exist throughout all chromosomes and these can be used to identify the location of a gene by seeking cosegregation of the gene of interest and some of these markers.

Restriction fragment length polymorphisms due to loss (or gain) of a restriction enzyme recognition site are also called **site polymorphisms** and usually have only two alternative fragments. A second type of RFLP exists where the number of repeated sequences (**tandem repeats**) between two recognition sites varies between chromosomes. These variable number of tandem repeat (VNTR) markers are extremely useful as most individuals generate different sized fragments from each member of a chromosome pair and the difficulty of fragments of identical size in a key individual (non-informativeness) is minimized. Figure 2.25 illustrates an example with a VNTR probe in a family with adult polycystic kidney disease. In

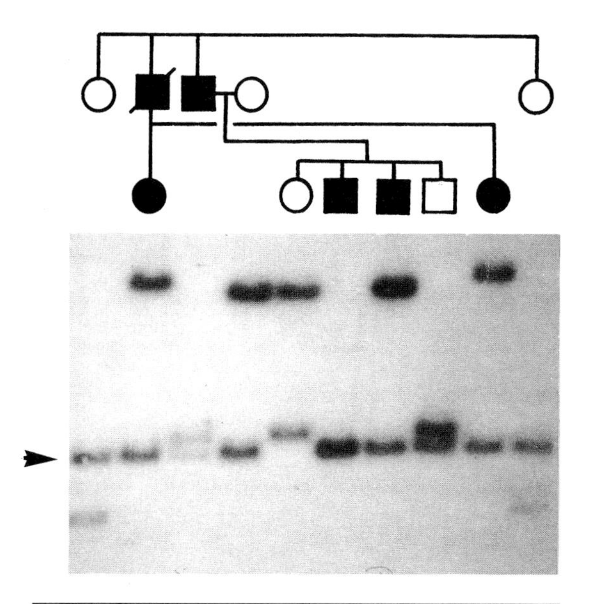

Fig. 2.25 Cosegregation of a VNTR fragment (arrowed) with the disease trait in a family with autosomal dominant polycystic kidney disease. Each affected person inherits the arrowed fragment.

this family the arrowed fragment shows complete cosegregation with the disease.

Variable number of tandem repeats can also be used to determine family relationships. In Fig. 2.26 the eldest 'daughter' has a fragment which is not present in either parent, which confirmed the suspicion of non-paternity. This approach can be enhanced by simultaneously studying multiple VNTRs (Fig. 2.27). The result is known as a DNA fingerprint and the pattern is unique for each person with approximately one-half of the fragments from the mother and one-half from the father. DNA fingerprinting is of value for the identification of the origin of tissue samples in forensic medicine and to help resolve family relationships in immigration and paternity disputes.

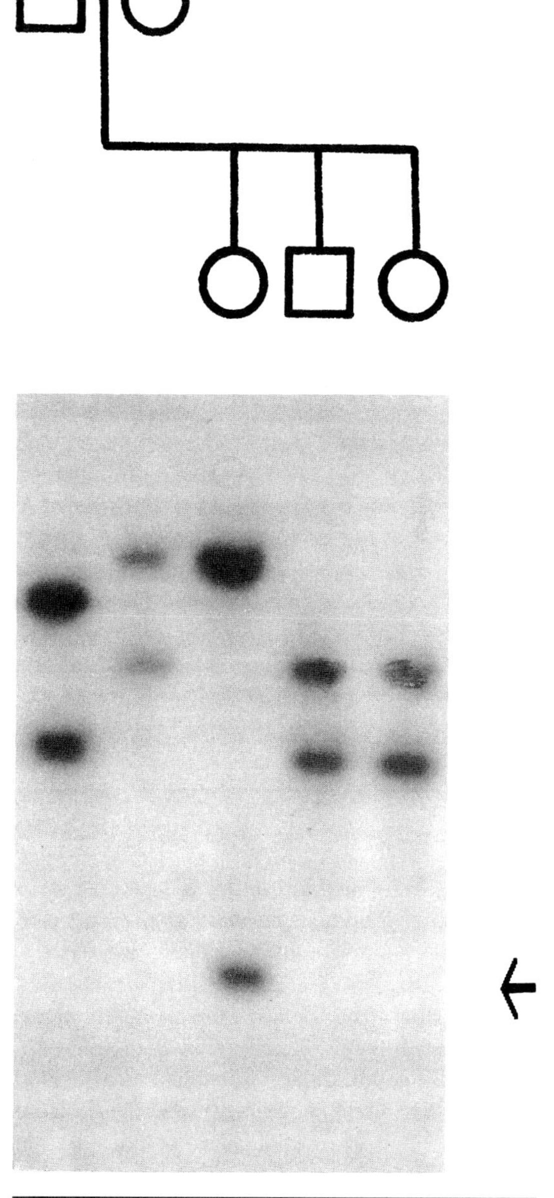

Fig. 2.26 Pedigree and results of DNA analysis with an autosomal VNTR probe. The eldest daughter has not inherited a paternal band, and an extra band is present which is not seen in the remaining family members.

Direct Mutation Detection

Gene tracking has the advantage of being useful in the absence of a knowledge of the molecular lesion

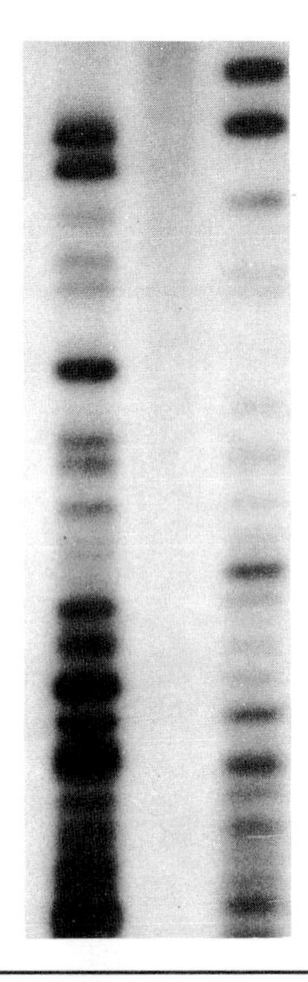

Fig. 2.27 DNA fingerprints from two sisters who inherit one half of each parent's variably sized fragments and thus have approximately one half of their bands in common.

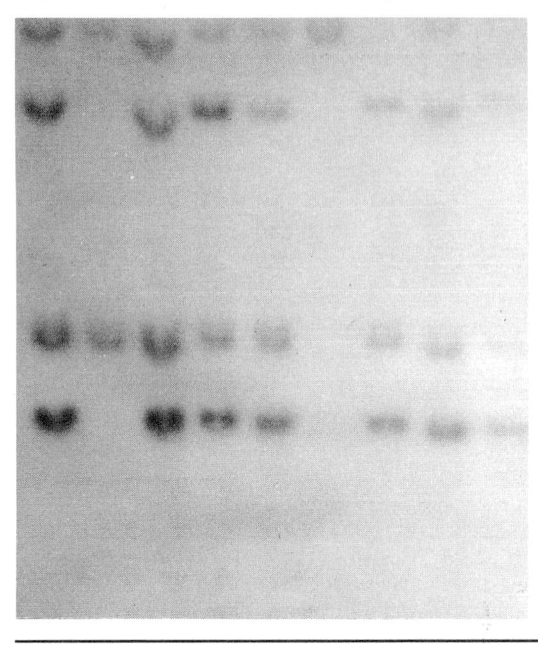

Fig. 2.28 Gene deletion in some boys with Duchenne muscular dystrophy. Note msising bands in lanes 2, 6, 7 and 9.

but it does have the disadvantages of errors due to recombination and non-paternity and the need to study several family members. An alternative approach is to identify the molecular lesion in an affected patient and then to examine family members at risk for the presence of this lesion. Molecular lesions in the single gene disorders include deletions and point mutations. Deletions can be detected by partial or total failure of hybridization to probes from the gene (Fig. 2.28).

Point mutations can be detected by one of three approaches: loss or gain of an RFLP (site polymorphisms); allele specific oligonucleotide probes; and genomic sequencing. Sickle cell disease always arises from a point mutation in the codon for the sixth amino acid from the N-terminal end of β-globin so that valine substitutes for glutamic acid (Fig. 2.29).

*Mst*II is a restriction enzyme which recognizes the sequence GGACTCC and, as indicated in Fig. 2.29, this recognition site is abolished in a β-globin molecule with the sickle cell mutation. Normal β-globin genes yield *Mst*II fragments of 1150 bp and 200 bp whereas a β-globin gene with the sickle cell mutation yields a fragment of 1350 bp. Thus digestion of a sample DNA with *Mst*II and probing with a β-globin DNA probe can distinguish between individuals who are homozygous normal, heterozygous or homozygous for sickle cell disease.

Allele specific oligonucleotide (ASO) probes are short (15–30 nucleotide) probes which have the complementary sequence to either the normal DNA or mutant DNA sequence at the point of interest. Under appropriate experimental conditions the presence or absence of hybridization with these probes will distinguish normals from heterozygotes and homozygous affected individuals (Fig. 2.29).

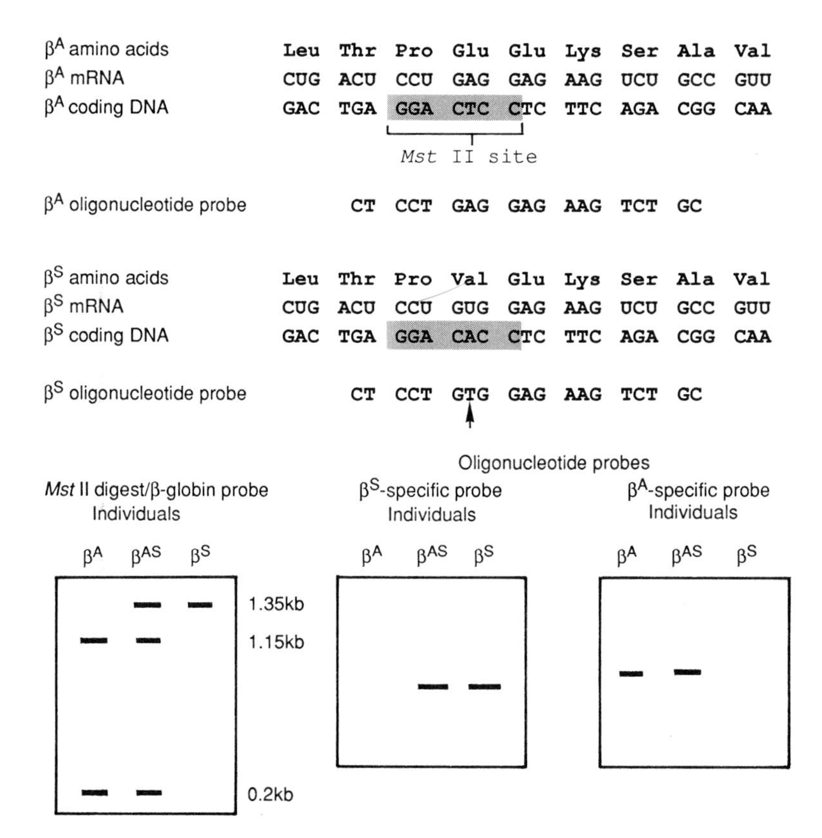

Fig. 2.29 Amino acid sequence and DNA sequence of normal β-globin and sickle β-globin. The difference can be recognized by failure of *Mst* II to cleave at the site of the sickle cell mutation or by allele specific oligonucleotide probes.

The third approach to direct detection is to use **genomic sequencing.** Formerly this would have been too time-consuming for routine clinical diagnosis but now it is possible to amplify sections of interest within genes rapidly using the *polymerase chain reaction (PCR)* and to determine their base sequence directly. The PCR consists of repeated rounds of localized DNA replication to produce an exponential increase in the number of copies of the target sequence. Two oligonucleotide primers are required which are complementary to flanking sequences of the target DNA segment (Fig. 2.30). The initial products are rapidly outnumbered by identical copies of the target DNA segment (short products). Amplification of more than one million fold can be routinely obtained from 30 or so cycles which take 2–3 hours in an automated procedure. Figure 2.31 shows a section of gene which has been amplified by PCR and sequenced.

The PCR can also be used to amplify DNA prior to cleavage with a restriction enzyme in order to demonstrate a particular RFLP. The advantage over standard Southern blotting is that a result is available in a few hours (as compared with 5–10 days) and the analysis can be performed on less than 1 μg of DNA (as compared with 5–10 μg). The disadvantage is that specific DNA primers are required at the beginning and end of each section of DNA to be amplified, and the sensitivity of the system means that many simultaneous controls are required to avert misinterpretation due to contamination.

Biochemical Analysis

Genes encode proteins and thus biochemical analysis of proteins can be a powerful tool in the detection of genetic lesions. Such analyses may be

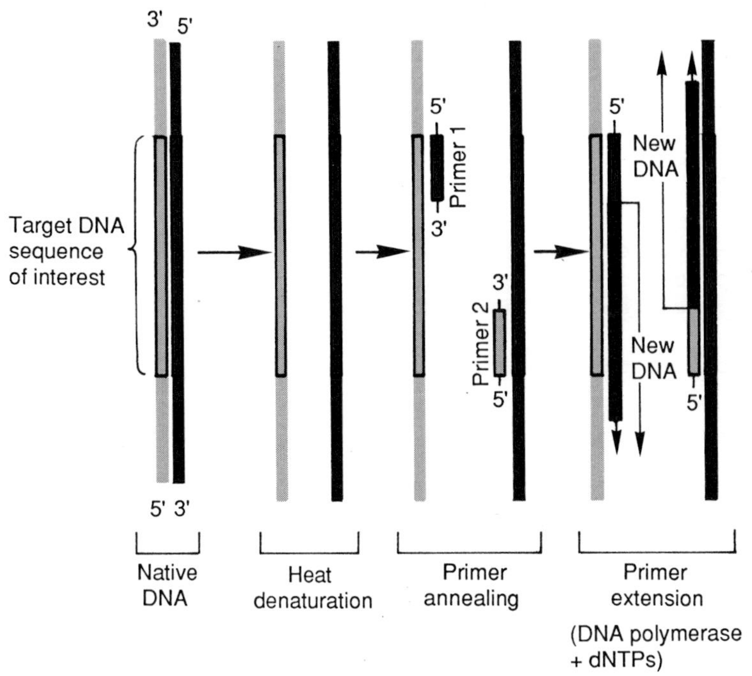

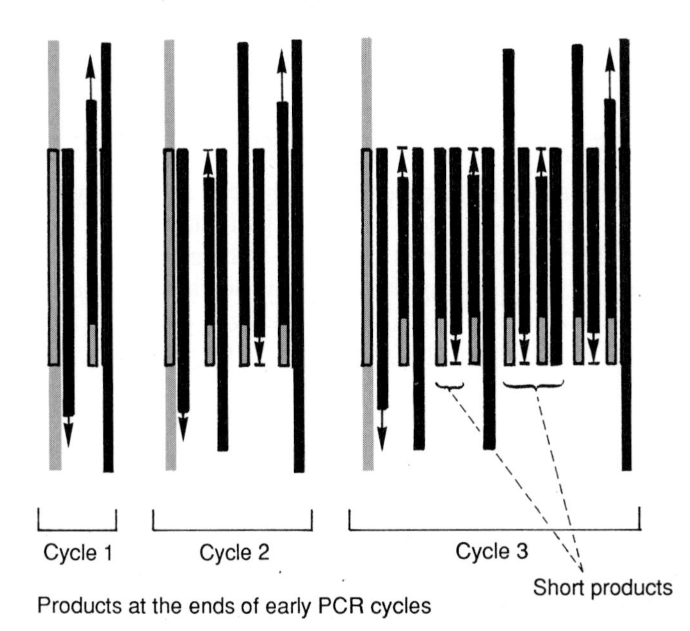

Fig. 2.30 Diagram of the steps involved in amplification of a DNA segment using the polymerase chain reaction (PCR).

quantitative with, for example, a reduction in level of activity of an enzymic protein (e.g. a 50% replication of hepatic phenylalanine hydroxylase in heterozygotes for phenylketonuria and low or no activity of this enzyme in homozygotes) or qualitative with differences in electrophoretic mobility (e.g. variants of α_1-antitrypsin) or ability to bind cofactors.

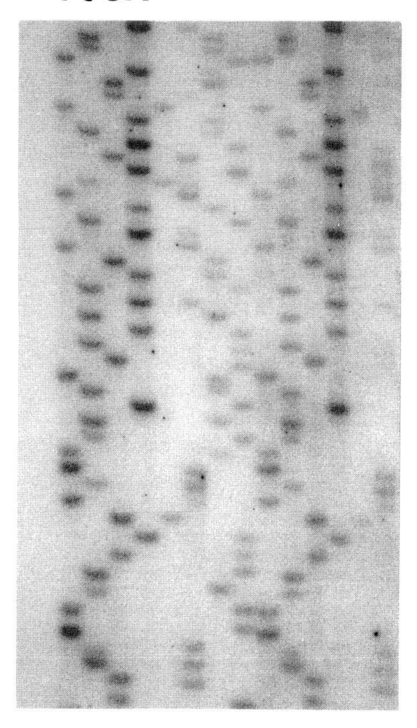

Fig. 2.31 Direct genomic sequencing following PCR amplification. The sequence is read off from the bottom and each lane corresponds to one of the four nucleotide bases (T, thymine; C, cytosine; G, guanine; A, adenine). The sequence of the first 20 bases derived from the four tracks on the left is TGGCCTTCCGAGTCT-TCCAC.

Molecular Pathophysiology of Genetic Diseases

This section considers the mechanisms of both origin and disease pathogenesis in the various types of genetic disorders.

Chromosomal Disorders

Chromosomal disorders are usually classified into numerical abnormalities, where the somatic cells contain an abnormal number of normal chromosomes, or structural aberrations, where the somatic cells contain one or more abnormal chromosomes. They may involve either the sex chromosomes or the autosomes and may occur either as a result of a germ cell mutation in the parent or more remote ancestor, or as a result of somatic mutation in which only a proportion of cells will be affected.

Numerical Aberrations

Somatic cells normally contain 46 chromosomes (diploid) and mature gametes contain 23 chromosomes (haploid). A chromosome number which is an exact multiple of the haploid number and exceeds the diploid number is called polyploidy and one which is not an exact multiple is called aneuploidy.

Aneuploidy

Aneuploidy usually arises from failure of paired chromosomes or sister chromatids to disjoin at anaphase of cell division (**non-disjunction**), although it may be due to delayed movement of a chromosome at anaphase (**anaphase lag**). By either of these mechanisms two cells are produced, one with an extra copy of a chromosome (**trisomy**) and one with a missing copy of that chromosome (**monosomy**). The cause of meiotic non-disjunction is not known but it occurs at increased frequency with increasing maternal age, with maternal hypothyroidism, possibly after irradiation or viral infection or as a familial tendency. The cause of mitotic non-disjunction is also unknown and predisposing factors have not been identified.

Table 2.7 shows example of common numerical chromosomal aberrations. In general aneuploidy is less serious for the sex chromosomes than for the autosomes. Autosomal monosomy usually results in early spontaneous miscarriage. Autosomal trisomies also tend to be miscarried and survivors show mental retardation and multiple congenital abnormalities. The mechanism by which the chromosomal imbalance causes its clinical effects is unknown.

Polyploidy

A complete extra set of chromosomes will raise the total number to 69, and this is called **triploidy**. This usually arises from fertilization by two sperm (dispermy), or from failure of one of the maturation divisions of either the egg or the sperm so that a diploid gamete is produced. Triploid pregnancies usually miscarry in early pregnancy.

Table 2.7 Examples of structural chromosomal aberrations

Karyotype	Comment
92,XXYY	Tetraploidy
69,XXY	Triploidy
47,XX,+21	Trisomy 21
47,XY,+18	Trisomy 18
47,XX,+13	Trisomy 13
47,XX,+16	Trisomy 16
47,XXY	Klinefelter syndrome
47,XXX	Trisomy X
45,X	Turner syndrome
49,XXXXY	Variant of Klinefelter syndrome

Structural Aberrations

Structural abberations all result from **chromosomal breakage**. When a chromosome breaks two unstable sticky ends are produced. Generally, repair mechanisms rejoin these two ends without delay. However, if more than one break has occurred, then as the repair mechanisms cannot distinguish one sticky end from another there is the possibility of rejoining the wrong ends. The spontaneous rate of chromosomal breakage may be markedly increased by exposure to ionizing radiation or mutagenic chemicals and is also increased in some rare inherited conditions. Chromosomal breakage is not randomly distributed and for all translocations the spontaneous mutation rate is one per 1000 gametes (which is about 100-fold greater than the mutation rate for individual gene loci). A number of different types of structural aberration are recognized (Fig. 2.32, Table 2.8).

A translocation is the transfer of chromosomal material between chromosomes. The process requires breakage of both chromosomes with repair in an abnormal arrangement. This exchange does not usually result in loss of DNA and the individual, who is clinically normal, is said to have a balanced translocation. The medical significance is that future generations are at risk because a balanced translocation carrier is capable of producing chromosomally unbalanced offspring.

Deletions usually arise from a loss of a portion of the chromosome between two break points or as a

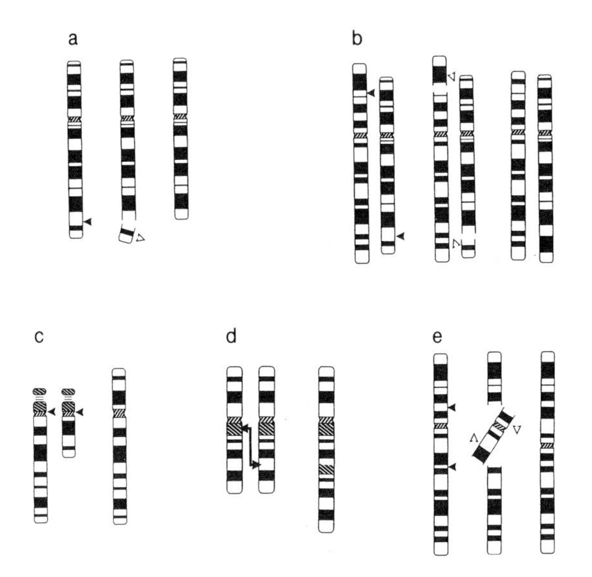

Fig. 2.32 Diagram of types of structural chromosomal abnormality: **a** deletion, **b** reciprocal translocation, **c** centric fusion or Robertsonian translocation, **d** duplication, **e** pericentric inversion (break points are arrowed in each case).

result of a parental translocation. The deleted portion lacks a centromere and will be lost at a subsequent cell division. A **ring chromosome** arises from breaks in both arms of a chromosome: the terminal ends are lost and the two proximal sticky ends unite to form a ring. As the smallest visible loss from a chromosome is about 4000 kb, individuals with visible deletions are rendered monosomic for large numbers of genes, and with autosomal deletions mental retardation and multiple congenital malformations are usual. Small deletions towards the limit of optical resolution are thus still clinically important and these are termed **microdeletions**,. These microdeletions remove multiple adjacent genes and range in size from the limit of optical resolution down to removal of a part of a single gene. These smaller microdeletions are not visible using light microscopy but can be revealed by DNA probes (see Fig. 2.28).

Duplication of a segment of a chromosome may originate by unequal crossing over during meiosis (Fig. 2.33) or as a result of a parental translocation or inversion. Duplications are more common than deletions and are generally less harmful. Indeed, tiny duplications at a molecular level (repeats) may play an important role in permitting gene diversification during evolution (e.g. the α- and β-globin gene clusters).

Inversions arise from two chromosomal breaks with inversion through 180 degrees of the segment between the breaks. If both breaks are in a single arm then the centromere is not included (**paracentric inversion**) whereas if the breaks are on either side of the centromere it is included (**pericentric inversion**). Generally this change in gene order does not produce clinical abnormality. The medical significance lies with the risk of generating unbalanced gametes.

Table 2.8 Examples of structural chromosomal aberrations

Karyotype	Comment
46,XY,t(5;10)(p13;q25)	Balanced reciprocal translocation involving chromosomes 5 and 10 (break points indicated)
45,XX,t(13;14)(p11;q11)	Centric fusion translocation of chromosomes 13 and 14
46,XY,del(5)(p25)	Short arm deletion of chromosome 5, *cri du chat* syndrome
46,X,i(Xq)	Isochromosome of Xq
46,XX,dup(2)(p13p22)	Partial duplication of the short arm of chromosome 2 (p13→p22)
46,XY,r(3)(p26→q29)	Ring chromosome 3 (p26→q29)
46,XY,inv(11)(p15q14)	Pericentric inversion of chromosome 11

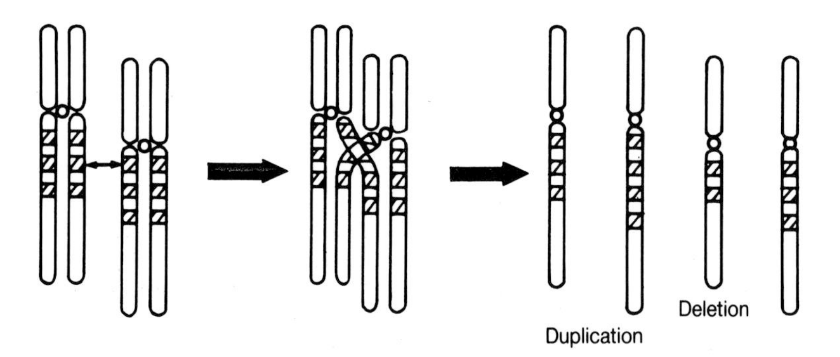

Fig. 2.33 Diagram to show malalignment with recombination resulting in chromosomes with duplications and deletions (unequal crossing over).

Single Gene Disorders

Single gene disorders result from mutations in one or both members of a pair of genes. These mutations are broadly divisible into length mutations with gain or loss of genetic material and point mutations with alteration of the genetic code but no gain or loss of genetic material.

Length Mutations

Length mutations include deletions, duplications and insertions. As indicated earlier, deletions can range from one base pair to several megabases (visible microdeletion) to many megabases (chromosomal deletion). Deletions can arise from chromosomal breakage, as a result of a parenteral translocation or inversion (which is itself caused by chromosomal breakage) or by unequal crossing over. The spontaneous rate of chromosomal breakage is markedly increased by ionizing radiation and by mutagenic chemicals. Unequal crossing over is especially likely to occur in areas with duplicated genes of similar sequence. This is exemplified by studies on the genes responsible for colour vision. There are three separate genes for the cone pigments blue (on chromosome 7), red and green (near the tip of the long arm of the X chromosome, Xq28). There is a single red gene on each X chromosome and one to three copies of the green genes. The red and green genes have 96% sequence homology, and unequal crossing over in the area can result in loss of gene function or in hybrid genes which produce pigments of altered function (Fig. 2.34).

Large deletions remove many adjacent genes (contiguous gene disorders) and these should be suspected if a boy has several X-linked disorders or if a patient with a single gene disorder has unexplained mental retardation and/or congenital malformations. Removal of all of a gene directly prevents transcription but smaller deletions can be equally serious by altering the reading frame of the messenger RNA (frame shift mutations, Table 2.9).

Duplications can also disrupt the reading frame and recently patients have been described where the structural gene was disrupted by an insertion.

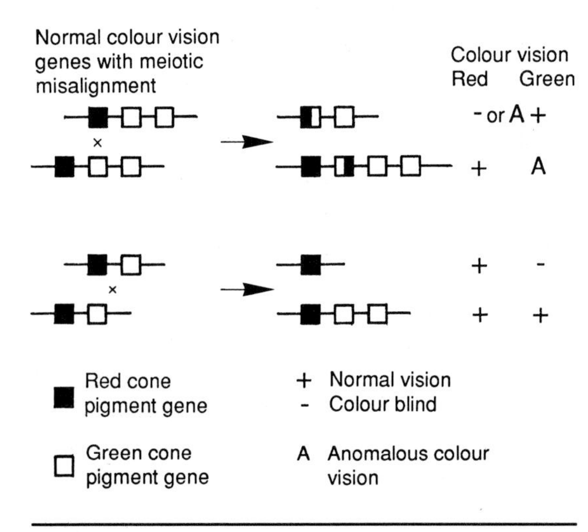

Fig. 2.34 Unequal recombination in the colour vision gene cluster resulting in loss of genes or creation of fused hybrid genes with altered action spectrums.

Table 2.9 Examples of DNA mutation

DNA base sequence	mRNA sequence	Amino acid sequence	Comment
CAA TTC CGA CGA	GUU AAG GCU GCU	Val-Lys-Ala-Ala	Normal sequence
CAA TTT CGA CGA	GUU AAA GCU GCU	Val-Lys-Ala-Ala	Point mutation with unchanged amino acid sequence
CAA CTC CGA CGA	GUU GAG GCU GCU	Val-Glu-Ala-Ala	Point mutation with amino acid substitution
CAA ATC CGA CGA	GUU UAG GCU GCU	Val-Stop	Point mutation with premature chain termination
CAA—TCC GAC GA	GUU AGG CUG CU	Val-Arg-Leu	Base deletion with frame shift
CAA TTT CCG ACG A	GUU AAA GGC UGC	Val-Lys-Gly-Cys	Base insertion with frame shift

Abbreviations as in Table 2.1.

These insertions were composed of repetitive DNA which is believed to be of ancestral viral origin. This suggests that intragenic insertion by retroviruses is another general mechanism in the causation of a proportion of single gene disorders.

Point Mutations

In a point mutation a single nucleotide base is replaced by a different nucleotide base. Because there are several codons for most amino acids (degeneracy of the genetic code), 25% of point mutations do not alter the amino acid encoded by that triplet (see Table 2.1) although in the remainder a different amino acid is substituted (Table 2.9).

Alteration of an amino acid codon to a chain terminator (**premature stop codon**) can prematurely stop transcription (5%). The other 70% of point mutations result in variant proteins which may have altered function and/or electrophoretic mobility (33%). Insertion or deletion of more or less than three (or a multiple of three) base pairs interferes with transcription by altering the reading frame of the messenger RNA so that a nonsense message is generated (**frameshift mutations**).

Most point mutations are spontaneous and unexplained; however, certain factors such as mutagenic chemicals and ionizing radiation can increase the rate. In the absence of such agents the mutation rate is in the order of one base pair substitution for every 10^9–10^{10} base pairs replicated. Methylated cytosine residues are relatively '**hot spots**' for mutations because deamination converts them to thymine. Neither methylated cytosine nor thymine is recognized as an abnormality by the usual DNA repair mechanisms and deamination of a methylated cytosine thus leads to a thymine substitution with substitution of an adenine for guanine on the opposite DNA strand.

Molecular Pathology of Single Gene Disorders

Determination of the molecular lesion in a single gene disorder is not just of academic interest since it allows the mutation to be tracked within a family in order to provide accurate genetic counselling. As more conditions are studied two important generalizations are becoming evident. Lesions can occur at any stage in the protein biosynthetic pathway (Fig. 2.35) and most conditions show a diversity of molecular lesions (heterogeneity of molecular pathology).

The β-globin gene is currently the best documented gene in respect of molecular pathology. In patients with β-thalassaemia over 90 different

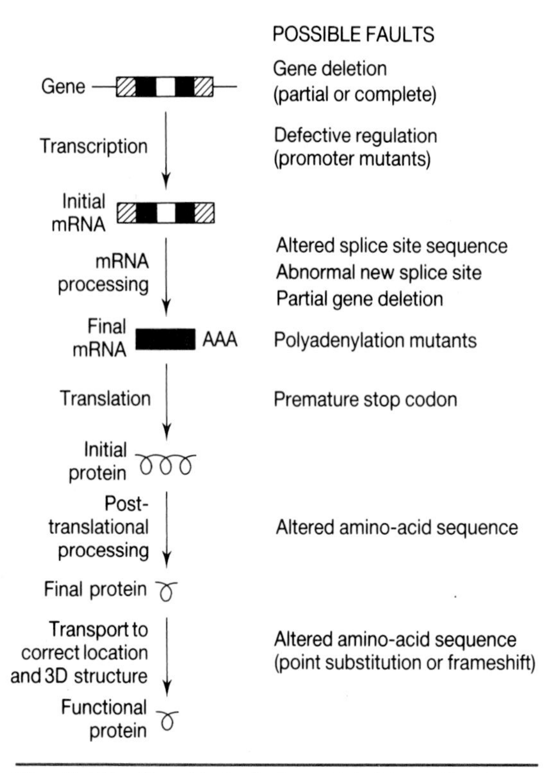

Fig. 2.35 Possible faults in protein biosynthesis.

molecular defects have now been described. Lesions have been documented at every level of the protein biosynthetic pathway including defective promoters. Of the known mutations, about 16% affect transcription, about one-half affect RNA splicing, and about one-third block translation. Both length and point mutations are observed, with the latter predominating.

In sickle cell anaemia all patients have an identical point mutation (see Fig. 2.29). This is believed to reflect selection at a population level for this particular mutation which confers resistance to falciparum malaria. In contrast, in certain conditions such as α-thalassaemia, red–green colour blindness, steroid sulphatase deficiency (X-linked ichthyosis) and Duchenne muscular dystrophy, length mutations (particularly deletions) are far more frequent than point mutations. In part, this excess is believed to reflect the structural similarity of adjacent genes in the α-globin cluster or the colour vision gene cluster and hence the ease of misalignment at meiosis and generation of small duplications and deficiencies if crossing over occurs (unequal crossing over).

As more conditions are studied, further exceptions will undoubtedly emerge but, for most conditions, a diversity of molecular pathology is to be expected.

Multifactorial Disorders

Multifactorial disorders, by definition, require the interaction of environmental and genetic factors. Generally, several genetic loci are inferred to have a role although for the majority of these disorders the number and nature of these loci is currently unknown. Twin and family studies indicate that multifactorial inheritance is involved in many common chronic disorders of adult life and many of the commoner major congenital malformations (Table 2.10). As indicated in Table 2.10 the contributing genetic loci are as yet unknown in the majority of these conditions, but DNA analysis using candidate genes has given a new impetus to research in this area. This is exemplified by studies on insulin dependent (type 1) diabetes mellitus. This was suspected to arise from a viral infection in a genetically susceptible host and the association with specific histocompatibility antigens DR3 and DR4 (Chapter 5) focused genetic attention on the major histocompatibility complex of genes which are clustered on the short arm of chromosome 6. A member of this gene cluster is DQ and at amino-acid position 57 of the DQ protein mutations which resulted in substitution of alanine, valine or serine appear to confer susceptibility, whereas aspartate appears to confer resistance to the disease.

Mitochondrial Disorders

Human mitochondria each have about 10 copies of a circular double stranded DNA molecule of 16 569

Table 2.10 Examples of multifactorial disorders (alphabetical order)

Condition	Frequency	Contributing genetic loci
Atopic disease	1/4	11q
Cleft lip and plate	1/1000	?
Cleft palate alone	1/1000	?
Diabetes mellitus (insulin dependent)	1/500	MHC
Diabetes mellitus (insulin independent)	1/50	?
Hypertension	1/10	?
Leprosy	Varies	MHC
Manic depression	1/10	?Xq, ?11p
Multiple sclerosis	1/2000	MHC, T cell receptor
Premature vascular disease	1/70	Fibrinogen, lipid pathways
Psoriasis	1/100	?
Pyloric stenosis (congenital)	1/300	?
Rheumatoid arthritis	1/50	MHC
Schizophrenia	1/100	?5q
Spina bifida	1–5/1000	?
Tuberculosis	varies	?

MHC, major histocompatibility complex.

bp. These mitochondrial chromosomes are self-replicating and encode several enzymes involved in oxidative phosphorylation. As the mitochondria are found in the cytoplasm they are transmitted in the ovum from a mother to all of her children.

A few clinically important disorders have now been discovered to result from mitochondrial DNA mutations. In Leber's hereditary optic neuropathy there is sudden irreversible loss of vision in early adulthood. In families so far studied two specific point mutations have been identified at nucleotide positions 9163 (in ATPase 6) and at nucleotide position 11 778 (in ND4 of complex I). In contrast, the mitochondrial myopathies (p. 876) usually have deletions or tandem duplications of variable size in the mitochondrial DNA. In the mitochondrial myopathies if the mutation is confined to skeletal muscle there is little risk to the offspring.

Somatic Cell Genetic Disorders

When a mutation is present in the fertilized ovum then this mutation will be transmitted to all daughter cells. If, however, a mutation arises after the first cell division then this mutation will only be found in a proportion of cells and the indvidual is a mosaic (two or more different genotypes in one individual). The mutation may be confined to the gonadal cells (gonadal mosaic, e.g. an unaffected parent with two children with a fully penetrant autosomal dominant trait) or to the somatic cells (somatic mosaic, e.g. a brown segment in an otherwise blue iris) or occur in a proportion of both. Cancer provides many examples of somatic cell genetic disorders in which molecular pathology has been demonstrated and it is suspected that other common disorders and ageing might have their basis in alteration of DNA in somatic cells.

Cancer Genetics (see Chapter 10)

Cancer affects about one in four of all adults at some stage in their lives and each tumour results from one or more mutations of the cellular DNA. In a small proportion of patients the first of these mutations is inherited and is thus present in all cells but in the remaining majority, the faults occur after birth in a restricted number of somatic cells. Two types of gene appear to be involved: tumour suppressor genes (anti-oncogenes) and oncogenes.

The tumour suppressor genes were discovered as a result of studies on the rare inherited forms of cancer, particularly retinoblastomas. Retinoblastoma is the commonest malignant eye tumour of childhood and in 20–30% of cases both eyes are affected. All of these bilateral cases and 15% of the unilateral cases are inherited as an autosomal dominant trait. The gene for this trait is localized to the proximal long arm of chromosome 13 (13q14) and in the tumour tissue this gene's messenger RNA and protein product are absent. An autosomal dominant trait implies a mutation in only one member of a pair of genes and for a tumour to occur a person who inherits a mutant gene must also develop a fault in the partner gene within a retinal cell. This second fault is often a deletion which can be of variable size but it may also arise from complete loss of the normal copy of chromosome 13 and resulting homozygosity for the mutant copy of 13 (Fig. 2.36).

In the non-inherited cases of retinoblastoma two separate mutations have to occur in the copies of chromosome 13 in a particular retinal cell. Hence, in contrast to the familial cases, bilateral involvement is most unlikely and age of onset tends to be later.

It is believed that neoplasia commonly has multiple steps in its pathogenesis and that the two steps seen in retinoblastoma might be unduly simple. The principle of loss of particular areas of a chromosome within tumour tissues, however, has wider applications and specific losses have now been demonstrated in multiple tumour types (Table 2.11). Demonstration of these chromosomal losses is technically very difficult using cytogenetic analysis, but is readily performed by DNA analysis which shows loss of heterozygosity for probes within the deleted region when compared with normal somatic tissues. Several tumours show similar chromosomal losses and

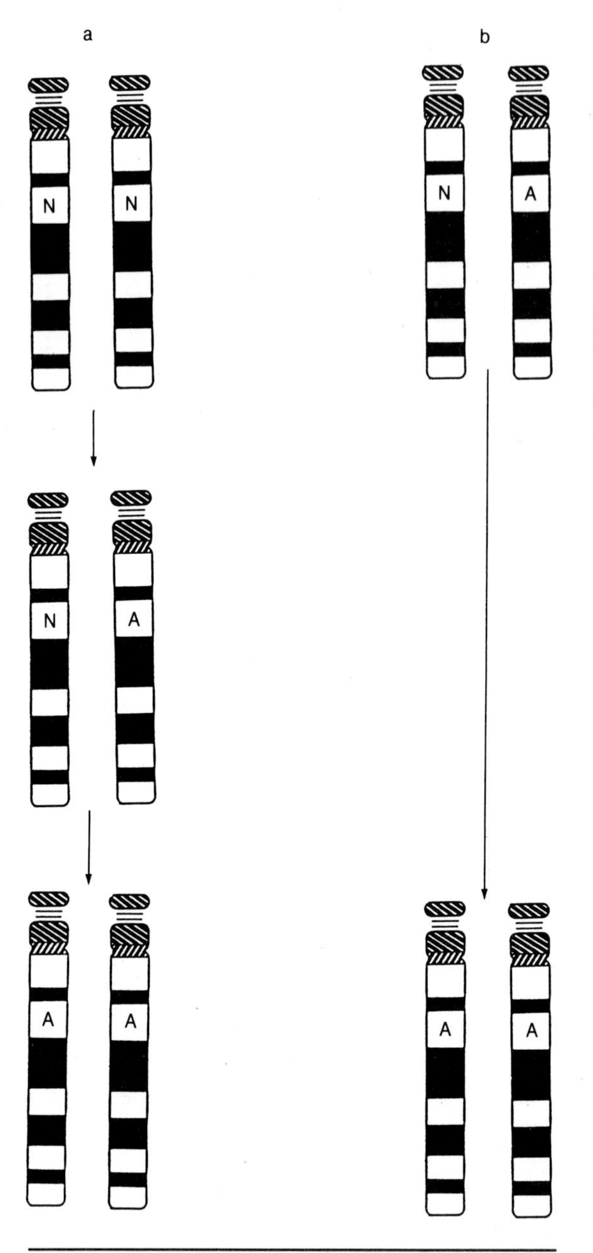

Fig. 2.36 Diagram of sporadic **a** and inherited **b** retinoblastoma. Copies of chromosome 13 are shown with either a normal (N) or an abnormal (A) gene.

Table 2.11 Examples of allele loss in human cancers

Tumour (alphabetical order)	Site of allele loss
Acoustic neuroma	22
Bladder carcinoma	11p
Breast carcinoma	11p, 13q
Colon carcinoma	5q, 17p, 18q, 22, others
Hepatoblastoma	11p
Hepatocellular carcinoma	11p, 4q
Insulinoma	11
Lung	
small cell	3p, 13q, 17p
other types	3p (occ. 13q, 17p)
Medullary thyroid carcinoma	1p
Melanoma	various
Meningioma	22
Osteosarcoma	13q
Phaeochromocytoma	1p, 22
Renal carcinoma	3p
Retinoblastoma	13q
Rhabdomyosarcoma	11p
Stomach carcinoma	13q
Wilms' tumour	11p

these areas are all believed to contain tumour suppressor loci.

Oncogenes were first discovered by molecular analysis of oncogenic retroviruses which cause cancer in mice, cats and monkeys. For example, the *Ras* oncogene is derived from the Rous sarcoma virus which causes a sarcoma in chickens. Each of these viral oncogenes (**v-oncogenes**) was actually derived from a normal host gene (which is not normally oncogenic) by recombination between it and the ancestral viral genome. Over 40 normal cellular copies of the oncogenes, the **proto-oncogenes** have now been isolated and mapped to human chromosomes (see Fig. 2.7). These proto-oncogenes can be activated to cause cancer by point mutation or through chromosome rearrangement.

Comparison of the DNA sequence in proto-oncogenes in tumour tissue with the other somatic tissues has revealed that specific point mutations can lead to different tumour types. For example in the H-*Ras* gene a glycine residue is normally present at position 12 but in some patients with bladder cancers, lung cancers or melanoma the tumour tissue shows a point mutation (GGC→GTC) with substitution of valine at position 12. This change is not inherited but is a somatic mutation within the cells which originate the cancer. Specific point mutations have also been identified at other positions within H-*Ras* and within other proto-oncogenes. Screening for these mutations within tumour tissue by DNA sequencing is laborious but specific oligonucleotide probes can be useful to detect specific common mutations. Tissues can also be screened for the presence of an activated proto-oncogene by showing that extracts of tumour DNA have the ability to transform a susceptible rodent cell line (NIH 3T3).

Human proto-oncogenes can also be activated

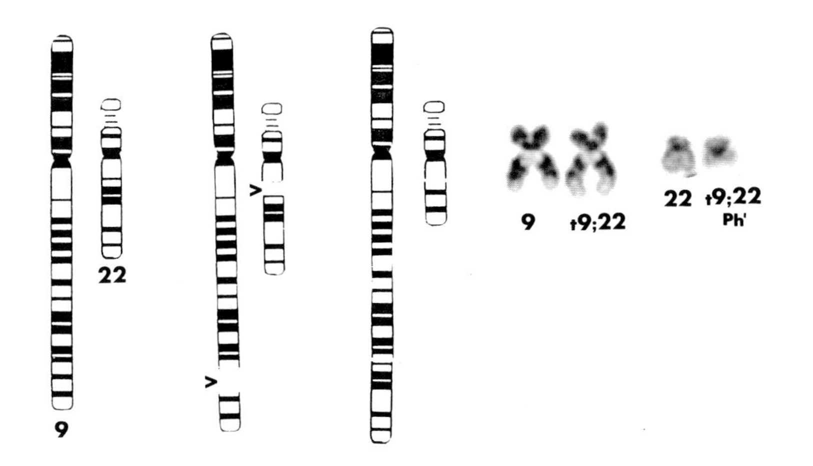

Fig. 2.37 Philadelphia chromosome (Ph') resulting from a reciprocal translocation between chromosomes 9 and 22 [(t(9;22) (q34;q11)].

through chromosome rearrangement. This is exemplified by chronic myeloid leukaemia (p. 628) and the *Philadelphia chromosome (Ph′)*. The majority of affected patients show this chromosome (a smaller than normal chromosome 22) in the malignant bone marrow cells and their products (but not in other tissues). It is actually a reciprocal translocation between chromosome 9 and 22 (Fig. 2.37). As a result of this translocation the *ABL* proto-oncogene is translocated from its normal site in 9q34 to chromosome 22q11 where it rearranges with a specific sequence called the breakpoint cluster region. The hybrid gene produces a novel protein in the leukaemic cells which is probably responsible for the neoplastic transformation. Another important example is found in Burkitt's lymphoma (p. 670). This is a B-cell malignancy characterized by specific chromosomal translocations involving 8q24 and either 14q32, 2p11 or 22q11. A proto-oncogene, *MYC*, which is normally located at 8q24 is transferred to 14q32 in the majority of cases and it appears that the *MYC* gene is activated by enhancers of the heavy chain immunoglobulin gene located in 14q32. In the other translocations it has been shown that parts of the light chain genes (kappa at 2p11 and lambda at 22q11) have been transferred to activate the *MYC* locus on 8q24.

Additional chromosomal changes occur frequently during the evolution of a cancer, increasing its malignancy and allowing it to spread locally and metastasize. These changes are often associated with amplification of proto-oncogenes or with the involvement of new proto-oncogenes. The number of copies of a particular proto-oncogene can be increased by the generation of multiple repeats, often in the form of extended, homogeneously stained chromosomal segments or in a series of tiny fragments termed double minutes.

Tumours arising from activation of proto-oncogenes are usually sporadic in contrast to conditions arising from loss of a pair of tumour suppressors which may have familial (autosomal dominant) counterparts. Tumour suppressor genes and proto-oncogenes have important functions for normal growth and development of cells and this is considered in more detail in Chapter 10.

Further Reading

Buyse, M. (ed.) (1990). *Birth Defects Encyclopedia.* Alan R. Liss, New York.

Connor, J. M. and Ferguson-Smith, M. A. (1991). *Essential Medical Genetics*, 3rd edn. Blackwell Scientific Publications Ltd, Oxford.

Davies, K. E. (1986). *Human Genetic Diseases: a Practical Approach.* IRL Press, Oxford.

Emery, A. E. H. (1984). *An Introduction to Recombinant DNA.* John Wiley and Sons, Chichester.

Emery, A. E. H. and Rimoin, D. L. (1990). *The Principles and Practice of Medical Genetics*, 2nd ed. Churchill Livingstone, Edinburgh.

McKusick, V. A. (1990). *Mendelian Inheritance in Man. Catalogs of Autosomal Dominant, Autosomal Recessive and X-linked Phenotypes*, 9th edn. John Hopkins University Press, Baltimore and London.

Schinzel, A. (1984). *Catalogue of Unbalanced Chromosomal Aberrations in Man.* de Gruyter, Berlin.

Weatherall, D. J. (1988). *The New Genetics and Clinical Medicine*, 2nd Edn. Oxford University Press, Oxford.

3

Disturbances of Body Fluids, Haemostasis and the Flow of Blood

The body fluids are divided into intracellular and extracellular compartments. Every cell is bathed in extracellular fluid from which it derives oxygen, nutrients, trace elements and hormones which regulate its activities, and into which the cell discharges its metabolic waste products. The extracellular fluid is divided into intravascular and interstitial fluids. The constituents of the interstitial fluid are constantly replenished by the blood flow. In this chapter we discuss how the balance between intracellular and extracellular fluid compartments is maintained and how it may be upset by disorders of blood flow. We outline the processes involved in maintaining the fluidity of the blood and the integrity of the vascular tree, and we consider how alterations in blood flow affect single cells, tissues and the whole organism.

Disturbances of Water and Electrolyte Balance

The water content of normal males is about 60% of total body weight and, because of their higher fat content, that of females is about 50%. In newborn infants, water comprises up to 70% of body weight. Body water is distributed between three compartments (Table 3.1). Thus, in a 70 kg man with a total body water of 42 litres, 30 litres would be intracellular and 12 litres extracellular; the latter is subdivided into about 3 litres of intravascular fluid, the plasma, and 9 litres of interstitial fluid. Although there is a constant exchange of water and small molecules between compartments, in health the volume and solute concentration of each compartment remain fairly constant. The volume of each compartment depends upon the osmolarity in each compartment and the oncotic pressure (colloid osmotic pressure) which affect the passive transfer of fluid between them.

Osmolality. The osmotic pressure created by a solution is proportional to the number of particles of solute that are present: it is not related to the sizes of the particles. This property is the osmolality of the solution and is expressed as mmol/kg. It is important to note that the number of particles that contribute to the osmolality is the sum of all the cations and anions present.

Table 3.1 Body content of water, sodium and potassium

	Water content (litres)	Sodium content (mmol)	Potassium content (mmol)
Extracellular fluid	12	2100	48
Plasma	3	525	12
Extravascular	9	1575	36
Intracellular	30	420	3300
Total	42	2520	3348

Note that an additional 1680 mmol of sodium are included in bone and collagen.

Oncotic pressure describes the pressure exerted by proteins across cell membranes. The extent of the oncotic pressure is small by comparison with the osmotic pressure and becomes of physiological importance in the capillary bed which is permeable to those particles (cations and anions) that exert osmotic pressure.

While the transfer of water between the compartments of the body is passive, the distribution of sodium and potassium between the intracellular and extracellular compartments depends on active transport mediated by cell membrane ATPases.

The concentration values of solutes are expressed as ratios between the amount of solute and the volume of solvent: in biological systems this is water. The concentration of a solute may fall either because the amount of the solute has fallen without a change in the volume of the solvent or the volume of solvent has risen without a change in the amount of solute. This has important practical repercussions when interpreting the results of measurements of solute concentrations in the body compartments: a reduced sodium concentration in plasma may mean that the plasma volume is expanded or the amount of sodium is low.

The External Balance of Water and Sodium

The total amount of body water remains constant because intake and loss are balanced. Intake is controlled by thirst. When water is lost the osmolality of the extracellular fluid, interstitial and intravascular, increases and stimulates osmoreceptors in the hypothalamus. The hypothalamic receptors control the osmolality of the blood within narrow limits. Urinary loss of water is regulated by arginine vasopressin (AVP, formerly called antidiuretic hormone). Arginine vasopressin is secreted by neurons in the hypothalamus, and stored in the posterior lobe of the pituitary gland where it is released into the blood. It acts on the renal collecting ducts and increases reabsorption of water. A fall in blood osmolality results in inhibition of AVP secretion and reduces water reabsorption by the distal nephron. Sodium loss is controlled by the glomerular filtration rate, the renin–angiotensin–aldosterone system, the adrenergic nervous system and atrial natriuretic peptides.

The renin–angiotensin–aldosterone system. Renin is a proteolytic enzyme secreted by myoepithelioid cells of the juxtaglomerular apparatus of the kidney. It is secreted in response to a fall in renal afferent arteriolar perfusion pressure, a fall in Na^+ concentration in the distal tubule or stimulation of the sympathetic nervous system. The juxtaglomerular apparatus consists of the renin-secreting cells of the afferent and efferent arterioles, the extraglomerular mesangium and the macula densa (Fig. 3.1). The macula densa is an aggregate of specialized tubular epithelial cells lining the part of the distal convoluted tubule adjacent to the glomerular arterioles. It is a sensor which controls the release of renin in response to the Na^+ concentration of the tubular fluid of each individual nephron. Renin cleaves angiotensin I from angiotensinogen, an α_2-globulin present in plasma and tissue fluids. Angiotensin I is inactive but is converted, mainly in the pulmonary circulation, to the octapeptide angiotensin II by angiotensin converting enzyme (ACE). Angiotensin II stimulates aldosterone secretion via receptors on the zona glomerulosa cells of the adrenal gland and has a potent pressor effect by producing peripheral vasoconstriction mediated by its receptors on vascular smooth muscle cells. Angiotensin II is degraded by aminopeptidases with the formation of small amounts of angiotensin III which also stimulates the release of aldosterone from the adrenal cortex.

Aldosterone stimulates reabsorption of sodium (and therefore water) by the distal renal tubules and, because it increases blood volume, may have a pressor effect. The increase in aldosterone secretion in response to a rise in renin is termed secondary hyperaldosteronism and is to be distinguished from primary hyperaldosteronism, in which an adrenal adenoma secretes excess aldosterone (p. 1100).

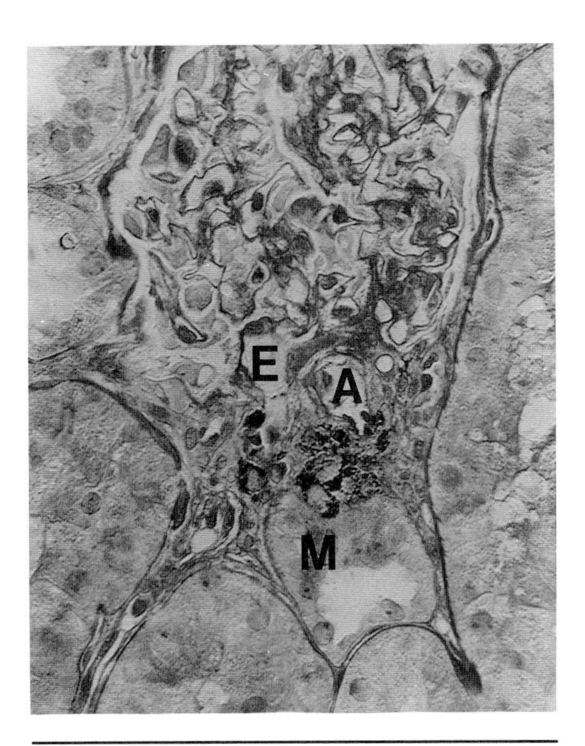

Fig. 3.1 The human juxtaglomerular apparatus showing the close anatomical relationship between the afferent arteriole (A), the efferent arteriole (E) and the macula densa (M). The transverse section through the distal tubule shows the columnar cells of the macula densa. The renin-containing myoepithelioid cells are identified by intracellular black staining granular immunoreactive renin. The section has been stained with a renin antiserum and a peroxidase antiperoxidase technique. ×252.

Atrial natriuretic peptide (ANP). Atrial distension due to expansion of intravascular volume releases ANP from atrial myocytes (Fig. 3.2) in which it is stored as a 126 amino-acid propeptide and from which it is secreted as an active 28 amino-acid peptide, ANP99–126. Atrial natriuretic peptide binds to receptors on vascular smooth muscle,

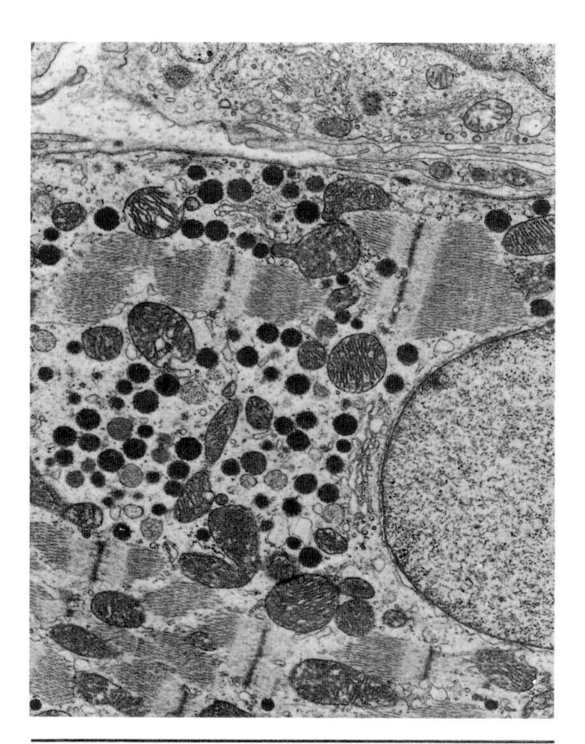

Fig. 3.2 An electron micrograph showing an atrial myocyte with a prominent Golgi apparatus and abundant endocrine granules which contain stored atrial natriuretic peptide.

the renal tubules, adrenal cortex and the brain; these receptors use cyclic GMP as a second messenger system. It causes vasodilatation, natriuresis and diuresis, inhibition of aldosterone secretion and suppression of AVP and renin release. Raised ANP levels occur in pregnancy, in chronic renal failure, congestive heart failure and in some patients with hypertension. Atrial natriuretic peptide is also synthesized in small amounts by ventricular myocytes and in the hypothalamic cardiovascular regulatory centres but its functional significance in these sites is uncertain.

Disturbances of water and sodium homeostasis. Because the intracellular and extracellular compartments are in osmotic equilibrium, changes in body water are distributed rapidly throughout the body's fluid compartments. However, in patients who lose or gain isotonic fluid, the principal changes occur in the extracellular compartment as there is little or no transfer of fluid between this compartment and the intracellular one. Thus, loss of isotonic fluid presents a more serious problem than loss of water, and requires urgent replacement.

The principal causes of water and sodium depletion and excess are set out in Table 3.2. Although some of these conditions may be associated with low plasma sodium concentrations this is not always the case. In some patients with acute loss of isotonic fluid, plasma sodium concentrations are normal, yet the patient may be severely hypovolaemic or even in shock. In patients with sodium and water retention, the plasma sodium may be normal, increased or even decreased.

The Internal Balance of Water and Sodium: Oedema

The capillary endothelium acts as a semipermeable membrane and is highly permeable to water and to almost all solutes in plasma with the exception of proteins. The passage of water across the walls of small blood vessels is determined by the balance between the hydrostatic and oncotic pressures. Normally, fluid is expelled from the arterial end of the microcirculation and re-enters at the venous end (see Fig. 4.3). An increase in the hydrostatic pressure or a fall in the plasma oncotic pressure will increase the net flow of fluid into the interstitial space. Fluid is constantly removed from the interstitial space by the lymphatics and accumulates to cause oedema only when the increase in flow cannot be accommodated by the lymphatic drainage. Thus, oedema may be caused by increased hydrostatic pressure, decreased plasma oncotic pressure or lymphatic obstruction.

Oedema may be localized or generalized. In generalized oedema, fluid may also accumulate in the serous cavities. In the peritoneal cavity this is called **ascites**, in the pleural cavity, hydrothorax or **pleural effusion** and in the pericardial sac, hydropericardium or **pericardial effusion**.

Table 3.2 Depletion and excess of water and sodium

Water	Sodium
Depletion	
Inadequate intake	Inadequate intake
Abnormal losses	Abnormal losses
Skin: sweating, fever	Skin: sweating, fever, burns
Kidneys: diabetes insipidus	Kidneys: osmotic diuresis
nephrogenic diabetes insipidus	diuretics
	mineralocorticoid deficiency (Addison's disease)
	Intestine: vomiting, diarrhoea, fistula
Excess	
Excessive intake	Excessive intake
Oral: polydypsia	Oral: sea water, salt tablets
Parenteral: hypotonic fluid	Parenteral: hypotonic sodium-containing fluids
Reduced loss	Reduced loss
Kidneys: overproduction of arginine vasopression (in syndromes of inappropriate secretion)	Kidneys: acute renal failure, secondary aldosteronism, Cushing's syndrome

When the oedema fluid has a low protein content, as in heart failure or the nephrotic syndrome (p. 894), it is called a **transudate**, in contrast to the protein-rich **exudate** which occurs in inflammation (p. 115).

Local Oedema

In acute inflammation arteriolar vasodilatation increases hydrostatic pressure in the microcirculation. Vascular permeability is also increased by chemical mediators or endothelial damage and contributes to the exudation of protein-rich fluid into the interstitial space. This is discussed in detail in the following chapter. Cerebral oedema which causes increased intracranial pressure (p. 811) and pulmonary oedema (p. 539), both of which may be fatal, are the most important clinical examples of local oedema.

Pulmonary oedema. The osmotic pressure of the plasma (25 mmHg; 3.32 kPa) is greater than the normal hydrostatic pressure in the pulmonary capillaries (8–10 mmHg; 1.06–1.33 kPa). Consequently, a considerable rise in the hydrostatic pressure is required to produce pulmonary oedema. Depending on the causal factors, pulmonary oedema may first be confined to the interstitium – 'interstitial oedema'; this gives rise to a characteristic radiological appearance. The fluid then escapes into the alveoli.

Hydrostatic pressure in the pulmonary microcirculation rises when the venous pressure is increased acutely, e.g. in left ventricular failure. Acute inflammation increases both hydrostatic pressure and vascular permeability and inflammatory oedema is pronounced in influenza and lobar pneumonia. Pulmonary oedema may also be part of generalized oedema, e.g. in renal disease, in overloading of the circulation by rapid transfusion of blood or fluids; pulmonary oedema is a complication of raised intracranial pressure by mechanisms which are not clear. In mitral valve stenosis (p. 506), chronic pulmonary venous congestion does not normally produce pulmonary oedema, probably because the pulmonary capillary bed is protected by increased tone of the pulmonary arterioles. However, pulmonary oedema may develop when physical exertion produces increased blood flow.

Oedema due to local venous congestion. A common example is the temporary oedema of the feet and ankles which develops on sitting for a long time. Leg movements help to pump venous blood to the heart and reduction in this function causes raised venous hydrostatic pressure. The commonest pathological cause of venous obstruction with oedema is deep venous thrombosis of the leg veins.

Oedema due to chronic lymphatic obstruction. Although the microcirculation acts as a semipermeable membrane, small amounts of protein normally escape into the interstitial fluid to be drained by the lymphatic system and returned to the plasma via the thoracic duct. Chronic lymphatic obstruction causes an accumulation of protein-containing fluid in the interstitium. For reasons which are not known, this causes growth of connective tissue. The swollen tissue becomes firm and does not 'pit' on pressure. Oedema from lymphatic obstruction is sometimes seen in the chest wall in breast cancer and is caused by permeation of the lymphatics by the cancer cells. Extended surgery for breast cancer which includes removal of the axillary lymph nodes and connective tissue, sometimes causes persistent and severe oedema of the whole of the arm and hand as a result of lymphatic obstruction. Fibrosis due to radiotherapy may contribute to this.

Lymphatic obstruction also occurs when the lymphatics or lymph nodes are chronically inflamed, for example in lymphogranuloma venereum (p. 331) and in filariasis (p. 1183).

Generalized Oedema

Generalized oedema is due to water and electrolyte (mainly sodium) retention but does not become apparent clinically until the accumulated fluid exceeds 5 litres. The principal mechanisms which lead to the formation of generalized oedema are as follows.

Hydrostatic factors. In cardiac failure interference with venous return to the heart results in increased hydrostatic pressure at the venular end of the microcirculation. Oedema develops because less fluid re-enters the capillaries. Reduced cardiac output and arterial blood flow stimulate AVP and renin secretion, secondary aldosteronism often develops and sodium and water retention occur. However, secondary aldosteronism is present in only 50% of patients with cardiac failure and a poorly understood form of renal sodium retention is present in the others.

Hypoproteinaemia. Albumin is principally responsible for plasma oncotic pressure. Oedema tends to occur when the serum albumin level falls below 25 g/l. Hypoalbuminaemia may be due either to loss of albumin as occurs in the urine in the nephrotic syndrome and other renal diseases (p. 894) and into the gut in protein losing enteropathies (p. 721), or to insufficient production in liver failure (p. 773) and malnutrition.

Nutritional (Famine) Oedema

Generalized oedema occurs in severe malnutrition, notably in **kwashiorkor** (p. 342). A combination of low plasma protein, a poorly understood increase in vascular permeability and the effects of deficiencies of vitamins and other essential dietary components are responsible.

Disturbances of Potassium Metabolism

The body contains about 3400 mmol of potassium of which only 60 mmol (about 2%) are extracellular. The external balance of potassium depends principally on dietary intake and renal excretion: only in severe diarrhoea does faecal loss become a significant route for potassium loss. The kidneys respond to variations in dietary intake of potassium by modifying secretion of potassium by the distal tubule. This is regulated by aldosterone and by the rate of sodium delivery to the distal tubules but there is also a passive component.

The internal balance of potassium depends on

Table 3.3 Principal causes of hypokalaemia and hyperkalaemia

Hypokalaemia	Hyperkalaemia
Excess renal loss	Excessive intake
Mineralocorticoid excess	Reduced renal loss
Diuresis: diuretics and osmotic diuresis	Fall in glomerular filtration rate:
Metabolic alkalosis	acute and chronic renal failure
Liquorice ingestion	Reduced tubular secretion:
Drug-induced	Addison's disease
Renal tubular acidosis	Shifts between extracellular and intracellular spaces
Gastrointestinal loss	Acidosis
Vomiting	Cell damage: haemolysis, trauma, burns, tumour cell necrosis
Diarrhoeal or stomal fluid loss	Hyperkalaemic periodic paralysis
K^+-secreting villous adenomas	Digoxin overdose
Shifts between extracellular and intracellular spaces	Diabetic hyperkalaemia
Acute alkalosis	
Insulin therapy	
Hypokalaemic periodic paralysis	

active and passive exchange between the intracellular and extracellular compartments. The cell membrane Na^+/K^+-ATPase actively transfers potassium into cells while sodium is pumped out, an activity which is stimulated by insulin. Passive transfer of potassium is affected by the pH of the extracellular fluid, acidosis promotes cellular potassium loss and alkalosis cellular potassium uptake. The principal causes of disturbed potassium metabolism are summarized in Table 3.3.

Hypokalaemia

Inadequate potassium intake may cause potassium depletion because the compensatory reduction in urinary potassium excretion in the distal tubule develops slowly. Mineralocorticoids, including aldosterone, increase the permeability of the tubular cells to potassium, causing increased loss in the urine. Diuretics which increase sodium loss into the tubular lumen at a site proximal to the distal tubule stimulate potassium loss by increasing the electrochemical gradient favouring the passive transfer of potassium into the tubular lumen. In chronic metabolic alkalosis and distal renal tubular acidosis, secondary aldosteronism contributes to the potassium losses, while in proximal renal tubular acidosis, bicarbonate loss results in increased luminal electronegativity and potassium loss.

Gastrointestinal loss is most often due to loss in diarrhoeal fluid. The most striking examples are in the 'secretory diarrhoea' in cholera (p. 707) and in response to vasoactive intestinal polypeptide (VIP) from pancreatic islet cell tumours. Rarely, potassium loss may be caused by large potassium secreting villous tumours of the colon which secrete potassium-rich mucus (p. 732).

Hypokalaemia can develop as a complication of insulin therapy in diabetic coma; insulin stimulates cellular uptake of potassium. In the rare condition of familial hypokalaemic periodic paralysis, episodes of hypokalaemia are associated with the ingestion of high carbohydrate meals. The cause of the excessive insulin-induced potassium shift in this syndrome are not known.

Clinical effects of potassium depletion. Concentrations of potassium of about 2.0 mmol/l may cause muscular weakness and, in more severe hypokalaemia, paralysis with respiratory failure develops. Hypokalaemia is accompanied by abnormalities in the electrocardiogram and cardiac arrhythmias may occur.

Hyperkalaemia

Excessive potassium intake is unusual but may be caused by miscalculated therapeutic intravenous injection or, rarely, by consumption of large volumes of fruit juice. Shifts of potassium from the intracellular to the extracellular space may cause acute increases in plasma potassium concentration but, in many cases, plasma levels do not reflect the total body potassium content.

Reduced renal excretion of potassium is a feature of both acute oliguric and chronic forms of renal failure. In chronic renal failure, however, significant hyperkalaemia only occurs when the glomerular filtration rate has fallen to very low levels and is usually associated with a metabolic acidosis. Hyperkalaemia occurs in acidosis and in extensive tissue destruction (e.g. soft tissue trauma, burns and haemolysis). Hyperkalaemia may develop in diabetic patients who have rapidly become hyperglycaemic. High plasma glucose levels increase extracellular fluid osmolality; this draws fluid into the extracellular space accompanied by passive diffusion of potassium. Lack of insulin and metabolic acidosis contribute to a failure of the return of potassium to the cells. In hyperkalaemic periodic paralysis, an autosomal dominant condition, sudden hyperkalaemia, often provoked by severe muscular exercise, results in muscle paralysis.

Clinical effects of hyperkalaemia. Hyperkalaemia lowers cell membrane potential and causes increased cardiac excitability. Very high potassium concentrations are life threatening and may lead to cardiac arrest. Intravenous glucose together with administration of insulin stimulates transfer of potassium into the intracellular compartment.

Haemostasis, Bleeding Disorders and Thrombosis

Blood is normally fluid within the vascular system but it rapidly forms a solid adherent plug at any site of vessel injury. In cases of minor endothelial cell injury the defect is quickly sealed by a platelet plug, but when injury is more severe the fluid blood is converted to a gel within the injured blood vessel by a process termed **thrombosis**. Solidification of the blood outwith the vascular system or within the vascular tree after death is usually referred to as clotting. A highly complex system of checks and controls prevents spontaneous haemorrhage on the one hand, and intravascular thrombosis on the other. This physiological balance is called **haemostasis**, and is the result of an interplay of four major components – the coagulation system, the fibrinolytic system, endothelial cells and platelets. This interplay of other components which balances the risk of thrombosis against the risk of haemorrhage has been termed the **thrombo-haemorrhagic balance**.

Coagulation

Blood coagulates as the result of activation of an enzyme cascade in which circulating inert precursors of procoagulant proteins are converted to their enzymatically active forms by a sequence of limited proteolytic reactions (Fig. 3.3). By convention, most coagulation factors are identified by Roman numerals. Confusingly, these numbers relate not to the order of activation but to the order in which the factors were discovered. Most factors

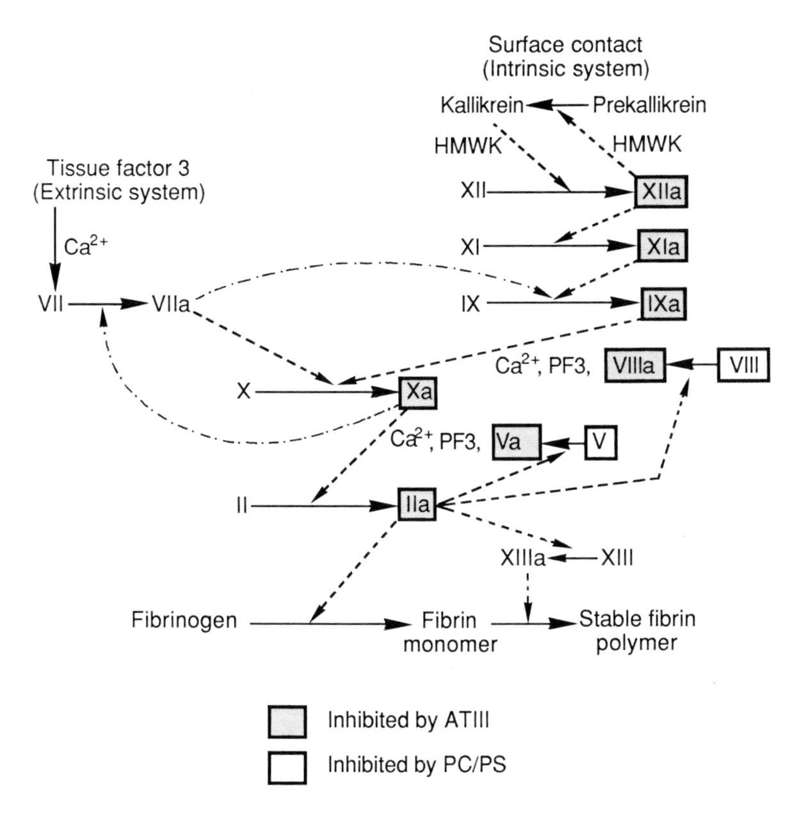

Fig. 3.3 Simplified coagulation cascade showing how conversion of inactive to activated (a) components by the intrinsic and extrinsic systems produces fibrin. The points at which the intrinsic and extrinsic systems interact (–.–.) and the points at which antithrombin III (ATIII) ▩ and protein C/protein S (PC/PS) □ regulate coagulation are also shown. Enzymatic activities are shown as arrows with interrupted lines (--->). HMWK – high molecular weight kininogen.

were also originally named but with the exceptions of Hageman factor (factor XII), tissue factor (factor III), fibrinogen (factor I), and prothrombin (factor II), their names are now used less frequently. They are listed in Table 3.4. Factors in their activated state are usually identified by the suffix 'a' e.g. factor Xa.

Table 3.4 Coagulation factors

I	Fibrinogen
II	Prothrombin
III	Tissue factor
IV	Calcium
V	Pro-accelerin, labile factor
VII	Proconvertin, serum prothrombin, conversion accelerator
VIII	Antihaemophilic factor
IX	Christmas factor
X	Stuart–Prower factor
XI	Plasma thromboplastin antecedent
XII	Hageman factor
XIII	Fibrin stabilizing factor

The end stage of blood coagulation is the conversion of fibrinogen into insoluble fibrin polymer; this is responsible for plasma changing from a sol into a gel. In the traditional view, coagulation is mediated by two pathways, the intrinsic and the extrinsic. The intrinsic pathway is triggered when blood comes into contact with any negatively charged non-endothelial surface. The extrinsic pathway is triggered by tissue factor which is released from damaged tissues; as shown in Fig. 3.3 this pathway bypasses the earlier stages of the intrinsic pathway, but both lead to the same final common pathway. This division between the intrinsic and extrinsic pathways is now considered to be artificial. There are interactions between the two pathways: both are necessary for normal haemostasis and deficiencies in one pathway cannot be totally compensated by the other.

Following endothelial injury the first step in the intrinsic pathway is the adsorption of the contact

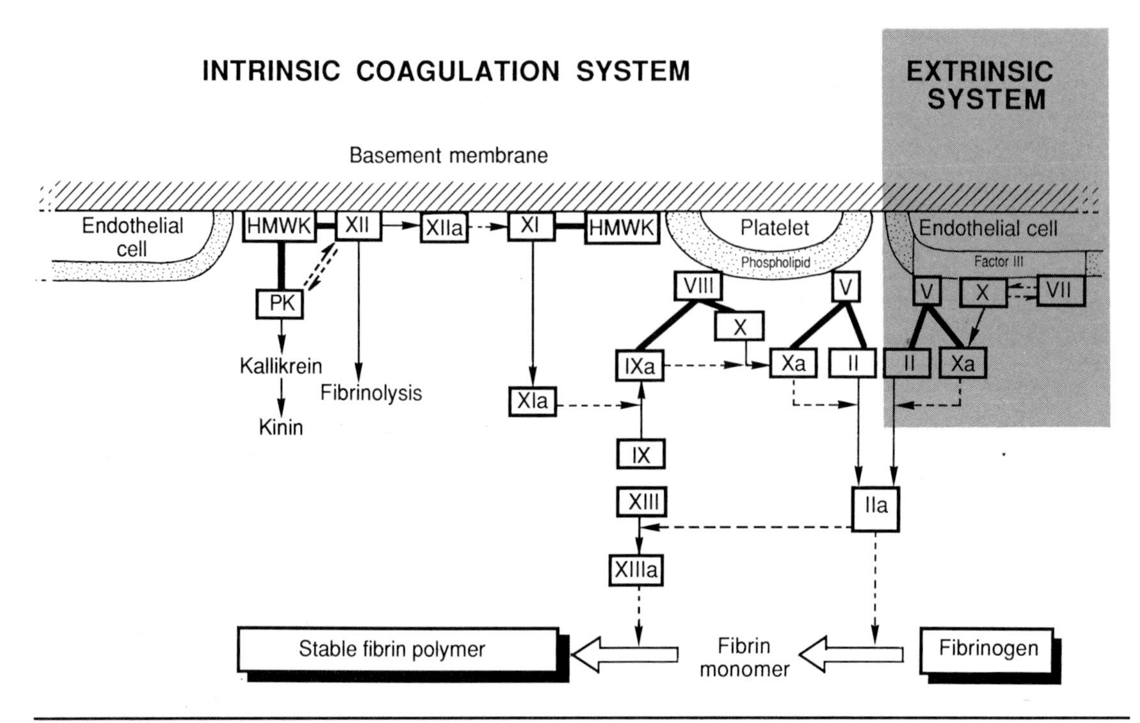

Fig. 3.4 The coagulation system. Damage to the endothelium exposes the basement membrane to which high molecular weight kininogen (HMWK) binds and contact activation of the intrinsic pathway occurs. The initial activation step is reciprocal activation between factor XII and prekallikrein (⇌). Surface activation continues as factors VIII and V become bound to the surface phospholipid of adherent platelets and bind factors IXa and X and Xa and II respectively. This produces thrombin (factor IIa) which converts fibrinogen to fibrin and activates factors XIII, VIII and V. The extrinsic system is activated simultaneously with the intrinsic system. Tissue factor III, present on the surface of damaged endothelial cells or in the subendothelial tissues, binds factors V, VII and X. Reciprocal activation (⇆) of factors VII and X occurs so that factors VIIa and Xa are formed. Factor Xa then binds to its cofactor, tissue factor-bound factor V, and proceeds to activate factor II (also bound to factor V) to form IIa-thrombin. Enzymatic activity is shown by interrupted lines.

factors, factor XII (Hageman factor), prekallikrein and high molecular weight kininogen (HMWK) (Fig. 3.4) on to the negatively charged subendothelial connective tissues such as collagen fibrils. Factor XII converts prekallikrein to the active enzyme kallikrein. Kallikrein is responsible for the activation of the kinin system (see Fig. 4.22) and also activates factor XII to the proteolytic enzyme, factor XIIa. Thus, a positive feedback loop is established (Fig. 3.4) so that after a lag-phase of several minutes significant amounts of factor XIIa are generated; which not only activates the next step in the coagulation cascade, but also activates the fibrinolytic system, which is responsible for the removal of thrombi. Thus, following contact activation, the coagulation, fibrinolytic and kinin systems are activated. Factor XI also binds to HMWK and is then converted to its active form, factor XIa, by factor XIIa. This initiates a series of amplification reactions including the conversion of factor X to factor Xa and eventually the conversion of factor II (prothrombin) to factor IIa (thrombin) which converts fibrinogen to fibrin (Fig. 3.3).

The extrinsic pathway is activated by tissue factor, an apoprotein–lipid complex which is present in cell walls. The initial step involves the binding of factor VII, factor X and calcium ions. Factor X becomes activated and then activates factor VII which then activates more factor X. Thus, a positive feedback loop in the activation of factors VII and X is established (Fig. 3.4). Once factor Xa is formed the formation of thrombin (factor II) and fibrin occurs as for the intrinsic pathway. Cross-pathway activation includes activation of factor VII by factor Xa and factor IX by factor VIIa.

The fibrinogen molecule consists of three pairs of disulphide-linked polypeptide chains. Thrombin cleaves small peptides from the N-termini of two pairs of the fibrinogen polypeptide chains to produce fibrin monomers which undergo rapid, spontaneous polymerization to form insoluble fibrin. These fibrin polymers are further strengthened by the action of factor XIIIa, a transamidase which cross-links adjacent molecules of polymerized fibrin. Factor XIII is converted to its active form by the action of thrombin. Thus thrombin has two major roles in coagulation, the conversion of fibrinogen to fibrin and the activation of factor XIII so that the fibrin cross-links can be stabilized. The stable fibrin polymer forms a scaffold for the cells involved in repair processes both in blood vessels and in the tissues.

Regulation of Coagulation

In addition to the positive feedback loops described above, amplification occurs at each stage of the coagulation process, because one molecule of enzyme can activate many molecules of substrate. Thus, in the absence of strict regulatory mechanisms the coagulation process, once activated, would continue until all the fibrinogen in the plasma was converted to fibrin. The two most widely investigated physiological inhibitors of coagulation are antithrombin III (ATIII) and the protein C/protein S system (Fig. 3.3). ATIII neutralizes thrombin and a number of other activated clotting factors (e.g. factor Xa, factor IXa, factor XIa and factor XIIa). Its speed of action is greatly enhanced by the presence of heparin and perhaps also by heparinoids produced by the vascular endothelium. Protein C and protein S are vitamin K dependent proteins synthesized in the liver, the latter also being synthesized by endothelial cells. Protein C is converted by thrombin to an activated form which, in conjunction with its cofactor protein S, inhibits factor Va and factor VIIIa. Patients who are congenitally deficient in any one of these inhibitors (ATIII, protein C or protein S) have a high incidence of thrombosis – usually venous and often recurrent. Other inhibitors of coagulation factors include C1-inhibitor (also an inhibitor of the classical pathway of complement activation), α_2-macroglobulin and α_1-antitrypsin.

Fibrinolysis

Thrombi must not only stem the leakage of blood from damaged vessels but must also be removed as healing takes place. Blood contains an enzymatic system which lyses thrombi and blood clots – the fibrinolytic system. This comprises an inactive proenzyme plasminogen which can be activated to the proteolytic enzyme plasmin by a number of plasminogen activators (Fig. 3.5). Although the main physiological substrate for plasmin is fibrin, plasmin also rapidly digests fibrinogen and coagulation factors V and VIII.

The fibrinolytic system is activated simultaneously with the intrinsic coagulation system by the contact system comprising factor XII, kallikrein and HMWK (Fig. 3.3). In addition there are two types of plasminogen activator which are

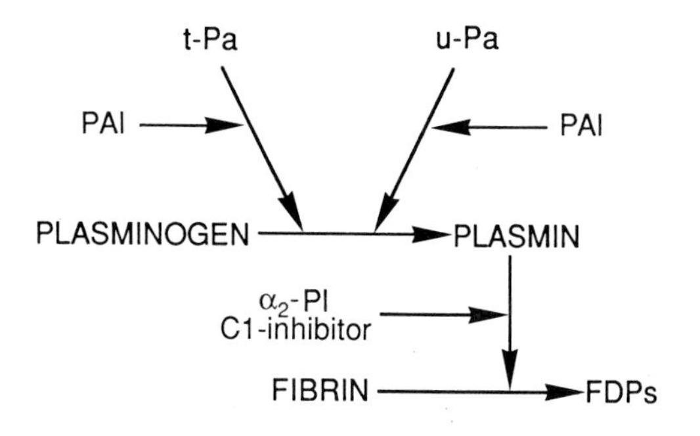

Fig. 3.5 Diagram of the fibrinolytic system showing activation of plasminogen by tissue plasminogen activator (t-Pa) and urinary plasminogen activator (u-PA). This converts plasminogen to the active enzyme plasmin which degrades fibrin to fibrin degradation products (FDPs). The system is regulated by inhibition of plasminogen activator inhibitors (PAIs) and by α_2-plasmin inhibitor (α_2-PI) and C1-inhibitor.

probably of greater importance *in vivo*. Tissue plasminogen activator (t-PA) is synthesized by endothelial cells and urokinase plasminogen activator (u-PA) is synthesized by a variety of cells including endothelial cells. When fibrin is formed, plasminogen and t-PA bind to it. Fibrin-bound t-PA converts fibrin-bound plasminogen to plasmin which in turn degrades fibrin. Thus normally, even as it is being formed, a thrombus contains within it the mechanism of its own destruction. This mechanism helps prevent extension of intravascular thrombi.

Urokinase plasminogen activator may also participate in the degradation of fibrin but its most important role is probably extravascular. Many cells (normal and malignant) have specific receptors for u-PA. Membrane-bound u-PA can convert plasminogen to plasmin and therefore provides cells with an efficient mechanism for extracellular matrix breakdown in, for example, tissue remodelling, following inflammation, tumour invasion and embryogenesis.

Regulation of Fibrinolysis

Fibrinolysis is controlled by two kinds of protease inhibitors in plasma – plasminogen activator inhibitors (PAIs) and inhibitors of plasmin, e.g. alpha-2 plasmin inhibitor (α_2-PI) and C1-inhibitor (Fig. 3.5). The main PAI in plasma is PAI-1. It is synthesized by endothelial cells and is also present in platelets. PAI-1 inhibits both t-PA and u-PA. Alpha-2-PI is the principal physiological inhibitor of plasmin. Its presence in plasma ensures that plasmin activity is confined to the site of fibrin formation.

Fibrinolytic activity prevents the development or spread of thrombi but overactivity would tend to make haemostatic plugs fragile. The fibrinolytic inhibitors, PAIs and α_2-PI ensure that premature lysis of thrombi does not occur before the vessel wall is repaired. Upset in this finely regulated balance between activation and inhibition of the fibrinolytic system would result, on the one hand, in an increased risk of haemorrhage and, on the other, in the development of thrombosis.

Digestion of fibrin by plasmin takes place in an orderly stepwise fashion and the fragments cleaved from fibrin polymers are released as fibrin degradation products (FDPs). Fibrin degradation products are cleared from the circulation by the mononuclear phagocyte system but this is a saturable mechanism and, if overwhelmed, FDPs may be detected in the blood and urine.

We have seen that there are control mechanisms at several stages of the coagulation and fibrinolytic systems. In addition, the fibrinolytic system is in dynamic equilibrium with the coagulation system, the two acting together to maintain an intact and patent vascular tree. Thus, the coagulation and fibrinolytic systems are both continuously active, the former augmenting platelet adhesion to endothelial defects by laying down fibrin where needed, and the latter preventing propagation of thrombus and removing fibrin deposits after they have served their haemostatic function.

Factors Involved in Coagulation and Fibrinolysis

Endothelial Cells

The endothelium has a key role in many pathological processes including inflammation, healing and repair (Chapter 4), in atherogenesis (p. 455), and in tumour growth and tumour spread (p. 384). Endothelial cells are heterogeneous (Figs 3.6 and 3.7) and synthesize and secrete numerous regulatory molecules (Table 3.5). Specialized endothelia are functionally important in the kidney, liver and other organs. Interactions between endothelial cells and soluble factors in the circulation are crucial to many metabolic processes. The role of the endothelium in regulating haemostasis is its most important physiological function.

Thrombi do not normally form in blood vessels

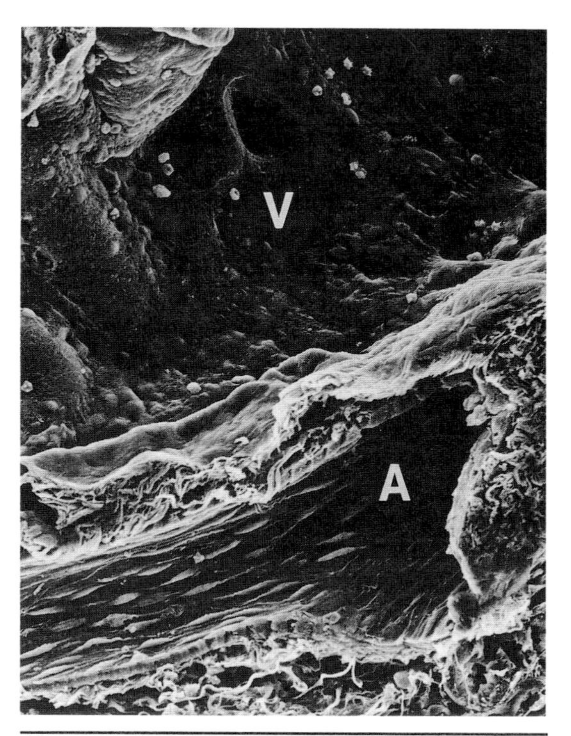

Fig. 3.6 A scanning electron micrograph showing an artery (A) and a vein (V). The arterial endothelial cells are aligned in the direction of blood flow due to the high shear stress. In contrast in the vein, where flow is slow, the endothelial cells adopt a cobblestone shape. These variations in endothelial morphology also reflect differences in function. ×1224.

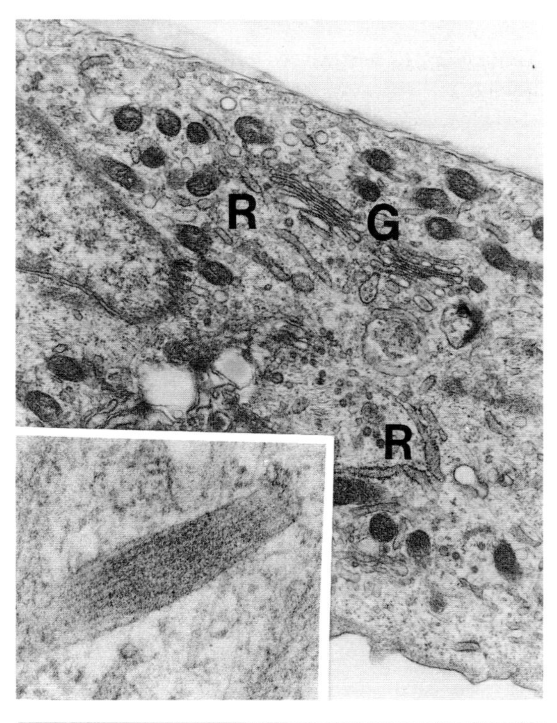

Fig. 3.7 A transmission electron micrograph of a cultured endothelial cell. The rough endoplasmic reticulum (R) is prominent and the Golgi apparatus (G) large. The insert shows a Weibel–Palade body. These contain the selectin GMP 140 (p. 16) and possibly other secretory products. ×11 160 and 28 080 (insert).

which have a healthy, undamaged endothelial lining. This is because the endothelial cell surface is antithrombotic and the endothelial cells prevent contact between the blood constituents and the prothrombotic vascular basement membrane. In addition, the endothelial cell secretes antithrombotic molecules (Table 3.5). Thrombomodulin is a glycoprotein which acts as the receptor for thrombin. When thrombin is bound to thrombomodulin it no longer converts fibrinogen to fibrin, factor V to Va or activates platelets, but instead acts as a specific activator of protein C.

Endothelial cells also exhibit prothrombotic activity: they synthesize von Willebrand factor, platelet activating factor (PAF) and fibronectin which mediate platelet adhesion and the coagulation factors V, VIII and III (tissue factor). These opposing functions of the endothelial cell contribute to the thrombohaemorrhagic balance (Fig. 3.8). Antithrombotic mechanisms predominate on the surface of normal endothelial cells and prothrombotic activity is minimal. However, damage to the endothelium leads to a shift in the thrombohaemorrhagic balance with increased prothrombotic activity and diminished antithrombotic mechanisms. Furthermore, endothelial cells retract in response to injury and expose the thrombogenic subendothelial connective tissues – collagen, elastin, fibronectin, thrombospondin, laminin and glycosaminoglycans. These, particularly collagen, promote platelet adhesion and activation and also provide a surface which initiates contact activation of the intrinsic coagulation pathway (Fig. 3.4).

Table 3.5 Endothelial cell products involved in haemostasis and blood flow

Product	Action
Regulation of coagulation	
Factor V Factor VIII Factor III (tissue factor) von Willebrand factor	Coagulation factors
Heparin-like molecules Thrombomodulin Protein S	Anticoagulation
Platelet activating factor Basement membrane collagens	Platelet activation
Prostacyclin ADPase EDRF (nitric oxide)	Platelet 'inhibition' (see text)
Tissue plasminogen activator (t-PA)	Promotes fibrinolysis
Plasminogen activator inhibitor (PAI)	Inhibits fibrinolysis
Regulation of blood flow	
Endothelin I* Angiotensin converting enzyme	Vasoconstriction
EDRF (nitric oxide) Prostacyclin	Vasodilatation

*The endothelins comprise a family of three peptides which have vasoconstrictor, bronchoconstrictor and growth promoting properties.

Platelets

Platelets circulate as discrete anucleate disc-shaped cells containing α granules, dense granules and lysosomes (Fig. 3.9). In addition to their role in coagulation they also are involved in acute inflammation (p. 139) and in atherogenesis (p. 453).

Platelets do not adhere to normal endothelium, but within seconds of endothelial cell damage, they adhere to exposed basement membrane (Fig. 3.10). Minor endothelial damage is sealed instantaneously by platelet adhesion, then this is followed by the growth of endothelium over the adherent platelets. More severe damage is associated with the formation of a larger platelet aggregate, the platelet plug, which may be sufficient to prevent bleeding. Three important sequential events occur during the formation of a platelet plug – adhesion, secretion and aggregation.

Platelet adhesion. Initial adhesion to endothelium is mediated by pseudopodia and depends on von Willebrand factor which connects platelet glycoprotein receptors (particularly GPIb) and collagen. Almost immediately, the platelets spread out and become more adherent. When damage is minimal this initial adhesion is followed by growth of endothelium over the adherent platelets. However, with more severe damage, the formation of a layer of adherent platelets is followed by the adhesion of more platelets so that layers of platelets are deposited on the initial layer, to form a platelet plug. The adhesion of platelets stimulates **platelet activation** which involves secretion and aggregation.

Platelet secretion. The platelet release reaction (p. 139) occurs soon after adhesion. Alpha granules contain fibrinogen, fibronectin, platelet derived growth factor (PDGF) and β-thrombomodulin. The dense granules contain Ca^{2+}, ADP, histamine and serotonin. Platelet factor 3 becomes activated and expressed on the platelet surface where it binds coagulation factors VIII and V which are cofactors in the activation of factors X and II respectively in the intrinsic coagulation pathway (Fig. 3.3). During platelet activation arachidonic acid metabolites, particularly thromboxane A_2 (TxA_2), are also formed.

Platelet aggregation occurs rapidly after adhesion and secretion. It is stimulated by TxA_2, ADP and thrombin. Initially, aggregation is reversible, but once the clotting system has been activated, thrombin combines with ADP and TxA_2 to induce platelet contraction and aggregation becomes irreversible. Fibrin polymer, formed by the action of

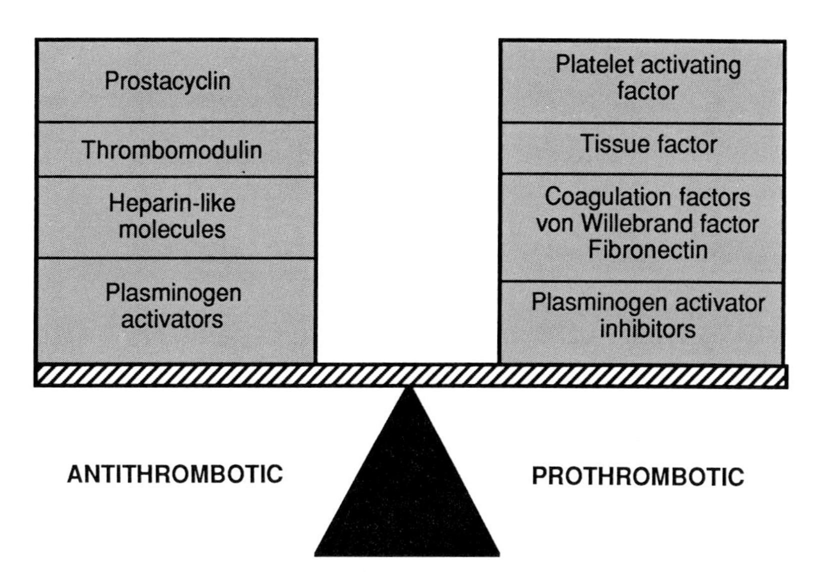

Fig. 3.8 The principal antithrombotic and prothrombotic products of endothelial cells. Multiple endothelial functions contribute to a dynamic balance which determines the local equilibrium between the tendencies for thrombosis and for haemorrhage.

thrombin on fibrinogen, binds to the original platelet plug and traps more platelets and erythrocytes, converting the platelet plug to a stable thrombus, tethered to its site of formation (Fig. 3.10).

Thromboxane and Prostacyclin Balance

Thromboxane (TxA_2) and prostacyclin (PGI_2) are metabolites of arachidonic acid (p. 140). Platelets synthesize TxA_2 while endothelial cells synthesize PGI_2 (Fig. 3.11). TxA_2 is a potent vasoconstrictor and platelet-aggregating agent, which is very unstable with a half-life of 30 seconds. PGI_2 has a half-life of approximately 2 minutes and is a powerful vasodilator and inhibitor of platelet aggregation. Small amounts of PGI_2 are produced continuously by normal endothelium but damage to the vessel wall results in increased production.

Endothelial damage has two apparently opposing effects: (1) exposure of subendothelial structures provokes platelet adhesion and aggregation which is limited by the increased endothelial production of endothelial derived relaxant factor (EDRF) and PGI_2 which act synergistically; (2) PGI_2 prevents platelet aggregation at a much lower concentration than is required to prevent platelet adhesion. Therefore, minor endothelial damage leads to platelet adhesion but not platelet aggregation.

Thus, there is a balance between the action of TxA_2 which stimulates platelet aggregation and PGI_2 and EDRF which inhibit platelet aggregation. Imbalance may lead to either thrombosis or haemorrhage.

Bleeding Disorders

***Haemorrhage** is the loss of blood from the circulation, usually due to trauma.* A tendency to spontaneous bleeding and to excessive bleeding in response to trauma is called a haemorrhagic diathesis. This may be due to quantitative or qualitative defects of platelets, a deficiency of one or more coagulation factors, or excessive fragility of blood vessel walls (Table 3.6). The bleeding disorders associated with excessive fragility of vessels are dealt with elsewhere as indicated in the table. Patients with bleeding tendencies often have haemorrhages in the skin and mucous membranes; tiny punctate haemorrhages are called **petechiae**, slightly larger ones **purpura** and the larger bruise-like haemorrhages are termed **ecchymoses**.

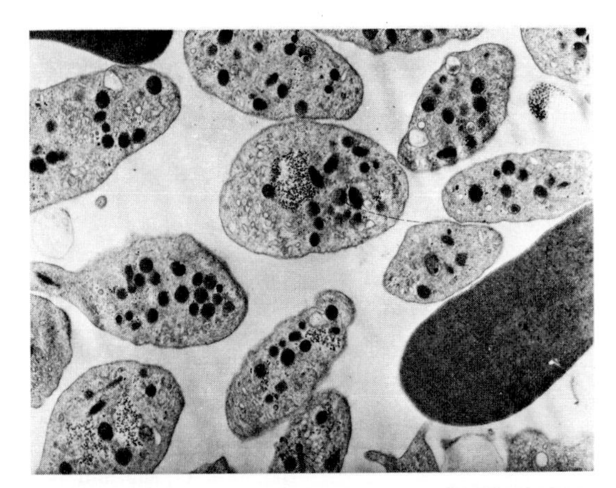

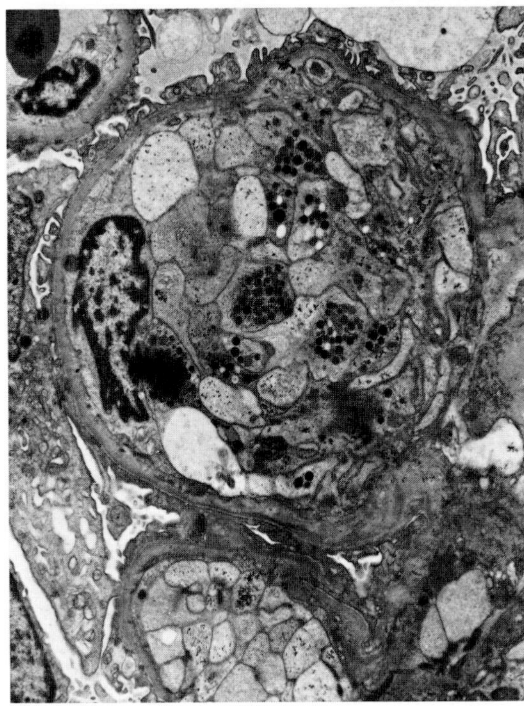

Fig. 3.9 Electron micrographs of platelets. Above, free platelets in suspension, showing the dense storage granules. ×8000. Below, two glomerular capillaries plugged by aggregated platelets, most of which have discharged their granules. ×3000.

Table 3.6 Bleeding disorders

Vascular fragility
- Inherited defect of capillary walls
  - Hereditary haemorrhagic telangiectasia
- Infections
  - Viral, e.g. measles
  - Rickettsial
  - Bacterial, e.g. meningococcal and other forms of septicaemia
- Inflammation
  - Henoch–Schönlein purpura
  - Hypersensitivity angiitis
- Lack of connective tissue support
  - Scurvy, Ehlers–Danlos syndrome, Cushing's syndrome/corticosteroid therapy

Platelet disorders
- Thrombocytopenia
  - Many causes (Chapter **00**)
  - Thrombotic thrombocytopenic purpura
- Impaired platelet adhesion
  - Bernard–Soulier syndrome
  - von Willebrand's disease
- Impaired platelet aggregation
  - Thrombasthenia
- Diminished platelet secretion
  - Storage pool deficiency
  - Cyclo-oxygenase deficiency
  - Thromboxane synthetase deficiency
  - Grey platelet syndrome

Deficiencies of coagulation factors
- Inherited
  - Factor VIII – haemophilia A
  - Factor IX – haemophilia B
  - von Willebrand's disease
  - Other deficiencies include factors, I, II, IV, V, VII, X, XI
- Acquired
  - Liver disease
  - Vitamin K antagonists, e.g. warfarin
  - Antibodies to coagulation factors, e.g. factor VIII, IX

Excessive intravascular coagulation
- Disseminated intravascular coagulation (consumptive coagulopathy)

Platelet Defects

Reduced platelet numbers, thrombocytopenia, is an important cause of spontaneous bleeding. In general the platelet count must fall to approximately 20 000/mm^3 for bleeding to occur. The causes of thrombocytopenia are discussed on p. 640. Inherited abnormalities of platelets which cause defective adhesion, aggregation or secretion are associated with excessive bleeding.

The Bernard–Soulier syndrome is an auto-

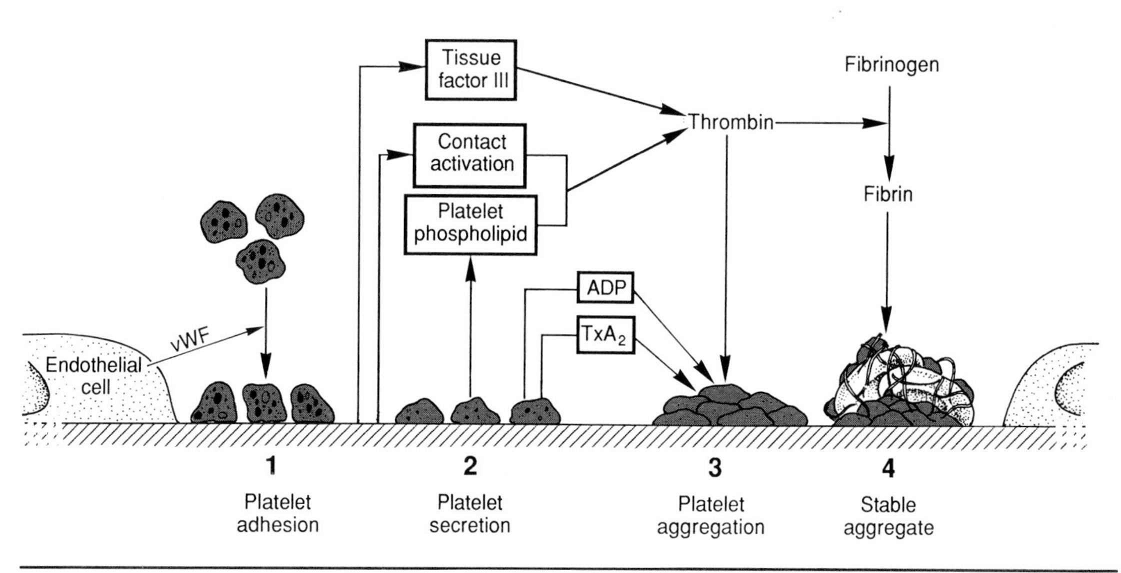

Fig. 3.10 Sequence of events in the formation of a platelet plug. (1) The damaged endothelium exposes basement membrane to which circulating platelets adhere in the presence of von Willebrand factor (vWF) released by the endothelial cell. (2) Following adhesion the platelets spread out and secrete their granule contents, and arachidonic acid metabolites are released. In terms of platelet aggregation, ADP and thromboxane A_2 (TxA_2) are important. While this is proceeding the coagulation system is activated by production of tissue factor and by contact activation so that prothrombin is converted to thrombin which then converts fibrinogen to fibrin. (3) Platelet aggregation is stimulated by ADP, TxA_2 and thrombin and facilitated by fibrinogen, as each fibrinogen molecule can bind to a number of platelets. (4) The platelet aggregate becomes more stable and tethered to the site of vascular injury by the formation of a stable fibrin network over the platelet aggregate. Passing blood cells are trapped in this network.

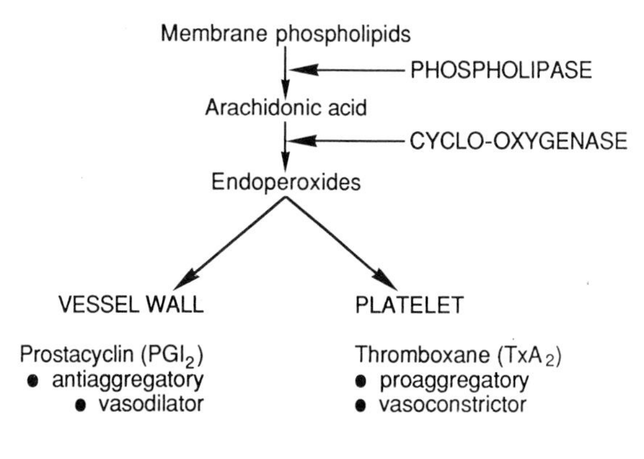

Fig. 3.11 The pathways of thromboxane and prostacyclin synthesis by the platelets and in the vessel wall.

somal recessive condition characterized by absence of the membrane glycoprotein Ib (GPIb), the platelet receptor for von Willebrand factor. These platelets cannot adhere to subendothelial collagen in the presence of normal amounts of functionally active von Willebrand factor.

In thrombasthenia, an autosomal recessive, there is a deficiency of two membrane glycoproteins GPIIb and GPIIIa which comprise the platelet receptor for fibrinogen and fibronectin and forms a second von Willebrand factor receptor. Thrombasthenic platelets will not aggregate, probably because they cannot be interconnected by fibrinogen or these other proteins. In addition to defective platelet aggregation patients with thrombasthenia show defective platelet spreading and clot retraction.

Defects of platelet secretion comprise a heterogenous group of disorders associated with a relatively mild bleeding tendency. Only in a proportion of cases is a hereditary component discernible. The disorders include primary defects of granule release associated with deficiency of the enzymes cyclo-oxygenase (p. 140) or thromboxane synthetase so that prostaglandins and thromboxane

A_2 cannot be synthesized, and deficiencies of the dense granules (storage pool disease) or α granules (grey platelet syndrome) are also described.

Acquired functional abnormalities leading to excessive bleeding are seen in uraemia and in 10% of patients taking aspirin; this drug inhibits the enzyme cyclo-oxygenase so that synthesis of prostaglandins and thromboxane is impaired.

In thrombotic thrombocytopenic purpura platelets adhere inappropriately to vascular endothelium. The patient becomes thrombocytopenic as platelets are 'consumed' in the platelet plugs which develop throughout the microcirculation. Patients present with renal failure and a combination of symptoms and signs of vascular occlusion and of bleeding and purpura due to the low platelet count.

Deficiencies of Coagulation Factors

These may be acquired or inherited. Acquired deficiencies usually affect multiple factors and may arise: (1) in liver disease (p. 745) – the liver is the major site of coagulation factor synthesis; (2) in vitamin K deficiency (p. 347), because factors II, VII, IX, X and proteins C and S require vitamin K for their synthesis; (3) in disseminated intravascular coagulation where excess consumption of factors occurs and (4) rarely, patients may develop acquired haemophilia, in particular haemophilia A or von Willebrand's disease, due to autoantibodies which interfere with the function of these clotting factors.

Inherited Disorders of Coagulation

Inherited deficiency of each of the coagulation factors has been documented. Most are autosomal recessive but classical haemophilia A (factor VIII deficiency) and haemophilia B (Christmas disease, factor XI deficiency) are X-linked.

Haemophilia A (classical haemophilia; factor VIII deficiency). This is the commonest hereditary bleeding disorder, affecting 1 in 10 000 UK males. Factor VIII is synthesized by the liver and circulates as a complex with von Willebrand factor. The factor VIII gene has been localized to chromosome Xq 2.8. A variety of deletions and point mutations in the factor VIII gene may be responsible for the deficiency. Identification of female carriers is achieved by analysis of common restriction fragment length polymorphisms within, or in linkage with, the factor VIII gene. Analysis of fetal DNA and measurement of factor VIII levels in fetal blood allow antenatal diagnosis.

The clinical severity of the disease usually parallels the severity of the factor VIII deficiency. This varies between families but tends to be similar within each kindred. Haemophilia is graded according to the factor VIII functional activity, and the diagnosis is made in patients with less than 30 units/dl. One unit of factor VIII is that amount which is present in 1 ml of fresh normal plasma. 'Severe' haemophiliacs have factor VIII levels of 0–1 u/dl, 'moderate' haemophiliacs levels of 2–5 u/dl and 'mild' haemophiliacs have levels over 5 u/dl. Mild haemophiliacs bleed excessively only after surgery, dental extraction or significant trauma.

Haemophilia B (factor IX deficiency or Christmas disease) is one fifth as common as haemophilia A. Factor IX is encoded by a gene located on the X chromosome (Xq 2.7) and is synthesized by the liver. The patterns of inheritance are the same as those of haemophilia A; the two forms can be distinguished only by the use of specific factor assays.

von Willebrand's disease. von Willebrand factor is a protein synthesized by endothelial cells as a monomer which polymerizes prior to secretion. After secretion it binds factor VIII and acts to promote platelet adhesion to collagen. Platelets have two receptors for von Willebrand factor: one is involved in adhesion of platelets to collagen while the other is involved in adhesion between platelets. It is usually described as being inherited as an autosomal dominant trait. In its most common form, the heterozygous form, the factor VIII activity and the von Willebrand factor activity are reduced either concordantly (type I von Willebrand's disease) or discordantly (type II von Willebrand's disease). These heterozygous forms of the disease are usually characterized by spontaneous mucous membrane bleeding, excessive bleeding from wounds and menorrhagia. In addition to these heterozygous forms of the disease, a type III von Willebrand's disease is recognized which probably represents a homozygous form of a 'recessive' type I von Willebrand's disease. In type III von Willebrand's disease all factor VIII and von Willebrand factor activities are very low and the patient presents with a severe bleeding disorder clinically similar to haemophilia. A condition rather similar to von Willebrand's disease, so-called pseudo-von Willebrand's disease, has been described. In this disorder it is believed that there is an abnormality in the platelets themselves which prevents normal adhesion to von Willebrand factor.

Clinical Features

Haemophilia A and B are virtually indistinguishable. Although the defects are present at birth, neonatal manifestations are uncommon; bleeding usually appears when the child begins to crawl. Characteristically, bleeding is episodic and may occur in joints (haemarthroses) or muscles; the former can be associated with considerable morbidity. Excessive external bleeding is much less common, and mucous membrane bleeding is unusual but intracranial bleeding is an important cause of death.

The use of plasma products, in particular factor VIII and factor IX concentrates, has been a major advance in the management of haemophilia. Antibodies to factor VIII and factor IX develop in some patients, inhibiting clotting activity and causing difficulties in the management of subsequent bleeding episodes.

Post-transfusion hepatitis largely due to hepatitis C virus (p. 754) is a potential complication of any blood product therapy, and the risk is heightened by the use of concentrates prepared from large plasma pools. A number of haemophiliacs have developed AIDS (acquired immune deficiency syndrome (p. 243)) as the result of infection with human immunodeficiency virus (HIV) in blood products given prior to the introduction of screening blood donors for HIV antibodies.

Disseminated Intravascular Coagulation

In disseminated intravascular coagulation (DIC) progressive activation of coagulation eventually results in failure of all components of haemostasis, hence, the other term for DIC is 'consumptive coagulopathy'. Disseminated intravascular coagulation may cause acute, sometimes lethal haemorrhage or a more chronic bleeding tendency.

Pathogenesis

Disseminated intravascular coagulation follows the massive or prolonged release of soluble tissue factors and/or endothelial derived thromboplastins into the circulation with generalized activation of the coagulation system. Tumours may release tissue factors as a result of necrosis or may produce thromboplastins. Endothelial damage not only causes the release of thromboplastins into the circulation, but synthesis of prostacyclin and protein S may be reduced and exposure of subendothelial collagen also activates the coagulation system. Massive activation of coagulation produces clumps of fibrin mesh throughout the circulation. The process consumes coagulation factors and also results in reduced levels of coagulation inhibitors (ATIII, PC) which are consumed by the activated clotting factors.

Thrombocytopenia is the result of aggregation of platelets by thrombin. These aggregates are either deposited in the damaged microcirculation or removed by the mononuclear phagocyte system.

Plasminogen activators are released from damaged endothelial cells, platelets or white cells and convert plasminogen to plasmin, which degrades fibrin so that fibrin degradation products (FDPs) appear in the blood. The extent to which fibrin is deposited in small vessels depends on the efficiency of this fibrinolytic response. However, activation of fibrinolysis is not entirely beneficial as plasmin digests fibrinogen, factor V and factor VIII, further reducing the levels of coagulation factors in the blood.

Clinical Features

Aetiology. DIC is never a primary event (Table 3.7). Approximately 50% of acute cases occur in obstetric practice (amniotic fluid embolism and placental abruption). Acute DIC frequently develops in severely hypoxic neonates. The other conditions most frequently associated with acute DIC are sepsis and shock in which the endothelium is damaged by hypoxia, acidosis or endotoxins. Acute DIC may complicate recovery from major surgery, severe trauma and fat embolism, severe burns or cardiac resuscitation. It is an inevitable accompaniment of the later stages of the various types of shock discussed later in this chapter. Acute pancreatitis (p. 793), acute intravascular haemolysis caused by an incompatible blood transfusion and venomous snake bites may also trigger acute DIC.

Chronic DIC may complicate some malignant tumours, particularly adenocarcinomas of the pancreas, lungs or stomach and acute myeloid leukaemia. Low-grade chronic DIC may also complicate a number of renal diseases and, in some of them, it may have a pathogenetic role (p. 930).

Table 3.7 Causes of acute and chronic disseminated intravascular coagulation

Acute	Chronic
Shock	Disseminated malignancy
Septicaemia	Carcinoma – pancreas, lung, stomach
Accidental trauma	Promyelocytic leukaemia
Burns	Liver disease
Acute intravascular haemolysis	Renal disease
Snake bites	
Acute pancreatitis	
Amniotic fluid embolism	
Placental abruption	
Septic abortion	
Neonatal respiratory distress syndrome	

Clinical effects. The risk of bleeding increases with the progressive consumption of platelets and clotting factors. Bleeding into the skin causes widespread petechiae and ecchymoses; the first sign may be excessive oozing of blood from venepuncture sites. Epistaxis, haematuria, and bleeding from the gums are also common. Massive gastrointestinal or pulmonary bleeding, or intracranial haemorrhage, both subdural and intracerebral, are common. Pulmonary bleeding causes breathlessness and tachypnoea and in these cases, chest radiographs show widespread pulmonary changes.

Thrombi may occlude small blood vessels anywhere in the body but the skin and the kidneys are particularly vulnerable. Ischaemic changes commonly affect the distal ends of fingers and toes and a spreading, haemorrhagic necrotic, gangrenous rash ('purpura fulminans') may develop. Peritubular and glomerular capillaries and the renal arterioles may all be occluded, causing or aggravating acute renal failure.

Thrombotic Disorders

Thrombosis *is defined as the formation of a solid or semi-solid mass from the constituents of the blood within the vascular system during life.* Coagulation is involved in the formation of all thrombi. Three major factors (Virchow's triad) predispose to thrombosis as follows.

Endothelial damage or altered endothelial function. Endothelial damage is the most important factor in thrombus formation. Good examples are the formation of thrombi on the endocardium overlying a myocardial infarction or on ulcerated atheromatous plaques in artery walls.

Slowing (stasis) and perturbation of blood flow. Slowing is important in the pathogenesis of venous thrombosis and of thrombus formation in the atria during atrial fibrillation and in aneurysms. Perturbation of blood flow is a factor in thrombosis. Increased blood viscosity as in polycythaemia (p. 633) causes stasis with thrombosis in small blood vessels. Stasis results in the loss of laminar blood flow and allows platelets to come into contact with, and adhere to the endothelium. Stasis also allows the local accumulation of activated coagulation factors. Turbulence causes reduction in endothelial PGI_2 and t-PA formation.

Changes in the composition of the blood favouring platelet aggregation and fibrin formation. Increased coagulability occurs after trauma, surgical operations, in late pregnancy and following delivery and in disseminated carcinomatosis. In many of these instances the platelet count is elevated and the platelets are more sticky; plasma levels of coagulation factors are increased while those of antithrombin III and protein C are reduced.

Increased coagulability complicates inherited deficiency of antithrombin III or protein C and urinary loss of antithrombin III in the nephrotic syndrome (p. 894). The development of autoantibodies to phospholipids (including anticardiolipin antibodies and the lupus anticoagulant) is increasingly recognized as an important cause of recurrent arterial and venous thrombosis. These antibodies occur in 10% of patients with systemic lupus erythematosus (p. 229) although they may also occur in isolation. Other factors associated with increased blood coagulability and therefore with thrombosis, include cigarette smoking, obesity, and the use of oestrogen-containing oral contraceptives.

Appearances and Composition of Thrombi

The composition of thrombus is determined by the rate of flow of the blood from which it forms. Thrombus forming in rapidly flowing blood, e.g. in an artery, consists mainly of aggregated platelets with some fibrin; it enlarges slowly and, because few red cells are entrapped, is firm and pale, varying from greyish white to pale red, and is commonly called pale thrombus. In contrast, thrombus forming in stagnant blood, e.g. adjacent to a complete occlusion of a blood vessel, resembles blood which has been allowed to clot *in vitro*: the thrombus is soft, dark red, gelatinous and consists of a meshwork of fibrin strands with entrapped red cells, leucocytes and platelets. Many thrombi comprise a mixture of pale and red areas, producing a laminated appearance (see Fig. 3.14).

Venous Thrombosis

Veins readily thrombose because blood flow is slow. Thrombosis of the leg or pelvic veins is the principal cause of pulmonary embolism an important cause of death. **Thrombosis of leg veins** usually starts in deep veins within the calf muscles (Fig. 3.12) from where it may extend progressively (propagate) to the posterior tibial, popliteal, femoral and iliac veins and occasionally extends to the inferior vena cava. Sometimes thrombosis may start more proximally than the calf, or separate thrombi may form in the calf and thigh veins. Propagation may be very rapid, especially when blood flow is slow, or alternatively, thrombosis may extend in stages (Fig. 3.13).

Deep venous thrombosis of the leg veins develops especially in immobilized patients and is particularly common after abdominal operations, severe injury, myocardial infarction, and in patients with cardiac failure. There is a higher incidence in middle-aged and elderly people. There is also an increased risk during the later stages of pregnancy and following childbirth. Thrombosis of

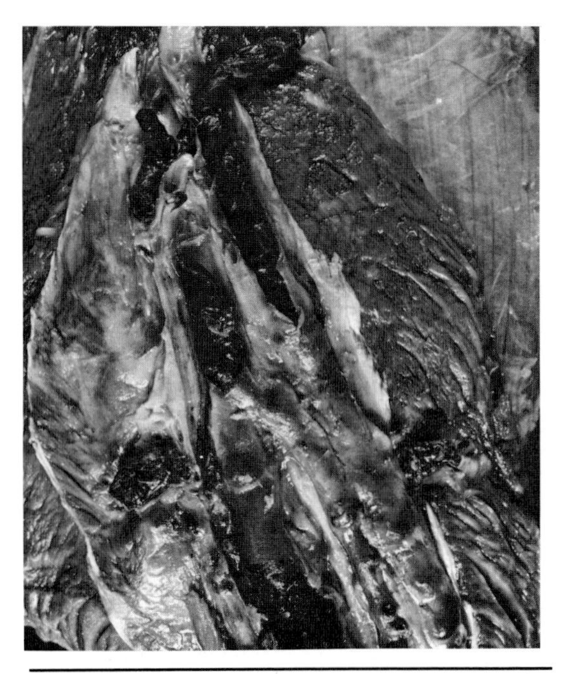

Fig. 3.12 Recently formed red thrombus in the deep veins in the muscles of the leg.

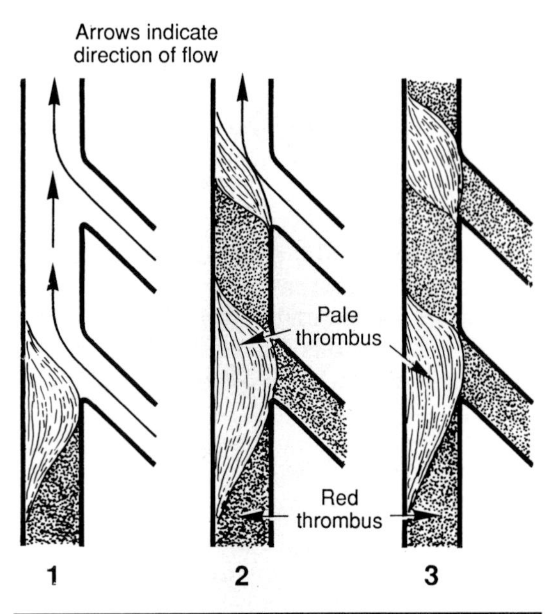

Fig. 3.13 Diagram of propagation of thrombus in a vein with tributaries. (1) The gradual build-up of thrombus composed mainly of fibrin and platelets eventually blocks the vessel. Coagulation of the stationary blood then forms red thrombus. (2) Slower deposition of thrombus from the flowing blood occurs at the junction of the next tributary. (3) The growing thrombus may then occlude this vessel with further formation of red thrombus.

pelvic veins is less common than leg-vein thrombosis. Thrombosis may form in the hypertrophied uterine veins after childbirth when the uterine blood flow diminishes considerably; extension to the internal and common iliac veins and pulmonary embolism may complicate pelvic vein thrombosis.

The coagulability of the blood increases immediately after trauma and during and for approximately 2 weeks following surgery. This explains why deep venous thrombosis often starts during or shortly after surgical operations and often extends rapidly to major veins during this period. Venous return from the lower part of the body is normally aided by the pumping action created by muscular movements of the legs and by use of the abdominal muscles and diaphragm in breathing. Inhibition of abdominal breathing and leg movements by postoperative pain are therefore contributory factors in venous thrombosis. Extensive deep venous thrombosis may cause tenderness of the calf muscles and oedema of the affected leg; however, in many patients the condition is undiagnosed.

The incidence of deep venous thrombosis and pulmonary embolism may be reduced by subcutaneous injection of small doses of heparin: in surgical patients this is most effective if started at the time of operation. Early mobilization of patients after operation, myocardial infarction and childbirth also reduces the risk.

Other predisposing factors for venous thrombosis include malnutrition, debilitating infections and wasting diseases such as cancer. In these instances it is sometimes called **marantic thrombosis** and in severely debilitated infants and young children it may affect the superior longitudinal sinus or renal veins. Venous thrombosis also tends to complicate haematological diseases, notably the myeloproliferative disorders (p. 633), in which there are excessive numbers of red cells, leucocytes and platelets. Inflammation of veins (phlebitis) also promotes thrombosis. **Migrating**

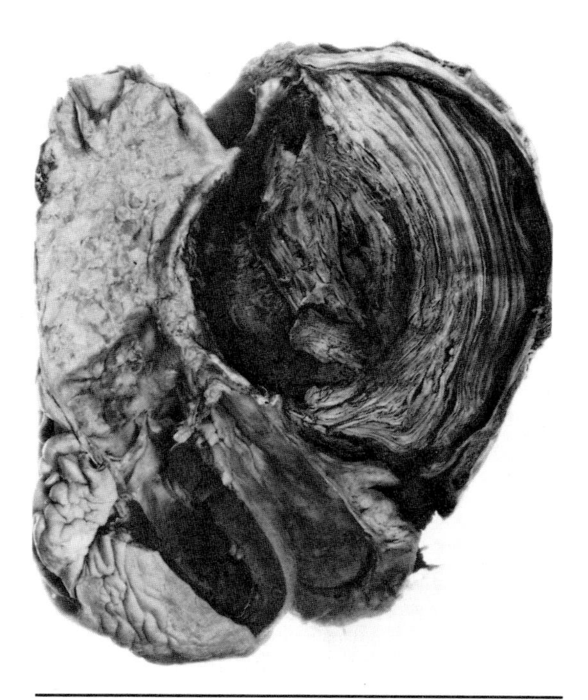

Fig. 3.14 A large aneurysm of the aortic arch; compare size of this with the heart (lower left). The aneurysmal sac has become largely filled by laminated thrombus.

thrombophlebitis, which affects various veins throughout the body, is usually of obscure aetiology, but is sometimes associated with cancer, particularly of the pancreas. In **septic venous thrombosis**, suppuration in the thrombus causes softening and fragments of infected thrombus may break away, giving rise to pyaemia (p. 296).

Arterial Thrombosis

The rapid flow of arterial blood prevents the occurrence of thrombosis unless the vessel wall is abnormal. In industrialized communities, atheroma is by far the commonest predisposing lesion. Atheromatous plaques produce turbulence and may also ulcerate; thrombi composed mainly of platelets and fibrin may then form on the ulcerated surface. These thrombi may narrow or occlude the lumen of arteries such as the coronary and cerebral arteries.

When there is localized dilatation (aneurysm) of the heart, aorta or other arteries, turbulence of the blood usually results in thrombosis. The thrombus may have a laminated appearance and may fill the aneurysmal sac (Fig. 3.14). Arterial thrombosis also complicates arteritis (p. 464) and in malignant arterial hypertension (p. 459) thrombosis follows necrosis of the walls of small arteries and arterioles.

Cardiac Thrombosis

Thrombi may form on the endocardium of the chambers and the valve cusps.

Atrial thrombosis is commonest in the auricular appendages (especially the right), and occurs most often in heart failure and in atrial fibrillation in mitral stenosis with atrial dilatation. In mitral stenosis (p. 506), the left atrium may become almost filled by thrombus. In the **ventricles** mural thrombus often forms on endocardium overlying an infarct – a patch of ischaemic necrosis of the heart wall (see Fig. 12.43).

Small platelet thrombi (vegetations) may form on the inflamed **heart valves** in acute rheumatic fever (see Fig. 12.58). In infective endocarditis, the cusps are colonized by micro-organisms and the vegetations are larger, softer and more friable and give rise to emboli (see Fig. 12.66). Thrombotic vegetations occur on normal endocardium, including the valves in chronic diseases associated with hypercoagulability (p. 514).

Capillary Thrombosis

Acute inflammation often causes thrombosis in capillaries and venules, due partly to endothelial damage and partly to haemoconcentration, the thrombi being composed mainly of packed red cells. In the Arthus reaction (p. 213) thrombosis of small vessels is also prominent. This is due to injury to the endothelium caused by release of toxic oxygen metabolites and enzymes by neutrophil polymorphs.

The Fate of Thrombi

Once formed, a thrombus may spread along the blood vessel by propagation (Fig. 3.13), or it may detach from the vessel wall to form an embolus. Thrombus is also removed and the processes involved are: (1) shrinkage of the thrombus by contraction of fibrin; (2) i.e. lysis by plasmin and the proteolytic enzymes of neutrophil polymorphs; (3) organization, involving digestion by macrophages and ingrowth of fibrovascular tissue; and (4) incorporation of thrombus into the vessel wall by growth of the endothelium over its surface – endothelialization. The relative importance of these processes depends on the type of thrombus and the site of its formation. Incorporation of arterial thrombus may contribute to the development and growth of atheromatous plaques; this is considered in detail on p. 453.

Occlusive venous thrombi are usually composed of red thrombus which contracts well. It may remain attached to the vessel wall, particularly at sites of endothelial damage with organization and ingrowth of granulation tissue. Retraction from the vessel walls or digestion by the local action of plasmin and possibly macrophages and neutrophil enzymes leads to the formation of small channels. Intimal endothelial cells proliferate and migrate to line these channels and also themselves create branching capillary channels which eventually join together. Thus a lumen may be restored – recanalization – leaving an eccentric thickened fibrovascular intimal plaque or a meshwork of fibrous strands marking the site of granulation tissue ingrowth with subsequent fibrosis. Occasionally, recanalization fails to occur. The thrombus is then replaced by granulation tissue which becomes increasingly collagenous, and the vein is eventually reduced to a solid, shrunken cord without a lumen. Dystrophic calcification of thrombi produces **phleboliths**, which are particularly common in pelvic veins.

Occlusive arterial thrombi are formed more slowly than venous thrombi and are pale, containing a higher proportion of platelets. Arterial endothelium is a relatively poor source of plasminogen activator and for these reasons the thrombus tends to remain attached to the arterial wall and its removal takes place mainly by organization. The newly formed capillaries anastomose and may develop into larger vessels extending through the length of the occlusion (Fig. 3.15). Unlike veins, however, recanalization seldom restores normal blood flow in arteries.

Mural thrombus. Granulation tissue grows in from the underlying heart wall and anchors the

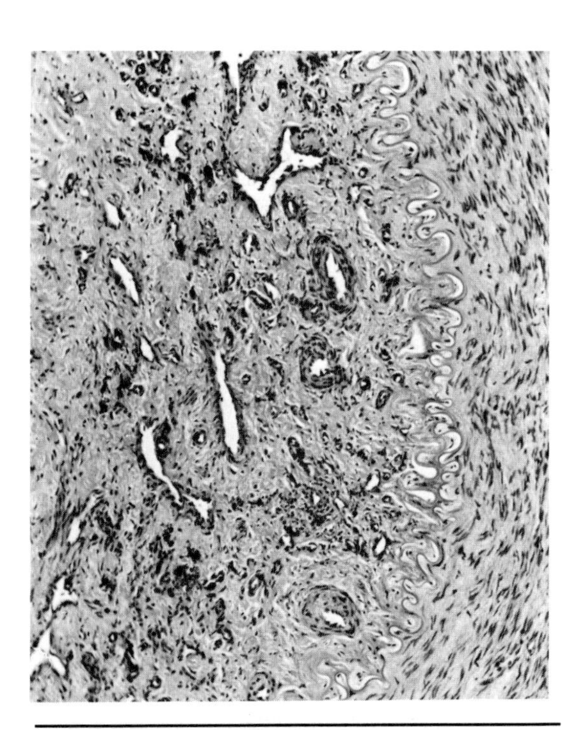

Fig. 3.15 Part of an artery showing the results of organization of thrombus. The lumen was originally to the left of the internal elastic lamina, which runs vertically near the right margin. The lumen is now filled with vascular fibrous tissue in which some of the new capillaries have enlarged and acquired muscle to become arterioles. ×115.

thrombus to the wall of the chamber. Large mural thrombi can persist for years without becoming fully organized, but because they become endothelialized, embolization occurs less frequently than would be expected.

Embolism

***Embolism** is the transference of abnormal material by the bloodstream with impaction in a vessel distant to the site of origin.* The impacted material is called an *embolus*. Clinically, by far the commonest embolus is a fragment of thrombus (thromboembolism). Platelet aggregates or fragments of material from ulcerating atheromatous plaques quite commonly form emboli in distal arteries. A fragment of tumour invading a vein may break off, producing an embolus; fat globules, bubbles of air or nitrogen, groups of parenchymal cells, amniotic fluid and infected foreign material are further examples of emboli. The site of impaction depends on the source of the embolus. Thus, emboli in the pulmonary arteries and their branches are derived from thrombus in the systemic veins or in the right side of the heart. Emboli in the systemic arteries are usually derived from thrombus formed in the left side of the heart and from thrombi or atheromatous debris from atheromatous plaques in the aorta or large arteries. Rarely, where there is a patent foramen ovale, an embolus may cross from the right to the left atrium and so to the systemic circulation – crossed or paradoxical embolism. Emboli originating in tributaries of the portal vein lodge in the liver.

Septic emboli are composed of thrombus infected with pyogenic bacteria. They may arise from septic thrombosis in a vein draining a suppurating infection or from the vegetation on heart valves in infective endocarditis (p. 511). At the site of impaction septic infarcts may progress to abscesses and rupture of the vessel may cause a so-called mycotic aneurysm.

Pulmonary Thromboembolism

The thrombi usually originate in the leg veins or, much less commonly, in the pelvic or other systemic veins or sometimes in the right side of the heart.

The effects of pulmonary embolism depend on the size of the embolus and on the state of the pulmonary circulation. A large thrombus, extending up to the femoral or iliac vein, may become detached *en masse* and block the outflow tract of the right ventricle, the main pulmonary trunk (Fig. 3.16) or both of its branches, causing sudden death by circulatory arrest. Less massive embolism, with occlusion of more than half the pulmonary arterial bed in previously healthy individuals, causes acute right ventricular failure by increasing

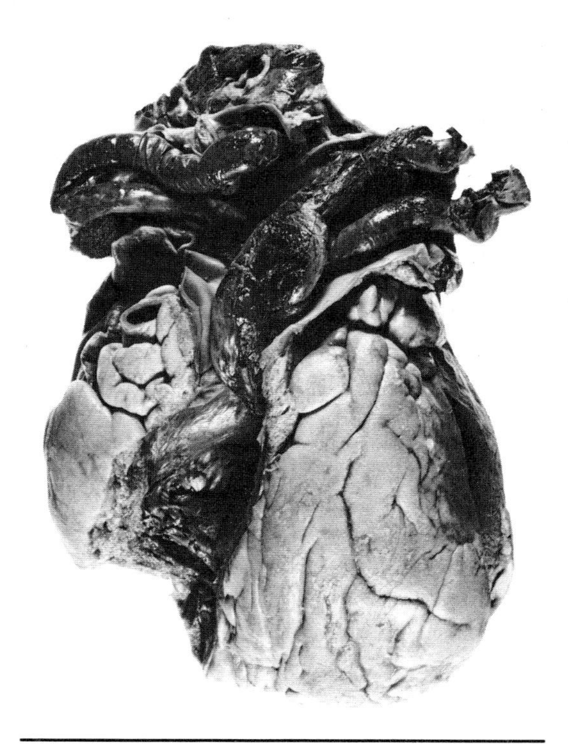

Fig. 3.16 Massive pulmonary embolism. Thrombus from the femoral vein has become detached and impacted in the pulmonary trunk and its right and left branches, causing sudden death.

the resistance to pulmonary blood flow. Lesser degrees of embolism may produce right ventricular failure in patients with pre-existing pulmonary hypertension or incipient heart failure. Occlusion of medium-sized or small pulmonary arteries only produces pulmonary hypertension if many vessels are occluded by a shower of small emboli or, rarely, by recurrent embolism over a period of months or years (p. 542). If the pulmonary circulation is normal, obstruction of medium-sized pulmonary arteries does not result in infarction, but if the circulation is impaired, e.g. by heart failure, infarction may result.

Only a small minority of pulmonary emboli are diagnosed *ante mortem*. Thus, the true incidence of pulmonary embolism is unknown. In ambulatory patients pulmonary emboli are usually small and produce few if any symptoms. They are rapidly removed by fibrinolysis, and because of the excellent collateral circulation, lung damage occurs only when cardiac failure is present.

Systemic Arterial Embolism

This causes blockage of an artery and the results vary according to the size of embolus and therefore the size of vessel occluded.

Atheromatous emboli. Emboli arise from thrombi which form on ulcerated atheromatous plaques. These can block a major artery. Advanced atheromatous plaques often crack or ulcerate and release lipid debris from their centre. This atheromatous embolism can be identified histologically by the presence of cholesterol crystals impacted in the distal arteries. Atheromatous embolism may complicate arterial catheterization and dilatation of a narrowed artery by balloon angioplasty (p. 523). Showers of emboli may cause abdominal pain, hypertension, renal failure or a vasculitis-like syndrome with a skin rash 'livido reticularis'. At autopsy histological evidence of atheromatous embolism can be found in the kidneys of 15% of an elderly population. Such embolism probably accounts for the ischaemic scars which are common in the kidneys of old persons, and smaller emboli could contribute to the nephron loss which occurs in old age and hypertension. Atheromatous embolism affects other arteries (e.g. the carotid and coronary arteries) and may be involved in cerebral and myocardial ischaemia.

Platelet emboli. Occasionally, loose aggregates of platelets circulate in the blood. These small aggregates may be responsible for transient ischaemic attacks with neurological signs and symptoms which occur in the elderly (p. 820). In the coronary circulation small platelet aggregates have been implicated in causing myocardial ischaemia (p. 492).

Fat Embolism

Following fractures of bone and other types of tissue injury globules of fat frequently enter the circulation. In most cases this is asymptomatic and the fat is removed. The **fat embolism syndrome** develops when extensive fractures of long bones are associated with laceration of fatty tissue and the entry of large amounts of fat into the circulation. Following the injury, there is a delay of about 24–48 hours during which the raised tissue pressure caused by the swelling of the damaged tissues forces fat into marrow sinusoids and veins. The features of the syndrome are dyspnoea, blood-stained sputum, tachycardia, mental confusion, a petechial rash and fever and sometimes cyanosis, coma and death.

Some of the fat passes through the pulmonary circulation and impacts in capillaries throughout the systemic circulation, where it causes widespread petechial haemorrhages in the skin and various tissues. The petechiae are more prominent on the upper trunk. Fat globules may be present in the urine and this is useful in diagnosis. In fatal cases, fat emboli are seen in the capillaries in many tissues (Fig. 3.17) and pericapillary haemorrhages and minute infarcts are often found in the brain, principally in the white matter. Thrombocytopenia and disseminated intravascular

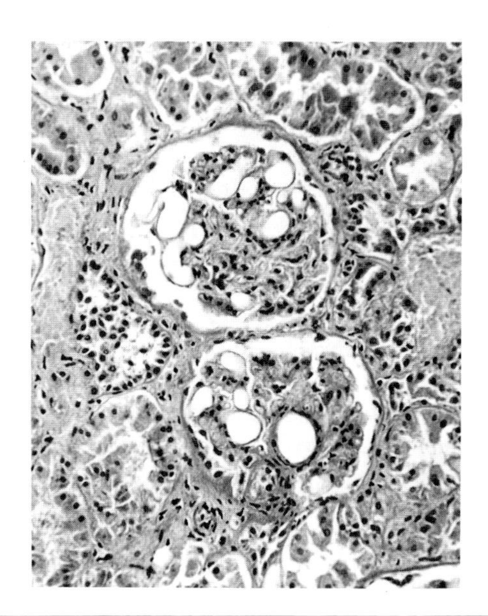

Fig. 3.17 Fat embolism of glomerular capillaries in a case of decompression sickness. Fat globules (dissolved out in processing the tissue) have impacted in glomerular capillaries and caused great distension. ×170.

coagulation develop in some patients and may contribute to haemorrhages. Over 80% of patients recover without residual disability.

Fat embolism may also complicate trauma to adipose tissue or a grossly fatty liver, major surgery, acute pancreatitis and decompression sickness (see below).

Amniotic Fluid Embolism

This is an unpredictable complication of labour which may complicate vaginal and caesarean delivery and abortions. Although rare, amniotic fluid embolism has a mortality of over 80%. Amniotic fluid containing fetal material enters the uterine veins probably via the placental bed. The mother becomes cyanotic, dyspnoeic and shocked and a few hours later, develops pulmonary oedema with diffuse alveolar injury similar to that seen in adult respiratory distress syndrome (p. 541). At autopsy, fetal squames may be found in the pulmonary circulation. Although mechanical obstruction of the pulmonary circulation may contribute to the clinical picture, the presence of fetal material causes disseminated intravascular coagulation. Humoral factors in the amniotic fluid may also produce pulmonary vasoconstriction and impair cardiac contractility.

Air Embolism

Air may enter the circulation through neck wounds which penetrate large veins because, in the upright position, their intraluminal pressure is lower than atmospheric pressure. Air may also enter veins during cardiothoracic surgery or when positive pressure is used in venous or arterial catheterization and in intravenous infusion of blood or fluids. Small volumes of air are rapidly absorbed without ill effect, but volumes of over 100 ml may cause acute distress and 300 ml or more may be fatal. Such large volumes become churned up with blood in the right side of the heart and the pulmonary circulation becomes blocked by froth.

Decompression sickness is a hazard when air is breathed at pressures greater than atmospheric pressure. The volumes of inhaled gases which pass into solution in blood and tissues are proportional to the atmospheric pressure. If the subject is then exposed rapidly to atmospheric pressure, as when a diver comes to the surface too quickly, or when there is sudden loss of pressure in a pressurized aircraft at altitude, the dissolved gases come out of solution (just as champagne effervesces on opening the bottle) and bubbles form in the blood and tissues. The bubbles consist largely of nitrogen which is less readily reabsorbed than oxygen or carbon dioxide. The effects depend on which vascular bed is predominantly affected. Muscle cramps (the 'bends'), cough ('the chokes') and dyspnoea are the commonest features. The central nervous system complications are the most serious. The spinal cord is particularly susceptible and paraplegia may result. Blockage of cerebral vessels leads to coma and sometimes to death. Fatty tissue absorbs large amounts of nitrogen and large bubbles may tear fat cells and produce embolism. In decompression sickness, the presence of bubbles and fat in the blood may activate plasma enzyme cascades causing DIC and shock. Recompression followed by slow decompression is the only effective form of treatment.

The chronic form of decompression sickness (Caisson disease) is associated with a long diving experience. It is characterized by bone necrosis affecting part of the shaft of the femur or humerus. In a minority of patients involvement of intra-articular bone may cause collapse of a joint, most often the shoulder or hip joint. The pathogenesis of these bone lesions is uncertain but ischaemic injury seems most likely.

Decompression barotrauma is not dependent on dissolved gases and thus is unrelated to the duration of a dive. It is likely to occur when a diver holds his/her breath during ascent or when a small airway is blocked. Rupture of lung tissue by expansion of trapped air may lead to pneumothorax, interstitial emphysema (escape of air into the tissues) of the mediastinum and neck, and entry of air into pulmonary veins. This last may cause air embolism usually to the brain producing neurological symptoms.

Abnormalities of Blood Flow

Disturbance of the flow of blood are intimately associated with diseases which affect the heart and blood vessels (Chapter 12). However, such disturbances have profound effects on most body tissues and a general account is given here.

In hyperaemia and congestion there is an excess volume of blood in organs or tissues. Hyperaemia is due to active dilatation of the arterioles, which increases blood flow. Congestion is due to passive failure of venous drainage of blood and, although there is excess blood in the tissues the flow is slow. Venous congestion is therefore considered later as an abnormality in which, in common with ischaemia and shock, there is reduced blood flow in tissues.

Hyperaemia and Increased Total Blood Flow

Local hyperaemia may be a response to physiological stimuli; for example in the gut following a meal and in skeletal muscle during exercise. Reactive hyperaemia follows transient blockage of the circulation. Local hyperaemia is one of the cardinal features of acute inflammation.

A generalized increase in blood flow is synonymous with increased cardiac output and there is often generalized hyperaemia. The commonest causes of increased blood flow are: (1) increased demand for oxygen due to an increase in metabolic rate, e.g. fever, hyperthyroidism and convalescence from severe injury; (2) hypoxic states, e.g. anaemia or impaired oxygenation of the blood by the lungs; (3) arteriovenous shunting which syphons off arterial blood, reducing its availability for tissue perfusion; (4) generalized inflammatory conditions of the skin; (5) liver failure, possibly due to accumulation of vasodilator substances normally metabolized by the liver (p. 775); and (6) extensive Paget's disease of bone (p. 958). In these various conditions there is increased cardiac output and if this is maintained for some time cardiac hypertrophy and eventually cardiac failure may ensue.

Decrease in Local Blood Flow

Ischaemia *means deficient supply of blood.* It occurs when blood flow to an organ or tissue has ceased (complete ischaemia), or is abnormally low (partial ischaemia). Arterial obstruction is a far more important cause than venous occlusion. The most important causes of complete arterial obstruction are thrombosis and embolism but atheroma, proliferation of the intima of small arteries and arterial spasm produce partial ischaemia.

Progressive narrowing of arteries, usually caused by atheroma, causes ischaemic atrophy of specialized cells with accompanying overgrowth of fibrous tissue, so that loss of function occurs. Cessation of blood flow is often associated with necrosis of the organ or part of the organ supplied by that artery. Tissue necrosis resulting from reduction or loss of blood supply is termed infarction and the area of dead tissue is called an infarct. Thus, in the heart, chronic myocardial ischaemia often causes fibrosis and angina pectoris while complete ischaemia results in myocardial infarction or sudden death (p. 488). The susceptibility to ischaemia is governed by two properties of the affected tissue, the anatomy and physiology of its blood vessels and the metabolism of the tissue.

The Susceptibility of Tissues to Ischaemia

Blood Supply and Collateral Circulation

The lung and the liver are resistant to ischaemia because they have a double blood supply; the bronchial arteries and the portal vein can each compensate for some of the effects of pulmonary or hepatic artery occlusion. Other tissues have a collateral blood supply due to arterial anastomoses; for example, in the presence of an intact circle of Willis one of the four neck arteries which supply the brain may be occluded without tissue damage. Also, in a person with a healthy vascular system, occlusion of a femoral artery will usually not cause permanent ischaemic damage to the tissues due to the arterial anastomoses in the legs. Dilatation of the other arteries creates increased flow through the collateral vessels which enlarge and eventually compensate for the reduced blood supply. Similarly, the bowel is supplied by mesenteric artery branches which form overlapping arcades. Blood is therefore supplied from adjacent branches when a distal vessel is occluded. In organs such as the kidney or spleen, the arterial territories do not overlap; these arteries are called **end arteries** and sudden occlusion will usually cause infarction. Similarly, the arteries in the brain beyond the circle of Willis are functional end arteries and occlusion of any of them produces cerebral infarction.

If arteries have gradually become narrowed by disease, a collateral blood supply may gradually develop and this may protect the tissues from sudden occlusion of one of the arteries. The collateral arteries enlarge and become thick-walled. Although the coronary arteries are end arteries, gradual narrowing of one can stimulate the development of collaterals from an adjacent artery (see Fig. 12.41). In general, however, in the presence of arterial disease there is an increased risk of ischaemic injury. In addition, when the arteries are narrowed, a sudden fall in blood pressure may cause infarction, e.g. boundary zone or watershed infarction in the brain (p. 821) or global infarcts in the heart (p. 497).

Tissue Metabolism and Ischaemia

The parenchymal cells of organs, which have a high metabolic rate, are relatively susceptible to both acute and chronic ischaemia, whereas the supporting tissues – fibrous and fatty tissue, bone and cartilage – are much less susceptible. Other important factors are the extent to which the cell depends on endogenous fuels rather than on exogenous fuel delivered by the blood, and the ability of the cell to metabolize anaerobically. Tissues without an immediate blood supply (e.g. cartilage), have a low metabolic rate and highly anaerobic metabolism and therefore have a high tolerance to hypoxia and ischaemia. On the other hand, the brain and the heart, which have high metabolic rates, highly aerobic metabolism and limited endogenous stores of fuel, tolerate hypoxia and ischaemia poorly.

Effects of Ischaemia on Cell Metabolism

The utilization of fatty fuels is an oxygen-requiring process. In ischaemias triglyceride cannot be oxidized and glycogen can only be catabolized to pyruvate because the mitochondrial oxidation of NADH to NAD^+ occurs too slowly. Pyruvate is then converted to lactate by lactate dehydrogenase, and the rise in intracellular lactate is one of the reasons for a fall in ATP. The reduced conversion of ADP to ATP causes a rise in ADP which is then converted to adenosine, xanthine and hypoxanthine. These metabolites diffuse out of the cell within minutes, causing a marked reduction of adenine nucleotides in the cell and the reduced energy supply leads to failure of the membrane ATPase cation pumps (Na^+/K^+; Ca^{2+}) which consume at least 25% of the cell's energy output (Fig. 3.18).

The highly reduced state of the mitochondrial electron transport systems and the action of enzymes such as xanthine oxidase create highly reactive free radicals and superoxide (p. 23) which may oxidize membrane lipids (lipid peroxidation) and the thiol groups of membrane proteins, leading to membrane damage.

Severe membrane damage leads to the loss of proteins from the cells and increased blood levels of some intracellular enzymes are used to confirm the occurrence of necrosis in the heart, liver and skeletal muscle. However, in ischaemia severe

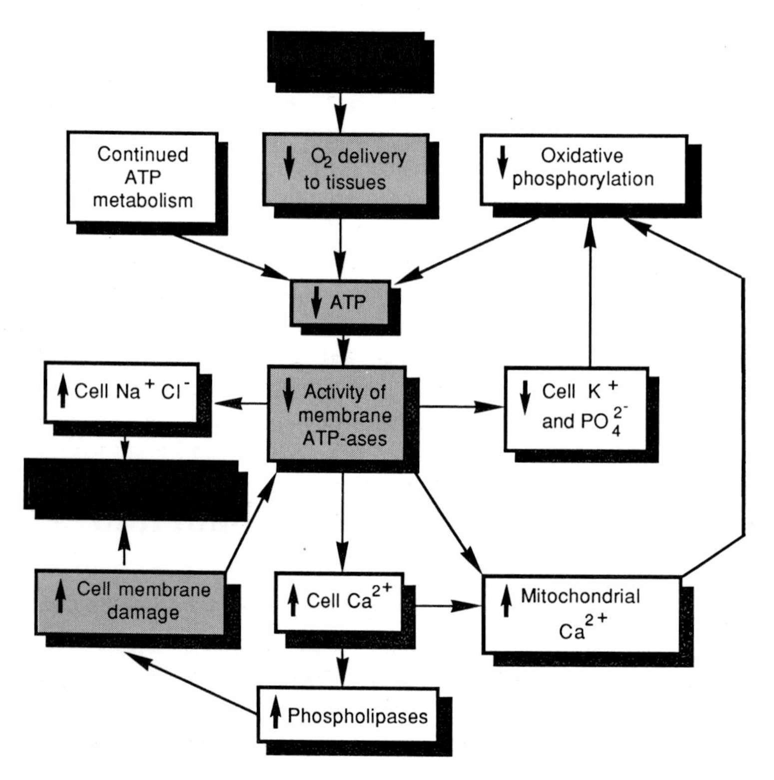

Fig. 3.18 A diagrammatic scheme of some of the pathways involved in ischaemia. The end result is cell swelling mainly due to increased membrane permeability and to failure of the cation pumps. The activation of phospholipase enzymes and their role in membrane damage is controversial.

membrane damage probably plays a less important role in cell necrosis than the loss of small molecules which are concerned with the energy supply. In cardiac myocytes, the intracellular concentration of creatine phosphate drops to zero within seconds of the onset of ischaemia; after 15 minutes the ATP concentration falls to 35% of normal and 50% of the total adenine nucleotides have been lost from the cell.

Reperfusion Injury

Restoration of flow after vascular occlusion may cause a paradoxical increase in cell injury. The formation of free radicals is increased when oxygen is supplied to cells which have raised level of NADH and hypoxanthine. Furthermore, because of the failure of Ca^{2+}-ATPase, cells are unable to control the levels of cystolic and mitochondrial calcium. Experimentally, reperfusion injury can be minimized by administration of the enzymes superoxide dismutase and catalase which dispose of free radicals, and by giving calcium channel blockers which slow the re-entry of calcium into cells. Reperfusion injury is thought to be responsible for the haemorrhages in some cerebral and myocardial infarcts. However, restoration of blood flow in a thrombosed coronary artery by giving streptokinase reduces long-term mortality, and the earlier the reperfusion the more beneficial the long-term effect. The effect of streptokinase administration on the extent of myocardial necrosis has not been determined.

Infarction

Tissue necrosis due to reduction or loss of blood supply is termed ***infarction***. An infarct is usually due to obstruction of one or more arteries by thrombosis or embolism. Occasionally, the blood flow may be stopped by occlusion of the draining veins and venous infarction may then occur. The term infarction, literally translated, means 'stuffing in', and was originally applied to infarcts in tissues in which good collateral circulation caused haemorrhage into the dying tissue. In most tissues an established infarct appears pale.

General Features

The size of an infarct depends upon the amount of tissue rendered ischaemic, the severity and duration of the ischaemia, and the susceptibility of the tissue cells to ischaemia. Infarcts may be red or pale and may undergo coagulative or colliquative necrosis (p. 25). Since hypoxic cells cannot maintain ionic gradients they absorb water and swell. Recent infarcts are therefore raised above the surface of the organ: the swelling of a large cerebral infarction may cause a fatal increase in intracranial pressure because the brain is confined by the skull.

In the days following infarction, the products of the dead cells diffuse out and promote an acute inflammatory reaction at the margin, with vascular congestion, oedema and migration of polymorphs and macrophages into the dead tissue. When an infarct extends to a coelomic surface, e.g. the pericardium, pleura or peritoneum, fibrin is often deposited on the surface and this is accompanied by a clear slightly turbid fluid exudate. This surface inflammation may give rise to pain and a 'friction rub' may be heard on auscultation when the roughened visceral surface slides over the parietal surface, e.g. during heart beats (pericardial friction 'rubs') or lung movement during respiration (pleural friction 'rubs'). The acute inflammation soon subsides, and organization (p. 131) begins; granulation tissue grows in from the margin and the infarct is gradually replaced by fibrous tissue. Eventually the site of the infarct is marked by a sunken fibrous scar. These features are illustrated by the following contrasting examples of infarction.

Myocardial infarction (p. 491). Myocardial infarction usually results from occlusive thrombosis supervening on atheroma of a major coronary artery. The dead myocardium undergoes coagulative necrosis and gradually becomes pale. Eventually, in patients who survive, a fibrous scar forms. Less commonly, infarction involves the inner (subendocardial) parts of the wall of the left ventricle: when the whole circumference is affected it is termed global infarction: such global infarction is caused by a drop in blood pressure in a patient with severe narrowing of all coronary arteries or their major branches by atheroma.

Cerebral infarcts may be pale or haemorrhagic. In contrast to other organs there is colliquative necrosis and the neural tissue breaks down to form a soft pulpy mass (see Fig. 18.17, p. 819). The debris is gradually removed by macrophages which become bloated with myelin (see Fig. 18.4b, p. 809). The residual cavity, once termed an 'apoplectic cyst' (see Fig. 18.18, p. 820) eventually contains clear fluid and is walled off by gliosis.

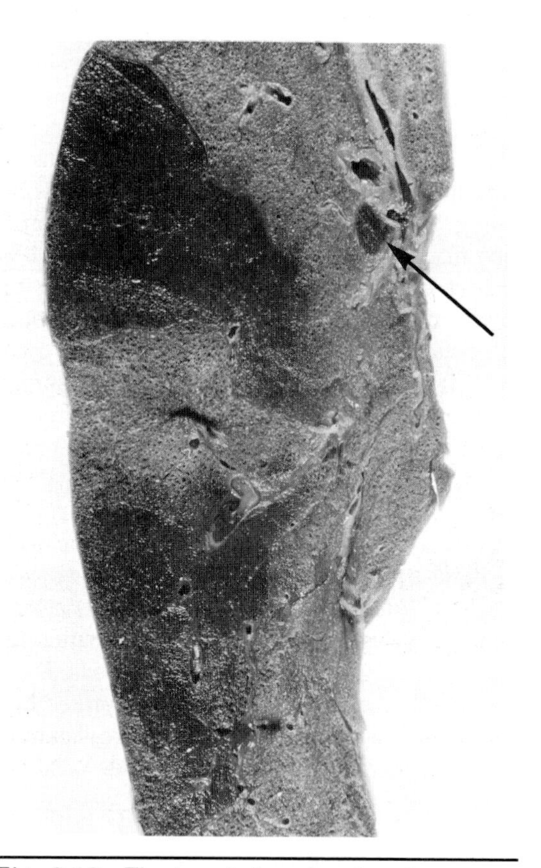

Fig. 3.19 The two dark wedge-shaped areas are haemorrhagic infarcts of lung, widening towards the pleural surface (left). A pulmonary artery is occluded by thrombus (arrow) beyond the apex of the upper infarct. ×1.3.

Lung infarcts are typically dark red and conical, with the base projecting slightly on the pleural surface (Fig. 3.19). They are firm and haemorrhagic because the bronchial arteries bleed into the dead tissue (Fig. 3.20).

Splenic infarcts are conical and subcapsular (Fig. 3.21). At first the infarcted tissue is dark red due to congestion, but after a few days it changes to pale yellow, before being slowly organized to leave a depressed scar. The enlarged spleen in sickle cell disease (p. 605) is particularly prone to infarction and this may involve the entire organ – so-called autosplenectomy. Similar infarcts occur in the kidney and, if large, may be complicated by transient hypertension due to release of renin (p. 464).

Intestinal infarction results from occlusion of a major artery, usually the superior mesenteric, or

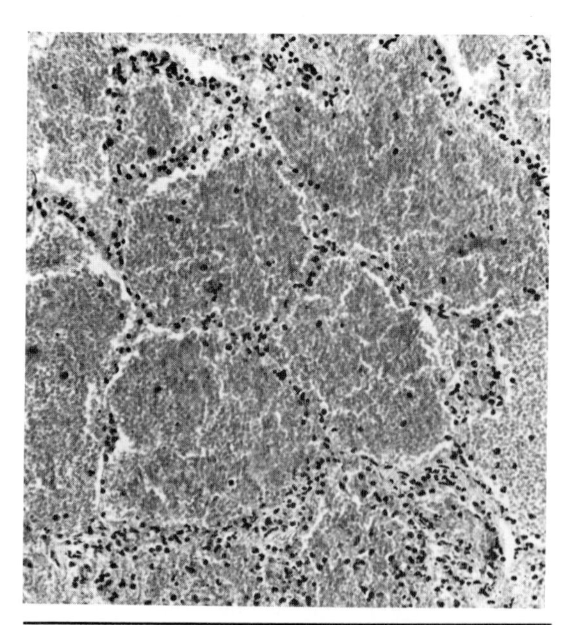

Fig. 3.20 Haemorrhagic infarct of lung showing alveoli filled with red cells. ×115.

from a drop in blood pressure when the mesenteric vessels are narrowed. The mesenteric veins may be mechanically occluded by twisting a loop of the gut (volvulus – p. 727) or strangulation in a hernial sac (p. 726) causing venous infarction of a bowel loop.

Liver infarction. Obstruction of the hepatic artery or its branches may cause infarction of the liver but obstruction of a branch of the portal vein is not followed by infarction because most of the oxygen supply is derived from the hepatic artery.

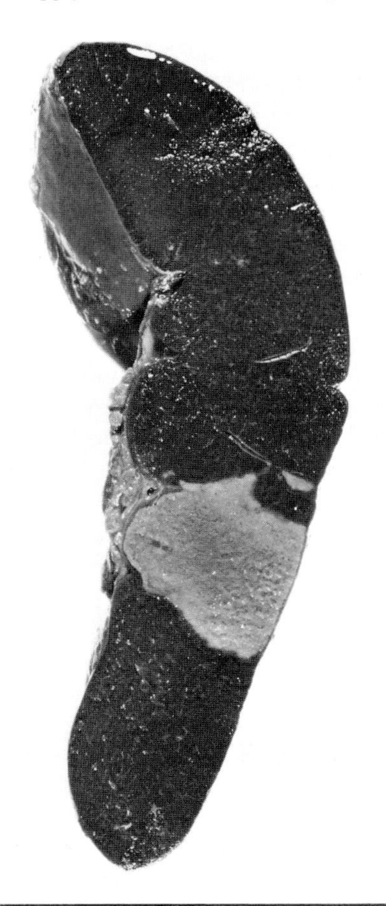

Fig. 3.21 Pale infarct of the spleen.

However, portal vein obstruction reduces the metabolic workload sufficiently to cause atrophy and loss of hepatic parenchymal cells. The sinusoids dilate and the lesion appears dark red and shrunken, a so-called red infarct (Fig. 3.22).

Venous infarction. Acute renal vein thrombosis causes infarction of the kidney and is fatal if bilateral. Marantic thrombosis of the superior longitudinal sinus in severely debilitated children may cause local haemorrhagic infarction of the cerebral cortex. Venous infarction of the gut has already been mentioned.

Septic infarction is usually restricted to infarcts caused by a septic embolus. The bacteria in the embolus invade the dead tissue and cause suppuration, initially at the margin, and then the infarct is converted to an abscess.

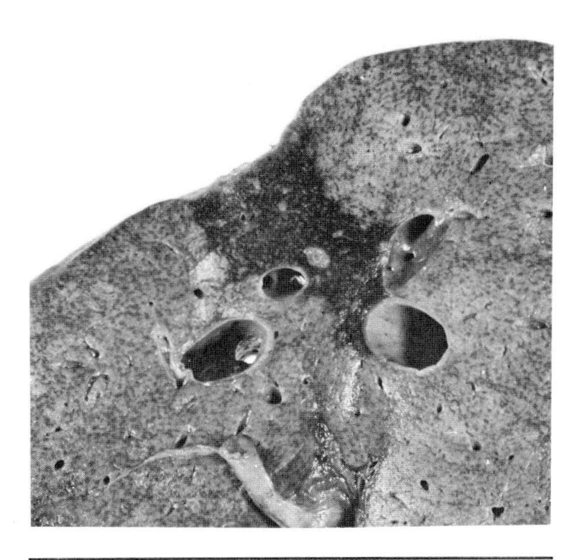

Fig. 3.22 A depressed red patch in the liver due to loss of parenchymal cells and sinusoidal congestion caused by thrombosis of a portal venous branch (not shown).

Decrease in Total Blood Flow

A chronic reduction in total blood flow is the main feature of chronic heart failure (p. 483). The functional impairment is usually progressive. Initially, cardiac output is inadequate when there is increased functional demand as in physical exercise; eventually, even at rest, there is inadequate output. The most important effects of heart failure are due to inadequate tissue perfusion. In addition, venous congestion and oedema develop. A sudden and severe fall in blood flow may give rise to shock.

Shock

***Shock** is the term applied to the complex series of changes which result from acute circulatory failure.* The three major types of shock are:

(1) **hypovolaemic shock** due to a reduced blood volume;

(2) **cardiogenic shock** due to a severe fall in cardiac output;

(3) **septic shock** associated with bacterial infection.

The features of **anaphylactic shock**, and the shock-like state of acute immune-complex disease, are described elsewhere (p. 209). Some causes of shock do not fall into these three main categories. Acute peritonitis due to escape of gastric juice into the peritoneal cavity from a perforated peptic ulcer, acute haemorrhagic pancreatitis (which is non-bacterial) and ingestion of many poisons can all cause severe shock. So-called neurogenic shock may complicate anaesthesia or spinal cord injury. Severe shock develops when incompatible blood is transfused accidentally. Although different mechanisms may be involved in all these conditions the end results, namely acute circulatory failure and its complications, are the same as those occurring in the three major categories.

In the early stages of shock, compensatory mechanisms maintain the blood supply to those organs with the most urgent perfusion requirements – the central nervous system, the kidneys and the heart. However, the compensated phase is achieved by severe reduction in the circulation through most other tissues. Unless tissue perfusion can be restored without undue delay ischaemic injury causes multi-organ failure and death.

Hypovolaemic Shock

The shocked patient is restless and confused, has a pale, cold, sweaty skin, often with peripheral cyanosis, a rapid weak pulse, a low blood pressure, increased rate and depth of respiration, and may become drowsy and confused and finally comatose.

The commonest cause is severe acute haemorrhage. In extensive burning with loss of 10% or more of the skin surface, hypovolaemia results from exudation of plasma from the damaged small blood vessels; the hypovolaemia develops more slowly than in haemorrhage and haemoconcentration is more pronounced. Hypovolaemic shock can also develop in severe dehydration as a result of vomiting and/or diarrhoea.

A normal healthy adult can lose 550 ml of blood, i.e. about 10% of the blood volume, without any significant symptoms; the blood volume is restored within a few hours by transfer of fluid from the extravascular compartment. Replacement of plasma protein takes a day or two, and restoration of red cells takes weeks. Loss of 25% of the blood volume (about 1250 ml) results in significant hypovolaemia over the subsequent 36 hours, while an unreplaced rapid loss of about 50% of the blood volume results in coma and death.

Early Compensatory Changes

Acute hypovolaemia causes a reduced central (systemic) venous pressure and a diminished venous return to the right atrium. The decreased cardiac filling causes a fall in stroke volume, and the cardiac output and arterial blood pressure fall. These changes trigger peripheral and central baroreceptors with consequent intense sympathico-adrenal stimulation, sometimes producing a 200-fold increase in the plasma levels of catecholamines. The heart rate increases to restore cardiac output and widespread arteriolar and venular constriction reduce tissue perfusion. The fall in renal perfusion stimulates renin secretion which in turn produces increased plasma levels of angiotensin II and aldosterone (p. 464). These agents amplify the effects of catecholamines: they cause sodium retention, increase systemic venous tone which increases central venous pressure, venous return to the heart and cardiac output. Angiotensin II also causes arteriolar and venular constriction particularly in the skin and splanchnic area, so that peripheral resistance is increased. Thus, even without treatment, the blood pressure may be partially or fully restored, although tissue perfusion is reduced.

The central nervous system, heart and kidneys are further protected because they **autoregulate** their own perfusion. In young persons cerebral and coronary blood flow are maintained close to normal levels at blood pressures down to about 50 mmHg, the lower limit of autoregulation. At this pressure, however, arteriolar relaxation is maximal and perfusion rapidly declines at lower pressures. In older patients with arteriosclerosis or in those with hypertension the lower limit of autoregulation may be 80–90 mmHg.

If less than 25% of the blood has been lost the blood volume can be restored by the compensatory mechanisms. Vasoconstriction of the arterioles is greater than that in the venules, so that the hydrostatic pressure in the capillaries is low and extravascular fluid enters the intravascular compartment. Aldosterone promotes retention of salt and water by the kidney, thus increasing volume in the extravascular compartment. Tissue perfusion is, nevertheless, precarious and in all save the mildest cases of hypovolaemic shock it is important to restore the blood volume by prompt intravenous administration of fluid. Blood transfusion is required when the loss exceeds 25% of blood volume. Isotonic saline is effective initially, but macromolecular solutions, such as plasma or dextrans, are required to maintain the osmotic pressure of the plasma and retain fluid in the circulation. The haematocrit should be maintained at 30% in order to minimize tissue hypoxia. Haemoglobin and haematocrit levels are not reliable guides to the degree of hypovolaemia during the first 36 hours, because haemodilution may not be complete. If cardiac function is normal, a low arterial pressure indicates hypovolaemia in early shock, but because of the high levels of circulating vasoconstrictors, blood pressure is not a reliable indicator of hypovolaemia. Central venous pressure gives a more accurate indication of hypovolaemia and should be monitored in all cases of severe shock.

Established Shock

The longer shock persists, the more complicated it becomes, and in advanced shock, hypovolaemia, cardiac insufficiency and bacterial infection are often combined. If shock persists, the widespread arteriolar constriction gradually passes off but venular constriction is more persistent. This leads to increased capillary hydrostatic pressure, loss of fluid into the extravascular space and a further fall in blood volume. At this later stage, the capillaries are congested with slowly flowing blood, producing cyanosis. The reduced blood supply to the tissues is aggravated by a number of factors (Fig. 3.23). Blood viscosity rises due to loss of intravascular fluid, and this leads to sludging of the red cells with the formation of rouleaux. Following haemorrhage, viscosity is further increased by a rise in plasma fibrinogen. Release of thromboplastin from hypoxic endothelium and tissue cells generates thrombin, which promotes platelet aggregation and occasionally this leads to DIC. Neutrophil polymorphs also adhere to the injured endothelium of small vessels and, especially in the lungs, they may contribute to tissue damage. Hypoxic injury to cells releases lysosomal enzymes and other secretory products into the blood. Proteolytic enzymes may activate the kinin and complement systems and thus further embarrass the circulation by causing vasodilatation and increased vascular permeability. Metabolic acidosis has a direct depressant effect on cardiac myocytes.

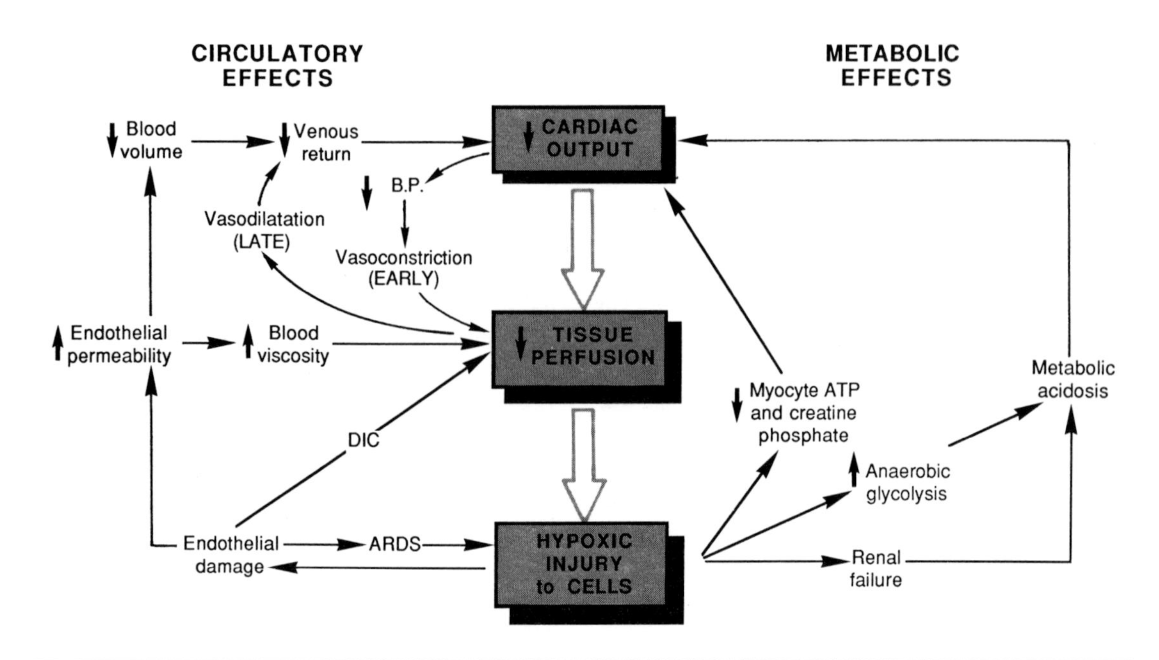

Fig. 3.23 The pathogenesis of shock: some of the circulatory and metabolic mechanisms which operate at a cellular level and tissue level. The diagram emphasizes the many 'vicious circles' involved and the central role of tissue perfusion in pathogenesis. ARDS, adult respiratory distress syndrome.

Myocardial depressant factor is released from the ischaemic pancreas and in addition to its cardiac effect it may damage cell membranes.

Cardiogenic Shock

Cardiogenic shock, due to severe acute reduction in cardiac output, is caused by cardiac catastrophes such as myocardial infarction, and less commonly, rupture of a valve cusp, or any cause of tamponade with haemopericardium (p. 520). The essential feature is 'pump failure'. Both the central venous pressure and the ventricular end-diastolic pressures are raised. The haemodynamic changes which develop are similar to those described for hypovolaemic shock and are triggered by the fall in blood pressure and the reduced tissue perfusion. The mortality rate approaches 80%. Surgical intervention, e.g. to replace a ruptured valve, is sometimes undertaken and aortic pumps have been used to assist the circulation prior to surgery.

Septic (Endotoxic) Shock

Septicaemia or severe localized infections may be complicated by shock in which hypotension is associated with early peripheral vasodilatation and a normal or sometimes increased cardiac output. This vasodilatation is in contrast to what happens in hypovolaemia and cardiogenic shock, but the overall effect is to reduce tissue perfusion. Septic shock may complicate infected burns or follow surgical procedures in infected patients. It may also follow simple instrumentation of the urogenital or biliary tract. Septic shock is particularly common in patients with immunodeficiency states, such as in leukaemia or lymphoma, and occurs as a complication of cytotoxic or immunosuppressive drugs therapy. Septic shock is particularly difficult to reverse, is often complicated by DIC and the mortality rate is over 50%. A monoclonal antibody to endotoxin has been produced and may prove to be of value in the treatment of these patients.

A similar, serious but rare condition known as

toxic shock syndrome is caused by exotoxins produced by *Staphylococcus aureus*. This syndrome was associated with the use of highly absorbent tampons during menstruation, facilitating growth of the organism in the menstrual blood. It may also complicate *Staphylococcus aureus* infections of the skin and other sites.

Aetiology and Pathogenesis

Septic shock is usually caused by Gram-negative bacteria which release endotoxin (p. 292). The organisms most commonly responsible include *Escherichia coli, Proteus, Klebsiella, Bacteroides* and, in cases of burns, *Pseudomonas aeruginosa.* It is caused much less commonly by exotoxins (p. 290) produced by Gram-positive bacteria such as staphylococci, streptococci or pneumococci.

The effects of endotoxin are mediated by a cascade of events. Activation of the complement, coagulation, fibrinolytic and kinin systems by endotoxin with subsequent activation of platelets and neutrophils is thought to play a significant pathogenetic role. Endotoxin also causes the sudden release of endothelial derived relaxing factor (EDRF – now known to be nitric oxide) and other vasoactive substances from endothelial cells. These factors may produce the early vasodilatation and contribute to a rapid fall in blood pressure. Macrophages are also stimulated and release a number of soluble mediators which may contribute to the haemodynamic disturbances. These mediators include interleukins, in particular IL-6, tumour necrosis factor (TNF), arachidonic acid metabolites and lysosomal enzymes and are discussed in detail in the next chapter.

Metabolic Disturbances in Shock

The hypoxia of shock interferes profoundly with cell metabolism. It prevents the entrance of pyruvic acid into the citric acid cycle, causing accumulation of lactic acid and acidosis. The hypoxic cells leak glucose leading to insulin-resistant hyperglycaemia and increased glycogenolysis. These metabolic disturbances, together with high levels of catecholamines, result in a rise of fatty acids and amino acids in the plasma. Impaired carbohydrate metabolism causes a fall in production of ATP so that energy is not available for many cell functions, including the membrane ATPases sodium pump. Potassium leaves the cells, sodium and water enter and cause cell swelling: these effects are sometimes termed the 'sick cell syndrome'. This causes a fall in serum but not whole body sodium and it is therefore necessary to avoid inappropriate administration of this ion.

Organ Function and Morphological Changes in Shock

All organs are affected in severe shock. In spite of the fundamental disturbances of cell function the morphological changes at autopsy, however, are often inconspicuous. Failure of autoregulation causes severe ischaemic damage with boundary zone infarction of the brain and subendocardial infarction of the heart.

Acute heart failure, first of the left and then of both ventricles, may develop in severe hypovolaemic or septic shock and is particularly common in older patients with pre-existing coronary artery disease. Inadequate myocardial perfusion produces focal necrosis or global infarction. Metabolic acidosis produces tachypnoea with increased respiratory effort in shock. Impairment of lung function occurs late with progressive reduction in gas exchange. In established shock pulmonary function may deteriorate rapidly due to a combination of causes – pulmonary oedema, alveolar collapse, intravascular and intra-alveolar fibrin formation and infection. These features, known collectively as **shock lung** or **adult respiratory distress syndrome (ARDS)** are discussed in detail on p. 541.

Below the lower level of autoregulation, perfusion of the kidneys is directly proportional to the blood pressure. Production of urine ceases at about 50 mmHg and if the pressure remains low for some hours, hypoxic injury leads to renal failure with **acute tubular necrosis**. The kidneys usually show cortical pallor and swelling (p. 921).

There may be gastrointestinal haemorrhage and, in DIC, more widespread small haemorrhages affect mucosal and serosal surfaces. Although DIC is common, fibrin thrombi are only occasionally histologically identifiable in small blood vessels. Fatty change and ischaemic necrosis of perivenular liver cells may be noted at autopsy but clinical liver failure in shock is uncommon. Hypotension may precipitate acute pancreatitis and this will aggravate shock. The adrenals occasionally show a combination of haemorrhage and necrosis (Waterhouse–Friderichsen syndrome), particularly in septic shock associated with meningococcal septicaemia (p. 1101).

The most severely affected organs in shock are the kidneys, the heart, the lungs and the brain. These patients require intensive care in specialized units. Because renal failure and cardiac failure are both treatable, respiratory failure is the commonest cause of death; there may be residual brain damage in some patients who recover.

Venous Congestion

When the heart fails to expel the blood arriving in the veins, the venous system dilates. Longstanding poor cardiac output also leads to an increase in blood volume (p. 488) most of which is accommodated in the veins, which consequently become engorged with blood. When venous congestion becomes chronic, tissue damage occurs. Left ventricular failure causing venous congestion occurs in the lungs, whereas right ventricular failure gives rise to systemic venous congestion. The term congestive cardiac failure is used when both chambers are in failure. Severe venous congestion is usually accompanied by oedema.

Pulmonary Venous Congestion

In venous congestion of the lungs the pulmonary venules and alveolar capillaries are engorged with blood. Acute pulmonary venous congestion results in pulmonary oedema. Red cells escape into the alveoli and the sputum may be blood-stained. Red blood cells are ingested by alveolar macrophages and the breakdown of haemoglobin causes accumulation of haemosiderin. These iron-laden macrophages, so-called heart failure cells, are a feature of chronic venous congestion. In the alveoli, the elastic and collagen fibres in the walls of alveoli become encrusted with iron released from macrophages. This causes fibrosis of alveolar walls which causes the lung to feel firmer and the deposition of haemosiderin gives a brown appearance – brown induration of the lung. Pulmonary venous congestion eventually causes pulmonary arterial hypertension which, if prolonged, causes structural changes in the pulmonary arterial tree (p. 542), right ventricular hypertrophy (cor pulmonale p. 487) and eventually, right ventricular failure. Thus, chronic left ventricular failure always leads to right ventricular failure.

Systemic Venous Congestion

This usually results from right sided heart failure (p. 487), and may be acute or chronic. Engorgement of the systemic veins is easily seen in the neck when the patient is in a recumbent position. In the capillary beds decreased blood flow causes excessive oxygen desaturation. The amount of reduced haemoglobin causes vascular tissues such as the skin to become blue in colour (cyanosis). Severe venous congestion is usually accompanied by oedema which is gravitationally distributed, affecting the lower half of the body.

In chronic venous congestion, the abdominal viscera may show structural changes. The liver is

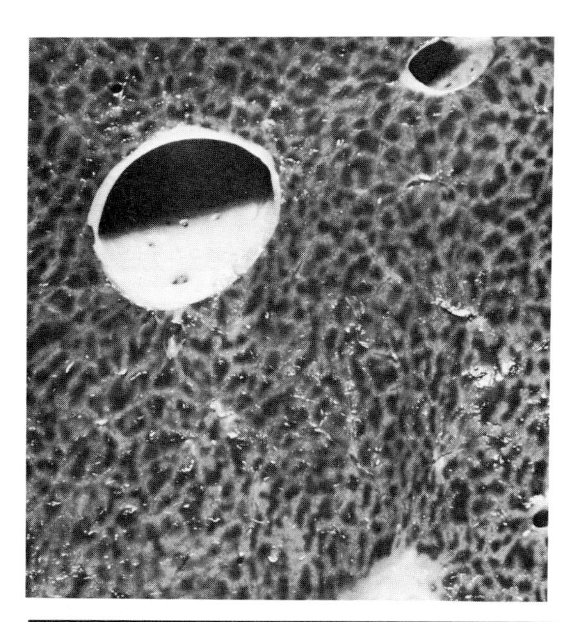

Fig. 3.24 The cut surface of the liver in chronic venous congestion. The congested perivenular zones are dark, and contrast with the pale (periportal) zones, giving a nutmeg-like appearance. ×1.8.

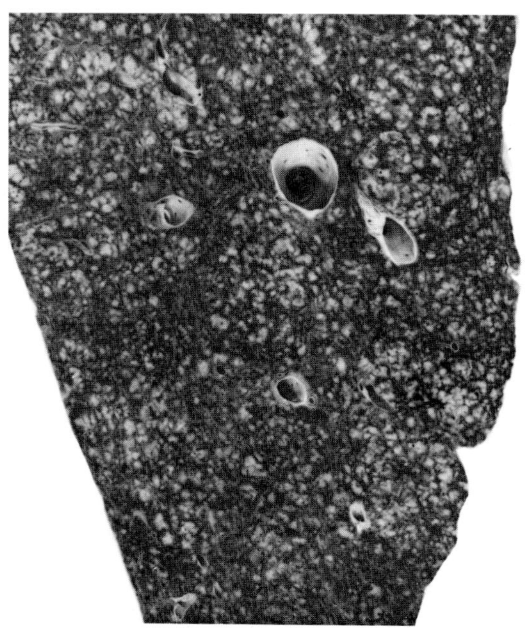

Fig. 3.25 Nodular regenerative hyperplasia of the liver in chronic venous congestion; the pale areas represent the regenerative nodules.

moderately enlarged and tender. Microscopically, the perivenular sinusoids are grossly distended with blood. The hepatocytes in the perivenular liver cell plates undergo atrophy due to pressure and chronic hypoxia, whereas the hepatocytes around the portal tracts are unaffected because they enjoy better oxygenation provided by the hepatic artery. Between the periportal and the perivenular areas the liver cells have an intermediate degree of hypoxia and sometimes show fatty change. This zonal variation in the effects of chronic venous congestion gives the liver a characteristic mottled appearance – nutmeg liver (Fig. 3.24). In long-standing cases, with recurrent episodes of congestive cardiac failure, fibrosis occurs in the areas of hepatocyte loss. The surviving hepatocytes undergo regeneration, producing nodular regenerative hyperplasia (Fig. 3.25). True cirrhosis does not occur. The spleen may be enlarged to two to three times its normal size and its firmness has led to the term 'cricket ball' spleen. Chronic congestion and hypoxia of the gut can cause malabsorption, while congestion of the kidneys causes mild proteinuria.

Further Reading

Aoki, N. (1989). Haemostasis associated with abnormalities of fibrinolysis. *Blood Reviews* **3**, 11–17.

Cowley, R. A. and Trump, B. F. (eds) (1982). *Pathophysiology of Shock, Anoxia and Ischemia*. Williams & Wilkins, Baltimore.

Mannucci, P. M. and Tripodi, A. (1988). Inherited factors in thrombosis. *Blood Reviews* **2**, 27–35.

Vane, J. R., Ånggard, E. E. and Botting, R. M. (1990). Regulatory functions of the vascular endothelium. *New England Journal of Medicine* **323**, 27–36.

Weston-Smith, S., Revell, P. and Savidge, G. F. (1989). Haemostasis associated with abnormalities of fibrinolysis. *Blood Reviews* **3**, 11–17.

4

Inflammation, Healing and Repair

Inflammation

The most important of the body's defence mechanisms is the inflammatory reaction. Inflammation, a term derived from the Latin *inflammare* meaning to burn, is the response of living tissues to cell injury. Its purpose is to localize and eliminate the causative agent, to limit tissue injury and then to restore the tissue to normality or as close to normality as possible. Thus, inflammation is a physiological response to injury, an observation made by John Hunter in 1794 who concluded: 'inflammation is itself not to be considered as a disease, but as a salutary operation consequent either to some violence or to some disease.'

As outlined in Chapter 1, tissue injury may be due to physical agents, chemical substances, microbial infections and immunologically mediated hypersensitivity reactions. In addition, tissue necrosis from any cause, e.g. ischaemia and anoxia, induces inflammation in adjacent living tissue. The inflammatory nature of a lesion is usually indicated by the suffix **-itis**. Thus inflammation of the appendix is appendicitis, of the liver hepatitis and so on. There are occasional historical exceptions: inflammation of the lung is traditionally pneumonia, not pneumonitis and of the pleura, pleurisy not pleuritis.

The acute inflammatory reaction is rapid in onset and lasts for days or a few weeks. Despite the multiplicity of causative agents the immediate tissue reaction is stereotyped. The local changes occur in the microcirculation, principally at the level of the capillary and post-capillary venule; these allow escape of plasma and plasma proteins (the fluid exudate), and white blood cells, polymorphonuclear granulocytes followed by monocytes and lymphocytes and accompanied also by platelets and erythrocytes (the cellular exudate). The stereotyped nature of these events is due to the release of chemical mediators which exert effects on the vascular endothelium, increasing vascular permeability, act as chemotactic agents for leucocytes and, in addition, are involved in the activation of leucocytes, allowing them to phagocytose and kill micro-organisms. The leucocytes and platelets disintegrate and release chemical agents which may cause further tissue injury. There is stasis of blood which is sometimes accompanied by thrombus formation, the resulting impaired blood flow further aggravating the initial injury. The cardinal signs of acute inflammation which were described by Celsus (30 BC–38 AD) – rubor (redness) color (heat), dolor (pain), tumor (swelling) – emphasize the importance of the changes in the microcirculation. The fifth manifestation – loss of function – was described much later by Virchow (1821–1902).

There are four possible outcomes to the acute inflammatory response: (1) resolution with a return of normal structure and function; (2) suppuration with abscess formation; (3) healing with regeneration of specialized tissues if this is possible or healing with the formation of fibrous tissue producing a scar; and (4) persistence of the causative agent with the inflammatory process becoming chronic.

Chronic inflammation persists for weeks, months or even years. It may be a sequel to acute (indeed as we shall see, there is some overlap between the features of acute and chronic inflammation) or it may be chronic *ab initio*. It is characterized by a cellular infiltrate in which the predominant cell types are lymphocytes and plasma cells together with monocytes which become macrophages and ingest and digest tissue debris and foreign material. In addition, there is proliferation of capillaries and fibroblasts in the adjacent area and there is an ingrowth of these into the injured tissue in an attempt to remove it and replace it by fibrous tissue. Depending on the tissue involved, there may be regeneration of the parenchymal cells. This is best exemplified in liver where a combination of fibrosis and regeneration of hepatocytes forming nodules results in cirrhosis (p. 764). As with acute inflammation these processes are in part controlled by chemical mediators collectively referred to as cytokines and which are secreted by lymphocytes and macrophages (p. 145). In contrast to the stereotyped nature of the acute inflammatory response, there is considerable variation in the patterns of chronic inflammation.

In the inflammatory response, which is essentially a protective response, there are complicated interactions involving the vascular system, the immune system and repair mechanisms. The response, however, may itself have injurious effects for the organ involved or for the host. In addition to local features there may also be generalized or systemic effects, the most obvious being changes in the regulation of body temperature and increased production of white blood cells by the bone marrow – leucocytosis. These systemic effects are also in part due to chemical mediators. Frequently there may be a need to intervene and try to limit the inflammation to the salutary process which Hunter perceived it to be. Such intervention includes drainage of an abscess, the use of antibiotics and the use of anti-inflammatory agents. A general scheme of the inflammatory process is given in Fig. 4.1, the individual events of which must now be examined in greater detail.

The Acute Inflammatory Reaction

The reactive changes in the first few hours after tissue injury involve three processes: (1) changes in vascular calibre and flow; (2) increased vascular permeability and the formation of inflammatory exudate; and (3) escape of leucocytes from blood vessels into extravascular tissue spaces.

These processes result in the accumulation of protein-rich oedema fluid, fibrin and leucocytes at the site of tissue injury. A knowledge of the normal microcirculation is essential for an understanding of the changes which occur in acute inflammation.

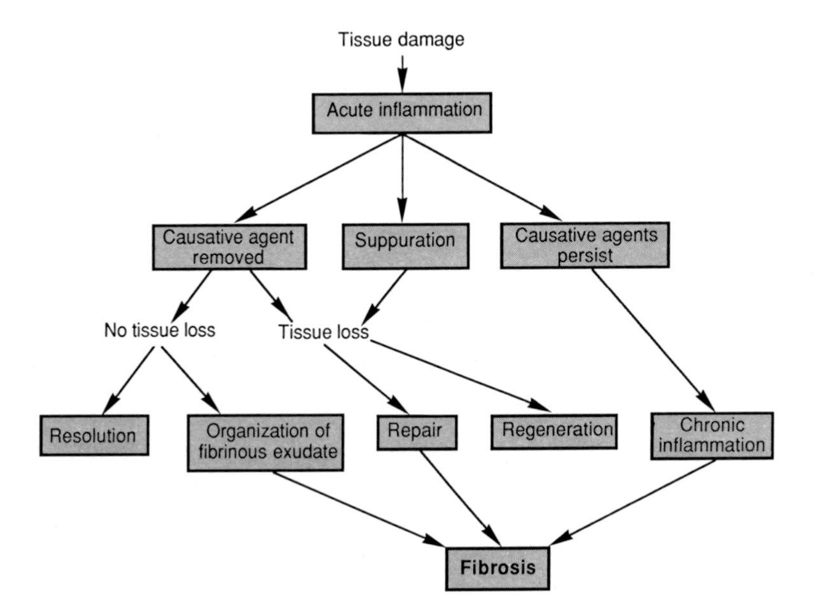

Fig. 4.1 The possible sequelae of acute inflammation.

The Normal Microcirculation

Blood enters the microcirculation through the arteriole, a vessel which has a narrow lumen and a thick muscular wall, and leaves by the larger, thin-walled venule. The metarterioles and capillaries connect the arterioles and venules. The metarterioles are surrounded by smooth muscle fibres which act as a precapillary sphincter and regulate blood flow through the capillaries. The capillary wall comprises endothelial cells supported by a basement membrane; smooth muscle fibres are absent. In many tissues the endothelium forms a continuous layer of uniform thickness all round the vessel. In other tissues, however, the endothelium is fenestrated: these include endocrine and exocrine glands, the kidney and intestinal mucosa and in the sinusoids of the liver, spleen and bone marrow large endothelial openings are present. Some capillaries are larger than others, and form preferential or thoroughfare channels. Under normal conditions the blood flows through the thoroughfare channels while flow through the main capillary bed is intermittent, and is regulated by contraction and relaxation of the precapillary sphincters. The small diameter of the capillary lumen causes the erythrocytes to pass along in single file, often becoming distorted, while in the wider arterioles and venules the laminar nature of blood flow ensures that the cellular elements of the blood move as a central closely packed column which is surrounded by a zone of cell-free plasma. This arrangement is called axial flow.

When tissue activity is increased, e.g. in muscular exercise, glandular secretion or intestinal absorption, the precapillary sphincters relax and the capillary bed opens up to meet the metabolic requirements. Blood flow in arterioles and venules is mainly regulated by nervous and humoral stimuli in addition to the intrinsic myogenic activity of the vessel wall. In the terminal vascular bed locally produced metabolites modulate flow by effects on precapillary sphincters and extrinsic factors are only of minor importance.

Changes in Vascular Calibre and Blood Flow in Acute Inflammation

Following injury there may be an immediate **transient constriction** of arterioles which is due to a direct vascular smooth muscle response to the injurious stimulus. However, this does not always occur and is of little importance. The next stage is a widespread dilatation of arterioles and venules and the opening up of many small vessels which had previously been carrying little or no blood – **active hyperaemia**. Blood flow through the injured area may increase as much as tenfold. Initially, flow through the dilated vessels is very rapid and as a consequence, flow becomes turbulent. After mild injury, rapid flow lasts only 10–15 minutes and then returns gradually to normal.

After the phase of increased blood flow, there is a **slowing of blood flow** which eventually leads to **stasis**. The main cause of stasis is the increased viscosity of blood in the microcirculation, and this occurs because the loss of fluid from the post-capillary venules (see next section) results in local haemoconcentration (increase in the haematocrit) as erythrocytes are retained within the vessels. Other factors which may contribute to stasis are (1) plasma leakage with increasing tissue pressure and compression of the small blood vessels, and (2) adhesion of leucocytes to the endothelium causing narrowing of the vessel lumens.

Increased Vascular Permeability and the Formation of the Inflammatory Exudate

The protein-rich fluid which leaves the blood vessels and accumulates at the site of tissue injury is called the inflammatory exudate. The relatively high protein content (35–50 g/1) contains most of the proteins which are present in plasma. On contact with the extravascular tissues, the coagulation system is activated and soluble fibrinogen is converted to insoluble fibrin within the inflamed tissues. The exudate is a rapid turnover pool, being formed by leakage from the microcirculation and being removed by lymphatic drainage (Fig. 4.2). The rate of formation of exudate is influenced by the rise in tissue pressure. In compact tissues or in those with fibrous capsules small volumes of exudate result in rapid increases in tissue pressure, while loose tissues or body cavities can accommodate large volumes of exudate without appreciable rise in tissue pressure.

The formation of an inflammatory exudate depends on the passage of fluid and protein across the walls of the small blood vessels of the microcirculation. Normally in these tissues, diffusion of small molecules occurs along concentration gradients and accounts for transport of materials including oxygen from the blood and waste products such as carbon dioxide from the tissues. For large molecules diffusion is too slow to be of importance. Ultrafiltration accounts for the bulk transfer of fluid and low molecular weight solutes (Fig. 4.3). Starling (1896) showed that this type of fluid transport is governed by the dynamic balance between hydrostatic and colloid osmotic pressures. Under normal circumstances the hydrostatic pressure at the arteriolar end of the capillary bed exceeds the plasma osmotic pressure (due mainly to albumin) so there is a net outflow of fluid. By the time the blood has traversed the microcirculation the intravascular hydrostatic pressure has fallen below the plasma osmotic pressure so that extravascular fluid is drawn into the blood vessels. The outflow and influx of fluid are approximately equal so that

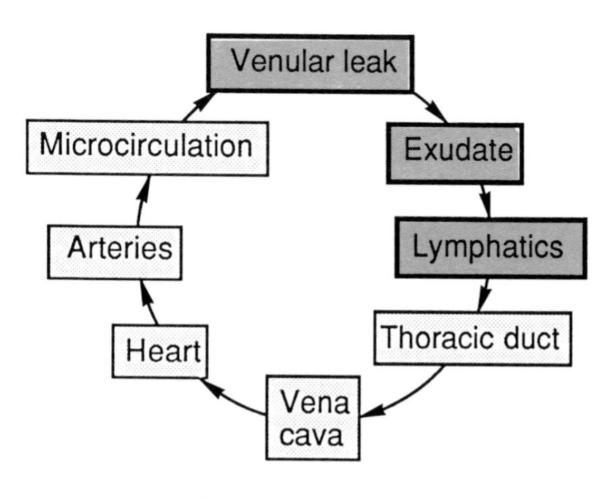

Fig. 4.2 Turnover of the inflammatory exudate.

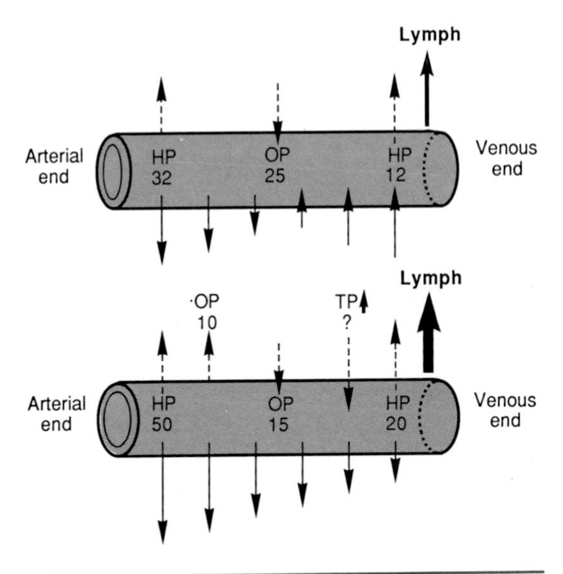

Fig. 4.3 Exchange of fluid by ultrafiltration across the wall of small blood vessels. HP and OP represent the difference between the hydrostatic and colloid osmotic pressures (mmHg) of plasma and extravascular space. The solid arrows indicate the net movement of fluid in and out of vessels along their length. The interrupted arrows indicate the direction of forces exerted by HP, OP and tissue pressure (TP). Upper figure, normal tissue: fluid movement across vessel wall approximates to equilibrium. Lower figure, acute inflammation: much more fluid leaves vessels than is returned to them. The values of HP and OP are approximations. In inflammation, HP may be less than indicated because of rise of TP and OP will also be reduced due to escape of plasma protein (via endothelial gaps) into the extravascular space which increases OP in the extravascular fluid (shown as 10 mmHg). The level of TP varies depending upon the nature of the tissue involved. In loose tissue TP will show no increase, whereas in tissues which are tightly tethered or have fibrous capsules TP can rise considerably (hence the question mark in this figure).

fluid does not accumulate in the extravascular tissues.

In inflammation, arteriolar dilatation results in increased intravascular hydrostatic pressure at the arteriolar end of the microcirculation. Although the hydrostatic pressure drops across the microcirculation, at the venule it still exceeds the plasma osmotic pressure. Thus, fluid leaves the vessels across the entire length of the microcirculation, with little or no reabsorption of extravascular fluid.

Although some protein escapes from small vessels in all normal tissues, it is minimal in those vessels which are lined by a continuous endothelium. Any protein which does reach the extravascular tissue is rapidly returned to the bloodstream by the lymphatics. By contrast, in inflammation large quantities of plasma proteins leave the blood vessels. Originally it was suggested that transport occurred across the endothelial cells in pinocytotic vesicles, but this theory has been largely discounted. It is now considered that in the absence of direct vascular injury, plasma proteins leave the blood vessels between the endothelial cells of post-capillary venules. Vasoactive mediators act on the endothelial cells, causing them to contract, leaving intercellular gaps through which proteins can pass (Fig. 4.4).

Studies of the time-course of vascular leakage have shown three characteristic patterns (Fig. 4.5):

(1) an *immediate transient response* occurring primarily in response to histamine. This may happen as an isolated event in cases of very mild injury or it may precede a phase of more prolonged leakage, such as that occurring in response to mild thermal injury. The immediate transient response begins within minutes of injury, peaks within 30 minutes and vascular integrity is restored within one hour.

(2) *delayed prolonged leakage*. This commonly occurs in response to mild degrees of physical injury such as thermal or ultraviolet burns, X-ray injury, chemical or bacterial toxins or delayed (type IV) hypersensitivity reactions. This type of leakage may be preceded by the immediate transient response. It usually begins after a latent interval of varying duration following the injury and may last many hours. Injury which evokes this type of response does not usually cause obvious tissue necrosis.

(3) the *immediate sustained reaction*, seen after severe injuries such as thermal burns, crushing injuries, the application of high concentrations of chemical or bacterial toxins. Leakage begins immediately and continues for many hours. This type of leakage is due to direct damage to the vascular endothelium of the capillaries (Fig. 4.6). Sometimes leakage also occurs from venules.

Emigration of Leucocytes

Recruitment of leucocytes to the site of tissue injury is an essential feature of the inflammatory response. The polymorphonuclear neutrophil leucocyte (the neutrophil) is the characteristic cell in the early stages of acute inflammation while the monocyte predominates in the later lesions. There are four important stages in the recruitment of cells into the damaged region: (1) margination of leucocytes including their adhesion to the endothelium of the post-capillary venule; (2) passage of the leucocytes through the vessel walls; (3) migration of leucocytes through the tissues to the site of injury; and (4) activation of the leucocytes to promote the phagocytosis of micro-organisms.

Margination of Leucocytes and Endothelial Adhesion

One of the best documented phenomena of acute inflammation is the adherence of leucocytes to the endothelial cells lining the post-capillary venule (Fig. 4.7). This phenomenon is called margination or pavementing as, instead of being present in the central column of cells, the leucocytes are seen at the periphery of the vessel lumen in contact with the endothelium.

Following tissue injury, alterations occur either in the vascular endothelium or in the leucocytes which promote adhesion between these two cell types. Although there is normally some contact between leucocytes and endothelial cells, the flow of blood dislodges any leucocytes which may adhere to the endothelial cells. It is probable that because of slowing of blood flow during acute inflammation, leucocytes sticking to endothelial cells are less likely to be dislodged. However, slowing of blood flow cannot be entirely responsible for this margination process as it begins during the phase of increased blood flow.

It is now known that the **selectins** and **leucocyte integrins**, examples of cell adhesion molecules discussed in Chapter 1, have an important role in leucocyte–endothelial cell interaction in acute inflammation and coagulation. The selectins include endothelial cell adhesion molecule 1 (ELAM-1), leucocyte adhesion molecule 1 (LAM-1) and platelet activation dependent granule external membrane protein (PADGEM) or granule membrane protein-140 (GMP-140). The earliest leucocyte margination appears to occur in response to the expression of GMP-140 on the endothelial cell membrane. Normally, this protein is stored within the Weibel–Palade granules of the endothelial cell but immediately following stimulation by histamine it is translocated to the endothelial cell membrane and acts as a receptor for neutrophils. Up-regulation of ELAM-1 expression on endothelial cells occurs in response to cytokines such as interleukin 1 and gamma interferon (p. 145). ELAM also mediates neutrophil adherence but is probably of greater importance once the inflammatory response has been established. There is specificity in leucocyte–endothelial interactions. For instance, neutrophils and occasionally monocytes and eosinophils adhere to the walls of inflamed venules, while lymphocytes, which express LAM-1, adhere to the high endothelial venules in normal lymphoid tissues and at sites of chronic inflammation. The leucocyte integrins include leucocyte function associated molecule-1 (LFA-1) whose ligands are the intercellular adhesion molecules 1 and 2 (ICAM-1 and ICAM-2). Up-regulation of ICAM-1 expression has been demonstrated in a number of inflammatory conditions, e.g. on hepatocytes in hepatitis and allograft rejection, keratinocytes in inflammatory dermatoses and on thyroid cells in autoimmune thyroiditis. Therefore, these receptor/ligand interactions are likely to be important mechanisms in inflammatory processes.

Leucocyte Emigration and Chemotaxis

Leucocytes escape from venules and small veins but only occasionally from capillaries. Emigration occurs by active amoeboid movement and it has been estimated that a neutrophil takes 2–9 minutes to pass through the vessel wall.

Once the leucocyte has stuck to the endothelial cell, it projects pseudopodia and migrates over the surface until an inter-endothelial cell junction is detected (Fig. 4.8). The leucocyte then insinuates itself between the endothelial cells, before penetrating the basement membrane. The basement membrane may form more of a barrier than the inter-endothelial junctions, as leucocytes are more often seen between endothelial cells and the basement membrane than passing between endothelial cells. During its passage from the lumen to the extravascular tissue the leucocyte disrupts both the inter-endothelial junction and the basement membrane, and although these defects are repaired rapidly, a few red cells may be forced through the gaps by intravascular hydrostatic pressure. The mechanisms of disruption and repair of endothelial cell junctions and the basement membrane are unknown.

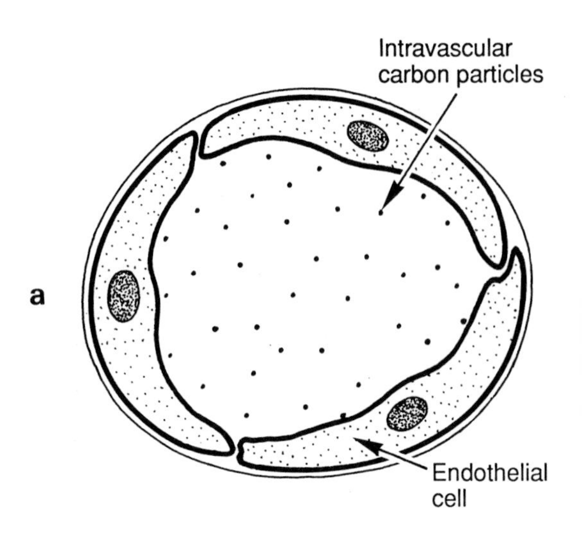

Chemotaxis. Certain bacterial products and inflammatory mediators (known as **chemotaxins**) are able to attract leucocytes towards them. This process is called chemotaxis and is mediated by the interaction of the chemotaxin with specific cell membrane receptors. This interaction stimulates the leucocyte to migrate along the chemical gradient in the direction of increasing concentration. Some inflammatory mediators are not chemotaxins but do stimulate the *random motility* of leucocytes without influencing their *directional motility*. Although chemotactic gradients have been shown to influence the direction and rate of leucocyte movement *in vitro*, the role of chemotaxis in leucocyte migration *in vivo* is uncertain. It is probable that chemotaxins act over extremely short distances (100 nm) to stimulate fine directional movement of phagocytic cells to their targets. Thus, the presence of chemotaxins in injured tissue could simply ensure leucocyte trapping and hence their accumulation.

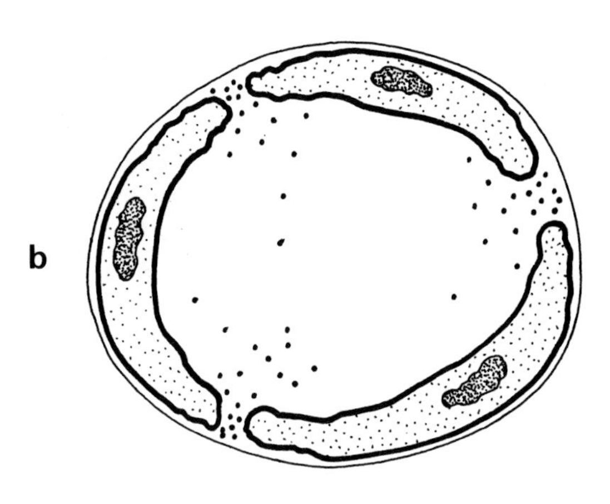

It is important to note that plasma exudation and leucocyte emigration are distinct events. Carbon labelling experiments have shown that massive leucocyte emigration can occur without any increased permeability in the same venule. Thus, it appears that a protein-tight seal can be maintained between endothelial cells and an emigrating leucocyte at all stages of its escape (Fig. 4.8).

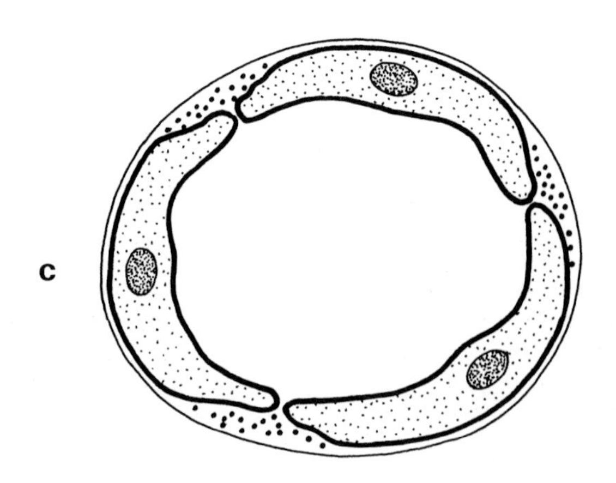

In acute inflammation neutrophils are the predominant cell within the first 24 hours. They begin to accumulate within minutes of injury while mono-

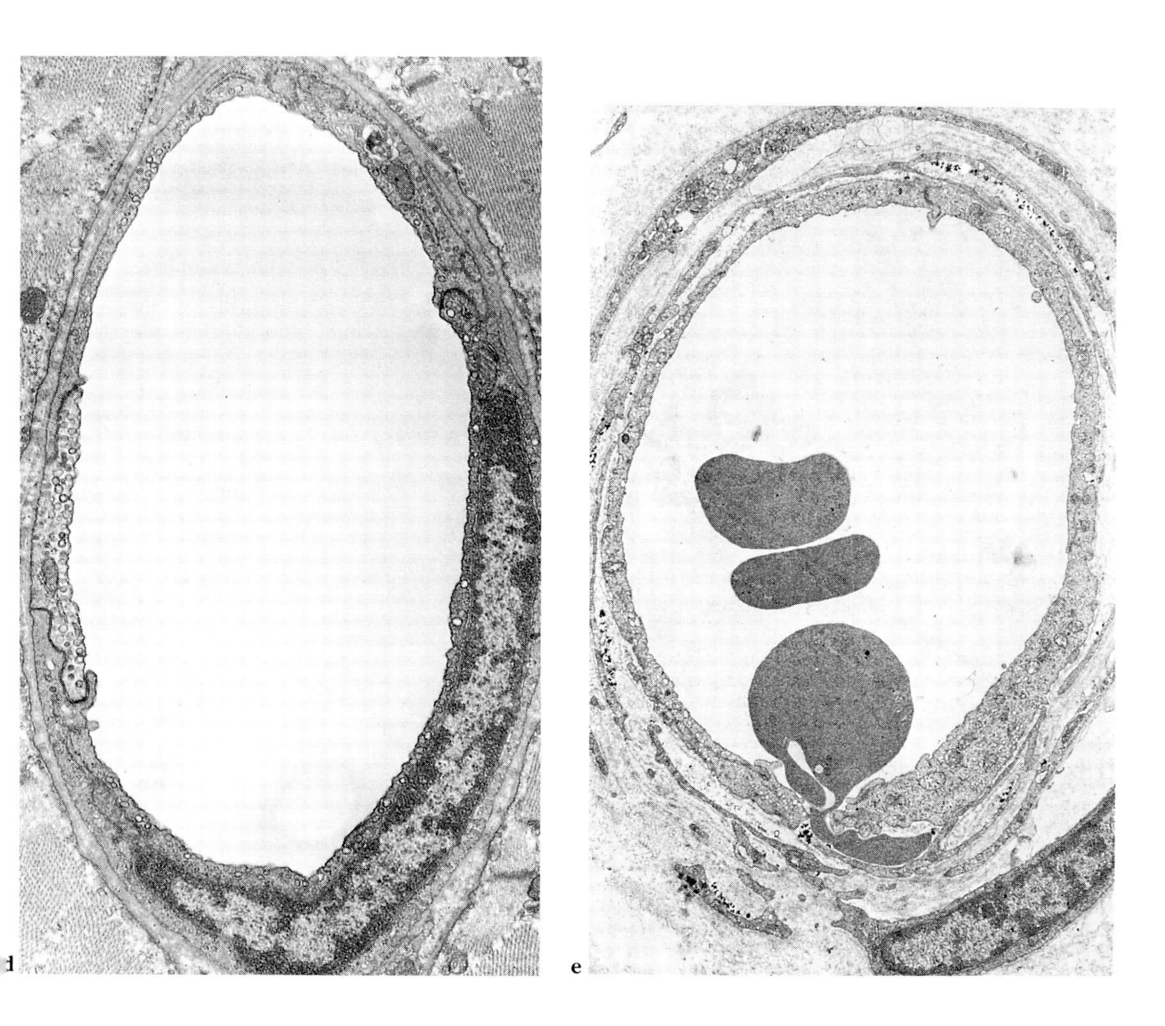

Fig. 4.4 Mechanism of increased vascular permeability in the absence of direct injury to the microcirculation. **a**, **b** and **c** are diagrams which show the sequence of events using carbon labelling. **a** Tightly closed inter-endothelial cell functions with intravascular colloidal carbon. **b** Histamine (and other mediators) induce endothelial cell contraction so that intercellular gaps appear and allow escape of plasma proteins (and colloidal carbon particles). **c** Once the effect of histamine has worn off the endothelial cells relax, the intercellular junctions re-form, and the carbon particles are trapped between the endothelial cells and the basement membrane. Plasma proteins pass through the basement membrane into the extravascular tissues. **d** and **e** are electron micrographs which show the same change occurring in living tissues. **d** Electron micrograph of small blood vessels in skeletal muscle. Note numerous pinocytotic vesicles in endothelial cell cytoplasm and the presence of three closed intercellular injections. ×10 000. (From Miles and Hurley, *Microvascular Research* 1983, **26**, 273.) **e** Electron micrograph of small venule in muscle 2 min after application of histamine solution. A large gap is present in endothelium of normal appearance. Carbon particles and portion of an erythrocyte lie within the gap. ×4500.

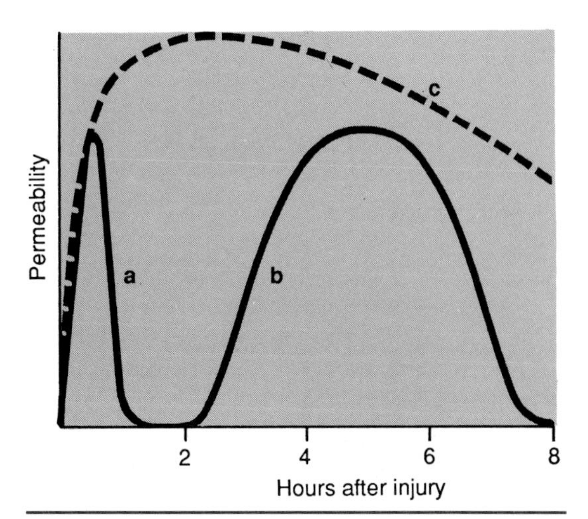

Fig. 4.5 The time-course of the three basic patterns of increased vascular permeability: **a** immediate transient – histamine type; **b** delayed prolonged; **c** immediate sustained – severe direct vascular injury. The time-course illustrated is for mild thermal injury. Other types of injury produce delayed-prolonged leakage with a different time-course.

cytes begin to accumulate later and do not become the predominant cell type until the inflammatory process has been in progress for at least 24 hours. However, this is not invariably true and is in part dependent on the nature of the causative agent. Thus, infection by certain bacteria provokes a sustained neutrophil polymorph infiltrate. In viral infections lymphocytes often predominate, and in certain parasitic infections the eosinophil polymorph predominates.

Activation of Leucocytes, Phagocytosis and Microbial Killing

Having escaped to the site of tissue injury the neutrophils must now undertake active service. They arise from the bone marrow and are released into the blood as end cells, i.e. incapable of further division. They have a short lifespan of 3–4 days. They have a typical multilobed nucleus and

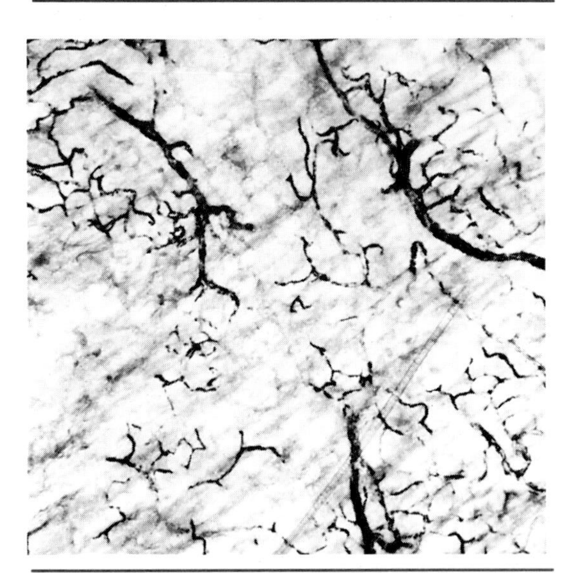

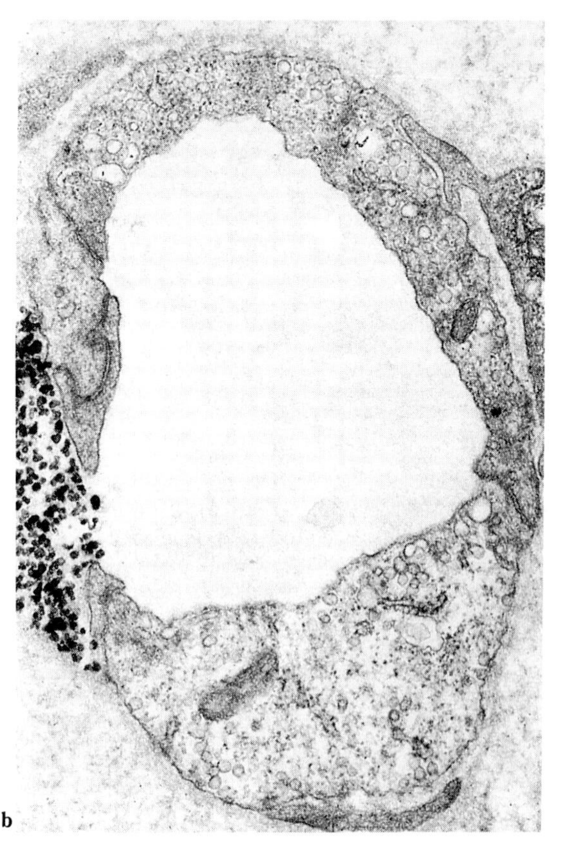

Fig. 4.6 **a** Carbon labelling following experimentally induced burn injury. Carbon deposits are visible in large and small venules, and also in capillaries which form a mesh on the surface of the muscle. Capillaries situated more deeply are also blackened but not visible at this plane of focus. ×28. **b** Electron micrograph of a capillary in rat muscle 3 h after mild thermal injury. An intramural deposit of carbon lies under a large gap in the endothelium which shows gross swelling and mild but definite evidence of injury. ×15 000.

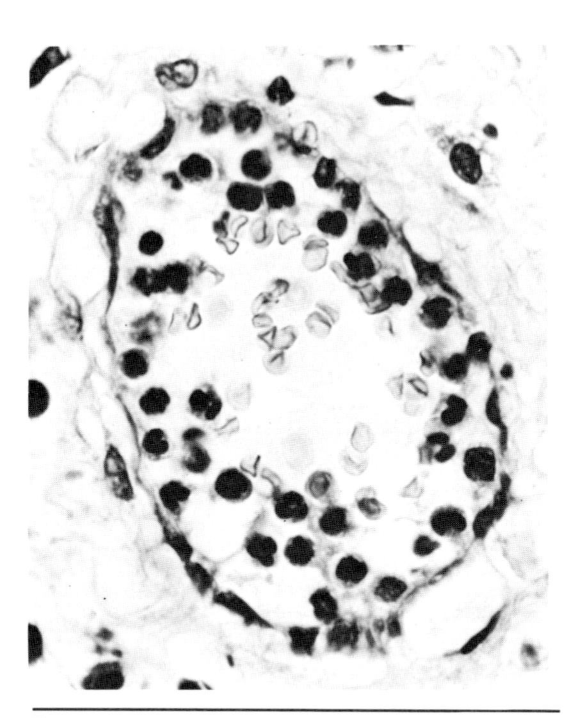

Fig. 4.7 Section of venule in acute inflammation, showing pavementing of neutrophils. ×1000.

possess three types of cytoplasmic granules, termed primary, secondary and tertiary, all of which contain enzymes (Fig. 4.9). Some of these enzymes are bactericidal while others are capable of degrading extracellular matrix proteins (Table 4.1). Many neutrophils die at sites of acute inflammation and release their enzymes which then digest cellular and tissue debris and extravascular fibrin. In sterile inflammation the main role of the neutrophil is the removal of insoluble tissue debris.

Phagocytosis. Phagocytosis (Fig. 4.10) is the process of engulfment and internalization by specialized cells of particulate material which includes invading micro-organisms, damaged cells and tissue debris. These phagocytic cells or phagocytes include polymorphonuclear leucocytes (particularly neutrophils), monocytes and tissue macrophages. Phagocytosis is enhanced if the material to be phagocytosed is coated with certain plasma proteins called **opsonins**, a process termed **opsonization**. Opsonins promote the adhesion between the particulate material and the phagocyte cell membrane. The three major opsonins are: (1) specific antibodies of IgG class; (2) the activated third component of complement (C3b) together with its inactivated form C3bi (p. 142); and (3) plasma fibronectin. Opsonization promotes phagocytosis because opsonins on the material to be phagocytosed are ligands for specific cell membrane receptors on the phagocytes. Thus, IgG binds to receptors for the Fc piece of IgG (Fc receptors), while C3b and C3bi are ligands for C3b and C3bi receptors respectively, and fibronectin binds to fibronectin receptors.

Once attached to the cell membrane of the phagocyte, the particle is engulfed by pseudopodia and enclosed in a membrane bound vesicle termed a **phagocytic vacuole**, or **phagosome**. The membrane lining the phagosome is the external cell membrane which becomes inverted during phagosome formation. As a result of fusion between the phagosome and lysosomes a **phagolysosome** is formed and the engulfed particle is exposed to the degradative lysosomal enzymes which are optimally active at a pH of about 5.0.

Microbial killing. The killing of micro-organisms by neutrophils depends upon oxygen-dependent and oxygen- independent mechanisms. **Oxygen-independent mechanisms** are mediated by some of the constituents of the primary and secondary granules (Table 4.1). It is probable that bacterial killing by lysosomal enzymes is inefficient and relatively unimportant compared with the oxygen-dependent mechanisms. The lysosomal enzymes are, however, essential for the degradation of dead organisms.

The **oxygen-dependent killing** of micro-organisms is due to H_2O_2, free radicals such as superoxide anion, $O_2^{\bar{\cdot}}$, and $OH^{\bullet}$ and possibly singlet oxygen, $^1O_2$. These are formed during the 'respiratory burst' (Fig. 4.11) which follows activation of cell membrane NADPH oxidase by phagocytosis. These events include increased oxygen consumption and activation of the hexose-monophosphate shunt. The respiratory burst can also be activated by low concentrations of chemotactic agents such as C5a or by bacterial lipopolysaccharides. Reduction of molecular oxy-

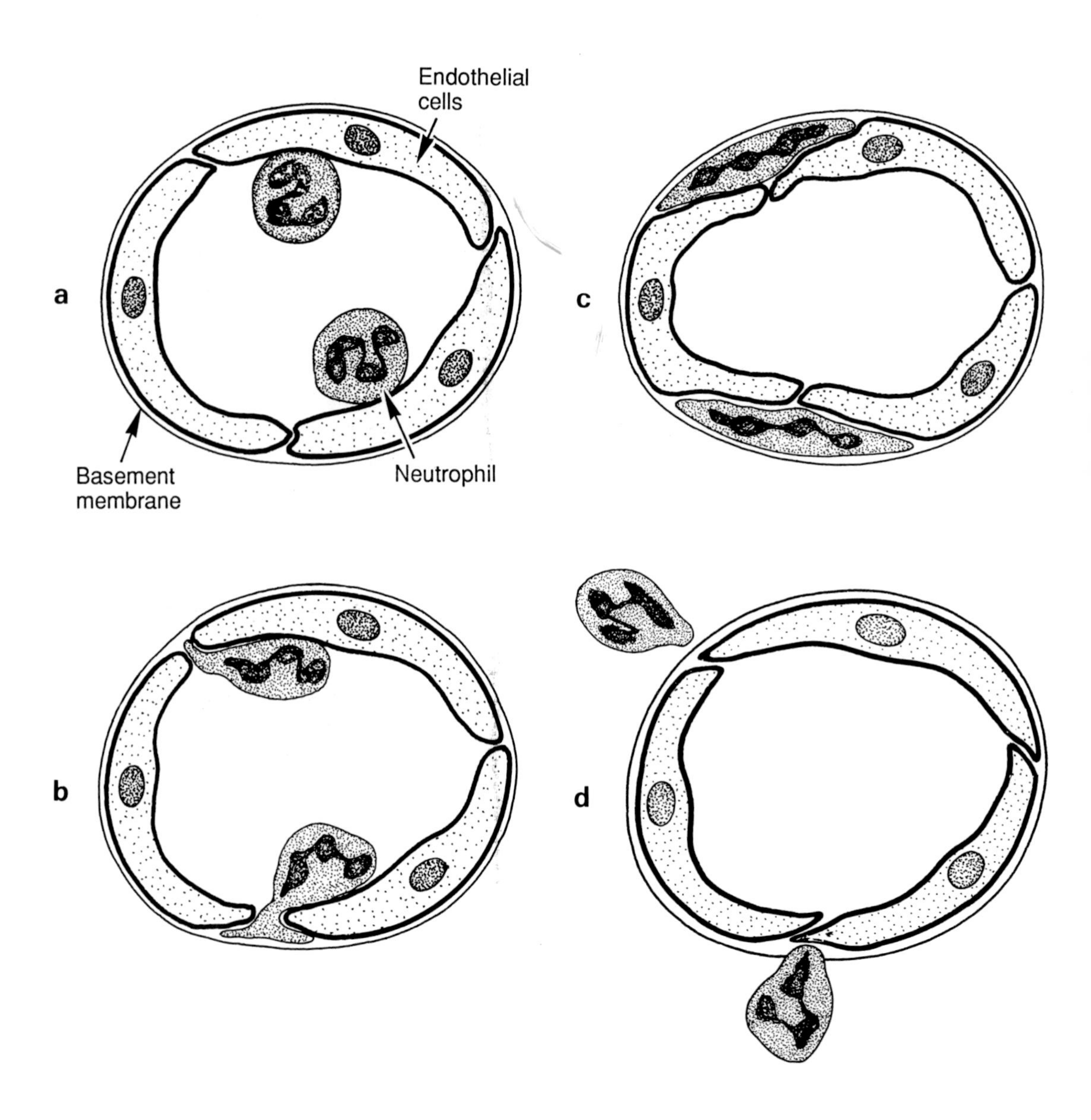

Fig. 4.8 a–d Diagram of events leading to escape of neutrophils from the post-capillary venule in acute inflammation. **a** Adhesion of neutrophils to endothelial cells (margination). **b** The neutrophil throws out pseudopodia to detect inter-endothelial cell junctions. **c** The neutrophil insinuates itself between endothelial cells and comes up against the basement membrane. **d** The neutrophil then passes through the basement membrane and enters the tissues where it migrates to the site of injury. **e–g** Electron micrographs of venules in inflamed muscle showing leucocyte margination and emigration. **e** A leucocyte is intimately apposed to vascular endothelium. A layer of densely stained material covers both endothelium and leucocyte but is absent in the area of contact between the two cells (lanthanum-alcian blue stain) ×9000. **f** A polymorph has inserted a pseudopod (→) into an intercellular junction in the endothelium of the venule. Endothelial-cell cytoplasm appears normal. ×9700. **g** A leucocyte passing through venular endothelium. Densely stained material covers both endothelium and the escaping cell except that part of the leucocyte which lies beneath the surface of the endothelium (lanthanum-alcian blue stain). ×9000.

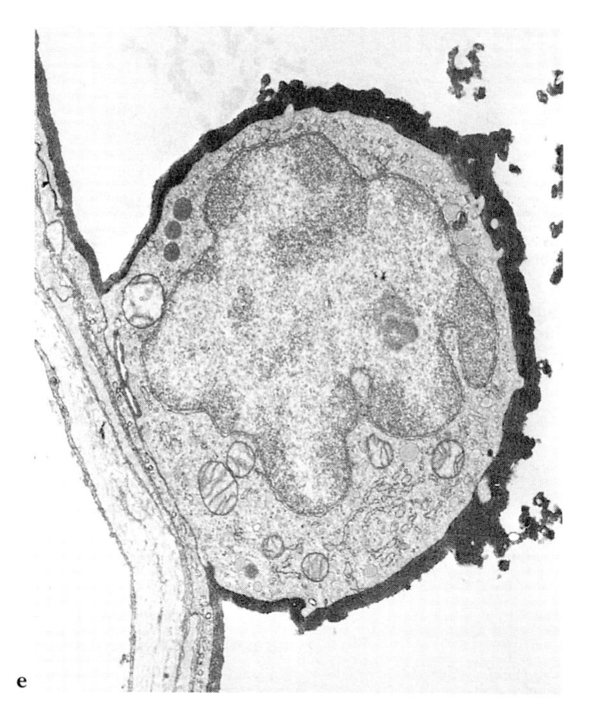
e

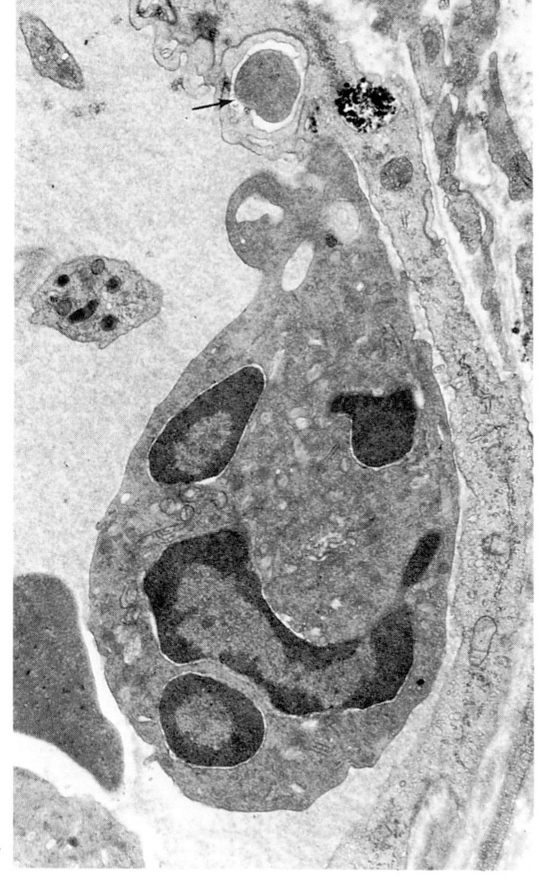
f

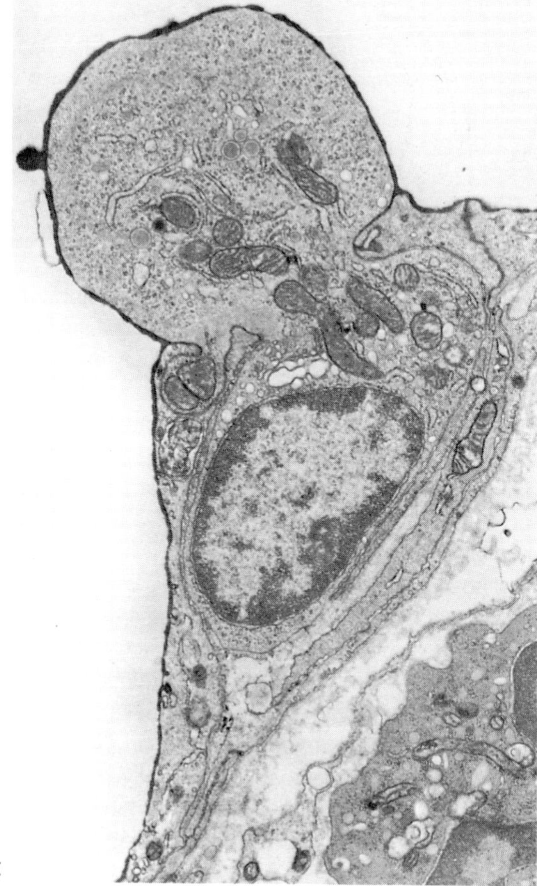
g

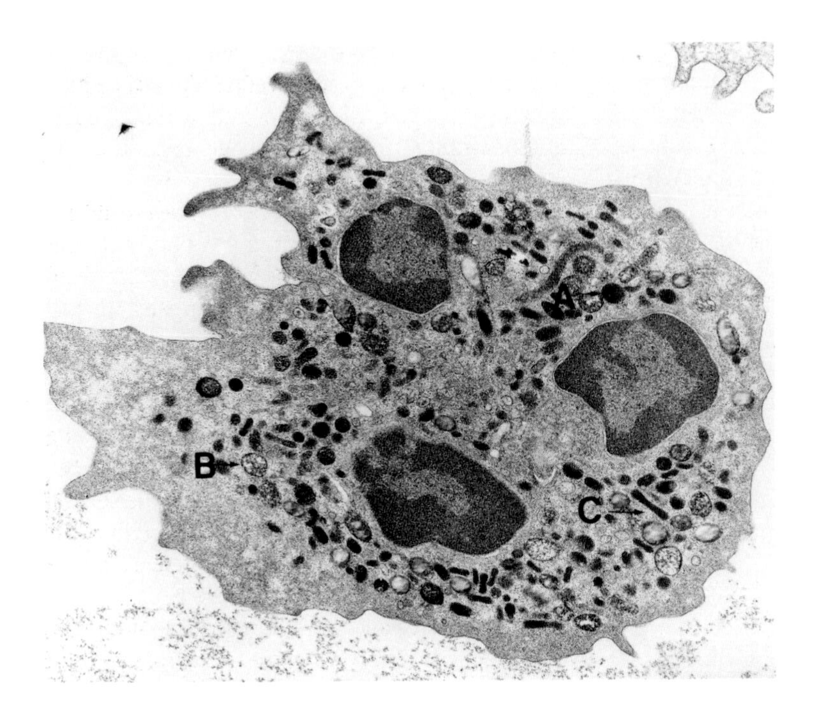

Fig. 4.9 Electron micrograph of neutrophil with different types of granules arrowed: primary granule (A), secondary granule (B), tertiary granule (C).

Table 4.1 Contents of polymorphonuclear leucocyte granules

Primary granules
Lysozyme
Myeloperoxidase
Phospholipase A_2
Elastase
Cathepsins
Acid hydrolases
Cationic protein
Secondary granules
Lysozyme
Phospholipase A_2
Collagenase
Lactoferrin
Alkaline phosphatase
Tertiary granules
Cathepsins
Gelatinase

gen to superoxide anion, O_2^-, by NADPH oxidase accounts for almost all of the increased oxygen consumption which occurs during the respiratory burst. In the phagosome, and on the cell surface, superoxide anion is converted to H_2O_2 by superoxide dismutase. Both superoxide anion and H_2O_2 are powerful bactericidal agents, and both can cause cell injury if they leak out of the phagosome. Glutathione peroxidase, a cytoplasmic enzyme, protects the cell by destroying H_2O_2 which leaks out of the phagosome.

The bactericidal activity of H_2O_2 involves the lysosomal enzyme myeloperoxidase which, in the presence of halide ions, converts H_2O_2 to hypohalous acid (the H_2O_2–halide–myeloperoxidase system). As chlorine is the most abundant halide in biological systems hypochlorous acid (HOCl), a powerful bactericidal agent, is usually produced. H_2O_2 may also be reduced (by the Haber–Weiss reaction) to form the highly reactive hydroxyl radical ($OH^\bullet$).

Apart from their bactericidal effects, these reactive oxygen metabolites, including singlet oxygen, are also capable of initiating injury to cells in the surrounding tissues. Such injury may be contributed to by the escape of lysosomal enzymes from neutrophil granules into tissue during phagocytosis. This unwanted 'side-effect' may play a role in the pathogenesis of several conditions such as adult respiratory distress syndrome (p. 541) and gout (p. 996). In gout, urate crystals which are phagocytosed by neutrophil polymorphs exert a toxic effect on lysosomal membranes and the acute inflammatory reaction in affected joints is due to the resulting release of lysosomal enzymes.

Morphological Features of Acute Inflammation

Although the phenomena of the early stages of acute inflammation always follow a basic pattern there is considerable variation in the macroscopic and microscopic appearances of acutely inflamed tissues. The variation depends, in part, on the relative magnitudes of the fluid and cellular responses to any particular type of injury, but more importantly on the nature and texture of the organ which is inflamed and on the degree of tissue damage produced by the injury which caused the inflammation. The histological features in the various systems are discussed in the systematic chapters and in addition reference is made to them in Chapter 8.

The appearances of mild acute inflammation in the skin form the basis of the cardinal signs and have already been described. More severe injury to the skin may cause local accumulation of exudate in the form of blisters, or loss of a patch of epidermis with the formation of an ulcer. An ulcer is defined as loss of continuity in an epithelial surface. Ulceration may occur in any epithelium; in some instances it is associated with chronic inflammation, notably peptic ulceration (p. 695) and ulcerative colitis (p. 711). Acute inflammation of a hair follicle, usually due to staphylococci, may present as a boil or furuncle in which there is a focal collection of neutrophil polymorphs and tissue debris producing pus – suppuration. A localized accumulation of pus, which is a creamy fluid, yellow or blood-stained and often viscous, constitutes an **abscess**.

The macroscopic characteristics of acute inflammation in serous membranes are very different from those in the skin. The pleura, pericardium and peritoneum are normally thin, shining and transparent. The first recognizable change in acute inflammation of a serous membrane is an enormous increase in the number of visible small blood vessels within the inflamed area, reflecting vasodilatation. Next, the inflamed membrane becomes dull due to deposition of fibrin on the serosal surface. At the same time, clear fluid with a low cell count (**serous exudate**) begins to accumulate in the appropriate cavity. As the inflammation continues, more and more fibrin is deposited until the inflamed surface becomes covered with an opaque creamy layer of fibrin which obscures the underlying tissues, including the still-dilated small blood vessels – fibrinous exudate. The exudate increases in volume and becomes **seropurulent**, i.e. progressively more opaque due to accumulation within it of flakes of fibrin and of neutrophils. If little exudate forms, or what does form is removed rapidly via lymphatics, the parietal and visceral serous layers become stuck together by fibrin. Separation of the adjacent layers imparts a characteristic rough irregular – so-called 'bread and butter' – appearance to the inflamed serous membrane (Fig. 4.12). In some acute bacterial infections, massive emigration of polymorphs results in a **purulent exudate** with pus formation.

Mild inflammation of a mucous membrane is typified by the common cold (coryza). The causal virus multiplies in the epithelial cells of the nasal mucosa and excites an acute inflammatory reaction. This leads to reddening (vasodilatation) and swelling (local accumulation of exudate) of the nasal mucosa, and to the nasal obstruction seen in the early stages of a cold. Some epithelial cells may be killed by the virus and desquamate, producing ulceration. Mucosal glandular cells are stimulated to secrete a thin mucous fluid and this, mixed with exudate leaking from areas of epithelial desquamation, forms the thin, irritant nasal discharge seen in

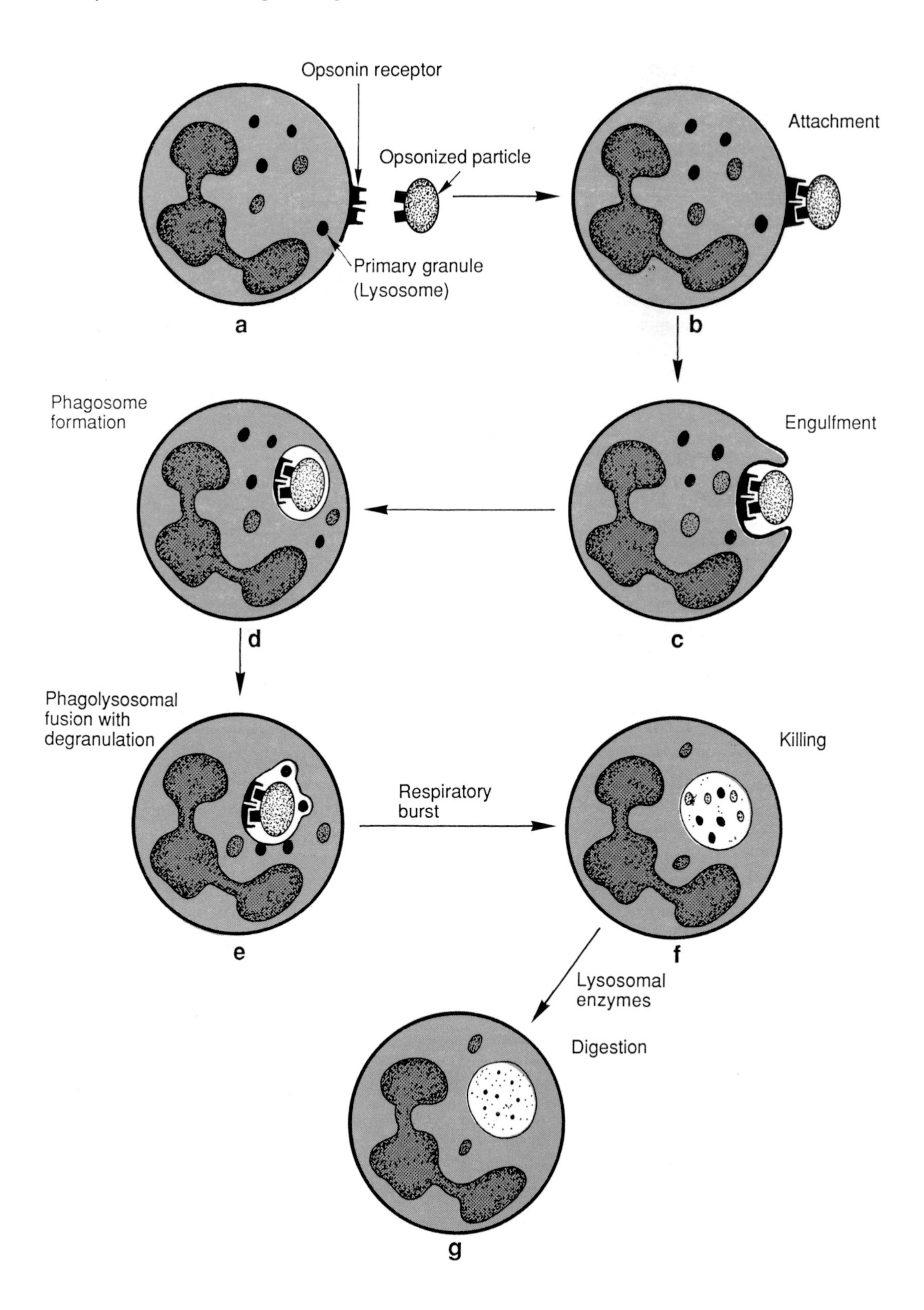
Opsonin receptor
Opsonized particle
Primary granule
(Lysosome)
a
Attachment
b
Phagosome
formation
Engulfment
d
c
Phagolysosomal
fusion with
degranulation
Respiratory
burst
Killing
e
f
Lysosomal
enzymes
Digestion
g

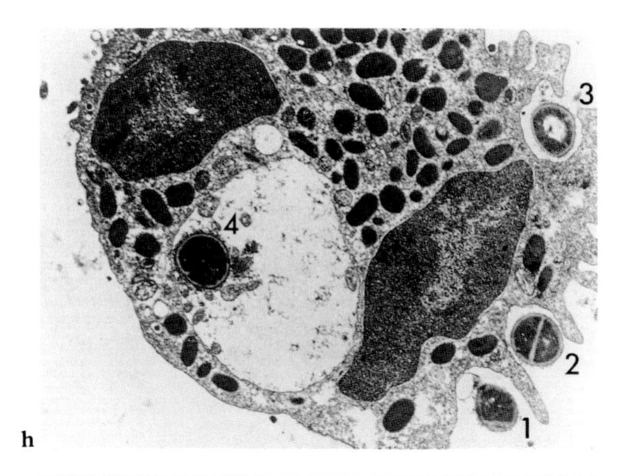

Fig. 4.10 Phagocytosis and killing of micro-organism. **a** The micro-organism is opsonized with antibody or complement. **b** The opsonized particle becomes attached to neutrophil membrane receptors for the opsonin. **c** Engulfment. **d** The opsonized micro-organism is internalized into a phagocytic vacuole (phagosome). **e** Fusion of the lysosomes (primary granules) with the phagosome allows the discharge of lysosomal enzymes into the phagolysosome and **f** triggers the respiratory burst which results in bacterial killing. **g** Lysosomal enzymes degrade the dead micro-organism. **h** Electron micrograph of phagocytosis and killing of *Staphylococcus aureus* by a neutrophil. 1, 2 & 3 are different stages of engulfment of micro-organisms leading to their presence in a phagolysosome (4).

the early stages of a cold. Bacteria may colonize and multiply within the bare areas of mucosa and aggravate the inflammation. The nasal discharge becomes increasingly purulent due to emigration of large numbers of neutrophil polymorphs until it consists of a mixture of mucous secretion and pus. When the infection is finally overcome, the inflammatory reaction ceases and the denuded areas of epithelium are restored by proliferation and migration of surviving epithelial cells. If the injury to a mucous membrane is severe enough to cause extensive epithelial necrosis, the dead cells separate and large shallow ulcers are formed. This more severe type of inflammation of mucous membranes is termed **pseudomembranous inflammation**; diphtheritic infection of the pharynx or larynx used to be the commonest example but nowadays this type of reaction is seen most often in the large bowel following infection with *Clostridium difficile* (p. 709). The basic elements of pseudomembranous inflammation are extensive confluent necrosis of surface epithelium and severe acute inflammation of underlying tissues. The fibrinogen in the inflammatory exudate coagulates within the necrotic epithelium and, together with neutrophil polymorphs, red cells, bacteria and tissue debris, constitutes the false (pseudo) membrane, which forms a white or cream-coloured layer over the surface of the inflamed mucosa.

Uncomplicated acute inflammation makes little difference to the macroscopic appearance of solid organs such as liver and kidney. These organs normally contain so much blood that vasodilatation is impossible to detect, and their dense texture and firm fibrous capsule ensure that very little exudate can accumulate without causing sufficient rise in tissue pressure to limit further leakage of fluid from small blood vessels. Only when acute inflammation is accompanied by large areas of tissue necrosis or has progressed to the formation of pus can it be recognized macroscopically with confidence in these vascular solid organs. Thus, in the kidney 'streaks' of pus may be evident in the medulla in acute pyelonephritis (p. 917) and in the liver, abscesses may develop as a feature of acute suppurative cholangitis (p. 769).

In contrast, since the lung is a collection of intercommunicating air-filled spaces, large amounts of inflammatory exudate can form and pass from alveolus to alveolus via airways and inter-alveolar pores without causing any rise in tissue pressure. Acute inflammation in the lung is therefore usually associated with the formation of a large volume of exudate. In lobar pneumonia alveoli within one lobe fill rapidly with exudate and inflammatory cells. The fluid component is subsequently resorbed by lymphatics, leaving a pale solid area of lung with a dry granular surface. Histologically, the alveoli are filled with fibrin and neutrophil polymorphs.

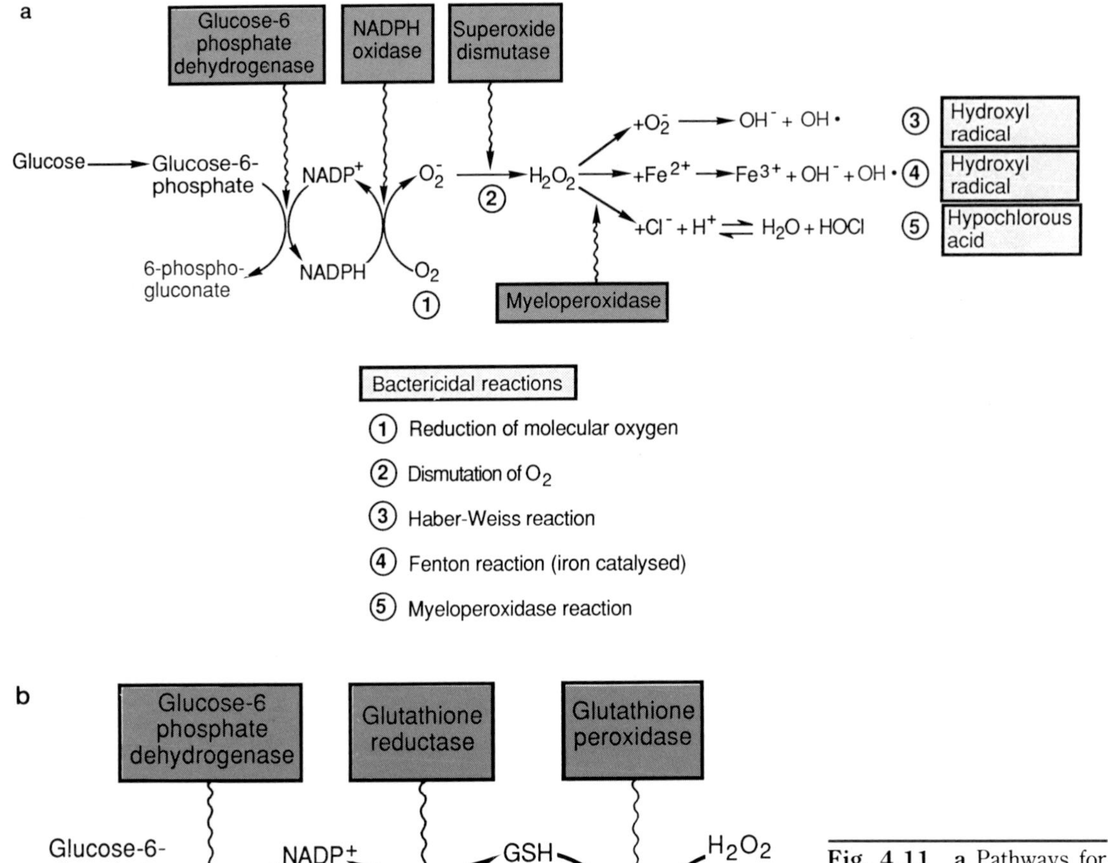

Fig. 4.11 **a** Pathways for oxygen-dependent killing of micro-organisms by neutrophils. **b** Mechanism for detoxification of hydrogen peroxide in neutrophil cytoplasm. GSH, reduced glutathione; GSSG, oxidized glutathione.

Effects of the Acute Inflammatory Reaction

It must by now be clear to the student that the acute inflammatory response is a complex, carefully modulated reaction. Before discussing in further detail how this is mediated, it is perhaps as well to pause and summarize the effects of acute inflammation. Inflammation is overwhelmingly beneficial; it helps to eliminate invasive micro-organisms, limits the injurious effects of irritating chemicals and bacterial toxins, and participates in the removal of necrotic cells and tissue debris. However, acute inflammation is not without its disadvantages, and in some instances it seems positively harmful. While many of the effects are observed in the localities of the tissue injury, these are often accompanied by systemic effects. Systemic effects may also accompany chronic in-

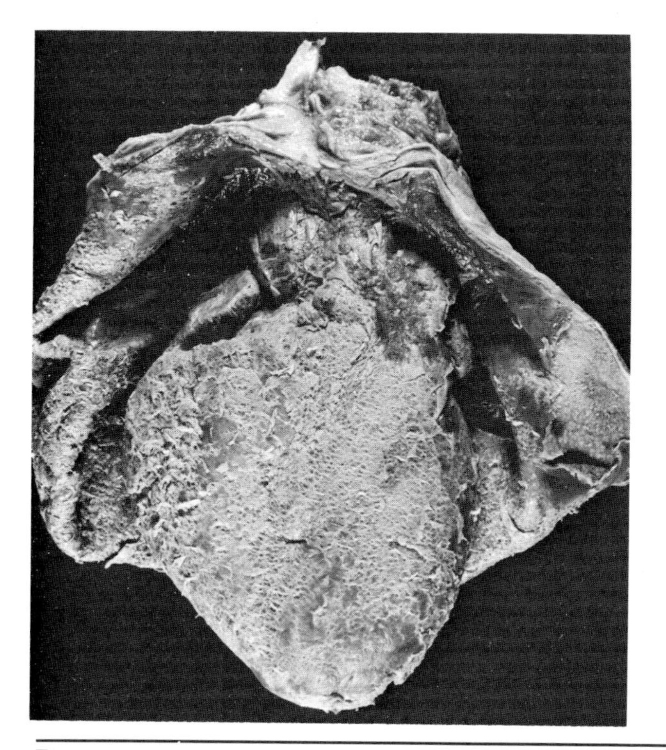

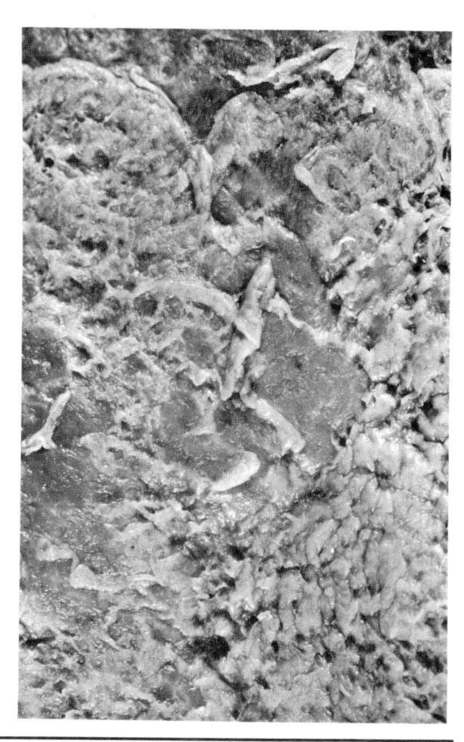

Fig. 4.12 Acute pericarditis; showing a thick, irregular deposit of fibrin on the pericardial surface. The appearance has been likened to that when a butter sandwich is pulled apart ('bread and butter' pericarditis). Left, ×0.7. Right, ×3.

flammation and this topic is therefore discussed later.

Beneficial Effects of Acute Inflammation

These are conferred partly by the flow of exudate through the inflamed tissues and partly by the phagocytic and microbicidal effects of emigrated leucocytes. The fluid exudate is protective in the following ways.

Dilution of toxins. The concentration of chemical and bacterial toxins at the site of inflammation is reduced by dilution in the exudate and by its removal from the site by the flow of the exudate from the venule through the tissues to the lymphatics.

Protective antibodies. Exudation results in the presence of plasma proteins at the site of inflammation. In an immune individual this will include antibodies. Thus, in acute inflammation due to infection, antibodies directed against the causative organism will react with them and promote their destruction by phagocytosis or by complement mediated lysis. Bacterial toxins are neutralized by specific antitoxins.

Fibrin formation. Fibrinogen in the exudate is converted to fibrin by the action of tissue thromboplastin. A network of deposited fibrin delays bacterial spread and may facilitate their phagocytosis by leucocytes.

Plasma mediator systems. Along with antibodies and fibrinogen, the exudate contains the proteins of the plasma mediator systems (complement, coagulation, fibrinolytic and kinin systems). This ensures a constant supply of mediators to maintain the inflammatory response.

Cell nutrition. The flow of inflammatory exudate brings with it glucose, oxygen and other nutrients to meet the metabolic requirements of the greatly increased numbers of cells. It also removes their soluble waste products via lymphatic channels.

Promotion of immunity. Micro-organisms and their toxins are carried by the exudate, either free or in phagocytes, along the lymphatics to the local lymph nodes where they stimulate an immune response with the generation of antibodies and the cellular mechanisms of defence (Chapter 5). The immune response occurs within a few days and may be maintained for years.

The beneficial role of leucocytes in phagocytosis and microbial killing has been dealt with above.

Harmful Effects of Acute Inflammation

Swelling of acutely inflamed tissues may have serious mechanical effects. For example, in acute laryngitis, obstruction to the lumen of the larynx may occur and interfere with breathing. Acute inflammation of tissues may impair function directly or may interfere with blood flow and so cause ischaemic injury. Examples include inflammation of the brain (encephalitis) or meninges (meningitis), both of which cause increased intracranial pressure which may lead to coma and death; also ischaemic necrosis of bone occurring during acute osteomyelitis (p. 963). In other instances inflammation may be regarded as inappropriate, e.g. type I hypersensitivity reactions (hay fever and asthma p. 208), type III hypersensitivity reactions (glomerulonephritis p. 896) and type IV hypersensitivity reactions (organ specific autoimmune diseases p. 227).

Subsequent Course of the Acute Inflammatory Reaction

Resolution

The optimal end result of an acute inflammatory reaction is complete restitution of the normal structure and function of an injured tissue, a process which is referred to as resolution. It requires: (1) removal of the inflammatory exudate, fibrin and cellular debris; (2) reversal of the changes in the microvasculature; and (3) replacement of any specialized cells lost as a result of the injury. This outcome will only be achieved if the injurious agent is removed. Furthermore, although some tissues show remarkable powers of regeneration, true resolution will generally only occur where there has been minimal necrosis of specialized cells or damage to the surrounding matrix.

When the injurious agent has been overcome, the release of chemical mediators of inflammation is reduced and consequently the stimuli for vasodilatation, increased vascular permeability and cellular recruitment are reduced. As vasodilatation subsides, the balance of hydrostatic and osmotic forces across the wall of small blood vessels returns to its normal resting state and some of the inflammatory exudate is reabsorbed into the venular end of the capillaries. However, the bulk of the fluid and all the protein in the exudate are removed through the lymphatics. Lymph drainage from an area of acute inflammation is greatly increased in both volume and protein content, and reactive changes develop in the draining lymph node (p. 651). Most of the infiltrating neutrophils die locally, but some leave by the lymphatics. As noted above, the release of reactive oxygen metabolites and enzymes by neutrophils during phagocytosis will produce further tissue damage and release of enzymes after their death contributes to their own digestion. Similarly, dead tissue cells undergo partial digestion by their own lysosomal enzymes as well as those released by neutrophils and macrophages.

As neutrophils disappear, monocytes and macrophages come to form an increasing proportion of the cells in the inflamed tissue, eventually replacing all the neutrophils. They are actively phagocytic and take up and degrade much of the debris of cells and tissues which have been destroyed in inflammatory lesions. This is often referred to as the **demolition phase** of inflammation, and in some of the mechanisms involved there is overlap with some of the features of chronic inflammation.

Most of the fibrin deposited in the extravascular spaces is broken down by fibrinolytic enzymes in the exudate and the soluble fibrin degradation products (FDPs) are removed by the lymphatics. A relatively small amount of fibrin is engulfed by macrophages. Plasmin is the principal compound responsible for the fibrinolytic activity of the inflammatory exudate. It exists as an inactive precursor, plasminogen. This is enzymatically activated by plasminogen activator which is present in plasma but may also be synthesized by macrophages. Certain bacteria also synthesize powerful fibrinolysins.

One of the best examples of virtually complete resolution is that seen in some forms of lobar pneumonia (e.g. pneumococcal pneumonia, p. 555). Here the presence of bacteria within alveoli elicits an acute inflammatory response with vasodilatation of the alveolar microvasculature, exudation of fluid and deposition of fibrin in the air spaces followed by the accumulation of neutrophil polymorphs. In spite of the intense inflammation, there is little associated damage to the alveolar walls. Some 72 hours after the initial changes, there is an influx of macrophages, heralding the onset of the demolition phase. These cells remove the fibrin and debris from degenerate polymorphs. They themselves subsequently leave via the lymphatics of the alveolar bed and the appearances can return virtually to normal.

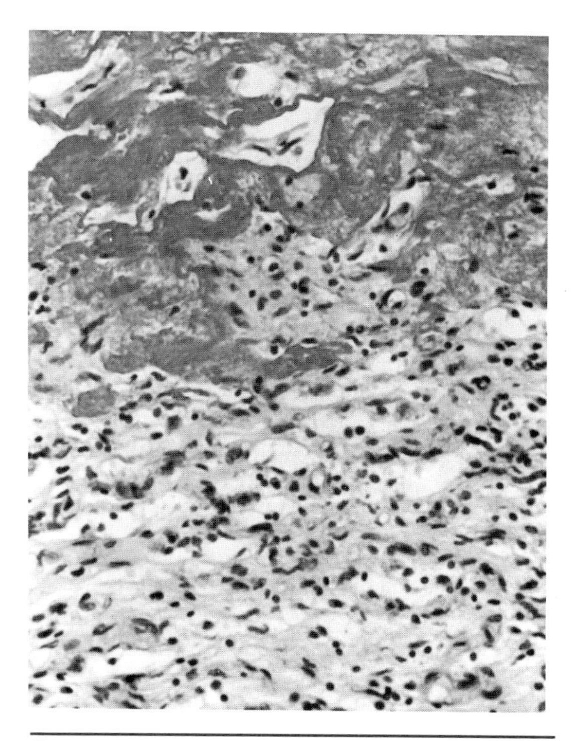

Fig. 4.13 A dense layer of fibrin on the pleural surface, showing organization, i.e. replacement by vascular granulation tissue, extending from the underlying pleura. ×250.

Healing by Fibrosis

Fibrosis, or scar formation, may result from acute inflammation in three circumstances.

(1) If heavy deposits of fibrin are formed during the early stages of acute inflammation they may not be removed completely within a few days by the fibrinolytic enzymes of the inflammatory exudate. Fibrin which is not removed undergoes a process called organization (Fig. 4.13). Macrophages migrate into the fibrin and are closely followed by ingrowth of new capillaries and fibroblasts – **granulation tissue**. This should not be confused with the term granuloma which refers to a form of macrophage response in chronic inflammation. The granulation tissue thus formed gradually changes to dense fibrous tissue. Organization of fibrin is a common sequel to acute inflammation of serous membranes, the synovial membrane of joints or the endothelium of heart valves. Adjacent surfaces initially glued together by fibrin become united by granulation tissue and eventually by firm, almost avascular fibrous tissue. Organization is also the process by which extravascular haematomas, intravascular thrombus and necrotic material are removed.

(2) If the injury causes death to a substantial amount of tissue, the mechanism of removal of the dead tissue depends on its nature. With highly cellular tissue, e.g. myocardium, the dead tissue is rapidly degraded by lysosomal enzymes, leaving a

deficit containing exudate, neutrophils and cellular debris which undergoes organization as just described and healing takes place by replacement fibrosis. Other dead tissue, e.g. fibrous tissue, is digested extremely slowly and, like dense deposits of fibrin, is also gradually replaced by organization with fibrous scarring.

(3) Progression of acute to chronic inflammation is always accompanied by fibrosis.

Suppuration

Suppuration, the formation of pus, is a common sequel of acute inflammation. Suppurative lesions are characterized by an exudate containing large numbers of neutrophils which, together with dead tissue cells, break down to form a thick, creamy, yellow or blood-stained fluid called pus. An **abscess** is a localized or discrete focus of pus. However, pus may occur diffusely in loose tissues or body cavities. Pus consists of living, dead and disintegrated neutrophils, living and dead micro-organisms and the debris of tissue cells, all suspended in the inflammatory exudate. Bacterial infection is the usual cause of suppuration and such bacteria are said to be pyogenic (pus forming) and include *Staphylococcus aureus, Streptococcus pyogenes, Streptococcus pneumoniae, Neisseria gonorrhoeae, Neisseria meningitides, Escherichia coli* and related Gram-negative bacilli.

The mode of development of an abscess can be appreciated by describing the events which follow infection by pyogenic bacteria, e.g. *Staphylococcus aureus* in the formation of a skin boil or furuncle. Initially, rapidly multiplying bacteria release toxins which damage tissue cells in the dermis. Both the toxins and the contents released from damaged cells provoke a severe inflammatory reaction. Eventually, when the toxin concentration is sufficiently great, the centre of the inflamed area dies. There is a massive influx of neutrophils into the oedematous tissues, but many of these cells die and release enzymes which produce rapid liquefaction of the dead tissue and within 48 hours of the onset of the infection, there is a ragged cavity filled with pus in the centre of an area of acutely inflamed tissue (Fig. 4.14).

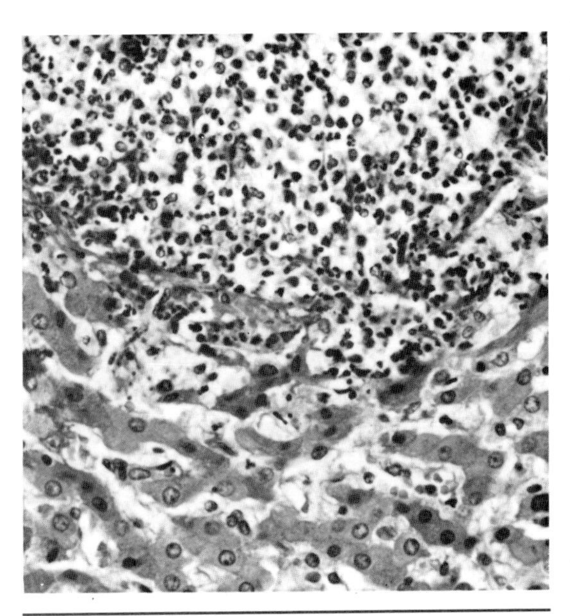

Fig. 4.14 Margin of an abscess cavity in the liver at an early stage in its formation. In the upper part of the field the liver tissue has been destroyed and digested, leaving a space filled with purulent exudate. ×250.

The continued proliferation of bacteria, with continued plasma exudation and accumulation of neutrophils, together with further neutrophil and tissue cell death, results in the size of the abscess cavity and the volume of pus increasing. Simultaneous with these changes, repair processes commence in the surrounding tissue and a layer of granulation tissue, the pyogenic membrane, begins to form around the abscess, separating it from the adjacent inflamed tissue. If the repair process is successful in limiting the extension of infection, the abscess eventually becomes lined by a well defined layer of granulation tissue with a thin band of collagen on the outer side. If the abscess does not burst or is not drained surgically, the layer of collagen thickens progressively. Inflammation in the surrounding tissue subsides, but neutrophils still escape into the abscess cavity from the newly formed blood vessels in the granulation tissue. In some cases this may proceed to abscess formation.

Abscesses may also form when pyogenic bacteria infect a body cavity. An example is acute appendicitis spreading to the peritoneal surface, where the inflamed part of the peritoneal cavity may become walled off from the rest of the peritoneal cavity by fibrinous adhesions. Fibrin glues the adjacent serous surfaces together and, aided by the omentum, a cavity containing the appendix, bacteria, inflammatory exudate and neutrophils is formed.

The contents of an abscess may be under considerable pressure, due to the rapid increase in the volume of the pus and the relatively unyielding surrounding tissues. Pressure accounts for most of the intense pain associated with an abscess. Because it is under pressure, pus tends to track along the line of least resistance and to be discharged on to a body surface, after which the abscess cavity collapses. Residual bacteria are eliminated by neutrophils and organization occurs with scar formation. Surgical drainage anticipates spontaneous discharge and thereby hastens the healing process.

Progression to Chronic Inflammation

Long continued tissue injury, such as persistence of micro-organisms in a focus of infection, results in progression of acute inflammation to chronic inflammation.

Chronic Inflammation

Inflammation is said to be chronic if it persists for weeks or months after the initial injury. The histological appearances of chronic inflammation differ from those of acute inflammation in two important respects: (1) there is frequently greater tissue destruction and the inflammatory infiltrate is characteristically a mixture of macrophages, lymphocytes, and plasma cells. Although neutrophils may be present (e.g. in chronic abscesses) they are much less prominent than in classical acute inflammatory reactions; and (2) the inflammatory reaction is usually more productive than exudative, i.e. the production of new fibrous tissue through formation of granulation tissue is more prominent than exudation of fluid. Chronic inflammation may arise in three ways as follows.

Progression from acute inflammation. When chronic inflammation supervenes on acute inflammation it almost always occurs against a background of persistent suppuration, for instance when an abscess remains undrained, or if foreign material is present within the inflamed area. If an abscess remains undrained the fibrous wall becomes thicker and more rigid and cannot collapse when drainage occurs. The residual cavity can only be replaced by ingrowth of granulation tissue from its walls. If due to inadequate drainage, pus stagnates within the abscess cavity, residual bacteria may multiply and reactivate the inflammatory process. Good examples of chronic abscesses are those which occur after delayed or inadequate draining of an empyema in the pleural cavity, or whenever an abscess forms in bone.

Foreign material which is driven in from outside (e.g. dirt, cloth, wood) may cause persistent suppuration, as may surgically implanted metallic or plastic prostheses. Indigestible, dead or damaged tissue may have the same effect as a foreign body. For instance, in boils and carbuncles, dermal collagen is damaged by bacterial toxins and is broken down only slowly by lysosomal enzymes. A piece of dead bone (sequestrum) in osteomyelitis is another example of a persistent endogenous 'foreign body'. The presence of a foreign body acts as a continuing inflammatory stimulus; its removal results in healing.

If a deep seated abscess continues to drain on to the skin or some other epithelial surface a sinus tract is formed. This has to be distinguished from a fistula in which a communication is formed between two epithelial surfaces, e.g. a gastrocolic fistula; such fistulae are also likely to be the site of continuing inflammation.

Recurrent episodes of acute inflammation. Some forms of chronic inflammation result from repeated bouts of acute inflammation. A good example of this is chronic cholecystitis (inflammation of the gallbladder) which is almost invariably associated with the presence of gallstones. In some patients the clinical picture is characterized by recurrent episodes of acute inflammation manifest by upper abdominal pain and systemic effects, fever and leucocytosis. Healing occurs between attacks but in time the histological appearances may show an admixture of acute and chronic inflammation. The term **continuing inflammation** is sometimes used to describe this situation.

***Chronic inflammation* ab initio.** Many types of injury may produce a chronic inflammatory reaction from the outset. Prolonged exposure to non-degradable but potentially toxic substances, such as silica or asbestos, is responsible for some examples. Certain micro-organisms, particularly those associated with intracellular infection (tuberculosis, leprosy, viruses), characteristically cause chronic inflammation. Fungal infections are also commonly associated with chronic inflammation. In other diseases characterized by chronic inflammation, such as rheumatoid arthritis and chronic inflammatory bowel disease, the cause is unknown, but immune mechanisms mediated by delayed (type IV) hypersensitivity reactions (p. 219) are thought to play an important pathogenetic role.

Morphological Features of Chronic Inflammation

The macroscopic features of chronic inflammation are extremely variable. Common forms which may be seen alone or in combination include: a chronic abscess; a persistent sinus; a chronic ulcer such as peptic ulcer of the stomach or a varicose ulcer; diffuse thickening of the wall of a hollow viscus such as in chronic cholecystitis or more localized thickening to form an inflammatory stricture of the bowel; a fistula; and chronic granulomatous inflammation which may be accompanied by caseation.

The microscopic features have already been outlined briefly but we must now deal with the many different cell types which may be present: macrophages and their derivatives (epithelioid cells and giant cells), lymphocytes, plasma cells, neutrophil and eosinophil polymorphs and fibroblasts. Indeed, the presence of a mixture of cell types is the most characteristic histological feature of chronic inflammation.

Macrophages are part of the mononuclear phagocytic system and are derived from bone marrow haemopoietic cells (Fig. 4.15). They circulate in the blood as monocytes and after leaving the circulation through post-capillary venules they become either free-tissue macrophages or fixed-tissue macrophages. The former migrate through the loose connective tissues of the peritoneum, lymphoid tissues, pulmonary alveoli and brain (microglia). In contrast, fixed-tissue macrophages stay in a single organ for most of their lifespan. These cells are present in the sinusoids of the liver (Kupffer cells), spleen and bone marrow and the lymphatic sinuses of lymph nodes. Osteoclasts of bone and the interdigitating dendritic cells of the lymphoid tissues and spleen are also probably derived from monocytes.

As stated above, monocytes are involved in resolution of the acute inflammatory response and are then removed by lymphatics. However, in chronic inflammation there is continued recruitment of monocytes from the circulation and this depends on the increased expression of adhesion molecules on endothelial cell membranes in response to cytokines such as interleukin 1 (IL-1) and the release of chemotactic factors such as C5a and leukotriene B_4. The prolonged survival of macrophages also contributes to the increased number of cells; if the causative agent is toxic to cells they may survive for only a few days but with some agents individual cells may survive for weeks or months. Local proliferation may also occur but is thought to be of only minor importance in most forms of chronic inflammation.

At sites of inflammation macrophages become 'activated' and this is predominantly in response to the cytokine interferon-γ. Activated macrophages (Fig. 4.16) are larger than resting macrophages, they show increased protein synthesis, have an increased content of lysosomal enzymes and increased phagocytic and bactericidal activities. A list of some macrophage secretory products which

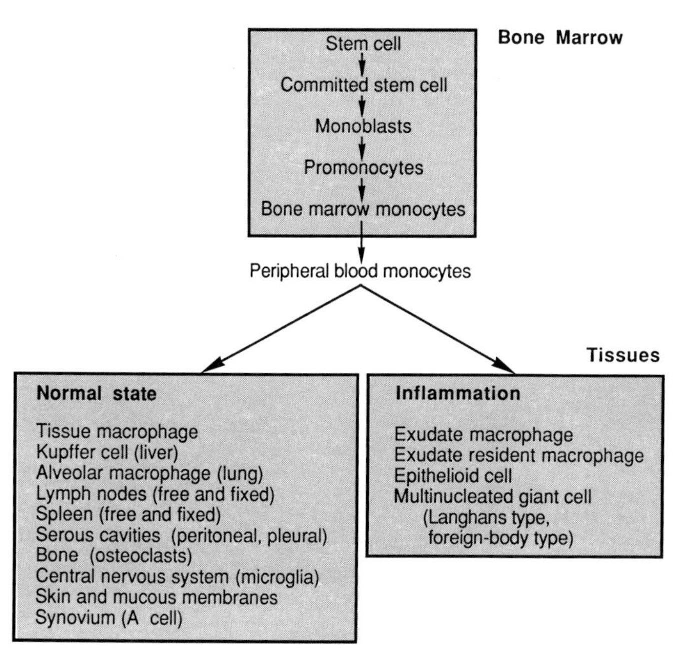

Fig. 4.15 Production of mononuclear phagocytes. Some of the progeny of multipotent stem cells in the bone marrow give rise to monoblasts which undergo division and become promonocytes which then in turn differentiate into monocytes in the bone marrow. After leaving the bone marrow, the monocytes circulate in the peripheral blood before entering the tissues where they differentiate into macrophages. In the normal state they become resident or tissue macrophages, but in inflammation they undergo activation to become macrophages and in some cases may become epithelioid or multinucleated giant cells. Exudate macrophages are monocytes which have migrated into an inflammatory lesion and become activated, whereas exudate resident macrophages are initially resident macrophages which have then been activated at the site of inflammation.

contribute to the inflammatory response is given in Table 4.2. The cytokines, particularly interleukin 1 (IL-1), are important mediators of leucocyte–endothelial cell interaction, they activate lymphocytes and contribute to modulation of the repair process.

Macrophages can engulf a far wider range of foreign materials than neutrophils and are much more efficient scavengers of inflammatory debris. Foreign body material and certain micro-organisms by virtue of their capsular proteins (e.g. mycobacteria and *Histoplasma capsulatum*) may survive in macrophages for long periods, resulting in phenotypic changes with the formation of epithelioid cells and giant cells as part of chronic granulomatous inflammation.

Other cell types. **Lymphocytes** and **plasma cells** are often present indicating a continuing immune response at the site of chronic inflammation. T lymphocytes secrete cytokines which are chemotactic for monocytes and which activate macrophages and fibroblasts. Lymphocytes migrate into areas of chronic inflammation through venules in which the endothelial cells have differentiated into high endothelial cells similar to those observed in lymph nodes and spleen (Fig. 4.17). The selectin LAM-1 which is expressed on the surface of lymphocytes is important in the lymphocyte–endothelial cell binding, a process similar to the neutrophil–endothelial cell binding which occurs in acute inflammation. Neutrophils may be present in large numbers, where there is persistent suppuration, chronic osteomyelitis for example, and in response to certain infections, actinomycosis, for example. Eosinophils are often conspicuous, especially in parasitic infections; they secrete major basic protein which is toxic to these organisms but also causes local tissue destruction. Fibroblasts, accompanied by capillaries, are present as part of the ongoing attempt to bring about healing and repair.

Chronic Granulomatous Inflammation

Certain forms of chronic inflammation are associated with a distinctive histological appearance.

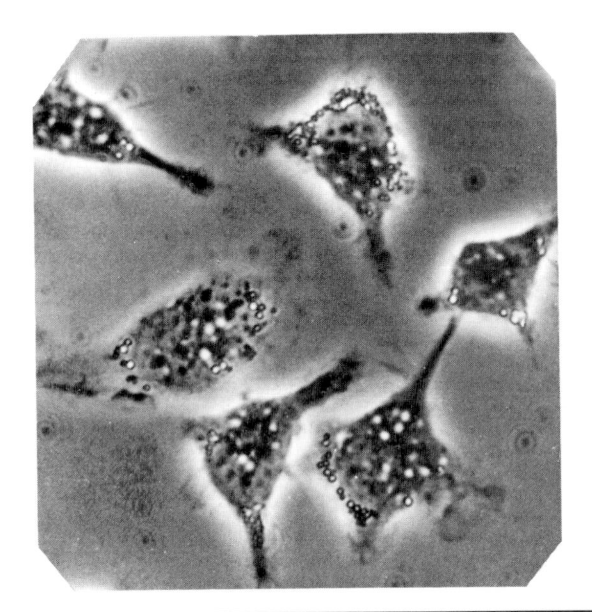

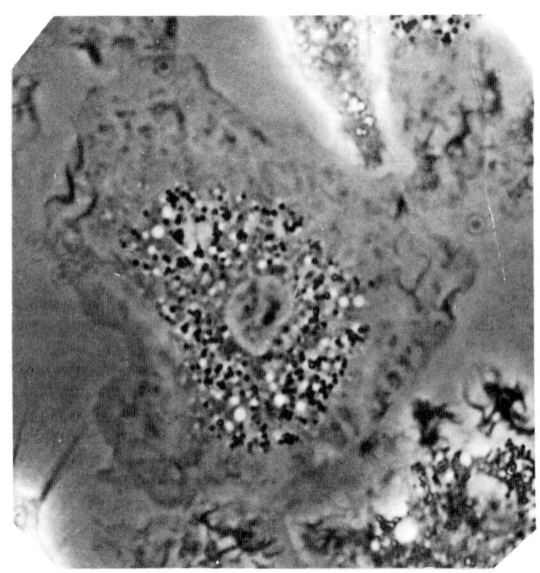

Fig. 4.16 Mouse peritoneal macrophages in culture, viewed by phase-contrast microscopy. Inflammatory exudate has been added to the culture shown on the right. Note the increase in size, content of (phase dense) lysosomes and (phase-lucent) vesicles and extensive cytoplasm 'ruffling' of the stimulated cell. ×960. (The late Professor W. G. Spector and Mrs Katherine M. Wynne).

This comprises an accumulation of modified macrophages, so-called epithelioid macrophages, arranged in small clusters or nodular collections or surrounded by a cuff of lymphocytes. Such aggregates are called **granulomas** and are the hallmark of granulomatous inflammation. Some of the macrophages may form giant cells and the term **giant-cell granuloma** may then be applied. In others there may be necrosis of tissue, **necrotizing granulomas.** In tuberculosis there is caseous necrosis characterized by the production of soft, white, cheese-like material, hence the name; the lesions are referred to as tuberculoid or **caseating granulomas.**

Other cells may be present including fibroblasts, plasma cells and occasionally neutrophils. However, it is the presence of epithelioid cells that is essential for a histological diagnosis of granulomatous inflammation. Epithelioid cells (Fig. 4.18) are so named because of their resemblance to epithelial cells. They have vesicular nuclei and abundant eosinophilic cytoplasm, con-

Table 4.2 Some secretory products of mononuclear phagocytes

Hydrolytic enzymes
Lysozyme
Collagenase
Elastase
Plasminogen activator
Lysosomal acid hydrolases
Arachidonic acid metabolites
Prostaglandins
Leukotrienes
Complement components
Many of both classical and alternative pathways
Oxygen metabolites
Hydrogen peroxide
Hydroxyl radicals
Superoxide
Cytokines
Interleukin 1 (IL-1)
Tumour necrosis factor α (TNFα)
Interleukin 6 (IL-6)

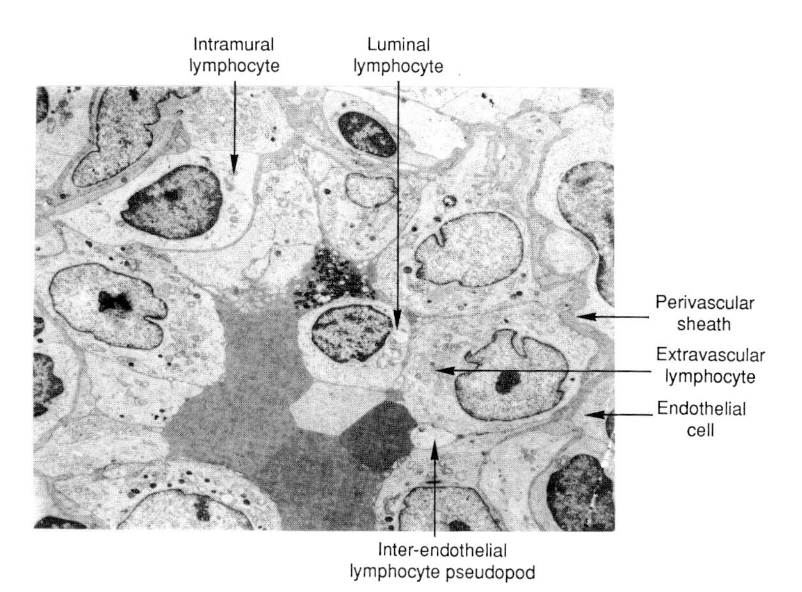

Fig. 4.17 Electron micrograph of high endothelial venules in chronic inflammatory tissue from a patient with Reiter's syndrome. (Dr Tony Freemont)

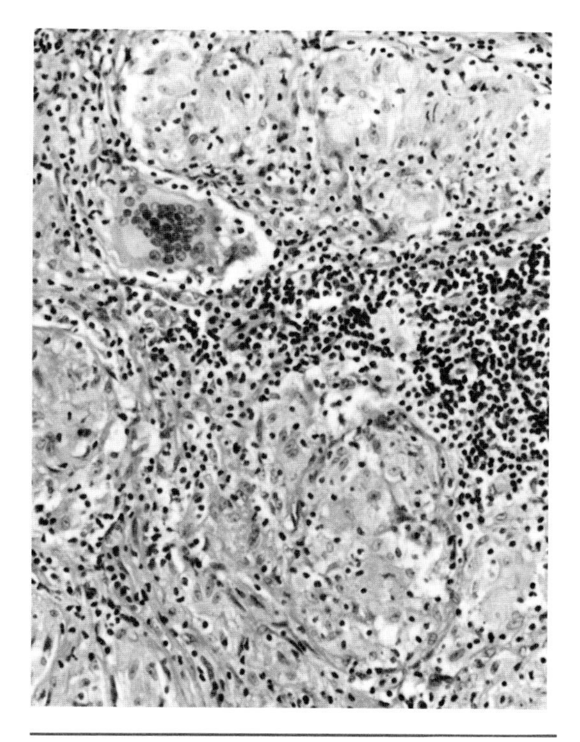

Fig. 4.18 Epithelioid cells.

taining a well developed secretory apparatus. The nature of the secretory material is not fully known but angiotensin converting enzyme (kininase II), acid phosphatase and mucopolysaccharides are present. They have limited phagocytic activity.

Giant cells may be very large with cytoplasm similar to that of epithelioid cells and contain multiple nuclei, often up to 100 per cell. They are found whenever there is material which macrophages find difficult to digest, such as foreign bodies, non-absorbable sutures or urate crystals in gouty tophi. They are also a characteristic feature of both tuberculosis (p. 300) and sarcoidosis (p. 313). Giant cells formed in the presence of indigestible material, **foreign-body giant cells** (Fig. 4.19a), have irregularly scattered nuclei. In the so-called **Langhans' giant cells** (Fig. 4.19b) seen in tuberculosis and sarcoidosis the nuclei are arranged peripherally in a horseshoe pattern; the centrioles are present in one area and cytofilaments radiate from this to the nuclei, a feature which may be recognizable on light microscopy as asteroid bodies. Giant cells arise by fusion of macrophages, perhaps by a simultaneous attempt

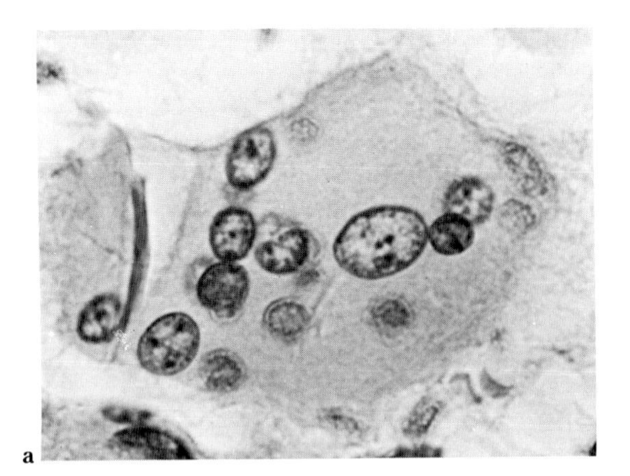

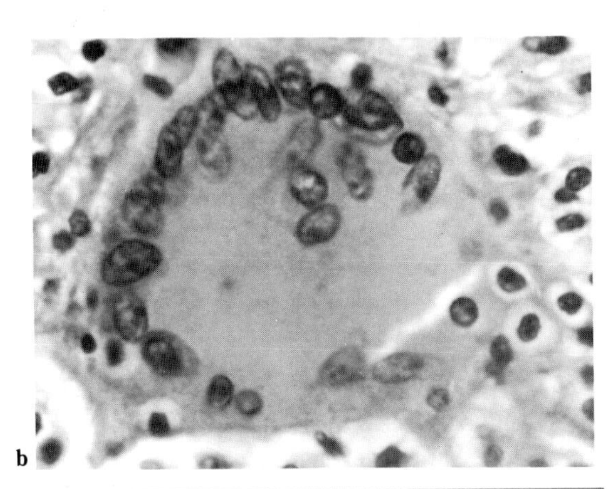

Fig. 4.19 Multinucleated giant cells formed by fusion of macrophages. **a** Foreign-body giant cell: the nuclei vary in size and are irregularly distributed, and the cell has engulfed a fragment of suture material. **b** Langhans' giant cell in a tuberculous lesion: note the peripheral arrangement of nuclei and abundant cytoplasm. ×750.

by two or more cells to engulf a single particle. They may be a form of biological 'accident' rather than a specific adaptation by macrophages.

The lymphocytes which are present within granulomas are predominantly CD4 positive T-helper/inducer cells whereas in the surrounding cuff CD8 positive suppressor/cytotoxic T cells are mainly present. The formation of granulomas is often, but not exclusively, a manifestation of a type IV hypersensitivity reaction and IL-1 and interferons are of importance in inducing this type of reaction. In AIDS patients, where there is a reduction of CD4 positive T-helper cells (p. 243), there is an impaired granulomatous response to mycobacterial infections.

Mediators of Inflammation

Sir Thomas Lewis in his classic paper in 1927 described the 'triple response' to injury. In this he noted that minor trauma to the skin was followed by the development of a red reaction (due to dilatation of the capillaries), a flare (extension of the red reaction to adjacent tissue) and whealing (due to local oedema). He postulated that neural mechanisms were responsible for the flare but that a diffusible 'H-substance' mediated the vascular changes. Since then a number of observations has suggested that the changes occurring in the inflammatory response were due to the production of chemical mediators in and around the area of damaged tissue. The three most important of these observations were: (1) acute inflammation occurs in denervated limbs; (2) the vascular changes of the inflammatory response occurred over a wider range than that of the original injury; and (3) the changes seen in the inflammatory response were essentially the same irrespective of the nature of the original injury. These mediators (Table 4.3) originate from tissue cells, circulating leucocytes and plasma proteins.

Cell-derived Mediators of Acute Inflammation

In addition to the cell types which we have discussed as part of the inflammatory reaction – neutrophils, monocytes, macrophages and lymphocytes – mast cells, basophils, platelets and endothelium are also important sources of chemical mediators. Furthermore, activation of mast cells, basophils and platelets also stimulates arachidonic acid metabolism with the synthesis of prostaglandins, leukotrienes and thromboxanes

Table 4.3 Some mediators of acute inflammation: sources and effects

Mediator	Source	Vasodilatation	Vascular leakage	Chemotaxis	Other effects
Histamine and serotonin	Mast cells, basophils and platelets	+	+	–	Leucocyte adhesion
Bradykinin	Kininogen	+	+	–	Pain
Fibrinopeptides	Fibrinogen	–	+	+	—
C3a	Complement system	–	+	–	Opsonic fragment (C3b)
C5a	Complement system	–	+	+	Leucocyte adhesion
Prostaglandins	Cell membrane	+	Potentiate other mediators	–	Pain, fever
Leukotriene B_4	Leucocytes	–	–	+	Leucocyte adhesion
Leukotriene C_4, D_4, E_4	Leucocytes, mast cells	–	+	–	Vasoconstriction
Lysosomal cationic proteins	Leucocytes	–	+	+	Immobilization of neutrophils
Lysosomal neutral proteases	Leucocytes	–	+	–	Tissue damage
Reactive oxygen metabolites	Leucocytes	–	+		Endothelial cell damage, tissue damage
Platelet activating factor	Leucocytes & other cells	–	+	+	
IL-1, IL-6 and TNFα	Macrophages & other cells	–	–	+	Acute phase responses; leucocyte adhesion

(Fig. 4.20). Cytokines are also cell-derived mediators of acute inflammation but because they are more characteristically involved in the pathogenesis of chronic inflammation they are dealt with separately.

Mast cells and basophils. Mast cells are present in most tissues and are particularly numerous around small blood vessels. Basophils migrate from the blood and can respond to chemotaxins. Both of these cell types contain storage granules. Degranulation occurs in response to a number of stimuli: (1) following cross-linking of antigen with surface bound IgE in type I hypersensitivity reactions (p. 208); (2) following the interaction of the complement system anaphylatoxins C3a and C5a with specific cell-membrane receptors; (3) trauma and tissue injury; and (4) chemical factors including IL-1 released by the other cell types present at the site of inflammation. Activation of mast cells (and other leucocytes) stimulates the production of platelet activating factor (PAF).

Platelets. The primary role of the platelet is the initiation of blood coagulation following injury to endothelial cells. Platelets lack a nucleus but possess three distinct types of granule – dense granules, α-granules and lysosomes, each of which contain a number of chemical mediators (Table 4.4). Platelets are activated by thrombin following activation of the coagulation system but in the inflammatory response they are also activated by coming into contact with collagen, by platelet activating factor (PAF), by antigen–

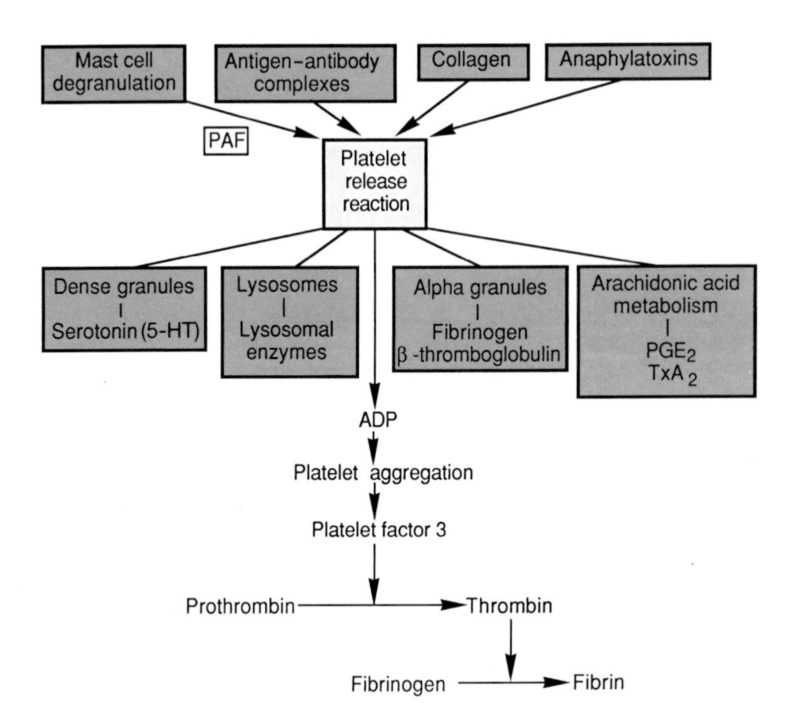

Fig. 4.20 The platelet release reaction. Different stimuli act on the platelet membrane to stimulate granule secretion and the formation of prostaglandins (PGE_2) and thromboxane (TxA_2). ADP released from the platelets acts on the platelet membrane to induce aggregation. Release of platelet factor 3 induces coagulation with the formation of fibrin.

Table 4.4 Source and mediators of acute inflammation produced by platelets

Dense granules	Serotonin Histamine Ca^{2+} Adenosine diphosphate (ADP)
α Granules	Fibrinogen and coagulation proteins Cationic proteins Platelet-derived growth factor
Lysosomes	Acid hydrolases
Prostaglandin synthesis	Thromboxane A_2

antibody complexes and the anaphylatoxins, C3a and C5a (Fig. 4.23). Activation of platelets comprises adherence, aggregation and degranulation with the release of granule contents.

Histamine and Serotonin (5-Hydroxytryptamine)

These vasoactive amines which are secreted principally by mast cells, basophils and platelets cause vasodilatation and increased vascular permeability. They act during the early stages of acute inflammation and histamine is principally responsible for the immediate transient phase of increased vascular permeability. The increase in vascular permeability is mediated by H_1-receptors on the post-capillary venules.

Platelet Activating Factor (PAF)

PAF is an acetylated lysophospholipid complex and probably comprises a group of mediators which induce platelet aggregation and degranulation; in addition, however, it increases vascular permeability, induces leucocyte adhesion to endothelium and stimulates the synthesis of arachidonic acid derivatives.

Arachidonic Acid Derivatives

These comprise the prostaglandins (PG) and the leukotrienes (LT); the metabolic pathways involved in their synthesis are outlined in Fig. 4.21. Prostaglandins and leukotrienes have functional roles in coagulation and haemostasis, and in the cardiovascular, respiratory, renal, endocrine and osteoarticular systems. They can be synthesized and released by many cell types and are not stored. Thus, in effect they resemble hormones, exerting local paracrine and autocrine effects following which they are inactivated.

Arachidonic acid is a 20-carbon polyunsaturated fatty acid that is derived from the diet or from linoleic acid. It is present in the cell membrane phospholipids and following an appropriate stimulus it is released (Fig. 4.21) by one of two phospholipases, of which phospholipase A_2 is the major one in inflammatory cells. The biologically active prostaglandins and leukotrienes are produced by intracellular cyclo-oxygenase and lipoxygenase respectively.

The exact prostaglandin produced depends upon the cell or tissue involved. Thromboxane A_2 and prostaglandin I_2 (prostacyclin) are the major prostaglandins of platelets and endothelial cells respectively and have an important role in haemostasis. PGD_2, PGE_2 and $PGF_{2\alpha}$ are synthesized by macrophages and neutrophils and cause vasodilatation. PGE_2 produces pain if injected intradermally and is involved in causing fever.

The derivatives of arachidonic acid are thus able to produce many of the features of the inflammatory response (Table 4.5). The anti-inflammatory effects of glucocorticoids and aspirin-like drugs is related to their ability to inhibit prostaglandin production (Fig. 4.21). Glucocorticoids induce the synthesis of a protein lipocortin (macrocortin, lipomodulin) which inhibits phospholipase A_2 activity, while aspirin-like drugs inhibit cyclo-oxygenase activity. At present there are no drugs which selectively inhibit the lipoxygenase pathway.

Table 4.5 Arachidonic acid metabolites as inflammatory mediators

Activity	Mediator
Vasodilatation	PGD_2, PGE_2, PGI_2, $PGF_{2\alpha}$
Increased vascular permeability	LTB_4, LTC_4, LTD_4, LTE_4
Leucocyte adhesion and chemotaxis	LTB_4
Pain	PGE_2, PGI_2

Plasma Mediator Systems

There are four plasma mediator systems which participate in the inflammatory response—the coagulation, fibrinolytic, kallirein–kinin and complement systems. Three of these are dependent upon activation of clotting factor XII (Hageman factor) for the expression of their activities. Contact of plasma with negatively charged foreign surfaces such as basement membrane, proteolytic enzymes, lipopolysaccharides and foreign bodies results in activation of Hageman factor. The cascades which are simulated by this are outlined in Fig. 4.22.

Coagulation and Fibrinolytic Systems

These are dealt with in detail in Chapter 3. Activation of the coagulation system results in the conversion of soluble fibrinogen to insoluble fibrin. Activation of the fibrinolytic system generates plasmin, and this is effected by plasminogen activator, derived from endothelial cells, and by kallikrein. Plasmin degrades fibrin to soluble fibrin degradation products, fibrinopeptides, which increase vascular permeability and are chemotactic for leucocytes. Kallikrein activates Hageman factor, thus forming a positive feedback amplification loop.

The Kinin System

The kinins are a series of vasoactive peptides of low molecular weight of which bradykinin, a nonapeptide, is best characterized. On a molar basis it is the most potent factor which increases vascular permeability. Kinins also cause vasodilatation and produce pain. Kinin activation is carefully regu-

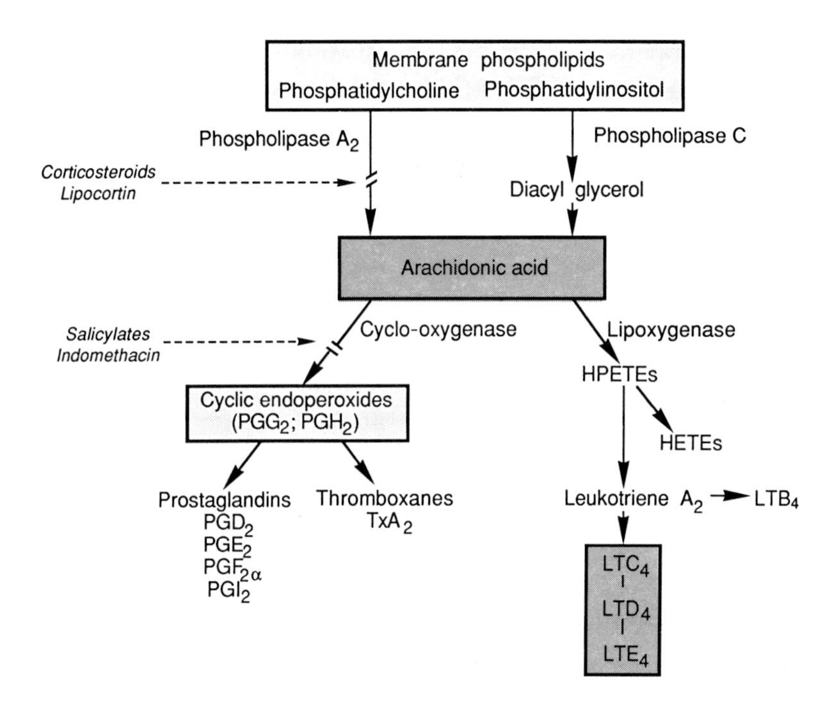

Fig. 4.21 Formation of arachidonic metabolites. Perturbation of the plasma membrane by receptor–ligand interactions or other stimuli results in the conversion of the membrane phospholipids phosphatidylcholine and phosphatidylinositol to arachidonic acid by the actions of phospholipase A_2 and phospholipase C respectively. Phosphatidylinositol is converted to diacyl glycerol which is then converted to arachidonic acid.

Arachidonic acid is metabolized by one of two pathways: the action of cyclo-oxygenase converts arachidonic acid to the unstable cyclic endoperoxides PGG_2 and PGH_2, which are then converted to prostaglandins, prostacyclin (PGI), or thromboxanes. The action of lipoxygenase metabolizes arachidonic acid to cyclic hydroperoxides (HPETEs) which are then converted to HETEs and leukotriene A_2 (LTA_2). Further metabolism of LTA_2 leads to the formation of LTB_4, LTC_4, LTD_4 and LTE_4. The latter three components are responsible for the activity ascribed to slow reacting substances of anaphylaxis – SRS-A (p. 206).

lated by carboxypeptidase N (kininase I) and angiotensin converting enzyme (kininase II) which inactivate kinins quickly.

Complement

The complement system comprises a group of 20 plasma proteins, which play important roles in host defence against bacterial infections and in the inflammatory response. The system can be activated by one of two independent pathways, the classical and the alternative (Fig. 4.23). Activation of either pathway results in the formation of multimolecular enzymes which activate the third (C3) and fifth (C5) components and generate a membrane attack complex which is capable of causing cell lysis. During activation a number of biologically active cleavage fragments, C3a, C4a and C5a, are released.

The classical pathway. The classical pathway is activated by agents such as antigen–antibody complexes containing IgG, (IgG_1, IgG_2 or IgG_3) or IgM antibody, by certain bacterial products and by viruses. Activation occurs when the first component (C1), which consists of three separate proteins (C1q, C1r, C1s), binds to the activating agent through the C1q subcomponent. Activated C1s ($C\bar{1}s$) activates the fourth (C4) and second

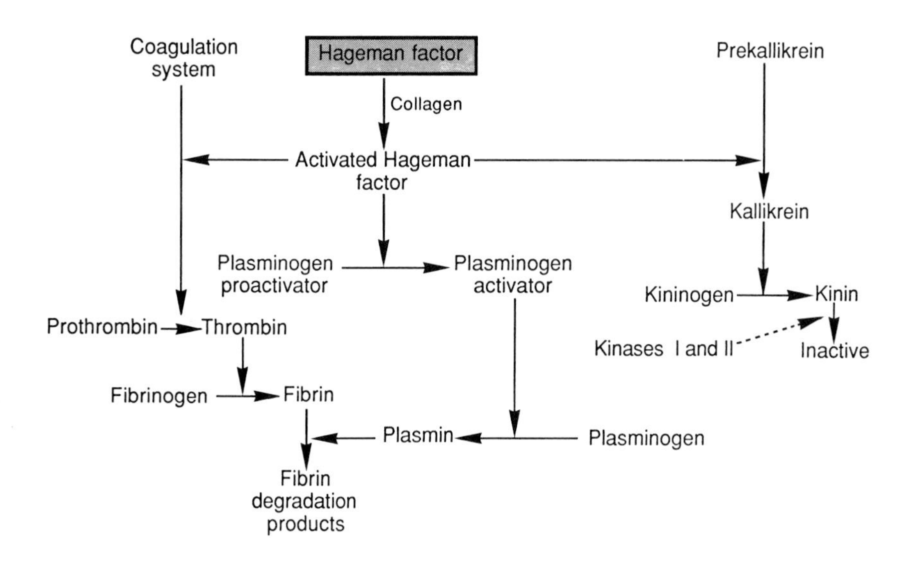

Fig. 4.22 Hageman factor-dependent pathways. Activation of Hageman factor (coagulation factor XII) by contact with collagen results in the acquisition of protease activity which is able enzymatically to activate the coagulation system, the fibrinolytic system and the kallikrein–kinin system. Kallikrein, an enzyme which converts kininogen to kinin, also amplifies the system by activating for Hageman factor. Kininases I and II inactivate kinins rapidly.

(C2) components. A small fragment, C4a, is released from C4 and the major part of the molecule C4b binds covalently to the surface of the activating agent. C2 binds to C4b and is also activated by $C\bar{1}s$.

The bimolecular enzyme C4b2a is the classical pathway C3 activating enzyme (C3 convertase), which activates C3 to release a small fragment C3a into the fluid phase, while the larger fragment C3b binds covalently to the activating agent. The multimolecular complex C4b2a3b is the classical pathway C5 convertase which activates C5 to release C5a into the fluid phase and allows the major part, C5b, to bind transiently to the surface of agent. C5b acts as a focus for the sequential binding of C6, C7, C8 and C9 to form the C5b–9 cytolytic membrane attack complex. This complex is highly hydrophobic and becomes inserted into cell membranes. On electron microscopic examination the complex appears as a hollow cylinder which spans the cell membrane (Fig. 4.24). Membrane disruption results in cell lysis.

The alternative pathway. The alternative pathway is activated by bacteria and other micro-organisms. C1, C2 and C4 are not involved but C3b is required for its initiation and is provided by continuous low-grade turnover of C3. Normally this C3b is degraded to C3bi by the control enzyme factor I and its cofactor, factor H. C3b which binds covalently to an activating surface escapes this regulatory effect, and instead binds factor B. The enzyme factor D then cleaves B to release the fragment Ba and leave the fragment Bb bound to C3b to form the unstable alternative pathway C3 convertase C3bBb. This enzyme is stabilized by the protein properdin (P) which binds to C3b. The complex C3bBbP is called the properdin-stabilized alternative pathway C3 convertase, and this activates C3 and C5 to stimulate formation of the membrane attack complex assembled in the same way as its classical pathway counterpart.

Anaphylatoxins. The peptides C4a, C3a and C5a are called anaphylatoxins. They cause smooth

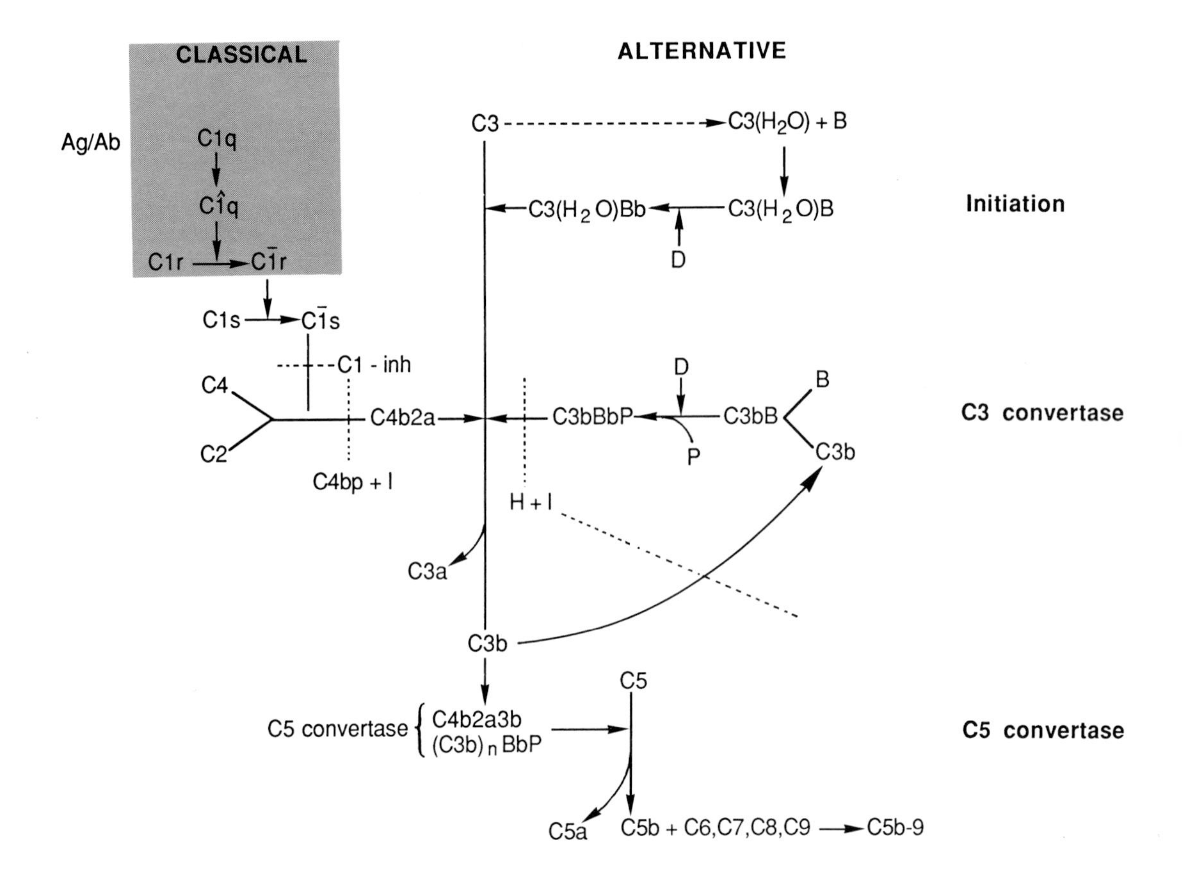

Fig. 4.23 Pathways for complement activation. Activation of either the classical (left) or alternative (right) pathways results in the generation of enzymes which activate the third (C3) and fifth (C5) components. The classical pathway is usually activated by antigen–antibody complexes which contain IgG (1, 2 or 3 subclasses) or IgM antibody. The first component (C1) binds to the Fc pieces of antibody (two molecules of IgG, one molecule of IgM) by the C1q subcomponent. A conformational change (denoted by the ^ initiates the conversion of C1r into its enzymatically active form, C1̄r, which then activates C1s by a single proteolytic cleavage. C1s cleaves the α chain of C4 to expose a thiolester bond in the larger cleavage product C4b which allows it to bind covalently (by ester or amide bonds) to the antibody molecule or the antigen. C2 binds to C4b and is in turn activated by C1̄s to form the classical pathway C3 convertase C4b2a, which activates C3 by cleaving the α chain to release C3a and allow C3b, the larger cleavage product, to bind covalently by means of its thiolester to the antigen–antibody complex. C3b which binds to C4b in C4b2a alters the specificity from C3 convertase to C5 convertase (C4b2a3b) which cleaves C5 to release C5a while C5b binds sequentially C6, C7, C8 and C9 to form the cytolytic membrane attack complex, C5b–9. The activity of C1 is regulated by C1 inhibitor which binds to the active sites of C1̄r and C1̄s. The activity of C4b2a and C4b2a3b is regulated by the enzyme factor I and C4b binding protein (C4bp). Factor I in the presence of C4bp degrades C4b so that the convertases cannot be formed. C4bp also binds to C4b to displace C2a from C4b to accelerate the delay of the convertase.

The alternative pathway positive feedback amplification loop is regularly undergoing low-grade fluid-phase turnover which is held in check by factor I and its cofactor, factor H. Factor I in the presence of factor H degrades C3b so that the alternative pathway convertase C3bBbP cannot form. Factor H also binds to C3b to displace Bb from the complex. The pathway is activated when C3b binds to the surface of micro-organisms (or other activators) to become resistant to the regulatory actions of factors H and I. Thus, convertase can be assembled unopposed on the surface of the activator. A molecule of C3b binding to the first C3b converts the C3 convertase to the C5 convertase $(C3b)_nBbP$). Thus, in non-immune individuals the alternative pathway allows micro-organisms to be opsonized by C3b and also promotes the assembly of the C5b–9 complex on their surfaces.

The initial turnover of the alternative pathway is believed to be stimulated by the low-grade hydrolysis of the thiolester of C3 to form a C3b-like molecule ($C3(H_2O)$), which can bind B and form a low efficiency C3 convertase ($C3(H_2O)Bb$) which is relatively resistant to the actions of factors H and I.

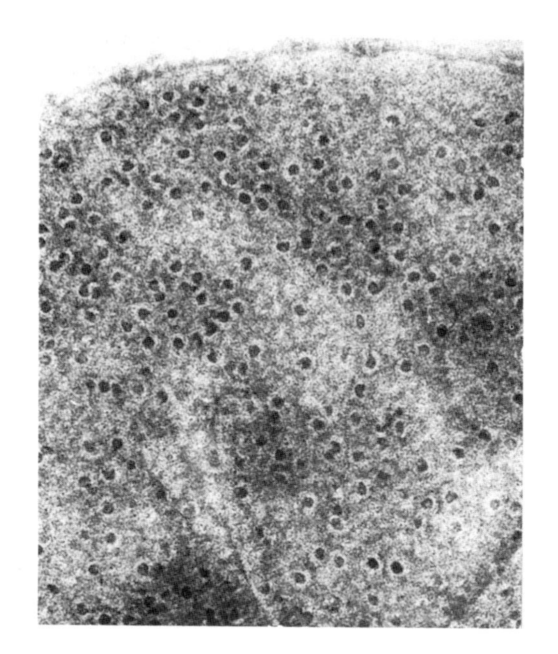

Fig. 4.24 Electron micrograph of membranes of complement-lysed erythrocyte. The characteristic 'doughnut' lesions have an outer diameter of 2 nm and an inner diameter of 1 nm.

muscle contraction, and increase vascular permeability. The latter effect is, at least in part, mediated by the secretion of histamine which occurs when anaphylatoxins interact with mast cells or basophils. C5a possesses the strongest and C4a the weakest anaphylatoxin activity. C5a, but not C3a or C4a, is a powerful chemotaxin for neutrophils, eosinophils, basophils and monocytes. C5a also stimulates neutrophil degranulation and superoxide production.

Cytokines

These are secretory products of T lymphocytes and macrophages. They have important roles in the normal immune response and in delayed (type IV) hypersensitivity. While they are discussed in greater detail in these sections they also are of significance in chronic inflammation and healing and repair. Interferon-γ is important in macrophage activation. Interleukin 1 (IL-1), a pleotropic cytokine, is a 15 kDa polypeptide which is essential for lymphocyte proliferation in response to antigen and stimulates fibroblast proliferation and collagen synthesis (paracrine effect), and is responsible for fever and some of the changes in hepatic protein synthesis (p. 149) which occur during inflammation (endocrine effects). Interleukin 6 (IL-6) is probably the major cytokine involved in the regulation of hepatic protein synthesis. Tumour necrosis factor α (TNFα), originally called cachectin, stimulates skeletal muscle and adipocyte catabolism and is thus responsible for weight loss in inflammation. It is also capable of killing normal cells and acts on the liver in the same way as IL-1. Both IL-1 and TNFα act on endothelial cells to upregulate the expression of adhesion molecules, thus promoting leucocyte–endothelial adhesion.

Other Cellular Mediators

The cytoplasmic granules of neutrophils and monocytes contain neutral proteases (collagenase, elastase, cathepsins) which are released at sites of inflammation and destroy matrix components including collagen, basement membrane and elastin. Plasmin generated by this action of plasmin activator also plays a significant role in degradation of the connective tissue matrix.

Neutrophils secrete a heterogeneous group of cationic proteins which increase vascular permeability by acting directly on the endothelial cell or indirectly by releasing histamine from mast cells. Neutrophil chemotactic factor, another cationic protein, is chemotactic for monocytes. Finally, cationic proteins have also been shown to inhibit the migration of other neutrophils and eosinophils.

The release of reactive oxygen metabolites by neutrophils and macrophages produces tissue damage as described earlier. Important targets for such damage include endothelial cells with resultant increase in vascular permeability and damage to protease inhibitors so that the activity of neutral proteases released from cells cannot be regulated. Oxygen metabolites may also damage other cells at sites of inflammation and also damage the matrix components.

Chemical Mediators and Inflammation – Biological Principles

A number of important principles regarding the inflammatory response can be stated.

(1) No single chemical mediator is responsible for any single feature of the inflammatory response. Thus, a defect in a particular mediator system will not prevent the acute inflammatory response occurring.

(2) There are very marked interactions between the different mediator systems so that discussion of the activities of one mediator system in isolation from the others is highly artificial. A good example of this is complement activation during which generation of anaphylatoxins may stimulate prostaglandin synthesis in mast cells.

(3) In virtually all mediator systems there are in-built regulatory mechanisms which ensure that the inflammatory response does not progress in an uncontrolled fashion.

Modulation of Inflammatory Cell Function

The functions of neutrophils, mast cells, basophils and platelets are influenced by 'second-messengers' including the intracellular levels of cAMP, cGMP, diacylglycerol and levels of free Ca^{2+} ions in the cytosol. These cell-signalling mechanisms have been discussed in detail in Chapter 1 and their complex interactions regulate cellular activity in a co-ordinated manner.

Agents which increase cAMP with resultant activation of cAMP dependent protein kinases reduce inflammation and function. Prostaglandins, e.g. PGE_2 or PGI_2, inhibit inflammatory cell function in this way. In clinical practice drugs such as theophylline act by increasing cAMP and are used to reduce the inflammatory response.

In contrast to the inhibition of inflammatory cell activity associated with increased cAMP levels, agents which increase cGMP, which activate (1) the phosphatidyl inositol cycle to generate glycerol or (2) inositol triphosphate to increase cytosolic Ca^{2+}, enhance inflammatory cell function.

Systemic Manifestations of Inflammation

In addition to the obvious local effects, inflammation is also associated with a series of systemic manifestations which are known collectively as the acute phase response (Table 4.6). The acute phase response is mediated in part by cytokines, in particular IL-1, IL-6 and TNFα, released primarily from macrophages at the site of inflammation, following exposure to a phagocytic stimulus, endotoxin, viruses or interferon-γ.

Pyrexia (Fig. 4.25). It has long been recognized that injection of dead bacteria or bacterial products induces fever. Such products are termed **exogenous pyrogens**, the best documented being endotoxin from Gram-negative bacteria. Endotoxins are lipopolysaccharides and their injection into rabbits induces fever within about one hour and this is followed by a refractory period in which further injections are ineffectual. Exogenous pyrogens act on leucocytes to produce an **endogenous pyrogen**, IL-1, which can be detected in plasma during the early stages of bacterial or viral infections. IL-1 acts on the thermosensory centres in the anterior hypothalamus, to raise the level of the thermostat. The temperature of the

Table 4.6 Features of the acute phase response

	Mediated by
Fever	IL-1, TNFα
Neutrophilia	IL-1, TNFα, C3e (a low molecular weight cleavage product of the C3 component of complement
Changes in plasma protein levels	
Hepatic synthesis increased	IL-6, IL-1, TNFα, IFN-γ
C-reactive protein	
Serum amyloid protein A	
Complement components	
Fibrinogen	
Haptoglobin	
Hepatic synthesis reduced	
Albumin	
Transferrin	
B-cell activation	IL-1, IL-6
Immunoglobulin synthesis	
Changes in plasma cation concentrations	
Zn^{2+} ↓	IL-1
Fe^{2+} ↓	
Cu^{2+} ↑	
Increased skeletal muscle protein catabolism	TNFα, IL-1

blood reaching this centre is then judged to be low, so that stimulation of the vasomotor centre results in peripheral vasoconstriction to reduce heat loss, and heat is generated by muscular contraction (shivering, clinically recognized as a rigor) and increased metabolic activity in the liver. Not only is the thermostat set high in fever, it is unstable, so that temperature fluctuations occur. A fall in temperature is accomplished by cutaneous vasodilatation and sweating.

Interleukin 1 acts on the thermosensory centre by stimulating the formation of PGE_2 which provides the secondary signal for elevation of body temperature. Aspirin and other cyclo-oxygenase inhibitors reduce body temperature in febrile individuals by blocking PGE_2 formation. The benefit of fever is not immediately obvious. However, it has been proposed that proliferation of some micro-organisms is impaired and that inflammatory and immune responses occur more efficiently at higher temperatures.

Leucocytosis, a two- to threefold increase in the peripheral blood leucocyte count, is a feature of acute inflammation. The increase is usually confined to the neutrophil population (neutrophil leucocytosis, **neutrophilia**). In addition to mature neutrophils, some immature forms (band forms) are also seen in the peripheral blood. Occasionally the circulating levels of these immature forms may be extremely high (40 000–100 000 cells/mm^3) and may mimic the blood picture of leukaemia. For this reason it is called a **leukaemoid reaction**. Specific mediators released by cells at the site of inflammation act on the bone marrow to increase proliferation of neutrophil precursors and also to accelerate the release of neutrophils from the bone marrow. Colony stimulating factors (CSFs), released from macrophages and activated T lymphocytes, also stimulate the proliferation of myeloid precursors in the bone marrow. Neutrophilia is a feature of most acute bacterial infections, while **lymphocytosis** (an absolute increase in the

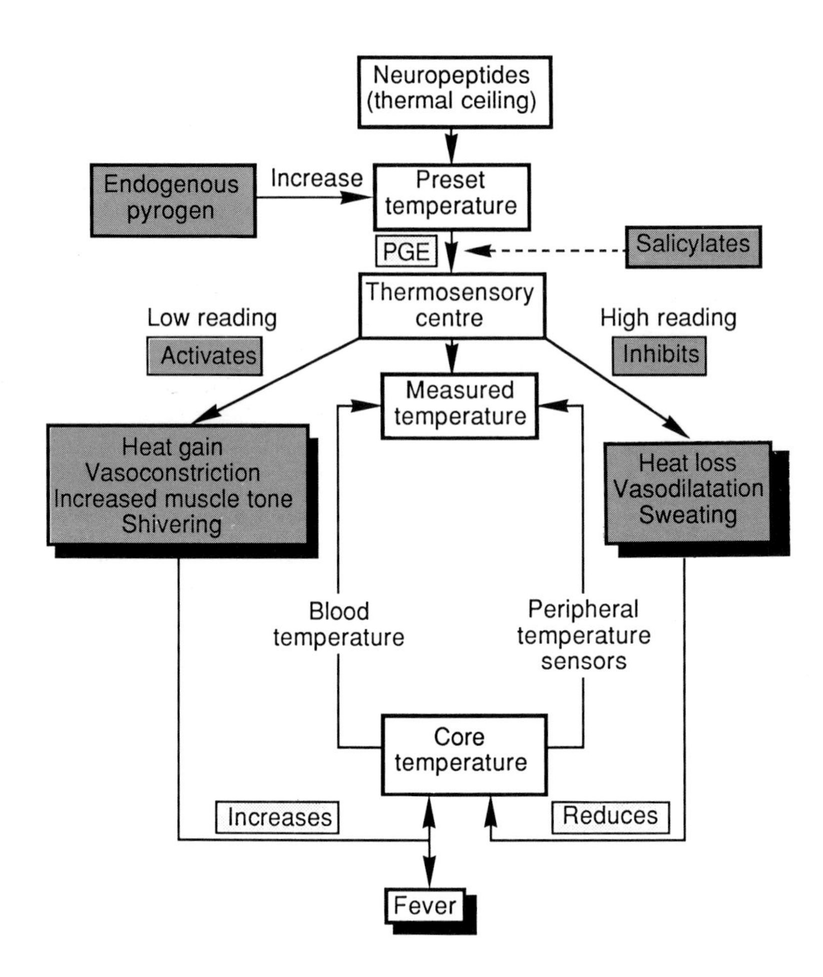

Fig. 4.25 Mechanism of regulation of body temperature and the production of fever. Under normal conditions the body temperature is set at 37°C under the influence of the thermoregulatory centre in the hypothalamus. The preset temperature is regulated by neuropeptides acting on this centre. The thermosensory centre measures the temperature of the blood which flows through it, so that if the blood temperature (and hence the body core temperature) is low, a series of events is triggered to prevent heat loss and to generate heat (left side). If the temperature of the blood is perceived as being too high, measures to reduce heat formation (inactivity and sleep) and increase heat loss are instituted (right side). In inflammation IL-1 is released from macrophages and other cells at the site of inflammation and circulates in the blood. It acts on the thermoregulatory centre to increase the set of the thermostat. The blood is then perceived as being too cold so shivering occurs. The effect of IL-1 on the thermoregulatory centre is dependent upon the local release of prostaglandin E_2. Salicylates and other prostaglandin synthetase inhibitors block the formation of PGE_2. Thus the preset temperature falls and the temperature of the blood is perceived as being elevated so that vasodilatation and sweating occur.

number of circulating lymphocytes) is characteristic of acute viral infections. **Eosinophilia**, an increase in the peripheral blood eosinophil count from the normal 1–3% of the total leucocytes to levels as high as 15%, is a feature of parasitic infections and allergic reactions. As a result of the increased number of circulating leucocytes more are available to leave the blood and enter the inflamed vessels.

In debilitated patients with chronic inflammation, **leucopenia**, a decrease in the total leucocyte count, may occur. Leucopenia is also a feature of infections such as typhoid fever and some protozoal infections.

Weight loss. Prolonged inflammation is associated with weight loss. It is also thought to be due to the actions of IL-1 and TNFα which increase catabolism in skeletal muscle, adipose tissue and the liver. Increased metabolism of endogenous fat and protein results in a negative nitrogen balance and ketoacidosis may occur. A high calorie diet is necessary to prevent weight loss.

Changes in hepatic protein synthesis. The serum level of albumin is reduced while levels of C-reactive protein, coagulation components, fibrinogen, complement components, serum amyloid A and other proteins involved in the inflammatory response are increased during acute and chronic inflammation. The switch from albumin synthesis to synthesis of proteins involved in the acute inflammatory response is due to changes in the hepatic synthesis rates of these proteins and is probably mediated by IL-1, IL-6 and TNFα.

Amyloidosis, affecting different organs and tissues, may occur as a complication of longstanding granulomatous or suppurative inflammation (p. 246).

Healing and Repair

When injury and any associated acute inflammatory response has resulted in necrosis of specialized cells and damage to the surrounding matrix, the host response must include attempts at replacement of the dead cells by healthy tissue. This response is referred to as **healing** and comprises two processes: (1) **regeneration of specialized cells** by proliferation of those surviving; and (2) **a connective tissue response** characterized by the formation of granulation tissue and its subsequent maturation. Some textbooks refer to this connective tissue response component as the repair reaction. The relative roles of these two processes varies between tissues and will also depend on the nature and severity of the injury. One of the key factors is the ability of surviving cells to divide. In some tissues, for example in the skin, there may be complete restoration of the architecture of the epithelium after healing, particularly if the injury is very superficial. At other sites where the specialized cells cannot regenerate, the healing process is dominated by the connective tissue response with the laying down of scar tissue (**fibrosis**). This is clearly a less satisfactory outcome for, although healing may have restored any structural defect in the tissue, it has impaired its function by replacing specialized cells with fibrous tissue.

The outcome is also affected by the nature, severity and duration of the injury. This is perhaps best illustrated in the liver. This organ shows a remarkable capacity for regeneration. In experimental animals up to 90% of the liver can be removed surgically and the remaining parenchyma will regenerate to the original mass and with a normal structure. In acute liver injury in humans, there may be massive zonal necrosis of hepatocytes with some collapse of the matrix and scar tissue development. However, in most cases of liver injury the hepatocyte regenerative response ensures restoration of liver architecture. By contrast, in chronic liver injury the amount of fibrosis may be quite substantial; when it is associated with regeneration, nodules of parenchyma are surrounded by bands of fibrous tissue, constituting hepatic cirrhosis (p. 764). Most of the conditions which lead to cirrhosis are characterized by persistent injury with chronic inflammation. It seems likely that the tendency for chronic inflammatory processes to produce fibrosis, which is seen in a number of organs, is related to a continuing production of macrophage and lymphocyte derived cytokines and growth factors which act as mediators of the healing process.

In this section we shall first deal with the general principles of the healing process before considering the best known and most intensely studied example, the healing skin wound. Finally, we shall look at examples of healing in other specialized tissues.

Healing: Regeneration

Proliferation of parenchymal cells is an integral part of the healing of an injured organ. The capacity for such regeneration varies between tissues. In some, such as the surface epithelium of the gastrointestinal tract, urinary tract or the skin, there is a continuous turnover of cells by programmed division of stem cells (p. 356). Such tissues are said to be composed of **labile cells** and are capable of substantial regeneration after injury providing that sufficient numbers of stem cells survive. The cells of the lymphoid and haemopoietic systems are further examples of labile cells. It should be appreciated that in the replacement of an injured epithelial surface, not only is there proliferation of surviving cells but also migration: this is seen particularly in skin wounds where keratinocytes migrate from both edges of the skin wound to cover the gap.

In other tissues, there is normally a much lower level of replication and there are few if any stem cells. However, the cells of such tissues (**stable cells**) can undergo rapid division in response to a variety of stimuli including various forms of injury. Quiescent stable cells are in G_0 of the cell cycle (p. 359) but when stimulated they may proceed into G_1 phase and on to cell division. Mesenchymal cells such as fibroblasts, osteoblasts and endothelial cells are stable cells which, as we shall see, can be stimulated to proliferate during healing. Other examples of stable cells include hepatocytes and renal tubular epithelium.

Finally, in some tissues the specialized cells are terminally differentiated and incapable of further replication (**permanent cells**). In this group are cardiac myocytes. There is virtually no capacity for replacement of these specialized cells and the healing process following injury in the myocardium is dominated by the connective tissue response.

Healing: the Connective Tissue Response

The connective tissue response component is referred to in some textbooks as the repair reaction. Before considering it in detail it is pertinent to discuss the composition of the extracellular matrix of connective tissue as many of its constituents play a major role in healing.

The Extracellular Matrix

The extracellular matrix is a complex of macromolecules which not only provides structural support for tissues but also modulates various functions of the constituent cells such as proliferation, differentiation, cell movement and attachment. This is achieved through complex cell–matrix interactions which depend on the expression of cell membrane receptors belonging to the integrin receptor family of adhesion molecules (p. 15).

The principal compounds which make up the extracellular matrix are collagens, structural glycoproteins, glycosaminoglycans, proteoglycans and elastin.

Collagen. The most abundant of the matrix proteins are the collagens which constitute a family of closely related, but genetically distinct proteins. Numerous collagens have been identified and characterized to varying degrees. The proteins share common structural properties which are unique to this family of molecules. Each is composed, at least in part, of a triple helical structure formed from three protein chains (α chains). Along a substantial length of the amino-acid sequence of these chains there is a repetitive triplet Gly-X-Y where X and Y can be any amino acid. Collagens are also rich in the amino acids hydroxyproline and hydroxylysine, which are formed by hydroxylation of proline and lysine residues in the newly synthesized polypeptide. This process requires a number of cofactors including ascorbic acid (vitamin C), ferrous ions and copper. Some collagens, e.g. type III, contain three identical α chains, while others such as type I are composed of two identical chains and one non-identical chain.

The principal cells involved in the synthesis of the collagens (and other extracellular matrix proteins) are fibroblasts and related cells such as osteoblasts. The proteins are synthesized on the endoplasmic reticulum of these cells as larger precursor forms of the individual α chains (pro-α chains). The sequence of events in collagen biosynthesis is outlined in Fig. 4.26. Secreted procollagen molecules are modified by the removal of peptides from the amino- and carboxy-terminal ends by specific peptidases. The resultant collagen molecules align to form collagen fibrils. These have a banded appearance on electron microscopy by virtue of the staggered arrangement of molecules in a fibril (see Fig. 4.28). This also contributes to the tensile strength of the fibrils; this is reinforced by cross-linking of individual collagen molecules by covalent bonding between lysine and hydroxylysine residues. The cleaved peptides are soluble and are rapidly removed. They can be detected in serum where they provide a measure of continuing collagen synthesis. Collagen fibres

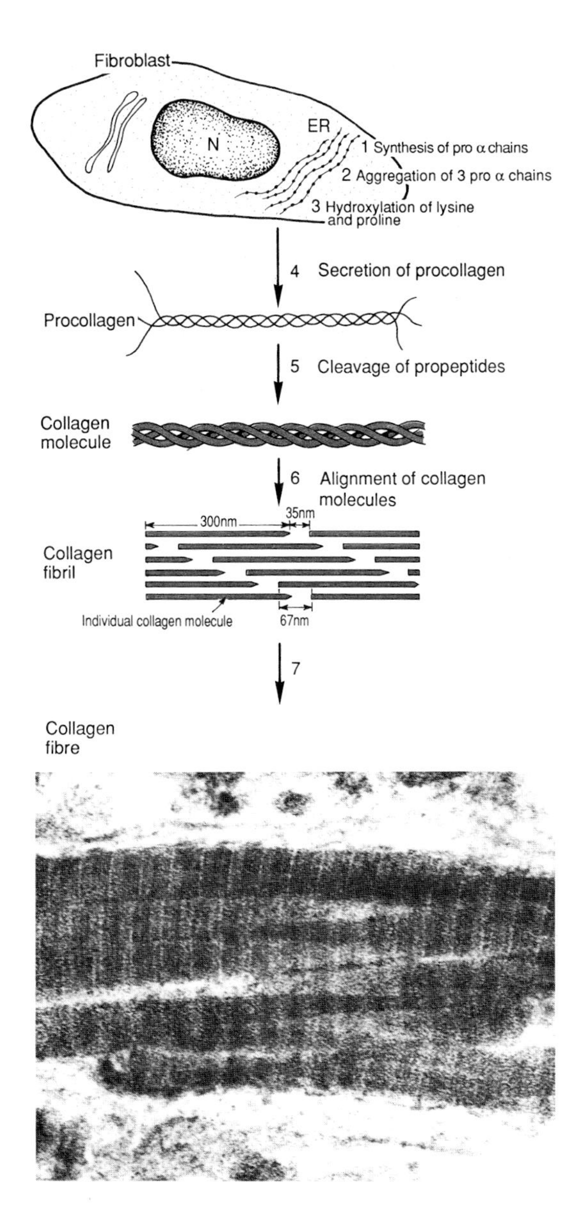

Fig. 4.26 Principal steps in biosynthesis of interstitial collagens: 1, Synthesis of pro-α chains in rough endoplasmic reticulum; 2, aggregation of three pro-α chains; 3, hydroxylation of lysine and proline residues; 4, secretion of procollagen molecule; 5, cleavage of propeptides; 6, alignment of collagen molecules to form fibrils; 7, aggregation of fibrils to form collagen fibre, seen here in longitudinal section and showing regular cross-banding. N, nucleus; ER, endoplasmic reticulum.

are formed by the aggregation of several collagen fibrils. Such fibres and possibly some individual fibrils often contain more than one collagen type; types I and III commonly coexist. The predominant type of collagen varies in different tissues; for example cartilage contains type II collagen almost exclusively (Table 4.7). Type IV collagen does not form fibrils and is found only in basement membranes. The most important collagens in healing are types I and III.

In all normal tissues there is continual collagen turnover, synthesis being balanced by degradation due to fibroblast and macrophage collagenases.

Structural glycoproteins There are several high molecular weight glycoproteins which function as matrix adhesion molecules (hence the term structural glycoproteins). The most abundant and best characterized is **fibronectin** which exists in two major forms, plasma and tissue fibronectin. This protein has binding sites for other matrix proteins such as collagen and also for cell surface integrins, this property enabling fibronectin to act as a link between cells and the matrix and to control the structure of the extracellular matrix. The site responsible for binding to the receptor comprises a sequence of three amino acids, Arg-Gly-Asp (RGD). It also has binding sites for fibrin, a feature which is probably of great importance in the initial stages of the healing process. **Laminin** is also involved in cell–matrix adhesion. This protein, however, is only found in basement membranes where it is closely associated with other proteins such as **collagen type IV** and **entactin**.

Glycosaminoglycans and proteoglycans. Glycosaminoglycans are a heterogeneous group of negatively charged polysaccharide chains. The most abundant are **hyaluronic acid**, **chondroitin sulphate**, **dermatan sulphate**, **heparan sulphate** and **keratan sulphate**. Like the collagens, the relative amounts of the various types varies from tissue to tissue. With the exception of hyaluronic acid, all of the compounds are covalently linked to a core protein to form proteoglycans. These molecules are long unbranched structures which occupy a large volume and are hydrophilic. They serve therefore to provide tissue turgor by attracting water and acting as a 'hydrated gel'. They also have the capacity to bind to collagens and fibronectin and may participate in the structural organization of the extracellular matrix.

Elastin. This protein forms the central core of elastic fibres. Elastin molecules are extensively cross-linked but, unlike many other proteins, they do not form a rigid tertiary structure but can oscillate between various forms to produce so-called random coils. This structure imparts the elastic fibres with the property of recoil after transient stretching. As one might expect, elastin and elastic fibres are most abundant in tissues in which there is a need for recoil, notably large arteries such as the aorta and in the dermis.

Table 4.7 Molecular form and distribution of the major types of collagen

Type	Predominant molecular form	Localization
I	$\alpha1[I]_2\ \alpha2[I]$	Major interstitial collagen (90% total collagen); skin, bone, cornea, tendon
II	$\alpha1[II]_3$	Cartilage, intervertebral disc, vitreous body
III	$\alpha1[III)_3$	Interstitial collagen; skin, internal organs
IV	$\alpha1[IV]_2\ \alpha2[IV]$	Basement membranes
V	$\alpha1[V]_2\ \alpha2[V]$	Minor interstitial collagen; similar distribution to III
VI	$\alpha[VI]\ \alpha2[VI]\ \alpha3[VI]$	Interstitial microfibrils; widespread distribution
VII	$\alpha1[VII]_3$	Anchoring fibrils at dermal–epidermal junction

Granulation Tissue*

With most forms of injury there is, in addition to loss of specialized cells, loss or damage to the surrounding matrix or connective tissue. The healing process that occurs is almost identical to that described above for healing by fibrosis following acute inflammation, i.e. organization of fibrin with formation of granulation tissue which subsequently matures into fibrous tissue. After injury at many sites, there is platelet aggregation and fibrin deposition with formation of blood clot. This is followed by an influx of macrophages, accompanied by proliferation of fibroblasts (Fig. 4.27), and an ingrowth of new blood vessels. The fibroblasts synthesize and secrete fibronectin and proteoglycans and these form the 'scaffolding' for rebuilding the matrix. Fibronectin binds to fibrin and acts as a chemotactic factor for the recruitment of more fibroblasts and macrophages. By day 5, collagen type III is the predominant matrix protein being produced. The turnover of collagen is even greater in an area of healing than it is in normal tissues and the chemical composition of the matrix undergoes rapid changes. Over a period of weeks type I collagen becomes the most abundant protein present and, at most sites, it is this component which is responsible for providing the tensile strength of the matrix in a scar.

Some of the fibroblasts involved in healing contain myofibrils which resemble those of smooth muscle cells (Fig. 4.28). There is evidence that these **myofibroblasts**, in addition to producing matrix proteins, have contractile properties and play a role in the contraction of wounds.

Coincident with fibroblast proliferation there is a proliferation of small blood vessels, a process called angiogenesis or neovascularization (Fig. 4.29). Proliferation of endothelial cells within pre-existing vessels in the surrounding connective tissue forms solid buds which subsequently develop a central lumen; this process is stimulated, in part, by fibronectin. Initially the vessels thus formed are rather fragile thin-walled capillaries (Fig. 4.30) but in time these mature to form arterioles and venules. In the early stages, the newly formed vessels tend to run at right angles to any surface and fibroblasts align themselves along their length. As the amount of interstitial collagen increases, there is a gradual change in the morphology of the fibroblasts. Initially large and plump, they subsequently become elongated and thinner; on electron microscopy their endoplasmic reticulum becomes less prominent. Furthermore, they are now aligned differently, according to the stresses that are imposed on the tissue. At the base of an ulcer, for example, these would lie parallel to the plane of the ulcer (Fig. 4.30b). At the same time, there is a process of **devascularization**, some vessels undergoing atrophy, others showing endarteritis obliterans (p. 441). For some considerable time there is continued

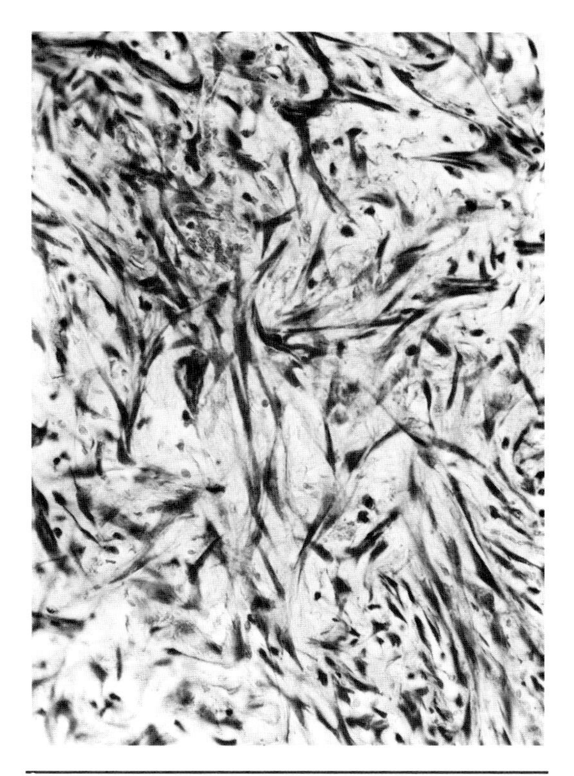

Fig. 4.27 Fibroblasts in a healing wound showing the characteristic shape and early formation of collagen fibrils. ×350.

*This should not be confused with the term granuloma which refers to a form of macrophage response in chronic inflammation (p. 135).

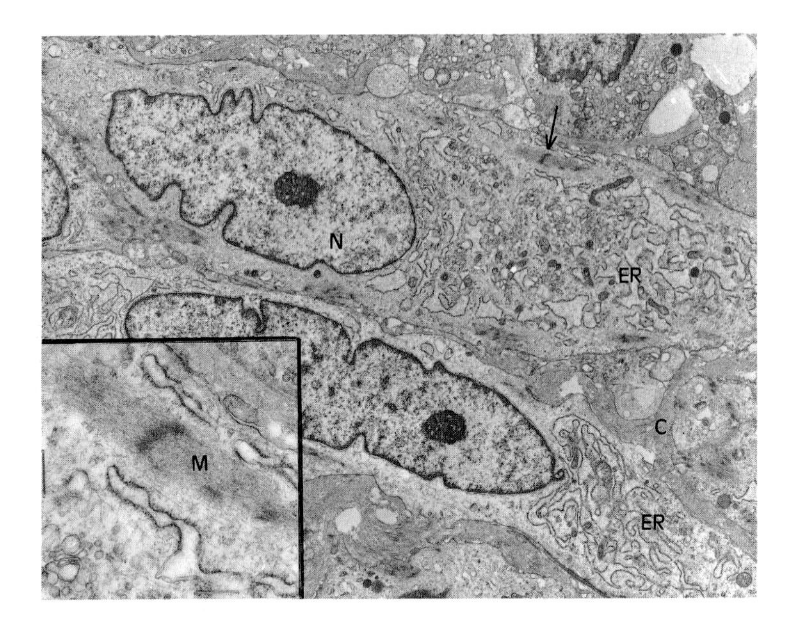

Fig. 4.28 Ultrastructural appearances of myofibroblasts. N, nucleus; ER, endoplasmic reticulum; C, extracellular collagen. Inset: the presence of well developed myofibrils (M) is a characteristic feature of these cells.

remodelling of the matrix, one of the effects of which is a gradual shrinkage of the scar.

Molecular Control of the Healing Process

It should now be clear that healing involves an orderly sequence of events which includes regeneration and migration of specialized cells, angiogenesis, proliferation of fibroblasts and related cells, matrix protein synthesis and finally cessation of these processes. These processes, at least in part, are mediated by a series of low molecular weight polypeptides referred to as **growth factors**. These molecules have the capacity to stimulate cell division and are recognized as playing a crucial role in the control of normal cell growth and differentiation as well as in a wide range of disease processes. The peptides bind to specific receptors on cell membranes, generate second messengers and initiate a series of intracellular events which result in cell proliferation. Here we briefly consider those growth factors which have been identified as possibly playing a role in the healing process (Table 4.8).

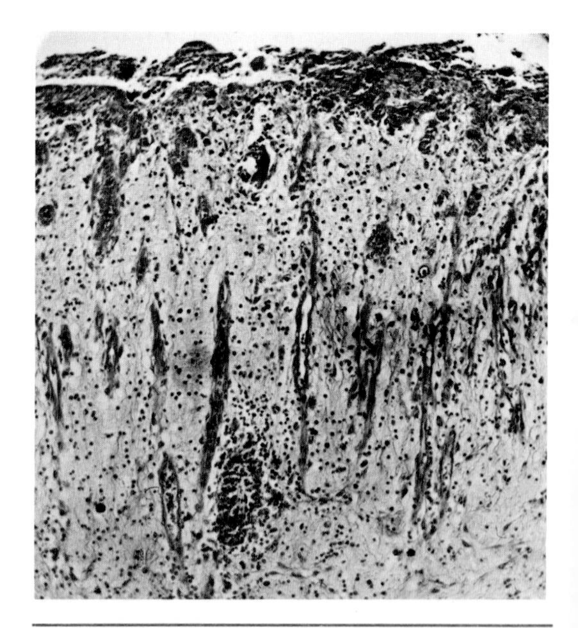

Fig. 4.29 Granulation tissue in healing skin wound showing the vertical lines of newly formed blood vessels (angiogenesis).

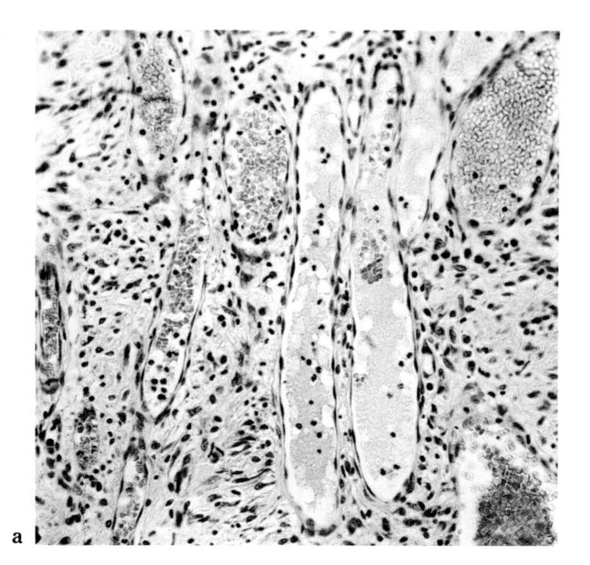

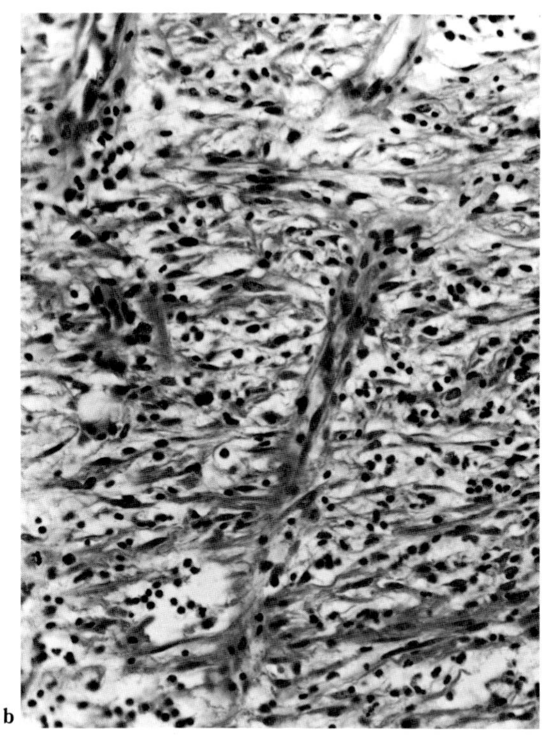

Fig. 4.30 a & b Changes in the composition of granulation tissue over time. **a** Initially the blood vessels are thin-walled capillaries which run at right angles to the wound surface; fibroblasts are aligned alongside the vessels. **b** At later stages there is devascularization and the fibroblasts become aligned differently.

Epidermal Growth Factor (EGF)/Transforming Growth Factor α (TGFα)

Epidermal growth factor (EGF) was one of the first growth factors to be identified. In most epithelial tissues, a membrane receptor for this peptide (EGF-R) is abundantly expressed. Current evidence, however, suggests that the natural ligand for this receptor is a peptide closely related to EGF, called transforming growth factor α (TGFα). This protein is synthesized by epithelial cells; its rate of synthesis increases in response to injury. This growth factor was initially termed a 'transforming' growth factor because of its capacity to induce phenotypic transformation in cultured cells. Another peptide, TGFβ, identified at the same time as TGFα, was found to have similar properties.*

* The designation 'transforming growth factor' refers only to one of the many diverse properties of these peptides. This label is perhaps a little misleading as it probably has little transforming activity *in vivo*.

Recent work suggests that in addition to being released by epithelial cells in response to injury a TGFα-like peptide may also be released by platelets during the early stages of the response. These peptides bind to EGF receptors on adjacent epithelial cells and stimulate their regeneration and migration (paracrine stimulation). Since epithelial cells such as keratinocytes and hepatocytes express both TGFα and EGF-R, such cells may also be stimulated by an autocrine loop. There is some evidence that TGFα may also be involved in the connective tissue response by stimulating the proliferation of fibroblasts and endothelial cells.

Transforming Growth Factor β

This peptide exists in three isomeric forms. The most abundant, $TGF\beta_1$, is found in highest levels in the α granules of platelets but is also expressed by a wide range of mesenchymal cells including activated macrophages. It is a potent fibroblast mitogen and may potentiate the effects of other

Table 4.8 Growth factors and cytokines in the healing process

Epidermal growth factor/transforming growth factor α	EGF TGFα	Regeneration of epithelial cells
Transforming growth factor β	TGFβ	Potentiates other growth factors; mitogenic for fibroblasts; enhances extracellular matrix formation; control of epithelial cell regeneration
Platelet-derived growth factor	PDGF	Chemotactic and mitogenic for fibroblasts and smooth muscle cells
Fibroblast growth factors	FGF	Mitogenic for fibroblasts; stimulates angiogenesis; regeneration of epithelial cells
Insulin-like growth factor I	IGF-I	Synergistic with other factors
Tumour necrosis factor α	TNFα	Stimulates angiogenesis

growth factors such as platelet derived growth factor. It also stimulates fibroblasts directly to increase their synthesis of extracellular matrix proteins. Furthermore, it appears to inhibit the synthesis of collagenases, the net effect being to promote matrix formation. It also acts as a 'negative growth factor' for epithelial cells by inhibiting cell replication, which is of importance in controlling regeneration in the healing responses.

Platelet Derived Growth Factor (PDGF)

Platelet derived growth factor, like TGFβ, is found most abundantly in the α granules of platelets and exists in several molecular forms. It may also be synthesized by macrophages and endothelial cells. The activity of PDGF was first identified when it was observed that cultured fibroblasts proliferated more rapidly in a medium containing plasma (in which platelets are present) than in one containing serum (from which the platelets have been removed). PDGF is also a potent mitogen for smooth muscle cells and may stimulate the migration of these cells to areas of injury together with fibroblasts and macrophages.

Fibroblast Growth Factors (FGF)

These factors were initially isolated from bovine brain and pituitary. Two forms were originally identified, acidic (aFGF) and basic (bFGF). These are now known to form part of a large family of related growth factors which are not restricted to neural tissue, but are synthesized by a large number of cells and stimulate proliferation in an equally wide range of cell types.

Basic FGF is present in macrophages and is a potent mitogen for endothelial cells and fibroblasts. FGFs are also mitogenic for some epithelial cells such as keratinocytes and may play a role in the regenerative component.

Other Peptide Growth Factors and Cytokines

A number of growth factors have been identified which are structurally very similar to the precursor form of insulin. Two such peptides have been well characterized, insulin-like growth factors (IGF), IGF-I and IGF-II. Unlike many of the other growth factors, IGFs are found in plasma. IGF-II appears to function as a generalized growth promoting agent during embryogenesis; IGF-I adopts this function in postnatal development, and may also act as a paracrine growth factor in healing. The precise mechanisms are unclear but the peptide may potentiate the actions of PDGF and TGFβ.

Tumour necrosis factor α is mitogenic for mesenchymal cells including fibroblasts and endothelial cells. Interleukin 1 stimulates the synthesis of extracellular matrix proteins by fibroblasts and is also mitogenic for these cells. There is also evidence that GM-CSF (p. 587) is mitogenic for myofibroblasts.

Interaction of Growth Factors

Much of our knowledge of these various factors is based on *in vitro* studies and their precise role *in vivo* is less certain. There is probably considerable interaction between the various growth factors and with other mediators such as prostaglandins. Furthermore, novel peptides are constantly being added to the list of growth factors, and growth factor-like activity is being identified in previously known molecules such as some neuropeptides (e.g. bombesin). Our understanding of this complex network of growth factors and cytokines is just evolving. Nevertheless, it is possible to construct a simplified working hypothesis for their role in healing based on experimental observations (Fig. 4.31). Growth factors may be derived from a number of sources following injury: (1) platelets, activated after endothelial damage; (2) macrophages or (3) lymphocytes recruited to the area of injury; (4) damaged epithelial cells; and (5) circulating serum growth factors. Some of the growth factors (TGFα, EGF) stimulate regeneration of surviving epithelial cells, while others (PDGF, TGFβ) mediate the further recruitment of macrophages. Several factors (TGFβ, PDGF, bFGF, IL-1) stimulate the proliferation and activation of fibroblasts and related cell types while others (TNFα, bFGF) mediate angiogenesis.

The healing process ceases when lost tissue has been replaced. The mechanisms regulating this process are not fully understood. Although cessation of epithelial regeneration may be explained by contact-inhibition, TGFβ acts as a growth inhibitor for both epithelial and endothelial cells and regulates their regeneration. Furthermore, a number of circulating peptides and prostanoids may regulate the connective tissue response in healing. Prostaglandins E_2 and interferon-α have been shown to inhibit fibroblast proliferation *in vitro*.

The availability of recombinant growth factors will allow further investigation of their properties and in addition raises the possibility of their use as therapeutic agents in clinical situations such as the healing of burns or other wounds.

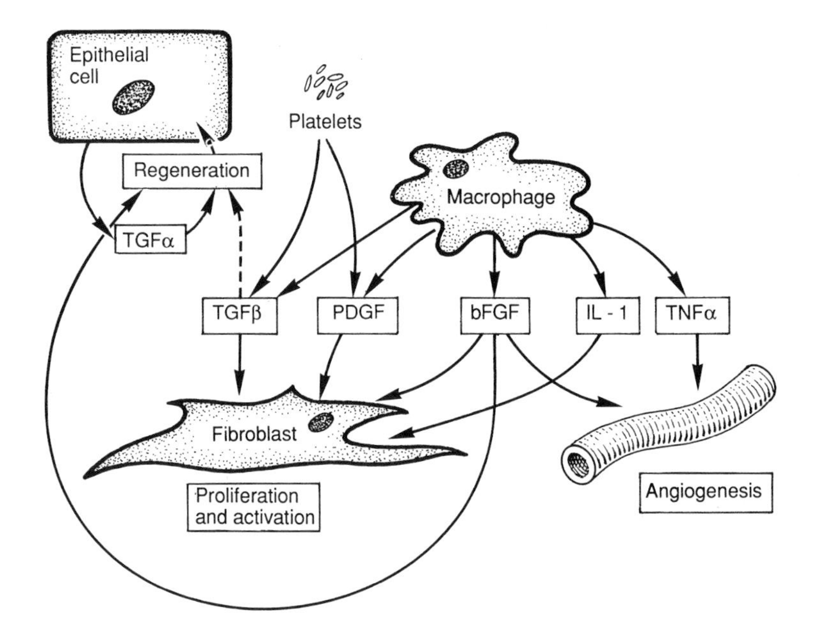

Fig. 4.31 Proposed role for some of the major peptide growth factors involved in healing. These molecules are derived from at least three sources: platelets, macrophages and epithelial cells. They stimulate (1) regeneration, (2) fibroblast proliferation and activation and (3) angiogenesis.

Healing of Skin Wounds

Healing by Primary Intention (Primary Union)

The simplest form of skin wound healing occurs when uninfected incisions and other clean wounds without loss of tissue are closed promptly by surgical sutures. This is referred to as healing by primary intention. It is a rapid process and contrasts with healing by second intention which occurs in an open wound (Fig. 4.32).

When an incision is made in the skin and subcutaneous tissue, blood escaping from cut vessels clots on the wound surface and fills the gap between the wound edges which, in sutured wounds, is narrow. Fibrin in the blood clot binds the cut surfaces together, while the dehydrated blood clot on the surface forms a scab which effectively seals the wound. In the first 24 hours, there is a mild inflammatory reaction at the wound edges with exudation of fluid, deposition of further fibrin and migration of neutrophil polymorphs followed by monocytes and lymphocytes. The blood clot is initially digested by released lysosomal enzymes and this process is aided from about the third day by macrophages.

The first tissue to bridge the incisional gap is the squamous epithelium of the epidermis. Within 24 hours, and extending from 3 to 4 mm around the wound edge, there is enlargement of the basal cells with some loss of their normally close adherence to the underlying tissue and with flattening of rete ridges. Two processes then contribute to the closure of the gap; (1) close to the cut edge, cells from the deeper part of the epithelium migrate out over the wound surface and become flattened to form a continuous advancing sheet; and (2) the stem cells in the basal layer of the epidermis and adjacent pilosebaceous follicles proliferate. While the advancing edge of the sheet of new epidermis consists of a single layer of flat cells, the older part at the periphery of the wound becomes stratified so that there is a gradient of thickness. The cells will only migrate over viable

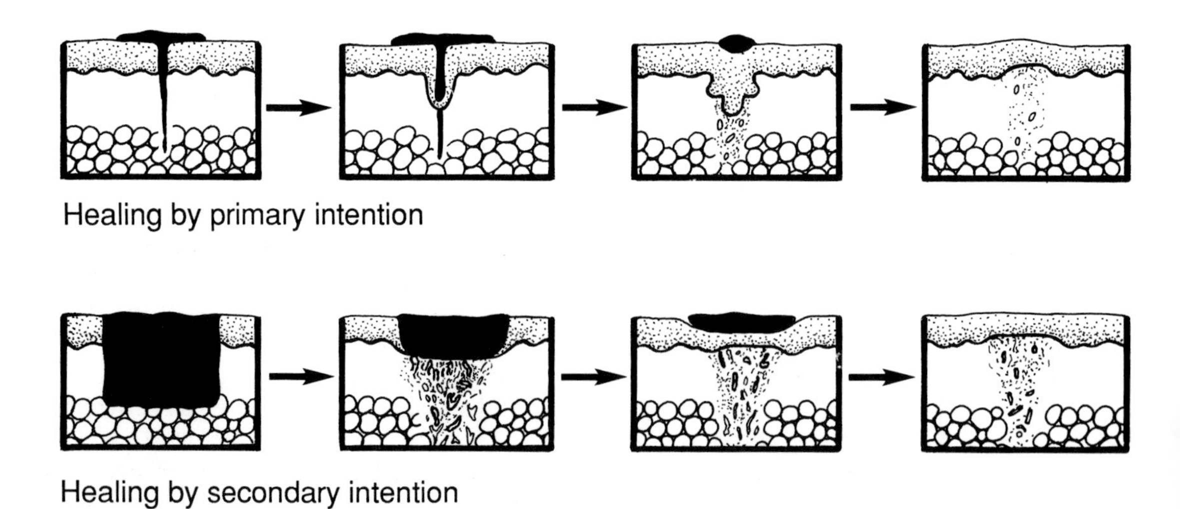

Fig. 4.32 Outline of stages involved in healing of skin wounds. Initially the wound fills with blood clot. This is followed by regeneration of keratinocytes and a connective tissue response (formation of granulation tissue) in the dermis. The basic mechanisms of healing by primary and secondary intention are similar. However, there is a greater connective tissue response in healing by secondary intention and the whole process is much slower.

tissue. They move beneath the surface blood clot and wound debris and down the cut edges of the dermis. Within 48 hours the wound may be bridged by epithelium which rapidly becomes stratified but does not form rete ridges. Any epithelium which has grown down into the dermis is later resorbed.

The dermis and subcutaneous tissues are repaired by the formation of granulation tissue. From about the third day, angiogenesis can be observed at the wound margins. The newly formed capillaries are very delicate, lacking a basement membrane, and behave as if acutely inflamed: they leak protein-rich fluid and neutrophils emigrate from them. Long, spindle-shaped fibroblasts begin to proliferate and migrate into the wound. They produce extracellular matrix proteins and the collagen fibres come to lie across the incision line and help to unite the cut edges from about the end of the first week after injury. By the third week the total amount of collagen in the wound has almost reached a maximum. At this stage the tensile strength of the wound is still low, but it increases over many months by replacement of some of the type III by type I collagen, by further intermolecular bonding between collagen fibrils, and by remodelling of the anatomical configuration of the collagen in response to mechanical stress.

Once the wound has healed the scar is commonly raised above the surface due to the underlying proliferative processes and is red as a result of increased vascularity. The blood vessels gradually decrease in number in the manner already described. Elastic fibres are formed much later than collagen. Sensory nerves may grow into the scar in about 3 weeks but specialized nerve endings such as Pacinian corpuscles do not reform. The end result of healing by first intention is a pale linear scar, level with the adjacent skin surface. Sometimes a hypertrophic scar or keloid forms (Fig. 4.33).

It should be appreciated that each suture tract is a wound, with haemorrhage, death of cells and injury to skin appendages, and in consequence there is a mild inflammatory reaction and fibroblast proliferation. Because the suture prevents closure of the surface epithelium the track is prone to infection and a 'stitch abscess' may occur. Epithelium also tends to grow down suture tracts from both ends. Often much of the epithelium is avulsed when stitches are removed but some may remain and occasionally give rise either to a small implantation cyst or to a marked inflammatory reaction to keratin.

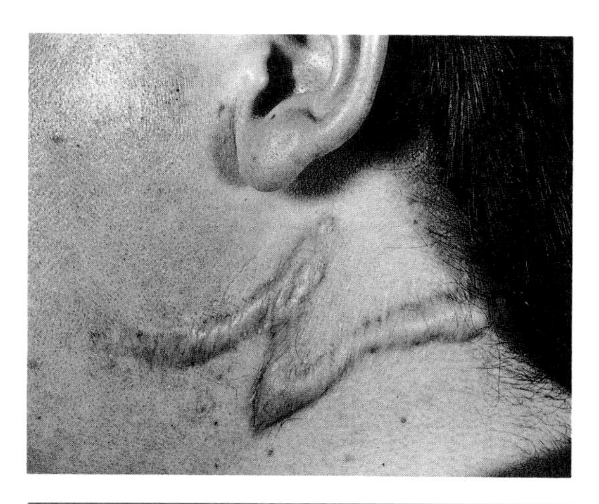

Fig. 4.33 Keloid scar which developed in a plastic surgery procedure (Z-plasty) for a traumatic wound on the neck. (Courtesy of Mr I. A. McGregor).

Healing by Secondary Intention (Secondary Union)

Healing of an open wound where there has been loss of tissue occurs by the formation of more substantial amounts of granulation tissue which grows from the base of the wound to fill the defect (Fig. 4.32). Healing takes much longer than when it occurs by first intention. As in the closed wound there is haemorrhage and exudation of fibrin from the cut surfaces. This is soon followed by a more intense inflammatory reaction with migration of neutrophils and subsequently of monocytes: these cells remove the fibrin and other debris. Epithelial cells at the margins enlarge and begin to migrate down the walls of the wound in the first day or two after injury. Migration and proliferation together produce a sheet of cells which advances in a series of tongue-like projections beneath any remaining blood clot or exudate on the wound surface. Since the denuded area is large, the advancing epithelial sheet does not completely cover the wound until the granulation tissue from the base has started to fill the wound space. As soon as the wound surface is covered, epithelial cell migration ceases and proliferation, stratification and keratinization are rapidly completed, though rete ridges are not re-formed. When the full thickness of the skin is destroyed by a burn, re-epithelialization is slow as the cells have to migrate beneath the thick layer of dead coagulated collagen. In contrast, in a burn which destroys only part of the skin thickness, in a superficial wound or at the donor site of a 'split thickness' skin graft, re-epithelialization is relatively rapid as proliferation of epithelium occurs from all the epithelial edges and also from the cut mouth of each pilosebaceous follicle.

Within a few days of injury the pre-existing vessels in the wound bed produce vascular sprouts which grow upwards, forming loops and coils near the wound surface (see Fig. 4.29). From these new, more permeable vessels small haemorrhages occur and neutrophils migrate, reinforcing those already present in the exudate on the wound surface and helping to keep down bacterial growth. This fibrovascular granulation tissue gradually fills the wound space and as epithelium grows over its surface the exudative inflammatory changes and the migration of neutrophils also subside. If epithelialization is delayed, e.g. by further trauma or infection, granulations may pout from the wound surface. Following healing, there is gradual retraction and disappearance of some of the new vascular channels and further cross-linking and remodelling of collagen which, over a period of months, becomes progressively less cellular.

Healing of an open, excised wound is aided by contraction of the surface area at sites where the skin is mobile and loosely attached to underlying tissue. However, the degree of passive contraction is related to normal skin tension and active contraction to bring the edges towards the centre of the wound is brought about by myofibroblasts. The term contracture is applied when healing produces distortion or limitation of movement of the tissues and is most often seen in patients who have had full thickness burns (Fig. 4.34). It may result either from excessive contraction of the wound itself or from scarring of the underlying muscle and soft tissue.

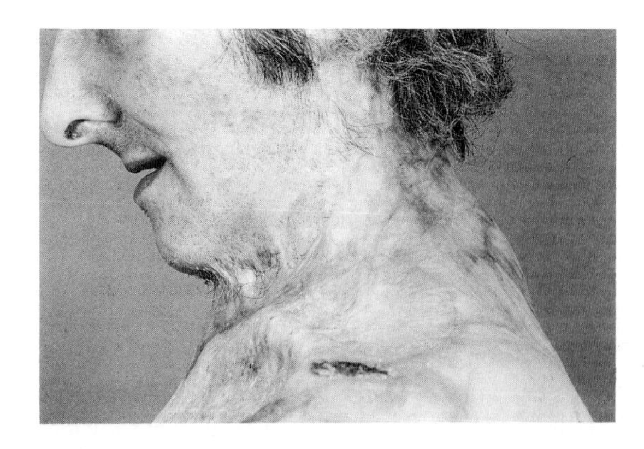

Fig. 4.34 Contractures following the healing of an extensive burn on the face and neck. (Courtesy of Professor W. H. Reid).

Factors Influencing Wound Healing

A number of factors can alter the rate and efficiency of healing. These can be classified into local and systemic factors (Table 4.9). Most of these factors have been established in studies of

Table 4.9 Factors known to impair healing

Local	Systemic
Infection	Nutrition
Poor blood supply	protein lack
Excessive movement	vitamin C deficiency
Presence of foreign body material	zinc deficiency
Ionizing radiation	Diabetes mellitus
	Corticosteroid treatment
	Haematological diseases, neutropenia
	Renal failure
	Tumour cachexia

skin wound healing but many are likely to be of relevance to healing at other sites.

The type and size of the wound are of great importance as is the site. Wounds in richly vascularized skin such as on the face will heal more rapidly than those at sites where the dermal blood flow is less, such as in pretibial skin. Local vascular insufficiency either as a result of venous stasis or a compromised arterial supply will prevent healing. Delayed healing will also occur if there is local infection. Irradiation will interfere with healing by inhibiting cell proliferation in both epithelial cells and mesenchymal cells. It is for this reason that adjuvant radiotherapy in the management of malignant tumours is often withheld until any surgical scar has been able to heal.

Wound healing will also be impaired if there is systemic infection; the reasons for this are probably multifactorial. Renal failure is associated with diminished capacity for healing although the precise mechanisms for this are uncertain.

Certain hormones, in particular corticosteroids, have an inhibitory effect if present at high concentrations. Inhibition may occasionally be seen in patients on therapeutic doses of steroids. Again the mechanisms are unclear; there appears to be effects on both regeneration and the connective tissue response. Wounds in steroid treated patients tend to have a scanty macrophage infiltrate with a consequent lack of macrophage-derived growth factors.

Protein calorie malnutrition (p. 342) impairs healing. Deficiency of vitamin C (scurvy) may have a similar effect because of its need as a cofactor in collagen synthesis. A considerable period of dietary insufficiency is required before scurvy is clinically apparent. However, patients with multiple injuries or extensive burns can rapidly become vitamin C deficient with consequent impairment of healing. Because vitamin C is involved in the intracellular hydroxylation of procollagen, one of the effects of deficiency is the secretion of collagen which subsequently shows less cross-linking than normal and is thus more readily degraded. Zinc is also required for normal collagen synthesis. Deficiency of this mineral in patients with severe burns or intestinal fistulae may contribute to impaired healing.

Fracture Healing

The basic processes involved in the healing of bone fractures bear many resemblances to those seen in wound healing. Primary union of a fracture virtually never occurs, healing by production of callus, a process analogous to healing by second intention being the rule. Unlike healing of a skin wound, however, the defect caused by a fracture is repaired not by a fibrous 'scar' tissue, but by specialized bone forming tissue so that under favourable circumstances the bone is restored nearly to normal.

Fracture healing can be considered in several stages: the immediate consequences of the injury, including haemorrhage and necrosis of bone; the formation of an immobilizing collar of external callus proceeding along with repair in the medullary cavity and cortex and union across the fracture gap; finally, remodelling of the healed fracture.

Immediate Consequences of Fracture

In patients with normal bone structure, considerable force is required to break a bone, and there is usually displacement of the bone ends. Blood vessels within bone, periosteum and soft tissue are torn, causing haemorrhage between the bone ends and within the adjacent tissues, sometimes in very large amounts; in addition bone and haemopoietic marrow around the fracture site are rendered ischaemic and undergo necrosis. Cortical bone usually suffers more extensive necrosis than medullary bone. When there is splintering of bone (a comminuted fracture) these fragments also undergo necrosis. Bone death is recognized histologically by loss of osteocytes from lacunae (p. 946). A local inflammatory response follows fracture, with hyperaemia, exudation of protein-rich fluid, and extravasation of neutrophil polymorphs, which are relatively few unless the fracture site becomes infected. This is common only in compound fractures where the overlying skin is torn, allowing direct bacterial contamination; on occasion infection follows internal fixation. A little later macrophages invade the fracture site and phagocytose blood clot and tissue debris.

Formation of Provisional Callus and Bony Union

External Callus

External callus can be thought of as a bandage of reactive tissue which is formed by the periosteum and immobilizes the bone fracture site.

Within a day or so of the fracture, there is rapid proliferation of osteoprogenitor cells of the inner layer of the periosteum overlying the viable cortex of each fractured bone end. Soon, highly cellular spindle-celled tissue surrounds the bone ends and extends into adjacent soft tissue and skeletal muscle. Mitotic figures are numerous, and a biopsy at this stage may readily be misinterpreted as a sarcoma if the pathologist is unaware of the history of recent fracture. The proliferating cells differentiate into osteoblasts which form osteoid and bone, and chondrocytes which produce cartilage. The periosteal reaction begins close to the fracture site and extends over a considerable length of cortex. In time the proliferation of osteoprogenitor cells diminishes and the fracture callus matures. Two enlarging cuffs of callus which are firmly anchored to the cortex advance towards each other and finally unite to bridge the fracture line (Fig. 4.35). The amount of cartilage which is formed in provisional callus varies greatly and is thought to be promoted by a poor blood supply and by shearing stresses. External callus in general, and cartilage in particular, tend to be abundant in poorly immobilized fractures, such as those of clavicle or ribs; a wedge-shaped mass of cartilage may overlie the fracture line and this gradually undergoes endochondral ossification.

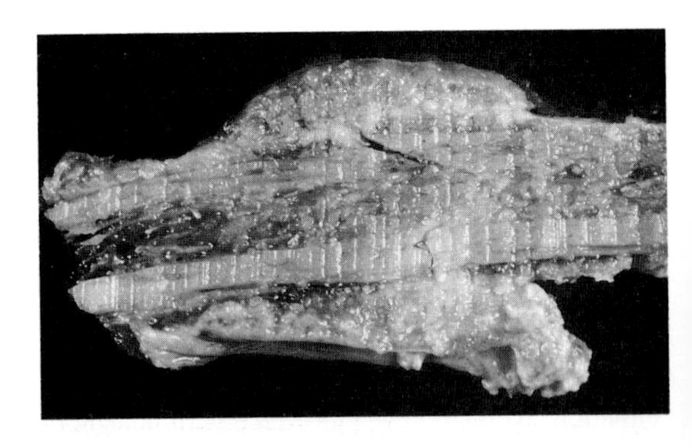

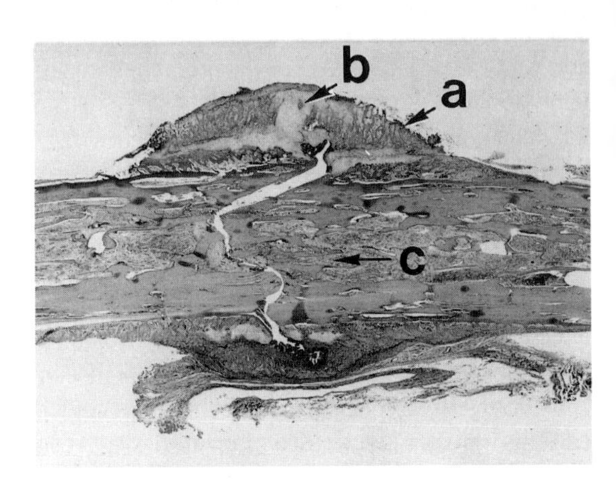

Fig. 4.35 Fracture healing. This segment of rib was excised from a woman of 22 who complained of a painful swelling of the chest wall of a few weeks' duration. The preoperative diagnosis was of a tumour of bone. Upper: the gross specimen shows an irregular fracture line involving both cortices and the medullary canal. The fracture is bridged by periosteal callus, which is particularly marked in the superior surface. Lower: histological examination shows that the periosteal callus consists of arcades of reactive bone (a) and a mass of cartilage (b) overlying the fracture line. There is also callus within the medullary canal (c). At this relatively early stage of fracture healing, the fracture gap remains unrepaired.

The amount of periosteal callus formed depends on the anatomical site and also on the degree of immobilization. External callus probably depends on surrounding skeletal muscle for its blood supply; thus little callus forms around fractures of the tibia which has a large subcutaneous border, and healing is often delayed. In intracapsular fractures (i.e. those within a joint capsule), such as subcapital fractures of the femoral neck, the periosteum is lacking and no external callus forms. Thus, healing of the fracture here depends largely on the formation of endosteal callus. This necessitates close contact between the bone ends and excellent immobilization which may be achieved by internal fixation.

Medullary and Cortical Repair

Healing within the medullary cavity involves vascular proliferation and revascularization of necrotic marrow, together with reactive new bone formation with osteoblasts proliferating and growing into the site of injury. Endosteal callus is less abundant than periosteal callus, and cartilage is rarely seen. In those sites, like the neck of femur where periosteum is absent, medullary callus is of particular importance in achieving bony union. When union is delayed, there is often a band of fibrous tissue in the marrow cavity at the fracture site.

Changes also occur in the cortex adjacent to the fracture site. There is increased osteoclastic resorption within viable cortex, with widening of the Haversian canals. This results in local osteoporosis and is at least partly a response to immobilization. Ingrowth of vessels from the living bone into necrotic cortex allows osteoclastic resorption of dead bone and replacement by viable new bone.

Healing of the Fracture Gap

The fracture gap is filled with bone in one of two ways. **Direct ossification**, which is rapid and effective, is brought about by osteogenic cells spreading from the medullary and periosteal callus. In contrast, **fibrous union** may occur initially, with the ingrowth of fibrous tissue which only much more slowly becomes ossified. This slower form of union occurs especially when there are unfavourable local conditions such as instability, separation or marked resorption of the bone ends, massive necrosis, a poor blood supply or infection.

Remodelling

When bony union has occurred across the fracture gap the newly laid down bone is reconstructed to restore full mechanical strength. The newly formed woven bone is resorbed and gradually replaced by lamellar bone. Most remaining necrotic bone is removed and replaced. The cortex is re-formed across the fracture gap and gradually medullary callus is removed with restoration of the marrow cavity. Once function has been regained, the bone is remodelled in response to mechanical stresses. If the fracture alignment is perfect, external callus is resorbed; if the fracture has united at an angle, new bone is incorporated on the concave side while resorption occurs on the convex, so that the bone becomes straighter. This process is particularly effective in children; in adults angulation is less well corrected. The whole repair process may take about a year, although the time varies from site to site. It is rapid and more complete in children.

Factors Affecting Fracture Healing

Both local and systemic factors affect fracture healing.

Local factors. Infection of the fracture site, interposition of soft tissue between the bone ends, and excess movement all tend to delay fracture healing. The presence of tumour deposits (pathological fracture) will also prevent or delay healing. A poor local blood supply, for example following irradiation, is also associated with difficulty in healing. Conversion to bone after fibrous union is sometimes very slow (**delayed union**), and occasionally fails to occur (**non-union**). In this case, the fibrous tissue becomes very dense and ultimately is converted to fibrocartilage. A linear split may develop and enlarge with formation of a lining similar to synovium, resulting in a false joint (**pseudoarthrosis**).

Systemic factors. Lack of vitamin C results in depression of collagen biosynthesis; as a result bone formation is deficient. Corticosteroids administered to animals with fractures delay healing, but it seems that they have little effect when given to patients in the usual therapeutic doses. In vitamin D deficiency abundant callus may form, but it fails to calcify and remains soft.

Complications of Fractures

Extensive haemorrhage, particularly likely in fractures of the femur and pelvis, may result in **hypovolaemic shock** (p. 106). **Fat embolism** (p. 98) may follow damage to marrow, when globules of fat enter from venules and impact in the microcirculation of the lungs, brain and kidney. As well as local bone necrosis which follows fracture, more extensive **osteonecrosis** (p. 961) may occur depending on local peculiarities of the blood supply. Thus, subcapital fractures of the femoral neck are often followed by osteonecrosis of the femoral head, and fractures of the carpal scaphoid are often complicated by necrosis of the proximal half of the bone. **Osteoarthritis** (p. 985) may result when the fracture line has involved the articular surface, with the production of an incongruity of the articular cartilage. In addition, malaligned fractures throw abnormal stress on the joint and may also cause osteoarthritis. The development of pseudarthroses has already been described.

Role of Mediators in Healing of Fractures

As with healing and repair in other tissues there is good evidence that growth factors, cytokines and arachidonic acid derivatives are important in fracture healing and remodelling. Interleukin 1, PDGF, EGF and PGE_2 all promote bone resorption and this, through the normal coupling between osteoclasts and osteoblasts (p. 947), is a stimulus to bone formation. These factors may act directly or by activation of macrophages with the release of substances such as osteoclast activating factor (OAF). Osteoblasts have receptors for and also produce TGFβ, and macrophage-derived growth factor(s) apparently specific for osteoblasts have been described in experimental studies.

Healing in Other Tissues

Neural Tissue

The response to injury differs between the central nervous system and the peripheral nervous system. Once mature nerve cells of the brain, cord or ganglia are destroyed, they cannot be replaced by proliferation of other nerve cells. Furthermore, there is only very limited regeneration of axons. Healing is restricted to a connective tissue response which involves microglial cells and astrocytes – gliosis. In contrast, peripheral nerves have considerable regenerative capacity and this topic is discussed fully in Chapter 18.

Muscle

When skeletal muscle fibres are injured, the sarcoplasm of necrotic fibres disintegrates and is phagocytosed by macrophages. The healing process that follows involves two processes. First, multinucleated sprouts form from the surviving ends of injured fibres. Second, there appears to be proliferation of mononucleated myoblasts. The final outcome of the healing process depends to a great extent on the degree of injury sustained by the surrounding endomysium. If this is intact, as occurs in toxic muscle damage associated with severe infections, then there may be complete restitution of the normal structure and function of the muscle. If, on the other hand, there is damage to the surrounding matrix, then the healing process is dominated by the connective tissue response with the laying down of scar tissue and consequent loss of function.

Healing in smooth muscle also tends to be characterized by a prominent connective tissue response. It should be noted, however, that smooth muscle at some sites (e.g. myometrium) does have a significant capacity for regeneration.

Cardiac muscle has limited capacity for regeneration. Myocytes destroyed by ischaemic injury, for example, are replaced by scar tissue. This may be accompanied by hypertrophy of surviving fibres. In some viral myocarditides, there may be preservation of the endomysium, analogous to the situation in toxic skeletal muscle injury and in this situation there may be limited regeneration of cardiac myocytes.

Further Reading

Babior, B. M. (1984). The respiratory burst of leukocytes. *Journal of Clinical Investigation* **73**, 599–660.

Burgeson, R. E. (1988). New collagens, new concepts. *Annual Review of Cell Biology* **4**, 551–7.

Clark, R. A. F. and Henson, P. M. (eds) (1988). *The Molecular and Cellular Biology of Wound Repair.* Plenum Press, New York.

Deuel, T. F. (1987). Polypeptide growth factors: roles in normal and abnormal cell growth. *Annual Review of Cell Biology* **3**, 443–64.

Hogg, N. (1989). The leukocyte integrins. *Immunology Today* **10**, 111–14.

Hynes, R. O. (1987). Integrins: a family of cell surface receptors. *Cell* **48**, 549–54.

Kelley, W. N., Harris, E. D., Ruddy, S. and Sledge, C. R. (1989). *Textbook of Rheumatology*, 3rd edn, Chapters 14–23. W. B. Saunders Co, Philadelphia, London and Toronto.

Nathan, C. F. (1987). Secretory products of macrophages. *Journal of Clinical Investigation* **79**, 319–26.

Osborn, L. (1990). Leukocyte adhesion to endothelium in inflammation. *Cell* **62**, 3–6.

Sevitt, E. (ed.) (1981). *Bone Repair and Fracture Healing in Man.* Churchill Livingstone, Edinburgh.

Sporn, M. B. and Roberts, A. B. (1986). Peptide growth factors and inflammation, tissue repair and cancer. *Journal of Clinical Investigation* **78**, 329–32.

Weiss, J., Victor, M., Stendhal, O. and Elsbach, P. (1982). Oxygen independent intracellular mechanisms. *Journal of Clinical Investigation* **69**, 959–70.

Whaley, K. (ed.) (1987). *Complement in Health and Disease.* MTP Press Ltd, Lancaster.

Williams, T. J. (1989). Vascular changes in inflammation and mechanisms of oedema formation. In *Textbook of Immunopharmacology*, p. 196, Dale, M. M. and Foreman, J. (eds). Blackwell Scientific Publications Ltd, Oxford.

5

The Structure and Function of the Immune System

The immune system has evolved as a defence against microbial infection and comprises two forms of immunity, specific and non-specific. The specific immune response against a particular micro-organism only protects against that organism and an account of this specific immunity forms the major part of this chapter. Nevertheless, several non-specific immune defence mechanisms exist and are of considerable importance in host defence against infection. Indeed, it is only if these non-specific responses are overcome that a specific immune response becomes necessary. These are dealt with in greater detail in Chapter 8 but are briefly summarized here.

Non-specific Immune Mechanisms

Mechanical. The intact skin and the epithelial layers of mucous membranes form a simple but effective barrier to microbial invasion. Most mucosae also employ mechanisms which assist expulsion of pathogens from the tissue. These include reflex activities such as coughing, sneezing or vomiting, as well as the constant upward movement of the mucus in the respiratory tract brought about by the beating of the cilia on the surface of respiratory epithelial cells. In the intestine, a similar function is fulfilled by the downward propulsion of luminal contents caused by peristalsis, while the constant flow of sterile urine serves to cleanse the urinary tract and tears serve a similar purpose in the eye.

Humoral. The fluids secreted by most body tissues contain factors which can kill or inhibit the growth of micro-organisms. **Sebum** released by the sebaceous glands of the skin is antibacterial, while blood and internal secretions such as tears, saliva and intestinal fluid are rich in the enzyme **lysozyme** and other antibacterial substances such as polyamines. Other protective proteins present in blood and other body fluids include complement components, C-reactive protein and interferons. Intestinal secretions contain additional factors of great importance in non-specific immunity, including gastric acid, pancreatic enzymes and bile salts whose presence normally makes the local environment hostile to most organisms.

Cellular. Many cell types contribute to non-specific defence of the body. These include leucocytes such as neutrophils, eosinophils and macrophages, which can phagocytose and kill infecting organisms. These and other cells such as mast cells and basophils can also produce soluble mediators which assist in the inflammatory response (Chapter 4). Finally, natural killer (NK) cells are a subpopulation of lymphocyte which can kill infected tissue cells in a non-specific manner.

These mechanisms all act rapidly during the early stages of an infection and can function in the absence of a specific immune response. However, many of them can also be initiated or amplified by components of the specific immune system interactions discussed below.

The Immune Response

The features of the specific immune response which distinguish it from the non-specific mechanisms described above are:

(1) **Specificity.** Infection with one micro-organism leads to protection only against that organism or a closely related organism.

(2) **Memory.** Once an immune response against a particular microbe has occurred, protection against a second infection with the same organism is usually lifelong, because the immune system possesses a rapid recall system known as immunological memory. This enables a quicker and larger response to occur on subsequent exposure (secondary immune response) and is the rationale for the ability of immunization to protect against infectious diseases.

(3) **Self, non-self discrimination.** An important feature of the specific immune response is the ability to discriminate between self-components and non-self (foreign). Although the body occasionally recognizes self-components as foreign and develops an autoimmune response, exposure to self-components during fetal life usually leads to a state of specific unresponsiveness known as **immunological tolerance**.

Specific immune responses are triggered by substances known as **antigens** and the resulting responses can be divided into humoral and cellular components. Humoral responses result in the synthesis of antibody molecules which react with the triggering antigen. Antibodies belong to a group of proteins known collectively as immunoglobulins. The protective effect of antibody can be transferred by injecting the serum of an immune individual into a non-immune individual (passive immunity). In contrast, the cellular immune response is independent of antibody production and can only be transferred by lymphocytes. The normal immune response to infection involves both forms of immunity and is a complex process involving cooperation between lymphocytes, macrophages and many other cell types.

Cellular Basis of the Immune Response

(Table 5.1)

All specific immune responses are dependent on lymphocytes. Antibodies are produced by the **B lymphocytes**, while cellular immune responses are initiated by **T lymphocytes**. All lymphocytes are derived from a common haemopoietic precursor in the bone marrow (fetal liver or yolk sac in prenatal life), before undergoing further maturation either in the bone marrow itself (**B lymphocytes**; B cells) or the thymus (**T lymphocytes**; T cells) (Fig. 5.1). These tissues are known as the **primary lymphoid organs**. Both the humoral and cellular immune response require a single resting or 'virgin' lymphocyte to bind to a unique antigenic determinant by a specific receptor and to give rise to large numbers of identical daughter cells which retain the antigen specificity of the initial progenitor. Collectively, these new cells

Table 5.1 Cells involved in immune responses

Accessory cell	Non-lymphocytic cell which functions as a modulator of immune responses or of lymphocyte function or development. Usually Ia-positive (see Ia antigens). In many cases, essential for T-helper cell activity in initiating immune responses. Many accessory cells resemble the mononuclear phagocytes in their physiological characteristics but others, e.g. dendritic cells, are not phagocytic.
Activated lymphocyte	An antigen-stimulated lymphocyte which is either proliferating (i.e. a blast form) or which is taking an active part in an immune response.
Antigen presenting cell	Non-lymphocytic cell that carries antigen and presents it to lymphocytes resulting in the induction of an immune response.
B lymphocyte (B cell)	A lymphocyte which is derived from bone marrow without passing through the thymus (cf. T lymphocyte). In birds B-lymphocyte maturation is determined by the bursa of Fabricius. B lymphocytes play a major role in humoral immunity. On stimulation by antigen they differentiate into antibody-forming plasma cells.
Cytotoxic T cell	Effector T-lymphocyte subset (usually CD8) which directly lyses target cells. Cytotoxic T lymphocytes kill virus-infected cells provided that the latter also carry syngeneic class I antigens (MHC restriction).
Dendritic cell	The term includes (1) follicular dendritic cell (see below) and (2) dendritic cells of the splenic white pulp and lymph node paracortex but which are accessory cells for T-cell activation.
Effector lymphocyte	Fully differentiated product of an antigen-stimulated lymphoblast which has a direct functional role in the immune response. Plasma cells are the 'lymphocytes effector' of the B-cell series.
Follicular dendritic cell	A cell found in the germinal centres of the lymph nodes and spleen. Possesses cytoplasmic processes which can retain antigen for long periods of time.
Immunoblast	Term used by histopathologists to refer to a lymphocyte which has been stimulated by antigen and which will differentiate into an effector cell. Thus in this terminology there is a distinction between lymphoblast and immunoblast, the former being allied to a cell undergoing lymphopoiesis.
Lymphoblast	A blast cell of the lymphoid cell series with a nuclear pattern characterized by fine chromatin and basophil nucleoli. Lymphoblasts are formed *in vivo* or *in vitro* following antigenic or mitogenic stimulation, and divide to form populations of effector lymphocytes. There are also many established lymphoblast lines in tissue culture.
Macrophage	Phagocytic cell of the mononuclear phagocyte system. Most macrophages are believed to be derived from blood monocytes which migrate into the tissues and differentiate there.
Memory cells	T cells and B cells which mediate immunological memory.
Natural killer (NK) cell	Lymphoid cell which kills a range of sensitive tumour cell targets in the absence of prior immunization and without antigen specificity. Distinguished morphologically by the presence of large intracytoplasmic granules visible under the light microscope (large granular lymphocytes).
Plasma cell	The end cell of the B-lymphocyte line, it is the major immunoglobulin-producing cell type and therefore the classical cell of humoral immunity. Present in lymphoid tissues and increased in numbers in the draining lymph node and at the site of entry of antigen following antigenic stimulation.
Resting lymphocyte	Small, quiescent lymphocyte in G_o phase of cell cycle. May not have previously encountered antigen (virgin lymphocyte) or may be a memory cell.
T-helper cell	A thymus-derived lymphocyte (usually CD4) whose presence (help) is required for the production of normal levels of antibody by B lymphocytes.
T lymphocyte (T cell)	Lymphocytes that are derived from the thymus. Play a major role (1) as antigen reactive cells and effector cells in cell mediated immunity and (2) by co-operation with B lymphocytes in antibody production (humoral immunity) against thymus dependent antigens.
T-suppressor cell	Subpopulation of T lymphocytes (usually $CD8^+$) which directly suppresses the immune response.
Virgin lymphocyte	Small resting lymphocyte which has never encountered antigen.

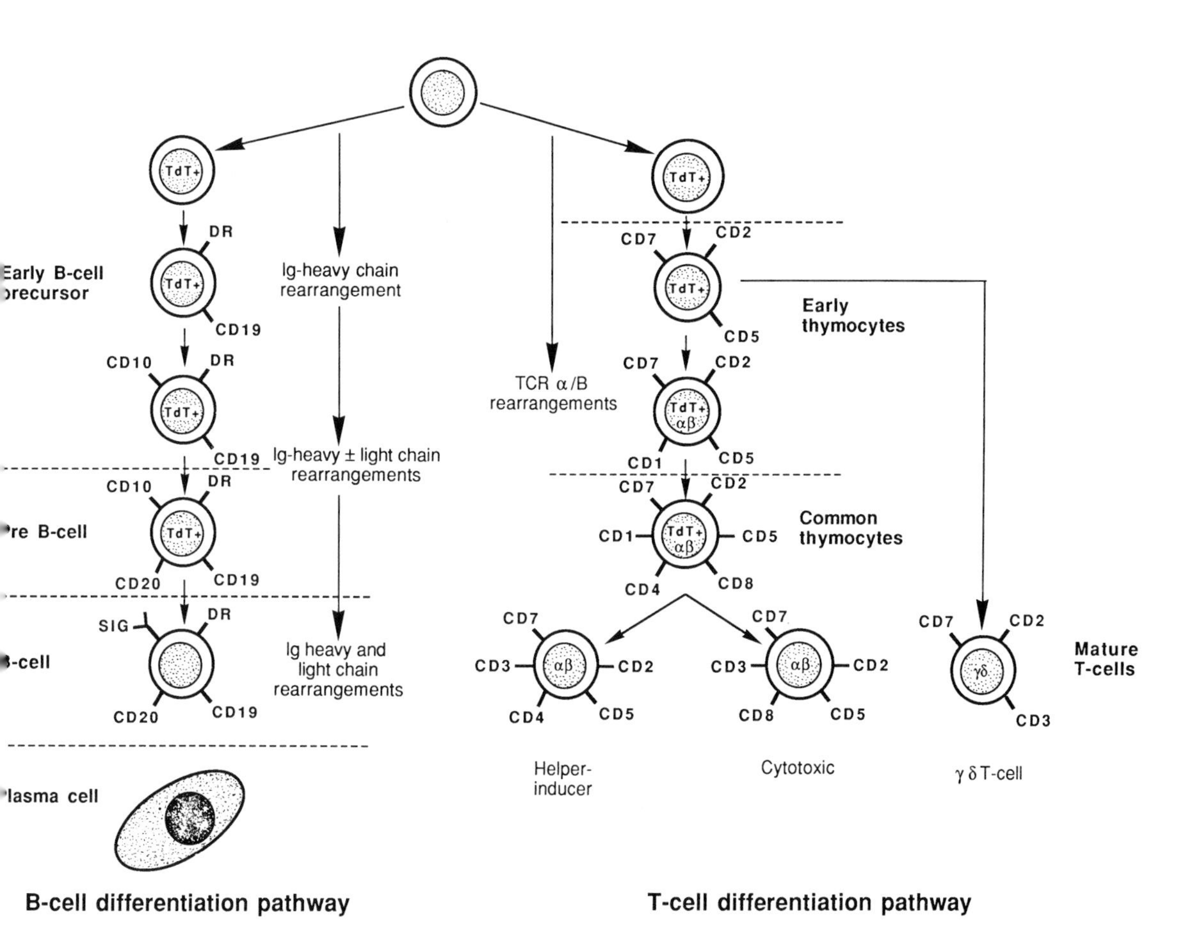

Fig. 5.1 Steps in the differentiation of B cells and T cells, TdT, terminal deoxynucleotide transferase which is found in immature cells and may be involved in the introduction of somatic mutations into immunoglobulin and T-cell receptor genes; Ti, T-cell receptor; CD antigens, cluster of differentiation antigens (see Table 5.6). Both T- and B-cell precursors arise from a common stem cell in the bone marrow. B-cell maturation occurs in the bone marrow while T-cell precursors migrate to the thymus where most of them complete their development. A small number of early thymocytes leave the thymus and differentiate into T cells in the peripheral lymphoid tissues.

comprise a **clone** and this clonal proliferation ensures that the immune response can be amplified rapidly without loss of specificity.

The development of T cell and B-cell clones involves a complex process of proliferation and differentiation and results in populations of committed effector cells, whose function is to bring about elimination of the antigen. In the B-cell system, these effector cells are antibody-producing **plasma cells**, while in the T-cell system, the effector cells are **cytotoxic T cells** and the **T cells which produce delayed-type hypersensitivity reactions**. T-cell differentiation also produces lymphocytes with regulatory functions (**helper** and **suppressor T cells**). In addition, clonal proliferation of both T and B cells results in populations of antigen-specific **memory cells** whose function is to respond rapidly when the appropriate antigen is encountered in the future and are thus responsible for the secondary immune response. The cellular events which occur during and after recognition of antigen occur in the **secondary lymphoid organs**, which include lymph nodes, spleen, tonsils, Peyer's patches and appendix.

Anatomy of the Immune System

Thymus

T cells are dependent on an intact thymus for normal development and function. The stromal elements of the thymus develop very early in fetal life as epithelial ingrowths of the endoderm of the 3rd and 4th branchial arches which become infiltrated by mesenchyme of ectodermal origin. Early in the second trimester the primitive stroma is populated by stem cells of haemopoietic origin and the organ takes on its characteristic appearance of individual lobules with an outer cortex and inner medulla (Fig. 5.2). The cortex has a dense network of epithelial cells, as well as containing macrophage-like cells and most of the lymphocytes found within the thymus. Cell suspensions from the thymus contain elements known as '**nurse cells**' which are clusters of lymphocytes and cortical epithelial cells, believed to be important in the process of T-cell differentiation. The cortex is an area both of intense lymphopoiesis and of considerable cell death. Indeed, it is calculated that 1% or less of the lymphocytes formed in the thymus survive to emigrate as mature T cells. The reasons for this apparently wasteful process are discussed on p. 200. The thymic medulla contains fewer lymphocytes, and shows less evidence of cell turnover. It contains bone-marrow-derived 'accessory' cells which are required for the final stages of T-cell development (p. 195).

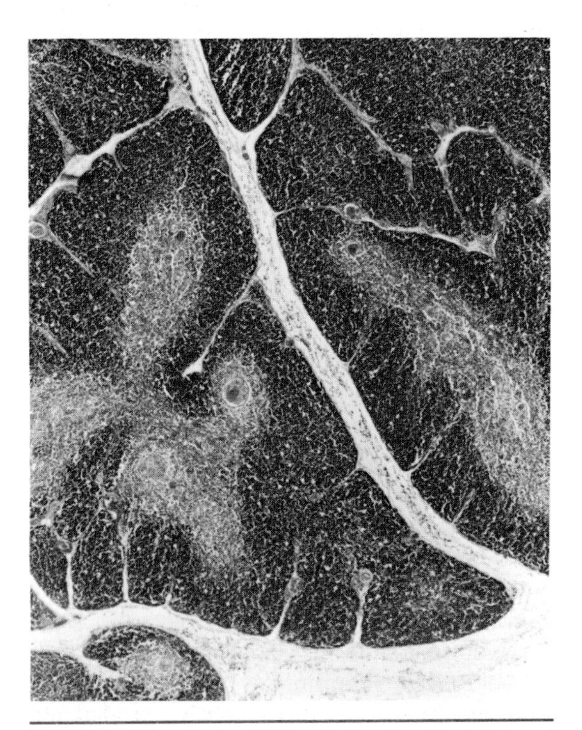

Fig. 5.2 Thymus in childhood, showing lobulation and division into cortex (darker areas) and medulla.

As a primary lymphoid organ, the thymus plays no part in the induction of an immune response to specific antigens. Its functions, which are entirely independent of antigen, are performed almost exclusively during fetal life or in the early neonatal period. It has long been known that congenital absence of the thymus (or thymectomy at birth) produces an almost complete deficiency in T-cell function. However, around birth, the thymus exports large numbers of T cells to the periphery and it plays little role after puberty, when most cell mediated immunity is effected by long-lived peripheral T cells.

Lymph Nodes

The lymph nodes have two major functions: (1) the interception and removal of foreign material in the lymph stream passing through them; and (2) the production of immune responses.

Normal Structure

A lymph node consists of superficial **cortex** and a central **medullary region** (Fig. 5.3). The framework of the node consists of a network of fine reticulin fibrils interspersed with lymph sinuses lined by reticulum cells. Most of the free cells in the node are lymphocytes. In the cortex, the lymphocytes are closely arranged, and the superficial part consists of foci, termed *primary follicles*. In a stimulated node, a focus of lymphopoiesis, the

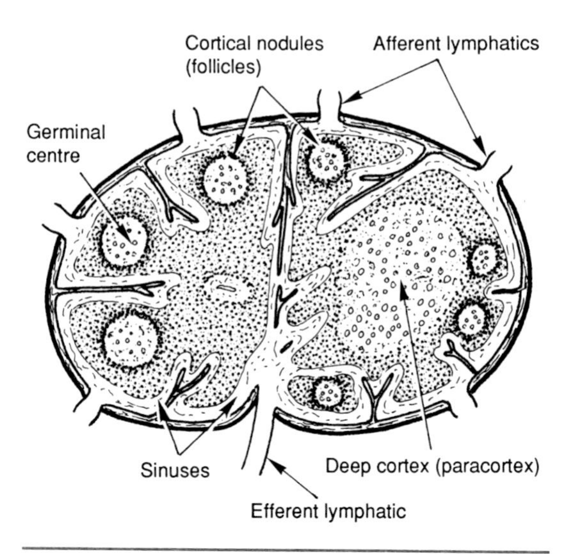

Fig. 5.3 Diagram of a lymph node, showing the superficial cortex with nodules and germinal centres, and on the right an ill-defined area of deep cortex.

germinal centre, develops within the primary follicles. These follicles are primarily populated by B cells although some helper T cells are also present. The follicular germinal centre cells comprise B lymphoblasts and follicular dendritic cells, which are involved in trapping and presenting antigen to B cells.

The deeper cortex, sometimes termed the *paracortex*, consists of ill-defined uniform areas of tissue lying between the superficial cortex and medulla. This area is also known as the **thymus dependent area** and is populated by T cells and interdigitating dendritic cells which present antigen to T cells. The paracortex also contains specialized blood vessels, known as **high endothelial venules** (HEV), which comprise the post-capillary venule region of the vasculature and which are important for the movement of lymphocytes into the lymph node from the bloodstream.

Lymph, arriving at the node by the **afferent lymphatics**, enters the peripheral sinus which surrounds the node and communicates at the hilum with the efferent lymphatic. From the peripheral sinus, lymph drains inwards to the medulla in sinuses which pass between the superficial cortical nodules and traverse the deep cortex. In the medulla, numerous lymph sinuses unite to form the efferent lymphatic.

Effects of Antigenic Stimulation

In response to local antigenic stimulus the lymph nodes draining that area of tissue show a large and rapid increase in blood flow, an increased accumulation of lymphocytes in the node and a reduction in emigration of lymphocytes in the efferent lymph. This process of 'shut-down' is probably initiated by the arrival in the node via the afferent lymphatics of antigen itself or of antigen-laden accessory cells, with subsequent activation of antigen-specific T cells and release of soluble mediators. Thereafter, the lymph nodes enlarge markedly due to proliferation of antigen-reactive lymphocytes. Activated T cells (T lymphoblasts) appear in the paracortex within 2 days and are most prominent around 5 days. During this period, many of these T lymphoblasts can be found leaving the lymph node in the efferent lymph, while others remain to develop into small, memory T cells, which then enter the recirculating pool.

After a short interval, these events in the thymus dependent area are followed by activation and proliferation of B lymphocytes in the follicular areas, with the subsequent appearance of germinal centres and plasma cells. In addition, some B lymphoblasts will develop into small recirculating memory cells. The primary roles of the germinal centre are to generate antibody-producing plasma cells and to act as a source of memory cells. These functions depend on the retention of antigen on the surface of follicular dendritic cells for long periods so that it is continuously presented to B-cells in the germinal centres.

Spleen

The anatomy of the spleen is described on p. 647. Its lymphoid compartment is found in the **white pulp (Malpighian bodies)** which is divided into T-cell and B-cell areas. T cells are found around the central arteriole in the **periarteriolar**

lymphatic sheath (PALS), while B cells are found in the peripheral follicles. The area between the red pulp and follicular areas is known as the **marginal zone** which is an important area for emigration of blood-borne lymphocytes. Resident B cells are also found in this area, but differ from B cells found in the true follicles by being non-recirculatory and having IgM, but not IgD on their surface. These B cells may be primarily concerned with immunity to thymus independent antigens (p. 199).

The white pulp of the spleen responds to antigenic stimulation exactly as described above for the lymph node. However, as the spleen is primarily concerned with blood-borne antigens, it has no afferent lymphatics or high endothelial venules.

Mucosal Associated Lymphoid Tissues

Most of the antigens encountered by an individual will arrive via mucosal surfaces. Therefore, these sites have evolved a large and complex lymphoid apparatus to protect their essential physiological functions. The mucosal associated lymphoid tissues (MALT), which contain most lymphocytes in the body, form a diffuse but discrete compartment of the immune system, discrete in that there is limited exchange between their lymphocytes and those of other tissues. Some of the cell types and immune mechanisms are unique to the MALT; for example, the immune system of the gut must at the same time protect itself from invasive pathogens but also become unresponsive to food antigens.

Mucosal associated lymphoid tissues are found in the gastrointestinal and respiratory tracts, the urogenital system and probably the breast and other exocrine glands, including salivary glands and lacrimal glands. Of these, the largest and best understood are the gut-associated lymphoid tissues (GALT), which consist of the **Peyer's patches, isolated mucosal lymphoid follicles, mesenteric lymph nodes** and **appendix**. These tissues of the GALT have the overall structure and appearance of all secondary lymphoid tissues, but in some species, Peyer's patches may also act as a primary lymphoid organ by producing B cells. Peyer's patches have an overlying epithelial layer which separates the lymphoid tissue from the gut lumen. This **dome epithelium** contains many lymphocytes and macrophages and appears to be a site for antigen uptake. A specialized population of cells within the dome epithelium, **micro-fold cells (M cells)**, seems particularly well suited to processing luminal antigen, with an array of membrane folds and pores replacing the usual microvilli (Fig. 5.4). Antigen absorbed by M cells enters the Peyer's patch very rapidly, where it is transferred to conventional accessory cells.

There are also many lymphoid cells scattered throughout the lamina propria and epithelium of the intestine. The lamina propria contains many T cells, B cells and plasma cells, as well as macrophages, mast cells and eosinophils. Approximately 90% of the plasma cells synthesize IgA class antibody and this accounts for most of the total daily production of immunoglobulins by an individual. The structure and functions of IgA are described on p. 181. Around 15% of the cells in the small intestinal epithelium are lymphocytes. These **intra-epithelial lymphocytes** (IEL) are virtually all T lymphocytes but, unlike other T cells, most express the CD8 subset marker. The functions of this large population of T cells are unknown.

Lymphocyte Recirculation
(Fig. 5.5)

The different compartments of the lymphoid system should not be considered to be static as there is continuous exchange of lymphoid cells between the different sites. This increases the possibility of the low number of antigen-specific lymphocytes of encountering antigen anywhere in the body. It also allows stimulated lymphocytes to follow their programmed differentiation pathways in discrete, specialized organs.

Small lymphocytes in the blood enter lymph

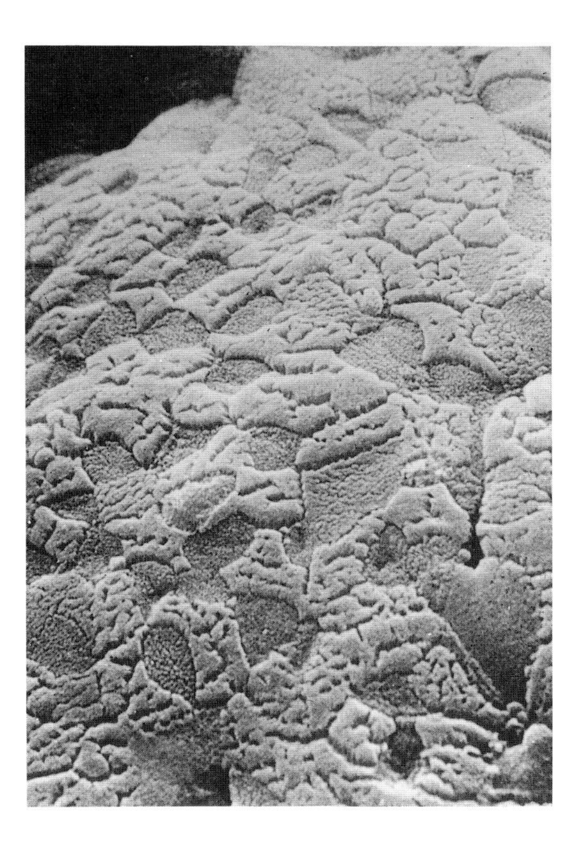

Fig. 5.4 Gut associated lymphoid tissue (GALT): Peyer's patch showing dome epithelium with microfold cells (M cells) which possess surface membrane folds and pores instead of microvilli.

nodes by passing through the HEV found in all secondary lymphoid tissues, except the spleen. The recognition of HEV by lymphocytes is probably mediated by specific 'homing' receptors on both the lymphocytes and the HEV. These include lymphocyte adhesion molecules and vascular cell adhesion molecules (p. 15). However, there may be distinct groups of such receptors on lymphocytes and on HEVs from different secondary lymphoid organs. After passing through the HEV into the paracortex, recirculating lymphocytes migrate to their appropriate compartment in the tissue, T cells to paracortical region and B cells to the follicular areas. Thereafter, the cells may remain in the lymph node or may exit into the efferent lymph via the medullary sinus and re-

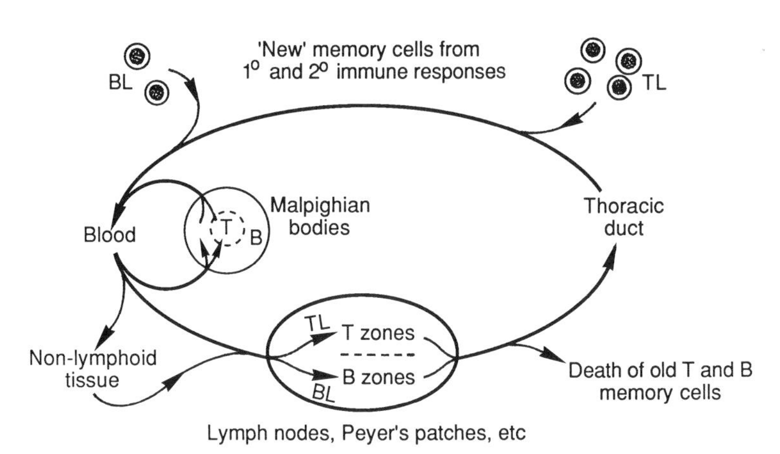

Fig. 5.5 The recirculation pathway of long-lived T lymphocytes (TL) and B lymphocytes (BL).

enter the venous system. In the spleen, similar migration from blood to lymph occurs, but the recirculating lymphocytes emerge from open-ended or 'leaky' capillaries in the red pulp or marginal zone to enter the organized white pulp.

Recirculating lymphocytes are characteristically long-lived cells, a high proportion being memory cells with a lifespan of several decades. The majority are T cells which appear to recirculate more efficiently and more rapidly than the smaller number of recirculating B cells. T lymphoblasts do not bind to HEV and do not recirculate through lymphoid organs. They accumulate in non-lymphoid tissues which are undergoing an inflammatory response. Thus, lymphocytes which have been stimulated in the bloodstream or lymph node will migrate rapidly back to the site of local antigen exposure.

Specialized Recirculation Routes

The mucosal lymphoid tissues appear to form a distinct compartment of the immune system with separate pathways for lymphocyte recirculation. B or T cells which have been activated in Peyer's patches or the mesenteric lymph nodes have a selective ability to migrate to the intestinal mucosa, whereas lymphoblasts from other lymphoid organs do not. Although this promotes seeding of IgA-committed B cells to their site of action in the intestinal wall, the selective migration also involves T cells and is therefore not IgA determined. There are no true HEV in the intestinal mucosa, but related structures may exist in this site to account for specific lymphocyte–vascular interactions.

Factors Affecting the Immune Response

The form taken by the immune response depends upon: (1) the nature of the antigen, the route by which it enters the body and the dose administered; and (2) the genetic constitution of the individual.

Antigens

An antigen is a substance which is capable of interacting with products of the specific immune response such as antibodies or antigenic receptors on lymphocytes. In general terms antigens are large molecules, usually of molecular weight exceeding 3 kDa, fairly rigid in structure, and either protein or carbohydrate, with or without other constituents, such as lipid. Antigen–antibody reactions are the result of stereochemical interactions between molecules of complementary configurations, analogous to the interaction of a lock and key. Although all antigens are capable of forming such interactions with products of the immune response, not every antigen can initiate an immune response after entry into the body. To do this, an antigen must be immunogenic. **Immunogens** are antigens which can trigger an immune response by cross-linking antigen-specific receptors on lymphocytes. An antigen may fail to be immunogenic either because it is not large enough to cross-link receptors or because the appropriate lymphocytes cannot respond to the triggering signal.

Although some small molecules, such as para-aminobenzoic acid (PABA) (Fig. 5.6), are not by themselves immunogenic, they may become so if they are attached to larger molecules, such as serum albumin. In these circumstances, the small molecule is said to be a **hapten**, i.e. a substance which can take part in a specific immunological reaction but which cannot by itself evoke an immune response.

Study of synthetic polypeptide and polysaccharide antigens has shown that recognition is dependent on the three-dimensional configuration of a few amino acids or monosaccharides. Nat-

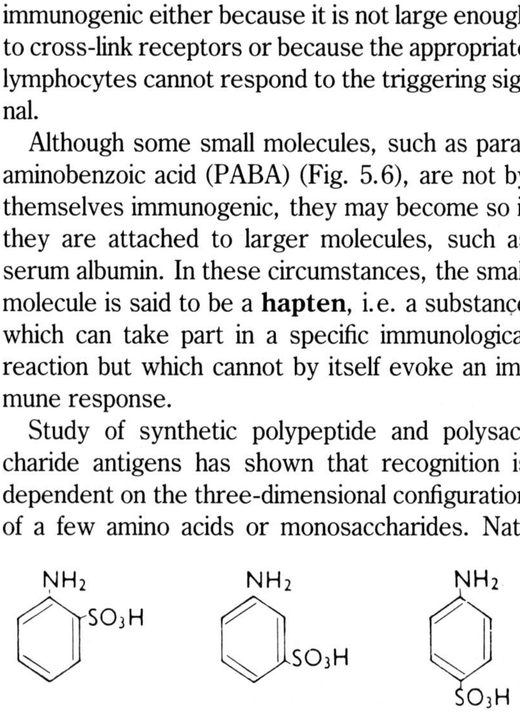

NH_2 SO_3H *ortho* — NH_2 SO_3H *meta* — NH_2 SO_3H *para*

Fig. 5.6 Isomeric forms of aminobenzene sulphonic acid.

urally occurring macromolecules contain several such sites which can be recognized by the immune system. Each of these sites is known as **an antigenic determinant** or **epitope**. Large, complex antigenic particles and living organisms such as bacteria, which contain a greater number and variety of epitopes, are more powerful immunogens than small soluble molecules. Alterations in only one amino acid or sugar chain in the antigenic determinant may result in a loss of reactivity with antibody or lymphocytes, illustrating the exquisite specificity of the immune response.

Route of administration of antigen. The route of antigen administration affects the immune response both quantitatively and qualitatively. This is probably due to antigen encountering different types of accessory cells involved in antigen presentation. The subcutaneous, intramuscular and intradermal routes usually produce strong immune responses, while intravenous administration of antigen normally results in a weak antibody response and is also liable to induce specific immunological tolerance (p. 201). Small amounts of ingested soluble antigens which escape digestion and are absorbed, usually induce immunological tolerance. However, living or particulate antigens stimulate active immune responses at mucosal surfaces. Mucosal immune responses are usually restricted to the surface which first encounters the antigen, while parenteral administration of antigen rarely stimulates mucosal immunity.

Dose of antigen administered. Generally speaking, the greater the dose of antigen administered, the greater the immune response. However, extremely low or high doses of antigen may induce immunological tolerance, low zone tolerance and high zone tolerance respectively.

Genetic Constitution of the Individual

The repertoire of specific immune responses which an individual can mount depends on several genetically determined factors. These include the various antigen binding sites found both on antibody molecules and on the cell surface receptors of T cells. Immunity to many pathogens may also be determined by genes which control non-specific immune factors, e.g. the phagocytic and degradative functions of macrophages. In addition, specific **immune response (Ir) genes** are located within the major histocompatibility complex (MHC) which is on chromosome 6 in man. Ir genes do not encode the antigen binding sites of antibodies or T cells, but influence the presentation of antigens to these cells.

Tissue Antigens

When cells or tissues from one individual are injected or transplanted into another, there is usually a prompt immune response which results in rejection of the graft. The more genetically dissimilar the individuals, the greater is the immune response which occurs. The terminology used to describe these genetically determined immune responses is summarized in Table 5.2.

When an antigen or tissue is derived from a species other than that of the immunized host, it is called a **heteroantigen** and the antibodies are heteroantibodies. Antibodies against bacteria are of this type. Injection or transplantation of one human with the red cells or tissue cells of another may result in an immune response to antigenic groups not shared by both individuals; for example, human red cells containing the rhesus antigen D (RhD positive cells) will induce the production of antibodies in a person whose own red cells do not contain this antigen (RhD negative). A similar situation exists for other red cell antigens and for human leucocyte associated (HLA) antigens. Antigens of this type which differ within a species are called **alloantigens** and the corresponding antibodies **alloantibodies**. In general, alloantigens are less likely to evoke an immune response than heteroantigens. An individual normally does not respond to the antigens of his own cells because during fetal life these tissue antigens induce specific immunological tolerance, rather than active immunity (p. 201). Thus, the injection of an individual with his own cells or tissues (**autoantigen**) does not normally produce an

Table 5.2 Terminology of antigens, antibodies and tissue grafts

Relationship between donor and recipient	Genetic terminology	Antibody antigen	Transplantation terminology
Same animal	—	Autoantibody Autoantigen	Autograft
Identical twins or same inbred strain	Syngeneic (Isogeneic)	—	Isograft
Same outbred species or different inbred strains	Allogeneic	Isoantibody Isoantigen	Allograft (Homograft)
Different species	Heterogeneic Xenogeneic	Heteroantibody Heteroantigen	Xenograft (Heterograft)

autoimmune response. When this does occur, it leads to a variety of autoimmune diseases which are considered further on p. 226.

The Major Histocompatibility Complex (MHC)

The major histocompatibility complex (MHC) comprises a series of genes encoding a group of highly polymorphic cell membrane glycoproteins. In man, these MHC antigens are called **human leucocyte associated antigens (HLA antigens)**, and their importance lies in the central role they play in immune recognition. The human MHC gene complex which is located on the short arm of chromosome 6, comprises three groups of genes, which are designated I, II and III (Fig. 5.7).

The class I antigens are found on all nucleated cells and are encoded by genes in the A, B and C

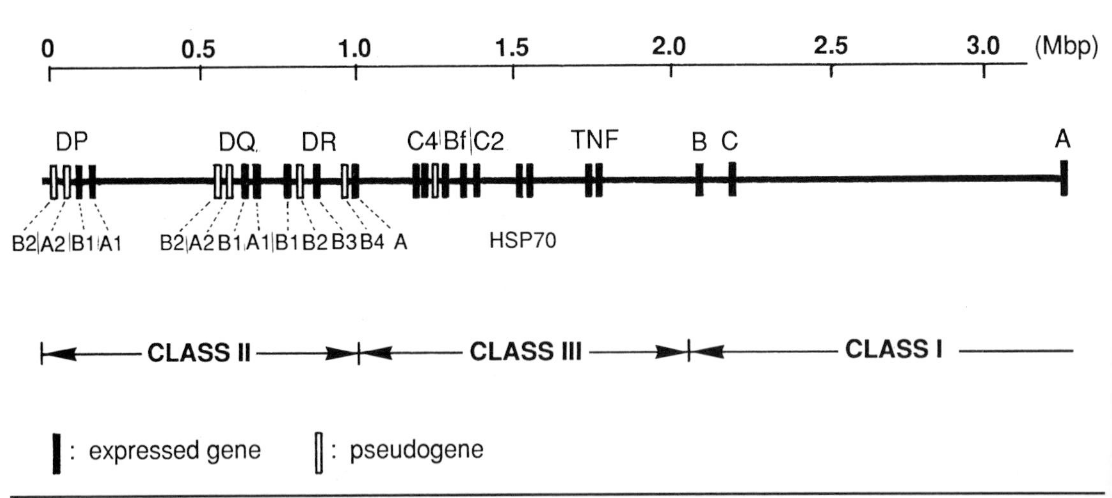

Fig. 5.7 Distribution of the MHC genes on chromosome 6 in man. The MHC region occupies approximately 3 × 10^6 base pairs (3 Mbp). The class I and class II regions are separated by the class III region which contains genes encoding C4, C2, factor B (Bf), heat shock protein 70 (HSP70) and tumour necrosis factors (TNFα and TNFβ). The genes of the class I and class II regions encode proteins which are involved in antigen recognition whereas those encoded by genes in the class III region are concerned with the effector arm of the immune response and the response of tissues to injury. Pseudogenes are genes which are not expressed.

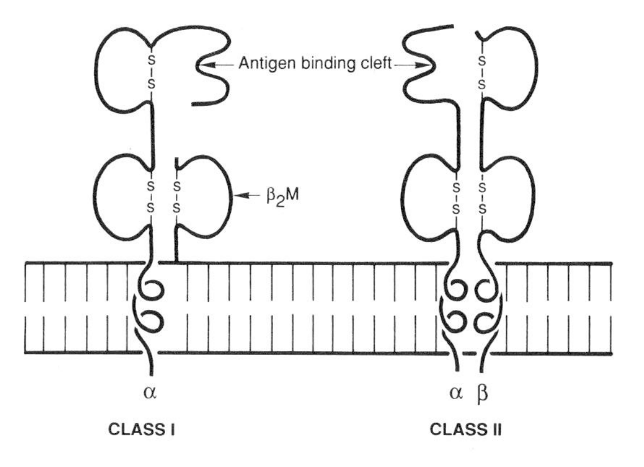

Fig. 5.8 Diagram of class I and class II MHC antigens. Class I MHC antigens consist of a variable α chain and an invariant β chain (β_2M, β_2 microglobulin). The former penetrates the cell membrane while the latter is non-covalently linked to the former and is not anchored to the cell membrane. The extracellular portion of the α chain is organized into discrete structural domains and contains the antigen binding cleft. Class II MHC antigens comprise α and β chains both of which are variable and penetrate the cell membrane. Both chains contribute to the formation of the antigen binding cleft.

regions of the HLA locus. These genes encode a 44 kDa transmembrane glycopeptide chain which is polymorphic and which is linked non-covalently to a smaller invariant chain, **β_2-microglobulin** (Fig. 5.8), encoded by a gene on chromosome 15. As class I alleles are expressed codominantly, tissues bear the antigens of both parents.

Class II antigens, sometimes referred to as Ia (immune associated) antigens, are encoded by genes in the HLA-D region which consists of at least three major loci, DP, DQ and DR. These antigens are expressed constitutively on B cells, macrophages and lymphoid dendritic cells and are involved in presentation of antigen to T cells. Some other cells can express class II antigens facultatively (Table 5.3) particularly when stimulated by interferon-γ. Class II antigens (Fig. 5.8) consist of two non-covalently linked transmembrane glycopeptide chains, α(34 kDa) and β(29 kDa), both of which are encoded on chromosome 6. Like the class I antigens, class II alleles are expressed codominantly.

The three-dimensional structure of class I MHC molecules has been described recently and class II is believed to be similar. On the surface of the class I molecule, two prominent stretches of α-helix form the side walls of a groove, whose floor is formed by a β-pleated sheet (Fig. 5.9). Short antigenic peptides (epitopes) are bound in the cleft and presented to specific T cells (p. 190). In the case of class I antigens, the heavy chain comprises the entire antigen binding cleft, while in class II antigens, both the α and β chains contribute equally.

Table 5.3 Constitutive and facultative expression of class II MHC molecules

Cells expressing class II constitutively
Dendritic cells
B lymphocytes
Thymic cortical epithelium
Cells with some normal expression which can be increased during inflammation
Macrophages
Intestinal epithelium
Normally class II MHC negative but inducible
T lymphocytes
Thyroid epithelium
Pancreatic B cells
Keratinocytes
Renal tubules
Endothelium

Detection of HLA Antigens

As each chromosome has three loci at both the human class I and class II regions, each individual can potentially express at least 12 different HLA antigens. As the MHC genes are closely linked, recombination during meiosis is unusual and so the genes on each chromosome are frequently inherited as entire sets (**extended haplotypes**). As a result, within the population, certain HLA antigens at one locus are associated with antigens from another locus more frequently than would be expected by chance. For instance HLA-A is commonly associated with HLA-B8 and DR3 while HLA-A2 is associated with B7 and DR2. This phenomenon is called **linkage disequilibrium**.

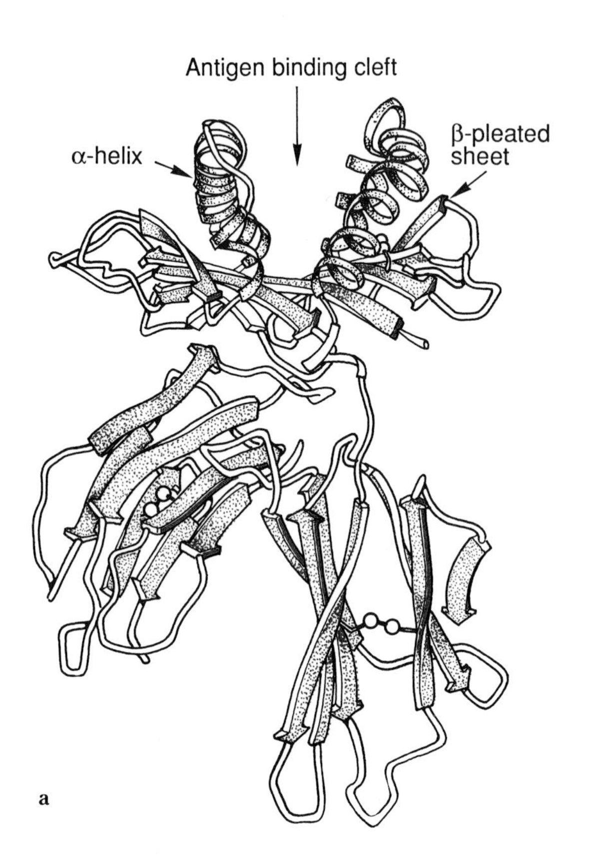

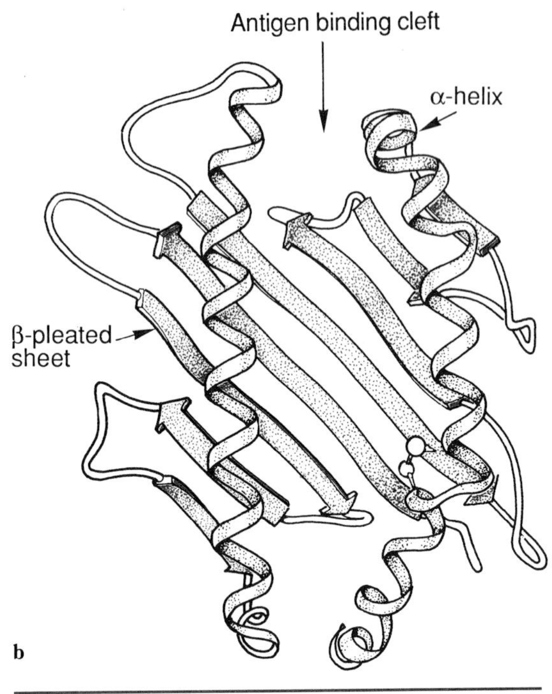

Fig. 5.9 Three-dimensional structure of a class I MHC molecule: **a** side view; **b** plan view. The α chain is organized into two runs of α-helices which are separated by a β-pleated sheet. The α-helices form the margins of the antigen binding cleft while the β-pleated sheet forms the floor.

Class I antigens are detected serologically using antisera in a complement-dependent cytolytic assay. The antigens are designated by the locus and a number, e.g. A1, A2, A3, B1, B3, C1, C12, etc. Of the class II antigens, DQ and DR are defined serologically as well as by the mixed lymphocyte reaction (MLR). In this assay the patient's lymphocytes are mixed with a panel of cells of known HLA specificity (typing cells). The patient's cells proliferate only if they are incompatible with the typing cells. DP antigens are also defined by an MLR but in this case the typing cells have to be primed previously against known DP antigens. These antigens can now be defined precisely on the basis of their nucleotide sequences.

HLA Antigens and Disease

There are several associations between HLA antigens and particular disease states (Table 5.4). The most impressive is in ankylosing spondylitis (p. 994), in which approximately 90% of patients express HLA-B27 antigens compared with 9% of the general population. Most autoimmune diseases are associated with particular HLA profiles. Most of these associations originally seemed to be with HLA-B8, DR2, DR3, or DR4 (Table 5.4), but it is becoming increasingly apparent that the significant associations are with the antigens of the DP or DQ loci. The earlier results reflected fortuitous effects of the linkage disequilibrium between individual HLA genes described above.

The immune system plays a direct pathogenic role in virtually all HLA-linked diseases, probably reflecting the role of class II genes in regulating immune responses to particular antigens. Certain class II MHC genes may predispose to the development of autoimmune disease either because of an unusual ability to present self-antigens to

Table 5.4 Associations between HLA and some diseases

Condition	HLA	Frequency (%) Patients	Controls	Relative risk
Idiopathic haemochromatosis	A3	76	28.2	8.2
	B14	16	3.8	4.7
Ankylosing spondylitis	B27	90	9.4	87.4
Reiter's disease	B27	79	9.4	37.0
Coeliac disease	DR3	79	26.3	10.8
	DR7	also increased		
Sjögren's syndrome	DR3	78	26.3	9.7
Idiopathic Addison's disease	DR3	69	26.3	6.3
Graves' disease	DR3	56	26.3	3.7
Insulin-dependent diabetes	DR3	56	28.2	3.3
	DR4	75	32.2	6.4
	DR2	10	30.5	0.2
Myasthenia gravis	DR3	50	28.2	2.5
	B8	47	24.6	2.7
SLE	DR3	70	28.2	5.8
Idiopathic membranous nephropathy	DR3	75	20.0	12.0
IgA deficiency in blood donors	B8	49	24.3	3.0
	DR3	81	24.6	13.0
Multiple sclerosis	DR2	59	25.8	4.1
Goodpasture's syndrome	DR2	88	32.0	15.9
Rheumatoid arthritis	DR4	50	19.4	4.2
IgA nephropathy	DR4	49	19.5	4.0
Hydralazine-induced SLE	DR4	73	32.7	5.6
Hashimoto's thyroiditis	DR5	19	6.9	3.2
Pernicious anaemia	DR5	25	5.8	5.4

mature T cells in immunocompetent individuals or because of an inability to inactivate autoreactive T cells during fetal life (p. 201). Another possibility is that certain microbial antigens might be similar to an HLA antigen (**molecular mimicry**). This could result in either a poor and hence prolonged immune response to an infection with that organism, or to an immune response which attacks not only the microbe but also the host cells.

Humoral Immunity

Antibody Structure

Antibody molecules have the special property of combining specifically with antigen. In so doing, they may cover up harmful areas on molecules of toxin, in which case they are said to be antitoxins, or their combination with cells such as bacteria may lead, with the help of complement, to death and lysis of the bacteria (bacteriolytic effect) or to phagocytosis by polymorphs and macrophages (opsonic effect). Chemically, antibodies belong to

Table 5.5 Physical and biological properties of human immunoglobulin classes

Property	IgG	IgA	IgM	IgD	IgE
Molecular form	Monomer	Monomer, polymer	Pentamer	Monomer	Monomer
Subclasses	IgG_1, IgG_2, IgG_3, and IgG_4	IgA_1 and IgA_2	None	None	None
Molecular weight	150 000	160 000	950 000	175 000	190 000
Serum concentration	1250 mg/dl	210	125	4	0.03
Antibody valence	2	2	10	2	2
Complement activation (classical pathway)	+ (IgG_1, IgG_2, IgG_3)	−	+	−	−
Cells to which binding occurs	Macrophages, neutrophils	None	None	None	Mast cells
Other properties	Secondary response. Placental transfer	Surface secretions	Primary response. B-cell antigen receptor	B-cell antigen receptor	Type I hypersensitivity. Parasite expulsion

the immunoglobulin (Ig) proteins of the plasma. There are five classes: **IgG, IgM, IgA, IgD and IgE** (Table 5.5).

All immunoglobulins are composed of one or more similar units, each unit consisting of two pairs of identical polypeptide chains (Fig. 5.10); one pair (the **heavy chains**) have a molecular weight which is approximately twice that of the other pair (the **light chains**). In turn each chain is composed of smaller subunits (**domains**) which have a similar overall structure and conformation, as well as a characteristic intrachain disulphide bond. Heavy chains differ structurally for each class of immunoglobulin, and the letters γ, μ, α, δ, ε, are used to indicate the heavy chains of IgG, IgM, IgA, IgD and IgE respectively. In contrast, there are only two types of light chain, κ and λ, in all classes, and each immunoglobulin molecule has either κ or λ light chains.

The antigen receptor on B cells is monomeric IgM (±IgD). Surface immunoglobulin is attached to the membrane by means of a hydrophobic transmembrane domain at the C-terminus of the heavy chain. During B-cell maturation the exon encoding the transmembrane domain is spliced to that encoding the C-terminus of the heavy chain so that

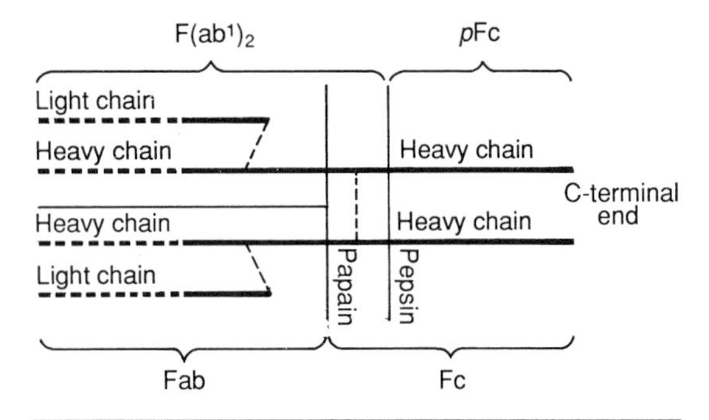

Fig. 5.10 Structure of a monomeric immunoglobulin molecule. In any particular molecule, the two light chains have an identical amino-acid sequence and so do the two heavy chains. Each immunoglobulin class has a distinctive Fc piece (C-terminal end of the heavy chains). The amino-acid sequences of the interrupted portions of the light and heavy chains (the N-terminal ends) vary greatly among immunoglobulin molecules, even of the same class, and constitute the specific antigen binding (Fab) sites, of which there are two on each molecule, each consisting of the N-terminal ends of a light and a heavy chain. The antigen binding region of the molecule is also known as the idiotype. The light interrupted lines represent disulphide bonds and the light continuous lines the sites of action of papain and pepsin, which divide the molecule respectively into two Fab and one Fc fragment, and one $F(ab^1)_2$ and two pFc^1 fragments.

mRNA encoding surface IgM is transcribed.

The specificity of antigen–antibody union depends on the antibody combining site having a complementary shape to the antigenic determinant, thus permitting the necessary close fit. The shape of the combining site is determined by the amino-acid sequence of the N-terminal ends of the heavy and light chains. In contrast to most other proteins, each one of which in a given individual is of uniform amino-acid sequence, the immunoglobulins show marked heterogeneity of their N-terminal domains (the variable regions), with variations running to millions. Most of this sequence variation occurs in three or four areas, the **hypervariable regions**. Each heavy and light chain pair is folded so that in the intact molecule hypervariable regions are exposed and in opposition, to constitute the antigen-combining site. This variety is responsible for the great range of antibodies which can develop in response to stimulation by an enormous number of different antigens.

Some idea of the specificity of antibody–antigen union can be gained from study of antibodies raised against chemically defined haptens. For example, antibody raised against *para*-aminobenzene sulphonic acid does not combine with the *ortho*-form but gives a weak reaction with *meta*-aminobenzene sulphonic acid (Fig. 5.6). The latter is called a cross-reaction and results from the production of some antibody molecules which fit the cross-reacting antigen sufficiently well to permit intermolecular attraction by the short-range forces mentioned above. The firmness of combination between the antigen-binding sites of antibody and an antigen (**affinity**) is dependent upon the closeness of fit. Antibodies may be of high or low affinity and cross-reactions are generally of low affinity.

Immunoglobulin G (IgG) is monomeric (Fig. 5.11). It is the most abundant immunoglobulin in the plasma and extravascular fluids. There are receptors for the Fc part of IgG antibodies (Fc receptors) on polymorphs and macrophages which facilitate adherence and phagocytosis of the corresponding antigens. IgG crosses the human placenta via Fc-γ receptors transferring passive immunity from mother to child. There are four subclasses of IgG (Fig. 5.11) which differ somewhat in their properties (Table 5.6).

Immunoglobulin M. Circulating IgM is a macroglobulin consisting of pentamers of the basic four-chain unit or monomer, which are linked by an additional polypeptide **J chain** (Fig. 5.11). IgM is the first class of antibody to be produced following the initial introduction of an antigen and is therefore the most important immunoglobulin in the primary immune response. Thus, the presence of IgM antibody to a micro-organism indicates recent or continuing infection by that organism. IgM has ten combining sites so that the strength of its binding to antigenic molecules is greater, i.e. it has high **avidity** for its corresponding antigen. IgM is also the most effective in complement activation (p. 142). Because of its size, IgM is largely confined to the plasma, where it has an important function in destroying micro-organisms. Monomeric IgM is present on B-cell membranes where it acts as an antigen receptor.

Immunoglobulin A (IgA) is the principal immunoglobulin produced at mucosal surfaces and is the second most abundant plasma immunoglobulin. It occurs in two principal forms: circulating IgA is monomeric, whereas IgA in secretions (**secretory IgA**) is a dimeric molecule. The components of these dimers are linked by a J chain, and during passage through mucosal epithelium, an additional protein, **secretory component (SC)** is added. A small proportion of serum IgA is dimeric but contains no secretory component. There are also two subclasses of IgA, IgA_1 and IgA_2, which are present in equal amounts in plasma, while IgA_2 predominates in secretions.

Dimeric IgA and its J chain are synthesized by plasma cells in the lamina propria of mucous membranes of the gut, the respiratory and urinary tracts, and is then secreted in large amounts into the lumens of these organs. This is achieved by two specific transport systems:

(1) Locally produced IgA gains access to the lumen by initially complexing with secretory component which acts as a receptor on the basal surface of epithelial cells and which has very high specificity for polymeric immunoglobulin, par-

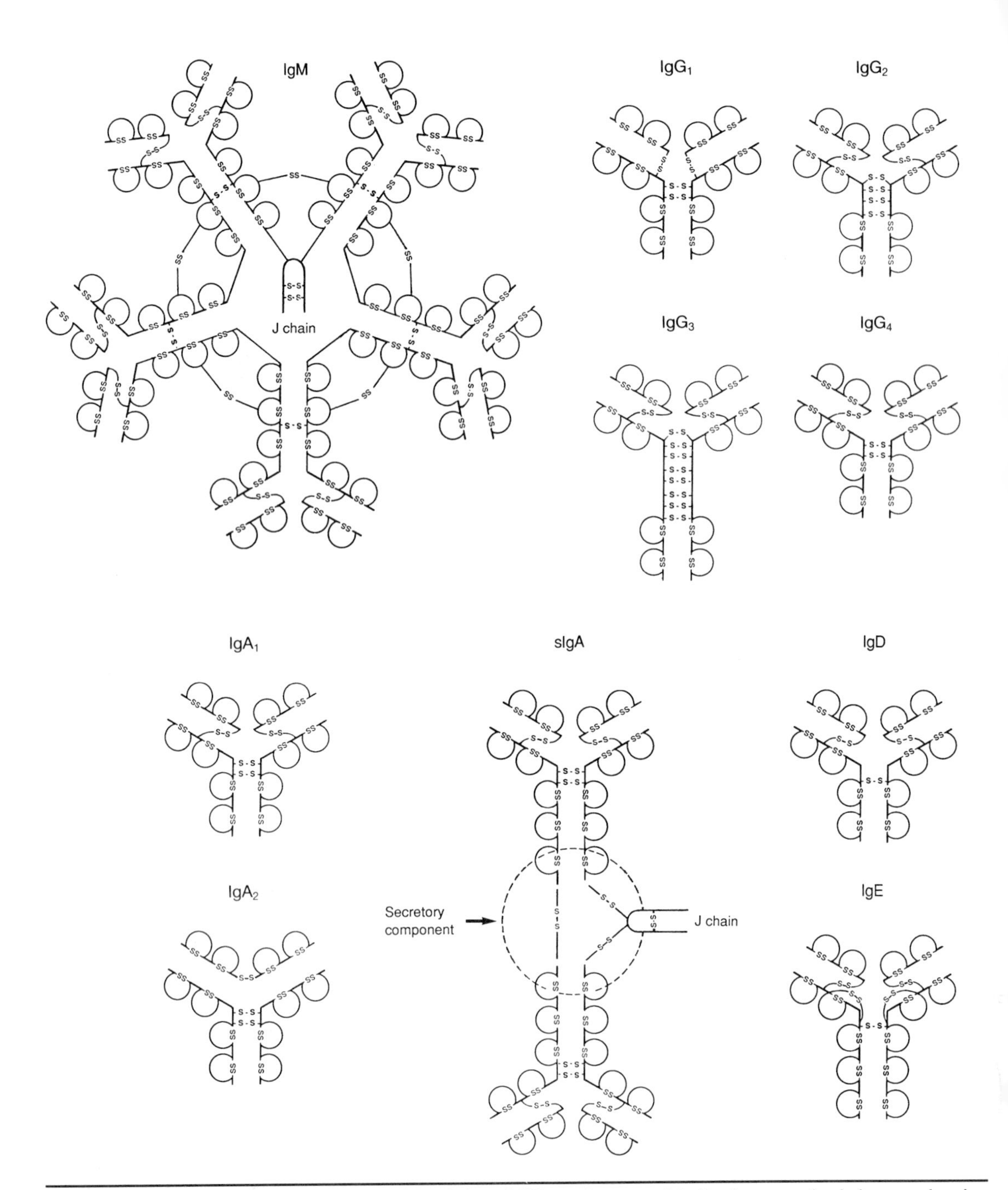

Fig. 5.11 Organization of the heavy and light chains of different immunoglobulin classes and subclasses, showing constant domains and disulphide bonds. IgM is pentameric, thus having ten antigen binding sites. Apart from secretory IgA (sIgA) which is dimeric and therefore has four antigen binding sites, the remaining immunoglobulins are monomeric and therefore have only two antigen binding sites. The relationship of the Fab regions of the IgG subclasses to the Fc piece, and the length of the hinge region are important in determining the ability of the subclass to activate complement or to bind to Fc receptors. Access of C1 or Fc receptors to the Fc regions of IgG_1, IgG_2 and IgG_3 is facilitated by the long hinge region in the case of IgG_2 and IgG_3, whereas the orientation of Fab regions of IgG_1 is such that access is simple. In contrast, the orientation of the Fab regions of IgG_4 is such that the Fc region is far less accessible so that C1 and Fc receptor binding are obstructed. Modified from Samter, E. D. M. Townage, D. W., Frank, M. M., Alister, K. F. and Claman, H. N. (1988). In: *Immunological Diseases*. Little, Brown and Co, Boston/Toronto.

Table 5.6 Properties of IgG subclasses

	IgG_1	IgG_2	IgG_3	IgG_4
% Total IgG in normal serum	65	23	8	4
Electrophoretic mobility	Slow	Slow	Slow	Fast
Combination with staphylococcal A protein	+++	+++	–	+++
Cross placenta	++	±	++	++
Complement activation (classical pathway)	+++	++	++++	±
Binding to monocytes	+++	+	+++	±

ticularly dimeric IgA (Fig. 5.12). The IgA dimer is then endocytosed and transported to the luminal surface. Here the secretory component is partially ligated and the freed IgA–SC complex is secreted into the lumen, where it is trapped in the mucous layer. In addition to its transport function, SC is believed to protect the IgA molecule from proteolysis. Of other classes of immunoglobulin only polymeric IgM can also be transported across the mucosal epithelium in this way.

(2) IgA also gains access to the gut lumen by a more indirect route (Fig. 5.13): dimeric IgA produced in the lamina propria escapes into the portal bloodstream, is removed by hepatocytes, and is then rapidly transported into bile after complexing with secretory component on their canalicular surface. This important mechanism not only explains the low proportion of dimeric IgA in serum but also the high serum IgA levels which occur in liver diseases.

The functions of secretory IgA are not fully understood. By attaching to the mucous layer on

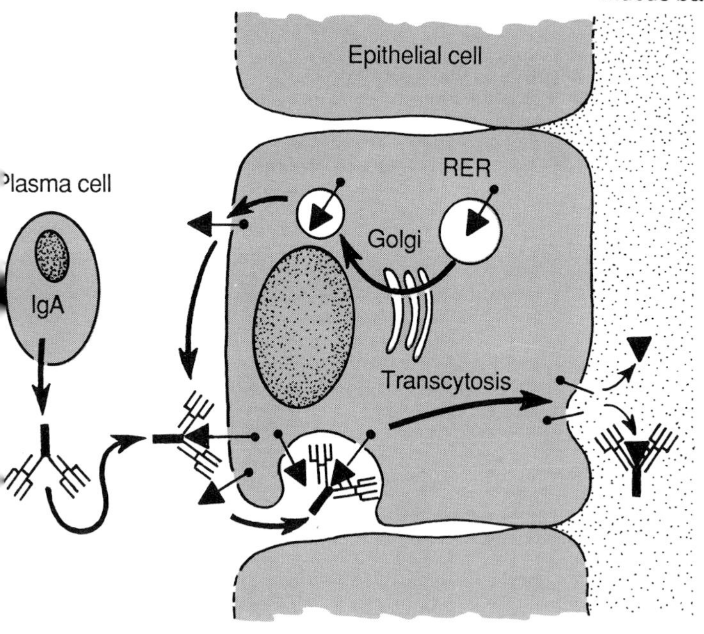

Fig. 5.12 Secretion of IgA across a mucous membrane. Monomeric IgA is synthesized by the plasma cell in the lamina propria, and two molecules are linked by the J chain to form IgA dimers. Following the complexing to free secretory piece (●—▶) which protrudes from the basal layer of the epithelial cell, the IgA-secretory piece complex is internalized and transported to the luminal surfaces. During secretion, part of the secretory piece (●—) is cleaved off the complex and recirculated though the RER and Golgi and re-expressed in its original form on the basal surface. Simultaneously, the dimeric IgA molecule complexed with a fragment of the secretory component (▶) is released into the lumen.

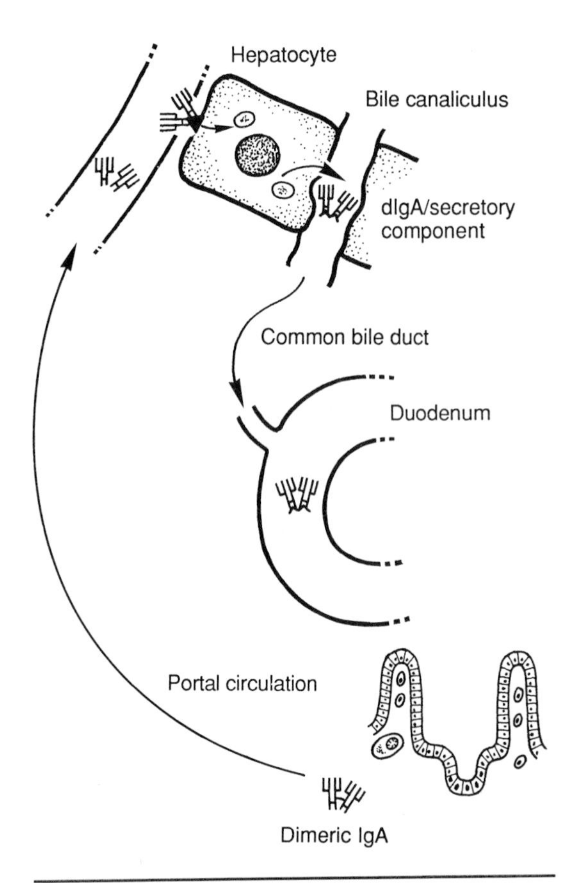

Fig. 5.13 Enterohepatic circulation of IgA. Some dimeric IgA (dIgA) from the gut escapes into the portal circulation and is transported to the liver where it binds to an IgA receptor on the sinusoidal surface of the hepatocyte. Following transport across the hepatocyte, IgA is secreted into the biliary canaliculus and then transported in the bile to the duodenum. This mechanism explains the presence of small amounts of polymeric IgA in the circulation and the high levels of IgA in liver disease.

the epithelium, it forms an important part of the mucosal barrier and may act as a non-inflammatory eliminator of pathogenic organisms. IgA does not activate complement but may have opsonic activity, as IgA receptors are present on neutrophils. IgA is also able to neutralize bacteria and viruses.

Immunoglobulin E (IgE) has the special property of attaching to mast cells and basophil leucocytes by means of its Fc fragment, leaving the specific combining sites exposed to combine with antigen. IgE antibody is involved in immediate (type I) hypersensitivity reactions (p. 205).

Immunoglobulin D. The biological properties of circulating IgD are unknown, but on B cells, where it is found together with IgM, it acts as an antigen receptor.

The Production of Antibody

Injection of an antigen to which an individual has not previously been exposed results in a **primary antibody response**, during which a small amount of specific IgM antibody appears in the blood about 7 days after the injection. Re-injection of the same antigen at a later date leads to a **secondary** or **anamnestic (remembering) response**, consisting mostly of large amounts of specific IgG. This secondary response occurs after about 4 days or so and may continue for some weeks thereafter.

The production of antibody requires proliferation and differentiation of B cells, a process which is accompanied by the enlargement of the responding cells to become lymphoblasts. These cells differentiate into memory B cells or plasma cells. The latter contain a large amount of rough endoplasmic reticulum, allowing them to synthesize and secrete large amounts of immunoglobulin (Fig. 5.14). Circulating immunoglobulins are largely produced by plasma cells in spleen, bone marrow and lymph nodes, but plasma cells are also abundant in the lymphoid tissues of mucosal surfaces and at inflammatory sites. Each plasma cell at any given time produces light chains (κ or λ but never both), together with heavy chains of only one immunoglobulin class. Furthermore, individual plasma cells produce antibody which binds to the same antigenic determinant which stimulated the parent B cell. An additional polypeptide, the **J chain**, is synthesized by plasma cells producing IgM and IgA.

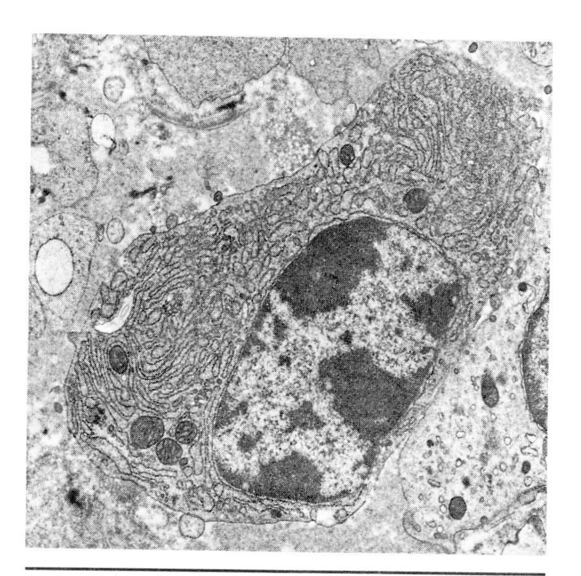

Fig. 5.14 Electron micrograph of a plasma cell in a lymph node, showing the eccentrically placed nucleus with the peripheral chromatin condensation and abundant rough endoplasmic reticulum in which immunoglobulin is being synthesized. ×1300.

The Origin of B Lymphocytes

In birds, the bursa of Fabricius develops as a lymphoepithelial organ in the wall of the hind gut and is invaded in embryonic life by haemopoietic stem cells which proliferate and differentiate into B (bursa-dependent) lymphocytes. These, in turn, enter the blood and help to populate the secondary lymphoid organs. In mammals, which have no bursa, it is believed that the haemopoietic tissues themselves are the site of production of B cells from stem cells (see Fig. 5.1) although they may also be formed in the gut associated lymphoid tissues.

Commitment of stem cells to B-cell differentiation occurs spontaneously and independently of antigen, probably in response to growth factors released from the stromal cells of the bone marrow. Lymphocyte progenitor cells destined to become B cells (see Fig. 5.1) express cytoplasmic μ heavy chains ($C\mu^+$ cells). Light chains are absent, so that complete antibodies are not formed at this stage and immunoglobulins cannot be detected on the cell surface. These are termed pre-B cells.

Light chain synthesis and the formation of complete immunoglobulin molecules in the cytoplasm occurs later. This is followed by the expression of immunoglobulin on the cell surface. The immunoglobulin initially expressed is monomeric IgM although this is followed by the concomitant synthesis and surface expression of IgD. These $sIgM^+$ $sIgD^+$ B cells which are termed **resting** or **'virgin'** B cells are now **committed** to recognize subsequently only the antigen for which their surface immunoglobulin is specific. They will respond to stimulation by antigen, differentiating into plasma cells. Throughout this maturation pathway, each B cell and its progeny (a clone) will synthesize only one type of light chain (κ or λ), and will retain antigen specificity.

Development of Specific Responsiveness and Diversity in B Cells

The specificity of antibody depends on the sequence of amino acids in the variable regions of the polypeptide chains, and so reflects the sequences of the bases in the DNA of the genes encoding immunoglobulins. Commitment implies that the genome of a B cell encodes one particular heavy chain variable region sequence and one light chain variable sequence. All the B cells of a proliferating clone are committed to produce the same antibody through many cell generations.

Diversity depends partly on the fact that the genome of the individual contains large numbers of alternative germline genes encoding the variable regions of the Ig chains (**V genes**) and partly on somatic mutations in the nucleotide base sequences during maturation. Each immunoglobulin chain is synthesized as a single unit, by translation of mRNA encoding the constant and variable regions of the whole chain. The mechanisms of gene selection responsible for the generation of antibody diversity is illustrated for heavy chain synthesis in Fig. 5.15 and is similar for light chains. The heavy chain V genes (V_H) alone do not encode the entire variable region, which also depends upon adjacent **diversity** (D) genes and **joining**

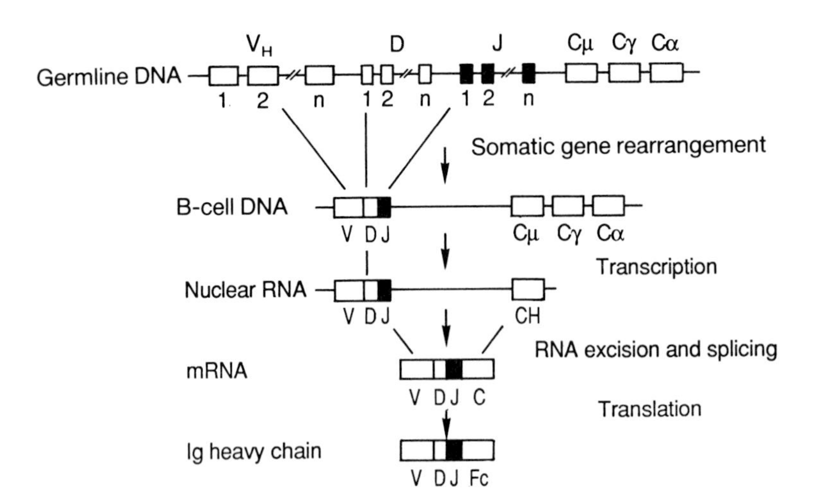

Fig. 5.15 Diagram of the rearrangement of the gene segments coding for heavy chain polypeptides during B-cell maturation. Variable (V), diversity (D) and joining (J) segments recombine at the DNA level during differentiation. VDJ_H–C_H recombination occurs by processing of the original transcription form of mRNA.

(J) genes, which encode their segment of the immunoglobulin which links the variable region to the constant region.

In the embryonic germline form, heavy chain genes exist as exons encoding variable (V_H), diversity (D) and joining (J) regions and the constant regions (C_H) of different classes of immunoglobulin, i.e. Cμ, Cγ, Cα, Cδ, Cε. These exons are separated by long intronic sequences. Differentiation involves rearrangement of this germline form, which is achieved by the formation and excision of loops of DNA. A single V_H gene is brought into continuity with one D gene and one J gene to form the single VDJ_H DNA configuration found in the differentiated B cell. A similar mechanism of somatic gene rearrangement brings a single V_L gene in apposition to a J_L gene to complete the VJ_L DNA configuration of the light chain variable region genes found in B cells. These rearrangements occur only on one chromosome of the pair and when completed, the immunoglobulin gene locus on the other chromosome is prevented from rearrangement (**allelic exclusion**).

The individual B cell now has a heritable commitment to the production of antibody of a specificity defined by its selected V, D and J genes. For the light chains there are approximately 1000 V_L gene segments and 10 J segments, giving a repertoire of 10^4 amino-acid sequences. The specificity of antibody depends on the variable regions of both light and heavy chains, and if we assume a similar variability (10^4) for the heavy chain, this gives a total repertoire of 10^8 different antibodies, which agrees fairly closely with most estimates based on analysis of the antibodies which develop in response to one particular antigenic determinant.

The Response of B Lymphocytes to Antigenic Stimulation

A virgin or a memory B cell responds to antigen via the immunoglobulin molecules inserted in its cell membrane with the Fab end of the molecules projecting outwards. These act as specific antigen receptors and their ligation results in their aggregation into clumps which coalesce into a single mass or 'cap' at one part of the surface. This results in internalization of the antigen–Ig complex, which initiates the pathway of differentiation into plasma cells. Antigen stimulates all those B cells which express specific surface immunoglobulin receptors capable of binding any epitope present on that antigen. Each of these cells gives rise to a clone of plasma cells producing its own distinctive antibody molecules (Fig. 5.16). The result is a mixture of diverse antibodies (**polyclonal**), some of which can bind the antigen more

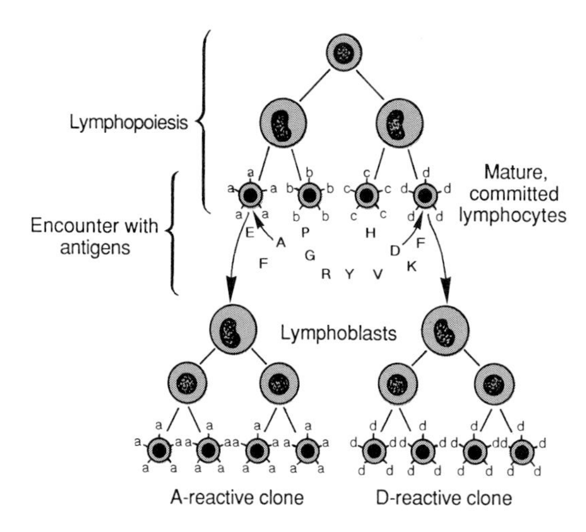

Fig. 5.16 The clonal selection theory of immune response. During lymphopoiesis, each developing T or B cell becomes committed to respond to a narrow range of antigenic determinants: this is reflected by the specificity of the antigen receptors (a, b, c, etc.) on its surface. For example, lymphocytes with hypothetical 'a' receptors can bind an antigen 'A', but not 'D' or 'E', etc. Binding of an antigen stimulates a lymphocyte to proliferate, producing a clone of lymphocytes with identical commitment.

firmly than others, but all of which exhibit exquisite specificity. If the antigen is administered repeatedly in small doses, it is bound preferentially by B cells with higher affinity receptors so that there is a progressive increase in the affinity of the antibody produced. This effect is increased during clonal expansion and differentiation, as point mutations accumulate in certain regions of the V region genes. This process of somatic mutation does not alter the VDJ germline genes themselves and has no effect on the overall specificity of the antibody molecule produced, but it ensures closer fit between antibody and antigen.

Heavy Chain Switching

During the immune response to many antigens, a change occurs in the heavy chain isotype of the secreted antibody. Early in the immune response, IgM predominates but later, IgG and IgA antibodies appear. The plasma cells secreting these latter antibodies are usually derived from clones which originally expressed surface IgM as their antigen receptor. This heavy chain '**switch**' is achieved by the formation and excision of a loop of DNA (similar to that observed in V gene rearrangements), bringing the VDJ_H gene complex into close proximity with the genes encoding $C\gamma$ or $C\alpha$, with the loss of the intervening C_H genes. This isotype switching is controlled in part by T-cell-derived mediators, including interleukins 4, 5 and 6.

Regulation of B-lymphocyte Activation

There are several mechanisms by which antibody production is regulated at the level of the B cell. For instance, binding of immune complexes containing IgG and antigen to either Fc receptors for IgG or via antigen-specific surface immunoglobulin provides an inhibitory signal for B cells. Other regulatory mechanisms include the production of anti-idiotype antibodies and regulatory T cells and are discussed later.

Monoclonal Antibodies

Because the specificity of antibody is retained during clonal proliferation, the antibody produced by a single clone is homogeneous or **monoclonal**. By means of cell-fusion techniques, it is possible to maintain continuously proliferating ('immortal') clones of antibody-producing cells. A mouse or rat is immunized with the antigen and after allowing time for the development of an antibody response, 'immune' spleen cells are fused with cells of a plasma-cell tumour (myeloma, p. 637), usually from an animal of the same species. The antibody secreting hybrid cells, 'hybridomas', are cloned and each clone secretes a monoclonal antibody. The technique depends on the hybrid cell inheriting the proliferative capacity of the myeloma cell and the capacity of the spleen cell to produce antibody of the desired specificity.

A monoclonal antibody reacts specifically with one particular epitope on the antigen. Unexpected reactivity with other antigens containing a similar epitope can occur. Despite this limitation monoclonal antibodies are extremely useful reagents in immunoassays. In addition they have been of considerable value in immunophenotyping cells in tissues and in suspensions, defining both cell membrane and cytoplasmic markers. This has been of particular value in defining clusters of differentiation (CD) antigens (Table 5.7) which are displayed by developing and mature cells of the haemopoietic system. The applications of this system to T cells are discussed in the next section.

Cell Mediated Immunity

T Lymphocytes

The various effector functions referred to as cell mediated immunity are dependent on T cells, which also play a central role in regulating the specific immune response and are responsible for stimulating many non-specific inflammatory mechanisms. T cells comprise about 70% of peripheral blood lymphocytes and there is considerable heterogeneity within this population (Table 5.8).

There are two main groups of **effector T cell**: (1) **cytotoxic T lymphocytes (CTL)** directly lyse appropriate target cells. They may also kill tumour cells and cells of grafted organs; (2) T cells which mediate **delayed-type hypersensitivity (DTH) responses** by the production of soluble mediators, cytokines, that recruit and activate non-specific inflammatory cells such as macrophages. Delayed-type hypersensitivity reactions are important in protective immunity against intracellular pathogens and are involved in allograft rejection and in autoimmunity.

There are thought to be at least two groups of **regulatory T cells**: (1) **helper T cells** (T_H) assist antibody production in response to most antigens. A related group of **'inducer' T cells**

Table 5.7 Cluster of differentiation (CD) markers on cells of the immune system

CD number	Alternative names	Distribution
1	T6	Thymocytes; dendritic cells
2	T11; EFRC receptor	All T cells; NK cells
3	T3	Mature T cells
4	HIV receptor	T_H subset of T cells; some monocytes/macrophages
5	—	T cells; subset of B cells
7	IgM receptor	Activated/immature T cells
8	—	Cytotoxic and ? T_s subset of T cells; some NK cells
11a	LFA-1 α chain	All leucocytes
11b	C3b-receptor α chain	Monocytes/macrophages; polymorphonuclear leucocytes; NK cells
11c	gp150/95 α chain	Monocytes/macrophages; polymorphonuclear leucocytes; NK cells
16	Fc γ receptor III	NK cells; monocytes/macrophages
18	β chain for CD11a,b,c	
19	—	B cells
23	Low affinity IgE receptor	B-cell subset
25	Tac; IL-2 receptor β chain	Activated T cells (some B cells, monocytes/macrophages)
28	—	T cells
29	VLAβ chain platelet GPIIa	Most leucocytes including subset of T cells
45	Leucocyte common antigen	All leucocytes
45RO	UCHL1	Subset of T cells; B cells
56	NKH1; Leu 19	NK cells
57	Leu 7; HNK-1	NK cells; some T cells

Table 5.8 Functional subsets of T lymphocytes

Subset		Phenotype	MHC restriction	Function
Cytotoxic (CTL; Tc)		$CD3^+4^-8^+$	Class I	Kills target cells
Helper	T_H1	$CD3^+4^+8^-$	Class II	Delayed-type hypersensitivity, inflammation. Secretes IL-2, IFN-γ, TNF
	T_H2	$CD3^+4^+8^-$	Class II	Assists antibody production. Secretes IL-4, IL-5
Suppressor		$CD3^+4^-8^+$	?	Immune regulation

seems to be responsible for the initial activation of effector T cells. **Suppressor T cells** (T_S) are thought to play a role in preventing autoimmunity and in regulating the overall level and persistence of protective immune responses.

Phenotypic Features of T Cells

It is impossible to differentiate between classes of lymphocytes on morphological grounds, but T cells, unlike B cells, lack surface immunoglobulin. T cells also have a surface receptor which allows them to bind sheep red blood cells. This ability to bind sheep red blood cells was at one time used to differentiate T cells from B cells, but a variety of T-cell-specific surface antigens can now be detected using monoclonal antibodies. Each of these antigens is assigned to a numbered **'cluster of differentiation' (CD)**, according to the system developed to annotate haemopoietic cell surface molecules (see Fig. 5.1).

In all species T cells can be identified by the presence of surface CD3 antigen which is associated with the T-cell receptor for antigen. CD2, the receptor for SRBC, and CD5 are also found on all T cells (pan T-cell markers), but they are also found on other lymphocytes (Table 5.7) and therefore cannot be used to identify T cells with certainty.

The vast majority (>95%) of mature T cells express either CD4 or CD8 molecules but never both. The primary role of these molecules is to direct the T cells to recognize foreign antigen when complexed with different classes of MHC molecules. The mutually exclusive T-cell subsets which are defined on the basis of CD4 or CD8 positivity are often assumed to be functional helper T cells ($CD4^+$) and cytotoxic/suppressor T cells ($CD8^+$) respectively. Although this relationship is generally true, helper cells have been demonstrated within the $CD8^+$ population and $CD4^+$ cytotoxic T cells also exist.

The expression of different forms of the leucocyte common antigen (CD45) have been used to discriminate between resting or virgin T cells, which express the CD45RA form and activated or memory T cells, which express the CD45RO form.

Antigen Recognition by T Cells

Structure of T-cell Receptor for Antigen (TcR)

The majority of peripheral blood T cells (circa 95%) carry a **T-cell receptor** (TcR) comprising a heterodimer formed by α and β chains linked by a disulphide bond (Fig. 5.17). Both chains have molecular weights of 40–45 kDa and comprise two immunoglobulin-like domains each with an intrachain disulphide bond and each with significant sequence homology to individual immunoglobulin chains. Each of the TcR chains has a cytoplasmic tail, a highly conserved transmembrane region and a distal extracellular domain **(V) domain** which varies much more between different T cells than the more proximal **constant (C) domain**.

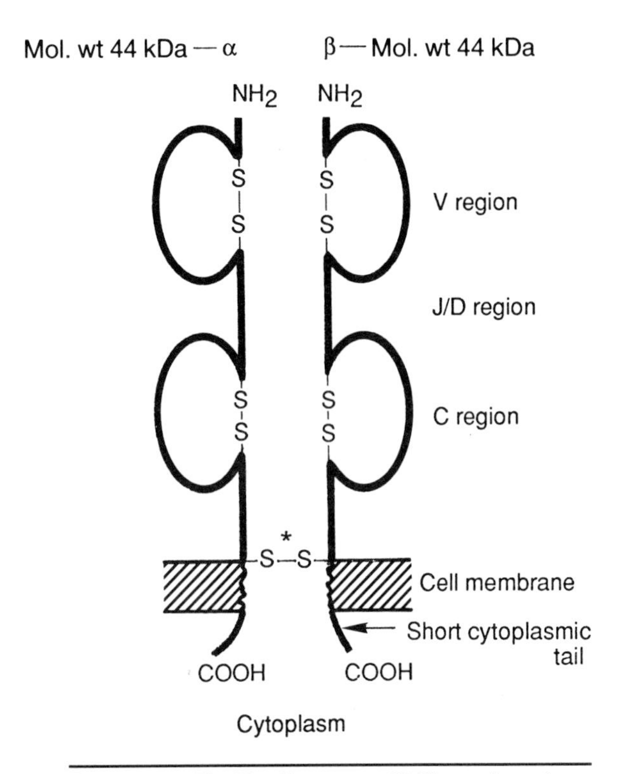

Fig. 5.17 The T-cell receptor (TcR) consists of two distinct polypeptide chains (α and β), which span the T-cell membrane. Each chain is organized into two constant domains with variable regions at the free end. These variable regions comprise the antigen binding site. The chains are held together by an interchain disulphide bond.

The overall organization of the TcR genes is very similar to that of the immunoglobulin loci and a similar strategy is used to create a large repertoire of antigen receptors from a relatively small number of components (Fig. 5.18). The α and β chains are each encoded by separate chromosomes. Each locus has one or more C genes which encode the constant (C) portion of the chain and, at some distance, an array of V genes which encode the distal variable regions. The intervening part of all the loci contains a variable number of **joining (J) regions.** Like immunoglobulin heavy chain genes, the β gene also has diversity (D) segments, but these are absent from the α locus.

During the process of rearrangement which produces a mature TcR from the diverse genetic elements, a selected V gene is spliced initially to a D gene (if available) and then to a J region. The resulting VDJ complex then rearranges with one of the C genes. Productive rearrangement of the TcRβ genes on one chromosome prevents rearrangement of the other allele (allelic exclusion), but this does not occur for the TcRα genes. Although there are relatively few TcR V region genes compared with the immunoglobulin locus, the diversity of the TcR repertoire is enlarged by the availability of a greater number of J and/or D regions to which each V region can be spliced. In addition there is greater flexibility in the exact residues which can take part in these rearrangements, leading to marked variation in the protein sequence at the VDJ region.

The remaining 5% of $CD3^+$ mature T cells do not express the αβ form of the TcR but have an alternative form of TcR comprising γ and δ chains. Most of the γδ T cells do not express CD4 or CD8 molecules and they appear to represent a separate lineage from αβ T cells. However, the γ and δ chains have the same overall protein structure as the α and β molecules. The function of γδ T cells is unknown, but they appear early in ontogeny and may show restricted tissue distribution.

MHC Restriction

T cells can bind to an antigen only when it is presented on the surface of another cell in the form of a complex with an MHC molecule. This so-called MHC restriction depends on the ability of T cells to bind syngeneic MHC molecules with low affinity. Although this reaction is relatively weak, it is strengthened when the MHC molecule is altered slightly by the presence of an antigenic peptide in the groove on the surface of the MHC molecule. The MHC molecule imposing this restriction varies with the T cell involved, but in all cases the TcR must interact both with the antigenic peptide and with the surrounding loops of the MHC molecule.

Class II MHC restriction. $CD4^+$ T cells recognize small antigenic peptides (10–15 amino acids) associated with MHC class II molecules (Fig. 5.19). **Accessory cells** internalize exogenous soluble antigen by pinocytosis and par-

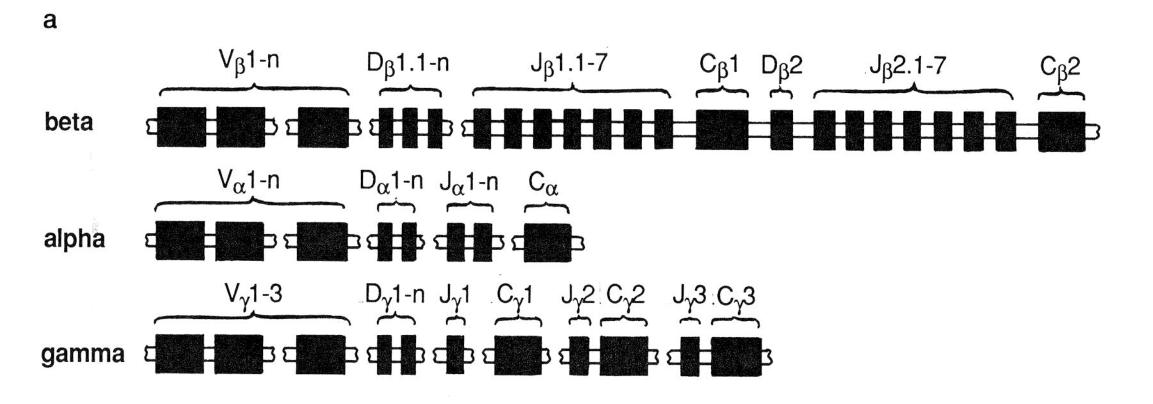

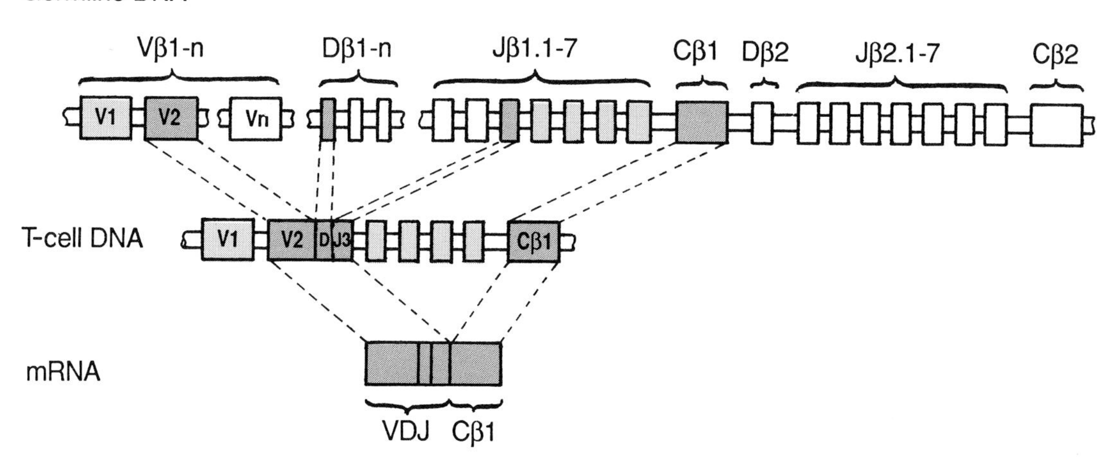

Fig. 5.18 **a** Organization of the genes encoding the α, β and γ chains of murine T-cell receptors. As in synthesis of antibody molecules, synthesis of the T-cell receptor depends upon the splicing of a randomly selected variable region exon to a D (diversity) region and a J (junctional) region exon. The VDJ segment is then spliced to the genes encoding the approximate constant regions. **b** Diagram of gene segments encoding T-cell receptor during T-cell maturation. Variable (V), diversity (D) and joining (J) segments in the germline DNA recombine during T-cell development by excising loops of DNA. Further processing occurs at the mRNA level so that a single VDJ C combination is expressed. (From Male, D., Champion, B. and Cooke, A. (1987). *Advanced Immunology*. Gower Medical Publishing, London.)

ticulate antigens by phagocytosis. This process may be entirely non-specific, but can be accelerated if antigen is opsonized by IgG or C3b, allowing uptake via specific receptors for these opsonins. The internalized antigen then enters endosomal vesicles, where it undergoes partial proteolysis by lysosomal or other acid-dependent proteases. The resulting peptides become associated with newly synthesized class II MHC molecules when the peptide-containing endosomes fuse with the Golgi bodies. The peptide–MHC complex is then transported to and inserted in the membrane of the accessory cell for recognition by $CD4^+$ T cells.

Class I MHC restriction. $CD8^+$ T cells recognize antigenic peptides containing 9–10 amino-acid

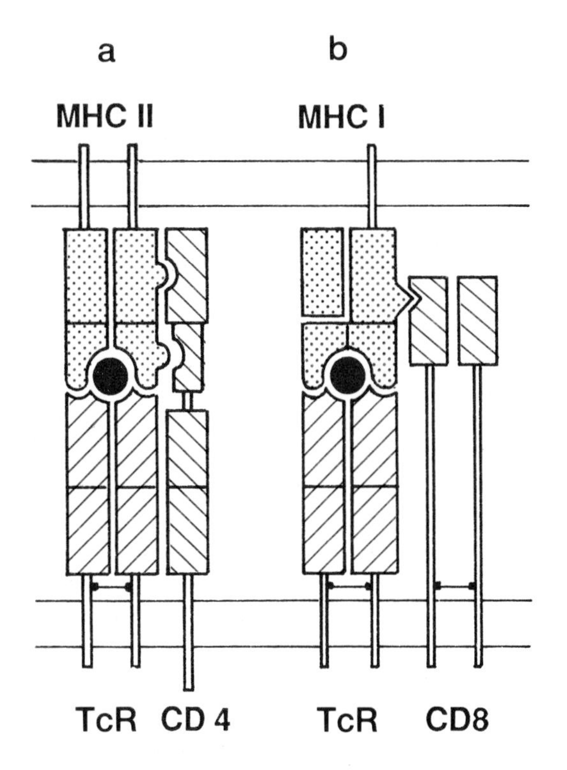

Fig. 5.19 MHC restricted antigen recognition by T cells. **a** The interactions between T-cell receptor and CD4 with the peptide MHC class II complex. **b** The interactions between T-cell receptor and CD8 with the peptide MHC class I complex. **c** In class II MHC restriction, an exogenous protein is internalized and degraded. The resultant peptides associate with newly synthesized MHC class II molecules and are expressed on the cell surface for presentation to $CD4^+$ T cells. **d** In class I restriction, peptides of a foreign antigen which are synthesized by the cell (e.g. microbial antigens) are complexed with newly synthesized MHC class I antigens, and expressed on the cell surface for presentation to $CD8^+$ T cells.

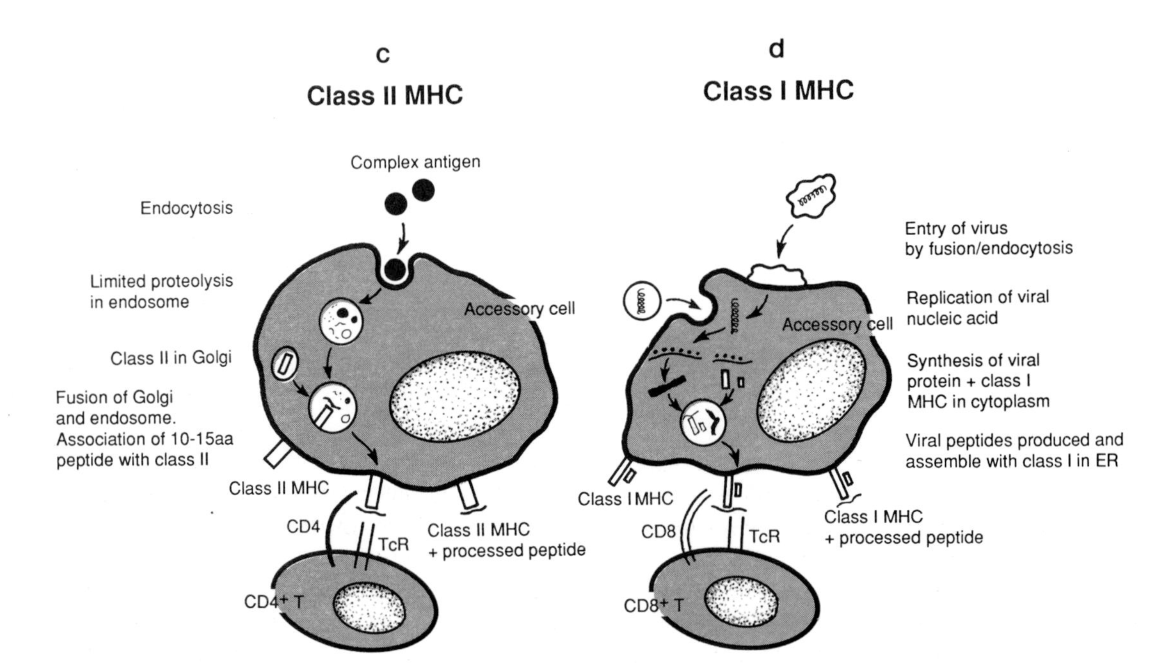

residues which are derived from proteins synthesized within the cell itself (e.g. viral proteins in a virus infected cell). These endogenous peptides enter the endoplasmic reticulum where they complex with newly synthesized class I MHC molecules and are transported to the cell membrane for recognition by CD8+ T cells (Fig. 5.19).

Nature of Antigen Presenting Cells

The role of **antigen presenting cells (APC)** is to produce antigenic peptides of appropriate size, conformation and physicochemical nature to enter the antigen presenting cleft in the MHC molecule. The antigen presenting cell provides the conditions necessary for T-cell activation by forming a stable link with the antigen-specific T cell and by producing co-stimulating factors.

The presence of class I MHC molecules on virtually all nucleated cells and their ability to associate with cytoplasmically derived proteins means that most metabolically active tissue cells are potentially capable of presenting antigen to CD8+ T cells. This is obviously beneficial when one considers that the principal role of these cells is to eliminate viruses which may potentially infect any cell type.

A limited number of cell types meet the more stringent antigen presenting cell requirements of CD4+ T cells. These antigen presenting cells must express class II MHC antigens and must be able to internalize and process complex antigens. They also produce co-stimulatory factors which T cells require for full activation, the best characterized of which is interleukin 1 (IL-1). The best characterized of these antigen presenting cells are the interdigitating dendritic cells found in the T-cell areas of lymphoid organs. These are bone-marrow-derived cells and have a characteristic morphology, with many cytoplasmic protrusions which interdigitate between surrounding lymphocytes. Although dendritic cells are characteristically found in organized lymphoid tissues, similar cells are found scattered throughout most other tissues. These tissue dendritic cells are often called 'passenger leucocytes' and are critically important in initiating the rejection of allografts (p. 223). One of the best characterized of the tissue dendritic cells are the Langerhans cells of the epidermis, which take up antigen applied to the skin and then migrate to the draining lymph node via the afferent lymphatics (Fig. 5.20). In the lymph node, the Langerhans cell differentiates into an interdigitating dendritic cell and only then becomes fully capable of activating T cells. A similar pathway is believed to operate at the gastrointestinal and respiratory mucosal surfaces which are exposed to large amounts of antigen.

Dendritic cells are not the only antigen presenting cells capable of activating CD4+ T cells and indeed have the major disadvantage of not possessing the lysosomal enzymes required to digest more complex antigens such as bacteria. This function seems likely to be fulfilled by conventional tissue macrophages, which are known to act as antigen presenting cells under appropriate circumstances. However, as macrophages only express class II MHC molecules when activated by T-cell derived mediators such as interferon-γ (IFN-γ), their main role in antigen presentation may be at sites of chronic inflammation.

B cells can also present antigen to CD4+ T cells. This may be essential for the induction of most primary immune responses. Always MHC class II positive, B cells can present a wide range of exogenous antigens after non-specific uptake as described above. However, antigen-specific B cells have the additional advantage of being able to concentrate their appropriate antigen on the cell surface by attachment to surface immunoglobulin. As a result, B-cell presentation of specific antigen to CD4+ T cells is estimated to be one thousand times more efficient than presentation of other non-specific antigens.

Many tissue cells including skin keratinocytes, gut epithelium, thyroid epithelium, renal tubules, pancreatic islets and vascular endothelium can be induced to express class II MHC antigens facultatively. This occurs in autoimmune conditions and other forms of immune mediated inflammation such as allograft rejection and graft-versus-host disease. It is thought that this facultative expression of class II MHC antigens may not be responsible for triggering an immune response but may play an amplifying role in the immunopathology by

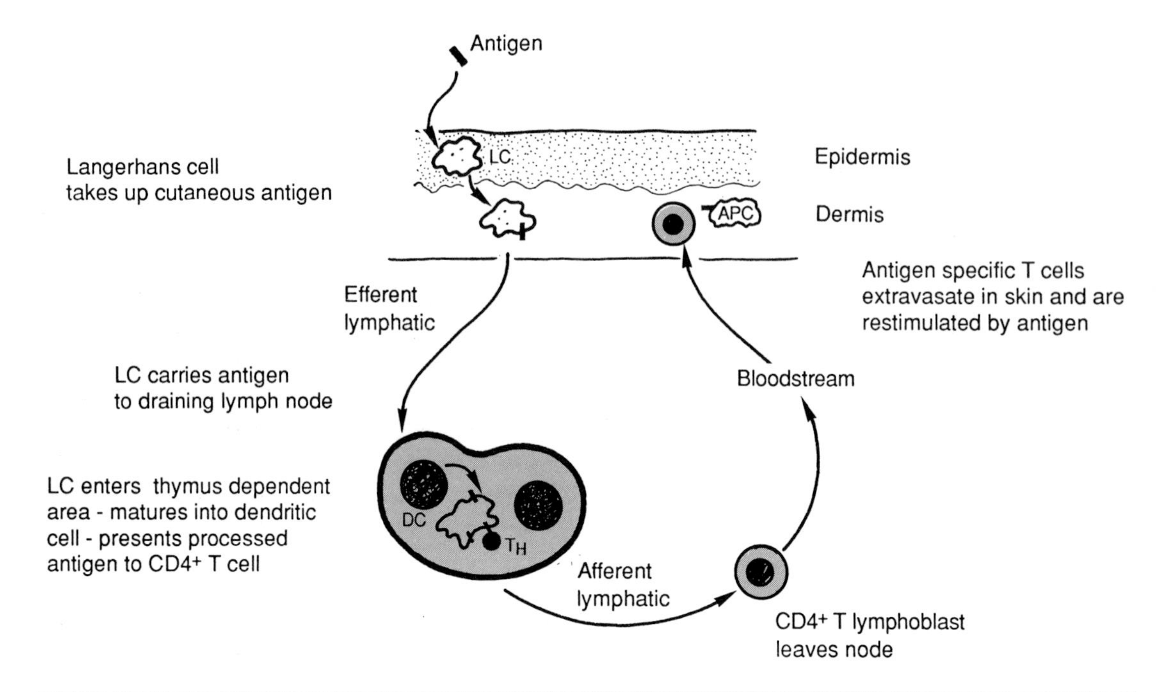

Fig. 5.20 Cell mediated immune response. Antigen in the skin is internalized by a tissue dendritic cell – Langerhans cell (LC) which processes the antigen and migrates to the regional lymph node. There it differentiates into an interdigitating dendritic cell (DC) and presents the antigen to $CD4^+$ T cell (T_H) and also provides the stimulus (IL-1) for proliferation and differentiation of the appropriate T cell. Antigen reactive clones of T cells then leave the regional lymph nodes by the efferent lymphatics, enter the bloodstream and finally reach the area of skin containing the antigen. There they are presented with antigen by antigen presenting cells (APC) and undergo activation.

further stimulating T cells. It has also been suggested that class II molecules expressed on tissue cells may regulate the inflammatory response by inhibiting T-cell activation. Normal thymic epithelial cells express class II MHC molecules constitutively, and this is essential for the maturation of T-cell precursors.

T-cell Activation
(Fig. 5.21)

Although the recognition of antigen and MHC by the TcR delivers the initial stimulus for T-cell activation, it is insufficient to induce T-cell proliferation. This requires the presence of certain non-specific co-stimulatory factors. One of these cytokines, interleukin 1 (IL-1), is produced by antigen presenting cells following its interaction with a T cell. Co-stimulation of antigen-reactive T cells is one of the most important activities of this pleotropic cytokine. Ligation of CD28 on the T cell is a further co-stimulating function of accessory cells. In $CD4^+$ T cells this sequence of events rapidly initiates the synthesis of a variety of further mediators, the most important being interleukin 2 (IL-2; T-cell growth factor) which is an absolute requirement for replication and full differentiation of T cells. The IL-2 producing T cell simultaneously expresses high affinity cell surface receptors for IL-2 and undergoes a period of autocrine stimulation. Secreted IL-2 also exerts a stimulatory paracrine effect on those neighbouring T cells which express IL-2 receptors and thus amplifies the local response. Interleukin 4 (IL-4), another T-cell derived mediator may have similar autocrine and paracrine effects on some T cells.

$CD8^+$ T cells are also dependent on IL-2 for

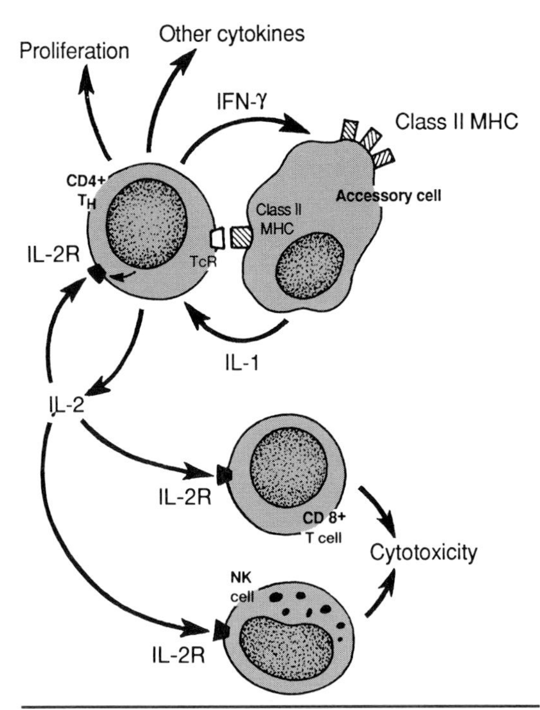

Fig. 5.21 Processes involved in T-cell activation. Antigen is presented by an accessory cell (MHC class II positive) to a $CD4^+$ T cell which undergoes proliferation and secretes a number of cytokines (including IFN-γ and IL-2) and expresses IL-2 receptors in response to the antigenic stimulus and IL-1. IFN-γ and other cytokines are important in the production of the delayed-type hypersensitivity response. IFN-γ synthesized by the $CD4^+$ T cell acts on the accessory cell (paracrine effect) to increase MHC class II expression which promotes antigen presentation. IL-2 acts on the IL-2 receptor of the $CD4^+$ T cell to augment the initial antigen/IL-1 stimulus (autocrine effect). IL-2 also acts to activate cytotoxic $CD8^+$ T cells and NK cells.

growth, but only a small proportion of $CD8^+$ T cells produce this cytokine. Therefore, the proliferation and differentiation of $CD8^+$ T cells usually requires the presence of IL-2-secreting $CD4^+$ T cells.

Role of Accessory Molecules in T-cell Activation

Apart from the recognition of the antigenic peptide–MHC complex, efficient T-cell activation requires a variety of other cell surface recognition molecules which amplify the initial antigenic trigger.

CD3 complex. The CD3 molecule and the TcR are always co-expressed on all mature T cells, both of the αβ and γδ classes. The CD3 molecule comprises a complex of 5–7 individual chains (γ, δ, ε, ζ, η). The CD3 γ, δ and ε chains are found on all T cells, while the ζ and η chains exist either as a heterodimer or a homodimer (Fig. 5.22). The CD3 chain is linked non-covalently in the cell membrane to either the β or δ chain of the TcR. The CD3 chains are entirely invariant and do not bind antigen, but several of the chains are phosphorylated during T-cell activation. CD3 appears to have a role in transducing the initial activation signal from the TcR and activating second messengers. In addition, the CD3 complex may help transport the TcR to the cell membrane.

The CD4 and CD8 molecules are invariant transmembrane proteins, the extracellular domains of which have structural homology with immunoglobulin chains. CD4 is a single chain protein of 55 kDa, while CD8 is a heterodimer comprising two 34 kDa chains. The CD4 and CD8 molecules have two roles in T-cell activation. Both bind directly to non-polymorphic regions of the appropriate MHC molecule on antigen presenting cells, thus stabilizing the initial interaction be-

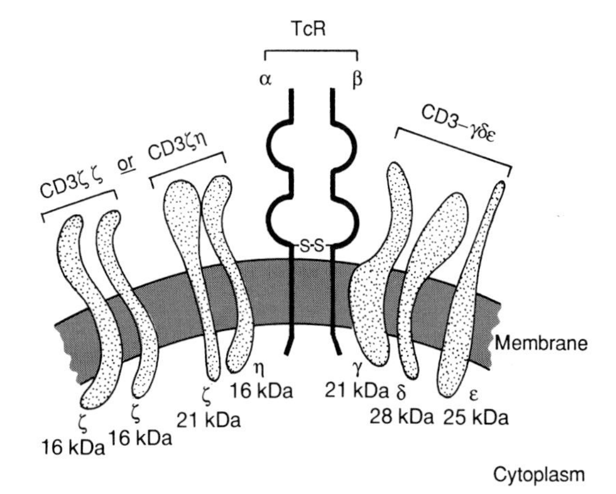

Fig. 5.22 CD3–TcR complex. The γδε chains are present in all T cells, in association with either the ζζ homodimer or the ζη heterodimer. The CD3 complex is non-covalently bound to the TcR and is involved in signal transduction following the binding of peptide–MHC complex by the TcR.

tween TcR and the antigen–MHC complex. In addition, after binding to the MHC molecules, CD4 and CD8 bind to the CD3–TcR complex and associate with a tyrosine kinase (p56 lck) in the T-cell membrane, to produce amplification of the initial activation signal.

Other accessory molecules. Several additional cell surface molecules have been implicated in T-cell activation (Fig. 5.23). **CD2** may form an additional signal transduction element and also increases the adhesion between T cells and antigen presenting cells by interacting with the integrin, leucocyte function antigen-3 (LFA-3). The integrin, leucocyte function antigen-1 (LFA-1) stabilizes the binding of T cells (and other lymphocytes) to accessory cells via its ability to interact with specific receptors such as intercellular adhesion molecules (ICAMs) on macrophages and other cells. LFA-1 is critical for virtually all T-cell functions. CD28 is a recently described molecule on the surface of T cells whose binding to receptors on accessory cells acts as a strong co-stimulating signal to the T cell.

Functions of Activated T Cells

T cells have two roles in the immune response, effector and immunoregulatory. Effector T cells which are responsible for the cell mediated immune response comprise two distinct groups the cytotoxic T cell (CTL) and the cytokine producing or delayed-type hypersensitivity (DTH) T cell.

Cytotoxic T cells comprise a population of fully differentiated, antigen-specific T cells whose function is to produce antigen-specific lysis of target cells by direct cell–cell contact. They frequently contain a few cytoplasmic granules and are usually, but not exclusively, **$CD8^+$ class I MHC-restricted** T cells.

By virtue of the expression of class I MHC on all nucleated cells and the ability of class I MHC to associate with endogenously synthesized peptides, $CD8^+$ cytotoxic T cells are important in the defence against viral infections of tissues. Furthermore, as many of the viral antigens recognized by cytotoxic T cells are synthesized early in viral replication, elimination of infected cells can occur before infectious virus can be released. A role for cytotoxic T cells in the rejection of allografts and the clearance of bacterial or parasite infections also seems likely, but is less well defined.

The exact mechanism used by CTL to produce target cell death is not yet clear. Initial recognition of the target cell by the TcR and ligation of the appropriate accessory molecules, causes an energy- and cation-dependent phase of intimate membrane–membrane contact. This is followed by polarization of cytoplasmic granules in the

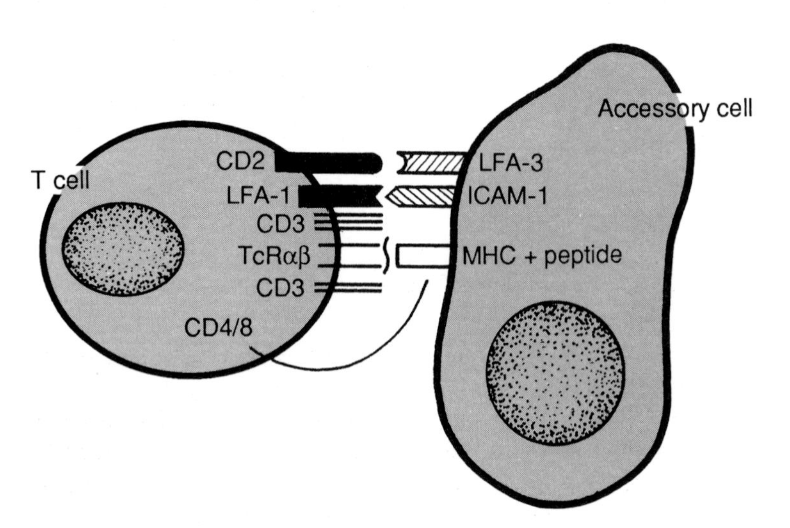

Fig. 5.23 Cell surface molecules involved in the interaction of T cells with antigen presenting cells.

cytotoxic T cell towards the target cell and delivery of a putative 'lethal hit'. This may be the release of granule-derived mediators, such as serine proteases or other toxic enzymes, or may be due to the release of non-specific toxic cytokines, including lymphotoxin (tumour necrosis factor β). Cytotoxic T-cell granules also contain a protein complex termed **perforin** which has homology with the ninth component of complement and polymerizes to form similar membrane pores in the target cell. However, it seems unlikely that membrane damage accounts for the lytic activity of cytotoxic T cells as the first abnormalities seen in the target cell are nuclear fragmentation and changes resembling those seen in apoptosis (p. 28). The cytotoxic T cell is resistant to its own lytic effects and after killing one target cell, is capable of recycling to kill many more.

Delayed-type hypersensitivity reactions (DTH). This is the second component of cell mediated immunity and is typified by the tuberculin skin reaction. Delayed-type hypersensitivity responses are characterized by a heavy infiltrate of T cells and macrophages and, as the name implies, develop slowly over a period of 24–48 hours (p. 219).

The basis of a delayed-type hypersensitivity reaction is much more complex than that of the cytotoxic T cells' response described above. In most cases, it is initiated by a population of **class II MHC-restricted CD4$^+$** T cells, whose principal function is to release an array of cytokines (Table 5.9) which, in turn, recruit and activate other inflammatory cells. These include macrophages, eosinophils, basophils and mast cells. The best understood of these cytokines is interferon-γ (IFN-γ) which is essential for the expression of an effective cell mediated immune response. IFN-γ activates macrophages, thus stimulating phagocytic activity; it increases the expression of class II MHC molecules and stimulates production of other inflammatory cytokines, including IL-1, tumour necrosis factor α (TNFα) and interferon-α/β (IFN-α/β). As a result, IFN-γ not only enhances the inflammatory and antimicrobial functions of macrophages but also increases their ability to process and present antigens to further T cells. IFN-γ also induces facultative expression of class II MHC antigens on tissue cells and has antiviral and antiproliferative properties.

The production of IFN-γ by effector T cells is accompanied by synthesis of lymphotoxin, TNFβ. Its activities overlap many of those of IFN-γ and the effects of the two mediators are frequently synergistic. TNFβ is a particularly potent cytostatic and cytotoxic agent, with a marked ability to produce apoptosis. Unlike IFN-γ, TNFβ does not induce class II MHC expression on cells, but both cytokines augment the expression of class I MHC molecules. TNFβ also shares many of the inflammatory and pyrogenic effects of IL-2 and TNFα which are produced by macrophages. Details of the sources and actions of these and other cytokines which play a role in DTH reactions are listed in Table 5.9.

In mice (but not yet in man) there is evidence that the CD4$^+$ T cells which mediate DTH may be distinct from the CD4$^+$ cells which act as helper T cells in the antibody response. The former cells (T_H1) secrete IL-2, IL-3, IFN-γ and TNFβ, while the latter (T_H2) secrete IL-3, IL-4 and IL-5.

The biological role of DTH is primarily in protection against persistent infections and microbes which can replicate within the lysosomes of macrophages. The production of cytokines underlies the ability of small numbers of antigen-specific T cells to evoke a marked inflammatory response against the limited amounts of antigen which escape from the lysosomes. However, the potent activation of these non-specific immune mechanisms carries the risk of unwanted tissue damage during an initially protective response.

Natural Killer Cells

This group of lymphocytes is capable of cytotoxic activity during cell mediated responses. Natural killer (NK) cells are medium-sized lymphocytes with several cytoplasmic granules ('large granular lymphocytes') and appear to use the same lytic mechanism as classical cytotoxic T cells.

Table 5.9 Principal cytokines of the immune system

Cytokine	Source	Functions
Interleukin 1	Mononuclear phagocytes, accessory cells, keratinocytes, thymic epithelium	T-cell co-stimulator; B-cell growth; inflammatory effects on, e.g. fibroblasts, endothelium, pyrogen
Interleukin 2	$CD4^+$ T lymphocytes	T-cell growth and differentiation factor; B-cell growth, NK cell activation
Interleukin 3	$CD4^+$ T lymphocytes	Haemopoietic stem cell growth; mucosal mast cell activation
Interleukin 4	$CD4^+$ T lymphocytes	B-cell growth factor; enhances IgE production; T-cell growth factor
Interleukin 5	$CD4^+$ T lymphocytes	B-cell growth and differentiation factor; enhances IgA production
Interleukin 6	Activated T cells, fibroblasts, mononuclear phagocytes, keratinocytes	B-cell switch/differentiation factor; inflammatory effects similar to IL-1
Interleukin 7	Bone marrow stromal cells	Early T-cell/B-cell growth
Interleukin 8	Mononuclear phagocytes, fibroblasts, endothelial cells, keratinocytes & others	Neutrophil chemo-attractant and activator; T-cell chemo-attractant
Interferon-α/β	Mononuclear phagocytes, fibroblasts	Antiviral; NK cell activation, cytoregulation; macrophage activation; cytostatic; B-cell regulation; enhances class II MHC expression
Interferon-γ	Activated T cells, NK cells	Activates macrophages and induces expression of HLA class II molecules on macrophages and many other cells; suppresses haemopoietic progenitor cells; activates endothelial cells; antiviral activity
Tumour necrosis factor α	Mononuclear phagocytes, activated T cells, NK cells	Similar inflammatory effects to IL-1; activates T cells, macrophages; acute phase response; anti-neoplastic cells—cytostatic/cytotoxic; synergistic with IFN-γ; induces expression of class I MHC
Tumour necrosis factor β (lymphotoxin)	$CD4^+$ T lymphocytes	Similar to tumour necrosis factor α

However, they differ from cytotoxic T cells in a number of ways. Although they possess T-cell markers, such as CD2 and occasionally CD8, they are $CD3^-$ and do not rearrange or express any TcR genes. Natural killer cell cytotoxicity is not MHC-restricted or antigen-specific and their activity can be demonstrated in normal individuals in the absence of specific immunization. Furthermore, no secondary response or enhanced activity can be demonstrated following immunization. Thus, NK cells appear to represent a third distinct lineage of lymphocytes.

It is thought that NK cell killing depends on their recognition of a group of differentiation antigens. They may be important as a first line form of immune surveillance against virus infections and may serve as non-specific regulators of lymphopoiesis and haemopoiesis. Natural killer cells can kill cells in the absence of antibody, but as they possess receptors for the Fc portion of IgG their lytic activity can be enhanced by linkage to target cells via specific antibody.

Regulation of the Immune Response

In addition to cytotoxicity and delayed-type hypersensitivity reactions, T cells are responsible for regulating other components of the immune response.

T–B-cell Cooperation in the Antibody Response

By virtue of an ability to activate B cells directly, certain unusual antigens can induce an antibody response in the absence of T cells. These thymus independent antigens are usually polymeric molecules containing multiple identical determinants on a rigid backbone, which allows them to cross-link surface immunoglobulin on the B cell. As thymus independent antigens include many bacterial surface molecules such as endotoxins, polymerized flagellin and pneumococcal polysaccharide, this type of T-cell-independent antibody response is of obvious importance in protective immunity.

Nevertheless, thymus-independent antigens are rare and normally induce only an IgM response. In order for these antigens to produce an IgG antibody response and in order to produce a humoral response to other antigens (i.e. thymus dependent ones) antigen-specific $CD4^+$ T cells are required. After immunization with a complex antigen, helper T cells recognize epitopes of 'carrier determinants' which are distinct from those recognized by the B cell (haptenic determinants). Thus, an efficient secondary antibody response to a hapten–carrier complex (e.g. dinitrophenyl–bovine serum albumin, DNP–BSA) can be generated by mixing T_H cells which have been primed only by the carrier (BSA) with B cells primed to the hapten (DNP) This mechanism allows a single population of carrier-specific T_H cells to help an antibody response to many different haptenic determinants on the same carrier molecule.

Close contact between specific T_H and B cells is generally required for the generation of an efficient antibody response. The simplest way to envisage this is to consider what happens when a specific B cell recognizes haptenic determinants on the intact antigen via its surface immunoglobulin. After internalization and processing the peptides generated are presented by the B cell as carrier determinants for the appropriate T_H cell. In other cases, T–B-cell co-operation requires the presence of an accessory cell which presents the same antigen to both T_H and B cells. Under these circumstances, the carrier determinants recognized by the T_H cells would be processed peptides complexed with class II MHC, while the haptenic determinants recognized by the B cell would be determinants present on intact antigen held on the accessory cell surface.

Role of T Cells in B-cell Differentiation

The requirement for T_H cells in antibody production reflects the fact that recognition of antigen by surface Ig is usually insufficient to trigger differentiation of the B cell into a plasma cell. In addition to IL-2 other T-cell derived mediators are required both to stimulate division of the triggered B cell and to promote synthesis and secretion of immunoglobulins (Table 5.9). The most important of these mediators are interleukins-4, 5 and 6. IL-4 acts mainly in the early stages of B-cell differentiation by initiating cell division of antigen-stimulated B cells and is involved in initiating immunoglobulin gene switching. It also appears to have the ability to enhance IgE production. **IL-5** enables an already stimulated B cell to progress through its complete growth and differentiation pathway and may be required for its final development into a mature plasma cell. IL-5 also has a selective effect on IgA production. **IL-6** acts on the last stages of plasma cell differentiation and may also selectively enhance IgA synthesis. In contrast, IFN-γ inhibits many of the effects of these mediators. Finally, IL-2 and the accessory cell product IL-1, are also important for early events in B-cell development.

Negative Regulation of the Immune Response

The role of the immune system is to protect against harmful pathogens but it is important that immune responses are controlled in order to prevent continued and progressive tissue injury. As a consequence many different negative regulatory mechanisms have evolved.

Idiotypic Networks

The antigen-combining sites of antibody molecules are unique to each antibody specificity. Because most antibodies appear after the immune system has matured fully, their antigen-binding sites themselves constitute a non-self antigen and are known as idiotypes. A further antibody response will stimulate the production of antibodies (anti-idiotypes) directed at these idiotypes. Anti-idiotypes may then interact with the surface immunoglobulin on the B cells, preventing the original antibody blocking further interaction with antigen and possibly providing a signal to switch off antibody production. The binding of anti-idiotypes to secreted antibody can also prevent its interaction with antigen and thus inhibit the recruitment of immune complex-dependent mediator systems. As the anti-idiotype antibody process could involve an infinite number of such idiotype–anti-idiotype interactions, it is capable of providing a complex negative feedback network. A corresponding system of TcR idiotypes and anti-idiotypes may exist to regulate the activity of T cells.

Suppressor T Cells

Virtually all models of immunoregulation have provided evidence for the existence of a population of T cells which can inhibit the function of B cells or other T cells. These suppressor T cells (T_S cells) have not only been implicated in regulating normal immune responses, but also in the maintenance of tolerance to autoantigens. In most cases, T_S cells are found to be $CD8^+$ T cells but they appear to differ from $CD8^+$ T cells with cytolytic activity. Despite a large body of evidence for the phenomenon of T-cell mediated immunosuppression, stable clones of antigen-specific T_S cells have not yet been propogated *in vitro*, which casts doubt on their existence. T-cell mediated immunosuppression may merely reflect inhibitory effects mediated by cytokines or other T-cell products.

T-cell Education

The thymus is responsible for the ability of T cells to recognize foreign antigens associated with self-MHC molecules and for their inability to mount immune responses against autoantigens. The mechanisms underlying these critical events in T-cell education are paralleled by changes in lymphocyte phenotype (see Fig. 5.1).

The lymphohaemopoietic stem cells which enter the thymus have no identifiable T-cell characteristics. Within the cortex the primitive T cells divide, probably in response to a signal delivered by cortical epithelial cells. The CD2 molecule is the first T-cell specific marker to be expressed. Shortly afterwards, the CD3 complex is synthesized and T cells expressing the receptor can be detected. β TcR genes then begin to rearrange and the β chain can be demonstrated intracellularly. The TcR α chain gene is the last to be rearranged and $\alpha\beta^+$ T cells only appear when this process is complete. At this stage, the immature T cells are $CD3^+$, but do not express either of the CD4 or CD8 subset markers ('double negative'). However, soon after the αβ TcR appears on the cell surface, each cell begins to express both CD4 and CD8 molecules ('double-positive' T cells). These $CD3^+$ $CD4^+$ $CD8^+$ T cells then migrate from the cortex to the medulla and differentiate into mature functional T cells with either the $CD3^+$ $CD4^+$ $CD8^-$ or $CD3^+$ $CD4^-$ $CD8^+$ phenotype. Around birth, a massive emigration of these mature T cells populates the peripheral immune system.

During this differentiation process, T cells become MHC restricted and learn not to recognize other self-antigens by processes of positive and negative selection. A population of immature T cells with a bias to recognizing self-MHC is first expanded but before they are capable of mounting a strong response to autoantigens, they are eliminated. Positive selection occurs when those T-cell precursors which randomly express TcR genes capable of recognizing self-MHC antigens receive positive signals for continued growth from cortical epithelial cells with the appropriate MHC. Thereafter, the maturing cells move into the medulla where a population of bone-marrow-derived accessory cells deliver a negative signal to those T cells which possess TcR with high affinity for peptides from self-proteins complexed with self-MHC molecules. This negative selection process results in complete elimination of all clones of self-reactive T cells (clonal deletion), thus preventing permanently the possibility of autoimmunity. As a result, the individual acquires a repertoire of mature T cells which cannot respond effectively to self-antigens, but which retains a bias towards recognizing self-MHC molecules. The mechanisms of clonal deletion are not known but cell death occurs by apoptosis.

Immunological Tolerance

An individual may sometimes fail to make a response to an antigen which, under other circumstances, would induce active immunity. This state of unresponsiveness is referred to as immunological tolerance.

Biological Significance of Immunological Tolerance

The inability to respond to autoantigens is critically important for preventing autoimmune disease. This '**self-tolerance**' depends primarily, as we have described, on the clonal deletion of self-reactive T cells in the fetal thymus. Developmentally determined unresponsiveness of autoreactive B cells may also be involved in the phenomenon of self-tolerance.

Tolerance may also be induced by certain immunization regimens in animals with a mature immune system. The ability of the immune system to develop this type of **acquired tolerance** may be necessary to prevent the development of hypersensitivity reactions during an initially protective response to pathogens. It is also beneficial to become tolerant rather than immunologically reactive to certain types of foreign antigen. For example, the oral administration of soluble protein antigens induces tolerance, oral tolerance, because an immune response to food antigens might provoke unwanted hypersensitivity reactions on subsequent antigen exposure.

Factors Influencing the Induction of Tolerance

Several host and antigenic factors can determine whether an encounter with antigen induces tolerance or immunity. Of these, the most important appears to be immaturity of the lymphocytes in the immune system. The susceptibility of the immature animal to the induction of tolerance is evidenced by the normally profound unresponsiveness to self-antigens which are encountered during fetal life. This phenomenon continues for a short time after birth, as evidenced by the fact that immunization of neonatal mice with allogeneic lymphocytes prevents them from rejecting skin grafts from the lymphocyte donor strain when these are applied in adult life (Fig. 5.24). Other factors which increase the possibility of inducing tolerance rather than immunity are the use of very high or very low doses of antigen (high zone and low zone tolerance), administration of soluble as opposed to particulate antigens, and the use of intravenous or oral routes of immunization. Finally, several immunomodulatory regimens are now being used to induce or maintain tolerance, notably in clinical transplantation practice. These include immunosuppressive drugs (cyclosporin A, FK506 and cyclophosphamide), total lymphoid irradiation and *in vivo* administration of antibodies directed at CD4 molecules on T cells.

Mechanisms of Immunological Tolerance

These are summarized in Table 5.10. Tolerance of self-antigens appears to be due to permanent elimination of autoreactive T-cell clones in the fetal thymus. Whether this reflects an unusual re-

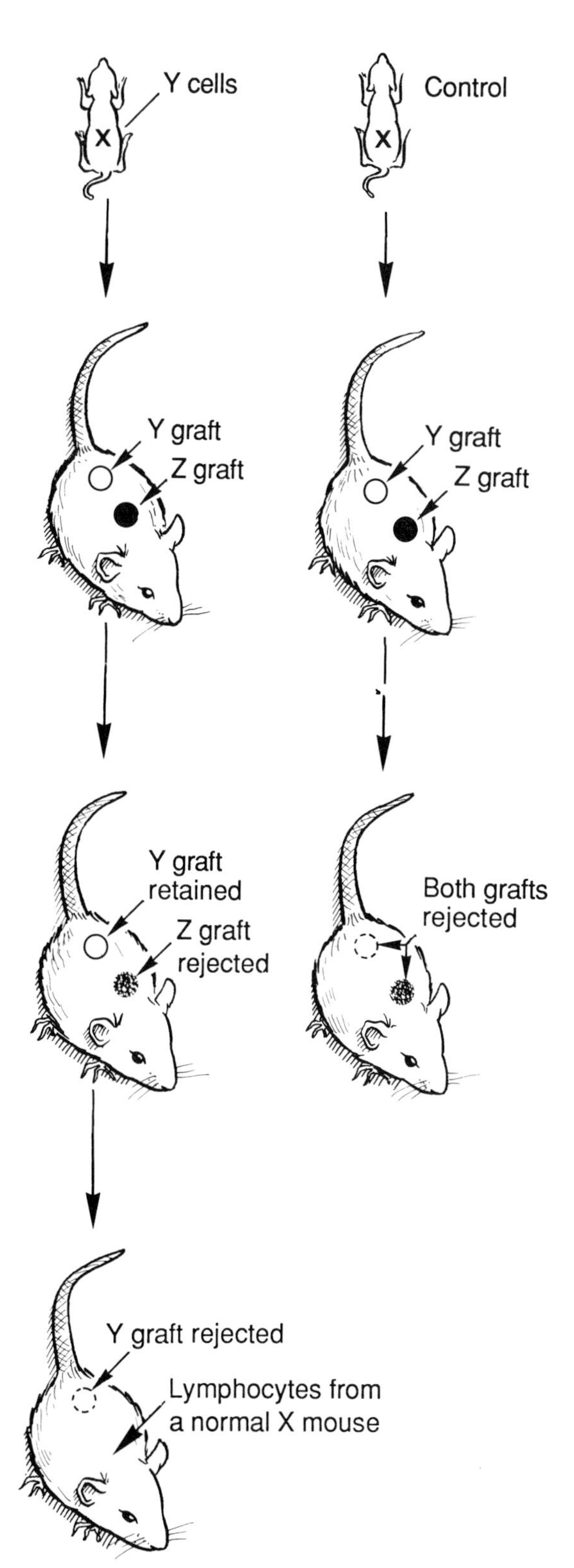

Table 5.10 Mechanisms of self-tolerance

Deletion of self-reactive T lymphocytes in thymus	
Functional inactivation (anergy) of self-reactive T cells	
Suppressor T cells	
Deletion of self-reactive B lymphocytes	
B-cell anergy	Direct inactivation
	Absence of self-reactive T_H

sponse of immature T-cells to antigen or is due to unusual mechanisms of antigen presentation in the thymus is not known. Clonal deletion of this nature probably does not account for regulation of autoreactive B cells or for the acquired forms of tolerance described above. In these situations, antigen-specific lymphocytes remain in the immune system, but have become functionally inert (**anergic**) after their first encounter with antigen. The anergic state reflects a direct effect of antigen on individual cells, in which partial activation is followed by refractoriness to restimulation. It occurs, either because the lymphocytes encounter an ineffective combination of the signals required for cellular activation or because the lymphocytes respond inappropriately to these signals. Another explanation is that effector T cells and B cells are rendered anergic due to the inhibitory effects of presumed T_S cells. Thus, in contrast to clonal deletion, in tolerance involving cellular anergy, antigen binding lymphocytes exist but do not become activated. A breakdown of the regulatory mechanisms may terminate the anergic state and allow the expression of autoreactive cells and the emergence of autoimmune disease.

Fig. 5.24 Immunological tolerance to allogeneic cells. A neonatal 'X' strain mouse (top left) injected with strain 'Y' cells becomes tolerant to 'Y' transplantation antigens, as shown by retention of a subsequent 'Y' skin graft. It rejects an unrelated ('Z' strain) graft normally. Injection of lymphocytes from a normal 'X' mouse results in rejection of the 'Y' graft. (In practice, injection of lymphocytes or haemopoietic cells is commonly used to induce tolerance in such experiments: this raises the complication of the graft-versus-host reaction (p. 225) which, for the sake of simplicity, has been ignored in this illustration.)

Further Reading

Longman, R. E. (1989). *The Immune System.* Academic Press, London.

Male, D., Champion, B. and Cooke, A. (1987). *Advanced Immunology.* Gower Medical Publishing, London.

Roitt, I. M. (1991). *Essential Immunology*, 7th edn. Blackwell Scientific Publications, Oxford.

Roitt, I. M., Brostoff, J. and Male, D. (1985). *Immunology.* Churchill Livingstone, Edinburgh/Gower Medical Publishing, London.

Samter, M., Townage, D. W., Frank, M. M., Alister, K. F. and Claman, H. N. (1988). *Immunological Diseases.* Little, Brown and Company, Boston/Toronto.

6

Diseases of the Immune System

Immunopathology is the study of diseases which have, or appear to have, an immunological basis. These diseases can be divided into three broad categories: (1) hypersensitivity reactions in which inappropriate activation of immune responses produces tissue damage; (2) autoimmunity in which immunity to self-antigens occurs; and (3) immunodeficiency diseases in which the individual is incapable of mounting a normal range of immune responses and as a result is unduly susceptible to infection.

Hypersensitivity Reactions

The purpose of the immune response is to protect against invasion by foreign organisms. However, in certain situations the introduction of an exogenous antigen or the presence of an endogenous antigen (self-antigen or autoantigen) elicits an unduly severe, tissue damaging, inflammatory hypersensitivity reaction. This reaction may be localized to the site of entry of the antigen, or may be generalized, affecting different organs and tissues. Occasionally, the systemic reaction may be severe with fever, shock, gastrointestinal and pulmonary disturbances and even fatal circulatory collapse.

Hypersensitivity reactions can be divided into four types depending on the mechanism of immune recognition involved and on the inflammatory mediator system recruited (Gell and Coombs classification; Table 6.1). Types I, II and III depend upon the interaction of antibody with the target, whereas in type IV reactions, recognition is achieved by antigen receptors on T cells. Because the mediator systems involved in the pathogenesis of antibody-dependent hypersensitivity reactions are already present in the cells found at the site of the antigen–antibody reaction, or are present in the plasma, they occur rapidly, often within minutes. In contrast, type IV hypersensitivity reactions rely on the recruitment, proliferation and activation of lymphocytes and macrophages. Thus, these take longer to evolve and have therefore been called delayed-type hypersensitivity reactions. Although the division of hypersensitivity reactions into four types is useful for classification purposes, it is important to emphasize that more than one type of hypersensitivity reaction may be involved in the pathogenesis of certain diseases.

Type I Hypersensitivity (Atopic or Anaphylactic Reactions)

Type I hypersensitivity reactions occur in approximately 10–20% of the population but some suggest the figure may be as high as 30–35%. Although in the majority of patients the symptoms are mild, a minority of patients suffer life-threatening systemic anaphylaxis.

Table 6.1 Gell–Coombs classification of immunologically mediated hypersensitivity reactions

Type	Recognition system	Cells/Mediators involved	Time of onset	Disease examples
I Anaphylactic	IgE	Mast cells Basophils	Immediate (min) + Late reaction	Anaphylaxis, atopic disorders
II Cytotoxic, cytopathic	IgG, IgM	Complement NK cells Neutrophil Macrophage	Immediate	Autoimmune haemolytic anaemias, haemolytic disease of the newborn, Goodpasture's syndrome, thyrotoxicosis
III Immune-complex disease	IgG, IgM, IgA	Complement Neutrophils	Intermediate (4–8 h)	Arthus reaction, farmer's lung, serum sickness, systemic lupus erythematosus, most types of glomerulonephritis
IV Delayed-type, cell mediated hypersensitivity	T lymphocyte	Cytokines from lymphocytes and macrophages Cytotoxic T cells	Delayed (24–48 h)	Contact dermatitis; allograft rejection; tuberculosis

Predisposition to Type I Hypersensitivity

The high familial incidence of type I hypersensitivity reactions, often spanning several generations, suggests a genetic predisposition, which is termed atopy. Within families atopy is linked with certain HLA haplotypes, but in the general population an association between atopy and a single HLA haplotype has not been found. Atopic individuals have higher serum IgE levels and produce more IgE in response to antigenic stimulation than normal subjects. It is, therefore, probable that a genetic factor, possibly HLA-linked, determines the intensity of IgE responses. However, IgE does have a protective role; individuals coming from countries in which parasitic diseases are endemic, have higher IgE levels than those living in developed countries. In these individuals IgE antibody production occurs as a defence mechanism against parasite antigens and type I hypersensitivity reactions may be involved in parasite expulsion.

Mechanisms of Type I Hypersensitivity

In order for a type I hypersensitivity reaction to occur the individual must previously have been exposed to the antigen (allergen) and must have responded by the production of IgE antibody. The mechanism of the early-phase of type I hypersensitivity reactions has been investigated intensively. Historically, it was shown that if the injection of an allergic patient's serum into the skin of a non-atopic individual was followed by the injection of the allergen into the same site, an immediate weal-flare response developed, the Prausnitz–Küstner reaction. This reaction, which can be elicited up to 3–4 weeks after the initial serum injection, is due to the passive transfer of IgE antibody (reaginic antibody)* from the allergic patient. IgE binds strongly by its CH2 and CH3 domains to specific high affinity membrane receptors (Fc_E receptors; Fc_ERI) on tissue mast cells and circulating basophils (Fig. 6.1). At least two types of mast cell exist, the connective tissue and the mucosal mast cell. They differ in the protease and peptidoglycan content of their granules. Although both types express Fc_ERI, the mucosal mast cell may not be involved in type I hypersensitivity reactions.

Activation and degranulaton of connective tissue mast cells or circulating basophils results from the binding of antigen to cell-bound IgE antibody. For mast cell activation to occur the IgE receptors must be cross-linked and thus, the antigen must be polyvalent. Mast cell activation is associated with degranulation, and activation of phospholipases A_2 and C (Fig. 6.1). Mast cell granules contain the preformed mediators histamine, heparin, neutrophil chemotactic factor, eosinophil chemotactic factor and proteases. The rapid secretion of these preformed mediators accounts for the immediate symptoms following exposure to allergens.

The biochemical steps involved in degranulation involve activation of phospholipase C as a result of Fc_ERI cross-linking. Conversion of phosphatidyl inositol to inositol triphosphate (ITP) and diacyl glycerol occurs, increasing intracellular calcium and activating protein kinase C respectively (p. 18). Lysphosphatidic acid, a 'fusogen', is formed and promotes fusion between the cell membrane and the membranes of storage granules so that exocytosis occurs.

The late-phase response to mast cell activation starts 2–6 hours after antigen exposure and may last 24 hours. It is caused by the newly generated lipid mediators and the accumulation of eosinophils and neutrophils in response to the release of chemotactic factors such as LTB_4.

Activation of phospholipase A_2 results in formation of arachidonic acid and the subsequent generation of prostaglandin D_2, thromboxane and leukotrienes B_4, C_4 and D_4. Prior to their precise characterization, these leukotrienes were known collectively as slow reacting substance of anaphylaxis (SRS-A). Platelet activating factor (PAF) is also released during mast cell activation.

*Reagin was the term applied originally by Prausnitz and Küstner to describe the antibody-like factor in the serum of atopic subjects. It is now known to be IgE.

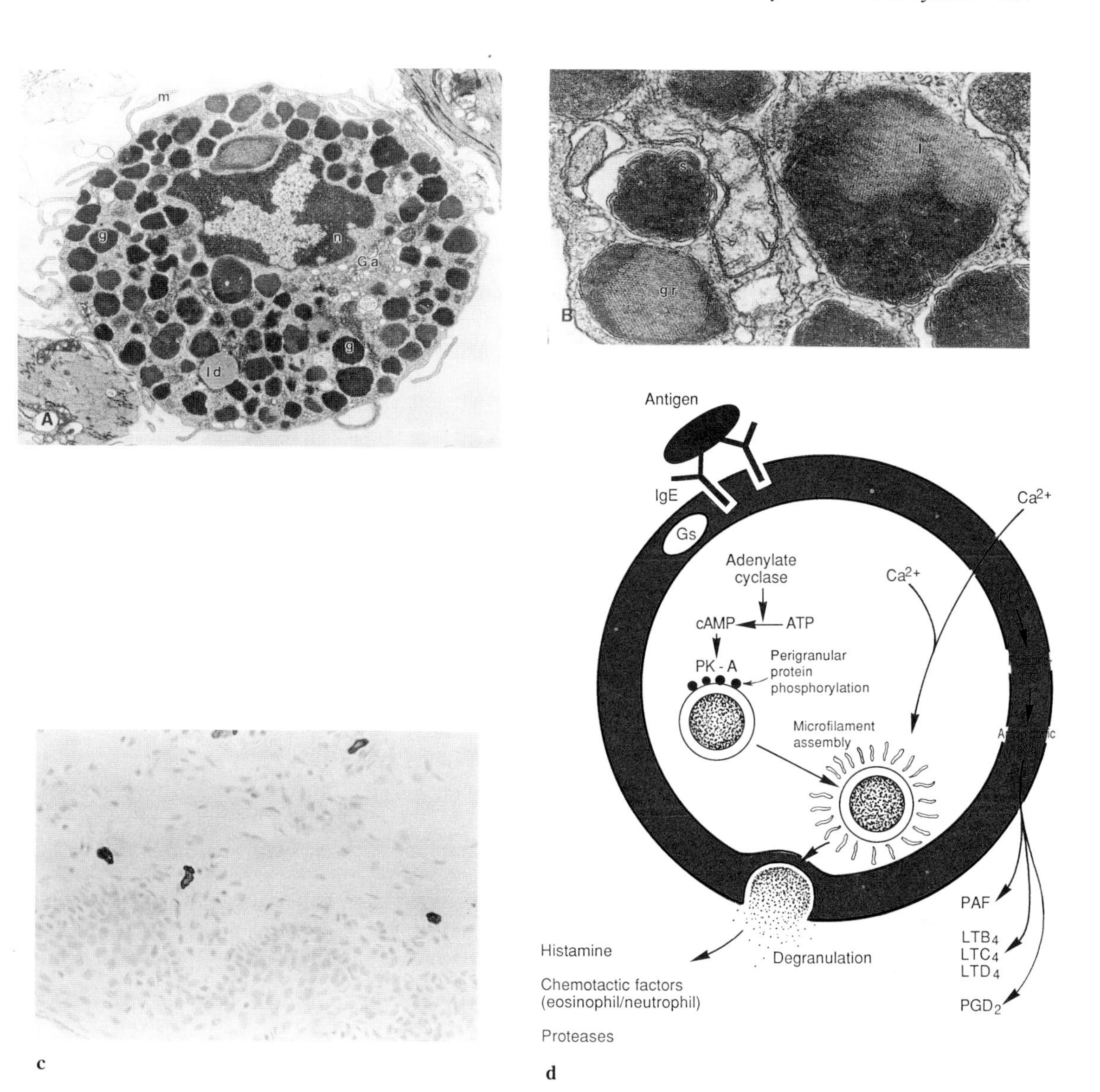

Fig. 6.1 **a** Low magnification transmission electron micrograph of a typical dissociated human foreskin mast cell. The cell contains a single nuclear profile (n), and many electron-dense secretory granules (g). Microplicae (m) or folds extend from the surface. There are a few lipid droplets (ld), and the Golgi apparatus (Ga) is near the nucleus. The filaments in the cytoplasm are intermediate filaments. ×8370. **b** A higher magnification micrograph shows the basic crystalline patterns seen in the mast cell granules: lattice (l), grating (gr), and scroll (s). ×30 225. **c** Mast cells in human skin stained immunocytochemically with a monoclonal antibody to human mast cell tryptase (Dr Andrew Walls). **d** Scheme of events occurring in a mast cell following cross-linking of IgE receptors by antigen. The two major second signals involved are (i) a transient elevation of cAMP levels which initiates degranulation; and (ii) activation of phospholipase A_2 (PLA_2) so that membrane phospholipids are converted to PAF, leukotrienes and PGD_2. Elevation of cytoplasmic free calcium (Ca^{2+}) is involved in activation of PLA_2 and in the assembly of microtubules and microfilaments which are involved in the movement of the granules to the cell surface.

(**a** and **b** are from Caulfield *et al.* (1990). *Laboratory Investigation* **63**, 502–10. Courtesy of authors and editors.)

The biological effects of these mast cell products have been described in relation to the acute inflammatory reaction (p. 139). They are responsible for the major features of localized atopic reactions – congestion (vasodilatation), oedema due to increased venular permeability and infiltration with eosinophil leucocytes. They also increase secretion of mucosal glands in hay fever and asthma and produce the bronchoconstriction of asthma which results from contraction of bronchial smooth muscle.

Eosinophils (Fig. 6.2) are the predominant cells in the tissue lesions of type I hypersensitivity reactions, and a peripheral blood eosinophilia is a common accompaniment of these disorders. It has been proposed that eosinophils regulate the activities of mast cell products. However, eosinophil cationic protein and major basic protein damage respiratory epithelium *in vitro* which suggests that these cells play a pathogenetic role in allergic tissue damage. Eosinophils also elaborate LTC_4 and PAF (p. 140).

The role of neutrophils in type I hypersensitivity reactions is controversial. However, as they are prominent in the tissue lesions of the late-phase responses and produce an array of inflammatory mediators and toxic oxygen products, they probably account for some of the tissue injury.

Eosinophils, neutrophils and macrophages possess low affinity membrane receptors for IgE, $Fc_{E}RII$, which are distinct from $Fc_{E}RI$. Binding of IgE to these cells may occur but whether this is important in the pathogenesis of type I hypersensitivity reactions is presently unknown.

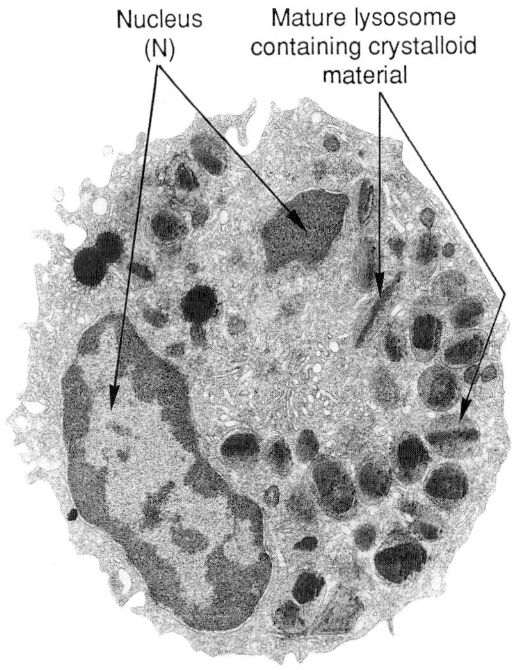

Fig. 6.2 Electron micrograph of an eosinophil showing one complete lobe and a portion of the second lobe of the nucleus (N). The cytoplasm contains numerous lysosomes and some of these (the more mature forms) contain electron-dense crystalloid material which is secreted when the cell is activated. (Prof. A. B. Kay).

Clinical Examples of Type I Hypersensitivity Reactions

The clinical features of type I hypersensitivity classically occur within minutes of exposure to antigen. In many patients this early phase may be followed after 2–6 hours by a recrudescence of symptoms, the so-called late phase.

Localized Type I Hypersensitivity

The commonest manifestations of atopy are **hay fever** and **extrinsic asthma**, which tend to run in families and are sometimes preceded by **atopic eczema** in infancy and childhood. The sufferer from hay fever develops acute inflammation of the nasal and conjunctival mucous membranes with sneezing, and nasal and lacrimal hypersecretion within minutes of exposure to the causal agent (**allergen**) – usually grass pollens. Similarly, an attack of asthma, with difficult, wheezing respiration due to narrowing of the airways by bronchospasm and mucous secretion, develops rapidly when the asthmatic inhales the allergen to which he is hypersensitive, e.g. house dust or animal dander. Atopic individuals, particularly in childhood, may also suffer from **'food allergies'** in which absorption of antigenic constituents of, e.g. milk or eggs, promotes an acute reaction in the gut with colicky pain, vomiting and diarrhoea. **Urticaria**, consisting of acute inflammatory lesions of the skin with wealing due to dermal oedema, is common in atopic subjects and also occurs alone as an acute or chronic condition.

Systemic Type I Hypersensitivity

Atopic patients sometimes develop **acute systemic anaphylaxis (anaphylactic shock)** with dyspnoea, urticaria, convulsions, and sometimes death. Fortunately, severe anaphylactic shock is rare, but it sometimes occurs as a hypersensitivity reaction to drugs, notably penicillin, and to the venoms of stinging insects, when the allergen is absorbed in large amounts so that significant levels are present in the blood.

Allergens in the blood bind to IgE antibody on the surface of circulating basophils. This activates them and degranulation and secretion of arachidonic acid metabolites occur. These metabolites are similar to those produced by mast cells although the lipoxygenase pathway (p. 142) is less active in the basophil. Thus, leukotrienes are formed in only small amounts as is prostaglandin D_2. Circulating antigen also leaves the bloodstream and activates tissue mast cells. The result is widespread urticaria, vasodilatation, causing severe shock, together with intense contraction of non-vascular smooth muscle, notably in the bronchial tree. The condition is a medical emergency and prompt intravenous injection of adrenaline is indicated.

Diagnosis of Atopy

Diagnosis of atopy depends upon an accurate clinical history, which may suggest that acute attacks result from exposure to a particular allergen. To confirm the state of hypersensitivity, dilute solutions of the suspected antigens are placed on the skin and pricked in with a needle. A positive result is indicated by a local weal and flare reaction, developing within minutes and lasting for 1–2 hours (Fig. 6.3). The results of skin tests may not always be helpful. For example, a large proportion of atopic individuals give positive reactions to a number of allergens so that the individual allergen which is responsible for a particular set of symptoms may not always be identified. Furthermore, some patients with obvious type I hypersensitivity diseases may have negative skin tests. Provocation tests, for example bronchial challenge by controlled inhalation of the suspected allergen in asthma, or nasal insufflation in a hay fever patient, may precipitate the symptoms. These tests should only be performed when resuscitation facilities are available.

In general, even in atopic individuals, serum levels of IgE are extremely low (<1 μg/ml). However, immunoassays to measure total serum

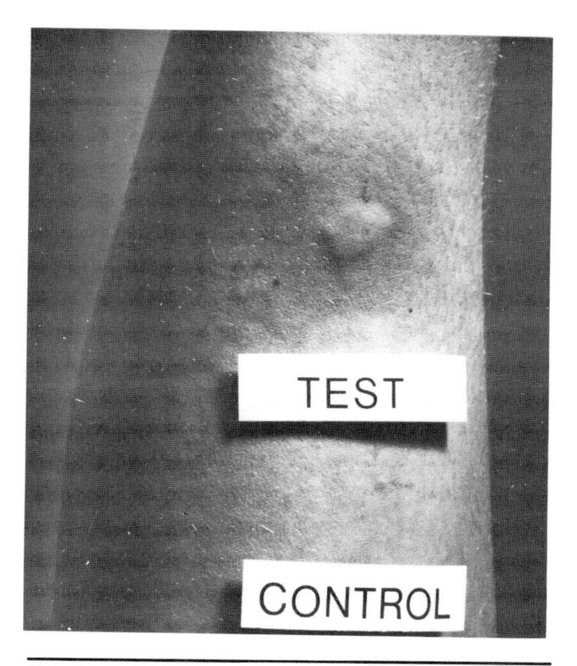

Fig. 6.3 Skin test showing immediate (type I) hypersensitivity reaction. The patient was an asthmatic and the test was performed by intradermal injection of an extract of house dust. Note the oedema and wide zone of reddening. Photograph taken 10 minutes after injection. (Dr Ian McKay.)

IgE and radioallergosorbent tests (RAST) of antigen-specific IgE antibody levels have been developed and may reveal elevated levels of total IgE or specific IgE antibodies. This has proved helpful in some patients in whom skin test results were equivocal.

Management of Type I Hypersensitivity Reactions

If the allergen can be identified it should be avoided if at all possible. Mast cell stabilization by disodium cromoglycate reduces mediator release and is useful for preventing early- and late-phase manifestations. Agents which increase intracellular cAMP levels reduce mast cell degranulation. These include the phosphodiesterase inhibitors, theophylline and other methyl xanthines or adenylate cyclase activators such as adrenaline or isoprenaline, which are β sympathomimetics. Antihistamines prevent the binding of histamine to H_1-receptors. Glucocorticoids have widespread effects on mediator formation and release, and on the inflammatory response.

Desensitization is performed by giving repeated subcutaneous injections of allergen, starting with minute doses and increasing gradually to larger doses until desensitization is achieved or a local or systemic allergic reaction occurs. Alternatively, less frequent injections of chemically modified allergens may be used. Desensitization is associated with the production of IgG antibody and this is then thought to bind to the allergen before it reaches IgE antibody on the mast cell. The procedure offers temporary relief to a proportion of patients, but as it is not without risk it should only be performed when resuscitation facilities are available.

Type II Hypersensitivity (Antibody-dependent Cytotoxicity)

This is mediated by antibodies usually of the IgG or IgM class, which are usually cytotoxic and which react with tissue components.

Mechanisms of Cytotoxicity

Cytotoxicity can occur as a result of complement activation, with the insertion of the C5b–9 membrane attack complex into the cell membrane (p. 142). For non-nucleated cells a single C5b–9 complex is sufficient to produce lysis, whereas nucleated cells, because of their ability to repair cell membrane rapidly, are more resistant and therefore multiple C5b–9 complexes are required for their lysis.

Complement also enhances destruction of antibody-coated cells by opsonization. During complement activation, activated C3, C3b, becomes covalently bound to the antibody-coated cells. Neutrophils and macrophages possess cell membrane receptors for C3b (complement receptor type I; CR1) and its inactivated form, iC3b (CR3). Thus, C3b promotes the adhesion between the phagocytic cell and the antibody-coated target and enhances its phagocytosis and intracellular destruction (Fig. 4.10).

In some instances **antibody-dependent cell mediated cytotoxicity (ADCC)** occurs and is due to the destruction of antibody-coated cells by phagocytic cells or large granular lymphocytes (NK cells, p. 197). ADCC depends upon the interaction of the Fc piece (CH_2 and CH_3 domains) of IgG antibody with Fcγ receptors. In the case of the NK cells, cytotoxicity appears to be produced by the secretion of granules (perforins) which produce cell membrane lesions which are similar to complement produced lesions (p. 145).

Clinical Examples of Type II Hypersensitivity Reactions

With few exceptions, the targets of cytotoxic antibodies are the cells of the blood. Such injury has been investigated mainly in man, in whom it may occur in a number of circumstances.

Cytotoxic Antibodies to Blood Cells

Autoantibodies. The classical example is autoimmune haemolytic anaemia in which red cell injury is brought about by autoantibodies of the IgG or IgM class, which recognize antigenic determinants on the red cell surface. IgG promotes the binding of red cells to the Fc receptors of macrophages in the splenic red pulp and of Kupffer cells in the liver. IgG and IgM antibody both activate complement (p. 142) which may lead directly to haemolysis or may promote phagocytosis and extravascular destruction of red cells by macrophages. IgM can also produce red cell agglutination, which leads to their sequestration and destruction in the red pulp of the spleen.

Autoimmune thrombocytopenic purpura is caused by an autoantibody which reacts with a surface component of normal platelets, while autoantibodies to leucocytes may be a cause of leucopenia.

Drugs may induce cytotoxic antibodies by binding to the cell membrane and acting as haptens, e.g. thrombocytopenia with sedormid, or by modifying cell membrane antigens so that they are recognized as foreign, e.g. haemolytic anaemia with α-methyldopa.

Isoantibodies (alloantibodies). Red blood cells carry numerous surface polymorphic antigenic constituents, the most important being the antigens of the ABO and rhesus (Rh) system. The A and B antigens of the ABO system are derived from an oligosaccharide, H substance, by the action of glucosyltransferases encoded by A and B genes respectively. Individuals who express both genes are AB positive, while those who express neither gene are group O and express H substance only. Individuals who are group A positive have anti-B in their serum, those who are B positive have anti-A, those who are AB positive have neither anti-A nor anti-B, while those who are group O produce both anti-A and anti-B. These antibodies are usually IgM and are called **isohaemagglutinins**. They are thought to arise as the result of the individual becoming immunized against antigens present on intestinal bacteria. Individuals do not form antibodies against ABO antigens which are present on their own erythrocytes. Transfusion of ABO incompatible blood results in rapid destruction of the transfused red cells, because of the presence of circulating isohaemagglutinins in the recipient.

The production of antibodies to rhesus (Rh) blood group antigens may also produce erythrocyte destruction. Although there are several Rh antigens, D is the most important. Approximately 85% of Caucasians are RhD positive and 15% are negative. Antibodies to the Rh antigens are only produced following blood transfusion or pregnancy. Transfusion of RhD positive red cells into an RhD negative individual results in the development of anti-RhD antibody of the IgG class. Subsequently transfused RhD positive red cells are destroyed rapidly in the spleen. The red cells are removed by binding to the Fc receptors of the splenic macrophages of the spleen, where they are subsequently destroyed. As the number of RhD antigens on the red cell surface is very low they are too far apart for two IgG molecules to come sufficiently close together to activate complement.

During labour (or abortion) some fetal red cells enter the mother's circulation and if she is RhD negative and the fetus is RhD positive, anti-RhD antibodies may be produced. Thus, in subsequent pregnancies, if the fetus is RhD positive these IgG class antibodies can cross the placenta and will destroy the fetal red cells, causing anaemia and perhaps death – hydrops fetalis (Fig. 6.4). The

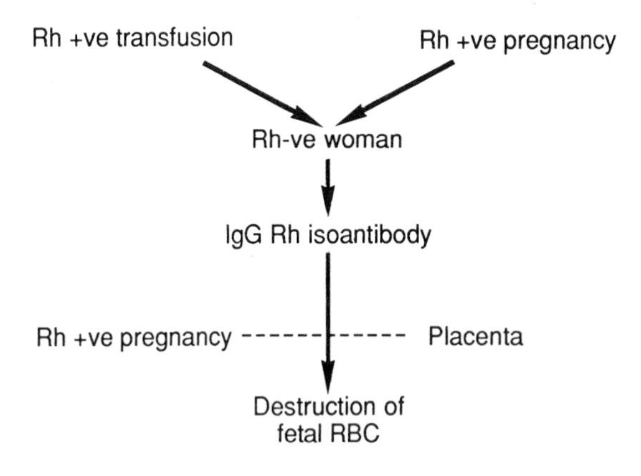

Fig. 6.4 Haemolytic disease of the newborn. Fetal red cell destruction is brought about by maternal isoantibody which has developed as a result of a previous Rh positive pregnancy or transfusion of Rh positive red cells.

development of RhD antibodies can be prevented by injecting RhD antibody within 48 hours of delivery of an Rh-incompatible child. The injected antibody binds to the circulating fetal red cells resulting in their sequestration in the spleen and before they provoke an immune response.

Leucocytes and platelets express HLA antigens (p. 176), but this is important in blood transfusion only if one wishes to supply one of these cell types to a deficient patient. Blood transfusion and pregnancy stimulate the development of anti-HLA and other antibodies and subsequently transfused platelets or leucocytes may be destroyed rapidly. Such isoimmunization is of importance if subsequent organ transplantation (e.g. of a kidney or heart) is performed. Maternal isoantibodies may cross the placenta and cause thrombocytopenia in the fetus. Immune responses of HLA isoantigens may also develop as a result of organ transplantation and are important in allograft rejection.

Autoantibodies to Antigens in Extravascular Tissues

Autoantibodies which react with intracellular components of tissue cells (e.g. anti-deoxyribonucleoprotein in systemic lupus erythematosus) are not a cause of tissue injury. Although autoantibodies to the surface constituents of tissue cells could initiate cytolysis by complement activation or ADCC, there is little evidence that this occurs *in vivo*.

There are, however, a few important examples of autoantibodies which react with cell surface receptors and have a profound effect on the target tissue cells. In primary hyperthyroidism (Graves' disease; p. 1090) an autoantibody which reacts with the TSH receptor of thyroid epithelium stimulates the cell to increased function and proliferation by activation of adenylate cyclase. This process is sometimes called 'stimulatory hypersensitivity'. In some patient with primary hypothyroidism (p. 1090) an autoantibody to the TSH receptor blocks signal transduction so that the signal to produce thyroid hormone is not received by the thyroid epithelial cell. A small proportion of patients with primary Addison's disease (autoimmune adrenal insufficiency) have antibodies which bind to the ACTH receptor on adrenal cortical cells and prevent the binding of ACTH (p. 1102). In myasthenia gravis (p. 879), an antibody to nicotinic acetylcholine receptors of skeletal muscle binds to the receptor and blocks the action of acetylcholine so that muscle weakness results (Fig. 6.5). In primary hyperthyroidism and myasthenia gravis the antibodies are of IgG class and if present in pregnant females they can cross the placenta and produce neonatal hyperthyroidism and myasthenia gravis respectively. A third example of a harmful autoantibody is found in a small proportion of sterile men; it reacts with spermatozoa and if present in sufficient concentration in seminal fluid it impairs their motility.

Finally, extracellular tissue injury may also occur as a type II hypersensitivity reaction. The best known example is a rare type of glomerulonephritis, Goodpasture's syndrome (p. 902), in which an autoantibody to the basement membrane of the glomerular and pulmonary capillaries develops. The antibody binds to the inner surface of the basement membrane, and complement activation occurs as in the Arthus reaction, to produce destructive inflammatory lesions in the glomeruli and lungs.

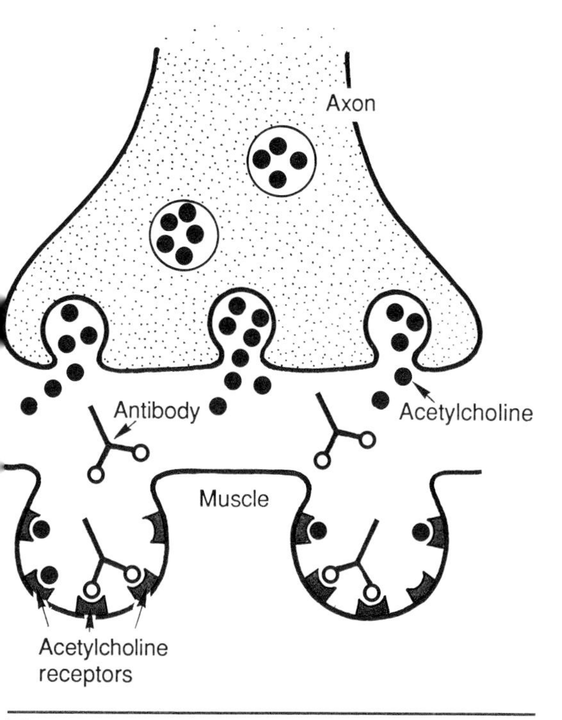

Fig. 6.5 Role of immunity in myasthenia gravis. Autoantibodies to the acetylcholine receptor bind to the acetylcholine receptors on the motor endplate. Not only do they compete with acetylcholine for the receptors but as a consequence of their binding, (1) the receptors are internalized which reduces their numbers and (2) complement activation occurs which damages the motor endplate.

Type III Hypersensitivity (Immune-complex Disease)

Type III hypersensitivity reactions occur as a result of the accumulation of antigen–antibody or immune complexes in tissues. Immune complexes are formed by union between IgG, IgM or IgA antibody and antigen, either locally in the tissues or in the circulation. Immune complexes formed in the tissues give rise to a localized inflammatory response, the Arthus reaction, while those which are formed in the circulation are widely distributed and give rise to a generalized reaction, commonly known as circulating, or systemic, immune-complex disease.

Localized Type III Reactions (The Arthus Reaction)

The Arthus reaction occurs at the site of injection of a soluble antigen and depends on the presence of precipitating antibody in the circulation. Insoluble antigen–antibody complexes are formed in and around the walls of post-capillary venules. The inflammatory reaction develops over 4–8 hours and may progress to tissue necrosis. The lesion shows the typical features of acute inflammation with congestion of small vessels, fluid exudation and marked margination and emigration of neutrophils. Platelet aggregation occurs and in severe cases, haemorrhage and thrombosis with necrosis extends from the walls of small vessels into the surrounding tissues.

These features depend upon complement activation. Complement activation by insoluble immune complexes results in the covalent binding of C3b to the surface of the insoluble complex leading to its dissolution (solubilization), allowing the smaller soluble complexes to diffuse out of the tissues. Complement activation also generates C4a, C3a and C5a, anaphylatoxins which produce acute inflammation by increasing vascular permeability and stimulating the emigration of neutrophils (Fig. 6.6). Neutrophils phagocytose the complexes by their Fcγ receptors and C3 receptors (CR1 and CR3) leading to the release of lysosomal enzymes, including neutral proteases, and of cationic proteins and toxic oxygen radicals. This produces tissue damage and the inflammatory reaction is then amplified by the production of kinins and other vasoactive peptides.

Sequestered (Planted) Antigens

There is experimental evidence that non-glomerular antigens in the blood may pass through

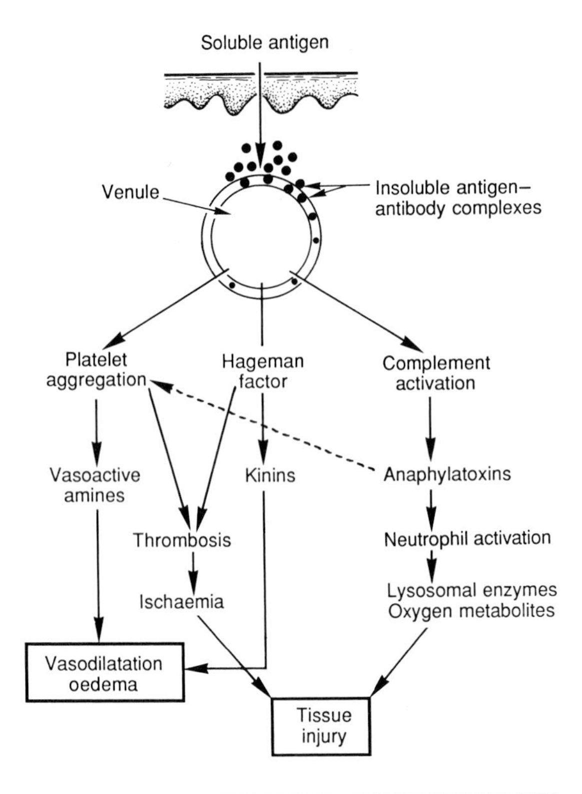

Fig. 6.6 The Arthus reaction. The formation of insoluble antigen–antibody complexes in the venule wall results in (1) platelet aggregation and (2) complement activation. Formation of anaphylatoxins during complement activation will also stimulate platelet aggregation. As a result of the inflammatory process resulting from (1) and (2), endothelial cell damage occurs and Hageman factor is activated, resulting in activation of the coagulation system and the formation of kinins. Tissue injury results from neutrophil activation and ischaemia.

the fenestrated glomerular endothelium and become bound to the capillary basement membrane. Here they may subsequently bind with circulating antibodies which also pass through the fenestrated endothelium, forming immune complexes and triggering an inflammatory response by activating complement and neutrophils. If an antigen was deposited widely in different tissues prior to the formation of antibody, the systemic distribution of the subsequent inflammatory reactions would be identical to those of systemic (circulating) immune-complex disease.

Systemic (Circulating) Immune-complex Diseases

Immune-complex formation is the normal consequence of an immune response to an antigen, and low levels of circulating immune complexes occur transiently in normal individuals without producing tissue injury. However, in some individuals circulating immune complexes are deposited in the walls of blood vessels, especially in the glomerular capillaries, where they cause tissue damage.

Experimental Circulating Immune-complex Disease

Acute serum sickness. This form of type III hypersensitivity reaction was demonstrated in rabbits following a single intravenous injection of a large soluble protein antigen, e.g. bovine serum albumin. No harmful effects occur until after several days when antibody is produced (Fig. 6.7). As antibody appears, it combines with antigen still present in plasma, to form immune complexes. Initially, complexes are formed in marked antigen excess, and are therefore small and soluble and do not activate complement. As more antibody is produced the antigen: antibody ratio shifts so that complexes are formed sequentially in slight antigen excess, at equivalence and then in slight antibody excess. These later formed complexes are relatively insoluble and have the capacity to activate complement.

In some tissues in which the endothelium is fenestrated (e.g. renal glomerulus, synovial membrane) immune complexes can leave the circulation and become deposited on the basement membrane. The deposition of complexes in blood vessels which are lined with continuous endothelium (e.g. skin, endocardium, large and medium-sized arteries) depends upon increased vascular permeability (Fig. 6.8), but the precise mechanisms involved are not clear. It is thought that degranulation of circulating basophils, through C3a or via the interaction of antigen with cell bound IgE antibody, stimulates release of the vasoactive

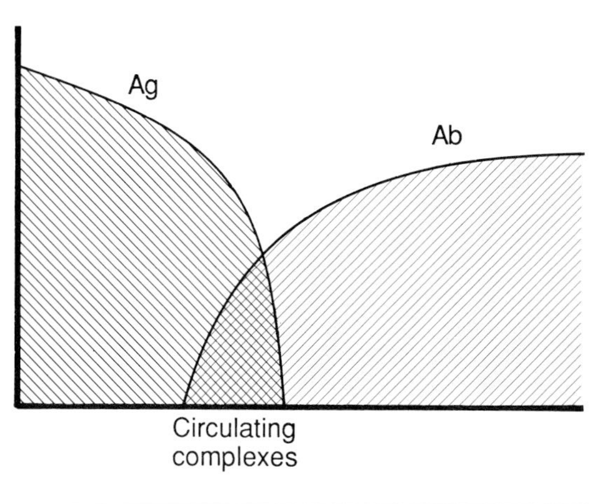

Fig. 6.7 Serum sickness reaction. The formation of antigen–antibody complexes in the circulation. Injection of antigen is followed after some days by the appearance of antibody in the plasma: during the next few days, the concentration of antigen falls sharply and antigen–antibody complexes are present in the plasma.

mediators and leukotrienes as well as PAF (p. 140). The latter compound stimulates the release of the vasoactive amine serotonin (5-HT) from platelets.

Once the immune complexes are deposited in the blood vessel walls they continue to activate complement so that an acute inflammatory reaction occurs, as has been described for the Arthus reaction. The reaction is extremely intense and when arteries are affected the lesions may extend through the full thickness of the vessel wall. Activation of complement and neutrophils results in phagocytosis of the deposited complexes within 48 hours and as antigen is eliminated from the circulation, complexes are no longer formed. Thus, experimental serum sickness is brief and self-limiting.

Chronic immune-complex disease. Chronic immune-complex disease can be induced experimentally by injecting rabbits intravenously with antigen on a daily basis. However, in this situation the complexes are localized exclusively in the glomerular capillaries and give rise to lesions resembling some of the different types of progressive glomerulonephritis seen in man (Chapter 19). For instance, membranous glomerulonephritis is associated with the subepithelial deposition of small circulating complexes, whereas lesions resembling proliferative and mesangiocapillary glomerulonephritis only occur in rabbits which produce precipitating antibody and form large, relatively insoluble, complement-activating immune complexes.

Factors Predisposing to Systemic Immune-complex Disease

Following immune-complex activation of the classical complement pathway, C3b which is generated, binds covalently to the complex in an attempt to prevent the formation of large insoluble complexes in the circulation. This process, known as prevention of immune precipitation, can be demonstrated *in vitro* by mixing antigen and antibody together, in the presence of normal human serum. Complexes formed in serum tend to remain soluble, whereas they precipitate when formed in the absence of serum, when complement activity has been destroyed by heat inactivation (56°C for 15 minutes) or when the serum is deficient in the early components of the classical pathway (C1q, C1r, C1s, C4, C2 or C3). Immune complexes rendered small and soluble by complement activation (i.e. complement reacted complexes) circulate in the blood and are removed and degraded by the macrophages of the liver and spleen. If, however, the complement reacted complexes remain large and relatively insoluble, due to the size or insolubility of the antigen, precipitation in blood vessel walls can be prevented by their binding of C3b receptors (CR1) on erythrocytes. In this way they can be transported to the liver and spleen for degradation by macrophages (Fig. 6.9). Thus, the three main defence mechanisms which protect against circulating immune-complex disease are: (1) complement mediated prevention of immune precipitation; (2) the erythrocyte transport mechanism; and (3) the macrophages of the liver and spleen.

These protective mechanisms can be circumvented in a number of ways (Fig. 6.10):

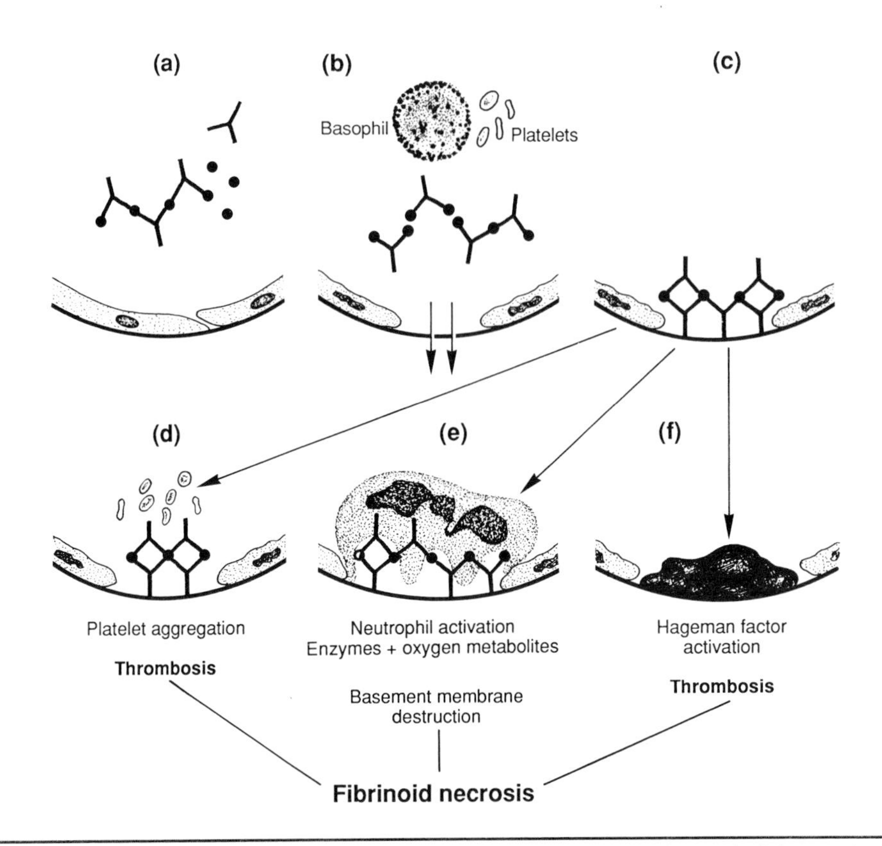

Fig. 6.8 Proposed mechanisms in the pathogenesis of immune-complex induced vascular injury. **a** Antigen (●) and antibody (⅄) bind in the circulation to form antigen–antibody complexes. **b** These complexes can trigger secretion of vasoactive mediators from circulating basophils and platelets by binding to Fc-γ receptors. In rabbits it has been shown that antigen binds to basophil-bound IgE antibody to trigger histamine secretion and the synthesis of platelet activating factor (PAF) which stimulates platelet activation and the secretion of platelet granules. **c** The vasoactive mediators released from basophils and platelets open up junctions between endothelial cells so that the antigen–antibody complexes are deposited on the basement membrane. **d** Deposited complexes induce platelet activation and aggregation by Fc-γ receptors. Thrombosis occurs. **e** Deposited complexes activate neutrophils via Fc-γ receptors. Enzymes and reactive oxygen metabolites cause basement membrane destruction. **f** Exposure of basement membrane and basement membrane damage results in Hageman factor activation with thrombosis. In addition, and not shown in the figure, complement activation occurs. C5a attracts neutrophils into the damaged area and the membrane attack complex directly damages the basement membrane. The end result is the characteristic appearance of fibrinoid necrosis.

(1) Persistent antigen exposure, either due to chronic infection with replicating organisms (e.g. plasmodia or *Mycobacterium leprae*) or due to continuous release of an autoantigen from damaged tissue (Table 6.2);

(2) Failure of the complement system to keep complexes small and soluble. Inherited deficiencies of each of the classical pathway components is associated with an increased risk of developing immune-complex disease. IgA activates complement poorly, if at all. Thus, complexes formed with IgA antibody are more likely to produce immune-complex glomerulonephritis;

(3) Low expression of CR1 on erythrocytes

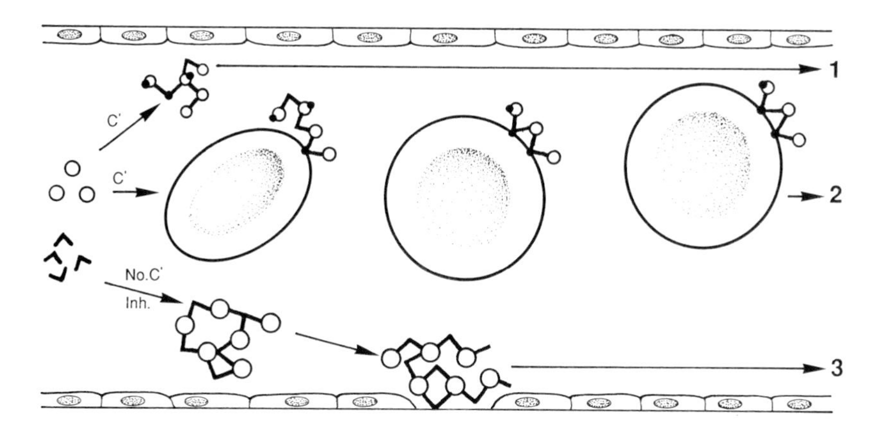

Fig. 6.9 Protection against development of immune-complex disease by complement. Antigen–antibody complexes formed in the microcirculation from antigen (o) and antibody (/\) will activate complement by the classical pathway. (1) If the antigen is small and soluble the complex remains small and soluble due to the deposition of C3b (•) on the antigen and antibody. Deposition of C3b on the antigen covers epitopes so that cross-linking cannot occur. C3b on the antibody prevents interactions between the Fc pieces of the antibodies which are involved in the rapid precipitation of complexes. Small soluble complexes circulate and are removed by the macrophages of the liver and spleen. (2) If the antigen is large and rather insoluble, the complexes remain relatively insoluble even after complement activation. Such complexes are potentially injurious. However, these complexes can be retained in the circulation by binding to C3b receptors (CR1) on erythrocytes and be transported to the macrophages of the liver and spleen for degradation. (3) When an individual has an inherited deficiency of a classical pathway complement component, has acquired hypocomplementaemia, if erythrocyte CR1 numbers are low, or if there is an inhibitor of complement activation in the blood, large insoluble lattices can form in the circulation and be deposited in the tissues to produce inflammation.

occurs in some patients with systemic lupus erythematosis (SLE). This reduces red cell capacity to transport complement reacted immune complexes.

(4) Failure of the macrophages of the liver and spleen to remove complexes from the circulation would theoretically be responsible for the production of immune complex disease. However, this only occurs following saturation of the mononuclear phagocyte system with a large immune complex load; it cannot be of aetiological significance.

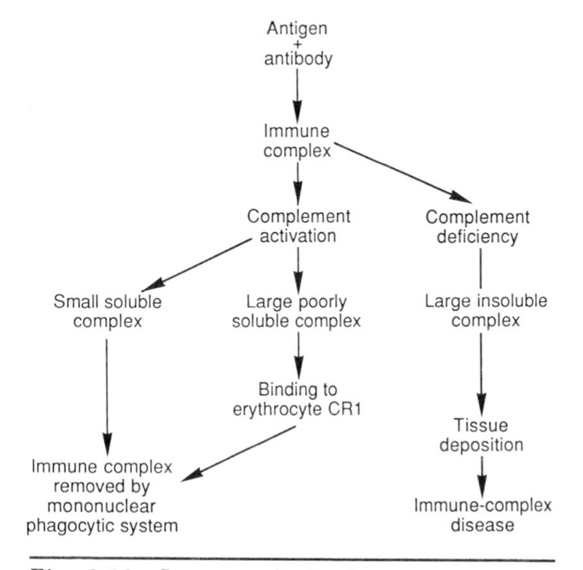

Fig. 6.10 Summary of role of complement in protection against immune-complex diseases.

Table 6.2 Antigens involved in type III hypersensitivity (immune-complex) diseases

Antigen		Clinical manifestations
Viruses	Hepatitis B	Polyarteritis nodosa Essential mixed cryoglobulinaemia
	Cytomegalovirus	Glomerulonephritis
	Dengue virus	Dengue haemorrhagic fever
Bacteria	β-Haemolytic streptococci	Post-streptococcal glomerulonephritis
	Strep, viridans	Bacterial endocarditis
	Staphylococcus	Shunt nephritis
	Mycobacterium leprae	Lepromatous leprosy
	Treponema pallidum	Jarisch–Herxheimer reaction
Parasites	*Plasmodium malariae*	Quartan malarial nephropathy
	Schistosoma mansoni	Schistosoma nephropathy
	Toxoplasma gondii	Toxoplasma nephropathy
Drugs	Gold, penicillamine	Membranous nephropathy
	Foreign serum	Serum sickness
	Monoclonal antibodies	
Autoantigens	DNA	SLE
	Renal tubular antigen	Membranous nephropathy
	IgG	Rheumatoid arthritis and cryoglobulinaemia
Tumour antigens		Tumour related nephropathy

Clinical Examples of Type III Hypersensitivity Reactions

Local Immune-complex Disease

The Arthus reaction in man was commonly seen when crude preparations of horse antitoxin globulin or whole antitoxin serum were administered for the prevention and treatment of diseases such as diphtheria or tetanus. The reaction occurred following the subcutaneous or intramuscular injection of antitoxin into immunized individuals.

Farmer's lung, a form of extrinsic allergic alveolitis, is a good example of the Arthus reaction. The farm worker inhales large numbers of spores of the bacterium *Micropolysporum faeni* which grows in mouldy hay. Soluble bacterial antigens are absorbed via the alveolar walls and stimulate antibody reproduction. Subsequent exposure to the organism induces an Arthus reaction in the alveolar walls. Many farm workers develop precipitating IgG class antibodies to *M. faeni* although few suffer farmer's lung on subsequent exposure. Present evidence suggests that IgE antibody may be necessary to cause farmer's lung and that the Arthus reaction is triggered by an initial type I hypersensitivity reaction which increases vascular permeability and allows IgG antibodies to escape through the vessel walls to come into contact with antigen. Extrinsic allergic alveolitis occurs in various occupations in which workers inhale dust containing proteins, fungi and other biological materials (p. 572).

Systemic Immune-complex Disease

Serum sickness due to the administration of crude antiserum or antilymphocyte globulin is now rare, but similar reactions can occur after the administration of drugs which confer antigenicity on plasma proteins.

With the exception of acute serum sickness and acute post-infectious glomerulonephritis, most circulating immune complex diseases in humans are chronic conditions.

Glomerulonephritis. Most forms of glomerulonephritis are due to the deposition of immune complexes in the glomerulus (Chapter 19). Acute glomerulonephritis following a throat infection develops when streptococcal antigen enters the blood and immune complexes are formed and deposited in the glomerular capillaries. Other infections, infestations, drug hypersensitivities and autoantigens which produce glomerulonephritis are listed in Table 6.2. However, in most types of human glomerulonephritis the nature of the antigen is unknown.

From experimental observations it is clear that the various patterns of glomerulonephritis depend on the size of the circulating complexes, the duration of and rate of their deposition. It is not clear why glomerular capillaries are unduly susceptible to deposition of circulating antigens and immune complexes. Part of the explanation may lie in the unusually high blood pressure within them, and their fenestrated endothelium.

Examples of 'planted' antigens which may result in immune complex formation within the glomerulus include DNA and endostreptosin, a protein of group A streptococci.

Other examples. Systemic lupus erythematosus is an example of a systemic immune complex disease while in rheumatoid arthritis it is thought the local formation of immune complexes within the joints plays a role in the pathogenesis of the inflammatory synovitis.

The focal lesions of polyarteritis nodosa (p. 464) and some other forms of arteritis may be the result of type III hypersensitivity reactions and immune complexes containing hepatitis B virus surface antigen have been implicated in a small proportion of cases. However, there is little evidence to support a pathogenetic role for immune complexes in most forms of vasculitis other than those which occur in systemic lupus erythematosus and rheumatoid arthritis.

The severe form of **dengue fever**, dengue haemorrhagic fever or dengue shock syndrome, occurs as a result of a second infection in a child who has already developed antibodies to the virus. The antibody resulting from the first infection cross-reacts with the second strain of virus but cannot neutralize it. Viral antigen–antibody complexes are therefore formed in the circulation with resulting shock, thrombocytopenia and mucosal haemorrhages.

Management of Type III Hypersensitivity Reactions

Avoidance or elimination of exogenous antigens will prevent the formation of immune complexes. If this is impossible, immunosuppression is used to reduce antibody production and therefore immune-complex formation. Plasma exchange may be used to remove circulating complexes and plasma mediators. Anti-inflammatory drugs (non-steroidal and corticosteroids) are used to reduce the degree of inflammation in the damaged tissues.

Type IV Hypersensitivity (Cell Mediated Immunity: Delayed-type Hypersensitivity)

Type IV hypersensitivity reactions are antigen-elicited cell mediated immune responses which produce tissue injury independently of the presence of antibody. Unlike the previous three types of hypersensitivity reactions, type IV reactions can only be transferred to a non-sensitized individual by using lymphocytes from a sensitized donor. The inflammatory lesion develops slowly, hence the term delayed-type hypersensitivity.

Mechanisms of Type IV Hypersensitivity

This has been described in detail in Chapter 5 (p. **000**), but a brief account will be given here. Antigen is processed and presented in the antigen presenting cleft of MHC class II molecules on antigen presenting cells. $CD4^+$ memory T cells recognize the processed antigen–MHC complex during their random circulation through the tissues. Contact between class II MHC-restricted $CD4^+$ memory T cells and their appropriate antigen complexed with class II MHC antigens leads to activation, clonal expansion and differentiation of the T cells. A number of cytokines are produced including interferon-γ, lymphotoxin (TNFβ) and macrophage chemotactic factors. The chemotactic factors attract macrophages to the site, interferon-γ activates them and stimulates the secretion of IL-1 and TNFα, enzymes and reactive oxygen metabolites. The cytotoxic effects of TNFα and TNFβ and the degradative effects of macrophage enzyme and oxygen metabolites produces extensive tissue necrosis at the site of delayed-type hypersensitivity reactions.

$CD8^+$ cytotoxic T cells are able to kill cells which present antigens in the antigen presenting cleft of class I MHC molecules. As these antigens are synthesized within the presenting cell, this mechanism is important in effecting the immune response to viruses. The mechanism of cytotoxicity is described on p. 196.

Morphological Features of Type IV Hypersensitivity

The best known example of a type IV reaction is the tuberculin reaction. This reaction forms the basis of the Mantoux and Heaf tests for tuberculosis. A small amount of soluble tuberculoprotein (purified protein derivative, PPD) is injected intradermally and, if the individual has developed cell mediated immunity to the tubercle bacillus as a result of infection or immunization with BCG (attenuated *Mycobacterium bovis*), an area of erythema and induration develops between 12 and 24 hours, peaks between 24 and 48 hours and then gradually recedes. In highly sensitized individuals, necrosis and ulceration may occur. Microscopically, the features at the site of a positive reaction comprise vascular congestion, accumulation of lymphocytes in and around small vessels, and swelling of collagen due to inflammatory oedema. At the height of the reaction there is intense perivascular infiltration with lymphocytes and occasional macrophages (Fig. 6.11).

Delayed-type hypersensitivity reactions in different diseases always contain lymphocytes, lymphoblasts and macrophages (which may transform to epithelioid cells or fuse to form giant cells) and may undergo necrosis. However, the histological appearances in different diseases vary considerably due to such factors as the direct injurious effects of bacterial toxins and to the presence of other hypersensitivity reactions.

Clinical Examples of Type IV Hypersensitivity Reactions

Cell mediated immune responses of the type IV variety are important in host defence against infection by intracellular organisms such as viruses, certain bacteria, fungi and protozoa. The destructive tissue lesions of tuberculosis, leprosy and syphilis are the result of cell mediated immune responses directed against the causal organisms. The skin rashes of smallpox, measles and herpes simplex (cold sore) are also due to cell mediated immune responses producing damage to virus infected cells. Delayed-type hypersensitivity is also important in allograft rejection, contact dermatitis against chemicals which bind to skin proteins or

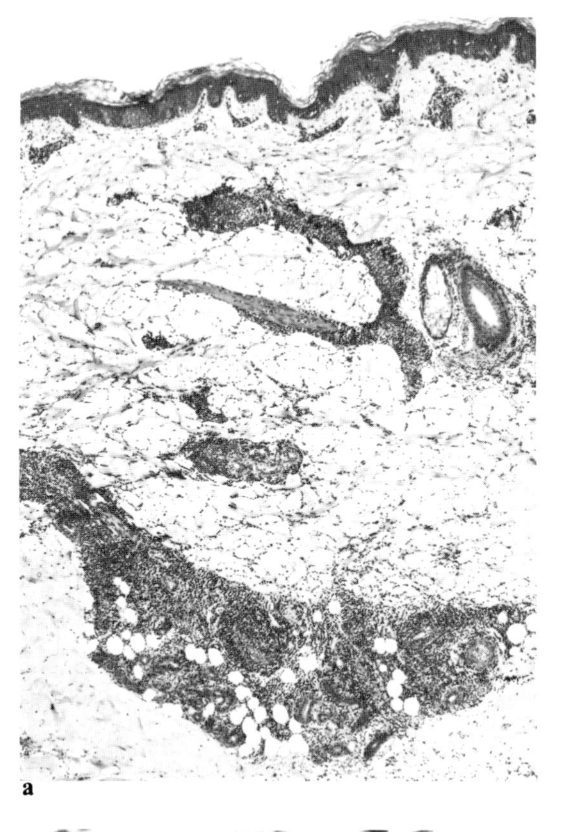
a

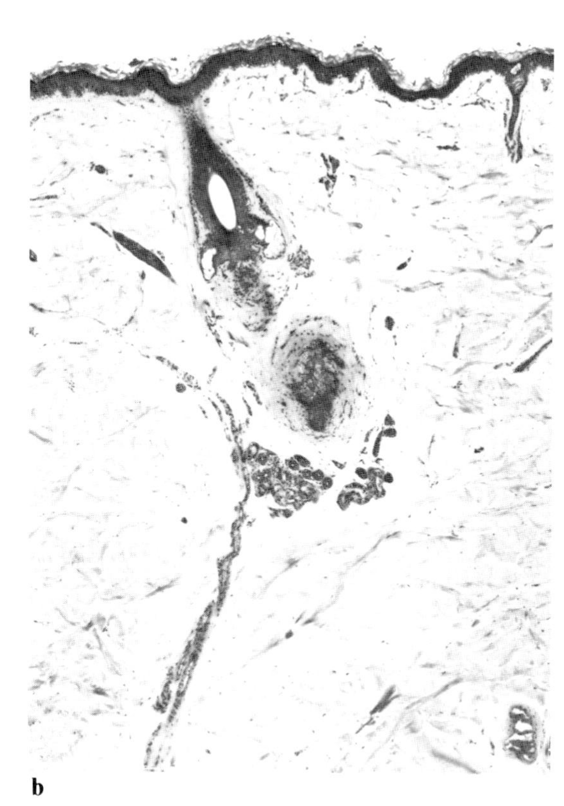
b

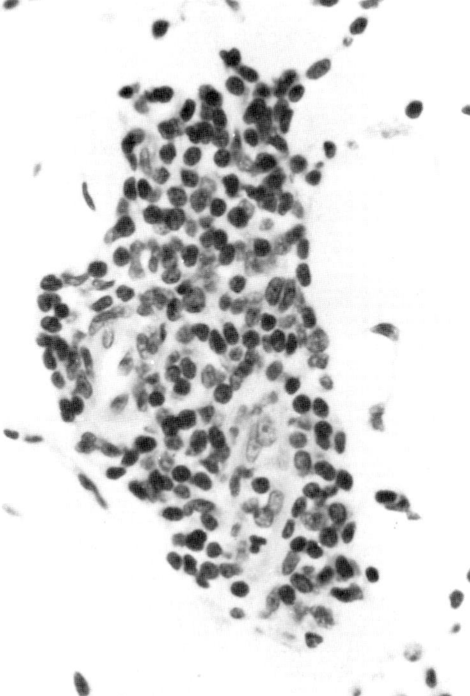
c

Fig. 6.11 Skin biopsies showing positive **a** and negative **b** Mantoux tests. Note the heavy cellular infiltrate around the sweat glands and pilosebaceous units in **a**. This distribution is determined by the vascularity of the skin appendages. ×40. At higher magnification **c**, the infiltrating cells are seen to be mostly lymphocytes, which are aggregated around the small blood vessels. ×470.

against chemically modified self-antigens, and in autoimmune disease (autoantigens).

Contact dermatitis, provides a classical model of type IV hypersensitivity occurring in patients exposed to a wide variety of agents. The agent binds to protein in the skin and forms a hapten–carrier complex. In the *induction phase*, the hapten–carrier protein complex is bound to the surface of epidermal Langerhans' cells, which then migrate to the dermis and regional lymph nodes. The antigen is presented to T cells in the lymph node or possibly in the dermis. T cells which are sensitized in the skin migrate to the paracortical areas of the draining lymph nodes and induce effector T cells. Usually induction to a skin sensitizer occurs over months or years of repeated exposure to small amounts of antigen, although it may occur within 7–10 days of the initial exposure. Re-exposure to the relevant antigen triggers the *elicitation phase* in which the effector T cells meet the antigen in the skin and set up a delayed-type hypersensitivity reaction.

The precise identification of the causal hapten depends upon a careful history and the use of patch tests in which the sensitizer is applied to the skin of the upper back, and covered for 48 hours. Positive reactions appear as areas of redness and induration at the test site and occur within 2–4 days of exposure (Fig. 6.12).

a

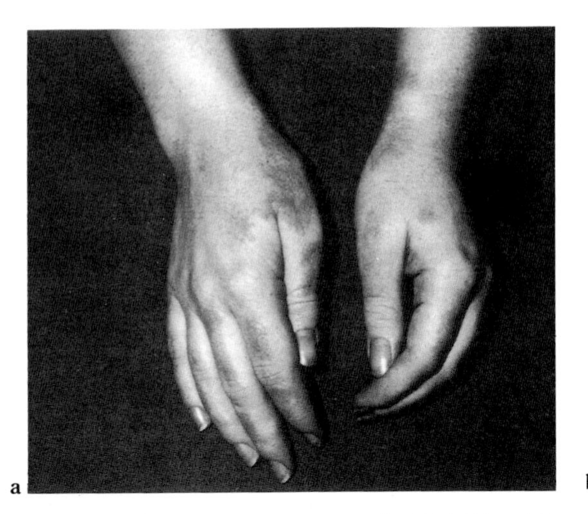

b

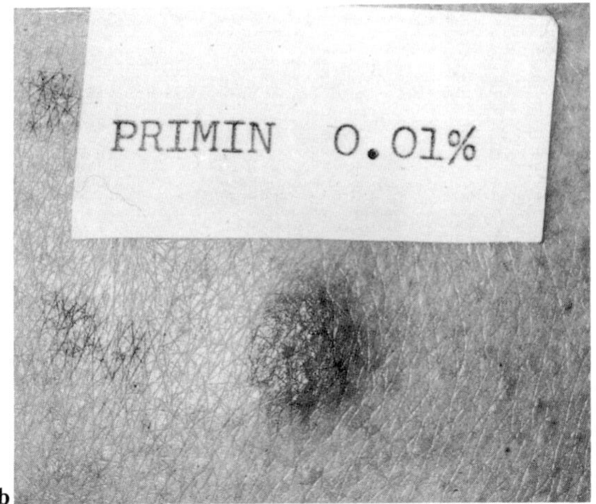

c

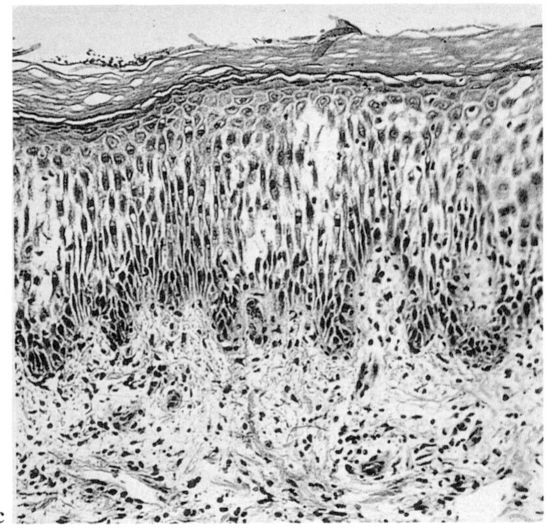

Fig. 6.12 **a** Primula dermatitis. **b** A positive patch test for contact hypersensitivity to primula. A patch containing Primin, the antigenic component of *Primula obconica*, was held in contact with the skin for 48 hours. A positive result is shown by erythema and induration, sometimes with vesiculation. **c** Contact dermatitis. Note oedema of epidermis and perivascular infiltration of lymphocytes in the dermis. The patient had developed hypersensitivity to chromium salts used as a hardener in cement. ×110.

Management of Type IV Hypersensitivity Reactions

Where possible, avoidance of environmental antigens (e.g. in contact dermatitis) or the elimination of infectious organisms by antibiotics or antifungal medication prevents the disease. Immunosuppressive drugs such as azathioprine and cyclosporin A which suppress cell mediated immune response are used in organ transplant recipients, and recently elimination of T lymphoblasts by specific monoclonal antibodies has been used with some success.

Tissue Transplantation

The replacement of diseased organs by healthy ones from another individual has been a major medical objective for many years. Autologous (from the same patient) skin grafts have been used successfully to treat burns. The epidermis of the graft extends to cover the denuded area and survives indefinitely. In contrast, allogeneic grafts (from another individual) become established but undergo necrosis within 2–3 weeks, a process called graft rejection.

Allograft Rejection

This is mediated by the host's immune response to the 'foreign' HLA antigens of the graft. Cell mediated and humoral immunity are both involved (Fig. 6.13), although their relative importance varies in different individuals. Vascular endothelium expresses both class I and class II MHC antigens and is the major target of the rejection response. However, increased expression of class I antigens and facultative expression of class II antigens on the parenchymal cells of the grafted organ may also result in tissue injury.

Cell Mediated Immunity

The importance of T cells in graft rejection is well documented. Donor HLA antigens may be presented in the graft or following transport to the regional lymph nodes. The most potent immunogens are 'passenger leucocytes' (donor lymphoid cells) transferred in the grafted organ, in particular dendritic cells rich in class I and II MHC antigens.

The recipient's $CD4^+$ T cells are stimulated by donor MHC class II antigens and $CD8^+$ T cells mature into cytotoxic T cells in response to donor class I antigens (Fig. 6.13). Secretion of IL-1 by antigen presenting cells is required to trigger $CD4^+$ T cells to proliferate and synthesize IL-2, IFN-γ and other cytokines (p. 198). Vascular permeability is increased and lymphocytes and macrophages accumulate in the graft. $CD8^+$ cytotoxic T cells damage class I bearing cells in the graft. Increased expression of cellular adhesion molecules (CAMs; p. 15 and p. 196) on the endothelial and parenchymal cells of the transplanted organ in response to IL-1 and TNFα, facilitates the interaction between recipient T cells and donor cells and therefore promotes the rejection process.

Antibody Mediated Immunity

Antibodies to donor class I or class II antigens are produced by recipients of allogeneic grafts. These antibodies react with MHC antigens, particularly on the endothelial cells and produce complement-dependent and antibody-dependent cell mediated

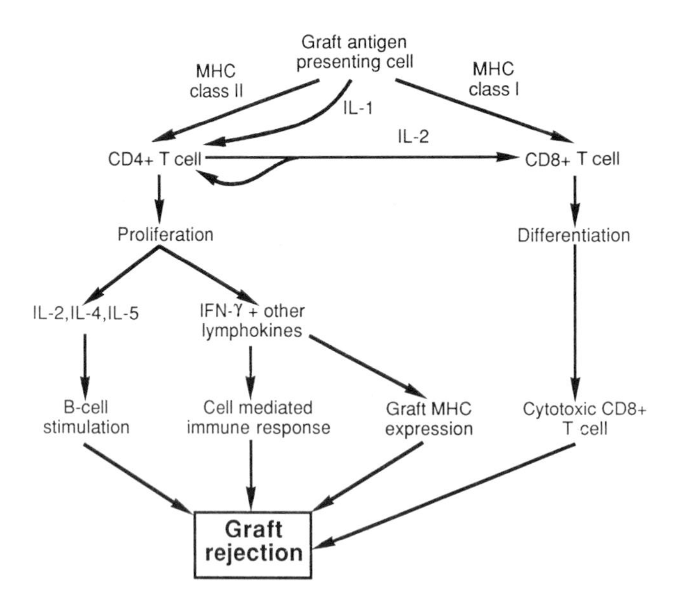

Fig. 6.13 Pathogenesis of allograft rejection. Antigen presenting cells in the graft present antigen to CD4+ T cells (MHC class II restriction) and CD8+ T cells (MHC class I restriction). The CD4+ T cells proliferate and differentiate and secrete cytokines which: (1) stimulate proliferation and differentiation of antigen specific B-cell clones to produce an antibody against transplantation antigens, (2) mount a cell mediated immune response against the graft and (3) increase MHC antigen expression by cells of the graft which promotes the rejection process. CD8+ T cells differentiate into cytotoxic T cells.

cytolysis. This rejection vasculitis is also in part due to activation of the coagulation, fibrinolytic and kinin systems along with platelet, neutrophil and NK cell activation. In addition, HLA antigens released into the blood may complex with antibodies and produce a type III hypersensitivity reaction.

Some transplant recipients who have previously been sensitized to donor HLA antigens because of blood transfusion, pregnancy, or infection with bacteria or viruses with HLA cross-reacting surface antigens, develop graft rejection within minutes of grafting. This hyperacute rejection is now extremely rare due to pretransplant screening for cytotoxic antibodies.

As a rule, the greater the genetic disparity between donor and recipient MHC antigens, the stronger and more rapid will be the rejection reaction. However, there is evidence that weaker transplant (non-MHC) alloantigens may influence the outcome. The best results of grafting are obtained when the donor is an HLA-identical sibling. In this regard it is worth re-emphasizing that MHC genes are inherited as extended haplotypes so that there is a 1:4 chance that an identical sibling will be found, assuming that both parents are heterozygous and neither shares a haplotype with the other. Although the introduction of cyclosporin A as an immunosuppressive drug has greatly improved the survival of mismatched tissue transplants, most authorities accept that HLA matching is still important, particularly at the DR and B loci. It is, of course, essential to ensure ABO blood group compatibility between donor and recipient.

The indications for kidney, liver, heart and lung transplantation are discussed in the appropriate chapters elsewhere in the book, together with the morphological factors which characterize rejection of these allografts.

Immunosuppressive Therapy

For many years azathioprine and prednisolone were the mainstay of immunosuppressive therapy. Neither acts specifically on cells involved in the rejection process and azathioprine acts on dividing cells. Thus, both drugs produced generalized immunosuppression with the result that infections with virulent pathogens and opportunistic micro-organisms such as cytomegalovirus, *Pneumocystis carinii* and various fungi were common. The introduction of cyclosporin A in the mid-1980s altered the picture dramatically. This fungal peptide prevents antigen-sensitive T cells in the G_0 from entering the G_1 phase and blocks transcription of lymphokine mRNA. Cyclosporin A does not appear to affect dividing cells of the bone marrow or gastrointestinal tract. In addition to T cells, cyclosporin appears to act on the antigen presenting dendritic cells and may stimulate development of specific T-suppressor cells. Fujimycin (FK 506), another fungal peptide which has been shown to be 100–1000 times more potent than cyclosporin A in experimental animals, is now being evaluated clinically.

Pretransplant blood transfusion has been shown to have a beneficial effect on the outcome of kidney transplantation. The mechanisms underlying this immunosuppressive effect are unclear, but may involve (1) the induction of antibodies to class I and class II MHC antigens or anti-idiotype antibodies which block recognition of graft cells by host T cells; or (2) the production of suppressor factors, some of which may be antigen specific.

Mouse or rat monoclonal antibodies which act on T-cell antigens, including CD3 (p. 195), the IL-2 receptor, and CD52 have been used with some success in small numbers of patients. One of the major problems with this approach is that the recipient produces antibodies to the monoclonal antibodies, reducing their efficacy and with a risk of precipitating immune-complex disease. Attempts to produce 'humanized' monoclonal antibodies (mouse variable regions and human constant regions) by genetic engineering are being undertaken. Perfusion of the allograft with monoclonal antibodies to the leucocyte common antigen (CD45) has been used, in an attempt to deplete the graft of antigen presenting dendritic cells.

Bone Marrow Transplantation

The indications for bone marrow transplanatation are discussed in Chapter 14. They include aplastic anaemia and adults with acute leukaemia. Children with leukaemia usually respond well to chemotherapy so that only a small proportion require bone marrow transplants. In adults with haemopoietic malignancies, bone marrow transplantation is usually used to treat those between 15 and 40 years of age, as older individuals are more prone to the development of graft-versus-host disease. In most cases bone marrow transplantation must be preceded by lethal irradiation of the recipient's bone marrow to destroy leukaemic cells or to create a graft bed in aplastic anaemia. Successful bone marrow transfer requires a high degree of HLA compatibility in order to avoid fatal graft-versus-host disease which may occur even with complete HLA matching.

Graft-versus-host (GVH) Disease

When lymphoid cells are injected into an allogeneic host, they are destroyed unless the host is immunologically deficient or tolerant and cannot mount a rejection reaction. In such a situation, the grafted cells may survive and mount an immune response against the host, producing a GVH reaction. This is a recognized hazard of allogeneic bone marrow transplant. GVH reactions can also occur in an immunosuppressed individual given T cells in a blood transfusion or a solid organ transplant.

Graft-versus-host disease presents in acute and chronic forms, the former occurring within 3 months and in up to 70% of bone marrow recipients. Mature T cells in the donor marrow respond to the host's HLA antigens and mount a cell mediated reaction to host cells. The major features of acute GVH are exfoliative dermatitis, diarrhoea and intestinal malabsorption, and cholestatic liver disease. Other features include fever, weight loss, anaemia and thrombocytopenia. Many of these effects are exacerbated by secondary infections which occur as a result of immunodeficiency brought about by the GVH reaction. Severe GVH disease is rapidly fatal. Treatment of the donor marrow to remove T cells reduces the risk of GVH disease but is associated with a higher incidence of recurrence of leukaemia. Treatment of recipients with cyclosporin A reduces the risk of GVH disease and methotrexate and corticosteroids are used to treat the established disease.

Chronic GVH disease occurs in up to 45% of individuals who have received a bone marrow transplant 3–15 months previously. The clinical features resemble those seen in the connective tissue diseases particularly Sjögren's syndrome and progressive systemic sclerosis. The role of HLA incompatibility is unclear, and the effects of treatment with immunosuppressive drugs and corticosteroids are unpredictable.

The Fetus as an Allograft

The fetus inherits MHC genes from both parents and this expresses paternal and maternal HLA antigens. The trophoblast, of fetal origin, is bathed in maternal blood and yet it is tolerated for 9 months. There is no depression of maternal immune responsiveness during pregnancy and specific immunological tolerance to the fetal alloantigens cannot be demonstrated. Indeed, a proportion of mothers develop an immune response to paternal antigens as shown by the presence of anti-HLA antibodies and cytotoxic lymphocytes. The factors preventing rejection of the fetus are unclear but may include: (1) the absence of class I and class II antigen expression by trophoblast, protecting the fetus from allogeneic attack; and (2) coating of the trophoblast by mucopolysaccharide which provides an 'immunological barrier'.

Autoimmune Diseases

A state of autoimmunity exists when an immune response has been generated against 'self' antigens (autoantigens), and an autoimmune disease is one in which this autoimmune response plays a pathogenetic role. Although a growing number of diseases has been classified as autoimmune, quite often the evidence is circumstantial, being based on the detection of autoantibodies in the serum. Autoantibodies are often found in apparently normal individuals, particularly the elderly, and may appear following certain types of tissue injury (e.g. autoantibodies to myocardium following myocardial infarction). It has been suggested that these autoantibodies help in the elimination of the products released from damaged tissues. Furthermore, during a normal immune response, the hypervariable region of antibodies stimulates an immune response and anti-idiotypic antibodies are produced. These autoantibodies may be important in the regulation of the immune response. Thus, the presence of circulating autoantibodies does not necessarily indicate the presence of autoimmune disease. In order to state with confidence that a disease is autoimmune one must be able to show that the autoimmune response is not secondary to tissue injury but has primary pathogenetic significance and that no other cause for the tissue injury exists.

Autoimmune diseases are classified into those affecting a single organ or tissue, the organ-specific autoimmune diseases, and those affecting many organs and tissues, the non-organ-specific group (Table 6.3).

Table 6.3 Classification of autoimmune diseases

Organ-specific	Intermediate	Non-organ-specific
Hashimoto's thyroiditis	Goodpasture's syndrome	Systemic lupus erythematosus
Primary myxoedema	Autoimmune haemolytic disease	Rheumatoid arthritis
Thyrotoxicosis	Autoimmune leucopenia	Dermatomyositis/polymyositis
Chronic atrophic gastritis	Idiopathic thrombocytopenia	Progressive systemic sclerosis
Pernicious anaemia	Pemphigus vulgaris	
Addison's disease	Pemphigoid	
Premature ovarian failure	Sympathetic ophthalmia	
Male infertility	Primary biliary cirrhosis	
Myasthenia gravis	Chronic active hepatitis	
Juvenile diabetes mellitus	Ulcerative colitis	
	Sjögren's syndrome	

Autoimmune diseases are traditionally divided into those which affect single organs or tissues (organ-specific) and those which affect many organs and tissues (non-organ-specific). However, these groups lie at opposite ends of the spectrum of autoimmune disease and in between there is an intermediate group which show features of both organ-specific and non-organ-specific autoimmune diseases.

Organ-specific Autoimmune Diseases

The organ-specific autoimmune diseases are characterized by chronic inflammatory cell destruction of a particular organ accompanied by the presence of autoantibodies which react specifically with normal cellular components of the target tissue (Table 6.4). The pathological features of the individual organ-specific autoimmune diseases are discussed in the appropriate systemic chapters. The pathogenetic processes involved are thought to involve type II and type IV hypersensitivity reactions.

The antigens involved are usually located on the plasma membranes of target cells (Table 6.4), except for Goodpasture's syndrome and pernicious anaemia. In the former the antigen is in the glomerular capillary basement membrane (Chapter 19). In pernicious anaemia the situation is a complex one. There is a megaloblastic anaemia (p. 615) due to the malabsorption of vitamin B_{12}. There is an associated gastric atrophy and antibodies to an antigen of the secretory canaliculi of the gastric parietal cells and to the gastrin receptor are present. The antibodies are responsible for the gastric atrophy, preventing the turnover of parietal cells by inhibiting their proliferation and maturation. Injury to the gastric mucosa is also produced by a type IV hypersensitivity reaction. In addition to immune injury to the gastric mucosa, antibodies to intrinsic factor are present in the circulation and the intestinal secretions. Both inhibit the absorption of vitamin B_{12}. One type of antibody binds to intrinsic factor, and prevents the formation of a vitamin B_{12}–intrinsic factor complex. The other binds to the vitamin B_{12}–intrinsic factor complex and prevents its absorption by the mucosal cells of the ileum.

Non-organ-specific Autoimmune Diseases

The non-organ-specific autoimmune diseases, often called the connective tissue diseases, are

Table 6.4 Organ-specific autoimmune diseases

	Disease	Autoantibodies to	Disease Mechanisms
Thyroid	Hashimoto's thyroiditis (HT)	Thyroglobulin Thyroid microsomes	Chronic inflammation of thyroid
	Graves' disease	As for HT. TSH receptor antibodies which have TSH action	Increased thyroid hormone production, hyperthyroidism. Some antibodies stimulate growth of thyroid
	Primary myxoedema	As for HT. TSH receptor antibodies which block TSH action	Block action of TSH on receptor, reduce growth stimulus. Reduced thyroid hormone production and thyroid atrophy
	Simple goitre	TSH receptor antibodies which stimulate growth	Enlargement of thyroid
Stomach	Chronic atrophic gastritis leading to pernicious anaemia	Gastric parietal cells microsomes surface	Chronic inflammation of gastric mucosa causes achlorhydria. Block action of gastrin to prevent proliferation and maturation of parietal cells – atrophy
		Intrinsic factor	Blocks interaction with vitamin B_{12}
		Intrinsic factor/B_{12} complex	Prevents absorption of intrinsic factor/B_{12} complex
Adrenal cortex	Addison's disease (idiopathic)	Adrenal cell microsomes	Chronic inflammation of adrenal cortex causes atrophy. Underproduction of glucocorticoids/ mineralocorticoids
		ACTH receptor	Inhibits binding of ACTH to receptor
Pancreatic islet cells	Diabetes mellitus (type I)	Antibodies to B cells	Chronic inflammation of islets – reduced insulin production
Skeletal muscle	Myasthenia gravis	Acetylcholine receptor	Reduce number of acetylcholine receptors by complement activation
		Cross-reactive antibodies to thymic epithelium and skeletal muscle	

Other organ-specific autoimmune diseases include premature ovarian failure (autoantibodies to steroid hormone producing cells), primary hypoparathyroidism (autoantibodies to cells of parathyroid gland), some cases of male infertility (antibodies to spermatozoa).

characterized by acute and chronic inflammatory lesions in many organs and by the presence of circulating autoantibodies, most of which react with normal constituents common to most cell types (Table 6.5).

Systemic Lupus Erythematosus

Systemic lupus erythematosus (SLE) is the classical example of a non-organ-specific autoimmune disease. It has a prevalence rate of 1:2 000 in the United States, affects females more commonly than males (9:1) and has a peak age of onset in the third decade. The aetiology of SLE is unknown, but both genetic and environmental factors have been implicated. The disease is HLA-associated, with HLA-A1, B5, B7, B8, DR2 and DR3 being most consistently associated. In addition, homozygous deficiency of the classical pathway complement components, especially C2 and C4, are frequently associated with SLE. Environmental factors which predispose to the development of SLE include drugs (drug-induced lupus – p. 417) and sex hormones. The importance of hormones is illustrated by the female preponderance, and the frequent disease exacerbations which occur in pregnancy and the puerperium.

Clinical Features

Arthralgia (joint pain) or non-erosive arthritis occur in almost all patients. Aseptic bone necrosis is uncommon and usually related to corticosteroid therapy. Myalgia (muscle pain) is common, but true myositis occurs in 5% of patients.

The skin is a commonly involved organ (p. 1121) with the classical malar rash occurring in 30–40% of patients. Other skin lesions include chronic discoid lupus, subacute cutaneous LE, alopecia and vascular lesions. Respiratory tract involvement may be manifest as pleurisy, with or without effusion, acute pneumonitis or diffuse interstitial pulmonary fibrosis. Cardiac involvement is frequent, with pericarditis with or without effusion, myocarditis, and Libman–Sacks endocarditis (p. 515). Inflammation of small blood vessels (vasculitis) (p. 464) is common and is often associated with peripheral neuropathy (p. 863). Central nervous system manifestations include a spectrum of psychiatric and neurological disorders, including dementia, depression, convulsions, migraine and strokes.

Glomerulonephritis is a common manifestation. The histological appearances are extremely variable. The mildest form reveals the presence of mesangial immune complexes. Other appearances include membranous, focal proliferative, diffuse proliferative and mesangiocapillary glomerulonephritis (p. 909). Recurrent venous and arterial thrombosis, thrombocytopenia and recurrent abortions are associated with the presence of the lupus anticoagulant. This is an antibody to the factor X clotting complex and is also often associated with anticardiolipin antibodies and false positive serological tests for syphilis. The clinical features associated with anticardiolipin antibodies and the lupus anticoagulant, the so-called anticardiolipin syndrome, may occur in the absence of other clinical features of SLE.

Haematological complications include haemolytic anaemia, leucopenia and thrombocytopenia.

Mechanism of Tissue Injury

Although antibodies to erythrocytes, leucocytes and platelets may be responsible for haemolytic anaemia, leucopenia and thrombocytopenia respectively, those which react with nuclear or cytoplasmic constituents are not cytotoxic. However, autoantigens released following cell death may interact with their respective autoantibodies and produce type III hypersensitivity reactions, which are characteristic of SLE. Native DNA–anti-DNA complexes are present in the renal and skin lesions of SLE. Anticardiolipin antibodies interact with platelet and endothelial cell membrane lipids to alter production of thromboxane A_2 and prostacyclin respectively (p. 142) and cause recurrent thrombosis.

Rheumatoid Arthritis

Rheumatoid arthritis (RA) is a chronic symmetrical inflammatory polyarthritis. The prevalence is remarkably uniform throughout the world, affecting 1–2% of the adult population. The peak onset is between the ages of 25 and 55 years, and females are affected more commonly than males. Apart from arthritis which is discussed on p. 988, extra-articular complications occur and the term rheumatoid disease has been applied to RA with extra-articular manifestations.

The rheumatoid nodule (p. 991) is the most common extra-articular feature occurring most commonly in the skin but also affecting other tissue, particularly in the eye (episcleritis p. 883) and the lung. Other complications include pericarditis, pleurisy, pleural effusion, fibrosing alveolitis and Caplan's syndrome (p. 572). Vasculitis is usually associated with skin ulceration and peripheral neuropathy but may affect any organ. Spinal cord compression due to subluxation of the atlanto-axial joint or sub-axial subluxation may be fatal. Lymphadenopathy and splenomegaly are due to reactive follicular hyperplasia (p. 648).

The main pathological feature in the joints is a chronic destructive inflammatory polyarthritis. Immune complexes are present in the synovial fluid, the synovial membrane and possibly the articular cartilage, and complement activation products have been detected in the synovial fluid.

The serum of most patients with rheumatoid arthritis contains rheumatoid factors which are autoantibodies directed against determinants on the Fc piece of IgG. These autoantibodies are usually of IgM class although IgG and IgA rheumatoid factors may also occur. The affinity of rheumatoid factors for IgG is low so that strong binding is only seen when multivalent IgG attachment is possible (Fig. 6.14). This occurs when IgG

Table 6.5 Autoantibodies commonly used in the diagnosis of non-organ-specific autoimmune diseases (connective tissue diseases)

	Rheumatoid factor	Antinuclear* antibody	Native DNA	Histone	Anti-Sr
Systemic lupus erythematosus (SLE)	20–30%	>95% H + S + M	40–60%	70%	20–30
Drug-induced LE	<25%	>95% H	–	>95%	–
Progressive systemic sclerosis	25–40%	70–90% S + N	–	–	–
CREST syndrome	25–30%	70–90% S + N	–	–	–
Polymyositis	30%	40–60% H + S	–	–	–
Mixed connective tissue disease	50%	>95% S	–	–	–
Sjögren's syndrome	80%	50–80% S + N	–	–	–

*Antinuclear antibody determined by immunofluorescence using frozen sections of rat or mouse liver as substrate. The patte
fluorescence are homogeneous (H) due to antibody to DNA–histone complex; nucleolar (N) due to antibody to nucleolar ribonucleopr
speckled (S) due to antibody to saline extractable antigens, membranous (M), also known as rim or shaggy, due to antibody to D

is aggregated by binding to antigen in an immune complex which could occur as a result of antibodies reacting with a specific infectious agent; however, none has yet been isolated.

IgG rheumatoid factors react with the Fc piece of adjacent IgG molecules so that a lattice of self-associating IgG rheumatoid factors is formed (Fig. 6.14). Such complexes are capable of inducing complement activation and inflammation. Thus, it appears that an intrasynovial type III hypersensitivity (Arthus reaction) may be responsible for the inflammatory process, although a type IV hypersensitivity reaction against synovial lining cells is also thought to be important.

Systemic Sclerosis

Systemic sclerosis is a disease of unknown aetiology characterized by excessive production of collagen in involved tissues. The term scleroderma is often used, as the most striking feature is induration and thickening of the skin. However, scleroderma is misleading as it includes a localized form of skin disease, scleroderma morphoea (p. 1122) and fails to take into account the multi-organ involvement which occurs in systemic sclerosis). Systemic sclerosis is further subdivided into the **CREST syndrome** in which cutaneous involvement is associated with visceral disease (**c**alcinosis, **R**aynaud's phenomenon, o**e**sophageal involvement, **s**clerodactyly, **t**elangiectasia), and **progressive systemic sclerosis** with extensive visceral involvement. Oesophageal and small intestinal involvement may result in dysphagia and malabsorption. Diffuse interstitial pulmonary fibrosis may lead to respiratory failure. Renal failure and hypertension are responsible for 50% of deaths. The predominant finding in the kidneys is narrowing of the interlobular arteries due to concentric intimal proliferation. Hypertension occurs

ti-RNP†	Anti-Ro†	Anti-La†	Scl 70†	Anticentromere	Jo-1†	Anticardiolipin antibody
40%	30–40%	15%	–	–	–	30%
–	–	–	–	–	–	–
15%	–	–	40–70%	<10%	–	–
10%	–	–	10%	90%	–	–
–	10%	–	–	–	25%	–
>95%	–	–	–	–	–	+
–	70–95%	60–90%	–	–	–	–

RNP, Ro, La, Scl 70 and Jo-1 are known as extractable nuclear antigens as they are extremely soluble in isotonic saline. They are all ıcleoproteins. Scl 70 is DNA topoisomerase 1, Jo-1 is histidyl-tRNA synthesase. Centromeric proteins are detected by anti-omere antibody.

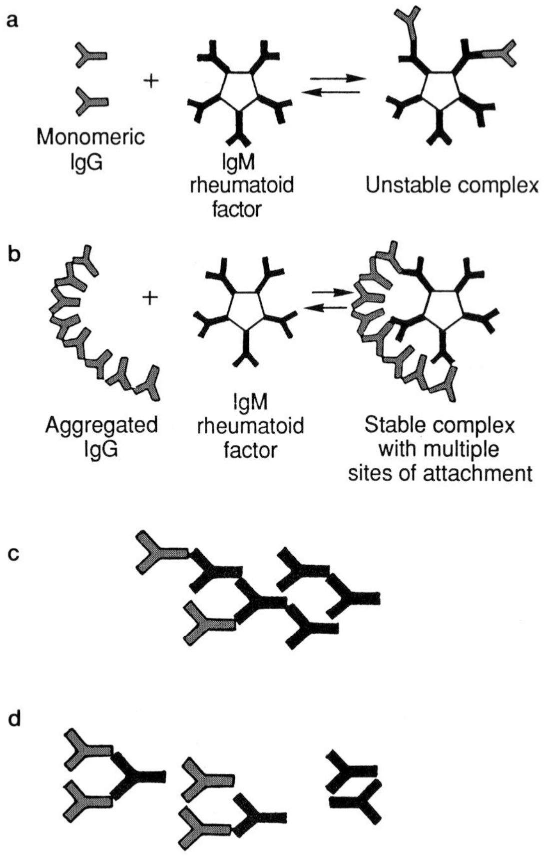

Fig. 6.14 Interactions of IgM rheumatoid factor with IgG. **a** The affinity of IgM rheumatoid factor for the Fc region of IgG is low so that it does not form stable complexes with circulating monomeric IgG. **b** However, if IgG is aggregated in the form of an antigen–antibody complex a single IgM rheumatoid factor molecule can bind to multiple IgG molecules. This produces a high affinity interaction so that stable complexes are formed. **c** and **d** Different ways in which molecules of IgG rheumatoid factor can associate with non-rheumatoid factor monomeric IgG or self-associate to form large complexes which are thought to play a major role in the pathogenesis of many of the extra-articular complications of rheumatoid arthritis, particularly the vasculitis.

in 30% of patients and in 25% of these it is malignant. In malignant hypertension fibrinoid necrosis of the arterioles occurs with thrombosis and infarction.

Polymyositis/ Dermatomyositis

This disease is characterized by inflammation of muscles, particularly proximal groups with pain, weakness and tenderness. Associated skin involvement occurs in 50–60% of cases (dermatomyositis) and is usually in the form of a photosensitive facial rash. A non-erosive arthritis occurs in 40% of patients. Other features include myocarditis, respiratory muscle weakness, and diffuse intestinal pulmonary fibrosis. Jo-1, an antibody to histidyl-tRNA synthetase, is present in the sera of 25% of patients, particularly those with coexistent diffuse interstitial pulmonary fibrosis. Antibodies to other tRNA synthetases occur, but far less frequently.

Mixed Connective Tissue Disease

Sometimes patients present with clinical features of more than one connective tissue disease, and a diagnosis of overlap syndrome or mixed connective tissue disease (MCTD) is then made. The clinical features usually include scleroderma-like features and myositis. The prognosis is better than in SLE because renal and cerebral involvement are uncommon. The major laboratory finding of note is high titre antibody to ribonucleoprotein, an extractable nuclear antigen.

Vasculitis

The term vasculitis indicates inflammation of any blood vessel (arteries, arterioles, capillaries, venules, veins), but it usually refers to arteritis or arteriolitis. Although vascular inflammation occurs in infectious diseases as a result of embolization, septicaemia or direct invasion, it is a frequent accompaniment of other connective tissue diseases. In addition there is a group of diseases in which vasculitis is the primary feature. There is no universally accepted classification of vasculitis but the most widely accepted is based on the size and type of vessel involved (p. 465). Vasculitis may affect any tissue of the body and involvement of individual tissues is discussed in the appropriate systemic chapter.

The best example is **polyarteritis nodosa**, an acute inflammatory disease which predominantly affects medium-sized arteries. Males are affected more commonly than females. The clinical features include muscle pains and tenderness, peripheral neuropathy, renal disease, hypertension, heart failure, pericarditis, myocardial infarction, asthma and pulmonary infiltrates, skin lesions and arthritis. Immune complexes containing the surface antigen of hepatitis B virus have been detected in the lesions of a small number of patients. Other viruses implicated include cytomegalovirus, hepatitis A, HTLV-1, HTLV-3, parvovirus and herpes zoster. However, it should be noted that in the vast majority of patients with polyarteritis nodosa and other vasculitic diseases, other than those complicating SLE and rheumatoid arthritis, there is little or no evidence to support a pathogenetic role for immune complexes.

Antineutrophil cytoplasmic antibodies (ANCAs) are found in a high proportion of the sera of patients with Wegener's granulomatosis (p. 468) and microscopic polyarteritis (p. 466) and are of major diagnostic significance. The antigens recognized by these antibodies appear to be myeloperoxidase and a serine protease.

Aetiology of Autoimmune Disease

Genetics

Individual organ-specific autoimmune diseases have a high familial incidence and there is a strong tendency for members of affected families and individuals to develop more than one such disorder. Thus, patients with Hashimoto's thyroiditis have a high incidence of gastric antibodies and may develop pernicious anaemia, while both thyroid and gastric antibodies are unduly prevalent in patients with autoimmune Addison's disease or primary hypoparathyroidism. Likewise, there is familial clustering of the connective tissue diseases, SLE, rheumatoid arthritis and Sjögren's syndrome (p. 681).

Although familial clustering could be due to a shared environmental factor such as an infective micro-organism, there is considerable evidence that the predisposition to autoimmune disease is inherited. The concordance of thyrotoxicosis is higher in monozygotic than in dizygotic twins. In most autoimmune diseases the genetic predisposition is defined by expression of particular HLA antigens, particularly those encoded by the genes of the class II region (p. 176). There is accumulating evidence for specific point mutations in DP, DQ and DR antigens in certain diseases which encode amino acids in the antigen presenting cleft. A good example is diabetes mellitus; over 90% of patients with type I (p. 799) are homozygous for a mutation in the antigen binding cleft of the DQβ gene, which results in the presence of an amino acid other than aspartate at position 57 of the DQβ polypeptide chain. Such mutations could trigger an autoimmune response by permitting the presentation of self-antigens to T cells. However, autoimmune diseases are not inherited in a Mendelian manner and so environmental factors must also be involved in their aetiology.

Autoimmune Responses

Facultative MHC Expression

The injection of tissue extracts alone does not provoke autoimmunity in animals. For an autoimmune response to occur the autoantigen must be processed and presented to an antigen-sensitive cell. In most organ-specific autoimmune diseases such as thyroiditis, Sjögren's syndrome, primary biliary cirrhosis and juvenile diabetes mellitus, HLA class II molecules are expressed aberrantly on the target cells. Such facultative expression, which occurs in response to cytokines such as IFN-γ, could assist in the presentation of cell surface autoantigens, although this probably occurs secondarily to the disease process.

The development of autoimmune responses usually involves the participation of both B and T cells. Most autoreactive lymphocytes (especially T cells) are deleted during ontogeny (p. 201), but lymphocytes of normal individuals have been shown to include B cells capable of binding and responding to particular autoantigens, e.g. thyroglobulin or DNA. Self-tolerance is thought to be maintained by the absence of self-reactive T_H cells or to the presence of antigen-specific T_S cells.

Autoimmunity could result from: (1) failure of certain MHC antigens to permit deletion of certain autoreactive T cells during ontogeny; (2) mechanisms which result in the bypass of T-cell tolerance; (3) disturbance of the balance between T_S and T_H cells; (4) facultative MHC expression (see above); (5) release of sequestered antigens.

Bypass of T-cell Tolerance

A number of mechanisms could result in the breakdown of T-cell tolerance.

Antigenic Modification

In most autoimmune diseases there is no evidence that antigens from affected tissues differ from those found in normal individuals. Nevertheless, autoimmunity can result from modification of an autoantigen by a drug. For example, the antihypertensive agent α-methyldopa stimulates a T_H-cell response which facilitates B cells to recognize the rhesus e antigen on the erythrocyte cell membrane as a hapten. The production of antibodies to the modified antigen produces a haemolytic anaemia. Likewise patients treated with hydralazine, isoniazid or procainamide tend to develop antibodies to nuclear constituents and may develop some of the features of rheumatoid arthritis or SLE, which disappear on withdrawal of the drug.

Partial proteolysis of autoantigens such as collagen, thyroglobulin and IgG exposes neoepitopes which increases their immunogenicity. Proteolysis by leucocyte enzymes could account for antibodies to collagen and IgG which are seen in many chronic inflammatory diseases such as rheumatoid arthritis.

Cross-reacting Antigens

Environmental antigens may stimulate autoimmunity because they resemble normal tissue constituents (molecular mimicry) and so induce the development of T cells and antibodies which cross-react with normal cellular constituents. The classical example is streptococcal pharyngitis, in which antibodies are produced to the streptococcal M protein and cross-react with M protein of the sarcolemma of cardiac muscle to produce the acute myocarditis of rheumatic fever. Another possible example is the immunological cross-reactivity between the glycoprotein D of the herpes simplex virus and certain bacterial antigens with the acetylcholine receptor. These cross-reactions may be important in the pathogenesis of myasthenia gravis (p. 879).

Heat shock proteins (HSPs) have been highly conserved during evolution so that there is antigenic cross-reactivity between bacterial and human HSPs. The HSP genes are expressed constitutively in most cells, but the levels of expression are increased dramatically during episodes of cellular injury. There is now good evidence that HSPs are major antigens of many micro-organisms. T cells and antibodies against shared bacterial and human HSPs have been detected in many individuals. When cells are damaged, intact HSP or HSP peptides, in association with MHC antigens, could be expressed on the cell membrane and be recognized by antibody or cross-reactive T cells. In rheumatoid arthritis, T cells isolated from the synovial fluid have been shown to respond to mycobacterial HSP-65, and HSP-65 has been shown to be expressed in the inflamed rheumatoid synovial membrane.

Sequestered Antigens

The release of sequestered antigens which are not normally exposed to the immune system may produce an autoimmune response. Release of crystallin from the lens of the eye during cataract extraction, or of antigens from the uveal tract due to trauma, is followed by autoimmune uveitis. Agglutinating antibodies to spermatozoa may be produced following testicular trauma or rupture of an epididymal retention cyst. However, the release of autoantigens into the circulation cannot be the only factor as other autoantigens (e.g. thyroglobulin and DNA) are always present in the plasma at low concentrations and B cells which bind these antigens specifically are also present. Furthermore, the release of autoantigens from injured tissue does not normally evoke an autoimmune response.

Polyclonal Activation of Lymphocytes

In infectious mononucleosis, B cells are infected with Epstein–Barr (EB) virus which induces polyclonal B-cell proliferation along with the production of IgM autoantibodies which tend to disappear as the infection subsides. The EB virus is acting as a polyclonal B-cell activator which bypasses the need for specific T-cell help by acting directly on B cells. Gram-negative lipopolysaccharide acts in a similar manner. A subpopulation of B cells which express the CD5 marker ($CD5^+$ B cells) are able to synthesize a variety of non-organ-specific autoantibodies including rheumatoid factor, anti-DNA antibodies and anticardiolipin antibodies. This subset could be a target for polyclonal activators.

In contrast to the autoantibodies which are produced by polyclonal B-cell activators, those which are present in autoimmune diseases are usually IgG, indicating a role for both T and B cells. The finding that most DNA autoantibodies and a proportion of thyroglobulin autoantibodies are either monoclonal or oligoclonal also shows that not all autoimmune responses are due to polyclonal B-cell activation.

Idiotype Bypass

During a normal immune response anti-idiotypic antibodies are produced which are involved in the regulation of the immune response (p. 200). There are at least two possible mechanisms whereby anti-idiotype responses induce autoimmunity.

Ligand mimicry. The antigen binding site of some anti-idiotypic antibodies carry the internal image of the antigen binding site of the original antibody which stimulated its production (Fig. 6.15). Thus, the structure of the binding site of the anti-idiotype may resemble that of the ligand and could bind to the receptor and mimic the action of the ligand. The production of anti-TSH receptor antibodies in thyrotoxicosis (Graves' disease, p. 1086) is a possible example.

Cross-reactive idiotypes. During an immune response to a microbial infection, anti-idiotype antibodies are produced. These anti-idiotypes recognize epitopes (idiotypes) on the variable region of the antibacterial antibodies. Idiotypes are often shared by clones of antibodies which recognize different antigens. Thus an anti-idiotype on an antibacterial antibody could trigger an autoimmune response by cross-linking the membrane immunoglobulin of an autoreactive B cell (Fig. 6.15). Triggering of T_H cells which recognize the anti-idiotype would be essential for the provision of a helper signal to the autoreactive B cell. Similarly, if a microbial antigen cross-reacts with an idiotype of an autoreactive B cell, an autoimmune response could be triggered (Fig. 6.15).

Helper–Suppressor Cell Imbalance

The expression of autoreactive T cells and B cells in normal individuals is thought to be controlled by T_S cells (but see p. 200). There is evidence that patients with SLE have a deficiency of T_S-cell activity, which would result in hyperglobulinaemia and the production of autoantibodies. Diminished T_S-cell activity occurs in some animal models of SLE (e.g. NZB × NZW F1 hybrid mice), while others have increased T_H-cell activity with the hypersecretion of T_H factors (e.g. MRL-1pr/1pr mice). A similar increase in T_H-cell activity is seen in some patients with SLE.

In conclusion, the aetiology of the two major

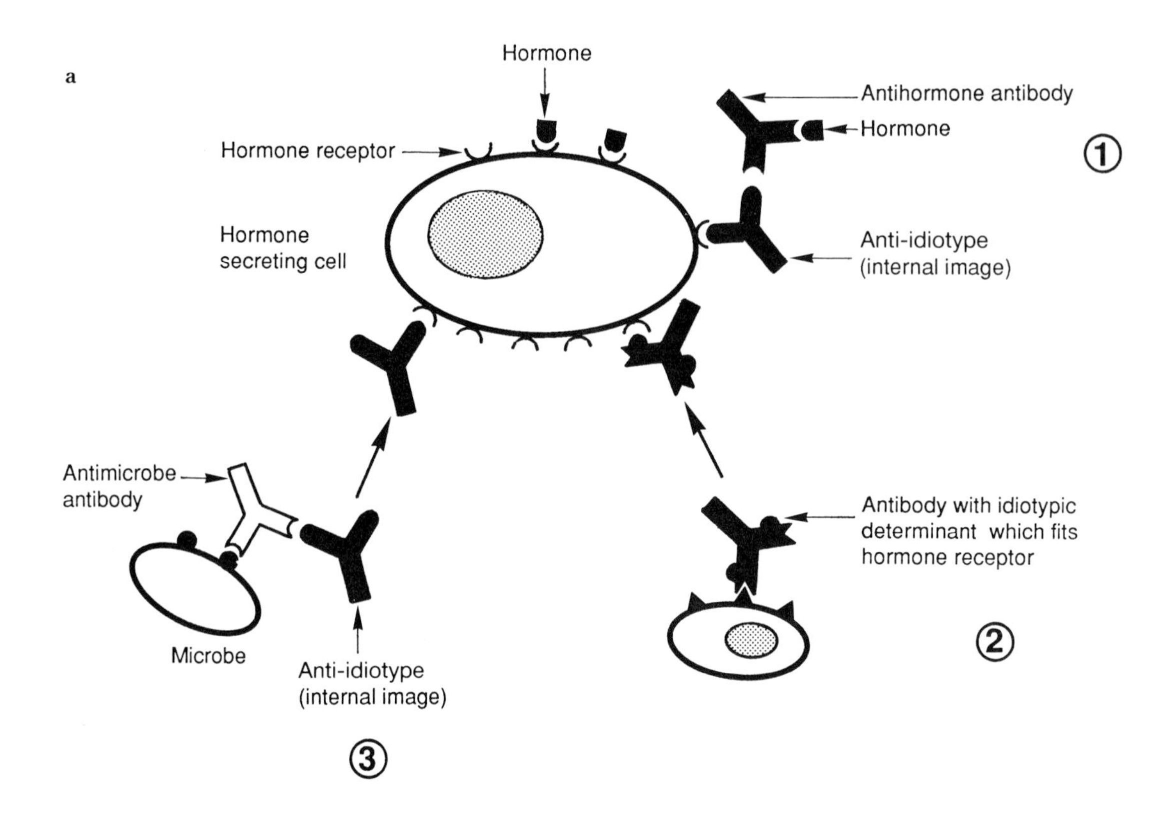
a
Hormone
Antihormone antibody
Hormone
Hormone receptor
①
Hormone
secreting cell
Anti-idiotype
(internal image)
Antimicrobe
antibody
Antibody with idiotypic
determinant which fits
hormone receptor
Microbe
Anti-idiotype
(internal image)
②
③

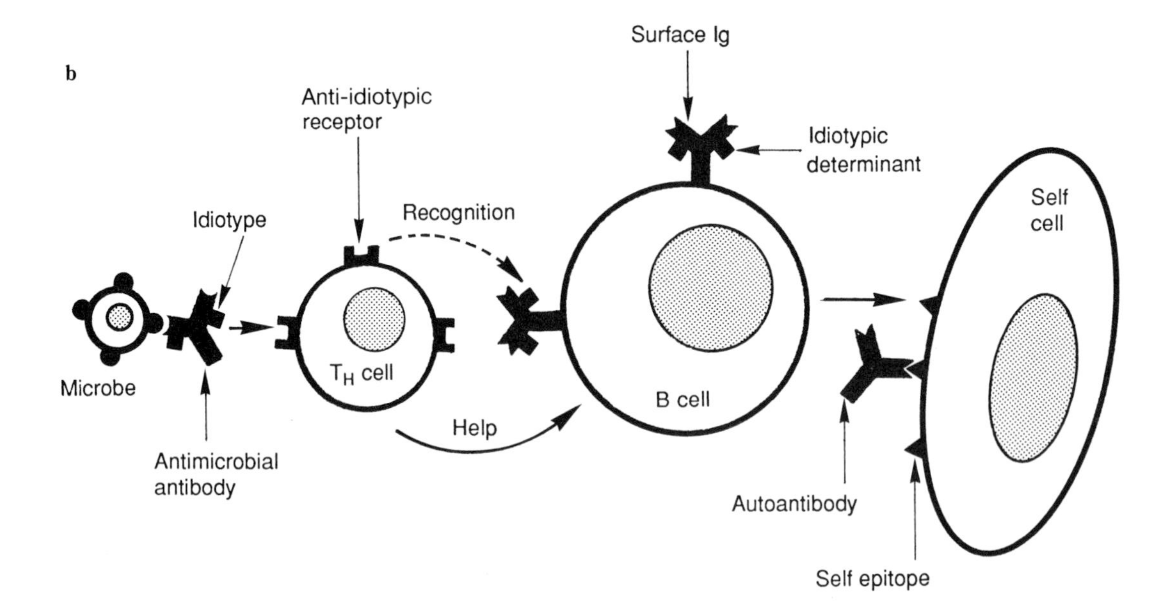
b
Surface Ig
Anti-idiotypic
receptor
Idiotypic
determinant
Idiotype
Recognition
Self
cell
Microbe
T_H cell
B cell
Help
Antimicrobial
antibody
Autoantibody
Self epitope

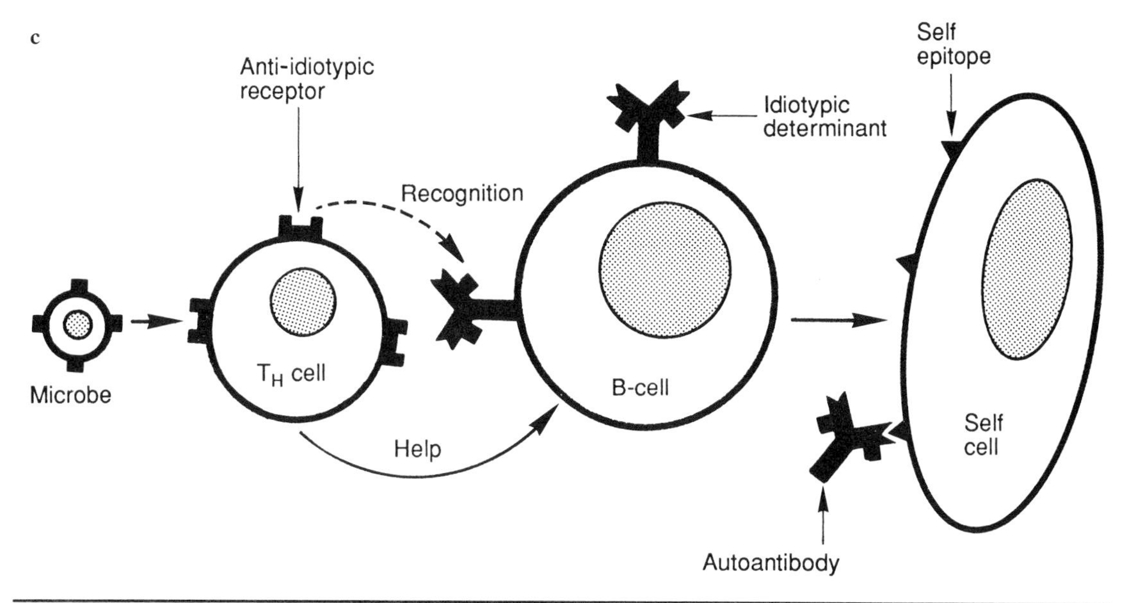

Fig. 6.15 **a** Possible ways in which antibodies to hormone receptors may be produced. (1) Antibody to the hormone provokes an anti-idiotype response and the anti-idiotype (which bears the internal image of the antihormone antibody) is recognized as hormone by the receptor. (2) An antibody to a microbial antigen bears an idiotype which is recognized as hormone by the receptor. (3) A microbial antigen is structurally similar to the hormone so that an anti-idiotype antibody which bears the internal image of the antimicrobial antibody is recognized as hormone by the receptor. **b** An antibody to a microbe bears an idiotype which is also expressed on an autoreactive B cell. Binding of the idiotype to a T-cell receptor which recognizes that idiotype provides a stimulatory signal to the autoreactive B cell. **c** A microbial antigen is recognized by a T-cell receptor which also recognizes an idiotype on an autoreactive B cell. Binding of the microbial antigen to the T-cell receptor provides the stimulatory signal to the autoreactive B cell.

types of autoimmune disease is obscure. The mechanisms underlying the organ-specific autoimmune diseases probably differ from those responsible for the non-organ-specific autoimmune diseases. Whatever the aetiology, genetic factors are involved, although their precise contribution has yet to be determined. As only a minor proportion of individuals who have inherited the genetic predisposition develop autoimmune disease, environmental agents must be involved.

Immunodeficiency

An individual is said to be immunodeficient if the immune system is compromised so that he/she is unduly susceptible to infections by microorganisms. Thus, the term immunodeficiency covers a group of disorders in which defects of specific immune responsiveness, neutrophil and macrophage function, complement or NK cells lead to impaired resistance to microbial infection.

The term primary immunodeficiency is applied to those disorders which usually become manifest in early childhood, and in most there is good evidence that the disease is genetically determined. Secondary immunodeficiencies occur when the immune system becomes defective as a result of a disease process or of immunosuppressive medication.

Primary Immunodeficiencies

As the development of the immune system is highly complex and each individual component has the potential to malfunction, it is not surprising that an extraordinarily large number of primary immunodeficiency syndromes has been described. Although primary immunodeficiencies are rare, early and accurate diagnosis is important as they are often life-threatening conditions and effective treatment for some is now available. There are a large number of syndromes but only a brief review of some of the more important ones in presented in this section. Deficiencies of specific immune responsiveness can be divided into those which affect both T cells and B cells, combined immunodeficiency, and those which affect either T cells or B cells. However, some deficiencies, e.g. Wiskott–Aldrich syndrome and ataxia telangiectasia, are difficult to classify on this basis.

Combined T-cell and B-cell Deficiencies

Severe Combined Immunodeficiency Disease (SCID)

This is a heterogeneous group of disorders which are characterized by gross functional impairment of both the cell mediated (T-cell) immune systems. A positive family history is obtained in almost 50% of cases and indicates either an X-linked or autosomal recessive pattern of inheritance.

Patients with SCID normally die of overwhelming infection within the first 2 years of life. Affected infants show delayed growth, recurrent bacterial and virus infections and often candidiasis of the mouth, larynx and skin. Response to antibiotics and chemotherapy is poor, and immunization with living virus is likely to prove fatal. Graft-versus-host disease can occur following transfusion of whole blood, or from the transfer of maternal lymphocytes to the fetus at the time of delivery. The SCID syndrome occurs as a result of a number of different mechanisms that lead to defects in cellular differentiation. The main types are as follows.

Reticular dysgenesis is the most severe form and is due to a haemopoietic stem cell deficiency as a consequence of which production of T cells, B cells and granulocytes is grossly impaired. These children die within the first few days of life as a consequence of the failure of both specific and non-specific protective mechanisms against infections.

'Swiss-type' SCID is due to failure of lymphoid stem cell development. Patients have severe lymphopenia with very few circulating B or T lymphocytes. The thymus is hypoplastic and deficient in Hassall's corpuscles and small lymphocytes. The lymph nodes are extremely small and without germinal centres, lymphocytes and plasma cells.

An unusual syndrome characterized by extremely low numbers of T cells and very low levels of IgG and IgA. The patients have normal or increased numbers of B cells and raised levels of circulating IgM. The defect may result from either a failure of stem cells to develop into T cells or to faulty development of thymic epithelium or defective production of thymic humoral factors. The low levels of IgG and IgA are thought to be due to lack of T_H cells.

Adenosine deaminase (ADA) deficiency affects half the patients with the autosomal recessive form of SCID (Fig. 6.16). As ADA catalyses the conversion of adenosine to inosine and deoxyadenosine to deoxyinosine in the purine metabolic pathway, this deficiency leads to accumulation of deoxyadenosine and its derivative, deoxyadenosine triphosphate, both of which are toxic to lymphocytes. Transfusion of ADA positive erythrocytes results in immunological improvement in a few patients. In the future, insertion of a normal ADA gene into the patient's own marrow cells may become the treatment of choice.

The bare lymphocyte syndrome. In this dis-

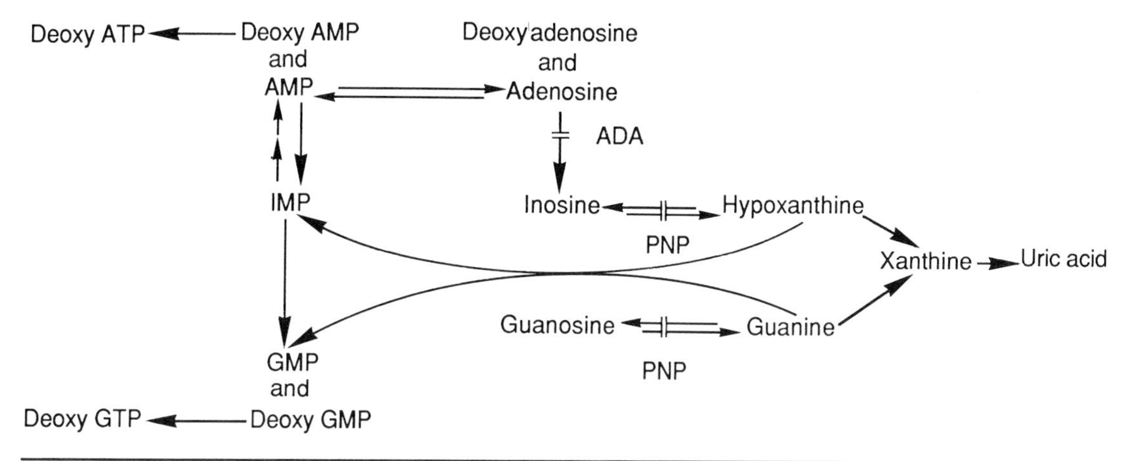

Fig. 6.16 Steps in purine catabolic pathway. One form of severe combined immunodeficiency is associated with a defect in adenosine deaminase (ADA) that catalyses the conversion of adenosine to inosine and deoxyadenosine to deoxyinosine. In purine nucleoside phosphorylase (PNP) deficiency, the enzyme PNP that catalyses the conversion of inosine to hypoxanthine and guanosine to guanine (and their deoxy derivatives) is absent or abnormal. ATP, adenosine triphosphate; AMP, adenosine monophosphate; IMP, inosine monophosphate; GTP, guanosine triphosphate; GMP, guanosine monophosphate; ADA, adenosine deaminase; PNP, purine nucleoside phosphorylase.

ease HLA antigens (either class I or class II) are not expressed. Patients with class I deficiency develop oral candidiasis, *Pneumocystis carinii* or bacterial pneumonia, septicaemia and diarrhoea. Class II deficiency is associated with increased infections and malabsorption. Cell mediated immunity is markedly depressed and immunoglobulin levels are very low, particularly IgA and IgG.

Ataxia telangiectasia. This autosomal recessive disease results in defective T- and B-cell function. Cerebellar ataxia develops at about 2 years of age and telangiectatic dilated small blood vessels appear later. Immunodeficiency develops slowly with depression of cell mediated immunity and low serum levels of IgA and IgE. Occasionally, IgG levels are reduced. The thymus is often poorly developed and lacks Hassall's corpuscles. Recurrent infections of the paranasal sinuses and lungs are common complications. The condition is fatal, often from the development of a lymphoma. The nature of the underlying defect is unknown, but it has been suggested that site-specific DNA breaks which are involved in the generation of active immunoglobulin and T-cell receptor genes, may not be repaired in ataxia telangiectasia. There is no curative therapy.

Deficiencies of T-cell Function

DiGeorge's syndrome is a rare example of selective T-cell deficiency which results from failure of the third and fourth branchial arches to develop. Thus the thymus, parathyroids, some parafollicular cells in the thyroid and the ultimobranchial body fail to develop. Affected infants exhibit total absence of cell mediated immune responses, hypocalcaemic tetany and congenital defects of the heart and great vessels. The peripheral blood lymphocyte count is often low and virtually all circulating lymphocytes are B cells. The thymus-dependent areas of the lymph nodes and spleen are depleted of lymphocytes. Serum immunoglobulin levels are usually normal, although serum levels of IgG and IgA may be reduced.

The condition affects both males and females and does not appear to have a genetic basis. In many cases the condition is rapidly fatal. Affected infants can deal with pyogenic bacteria but suffer from opportunistic infections such as *Pneumocystis carinii* and from fungal and virus infections. Immunization with live vaccines may give rise to severe fatal systemic infections. In those infants who survive the neonatal period immunoglobulin production appears normal, although specific antibody responses are impaired, probably because of lack of T_H cells. In some patients transplantation of fetal thymus has been successful.

Complete absence of the thymus is rare and partial DiGeorge's syndrome is commoner. These patients have an extremely small, but histologically normal thymus. T-cell numbers are low at birth (<10% of peripheral blood lymphocytes) but increase with age, so that by 5 years T-cell function is usually normal.

Nezelof's syndrome is transmitted as an autosomal recessive or X-linked recessive and is due to thymic hypoplasia, but the parathyroid glands and cardiovascular system are normal. B cells and immunolgobulin levels are usually normal.

PNP deficiency. This T-cell deficiency is due to lack of the enzyme purine nucleoside phosphorylase (PNP) (Fig. 6.16). This enzyme catalyses the conversion of inosine to xanthine and of guanosine to guanine in the purine catabolic pathway. In PNP deficiency, deoxyguanosine accumulates, and is phosphorylated to deoxy-GTP which inhibits ribonucleotide reductase so that deoxy-GTP depletion occurs. Thus, DNA synthesis in T cells is diminished and severe T-cell deficiency occurs with particular susceptibility to cytomegalovirus and varicella infection. Autoimmune blood dyscrasias, lymphomas and neurological disease with spasticity and limb weakness occur. B-cell numbers, immunoglobulin levels and antibody production are normal.

Wiskott–Aldrich syndrome is X-linked and is characterized by thrombocytopenia, eczema and recurrent infections. The progressive depletion of lymphocytes in the blood and in the T-dependent areas of the lymphoid tissues, is associated with declining cell mediated immunity. Although blood group isoantibodies are absent, serum levels of IgA and IgE are raised, while IgG is usually normal and IgM is decreased. Antibody responses to polysaccharide antigens are poor. Patients are prone to develop lymphoreticular neoplasms and early death is the rule. The defect is thought to be due to a deficiency of a cell membrane glycoprotein (sialophorin) on the T cells and platelets of patients. As sialophorin is encoded on chromosome 16 it has been suggested that the locus on the short arm of the X chromosome encodes a sialophorin regulatory element. Bone marrow transplantation may correct all the abnormalities.

Deficiencies of B-cell Function

Infantile X-linked agammaglobulinaemia (Bruton-type agammaglobulinaemia) is characterized by virtual absence of serum immunoglobulins. The disease is due to a failure of B cells to produce immunoglobulin. Circulating B cells are absent, although pre-B cells, containing intracytoplasmic μ chain only, are present in the bone marrow. The disorder is thus due to a failure of maturation of pre-B cells.

Clinically the disease presents about 8–9 months of age, once the child's maternal IgG has been catabolized. Septicaemia and recurrent pyogenic infections (*Staphylococcus aureus*, *Haemophilus influenzae*), are common and affect the skin, the respiratory system and the meninges. Persistent diarrhoea is due to intestinal infection with *Giardia lamblia* or enteroviruses. Fungal and most viral infections are generally handled normally, although there is undue susceptibility to enterovirus infections in hypogammaglobulinaemic patients which may cause chronic meningitis and myositis. Chronic polyarthritis due to infection with mycoplasma resembling rheumatoid arthritis is common.

The diagnosis depends upon demonstrating the near absence of serum IgG (below 0.5 g/l), IgM and IgA (below 3×10^{-2} g/l), although deficiency of IgG cannot be demonstrated until maternal IgG has fallen to a low level. The thymus is normal, the tonsils are rudimentary and the lymph nodes show absence of germinal centres. Plasma cells are not detected in any of the lymphoid tissues. Cell mediated immune responses are normal but blood group isohaemagglutinins are absent, and antibodies are not made in response to immunization.

There is rarely a family history. Occasionally an autosomal recessive form of the disease occurs in females. Regular administration of immunoglobulin parentally prevents infections, hence it is important to make the diagnosis early in life.

Transient hypogammaglobulinaemia is familial and affects both males and females. It is more severe in premature infants, as maternal IgG mainly crosses the placenta in late pregnancy. It presents similar clinical and morphological features to X-linked agammaglobulinaemia, but it disappears within the first 3 years of life. The deficiency usually affects IgG alone.

Common Variable Immunodeficiency

This represents a heterogeneous collection of disorders, which may be congenital or acquired, sporadic or familial. All patients have hypogammaglobulinaemia, usually affecting all immunoglobulin classes, but occasionally IgG alone is affected. Cell mediated immune responses are impaired in 30% of patients. Like patients with X-linked agammaglobulinaemia, those with common variable immunodeficiency suffer from recurrent bacterial infections and giardiasis, but echovirus infections are less common. Patients have a high incidence of autoimmune diseases (e.g. rheumatoid arthritis, pernicious anaemia, haemolytic anaemia) and lymphoreticular malignancy.

A few patients have virtually no circulating B cells, due to a failure of stem cells to mature into B cells. However, the majority have a defect in the terminal maturation of B cells into plasma cells. The B cells of a minority of patients are able to synthesize, but cannot secrete immunoglobulins. Histologically, the B-cell areas of the spleen and lymph nodes and gut are hyperplastic.

Selective IgA Deficiency

This is common, occurring in 1 in 600 individuals. Usually it is asymptomatic, although a minority of patients suffer from recurrent bacterial infections of the respiratory, gastrointestinal or genitourinary tracts, coeliac disease, autoimmune disease (especially systemic lupus erythematosus or rheumatoid arthritis), or respiratory tract allergy. It has been suggested that those patients who develop infections are also deficient in the IgG_2 and IgG_4subclasses.

The nature of the defect appears to be an inability of the majority of IgA-positive B cells to mature into IgA-secreting plasma cells. Antibodies to IgA are present in 40% of IgA-deficient individuals, who, if transfused with whole blood or plasma, or are given immunoglobulin replacement therapy, develop severe, sometimes fatal, anaphylactic reactions.

Isolated deficiencies of IgM, IgG and IgG subclasses may also occur and usually present with recurrent bacterial infections.

Phagocytic Cell Defects

Chronic Granulomatous Disease (CGD)

This disease may be inherited in an X-linked or an autosomal recessive manner. Neutrophils and monocytes fail to activate the oxidative phosphorylation pathways and do not generate bactericidal reactive oxygen intermediates (p. 124). As a consequence there is an inability to kill bacteria, although phagocytosis occurs normally. From early childhood patients suffer from recurrent and chronic infections, with extensive suppuration and granulation tissue formation, particularly in skin, bones and viscera. The causative organisms are usually staphylococci, Gram-negative bacteria and certain fungi.

The phenotypic expression of CGD may be the result of one of a number of disorders of oxidative metabolism. Deficiency of glucose-6-phosphate dehydrogenase and of glutathione peroxidase may be associated with CGD. In most of the patients with the X-linked form of the disease, cytochrome *b*-245, an essential component of the electron transport chain which is coupled to the enzyme NAD(P)H oxidase, is absent. In patients with the autosomal recessive variety, cytochrome *b*-245 is present, but a protein which is the substrate for a phosphorylation reaction is missing, and as a result electron transfer cannot occur. The enzyme defect can be detected *in vitro* by failure of monocyte and neutrophils to reduce the yellow dye nitroblue tetrazolium (NBT) to an insoluble blue-black formazan precipitate.

Myeloperoxidase Deficiency

Patients with this disorder fail to make hypochlorous acid (p. 124) and so demonstrate a bactericidal defect. As they can still form hydroxyl ion there may be no undue susceptibility to bacterial infections. However, there may be a susceptibility to systemic candidiasis.

Chediak–Higashi Syndrome

This is an autosomal recessive disease characterized by recurrent pyogenic infections which can be fatal. There is a failure of neutrophils to kill phagocytosed bacteria. The neutrophils contain giant lysosomes which do not function normally. NK cell function is also absent.

In the **lazy leucocyte syndrome** there is an intrinsic defect of neutrophil motility so that the cells cannot respond to a chemotactic stimulus.

Deficiency of Leucocyte Adhesion Molecules

Adhesion of neutrophils to endothelial cells and phagocytosis depend upon the expression of the surface adhesion molecules LFA-1, MAC-1 (CR3 – the iC3b receptor) and p150:95 (p. 15). These molecules possess a common β chain but each has a distinct α chain. The β chain has a transmembrane domain which anchors the molecule to the cell membrane.

In leucocyte adhesion protein deficiency there is a failure to synthesize the common β subunit so that none of the three adhesion molecules is expressed. Patients suffer from severe bacterial infections as neutrophils and macrophages cannot emigrate from post-capillary vessels. There is also failure of wound healing. As some of the molecules are also involved in lymphocyte function, patients also have reduced T-cell and NK-cell mediated cytotoxicity and impaired antibody production.

Complement Deficiencies

Deficiencies of almost all the complement components have been described. With the exception of C1-inhibitor deficiency (autosomal dominant) and properdin deficiency (X-linked) all are inherited as autosomal recessive disorders. The commonest deficiency is thought to be C2 deficiency, with 1% of the population being heterozygotes. Immune complex diseases such as systemic lupus erythematosus occur commonly in patients with deficiencies of the classical pathway components (C1q, C1r, C1s, C4, C2 and C3) as these interact with antigen–antibody complexes to keep them small and soluble and so preventing them from being deposited in and around blood vessels.

Recurrent bacterial infections are common complications of most complement deficiencies. Patients with C3 deficiency cannot opsonize or lyse bacteria and suffer from recurrent severe pyogenic infections (pneumonia, meningitis, septicaemia). Patients with a deficiency of C5, C6, C7, C8 or C9 appear to have a predisposition to develop recurrent neisserial bacteraemia, while patients with properdin deficiency tend to develop fulminant meningococcal septicaemia with a mortality rate of 75%.

C1-inhibitor deficiency is associated with recurent spontaneous episodes of subcutaneous and submucous oedema (hereditary angio-oedema), due to uncontrolled activation of C1. Circumscribed areas of subcutaneous oedema develop, often in response to minor trauma, and submucous oedema may give rise to life-threatening laryngeal obstruction or to recurrent episodes of abdominal pain, which may lead to unnecessary laparotomy. Treatment with impeded androgens (e.g. danazol) results in increased serum levels of C1-inhibitor to a level which is sufficient to control complement activation. This occurs as a result of increased transcription of the normal gene. Antifibrinolytic agents may control the disease and purified C1-inhibitor concentrate may be used to treat acute attacks.

Secondary Immunodeficiencies

These are conditions in which the immune system develops and functions normally but becomes defective as a result of disease processes or immunosuppressive agents. Examples include malnutrition, certain infections, various forms of cancer and renal failure.

Protein-calorie deficiency is probably the commonest cause of immunodeficiency world wide. Lack of protein leads to depressed cell mediated immunity, and hypocomplementaemia (p. 342). Impaired cell mediated immunity occurs in some bacterial and protozoal infections in which there is extensive colonization of macrophages, e.g. leprosy (p. 308) and leishmaniasis (p. 1148). T-cell function is also depressed in sarcoidosis (p. 313). In advanced malignancy, depression of both T-cell and B-cell immunity occurs, particularly in patients with lymphoid malignancies and leukaemia. Certain acute viral infections, particularly infectious mononucleosis and measles, produce temporary impairment of cell mediated immunity. The acquired immunodeficiency syndrome (AIDS) is due to infection with the human immunodeficiency virus (HIV).

Acquired Immunodeficiency Syndrome (AIDS)

In the past decade AIDS has become a major health problem throughout the world. The WHO statistics showed that on 1 July 1989 there were 167 373 patients reported to have full blown AIDS. Of these, 95 561 were in the USA, 29 906 in Africa and 22 708 in Europe. It is estimated that there are 5 million people in the world who are infected. The disease is caused by the human immunodeficiency virus (HIV), a retrovirus of which there are two known strains, HIV-1 and HIV-2 (Fig. 6.17). The former is the principal causative agent of AIDS in North America, Europe and Central Africa, while the latter is an additional cause in West Africa. Unlike other members of the retrovirus family which transform infected cells, HIV-1 and HIV-2 are cytolytic for T cells. Structurally, HIV-1 and 2 are more closely related to lentiviruses than to the human transforming retroviruses. The lentiviruses include feline immunodeficiency virus (FIV) and simian immunodeficiency virus (SIV), are all cytopathic and produce slowly progressive fatal diseases.

$CD4^+$ T cells, and monocytes and macrophages which also bear the CD4 antigen, become infected because the CD4 antigen acts as a virus receptor. The HIV-1 envelope glycoprotein, gp120, binds to CD4 and allows the virus to enter the cell. Once in the cell, viral DNA (Fig. 6.18) is synthesized from viral RNA by reverse transcription. In some cells, the HIV-1 DNA is integrated into the host genome, but in others, large amounts of unintegrated proviral DNA accumulate.

Virus replication may occur in T cells in which HIV-1 DNA has been integrated (productive infection), and ultimately leads to cell death (cytopathic effect). However, in some T cells containing integrated HIV-1 DNA, the virus does not replicate (latent infection), but once the T cell is activated by antigenic stimulation, possibly by other viruses such as cytomegalovirus, hepatitis B, EB virus or herpesvirus, replication occurs. Latency may last for months or years, and accounts for the long and

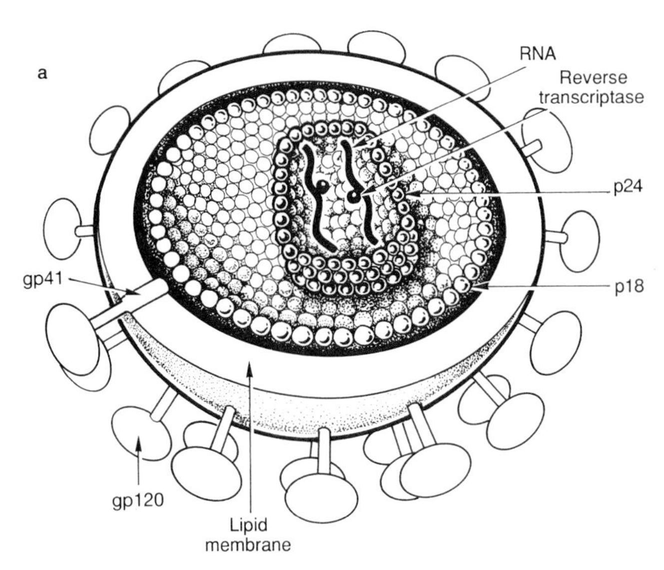

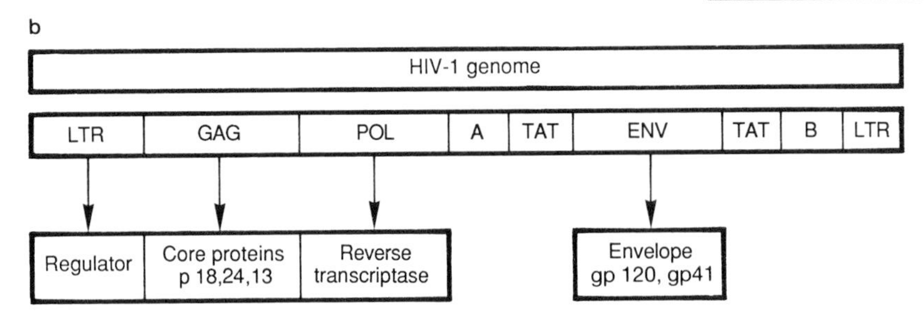

Fig. 6.17 **a** Cross-section of HIV-1 virion which is a sphere of approximately 100 nm in diameter. The lipid layers are derived from the host cell. The viral glycoprotein gp41 spans the membrane while gp120 protrudes into the environment. This protein/lipid coat covers the core which consists of two protein shells, the outer containing the core protein p18 and the inner the core protein p24. The RNA genome and reverse transcriptase are contained within the inner shell. **b** Diagram of HIV genome which contains the GAG sequence which encodes the core proteins p18, p24 and p13 and POL which encodes reverse transcriptase. A and B contain genes *vif* and *vpr*, the former of which is responsible for the production of infectious virus. TAT is involved in the upregulation of HIV synthesis by anti-repression mechanisms, ENV encodes the envelope glycoproteins gp120 and gp41. LTR comprises a series of long terminal repeat units which contain regulatory genetic elements.

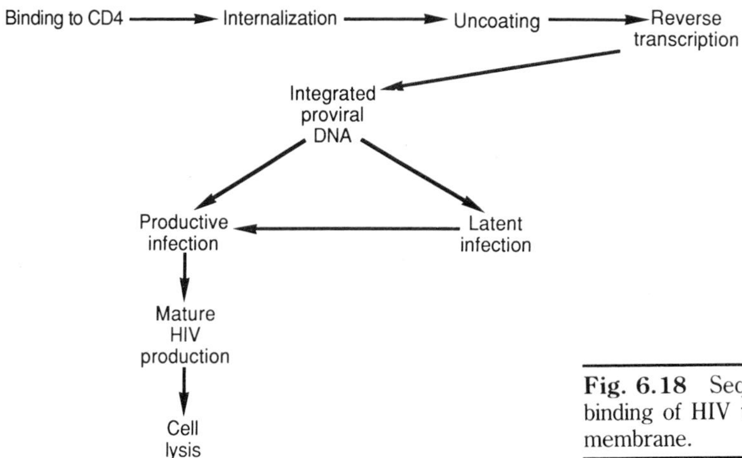

Fig. 6.18 Sequence of cellular events following the binding of HIV to the CD4 antigen in the target cell membrane.

often variable incubation period of AIDS. Although monocytes and macrophages may also become infected, they are resistant to the cytopathic effects of the virus and may thus be the major reservoir of the virus in HIV infected individuals.

Transmission of HIV-1

Venereal transmission of HIV-1 by anal intercourse is the main mode of transmission in male homosexuals and bisexuals. Heterosexual transmission is becoming more common in Europe and North America and is thought to be the main mode of transmission in Africa. Infected males are thought to transmit the virus in infected lymphocytes in their semen, the infected seminal fluid entering the recipient's body through abrasions in the rectal mucosa. During vaginal intercourse it is thought that the virus penetrates the vaginal mucosa. Female to male transmission occurs, probably as a result of the virus being present in vaginal and cervical secretions and in monocytes and endothelial cells of the submucosa of the uterine cervix.

Parenteral transmission of HIV-1 occurs predominantly in intravenous drug users although haemophiliacs have been infected by receiving contaminated factor VIII concentrate produced from large pools of individual plasma donations; infection of recipients of isolated blood transfusions has also occurred. The problem of transmission of HIV-1 by blood concentrates and blood transfusion has been reduced by screening all blood donations for HIV-1 antibody, and by heat-treating blood concentrates. However, as false negative results occur occasionally and antibody tests are negative for up to 4 months in the latent period between the time of infection and the appearance of antibody, the potential for virus transmission by this route persists.

Transmission of HIV-1 from infected mothers to the fetus may occur transplacentally. Infection with infected blood or amniotic fluid during delivery, or through ingestion of infected breast milk, are other possible routes whereby babies can be infected. Diagnosis of HIV-1 infection of the child in the first few months of life is difficult as maternal antibodies cross the placenta.

Immunological Features

(Fig. 6.19)

The earliest immunological abnormality is a rise in the number of $CD8^+$ T cells which occurs at the time of seroconversion. This is common in many virus infections. Following this there is approgressive decrease in the number of $CD4^+$ T cells due to their destruction by HIV. The absolute number of $CD4^+$ cells is the best index of the disease stage. In the AIDS related complex (ARC) the number is generally below 400/mm^3 (lower limit of normal 450–500/mm^3), while major infections usually do not occur when the count is above 200/mm^3.

Destruction of $CD4^+$ T cells leads to a progressive lymphopenia. Normally the ratio of $CD4^+$ T cells to $CD8^+$ T cells is approximately 2, whereas in AIDS patients it is reversed and may be down to 0.5. However, conversion of the ratio is

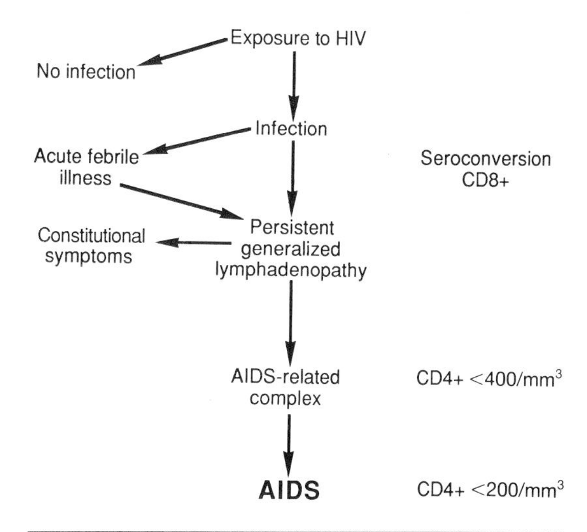

Fig. 6.19 Sequence of events following exposure of the individual to HIV. Clinical features to the left and serological and cellular changes to the right. An infected individual may experience an acute febrile episode (during which the number of $CD8^+$ T cells increases) or he may not experience any symptoms. After a latent period of variable length some patients experience constitutional symptoms and have persistent generalized lymphadenopathy. When the number of $CD4^+$ T cells in the blood has fallen below 400/mm^3, the AIDS related complex (ARC) may occur. The full blown picture of AIDS occurs when the $CD4^+$ T-cell count is below 200/mm^3.

not diagnostic for AIDS. Cell mediated immune responses and the proliferative responses of T cells to antigens and mitogens are impaired, and there is decreased natural killer (NK) activity. Despite diminished antibody responses to specific antigens, hypergammaglobulinaemia occurs due to polyclonal B-cell activation which may be due to intercurrent virus infection (e.g. cytomegalovirus, EB virus) or to the HIV envelope glycoprotein, gp120, which is structurally homologous to neuroleukin, a B-cell activator. Reduced antibody responses may be the result of reduced numbers of T_H cells or because of an intrinsic B-cell defect.

Clinical Features (Fig. 6.19)

Most, if not all patients who become infected with HIV-1 will develop AIDS although the incubation period may be extremely long. It has been estimated that about 25–35% of infected individuals will develop AIDS in 5–7 years. Up to half of the patients will suffer a febrile illness similar to infectious mononucleosis during the incubation period before seroconversion occurs. Persistent generalized lymphadenopathy with mild constitutional symptoms develops in some patients following this febrile illness but it also may occur in the absence of preceding symptoms.

AIDS-related complex (ARC) comprises persistent fever lasting longer than 3 months, weight loss, diarrhoea, leucopenia and anaemia. The $CD4^+$ T-cell count is lower than $400/mm^3$. Rapid and pronounced falls indicate those patients going on to develop AIDS.

The clinical features of full blown AIDS are either due to the secondary immunodeficiency or to the direct effects of infection of particular tissues. As a result of the immunodeficiency, patients develop opportunistic infections such as *Pneumocystis carinii* pneumonia, cytomegalovirus infection, candidiasis, toxoplasmosis and atypical mycobacterial infections. $CD4^+$ T-cell counts are below $200/mm^3$. Malignant disease is common, particularly Kaposi's sarcoma (p. 1140), non-Hodgkin's lymphoma or primary lymphoma of the brain. Kaposi's sarcoma occurs primarily in homosexual and bisexual males and is unusual in intravenous drug abusers.

The central nervous system is a major target for HIV infection and patients may develop dementia, myelopathy or peripheral neuropathy. HIV is thought to enter the brain by infected monocytes, although direct infection of neurons, oligodendrocytes and astrocytes may occur, as these cells express the CD4 antigen. Infection of endothelial cells in the intracerebral blood vessels may lead to changes in permeability and allow HIV to enter the brain tissue.

Treatment

Dideoxynucleoside 3′-azido-3′-deoxythymidine (AZT), a potent chain terminating inhibitor of HIV reverse transcriptase, inhibits HIV replication *in vitro*. In AIDS patients it appears to produce partial restoration of immune function. Recent studies performed with AZT in HIV antibody positive individuals suggest that AZT slows the progression of the disease so that the latent period is prolonged so that the proportion of patients developing clinical features of HIV infection in a particular time is reduced.

Amyloidosis

Amyloid is an insoluble proteinaceous material of varying chemical composition which may be deposited in the extravascular matrix of one or several organs. As a consequence organ function is impaired, leading to a broad spectrum of clinical manifestations. Amyloidosis, therefore, represents a number of disorders, sometimes referred to as the β fibrilloses, and is classified on the basis of the chemical composition of the fibrils (Table 6.6). The fibrils show a common structural configuration, arranged as antiparallel β-pleated sheets, hence the alternative name.

Systemic amyloidosis may occur:

Table 6.6 Classification of amyloidosis

Type	Source of fibrillary protein	Disease/disorder
AL	Ig light chains	Primary amyloidosis
AL	Ig light chains	Multiple myeloma, immunoblastic lymphoma,
AH	β_2-microglobulin	Chronic renal failure with haemodialysis
AA	SAA	Chronic infection, chronic inflammation, renal carcinoma, Hodgkin's disease
AA	SAA	Familial Mediterranean fever
AF	Prealbumin	Familial amyloidotic polyneuropathy, familial Danish amyloidosis and other types
ASc_1	Prealbumin	Senile systemic amyloidosis
ASc I	Atrial natriuretic peptide	Senile cardiac amyloidosis
ASb E (A4 Protein)	?	Alzheimer's disease + other forms of presenile dementia
AE	Procalcitonin or insulin	Endocrine tumours, e.g. medullary carcinoma of thyroid, B-cell tumour of pancreas

(1) in association with plasma cell and B-cell dyscrasias in which the fibril is amyloid light chain (AL) and the related serum protein consists of immunoglobulin light chains;

(2) as a result of long-standing chronic inflammatory processes in which the fibril is amyloid A (AA) and the related serum protein is serum amyloid A (SAA);

(3) in heredofamilial forms including familial Mediterranean fever in which the fibril biochemically resembles (2) and other forms in which there is heterogeneity of the fibril and the related serum proteins are genetic variants of prealbumin (transthyretin); and

(4) as the senile form affecting up to 30% of the elderly and in whom the fibrils are related to prealbumin. Localized forms of amyloidosis may occur in a number of organs and lesions (Table 6.6).

Composition of Amyloid Deposits

Amyloid consists of the following components:

(1) Rigid non-branching protein fibrils (Fig. 6.20), 7.5–10 nm in diameter and of variable length, which have a hollow core. They comprise approximately 90% of amyloid tissue and constitute the peculiar β-pleated component of amyloid which is responsible for its staining and other physicochemical properties.

(2) Rod-like aggregates of a pentagonal doughnut-shaped glycoprotein 10 nm in diameter, amyloid P-protein (component P) which comprises 10% of amyloid tissue and is present in all but the central nervous system forms of amyloid. Component P is synthesized by the liver, circulates as

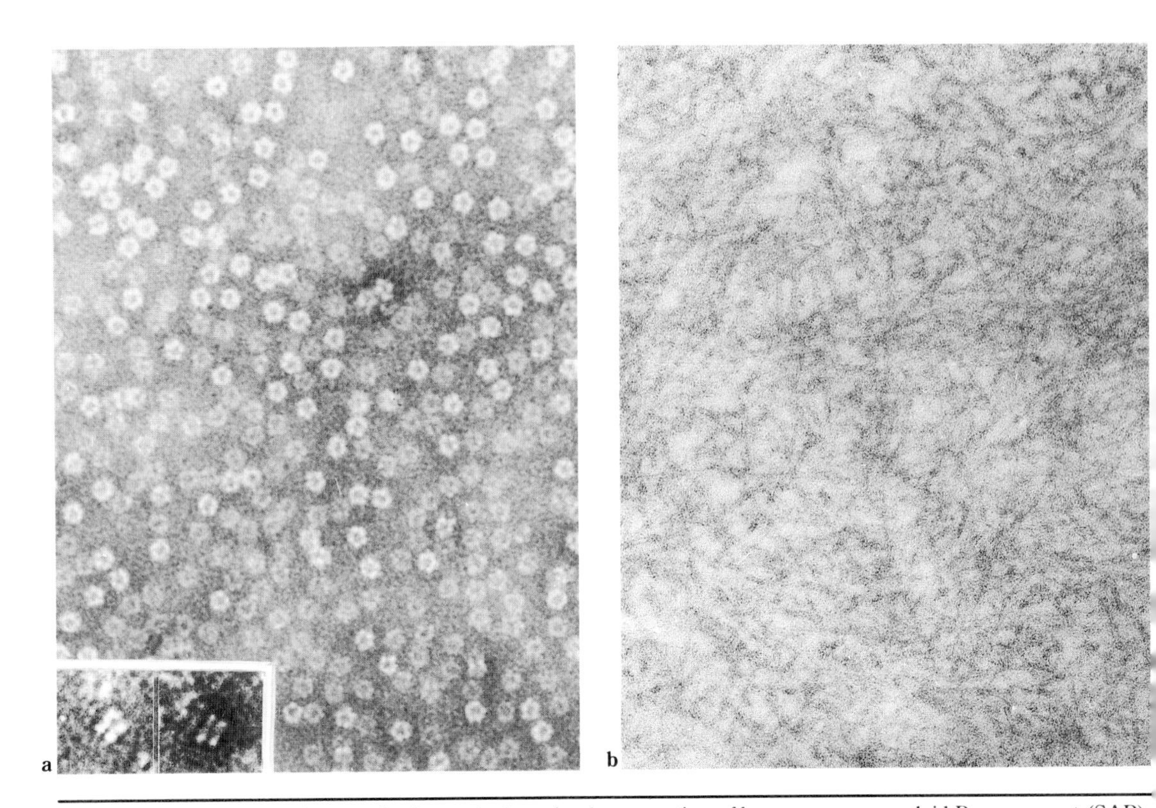

Fig. 6.20 **a** Electron micrograph of negatively stained preparation of human serum amyloid P component (SAP). Most molecules are seen face-on and have the typical five sided doughnut-like appearance. ×320,000. The inset (higher magnification) shows the side-on view of these molecules which appear as dimers of a disc-like molecule. **b** Electron micrograph of amyloid showing bundles of rigid non-branching fibroids.
(**a** is from Pepys, M. B. and Baltz, M. L. (1983). *Advances in Immunology* **34**, 141–212. Courtesy of the authors and editors.)

serum amyloid P (SAP) and is chemically closely related to C-reactive protein. Component P is a constituent of normal basement membrane and of the microfibrillary network of elastic fibres.

(3) A small amount of glycosaminoglycan, usually heparan sulphate. In addition lipoproteins, fibrin, complement proteins and other plasma constituents are present in trace amounts.

Proteins of the Amyloid Fibrils (Table 6.6)

AL amyloid. The first amyloid proteins to be isolated and to have their amino-acid sequence determined were from patients with multiple myeloma or with primary amyloidosis. The fibrils consist of the variable region of immunoglobulin light chains, usually λ but sometimes κ chains. Although deposits from different organs of the same individual have the same amino-acid sequence, deposits from different patients have different amino-acid sequences. AL protein is found in the amyloidosis which develops in 10–15% of patients with multiple myeloma and a proportion of patients with B-cell neoplasms (p. 636). It is also present in the deposits of patients with primary amyloidosis, and usually all of these patients have monoclonal immunoglobulins or free light chains or both in their blood or tissue. Thus in primary AL amyloidosis an underlying B-cell abnormality is present.

AA amyloid. The protein present in the fibrils of AA amyloid is identical in all patients and is derived from the amino-terminal two-thirds of an acute-phase protein, serum amyloid A protein (SAA), which is synthesized by the liver as an apoprotein and circulates in a complex with high density lipoprotein. Serum AA levels may increase up to 1000-fold during an inflammatory response. AA protein is found in the amyloid deposits which occur secondarily to long-standing inflammation, in the deposits associated with malignant disease (e.g. Hodgkin's disease, renal carcinoma) and also in the amyloid of familial Mediterranean fever.

A prealbumin (AF protein). Prealbumin, synthesized by the liver, serves as a transport protein for thyroid hormones and retinol (vitamin A) hence its other name, transthyretin. The fibrillary proteins isolated from patients with familial amyloid polyneuropathy are inherited variants of prealbumin. The best characterized variant has a valine residue substituted for methionine at position 30 (Portuguese familial amyloid polyneuropathy), although substitutions at other sites (e.g. position 33 in the Jewish form of the disease) have been documented. The Danish form of hereditary amyloidosis, which is not associated with polyneuropathy, has methionine substituted for a leucine residue at position 111. A derivative of normal prealbumin is present in the deposits of isolated cardiac amyloidosis and in the systemic amyloidosis of ageing.

AE proteins (endocrine amyloid deposits). Amyloid deposits in neoplastic or degenerative disorders of endocrine glands contain fibrils which appear to be derived from locally synthesized polypeptide hormones or their prohormone precursors. The fibrils of the amyloid deposits in medullary carcinoma of the thyroid (a malignant tumour of calcitonin secreting C cells) contain a fragment of precalcitonin, and those which occur in insulin secreting tumours (insulinomas), or in the pancreatic islets in diabetes mellitus contain amylin, a calcitonin-related peptide. Amyloid deposits may also occur in bronchial carcinoids, carotid body tumours, parathyroid adenomas, phaeochromocytomas, pituitary adenomas and gastrinomas but the precise nature of the AE protein in these has not been defined.

ASb proteins (amyloid senile cerebrovascular deposits). Amyloid deposits are present in the neuritic plaques, neurofibrillary tangles and the blood vessels of individuals with Alzheimer's disease and with dementia of Alzheimer's type (p. 843). Similar lesions are seen in patients with Down's syndrome. A 4 kDa protein (A4 protien) has been isolated from the plaques and shown to be a fragment of a larger, probably intramembranous protein. The gene encoding A4 protein has been localized to chromosome 21. The A4 protein is synthesized locally within the central nervous system and is not derived from a serum precursor protein.

ASc proteins (senile amyloidosis). ASc protein forms the fibrils in generalized senile amyloidosis while ASc I, which is derived from atrial natriuretic peptide, forms the fibrils in senile cardiac amyloidosis.

AH proteins (haemodialysis-associated amyloid deposits). In patients on long-term haemodialysis who develop focal amyloid deposits in joints and periarticular tissues the amyloid fibrils are derived from β_2-microglobulin (p. 934).

Morphological Features of Amyloid

In all organs amyloid is deposited close to or within the walls of blood vessels. Lugol's iodine stains deposits deep brown and can be used to demonstrate amyloid both macroscopically and microscopically. In histological sections stained by haematoxylin and eosin, amyloid appears as a homogeneous refractile eosinophilic deposit. The deposits exhibit metachromasia using dyes such as methyl violet and crystal violet. In polarized light amyloid stained by Congo red or Sirius red shows an apple-green birefringence, and this provides the most reliable of the traditional methods for demonstrating amyloid (Fig. 6.21). Thioflavine T

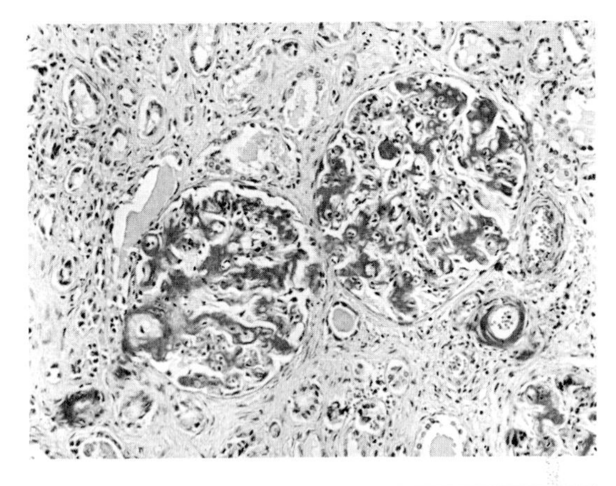

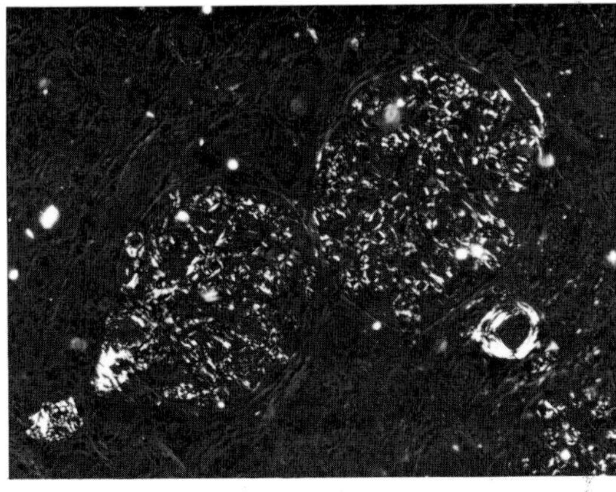

Fig. 6.21 The kidney in amyloidosis, stained by Congo red. The glomerular capillaries and arterioles are affected. Above, viewed by ordinary light: the amyloid is seen as homogenous material. Below, viewed through crossed polarizing films, showing birefringence of the amyloid. ×105.

binds to amyloid and its presence is demonstrated by fluorescence microscopy. Immunostaining with antibodies to AA and AL protein will distinguish between the two common types of amyloid.

On electron microscopy (Fig. 6.20) the typical fibrillary pattern is evident. Individual fibres are made up of two to five intertwining 2.5–3 nm filaments. The rods of stacked pentagonal component P radiate perpendicularly from the fibres. The fibres have a tendency to aggregate into groups of parallel arrays each of which has a different orientation. This structure orientates dyes such as Congo red and Sirius red and is thus responsible for the ability of amyloid to rotate polarized light and produce birefringence.

The β-pleated configuration of the protein fibrils has been characterized by X-ray crystallography and infra-red spectroscopy. The unusual β-pleated structure contrasts with the α helical arrangement of amino-acid chains which characterize other fibrous proteins.

Pathogenesis of Amyloid
(Fig. 6.22)

Partial degradation of immunoglobulin light chain or of apo-SAA by macrophage protease plays a key role in AL and AA amyloid respectively. In AL amyloid the variable region polymerizes to form the amyloid fibril. It is probable that only certain light chain molecules can form amyloid fibrils as amyloidosis occurs in a minority of patients with multiple myeloma.

In AA amyloid, denaturation of the circulating complex releases apo-SAA which has an identical amino-acid sequence to the AA protein in the deposits. Hepatic synthesis of apo-SAA, in common with that of other acute-phase proteins, is stimulated by interleukin 1 (IL-1) which is released from macrophages and other cells. The precise reason why only some individuals with raised SAA levels develop amyloidosis is not known.

Transthyretin and β_2-microglobulin do not undergo proteolysis before forming fibrils. The role of P component in the pathogenesis of the amyloid lesion is not understood, but it may play an essential role in the conversion of protein fragments into fibrils.

Clinical Features

The clinical classification of amyloidosis is useful and is based on the clinical presentation of the patient (Table 6.6). Primary, secondary and familial amyloidosis are examples of systemic amyloidosis which may affect the heart and kidney

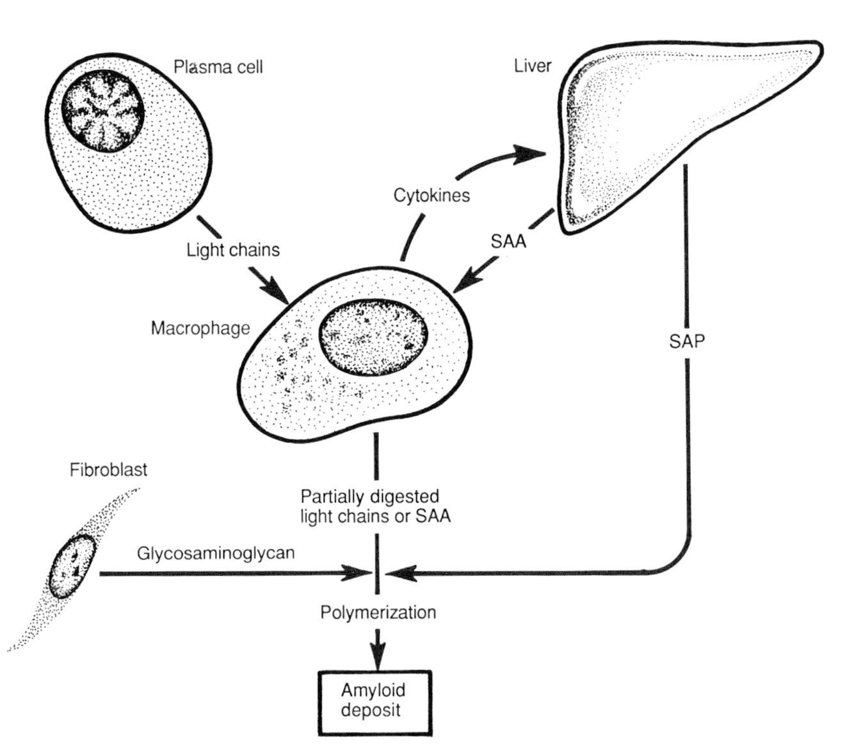

Fig. 6.22 Pathogenesis of AL and AA amyloid. Partial proteolysis of light chains or SAA by macrophages is thought to be important in the pathogenesis of these types of amyloid. However, in other types of amyloid (e.g. AF and AH types) proteolysis is not required. The liver and fibroblasts play a role in synthesizing SAP and glycosaminoglycans respectively. Cytokines (e.g. interleukins 1 and 6) tumour necrosis factor α synthesized by macrophages act on the liver to increase synthesis of SAA and SAP.

leading to cardiac failure and renal failure respectively, and in addition the liver, spleen, gastrointestinal tract, tongue and subcutaneous tissues.

The detailed morphological appearances and the clinical features of amyloid are discussed in the appropriate systematic chapters.

Primary amyloidosis occurs in the absence of any preceding disease. Secondary amyloidosis complicates a pre-existing disease such as multiple myeloma and other B-cell dyscrasias, other malignancies, chronic inflammatory diseases (e.g. rheumatoid arthritis, tuberculosis, lung abscesses, osteomyelitis, Crohn's disease) and chronic haemodialysis.

Familial amyloidosis occurs in several forms. In familial Mediterranean fever, an inherited disorder of glucocorticoid metabolism occurring principally in Sephardic Jews, recurrent inflammation of the serous cavities occurs. Other forms of familial amyloidosis, including familial amyloid polyneuropathy which occurs in Scandinavia, Portugal and Japan, and Danish familial cardiac amyloidosis which is not associated with polyneuropathy, are all associated with point mutations in prealbumin, the precursor of the amyloid fibrils in these patients. The prognosis is variable. Generalized amyloidosis is almost always fatal. Renal failure is the commonest cause of death but cardiac failure and, rarely, liver failure also occur. The average survival from the time of diagnosis of primary amyloidosis is approximately 14 months, while that for myeloma-associated amyloidosis may be as low as 4 months. The prognosis of amyloidosis secondary to chronic inflammatory conditions depends on the underlying disease and the rate of progression of amyloidosis. There are reports of clinical recovery following the control of the underlying disease.

Further Reading

Chapel, H. and Heaney, M. (1988). *Essentials in Clinical Immunology*, 2nd edn. Blackwell Scientific Publications, Oxford.

Lachmann, P. J. and Peters, P. A. (1982). *Clinical Aspects of Clinical Immunology*, 4th edn. Blackwell Scientific Publications, Oxford.

Pepys, M. B. and Baltz, M. (1983). Acute phase proteins with special relevance to C-reactive protein and related proteins (pentraxins) and serum amyloid A protein. *Advances in Immunology* **34**, 141–212.

Samter, M., Talmage, D. W., Frank, M. M., Austen, K. F. and Claman, H. N. (1988). *Immunological Diseases*. Little, Brown and Co., Boston Toronto.

7

Metabolic Disorders

The diseases discussed in this chapter are a heterogeneous group of disorders affecting the metabolism of a wide variety of molecules including carbohydrates, lipids, mucopolysaccharides and amino acids. Each is an inherited defect of a single gene usually coding for an enzyme involved in a metabolic pathway, or a protein responsible for transport of a substance across cell membranes. In these the mutation is usually located within the exons coding for the protein, resulting in the production of a polypeptide of abnormal amino-acid sequence. Other mechanisms may also result in abnormal enzyme activity; a mutation may lie in a controlling sequence causing diminished transcription of messenger RNA and thus reduced synthesis of a normal protein. There may be defective splicing of messenger RNA, with loss of one or more exons, also resulting in an abnormal protein. Post-translational modification, e.g. glycosylation, may be abnormal and defects in packaging (e.g. mucolipidosis type II) and failure of secretion of enzymes (e.g. α_1-antitrypsin deficiency, p. 772) may occur. Thus, many different mechanisms may cause defects.

These diseases are defined on the basis of the defect and on its phenotypic expression, i.e. the biochemical and pathological features which are present in affected individuals. There is often considerable heterogeneity in the expression of any defect depending on whether there is total or partial deficiency of an enzyme. Those mutations affecting critical regions of the molecule, e.g. substrate binding sites, will usually result in more severe disease than those in less important regions. Although a few disorders are autosomal dominant in inheritance, the large majority are recessive. In recessive conditions, the disease in homozygotes is usually severe, while heterozygote 'carriers' may be normal, may have an asymptomatic biochemical abnormality, or a mild form of the disease. The clinical manifestations of some disorders are entirely due to the genetic abnormality, while the clinical features of others only become manifest in response to some environmental stimulus. Metabolic pathways dependent on the enzyme are usually blocked; this results in absence or relative lack of the metabolic products, accumulation of the enzyme substrate or the development of alternative metabolic pathways. Very unusually, the activity of the enzyme may be increased. Defects in lysosomal, mitochondrial and peroxisomal enzymes are recognized. Also included are diseases affecting transport mechanisms involving plasma, mitochondrial or lysosomal membranes.

A number of the more common metabolic disorders are dealt with in the appropriate systemic chapters, e.g. the inherited coagulation deficiencies, Wilson's disease and diseases of iron overload. The less common disorders are reviewed here, some in a little detail and others briefly summarized.

Disorders of Carbohydrate Metabolism

Diabetes mellitus is discussed in Chapter 17.

Glycogen Storage Diseases (GSD)

This term refers to a group of disorders characterized by excessive accumulation of glycogen of normal or abnormal structure in various tissues including the liver, heart, skeletal muscle, kidneys, erythrocytes and leucocytes (Table 7.1). In each disorder a defect has been identified in an enzyme involved in glycogen metabolism (Fig. 7.1). The diseases together affect less than 1 in 50 000 live births. With the exception of type IX B, which is X-linked, all are inherited as autosomal recessive.

Most patients present in childhood. The clinical features are variable. Involvement of the liver leads to hepatomegaly and sometimes to liver failure. The heart may be enlarged and the child may die of cardiac failure. In some forms skeletal muscle alone is affected and myopathy results. Leucopenia or abnormal leucocyte function may result in recurrent infections. Convulsions may accompany severe metabolic disturbance including hypoglycaemia, lactic acidosis and hyperuricaemia.

***GSD type IA* (von Gierke's disease)**, due to deficiency of glucose-6-phosphatase, usually presents in infancy with massive hepatomegaly. There is hypoglycaemia often precipitated by intercurrent infections; this may be accompanied by severe lactic acidosis with seizures and sometimes death. Hypertriglyceridaemia and hyperuricaemia occur frequently and may lead to xanthomas and gout. On liver biopsy, the hepatocytes are swollen and vacuolated, and contain excess glycogen. Despite this, liver function tests are usually normal. Hepatic adenomas may develop in adulthood. Excess glycogen is also present in the epithelium of the proximal renal tubule and there may be aminoaciduria (Fanconi's syndrome). Absence of glucose-6-phosphatase activity can be demonstrated in liver and jejunal biopsies. The aim of treatment is to maintain normoglycaemia.

In **types IB and IC**, glucose-6-phosphatase activity is normal but there is defective transport of glucose-6-phosphate across microsomal membranes. In type IB, an accompanying neutropenia results in recurrent infections.

***GSD type II* (Pompe's disease)** results from deficiency of the lysosomal enzyme α-glucose-1, 4-glucosidase (acid maltase). It was the first lysosomal storage disorder to be clearly defined. Glycogen accumulation is seen particularly in the

Table 7.1 The glycogen storage disorders

	Enzyme affected	Major site of storage	Clinical features
IA (von Gierke's)	Glucose-6-phosphatase	Liver, kidney, intestine	Hypoglycaemia with seizures, hepatomegaly
IB,C	Glucose-6-phosphate translocases		Type IB – neutropenia with infections
II (Pompe's)	α-glucose-1,4-glucosidase (acid maltase)	Heart, skeletal muscle, liver	Cardiac failure, hepatomegaly
III	Amylo-1,6-glucosidase (debranching enzyme)	Liver and heart muscle (IIIA); liver or heart muscle (IIIB)	Mild hypoglycaemia, hepatomegaly, myopathy
IV (amylopectinosis)	Alpha-1,4-glucan-6-glycosyltransferase (branching enzyme)	Liver, heart	Cirrhosis
V (McArdle's)	Muscle phosphorylase	Skeletal muscle	Myopathy
VI (Her's)	Hepatic phosphorylase	Liver, skeletal muscle	Mild hepatomegaly
VII	Phosphofructokinase	Skeletal muscle	Muscle weakness; resembles type V
VIII	Phosphorylase	Liver, brain	Hepatomegaly; progressive mental deterioration
IX A*	Phosphorylase β kinase (autosomal recessive)	Liver, muscle	Resembles types I and III but symptoms are milder
IX B*	Phosphorylase β kinase (X-linked recessive)		
X	Phosphorylase kinase	Liver, muscle	Hepatomegaly; mild muscle cramps
XI	Not known	Liver, kidney	Renal tubular dysfunction
O	Hepatic glycogen synthetase	Deficient in liver glycogen	Prolonged hyperglycaemia

*Sometimes classified as subgroups of type VI.

heart (Fig. 7.2), skeletal muscle, the liver (both hepatocytes and Kupffer cells) and in motor nuclei of the brain stem and spinal cord. Severe cases develop cardiac failure in infancy; the heart is hypertrophied and the myocardial cells, including those of the conducting system, are enlarged, vacuolated and contain abundant lysosomal glycogen. Skeletal muscle fibres are also enlarged, and there may be striking muscle weakness. Juvenile and adult variants which are less severe are also described. Prenatal diagnosis may be made by identifying glycogen within the lysosomes of amniocytes.

In ***GSD type III*** there is deficiency of the 'debranching' enzyme amylo-1,6-glucosidase. The clinical features of hypoglycaemia and hepatomegaly resemble those of type I but in addition cardiac and skeletal muscle may be affected. The disease is less severe than type I and the long-term prognosis is favourable. The excess accumulation of the abnormal glycogen produces a

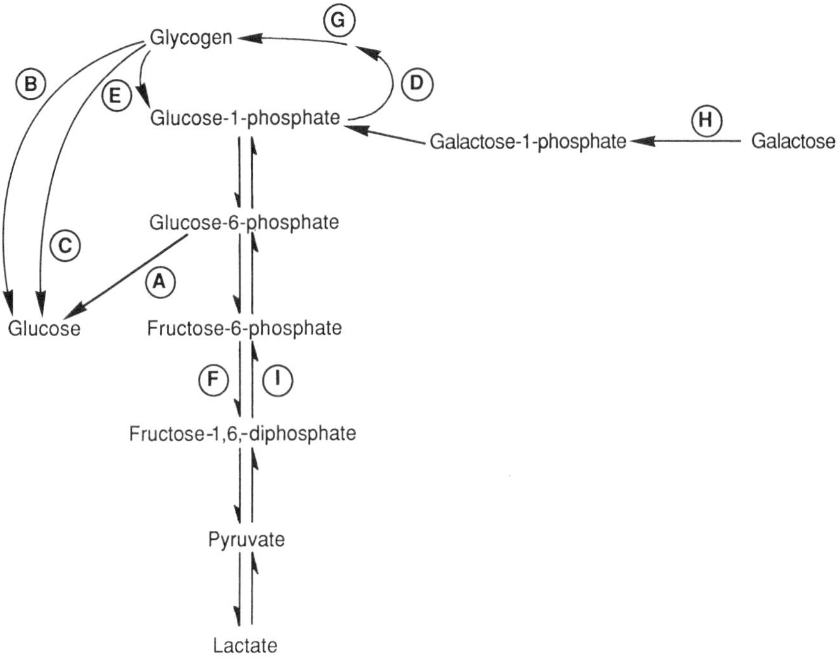

Glycogen (G)
(B) (E) Glucose-1-phosphate (D)
Galactose-1-phosphate (H) Galactose
Glucose-6-phosphate
(C) (A)
Glucose Fructose-6-phosphate
(F) (I)
Fructose-1,6,-diphosphate
Pyruvate
Lactate

Fig. 7.1 Glycogen metabolism. In this outline of glycogen metabolism, letters A–I indicate those enzymes which are defective in glycogen storage diseases and some abnormalities of fructose and galactose metabolism. A, glucose-6-phosphatase associated with GSD IA; B, α-1,4-glucosidase – GSD II; C, debranching enzyme – GSD III; D, branching enzyme – GSD IV; E, phosphorylase – GSD V, VI, VIII; F, fructokinase – GSD VII; G, glycogen synthetase – GSD 'O'; H, galactose-1-phosphate uridyltransferase – galactosaemia; I, fructose-1,6-diphosphatase, F1–6 diphosphatase deficiency.

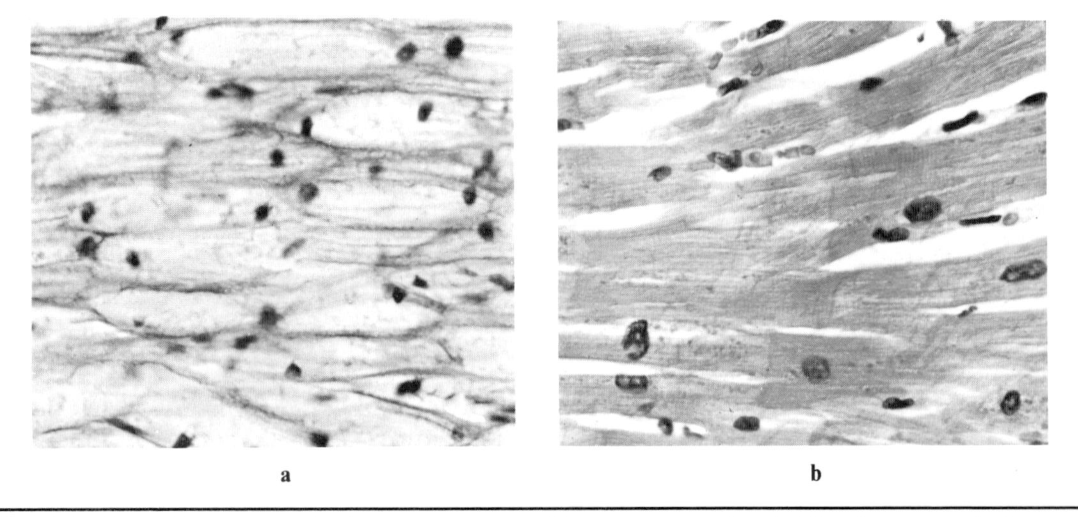

Fig. 7.2 Myocardium in Pompe's disease **a**, compared with normal myocardium **b**. The affected muscle fibres are distended with glycogen which does not stain with eosin but gives them a vacuolated appearance. ×460.

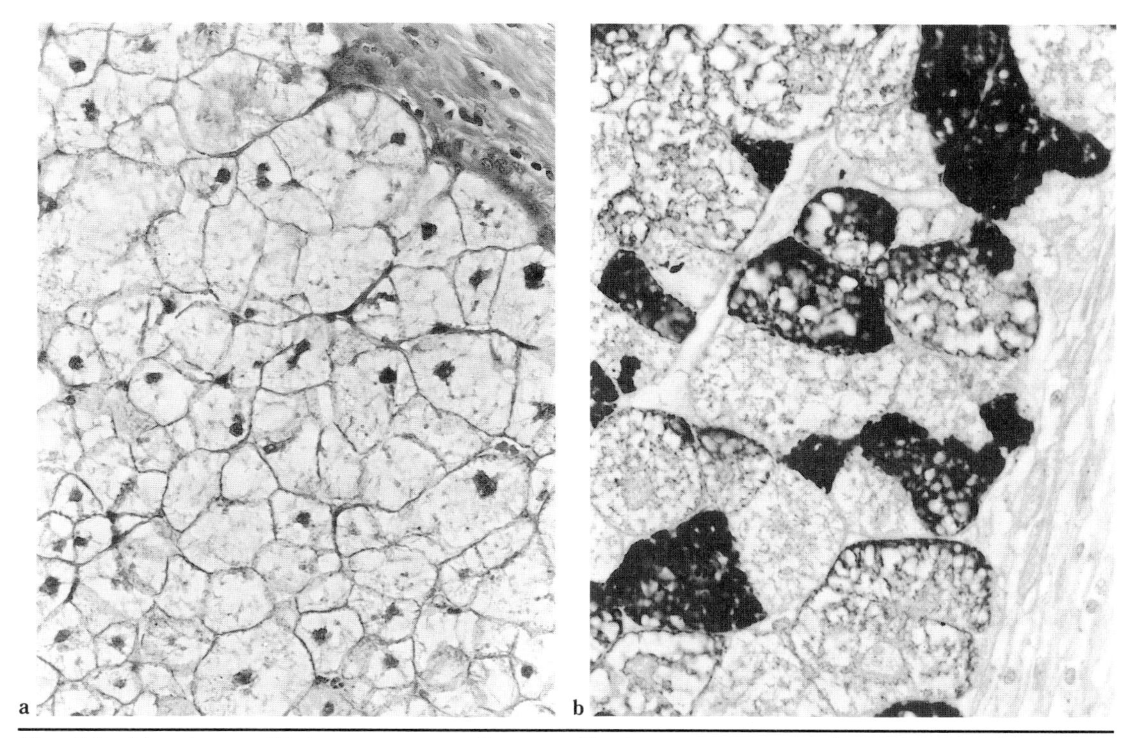

Fig. 7.3 Liver in type III glycogen storage disease. **a** The hepatocytes are swollen and their outlines sharply defined. ×98. **b** On PAS staining the abnormal accumulation of glycogen produces intense staining in some hepatocytes, in others the staining pattern is less intense and more diffuse. ×350.

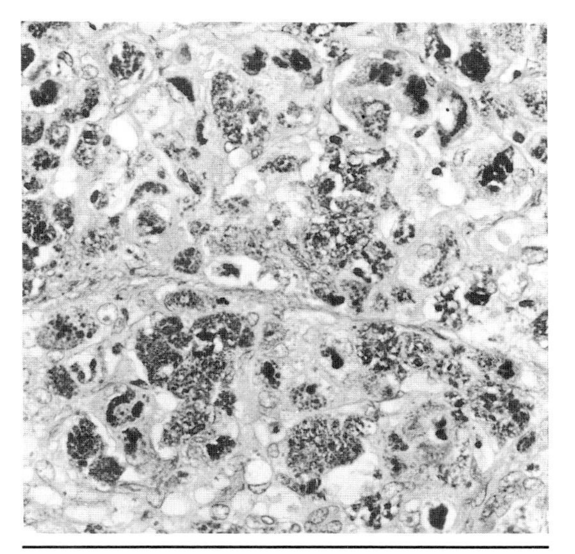

Fig. 7.4 Liver in type IV glycogen storage disease. Within hepatocytes there are diffuse aggregates of insoluble PAS positive diastase resistant glycogen, abnormal because of absence of the branching enzyme. PAS/diastase ×245.

vacuolated 'plant-cell'-like appearance of hepatocytes (Fig. 7.3). The diagnosis can be made by demonstrating excess glycogen in erythrocytes.

GSD type IV, due to deficiency of the 'branching' enzyme alpha-1,4-glucan-6-glycosyltransferase, is very rare. The affected tissues contain coarse aggregates of an abnormal form of glycogen (Fig. 7.4) with few branch points (long-chain length amylopectin) which is PAS positive even after diastase digestion but can be digested with pectinase. Cirrhosis with portal hypertension develops rapidly, leading to death in infancy.

In ***GSD type V***, muscle phosphorylase deficiency prevents release of glucose from glycogen. In these patients exercise intolerance with muscle weakness, muscle pain and sometimes muscle cramps are noted in late childhood. Myoglobinuria may occur and serum creatine kinase levels are elevated even at rest. Strenuous muscle exercise must be avoided. Oral administration of glucose will improve the symptoms.

In ***GSD type VI*** there is clinical evidence of muscle fatiguability. In this disorder skeletal muscle cannot metabolize glucose; the symptoms are similar to type V but are more severe and are not relieved by oral glucose. Erythrocytes are also affected, have a shortened half-life and there is a mild haemolytic anaemia.

Glycogen synthetase deficiency is sometimes known as GSD type O. Synthesis of glycogen from glucose-1-phosphate is greatly impaired. The liver contains increased lipid and very little glycogen; hyperglycaemia and seizures are common.

Other Abnormalities of Carbohydrate Metabolism

Galactose

Galactose is ingested as the disaccharide lactose which is the main carbohydrate present in milk. **Galactosaemia**, an autosomal recessive condition, may result from a deficiency of any of three enzymes involved in galactose metabolism – galactose-1-phosphate uridyltransferase (by far the commonest), galactokinase and uridine-diphosphate galactose-4-epimerase. The clinical features vary, depending on which enzyme is abnormal. On exposure to dietary lactose, usually in the first few days of life, there is accumulation of galactose and galactose-1-phosphate which are highly toxic. There is failure to thrive, with severe vomiting and diarrhoea. Severe liver injury develops within weeks, resulting in jaundice, hepatomegaly and ultimately cirrhosis. Cataract and neuronal injury may also occur. A diet free from lactose is required throughout childhood, and probably this is best maintained for life.

Fructose

The daily intake of fructose, as sucrose or the free monosaccharide, is about 100 g. It is metabolized in the small intestine, liver and kidney. Three defects of metabolism are known, all inherited as autosomal recessive.

Hereditary fructose intolerance is due to deficiency of fructose-1,6-diphosphate aldolase in the liver, kidney and gut. Ingestion of fructose leads to transient hypoglycaemia, vomiting and diarrhoea. There is failure to thrive and, with continued exposure, hepatomegaly and hepatic failure may develop. The liver shows fatty change, mild hepatitis and, in advanced cases, fibrosis which can progress to cirrhosis. A diet free of fructose is required; the prognosis is then excellent.

Fructose-1,6-diphosphatase deficiency is a severe disorder of gluconeogenesis. The clinical features develop soon after birth and include hepatomegaly, hypoglycaemia and lactic acidosis often precipitated by infection and producing hyperventilation, convulsions and coma. Liver biopsy shows marked fatty change and the enzyme deficiency is demonstrated on the biopsy material. Again a fructose-free diet is curative.

Essential fructosuria is a benign asymptomatic disorder due to hepatic fructokinase deficiency and is discovered on routine urine analysis.

Disorders of Lysosomal Storage

These comprise a large group of inherited diseases in which there is an abnormal accumulation of enzyme substrates within lysosomes. This has already been discussed for type II glycogen storage disease in which there is an enzyme defect; excess accumulation of amino acids may also occur, e.g. cystine in cystinosis (p. 271) due to a defect in lysosomal membrane transport. In addition, lysosomal storage may be induced by drugs which interfere with enzyme function. Thus amiodarone (and other drugs) causes a secondary form of phospholipidosis which involves alveolar macrophages, hepatocytes and other cells. It is in part due to binding of phospholipids in lysosomes by the cationic amphiphilic amiodarone molecule and in part due to inhibition of phospholipase A by this drug.

In this section, we discuss those disorders in which there is interference with the degradation by complex enzymatic systems of large molecules of many types. They are classified according to the type of substance which accumulates in the affected cells and includes various lipids, mucopolysaccharides and glycoproteins. They are all autosomal recessive disorders except for Hunter's disease and Fabry's disease which are X-linked. Some disorders affect almost all cell types while others are confined to only one, such as the neuron; these are sometimes referred to as neuronal storage diseases and are discussed in Chapter 18.

The Sphingolipidoses

These are characterized by the accumulation of various forms of sphingolipid, which are intermediates in glycolipid degradation (Table 7.2).

Gaucher's disease is the commonest lysosomal storage disorder and occurs in acute, subacute and chronic forms. There is a clinical overlap in these subtypes, but within any one family all affected individuals display the same form. In all types the enzyme glucocerebroside-β-glucosidase is deficient and glucocerebroside (glucosylceramide) accumulates preferentially within macrophages of the mononuclear phagocyte system. In the more common chronic (type I) form some enzyme activity is present. Patients present in childhood and survive into adulthood or may present in adulthood. Usually there is hepatosplenomegaly, while bone marrow involvement leads to anaemia. The long bones are deformed with flared metaphyses, and osteonecrosis (p. 961) may occur. In the acute (type II) form there is no residual enzyme activity, and the disease presents in infancy

Table 7.2 The major forms of sphingolipidoses

	Enzyme defect	Stored substance
Gaucher's disease	Glucocerebroside-β-glucosidase	Glucocerebroside (glucosylceramide)
Niemann–Pick disease		
Types A and B	Sphingomyelinase	Sphingomyelin, cholesterol and glycolipid
Types C and D	Uncertain	
G_{M1} gangliosidosis	β-Galactosidase	G_{M1} gangliosides
G_{M2} gangliosidosis		
Tay–Sachs disease	Hexosaminidase A	G_{M2} gangliosides and related glycolipids;
Sandhoff disease	Hexosaminidase A and B	oligosaccharides also in Sandhoff disease
Fabry's disease	α-Galactosidase	Ceramide trihexosides
Farber's disease	Acid ceramidase	Ceramide
Krabbe's leucodystrophy*	Galactocerebroside-β-galactosidase	Galactocerebroside (galactosylceramide)
Metachromatic leucodystrophy*	Arylsulphatase A	Galactocerebroside sulphate

*See Chapter 18.

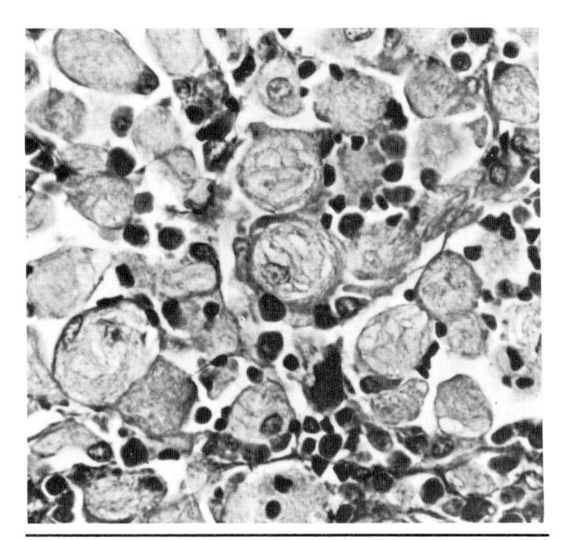

Fig. 7.5 Section of spleen in Gaucher's disease, showing the characteristic large cells with striated and vacuolated cytoplasm. ×440.

with hepatosplenomegaly, failure to thrive and progressive neurological impairment leading to death within 2 years. In type III brain involvement is less marked.

In all forms of the disease most organs contain numerous Gaucher cells. These are large, 20–100 μm in diameter and have a characteristic fibrillary cytoplasm described as 'crumpled silk' with strands of PAS positive glucocerebroside (Fig. 7.5). Variable degrees of fibrosis may occur.

Niemann-Pick disease is particularly prevalent in the Jewish race. Several forms are recognized, but within these there is considerable heterogeneity. In type A, which includes 70% of all cases, children in the first few weeks of life develop hepatosplenomegaly, lymphadenopathy and progressive deterioration in cerebral function. In half the cases a 'cherry-red' spot is seen at the macula, resembling that seen in Tay–Sachs disease. Occasional patients present with neonatal hepatitis. In type B, the disease presents later in infancy, with hepatosplenomegaly and pulmonary infiltration while the central nervous system is spared. Uncommonly, asymptomatic cases are discovered in adulthood because of hepatosplenomegaly or the presence of foam cells in the marrow.

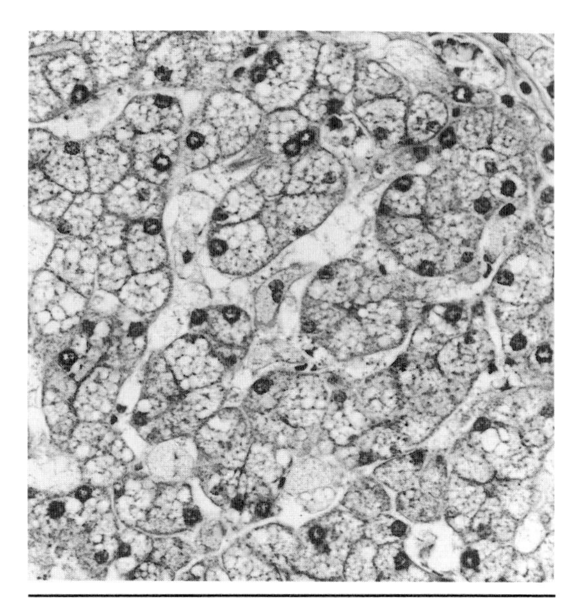

Fig. 7.6 Niemann–Pick disease type A. The accumulation of sphingomyelin in both hepatocytes and Kupffer cells gives a coarse, vacuolated foamy appearance to the cytoplasm. ×245.

In both types A and B, deficiency of sphingomyelinase leads to the accumulation of sphingomyelin. Macrophages throughout the mononuclear phagocyte system, hepatocytes and, in type A disease, neurons within the central and peripheral nervous systems, have vacuolated and foamy cytoplasm (Fig. 7.6). Involvement of the gut may lead to malabsorption and diarrhoea. In type A the brain is atrophic with gliosis and secondary demyelination. Death usually occurs within the first 2 years of life.

In types C and D Niemann–Pick disease the levels of sphingomyelinase are normal and the precise enzyme defect is unknown. The accumulation of sphingomyelin is less marked and cholesterol and other lipids are also stored in excess. These groups usually present in juveniles with varying neural and visceral involvement leading to progressive mental deterioration and hepatosplenomegaly.

G_{M1} gangliosidosis due to deficiency of β galactosidase occurs in two forms; the generalized, infantile form (type I) is characterized by deposition of the ganglioside G_{M1} in the brain and various

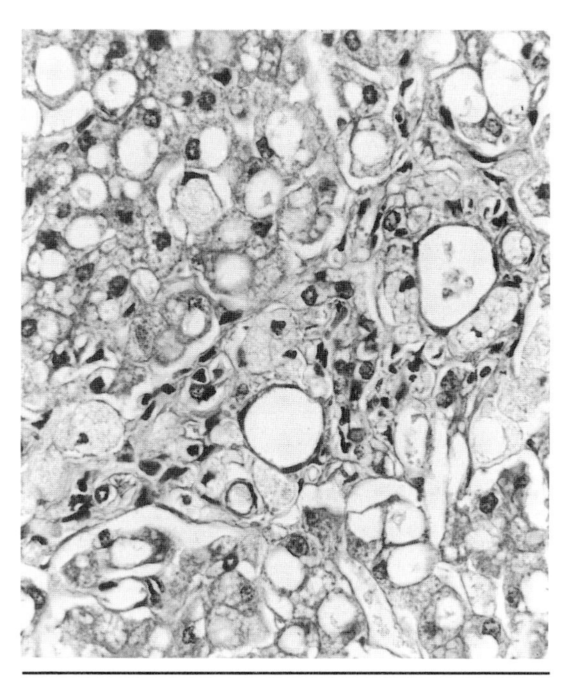

Fig. 7.7 Liver in G_{M1} gangliosidosis. Some hepatocytes have vacuolated cytoplasm. Kupffer cells and macrophages within the portal tract also contain ganglioside G_{M1} and are vacuolated. ×350.

viscera, leading to mental retardation, blindness and hepatosplenomegaly (Fig. 7.7). Most children die before the age of 2 years. In the juvenile form (type II) the viscera are usually not involved and slowly progressive neurological deterioration occurs, with death in later childhood. The neurons and affected parenchymal cells in other organs are enlarged with vacuolated cytoplasm.

In ***G_{M2} gangliosidosis*** G_{M2} gangliosides accumulate within the brain as a result of hexosaminidase A deficiency. Infantile Tay–Sachs disease is the most severe form in which progressive neurological deterioration leads to dementia within the first year of life and death in 2–3 years. The child becomes totally blind and ophthalmoscopy demonstrates a typical macular cherry-red spot. Tay–Sachs disease occurs predominantly in Ashkenazi Jews with an incidence of 1 in 2000 live births. In the non-Jewish form of G_{M2} gangliosidosis (Sandhoff disease) there is deficiency of both hexosaminidase A and B. The clinical features are identical. Milder forms of the G_{M2} gangliosidoses may present in childhood or early adult life.

Fabry's disease is X-linked, and female carriers may show a mild form of the disease. Glycosphingolipids are deposited as crystals within endothelial and smooth muscle cells of blood vessels (Fig. 7.8) and within the mononuclear-phagocyte system. The crystals show Maltese cross birefringence when viewed in polarized light. Patients usually die between 35 and 45 years from cardiac or renal failure or cerebrovascular disease. Renal transplantation has been successfully carried out. Cutaneous angiokeratomas appear in childhood and increase in number through adult life. A clinically distinct feature is the 'Fabry crisis', a brief or prolonged episode of excruciating pain in the hands and feet, thought to be due to involvement of the autonomic nervous system.

The Mucopolysaccharidoses (MPS)

This is a group of disorders characterized by the intracellular deposition and increased urinary excretion of mucopolysaccharides (glycosaminoglycans). The specific enzyme defects and deposited mucopolysaccharide of each disease are summarized in Table 7.3. The mucopolysaccharides accumulate in cells of the mononuclear phagocyte system, vascular endothelium and smooth muscle cells, fibroblasts, parenchymal cells and neurons (Fig. 7.9). In all cases prenatal diagnosis can be made by amniocentesis or chorionic villus sampling (Fig. 7.9).

Type I MPS (Hurler's syndrome). Affected children are dwarfed and have a characteristic facial appearance which gave rise to the old name of **gargoylism**. The head is enlarged, with prominent supraorbital ridges, the nose is broad, the lips are thick and the tongue enlarged (Fig. 7.10). The

Table 7.3 The mucopolysaccharidoses

	Enzyme defect	Storage/urinary product
I-H (Hurler)	α-L-Iduronidase	Dermatan sulphate, heparan sulphate
I-S (Scheie)		
II (Hunter) (X-linked)	Iduronate sulphamidase	
III (Sanfilippo) – types A to D	(A) Heparan sulphate sulphamidase (B) α-*N*-Acetylglucosaminidase (C) Acetyl CoA: aminodeoxyglucoside *N*-acetyltransferase (D) *N*-Acetylglucosamine-6-sulphatase	Heparan sulphate
IV (Morquio) – types A and B	(A) *N*-Acetylgalactosamine-6-sulphatase (B) β-Galactosidase	Keratan sulphate
VI (Maroteaux–Lamy)	*N*-Acetylgalactosamine-4-sulphatase (arylsulphatase B)	Dermatan sulphate
VII (Sly)	β-Glucuronidase	Dermatan sulphate and heparan sulphate

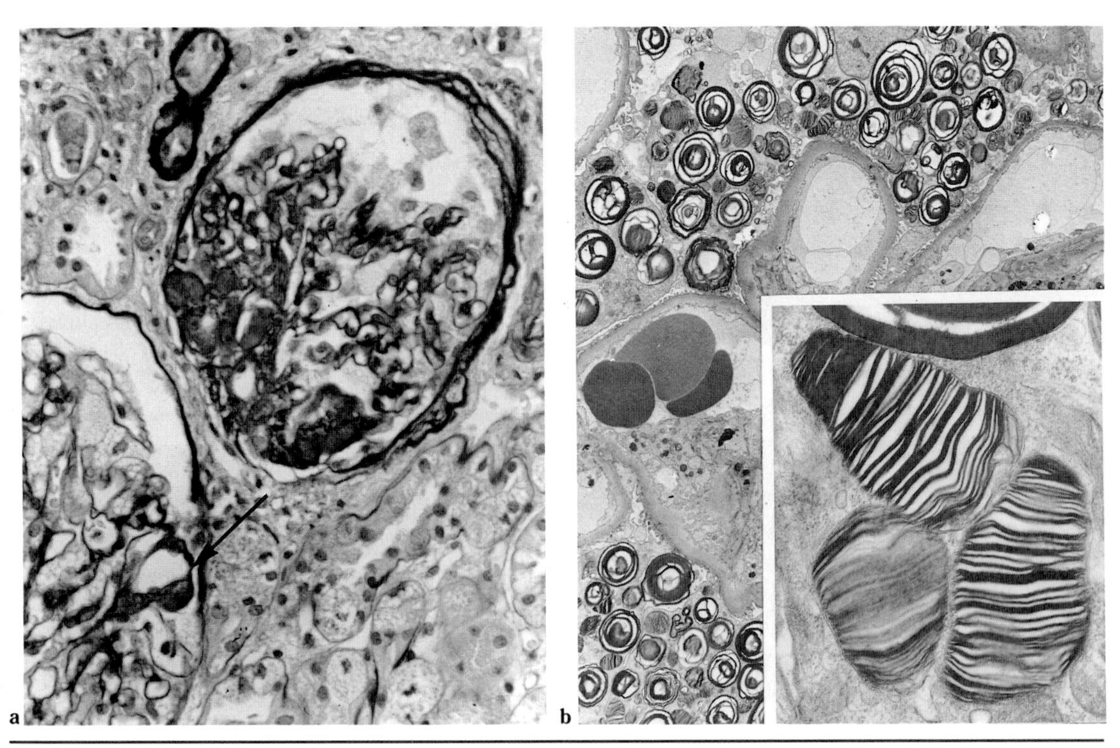

Fig. 7.8 Fabry's disease. **a** Renal biopsy showing ceramide trihexoside accumulation in glomerular endothelial cells: in the upper glomerulus numerous groups of cells are affected, whereas in the lower one a single capillary tuft is involved (arrow). PAS ×245. **b** On electron microscopy numerous dense laminated inclusions are present in endothelial cells; some inclusions have a striking 'zebra-like' appearance (inset). ×2000 (inset ×20 000).

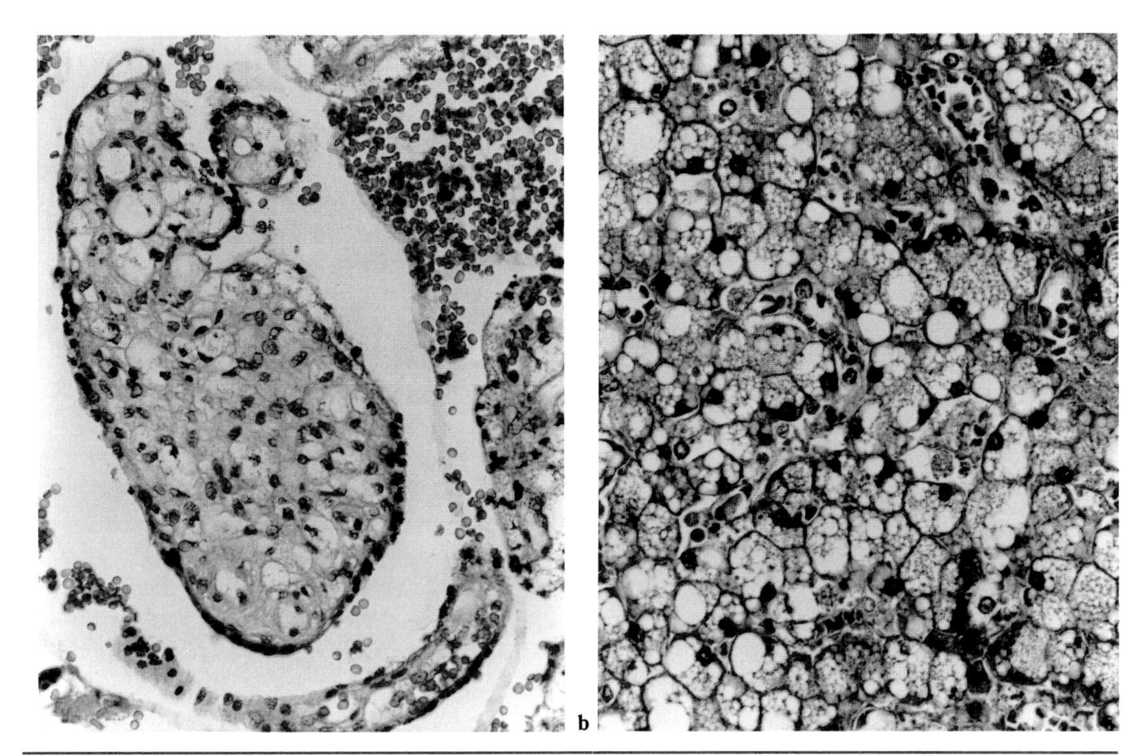

Fig. 7.9 **a** Mucopolysaccharidosis type II (Hunter's syndrome). Placental tissue showing a swollen villus within which there are numerous distended vacuolated cells laden with mucopolysaccharides. ×200. **b** Liver in Hurler's syndrome: the hepatocytes are swollen and vacuolated. ×294.

cornea becomes opaque due to the deposition of mucopolysaccharides and blindness may result. Hepatosplenomegaly and skeletal deformity are common; the vertebrae are of abnormal shape and there is often kyphoscoliosis. The limb bones are broader and shorter than normal, and the sutures of the skull are widened. Mental retardation is almost invariable. Death occurs in childhood from respiratory infection or from cardiac failure due to aortic valvular disease or myocardial ischaemia because of coronary artery involvement. Bone marrow transplantation replaces the defective enzyme and halts progression of the disease, but the mental and skeletal changes are not reversed.

Scheie's syndrome, a clinically mild disease, is due to the same enzyme defect as Hurler's syndrome. The main features are joint stiffness, aortic valve disease and corneal opacification. Mental and physical development are normal. A form with features intermediate between Hurler's syndrome and Scheie's syndrome (type I H/S) has been described.

Type II MPS (Hunter's syndrome) is an X-linked recessive disorder similar to type I, but rather less severe. Corneal opacification does not occur, but deafness may develop. Severe (type A) and mild (type B) forms are recognized.

Type III MPS (Sanfilippo syndrome), consists of four biochemically distinct subgroups. In all these, however, heparan sulphate accumulates. The brunt of the disease falls on the nervous system, and mental deficiency is severe.

Type IV MPS (Morquio's syndrome) presents after infancy, with severe skeletal deformities and dwarfism. The base of the skull is often flattened (platybasia) and there is deformity and fusion of vertebrae producing spinal cord compression. Intellect is usually normal.

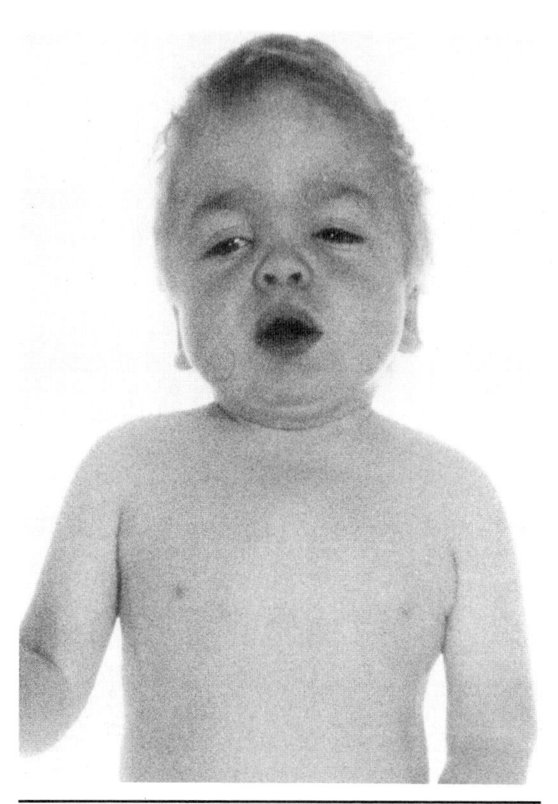

Fig. 7.10 Young male with type I mucopolysaccharidosis (Hurler's syndrome). The head is swollen, there are prominent supraorbital ridges and a peculiar vacant expression. (By courtesy of Professor Forrester Cockburn.)

The Mucolipidoses (ML)

These conditions are extremely rare (Table 7.4). As indicated in Chapter 1 ML-II and ML-III are the result of an abnormal lysosomal enzyme transport system. The defect prevents addition of a mannose-6-phosphate recognition marker to lysosomal enzymes in the RER; without this marker, the enzyme cannot be packaged into lysosomes and so there is an 'enzyme lack'. In ML-II, the numerous inclusion bodies composed of fibrillary and granular material which accumulate within membrane-bound vacuoles in fibroblasts and other mesenchymal cells give rise to the term I-cell disease. Less prominent inclusions are seen in ML-III.

The Glycoproteinoses

This is a group of lesions characterized by deficiencies of enzymes involved in the degradation of the oligosaccharide side chains of glycoproteins. They include sialidosis (formerly mucolipidosis type I), mannosidosis, fucosidosis and aspartylglycosaminuria. Oligosaccharides are present in the urine and in each biochemical type there is a distinctive pattern of excretion. The clinical features vary but often resemble those of Hurler's syndrome. They include abnormal facies, mental retardation, hepatosplenomegaly and, in most types, vacuolated lymphocytes are present in the circulation.

Table 7.4 The mucolipidoses

	Enzyme defect	Clinical features
II (I-cell disease)	Uridine diphosphate-*N*-acetylglucosamine: lysosomal enzyme precursor *N*-acetylglucosamine phosphate transferase	Hurler-like
III (Pseudo-Hurler polydystrophy)		Hurler-like; much milder than II
IV	Uncertain; possibly ganglioside sialidase	Psychomotor retardation; severe visual impairment

Mucolipidosis type I is now classified as sialidosis (a glycoproteinosis).

Disorders of Lipoprotein and Lipid Metabolism

Lipids are transported in the plasma as spherical particles in which protein molecules (apoproteins) render the lipids soluble. These lipoproteins have different electrophoretic mobility and are of varying size, diminishing size being associated with increasing density. They are of differing composition (Table 7.5). Hydrophobic (non-polar) lipids, triglycerides and cholesteryl ester form the core of the particles and are enclosed by a layer of apoprotein, small amounts of cholesterol and hydrophilic (polar) phospholipids. Disturbances of lipoprotein and lipid metabolism are intimately associated with atheroma and cardiovascular disease and further details of their metabolism and composition are to be found in Chapter 12. In this section the molecular defects and other diseases associated with disturbance of lipoprotein and lipid metabolism are reviewed (Table 7.6).

Abnormalities of Apoproteins

Apo B Proteins

The two apo B proteins, B-100 and B-48, are products of a single gene located on the short arm of chromosome 2 (the terminology reflects the relative molecular weight of these and similar proteins; apo B is ranked as 100 and smaller molecules are ranked numerically). Apo B-100 and apo B-48 are the predominant apoproteins in very low density (VLDL) and low density (LDL) lipoproteins and in chylomicrons respectively and have an essential role in their secretion in the liver and intestine. There are a number of syndromes related to total absence of both B-100 and B-48 (abetalipoproteinaemia), partial lack of both (various hypobetalipoproteinaemias) and absence of either B-100 or B-48 in isolation.

Table 7.5 Features of the various lipoproteins

Particle	Diameter (nm)	Approximate triglyceride/ cholesterol ratio and cholesterol content (%)	Apolipoprotein
Chylomicron	80–1200	20:1 (<5%)	A-1, A-2, A-4, B-48 and C
Very low density lipoprotein (VLDL)	30–80	3:1 (25%)	B-48, C, E
Intermediate density lipoprotein (IDL)	25–35	2:3 (40%)	B-100, E
Low density lipoprotein (LDL)	15–25	1:5 (65%)	B-100
High density lipoprotein (HDL)	5–15	1:4 (<20%)	A-1, A-2, C

Table 7.6 Summary of apoprotein, enzyme and receptor defects in lipoprotein and lipid disorders

	Defect	Clinical features*
Apoprotein abnormalities		
Apo B-100 and apo B-48 absence or partial lack of both Apo B-100 absence Apo B-48 absence	Heterogeneous including abnormalities of processing and secretion; truncated lipoprotein molecule	Abetalipoproteinaemia and hypobetalipoproteinaemia with malabsorption, visual deterioration, haemolytic anaemia and spinocerebellar ataxia
Apo C-II deficiency†	Structural defect in the protein	Type I hyperlipidaemia; hypertriglyceridaemia, pancreatitis, xanthomas
Apo A-I (Milano)	Single amino-acid substitution	Reduced HDL
Apo A-I + apo C-II deficiency	Rearrangement in apo A-I gene and apo C-II gene in some kindreds	May be associated with very low HDL levels (see text – Tangier disease)
Apo E variants	Single amino-acid substitutions	Type III hyperlipidaemia; elevation of plasma cholesterol and triglycerides; early atheroma
Lipoprotein enzyme deficiencies		
Lecithin cholesterol acyltransferase (LCAT) deficiency	Gene mutation; absent or inactive enzyme	Corneal opacities, mild hypertriglyceridaemia, and reduced levels of HDL
Hepatic lipase deficiency	Unknown	Type IV hyperlipidaemia; mild elevation of IDL and HDL
Lipoprotein lipase deficiency Lipoprotein lipase inhibitor	Unknown Circulating inhibitor of lipoprotein lipase	Type I hyperlipidaemia; hypertriglyceridaemia, pancreatitis, xanthomas
Receptor defects		
LDL receptor	Many mutations produce 4 classes of defect:	
	(1) Absence of receptor synthesis (2) Receptor secretion blocked between RER & Golgi (3) Defective receptor binding (4) Defective clustering of receptors in coated pits	Type II hyperlipidaemia; severe elevation of LDL, premature atheroma

*The various types of hyperlipidaemia are discussed in Chapter 12.

†Apo C-II is an essential co-factor for lipoprotein lipase and a deficiency of either causes type I hyperlipidaemia.

Abetalipoproteinaemia

Abetalipoproteinaemia is associated with absence of chylomicrons, VLDL and LDL from the plasma. There are complex 'compensatory' changes affecting other lipoproteins but essentially these patients have markedly reduced plasma cholesterol and triglycerides. The clinical features include malabsorption of fat and fat-soluble vitamins from birth, associated with the accumulation of lipid within vacuoles in the duodenal and proximal jejunal mucosa (p. 724). An abnormality of red cell shape, acanthocytosis (Fig. 7.11), results from disturbance in the lipid composition of the erythrocyte membrane, and causes reduced red cell survival with a haemolytic anaemia. The anaemia is aggravated by deficiency of iron and folate because of malabsorption. Neuromuscular disorders, in particular spinocerebellar ataxia, are associated with neuronal loss in the spinal ganglia and consequent posterior column degeneration. These lesions are in part due to lack of vitamin E. Retinal degeneration with loss of photoreceptors and pigment epithelium occurs, possibly due to lack of vitamins A and E. Accumulation of lipofuscin pigment produces ophthalmoscopic changes similar to that seen in retinitis pigmentosa (p. 881).

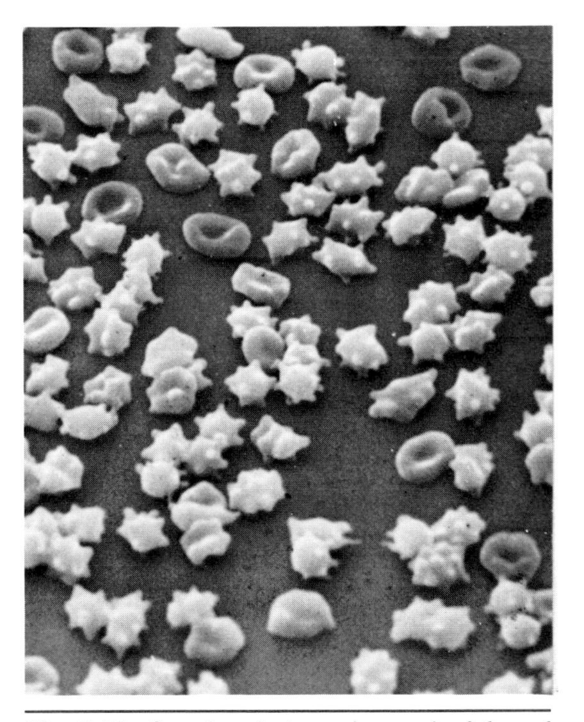

Fig. 7.11 Scanning electron micrograph of the red cells in a patient with abetalipoproteinaemia. Most of the red cells show the deformity of acanthocytosis; a few show the appearance of normal biconcave discs.

Apo E Protein

Abnormalities of apo E protein cause type III hyperlipidaemia in which there is increased plasma cholesterol and triglycerides. The patients have an increased incidence of premature atheroma, and are obese with xanthomas on the palms and tendons. A number of apo E variants have been described involving substitution of a single amino acid. Chylomicron and VLDL remnants (β-VLDL) are present in the plasma and the latter are taken up by macrophages with xanthoma formation.

Other Apoproteins

Apo A-I and A-II are associated with high density lipoproteins (HDL). Single amino-acid substitutions in apo-A-I, and deficiencies of apo A-I and apo A-II may result in very low levels of plasma HDL, a risk factor for ischaemic heart disease. Low levels of HDL also occur in association with deficiency of lipoprotein lipase, its essential co-factor apo C-II and lecithin cholesterol acyltransferase (LCAT).

In ***Tangier disease*** there is absence of plasma HDL and very low plasma cholesterol levels but raised triglyceride levels. There are low levels of some apo A proteins, but the precise defects are not known. Cells of the mononuclear phagocyte system take up large amounts of cholesterol ester and have abundant foamy cytoplasm (Fig. 7.12). The spleen, lymph nodes and tonsils are enlarged; the tonsils are bright yellow and this feature is pathognomonic. Neuropathy may result from lipid accumulation in Schwann cells.

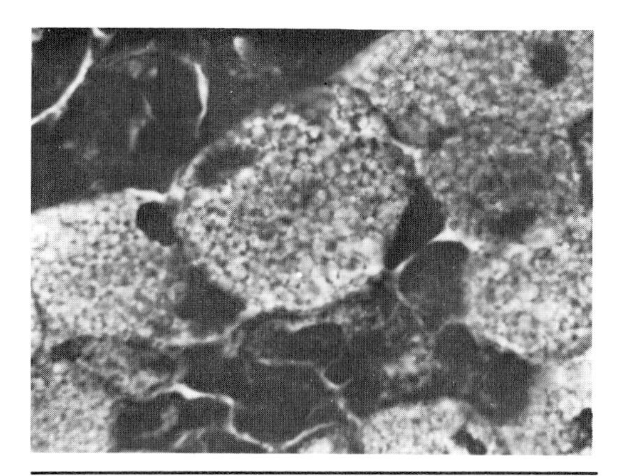

Fig. 7.12 Foamy cells in Tangier disease – macrophages distended with multiple fine droplets of doubly refractile lipid. Photographed through crossed polarizing filters. ×500.

Enzyme Defects

Lipoprotein lipase deficiency results in accumulation of chylomicrons in the circulation with very high plasma triglyceride levels producing a milky plasma. A similar clinical picture is seen in apo D-II deficiency and also in a very rare familial disorder associated with the presence of an inhibitor lipoprotein lipase. Patients present in childhood with recurrent episodes of pancreatitis, cutaneous xanthomatosis and hepatosplenomegaly. There is no predisposition to atheroma and a low fat diet is clinically 'curative'.

In ***lecithin cholesterol acyltransferase (LCAT) deficiency*** cholesterol cannot be esterified resulting in increased levels of triglyceride in the plasma, within VLDL and LDL, and there are low levels of HDL. Patients develop corneal opacities, early-onset atheroma and cutaneous xanthomas. There are abnormalities of red cells with anaemia, and foamy histiocytic deposits in marrow, spleen and glomeruli. Renal failure can occur.

LDL Receptor Defects

The mechanisms involved have been discussed in Chapter 1 and the four classes of defect are summarized in Table 7.6. These are associated with marked elevation of plasma LDL and consequently of plasma cholesterol. There is a high incidence of early-onset atheroma with subcutaneous and tendinous xanthomatosis and prominent arcus corneae. Homozygotes have four to five times normal plasma cholesterol levels and die of ischaemic heart disease within the first three decades. In heterozygotes cholesterol levels are two to three times normal from birth, and ischaemic heart disease develops usually after 30 years of age. The heterozygous frequency is one per 500, and one in a million of the population is homozygous.

Disorders of Amino-acid Metabolism

The large number of genetically transmitted abnormalities which affect the metabolism of amino acids fall into two major groups, both of which are almost always inherited as autosomal recessive traits. In one group the transport of amino acids across cell membranes is affected. These are described in the next section of this chapter. In the second group enzymes involved in amino-acid metabolism cause the accumulation of the enzyme substrate and also of products of alternative metabolic pathways. Many of these substances are toxic and may induce organ damage. In addition, lack of the normal product of the enzymatic reaction may lead to lack of an important end product; thus, in albinism, the formation of melanin pigment is diminished, sometimes due to deficiency of the enzyme tyrosinase.

Phenylalanine and Tyrosine

The normal metabolic pathways involved in the metabolism of these amino acids are summarized in Fig. 7.13.

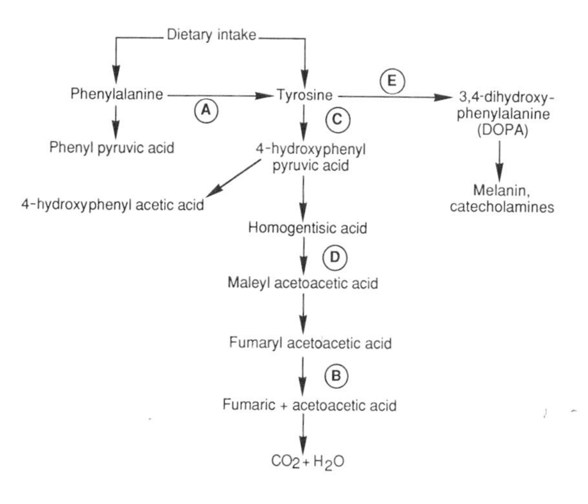

Fig. 7.13 Outline of phenylalanine and tyrosine metabolism. Enzyme defects are indicated as follows: A, phenylalanine-4-mono-oxygenase resulting in phenylketonuria; B, fumaryl acetoacetic acid hydrolase – tyrosinaemia type I; C, tyrosine aminotransferase – tyrosinaemia type II; D, homogentisic acid oxidase – alkaptonuria; E, tyrosinase – albinism (some variants).

The Hyperphenylalaninaemias (Phenylketonuria)

Phenylalanine is an essential amino acid, the daily requirement for which is estimated at 200–750 mg. Hyperphenylalaninaemia can occur as a result of deficiency of the enzyme phenylalanine 4-mono-oxygenase (phenylalanine hydroxylase): there are less severe variants with some enzyme activity in which phenylketonuria does not occur. The estimated worldwide incidence of phenylketonuria is 100 per million live births, an incidence which is higher in the United Kingdom particularly in those of a Celtic background, with 190 per million live births. Much less commonly (one per million live births) deficiencies in other enzymes involved in phenylalanine metabolism may lead to hyperphenylalaninaemia.

As a result of the enzyme deficiency conversion of phenylalanine to tyrosine is inhibited. This results in increased blood levels of phenylalanine and in the formation of phenyl ketones such as phenylpyruvate and phenylacetate, hence the term phenylketonuria. This is a good example of a genetic disorder in which an environmental factor, in this case dietary, is essential for the disease to become manifest.

Clinically, patients present in early childhood with psychomotor delay which, if untreated, progresses to profound mental handicap. The child is often hyperkinetic and seizures occur in about half the cases. Excess phenylalanine is thought to be responsible for these neurological effects. Affected individuals are often pale skinned with fair hair and blue eyes, probably reflecting interference by phenylalanine in melanin synthesis. Pathologically, there is impaired myelination and neuronal development. The fetus of mothers with inadequate dietary control or partial deficiency of phenylalanine hydroxylase may be affected by maternal hyperphenylalaninaemia.

The Guthrie screening test will detect hyperphenylalaninaemia in neonates; as yet no generally applicable test is available for prenatal diagnosis, but it is thought that linkage analysis based on DNA restriction fragment length polymorphism may allow antenatal detection in families where a known defect exists. Treatment consists of a diet free from phenylalanine. Since most proteins contain phenylalanine the diet has to be carefully prepared so as to ensure an adequate calorie intake and adequate amounts of essential amino acids and trace elements. There is some evidence that restriction need not be continued after the age of 10, but this is still debatable. Clearly it is essential to restrict the diet of pregnant women in order to protect the fetus.

Tyrosinaemia

The enzyme deficiencies which may result in tyrosinaemia and tyrosinuria are outlined in Fig. 7.13.

Tyrosinaemia, type I is due to a deficiency of fumaryl acetoacetase hydroxylase with the accumulation of fumaryl acetoacetate and elevated plasma levels of tyrosine and methionine. The acute form presents in the first few weeks of life, with vomiting, diarrhoea, oedema and hepatomegaly and, if untreated, death from liver failure occurs in a few months. The renal tubular epithelium is damaged and aminoaciduria (Fanconi syndrome) develops. Hypoglycaemia occurs as a consequence of hyperplasia of the islets of Langerhans. A chronic form exists where the clinical features are similar, but it progresses more slowly and hypophosphataemia with rickets becomes a prominent feature.

Most patients die in childhood, although a diet low in tyrosine and phenylalanine may limit the progression of the disease. There are distinctive abnormalities in the liver (Fig. 7.14) with fatty change, pseudoglandular transformation, chronic hepatitis, fibrosis and prominent nodular regeneration; primary liver cell carcinoma occurs in up to 40% of cases. Liver transplantation has been beneficial in a few cases but the renal complications are not prevented.

In ***tyrosinaemia, type II***, tyrosine accumulates, with the formation of needle shaped intracellular crystals, as a consequence of tyrosine aminotransferase deficiency. Mental handicap, hyperkeratosis of the skin, and corneal ulceration and conjunctivitis occur early in life. Dietary restriction is required to maintain low blood tyrosine levels.

In **tyrosinosis** (asymptomatic tyrosinaemia), tyrosine and the metabolite 4-hydroxyphenylpyruvate accumulate in the plasma.

Alkaptonuria (Ochronosis)

Alkaptonuria is the result of deficiency of homogentisic acid oxidase. Homogentisic acid accumulates and is excreted in the urine which darkens on oxidation. In addition homogentisic acid polymerizes to form a brown black melanin-like pigment which is deposited particularly in fibrous tissue and cartilage. The cross-linking of collagen in the articular cartilage is inhibited and premature osteoarthritis develops (p. 986).

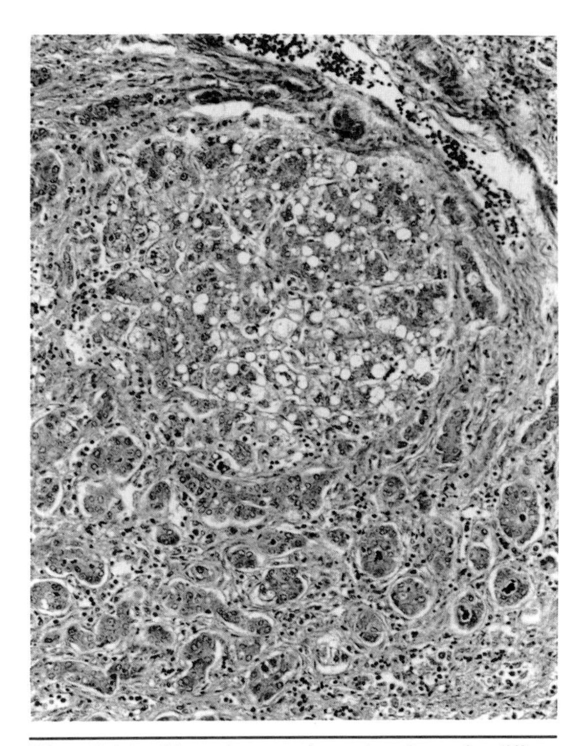

Fig. 7.14 Liver in tyrosinaemia: there is diffuse fibrosis and the liver cells show pseudoglandular transformation surrounding bile concretions: there is also well defined nodular transformation. ×98.

Albinism

This term refers to a heterogeneous group of inherited conditions characterized by defective synthesis of melanin. The world prevalence is approximately 1 in 20 000. The abnormality may affect both the skin and the eye (oculocutaneous albinism – OCA) or predominantly the eye (ocular albinism – OA). In some patients there is a defect in tyrosinase activity.

The major problems associated with albinism are an increased risk of sun induced skin tumours, particularly squamous carcinomas, and visual abnormalities. Optic neuronal pathways are abnormal, in particular the decussation of fibres in the optic chiasma, and binocular vision is often very limited. Visual acuity and distant vision are also usually impaired.

Disorders of Membrane Transport Systems

These disorders may be the result of defects in the membranes of organelles or of the plasma membrane itself. Transport of various molecules may be affected: of glucose and other sugars leading to renal glycosuria and malabsorption of glucose and galactose; of amino acids leading to aminoaciduria or, in cystinosis, to lysosomal accumulation of cystine; of phosphates leading to hypophosphataemic rickets (p. 953); of electrolytes such as Cl^- in cystic fibrosis; and of various peptides and low molecular weight proteins in Fanconi's syndrome.

Defects of Amino-acid Transport

Amino acids pass freely into the glomerular filtrate, and are almost entirely reabsorbed by active transport by the epithelial cells of the proximal convoluted tubule. Inherited defects in renal handling may be due to abnormalities of specific transport molecules for individual amino acids (e.g. tryptophan), or groups of similar amino acids (e.g. neutral amino acids). These specific defects must be distinguished from generalized aminoaciduria which may be primary or secondary. Other inborn errors (e.g. galactosaemia and Wilson's disease) induce aminoaciduria due to the toxic effect of a metabolite on the renal tubules. Drugs may also interfere with tubular transport function and cause aminoaciduria. The Fanconi syndrome comprises generalized aminoaciduria, renal glycosuria, hyperphosphaturia, rickets or osteomalacia, hypokalaemia, one type of renal tubular acidosis and renal loss of various peptides and low molecular weight proteins. The various syndromes are summarized in Table 7.7.

Hartnup Disease

In this autosomal recessive disorder the defect lies in the transport system for neutral amino acids (including alanine, serine, leucine, tryptophan) and may affect both the renal tubules and the small bowel or each of these systems separately. Amino-acid transport in other organs is normal. Affected individuals may be asymptomatic or may develop a pellagra-like syndrome (p. 349) with photosensitivity skin reactions, cerebellar ataxia and neuropsychiatric disturbance including major psychoses. There is sometimes mental retardation. Malabsorption and increased urinary secretion of tryptophan are thought to lead to tryptophan deficiency and hence niacin deficiency with clinical features resembling pellagra. Other than contributing to tryptophan deficiency, the aminoaciduria has no clinical consequences. Nicotinamide replacement therapy may improve the pellagra-like effects but does not affect the basic defect.

Cystinosis

In this autosomal recessive condition cystine accumulates and forms crystals within lysosomes in most body tissues (Fig. 7.15). There is normal absorption and renal excretion of cystine; although lysosomal uptake of cystine is normal, lysosomal

Table 7.7 Causes of aminoaciduria

A **Specific aminoacidurias**	Transport defect for	Clinical features
Hartnup disease	Neutral amino acids	Photosensitivity, neuropsychiatric manifestations
Blue diaper syndrome	Tryptophan	Urinary tryptophan metabolites oxidized to indigo blue; growth retardation may be seen
Familial iminoglycinuria	Glycine, proline, hydroxyproline	Probably harmless biochemical abnormality
Lysinuric protein intolerance	Dibasic amino acids (lysine, ornithine, arginine)	Failure to thrive, hyperammonaemia, neutropenia, mental handicap
Cystinuria	Cystine and dibasic amino acids	Urinary 'cystine' stones

B **Generalized aminoacidurias**

Primary (idiopathic)

Secondary due to inborn errors of metabolism including:
galactosaemia; tyrosinaemia type I; glycogen storage disease type I; cystinosis; hereditary fructose intolerance; Wilson's disease; congenital renal tubular acidosis

Acquired, secondary to:
renal diseases (p. 924); drugs and heavy metals (p. 922); malignant disease, e.g. multiple myeloma.

clearance is impaired. The clinical manifestations are heterogeneous; in severe cases renal impairment with progressive glomerular damage leads to death in the first decade of life, while a benign form is found in which crystals are found in small amounts in only a few tissues such as the cornea. Transplantation can correct the renal disease but cystine accumulation in the retina and cornea, in endocrine glands and in the brain leads to blindness, diabetes mellitus and hypothyroidism or cerebral atrophy.

Cystic Fibrosis (Mucoviscidosis)

Cystic fibrosis is a disorder characterized by the production of abnormally viscid secretions by exocrine glands including the pancreas, the intestine and the mucus-secreting glands of the respiratory and gastrointestinal tracts. There are also secretory abnormalities involving the sweat glands, liver, salivary glands and glands of the reproductive organs. The consequences of blockage of ducts by inspissated secretions include atrophy of secretory acini with exocrine failure, and retention of secretions predisposing to bacterial infection. Thus pancreatic involvement leads to malabsorption, while recurrent respiratory infections are the commonest cause of death, usually in adolescence or early adult life.

Inheritance. Cystic fibrosis is autosomal recessive and the commonest genetically transmitted disorder in Caucasians, affecting approximately one in 2000 live births. The prevalence of heterozygous carriers, who are usually asymptomatic, is around one in 25.

Clinical Features

Because of its high incidence cystic fibrosis is an important cause of pulmonary and gastrointestinal

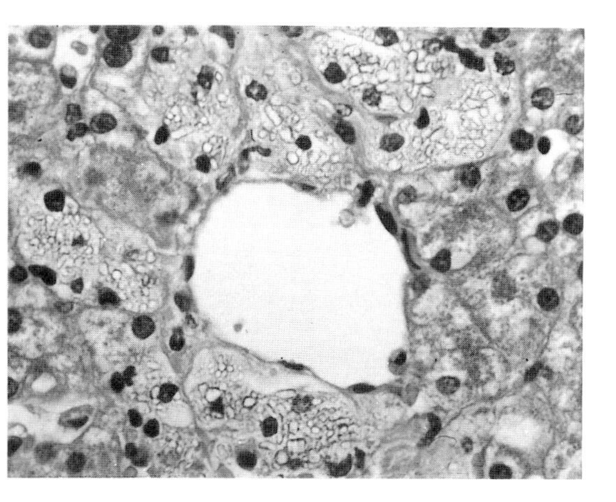

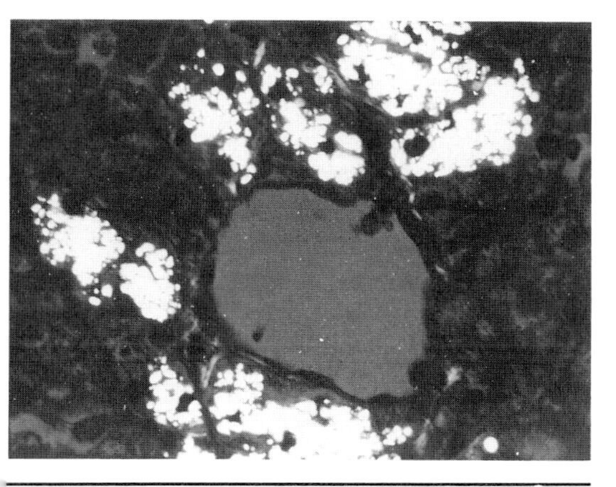

Fig. 7.15 Liver in cystinosis: cystine crystals are present within Kupffer cell aggregates (upper) and demonstrate brilliant birefringence when viewed under polarized light (lower).

dysfunction in infancy and childhood. It usually presents in infancy with repeated respiratory infections, failure to thrive, and malabsorption with steatorrhoea. In 10% of patients thick intestinal secretions cause obstruction of the terminal ileum in the neonatal period. This condition, known as meconium ileus, may also occur *in utero*, causing perforation of the intestine and meconium peritonitis. Some cases of cystic fibrosis are identified because of a family history. In some children the disorder does not present until adolescence, usually with pulmonary disease but occasionally with ileal obstruction or chronic constipation. Children often develop rectal prolapse. Nasal polyps are very common. The most reliable test for cystic fibrosis is the demonstration of elevated concentrations of chloride (and sodium) in the sweat; in a child with appropriate clinical manifestations a chloride level above 60 mmol/1 is diagnostic. A very small percentage of patients have lower or normal levels.

The most important pulmonary pathogens are *Pseudomonas aeruginosa* and *Staphylococcus aureus*. In the past most children died in infancy from respiratory infection. The frequency and severity of chest infection are reduced by intensive physiotherapy and postural drainage. However, pulmonary disease with cor pulmonale remains the major cause of death.

Steatorrhoea, impaired protein digestion and a consequent failure to thrive are the result of exocrine pancreatic dysfunction. The fat loss in the stool is often profound and may cause deficiency of the fat-soluble vitamins, A, D, E and K. Oral supplements of pancreatic enzymes and vitamins diminish the severity and prevent the consequences of malabsorption. Islet cell failure with diabetes mellitus is uncommon in infancy, but disturbed carbohydrate metabolism may affect 10–20% of adult survivors some of whom may require insulin replacement.

The majority of patients now survive into adult life and 25% into early middle age. As a result, involvement of other organs has become more important clinically. Thus, secondary biliary cirrhosis with liver failure affects approximately 10% of patients surviving into the third decade. Sexual maturation occurs but there is a high incidence of infertility, contributed to by abnormalities of the vas deferens, epididymis and seminal vesicle in the male, and by increased viscosity of the cervical mucus in the female. However, normal pregnancy can occur and milk secretion is normal.

Heart–lung and liver transplantation offer hope of prolonged survival to long-term patients with respiratory failure or secondary biliary cirrhosis; the donor organs do not develop cystic fibrosis.

Pathology

The lung shows the most dramatic consequences of cystic fibrosis. In infancy the ducts of mucous glands and the bronchi become filled with thick tenacious mucus. Inevitably secondary bacterial infection results; inflammation causes damage to the walls of bronchi which dilate, causing bronchiectasis. There is often extensive squamous metaplasia of the respiratory epithelium. Bronchopneumonia and lung abscesses may develop. Pneumothorax may occur, due to rupture of distended air sacs into the pleural space. If there is pulmonary hypertension the pulmonary arteries show the typical changes (p. 543). The ducts of the pancreas are blocked by secretion and there is atrophy of the exocrine glands with fibrosis. In long-standing cases, the exocrine pancreas largely disappears and is replaced by fibrofatty tissue containing surviving islets of Langerhans.

Fatty change is the most common hepatic manifestation of cystic fibrosis, but a much more specific abnormality is **focal biliary fibrosis**. In these foci numerous cholangioles are dilated and contain inspissated secretions (Fig. 7.16). In time, secondary biliary cirrhosis (p. 769) may supervene. There is an increased prevalence of gallstones in children. There is no morphological abnormality of sweat glands.

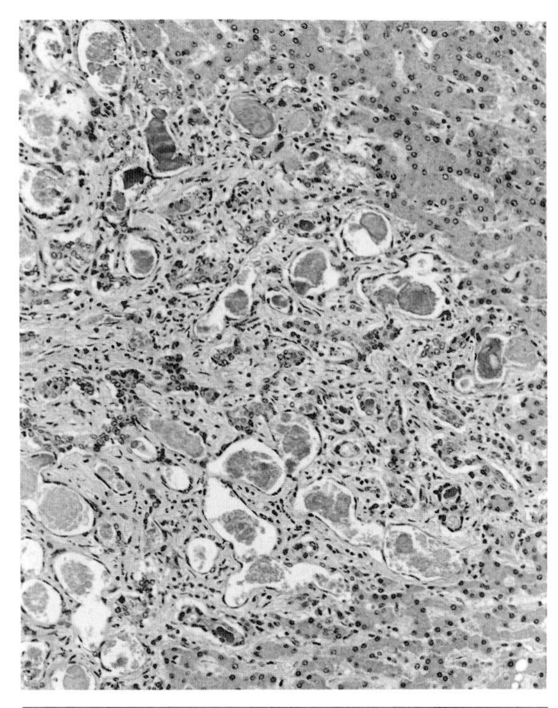

Fig. 7.16 Autopsy liver from 16-year-old child with cystic fibrosis: the liver was irregularly scarred. On microscopy numerous distended cholangioles containing inspissated concretions are present around a portal tract. ×245.

Aetiology

Transport of chloride ions across the cell membranes of epithelial cells is abnormal in cystic fibrosis. Sodium and chloride are excreted in normal quantities into sweat, although the secretory coil is insensitive to β-adrenergic stimulation with a lack of response to cAMP induction. However, normal reabsorption of chloride ions by the cells of the sweat duct does not occur, resulting in the pathognomonic high levels of chloride in the sweat. In other epithelia such as the respiratory tract, the cells are impermeable to chloride ions whose secretion is defective. As a consequence secretion of water is also diminished, leading to abnormally viscid mucus.

The cystic fibrosis gene has been mapped to the long arm of chromosome 7 (7q31), and the gene identified and sequenced. It is thought to code for a protein of 1480 amino acids, the cystic fibrosis transmembrane conductance regulator (CFTR). Several mutations in the CF gene have been identified, most of which occur in a highly conserved region which is thought, on the basis of a computer prediction of the structure of the CFTR, to code for a nucleotide binding fold. The most common mutation (D508) is a deletion of the codon for phenylalanine at position 508. The frequency of the D508 mutation varies among different populations (90% of patients in Denmark, 40% in Italy).

Sequence homology suggests that CFTR is a member of a superfamily of ATP dependent transport proteins which includes P glycoprotein, responsible for multidrug tumour resistance (p. 423). It is not clear whether the CFTR is itself a chloride channel or regulates other chloride channels. Abnormal chloride ion transfer in cultured cystic fibrosis cells can be corrected by expression of a normal CFTR gene introduced by a viral plasmid. Although the precise function of the CFTR is not yet clear, knowledge of its sequence allows antenatal diagnosis in affected families and raises the possibility of gene therapy to correct the defect.

Other Metabolic Disorders

Disorders of Purine Metabolism

The major clinical disorder associated with abnormal purine metabolism is gout (p. 996). Although there is often a familial predisposition to gout, very few cases are due to specific enzyme defects, the nature of the metabolic abnormality being unknown in the large majority. Abnormalities of hypoxanthine guanine phosphoribosyltransferase and phosphoribosyl pyrophosphate synthetase, both of which are X-linked, are associated with primary hyperuricaemia and gout. Gout may sometimes be a secondary manifestation of other inborn errors of metabolism, e.g. glycogen storage disease type I.

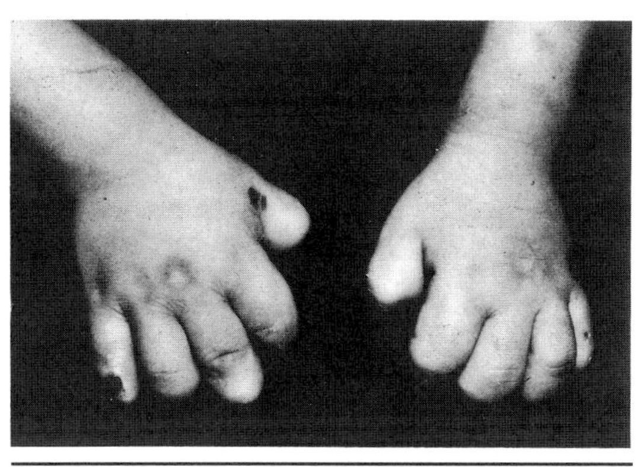

Fig. 7.17 Lesch–Nyhan syndrome: severe self-mutilation in a young child. The tips of the thumb and the fingers having been chewed off. (By courtesy of Professor Forrester Cockburn.)

Hypoxanthine guanine phosphoribosyltransferase (HGPRT) transfers a phosphoribosyl group to hypoxanthine with the production of inosine-5-phosphate; this is a salvage pathway to re-utilize hypoxanthine, a purine breakdown product, for further purine synthesis. Deficiency of the enzyme leads to increased *de novo* purine synthesis and also excess production of uric acid, the final product of purine catabolism. The genetic lesions are heterogeneous. The defect may be complete, leading to the Lesch–Nyhan syndrome, or partial leading to severe gout.

The Lesch–Nyhan syndrome is characterized by hyperuricaemia, and a neurological disorder with choreoathetosis, spasticity, mental retardation and often severe self-mutilation (Fig. 7.17). There is growth failure, sometimes a macrocytic megaloblastic anaemia and evidence of impaired B-cell function. Neurological abnormalities are usually apparent in infancy, although the episodes of self-mutilation may start at any time in childhood. Hyperuricaemia leads to renal calculi and gouty arthritis and often to death from renal failure with interstitial nephritis (p. 925). Asymptomatic carrier females can be detected biochemically, and amniocentesis and culture of amniotic cells allow prenatal diagnosis. Partial HGPRT deficiency is associated with the development of uric acid renal calculi and arthritis in adolescence, but usually without the neurological features of the Lesch–Nyhan syndrome.

Phosphoribosyl pyrophosphate synthetase (PRPPS) catalyses the addition of a pyrophosphate group to ribose-5-phosphate; the product is then complexed to a purine base to synthesize a purine nucleotide. **Increased activity*** of the enzyme increases purine synthesis and is associated with severe gout. The precise molecular defect varies between different patients; in some the enzyme is insensitive to negative feedback by purine ribonucleotides, in some the enzyme has increased activity and in others increased affinity for the substrate. Heterozygotes also show increased purine synthesis, but remain asymptomatic.

* A genetically determined increase in enzyme activity causing a metabolic disease is extremely rare.

Other Disturbances of Purine Metabolism

Deficiency of the enzyme adenosine deaminase (ADA) occurs in about half of the cases of the autosomal recessive severe combined immunodeficiency syndrome (p. 238). Deficiency of purine nucleoside phosphorylase (PNP) is associated with isolated T-cell immunodeficiency (p. 239).

Hereditary xanthinuria is due to a deficiency of xanthine oxidase which catalyses the oxidation of hypoxanthine through xanthine to uric acid. As a result there is excessive urinary excretion of hypoxanthine and xanthine; production of uric acid is diminished and both serum and urine concentrations are very low. Many patients are asymptomatic, while others develop xanthine calculi with renal colic, and a crystal synovitis. It should be noted that allopurinol, the major drug used in the treatment of hyperuricaemia, is a xanthine oxidase inhibitor.

Disorders of Porphyrin Metabolism

The porphyrias are a group of disorders due to enzyme defects in the biosynthetic pathway of haem, the iron containing respiratory pigment. Haem synthesis involves a series of eight enzymes (Fig. 7.18) commencing with the combination of glycine and succinyl CoA, with subsequent production of intermediary porphyrins and finally the incorporation of Fe^{2+}. Defects involving seven of these enzymes have been demonstrated.

The classification of the porphyrias (Table 7.8) is dependent on three factors: the major sites of porphyrin synthesis (principally the liver or bone marrow), the various types of intermediate metabolites which accumulate, and the clinical features. The incidence and geographical distribution of the porphyrias vary considerably. Some are extremely rare. Patients may present with neurological symptoms including peripheral neuropathy, severe abdominal pain and neuropsychiatric disturbances; with bullous photosensitive skin reactions; with hepatic disorders including haemosiderosis, fibrosis and sometimes cirrhosis; or with a combination of these. Acute episodes may be spontaneous or are often provoked by a vast range of drugs, alcohol, intercurrent infection or by hormonal changes in pregnancy or premenstrually. The diagnosis is established by measuring enzyme activity and the presence and levels of intermediary metabolites in red cells, liver and other tissues, together with the pattern and levels of metabolite excretion in the urine and faeces.

Porphyria cutanea tarda is the most common of the porphyrias. In the inherited form the en-

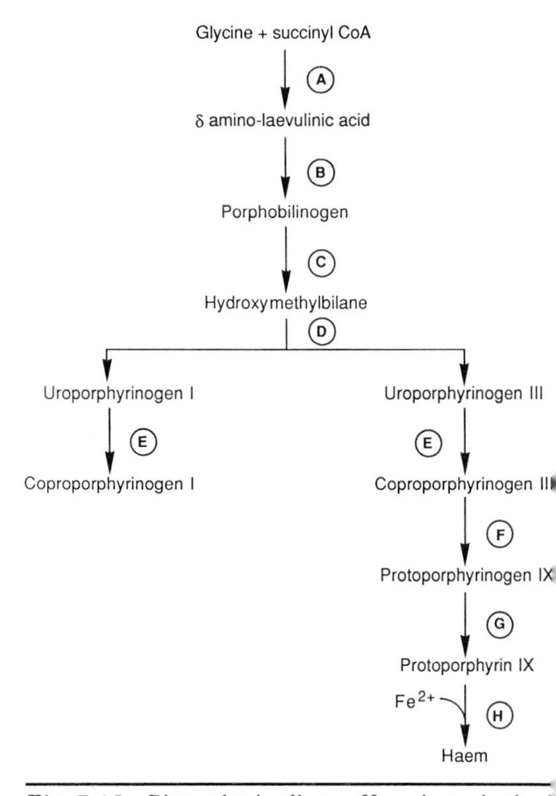

Fig. 7.18 Biosynthesis of haem. Haem is synthesized from glycine and succinyl CoA by a series of 8 enzymes, designated A–H in this figure and defined in Table 7.8. With the exception of ALA synthetase (A), a deficiency of each enzyme has been described resulting in a different form of porphyria.

Table 7.8 The porphyrias

Hepatic		
Acute intermittent porphyria (AIP)	Porphobilinogen deaminase (C)†	Abdominal pain, neuropathy, psychiatric disturbance. Attacks precipitated by drugs, alcohol and hormones
Hereditary coproporphyria (HCP)	Coproporphyrinogen oxidase (FF)	Similar to AIP but usually milder. Sometimes photosensitivity
Erythropoietic		
Congenital erythropoietic porphyria (CEP)*	Uroporphyrinogen III cosynthetase (D)	Severe dermatosis, anaemia. Present in infancy and reduced life expectancy
Erythropoietic protoporphyria (EPP)	Ferrochelatase (H)	Dermatosis in childhood. Hepatic cirrhosis and gallstones in a minority of cases
Porphyria cutanea tarda (PCT)	Uroporphyrinogen‡ decarboxylase (E)	Photosensitivity. Hepatic haemosiderosis with fibrosis leading to cirrhosis develops in 25% of patients
Variegate porphyria (VP)	Protoporphyrinogen oxidase (G)	Acute symptoms as in AIP. Photosensitivity
Hepatic erythropoietic porphyria (HEP)*	Uroporphyrinogen¶ decarboxylase (E)	Indistinguishable from CEP

*Autosomal recessive, others dominant.
†These letters compared to those in Fig. 7.18 and indicate the site in the haem synthesis pathway at which the enzyme acts.
Three patients with δ-aminolaevulinic acid dehydratase deficiency (B) have been reported in which abdominal pain and neuropathy were features.
‡Homozygous deficiency.
¶Heterozygous deficiency.

zyme defect affects all tissues and usually presents in childhood. In the sporadic form, which occurs mainly in adults, the enzyme deficiency affects only the liver. Precipitating factors include alcohol, oestrogen and drugs; in addition haemodialysis for renal failure may unmask the disease.

Acute intermittent porphyria presents clinically in only 10–15% of affected individuals, the disease remaining latent in the others. In acute attacks abdominal pain and vomiting are frequent. Sensory and motor peripheral neuropathy may lead to respiratory muscle paralysis. Hypertension and left ventricular failure can develop. Psychiatric manifestations may vary from mild mood disturbance to psychotic episodes.

Variegate porphyria affects approximately 0.1% of the white population of South Africa, particularly those of Dutch origin; many cases can be traced by family trees from individual Dutch settlers in the seventeenth century. The term variegate is applied because the disease may present with neural and visceral symptoms, with cutaneous photosensitivity or with both these features.

Peroxisomal Disorders

Peroxisomes (also known as microbodies) are so named because of their ability to form hydrogen peroxide. These membrane bound organelles have a role in the metabolism of some phospholipids, cholesterol, bile acids, medium and long chain fatty acids and some amino acids. A number of clinical disorders, including Zellweger's syndrome and infantile disease, are due to absence of peroxisomes or deficiency of peroxisomal enzymes with a total incidence of about 8 per million live births.

Zellweger's syndrome is characterized by: facial abnormalities with a high forehead, a depressed nasal bridge and shallow orbital ridges; muscular weakness and hypotonia with an absent Moro reflex; abnormalities of the eyes with cataract formation; neurological abnormalities with failure of normal neuronal migration; diffuse hepatic fibrosis proceeding to cirrhosis; and adrenal atrophy with accumulation of long-chain fatty acids. The majority of patients die in the first few weeks, but some live longer and show severe growth failure. Peroxisomes are absent in the liver and they are markedly reduced in other organs. The primary defect may be a failure of production or assembly of the peroxisomal contents rather than the peroxisomal membrane. Accumulation of long-chain fatty acids and of intermediate metabolites of bile acid are among the biochemical abnormalities.

Further Reading

Scriver, C. R., Beaudet, A.L., Sly, W. S. and Valle, D. (1989). *The Metabolic Basis of Inherited Disease*, 6th edn. McGraw-Hill Information Series Company, New York, London.

Wigglesworth, J. S. and Singer, D. B. (1991). *Textbook of Fetal and Perinatal Pathology*. Blackwell Scientific Publications, Oxford and London.

8

Microbial Infections

Host Organism Reactions

Throughout evolutionary development, many species have adapted to a parasitic existence, living in or on the surface of a host of another species from which they derive warmth, nourishment and mobility. The relationship is not necessarily harmful to the host and may be advantageous. For example, various relatively harmless bacteria colonize the skin of man and help to exclude more harmful bacteria, while reabsorption of bile pigment from the gut and the production of vitamin K depend largely on the metabolic activities of the intestinal bacterial flora. These normal inhabitants of the skin and mucous membranes are called **commensals**. Other parasites, termed **pathogens**, are less well adapted and may, by injuring the host, severely endanger their own survival: they include microorganisms – viruses, bacteria, fungi and protozoa – and also metazoa of various sizes. The term **pathogenicity** indicates the capacity of a particular microorganism to cause disease whereas **virulence** describes the degree of pathogenicity measured by the severity of the ensuing infection.

Although it is important to distinguish between commensals and pathogens, the distinction is not absolute, for many commensals **(potential**

pathogens) are only harmless so long as they are kept at bay by the host's defence mechanisms. In immunodeficiency states, for example, various normally harmless microbes may cause **'opportunistic' infections**. Similarly, a breach of local defence mechanisms, even in a normal individual, may allow commensals to cause severe infections, an example being *Escherichia coli*, which normally inhabits the gut: this bacterium may be introduced into the urinary tract by catheterization of the bladder, and may then cause severe acute pyogenic infection, even extending into the kidneys (p. 917). Local abnormalities in the host may also predispose to injury by commensals: for instance, heart valves which have been scarred and distorted by rheumatic fever are readily colonized by *Streptococcus viridans*, a bacterium which lives in the mouth and finds its way into the blood following tooth extraction or when the teeth are brushed vigorously. In normal individuals it is quickly eliminated, but it can settle and multiply in the distorted valve cusps, causing infective endocarditis. Because the distinction between pathogens and commensals is not sharp, it is helpful to use the term infection to indicate the presence of a microorganism in a part of the body where it is normally absent, and where, if allowed to multiply, it is likely to stimulate a host response and cause **infective disease**. Following invasion, the microorganisms may be eliminated without causing obvious disease (subclinical infection) or clinical disease of any grade of severity may follow. The outcome depends on the complex balance between the aggressive mechanisms of the microorganism and the defences of the host.

Non-specific Defence Mechanisms

The skin and mucous membranes are exposed to many different types of microorganisms present in expired droplets in the air, in dust particles, and in food and water. They have properties which render them suitable for the survival and sometimes multiplication of certain organisms, but inhospitable to others. In some instances, the requirements of a particular microbe for growth *in vitro* help to explain its colonization of particular parts of the surface of the body, but many of the factors determining such colonization are still unknown, and indeed the predilection of certain bacteria for a particular host species is, in most instances, quite unexplained. Nevertheless, certain factors are known to be of great importance in limiting or preventing invasion by many types of microbes and these must be considered briefly.

Barriers to Invasion

Mechanical Barriers

The keratinized layer of the epidermis is an excellent mechanical barrier to microbial invasion and provided it is kept clean and dry, direct invasion is extremely unlikely. Penetration may however occur when dirt is allowed to accumulate on the skin, particularly in moist warm areas subject to friction such as the axillae and submammary folds. In many skin diseases which result in exudation with loss or sogginess of the keratin layer, bacterial and fungal infections are common complications. The conjunctival, oral, respiratory tract and gastrointestinal mucosae, covered as they are by a film of mucous or serous secretion, also present a formidable barrier to many microorganisms although some can readily infect epithelium, e.g. influenza virus and rhinoviruses.

Wounds and ulcers of the skin and mucous membranes open up pathways for bacterial invasion. Burns are particularly liable to become heavily infected because the dead superficial tissue provides a good medium for *Streptococcus pyogenes, Pseudomonas aeruginosa* and many other bacteria. In the mouth, tooth extraction and tonsillectomy inevitably lead to bacterial invasion, and tonsillectomy has been shown to predispose to invasion by the virus of poliomyelitis in the postoperative period. Vitamin A and vitamin C deficiency also impair the resistance of the mucous membranes and skin to bacterial invasion.

Some parasitic organisms have evolved a life cycle in which they multiply in insect vectors and are introduced to man and other hosts by an insect bite, thus penetrating the major barrier of skin. Examples include the protozoa which cause nalaria, the metazoan filarial worms and the virus of yellow fever, all of which are transmitted by nosquitoes. *Yersinia pestis*, the cause of bubonic plague (the Black Death), is transmitted by the flea of the black rat and the rickettsia which causes yphus are spread by lice. Rabies virus enters the issues by the bite of a rabid animal.

Glandular Secretions

The secretions of glands opening on to the skin surface play an important role by maintaining the ntegrity of the skin and also by providing an environment in which many types of bacteria cannot survive for long. The acidity of the sweat and he long-chain unsaturated fatty acids produced by he action of commensal bacteria on sebaceous secretion both exert a selective bactericidal effect and consequently the bacterial flora of the skin surface tends to be rather constant. It has been shown that some types of pathogenic bacteria when placed on the skin are virtually all destroyed within an hour or two. The secretions of mucous membranes possess similar qualities. **Lysozyme**, an enzyme which digests the mucopeptide of bacterial cell walls, is present in high concentration in acrimal gland secretions and probably exerts an mportant protective effect in the conjunctival sac: t is secreted also by the salivary and nasal glands but in much smaller amounts. **Secretory IgA antibodies** are present in saliva, tears, intestinal contents, respiratory tract mucus, milk and urine (p. 181) and are important in the prevention of nvasion by certain viruses, although their significance in relation to bacterial invasion is less certain. They may render bacteria susceptible to the ytic action of lysozyme and may also activate complement by the alternate pathway.

The acidity of the gastric juice is effective in illing most types of microorganism ingested in ood or water, but hypochlorhydria due to chronic gastritis or other causes is common. In general, hose microbes which cause intestinal infections, such as the salmonellae, dysentery bacilli and nteroviruses, are relatively acid-resistant. *Entamoeba histolytica*, the cause of amoebic dysentery, produces cysts which resist the gastric juice nd pass through the stomach before hatching out and invading the wall of the colon.

The normal acidity of the urine contributes to the defences of the urinary tract against infection, while some IgA is secreted by the urothelium and may help to eliminate bacteria.

Secretion Currents

The continuous flow of tears over the surface of the conjunctiva has an important effect in the removal of contaminating bacteria which are carried rapidly into the nasopharynx. In the nose and mouth also, the secretions covering the mucosa flow towards the pharynx and hence to the stomach, carrying with them residual food particles, bacteria, etc. The importance of the saliva is illustrated by the oral infections and severe dental caries which accompany loss of salivary secretion in Sjögren's syndrome (p. 681). The lacrimal secretion is also diminished and conjunctival infections result. The importance of removal of contaminating bacteria by the saliva may explain the common occurrence of infection in the crypts of the tonsils and also in the periodontal sulci, for once bacteria gain entrance to these spaces they are out of the main stream of salivary flow.

In the respiratory tract there is a continuous flow of mucus upwards over the surface of the bronchial and tracheal mucosa: inhaled particles are caught up and removed in this stream and the air is almost sterile by the time it reaches the respiratory bronchioles. This defence mechanism is dependent on a normal production of mucous secretion and on the integrity of the ciliated respiratory epithelium. Most of the microorganisms capable of invading the respiratory mucosa in spite of mucociliary flow are enabled to do so by having surface components which allow them to bind to respiratory epithelium: such organisms include influenza viruses, *Mycoplasma pneumoniae* and *Bordetella pertussis*. Other microorganisms are less likely to cause respiratory infections unless the mucosa is first damaged. Such damage may be caused by the influenza virus. The integrity of the respiratory mucosa is also seriously impaired in chronic bronchitis, most commonly due to cigarette smoking but also to atmospheric pollution: this leads to metaplasia, the ciliated epithelium being replaced by goblet cells in the smaller bronchi. There is increase in the amount of secretion, which also becomes more viscous and tends to stagnate and become infected.

Intestinal pathogens, such as the salmonellae of 'food poisoning' and the shigellae of bacillary dysentery, induce an acute inflammatory reaction in the intestinal mucosa: diarrhoea results from the increased peristalsis and exudation and repeated evacuation of the gut helps to get rid of the offending bacteria.

The flow of the urine is of importance in preventing growth and spread of any bacteria gaining entrance to the urinary tract by the urethra, and any abnormality resulting in stagnation of urine or incomplete emptying of the bladder, particularly if chronic (e.g. obstruction by an enlarged prostrate), predisposes to infection.

Bacterial Commensals

In spite of the defence mechanisms described above, the skin, mouth, nasal cavity, conjunctival sac, intestines and vagina are all colonized by bacteria of various types. The local environment provided by each of these various surfaces favours the survival of particular types of bacteria and thus, each regional surface develops its own flora. In their usual site of colonization, most of these commensals are non-pathogenic and they tend to prevent the establishment of other types of micro-organism, including pathogens, by competing for nutrients and by release of metabolic products which are toxic to other organisms. Some bacteria secrete bacteriocins, proteins usually having enzymatic activity which, if absorbed by specific receptors on closely related bacteria, cause the death of the recipient strains.

In normal circumstances the commensal bacterial flora is remarkably stable but if disturbed, colonization by pathogens may result: hence the occurrence of fungal infections of the pharynx in patients on antibiotic therapy, and the possible production of lesions by the toxin of *Clostridium difficile* in pseudomembranous colitis, when the normal flora is depressed by broad spectrum antibiotics. 'Seeding' of the gut with non-pathogenic bacteria has been partly successful in preventing the overgrowth of pathogens in neonates and in patients treated by antibiotics.

Phagocytes

Macrophages are widely distributed in all epithelia surfaces. Phagocytic cells also migrate on to the surface of various mucous membranes: for example, neutrophil polymorphs pass through the thin epithelium lining the depths of the tonsillar crypts and macrophages pass into the alveoli of the lungs In both these sites the migrant cells have been shown to phagocytose particles on the surface o the mucosa and this may play a role in preventing invasion.

Types of Infections

Within living memory, infective disease was the major cause of death throughout the world, and the elimination or reduction in the incidence of man important infections largely accounts for the greatly increased lifespan in technologically advanced communities. Various factors have contributed to this decline of serious infections: the include improved standards of community and personal hygiene, better nutrition and housing prophylactic immunization and antimicrobial chemotherapy.

Despite these major advances, infective disease is still of considerable importance: it remains the principal cause of death in many tropical and subtropical countries where, in addition to bacteria and viral infections, protozoal and metazoal parasites account for a great deal of illness. Even i countries where infections have been greatly reduced, many problems remain. The common col is as common as ever, and upper respiratory viru infections are the major cause of absenteeism fro school, office and factory. The rise in the volum and speed of world travel has increased greatly th risk of epidemics of influenza, cholera, etc. Th widespread use of antibiotics has resulted i the spread of resistant pathogenic bacteria, particularly in hospitals. The pattern of communicabl disease is changing constantly. Some disease once common are now rare in the Western worl (e.g. diphtheria, poliomyelitis) and the incidence c tuberculosis has declined markedly. Howeve new and important infections have emerged. These are either diseases previously unrecognized because the causal organism had not been identified or totally new infections not present in the past. Examples of the former are campylobacter enteritis, now the commonest form of infective diarrhoea in the UK, and Legionnaires' disease. The acquired immune deficiency syndrome (AIDS) due to the human immunodeficiency virus (HIV) falls into the latter category. Another interesting and increasingly important group are the 'opportunistic' infections encountered in immunocompromised patients and in association with surgical prostheses which are caused by organisms usually considered to be of low pathogenicity.

There are, moreover, a number of important diseases which may eventually prove to be due to infection, for example rheumatoid arthritis, multiple sclerosis, ulcerative colitis and sarcoidosis. Viruses are probably important causal factors of various lymphoid neoplasms, the evidence being strongest in adult T-cell leukaemia/lymphoma and Burkitt's lymphoma (p. 391). It is also possible that hepatitis B virus is a major causal factor of liver cell cancer (p. 778).

The rest of this chapter is a brief account of the general properties of bacteria and viruses and the infections they cause. Special features of infection of the lungs, kidneys, brain and other organs are described in the appropriate systemic chapters. Diseases caused by protozoan and metazoan parasites are described in Chapter 25.

Bacterial Infections

General Properties of Bacteria

Bacteria are unicellular microorganisms with a rigid cell wall which determines their shape (Fig. 8.1). This may be spherical, cylindrical or helical to produce cocci, bacilli or spirochaetes, respectively. The short diameter of the bacterial cell is of the order of 1 μm. There are fundamental differences between the relatively primitive **prokaryotic** bacterial cell and the more complex **eukaryotic** cells of fungi, protozoa, plants and animals. The principal distinguishing features of the prokaryotic cell are that:

(1) the nucleus is composed of a single chromosome which is not surrounded by a nuclear membrane to separate it from the cytoplasm.

(2) the rigid part of the cell wall is composed of a cross-linked mucopeptide–**peptidoglycan**.

(3) the respiratory enzymes are not organized into structures that correspond to mitochondria.

Cell Wall

The organization of this structure (Fig. 8.2) determines the Gram-staining reaction of the bacterium. Gram-positive bacteria have a thick peptidoglycan layer in which the mucopeptide is associated with teichoic acids. In Gram-negative bacteria the wall is more complex: the peptidoglycan layer is thinner and separated from a surrounding outer membrane by the periplasmic space. The outer membrane contains proteins, some of which form porins through which certain hydrophilic molecules are transported: hydrophobic molecules are excluded. Lipopolysaccharides are present on the cell surface with the lipid end of the molecule embedded in the outer membrane.

The cytoplasmic membrane which is composed of proteins buried in a phospholipid bilayer lies inside and is supported by the cell wall. It is involved in the passive diffusion and active transfer of substances into, and out from, the cytoplasm. Bacterial cytoplasmic membranes lack cholesterol which is normally present in their animal-cell equivalents. **Mesosomes** are convolutions of the cytoplasmic membrane which are involved in DNA segregation during cell division. They also contain

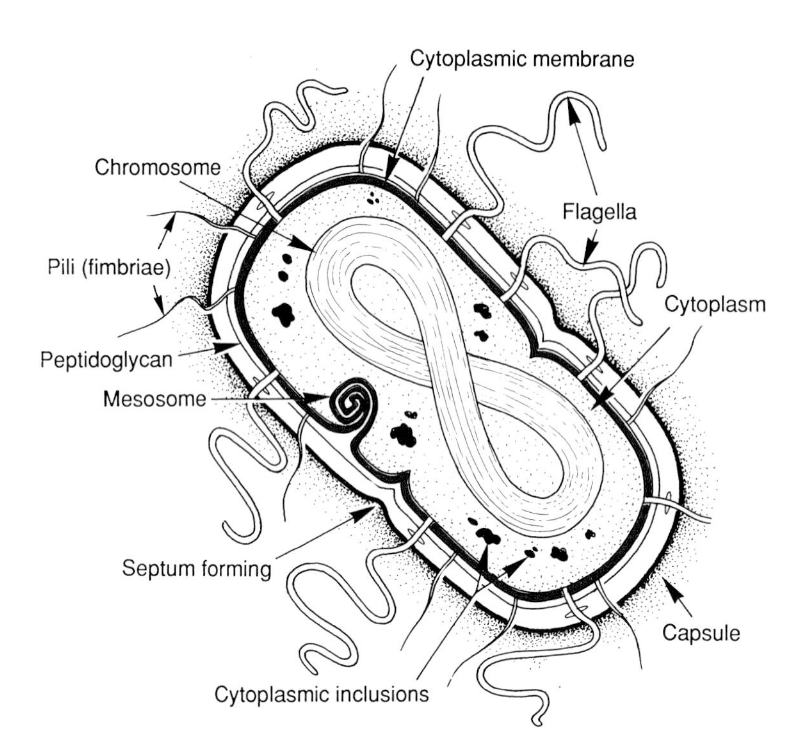

Fig. 8.1 Diagram to show the structure of a bacterial cell.

respiratory enzymes and perform a function akin to the mitochondria of eukaryotic cells.

Structures external to the cell wall present in some bacteria include:

(1) layers of gelatinous material, usually polysaccharide but sometimes protein, which may be organized into a demonstrable **capsule** or a thinner **microcapsule** which is invisible with the light microscope, or may exist as loose amorphous slime. These act to protect the cell against noxious agents and during infection inhibit the phagocytic activity of host-defence cells.
(2) **flagella**, long thin filaments composed of contractile protein which originate in the cytoplasmic membrane, are responsible for motility. They are found in many bacilli but few cocci, and their number (ranging from 1 to 20 per cell) and distribution are characteristic of the individual species. Many non-motile pathogens (e.g. streptococci) are as invasive as those that are motile and the possession of flagella does not confer the ability to penetrate tissues.
(3) **fimbriae** (or **pili**), short filaments composed of protein that project from the cell wall of many Gram-negative bacteria, are associated with the ability to adhere to surfaces including animal cells. The adhesive property of fimbriae can be demonstrated by the ability of fimbriate bacteria to agglutinate red blood cells. This haemagglutination may be inhibited by mannose, and mannose-sensitive adhesions are the commonest kind: other types of fimbriae are mannose-resistant. *Sex fimbriae* are involved in the transfer of DNA from one bacterium to another during conjugation.

Intracellular Contents

The cytoplasm of bacterial cells contains **ribosomes**, the site of protein synthesis, and various types of **inclusion granules** which are stores of reserve energy composed of volutin (polymetaphosphate), lipid or polysaccharide.

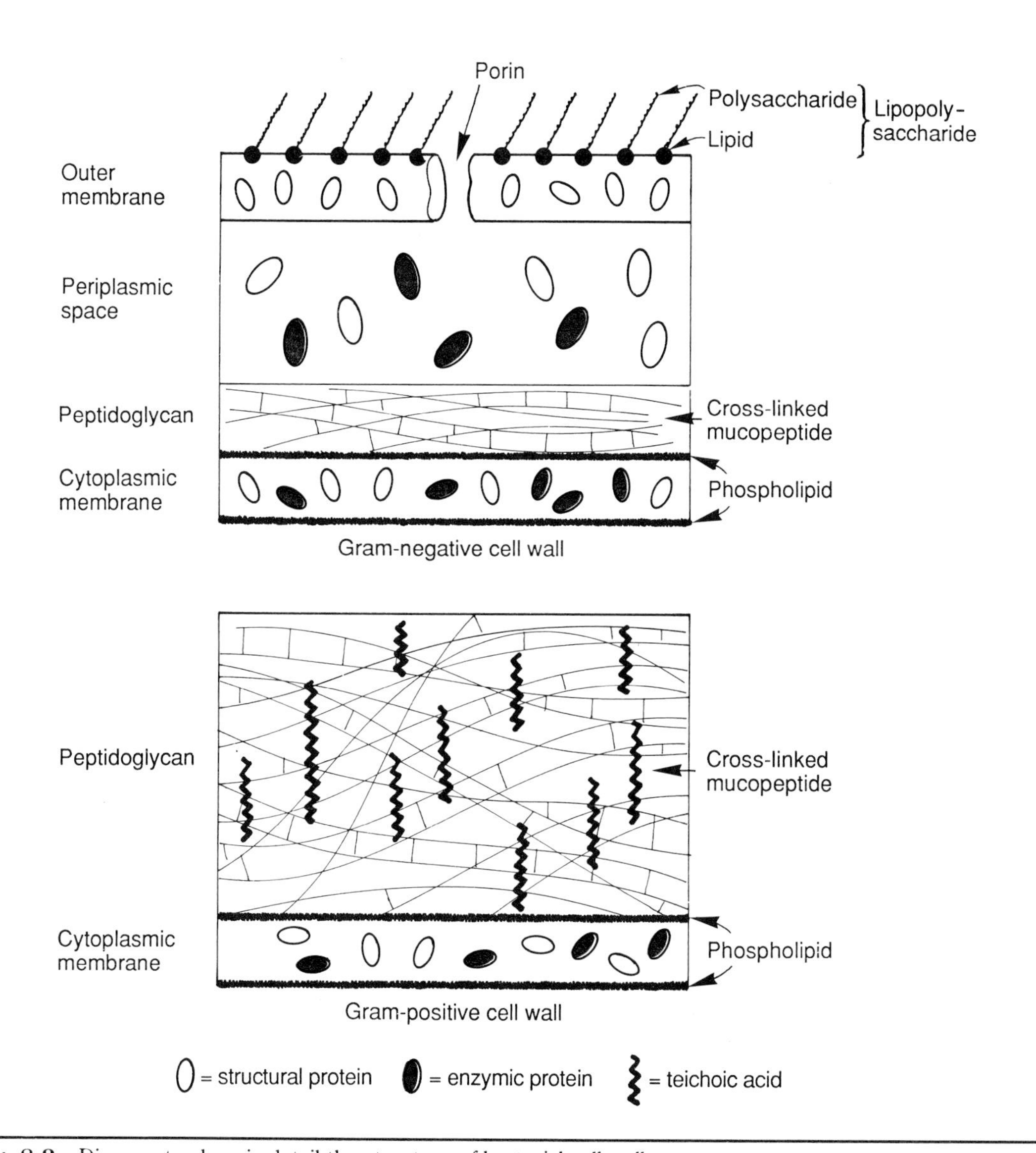

Fig. 8.2 Diagram to show in detail the structure of bacterial cell walls.

The '**nucleus**' consists of a single closed circle of tightly coiled DNA which contains all the essential genes. It lacks histones and a nuclear membrane. Bacteria may, from time to time, contain much smaller extranuclear circlets of double-stranded DNA which encode non-essential functions. These are known as **plasmids** and, by replicating along with the genome, are able to maintain themselves in the cytoplasm for many generations.

Bacterial Reproduction

Bacteria reproduce by simple **binary fission**. Depending on the species, the daughter cells either separate or remain in contact to form characteristic pairs, chains or clusters.

Bacteria can be grown on inanimate culture media: under ideal conditions *in vitro* many bacteria can divide and double in number every 20–30 minutes. After some hours of this exponential (logarithmic) growth, very large numbers of cells have been formed but as essential nutrients become depleted, a stationary phase is reached. Reproduction of pathogens *in vivo* is slower. The basic metabolic processes of bacteria are remarkably similar to those of higher plant and mammalian cells. The subtle differences which are present, however, are essential for the selective toxicity of antimicrobial chemotherapeutic agents on bacterial pathogens.

Spores

Some bacteria when exposed to adverse conditions develop into dormant resistant structures – **spores** – in order to ensure survival. Spore-forming bacteria of medical importance include aerobic Gram-positive bacilli of the genus *Bacillus* and anaerobic Gram-positive bacilli of the genus *Clostridium*. Each spore originates from a single bacterial cell and when environmental conditions improve can germinate to revert to the *vegetative form*.

Genetic Variation in Bacteria

Since bacteria reproduce asexually by binary fission, all daughter cells are normally identical. Genetic variation, however, does take place as a result of either **mutation**, the commonest cause, or **gene transfer**. Three mechanisms of gene transfer are recognized.

Transformation (Fig. 8.3). A fragment of extracellular free DNA released from a dead cell is taken up by a living bacterium of the same or a closely related species and incorporated into the genome. After recombination the transformed cell expresses the new genes. This was first demonstrated in *Streptococcus pneumoniae* by transformation of a gene encoding production of capsular material. Subsequently it has been shown to occur in *Haemophilus influenzae, Bacillus* species and some other bacteria. Essentially a laboratory manipulation, it is not certain that this mechanism operates in nature.

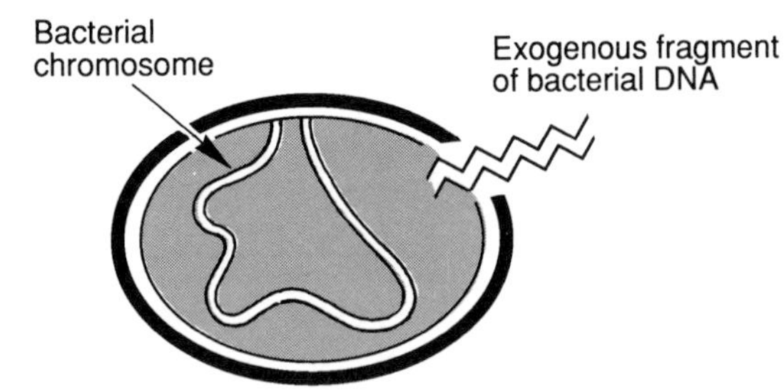

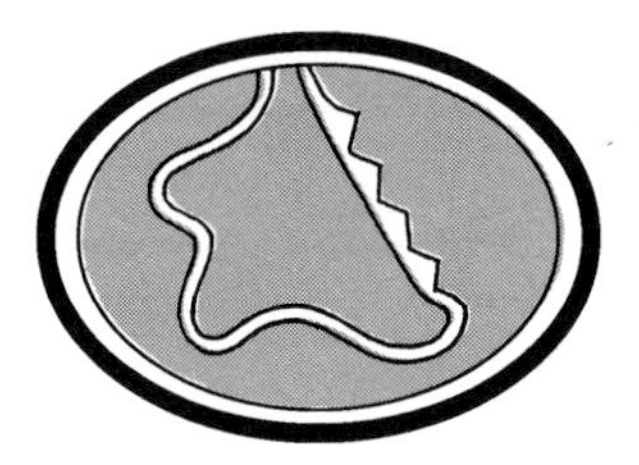

Fig. 8.3 Gene transfer by transformation.

Transduction. Bacteriophages are viruses which infect bacteria. When **virulent** they multiply within the cells and after reassembly, cause bacteriolysis with liberation of phage virions ready to infect other cells. Sometimes, by accident, a particle is formed at reassembly containing a fragment of DNA from the bacterial genome instead of viral DNA. On infection of another bacterium this DNA may become incorporated into the genome of the new host cell. This process is known as transduction (Fig. 8.4) and can only take place between closely related strains because each phage has a limited host range.

When **temperate** they enter into a stable latent relationship with the infected bacterium and the viral DNA (prophage) is integrated into the host cell genome and replicates with it. This phenomenon is called **lysogeny** and the phage genes may result in the bacterium exhibiting new

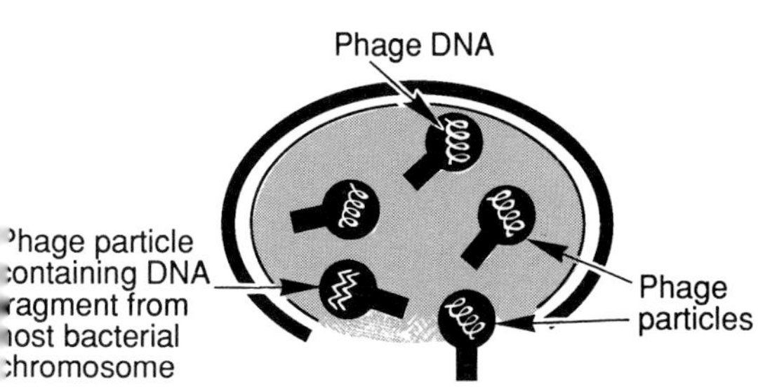

Phage-infected bacterium lyses to release new phage particles

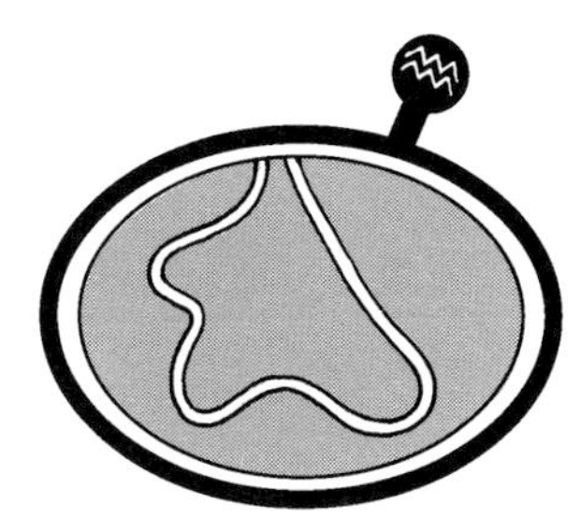

Phage carrying bacterial DNA fragment enters recipient bacterium

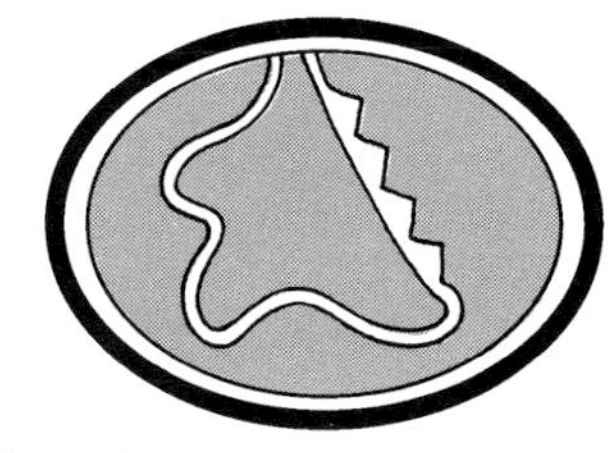

Bacterial DNA from phage recombines into chromosome of recipient bacterium

Fig. 8.4 Gene transfer by transduction.

properties as the result of **lysogenic conversion**. These new characteristics will continue to be expressed for as long as the prophage remains in the genome.

Conjugation (Fig. 8.5). Some, but not all, plasmids can be transferred to other bacteria. Self-transmissible plasmids contain **transfer promotion (tra) genes** as well as those that encode other properties. *Tra* genes control the development of sex fimbriae which attach the donor to the recipient cell, and when this contact has been made, a copy of the whole plasmid can be transferred from one cell to the other by conjugation. Plasmids can be transferred between unrelated bacteria of different genera, a major mechanism by which bacteria, especially enterobacteria, acquire additional genes.

Pathogenic Mechanisms of Bacteria

Some infections, such as those caused by the pyogenic cocci *Streptococcus pyogenes* and *Staphylococcus aureus*, are accompanied by local acute inflammation. Other bacteria invade silently: *Treponema pallidum*, the cause of syphilis, spreads widely through the body before the appearance of the primary lesion at the site of entry; *Salmonella typhi*, following ingestion, penetrates the small intestine and multiplies in the mesenteric lymph nodes before the bacilli enter the bloodstream via the thoracic duct to settle in the mononuclear phagocytes of liver, spleen and bone marrow. After further multiplication in these organs there is a secondary septicaemia which coincides with the onset of a febrile illness. In both of these diseases there is a symptomless incubation period in the order of 2–3 weeks between the acquisition of the pathogen and the development of clinical symptoms. It is easier to understand the relatively straightforward host-organism reactions that take place in a pyogenic soft tissue infection than it is to explain the complex patterns that characterize syphilis, typhoid, brucellosis, malaria and many other diseases caused by microorganisms.

It still remains a mystery why some bacteria are attracted to and cause infection in certain tissues. Both *Strep. pneumoniae* and *Neisseria meningitidis* inhabit the nasopharynx as potential pathogens but show very different disease associations; the former is likely to descend and invade the respiratory tract whereas the latter has an affinity for the meninges which it probably reaches via the bloodstream. Invasiveness, adhesion and toxigenicity

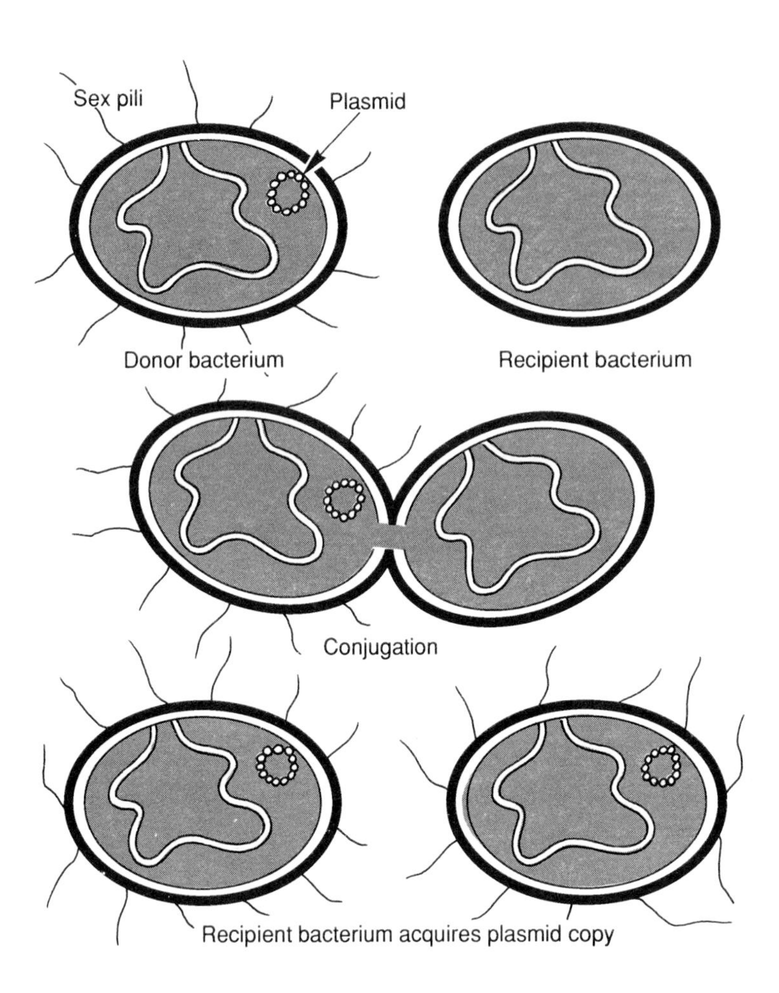

Fig. 8.5 Gene transfer by conjugation.

are recognized as important mechanisms in microbial pathogenicity.

Invasiveness

The ability of bacteria to spread and multiply within previously healthy tissue is called invasiveness. This is often the result of a resistance to the phagocytic activity of polymorphs and macrophages. Some bacteria secrete exotoxins (p. 290) which kill phagocytes. Examples are the haemolysins and leucocidins of *Strep. pyogenes* and *Staph. aureus* which may act by damaging the lysosomes of the phagocyte with the release of enzymes into the cytoplasm and resultant self-destruction of the cell. The most important property, however, is the capacity to inhibit adsorption to and subsequent ingestion by the phagocyte. This depends on the possession of antiphagocytic substances on the surface of the bacterial cell. These may be present as visible capsules composed either of polysaccharide, as in *Strep. pneumoniae, H. influenzae, Klebsiella pneumoniae*, or of polypeptide as in *Bacillus anthracis*. In other bacteria, a thinner microcapsule exists, such as the M protein of *Strep. pyogenes* or the polysaccharide capsular (K) antigens found in some enterobacteria; the Vi antigen of *Salmonella typhi* is another example of this. *Ps. aeruginosa* is characteristically surrounded by an extracellular polysaccharide slime. All these surface structures enable the bacterial cell to resist phagocytosis and are related closely to virulence. However, phagocytosis proceeds if the bacterium is coated with specific antibody, or complement (opsonization, p.

121). An unusual escape mechanism is the secretion of protein A by *Staph. aureus*. This substance binds to the Fc piece of IgG antibody and is believed to prevent the binding of opsonized cocci to phagocytic cells.

Following phagocytosis the usual outcome is death of the bacterium, but a few microorganisms are able to resist intracellular killing. An example of this is provided by *N. gonorrhoeae* which, although readily phagocytosed, may kill the polymorph and multiply within it (Fig. 8.6). Survival and multiplication within macrophages is typical in infections due to *Mycobacterium tuberculosis, Mycobacterium leprae, Listeria monocytogenes* and *Brucella* species. Indeed, it is an essential step in the development of the diseases they produce, because it not only enables the pathogen to be disseminated within the host but also determines the nature of the immune response.

Invasiveness is sometimes related to the local release of exotoxins or other factors that increase the potential of the bacterium to penetrate and multiply (**aggressins**). The pathogenic clostridia responsible for gas gangrene produce an array of exotoxins that cause tissue damage. The alpha-toxin of *Clostridium perfringens (welchii)* is a phospholipase which causes cell lysis due to lecithinase action on the lecithin found in cell membranes. Other toxins of *Cl. perfringens* include a collagenase, a proteinase and a deoxyribonuclease. *Strep. pyogenes* elaborates a fibrinolytic exotoxin, streptokinase, and in addition hyaluronidase. Hyaluronidase (also formed by *Cl. perfringens*), which dissolves the hyaluronic acid cement substance of connective tissue, is an example of an aggressin.

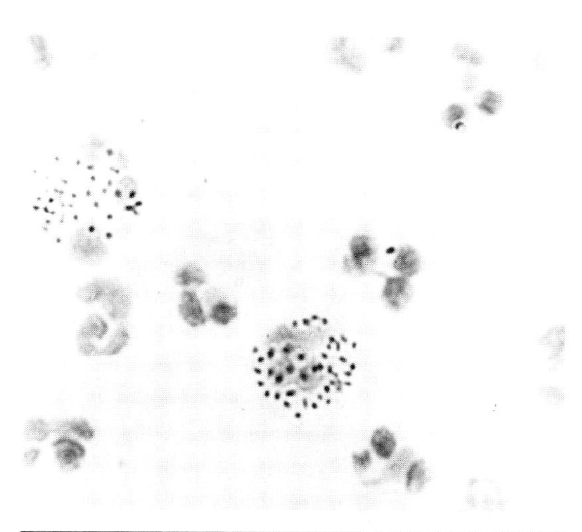

Fig. 8.6 Smear of urethral exudate in acute gonorrhoea. Two polymorphs contain large numbers of gonococci, and show degenerative changes. Other polymorphs contain few or no bacteria and appear relatively healthy. Gram stain ×1200.

Staph. aureus produces a number of locally active exotoxins (e.g. fibrinolysin, leucocidin, haemolysins), hyaluronidase and its characteristic aggressin, coagulase. This enzyme has thrombin-like activity and converts fibrinogen to fibrin. There are conflicting views on the significance of this action *in vivo*. Formation of a fibrin mesh at the site of infection has been regarded by some as a localizing factor, whereas others consider that fibrin is precipitated around the cocci and that this inhibits phagocytosis and promotes tissue invasion.

Adhesion

The ability of bacteria to adhere to mucosal epithelial cells, and which is usually associated with fimbriae, is another factor related to virulence. The attachment of *N. gonorrhoeae* to epithelium is mediated by fimbriae. Fimbriate strains caused infection when inoculated into the urethras of male volunteers whereas non-fimbriate strains did not.

Some strains of *Escherichia coli* can cause gastroenteritis and a number of different pathogenic mechanisms are recognized. Enteropathogenic *E. coli* (EPEC), the classical cause of epidemic infantile diarrhoea in former years, usually possess mannose-sensitive fimbriae which are said to be responsible for the typical profuse proliferation of bacilli in the upper small intestine. However, since such fimbriae are also present in most non-enteropathogenic strains of *E. coli*, they cannot be regarded as a specific pathogenic factor. The diarrhoea caused by enterotoxigenic *E. coli* (ETEC), which affects infants in the tropics and travellers from temperate countries to the third world, is the result of enterotoxin production. Symptoms are mild unless the strain also develops a colonization factor antigen (CFA), a mannose-resistant fimbrial adhesin, which promotes attachment of the bacilli to the intestinal epithelium.

The pathogenic potential of some *E. coli* strains responsible for urinary tract infection, especially those associated with pyelonephritis in children, is said to depend on yet another type of mannose-resistant fimbria. The attachment of these so-called P-fimbriae to urothelium prevents the bacilli from being flushed out by the flow of urine. The receptors for P-frimbriae, the glycosphingolipids of the P blood group system, are present in the kidney, particularly in the tubular cells as well as on urothelial cells.

Toxigenicity

Toxins are of two main types, exotoxins and endotoxins (Table 8.1, Fig. 8.7).

Exotoxins

Exotoxins are mostly secreted by living bacteria, although in some instances they are released only when the bacterium dies. They are simple proteins, are often extremely potent, and vary considerably in their biological effects upon the host. They are antigenically specific and their biological activity is usually neutralized by union with antibody. Many pathogenic bacteria produce a number of different exotoxins when cultured *in vitro*. Thus, *Strep. pyogenes* and *Staph. aureus* produce toxins which damage cell membranes and kill neutrophil polymorphs and macrophages. These are some of the factors responsible for local invasiveness, a characteristic of pyogenic cocci (p. 293). *Vibrio cholerae*, a curved Gram-negative bacillus, releases an enterotoxin which activates adenylate cyclase within the cells of the intestinal epithelium and this in turn raises the level of cAMP. The result is a massive outpouring of water and electrolytes into the lumen of the gut, which may lead to hypovolaemic shock.

Other exotoxins direct their effects on targets distant from their site of production. Some strains

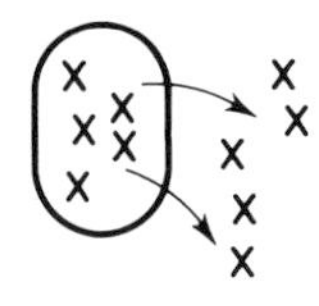

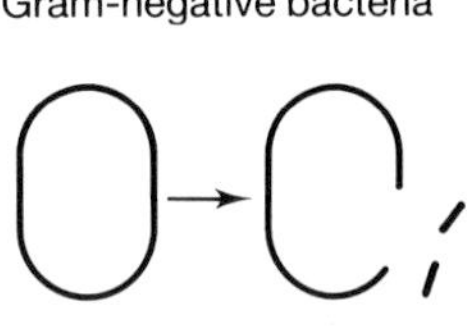

Fig. 8.7 Bacterial toxins. (Dr A. C. McCartney.)

Table 8.1 Characteristics of bacterial toxins

Exotoxins	Endotoxins
Usually produced by Gram-positive bacteria	Produced by Gram-negative bacteria
Diffuse out of intact bacteria	Released by death or disruption of the bacteria
Protein	Lipopolysaccharide–protein macromolecules
Heat labile (inactivated by 70–100°C)	Heat stable (not destroyed at 100°C)
Form toxoids	Do not form toxoids
Activity neutralized by antitoxin	Difficult to neutralize activity with anti-endotoxin
Exert a specific and restricted biological effect	Produce a vast array of biological effects
Extremely potent	Less potent

of *Strep. pyogenes* produce erythrogenin, a toxin which causes vasodilation of the small blood vessels in the skin, and is responsible for scarlet fever. The local streptococcal infection is usually in the throat, but the toxin is the cause of the generalized erythematous rash. Intradermal injection of erythrogenin results in local erythema unless the subject has circulating antitoxin. This is the basis of the Dick test for immunity to scarlet fever. Similarly, injection of antitoxin locally results in blanching of the skin in a patient with scarlet fever, and has been used as a diagnostic procedure, the Schultz–Charlton test. Some exotoxins are injurious to virtually all types of host cell and their effects thus depend on their concentration and distribution. *Corynebacterium diphtheriae*, the cause of diphtheria, causes local tissue injury in the pharynx, the site of infection (p. 529). However, it secretes a toxin for which most cells have receptor sites. This toxin catalyses the formation of ADP ribose which blocks a ribosomal transpeptidase necessary for the formation of peptide bonds. Protein synthesis is, therefore, inhibited. Clinically, neurological and cardiac symptoms develop and, in severe cases, death often results from myocardial injury (Fig 8.8).

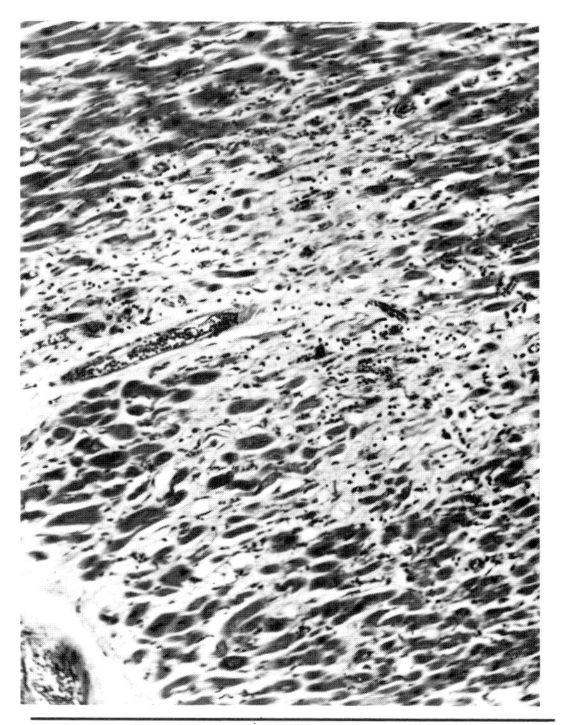

Fig. 8.8 Heart muscle in fatal diphtheria, showing destruction and disappearance of muscle fibres and a light inflammatory cell infiltrate. ×115.

Some bacteria produce toxins which act specifically on one type of tissue. For example, the major toxin of *Clostridium botulinum* is absorbed from the gut, circulates in the bloodstream, and enters the motor nerve endings at neuromuscular junctions, where it inhibits the release of acetylcholine to produce a flaccid paralysis which usually leads to death from respiratory failure. *Cl. botulinum* does not invade living tissues. Its heat-resistant spores contaminate preserved foods, in which the bacterium grows in anaerobic conditions and produces its toxin. Botulism is caused by eating preserved fruits, vegetables, meat, sausages, fish, etc. containing the toxin and is thus due to inadequate sterilization of such foods during their preparation.

Another neurotoxin is produced by *Clostridium tetani*. This organism is a commensal of the intestine of various mammals, including domestic animals. Its spores contaminate the soil and infect dirty wounds, where they germinate to form vegetative bacilli which grow in the anaerobic conditions of dead tissue and foreign material soaked with blood and exudate. The toxin, released from the bacilli, enters nerve fibres and passes along the axons both locally and generally (after dissemination in the blood), to reach the spinal cord, where it inhibits the release of glycine, the major inhibitory agent at synapses on the anterior horn cells. This results in increased tone of the skeletal muscles and a central excitatory state with attacks of generalized spasm of the voluntary muscles.

It is often difficult to determine the importance of particular bacterial toxins. Not only are many toxins produced by a single strain of bacteria but different samples of a toxin, even in highly purified form, may have different biological properties. Toxins also vary greatly in their effects on hosts of different species and experimental observations on animals are not necessarily applicable to man. Finally, production or non-production of toxin by bacteria growing *in vitro* does not necessarily indicate a similar behaviour *in vivo*. It is a feature of exotoxins that their biological effects are neutralized by the corresponding antitoxin and in some instances, e.g. diphtheria and tetanus, prior administration of the antitoxin or active immunization by injection of toxoid (inactivated toxin which retains its immunogenicity) will protect against the disease.

The expression of some exotoxins is controlled by the integration of a virus (prophage) into the bacterial chromosome (a process known as lysogenic conversion). The outstanding example is *C. diphtheriae*, the toxin of which is only produced by lysogenic bacteria containing the prophage toxigenic gene. Other examples include the erythrogenic toxin of some strains of *Strep. pyogenes* and the neurotoxins of some strains of *Cl. botulinum*.

Endotoxins

Endotoxins are constituents of the cell wall of Gram-negative bacteria and are released mainly when bacteria die. They are complexes of phospholipid (lipid A) and polysaccharide and are often referred to as bacterial lipopolysaccharides (LPS). The endotoxins produced by different bacteria differ in their antigenicity but they all have the same biological effects, which are due mainly to lipid A.

Compared with many exotoxins, endotoxins exhibit relatively weak cytotoxicity, although in severe Gram-negative bacterial infections they injure parenchymal cells of the various organs. In addition, they induce the following changes.

(1) discharge of lysosomal granules from neutrophil polymorphs, with escape of their contents to the exterior. This is rapidly followed by death of the degranulated polymorphs.
(2) stimulation of leucopoiesis and release of young neutrophil polymorphs from the marrow into the blood.
(3) activation of monocytes, with increased motility, phagocytic capacity and increased synthesis and secretion of their lysosomal enzymes.
(4) stimulation of monocytes and macrophages to synthesize and secrete endogenous mediators such as tumour necrosis factor, interleukin 1, colony stimulating factor, interferon, etc.
(5) activation of factor XII with consequent triggering of the coagulation, kinin and fibrinolytic cascade systems of the plasma.
(6) aggregation of platelets and triggering of the platelet release reaction.
(7) activation of the complement system by both the classical and the alternative pathways.

It will be apparent from Chapter 4 that these various activities result in the production of the many potential mediators of the acute inflammatory reaction, and when a small dose of endotoxin is injected locally, e.g. intradermally, it induces acute inflammation which lasts for a few hours. Presumably this reaction is triggered by the cytotoxic effect of endotoxin. Once initiated, the reaction is augmented by the products of neutrophil polymorphs, macrophages and platelets, activation products of the cascade systems and enzymes released from damaged tissue cells. When larger amounts of endotoxin are injected intravascularly, a systemic reaction results, characterized by fever, headache, vomiting and endotoxic ('septic') shock, the features of which are described on p. 106.

Endotoxins are polyclonal B-cell activators and stimulate B cells to differentiate and secrete specific antibodies, thus bypassing the need for T-helper cells (i.e. they are thymus independent antigens, p. 199).

Acute Bacterial Infections

The several processes which constitute the acute inflammatory reaction have been described in Chapter 4. They are basically the same in all acute inflammatory reactions, including those due to bacterial infections, but they differ in detail depending on the properties of the causal agent and the special features of the tissue involved. In some lesions for example, inflammatory oedema may be unusually severe, whereas in others emigration of polymorphs or fibrin deposition may be predominant. In consequence of these variations, some acute inflammatory lesions due to infections present sufficiently characteristic appearances to warrant the use of such descriptive terms as catarrhal, pseudomembranous, serous, haemorrhagic and pyogenic (suppurating) inflammation. Infections causing some of these types of inflammation, and also the special features of gangrenous infection, are considered below.

Catarrhal inflammation. This is characteristic of relatively mild infection of a mucous membrane, as occurs in the majority of viral infections of the nose and throat, including the common cold, and in the trachea and bronchi in mild cases of influenza. Examples of catarrhal bacterial infection include 'food poisoning' caused by salmonellae (excluding typhoid and paratyphoid fevers), in which the mucosa of the stomach and intestine are involved (gastroenteritis) and the milder forms of bacillary dysentery, which is an acute colitis. Microscopically, there is some loss of surface epithelium, inflammatory oedema of the underlying connective tissue, and infiltration with neutrophil polymorphs. Increased secretion of the mucosal glands, together with exudate, produces a thin watery discharge from the mucosal surface, which in some instances, e.g. the common cold, becomes mucopurulent before the original infection and secondary bacterial infection are overcome. After a single attack, the mucosa returns to normal but repeated or chronic infection can result in metaplasia of the surface epithelium and scarring of the underlying tissue, as occurs in the paranasal sinuses and the larynx.

Pseudomembranous inflammation occurs when infection of a mucous membrane is severe enough to cause superficial necrosis. The dead tissue becomes impregnated and coated with fibrin from the inflammatory exudate to form a pseudo- (i.e. non-living) membrane. It is caused by bacteria which are of low invasive capacity but produce potent exotoxins; the classical examples are diphtheria (now uncommon in immunized communities), which may affect the nose, throat or larynx and severe forms of bacillary dysentery. Such changes occur in the more recently described pseudomembranous colitis caused by *Cl. difficile* (p. 709). Polymorphs accumulate at the junction of the living and dead tissue, where their digestive enzymes result in detachment of the pseudomembrane, leaving a raw surface which becomes re-epithelialized, sometimes with loss of mucosal glands and some scarring.

Serous inflammation occurs on the walls of serous cavities and is characterized by the production of a thin watery exudate. Later, as the fibrin becomes deposited on the serous surface, the term fibrinous inflammation is applied. Haemorrhagic inflammation indicates that the exudate is blood-stained due to the presence of red blood cells.

Pyogenic or suppurative inflammation. This is caused by invasive bacteria which produce potent exotoxins affecting all types of cells and promote considerable emigration of neutrophil polymorphs, resulting in formation of pus, either in a body cavity or in spaces formed by toxic necrosis of tissue and digestion of the dead tissue by neutrophil polymorphs. The causal bacteria are termed pyogenic (pus-forming) and include *Strep. pyogenes, Strep. pneumoniae, Staph. aureus, N. meningitidis, N. gonorrhoeae, Ps. aeruginosa (Ps. pyocyanea), Proteus* species, *Bacteroides* and invasive strains of *E. coli.* Various species of *Bacteroides*, the anaerobic bacilli present in enormous numbers in the colon, are frequently present in pyogenic infections of the abdomen and female genital tract, commonly accompanied by *E. coli.*

Suppuration indicates that infection has progressed to a stage where the defence mechanisms are rendered largely ineffective, because influx of exudate into an abscess gradually diminishes as the pressure rises and the beneficial effects of a continuous flow of exudate are thus lost. As a result, bacteria continue to multiply in the pus and their toxins cause necrosis of the surrounding tissue, with increase in size of the abscess. Accordingly, suppurating infection tends to persist and, even if the infection is eventually overcome, maturation of the large amount of granulation tissue formed may result in considerable scarring. Sometimes a hard mass results from calcification of the inspissated pus. More often, the abscess eventually ruptures on to a surface and the pus is discharged. When this happens, the pressure is relieved and flow of exudate recommences with either elimination of the infection and healing with scarring, or a persistent sinus discharging pus. Antibiotic therapy may eliminate the infection in a small abscess, but in a larger one it may not be possible to achieve a sufficient concentration of antibiotic in the stagnant pus, and surgical drainage is usually necessary to promote elimination of the infection before extensive tissue destruction has occurred.

Perhaps the commonest example of an abscess is a **boil (furuncle)** (Fig. 8.9). It occurs most often in the dense dermal connective tissue at the back of the neck. The causal organism, *Staph. aureus*, invades via the hair follicles or sebaceous ducts and sets up an acute inflammatory swelling. It spreads locally in the dermis and necrosis of a patch of skin at the centre of the lesion results from toxic action: neutrophil polymorphs migrate from the surrounding inflamed tissue and digest the periphery of the necrotic 'core', which thus becomes separated from the lining tissue by a layer of pus. When separation is complete, the core is discharged, leaving an ulcer. This is usually followed by elimination of the staphylococci, and the ulcer heals, leaving a pitted scar. In some instances, particularly in individuals with impaired resistance to infection, e.g. untreated diabetics, the infection may spread extensively in the dermal and underlying soft tissue of the neck, giving rise to a **carbuncle** consisting of a complex isolated abscess, or several separate abscesses, with multiple discharging sinuses. Suppuration in a serous cavity presents the same general features as an abscess developing in a solid tissue and the principles of treatment are the same.

Bacterial Infection of the Blood

Only very rarely are bacteria present in the blood in sufficient numbers to be detected by direct

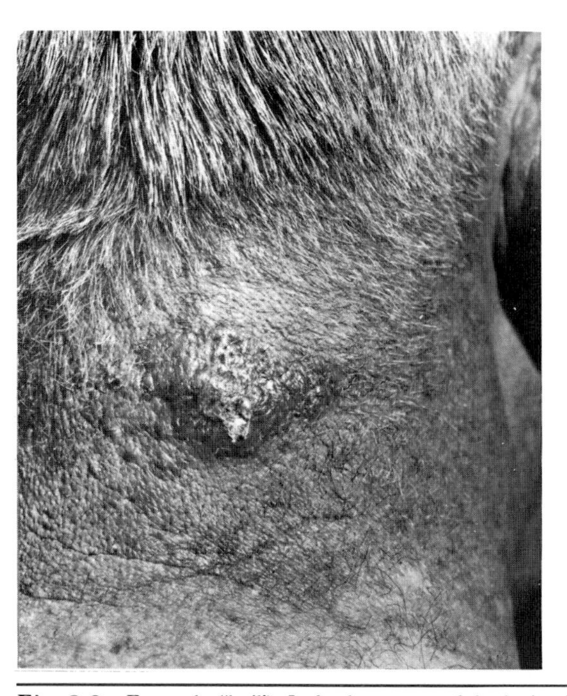

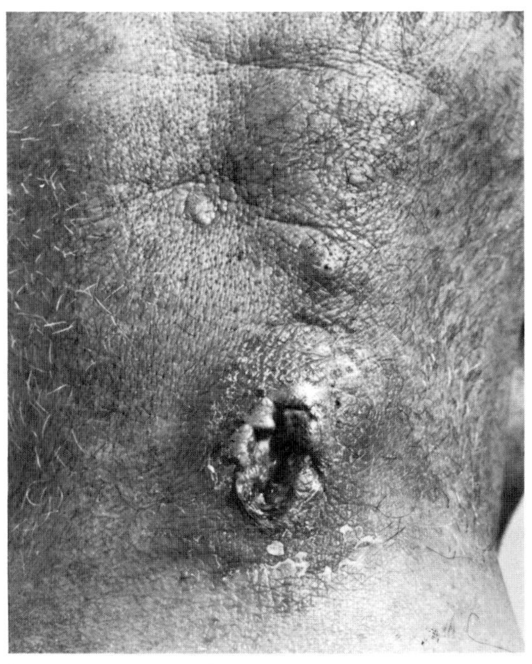

Fig. 8.9 Furuncle ('boil'). Left, the centre of the lesion is necrotic and about to be discharged. Right, the necrotic core has been discharged, leaving a ragged ulcer. ×1.

microscopy, blood culture being necessary for their detection. It is customary to classify the presence of bacteria in the blood into bacteraemia, septicaemia and pyaemia. The distinction between the three is not sharp, but they are none the less useful terms.

Bacteraemia. Small numbers of bacteria of low virulence are present from time to time in the blood of normal subjects, or in individuals with minor, often subclinical lesions. *Strep. viridans* may be cultured from the blood after vigorous brushing of the teeth, particularly if there is dental sepsis. It is also likely that intestinal bacteria enter the portal circulation occasionally. Because of its high content of antibodies and complement and the large numbers of circulating phagocytes and sinus-lining macrophages in the liver, spleen, etc., the blood is a hostile environment to most micro-organisms, and although bacteria may multiply in local infections, those entering the blood are usually destroyed rapidly. Even in more serious and extensive localized infections, such as pneumococcal pneumonia, or *E. coli* infections of the urinary tract, bacteria can sometimes be detected by blood culture, but usually they fail to multiply significantly in the blood and disappear from it when, or even before, the local infection subsides. This applies also to the bacteria which enter the bloodstream as a regular feature of certain diseases, for example typhoid fever and brucellosis (undulant fever).

Bacteraemia is of some importance, for whenever they enter the blood, bacteria may settle in various parts of the body and cause lesions, for example suppurative meningitis or arthritis in pneumococcal pneumonia, periostitis due to *Salmonella typhi* in typhoid fever and endocarditis by *Strep. viridans.*

Septicaemia means the presence and multiplication of bacteria in the blood, and is applied especially to the rapid multiplication of highly pathogenic bacteria, e.g. the pyogenic cocci or the plaque bacillus, *Y. pestis*. The term thus implies a serious infection with profound toxaemia, in which the bacteria have overwhelmed the host defences. In some instances it is difficult to distinguish between bacteraemia and septicaemia. For example, invasive strains of *E. coli* cause infections of the peritoneal cavity, urinary and genital tracts: blood infection may occur, particularly as a complication of generalized peritonitis, but it is often not clear whether the bacteria are multiplying in the blood or are continuously entering it, e.g. from the infected peritoneum.

Multiple small haemorrhages may occur in septicaemia (Fig. 8.10), due either to capillary endothelial damage from the severe toxaemia or to multiple minute metastatic foci of bacterial growth. The number of neutrophil polymorphs in the blood may be raised, although in overwhelmingly severe septicaemia they may be diminished and show toxic degranulation. The spleen is often enlarged and congested, and may contain large numbers of neutrophils. If the septicaemia is not rapidly fatal,

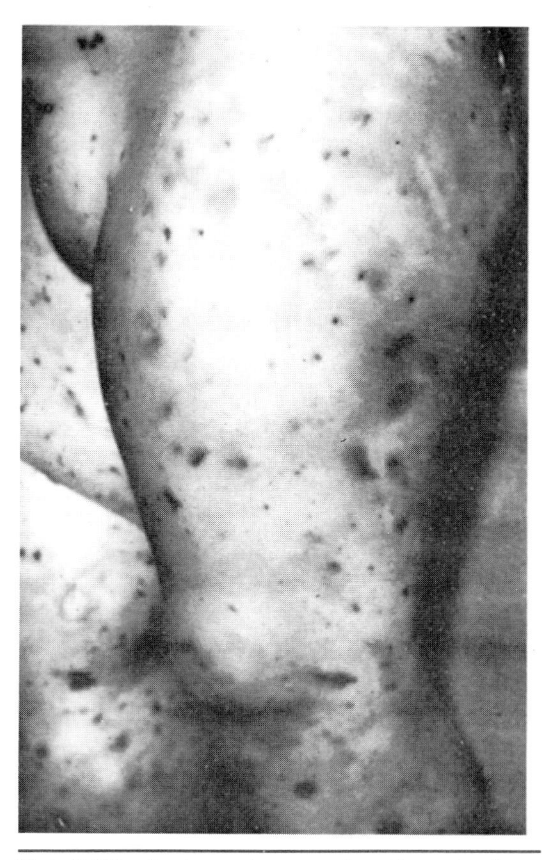

Fig. 8.10 Acute meningococcal septicaemia, showing the haemorrhagic rash.

foci of suppurating infection may develop in various parts of the body as a result of local invasion by blood-borne bacteria.

Pyaemia. In localized pyogenic infections toxic injury to the endothelium of veins involved in the lesion may result in thrombosis: bacteria may invade and multiply in the thrombus, which then becomes heavily infiltrated by neutrophils and broken down by their digestive enzymes. Small fragments of the softened septic thrombus may then break away and be carried off in the blood (pyaemia – literally, pus in the blood), where they become impacted in small vessels. They cause local injury both by obstructing the vessels and by the release of toxins from their contained bacteria: a combination of necrosis, haemorrhage and suppuration results, with formation of multiple **pyaemic abscesses** in the various tissues, their distribution depending on the site of the original septic thrombosis. Fragments of infected thrombi released into the circulation may impact in arteries, causing correspondingly larger foci of necrosis and suppuration (**septic infarcts**).

Pyaemic abscesses are typically surrounded by a zone of haemorrhage. Microscopy of an early lesion may show a central zone of necrosis, usually containing huge numbers of bacteria, which is surrounded by a zone of suppuration and an outermost zone of acutely inflamed, often haemorrhagic tissue. As the lesions progress, the necrotic tissue is digested, and apart from their multiplicity and widespread distribution, the lesions become indistinguishable from non-haematogenous abscesses.

Septic thrombosis of systemic veins results especially, but not exclusively, in pyaemic abscesses in the lungs, while septic thrombosis in pulmonary veins results in pyaemic abscesses mainly in the systemic arterial distribution. In acute bacterial endocarditis, in which septic thrombus forms on the infected valve cusps, the distribution of pyaemic lesions depends on the particular heart valve(s) involved. Septic thrombus of a portal venous tributary, e.g. in acute appendicitis, gives rise to **portal pyaemia**, with abscesses mainly in the liver. Inevitably, bacteria are released from septic thrombus in pyaemia and frank septicaemia commonly supervenes.

Septicaemia and pyaemia were formerly most often due to the pyogenic cocci. Their incidences have been greatly reduced by antibiotic therapy, and bacterial infections which are less readily eliminated by antibiotics have increased in relative importance. Invasive strains of *E. coli* with virulence factors conferred on them by plasmids are now the commonest cause of blood infections in general hospital practice. In states of lowered resistance to bacterial infection, e.g. agranulocytosis and immunodeficiency (including therapeutic immunosuppression), blood infection is a particular hazard. Bacteria which are normally of relatively low resistance may cause septicaemia and pyaemia in immunocompromised individuals.

The Common Pyogenic Bacteria

Pyogenic infections in man are most commonly caused by *Staph. aureus* and *Strep. pyogenes* both of which are Gram-positive cocci.

Staph. aureus is the usual cause of skin sepsis such as pustules, boils, carbuncles and wound infections including postoperative infections. These infections, which are associated with the discharge of thick creamy pus, characteristically remain localized although suppurating lymphadenitis may develop in the draining nodes and occasionally, there may be progression to septicaemia and pyaemia. Infections such as pneumonia, usually secondary to a respiratory viral infection (classically influenza), osteomyelitis and endocarditis are less common. In addition to these pyogenic infections there are a number of disease syndromes with clinical manifestations mediated by specific staphylococcal toxins. Examples are:

(1) **staphylococcal food poisoning** characterized by vomiting and sometimes diarrhoea, within a few hours of eating contaminated food in which *Staph. aureus* has formed an enterotoxin.
(2) **toxic epidermal necrolysis** (Ritter–Lyell's disease) a condition seen predominantly in neonates due to the elaboration of epidermolytic toxins A and B in the infected skin with

the result that large areas desquamate and appear 'scalded'.
(3) **toxic shock syndrome** caused by the release of toxic shock syndrome toxin-1 usually from staphylococci multiplying in tampons during menstruation. Clinically there is fever, collapse and a skin rash with desquamation.

Almost all strains of *Staph. aureus* responsible for hospital infections and the majority encountered in general practice are resistant to penicillin and sometimes to other antibiotics. Strains associated with outbreaks of hospital infection possess the properties of communicability, the ability to spread easily from person to person, and virulence. Such strains wax and wane: throughout the world many hospitals suffered a staphylococcus plague in the 1950s and early 1960s but epidemic staphylococci then disappeared for more than a decade. The re-emergence of hospital staphylococcal infection as a major problem in the 1980s has been associated with the appearance of strains resistant to methicillin and numerous other drugs, so-called methicillin- (or multiply) resistant *Staph. aureus* (MRSA).

Phage typing has proved of great value in the investigation of the epidemiology of such outbreaks: it is performed by testing the susceptibility of *Staph. aureus*, isolated from various sources, to the lytic effects of a panel of bacteriophages. Patients with wound infections and other septic lesions are the important sources of infection, but in addition there are inapparent reservoirs of staphylococci. These include symptomless carriers in whom the commonest carriage site is the anterior nares. Some, but not all, carriers have the ability to shed the organism heavily into surroundings. Some patients disperse large numbers of staphylococci from colonized superficial lesions, e.g. ulcers which do not appear inflamed.

Strep. pyogenes commonly produces acute pharyngitis and tonsillitis and local spread may cause otitis media and mastoiditis. Other infections associated with this organism include inflammation of the subcutaneous connective tissues, **cellulitis**, **impetigo**, pustular lesions, usually of the face, and **erysipelas**, a spreading infection of the dermis producing a raised, red, painful lesion of the skin, usually of the face, with a well defined margin. Formerly, *Strep. pyogenes* was a very common and important cause of fatal peritonitis or septicaemia arising from infection of the genital tract following childbirth. It was also a cause of fatal septicaemia resulting from a minor injury, e.g. a finger prick sustained by the surgeon or pathologist dealing with a streptococcal infection. Aseptic and antiseptic techniques and the use of antibiotics have, however, greatly diminished the incidence of serious and fatal streptococcal infections. *Strep. pyogenes* has not been observed to develop resistance to penicillin and this agent remains the drug of choice for treating streptococcal infections. The organism does not readily withstand drying and spread is either by contact or via respiratory droplets from an infected source. A proportion of infections can be traced to nasal and throat carriers who are usually symptom free. Some strains of *Strep. pyogenes* produce a prophage-determined erythrogenic toxin and cause an acute pharyngitis accompanied by an erythematous skin rash (scarlet fever). Immunologically mediated late sequelae of streptococcal pharyngitis are rheumatic fever (p. 501) and post-streptococcal glomerulonephritis (p. 899).

The differences between infections due to staphylococci and streptococci are partly explained by their different toxins. The tendency for staphylococcal infections to remain localized is possibly due to the production of coagulase which clots fibrinogen, producing a deposit of fibrin which may help to limit spread of the organisms. The spread of streptococcal lesions is thought to be due to the production of hyaluronidase, which digests hyaluronic acid and thus liquefies the ground substance of connective tissues.

Strep. pneumoniae, also a Gram-positive coccus, is the commonest cause of acute bacterial pneumonia and infections caused by it may be complicated by bacteraemia or septicaemia and metastatic blood-borne lesions, e.g. suppurative meningitis or arthritis. A major factor in the pathogenicity of *Strep. pneumoniae* is its capsular polysaccharide which inhibits phagocytosis. Non-capsulated (rough) forms of *Strep. pneumoniae* are non-pathogenic. There are over 80 serotypes of this organism, classified by the antigenicity of their capsule. The most virulent is type 3, which has the thickest capsule.

Bacteria belonging to the genus *Neisseria* are Gram-negative cocci and the two recognized pathogens, *N. meningitidis* and *N. gonorrhoeae* are both responsible for pyogenic infections. *N. meningitidis* (meningococcus), colonizes the nasopharynx silently, and produces a septicaemia or bacteraemia with the subsequent development of meningitis. The septicaemia is often associated with a haemorrhagic rash (Fig. 8.10) and severe endotoxic shock with acute haemorrhagic adrenocortical necrosis (Waterhouse–Friderichsen syndrome) (p. 110).

N. gonorrhoeae (gonococcus) is transmitted by coitus and is the cause of gonorrhoea. In the male, it affects initially the anterior urethra and its glands, but unless treated effectively progresses to the posterior urethra and vas deferens, where it causes prostatitis, seminal vesiculitis and epididymitis: these latter lesions are more difficult to eliminate and may become chronic. In women, the gonococcus colonizes first the glands of the urethra, vagina and endocervix. As in the male, the early infection is easily cured, but it may be virtually symptomless and if allowed to progress it commonly causes salpingitis which is more difficult to treat. Gonococcal lesions are typically pyogenic. The gonococcus has the unusual property of multiplying within neutrophil polymorphs, which gives a characteristic appearance in smears and aspirates of the lesions (Fig. 8.6), but the microorganisms may be scanty and culture may be necessary for diagnosis. Gonococcal virulence and the site of infection are determined partly by the possession of surface fimbriae. Gonococcal septicaemia (with a skin rash resembling that of meningococcal septicaemia), arthritis, endocarditis and meningitis occur occasionally. Strains of gonococci resistant to penicillin due to the production of a β-lactamase are still relatively uncommon in the UK but they now cause a significant proportion of infections elsewhere, particularly in the Far East and parts of Africa. Late effects include posterior urethral stricture in men, an increased risk of tubal pregnancy in women, and sterility in both sexes. Subclinical infection is particularly prone to occur in women, and is important in the spread of the disease. Infection of the infant during delivery results in ophthalmia neonatorum, a purulent conjunctivitis which, untreated, can cause blindness.

There are a number of Gram-negative bacilli, normally present as intestinal commensals, which are important pathogens outside the gut. These include aerobic enterobacteria ('coliforms') such as *E. coli, Proteus* species and *Klebsiella* species and anaerobic non-sporing Gram-negative bacilli belonging to the genus *Bacteroides*. Singly, but more often in combination, they are the usual cause of pyogenic infection of the abdomen, e.g. appendicitis and peritonitis, and they are also a cause of gynaecological sepsis. Aspiration of similar bacteria from the nasopharynx may result in pneumonia and lung abscess. The coliforms are responsible for most urinary tract infections which are often accompanied by pyuria.

The habitat of *Ps. aeruginosa*, a strictly aerobic Gram-negative bacillus, is also the intestinal tract but in addition it is found in water and it is also able to flourish in most environments such as sink waters and aqueous solutions which provide important reservoirs of this organism in hospital. The organism produces the pigment pyocyanin as well as fluorescein and these together result in its infections being characterized by 'blue' pus. The most important pseudomonas infections are encountered in patients with serious underlying conditions (e.g. burns, malignancy), or subjected to invasive procedures (e.g. indwelling urinary tract catheterization, respiratory tract intubation).

All of the Gram-negative bacilli can be found in wounds, bedsores, burns and various ulcers, sometimes as secondary invaders, and it is often difficult to determine whether they are present as pathogens or merely as colonizers. Serious Gram-negative sepsis may progress to septicaemia and endotoxic shock (p. 108).

Gangrene

Definition. *The term gangrene means digestion of dead tissue by bacterial action.* Many types of bacteria, often present in various combinations, may participate, and breakdown of tissue protein, carbohydrates and fat may result in simple end products including the volatile compounds and gases which give the foul odour of putrefaction. The same changes are observed *post mortem* and in putrefaction of meat, etc. Gas production may give rise to emphysematous crackling on palpation. The changes in colour, dark-brown or greenish-brown and sometimes almost black, are due to changes in haemoglobin and are more conspicuous when the dead tissue contains a lot of blood.

Gangrene may be either primary or secondary. The difference lies in the cause of the tissue necrosis. Primary gangrene is brought about by infection with pathogenic bacteria which both kill the tissue by secreting potent exotoxins and then invade and digest the dead tissue: this will be considered here. In secondary gangrene (p. 26), necrosis is due to some other cause, usually loss of blood supply from vascular obstruction or tissue laceration and saprophytic bacteria then digest the dead tissue.

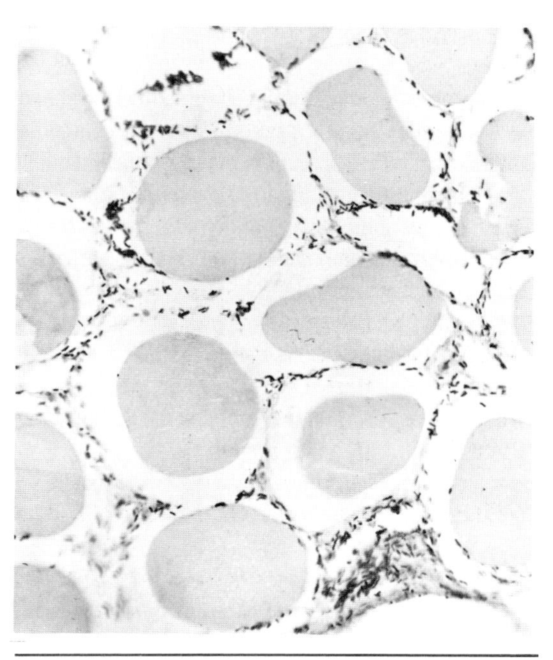

Fig. 8.11 Skeletal muscle in gas gangrene. The muscle fibres are necrotic and their nuclei have disappeared. Large numbers of *Cl. perfringens* are present in the dead tissue, mainly in the endomysium. ×400.

Primary Gangrene

This includes gas gangrene which results from infection with specific bacteria and gangrene brought about by various other bacteria.

Gas gangrene is caused by a group of anaerobic Gram-positive sporulating bacilli, the clostridia, of which the three most important are *Cl. perfringens (Cl. welchii)*, *Cl. oedematiens (Cl. novyi)* and *Cl. septicum*. These organisms are intestinal commensals in man and animals: their spores are widespread in soil and are liable to contaminate wounds. They are able to flourish in dead tissue found in lacerated wounds, such as those caused by road accidents and by shrapnel. In an anaerobic environment, the clostridia produce exotoxins. These diffuse into and kill the adjacent tissues which in turn are invaded, so that the process spreads rapidly, particularly along the length of the skeletal muscles (Fig. 8.11). Gas gangrene is most often due to several different clostridia one of which is usually *Cl. perfringens*. Before the muscle and other tissues are killed, they become intensely oedematous, are extremely painful and appear swollen and pink. Microscopically, emigration of leucocytes is minimal. Among a number of toxins, *Cl. perfringens* produces lecithinase which, by its action on phospholipids, lyses cell and mitochondrial membranes, hyaluronidase and collagenase. *Cl. perfringens* ferments sugars, producing H_2 and CO_2 which collect as bubbles in the dead tissues, rendering them crepitant on palpation. The dead tissues are commonly invaded by a mixture of other organisms present in the original wound and these may play a major role in putrefaction. Gas gangrene may complicate intestinal lesions, e.g. appendicitis or strangulation, as clostridia are present in the intestine. It also occurs as a puerperal infection of the uterus from contamination via the perineum. In addition to the rapidly spreading local lesion, gas gangrene is accompanied by acute haemolysis and a severe toxaemia: death results from peripheral vascular collapse. Spread by the bloodstream may occur as a late, usually terminal event. In consequence, all the tissues at autopsy may contain large numbers of clostridia and show extensive digestive changes.

Lacerated wounds must be treated by early excision of devitalized tissue to prevent clostridial infections. Antibiotics, especially penicillin, have also contributed greatly to the prevention of gas gangrene by inhibiting the growth of clostridia. Once gas gangrene has developed, all the affected tissue must be excised.

The clostridia of gas gangrene may also cause infection of subcutaneous tissue (cellulitis) without affecting the underlying muscle, or may grow in dirty wounds, producing a foul discharge but without invasion of the surrounding tissue.

Other Examples of Primary Gangrene

Meleney's postoperative synergistic gangrene is a slow spreading infection of the skin and subcutaneous tissue of the chest or abdominal wall which, as it progresses, leaves the central zone gangrenous. The lesion may spread relentlessly to involve much of the trunk. A number of different combinations of bacteria acting synergistically have been held responsible.

Noma (cancrum oris) is a gangrenous condition occasionally seen in poorly nourished children and tends to complicate debilitating infections: it begins on the gum margin and spreads to the cheek, where an inflammatory patch of dusky red appearance forms and then becomes darker in colour and ultimately gangrenous. The condition is caused by *Bacteroides* species together with *Borrelia vincenti* which are normally present in the mouth.

Chronic Bacterial Infections

Many chronic infections of global significance induce granulomatous inflammation (p. 135). The agents include bacteria, fungi, protozoa and worms. A consistent feature of granulomatous inflammation is the tendency to fibrosis and subsequent scarring and deformation of tissues. Cytokines such as interleukin 1 (IL-1), secreted from macrophages, stimulate fibroblasts to lay down collagen, much of which is then permanent. In several diseases such as tuberculosis, sarcoidosis and schistosomiasis, major chronic clinical effects derive from widespread scarring in various organs.

Mycobacterial Diseases

Of the dozens of mycobacterial species identified, most are environmental saprophytes and only a few are significant causes of disease in man. The two most important, *M. tuberculosis* and *M. leprae*, are unusual in that their prime habitats are the cells of human tissues. The organisms are aerobic Gram-positive bacilli with a waxy cell wall which renders them difficult to stain. Once the stain has penetrated the cell wall, however, it is difficult to remove. Mycobacteria are referred to as acid- and alcohol-fast bacteria (AAFB) since they resist decolorization by mineral acids and alcohol as in the Ziehl–Neelsen staining methods. *M. tuberculosis* grows slowly in culture (it divides no faster than every 18 hours). It is highly pathogenic when injected into guinea-pigs, and this is still occasionally used as a diagnostic method.

Mycobacterium tuberculosis infection

The term 'tuberculosis' is generally restricted to disease caused by *M. tuberculosis* and *M. bovis*. Other mycobacterial infections (so-called 'atypical' or non-tuberculosis mycobacteria) may produce clinicopathologically similar diseases (see below,

'Other mycobacterioses') but it is preferable to specify these infections according to the causal agents.

Formerly one of the great killing diseases in temperate climates, the incidence of new clinical cases of tuberculosis in the UK has fallen to about 10/100 000 people per annum, and the fatality rate is now less than 10%. The decline in incidence is related to improved hygiene and social conditions, and to the prevention of transmission of tuberculosis via cows' milk. Medical therapy and BCG vaccination have been less important epidemiologically. However, in many developing countries tuberculosis is still the major chronic infectious disease, with incidence rates often over 200/100 000 people per year, and mortality rates up to 50%.

Acquisition of Tuberculosis

M. tuberculosis infection is usually acquired by inhalation of bacilli from the respiratory secretions of people with 'open tuberculosis'. The organism may survive for weeks in dried secretions in the environment. Much less commonly, tuberculosis can be contracted by drinking cows' milk which is infected with *M. bovis*. Both species of mycobacteria are equally pathogenic.

Susceptibility to Infection

The degree of exposure depends on the prevalence of open tuberculosis in a community. The likelihood of developing tuberculosis following exposure depends upon a number of factors.

Race. Certain ethnic groups such as North American Indians, black Africans and Asians are much more susceptible to tuberculosis than others. Since tuberculosis has probably behaved as an epidemic with a time scale measured in centuries, such differences may only reflect a less adapted coexistence with the infection compared with Europeans, due to more recent exposure to the disease.

Age. Young children and old people are more susceptible than young adults. This probably reflects the imperfect function of the immune system at the extremes of age.

Immunological and other host defence factors. Since *M. tuberculosis* is an intramacrophage parasite, the function of these cells determines the outcome of infection. Immunocompromised people are more liable to suffer tuberculosis; the causes include steroid therapy, immunosuppressive drugs, HIV infection, diabetes, cirrhosis and malnutrition. Individuals with damaged lungs, e.g. from silicosis, are similarly at risk.

Previous exposure to mycobacteria. This comes from the use of BCG vaccination and from environmental mycobacteria. Bacille Calmette-Guérin (BCG), an attenuated strain of *M. bovis* which is used to provide a primary infection of low virulence, stimulates immunity to *M. tuberculosis*. The degree of protection against clinical tuberculosis provided by BCG varies from 0 to 80% depending on the region studied (in the UK, the protection conferred by BCG vaccination is considered to be at the upper end of this range). The reasons for this regional variation are unknown.

BCG is a live vaccine which produces a local short-lived primary complex infection (see below) with lymphadenopathy. Symptomatic complications are unusual, and disseminated disease occurs rarely, usually in children with inherited immunodeficiencies.

Events Following Tissue Infection with M. tuberculosis

The characteristic response to mycobacterial infection is the formation of an epithelioid cell granuloma (often called a 'tubercle'), which usually undergoes caseous necrosis. The initial host response to the presence of *M. tuberculosis* is an influx of neutrophil polymorphs, but these are unable to kill mycobacteria. Macrophages then phagocytose and digest bacilli and present antigens to T cells. The size of the cellular reaction increases as more macrophages are recruited, but unactivated macrophages are generally unable to kill the multiplying mycobacteria. The bacilli can activate macrophages directly, but more important in this regard are lymphokines such as interferon-γ secreted by CD4+ T cells. The macrophages mature into epithelioid cells and some fuse to become Langhans' giant cells (Fig. 8.12). Epithelioid cells are less able to phagocytose material, but are more efficient killers of intracellular organisms. Tuberculous granulomas fuse to form masses visible to the naked eye. Typically, the centre of the granuloma undergoes necrosis: histologically it is acellular and amorphous, staining pink with standard haematoxylin and eosin stains. Macroscopically, this necrosis is solid and white or yellowish in colour, resembling hard cheese, hence the term 'caseous' necrosis. Caseation is not diagnostic of tuberculosis, for other granulomatous infections such as histoplasmosis also cause similar lesions, but its presence should always suggest tuberculosis (Fig. 8.13).

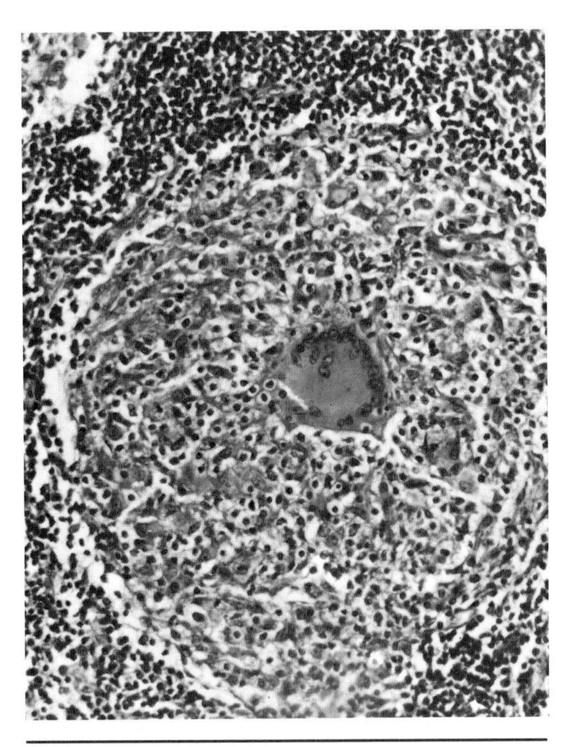

Fig. 8.12 An early tubercle, consisting mainly of epithelioid cells, some of which have fused to form a Langhans giant cell. Lymphocytes are scattered among the epithelioid cells and are numerous around the periphery. ×174.

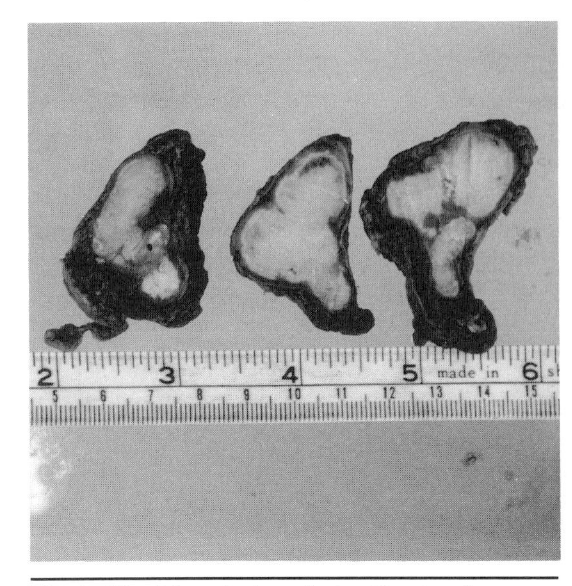

Fig. 8.13 Adrenal tuberculosis with extensive caseation. Ruler shows inches and centimetres.

The cause of this necrosis, which is a mass of macrophages, is uncertain, but it is related to hypersensitivity. Activated macrophages manufacture proteases and toxic oxygen radicals in order to kill phagocytosed infectious agents; and these secreted chemicals may kill the cells. Tumour necrosis factor α (TNFα), a cytokine which is secreted by macrophages, is likely to be important in granuloma necrosis. Finally, the necrosis of large masses of granulomatous tissue (e.g. centimetres or more across) may result in part from ischaemia as granulomas involve blood vessels and obliterate their lumina. *M. tuberculosis* is usually said to be a non-toxic organism, but if present in vast numbers it may be a direct cause of necrosis.

The advent of caseation necrosis roughly corresponds with the acquisition of delayed hypersensitivity to tuberculin as measured by skin tests (see below). This implies an association between antigen recognition by lymphocytes with macrophage influx in the skin, and lymphocyte-mediated macrophage activation in granulomas.

Tuberculosis is classically divided into two phases, primary and post-primary. This follows from the different patterns of host respones to *M. tuberculosis* infection upon a second exposure.

Although in clinical practice this distinction may be blurred, it is none the less a helpful concept for understanding the complex events that characterize this disease.

Primary Tuberculosis

The usual manner of first infection to *M. tuberculosis* is the inhalation of bacilli during childhood. The bacilli pass into the alveoli in the peripheral (subpleural) parts of any lobe of the lung and initiate the granulomatous inflammation described above. During the initial macrophage reaction, bacilli pass along lymphatics to the hilar lymph nodes and induce a similar necrotizing granulomatous inflammation there. The combination of subpleural and hilar node tuberculous lesions is the 'primary complex' (often called a 'Ghon focus') (Fig. 8.14).

Whilst the primary complex evolves, there is a tuberculous bacteraemia (leakage of mycobacteria into the bloodstream from the hilar node) and the patient may have a fever and develop the skin lesions of *erythema nodosum* (a local hypersensitivity reaction to *M. tuberculosis* antigens in the subcutaneous tissue). However, the majority of people with a primary complex are asymptomatic. In about 90% of infections, the primary complex heals: the bacilli cease multiplication and the granuloma mass resolves to leave a fibrous scar in lung and lymph node. In due course, the fibrous tissue may calcify (dystrophic calcification), and even ossify, leaving evidence of previous tuberculosis on chest X-rays. The sequelae in the remaining 10% of primary infections are shown diagrammatically in Fig. 8.15.

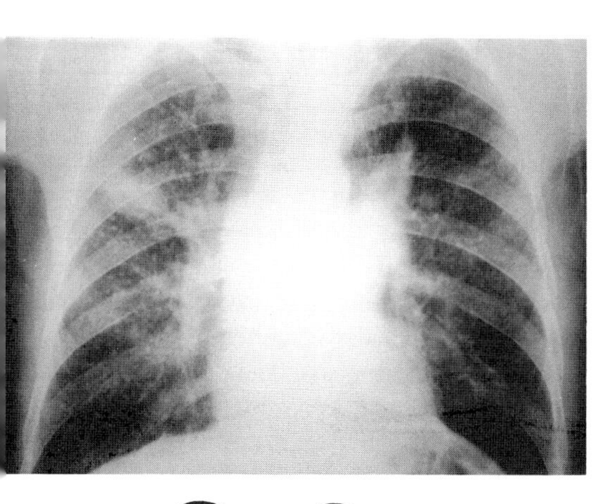

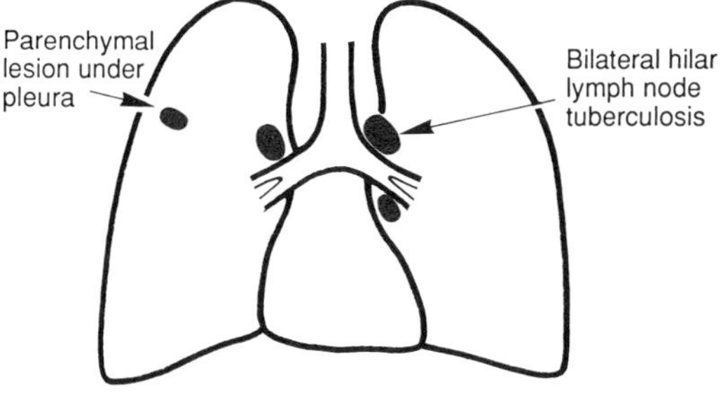

Fig. 8.14 Tuberculous primary complex. Chest X-ray; explanatory diagram shown below.

The subpleural focus may discharge bacilli or antigen into the pleural cavity, and the hypersensitivity inflammation results in a pleural effusion. This is a common presentation in adolescents infected with *M. tuberculosis* for the first time. Progressive primary tuberculosis occurs in a minority of cases. In these patients the primary lung lesion does not heal but expands to produce a tuberculous pneumonia, which is usually fatal unless treated. Sometimes the hilar node lesion expands to obstruct a bronchus with resulting lobar collapse. Occasionally the tuberculous node may erode into the bronchial wall and discharge infectious material into the bronchi and cause tuberculous bronchopneumonia. Finally, heavy tuberculous bacteraemia and miliary tuberculosis may occur (see below).

Tuberculous Bacteraemia and its Sequelae

The bacteraemia that occurs early in infection results in seeding of bacilli in macrophages in many organs of the body. These include the cerebral cortex, renal cortex, bone and joints, fallopian tubes, adrenal glands, lungs, bladder and epididymis; these lesions are not always macroscopically evident. Although bacilli may persist in these sites for years or decades without evidence of disease, their subsequent reactivation produces destructive, necrotizing granulomatous disease, sometimes known as 'end-organ tuberculosis'. Ex-

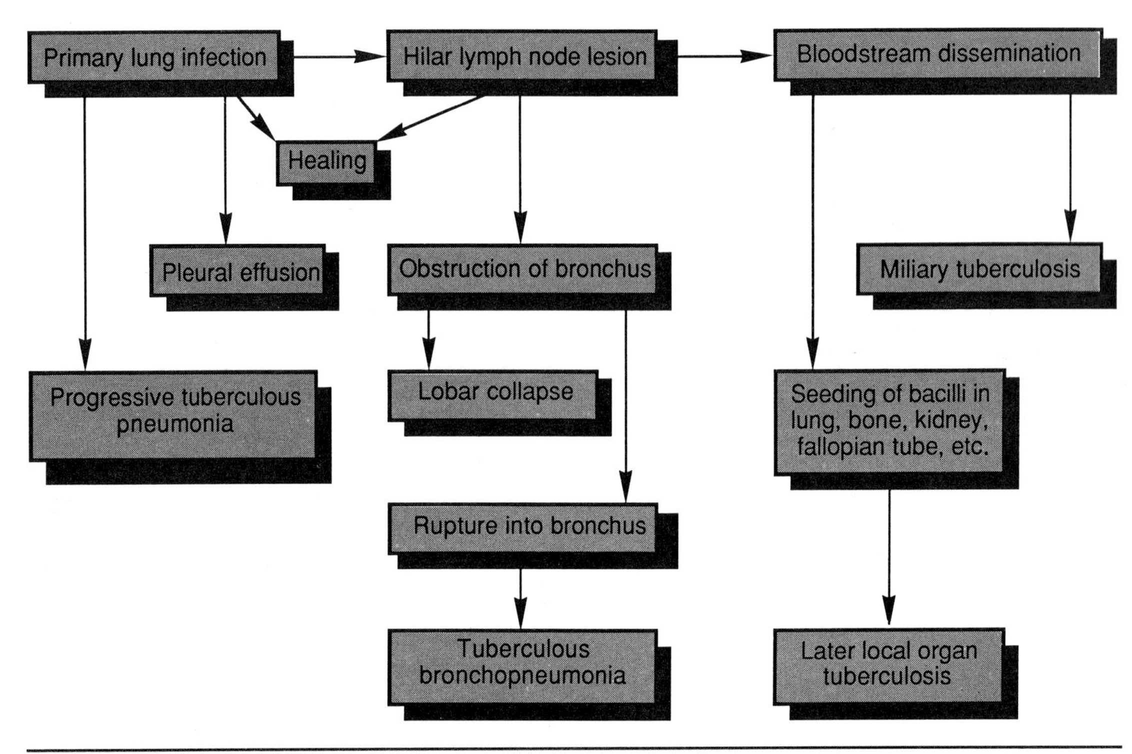

Fig. 8.15 Diagram of the sequelae of a primary infection with *Mycobacterium tuberculosis*.

amples are: (1) 'tuberculoma' of the central nervous system (p. 826), which in tropical countries is a commoner cause of cerebral space-occupying lesions than primary brain tumours; (2) adrenal tuberculosis with destruction of the functioning gland tissue, with resulting hypoadrenalism (Fig. 8.13); (3) tuberculous inflammation and obstruction of the fallopian tubes with resultant infertility; (4) destruction and collapse of vertebrae (Pott's disease) with resulting compression of the spinal cord (p. 966).

Large necrotic tuberculous lesions may be invaded by polymorphs and undergo liquefaction. Such lesions are often called 'cold abscesses', because they are not accompanied by the intense acute inflammation of a pyogenic bacterial infection.

Miliary Tuberculosis

If the tuberculous bacteraemia is heavy, via a massive leak of caseous material from a node into the bloodstream, widespread miliary tuberculosis results (Latin 'milium' – millet seed). Numerous 1–2 mm diameter spots (granuloma aggregates) are seen throughout the lungs (Fig. 8.16), liver, spleen and lymph nodes. The meninges are often involved with pronounced exudation and cellular infiltration, particularly over the basal part of the brain. The cerebrospinal fluid protein is very high so that the CSF may even clot on standing. Tuberculous meningitis is fatal unless treated. After curative therapy, the organization of the exudate may result in meningeal fibrosis with subsequent cranial nerve palsies and hydrocephalus.

Intestinal Primary Infection

In Britain, cows' milk was commonly infected with *M. bovis* or *M. tuberculosis* until pasteurization eradicated the problem. Upon ingestion, the bacilli produce primary complex tuberculous lesions similar to those in the lung. The initial site may be in the gums with lymphatic spread of bacilli to the cervical lymph nodes. In the intestine, the commonest location of the primary lesion is the

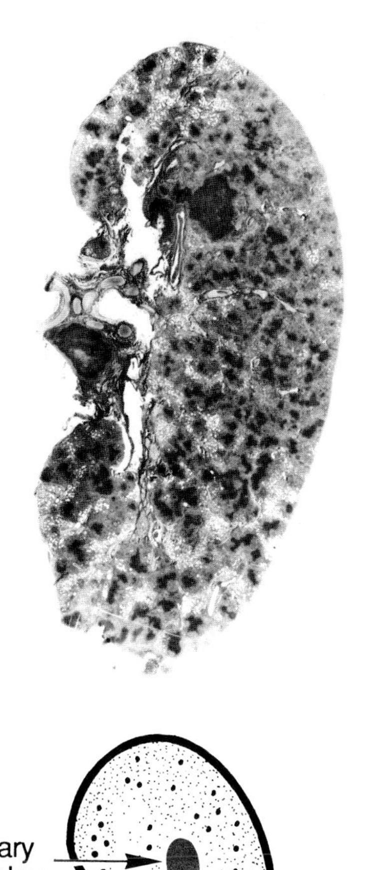

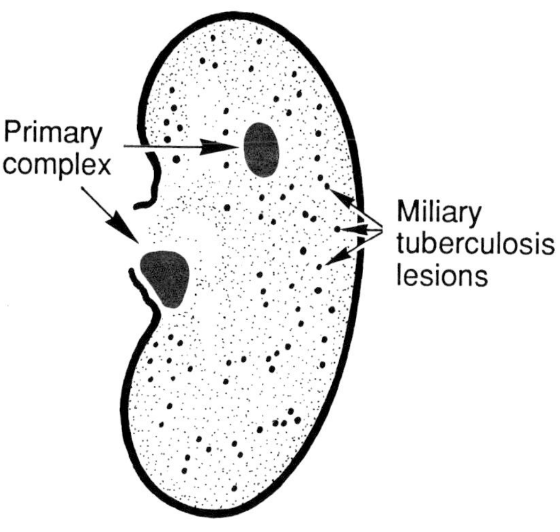

Fig. 8.16 Primary tuberculous lung infection that has progressed to miliary tuberculosis: slice of lung; explanatory diagram shown below.

ileocaecal region, with local mesenteric node involvement. The mucosa ulcerates, and the intestinal wall thickens with granulomatous inflammation. Bacteraemia with its complications may occur.

Post-primary (Adult) Tuberculosis

The pathology of pulmonary tuberculosis in adults is significantly different from that in children. People previously exposed to *M. tuberculosis* have developed hypersensitivity to its antigens, and react more rapidly when they are encountered again. Experimentally, this is shown as the Koch phenomenon (Robert Koch identified *M. tuberculosis* in 1882).

The Koch phenomenon. When live *M. tuberculosis* is injected subcutaneously into a hind leg of a guinea-pig for the first time, a tuberculous nodule develops at the injection site after a week or two. The regional lymph nodes become tuberculous and eventually the animal will die of disseminated disease. If a second subcutaneous injection of bacilli is given into the other hind limb 4–6 weeks after the first, the host response is quite different. A nodule develops within days, ulcerates, sloughs off and heals. The regional lymph node does not become tuberculous. Thus, the local tissue response to the second infection with *M. tuberculosis* is more rapid than the first; the macrophages are more able to inhibit multiplication of bacilli and prevent their spread into lymphatics. The rapidity of tissue necrosis indicates a greater hypersensitivity to the organism. A similar necrotizing tissue response occurs if the second injection is tuberculoprotein rather than live bacilli. The phenomenon is an example of the development of delayed type (type IV) hypersensitivity.

Post-primary Pulmonary Tuberculosis

This is the most important form of tuberculosis, being the commonest clinical presentation with patients who excrete bacilli into the environment to infect other people. Conventionally the term is used for lung infection occurring 5 years or more after a primary infection.

Some 5–10% of people who have inapparent tuberculosis in childhood develop active pulmonary disease later in life. The origin of this infection may be exogenous (i.e. a new or a re-infection) or endogenous (i.e. a reactivation of bacilli remaining inside the body). By examination of the phage types of *M. tuberculosis* in primary and post-primary tuberculosis, it is known that both processes can occur. In practice, in areas of the world where tuberculosis is uncommon, post-primary cases are probably reactivation phenomena, whereas both processes operate where tuberculosis is common (e.g. the tropics). Adults who acquire pulmonary tuberculosis for the first time (i.e. no childhood exposure) usually manifest the post-primary pattern of disease rather than the childhood pattern. This must indicate a difference in the way the host immune system recognizes and deals with mycobacteria at different ages.

Post-primary pulmonary tuberculosis (p. 563) is typically a cavitating and fibrosing lesion. It is usually located in the upper lobes near the apex (Fig. 8.17). The granulomatous process destroys the lung tissue which is replaced by fibrous tissue. When the lesion enlarges to involve an airway, the necrotic material is discharged and coughed up, leaving a cavity. The predisposition for apical disease may result from the location of dormant infection: there is evidence that bacilli seed haematogenously to the apical zones during a primary infection. The hilar nodes do not become significantly involved by tuberculosis as happens in the primary infection. The restriction of the infection to the lung, and its more aggressive and destructive nature are analogous to events in the Koch phenomenon.

Bacilli coughed up and swallowed may infect the small intestine. The inflammation involves the Peyer's patches, and ulceration is typically circumferential. Healing distorts the bowel and may cause a stricture.

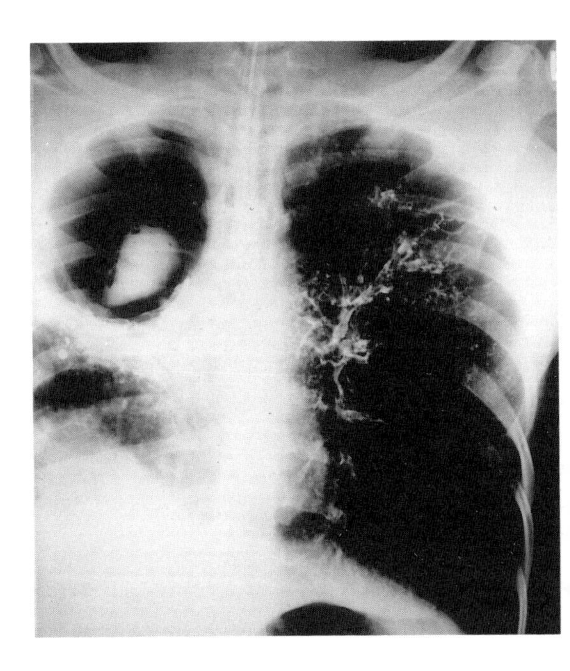

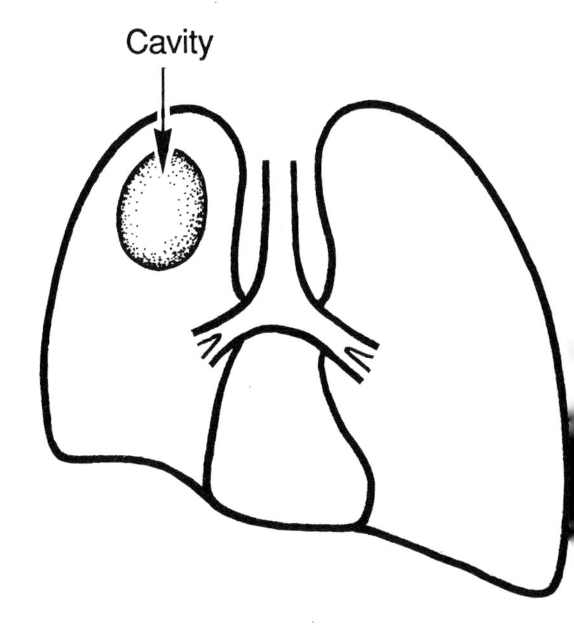

Fig. 8.17 Post-primary pulmonary tuberculosis. Chest X-ray of patient with a large tuberculous cavity in the right upper lobe. In the cavity is some contrast material from a bronchogram. The diaphragm is raised because the diseased lung has shrunk. Explanatory diagram shown below.

Extrapulmonary Tuberculosis

Many of the tuberculous lesions which develop in adults outside the lungs are reactivated foci which have been seeded during a primary infection. Typical sites include the bones and kidney. In tuberculous lymphadenopathy, another common presentation, the nodes may discharge into the skin, forming a tuberculous sinus ('scrofula'). Tuberculous pericarditis may develop from haematogenous seeding or by infection from a contiguous hilar lymph node. The type of pericarditis varies from effusion to a cellular exudative response with caseous granulomas. Healing of the latter process results in fibrosis and possibly calcification with constrictive pericarditis (p. 520).

It is notable that in immigrant groups from regions where tuberculosis is very common the patterns of presentation of tuberculosis are more atypical than the classical primary and post-primary pulmonary lesions. In the UK this is especially seen in immigrants from the Asian subcontinent, who tend to present with extrapulmonary lesions in greater numbers than do Caucasian adults, who usually present with pulmonary tuberculosis.

Healing and Chemotherapy of Tuberculosis

Before chemotherapy for tuberculosis, the disease was not necessarily fatal. It waxed and waned with episodes of increased inflammation and healing. Large caseous lesions became walled off by dense fibrous tissue, and much tissue distortion occurred. Effective chemotherapy permits more effective resolution; granulation tissue replaces the necrotic mass and fibrosis is less. Early lesions may clear up completely, and chronic fibrocaseous pulmonary lesions are transformed to smooth-walled cavities lined by epithelium.

Diagnosis of Tuberculosis

Diagnosis of pulmonary disease rests on detecting bacilli in the sputum. Smears of sputum are stained with a Ziehl–Neelsen method (or the fluorescent auramine stain) and examined microscopically. In suspected cases, culture of sputum (or tissue) samples for *M. tuberculosis* should be performed. Even if sputum examination is negative, culture may be positive. Moreover, it permits identification of the species of mycobacterium (not all cases are due to *M. tuberculosis* – see below) and enables drug sensitivity testing. Biopsy and culture of liver and bone marrow may be useful in diagnosing tuberculosis. Even in post-primary disease, granulomas may be found as small numbers of bacilli are shed into the circulation.

Tuberculin Skin Testing

Delayed hypersensitivity skin tests for tuberculosis use PPD (purified protein derivative, tuberculoprotein), a preparation of protein from killed bacilli or culture medium containing *M. tuberculosis*. The solution of antigen is injected intradermally in the Mantoux and Heaf tests, and the skin site examined after 48 hours.

An erythematous papule, which is graded according to diameter, represents a positive test and demonstrates hypersensitivity to mycobacterial antigens. Histologically, the papule comprises lymphocytes and macrophages around dermal vessels. In a suspected case this can provide support for a diagnosis of tuberculosis. However, skin test positivity also results from previous BCG vaccination and exposure to other mycobacteria. Generally, a strongly positive reaction raises the possibility of active disease. However, some clinical cases of primary tuberculosis are skin test negative, and in the elderly patient with severe tuberculosis, skin tests may also be misleadingly negative.

Hypersensitivity to tuberculin is not equivalent to resistance (immunity) to tuberculosis infection. Experimentally, it is possible to dissociate the two phenomena: guinea-pigs may be rendered hypersensitive to *M. tuberculosis* antigens by injecting tuberculoprotein, without improving their resistance to live organisms. Conversely, injecting bacilli extracted in methyl alcohol confers partial resistance to subsequent challenge without inducing hypersensitivity. Despite this, hypersensitivity and immunity usually coexist – hence the continued use of BCG vaccination in many countries.

HIV and Tuberculosis

The reduced numbers of $CD4^+$ T cells in patients with AIDS reduces cell mediated immunity and increases susceptibility to a number of infections including tuberculosis. The pattern of HIV-associated tuberculosis often resembles aggressive primary disease. Widespread tuberculous lymphadenitis and multiple lesions in the lung and liver are seen. Histologically, there is severe granular necrosis rather than true caseation, and vast numbers of bacilli are present in the lesions (Fig. 8.18).

This type of pathology is not confined to HIV-infected people. Elderly people, and patients with leukaemia or other malignant diseases, may develop an occult illness where several organs (e.g. lung, bone marrow, spleen) appear affected. There may be little fever, and the white blood count may be low. Tuberculin skin tests are negative. Yet, as revealed by biopsy or autopsy, there is widespread tuberculosis. This is termed 'non-reactive' or 'anergic' tuberculosis, and is probably the same process seen in AIDS patients.

Conclusion and Summary

The pathology of tuberculosis is given here in some detail as the prototype of chronic infectious granulomatous diseases. It shows the effects of a virulent intracellular parasite which may be contained by cooperation between macrophages and T cells. Except in cases of immunosuppression, where the toxic effects of numerous bacilli become evident, the lesions of tuberculosis are due to the host's hypersensitivity reaction to *M. tuberculosis* antigens. Tuberculosis is unpredictable in its sequelae. Once someone is infected with *M. tuberculosis*, the bacilli are likely to remain in the body, perhaps for the entire lifespan of the individual.

Leprosy (Hansen's Disease)

Leprosy is a chronic disease caused by infection with *M. leprae* and affects primarily the peripheral

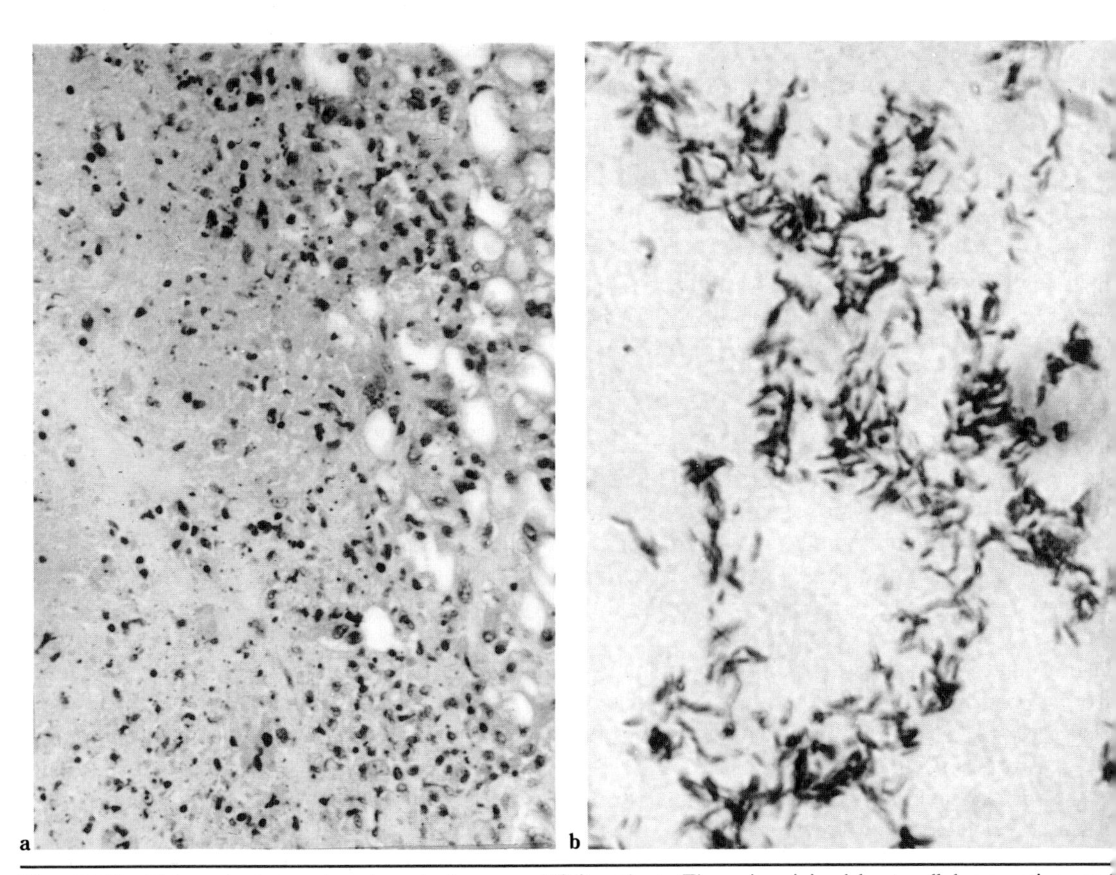

Fig. 8.18 Tuberculosis in a lymph node from an AIDS patient. There is minimal host cellular reaction, and numerous bacilli in the necrotic tissue: **a** H & E; **b** Ziehl–Neelsen stain.

nervous system and skin. As a result of nerve damage there may be paralysis, deformity and ulceration. About 12 million people in tropical and warm temperate climates have leprosy, although many more have been infected without developing the disease.

The leprosy bacillus has not yet been grown in culture. The mouse footpad supports growth and the nine-banded armadillo can become infected naturally and develop a disseminated form of the disease. *M. leprae*, which has a long dividing time of about 12 days, colonizes the cooler parts of the body.

Patients with the lepromatous form of the disease (see below) may excrete over 10 million bacilli per day from the nose into the atmosphere and undiagnosed patients are the main source of infection. The mode of transmission is not known. The bacilli probably enter via the respiratory tract, disseminate haematogenously and grow particularly in the dermal nerves.

The consequences of infection depend on the immune status of the host. Leprosy represents the best example of an infectious disease that has an immunopathological spectrum of clinical and histopathological manifestations which depend on the host's immune response. The bacillus is killed intracellularly by macrophages activated by specifically primed T cells; acquired resistance to *M. leprae* therefore depends on the cell mediated immune response. Antibody has no protective effect. The bacillus itself is non-toxic and lesions are produced either by evoking a potentially destructive granulomatous reaction or by interference with the metabolism of cells (e.g. Schwann cells) by colonization with huge numbers of bacilli.

Types of Leprosy

The incubation period for clinical leprosy is measured in years. Most of those infected have innate resistance and the bacilli are destroyed before they multiply significantly. However, the small number of surviving bacilli that survive multiply in Schwann cells and evoke a lymphocytic and macrophage response. The early form of leprosy is known as **indeterminate leprosy** and presents clinically as a hypopigmented, anaesthetic macule anywhere on the body. Occasional bacilli are present in dermal nerve fibres and most patients with this lesion eliminate the bacilli without treatment. About a quarter progress to **determined leprosy**, the bacilli continuing their multiplication and spreading beyond the dermal nerves.

The type of leprosy that results depends on the degree of immunity. A proportion of those infected fail to develop cell mediated immunity to *M. leprae* and this results in **lepromatous (multibacillary) leprosy** in which bacilli are present in large numbers in the affected tissues. This defect of immunity is antigen-specific, possibly mediated by suppressor T cells, so that patients do not suffer from opportunisitic infections. Conversely, those with a high degree of cell mediated immunity develop **tuberculoid (paucibacillary) leprosy** with scanty bacilli in the tissues. A proportion of patients do not progress initially into typical tuberculoid or lepromatous leprosy but develop an intermediate, unstable form of disease, **borderline leprosy**. Without treatment, they move eventually along the immunopathological spectrum toward lepromatous or, less commonly, tuberculoid leprosy (Fig. 8.19). The proportions of paucibacillary to multibacillary patients vary considerably around the world.

Lepromatous leprosy. The dermal lesions consist of symmetrical nodules and diffuse coarsening and thickening of the skin over much of the body. The eyebrows are lost and the classic 'leonine facies' may develop (Fig. 8.20). Histologically, the dermis is filled with rounded macrophages stuffed with bacilli which often form clumps termed **globi** (Fig. 8.21). An untreated case may have 10^7 bacilli per gram of skin, but most organisms are dead and fragmented. Lymphocytes are scanty or absent. The dermal nerves are infiltrated by bacilli-laden macrophages and Schwann cells are heavily parasitized by bacilli. Eventually the nerves undergo fibrosis. Since this affects sensory nerves particularly, the extremities become anaesthetic in a glove-and-stocking distribution and are readily traumatized. This is the main reason for the atrophy and loss of digits and toes seen in advanced cases. Lepromatous leprosy is a systemic disease, the bacilli spreading by the bloodstream to the

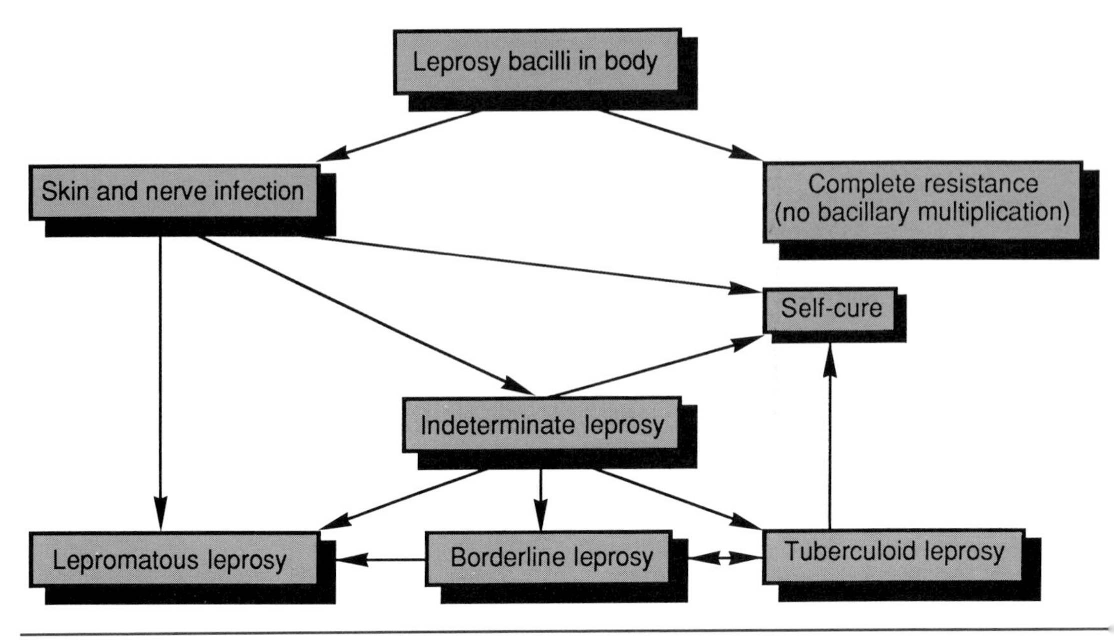

Fig. 8.19 The various patterns of untreated *Mycobacterium leprae* infection.

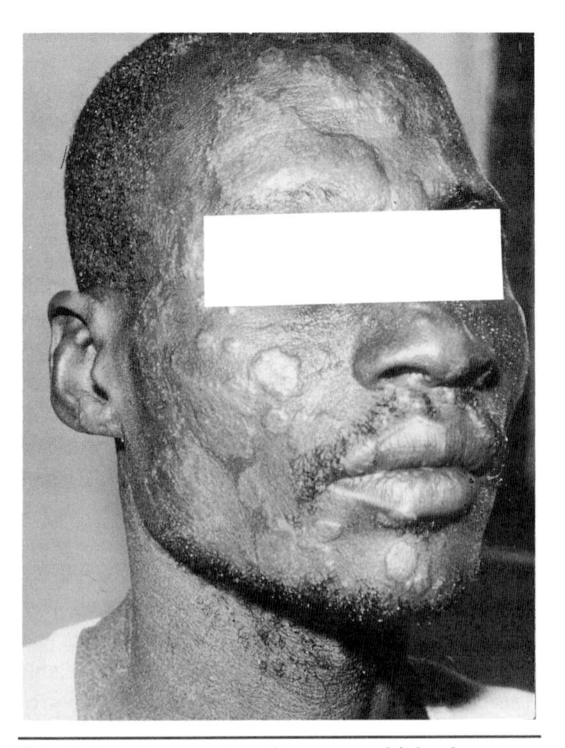

Fig. 8.20 Lepromatous leprosy: multiple plaques on the face.

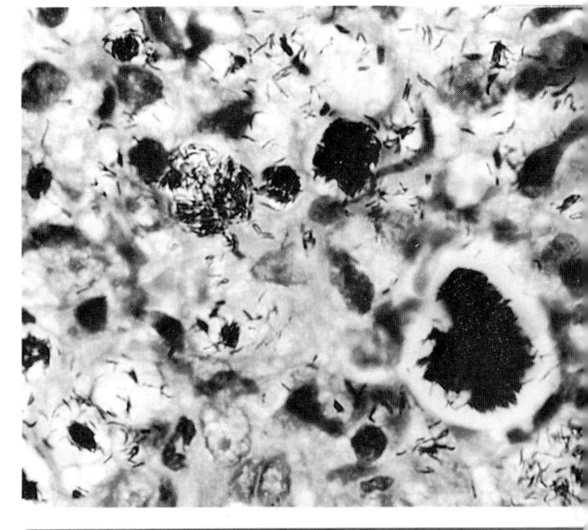

Fig. 8.21 Lepromatous leprosy. Abundant bacilli are seen, many of them in agglomerated clumps or 'globi' Wade–Fite stain for acid-fast bacilli ×1000.

nasal mucosa, larynx, lymph nodes, liver, eyes bones and testes. These multibacillary lesions can cause iritis, osteitis and bone erosion, blocked nose, laryngeal mucosal thickening with hoarse voice and orchitis. In the testes, the lesions may heal with fibrosis resulting in hypogonadism, so that gynaecomastia is sometimes seen. In long-standing cases, secondary amyloidosis is often a serious complication. In the absence of treatment patients with lepromatous leprosy will not recover cell mediated immunity and the bacilli multiply progressively.

Tuberculoid leprosy. This form is limited to the skin and peripheral nerves. The lesions are asymmetric and fewer and smaller than in lepromatous leprosy. They are annular, flat and anaesthetic, and peripheral nerves are often palpably enlarged, e.g. the median nerve at the wrist and the ulnar nerve at the elbow. Histologically, the lesions consist of epithelioid cell granulomas in the dermis and cutaneous nerves (Fig. 8.22). Severe nerve damage results from the destructive effect of the fibrosing granulomas. The larger peripheral nerves may also be seriously damaged during leprosy reactions (see below), and the intraneural granulomas may undergo caseous necrosis (the only situation where leprosy granulomas become necrotic). Consequently, there is paralysis, claw hands, foot drop, claw toes and anaesthesia. Ulceration of the skin and secondary infection with cellulitis and osteomyelitis may follow.

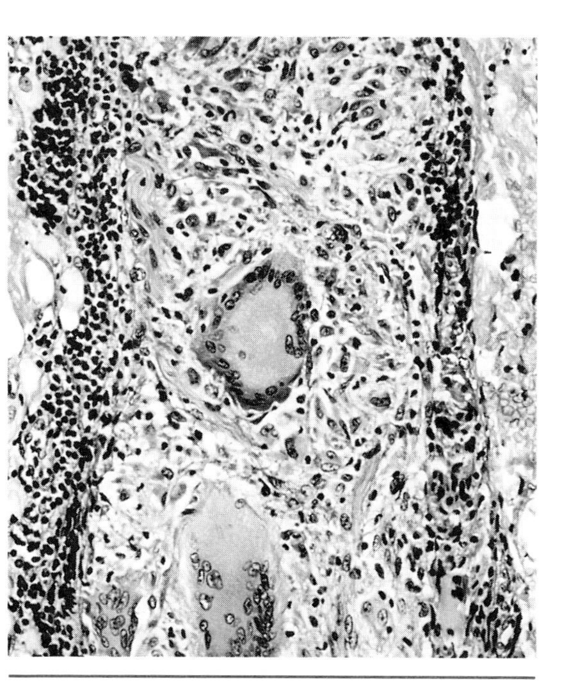

Fig. 8.22 Tuberculoid leprosy. A deep dermal nerve shows infiltration by epithelioid cells and Langhans giant cells and a peripheral lymphocytic infiltrate. This granulomatous reaction destroys the nerve and causes anaesthesia. ×250.

Borderline leprosy. Clinically and pathologically, this has mixed features of tuberculoid and lepromatous leprosy, with numerous erythematous skin papules containing moderate numbers of bacilli and a diffuse epithelioid-cell infiltrate in the dermis.

Some of the features of the different types of leprosy are shown in Fig. 8.23.

Diagnosis of Leprosy

Slit-skin smears are used in the diagnosis of leprosy: fluid from an incised skin lesion is treated by a modified Ziehl–Neelsen stain for acid-fast bacilli. Many bacilli are seen in lepromatous and borderline cases, but very few, or none in indeterminate and tuberculoid lesions. Scrapings from the nasal mucosa in lepromatous patients also reveal abundant bacilli.

The **lepromin skin test** is an index of cell mediated immunity to *M. leprae* and is performed by injecting heat-killed *M. leprae* intradermally. A positive reaction (the **Mitsuda reaction**) occurs within 4 weeks as an erythematous nodule in patients with tuberculoid or indeterminate leprosy. The reaction does not occur in lepromatous leprosy, and a positive result is of little diagnostic value because it may result from exposure to other mycobacteria and from self-cured subclinical *M. leprae* infections. In lepromatous leprosy, there is a raised serum IgG level, a high titre of antibody to *M. leprae* antigens and often antinuclear autoantibodies and a false-positive screening test for syphilis.

Leprosy Reactions

Two types of acute immunologically mediated reactions may be seen in leprosy patients, usually occurring after commencing antimicrobial therapy.

Erythema nodosum leprosum occurs at the lepromatous end of the leprosy spectrum when

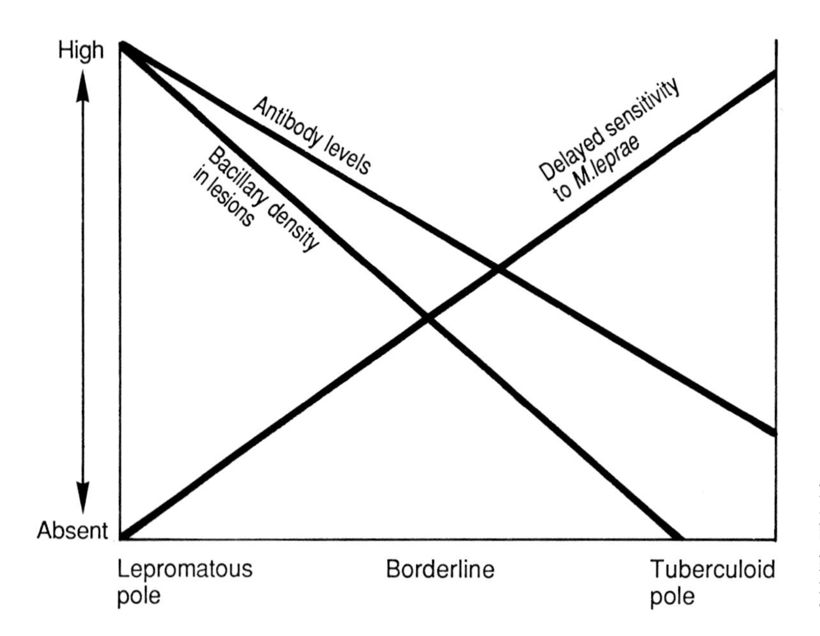

Fig. 8.23 Immunological and bacteriological features along the pathological spectrum of leprosy.

initial drug treatment kills large numbers of *M. leprae* and releases antigenic material. As the antibody titre is usually high, immune complexes are formed locally and induce crops of painful inflammatory papules along with fever and malaise. Histologically, the tissues show oedema, polymorph infiltration and vasculitis. The features are thus those of a mild Arthus-type reaction (p. 213). Circulating immune-complex diseases (p. 214) may occur with an acute generalized reaction, glomerulonephritis, polyarthritis and iritis.

Delayed hypersensitivity reactions occur in borderline patients who are immunologically unstable. Their degree of cell mediated immunity is liable to change, and as treatment reduces the amount of *M. leprae* antigen, T-cell mediated macrophage activation increases. There is cellular infiltration and oedema of the tissue granulomas so that swollen erythematous papules develop in the skin. The nerves become inflamed and may undergo necrosis and formation of 'cold abscesses' causing paralysis.

Relapse and Causes of Death

Inadequate treatment or the development of drug resistance may permit the disease to relapse. This is seen as growth of the skin nodules, which then contain innumerable leprosy bacilli.

Leprosy patients usually have a normal lifespan and die from other causes. The main fatal consequence of leprosy is renal failure from amyloidosis. Proper bactericidal drug therapy arrests and cures the disease. However, it cannot reverse the complications that derive from permanent nerve damage.

Other Mycobacterial Infections

Several non-tuberculosis mycobacterial infections can produce serious disease in man. The commonest are caused by *M. avium-intracellulare* and *M. scrofulaceum*.

M. avium-intracellulare (MAI)

Mycobacteria of this complex live in the soil and water, and are constantly imbibed and inhaled. Three clinical patterns are important.

(1) In adults MAI may cause pulmonary disease which closely resembles post-primary tuber-

culosis. In developed countries MAI accounts for 1–10% of apparent pulmonary tuberculosis cases (in tropical countries, pulmonary tuberculosis is virtually always caused by *M. tuberculosis*). Many patients have a predisposing pulmonary condition such as chronic obstructive airways disease, silicosis, rheumatoid disease and even inactive old tuberculosis. There is cavitation and fibrosis, and a similar histopathology to classical tuberculosis.
(2) In children, mycobacterial cervical lymphadenitis is a common condition: usually the submental and anterior triangle nodes are diseased. In contrast to the situation in the tropics, and in immigrants from the tropics, where *M. tuberculosis* is the major cause of mycobacterial lymphadenitis, in developed countries non-tuberculosis mycobacteria such as MAI are more often the cause. The organisms presumably invade via the oral cavity and pass to the local nodes to produce a caseating, granulomatous lymphadenitis, which commonly discharges through the skin. It is indistinguishable histologically from *M. tuberculosis* infection. However, unlike the latter, excision and drainage of the lesion is sufficient treatment, without the need for chemotherapy. The inflammation heals with some scarring.
(3) In patients with defective cell mediated immunity, MAI causes a disseminated infection of macrophages throughout the body. In developed countries, between 5% and 25% of AIDS patients have disseminated MAI infection. In these patients, the expected granulomatous reaction to the mycobacteria either does not develop or is not sustained, and macrophages become filled with bacilli, resembling lepromatous leprosy. There is little tissue necrosis as MAI is not toxic. The affected organs, typically the intra-abdominal lymph nodes, liver and spleen, enlarge due to the hyperplasia of MAI-infected macrophages (Fig. 8.24).

Mycobacterium scrofulaceum

This species is important as a common cause of cervical lymphadenitis in children, with similar pathology to MAI infection at that site.

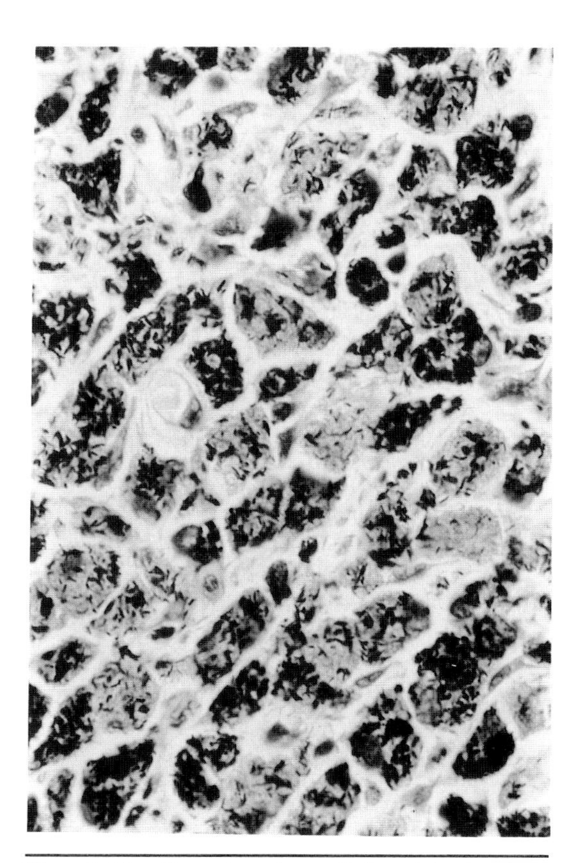

Fig. 8.24 *M. avium–intracellulare* infection in a lymph node from an AIDS patient. There are numerous bacilli inside macrophages, but no necrosis. Ziehl–Neelsen stain.

Sarcoidosis

This disease, of unknown aetiology, is characterized by multiple granulomatous lesions which may affect lymph nodes, lungs, skin, spleen, eyes, salivary glands, liver and bones, particularly of the hands and feet. It has a worldwide distribution, but with great geographical variation in incidence. It occurs over a wide age range, but is most common in young adults and is much more common in blacks than whites in the USA, and in immigrants than natives in Great Britain. The highest reported incidence is in Sweden.

The disease most commonly gives rise to enlarged mediastinal and pulmonary hilar lymph nodes, often without symptoms, but sometimes accompanied by fever. Other groups of lymph nodes are often affected and widespread minute lesions in the lungs may present an X-ray picture resembling that of miliary tuberculosis. Sarcoid lesions also occur in the skin and occasionally *erythema induratum* (p. 1124) develops and may be the presenting clinical feature. Microscopically, the sarcoid lesions consist of tubercle-like follicles composed of epithelioid cells with occasional Langhans giant cells and with fewer lymphocytes than in tuberculosis (Fig. 8.25). The giant cells may contain curious calcium-rich star-shaped or conchoid inclusions (asteroid or Schaumann bodies). Unlike tuberculosis, the lesions do not undergo caseation although there may be a little central necrosis.

The course of the disease is unpredictable: it may be acute or chronic and temporary or permanent remission may occur spontaneously. It can cause blindness by involving the uveal tract. It is occasionally fatal, usually as a result of diffuse fibrosis of the pulmonary lesions with consequent right ventricular heart failure, or as a result of intercurrent infection. Hypercalcaemia may develop with consequent renal damage.

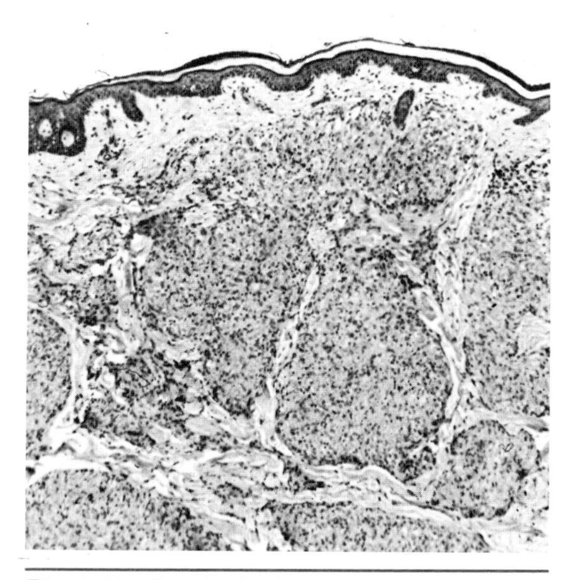

Fig. 8.25 Sarcoidosis of skin. The lesions consist of aggregates of epithelioid cells with relatively few lymphocytes. In contrast to tuberculosis, there is little or no necrosis. ×80.

Diagnosis

Non-caseating epithelioid-cell granulomas, with or without giant-cell inclusions, are not diagnostic of sarcoidosis: they occur in various conditions including tuberculosis, various fungal infections, syphilis, brucellosis and berylliosis. The diagnosis of sarcoidosis thus depends also on the clinical features, the distribution of the lesions, and on excluding the above possibilities.

Intradermal injection of a sterile suspension prepared from sarcoid lesions (**Kveim test**) into most patients with sarcoidosis leads to the development of a local lesion, which becomes maximal in about 6 weeks and has the histological features of sarcoidosis. False-positive results may occur in other conditions, notably Crohn's disease (p. 713). Cell mediated immunity is depressed in patients with sarcoidosis, as shown by a negative tuberculin test, even in those patients known to have been previously positive. T-cell numbers and function are depressed while antibody production is normal or increased.

Aetiology

The sarcoid lesion, consisting of epithelioid cells and lymphocytes, is itself suggestive of a delayed hypersensitivity reaction, although no specific exogenous agent has been shown to be involved. Subsequent development of tuberculosis has been observed in some patients, but sarcoidosis seems unlikely to be a modified form of tuberculosis, because depression of delayed hypersensitivity (as in sarcoidosis) would be expected to be associated with a florid form of tuberculosis with large numbers of *M. tuberculosis* in the lesions. Furthermore, the condition is often improved by administration of corticosteroids.

Other Bacterial Infections

Syphilis

Syphilis is a systemic infection caused by the spirochaete *Treponema pallidum*, which is transmitted mainly by sexual intercourse (venereal syphilis), and less commonly via the placenta (congenital syphilis) or by accidental inoculation from infectious material.

The name 'syphilis' derives from a poem composed in AD 1530 by Girolamo Frascatoro, a Veronese physician, in which Syphilis (a swineherd) offends Apollo and is afflicted with the disease. The origin of the infection is unclear. It may have been brought back by Columbus' sailors from the New World (the Columbian theory); alternatively, it may have occurred as the result of a change in the host-parasite relationship of an already existing treponemal infection such as yaws or pinta (see below) which were prevalent in Africa and Asia (the unitarian theory). Either way, it is certain that towards the end of the fifteenth century, a pandemic of venereal syphilis swept through Europe with high mortality. Now, even untreated syphilis has a low mortality; an example of the way in which 'new' infections may gradually lose their severity over time as the host adapts and builds up resistance (there are parallels here with influenza and tuberculosis).

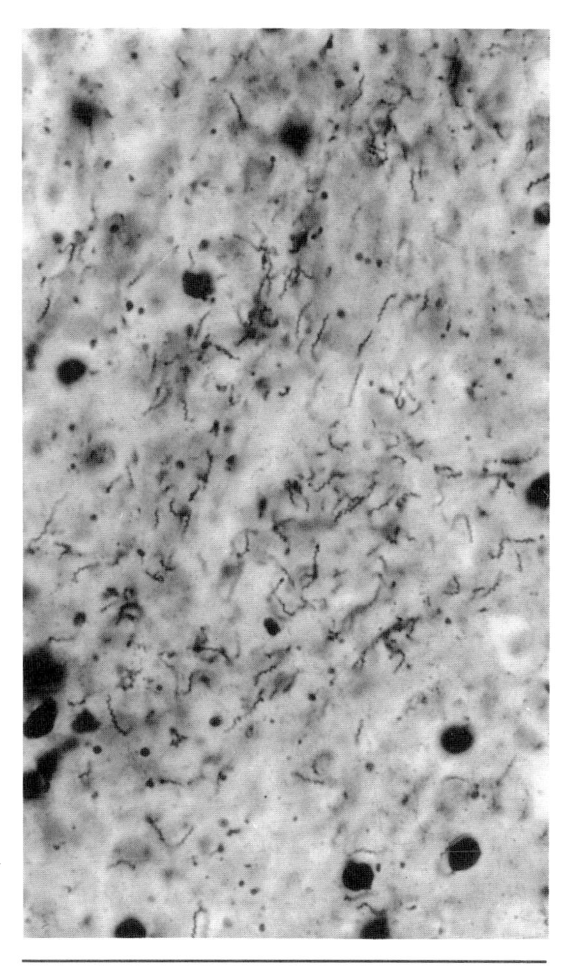

Fig. 8.26 Large number of spirochaetes in the liver of a fetus who died of congenital syphilis. ×1000.

General Features

Treponema pallidum is a spirochaete 4–14 × 0.2 μm in length (Fig. 8.26) which cannot be grown in culture. Various other mammals can be infected, such as monkeys and rabbits, with resulting chronic infection. The venereal infection has a current incidence of approximately 10 cases per 10^5 population per annum in the UK, but is notably common in homosexuals. The organism is delicate, susceptible to drying and does not survive long outside the body. It invades mucosae directly, possibly aided by surface abrasions. Following intercourse with an infected person, a primary lesion, an ulcer known as the chancre, develops at the site of infection, usually the external genitalia, but also lips and anorectal region (according to sexual practice). Within hours of infection, spirochaetes disseminate via lymphatics and bloodstream, and there is local lymph node enlargement. Thereafter the disease is unpredictable, and the major possible events and their time scales are shown in Fig. 8.27.

Conventionally syphilis is divided into sequential stages. After the primary chancre heals, in a proportion of untreated patients the disease progresses to the secondary stage with widespread

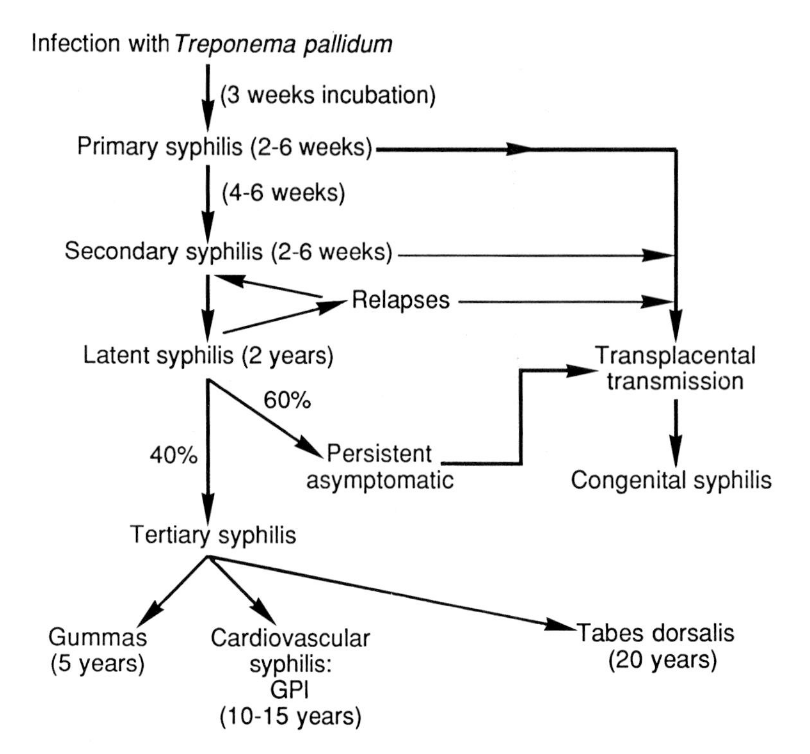

Fig. 8.27 The sequence of clinicopathological events in untreated venereal syphilis. Some typical time scales and proportions are indicated.

skin, mucosal and visceral lesions. These subside spontaneously, and the patient enters the latent stage without clinical features but still infected and antibody positive. Some patients relapse with renewed secondary stage lesions; others will remain asymptomatic (latent) indefinitely. About 40% of untreated patients develop tertiary syphilis over subsequent years and decades. These lesions affect skin, bones, cardiovascular system and central nervous system particularly. Effective chemotherapy with penicillin will abort the infection at any stage, but cannot reverse permanent pathological damage.

Patients with active primary and secondary syphilis are infectious to others. Infectivity declines about 2 years after infection, but patients in the latent asymptomatic stage may still have episodes of transient spirochaetaemia which may cause congenital syphilis in pregnant females.

The Pathology of Syphilis

The following is a brief account of the pathology and pathogenesis of syphilis. Further descriptions are found in the chapters on the cardiovascular system and the central nervous system.

Histologically, the early lesions of syphilis are characterized by an intense plasma cell infiltrate, small vessel proliferation, capillary endothelial cell hypertrophy and abundant spirochaetes. The proliferation of the intima of small arteries, causing reduction in the lumen, is referred to as *endarteritis obliterans*; the accompanying perivascular inflammation as *periarteritis* (Fig. 8.28). In the later lesions, the spirochaetes are scanty or nondemonstrable, and the host reaction becomes granulomatous, with necrosis.

The primary chancre

This appears as a hard, erythematous nodule about 1 cm in diameter (Fig. 8.29) with regional lymph node enlargement. The centre of the chancre ulcerates, with a clean rim, and it usually does not become secondarily infected. The ulcer is painless, persists for some weeks, and heals. In women, a chancre develops on the vulva, or the cervix (where it may be unnoticed). Anal inter-

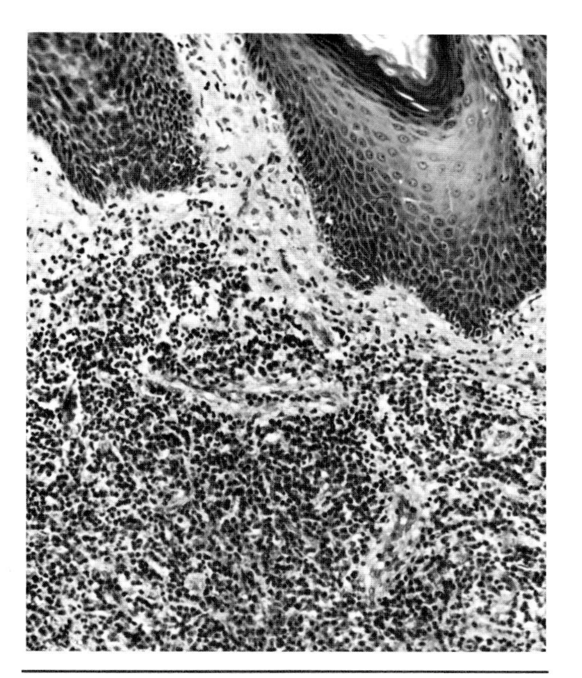

Fig. 8.28 Primary chancre. Small vessel proliferation and dense lymphocytic and plasmacytic perivascular infiltrate. The epidermis is hyperplastic. ×120.

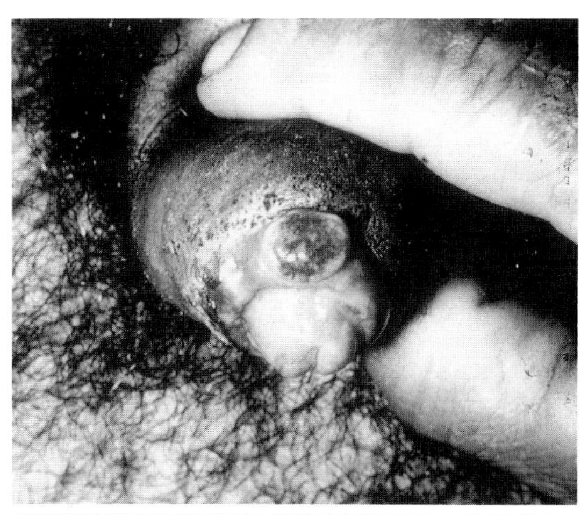

Fig. 8.29 Primary chancre on the penis. Ulcerated foreskin.

course produces anorectal lesions with a rectal discharge due to treponemal proctitis. Histologically, there is vascular proliferation, a predominantly plasma cell infiltrate and deposition of mucopolysaccharide-rich oedema fluid in which spirochaetes are abundant. Following ulceration, epithelial hyperplasia occurs. The lesion heals via granulation tissue, with minimal scarring. The lymph nodes show both follicular and T-cell zone hyperplasia.

Secondary lesions

There is always a widespread erythematous skin rash and generalized lymphadenopathy. Other typical lesions include **mucous patches** ('snail track ulcers') on the pharynx and genitalia; and **condylomata lata** – papular lesions in moist areas such as axillae and perineum. A low-grade meningitis is common. Uveitis, hepatitis and, occasionally, immune-complex mediated nephrotic syndrome are also seen. These lesions represent activity in sites where spirochaetes have lodged during the primary infection. They heal spontaneously. Histologically, the inflammation and vascular lesions are similar to those of primary syphilis; spirochaetes are again plentiful. Recurrent episodes (relapses) may show a more granulomatous histology in skin lesions.

Tertiary lesions

These appear irregularly over succeeding years (see Fig. 8.27) and may cause serious and permanent damage by means of chronic inflammation. In historical studies of untreated syphilis, about 25% of patients died directly of late syphilis. The three basic forms of tertiary syphilis are the gumma, the cardiovascular lesions, and neurosyphilis, with approximate frequencies in untreated patients of 16%, 10% and 7% respectively. The lesions result from activation of inflammation at the sites where spirochaetes lodge.

Gummas are necrotic masses of variable size that appear most often in skin, liver, testes and bones. They are destructive, causing for example collapse of the bridge of the nose and palatal perforation, and persistent ulcers in the skin. Osteitis and periostitis may lead to thickening and deformity of long bones, such as the 'sabre tibia'. Multiple liver gummas produce hepatomegaly and the ensuing scarring may distort the gross appearances ('hepar lobatum'). Histologically, gummas consist of parenchymal necrosis with surrounding granulomatous response, often with giant cells. They resemble tuberculosis lesions macroscopically and microscopically, but are usually harder in texture.

Cardiovascular syphilis. The lesions include aortitis, aortic valve regurgitation, aortic aneurysm and coronary ostia stenosis. The aortitis affects the proximal aorta, which has intimal plaques and longitudinal grooves; the 'tree barking' appearance is the result of medial scarring and secondary atherosclerosis. The medial lesions are endarteritis and periarteritis of the vasa vasorum in the wall of the aorta. Granulomatous inflammation is often seen as well as a plasma cell infiltrate, and the effect is destruction of elastic and muscle layers in the aorta. In time, the aorta may dilate to form an aneurysm and eventually rupture, classically at the arch.

Similar dilatation at the aortic ring causes functional aortic valve regurgitation. Additionally, the valve cusps become inflamed, thickened and fibrosed, their edges rolled and retracted. At the site of the coronary artery ostia, the intima becomes thickened, which may occlude the ostia and cause coronary insufficiency.

Neurosyphilis comprises meningovascular disease, general paralysis of the insane, and tabes dorsalis. The meningeal blood vessels show a periarteritis with lymphocytes and plasma cells. Small gummas may also be seen in the meninges, resembling tubercles. Syphilitic endarteritis of medium-sized arteries may cause ischaemic cerebral lesions. More commonly, the consequences of meningovascular syphilis are cranial nerve palsies and hydrocephalus. **Tabes dorsalis** is degeneration of the posterior columns of the spinal cord and of the dorsal nerve roots. It is accompanied by meningitis. The standard explanation for the pathogenesis of tabes dorsalis is that inflamation and fibrosis of the dorsal nerve roots causes their atrophy.

In **general paralysis of the insane** (GPI) the meninges are white and thickened and associated with underlying gyral atrophy. The early stages are a meningoencephalitis, with spirochaetes in the cerebral cortex, perivascular lymphocytes and plasma cells, proliferation of astrocytes and microglial cells, and degeneration of neurons. At the end stage, there is minimal inflammation and no spirochaetes are seen.

Congenital syphilis

Following transplacental infection of the fetus, lesions do not develop until after the fourth month of pregnancy, since fetal immunological competence only commences then. The outcome depends in part on the infective dose (i.e. the degree of maternal spirochaetaemia) and hence, the stage of maternal infection. In the primary and secondary stages, the fetus is heavily infected and may die of hydrops *in utero* or shortly after birth. There is hepatosplenomegaly. The viscera are heavily infected with spirochaetes (see Fig. 8.26) with foci of necrosis, and organs such as the liver and pancreas show diffuse fibrosis. The lungs are pneumonic with interstitial fibrosis. Enchondral ossification of long bones is disturbed, with characteristic widening of the growth plate. The placenta is heavy, pale and shows a plasmacytic villitis.

In subsequent pregnancies (i.e. after the maternal second stage of infection), the effects are progressively less severe. The child may have less dramatic visceral disease, and manifest papular rashes on skin and mucosae such as the nose, causing 'snuffles'. These are histologically similar to lesions of secondary syphilis. Later, a characteristic deformity appears in the incisor teeth, which are peg-shaped with notched edges (Hutchinson's teeth). Still later, neurosyphilis may develop, as may interstitial keratitis, leading to corneal opacity and blindness. Children infected *in utero* who are seropositive but show no lesions until two or more years after birth are classified as having late congenital syphilis. Some infected children never develop lesions but remain seropositive for life. Routine serotesting and treatment of pregnant women has greatly reduced the incidence of congenital syphilis.

Pathogenesis of Syphilitic Lesions

The primary and secondary lesions of syphilis occur at sites of local proliferation of *T. pallidum*. The organism does not produce toxins and is not cytopathic in macrophage culture. The initial inflammatory response is lymphocytic and plasmacytic, indicating an immune response. There appears to be a serum factor in early syphilis which temporarily suppresses cell mediated immunity. The extent to which the primary chancre is caused by immunopathology, or is the result of ischaemia from endarteritis obliterans, is uncertain.

Although patients with primary syphilis of more than 2 weeks' duration cannot be re-infected by a challenge, antibodies do not provide immunity in experimental infection. They may play a role in gradually reducing the numbers of organisms. The later gummatous lesions contain few spirochaetes and are granulomatous, indicating the development of cell mediated immunity, which probably controls treponemal multiplication. The cause of the necrosis in gummas is probably similar to that seen in tuberculosis.

Diagnostic Tests for Syphilis

In primary and early secondary syphilis, where spirochaetes are plentiful in the lesions, immediate diagnosis can be made by the examination of smears by dark-ground microscopy. In other circumstances, and in later syphilis where organisms are scanty or absent, the diagnosis is made serologically. Two types of antibody tests are used: those that detect non-specific antibodies, and those that detect specific antibodies against antigenic components of the treponemes.

The non-specific antibodies are autoantibodies against lipoidal antigens of human and other mammalian tissues. Cardiolipin, an alcohol extract of ox heart muscle, is used as the antigen. The prototype serology test was the complement fixing Wassermann reaction (WR); now the rapid plasma reagin (RPR) and venereal disease research laboratory (VDRL) methods are standard, and the VDRL can be quantified to give titres. Either the antigens that induce lipoidal antibody are components of *T. pallidum* (and the serology is therefore a cross-reaction), or they are material released from host tissues by the damaging effect of the infection itself. Lipoidal antibody is detected 7–10 days after the primary chancre develops, and is present so long as there is active disease; i.e. these reagin tests may become negative during the latent phase and usually become negative after successful treatment.

Several infections unrelated to treponemal infection (e.g. malaria) can produce a short-lasting biological false-positive reaction (BFP) with lipoidal antibody tests, while persistent BFP is seen in some people with autoimmune disease, notably systemic lupus erythematosus.

The specific tests which detect antibodies to *T. pallidum* components are:

(1) the *T. pallidum* immobilization test (TPI) where antibody stops live treponemes moving; now used infrequently;
(2) the *T. pallidum* haemagglutination assay (TPHA), where sheep red cells coated with *T. pallidum* extract are agglutinated by antibody;
(3) the fluorescent treponemal antibody test (FTA-Abs) where antibody binds to treponemes fixed on the test slide and is detected by indirect immunofluorescence.

These specific tests become positive in primary syphilis and remain so indefinitely, irrespective of disease activity or treatment.

The lipoidal antibody tests are used for screening, and the specific tests for confirmation.

Other Treponematoses

There are several other treponemal diseases, now uncommon globally, related to syphilis: yaws (*T. pertenue*), pinta (*T. carateum*) and endemic syphilis (also called bejel – *T. pallidum*). None of the organisms can be cultured *in vitro*; they all induce antibody responses identical to those of venereal syphilis; the treponemes are morphologically identical and studies of DNA indicate that *T. pallidum* and *T. pertenue* are identical. In fact the diseases are distinguished only in their clinical features in man and by the patterns of infection in experimental animals. Visceral lesions are rare, in contrast to venereal syphilis. The routes of infection (cutaneous, non-venereal contact) and the age of the host are relevant. Yaws and endemic syphilis are infections of children; pinta is seen in young adults. Yaws, still seen in Africa, produces warty skin lesions and destructive bone lesions, similar pathologically to secondary syphilis and gummatous osteitis respectively; deep skin ulcers also occur.

Actinomycosis

This disease is produced by organisms which are normal commensals in the mouth, gut and female genital tract. Only occasionally do they invade the tissues to produce infection. The actinomycetes are Gram-positive branching bacteria which grow in the tissues to produce characteristic radiate colonies, sometimes visible macroscopically. In man, the microaerophilic *Actinomyces israelii* is the chief pathogen but occasionally other species and similar aerobic organisms (*Nocardia*) are involved. In bovines, in which actinomycosis due to *Actinomyces bovis* is common, the lesions are localized and large granulomatous masses occur, especially in and around the jaw.

In man the disease is most common in young adult males, producing lesions of a more suppurative type. In more than 50% of cases the mouth or jaws are affected, the parasite gaining entrance from a tooth socket following extraction, from a carious tooth or after maxillofacial injury. In abdominal actinomycosis the appendix or caecum is normally involved and infection usually follows surgery or perforation of a viscus. Pulmonary disease most commonly results from aspiration of oropharyngeal secretions and produces an indolent pneumonia with cavitation and empyaema. Pelvic actinomycosis, involving the fallopian tubes and ovaries, is associated with the prolonged use of intrauterine contraceptive devices (IUCDs). Actinomyces-like organisms can be demonstrated in Papanicolaou-stained cervical smears from many women with IUCDs, but invasive disease is rare. Cervical cytology rapidly returns to normal when the IUCD is removed.

The lesion is usually characterized by chronic suppuration with formation of multiple abscesses, each containing one or more colonies of the organism – the so-called honeycomb abscesses. Fibrous septa between the abscesses are lined by granulation tissue which contains many foamy cells, macrophages laden with lipid, giving the lining of each abscess a yellowish colour. In the centre is pus containing actinomyces colonies, which are sometimes visible by naked eye as small, yellow, brown or grey, gritty granules ('sulphur granules'). Lesions of the face and neck, originating about the jaw, may produce much granulation tissue in which many small foci of suppuration persist and discharge through the skin, resulting in multiple sinuses. The infection spreads directly through the tissues, disregarding tissue planes, but does not usually involve the regional lymph nodes. If untreated, it tends to invade the bloodstream, giving rise to pyaemia with secondary abscesses in the liver, lungs and brain. Actinomycetes are also responsible for some cases of mycetoma (p. 333).

Mycoplasmal Infections

Mycoplasma are very small filamentous or coccobacillary micro-organisms which lack a rigid cell wall containing peptidoglycan but can be grown in cell-free media and are classed as bacteria. They are distributed widely and are pathogenic to many animal and plant species. In man only one species, *Mycoplasma pneumoniae*, has been shown conclusively to be pathogenic, although other mycoplasmas have been isolated from the lesions of various other diseases. A major difficulty arises from their ubiquity and the consequent contamination of culture media; they can pass through bacteria-retaining filters and are also liable to contaminate cell cultures used in virology and for other purposes.

Mycoplasma pneumoniae is the cause of one form of 'non-bacterial' pneumonia, which is endemic in most parts of the world and also occurs as outbreaks, particularly in school age children and young adults. The organism disseminates in the body and may cause a meningoencephalitis. The immune response includes the production of an antibody which cross-reacts at low temperatures with a human red cell antigen, and, in some cases is responsible for acute haemolysis.

Because mycoplasma lack peptidoglycan in their cell wall, infections due to them are not affected by antibiotics which interfere with cell wall synthesis, e.g. the penicillins.

Viral Infections

General Properties of Viruses

Viruses are fundamentally different from all other pathogens. In essence they are parasitic nucleic acids, which are absolutely dependent on the metabolic machinery of the host cell for much of their replication. Their nucleic acids encode only for the components of synthetic pathways not found in the host and for the proteins which coat the virus nucleic acid molecule to form the virus particle, or virion.

The functions of the virion (Figs 8.30 and 8.31) are fourfold:

(1) It protects the virus nucleic acid genome from hostile environmental factors when it is being transmitted from host to host and from cell to cell. These factors include nuclease enzymes and ultraviolet irradiation.
(2) The virion optimizes the initiation of infection. Virus encoded proteins on the surface of

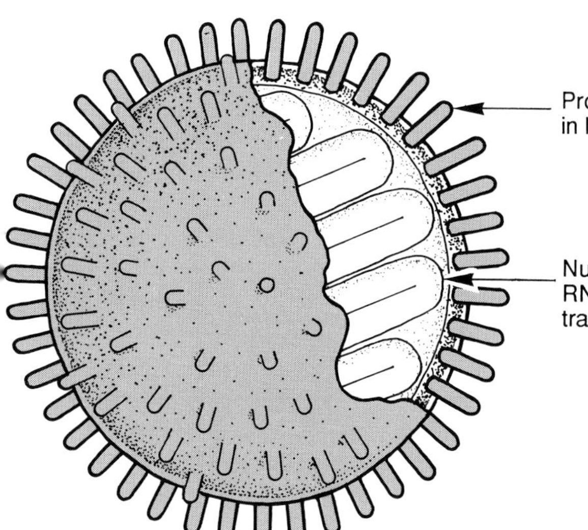

Fig. 8.30 Diagram of enveloped virion showing arrangement of external proteins and internal nucleoprotein. Measles virus (with haemagglutinin and fusion protein spikes) and influenza virus (with haemagglutinin and neuraminidase spikes) have this type of virion structure. Both viruses have a nucleoprotein which contains a single RNA molecule (measles virus) or 8 different RNA segments (influenza virus).

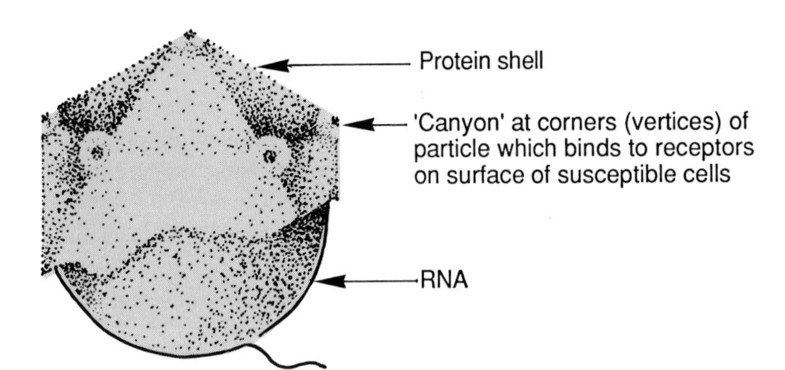

Fig. 8.31 Diagram of poliovirus virion.

the virion bind avidly to specific receptors on the cell surface and enable viruses to target particular cells for infection. Well studied examples are the haemagglutinin protein of influenza virus, which binds to terminal sialic acid molecules of glycoproteins on the surface of host cells, and the surface protein of the human immunodeficiency virus, gp160, which binds to the CD4 molecule on the surface of T-helper-inducer ($CD4^+$) lymphocytes (p. 197).

A further example is the fusion (F) protein of measles virus which is a spike-like glycoprotein, protruding from the virion envelope. After absorption to the host cell, mediated by the virion haemagglutinin, the F protein causes the virion envelope to fuse with the cell membrane, to allow the virion nucleoprotein to enter the cell.

(3) The virions of many – but not all – viruses carry out tasks required for the initiation of macromolecular synthesis, which cannot be performed by the host cell. Thus, the virions of viruses with negative-sense single stranded RNA genomes carry a transcriptase enzyme which is transferred into the host cell to initiate macromolecular synthesis by making complementary copies of the virus genome. The host cell will recognize only these complementary RNA copies as being biologically active. The measles virus nucleoprotein is a typical example of this: it contains transcriptase molecules and the genome of the virus.

(4) The virion also acts as a structural and a functional support package for the delivery of the virus genome into the host cell. This is particularly important for viruses whose genomes are made up of a number of different nucleic acid molecules, known as genome segments. Their virions are assembled in such a way that each particle contains the correct complement of segments. Examples of viruses with segmented genomes include influenza virus and rotaviruses.

Viruses are classified according to the type, structure and size of nucleic acid found in the virion, and the structure of the virion itself. Virion nucleic acids may be either RNA or DNA but not both. The nucleic acids may be double- or single-stranded, may encode for few or many gene products and may be contained in the virion as a single molecule, or in the case of some RNA virus families, as a number of segments. Virions may take the form of a protein shell made up of symmetrically arranged subunits which surround the nucleic acid or nucleoprotein complex. In addition there may be a membranous envelope, containing components derived from host cell membranes and virus-coded proteins, which, in turn, surrounds the nucleoprotein complex containing the virus genome.

The nature of the virus genome is extremely important in determining the impact that infection can have on the host. DNA viruses that replicate in the host nucleus can set up long-term relationships with the host at the cellular level, as their genomes – intact or in part – can either integrate themselves into host chromosomes or maintain themselves in the host nucleus. This relationship may result in persistent and latent infections, or long-term alterations in the host genome leading to malignant change. The role of viruses in neoplasia is considered in Chapter 3. RNA viruses cannot establish long-term association with their hosts in this way, as RNA molecules cannot physically link with host chromosomes or be replicated in the host nucleus by host enzymes. Retroviruses, the family which contains the human immunodeficiency virus (HIV), escape the molecular constraints of having an RNA genome in their virions by using their reverse transcriptase enzyme to copy this RNA into DNA in the early stages of infection; hence the name retrovirus. They are therefore best regarded as DNA viruses that happen to have their genomes in RNA form and are capable of setting up lifelong associations with the host.

The RNA polymerases which replicate the genomes of RNA viruses differ from the complex of enzymes responsible for DNA synthesis in that they lack a proof-reading function. RNA genome synthesis is, therefore, about a million-fold more error prone than DNA genome synthesis. This has profound consequences. First, it causes RNA virus genomes to be restricted in size (the largest RNA virus has only about 12 genes), to minimize the risk of multiple errors occurring at each replication event. Second, and more important in practical terms, it means that RNA viruses have very high mutation rates. Many of them exploit this property to evade specific immune defences of the host by rapid and frequent changes in their antigenic structure.

Effects of Infection on the Host

Most virus infections are mild and self-limiting, which is easy to understand from the evolutionary standpoint: it would not be in the interests of a virus, as an obligate parasite, to cause the extinction of its host and so host and virus have co-evolved to levels of resistance and virulence optimal for the maintenance of their respective population numbers. The only example of this which has been studied in real time is the evolution of myxomatosis in Australia, an 'experiment' with which the student is probably familiar. The virus that causes this infection is resident in South America where it causes a benign local fibroma in its natural host, the rabbit *Sylvilagus brasiliensis*. However, in the European rabbit, *Oryctolagus cuniculus*, it causes a generalized infection with a very high mortality rate. Field trials to test its efficacy in reducing the European rabbit population were carried out in Australia in 1950. The virus escaped, causing enormous epidemics in succeeding years with a case mortality rate greater than 99%, infected rabbits surviving for less than 13 days. Within 3 years, however, virus isolates from epidemics had become much less virulent, with mortality rates of 70–95% and survival times of 17–28 days. Changes in the resistance of the rabbit also occurred, mortality rates of infection falling to 25% following challenge with strains of virus with modified virulence and symptomatology becoming less severe. In myxomatosis, therefore, natural selection favoured virus strains with intermediate virulence because such strains are transmitted more effectively than highly virulent strains which kill their hosts too quickly, and non-virulent strains, which are poorly transmitted.

Most of the exceptions to the rule that virus infections are mild fall into two categories. First, a few virus species are inherently and consistently highly virulent for man and cause infections with a high mortality. Second, host deficiencies or other special factors, particularly the inability to mount or maintain a specific immune response, lead to greater cell and tissue damage following infections with viruses that are normally mild in their effects. Highly virulent viruses usually have one or two distinctive attributes. Most do not have man as their primary host but are transmitted from animal reservoirs, often by insect vectors. Second, many highly virulent viruses appear to have only recently come into contact with their host.

The biology of yellow fever virus provides good examples for both categories. This virus causes a severe hepatitis in man with liver cell necrosis. Its principal vertebrate hosts are monkeys in Africa and South America, and it is transmitted to man or from man to man by mosquitoes. The virus is thought to be African in origin, and infection of African monkeys infrequently results in illness or death. In contrast, infections in South American monkeys have a high mortality. This is considered to reflect the relatively recent introduction of the virus into the New World, possibly at the time navigation was established between Africa and America during the sixteenth century. Other examples of viruses which cause infections with high mortality rates are the rabies virus, which is transmitted to man by the bite of a rabid animal to set up a uniformly fatal dead-end infection (so-called because the virus is not transmitted any further but dies with its human host) and the human immunodeficiency virus, which almost certainly evolved from a monkey virus sometime in the last 20–30 years. Infection with HIV does not cause death directly but as a result of producing a severe secondary immune deficiency after an incubation period of a number of years. Progression to the acquired immune deficiency syndrome (AIDS) is characterized by the development of a variety of opportunistic infections (p. 243).

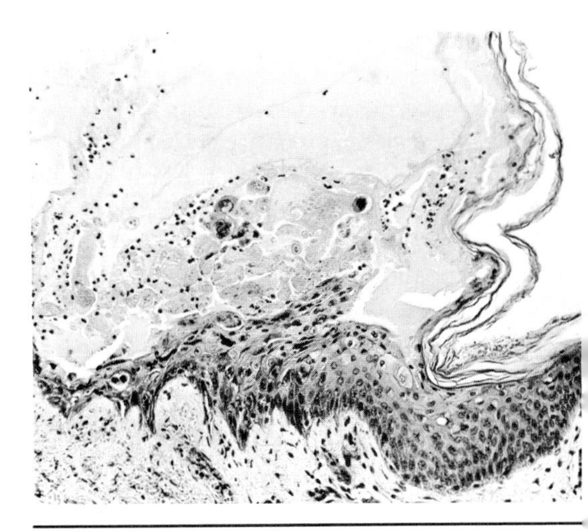

Fig. 8.32 Part of a vesicular skin lesion in varicella, illustrating virus-induced cell injury. The virus has replicated in the epidermal cells, resulting in cell death. The resulting epidermal defect has then become distended with inflammatory exudate, forming the vesicle. Note the swelling and hyperchromatic nuclei of the colonized epidermal cells, lying free in the vesicle and in the underlying epidermis. ×96.

Effects of Infection at the Cellular Level

The lesions in virus infections are caused by direct invasion of body tissues with subsequent cell damage due to the effect of virus replication in the host cells (Fig. 8.32). Viruses differ from bacteria in that they do not produce toxins which can act at a distance. The amount and type of damage caused by any particular virus is dependent on the types of cell that the virus infects, its effect on those cells, and the outcome of the competitive processes of virus growth and spread and the neutralizing effects of host defences. The response of the host to infection may also cause tissue damage and symptomatology through the inflammatory response and the specific immune response directed against virus-infected cells.

The events which occur during infection are:

(1) adsorption of the virion to the cell surface,
(2) entry of the virion into the cell and its uncoating,
(3) virus-induced macromolecular synthesis (transcription of virus messenger RNA, its translation into virus proteins, and the synthesis of virus genome), and
(4) virion assembly and release (Fig. 8.33).

The distribution of receptors for virus adsorption is particularly important in defining target cells, but the many factors which are essential for determining macromolecular synthesis have only been partially defined.

A dramatic example which links particular features of the virus-cell interaction with the pathogenesis of infection is provided by human parvovirus. This virus belongs to a large family of viruses which all have a very small single-stranded DNA genome and so have a very limited coding potential. Some types require gene products which are not encoded by their own genome and so can only infect cells which are already infected with another larger DNA virus (e.g. adenovirus). Human parvovirus causes erythema infectiosum (a common and trivial disease of childhood), arthritis, aplastic crises in patients who already suffer from chronic haemolytic anaemia, and hydrops fetalis as

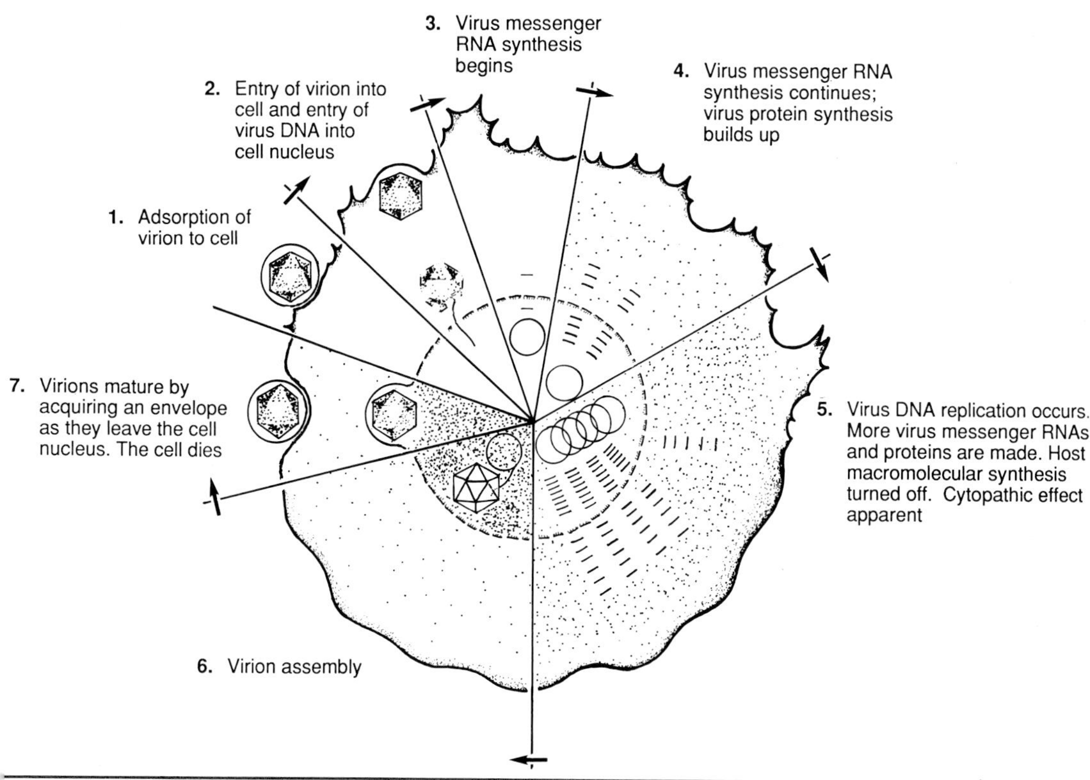

Fig. 8.33 Diagram showing the events which occur during the growth of herpes simplex virus. In latent infections the growth of the virus is arrested at stage 3. The events shown here are typical for most other viruses except that: **a** Genome synthesis and virion assembly of most RNA viruses takes place in the cytoplasm. **b** Most enveloped viruses acquire a lipid bilayer from cytoplasmic membranes.

a result of intrauterine infection. Because of its limited coding potential and consequent dependence on host enzymes for DNA synthesis, it appears that the virus can only grow in dividing cells. Its main target cell is the erythrocyte precursor. In patients with haemolytic anaemias these cells are dividing more rapidly than normal to compensate for the short red cell lifespan, and so they form a particularly favourable target for the parvovirus. The reduction in their numbers caused by the infection leads, for a time, to a virtual cessation of red cell production. Likewise, the targeting of rapidly dividing erythroid precursors by the virus in the fetus can cause a very severe anaemia with hydrops fetalis.

The events which follow virus-induced macromolecular synthesis are also important determinants of the ability of a cell to produce infectious virus particles. Post-translational processing of virus proteins often occurs; limited proteolysis is particularly important. For example, the influenza haemagglutinin (HA) and the fusion (F) protein of parainfluenza viruses are synthesized as single polypeptides, but must be cleaved to promote the fusion of the virion envelope with the cell membrane, an essential early event in the next cycle of infection. In contrast, in cells lacking the appropriate proteases, virions are assembled but the particles that bud from the cell are non-infectious.

Replication of viruses causes lethal damage to host cells in two main ways. First, many kinds of virus turn off host macromolecular synthesis during their growth cycle. This is an irreversible process which inevitably results in cell death. Second, those viruses which are assembled in the cell cytoplasm can only be released by causing cell disintegration. Little is known about how viruses cause cells to disintegrate but structural components of the virion are probably important. Viruses use several different mechanisms to dominate macromolecular synthesis in the infected cell and turn off host protein and nucleic acid syntheses. Large DNA viruses like herpesviruses, encode factors which rapidly degrade host mRNAs, while some viruses cause the degradation of the initiation factors which are required for the translation of host mRNAs. Other viruses compete effectively with the host by transcribing mRNAs in much greater abundance than host cell mRNAs, thus dominating the cell, or by producing mRNAs with structural features which are favoured over host molecules. Thus, the influenza virus mRNA competes extremely efficiently for host translation–initiation factors, while poliovirus mRNA initiates translation more efficiently than does host mRNA.

Distribution of Lesions in Virus Infections

In some instances the main lesion is at the site of the initial infection. For example, the virus responsible for influenza gives rise to localized infection which spreads rapidly throughout the mucosa of the larger air passages of the upper respiratory tract.

After an incubation period of between 1 and 4 days, tracheobronchitis with involvement of the small airways ensues. Columnar ciliated cells become vacuolated, lose their ciliae and desquamate. Mucus-producing epithelial cells are also lost, leaving either a single-cell thick basal layer or an exposed basement membrane. Submucosal accumulations of neutrophils and mononuclear cells appear with oedema and hyperaemia. After a few days the epithelium starts to regenerate but full recovery from tissue damage may take several weeks.

Viraemia and replication of influenza virus in organs other than the respiratory tract have only rarely been demonstrated, and the life threatening forms of the disease are its pulmonary manifestations, either primary viral pneumonia or, more commonly, secondary bacterial pneumonia. In primary viral pneumonia the disease process affects the alveoli. Their epithelial lining is destroyed and their oedematous walls become covered with a hyaline membrane. Secondary pneumonia is akin to bacterial sepsis. Epithelial damage removes defences and allows organisms like *Staph. aureus*, otherwise hardly ever a respiratory pathogen, to cause a devastating and often overwhelming pneumonia.

In many virus infections the initial infection is clinically silent, but the virus invades various other tissues and organs and produces characteristic lesions in them. Thus, in childhood fevers such as measles and varicella, the initial infection is probably in the mouth, pharynx and upper respiratory tract where the virus replicates. From there the virus spreads widely, via the blood (viraemia) and lymphatics to invade many other tissues. Lymphocytes become infected and act as vectors for virus transport to other sites. The virus also grows in cells of the mononuclear phagocyte system. Clinical manifestations of the involvement of these cells during the incubation period are the development of leucopenia with a relative lymphocytosis, and impaired cell mediated immunity with temporary loss of delayed hypersensitivity to tuberculin. When symptoms appear, 9–11 days after infection, virus replication is taking place in cells in many organs including the conjunctival, respiratory, alimentary and urinary tract mucosae, the lymphatic system, small blood vessels and the central nervous system; electroencephalographic changes occur in about half the children who suffer from measles, and the CSF lymphocyte count is increased in 10%.

The rash of measles results from an interaction between sensitized T cells and virus-infected cells in small blood vessels. In individuals with defects in cell mediated immunity, the rash does not appear and a progressive disease develops. In these patients the virus replicates unchecked in kidneys and brain, and in the lungs a giant-cell pneumonia may develop. Individuals with normal immune responses, however, can also suffer serious and sometimes fatal complications. Symptomatic encephalitis develops a few days after the appearance of the rash in approximately one out of every thousand previously healthy children. Virus is difficult to demonstrate in the brain and a perivascular lymphocytic infiltrate and the occurrence of demyelination suggest that autoimmune mechanisms may be operating.

Quite distinct from acute encephalitis is the rare, late complication of subacute sclerosing panencephalitis (SSPE). This develops many years after the acute disease. During this long latent period, virus has persisted but has become defective, as infected cells no longer synthesize some of the structural components of the virus particle, particularly the M protein, which is normally found on the inner side of the virion envelope. Because of this defect, infected cells no longer produce complete infectious virus particles. However, as direct cell-to-cell transmission can still occur, the virus spreads slowly through the brain, causing a generalized encephalitis affecting both the white and grey matter. A vigorous local immune response leads to production of large amounts of antibody. Serum titres are 10–100 times higher than those normally occurring post-infection and oligoclonal antibodies are found in the cerebrospinal fluid. Because of the mode of virus spread in the childhood fevers, the incubation period between initial infection and appearance of symptoms is 12–21 days. Poliovirus also spreads in a complex fashion within the body: following ingestion of the virus, there is an initial infection of the Peyer's patches in the small intestine. The virus then spreads to the regional lymph nodes and in many instances produces viraemia. In a few individuals, (e.g. about 1% of those infected with poliovirus type 1) the organism invades the anterior horn cells of the spinal cord, causing paralytic poliomyelitis. The intestinal infection, which is clinically silent, confers immunity against subsequent infection. Both circulating antibody and IgA antibody in the gastrointestinal secretions are produced.

Latent Virus Infections

Herpes simplex virus remains latent within the trigeminal ganglion but can become activated as a result of pneumonia or other febrile illness to produce vesicles around the mouth. Varicella virus also commonly remains latent, and may subsequently become active and replicate within the cells of the dorsal root ganglia to produce an attack of herpes zoster (p. 831).

Slow Virus Infections

These may be defined as infections caused by unconventional agents and having a long incubation period, in some instances years, and a prolonged and progressive course. Such diseases occur in certain animals, e.g. Aleutian disease of the mink, and it seems very likely that kuru and Creutzfeldt–Jacob disease (p. 833) are examples in man. Scrapie, a widespread slow virus disease in sheep, is most unusual in the remarkable resistance of its causal agent to heat and viricidal chemicals. The agents responsible for these diseases appear to be infectious, but they are smaller than the known viruses and the term prion has been applied to them.

Host Defences Against Viral Infections

Three phases of response to infection are mounted by the host.

(1) An immediate, non-specific response by natural killer (NK) cells (p. 197), which attack virus infected cells, is followed within a few hours by a second largely non-specific response mediated by interferon.

(2) Interferon is released from cells in response to virus infection and when taken up by other cells, makes them refractory to virus infection. Interferons also activate NK cells. Although the production of interferons is induced by virus, they are encoded by genes of the host cell genome. Interferons are classified into three types, α, β and γ. Interferons α and β are synthesized by viral-infected cells: the stimulus for their production is the presence in the cell of double stranded RNA, formation of which is a

feature of both DNA and RNA viruses. Cells can be induced to secrete interferon by double stranded synthetic polyribonucleotides. Interferon-γ, which is produced by activated T cells (p. 198), activates macrophages.

Interferons do not protect the virus-infected cells producing them: they attach to receptors on adjacent uninfected cells and inhibit the translation of viral mRNA proteins when these cells become infected. Interferons are species-specific but inhibit virtually all viruses. Interferon production, therefore, is a major factor in bringing about recovery from acute virus infections.

(3) After 4 days or so the third, an immune response to the virus, commences. Activated specific cytolytic T cells attack virus-infected cells and antibody directed against certain virion surface antigens can neutralize virus infectivity. While this may play a role in terminating infection by interrupting virus spread in the host, a more important function is to protect against re-infection. The presence of antibodies in people who have experienced a virus infection can be demonstrated by various *in vitro* tests for antibody such as complement fixation, immunofluorescence and enzyme-linked immunoassay – ELISA.

Our understanding of the relative role of specific defence mechanisms in virus infections has come in part from a study of inherited and acquired immunodeficiency states (p. 237). Patients with defective antibody production have an increased incidence of certain bacterial infections but handle most viruses normally. However, poliovirus and some related viruses may produce chronic persistent infections of the central nervous system. Complement deficiencies and defects of phagocytic function do not seem to predispose individuals to virus infections. Impaired T-cell function is frequently associated with severe virus infections, particularly with the herpesviruses (herpes simplex, cytomegalovirus and varicella zoster virus). These viruses normally cause mild and self-limiting infections (cold sores, chickenpox), persist in a latent form after the primary infection for the lifetime of their host and cause clinically manifest infections infrequently thereafter. The incidence of reactivations and the severity of such infections is much increased if T-cell function is depressed, probably because of inability of the remaining T cells to eliminate virus-infected cells.

Other host factors also affect the severity of virus infections. Measles virus causes an infection with high mortality in third world countries where malnutrition and intercurrent infections are common. These are considered to be important factors although the precise physiological and molecular reasons for the abnormal host response have not been worked out. Similarly, the high mortality of influenza in people older than 65, and in those who have pre-existing cardiovascular and pulmonary disease, has not yet been explained fully at the cellular level.

Active immunity can be produced readily by the administration of attenuated viruses, e.g. Sabin poliovirus vaccines, and also – although somewhat less effectively – by inactivated viruses, e.g. influenza and rabies vaccines. Naturally acquired immunity after virus infection is generally life-long and is due to the development of neutralizing antibodies. However, in a few virus diseases, re-infections or repeated infections are common. This may be due to the existence of numerous serologically distinct strains of virus, e.g. the common cold, or to the virus undergoing antigenic variation, e.g. influenza. In the case of certain viruses, and especially herpes simplex and herpes zoster viruses, reactivation of virus, despite the presence of circulating antibody, is not uncommon. Such recurrences are due to the ability of these viruses to remain latent, probably in the form of integrated DNA as **provirus** within the neurons of sensory ganglia. Reactivation takes place with axonal spread down sensory nerves, to produce vesicles in the area of skin supplied by the sensory nerves affected.

Rickettsial Infections

The rickettsiae are micro-organisms of various shapes, smaller than bacteria but resembling them in their structural and metabolic features, including formation of a cell wall. They are obligatory intracellular parasites and infect many species including arthropods, birds and mammals. Several species of rickettsiae cause disease in man (Table 8.2): in most instances they enter the body by the bites of infected ticks or mites, or from infected louse or flea faeces being scratched into the skin. The organisms enter and multiply in the endothelium of capillaries and other small blood vessels. At first they are localized to the site of infection, but blood dissemination occurs during the incubation period and endothelial involvement then becomes widespread. Capillary obstruction occurs from endothelial swelling or thrombosis, with resultant necrosis in heavily involved tissues, and a mixed inflammatory cell reaction develops, including neutrophil polymorphs, macrophages, lymphocytes and plasma cells.

The rickettsial diseases include **endemic (murine) typhus**, caused by *Rickettsia mooseri* and transmitted by the rat flea; **epidemic typhus** (*R. prowazekii*) and **trench fever** *(R. quintana)* which are spread by the body louse: the **spotted fever** group (*R. rickettsii, R. akari*, etc.) transmitted from various animals by the bites of infected ticks or mites, and finally **scrub typhus** (*R. tsutsugamushi*), transmitted from rodents by a mite. Epidemic and endemic typhus occur worldwide. The epidemic disease occurs in crowded louse-infested communities and is common in times of war, earthquakes and other major disasters. Man is the only known reservoir of infection of *R. prowazekii* which can only persist for years as a latent infection and cause relapse ('recrudescent typhus' or Brill–Zinsser disease): such cases are responsible for fresh outbreaks.

The rickettsial diseases vary in their severity and pathological detail: in all, the small blood vessels are involved and lesions tend to result especially in the brain, heart and skin. Diagnosis is usually made by demonstrating a rising titre of antibody, either in the patient or in laboratory animals inoculated with the patient's blood. Only *R. quintana* has been cultured successfully in cell-free media.

Q fever is a typhus-like illness caused by *Coxiella burnetii* which closely resembles the rickettsiae. However, it is capable of both intracellular and extracellular growth and it is resistant to drying. It is a parasite of domesticated animals of worldwide distribution and man is infected by inhalation of droplets while attending to animal births or by drinking infected milk. Q fever usually presents as a 'non-bacterial' pneumonia, although lesions may occur in the brain and other organs. *Cox. burnetii* may also colonize the valves of the heart, producing an infective endocarditis. Diagnosis is usually based on a rising titre of antibody, but the demonstration of *Cox. burnetii* in the blood by guinea-pig inoculation is sometimes necessary.

Chlamydial Infections

The chlamydiae are a group of small micro-organisms related to Gram-negative bacteria. They are obligatory intracellular parasites. The vegetative form multiplies by binary fission, and infection is spread by a smaller, compact, spore-like form (elementary body) which can survive, but not divide, extracellulary. They are susceptible to some antibiotics.

The genus *Chlamydia* is divided into three species. All infect man, although one species, *Chlamydia psittaci*, occurs primarily in birds and various mammals, with human diseases such as psittacosis – a respiratory infection – occurring after contact with infected birds. A related strain responsible for enzootic abortion of ewes may cause human abortion. *Chlamydia pneumoniae* is a

Table 8.2 Rickettsial diseases

Disease	Agent	Geographic distribution	Transmission	Mammal	Prominent clinicopathological features
Spotted fever group					
Rocky mountain spotted fever	*R. rickettsii*	Western hemisphere	Tick bite	Wild rodents/ dogs	Infection of endothelia and vascular smooth muscle. Centripetal rash. Eschar rarely seen*
Fievre Boutonneuse	*R. conorii*	Africa, Europe, Middle East, India	Tick bite		Prominent eschar
Queensland tick typhus	*R. australis*	Australia	Tick bite	Mammals/wild rodents	Centripetal rash. Eschar common
North Asian tick-borne rickettsioses	*R. sibirica*	Siberia, Mongolia	Tick bite	Wild rodents	Centripetal rash. Eschar common
Rickettsial pox	*R. akari*	USA, Russia, Africa	Mite bite	House mice and other rodents	Milder than Rocky Mountain spotted fever. Papulovesicular rash. Prominent eschar
Typhus fever group					
Endemic (murine) typhus	*R. mooseri*	World wide	Rat/flea faeces	Small rodents	Endothelial infection. Centrifugal haemorrhagic rash
Epidemic typhus	*R. prowazekii*	World wide	Body louse faeces	Humans	As above but more severe with higher mortality
	R. canada	N. America	Tick bite		
Flying squirrel typhus	*R. prowazekii*	S.E. United States	Fleas, lice of flying squirrel	Flying squirrel	As for endemic typhus
Brill–Zinsser disease	*R. prowazekii*	World wide	Late recrudescence years after original attack of epidemic typhus		As for epidemic typhus but lower mortality
Scrub typhus	*R. tsutsugamushi*	Asia, Australia, Pacific Islands	Trombiculid mite (chigger) bite	Wild rodents	Eschar common. Lymphadenopathy
Other rickettsial diseases					
Q Fever	*Cox. burnetii*	World wide	Droplet inhalation	Small and domestic mammals, e.g. cattle, sheep or goats	Fever, pneumonia, ring granuloma. No eschar or rash

* Black or dark scales at site of tick bite

recently recognized species which has also been called the TWAR (Taiwan acute respiratory) agent. It causes upper respiratory tract infections and pneumonia. Different serotypes of the third species, *Chlamydia trachomatis*, cause a wide spectrum of infections. Multiple cycles of kerato-conjunctivitis lead to visual impairment and blindness (trachoma). This is still common in some developing countries (p. 882). World wide the organism causes sexually transmitted infections – clinically resembling those caused by *N. gonorrhoeae* – and lymphogranuloma venereum. It also causes conjunctivitis and pneumonia in the neonate.

The initial reaction to chlamydial infection is granulomatous, with accumulation of macrophages and lymphoid cells. There is tissue necrosis and scarring may occur. In lymphogranuloma venereum, a small ulcerating primary lesion develops in the genitalia, but the draining lymph nodes become grossly involved and prolonged suppuration and extensive scarring result.

Both humoral and cell mediated immunity develop in chlamydial infections, the latter probably being the more important in the elimination of the infection. These diseases are considered more fully in the appropriate systemic chapters.

Fungal Infections (Mycoses)

Fungi are primitive eukaryotic micro-organisms which are now usually classified as neither plant nor animal. They are mainly saprophytic and make an important contribution to the breakdown of animal and plant tissues. Only a few of the many known species are pathogenic to man and most cause superficial, mild lesions.

Morphologically, some pathogenic fungi are dimorphic: that is they may assume a yeast-like form (single rounded cells which multiply by budding) or a hyphal form (branching filaments that interlace to make a mycelium or mould, and produce spores). The form assumed depends on the environs of the fungus. In human tissues, the pathogenic species are usually either yeasts or hyphae, which aids their histological distinction.

Fungal infections may be environmental in origin, though some species are normally benign commensals, such as *Candida albicans* which is acquired at the time of birth. Broadly speaking, fungal diseases are classified into three groups, depending on the species of fungus and the parts of the body affected.

(1) **Superficial mycosis**, e.g. tinea (dermatophytosis or ringworm) and candidiasis. The fungus infiltrates the cornified layers of the skin. The host reaction is marked and destruction of epidermis and skin appendages may be severe.
(2) **Subcutaneous mycosis**, e.g. mycetoma. After inoculation by traumatic implantation from contaminated vegetation, the fungi may remain localized in the subcutis or slowly spread locally. Visceral dissemination is rare. The host reaction ranges from suppuration to epithelioid-cell granuloma formation.
(3) **Systemic mycosis**, e.g. systemic candidiasis, histoplasmosis, mucormycosis, aspergillosis and cryptococcosis. With the exception of candidiasis these are basically respiratory diseases, as inhalation of the fungus causes the primary lesion. Later, dissemination to lymph nodes, liver, bones, adrenals, etc. may occur, depending on host resistance. For example, histoplasmosis behaves like tuberculosis, with a primary lung complex healing and, in a proportion of patients the development of chronic infection.

Resistance to invasive mycosis is effected mainly by cell mediated immunity. Immunocompromised patients are particularly liable to mucosal candidiasis and to disseminated *Cryptococcus* infection. Resistance to invasive *Aspergillus* infection requires polymorphonuclear leucocytes; hence its frequency in leukaemic patients.

In superficial infections, diagnosis can often be made from the clinical appearance of the lesions supported by microscopy of the skin or mucosal infections. In subcutaneous and systemic mycoses, biopsy and culture of the tissue (and sometimes blood culture) may be necessary.

Candidiasis

Candida albicans is normally present in the mouth and intestines and on the surface of moist skin. Defective host defence permits the fungus to invade superficially or deeply: inherited immunodeficiency states, agranulocytosis, leukaemias, antibiotic administration, immunosuppressive therapy, diabetes mellitus and pregnancy are examples of states that predispose to candidiasis.

In **mucosal candidiasis** the oral or vaginal mucosa is involved, with formation of white plaques (thrush) at sites of fungal growth. Histologically, there is a characteristic combination of budding yeasts and hyphae in the epithelium with a polymorph and lymphocytic reaction beneath. During pregnancy, the lowered vaginal pH promotes the growth of the fungus, causing a vaginitis. At autopsy of patients dying of leukaemia, thick plaques of oesophageal candidiasis are frequently seen. Oral candidiasis is a common early manifestation of AIDS. **Mucocutaneous candidiasis** is a destructive condition which may involve the entire skin surface, nails and mucous membranes. The fungus proliferates in the epithelium which becomes hyperplastic and hyperkeratotic, and a chronic granulomatous inflammation is seen in the underlying tissues.

Severe immunodeficiency states can lead to **systemic candidiasis**. Blood culture may be positive and the heart valves, lungs, liver and kidneys are commonly affected. In the kidney, there are multiple small abscesses resembling those seen in pyaemia and containing proliferating fungus in hyphal and yeast forms.

Aspergillosis

Spores of *Aspergillus* are ubiquitous in the atmosphere and many species infect man, although by far the commonest is *Aspergillus fumigatus*.

The fungus causes four different types of pulmonary disease (p. 565): inhalation of spores may result in **bronchial asthma** from type 1 (atopic) hypersensitivity or **acute allergic alveolitis** from type 3 (immune-complex) hypersensitivity. The fungus can colonize old tuberculous or bronchiectatic cavities, in which it may form a large colony ('**aspergilloma**'); or it may actually invade the lung tissue to produce a haemorrhagic and necrotizing **pneumonia**. This last condition tends to occur in immunodeficient or immunosuppressed individuals, in whom the fungus may also invade the walls of the pulmonary veins, causing local thrombosis, and become disseminated by the bloodstream: infection of the heart valves may result in large vegetations.

Histoplasmosis

Histoplasmosis is primarily a pulmonary disease. The fungal spores are present in the soil and in the faeces of chickens and bats, and infection results from their inhalation. It is a global disease, with a high prevalence in the USA. About 95% of infections are asymptomatic: as in tuberculosis, the primary lesion is a focal pulmonary granuloma that heals with fibrosis and calcification; the skin test (with histoplasmin) becomes positive. This test for cell mediated immunity is positive in a high proportion of inhabitants of endemic areas.

A small proportion of infected people develop an acute symptomatic pneumonia or a chronic cavitating pulmonary disease which resembles tuberculosis. Disseminated histoplasmosis, with a high mortality, is seen in the elderly and in those with defective immunity. The lymphoreticular system, bones and adrenals are involved, causing enlargement of the liver, spleen and lymph nodes. The adrenals may be destroyed by the process and histoplasmosis is a recognized cause of Addison's disease.

Microscopically, yeast-like bodies of 2–5 μm diameter are seen in macrophages (Fig. 8.34) and there are usually epithelioid-cell granulomas with or without caseation.

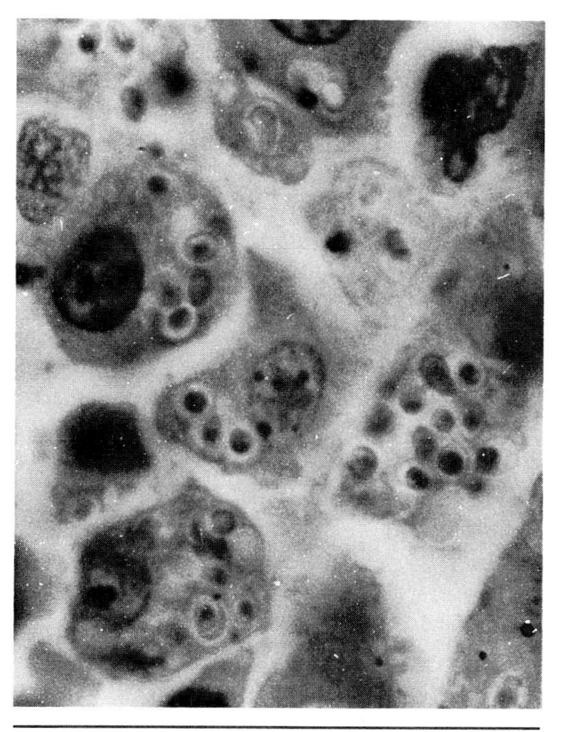

Fig. 8.34 Histoplasmosis. From the adrenals in a fatal case of disseminated histoplasmosis. The macrophages contain numerous small yeast-like cells of *Histoplasma capsulatum*. ×1500.

Cryptococcosis

Cryptococcus neoformans is a ubiquitous fungus, most abundant in pigeon droppings. It is a yeast cell with a thick mucoid capsule. When inhaled, it can cause a diffuse or focal lung lesion. The diffuse (hyporeactive) form is a mucoid pneumonia that grossly may be mistaken for a *Klebsiella* pneumonia (p. 557) or a bronchoalveolar carcinoma (p. 581). The focal lesion is often an incidental finding, seen on chest X-ray as a 'coin lesion'. The host reaction to cryptococci ranges from virtually nil to a necrotizing granulomatous pneumonia. The mucoid nature of the lesion derives from the capsule of the fungus.

The fungus disseminates by the blood to other organs, including the bones, lymph nodes and particularly to the meninges where it causes a gelatinous meningitis with a variably slight or granulomatous reaction in which the budding cryptococci are seen. This form of the disease is usually a complication of severe immunodeficiency, and cryptococcal pneumonia and meningitis are frequent opportunistic infections in HIV-infected people.

Mycetoma (Maduramycosis)

This is a chronic suppurative infection of the subcutaneous tissues following traumatic implantation of a causative agent. The condition usually affects the limbs and results in gross swelling, fistulous tracks to the skin and eventually invasion and destruction of bone. The causal agents of mycetoma can be either fungi (of which more than a dozen species are known, including *Madurella mycetomatis*) or actinomycetes, which include *Actinomadura*, *Nocardia* and *Streptomyces* species. The aetiological distinction is important since drugs are effective in actinomycetomas but not in fungal mycetomas.

The lesions are similar to those of actinomycosis (p. 320). They consist of multiple intercommunicating abscesses and sinuses lined by granulomatous tissue. They occur in the soft tissues and bones, usually of the foot and leg (Fig. 8.35). The condition is chronic and massive subcutaneous fibrosis results. Grain-like colonies of the causal agent, visible to the naked eye, are present in the abscesses and in pus discharged from the sinuses. The hyphae of fungal colonies are often embedded in cement-like material which impedes the entry of antifungal drugs.

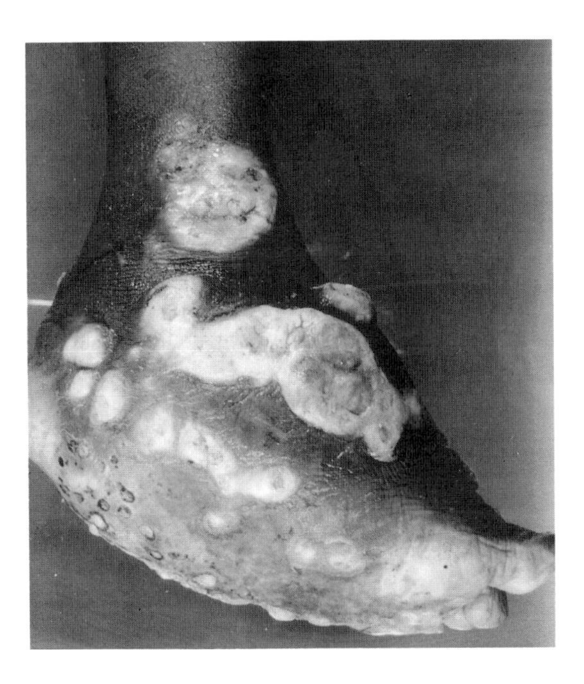

Fig. 8.35 Madura foot: mycetoma affecting the subcutaneous tissues of the foot.

Mucormycosis

This is caused by *Rhizopus oryzae*, previously known as *Mucor oryzae*, one of the zygomycete fungi which have characteristically wide, branching hyphae up to 25 μm across. Virtually all victims of mucormycosis are patients with uncontrolled diabetes mellitus in a state of ketoacidosis. The primary site of infection is the nasal turbinates. The clinical features involve sinusitis, inflammation of the orbit with proptosis, and meningoencephalitis, resulting from invasion of the fungus through the cribriform plate.

Rhizopus induces a florid acute inflammatory reaction and causes extensive necrosis. Further tissue damage results from its propensity to invade blood vessel walls with consequent thrombosis. Cavernous sinus thrombosis and pituitary infarction are commonly seen in fatal cases. Mucormycosis is the most fulminant of all mycoses, death usually occurring within a few days of diagnosis.

Antimicrobial Agents

Antiseptics are general poisons which affect both microbial and mammalian cells. Apart from topical application, toxicity prevents their use in the treatment of infections. Antimicrobial agents can be used therapeutically because they are able to kill or inhibit the growth of a micro-organism without harming the cells of the host. Their activity is directed at specific targets in the microorganism and which are either absent from the host cell or much more susceptible than the mammalian equivalent. This accounts for the **selective toxicity** which is a prerequisite for a useful drug.

Antibacterial Agents

Mode of Action

These drugs act at many varied sites within the bacterium but, of necessity, all exploit the essential differences between bacterial (prokaryotic) and mammalian (eukaryotic) cells. Penicillins and cephalosporins, both β-lactam agents, inhibit bacterial cell wall synthesis; aminoglycosides (e.g. streptomycin, gentamicin), macrolides (e.g. erythromycin) and tetracyclines all interfere, in different ways, with ribosomal function; polymyxins disrupt the cytoplasmic membrane; sulphonamides and trimethoprim act sequentially on the metabolic pathway for folic acid; quinolones (e.g. nalidixic acid, ciprofloxacin) prevent DNA replication during cell division.

Resistance

Primary resistance is an intrinsic property of the bacterium. It determines the usual spectrum of a drug because some bacteria are normally sensitive and others normally resistant to its action.

Acquired resistance is the result of genetic change and is due to either mutation or gene transfer. Gene transfer by transduction (p. 286) is the way in which resistance to penicillin, and some other antibiotics, is acquired by previously sensitive strains of *Staph. aureus*. Gene transfer by conjugation (p. 287) involves plasmids (p. 285) and is an extremely important way in which resistance is transmitted, not only within a bacterial species but also between related organisms such as the enteric Gram-negative bacilli. For example, resistance to one or more antibiotics can be transferred in the intestine from commensal *E. coli* to pathogenic *Salmonella* species on a single plasmid.

Resistance Mechanisms

These genetic changes result in the organism acquiring means which enable it to withstand the effect of the antibacterial agent. Such mechanisms include:

(1) **drug inactivation** due to the development of bacterial enzymes, e.g. β-lactamases which destroy the β-lactam ring essential for the antibacterial action of penicillins and cephalosporins; acetylating, adenylating and phosphorylating enzymes which modify aminoglycosides.
(2) **drug exclusion** when a permeability barrier forms to prevent the antibiotic reaching its target site. This is usually associated with low level resistance to several drugs, e.g. pneumococcal resistance to penicillin or erythromycin, and less often with high level resistance to a single agent, e.g. tetracycline.
(3) **alteration in the target site or metabolic pathway** in the bacterium so that it is no longer susceptible to the drug, e.g. in trimethoprim resistance the acquisition of a plasmid coding for a new enzyme results in the creation of an alternative pathway for the metabolism of folic acid which is unaffected by the drug.

Spread of Resistant Strains

Resistance is important only if it is of advantage to the bacterium. This happens in the presence of the antibiotic which, by exerting a **selective pressure**, favours the survival of resistant bacteria and allows them to flourish at the expense of sensitive strains. Therefore, it is not surprising that antibiotic-resistant strains are especially common in hospital because of the heavy use – and sometimes abuse – of these drugs to treat and prevent infection. Control of the emergence and spread of resistance requires the implementation of policies in the use of antibiotics not only in managing patients but also in animal husbandry, where antibiotics are sometimes incorporated as growth-promoting agents in animal foodstuffs.

Antiviral Agents

Mode of Action

An antiviral agent must favour the inhibition of virus functions without adversely affecting host cellular processes. Few drugs have been found to match these requirements, and those currently available are limited more by their cellular toxicity than any deficiency in antiviral potency.

Antiviral drugs have been developed either by the screening of large numbers of organic and inorganic compounds for *in vitro* activity against a wide range of viruses, or by chemical synthesis of nucleoside analogues with specific enzyme targets in mind.

An antiviral may be effective because of its ability to alter: (1) virus absorption to cellular receptors; (2) virus entry and uncoating; (3) transcription and translation of the viral genome with specific reference to the inhibition of viral polymerases; (4) virus assembly and release from the infected cell; and (5) the cellular nucleoside pool.

Organic and Inorganic Compounds

Amantadine and the newer analogue rimantadine inhibit the uncoating of influenza A strains during the initial stages of cellular infection. Their use as antiviral agents is restricted to prophylaxis rather than the treatment of established infections.

Phosphonoformate compounds are pyrophosphate analogues that inhibit phosphorylation of nucleotides by viral polymerases. Antiviral activity is broad spectrum including the DNA polymerases of all herpes viruses and the RNA polymerases of influenza viruses. The reverse transcriptase of several retroviruses including human immunodeficiency virus (HIV) is also inhibited.

Nucleoside Analogues

Nucleoside analogues interfere with viral polymerase activity by nucleoside competition and analogue insertion, leading to premature chain termination and incomplete gene transcripts. Idoxuridine (IDUR) and trifluorothymidine (TFT) are iodinated and halogenated thymidine analogues respectively. Both are used as topical agents against primary or recurrent superficial herpetic infections. Adenosine arabinoside, an adenine analogue, and acyclovir, an analogue of guanosine, are potent antiherpetic agents inhibiting viral DNA polymerase, and can be used systemically. Acyclovir also inhibits a virus specific thymidine kinase required for phosphorylating nucleosides in herpes-infected cells. The high therapeutic index and low toxicity attributed to acyclovir therapy results from the virus-specific preferential activation of antiviral metabolites within infected cells. A newer analogue of acyclovir, ganciclovir, has useful anticytomegalovirus activity. Azidothymidine, used against HIV, is a thymidine analogue which inhibits virus-specific reverse transcriptase. The ability to target non-cellular, virus-specific enzyme limits toxicity, an undesirable but inevitable feature of all nucleoside analogues.

Ribavirin, a synthetic triazole nucleoside, inhibits a wide range of DNA and RNA viruses by altering nucleoside pools and messenger RNA formation. Its use has been largely against respiratory viruses including respiratory syncytial virus.

Resistance

Acquired resistance by viruses during antiviral therapy has been well documented with almost all drugs that have been extensively tested. Point mutations in the virus genome are largely responsible for acquired resistance. Acyclovir resistant strains may be either thymidine kinase deficient or DNA polymerase resistant or both. However, these strains are only seen after prolonged treatment and appear to have a lower pathogenic potential for transmission, latency and clinical expression.

Interferons

The endogenous interferons α, β and γ are naturally produced during acute virus infection and act to limit further spread by inducing an antiviral state in other cells. Although attempts to manufacture interferons in *in vitro* systems were effective, they were expensive and difficult to purify. The advent of genetically recombinant interferons has made these substances readily available for antiviral, immunomodulatory and anti-proliferative use. Recombinant interferons have shown clinical efficacy against the common cold viruses, chronic hepatitis B virus infection, intractable genital warts and juvenile laryngeal papillomatosis. Although not in common usage, these substances are likely to have an important place in future antiviral strategies, particularly where synergism with other antiviral agents can lead to an increase in antiviral potency and a reduction in undesirable side-effects.

Further Reading

Chandler, F. W., Kaplan, W. and Ajello, J. (1989). *A Colour Atlas and Textbook of Histopathology of Mycotic Diseases*, 336pp. Wolfe Medical, London.

Christie, A. B. (1987) *Infectious Diseases: Epidemiology and Clinical Practice*, 4th edn, 1033pp. Churchill Livingstone, Edinburgh.

Collee, J. G. (1981). *Applied Medical Microbiology* (Vol. 3 of *Basic Microbiology*), 158pp. Blackwell Scientific, Oxford.

Davis, D., Dulbecco, R., Eisen, H. N. and Ginsberg, H. S. (1990). *Principles of Microbiology and Immunology*, 4th edn. Harper and Row, New York.

Editorial (1982). Genetics of resistance to infection. *Lancet* **1**, 1446–7.

Freeman, B. A. (ed.) (1982). *Burrow's Textbook of Microbiology*, 22nd edn. Saunders, Philadelphia, London and Toronto.

Jopling, W. H. and McDougall, A. C. (1988). *Handbook of Leprosy*, 4th edn, 180pp. Heinemann Medical, London.

Levy, S. B. (1982). Microbial resistance to antibiotics. *Lancet* **2**, 83–8.

Lucas, S. B. (1988). Histopathology of leprosy and tuberculosis – an overview. *British Medical Bulletin* **44**, 584–99.

Mims, C. A. (1989). *The Pathogenesis of Infectious Disease*, 3rd edn, 342pp. Academic Press, London.

Parker, M. T. P. and Collier, L. (eds) (1990). *Topley and Wilson's Principles of Bacteriology, Virology and Immunity*, 8th edn, 5 vols. Edward Arnold, London.

Sleigh, J. D. and Timbury, M. C. (1981). *Notes on Medical Microbiology*, 438pp. Churchill Livingstone, Edinburgh.

Timbury, M. C. (1991). *Notes on Medical Virology*, 9th edn, 196pp. Churchill Livingstone, Edinburgh.

Tyrrell, D. A. J., Phillips, I., Goodwin, S. C. and Blowers, R. (1979). *Microbial Disease: the Use of the Laboratory in Diagnosis, Therapy and Control*, 340pp. Edward Arnold, London.

Zak, K., Diaz, J. L., Jackson, D. and Heckel, J. E. (1984). Antigenic variation during infection with *Neisseria gonorrhoeae*: detection of antibodies to surface proteins in sera of patients with gonorrhoea. *Journal of Infectious Diseases* **149**, 166–74.

9

Nutritional Disorders

The importance of nutrition in disease has been recognized throughout the history of medicine. However, the fundamental requirements for food and water are sometimes not given the priority which they deserve. The object of this chapter is to describe some aspects of the relationship between nutrition and disease. The basic principles are as follows:

(1) The total nutritional requirements of an individual comprise the basal nutritional requirement together with any additional or adaptive requirements brought about, e.g. by a disease process, convalescence from disease, pregnancy, lactation or growth requirements in children.

(2) Nutritional requirements are met by oral intake unless artificial nutritional support procedures are necessary. The effectiveness of oral intake is dependent upon the availability of the appropriate food, and the patient's ability to eat and absorb the diet.

(3) If the total nutritional intake is adequate, normal tissue function will ensue unless specific disease related problems are present.

(4) If the total nutritional intake is inadequate, deficiency syndromes of either a general or specific nature will develop. These deficiency states may lead to further problems such as anorexia and changes in immune status with increased susceptibility to infections. These alterations may then further widen the gap between nutritional intake and requirements.

(5) If the nutritional intake is excessive, obesity or toxicity may develop.

Normal Dietary Requirements

Man is omnivorous but there are considerable geographical variations in diet composition, e.g. staple diets which may largely comprise wheat, maize, rice or cassava. There are also cultural aspects of food preparation and different social and economic factors which influence adequate nutritional requirements. Despite this, however, a normal diet can be defined as one in which the content of the various nutrients is sufficient to maintain optimal growth and function of all the body tissues. The dietary requirements in health are reasonably well established and tables of national guidelines have been published. Provided certain intakes of carbohydrate, protein, fat, vitamins, minerals and trace elements are achieved, fairly wide ranges of intake are acceptable. In general, even though there is more concern about underprovision rather than overprovision of food, obesity and other diseases of excess are prevalent in many countries. The roles and approximate daily requirements of essential nutrients are summarized in Tables 9.1 and 9.2. The nutrients have been classified either as macronutrients, namely protein, carbohydrate and fat, or micronutrients such as vitamins, minerals and trace elements.

Table 9.1 Important biological roles of various nutrients

Nutrient	Important biological roles
Macronutrients	
Their roles are numerous and well known	
Micronutrients	
Vitamin A	Visual integrity: cell differentiation
Vitamin D	Control of calcium and phosphorus metabolism
Vitamin E	Antioxidant
Vitamin K	Integrity of coagulation cascade
Vitamin B_1	ATP synthesis; cell membrane integrity
Vitamin B_2	Redox reaction co-factor
Vitamin B_6	Amino-acid and lipid metabolism
Vitamin B_{12}	DNA synthesis
Vitamin C	Reducing agent critical to collagen synthesis
Folate	DNA synthesis
Calcium	Skeletal rigidity, muscle function; regulation of cell metabolism
Chromium	Regulation of glucose metabolism
Copper	Aerobic metabolism; iron handling, collagen synthesis
Fluoride	Dental protection
Iodine	Thyroid hormone synthesis
Iron	Cellular respiration
Magnesium	Growth control; muscle function
Phosphorus	Bone metabolism; cardiac, respiratory and neurological function
Selenium	Antioxidant
Zinc	Protein, nucleic acid and membrane metabolism

Metabolic Effects of Starvation

There are many causes of inadequate nutritional intake, and these are summarized in Table 9.3. Whatever the underlying cause the end result is a reduced dietary intake which is inadequate for most requirements. The nutritional lack may be

Table 9.2 Daily requirements of various nutrients

Nutrient	Daily requirement*	
	Male (70 kg)	Female (55 kg)
Macronutrients		
Protein	55 g	45 g
Fat	Minimum is 5% of total calories ideally as polyunsaturates	
Carbohydrate	Minimum is sufficient to ensure total caloric intake of 31–35 kcal/kg body weight when added to caloric value of fat	
Micronutrients		
Vitamin A	700 μg	600 μg
Vitamin D	0–10 μg	0–10 μg
Vitamin E	4 mg	3 mg
Vitamin K	70 μg	60 μg
Vitamin B_1	1000 μg	800 μg
Vitamin B_2	1300 μg	1100 μg
Vitamin B_6	1400 μg	1200 μg
Vitamin B_{12}	1.5 μg	1.5 μg
Vitamin C	40 mg	40 mg
Folate	200 μg	200 μg
Calcium	700 mg	700 mg
Chromium	25 μg	25 μg
Copper	1200 μg	1200 μg
Fluoride	50 μg/kg	50 μg/kg
Iodine	140 μg	140 μg
Iron	9 mg	15 mg
Magnesium	300 mg	270 mg
Phosphorous	550 mg	550 mg
Selenium	75 μg	60 μg
Zinc	9.5 mg	7 mg

During pregnancy and lactation daily requirements of nutrients increase, in some cases by up to 100%.

* The values quoted are those of the United Kingdom (1991; HMSO), and are generally lower than those of the United States (1989; National Academy of Sciences).

Table 9.3 Causes of reduced food intake which may lead to protein-energy malnutrition

Infection
Starvation/famine
Unbalanced dietary intake
Malabsorption syndromes
Diseases leading to loss of nutrient, e.g. via gastrointestinal tract
Malignant disease
Inborn errors of metabolism
Specific diseases affecting liver and kidney
Psychological problems

Pregnancy and lactation will act as aggravating factors in many instances.

aggravated by normal increased physiological demands, e.g. growth in children, pregnancy and lactation. Conversely, energy requirements decline with age as a result of reduction in muscle activity and muscle mass with an increase in body fat which is metabolically less active.

The mechanisms of adaptation to an inadequate nutritional intake are of fundamental importance to survival. The changes depend on the duration of starvation and are described below and summarized in Fig. 9.1.

(1) Throughout the starvation period, the tissues continue to utilize glucose as an energy substrate. This leads to a fall in blood glucose followed by a decrease in insulin secretion.

(2) To offset this hypoglycaemia, hepatic glycogen is broken down to glucose. This mechanism can only continue for about 16 hours as hepatic glycogen stores are limited. Although there are approximately 350 grams of glycogen in muscle compared with only about 90 grams in liver, muscle glycogen cannot be mobilized to sustain blood glucose since muscle lacks the enzyme glucose-6-phosphatase. This ensures that muscle glycogen is retained for use by the muscle itself in severe stress situations.

(3) When hepatic glycogen stores are exhausted, increased hepatic gluconeogenesis takes place, utilizing amino acids as substrate. The amino acids are derived from the breakdown of protein, especially muscle protein, and there is a resulting increase in urinary urea excretion.

(4) Increased fat catabolism occurs in adipose tissue with release of fatty acids which become increasingly important energy sources in many tissues.

(5) Ketone bodies derived from fatty acid metabolism accumulate, since the limited carbohydrate supply induced by starvation impairs full oxidative destruction of ketones in the citric acid cycle. The ketone bodies can be utilized as a source of energy by nervous tissue, especially the brain.

(6) As the brain and other tissues increasingly use ketone bodies, glucose requirements are reduced. In addition, ketone bodies directly reduce glucose utilization by muscle. The rate of gluconeogenesis can therefore decrease, protein catabolism is reduced and urine urea concentration falls to low levels.

(7) In advanced starvation the acidosis caused by the accumulation of ketone bodies leads to an increased requirement to excrete hydrogen ions in the kidney. In order to buffer the urine the kidney deaminates glutamine, so allowing the excretion of hydrogen ions as ammonium cations. The deaminated glutamine can then be used as a substrate for gluconeogenesis in the kidney.

Individuals who are adapted to a reduced nutritional intake often have a lower than normal daily energy expenditure, as a result of reduced physical activity and a reduction of up to 25% in their metabolic rate. It is thought that this alteration in basal metabolic rate is in part due to the reduced conversion of thyroxine (T4) to tri-iodothyronine (T3) and to an increased rate of conversion of T4 to reverse T3, the inactive form of T3 (p. 1085).

The result of these adaptations is that the major energy stores of the body are mobilized in a way which spares protein breakdown and permits maximum survival. The adipose tissue stores, which usually amount to 9–15 kg, provide energy for approximately 40–70 days. The total body protein content of approximately 9–11 kg contains 3–4 kg of muscle protein. Since survival requires the retention of at least half of this, and provided that the rate of muscle protein breakdown is reduced to about 20 grams per day, muscle stores will allow survival for approximately 75 days.

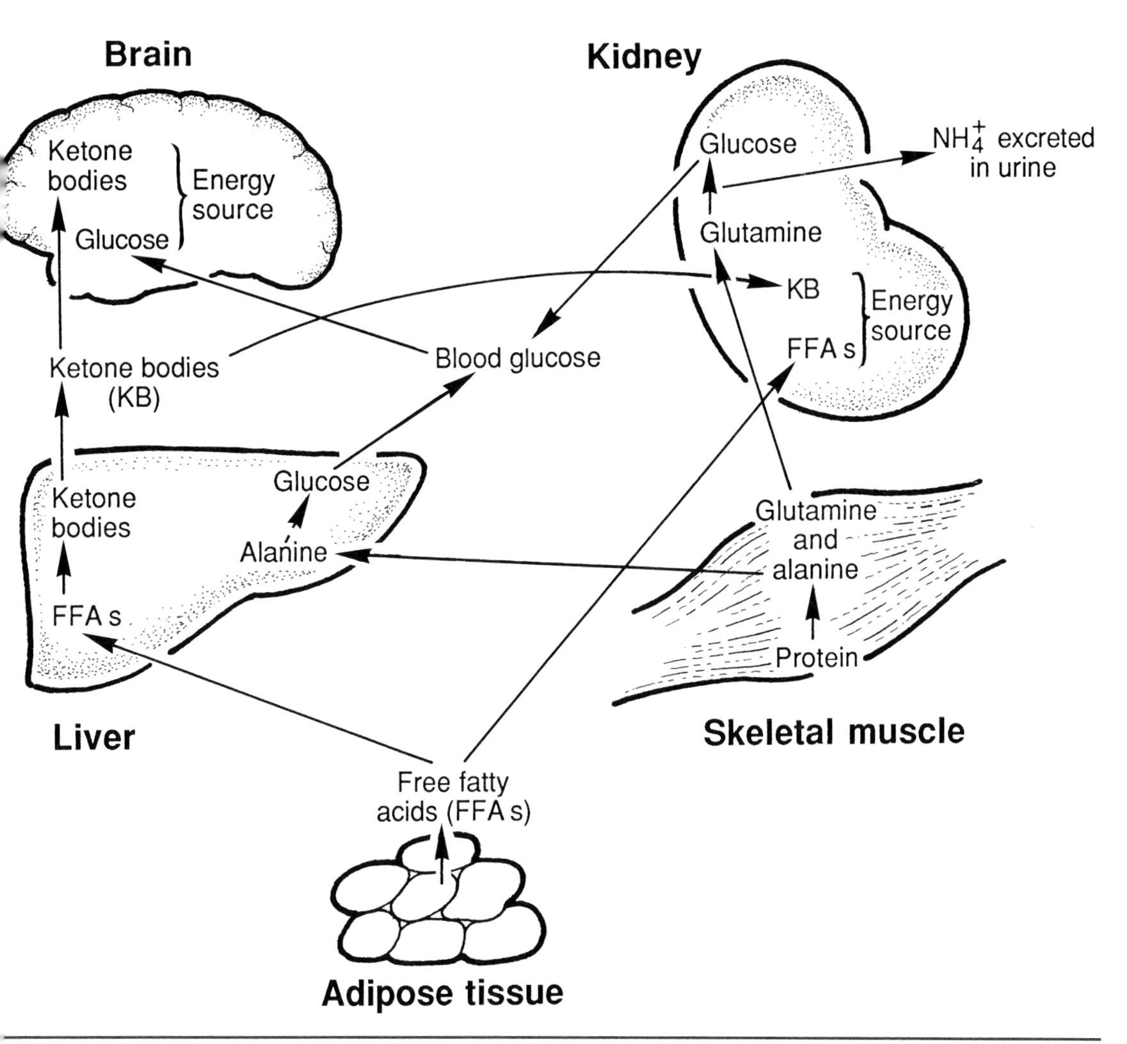

Fig. 9.1 Biochemical changes that occur in starvation and which are discussed in detail in the text. The figure summarizes the situation after approximately 24 hours of starvation when liver glycogen stores are exhausted. Protein catabolism and gluconeogenesis are maximal between day 1 and day 3 of a period of starvation.

Deficiency States Associated with Individual Nutrients

Nutrient deficiencies can be classified into type I and type II. Type I deficiency is characterized by specific signs or symptoms due to reduced tissue concentrations of the nutrient. This occurs in deficiency of iron, iodine or the B vitamins. By comparison, type II deficiency leads to a reduction in growth rate as the main effect, with characteristic tissue changes only occurring late in the development of the condition. Examples of this are protein-energy malnutrition and zinc deficiency. Since the rate of tissue development and growth are rapid in early life, deficiency states are often more common and the effects of deficiency more severe in infancy and early childhood. Although a comprehensive description of the results of deficiency of every nutrient is beyond the scope of this chapter a description of a number of important or characteristic deficiency states will be given.

Protein-energy Malnutrition

The main clinical effect of severe starvation is the syndrome of protein-energy malnutrition. In adults, this is characterized by the loss of adipose tissue as measured by skinfold thickness and the loss of tissue protein, especially skeletal muscle mass (Fig. 9.2). The skin becomes thin and inelastic and the hair becomes dry and falls out easily. Many changes designed to save protein and energy occur. Heart rate falls, blood pressure is reduced and basal metabolism is lowered. There is endocrine dysfunction causing amenorrhoea. On a worldwide basis protein-energy malnutrition in adults is due most commonly to an inadequate food supply. In Western societies, however, it is generally caused by chronic organic disease, postoperative inability to maintain an adequate nutritional intake and is also seen in anorexia nervosa.

In children, protein-energy malnutrition is usually classified as marasmus or kwashiorkor. **Marasmus** tends to be a disease of infancy often resulting from early weaning on to a diet which is deficient in protein and calories. The main features are growth retardation and wasting due to loss of fat and skeletal muscle mass. Oedema is usually absent. Associated deficiencies of vitamins and trace elements are common. By comparison, **kwashiorkor** tends to occur in older children (18–24 months) who have been weaned abruptly on to a high carbohydrate, low protein diet. This causes growth failure and loss of skeletal muscle mass but subcutaneous fat is preserved. Generalized oedema or localized limb oedema is an invariable and characteristic feature. Severe skin exfoliation, due primarily to Zn deficiency, leads to

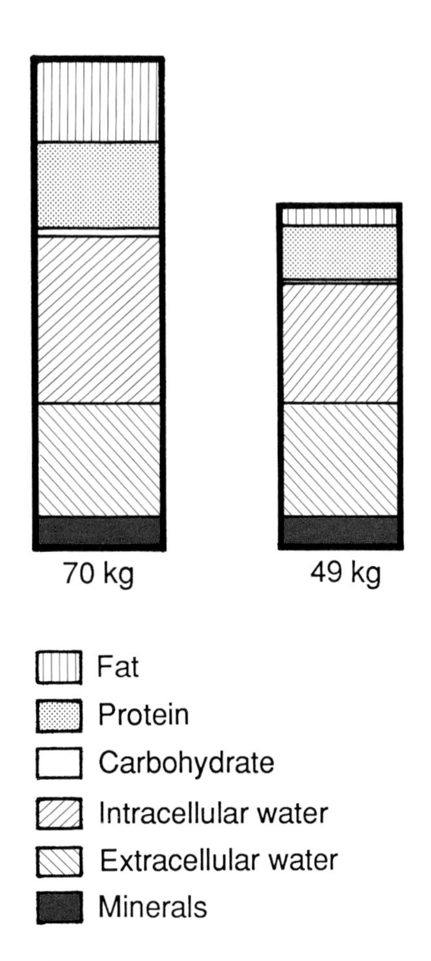

Fig. 9.2 Changes in body composition in an adult man after a prolonged period of inadequate nutrition. The reduction in fat and protein content accounts for a large proportion of the total reduction in body mass. As a percentage of total body mass before and after starvation, the intracellular water content remains virtually unaltered; however, as total body mass falls intracellular water content must also fall.

a variety of lesions. The hair becomes straight, friable and discoloured because of atrophy of the follicle roots. There is usually hepatomegaly due to fat accumulation and there is impaired synthesis of albumin and transferrin. Anaemia results from folic acid, iron or copper deficiency. Affected children are apathetic and irritable. Vitamin deficiency, especially of vitamin A, my coexist. Kwashiorkor and marasmus represent the extreme ends of the spectrum of protein-energy malnutrition. A range of hybrid states exists between these extremes as typified by '**oedematous marasmus**' and '**wasted kwashiorkor**'.

In protein-energy malnutrition there is a marked predisposition to intercurrent infections, tuberculous and viral infections being particularly common. In addition, organisms which are normally non-pathogenic may overgrow the gastric and intestinal mucosae producing chronic diarrhoea and often gaseous distension. The increased risk of infection appears to be due, at least in part, to the effects of malnutrition on the immune system. Reduced T-lymphocyte counts, impaired delayed hypersensitivity responses, reduced antibody responses, reduced concentrations of complement components (especially C3), and impaired neutrophil bactericidal activity all occur. An important consequence of intercurrent infection is that nutritional requirements are increased during the period of infection, thereby aggravating the malnourished state.

The metabolic basis of the features in these malnutrition syndromes is complex. An undue emphasis has been placed on the protein lack but it is now clear that there are deficiencies of numerous other factors. In addition to the inadequate intake there is also inappropriate loss of nutrients, and superadded infections further complicate and aggravate this situation. The treatment and management of affected children is complex and outwith our remit. Essentially, however, it is directed towards the control of infection, the replacement of nutrient deficiencies and the provision of an adequate diet to ensure normal growth and development.

Although protein-energy malnutrition is endemic in some parts of the world it is important to remember that industrial societies are not exempt from it. For example, marasmus commonly affects infants and children of impoverished families in industrialized countries. Furthermore, alcoholics, persons in long-term institutional care and patients maintained postoperatively on intravenous glucose solutions are at risk of developing a 'kwashiorkor-like' syndrome.

Effect of Diseases on Nutritional Status

In this section we look briefly at the nutritional problems which may be associated with disease in a number of organs. Metabolic diseases arising from inborn errors of metabolism are discussed in Chapter 7.

Injury and Infection

Injury and infection are associated with increased mobilization of the body stores of energy and protein. Although the precise mechanisms controlling this hypercatabolic response to injury are not fully understood, current evidence indicates that the combined actions of two main groups of mediators are involved. The first group comprises hormones, glucocorticoids, adrenaline and glucagon, which mobilize carbohydrate and fat stores as sources of energy. The second comprises the cytokines interleukin 1 (IL-1), IL-6 and tumour necrosis factor α (TNFα) which induce fever, stimulate the metabolic rate, increase hepatic acute phase protein synthesis (p. 146) and increase skeletal muscle protein breakdown. Protein catabolism is therefore used to support acute phase protein synthesis and gluconeogenesis in the liver. The net result is an increased supply of glucose to the tissues, contrasting with the situation during episodes of starvation in which glucose supply is decreased. The increased glucose production in the liver also facilitates the synthesis of glycoproteins, many of which are acute phase reactants (p. 147). As these mechanisms are hormonally driven they will continue even in the presence of insufficient dietary intake, i.e. in the presence of starvation. This results in acutely ill patients who cannot eat, rapidly depleting their body stores of fat and protein within a few weeks. The magnitude of the catabolic response depends on the severity of the injury or illness.

Patients in a hypercatabolic state require provision of extra energy substrates and protein. The increased energy requirements amount to about 10% for an abdominal surgery procedure such as a cholecystectomy, 25% for major surgery complicated by sepsis, and 50–100% extra may be required in severe accidental trauma such as widespread full-thickness burns. Protein requirements may also be substantially increased, and it may be impossible to maintain nitrogen balance since protein catabolism exceeds synthesis. Provision of a good quality protein intake, based upon urinary nitrogen losses together with an adequate energy intake, is necessary to minimize the overall net loss of muscle protein.

Malignant Tumours

Most patients dying of cancer have evidence of protein-energy malnutrition or 'cancer cachexia'. In many, it is so severe that death is largely due to malnutrition, often complicated by intercurrent infection.

The pathogenesis of cancer cachexia is multifactorial (Fig. 9.3) but is very poorly understood and depends partly upon the type of tumour. In most patients there is reduced food intake, most commonly due to anorexia but sometimes due to mechanical obstruction in the upper gastrointestinal tract. Reduced absorption from the gut is common, especially following radiotherapy or chemotherapy. Diversion of nutrients to a rapidly growing tumour is theoretically possible but is rare in man. In some patients there is weight loss even in the presence of an apparently adequate energy intake. This has led to the concept that there may be a more fundamental metabolic derangement in cancer patients, such as a reduced utilization of nutrients or an increased metabolic rate similar to that occurring in response to trauma. Tumour necrosis factor α (TNFα, formerly known as cachectin (p. 198), is a product of macrophages and activated T cells and causes increased mobilization of adipose tissue, probably by inhibiting lipoprotein lipase. It may have a role in the increased loss of fat in patients with neoplastic disease.

Gastrointestinal Disease

Gastrointestinal disease affects nutritional requirements in varied ways. The many causes of malabsorption and the syndromes which may result are discussed in detail in Chapter 15. In addition, acute gastrointestinal diseases requiring surgical intervention leads to a catabolic response with increased nutritional requirements.

A number of the malabsorption syndromes can be adequately treated, e.g. gluten-sensitive enteropathy by the withdrawal of gluten from the diet

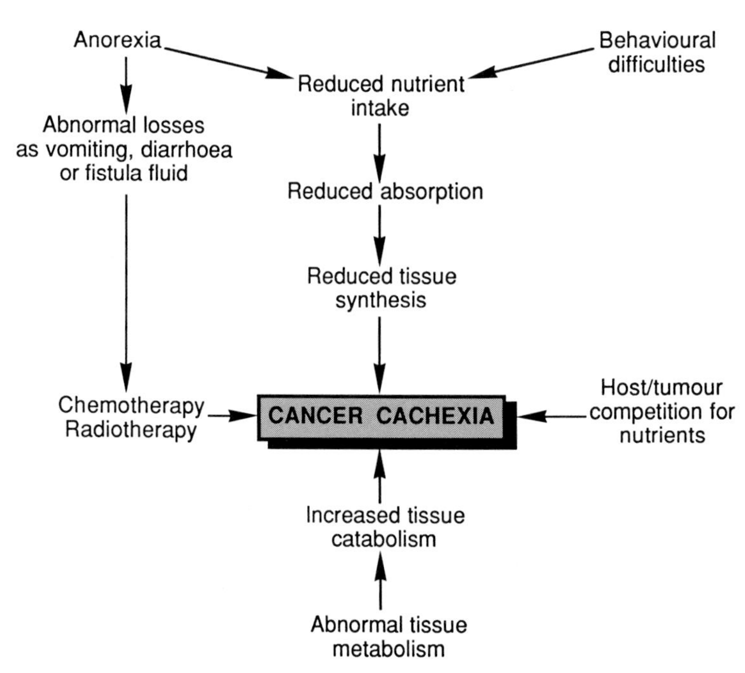

Fig. 9.3 Factors involved in the pathogenesis of cancer cachexia.

(p. 723). In other instances, however, e.g. a patient with an enterocutaneous fistula, enteral feeding by nasogastric or nasojejunal tube may be required, while in a patient with a short gut syndrome parenteral nutrition may have to be instituted. The nutritional problems associated with these forms of treatment are complex.

Renal Disease

Nutritional requirements in renal disease depend upon the severity of the illness and whether dialysis is being used. In patients with acute renal failure, energy needs will usually be increased as a result of the underlying illness and increased protein requirements will be necessary if there has been traumatic injury. In chronic renal failure not requiring dialysis, energy requirements must be met but protein intake should be restricted to reduce urea production. In patients undergoing regular dialysis, strict dietary control of protein is not required; potassium intake usually has to be restricted.

Liver Disease

Liver disease leads to important changes in nutritional requirements since the liver is the major nutrient processing organ in the body. In acute hepatitis a high carbohydrate, low fat and low protein diet is required, the level of protein depending upon the liver's ability to synthesize urea. In chronic liver disease with hepatic failure an important dietary measure is to reduce sodium intake, hence minimizing oedema and ascites. There are also complex disturbances involving protein metabolism in particular, but also carbohydrates and fat together with effects on fat soluble vitamins. Many of the features of hepatic encephalopathy are thought to be due to the profound metabolic disturbance which these patients manifest (p. 743).

Pulmonary Disease

Many forms of severe chronic respiratory disease are associated with protein-energy malnutrition. This may result from the increased work involved in breathing, and from difficulty in chewing and swallowing when breathing itself is difficult. Patients may benefit from a diet with an increased fat content and a reduced carbohydrate content, since this reduces the rate of CO_2 production for a given energy expenditure and so less CO_2 has to be lost from the lungs.

Vitamins

It is convenient to divide the vitamins into fat soluble and water soluble categories. Vitamins A, D, E and K comprise the former whereas the B group vitamins and vitamin C are water soluble. The B vitamin complex has a number of constituents; however only thiamine (B_1), riboflavin (B_2, niacin and pyridoxine (B_6) will be dealt with in detail. Folate and cobalamin (B_{12}) are discussed in Chapter 15. No well defined clinical deficiency state has been defined for biotin in adults or for pantothenic acid.

In the following paragraphs each vitamin is dealt with separately, but it has already been made clear that vitamin deficiency and other nutritional deficiency states commonly occur in combination. The factors which may be involved in causing vitamin deficiency states are summarized in Table 9.4.

Table 9.4 Factors which may be responsible for vitamin deficiency states

Reduced dietary intake
Availability from diet
e.g. may be destroyed during food storage or in cooking
Impaired gastrointestinal absorption
e.g. loss of fat soluble vitamins in hepatic and pancreatic disease
competitive loss to gastrointestinal organisms, e.g. B_{12} and folic acid (p. 723)
Impaired production by gastrointestinal organisms, e.g. vitamin K deficiency in neonates
Increased metabolic demands
Iatrogenic
e.g. impaired vitamin K synthesis following sterilization of the gut
impaired absorption or utilization by drug antagonists (cholestyramine and vitamin D) or analogues (isoniazid and vitamin B_6 pyridoxine)

The severity of the clinical syndromes is related to the severity and duration of the vitamin deficiencies; some, but not all, of the effects are reversible with vitamin replacement.

Fat Soluble Vitamins

Vitamin A

Retinol, a vitamin A derivative, is a constituent of rhodopsin, a pigment which is bleached by light. Vitamin A is therefore required for synthesis of rhodopsin and impaired dark adaptation is a relatively early manifestation of deficiency. Vitamin A is also essential for cellular differentiation in mucus-secreting epithelia. In deficiency states the epithelial surfaces most commonly affected are the mucous membranes of the eye, the respiratory, gastrointestinal and genitourinary tracts and the lining epithelia of the pancreatic ducts and sweat glands. These undergo epithelial metaplasia which has particularly serious clinical consequences for the eye. Initially, there is squamous metaplasia of the conjunctiva (xerophthalmia) leading to corneal drying and wrinkling. This in turn predisposes to corneal ulceration and liquefaction (keratomalacia) with subsequent scarring and blindness. It is estimated that in Asia alone approximately 250 000 children become blind annually due to vitamin A deficiency. Loss of mucus secretion in the major airways severely compromises mucociliary clearance and results in recurrent respiratory infections. Renal stone formation round keratin debris and obstruction of small pancreatic ducts by shed squames with resultant pancreatitis are other recognized clinical sequelae.

Hepatic, biliary and pancreatic dysfunction leading to severe fat malabsorption represent the largest group of causes of vitamin A deficiency in industrial nations and malnutrition is far less important. The relationship between vitamin A and the development of cancer in humans is controversial. Current evidence suggests that vitamin A may induce resolution of premalignant states such as actinic keratosis, laryngeal papillomatosis, bronchial and urinary epithelial metaplasia, preventing their progression to cancer. No direct causal relationship has, however, been demonstrated between vitamin A deficiency and the development of cancer.

Vitamin D

Vitamin D can be regarded both as a vitamin and as a hormone. Its main biological functions are to maintain normal plasma levels of calcium and phosphate, a task it achieves with the help of parathyroid hormone. There are three main sites of action: (1) the gut, where it stimulates independently the absorption of calcium and phosphate; (2) the kidneys, where it stimulates parathyroid hormone-dependent reabsorption of calcium by the distal convoluted tubule; and (3) bone, where it stimulates the mobilization and release of calcium, a function it shares with parathyroid hormone. Vitamin D, calcium and phosphate metabolism are therefore very closely linked.

In humans, vitamin D is derived from dietary sources and from endogenous synthesis. Endogenous synthesis occurs in the skin where exposure to sunlight converts the abundant precursor 7-dehydrocholesterol to vitamin D. Up to 80% of an individual's daily needs can be synthesized in this way, making the dietary contribution relatively easily attained even on a less than perfect diet. Fish oils, vegetables and cereals all contain significant quantities of vitamin D.

Vitamin D deficiency causes rickets in children and osteomalacia in adults and the pathological features of these diseases are fully discussed in Chapter 23. Pure dietary deficiency as a cause of rickets or osteomalacia is uncommon in industrial countries because of endogenous synthesis. Only the very young and the very old are at risk, through poor diet and lack of exposure to the sun. In industrial countries other causes of deficiency take on greater importance. These include:

(1) vitamin D malabsorption, the commonest cause and due mainly to small intestinal, biliary or pancreatic dysfunction;

(2) impaired vitamin D metabolism in hepatic or renal diseases (p. 949) when there is interference with vitamin D hydroxylation;

(3) type I vitamin D-dependent rickets in which there is a specific defect in 1-hydroxylation, an

autosomal recessive inherited abnormality; and

(4) type II vitamin D-dependent rickets caused by end-organ resistance to vitamin D.

Vitamin E

Vitamin E consists of eight closely related fat soluble compounds the most active of which is alpha-tocopherol. All eight possess potent antioxidant properties which enable them to neutralize the free radicals generated by many cellular redox reactions. Vitamin E minimizes free radical induced membrane lipid peroxidation, a protective role which is particularly important in the nervous system and in preventing red cell lysis. It has been suggested that vitamin E has a role to play in protecting against lung damage caused by inhaled oxidants.

A wide range of foodstuffs including eggs, meat, fish, chicken, vegetables, cereals and nuts contain substantial quantities of vitamin E. It is therefore unusual for deficiency to result from pure dietary lack other than in situations of malnutrition. In industrial countries the main cause of vitamin E deficiency is fat malabsorption. Abetalipoproteinaemia, a rare autosomal recessive disease, can produce severe vitamin E deficiency since lack of this protein markedly reduces vitamin E transport in the plasma.

Vitamin E deficiency causes a peripheral neuropathy due in part to axonal degeneration in peripheral nerves and in the posterior columns of the spinal cord with resultant loss or necrosis in the dorsal root ganglia. Retinopathy with impaired vision and generalized or ocular muscle weakness have also been reported.

Vitamin K

Vitamin K is required for the hepatic synthesis of four blood clotting factors, factor II (prothrombin), factor VII, factor IX and factor X. The dietary requirements for vitamin K in adults are very low for two reasons. First, vitamin K is synthesized by intestinal bacterial flora; absorption from this source alone comes close to meeting the daily requirements for many individuals. In addition, the vitamin is very efficiently recycled in man. Dietary vitamin K deficiency is therefore uncommon.

Vitamin K deficiency occurs in the neonate whose requirements greatly exceed those of an adult and in patients receiving broad spectrum antibiotics which have sterilized their gut, resulting in loss of endogenous vitamin synthesis. Patients with severe, prolonged fat malabsorption, and those patients receiving coumarin anticoagulants which block the recycling of vitamin K, may become deficient. The clinical manifestations are of haemorrhage, due particularly to the hypoprothrombinaemia. Ecchymoses, gingival bleeding, haematuria, melaena and haematemesis occur in all age groups. In neonates, intracranial haemorrhage is particularly serious. Provided liver function is normal the coagulation defect can be effectively reversed by parenteral administration of vitamin K.

Water Soluble Vitamins

Thiamine (vitamin B_1)

Thiamine, as thiamine pyrophosphate, has three vital roles in humans: (1) it is a cofactor for oxidative decarboxylation reactions which are required for the synthesis of ATP; (2) it is an essential cofactor of the pentose phosphate pathway; (3) it is essential for maintenance of the integrity of cell membranes. This third role appears to be particularly important in neurons as it is essential for nerve conduction, particularly through peripheral nerves.

Thiamine is found in a wide range of foodstuffs, so pure dietary deficiency occurs only when there is very poor dietary intake. This is encountered in particular where the staple diet is polished rice, as the thiamine is lost during processing. In industrial countries thiamine deficiency may develop in chronic alcoholics, in patients on long-term parenteral nutrition, malnourished children of underprivileged families and in patients with severe malabsorption or intractable diarrhoea. Furthermore, any disease which produces a marked increase in catabolism also significantly increases thiamine requirements and may convert subclinical thiamine deficiency into symptomatic disease.

The principal clinical effects of thiamine deficiency fall into three categories: (1) polyneuropathy or dry beriberi; (2) cardiac dysfunction or wet beriberi; (3) central nervous system dysfunction or the Wernicke–Korsakoff syndrome. Each of these effects may present in isolation but they may occur in combination, and when all three are present they often appear as in the order shown. Polyneuropathy results from myelin degeneration affecting motor and sensory fibres as well as spinal reflex pathways. The feet and legs are most commonly affected with symmetrical foot-drop, altered sensation and tenderness of the leg muscles. Proximal progression to involve the trunk, upper limbs and even the dorsal columns of the spinal cord can occur.

In wet beriberi there is severe oedema due to venous congestion. There is generalized peripheral vasodilatation and arteriovenous shunting resulting in a high output cardiac failure (p. 484). There is biventricular cardiac enlargement with dilatation and, terminally, a flabby myocardium. Less commonly acute thiamine deficiency can lead to low cardiac output with hypotension, lactic acidosis and a high mortality rate; a syndrome called Shoshin beriberi.

The Wernicke–Korsakoff syndrome is most commonly seen in chronic alcoholics. There are two related, often coexisting, components to the syndrome namely Wernicke's encephalopathy and Korsakoff's psychosis. The former is characterized by ataxia, nystagmus, ophthalmoplegia and progressive dementia. In Korsakoff's psychosis there is severe mental dysfunction, the cardinal signs being retrograde amnesia, an inability to learn new information and confabulation. It often only becomes apparent following thiamine induced resolution of Wernicke's encephalopathy, but it should not be regarded as a separate disease entity. The lesions which occur in the brain are described on p. 842; the most striking abnormality is atrophy of and haemorrhage into the mamillary bodies.

On a worldwide basis up to 20% of patients with severe thiamine deficiency die of the disease, particularly due to the cardiac abnormalities. There is no clear explanation for the cardiovascular and neurological selectivity of the effects of thiamine deficiency.

Riboflavin (vitamin B_2)

Riboflavin is an important constituent of a number of enzymes (flavoproteins) essential for normal cell metabolism. Flavin mononucleotide and flavin adenine dinucleotide act as coenzymes for many hydrogen transfer or redox reactions such as the first step in the oxidation of fatty acids by acyl-CoA dehydrogenase.

Riboflavin is widely distributed throughout the animal and plant world with high concentrations in milk, liver, kidney and a wide range of vegetables. Cereals are a poor dietary source. It is relatively heat-stable and therefore survives cooking. It is absorbed from the jejunum by a specialized transport mechanism.

Deficiency of riboflavin occurs in severe malnutrition. Pregnancy and lactation may produce a mild deficiency state due to increased requirements. The clinical features of riboflavin deficiency comprise cheilitis, glossitis, seborrhoeic dermatitis and interstitial keratitis of the cornea. The glossitis can be very marked with a glazed, shiny atrophic tongue showing a characteristic magenta colour. The seborrhoeic dermatitis involves the nasolabial folds and cheeks. Capillaries and inflammatory cells invade the cornea leading to opacities, eventually with ulceration and scarring.

These various disorders are not individually diagnostic of riboflavin deficiency, but their occurrence in combination should suggest the diagnosis. Riboflavin replacement therapy results in resolution of the mucosal and dermatological changes. Ocular damage is likely to persist.

Niacin (nicotinic acid)

The main biochemical role of niacin is in oxidative metabolism as a constituent of the two coenzymes, nicotinamide adenine dinucleotide (NAD) and nicotinamide adenine dinucleotide phosphate (NADP). NAD is an essential coenzyme for a number of dehydrogenases involved in fat, carbohydrate and amino-acid metabolism, whereas NADP is active particularly in the hexose-monophosphate shunt of glucose metabolism. Niacin is derived both from the diet and from endogenous synthesis. The main dietary sources are vegetables and cereals. Tryptophan, found in meat, egg and milk proteins, is the substrate for endogenous synthesis.

An adequate diet or a diet composed largely of maize or millet may lead to deficiency. Maize contains a substantial quantity of niacin, but is a very poor dietary source since the niacin is chemically complexed, preventing absorption. This form of dietary niacin deficiency affects many people in certain areas of India. Another form of niacin deficiency occurs in Africa and areas of Asia where millet is the staple diet. Millet contains high levels of leucine which inhibit endogenous niacin synthesis from tryptophan. Niacin deficiency in industrial societies is largely confined to malnourished alcoholics, and patients with severe, prolonged debilitating illnesses, and to food faddists with an inadequate protein intake. Rarely, niacin deficiency is seen in the carcinoid syndrome due to sequestration of tryptophan by tumour cells to produce serotonin. Deficiency also occurs in Hartnup disease (p. 271), an uncommon inherited defect in the absorption of aromatic amino acids including tryptophan.

Niacin deficiency causes pellagra (literally meaning rough skin), characterized by the three Ds of dermatitis, diarrhoea and dementia. In addition, severe fatigue and weakness are usually experienced. The dermatitis is classically symmetrical in distribution, affecting the dorsum of the hands (so-called glove dermatitis), the face, neck, arms and feet. Initially the affected areas become erythematous and a burning sensation is experienced. Later the skin becomes scaly with irregular pigmentation. Stomatitis and glossitis with a raw red beefy tongue may also occur. Diarrhoea results from widespread mucosal atrophy with ulceration and inflammation, particularly affecting the oesophagus, stomach and colon. The neurological abnormalities range from depression or insomnia to tremor, rigidity, paraesthesiae and paresis. Neuronal degeneration in the brain and posterior column degeneration in the spinal cord resemble the effects of vitamin B_{12} deficiency. If severe, an encephalopathy may result.

Niacin therapy leads to rapid improvement in the dermatitis, diarrhoea and the mental state. Neurological symptoms due to neuronal loss persist.

Pyridoxine (vitamin B_6)

The metabolically active form of vitamin B_6 is pyridoxal-5-phosphate which is essential for the normal biochemical handling of many amino acids and lipids. It acts as a coenzyme for amino-acid decarboxylation, deamination, transamination, transulphuration and desulphuration. In addition, haem synthesis, stabilization of muscle phosphorylase and normal nerve conduction all depend upon its presence.

A normal mixed diet provides abundant vitamin B_6 since it is widely distributed in animal and vegetable foods. Pure dietary deficiency is uncommon but may occur in infants and in the elderly. Pregnancy and lactation can render the mother and, subsequently, the infant deficient in pyridoxine. In chronic alcoholics an increased risk of deficiency results from the accumulation of an alcohol metabolite which displaces pyridoxal-5-phosphate from its normal sites of action, thus enhancing its degradation. Prolonged use of therapeutic agents known to inactivate vitamin B_6 may cause deficiency, good examples being penicillamine and isoniazid.

The clinical changes seen in pyridoxine deficiency closely resemble those described for riboflavin deficiency, namely cheilitis, glossitis and seborrhoeic dermatitis. Peripheral neuropathy and, on occasions, convulsions may occur. Complete clinical resolution results from vitamin B_6 administration.

Ascorbic Acid (Vitamin C)

Ascorbic acid is present in all living tissues, where it has a vital role to play as a reducing agent in many hydroxylation reactions. One of the best characterized of these is the hydroxylation of proline and lysine residues in procollagen, a process essential for cross-linking and stabilization of the triple helical structure of mature collagen (p. 151). In vitamin C deficiency the production of structurally abnormal collagen lacking tensile strength is central to the development of many of the clinical changes. Ascorbic acid is also important in noradrenaline synthesis, the degradation of cholesterol and the absorption of iron by maintaining it in the ferrous state.

Vitamin C deficiency or scurvy is no longer a major problem on a worldwide basis, as a result of its abundance in a wide range of foods. Deficiency is most likely to occur in individuals who have a poor dietary intake of fruit and vegetables. The elderly, food faddists and chronic alcoholics are particularly at risk. If deficiency occurs in infants or children the effects, although biochemically identical to adults, are far more dramatic because of the requirements for good quality collagen during growth. Skeletal changes in children are very prominent due to the failure to synthesize sufficient amounts of bone. Both membranous and endochondral ossification are severely impaired. The reduced amounts of osteoid which form are normally mineralized; however, the end result is poor quality bone which is subject to fracture and easily deformed by stress. Indrawing of the sternum can occur due to poor quality bone formation at the costochondral junctions. The subluxed costochondral junctions now protrude forward, giving a beaded appearance down each side of the chest, forming the so-called 'scorbutic rosary'. Failure of dentine formation as a consequence of disrupted collagen synthesis results in teeth that loosen and may fall out.

The second major clinical consequence of scurvy is haemorrhage. Blood vessel walls, particularly those of capillaries and venules, become fragile. This results in skin purpura and ecchymoses, subperiosteal bleeding, intra-articular haemorrhage and bleeding from the gingival mucosa. Intracranial haemorrhage, which is fortunately less common, can be fatal. Other important features of scurvy include impaired wound healing, anaemia secondary to abnormal iron metabolism and haemorrhage and finally, a characteristic plugging of hair follicles accompanied by perifollicular haemorrhages.

Both adults and children with scurvy respond well to vitamin C therapy. All the abnormalities except established skeletal deformities resolve.

Minerals and Trace Elements

There are a number of elements which are essential components of many of the body's enzymes, but which are required in very small amounts (Table 9.2) and most of which constitute less than 0.01% of body weight. This includes the so-called essential trace elements, iron, copper, iodine, fluorine, chromium, cobalt, selenium and zinc. Calcium and magnesium are required in larger amounts. These minerals are widely distributed in the diet but deficiency syndromes have been recognized and are briefly reviewed in this section.

Iron

Iron in the body is largely concerned with the processes of cellular respiration. An iron porphyrin (haem) group forms an essential component of haemoglobin, myoglobin, the cytochromes, catalase and peroxidase. In total this accounts for approximately 70% of total body iron. Non-haem iron forms the remainder, most of which is protein bound as the storage proteins ferritin and haemosiderin. Iron intake in a normal mixed diet is usually adequate to meet the widely differing needs of most individuals. The greatest need for iron is during the first two years of life, during adolescence and throughout a woman's childbearing years. By comparison, the dietary needs of a healthy adult male or a healthy postmenopausal female are small.

The efficiency of iron absorption from the gut varies around 10%. Haem iron, as found in meat and fish, is far better absorbed than the inorganic dietary iron present in cereals and vegetables. Furthermore, other dietary constituents markedly affect iron absorption. Ascorbic acid, citric acid, sugars and amino acids enhance absorption, whilst vegetable products rich in phosphates, oxalates, phytates and tannates cause a marked reduction.

Iron deficiency is probably the most common

single nutrient deficiency in the world and is most frequently the result of excess loss due to blood loss. The most important effect is the development of a hypochromic microcytic anaemia, although this is a relatively late occurrence. Depletion of iron stores followed by defective function of a range of iron dependent enzymes precedes the development of anaemia. This disruption of enzyme function explains the range of symptoms which may be seen in the absence of anaemia. They include (1) an increased susceptibility to infection as a result of impaired cell mediated immunity and defective neutrophil bactericidal function: (2) reduced capacity for physical activity; (3) abnormal thermoregulation; and (4) mild derangement of cognitive functions.

The causes of iron deficiency can be considered under the following headings:

(1) an absolute dietary deficiency, a problem in developing countries where the diet contains a large proportion of cereals and vegetables and the iron content is largely inorganic and less readily absorbed;

(2) a relative dietary deficiency when physiological demand exceeds dietary supply as in pregnancy and in growing infants and children;

(3) reduced iron absorption as a result of anatomical or functional disorders of the gut, particularly the small bowel, e.g. coeliac disease, extensive Crohn's disease and others;

(4) excessive iron loss, the major cause of which is chronic blood loss.

The effects of iron deficiencies on the haematological system are discussed in detail in Chapter 14 and diseases associated with iron overload in Chapter 17.

Calcium

Calcium is the most abundant mineral in the body with a total content of approximately 1300 grams in a 70 kg man. About 99% of this is found in the skeleton, where it ensures rigidity and acts as a reservoir for maintaining tissue and extracellular calcium ion concentrations. The contraction/relaxation cycle of skeletal and cardiac muscle and normal neuronal excitation and neuromuscular transmission depend on ionized calcium. Calcium plays an important role in the regulation of cell metabolism and in the activation of many complex enzyme systems.

Milk and dairy products are the richest sources of dietary calcium. Significant amounts are also present in eggs, pulses, nuts and vegetables such as cabbage and cauliflower. Calcium homeostasis is largely maintained by the balanced effects of vitamin D and parathyroid hormone on gut, kidney and bone. The main disorders affecting calcium metabolism are due to abnormal vitamin D or parathormone levels. Serum calcium is also affected by calcitonin and parathyroid hormone related peptide (PTHrP).

Dietary calcium deficiency is relatively uncommon except in severe malnutrition or where requirements are greatly elevated, e.g. during marked bone growth in children and in women who have repeated pregnancies. Hypocalcaemia leads to increased neuromuscular irritability and tetany which can be rapidly corrected by intravenous calcium administration.

Magnesium

The body contains approximately 20 grams of magnesium of which 70% is complexed with calcium and phosphate in bone. It is the most abundant divalent cation in the intracellular fluid compartment, where it activates numerous enzyme systems including those involved in energy pathways such as the phosphate group transfer reactions. In the extracellular fluid it has an important role to play in maintaining normal neuromuscular and nervous transmission. Approximately one-third of dietary magnesium is absorbed with homeostasis being maintained by regulation of urinary excretion.

Hypomagnesaemia usually results from increased gastrointestinal fluid losses such as occurs in severe diarrhoeal illnesses or from an intestinal fistula. Since magnesium is widely distributed in food, dietary deficiency is uncommon. Clinically, magnesium deficiency manifests itself as muscular weakness, muscle irritability, tetany, cardiac arrhythmias and sometimes behavioural disturbances.

Other Trace Elements

Copper is an essential constituent of several metalloenzymes which are involved in a number of key metabolic pathways: (1) cytochrome *c* oxidase and superoxide dismutase, which are required to maintain normal aerobic metabolism: (2) caeruloplasmin which acts as a peroxidase and oxidizes ferrous iron to ferric iron, so increasing iron availability for haem synthesis; (3) lysyl hydroxylase which is essential for cross-linking of collagen and elastin; (4) tyrosinase which ensures effective melanin production; (5) dopamine beta-hydroxylase which ensures effective neurotransmitter generation in the central nervous system. In addition, copper also appears to be necessary for the proper maintenance of myelin by mechanisms which are poorly understood.

Copper homeostasis is achieved by regulation of its absorption from the gut. The main route of excretion is active transport into the bile and loss in the faeces, and a very little is excreted in the urine. Copper deficiency is relatively uncommon, occurring only when there is severe generalized malnutrition. It is mainly seen in premature infants, in individuals on long-term intravenous nutrition, in severe malabsorption and in other causes of prolonged diarrhoea. In Menkes' kinky-hair syndrome, a rare X-linked recessive disorder, there is defective copper absorption.

Copper deficiency leads to a hypochromic microcytic anaemia and neutropenia; defective bone formation, with osteoporosis, costochondral cartilage cupping and flaring of the metaphyses of long bones with pathological fracture; subperiosteal haemorrhage; hypopigmentation; and disruption of central nervous system function with hypotonia and psychomotor dysfunction.

Wilson's disease or hepatolenticular degeneration, a metabolic disorder, results from copper overload and is discussed in Chapters 16 and 18.

Zinc is a vital constituent of over 200 metalloenzymes which are necessary for normal protein, nucleic acid and cell membrane metabolism. It is particularly important in ensuring normal growth, tissue repair and wound healing, and in reproduction. Homeostasis is maintained largely by regulating absorption.

Zinc deficiency may occur as a result of inadequate dietary intake, impaired absorption or excessive losses. Inadequate oral intake is relatively uncommon since zinc is present in a wide range of foods. However, patients who have to be maintained on synthetic enteral or parenteral diets are at risk of developing a deficiency state unless zinc supplementation is undertaken. Inhibition of zinc absorption by phytates and high fibre concentrations is well recognized, and deficiency has been reported in countries where the diet largely comprises unrefined cereals. Impaired zinc absorption may occur because of an inherited lack of a zinc binding protein (metallothionein) in the intestinal mucosa. Finally, excessive loss of zinc in fistula fluid or exudates may cause zinc deficiency.

Clinically, zinc deficiency produces a number of well recognized features: (1) hypogonadism and infertility; (2) impaired wound healing; (3) a distinctive but not diagnostic skin rash, **acrodermatitis enteropathica**, occurring on the hands and feet and around the eyes, mouth, nose, and anus; (4) growth retardation in children; (5) anorexia; (6) diarrhoea; (7) impaired night vision due to interference with vitamin A metabolism; (8) depressed mental function.

Selenium is an essential constituent of the enzyme glutathione peroxidase which protects membrane lipids and other cell constituents from oxidative damage by free radicals. Selenium is widely distributed in food and is well absorbed from the upper gastrointestinal tract. Selenium deficiency has been observed in two situations:

(1) in certain parts of China, the selenium content of the soil, water and food is low and a clinical deficiency state develops mainly in children and in women during their reproductive years. Affected individuals develop a congestive cardiomyopathy called Keshan disease;

(2) patients receiving prolonged parenteral feeding develop a skeletal muscle myopathy which

resolves on administering selenium. Similar muscle disorders can be produced in selenium-deficient animals. Some patients have also developed cardiomyopathy.

Chromium is widely distributed in the body and is involved in carbohydrate and lipid metabolism, potentiating the action of insulin. Chromium deficiency in man has been observed following long-term intravenous nutrition and causes glucose intolerance, neuropathy, high plasma fatty acid concentrations and impaired nitrogen balance.

Diseases due to Excess Dietary Intake

Obesity

In Western countries obesity represents the single most important result of nutritional excess. It is defined as an excess amount of body fat in relation to that required for health. However, it is clear that this is a somewhat arbitrary definition and the standard fat content required for health in adults will show considerable geographical variation. In addition, there are as yet no accurate means of measuring body fat; densitometry and measurement of skin fold thickness at standard anatomical sites are among the more accurate. A number of detailed analyses have been made in which body weight has been related to height and norms established for age and sex. Overweight, may then be defined when weight is 10% above the upper limit for these norms and obesity, when weight is 20% above the upper limits. The currently most common method of assessing obesity is calculation of the body mean index (BMI), the ratio of weight (kg) to height^2 (m). Values less than 25 are regarded as non-obese and those greater than 40 indicate severe obesity.

Obesity reflects an imbalance between the intake and the expenditure of energy. The reasons for this imbalance may be: (1) prolonged excessive energy intake due to lifestyle or psychological factors; (2) reduced energy expenditure due to inadequate physical activity: (3) reduced dietary thermogenesis. Dietary induced thermogenesis is the normal increase in resting energy expenditure in response to food. A reduction in this may explain the particular tendency of certain individuals to develop obesity compared to others with a similar lifestyle; and (4) endocrine abnormalities such as Cushing's syndrome or hypothyroidism.

It is now accepted that marked obesity causes excess morbidity and mortality because of its association with a number of diseases, the most important of which are hypertension, hyperlipidaemia leading to atheroma, type II (non-insulin dependent) diabetes mellitus, heart disease, cholelithiasis and osteoarthritis. A male who is 20% overweight, has a 25% excess mortality risk, but the increased risk for women is less. A complex interplay often occurs between the different diseases associated with obesity and the observed excess morbidity and mortality. A good example of this is in the relationship between obesity and heart disease. Hypertension has been clearly associated with obesity. The increased risk of heart disease is due to a combination of hypertension leading to left ventricular hypertrophy, together with hyperlipidaemia and type II diabetes, predisposing to coronary artery atheroma and ischaemic heart disease.

The association between obesity and cholelithiasis, particularly in women, is well established (p. 786). It is worth mentioning that obesity makes surgery technically more difficult and, in addition, postoperative complications such as deep venous thrombosis, bed sores and respiratory complications are more likely. In extreme obesity a hypoventilation syndrome (Pickwickian syndrome) may occur and may in part be due to mechanical impairment of ventilation (p. 538). The role of obesity in causing increased 'wear and tear' in large joints is a well accepted causal factor in osteoarthritis (p. 985). There is also a purported association between obesity and endometrial carcinoma (p. 1022).

Vitamin A Toxicity

Acute vitamin A toxicity in adults was reported in Arctic explorers who ate polar bear liver. Drowsiness, headache, vomiting, itching and desquamation of the skin occurred. Acute toxicity is however very uncommon. By comparison, chronic toxicity occurring predominantly in food faddists or from excessive dietary supplementation is better characterized. The main clinical effects of chronic toxicity are anorexia, nausea, vomiting, dry skin, pruritus, hair loss, headache, visual upset and hepatomegaly. Vitamin A is stored in the fat-containing (Ito) cells in the liver (p. 763) and chronic toxicity causes hepatocyte necrosis, fibrosis, sinusoidal dilatation and may lead to non-cirrhotic portal hypertension. The effects on children and adults are generally similar, but in children bony changes in the form of premature closure of the fontanelles and subperiosteal new bone formation occur. Very recently, attention has been focused on the possible teratogenic effects of excess vitamin A, and it has been suggested that substances rich in vitamin A should be avoided in the first trimester of pregnancy.

Vitamin D Toxicity

Chronic vitamin D toxicity may occur in patients with renal osteodystrophy who receive very large doses of synthetic vitamin D analogues. Vitamin D toxicity was sometimes seen in British children in the 1950s when over-fortification of milk products with vitamin D took place. In addition, toxicity may occur in the so-called milk-alkali syndrome, associated with milk and alkali ingestion for peptic ulcer symptoms. Clinically, toxicity causes hypercalcaemia with anorexia, nausea, constipation, abdominal pain, metastatic calcification and renal calculi. Acute vitamin D toxicity is very rarely seen.

Further Reading

Committee on Dietary Allowances, Food and Nutrition Board. (1989). *Recommended Dietary Allowances*, 10th edn. National Academy of Sciences, Washington, DC.

Kinney, J. M., Jeejeebhoy, K. M., Hill, G. L. and Owen, O. E. (1988). *Nutrition and Metabolism in Patient Care*. W. B. Saunders, Philadelphia.

McLaren, D. S. (1981). *A Colour Atlas of Nutritional Disorders*. Wolfe Medical Publications Ltd, London.

McLaren, D. S. and Meguid, M. M. (1988). *Nutrition and its Disorders*, 4th edn. Churchill Livingstone, Edinburgh.

Panel on Dietary Reference Values of the Committee on Medical Aspects of Food Policy (1991). *Dietary reference values for food energy and nutrients for the United Kingdom*. HMSO, London.

Shils, M. E. and Young, V. B. (1988). *Modern Nutrition in Health and Disease*, 7th edn. Lea & Febiger, Philadelphia.

Waterlow, J. C. (1981). Nutrition of man. *British Medical Bulletin* **37**, 1–103.

10

Growth and Neoplasia

Normal Control of Cell Proliferation in Tissues

Tissues are societies of cells. Within these societies there is always a subpopulation whose function corresponds closely to that of the tissue as a whole – e.g. hepatocytes in the liver, or keratinocytes in epidermis – and these are called parenchymal cells. Almost all tissues also contain blood vessels, lymphatics and nerves, running within tracts of interstitial connective tissue, and this is called stroma. The normal growth and maintenance of tissues requires that birth, differentiation and loss of cells in both parenchyma and stroma are regulated and co-ordinated. This chapter is about the principles underlying these important processes, and the pathology which results from them when they become disordered.

Stem Cells and Lineages

In both parenchyma and stroma most cells arise through proliferation and differentiation. The precursor cells from which a tissue is built, and on which the continuing life of a renewing tissue depends, are called **stem cells**. The characteristic feature of stem cells, which makes them different from all other cells in a tissue, is that they possess concurrently the capacities for self-renewal and lineage generation. **Self-renewal** is the process by which cell division yields at least one daughter identical to the original dividing cell. **Lineage generation** is the production of families of mature cells, characteristic of the tissue in question, through division and differentiation of their precursors. In most tissues, parenchyma and stroma have separate stem cells of their own.

Figure 10.1 shows one daughter of a dividing stem cell retaining stem cell characteristics, while the other becomes committed to lineage generation. Note that this daughter has ceased to be a stem cell, since its descendents are no longer identical to the original ancestral cell, but are progressing down a differentiation pathway, at least some steps of which are irreversible. Despite the many divisions which the lineage-generating cells may undergo, the key property of self-renewal to create another stem cell has been lost. Asymmetric divisions of the stem cell like this would be capable of sustaining the life of the tissue, since there is always one daughter which perpetuates the stem cell function. Stem cells do not always divide in this balanced way. Both daughters may retain stem function, or both may lose it. If most of the stem cell divisions in a tissue take this latter form, the tissue as a whole begins to lose the capacity for renewal.

Sometimes it is convenient to think of the cells of a tissue as falling into functionally defined compartments. Thus the '**stem cell compartment**' would contain the stem cells, and feed into a '**transit**' or '**amplification compartment**', characterized by cells engaged in the proliferation and differentiation of lineage generation. Cells in which division has ceased may continue to differentiate, but their fate is ultimately to die, and hence they are said to be in the '**terminal differentiation compartment**'. The rate at which cells pass from one compartment to the next varies from tissue to tissue, as does the proportion of cells in each compartment. Before specific examples are given, however, three important generalizations can be made.

First, contrary to intuition, stem cells usually divide infrequently. Most of the cell production of a tissue takes place in the transit compartment. Stem cells therefore constitute only a small minority of the cells in the tissue: they can be very inconspicuous despite their vital significance. Second, quite small changes in the number of divisions undertaken by cells in the transit compartment can have profound effects on the tissue composition, structure and function. For instance, in the bone

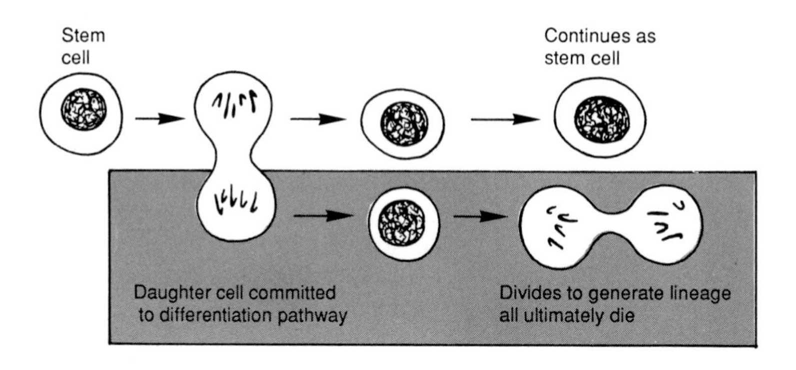

Fig. 10.1 Scheme of stem cell division in a continuously renewing cell population.

narrow, mature neutrophils are terminally dif-erentiated and ready for release into the blood-stream, whereas most of the earlier cell divisions elong to the transit compartment. Addition of just ne extra cell division to the transit pathway as a hole doubles the number of neutrophils ready for elease. Third, the cells of the terminal differentia-ion compartment often constitute the majority of he cells in the tissue; depending on the tissue in uestion, their lifespan from the last transit cell ivision can be days, months or years.

In practice, these compartments are much more han theoretical concepts. They are situated in articular locations in each tissue. For example, in *kin* (Fig. 10.2), the stem cells lie in the basal ayer, but not all basal cells are stem cells. The pidermal proliferative unit is a hexagon, with a tem cell at its centre, and daughter cells at the pices. Consecutive stem cell divisions distribute new daughter cells to the apices of the hexagon, displacing existing cells upward to more superficial layers of the epidermis. The size of the transit compartment probably varies from site to site, but as the keratinocytes enter terminal differentiation, they flatten and enlarge to occupy the entire surface projection of the hexagon. Progressive displacement towards the surface eventually leads to shedding of the familiar, hexagonal-shaped squames.

In the crypts of the *small intestine*, stem cells lie one or two cell positions above the crypt base. Most of the dividing cells lining the lower two-thirds of the crypt are in the transit compartment, whilst the remaining upper crypt and villus cells are terminally differentiated. Paneth cells derive from the same stem cells as the crypt and villus cells but, for reasons that are not clear, develop only in the lowest positions of the crypt. This

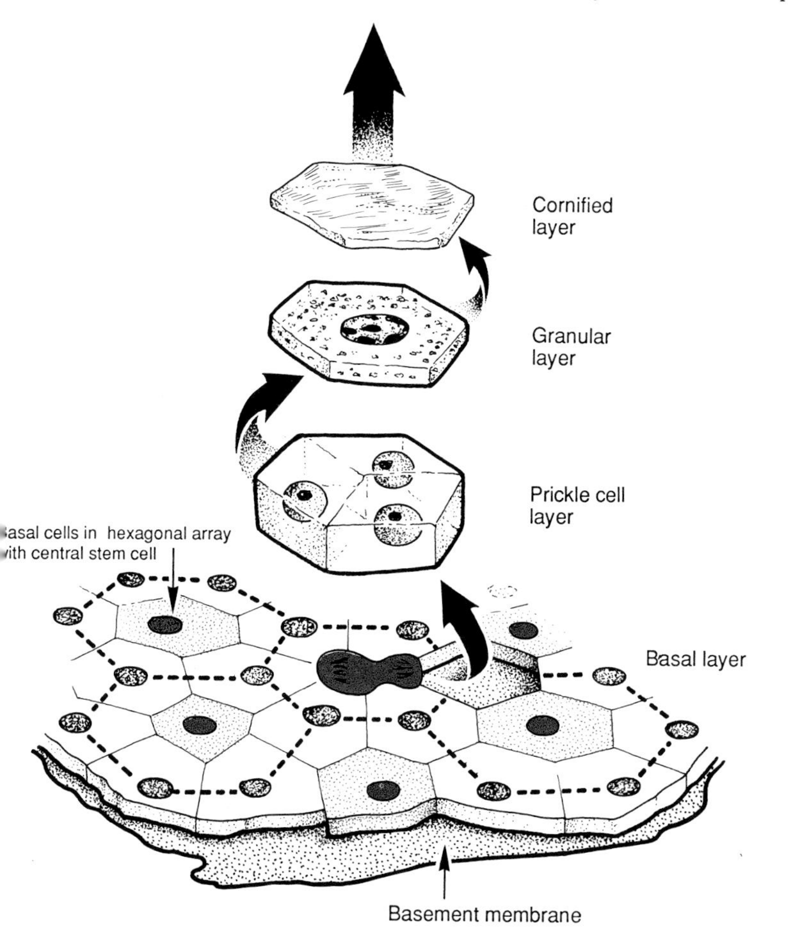

Fig. 10.2 Diagram of cell organization in epidermis. The basic structure is a hexagon, which in the basal layer has a central stem cell and daughter cells at each apex. Only one hexagon is shown in each of the layers represented above the basal layer. Cells from the apices of the basal layer hexagon move up to suprabasal layers, and their place is taken by division of the stem cells. As the cells move upwards they enlarge and flatten. Ultimately the cornified cells which are desquamated have the same surface area as the basal hexagon.

tissue design determines the morphological changes in the mucosa in response to different toxic agents (Fig. 10.3).

Stem cells are particularly sensitive to ionizing radiation. The immediate structural changes following radiation may be quite minor (because the stem cells are a small percentage of the total mucosal population), but as cells continue to mature through the transit and terminal differentiation pathway, they are not replaced, and the mucosa undergoes atrophy, and eventually ulceration, with a time course matching that of the normal transit time from crypt base to villus tip (3–5 days). In contrast, agents which are toxic to the mucosal cells lining the villi produce selective loss of the terminally differentiated compartment, with a compensatory expansion of the transit cells of the crypt. This is seen in persons who have a hypersensitivity to gliadin, a constituent of the wheat protein gluten, and who develop gluten sensitive enteropathy or coeliac disease (p. 723).

Study of cell generation in *bone marrow* has provided many insights into the way the local microenvironment regulates the development of cell lineages (p. 587). A polypeptide called stem cell factor, which supports the proliferation of haemopoietic stem cells, is synthesized by the 'stromal' cells of marrow: endothelium, fat cells, osteocytes and fibroblasts. There are also factor (e.g. granulocyte monocyte-colony stimulatin factor, GM-CSF) generated by terminally dif ferentiated myeloid cells, which promote or inhibi cell proliferation in the transit compartment and s regulate the production of cells in response t need. Similarly, feedback control can be exerte through circulating hormones. An example is th peptide hormone erythropoietin, released fro cells of the renal cortex in response to hypoxia which expands the production of cells of th erythroid series.

Perhaps the most complex system of tissu regulation is found in the *lymphoid system*. Detail of how lymphocyte production is adjusted to mee need are given in Chapter 16, but we can note her how the same principles pertain as have bee outlined already: stem cells are relatively rare, an divide infrequently; the rapid development of par ticular lineages involves cells in the transit path way; within lymph nodes, specific locations ar occupied by cells in particular phases of matura tion; and regulatory signals include locally activ factors released in the microenvironment (cyto kines), or exposed on the surface of cells durin cell-to-cell interaction (e.g. processed antigens MHC epitopes).

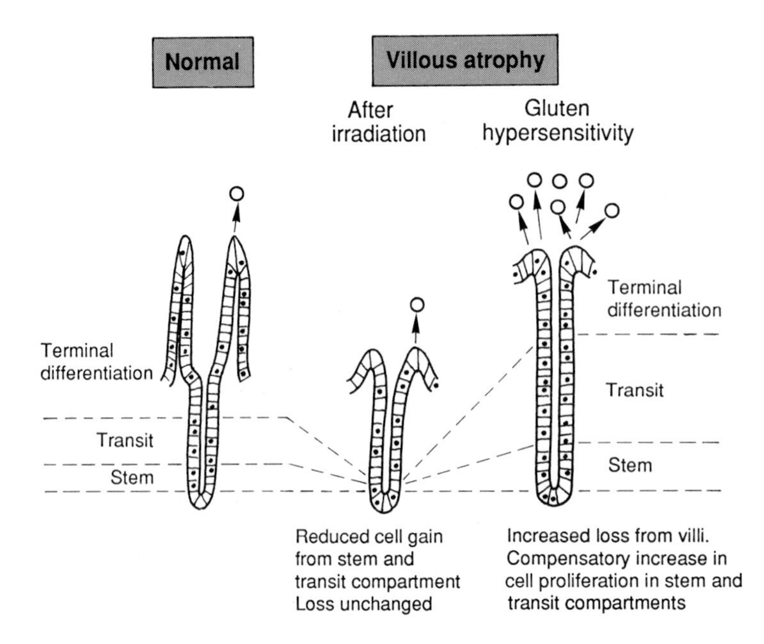

Fig. 10.3 Patterns atrophy of small intestir mucosa.

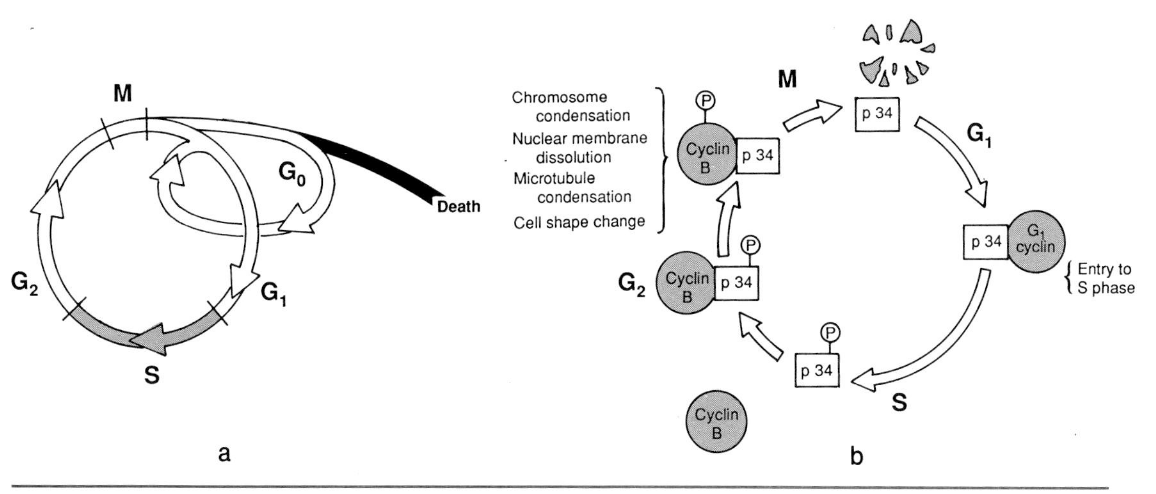

Fig. 10.4 **a** Scheme of the cell cycle and related non-proliferative states. **b** Regulation of the cell cycle.

Regulation of Cell Proliferation

Cells engaged in proliferation pass through four phases which together constitute the **cell cycle** (Fig. 10.4a). In G_1 preparation is made to enter DNA synthesis. In S, DNA synthesis occurs. In G_2, the cell assembles the machinery for distributing the newly replicated chromosomes equally to the two daughter cells which are generated in M, mitosis. Although it lasts only one-half to one hour, mitosis involves more changes in cell structure than all the rest of the cycle. Chromosomes condense, the nuclear envelope dissolves, and the cell loses most of its previous contacts, adopting a rounded shape. Microtubules polymerize from centres in the kinetochores (specialized portions of the chromosome centromeres) and the centrioles, which at this stage have come to lie at opposite poles of the cell. The kinetochores then move along the microtubules (they possess an ATP-driven motor which effects this), so drawing the chromosomes apart. At the same time the cell adopts a dumb-bell shape and cleaves in two, the chromosomes decondense and the nuclear envelope reforms around them in the two new daughter cells.

A great many cells in normal tissues, however, are in none of these phases. Some are in a non-proliferating state called G_0, or growth arrest, from which they can be activated to enter the cell cycle in G_1. Others can no longer enter the cycle; they are committed to terminal differentiation and death. The process whereby cells are stimulated to move from one phase of the cycle to the next is called cell cycle control. In contrast, the control of entry to the proliferative state from G_0 is called growth control. The regulation of cell death is also very important in determining the overall pattern of growth in a tissue.

Cell Cycle Control

Several of the key elements of cell cycle control are now known (Fig. 10.4b). In particular, the transition from G_2 to M is critically dependent on the activity of a cellular phosphokinase called **mitosis promoting factor** (MPF). MPF is a heterodimer, one component being a 34 kDa protein ($p34^{cdc2}$ kinase)* which contains the kinase

*The history of the unravelling of cell cycle control is recent, brilliant and dependent on cross-fertilization between different fields. Unfortunately this has had the effect of making the terminology a little clumsy. MPF was first discovered as a progesterone-induced protein in amphibian oocytes, in which it could be manipulated by microinjection. MPF was initially 'maturation promoting factor' because it released the oocyte out of its arrest in meiotic prophase, to become a mature ovum. *cdc2* is the code name for a yeast gene, identified by mutations which interrupted the normal *c*ell *d*ivision *c*ycle in these primitive eukaryotes. p34 designated a cell protein, which turned out to be identical to the produce of the *cdc2* gene. We shall call this protein p34 kinase for simplicity.

domain, the other a 62 kDa protein called cyclin B. The synthesis rates of both p34 kinase and cyclin B are surprisingly even throughout the cell cycle, but p34 kinase undergoes dephosphorylation just before M, and variations in the degradation rate of cyclin B ensure that its concentration rises steadily to a maximum at the same time, and falls precipitously in late M, around the onset of anaphase. Cyclin B becomes phosphorylated at around the same time as p34 kinase is dephosphorylated. The complex of dephosphorylated p34 kinase and phosphorylated cyclin is essential for entry to mitosis, perhaps because the substrates of its kinase activity include histone H_1 (contributing to chromosome condensation), lamins (the proteins of the nuclear envelope, which depolymerase on phosphorylation causing dissolution of the nuclear membrane), caldesmon (an inhibitor of actinomyosin ATPase) and the protein product of the cellular proto-oncogene c-*src*. The last two together probably mediate the changes in cell shape. Although MPF is clearly a central molecule in the initiation of mitosis, it is itself regulated by a cascade of phosphorylation and dephosphorylation reactions. The cellular proto-oncogenes c-*mos* and c-*fms* are amongst the genes involved in this cascade.

The p34 kinase is also rate-limiting in the other major control point in the cell cycle, the transition from G_1 to S. Here it forms a complex with another cyclin, perhaps cyclin E. Other cyclin-p34 complexes form during the cell's progress through S-phase. The switching of p34 kinase from one cyclin complex to the other, and the related modifications of phosphorylation status of the complexes, regulate the ordered movement around the cycle.

The processes involved in the S-phase itself are also becoming clear. At several thousand sites across the genome, DNA replication is initiated through the binding of a 'molecular machine' to favourable sequences in DNA. Within these **origins of replication** there is an AT-rich motif which facilitates unwinding of the two strands of the double helix. The molecular machine that undertakes DNA replication (Fig. 10.5) includes a helicase, which unwinds the strands, two DNA polymerases to catalyse replication of each strand, and several cofactors, one purpose of which is to ensure that replication of the leading and lagging strands are closely correlated. Some of these cofactors (e.g. the accessory protein for DNA polymerase delta, PCNA) appear selectively in proliferating cells and hence can be used as immunocytochemical markers for proliferating cells in tissues.

The replicative machine appears not to travel along the double helix in the manner of a car moving along an assembly line during its manufacture. Rather, the DNA is reeled through fixed replication sites, which are probably part of the protein skeleton of the interphase nucleus. The replication sites are distributed close to the nuclear periphery, and this raises the question whether they are thus favourably positioned to respond to incoming signals from the cytoplasm.

Cell Growth Control

Cells move from the quiescent G_0 state into G_1 in response to specific stimuli. The best known of these are locally active peptides and glycoproteins called **growth factors**. Some growth factors act on a wide spectrum of cell types; examples include platelet derived growth factor (PDGF), the somatomedins or insulin-like growth factors (IGFs) and the acidic and basic fibroblast growth factors (a- and b-FGF) which, despite their name, stimulate proliferation in many cells in addition to fibroblasts. Epidermal growth factor (EGF) acts predominantly on epithelial cells. Tumour-derived growth factor alpha (TGFα) is a closely related peptide. It was first identified in tumour cell culture supernatants but is now known to be produced by normal cells, including skin keratinocytes. It is clear that there are a great many growth factors with yet more specific target cell specificities, although the majority appear to belong to molecular 'superfamilies' of which the above are prototypes. Further, some factors have the opposite effect and inhibit proliferation of certain target cells (e.g. TGFβ). Many familiar hormones also exert positive or negative growth factor activity on their target cells (e.g. thyroid

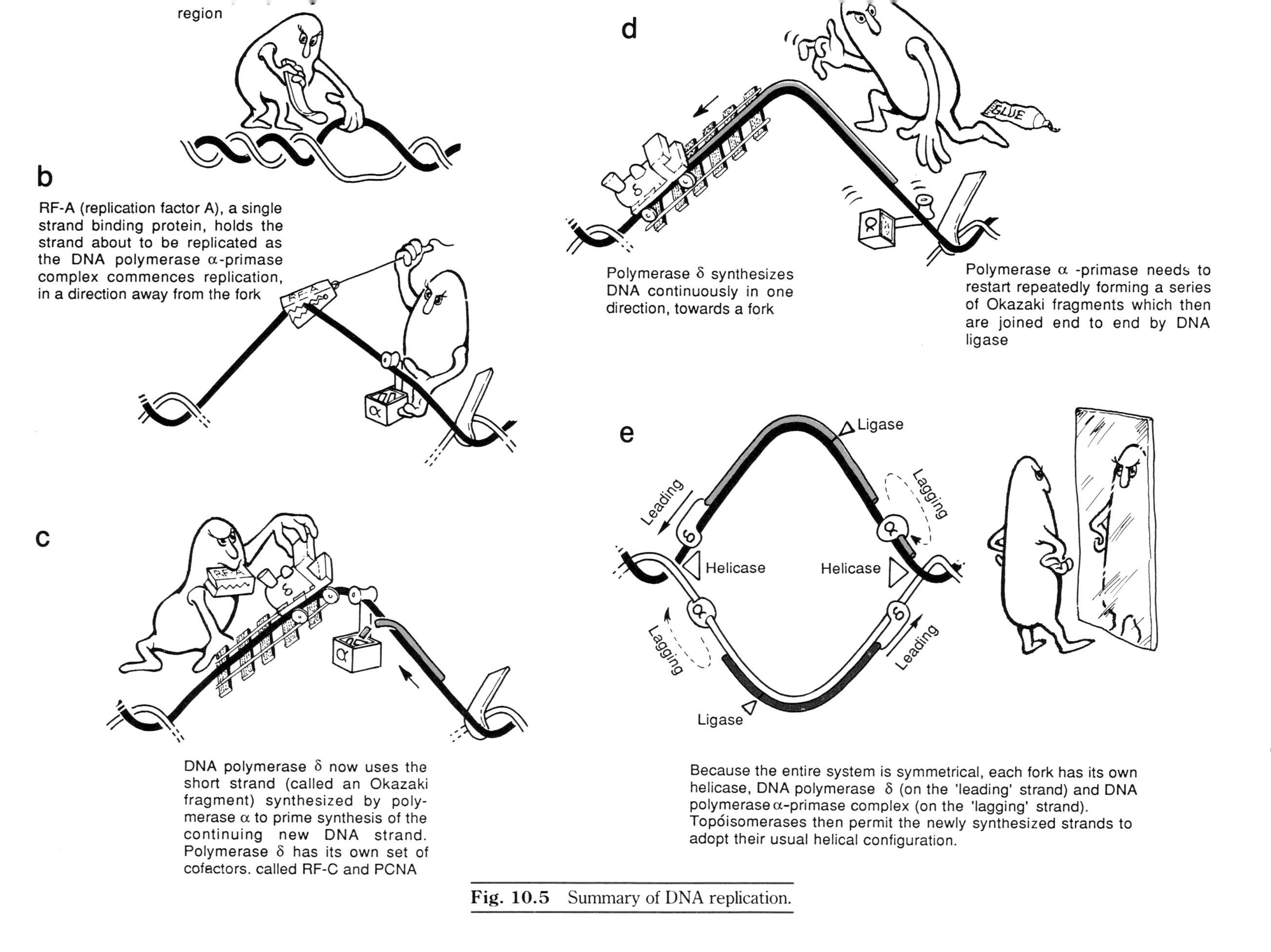

Fig. 10.5 Summary of DNA replication.

hormone on thyroid epithelium, progesterone on mammary epithelium).

Growth factors influence their target cells by binding to specific receptors. Sometimes they stimulate their target cells to synthesize and display receptors to other factors, so rendering the cell capable of response to proliferative stimuli to which it was previously inert. An example is the effect of IL-1 (a cytokine with actions on a great many cell types) in inducing IL-2 receptors in T lymphocytes. In this way complex interactions in growth control can be built up in tissues, creating interdependence between parenchyma and stroma, or between juxtaposed sets of parenchymal cells.

The interdependence of stroma and parenchyma is made even more intimate through the role of the extracellular matrix. Glycosaminoglycans of the matrix have the capacity to bind and stabilize specific growth factors in active form. This means that certain microenvironments, defined by their stromal elements, afford strong local growth factor stimuli specific for certain cell types. In this way, the microenvironment of the bone marrow sinusoids is enriched in IL-3 and GM-CSF, major growth factors sustaining haemopoietic differentiation in the stem cells which lie adjacent. Similarly, b-FGF, a potent angiogenic factor, is bound in active form by the basement membrane of endothelia.

It is far from clear how growth factor stimulation eventually produces activation of quiescent cells so that they can enter the cell cycle. Many of the growth factor receptors have inducible tyrosine kinase activity, and engagement of the receptor thus activates protein phosphorylation cascades within the stimulated cell. One immediate result of this is the activation of transcription of an important set of genes called **immediate early genes**, including c-*fos*, *jun*-B, and c-*myc*. The products of these genes in turn alter the patterns of transcription, so they can be considered as switches, turning on new activities throughout the cell. As they are of great importance in carcinogenesis, they will be described in more detail later.

Certain cell types, cultured *in vitro*, show a sequential series of activation events as they move from G_0 into G_1 and S. Growth factors which permit exit from G_0 do not always ensure entry to S. This has led to attempts to classify growth factors as **competence factors**, which permit exit from G_0, and **induction factors**, which have no effect on G_0 cells, but move cells into S once they have been made competent. It is not clear how important these distinctions are in real life within tissues, but the observations emphasize the complexity of growth control and the multiple potential control points in the process of cell replication.

There are also specific signals for returning cells to the G_0 state. One results from direct electrical coupling between adjacent cells by means of gap junctions. This is responsible for the growth arrest of non-neoplastic cells in culture when they reach a characteristic critical density – a phenomenon known as contact inhibition or **topo-inhibition.** Very little is known about the intracellular mechanisms which effect re-entry to G_0, but it seems to be an actively regulated process. New genes (**growth arrest genes**) are transcribed around the time when the cell leaves the cycle, but the function of their products is still incompletely understood.

Cell Death

Although cell death is often a pathological event, it is also used as a control point in the regulation of tissue populations. Under these circumstances it is effected by the process of **apoptosis** which tends to affect single cells and has been described in detail in Chapter 1 (p. 28). By apoptosis, large numbers of cells can be removed unobtrusively from within tissues. The initiation of apoptosis is regulated by growth factors, some turning it on whilst others delay or prevent it. The proto-oncogene *bcl-2* appears to be an important intracellular negative regulator of apoptosis in lymphocytes, and it is probable that other proto-oncogenes are involved in the regulation of apoptosis in other cell types.

Abnormalities of Growth

Tissues respond to chronic growth stimuli in stereotyped ways. Hypertrophy, hyperplasia and metaplasia have been discussed in Chapter 1 but are mentioned again here to contrast them with neoplasia.

Hypertrophy and Hyperplasia

Hypertrophy is the increase in size of a tissue or organ through increase in the size of the constituent cells.
Hyperplasia is the increase in organ or tissue size through increase in cell number. Both are reversible on removal of the growth stimulus. It is not clear how the decision between hyperplasia and hypertrophy is made. In simple eukaryotic cells like yeasts a critical size must be reached before cell division is initiated. There is some evidence for a similar mechanism in mammalian tissues, but cell size is unlikely to be the only factor involved.

The definitions above tend to conceal the fact that hypertrophy and hyperplasia are not merely quantitative changes in cell size and number. Frequently there is also evidence of altered cell organization and differentiation. In glandular tissues the secretory epithelium becomes taller, the glands themselves become more convoluted, and the epithelium undergoes invagination into the lumen to create papillary structures unlike anything in the unstimulated tissue (Fig. 10.6). In myocardium, chronic stimulation (e.g. by the increased workload which occurs in hypertension) leads not only to hypertrophy of muscle fibres, but to mitogenic stimulation of precursor cells which differentiate to fibroblasts. The resulting mixture of thick myocardial fibres and diffusely distributed fibroblasts is characteristic (p. 487).

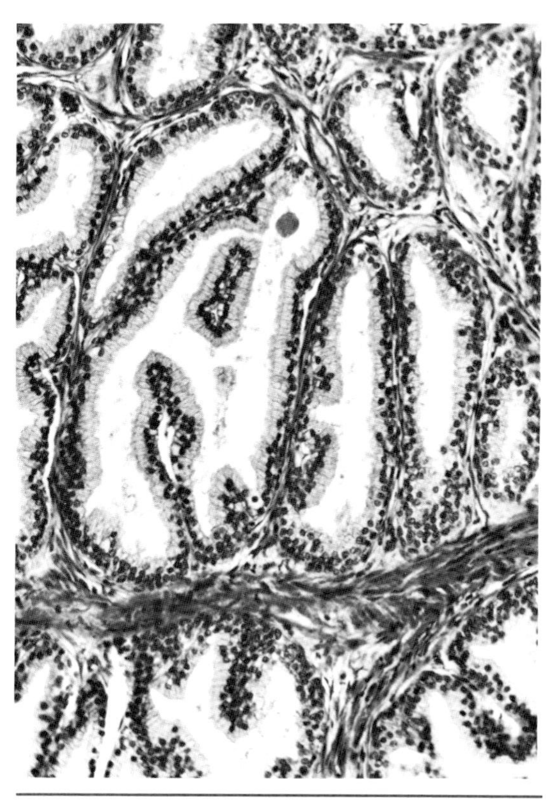

Fig. 10.6 Section of an enlarged prostate, showing hyperplasia of the glandular epithelium.

Hamartoma

Hamartomas are local malformations in which cell types normal to the affected part of the body are present in abnormal proportion. They are usually present from birth and growth is not progressive. Examples include the familiar 'mole' in the skin, properly called a cutaneous naevus, in which intradermal melanocytes are present in abnormally high frequency. The much rarer pulmonary hamartoma (p. 578) comprises a nodule of cartilage, smooth muscle and respiratory epithelium, all normal tissues in the lung, but in this lesion forming a disorderly mass that can be mistaken for more ominous pathology on X-ray.

Metaplasia

Metaplasia is the replacement of a normal, differentiated cell type by another that is inappropriate at that anatomical site. The switching of cell type in metaplasia always involves rather limited options. Thus, bronchial respiratory epithelium, on chronic irritation by tobacco smoke, often is replaced by a stratified squamous epithelium; stomach, particularly around foci of chronic inflammation, may develop the cytological features and organization of small intestinal mucosa; and the transitional cell epithelium of the bladder may undergo metaplasia to either a squamous or a mucus-secretory cell type. Amongst developmental biologists, a very similar phenomenon is called 'transdifferentiation', and is clearly the result of cell expression of a normal but inappropriate differentiation programme. Although metaplasia can sometimes result from exposure to substances that also cause cancer, it is – unlike cancer – a reversible change.

Neoplasia

Neoplasia is the process of tumour growth. The terms tumour and neoplasm are formally synonymous in pathology. The notable British pathologist, Rupert Willis, defined a tumour as '*an abnormal mass of tissue, the growth of which exceeds and is unco-ordinated with that of the normal tissues, and persists in the same excessive manner after cessation of the stimuli which evoked the change*'. In this definition, Willis incorporated several vital distinctions between neoplasia and other types of growth. First, the growth is **abnormal**. At many points in normal development groups of cells appear which proliferate more rapidly than their neighbours, and sometimes may also show novel properties such as the ability to infiltrate into adjacent structures. An example of this is the trophoblast. But this tissue is normal, and ultimately the fact that its growth is closely regulated becomes obvious. The **excessive and unco-ordinated** growth of neoplasms contrasts with that of hamartomas, which (although abnormal tissue masses), remain – usually throughout life – in a constant relationship with surrounding tissue. Neoplastic growth **persists** after removal of the initiating stimulus. Willis meant this to distinguish neoplasia from hyperplasia, and the cellular proliferation seen in inflammation and healing, which are all reversible. He was impressed by the many observations, clinical and experimental, in which single exposures to carcinogenic substances led to development of tumours years later, when the substances themselves must have long since gone.

There are some minor problems with this definition. In a later section we will see that the 'provoking stimulus' leaves within the new tumour cell a permanent genetic change, and sometimes that genetic change is itself part of the provoking stimulus, as in viral carcinogenesis. There is also evidence that some tumours need not grow progressively, or may even regress spontaneously. Furthermore, neoplasia can be a property of single cells, which strictly speaking does not fit with the intuitive notion of a 'mass of tissue'. None the less, the definition is a useful one. Most people who have to deal with human tumours are only too familiar with their potential for uncontrolled, irreversible growth.

Benign and Malignant Tumours

Tumours are divided into two classes, benign and malignant (Table 10.1). The critical distinction is their mode of growth. Benign tumours grow by **expansion**, compressing or displacing surrounding normal tissue, but malignant tumours grow by local **infiltration**, destroying the tissue through which they invade (Fig. 10.7). Benign tumours grow at their site of origin only, but malignant tumours may spread to distant sites, by the bloodstream, in the lymphatics, or across tissue spaces

Table 10.1 Summary of differences between benign and malignant tumours

	Benign	Malignant
Mode of growth	Expansion Remain localized	Infiltration and metastasis by lymphatics, blood vessels, and across tissue spaces
Rate of growth	Slower	Faster
Histological features	Similar to tissue of origin Nuclei normal Cells uniform in shape and size	Many differ from tissue of origin Nuclei enlarged, often with prominent nucleoli (pleomorphism) and abnormal mitotic figures Cells variable in shape and size (pleomorphism)
Clinical effects	Local pressure effects Hormone secretion Cured by adequate local excision	Local pressure and tissue-destructive effects Inappropriate hormone secretion Not cured by local excision because of metastases Non-metastatic metabolic and neurological complications

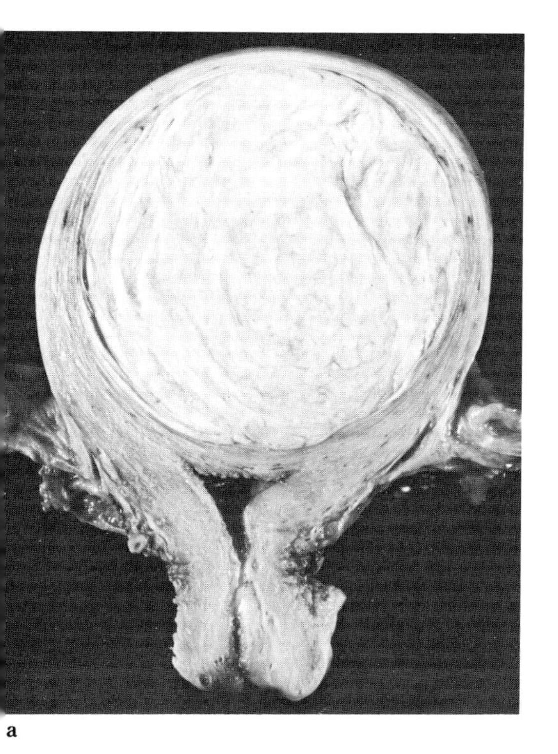

a

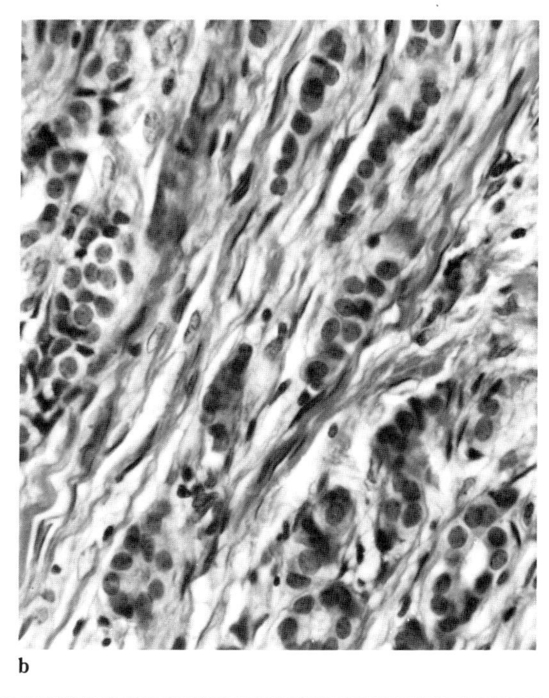

b

Fig. 10.7 **a** Growth by expansion in a benign tumour. This uterus contains a huge leiomyoma (sometimes called a 'fibroid') at its fundus. The tumour has expanded slowly, in a spherical shape, displacing the surrounding normal tissue but not destroying it. **b** Growth by infiltration. The cells of this carcinoma of breast – in small groups and chains – are growing through the surrounding connective tissue. The remote ductular origin of this tumour is hinted at by the glandular structures at the bottom right.

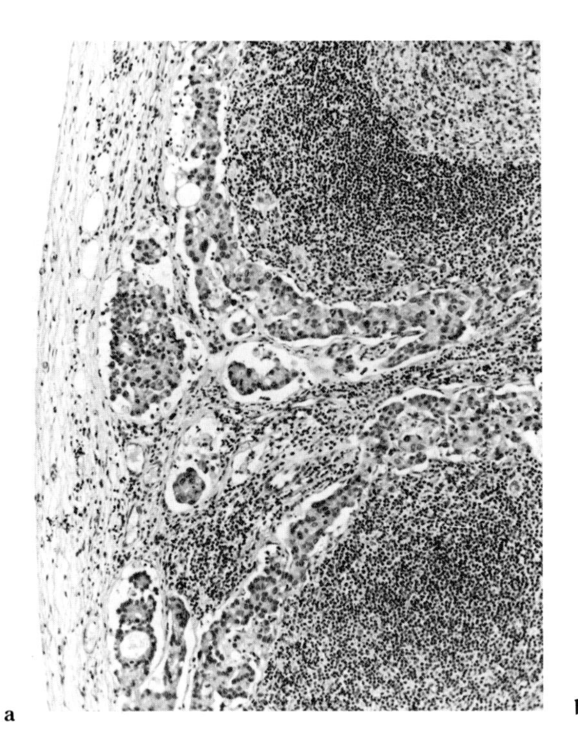

a

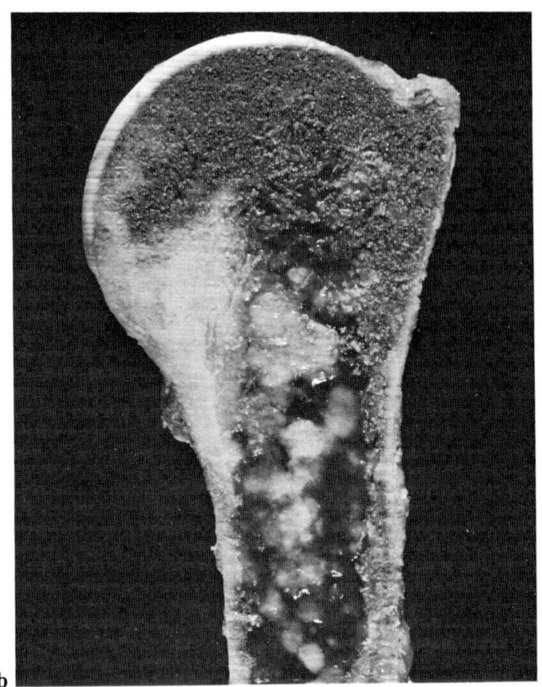

b

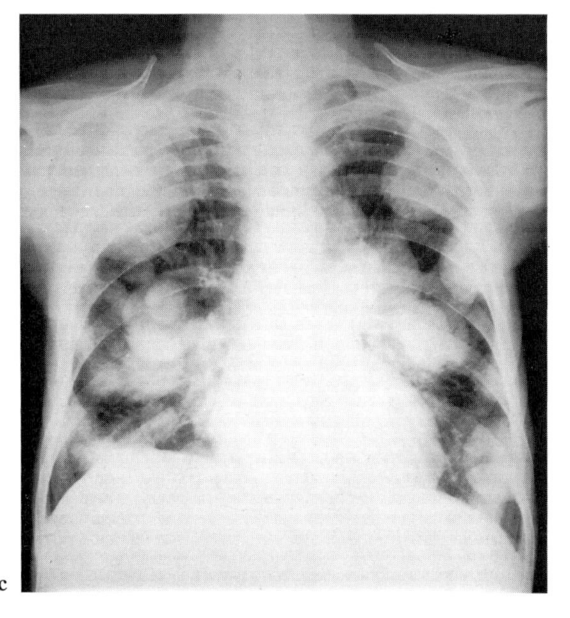

c

Fig. 10.8 **a** Metastasis by lymphatics. The acinar structures of this adenocarcinoma can be seen in the subcapsular sinus of a lymph node, and infiltrating around the lymphoid follicles of the node's cortex (seen at top and bottom right). **b** Metastasis by blood spread. The medullary cavity of this humerus is full of white tumour nodules, metastases of a breast carcinoma. **c** Metastasis by blood spread. The multiple radio-opaque round masses in the lung are deposits of metastatic sarcoma from a primary in the thigh.

such as the peritoneal or pleural cavities, or the cerebrospinal fluid space. This extremely important and dangerous property of malignant tumours is called **metastasis**, and the secondary tumours which grow at the distant sites are metastases (Fig. 10.8). In general, metastases are faithful copies of the primary tumour in terms of cell structure, although they may differ in more subtle ways as discussed later. Malignant tumours also tend to have a faster rate of growth than benign tumours. As a result, benign and malignant tumours have different clinical effects. By virtue of

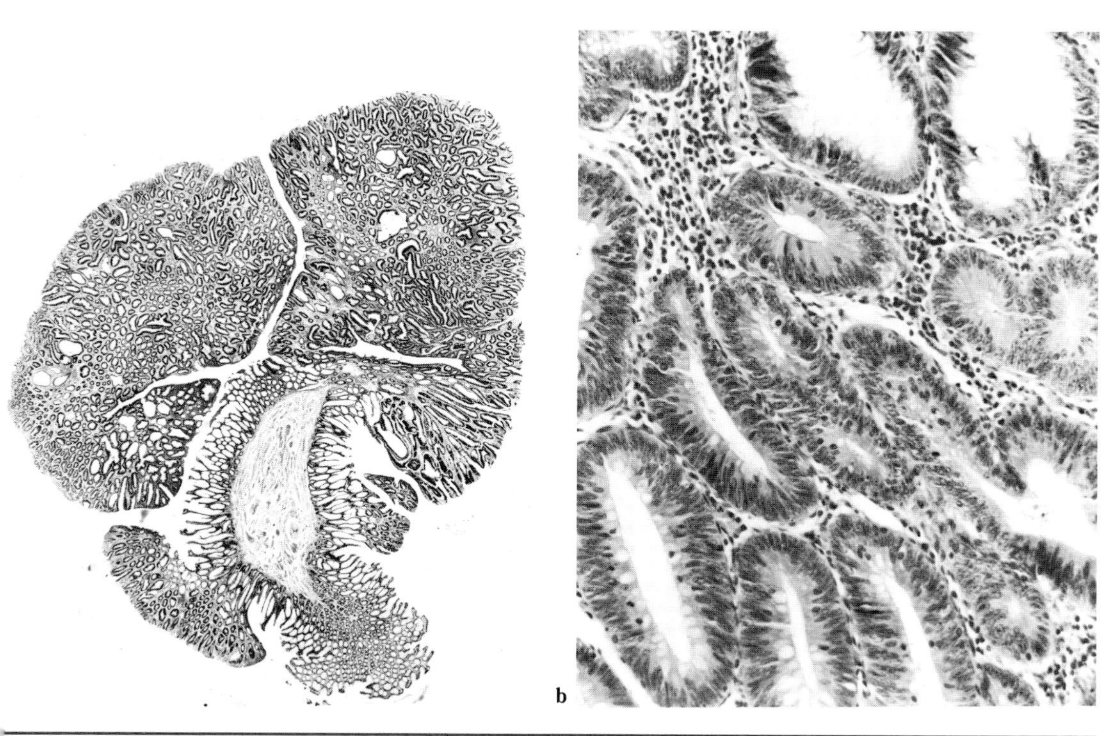

Fig. 10.9 **a** Tubular adenoma of the colon. The stalk, lined with normal colonic mucus-secreting glands, is seen in section in the middle of the picture. Near the top of the picture are the cellular but essentially well organized glands of the adenoma. **b** Histology of a colonic tubular adenoma. Although there is some loss of mucus secretory function, and the cells are very tightly packed together, they remain well organized, with basal nuclei and regular glandular array.

their position, benign tumours may cause symptoms by compression of adjacent structures, or in certain specific circumstances they may secrete hormones which contribute to the manifestations of disease. In contrast, malignant tumours always have the potential to cause death as a result of their aggressive growth behaviour.

The criteria given above are the 'gold standards' for distinguishing benign from malignant tumours, but they are essentially retrospective. Using these alone, tumours could only be classified after they had revealed their full capacity for abnormal behaviour. From the standpoint of both the clinician and the cell biologist, it is essential to differentiate benign from malignant tumours at a much earlier stage in their history, and therefore additional criteria are required. Critical information can often be provided from study of the morphology of the tumour cells. Histologically, benign tumours usually bear a close resemblance to their tissue of origin, whereas malignant tumours often are less well differentiated (Fig. 10.9). The cells of malignant tumours tend to be crowded more tightly together, and show an array of new cytological features. There is greater variety in size, shape and polarity (**pleomorphism**) and denser, coarser chromatin staining (**nuclear hyperchromatism**). Often the nucleoli of malignant tumours are abnormally large, numerous and intensely staining. The **mitotic index** is usually higher in malignant tumours, and the presence of tripolar mitoses, broken chromosomes, or otherwise **abnormal mitotic figures** is a strong indication of malignancy. These cytological features are sometimes grouped together under the umbrella term of **atypia**, whilst the coincidental disorganization of tissue structure is often called **dysplasia**. The changes in cell structure and tissue organization can be so extreme in malignant tumours that it is difficult to discern resemblance

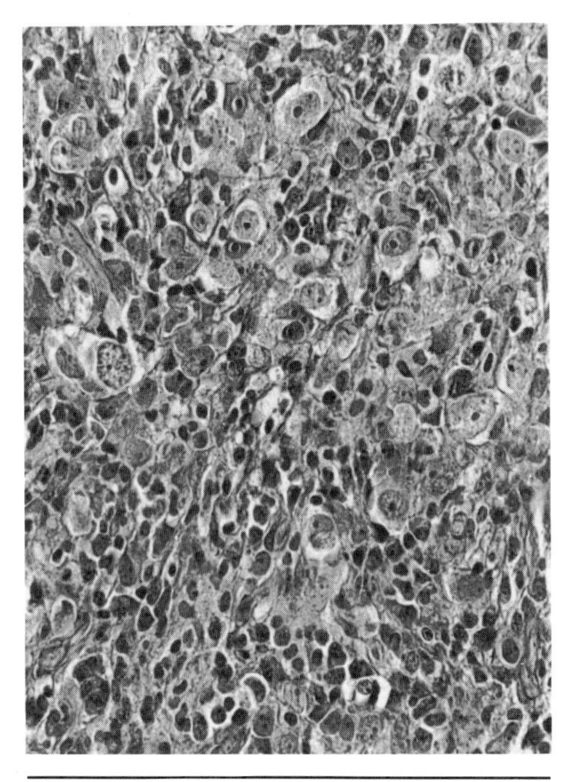

Fig. 10.10 An anaplastic malignant tumour, the histogenesis of which is not obvious. Immunohistology using monoclonal antibodies to epithelial cell markers showed it to be a carcinoma.

to the tissue of origin, or indeed any other normal differentiated tissue. Such malignant tumours are described as **anaplastic** (Fig. 10.10).*

The distinction between benign and malignant tumours is of fundamental importance, and has a major effect on the patient's future and the type of treatment that is appropriate. Because so much of the distinction depends upon assessment of morphological criteria, strenuous efforts are made to secure tumour tissue for diagnosis. Depending on its site, such tumour tissue can be obtained by endoscopic or open biopsy. Alternatively, dispersed tumour cells can be gathered from superficially positioned tumours, by scraping (as in the cervix) or brushing (as in the bronchus), or after natural exfoliation from the tumour surface into sputum or body fluids such as peritoneal fluid or urine. Cells can also be aspirated through a long fine needle from deep-seated tumours – fine needle aspiration (FNA).

* It is important to emphasize that, despite their consonance, the terms anaplasia and dysplasia are not in the same class as neoplasia, metaplasia and hyperplasia. Neoplasia, metaplasia and hyperplasia are **processes**, but anaplasia and dysplasia are merely **descriptive morphological terms**, which conveniently summarize the appearances of tissues in the light microscope.

Clinical Pathology of Tumours

The Basis of Tumour Nomenclature

All tumours have names. This section aims to show how these names encode important features of the tumours' characteristics: what sort of cells they derive from, how they are likely to behave, how they appear in the microscope, what special products they contain or secrete. The names transfer essential information between clinicians concerned with patient management, pathologists making the microscopic diagnosis, and cell biologists and epidemiologists studying the intrinsic nature of the tumour cells, their origins and their effects on people and populations. Tumour nomenclature is therefore a subject of great importance. In general it is systematic, and can be worked out by following a few rules (Table 10.2). As elsewhere in medical nomenclature, however, there are inconsistencies, many the result of historical usage. Tumour nomenclature usually has a histogenetic and a behavioural component. The histogenetic component gives information about the type of cell from which the tumour has arisen, or at any rate the predominant cell type of which it is presently constituted. The behavioural component tells whether the tumour is benign or malignant. Thus, *carcinomas are malignant tumours of epithelial origin, whereas sarcomas are malignant tumours of mesenchymal origin* (Fig. 10.11). Most

Table 10.2 Some examples of tumour nomenclature

Cell or tissue type	Benign	Malignant
Epithelial tumours		
Surface	Papilloma	Carcinoma (various types)
Glandular	Adenoma	Adenocarcinoma
Non-epithelial and mixed tumours		
Connective tissues		
adipose	Lipoma	Liposarcoma
fibrous	Fibroma	Fibrosarcoma
cartilage	Chondroma	Chondrosarcoma
bone	Osteoma	Osteosarcoma
smooth muscle	Leiomyoma	Leiomyosarcoma
striped muscle*		Rhabdomyosarcoma
Neuroectodermal		
glial cells*		Gliomas
nerve cells	Ganglioneuroma	Neuroblastoma Medulloblastoma
retinal cells*		Retinoblastoma
melanocytes*		Malignant melanoma
meninges	Meningioma	Malignant meningioma
Schwann cell	Neurofibroma	Neurofibrosarcoma
Haemopoietic and lymphoreticular*		Leukaemia and lymphoma (various types)
Germinal and embryonal cells	Benign teratoma	Malignant teratoma Dysgerminoma Seminoma
Placenta*		Choriocarcinoma

*Note that not all malignant tumours have a benign counterpart; similarly there are some types of benign tumour for which a malignant counterpart is rare or unknown.

benign tumours have names with the suffix **-oma**, preceded by a term indicating the tissue of origin. Hence, an **adenoma** is a benign tumour of glandular origin, a **chondroma** is a benign tumour of cartilage, and a **leiomyoma** is a benign smooth muscle tumour. Frequently it is useful to add further descriptive terms that specify the tumour's differentiation more exactly. A **squamous carcinoma** is a malignant epithelial tumour in which at least some cells show progressive keratinization (Fig. 10.12a), a **transitional cell carcinoma** arises from and expresses the differentiated features of urothelium, a **mucoid adenocarcinoma** is a malignant tumour of glandular epithelium in which the tumour cells lie within lakes of the mucin they secrete (Fig. 10.12b).

With the advent of immunocytochemistry it is now possible to define certain protein and polypeptide products within tumour cells. Benign tumours can exert potent and characteristic clinical effects if they secrete hormones, and for this reason there is a tendency to incorporate the name of the hormone into the name of the tumour, giving **insulinoma, glucagonoma**, and even **VIPoma**, all epithelial tumours of the peptide hormone secreting cells in the pancreatic islets.

Sometimes it is impossible for the nomenclature to express histogenesis precisely, for the straightforward reason that the histogenesis is not known. Many common lung tumours, for example, are clearly malignant, but do not appear similar in differentiation to any normal cell type in respiratory epithelium. These tumours require some form of specific nomenclature: they do not behave

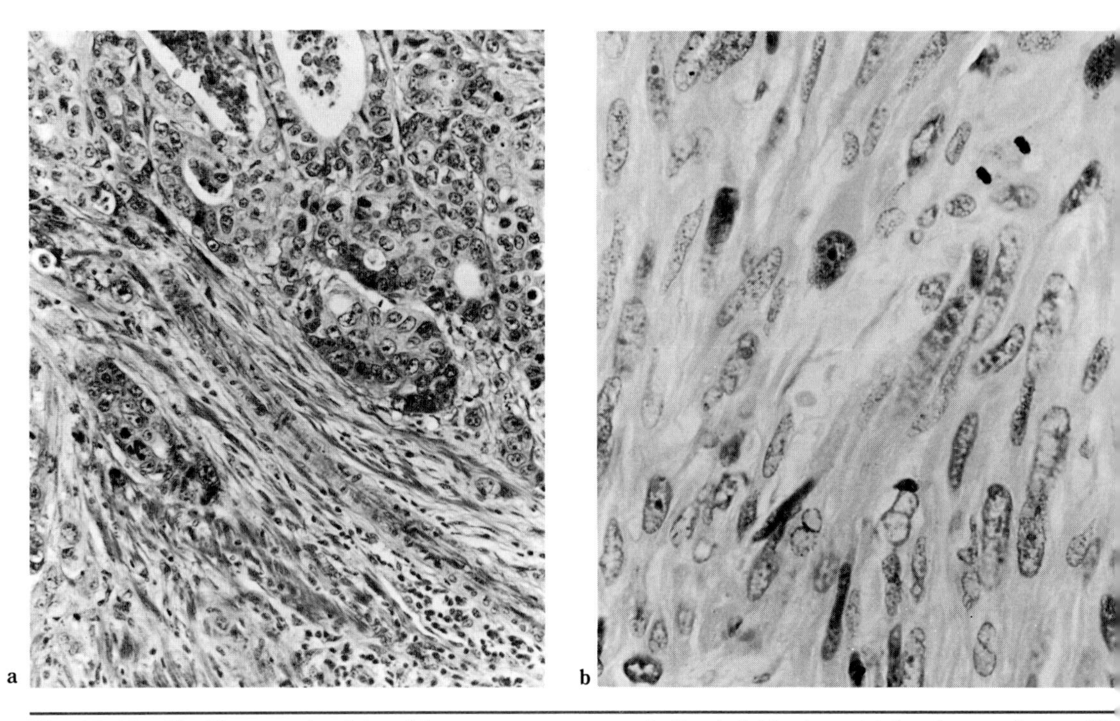

Fig. 10.11 The histogenetic origins of these tumours are revealed by their histology. (**a**) An adenocarcinoma. The cells near the top of the picture are still forming glandular structures, but they are infiltrating into bundles of normal smooth muscle (in this case in the wall of the rectum) at the bottom left. (**b**) A leiomyosarcoma. The cells are arranged in fascicles as is usual in smooth muscle, but the malignant nature of this tumour is revealed by the nuclear pleomorphism and mitotic activity. There is an anaphase in the top right hand corner.

in the same way as either squamous or adenocarcinomas, the other major tumour types at this site. Moreover, they may be a heterogeneous group, differing amongst themselves in prognosis and perhaps also in the most appropriate management. Microscopy suggests they can be classified on the basis of the size of the predominant cell type. Such tumours are therefore named simply on the basis of the available morphological features which allow them to be distinguished both from the lung tumours of more obvious histogenesis and from one another. In this way, a set of terms is built up which, although blandly descriptive, has specific meaning for tumours at this site: as well as squamous carcinomas and adenocarcinomas of lung there are **small cell lung cancers**, and **large cell lung cancers** (Fig. 10.13). It is recognized that this type of descriptive terminology may group together tumours of different histogenesis, but at present there is no better alternative.

Unfortunately, there are several important tumours that bear time-honoured names out of step with this logical scheme. **Gliomas** are tumours of the astrocytes or oligodendrocytes in the central nervous system. Some have a relatively benign growth pattern, and can be cured by surgery, but many are highly malignant tumours, despite the simple '-oma' suffix. **Teratomas** are tumours of primitive germ cell origin. They retain the capacity to differentiate towards all three embryological germ layers (endoderm, ectoderm and mesoderm). Ovarian teratomas are usually benign cystic tumours, containing a fascinating mixture of tissues, often set in close relationship to one another in a manner that recalls the histology of normal organs. Epidermis, respiratory and gas

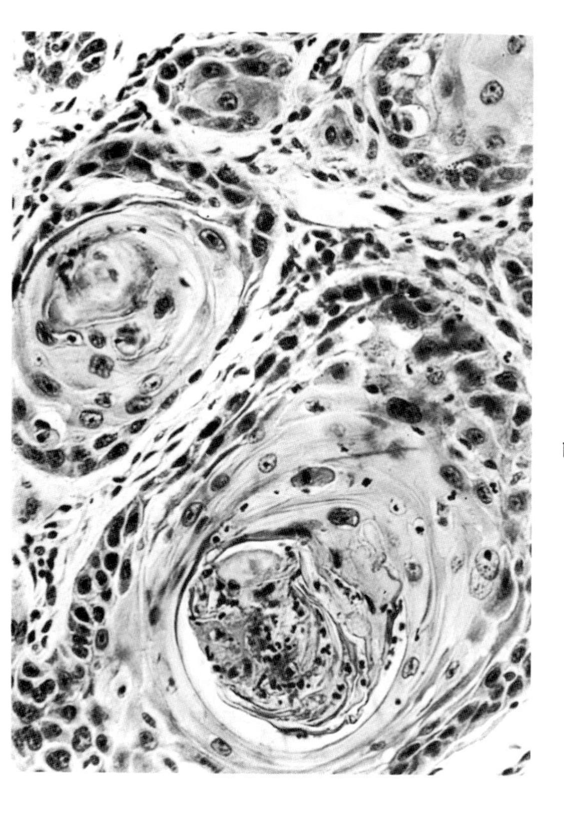

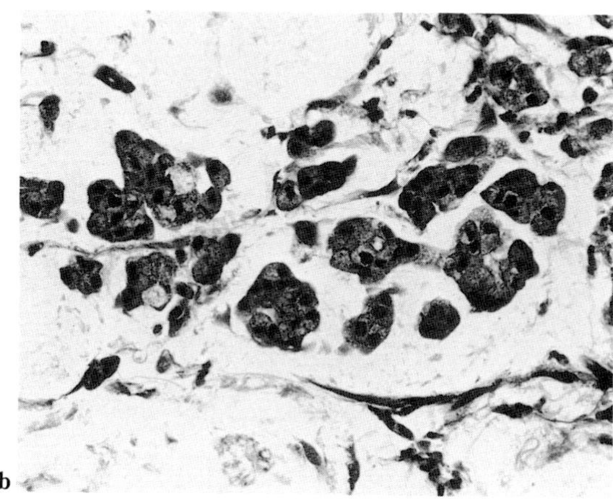

b

Fig. 10.12 **a** Shows portions of a squamous carcinoma. The cells form spherical structures with a recognizable basal layer on the outside, differentiating inwards to a mass of keratinized squames at the centre. **b** Shows a mucoid adenocarcinoma. The cells are in small, darkly staining groups, surrounded by the mucin which they secrete.

trointestinal epithelium, thyroid, bone, muscle and brain can be recognized in a jumbled mosaic. Testicular teratomas, on the other hand, are almost always malignant, and contain few cells with recognizably normal differentiation.

Lymphomas are tumours of the immune system. Again the simple '-oma' suffix is completely deceptive, since they are always malignant proliferations of lymphocytes. This is not the only problem of nomenclature affecting these tumours, as reference to Chapter 16 will clearly show. **Myeloma, multiple myeloma**, and **myelomatosis** are interchangeable terms describing a malignant proliferation of plasma cells, which usually arises in bone marrow and may destroy adjacent bone. **Leukaemias** are malignancies in which the normal circulating leucocytes are progressively replaced by large numbers of cells of a single lineage – lymphocytic, myeloid (granulocytic) or monocytic. The term leukaemia itself draws attention simply to the presence of large numbers of white cells in the circulating blood, and the diagnosis usually depends on examination of a blood film and bone marrow smear. There is extensive overlap, however, between lymphocytic leukaemia and lymphoma. Most lymphomas begin within lymph nodes, but eventually pass into a phase in which the abnormal lymphocytes appear in numbers in the bloodstream and so create a lymphocytic leukaemia. Similarly, many lymphocytic leukaemias are associated with enlarged lymph nodes packed full of neoplastic lymphocytes, features that qualify for the name of lymphoma.

Several tumours of children also have names which do not fit into the simple scheme described above. These tumours consist of poorly differentiated cells which seem to represent abnormally proliferating variants of the primitive cells of retina (**retinoblastoma**), kidney (**nephroblastoma**), and neurons of the autonomic and central nervous system (**neuroblastoma** and **medulloblastoma**).

One final important example of a malignant tumour with an anomalous name is **melanoma**, or perhaps more clearly **malignant melanoma**.

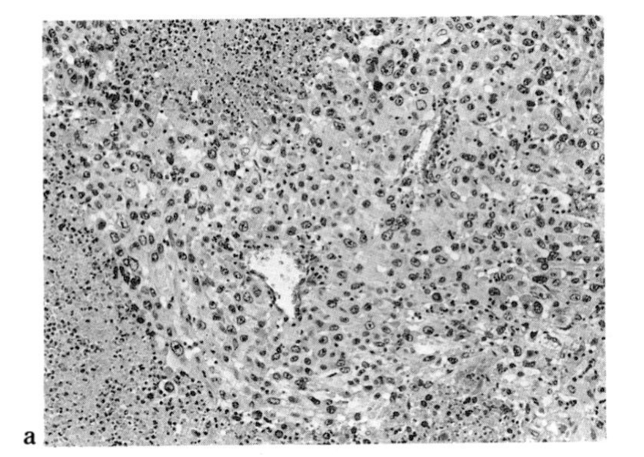

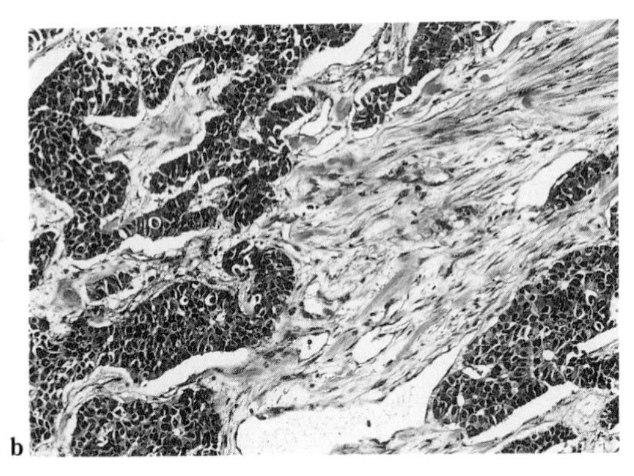

Fig. 10.13 Large cell carcinoma **a** and small cell carcinoma **b** of lung. Both photomicrographs are at the same magnification. The difference in tumour cell size between **a** and **b** is prominent, but neither tumour shows obvious differentiation towards squamous or glandular structures: hence the nomenclature. Note the additional features of tumour growth in these pictures. In **a** the tumour is growing in a cord around a thin walled blood vessel; distant from this supply of oxygen and nutrients, there is necrosis. In **b** the tumour cells are invading lymphatic channels.

This is a malignant tumour of melanin-synthesizing cells of retina or epidermis. There is no benign counterpart. Many melanomas, however, derive from the cells of pigmented naevi ('moles'). As we have seen above, these are hamartomas. It can be justly argued that the term hamartoma itself is deceptive, as these are not true tumours at all but local malformations. Similarly, the term haematoma describes a swelling due to extravasation of blood and, despite the '-oma' suffix, has nothing to do with tumours, benign or malignant.

Pre-invasive Malignancy

Names are good at distinguishing things from each other, but poor for describing elements within a continuum. The properties of established tumours do differ radically from those of normal tissue, and it is relatively easy to express this clearly by the nomenclature discussed above. Recently, however, cancer screening programmes have emphasized the prevalence of lesions which appear to be early stages in the development of tumours. They share some cytological properties with infiltrative tumours, but have not yet begun to infiltrate themselves. The implication is strong that they might do so if left for long enough, although we cannot say how long that would be. Nor is it possible to determine how far they have evolved from normality in terms either of time or biological events, or whether any of these events are reversible. Clearly, these lesions need names of their own, despite (or perhaps because of) these uncertainties.

The epithelium of the uterine cervix, for example, is the site of origin of squamous carcinomas, which infiltrate into the underlying connective

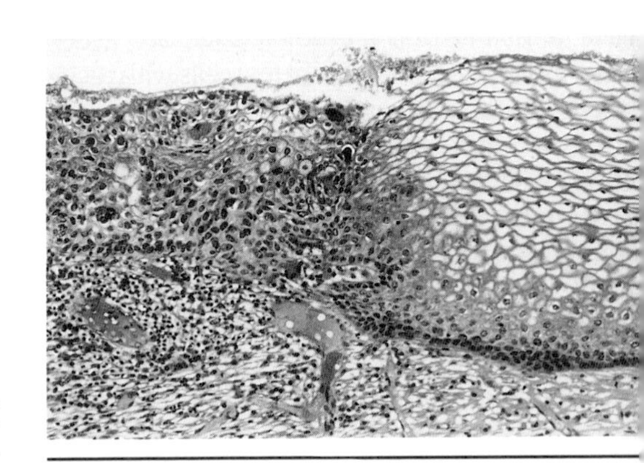

Fig. 10.14 Cervical intraepithelial neoplasia. Note the abrupt transition in the middle of the picture. To the right, the epithelium is more normal, with clear maturation of cells from the basal layer (where they are cuboidal) to the surface (where they are flat with tiny pyknotic nuclei). To the left, the epithelial cells show lack of maturation: near the surface there are still many cuboidal cells, containing relatively large nuclei, and the polarity of the cells throughout the epithelium is disordered.

issue and may eventually metastasize. A far ommoner lesion at this site, however, is an bnormality of growth entirely restricted to the pithelium. The cells show many cytological eatures normally expected within malignant umours, such as cellular overcrowding, hyper-hromatic nuclei and nuclear pleomorphism (Fig. 10.14). There is disturbance of the orderly se-quence of changes in cell shape, size and orienta-ion which is normally seen as cells mature and nove outwards from basal layer to surface. Cells nay become laden with keratin at an inap-ropriately deep level in the epithelium and, con-ersely, cell proliferation may not shut off in the isual way after the cells have left the basal layer so hat mitotic figures appear nearer the surface than ormal. Despite these manifestations of abnormal ell behaviour, the changes are all within the nor-nal confines of the epithelium; the basement nembrane is not breached. Since there is neither nfiltration nor metastasis, the term carcinoma, vithout qualification, would be inappropriate. Yet here is evidence that a proportion of these le-sions, if left undisturbed for months or years, may eventually evolve into classical infiltrating, malig-nant tumours. Accordingly, the term **cervical ntra-epithelial neoplasia (CIN)** is applied to his combination of disturbed surface maturation, nuclear and cytoplasmic pleomorphism and in-creased cellularity, wholly restricted to the epi-helium itself. Intra-epithelial neoplasia occurs at other sites also, such as the vagina and the squamous epithelium of the larynx. An entirely analogous phenomenon can appear within mucous-secreting epithelia. The older term **carcinoma *in situ*** is still used to describe some of these lesions.

Grading and Staging of Tumours

In describing malignant tumours, it is usually help-ful to supplement the basic histogenetic and be-havioural terminology with information on tumour grade and stage. **Grading** is an attempt to assign a rough numerical value to the extent of histological deviation from normal. Thus, a grade 1 tumour would show less cytological abnormality than a tumour of grade 3. Frequently, histological grade correlates with the potential aggressiveness of the tumour. **Staging** is an exercise in which clinical and histopathological information is combined to describe the extent of tumour spread. The most widely applicable staging system (**TNM**) formally incorporates the extent of local infiltration by the **tumour**(T), the involvement of local lymph **nodes**(N), and the presence of distant **meta-stases**(M). The precise meanings of the T numer-ical stages vary with the tumour site, but T0 is intra-epithelial neoplasia, and T3 is the most widely infiltrating stage. Thus a bladder carcinoma may be staged T3 N1 M0, implying that it has infiltrated through the detrusor muscle of the blad-der wall, and is present in local lymph nodes, but there is no clinical or radiological evidence of distant metastases.

The Importance of Tumour Nomenclature

Good nomenclature must be stable, so that trans-fer of essential information between clinicians, pathologists and others interested in the biology and epidemiology of tumours can proceed smoothly. It must be discriminating, so that dif-ferent biological entities are clearly separated, but it should not be over-divisive, creating useless complication. And it cannot be wholly static, for it must be able to incorporate new concepts. The past 20 years have witnessed a revolution in our understanding of the lymphomas and leukaemias, such that it has become worthwhile to treat certain classes of these disorders very intensively, as the chances of complete cure thereafter are high. Much of this new assurance comes from clear identification of tumour subclasses, often as a result of technical innovations in immuno-phenotyping and molecular genetics. These inno-vations in turn derived from more fundamental studies of the biology of the normal lymphoid system. Tumour nomenclature and classification therefore, must remain adaptable, evolving along with advances in basic and clinical science.

The Size of the Cancer Problem

In the UK, cancer accounts for about 25% of all deaths. Only ischaemic heart disease exerts a greater toll. Cancer deaths are strongly age-related, being increasingly common after the age of 50. Cancer is also common relative to other causes of death in children under the age of 10, although death from any cause is of course rare in this age group. Here the tumours are quite different from the common adult carcinomas of bronchus, breast and bowel. There is a relatively high incidence of acute leukaemias, together with types of solid tumour which are very rare in older people, such as neuroblastoma, retinoblastoma, medulloblastoma and nephroblastoma.

Cancer incidence and mortality show type-specific patterns (Fig. 10.15). Thus, squamous and basal cell carcinomas of skin, for example, are common tumours, but they are usually completely cured by surgery, so their mortality is practically nil. Carcinomas of the colon and rectum, in contrast, frequently appear amenable to surgery, but around half of these prove fatal in 5 years, usually because of the growth of metastases whose existence was not appreciated at the time of operation. For the remainder, survival for 5 years after operation generally implies cure. Carcinoma of the breast also carries a mixed prognosis, but unlike colorectal tumours, recurrence continues over 15 years or more after surgery. At the other end of the spectrum lies small cell lung cancer, for which treatment is seldom curative. Here, incidence and mortality are numerically identical; indeed most patients die within 6 months of the diagnosis.

There are sometimes striking temporal and geographic changes in the incidence of certain types of cancer (Fig. 10.16). From the late 1940s until very recently, for example, male mortality from small cell lung carcinomas rose relentlessly. Cancer of the uterine cervix is now affecting a younger age group of women than 20 years ago. Hepatocellular carcinoma is a relatively uncommon type of cancer in the West, but is a major cause of death in China and parts of Africa. These epidemiological patterns are most important clues to the causes of human cancer.

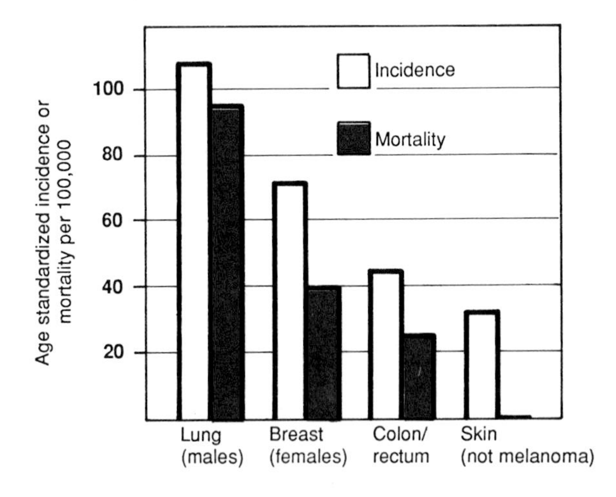

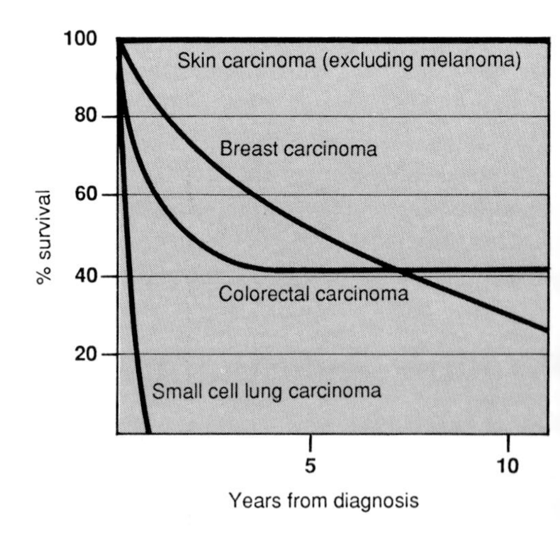

Fig. 10.15 **a** Comparison of incidence and mortality of malignant tumours at different sites. This gives an overall impression of the size of the problem which these cancers present, and the effectiveness, or otherwise, of treatment. **b** Survival, following treatment, of patients with different types of malignant neoplasm. This gives additional information to **a**: the clinical course, even of uniformly fatal tumours, varies widely.

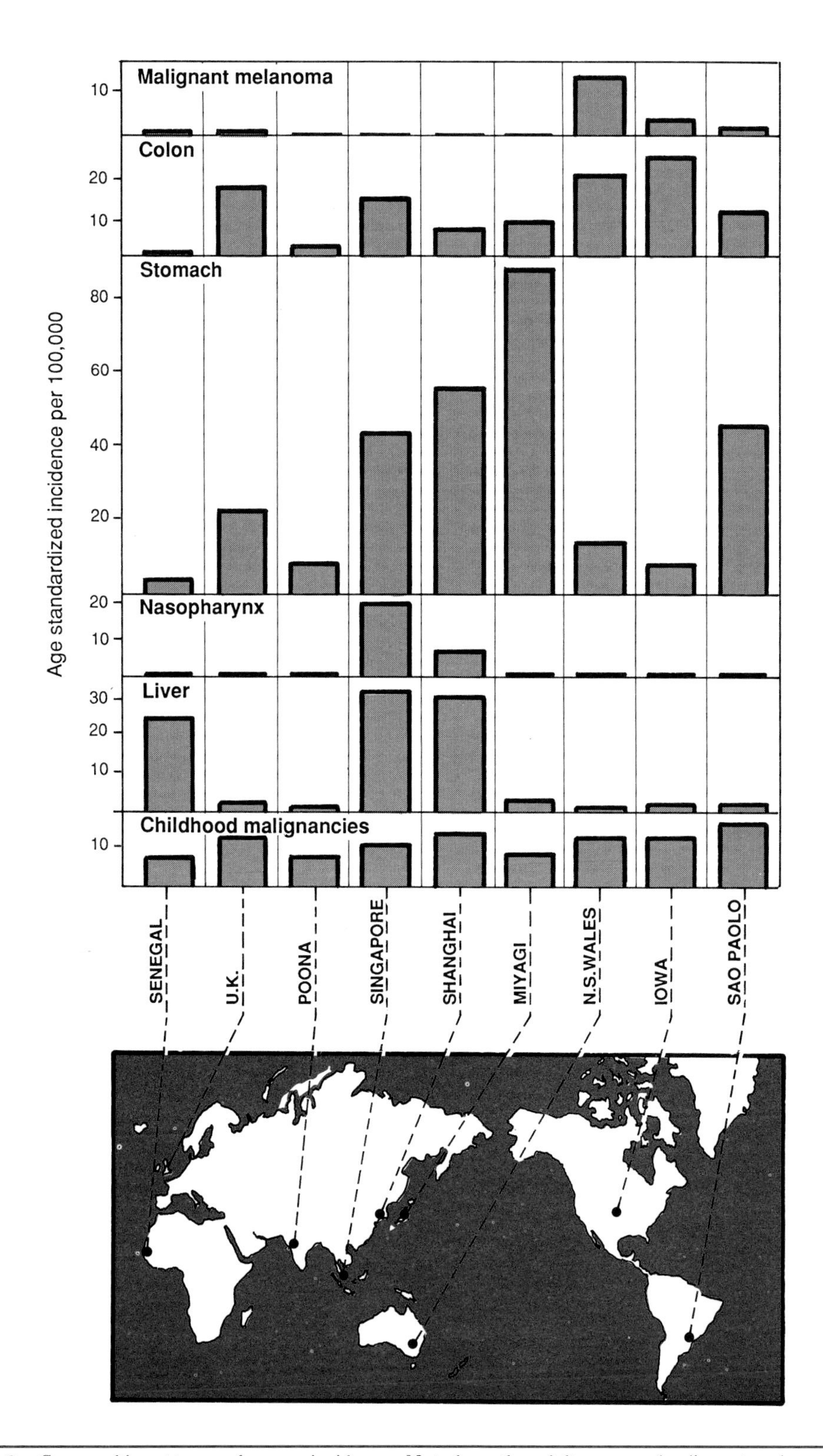

Fig. 10.16 Geographic patterns of cancer incidence. Note how the adult cancers (malignant melanoma, and carcinoma of colon, stomach, nasopharynx and liver) show large differences in incidence in different countries, but childhood malignancies show a more even distribution. Presumably this reflects the more significant role of environmental carcinogens in adult malignancies.

Clinical Effects of Tumours

Tumours do not necessarily produce symptoms of illness. In the past few years a great many people have been found, through screening programmes, to harbour early malignant tumours of cervix and breast. Most of these women had no symptoms attributable to their cancers, which were detected as tiny foci of radio-opacity in mammograms, or through the presence of abnormal cells in cervical smears. None the less, tumours can produce a great range of clinical effects, and these are important partly because their recognition leads to diagnosis and treatment, and partly because treatment of the symptoms of cancer does relieve suffering and sometimes is all that can be done.

Local Effects

Both benign and malignant tumours occupy space. In the midst of loose, connective tissue, or adipose tissue (e.g. breast), this has little immediately adverse effect, although the tumour will become a palpable mass. In firmer tissues, or those encased in bone, such as the brain, the expanding tumour compresses adjacent tissue, sometimes with perceptible disturbance in its function.

Expansile growth can also cause obstruction of adjacent ducts, by compression from outside. Alternatively the tumour may grow into the lumen of an organ like the trachea or oesophagus, and cause obstruction there directly. Obstruction produces stasis upstream, and this is often associated with infection. In addition to these obstructive effects, malignant tumours also cause local destructive infiltration with commensurate loss of function.

Vascular effects can be prominent. Many carcinomas bleed from their surfaces, and such chronic blood loss can produce iron-deficiency anaemia. Sometimes the space-occupying effects can intensify with a suddenness quite unlike the previous growth of the tumour, because of haemorrhage within the tumour itself. In strategically positioned tumours, such as those in the pituitary or thyroid gland, this haemorrhage can provide dramatic clinical effects.

Disturbances in Blood Coagulation

For reasons to be discussed, blood flow within tumours is often erratic, and the endothelium is abnormal and liable to injury. Moreover, some tumours release thromboplastins into the perfusing blood. These factors combine to make the blood flowing through tumours particularly susceptible to thrombosis. Occasionally, thrombus may extend along a major vein draining the tumour, a situation found classically in renal carcinoma, where the thrombus is often intermixed with tumour growing along the renal vein towards the inferior vena cava. A different clinical picture is seen in migratory thrombophlebitis, where there are multiple or repeated peripheral venous thrombotic events in association with a tumour at a distant site, often pancreatic carcinoma. Presumably thromboplastins are released from the tumour into the general circulation. Such thromboses can embolize to the lung. Of course, venous thrombosis and pulmonary embolism occur in cancer patients for more prosaic reasons also, such as immobility, or recent major surgery.

Sometimes the continuous activation of components of the coagulation system by tumour products leads to a depletion of these from the bloodstream – a chronic form of disseminated intravascular coagulation (p. 91) that may increase the tendency for spontaneous bleeding. This clinical sign is also a feature of leukaemias, where it is due to thrombocytopenia, the result of disturbance in the regulation of megakaryocyte maturation in the bone marrow because of the enormous expansion of the neoplastic lineage.

Metastatic Effects

Most cancer deaths after treatment are due to metastasis rather than failure to control the tumour at the primary site. The effects of metastases repeat those of the primary tumour, but at multiple sites, most commonly in lymph nodes, liver, lung, bone marrow and brain. Few sites are free from risk, although metastases to the spleen from non-haematological malignancies are very unusual. Metastases in bone marrow are particularly trying to the patient, because they cause bone pain which is often intractable, and may lead to pathological fracture. Another ominous condition is metastatic involvement of pleural and peritoneal cavities. Presumably because of the unusual vasculature of tumours, such metastases engender a vigorous exudation of protein-rich fluid from the mesothelium lining these serous cavities (malignant pleural effusion, malignant ascites), with clusters of tumour cells growing in suspension as well as attached to the mesothelium.

Non-metastatic Systemic Effects

Many of the effects of tumour growth which have been described have predictable systemic sequelae: chronic blood loss leads to iron-deficiency anaemia, anorexia produces weight loss and even marginal vitamin deficiency, immobility produces some degree of calcium mobilization from bone. However, there is a series of systemic effects of neoplasia which are not attributable to these causes.

Tumour cachexia is a syndrome of weight loss, associated with loss of depot fat and catabolism of muscle protein which can be the principal symptom of patients with certain tumours, far in excess of the degree predicted on the basis of tumour size alone. These effects are the result of secretion of interleukin 1 (IL-1) and tumour necrosis factor (TNF), probably by macrophages within the tumour, and perhaps of other, less well characterized tumour products.

A further, much rarer series of non-metastatic, systemic effects include endocrine, neurological and dermatological syndromes. The endocrine syndromes are the result of secretion of peptide hormones by the tumour itself. The commonest example is secretion of ACTH and neurohypophyseal peptides from small cell carcinomas of lung. This produces a cushingoid state with prominent potassium wasting. Secretion of ACTH peptides by small cell lung carcinoma may be almost universal, but often the peptides are incomplete and biologically inactive. The neurological syndromes are incompletely understood, but result from selective death of particular groups

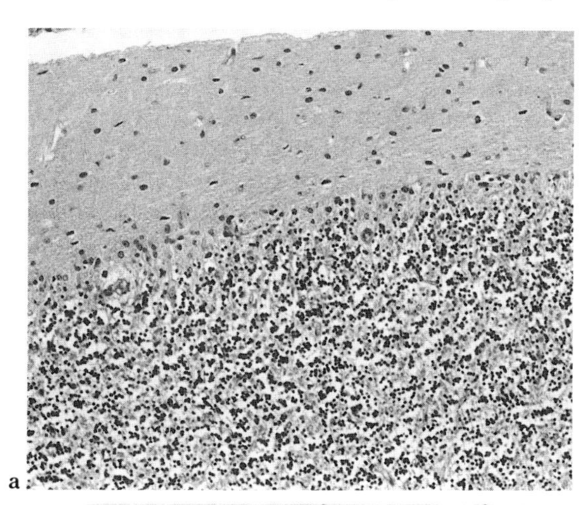

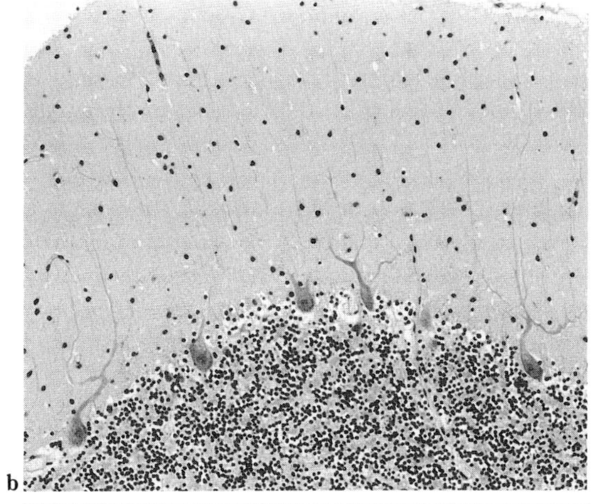

Fig. 10.17 Non-metastatic systemic effect of malignancy. Over a 6-week period, this man lost his sense of balance and became confined to a wheelchair. Chest X-ray revealed the cause of his problem – a tumour at the hilum of the right lung. He died shortly afterwards, and autopsy showed almost total loss of cerebellar Purkinje cells (**a**; compare with the normal cerebellar cortex, **b**). There were no other neuropathological abnormalities. The primary tumour was a small cell carcinoma of lung. (Kindly provided by Dr P. V. Best)

of neurons. There is only minimal reaction in the adjacent tissue. In one bizarre syndrome, for example, severe ataxia is caused by loss of cerebellar Purkinje cells (Fig. 10.17). Motor and sensory neuropathies are more common. An autoimmune aetiology has been suggested, but it is more probable that the neuron death is caused by neuron-specific growth regulatory factors released by the tumour. The dermatological syndromes include dermatomyositis (an inflammatory vasculitis involving skin and muscle), and acanthosis nigricans, in which there is increased melanin deposition and growth of skin tags in the axillae and groins.

Tumour Progression

Tumour progression is a term used to describe the stepwise acquisition of more aggressive properties by a tumour during its growth. Thus benign tumours may become malignant, intra-epithelial neoplasia can develop the ability to penetrate basement membrane and grow by infiltration, carcinomas previously sensitive to certain drugs may become resistant, and leukaemias which have persisted for years in chronic, apparently stable form, can evolve into acute, rapidly fatal disease. Tumour progression is a manifestation of the fact that tumours consist of genetically unstable, proliferating cells. Subpopulations with new properties are constantly generated, and if they possess growth advantage, quickly adopt a leading role in defining the tumour's character. The basis of this instability is discussed later.

Tumour Responses to Therapy

Surgery is the mainstay of cancer therapy. Many common primary tumours can be cured completely by surgical removal, and sometimes isolated metastatic nodules can be profitably excised too. Even in the presence of multiple metastases, removal of the primary tumour may help to relieve acute symptoms (e.g. colonic obstruction) and so 'buy time' that can be valuable to the patient and relatives.

Radiotherapy, chemotherapy and hormone therapy are used with increasing sophistication and specificity. Many leukaemias are treated exclusively by these modalities, and some (particularly in childhood) can be completely cured. Around half of breast cancers and many prostate cancers respond very well to hormone therapy, usually in conjunction with other measures. Some tumour types, e.g. choriocarcinoma, are outstandingly sensitive to chemotherapy. On the few occasions when such successfully treated tumours have been studied during their regression, histology has shown a mixture of apoptosis and necrosis in the tumour cells, the latter presumably because of collapse of vascular supply, or perhaps direct kill by the chemotherapeutic agent. The more general situation, however, is for the non-surgical modalities to control tumour growth for a short time only. It is instructive to briefly consider why this success should be so short-lived.

Radiotherapy kills cells most efficiently when they are proliferating and when the prevailing oxygen tension is high. Unfortunately, many tumours contain large numbers of cells reversibly arrested in G_0, and in most there are hypoxic regions. In fact, the hypoxic regions usually contain the arrested cells. As a result, satisfactory killing of all tumour cells is seldom possible without causing devastation to surrounding normal tissue, which also contains proliferating cells and is well oxygenated. Sometimes simple solutions to this problem can be found. The radiation source can be placed within a small tumour. In this way, pituitary tumours can be treated by yttrium-90 seeds positioned inside them, and some thyroid carcinomas can be treated with iodine-131 because they concentrate the isotope within their cells. Conversely, a beam of external radiation can be rotated around the patient so that the tumour itself receives a higher dose than adjacent tissue. These measures fail in most common malignant tumours, a residue of G_0 cells lives on. After treatment, these cells enter the proliferation cycle almost synchronously. As a result, even while a tumour appears to be regressing, and at a time when many of its cells are dead, there is a growth spurt amongst cells that previously were not dividing at all. In conventional protocols, radiation treatments are fractionated and widely spaced in time, to permit recovery of normal tissues and so minimize side-effects, but this also fosters swift regrowth of the tumour from cells that were in G_0 at the time of irradiation. Awareness of these problems has led to introduction of new treatment schedules in which repeated doses of radiation are delivered over a short period of time. This ensures that the residual tumour cells are irradiated as they regain radiation sensitivity on re-entering the cell cycle.

Very similar considerations apply to chemotherapy. Many of the available drugs kill cells because they interfere with specific metabolic events in the cell cycle. Hence, despite dramatic early regression, some tumour cells survive to proliferate later. There has been emphasis therefore on the development of drugs that kill non-replicating cells, destroy their competence to enter the cell cycle, or at any rate interfere with cell replication in a way that is not cycle phase specific. Amongst such new drugs is cisplatin, which binds directly to DNA, so reducing its capacity to act as a template in transcription or replication. Bleomycin intercalates between the DNA strands and engenders reactive oxygen intermediates there, which cause double-strand cleavage. The etoposides inhibit topoisomerase 2 in the midst of its cleavage-ligation cycle, a function necessary for maintaining the integrity of DNA and its accessibility as a template.

Unfortunately, there are many mechanisms whereby tumour cells possess or acquire resistance to chemotherapy. P170 is a membrane glycoprotein (often called P glycoprotein) which constitutes an export system for many intracellular molecules, including several anticancer drugs. The gene encoding P glycoprotein is expressed in many types of tumour (notably carcinomas of colon, rectum, kidney and pancreas) and renders them resistant to these drugs, since it ensures low intracellular concentrations. For this reason this gene is called *mdr* (for *m*ultiple *d*rug *r*esistance).

Tumour cells treated with drugs that affect topoisomerase 2 often develop mutations in this enzyme, and this confers resistance. Presumably the mutations reduce drug binding but not the enzymic function of the topoisomerase. Amplification of the gene coding for dihydrofolate reductase underlies a mechanism of acquired resistance to methotrexate, an inhibitor of this enzyme. Sometimes there are so many copies of the amplified gene that an unusual homogeneously staining region (HSR) appears in the appropriate chromosome, or even a distinct new minichromosome (called a double minute).

Generation of intracellular reactive oxygen intermediates is a mechanism shared by many anticancer drugs. Resistance to such drugs can be acquired through increased expression of genes that code for oxygen-scavenging systems such as glutathione, or the enzyme glutathione S-transferase.

Finally, one of the most effective agents in the treatment of breast cancer is hormone therapy with the oestrogen antagonist, tamoxifen. Carcinomas that do not possess oestrogen receptors are resistant to tamoxifen, and resistant subclones can develop within previously sensitive tumours, if they lose or fail to express their oestrogen receptor gene.

Illustrative Case Histories

Some concept of the variety of clinical presentation of tumours is given in Table 10.3 and three illustrative case histories.

Case 1

A 40-year-old woman complained of loss of energy and headache. Her menstrual periods had stopped and her brother, home from 4 years' work overseas had been shocked by the change in her facial appearance. Her jaw and nose were larger, as were her hands. Skull X-ray revealed an enlarged pituitary fossa. Tests showed thyroid insufficiency, depressed adrenocortical responses, and low levels of gonadotrophins. Growth hormone levels were high and had lost the normal diurnal variation.

Table 10.3 Some common presenting symptoms and signs of malignant tumours

Site of primary tumour	Symptoms and signs
Lung	Chronic cough Haemoptysis Persistent pulmonary infection (secondary to obstruction) Persistent radiological shadow
Breast	Palpable lump
Colon and rectum	Change of bowel habit Blood PR; persistently positive FOB Iron-deficiency anaemia Signs of large bowel obstruction
Prostate	Difficulties in micturition
Bladder	Haematuria
Kidney	Haematuria Ureteric colic (passage of clots) Polycythaemia Often silent or presents with metastases
Pancreas	Pain radiating to back Obstructive jaundice Thrombophlebitis Often silent
Endometrium	Menorrhagia Post-menopausal bleeding
Ovary	Palpable abdominal mass Often silent

PR, per rectum; FOB, faecal occult blood test.

A growth-hormone-secreting adenoma was diagnosed; fragments of adenoma and atrophic normal pituitary gland were removed by suction via a trans-ethmoidal surgical approach (Fig. 10.18). The patient made an excellent recovery, but required continuous hormone replacement therapy (thyroxine and glucocorticoid). Plasma growth hormone concentrations fell to low levels, but unfortunately her facial features changed little.

This woman had a benign adenoma of growth-hormone-secreting cells. Despite its benign growth characteristics it caused major symptoms because of (1) uncontrolled secretion of growth

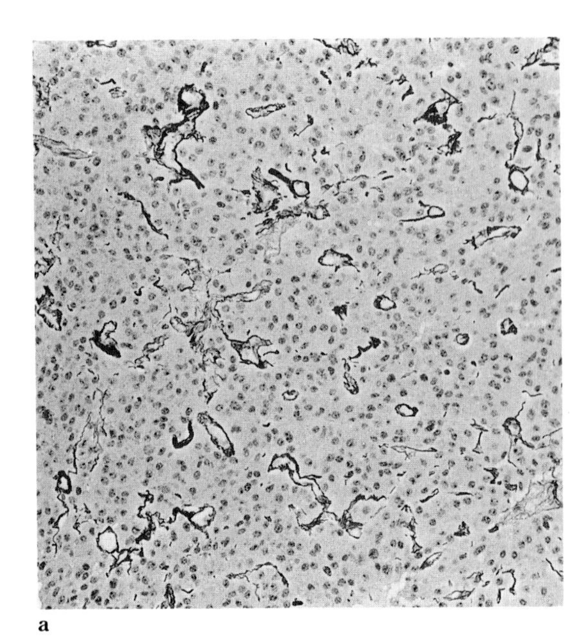

a

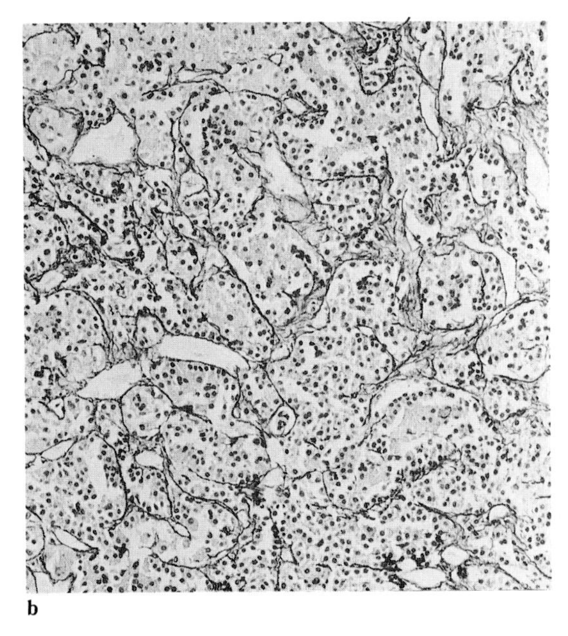

b

Fig. 10.18 **a** The pituitary adenoma, **b** a portion of the residual normal gland at the same magnification. The sections are stained to show, in addition to the cells, the argyrophil fibres in connective tissue. Such fibres surround each normal acinus, but in the adenoma are found only around blood vessels. Otherwise the cytological appearances of the adenoma are very similar to normal, although the adenoma cells are larger.

hormone and (2) occupancy of space, in the restricted volume available in the pituitary fossa, leading to atrophy of the residual normal gland (endocrine hypofunction), and tension in the tentorium sellae (headache).

Case 2

A 50-year-old single lady went to a breast screening clinic. On the mammogram a small radio-opaque region was found in the left breast (Fig. 10.19a). Fine needle aspiration cytology confirmed that the lesion was malignant. Mastectomy was performed followed by local radiotherapy and a course of tamoxifen. Histologically the tumour was a ductal carcinoma with an intraductal component (Fig. 10.19b). She remains tumour free 10 years later.

This case history shows how major malignant tumours can be picked up early on a screening programme and how with vigorous treatment a good response may be obtained.

Case 3

A 70-year-old man complained of chronic epigastric pain. He had lost a stone in weight. Initially he was treated for peptic ulcer, as it was thought his symptoms were due to this. There followed an acute episode of calf and leg pain, and a second attack of pain in the shoulder a few days later. In both, the pain localized to tender, inflamed subcutaneous veins. He was admitted to hospital where X-ray investigations, including a barium meal, were unhelpful, but a CT scan showed a pancreatic mass, and ultrasonic scan of the liver showed nodules in both lobes. In the course of his hospital stay he became jaundiced. He became progressively weaker, contracted bronchopneumonia, and died 10 days after admis-

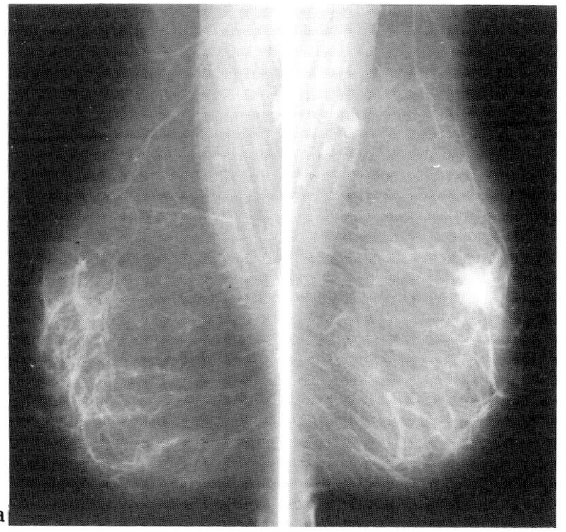

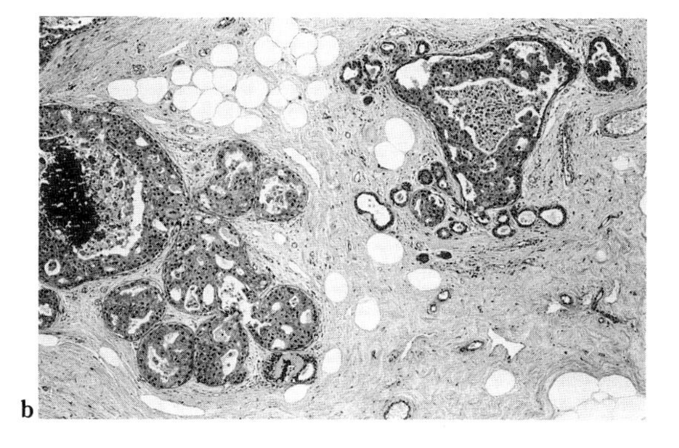

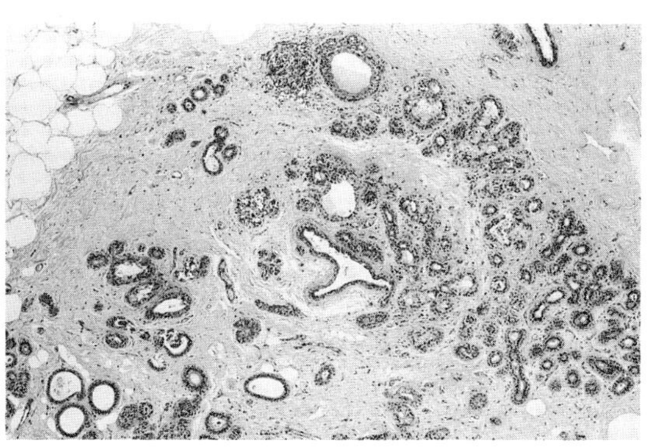

Fig. 10.19 **a** Early cancer as detected by breast screening. The right breast (to the left of the picture) is normal but in the left breast (to right of the picture) there is an irregular radio-opaque lesion corresponding to the tumour. The opaque areas in the upper central part of the picture represents the pectoral muscles. (Kindly provided by Dr Hilary Dobson). **b** The tumour had both invasive and intraductal components. The intraductal lesion is illustrated. Note the way in which ducts are lined by cells with nuclear pleomorphism. Necrotic material also fills the centre of the duct, and some of it is calcified. This is responsible for the fine stippled radio-opacities that often provide the first evidence for carcinoma in the mammogram. **c** Shows, for comparison, a portion of more normal breast nearby.

sion. At autopsy he had an adenocarcinoma of pancreas with hepatic secondaries (Fig. 10.20).

This case history shows how some malignant tumours can be clinically occult until late in their course. In retrospect, the epigastric pain was attributable to local infiltration by the pancreatic carcinoma, and the migratory thrombophlebitis – responsible for his arm and leg pain – was a non-metastatic systemic effect. The jaundice resulted from bile obstruction. Terminal bronchopneumonia is very common in debilitated, cachectic patients with advanced cancer.

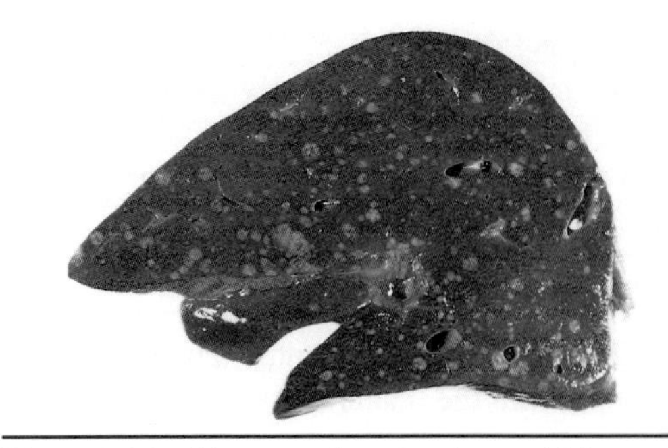

Fig. 10.20 Liver section showing multiple tumour metastases.

The Cell Biology of Tumours

Clonal Origin

Do tumours start as single abnormal cells, or must a 'field' of adjacent cells be rendered abnormal first? The question can be partly resolved by exploiting X-chromosome mosaicism to study tumour clonality. In females, one of the two X chromosomes is inactivated at an early stage in embryogenesis (this is called lyonization, see p. 54). The inactivation is essentially random, so that some cells inactivate the sperm-derived, and others the ovum-derived X, and because it occurs early in development, all normal tissues are composed of a fine-grain mosaic of both cell types. This mosaicism can be demonstrated in histological sections, stained with antibodies specific to isoenzymes coded for by X-linked genes. It can also be demonstrated by restriction fraction length polymorphism (RFLP) analysis, using probes to polymorphic sequences on the X chromosome. Although all cells retain the sequences of both X chromosomes, the sequences of the inactivated X are heavily methylated, and so can be distinguished by choice of restriction enzymes which do not cleave at methylated sites. In contrast to normal tissues, however, almost all tumours fail to show X-chromosome mosaicism, even when examined at an early stage of growth. It can readily be shown that the loss of mosaicism is not due to some intrinsic protection against tumorigenesis conferred by a particular X chromosome. The loss of mosaicism in tumours demonstrates, rather, that all the parenchymal cells of the tumour derive from a single element of the mosaic. The most reasonable conclusion is that tumours arise from single, altered cells.

Tumour clonality can be useful in diagnosis. Reactive lymphocyte proliferation is sometimes difficult to distinguish from lymphoma. B-cell lymphomas, however, are monoclonal and express only one immunoglobulin light chain type, whereas reactive B cells express both, a distinction readily perceived by immunocytochemistry. Similarly, myelomas generate monoclonal immunoglobulin chains in vast quantities, and these are readily detectable in serum, or even in urine, where they appear as the Bence Jones protein. More recently, monoclonality has been exploited to detect relatively small numbers of neoplastic T cells in tissue biopsies. Non-neoplastic T-cell populations include hundreds of different clones, each with a unique rearrangement of the T-cell receptor gene locus. In contrast, in a clonal, neoplastic population there is only one type of rearrangement, shared by all the cells. The difference can be visualized by DNA gel electrophoresis, in which the pluriclonal rearrangement appears as a smear, and the monoclonal one as a discrete band. These differences are conveniently demonstrated by selectively amplifying the rearranged region using the polymerase chain reaction – PCR (p. 61).

Some rare skin tumours, however, consistently reveal mosaicism. Amongst them are neurofibromas, in which a mixture of different cell types is obvious histologically. Such tumours may include two elements, a truly clonal neoplastic cell line, and a population of non-neoplastic cells which are induced to proliferate amongst them. Interaction between the two cell types may be obligatory for growth of both.

Transformation and Immortality

Cells from both normal tissues and tumours can be cultured *in vitro* in conditions which permit their proliferation. In the simplest version of the methods, the cells grow as monolayers, attached to the flat base of the culture vessel, and overlain by medium. It is possible to develop cultures which are homogeneous in cell type, and in this way tumour cells can be observed without the admixture of stroma which occurs *in vivo*. It was quickly discovered that cultured tumour cells and non-neoplastic cells tend to differ in three major properties: the transformed phenotype, immortality, and tumorigenicity when transferred to suitable experimental animals.

Non-neoplastic cells, seeded into culture vessels at low density tend to crawl about on the vessel base, dividing as they go, until all the space is occupied. Cell division then ceases (topo-inhibition or contact inhibition) and the cells lie in contact with each other, their membranes aligned to create an even, flat pavement. Proliferation can be temporarily re-initiated by supply of more growth factors (usually in the form of a serum supplement to the medium). Without this, even when surrounded by media rich in glucose, amino acids, minerals and vitamins, the cells remain arrested in G_0. Non-neoplastic cells also remain in G_0 unless permitted to attach to the dish base or some other solid substratum. Similarly, healthy, replicating cells revert to G_0 if suspended in medium rendered semisolid by incorporation of agar or methylcellulose. In contrast, tumour cells tend to behave in an entirely different way. They fail to show topo-inhibition, and continue to proliferate even in confluent cultures, lying across each other in a haphazard arrangement (Fig. 10.21). Their growth is independent (or much less dependent) of additional growth factors, and in suspension in semisolid medium they proliferate to form colonies (clones) of cells. This constellation of features is called the **transformed phenotype**. It has a close, although not absolute relationship with **tumorigenicity**. Thus, cells with the transformed phenotype tend to grow as tumours when injected into immunosuppressed mice. (The immunosuppression is necessary to avoid a straightforward immune-mediated rejection of what is essentially a

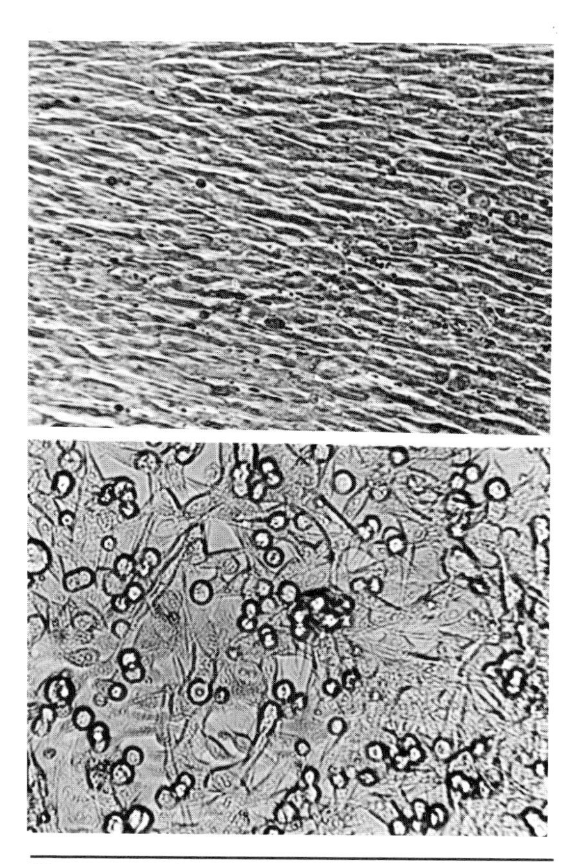

Fig. 10.21 Cell transformation *in vitro*. The fibroblasts in the upper figure are growing in parallel arrays, but in the lower figure have adopted a transformed morphology, lying across each other, and often becoming rounded.

graft of foreign tissue.) Moreover, monolayers of non-neoplastic cells, exposed to carcinogens *in vitro*, sometimes develop foci with the transformed phenotype, and cells from such foci may now prove to be tumorigenic.

The life of cultured cells can be perpetuated by removing them from the dish base and reseeding in a fresh dish at lower concentration. Non-neoplastic cells, however, reach a point of 'crisis' after 30–50 serial passages of this sort: usually quite abruptly their capacity for continuing replication ceases. This is sometimes called the Hayflick limit, after its discoverer. Hayflick recognized that after prolonged culture tumour cells behave differently. They either show no crisis, or emerge from it to grow even more readily. This capacity for indefinite replication *in vitro* is called **immortality**, and stocks of cells which can be passaged continuously are called cell lines. The cells of such lines can of course be killed by toxic agents, but if suitably subcultured they can long outlive the patients from which they came or the investigators working with them. Immortalized cells do not always show a transformed phenotype, nor do cells with either of these properties always engender tumours in immune suppressed animals. These changes, therefore, probably represent sequential steps in the evolution of aggressive growth properties.

Tumour Blood Supply

Although much can be learned about the cell biology of tumours by studying their growth *in vitro*, real tumours grow in tissues and therefore the tumour parenchyma must establish a special relationship with the pre-existing non-neoplastic stroma. In particular, tumours cannot grow beyond a few million cells (or a millimetre or so in diameter) without a dedicated blood supply. Tumour cells, and perhaps also the macrophages which infiltrate amongst them, release **tumour angiogenic factors**, notably growth factors of the b-FGF family, TGFα and β, arachidonic acid metabolites and a molecule with RNAse-like structure called angiogenin. As a result, a network of thin-walled vessels with actively proliferating endothelium spreads within the growing tumour, fed from leashes of small arteries which spring from the original local circulation. Although the non-neoplastic stroma responds to angiogenic signals from the tumour cells, any regulatory signals in the reverse direction seem to go unheeded. Thus, proliferation of tumour cells may outstrip the capacity of the new vessels to supply adequate oxygen and nutrient. The resulting patchy necrosis is characteristic of rapidly growing malignant tumours.

This pattern of tumour vasculature has important implications for tumour therapy. The aims of chemotherapy and radiotherapy in the past have been to destroy the tumour cells directly. The tumour endothelial cell may provide a useful alternative target, since it has been estimated that one endothelial cell may provide the interface for supply of nutrient and oxygen to over a thousand tumour cells. The success of new modes of cancer therapy (and some more established ones like hyperthermia) may depend upon critically damaging these endothelial cells.

Tumour Markers

Tumour cells frequently synthesize molecules which would be relatively unusual in the normal tissues from which the tumours arose. Often these molecules result from expression of genes which are silent in the majority of cells in adult tissues, but active at some stage in the normal development of the cell lineage in question. **Alpha-fetoprotein** is a 65 kDa serum protein secreted in easily detectable quantities by most hepatocellular carcinomas and yolk-sac tumours. Alpha-fetoprotein is present in normal adult blood at very low levels only, but it is secreted by regenerating hepatocytes, and also – in the fetus – by hepatocytes and other cell types. Similarly, **chorionic gonadotrophin** is a useful and fairly specific marker for trophoblastic tumours. The cells of many colorectal carcinomas shed from their surface a 180 kDa, heavily glycosylated protein called **carcinoembryonic antigen** (CEA). CEA, however, is also a product of normal mucus-secreting epithelial cells. It is secreted during regeneration of ulcerated mucosa, and also by the fetal gastrointestinal tract. CEA is therefore not truly a tumour-specific product, but it has some usefulness as a tumour marker in particular situations; being readily measured in the blood, it affords a convenient way to monitor local recurrence or the growth of metastases after treatment of a CEA-secreting primary tumour.

A further instructive example of tumour markers comes from the lymphomas. As normal T and B cells mature, their surfaces express a changing pattern of glycoproteins, many of which can be recognized histologically by use of specific monoclonal antibodies. The apparently unusual cell phenotypes found in most lymphomas correspond closely to phases of normal maturation. Because of clonal expansion in tumour growth, the **lymphoma phenotypes** are displayed by large numbers of cells (p. 662). In this way they are distinctive and therefore useful in diagnosis, but they need not be exclusively found in neoplastic cells. Probably the unusual phenotypes of many carcinoma cells also mirror features of minority cell types in the stem and transit compartments of non-neoplastic epithelia.

A similar explanation may account for apparently bizarre tumour products, such as ACTH or neuropeptide secretion by small cell carcinomas of lung. These peptides are normally products of cells which are embryologically related to cells in the respiratory mucosa. It is not difficult to devise theories which interpret their expression merely as rearrangements of normal differentiation pathways.

The tumour markers discussed in this section represent expression of normal genes. They are found on or secreted by the cells of particular tumours in readily measurable quantities, and so help in tumour diagnosis, detection or quantification. But they do not make a normal cell into a tumour cell. Genes which possess that dire property do exist, but are usually expressed at much lower levels. They are discussed later in this chapter.

Aggressive Growth

The growth of benign tumours is expansile. It requires – at least in theory – no more than a sustained increase in cell proliferation, or a decrease in cell loss. In contrast, malignant tumours infiltrate through surrounding tissues and grow as metastases in distant organs – aggressive behaviour that implies the acquisition of new cellular properties. Amongst these are increased motility, altered adhesion and the ability to cross existing tissue boundaries, most of them constituted of extracellular matrix (ECM). These properties permit local infiltration and invasion of blood vessels and lymphatics. Growth of distant metastases also requires that the tumour cells arrest, survive and proliferate within the target organ. These and other factors contributing to tumour aggressiveness are summarized in Fig. 10.22.

Tumour Cell Motility and Adhesion

Motility is a feature of almost all living cells, but usually is inhibited when close contact is made between similar cells, or between cells and a suitable substratum. Little is known about the factors that control motility. One agent (**autocrine motility factor**) is released by transformed cells into their culture medium, and appears to stimulate their motility. Cells sense the contacts they make with their immediate environment through **specific adhesion molecules** such as the integrins (p. 15). These transmembrane molecules (e.g. the receptors for laminin, vitronectin or fibronectin, components of basement membrane) have an extracellular receptor domain and a cytoplasmic domain in close proximity to anchor points for the actin filaments responsible for cell movement. Malignant tumour cells of several different types appear to express abnormally high levels of unoccupied laminin receptors. Moreover, motility and adhesion *in vitro* and the ability to form metastases *in vivo* are

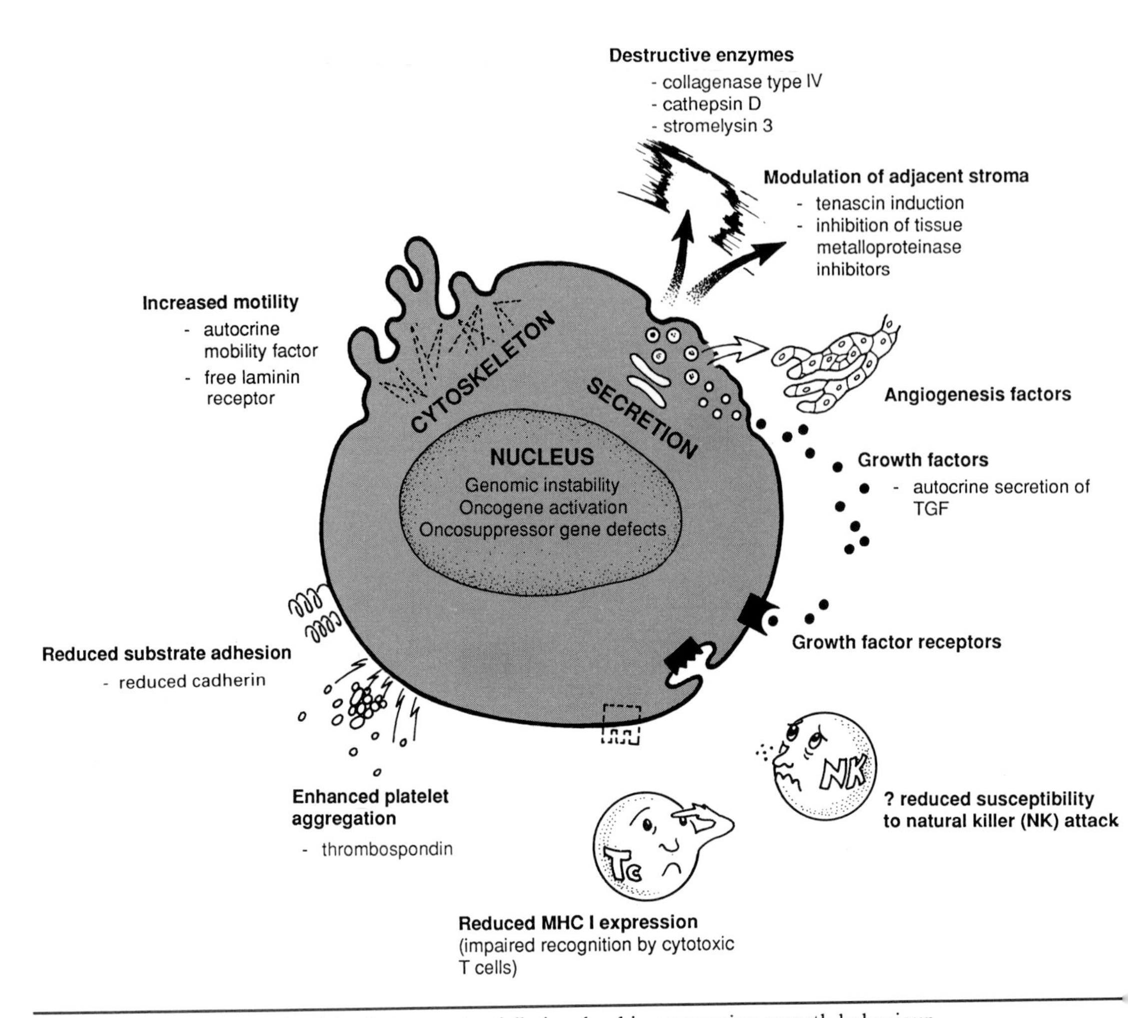

Fig. 10.22 Summary of cellular factors potentially involved in aggressive growth behaviour.

inhibited by blockade of the integrin receptor sites. This can be done experimentally by the peptides Arg-Gly-Asp-Ser (RGDS) or Tyr-Ile-Gly-Ser-Arg (YIGSR) which mimic recognition motifs present on many ECM molecules.

In many metastatic human carcinomas, there is reduced expression of E-cadherin, a calcium-dependent cell adhesion molecule that is a component of adherens junctions between epithelial cells. In contrast, many actively metastatic cells show increased expression of a splice variant of another presumed adhesion molecule, CD44.

Mechanisms of Invasion

Several different mechanisms contribute to invasion of the ECM. Like normal epithelial cells, the cells of carcinomas direct the synthesis of basement membrane adjacent to them, but the membranes that they lay down are frequently defective in composition or polarity and so may fail to provide the appropriate signals for growth arrest. Many tumour cells also release type IV collagenase, a protease specific for the collagen of basement membrane. Several other matrix-degrading enzymes may be associated with tumour invasion including glycosidases and the proteases cathepsin D, stromelysin 1 and 2, type I collagenase and plasminogen activator. Normal tissues contain inhibitors of these proteases (designated tissue inhibitors of metalloproteases, TIMP) and some tumour cells secrete inhibitors of these. Correlation with aggressive growth is imperfect, however, and the clinical behaviour of human tumours cannot yet be predicted on the basis of any of these tumour products.

A different type of mechanism is exemplified by the protease stromelysin 3. This is a product of stromal fibroblasts which appears to play a physiological role in the involution of unwanted tissue during fetal development. Normal adult stromal cells synthesize little or no stromelysin 3, but secretion is induced by factors released by malignant cells, including PDGF and the TGFs, and its presence in the stroma of human breast tumours correlates strongly with infiltrative growth.

Tumour cells may also modify the quality of the ECM synthesized by surrounding stromal fibroblasts. An example is the high concentration of tenascin found in the stroma of many breast carcinomas, but rare in normal breast. Cells adhere less strongly to tenascin than to fibronectin and other ECM molecules. In this way the tumour cells themselves may influence the composition of the substratum along which they crawl and so may facilitate their transit through existing tissue boundaries.

Selectivity of Metastasis

The factors that determine the frequency with which local lymph nodes are affected by metastatic tumour are not well known. It seems probable, however, that lymph node involvement is in direct proportion to the number of tumour cells reaching the node. In contrast, blood-borne metastasis is clearly a selective process. In animal experiments only a small proportion – probably a fraction of 1% – of malignant cells injected into the bloodstream eventually give rise to metastatic tumour masses. Autopsy studies show that the relative frequency of secondary tumours in different organs is not related in any simple way to their blood flow. Moreover, primary tumours of differing site and type tend to metastasize preferentially to different organs (Fig. 10.23). Animal experiments confirm the non-random nature of blood-borne metastasis. The cells which proliferate at metastatic sites are selected subclones from those in the primary tumour, and not necessarily identical to the majority of cells there. Secondary tumours recovered from one organ have an increased chance of homing to the same organ when passaged to another animal. These observations underlie the long-held view that there is a **seed and soil** relationship between tumour cells and their site of metastasis. The factors responsible for this relationship are still poorly defined, nor is it clear what determines lymphatic as opposed to vascular metastasis, but some generalizations are emerging.

Arrest of the tumour cells as tiny emboli within the microcirculation is an obvious prerequisite for growth at secondary sites. It is facilitated by deposition of platelets, fibrin, and thrombospondin on the tumour cell surface. The stimulus for this may be provided by some of the many differences recorded between tumour and normal cell surfaces, in terms of charge, lectin-binding sites, and

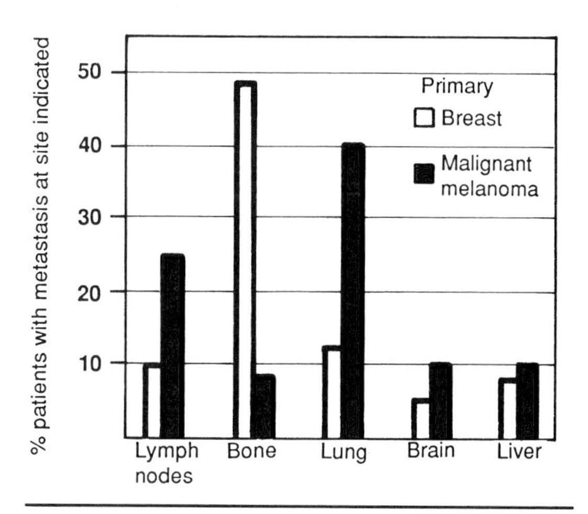

Fig. 10.23 In this autopsy analysis cases were included only if there were metastases to **one** site: thus in 10% of the breast carcinoma cases there were metastases only to lymph nodes, contrasting with 25% for malignant melanomas. This kind of analysis sharpens the focus on organ selectivity in metastasis.

glycolipid and glycoprotein profile. Some tumour cells may also bear specific surface molecules (addressins) or cell adhesion molecules (p. 15) which bind selectively to homing receptors (selectins) on the endothelia of particular tissues.

Survival and proliferation of metastatic cells has much to do with the local growth factor environment at the target site. One consequence of platelet activation around the metastatic cell is a high concentration of platelet growth factors (PDGF and TGFα). Tumours with a high stromal content at their primary site usually induce a similar stroma as metastases, and this may also provide some of the local environment they flourish in.

Are there genes that specifically confer or inhibit aggressive, metastatic growth? Obvious candidates include combinations of growth factor and growth factor receptor genes that would permit autonomous stimulation. Thus, an epithelial cell that both produced and could respond to EGF might proliferate independently of the supply of this factor from other sources. Experiments with rodent tumours suggest that the *ras* oncogene promotes metastasis, perhaps because amongst its many cellular effects it induces autocrine secretion of TGFs. One way to find genes relevant to aggressive growth is to compare the mRNA species from highly and poorly metastatic cell lines. Early results suggest that there are indeed metastasis-associated genes, some over- and some underexpressed in the more aggressive cells. Moreover, at least one such gene, coding for a nucleotide diphosphate kinase, underexpressed in highly metastasizing animal tumours, is also underexpressed in actively infiltrating human breast carcinomas. At this stage, it is not possible to say whether the negative correlation with aggressive growth is cause, effect or coincidence.

Host Reactions to Tumours

The notion that immunosurveillance against tumour cells might prevent their growth in man is attractive but unsubstantiated. Expression of MHC class I surface epitopes is decreased in many human tumour cells. One possible interpretation of this is that growth advantage is acquired by cells which are less likely to be recognized by the immune system. Some confirmation for this view comes from work on animal cells. In these, MHC class I expression is lost after transformation by adenovirus, and the transformed cells become poorer targets for cytotoxic T-lymphocyte recognition and attack, presumably because they can no longer present their antigens effectively for recognition. The significance of these results is obscure, however, as the transformed cells are also killed more readily by natural killer (NK) cells. In human tumours, there is no correlation between the extent of MHC class I expression and any aspect of aggressive growth.

Natural killer (NK) and lymphokine-activated killer (LAK) cells inhibit growth of animal tumours and are found within human tumours. Some of the clinically beneficial effects of interferon therapy may be attributable to stimulation of NK cell, and IL-2 (a stimulator of LAK cells) is currently being tested as a 'biological response modifier' in tumour therapy. Even in experiments *in vitro*, however, the effect is weak and difficult to detect unless the killer cells are present in high numbers. These non-specific immune defence mechanisms may therefore be of value in limiting the spread of metastases, where tumour cell numbers are small, but are unlikely to affect the growth of established tumours.

Immunosuppression is associated with clear increases in susceptibility to certain tumours. Skin carcinomas occur in high frequency in the chronically immunosuppressed recipients of renal transplants, and AIDS patients are at risk of lymphomas. This does not mean, however, that the cells of these tumours would normally be the targets of an immune reaction. As will be discussed later, it is probable that an oncogenic virus plays a role in the pathogenesis of both these tumours, and hence the protective role of the immune system may be the conventional one of limiting viral infection.

Genetic Instability

Genetic instability is one of the outstanding properties of neoplastic cells. Amongst the expanding (and initially monoclonal) population of a growing tumour, cells appear with further genetic changes and new properties. If these cells have gained growth advantage through the genetic change, in the course of time they eventually become the majority type of the tumour at the site. This underlies the phenomena of tumour progression, including the very important steps by which malignant tumours may evolve out of benign ones. It also explains the observation that metastases, although almost always similar to their primary tumours histologically, can have subtly different behaviour from the majority of cells that remain at the primary site.

Two types of genetic abnormality appear in tumours. The first is localized to the specific, cancer-related genes which are discussed in the next section of this chapter. The second is a major error in chromosome number (aneuploidy). Aneuploidy is very common in malignant tumours, though it is rare in benign ones. Initially the cell becomes tetraploid as a result of uncoupling of chromosome replication from cell division. Later, the chromosomes partition unequally (non-disjunction) and some may be lost. These steps may be repeated many times in different cells of a growing tumour, so engendering a series of subclones with different chromosomal constitution and DNA content. Gene specific defects and aneuploidy often coexist, yielding cells with differing doses of defective and normal genes (Fig. 10.24). The next section seeks to show why the dosage of cancer-associated genes is so significant in determining the phenotype of the cancer cell.

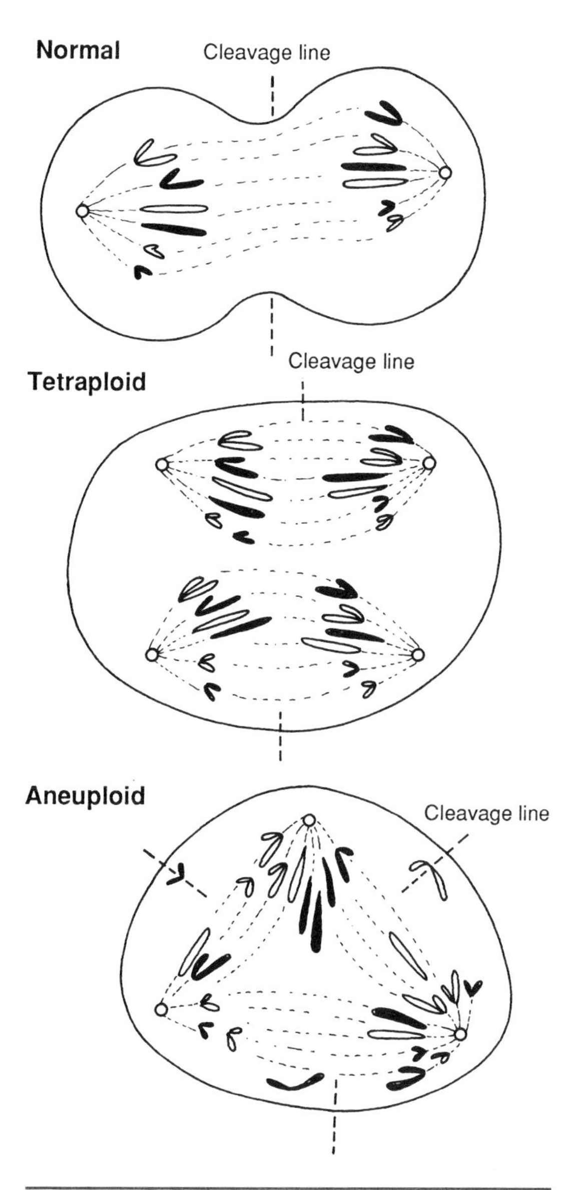

Fig. 10.24 Generation of aneuploidy. Normal cell division is organized so that division of the cell into two follows separation of the chromosomes at the end of telophase. Should this not occur, a tetraploid cell results, with two complete sets of chromosomes. By a number of possible mechanisms, this situation alters to an aneuploid state. In the example shown, only 3 centrosomes develop. In the 'free for all' chromosome separation that results, some daughter cells end up with extra chromosomes, some with deficiencies, and some individual chromosomes are lost.

The Molecular Biology of Tumours

Underlying the neoplastic phenotype are discrete, specific molecular events. Early evidence for the nature of these events came from studies on experimental carcinogenesis. Three broad classes of agent cause tumour growth in animals or induce transformation and immortalization *in vitro*: chemical carcinogens, viruses, and ionizing and ultraviolet radiation. Use of each has provided different insights into the critical changes which occur as normal cells become neoplastic.

Radiation Carcinogenesis

The carcinogenic effect of ionizing radiation is one of the clearest demonstrations that carcinogens effect irreversible changes within their target cells, so that neoplastic growth persists long after the removal of the initial carcinogenic stimulus itself. The nature of the critical changes induced by ionizing and ultraviolet radiation is almost certain to be damage to DNA. Although other molecules are damaged by radiation, only the DNA changes have been proven to remain in the target cell years later. Ionizing radiation causes single- and double-strand cleavage of DNA. Repair of the former, particularly in rapidly dividing cells, is error-prone and introduces single base mutations. Double-strand cleavage produces chromosome breakage, and attempts to repair multiple breaks simultaneously lead to inappropriate recombination events such as translocation or interstitial deletion.

Ultraviolet light is not sufficiently energetic to cause ionization, but generates pyrimidine dimers in DNA, which lead to inappropriate base substitution during replication, or in error-prone repair. Perhaps the most convincing evidence that this DNA damage is important for carcinogenesis comes from clinical observations in patients with xeroderma pigmentosum. This rare disorder is due to inherited deficiency of one of several DNA repair enzymes, and the affected patients fail to repair UV-induced damage efficiently. These patients have a greatly increased risk of skin carcinoma developing in parts exposed to the sun.

Chemical Carcinogenesis

Chemical carcinogens are of two types. **Inducers** are tumorigenic (or immortalize and cause transformation of cells *in vitro*) on their own, whereas **promoters** are ineffective on their own but greatly enhance the action of inducers. Promoters are effective only if administered shortly before, at the same time as, or later than, an inducer. Inducers are effective, in contrast, even if given many months before promoters. Moreover, animals treated systemically with an inducer develop tumours at the site of a later application of a promoter. Promoters therefore seem to unmask stable cellular changes already effected by inducers.

There is powerful evidence that these stable changes are DNA mutations. Thus, all inducers are either mutagenic themselves, or are metabolized to mutagenic compounds by cellular enzymes such as the cytochrome P450 oxidase system. Manipulation of the activity of this system can cause corresponding changes in the carcinogenicity of an inducer. Further, the tumours which develop are clonal expansions of cells bearing mutation of types characteristic of the inducer originally applied.

Two groups of inducing agent can be distinguished on biochemical grounds. **Direct carcinogens** (e.g. ethylmethane sulphonate, nitrosomethylurea) are active in the form in which they are administered, causing mutation by alkylation or acylation of DNA nucleotides. They tend to be rather weak carcinogens, probably because they react with abundant protective intracellular molecules, such as glutathione, before they meet DNA. **Metabolically activated carcinogens** are administered as 'procarcinogens' and generate short-lived but highly reactive intermediates in the course of intracellular metabolism. Many potent carcinogens are in this group. Amongst them are polycyclic aromatic hydrocarbons (e.g. benzopyrene), the fungal product aflatoxin B_1, and vinyl chloride – all of which generate reactive **epoxides** through metabolism by the cytochrome P450 system. Other metabolically activated carcinogens include aromatic amines (e.g. 2-naphthylamine), nitrosamines (e.g. *N*-methyl-N^1-nitro-*N*-nitrosoguanidine, MNNG) and dimethylhydrazine, a derivative of cycasin, the naturally occurring carcinogen in cycad nuts. These agents react with DNA bases (especially the O_6 of guanine or O_4 of thymine) to form bulky **adducts,** which yield single base mutations during repair or replication. Polycyclic aromatic hydrocarbons tend to generate G to T trans-versions such as are frequently found in cancers of the respiratory tract, whereas G to A transistions are commoner in the gastrointestinal tract tumours and are presumably caused by other agents.

Much less is known of the mechanism of action of promoters. The most studied is a derivative of croton oil called tetradecanoyl phorbol acetate. This is an analogue of the natural second messenger diacylglycerol, and (like it) stimulates protein kinase C (PKC). There are so many florid cellular effects of overstimulation of PKC that it is difficult to tell which are the most important in carcinogenesis, but they include stimulation of cell proliferation, gene amplification, and modification of cell-to-cell communication.

Although there are many other chemical carcinogens whose mode of action is obscure (Table 10.4) these examples emphasize the significance of DNA mutation, and also show that two or more dissimilar events may interact with the target cell before it adopts the neoplastic phenotype.

Viral Carcinogenesis

Although viruses are foreign elements in cells, they afford unique insights into cellular gene activity. This is because their genomes are much smaller and therefore more readily analysed than those of eukaryotic cells, and the products of their genes copy, caricature or replace the functions of normal cellular proteins. The functions of each part of the viral genome can be analysed by studying the effects of site-directed destructive mutations. Alternatively, temperature-sensitive mutants can be studied, in which viral gene expression is regulated by the experimenter, through altering the ambient temperature of the cells which harbour the virus. Individual viral genes can be cloned and their effects on the cell studied in isolation from the rest of the viral replication cycle.

Viruses which can cause tumours in animals include DNA viruses from the papova-, adeno- and herpes groups, and many retroviruses (i.e. RNA viruses which integrate a DNA copy of their genome into the host cell chromosomes). All the tumorigenic (oncogenic) DNA viruses contain compact genomes in which the genes are transcribed from overlapping reading frames. Each virus type possesses at least one gene which is responsible for the transforming potential of the virus as a whole. Some of these transforming genes are listed in Table 10.5. They are uniquely viral, different from each other and homologous in sequence to no known cellular genes. The precise functions of the transforming gene products are not clear in every case. T antigen drives DNA replication of its host cell, taking over the function of the endogenous helicase at the replication fork and binding DNA polymerase α. The latent membrane protein (LMP) of EBV has a sixfold membrane-spanning domain suggestive of an ion channel or (perhaps) a growth factor receptor. Another very important property of the nuclear transforming proteins of these viruses is their tight binding to specific endogenous nuclear phosphoproteins such as p53 and *RB-1*, to be discussed below.

All retroviruses have RNA genomes which are reverse-transcribed to DNA by a viral polymerase which then integrates into a host cell chromosome. The DNA copy, called the provirus, has a characteristic structure (Fig. 10.25) in which a repeated sequence (containing transcriptional enhancer and promoter elements) flanks three genes, coding for the viral core protein (*gag*), envelope protein (*env*) and reverse transcriptase (*pol*). Amongst the tumorigenic retroviruses there are many which induce tumours in their hosts within 3 weeks of

Table 10.4 Some common carcinogens

Compound	Environment association	Tumour type
Direct carcinogens		
Ethylmethane sulphonate	Weak, experimental carcinogens	
Indirect carcinogens		
Polycyclic aromatic hydrocarbons Benz(a)anthracene Dimethylbenzanthracene Benzo(a)pyrene	Combustion of organic compounds, including environmental pollution from coal and petrol burning; cooked foods; tobacco smoke	Lung Colon
Aromatic amines 2-Naphthylamine	Dye & rubber manufacture	Bladder*
Azo dyes Dimethylaminoazobenzene	Dye industry	Bladder*
Aminofluorenes Acetylaminofluorene	Insecticides (now withdrawn)	Bladder* Liver
Nitrosamines Dimethylnitrosamine *N*-methyl-*N*′-nitro-*N*-nitrosoguanidine (MNNG)	Foodstuffs	Liver
Alkylated hydrazines Dimethylhydrazine	Cycad nuts	Liver Colon
Vinyl chloride monomer	Plastics industry from polymerization vats	Liver (angiosarcoma)*
Aflatoxins	Mouldy nuts and cereals	Liver*
Unknown mechanisms		
Metals Cadmium Chromium Nickel	Various industrial exposures	Prostate, Lung*, Respiratory sinuses*
Asbestos	Construction industry	Lung* (including mesothelioma*)

Some of the associations of carcinogens with particular tumours are based on strong epidemiological evidence, including intervention studies (where the agent is taken away with beneficial effect) and backed up by experimental studies. Others depend upon weaker epidemiological linkage or experimental work alone. The strongest associations are marked with an asterisk (*). Industrial use of these well established carcinogens is now very tightly regulated.

Table 10.5 Some oncogenic DNA virus products

Virus	Transforming protein	Activities within host cell
SV40	T antigen	Helicase; binds p53 and Rb protein
Adenovirus	E_{1a}	Binds Rb protein
	E_{1b}	Binds p53
Human papillomavirus (HPV)	E_6	Binds p53
	E_7	Binds Rb protein
Epstein–Barr virus (EBV)	EBNA-2	? Transcription regulator
	LMP	? Membrane receptor or ion channel

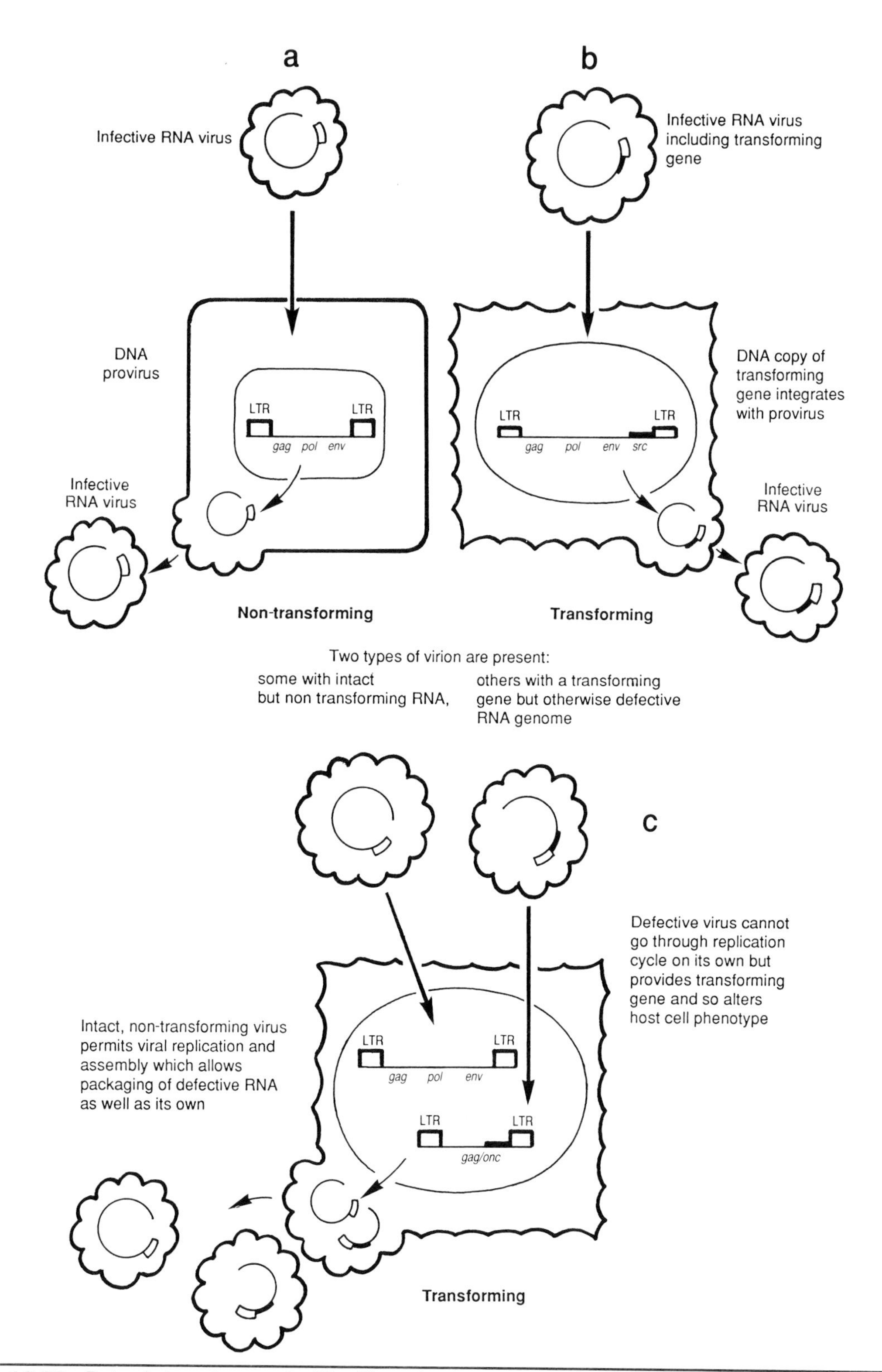

Fig. 10.25 Retroviral carcinogenesis. The life cycle of a non-transforming retrovirus is shown in **a**. In **b** the retroviral genome includes a transforming gene – *src*. **c** shows the situation in most of the rapidly transforming retroviruses: the transforming gene is transmitted in a retroviral genome which is defective in some viral functions: these are supplied by non-transforming 'helper' virions present in the same inoculum.

infection. These rapidly tumorigenic viruses possess a further gene, uniquely responsible for the viral transforming function. Other retroviruses induce tumours only after several months. These slowly tumorigenic viruses do not possess an extra transforming gene, but when virus is recovered from the tumours that eventually do grow, it is found to have acquired (and usually modified) a gene from the host cell.

Study of oncogenic (tumorigenic) retroviruses thus defined a large number of different viral genes, associated with particular animal tumours. By convention, they were given three-letter names which reflected the tumours they caused. Thus *src* is the transforming gene of the famous avian sarcoma virus (a rapidly tumorigenic retrovirus discovered by Peyton Rous in 1908 and the first proven example of viral oncogenesis); *ras* is the transforming gene of a rat sarcoma virus; and *myb* and *erb* A and B are transforming genes of viruses causing haemopoietic tumours in chickens – myeloblastosis and erythroblastosis respectively.

In summary, the outstanding contribution of viral carcinogenesis to the molecular biology of cancer was the identification of specific transforming genes. Although cancer cells clearly differ from non-neoplastic cells in a great many properties, the differences – at any rate in viral carcinogenesis – could be accounted for by the activity of a small number of such genes.

Cancer Genes

When molecular biological techniques were applied to human tumours, sweeping new generalizations began to appear, that rationalized these observations in radiation, chemical and viral carcinogenesis. The critical mutations, deletions or translocations of chemical and radiation carcinogenesis were shown to occur within a defined set of cancer-related genes; some of these genes are closely related to retroviral transforming genes; others code for the same nuclear proteins that are bound by the transforming proteins of DNA tumour viruses; sequential genetic events interact in a complementary way; and all these changes occur in common human tumours.

Two types of genes show distinctive and apparently causal changes in cancer: oncogenes and oncosuppressor genes.

Oncogenes

The discovery of cellular oncogenes depended upon the development of methods by which purified DNA could be inserted directly into target cells *in vitro*. This can be done by microinjection, by coprecipitating the DNA with fine particles (usually calcium phosphate crystals) which are then taken into the cell by endocytosis, or by presenting it within microscopic lipid vesicles which fuse with the cell membrane. A small proportion of the DNA applied by these routes becomes stably integrated within the chromosomes of the target cells. Experiments of this design (Fig. 10.26) showed that DNA from cancer cell lines could confer tumorigenicity and the transformed phenotype upon previously non-tumorigenic target cells. Moreover, the DNA of the target cells themselves acquired transforming ability in the process. The transforming ability was shown to reside within specific genes – oncogenes – present in the DNA of the original tumour cell line but not that of the non-tumorigenic target cells. Transfer of these genes alone was sufficient to confer tumorigenicity to the target cell and transforming ability to its DNA.

In a dramatic fusion of previously divergent themes in cancer research, it was then shown that these oncogenes bear close homology to the transforming genes of retroviruses. Yet it is clear that they are true endogenous cellular genes, and not of retroviral origin, since they possess introns (which retroviral genes do not) and lack the terminal repeat sequences characteristic of retroviruses. Moreover, these cellular oncogenes are slightly altered versions of a group of entirely normal cellular genes concerned with the regulation of cellular growth. These normal genes (which usually are not transforming, when transferred

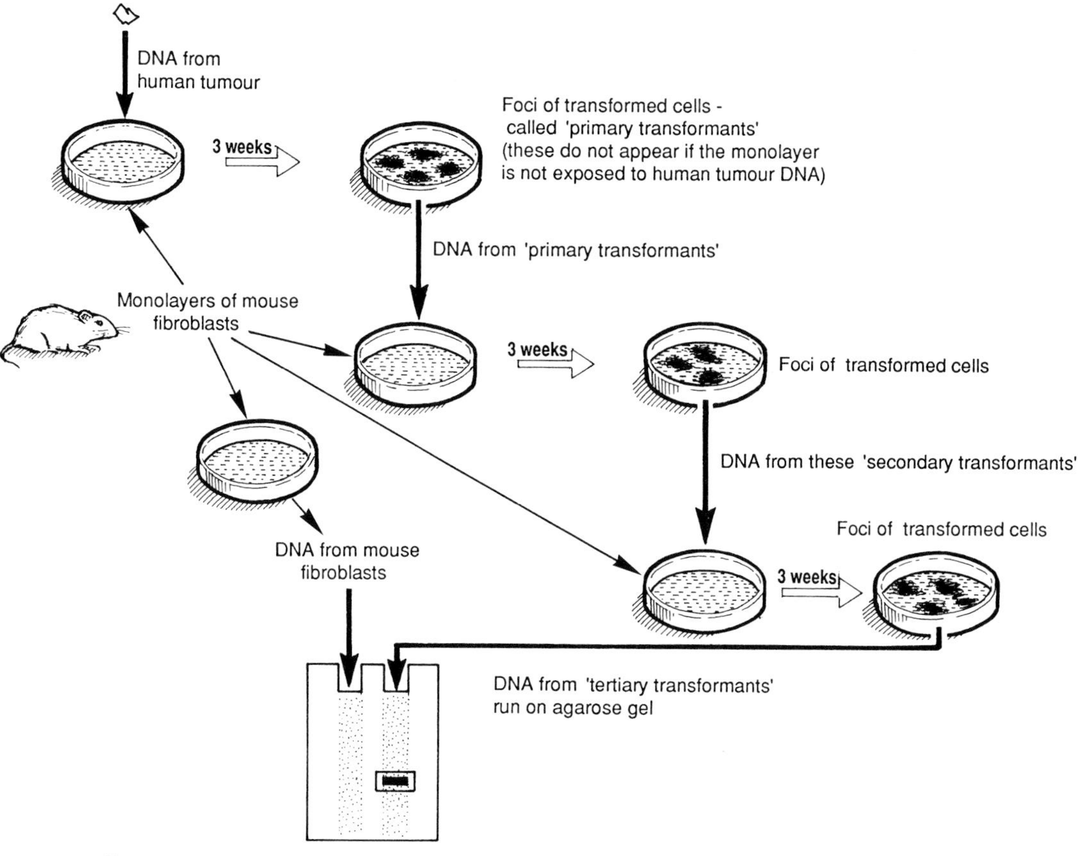

Fig. 10.26 An experiment to detect oncogenes in human tumour DNA.

from cell to cell) are called **proto-oncogenes**, to distinguish them from their transforming counterparts, the **cellular oncogenes** (c-*onc*) and the homologous **viral oncogenes** (v-*onc*).

The process whereby proto-oncogenes are changed to oncogenes is called **activation** (Fig. 10.27) and involves changes in the nucleotide sequence of the genes themselves or of DNA in their immediate vicinity. Activation can result from mutations, which either change critical nucleotides or effect truncation of important regulatory parts of the genes. Sometimes the proto-oncogene is amplified, so that many copies lie in tandem, with resulting excess production of transcripts. Excessive transcription can also follow changes in the environment of the proto-oncogene. Thus, chromosomal translocation can place a previously silent proto-oncogene under the control of some normally far distant transcriptional enhancer. This process appears to be a common feature in the development of B- and T-cell neoplasms, the proto-oncogene being juxtaposed either to T-cell receptor or immunoglobulin splice sites (Table 10.6). Viral integration can have the same effect, by inserting the strong viral transcriptional enhancers next to a proto-oncogene. Although this has been demonstrated in experimental animals, there are so far no examples in man, although the

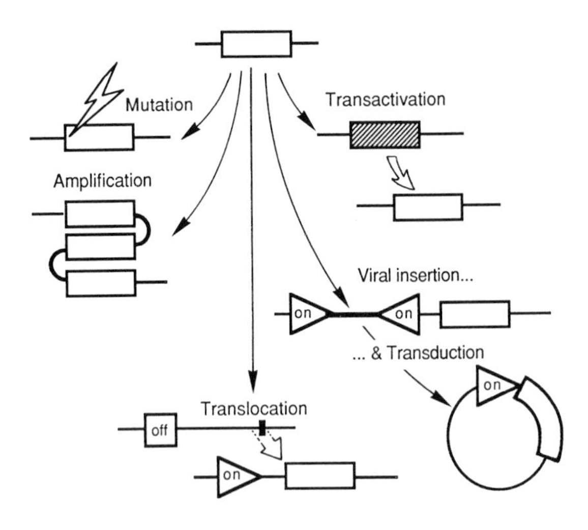

Fig. 10.27 Mechanisms of proto-oncogene activation.

human genome does contain several integrated retroviral-like genomes. The complementary situation is viral transduction, where a virus acquires a cellular oncogene within its own genome. Transduction is well documented in retroviruses. It is the basis for the similarity between v-*oncs* and c-*oncs*, and the appearance of modified cellular genes within the variants of slowly tumorigenic retroviruses recovered from the tumours which they eventually induce.

It is clear that oncogene activation provides the key to many problems in carcinogenesis. Chemical carcinogens and ionizing radiation cause mutations within – and activate – oncogenes in their target cells. These agents must also cause mutations at many other genetic loci, but the observation that tumours are frequently clonal expansions of cells bearing mutated oncogenes emphasizes the critical nature of oncogene activation in carcinogenesis. Slowly tumorigenic retroviruses activate oncogenes by integration nearby, whilst rapidly tumorigenic retroviruses carry into the infected cell their own version of an activated oncogene. None the less, oncogenes are not the only – and perhaps not even the most important – genes associated with carcinogenesis.

Oncosuppressor Genes

Oncosuppressors are genes whose expression appears to prevent neoplasia. Inactivation events in oncosuppressor genes therefore predispose to cancer. Oncosuppressors have been identified by three routes: studies on transmission of cancer susceptibility in human cancer families, mapping of regions where alleles are consistently lost in sporadic human tumours and experimental analysis of reversion of the neoplastic phenotype *in vitro*.

In certain human cancer families tumour susceptibility is inherited as a mendelian dominant trait. Outstanding examples are familial retinoblastoma and familial adenomatous polyposis. As outlined in Chapters 2 and 18, familial retinoblastoma affects children, the retinal tumours usually being multiple and bilateral. These children are at risk of developing primary tumours at many other sites also, notably osteosarcomas. Familial adenomatous polyposis (p. 733) is a condition in which benign adenomas of the colon and rectum appear progressively throughout the second and third decades of life. Formal clinical definition requires more than 100 adenomas in the colorectal mucosa, but often the number exceeds 1000. By the age of 40, the risk that at least one of these will have become malignant is 100%. These patients are also prone to other tumours, especially benign osteomas in the mandible, adenomas and carcinomas in the duodenum, and non-metastasizing proliferations of connective tissue called desmoid tumours.

The inheritance of tumour susceptibility has been traced to the *RB-1* gene (which lies within chromosome band 13q14) for familial retinoblastoma, and *APC* (in 5q21) for familial polyposis. Affected members of the cancer families inherit one defective copy of the gene, which is therefore present in all their cells (Fig. 10.28). Malignant tumours develop from cells which lose the residual normal copy by virtue of a second genetic event, the result of spontaneous mutation or carcinogen exposure. In physical terms, the inherited defect is almost always a small lesion: a point mutation or microdeletion. Presumably, in the germline, larger chromosomal defects affecting adjacent genes would be incompatible with

Table 10.6 Translocations commonly observed in haematological malignancies

Tumour type*	Translocation	Comment
CML	t(9;22) (q34;q11)	c-*abl* (9q34) and *bcr* (22q11) (the 'Philadelphia' chromosome)
Burkitt's lymphoma (also other B-cell leukaemias)	t(8;14) (q24;q32) t(2;8) (p12;q24) t(8;22) (q24;q11)	c-*myc* (8q24) and IgH (14q32) c-*myc* (8q24) and Igκ (2p12) c-*myc* (8q24) and Igλ (22q11)
ALL	t(4;11) (q21;q23) t(1;19) (q23;p13)	c-*ets* (11q23) c-*ski* (1q23) and ? insulin receptor (19p13)
ANLL	t(9;11) (p21;q23)	c-*ets* (11q23) and IFN gene cluster (9p21)
T-ALL	t(8;14) (q24;q11)	c-*myc* (8q24) and TCRα (14q11)
NHL (diffuse)	t(11;14) (q13;q32)	IgH (14q32) and *bcl*-1 (11q13)
NHL (follicular)	t(14;18) (q32;q21)	IgH (14q32) and *bcl*-2 (18q21)

*CML, chronic myeloid leukaemia; ALL, acute lymphoblastic leukaemia; ANLL, acute non-lymphoblastic leukaemia; T-ALL, T-cell acute lymphocytic leukaemia; NHL, non-Hodgkin's lymphoma.

normal development. In contrast, the 'second hit' occurs only in the tumour cells, and can be part of a much larger abnormality, such as a translocation or deletion of part or all of a chromosome arm. These large abnormalities cause loss of many alleles and are therefore relatively easy to identify by RFLP analysis.

Allele loss at oncosuppressor loci also occurs in sporadic tumours. In sporadic retinoblastoma, both copies of *RB-1* are inactivated, usually through a combination of relatively large chromosomal lesions with microdeletions or point mutations. Consistent, locus-specific allele losses appear in a high proportion of all the commonest human tumours (Table 10.7). In many of these, proof is lacking that the residual, retained alleles include a mutated, or otherwise defective cancer gene, but it is reasonable to assume that these allele losses mark the sites of new oncosuppressor genes.

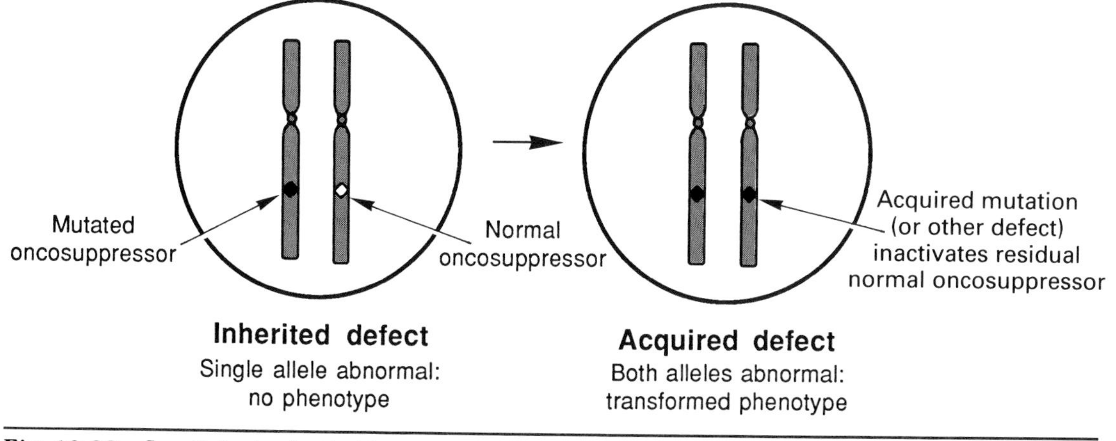

Fig. 10.28 Genetic basis of retinoblastoma.

Table 10.7 Common sites of chromosome abnormality in solid tumours

Tumour type	Chromosome abnormality	Probable gene involved
Small cell lung cancer	del 3p14–23	Undefined 3p oncosuppressor
	del 17p	p53
	del 13q14	*RB*
Colorectal carcinoma	del 17p13	p53
	del 18q15–22	*DCC*
	del 5q21	*APC*
Breast carcinoma	del 17p13	p53
	del 13q14	*RB*
	del 11p13	? Wilms' gene
Bladder carcinoma	del 11p13	? Wilms' gene
Wilms' tumour	del 11p13	Wilms' gene
Renal carcinoma	del 3p11–21	Undefined 3p oncosuppressor
Malignant melanoma	del 6q11–27	?
	del 1p11–22	?
	t(1;19) (q12;q13)	?
Salivary adenoma	t(3;8) (p21;q12)	?
Uterine leiomyoma	t(12;14) (q14; q23)	?
Lipoma	Translocations involving 12q13	
Meningioma	del 22q	

A locus frequently lost in a wide variety of tumours is on the short arm of chromosome 17 (17p13). The oncosuppressor at this site codes for a protein called p53. As expected, the residual, retained p53 gene usually contains point mutations which inactivate its oncosuppressor function. Moreover, by analogy with retinoblastoma, there exists a very rare familial cancer syndrome (the Li–Fraumeni syndrome) in which a point mutation in the p53 gene is transmitted in the germline and is responsible for increased susceptibility to carcinoma of breast, soft tissue sarcomas and other tumours. The biology of p53 is made more subtle, however, through the fact that the products of certain mutations have novel functions of their own. One is to complex with wild-type, non-mutated p53 protein, thus removing it from its normal action site in the cell, whilst the other appears to be a direct oncogenic action (Fig. 10.29). Both of these properties imply that only one 'hit' – a single mutation affecting only one copy of the p53 gene – may be competent to transform the target cell. In practice, point mutations in p53, with or without corresponding allele losses in 17p13, are frequently observed in many types of human cancer.

Another potential oncosuppressor is *NF-1*, the gene on chromosome 17q associated with neurofibromatosis (p. 868). This mendelian dominant condition is characterized by multiple skin neurofibromas, some of which become sarcomas. Rarely, other tumours also arise (e.g. phaeochromocytoma). A mutation in *NF-1*, carried in the germline, is responsible for inheritance of neurofibromatosis. It has not yet been possible to demonstrate allele losses at *NF-1* in the tumours (because of their genetic mosaicism), so the status of *NF-1* as an oncosuppressor is still to be proven.

The ability to effect reversion of the tumour phenotype was, historically, the first evidence for the existence of oncosuppressor genes, and remains the ultimate test of their function. In early experiments *in vitro*, Sir Henry Harris fused malignant with non-malignant cells, so that the resulting cells possessed all the chromosomes of both. He showed that the products of such fusions lacked malignant properties, but regained them after loss of certain normal chromosomes. More

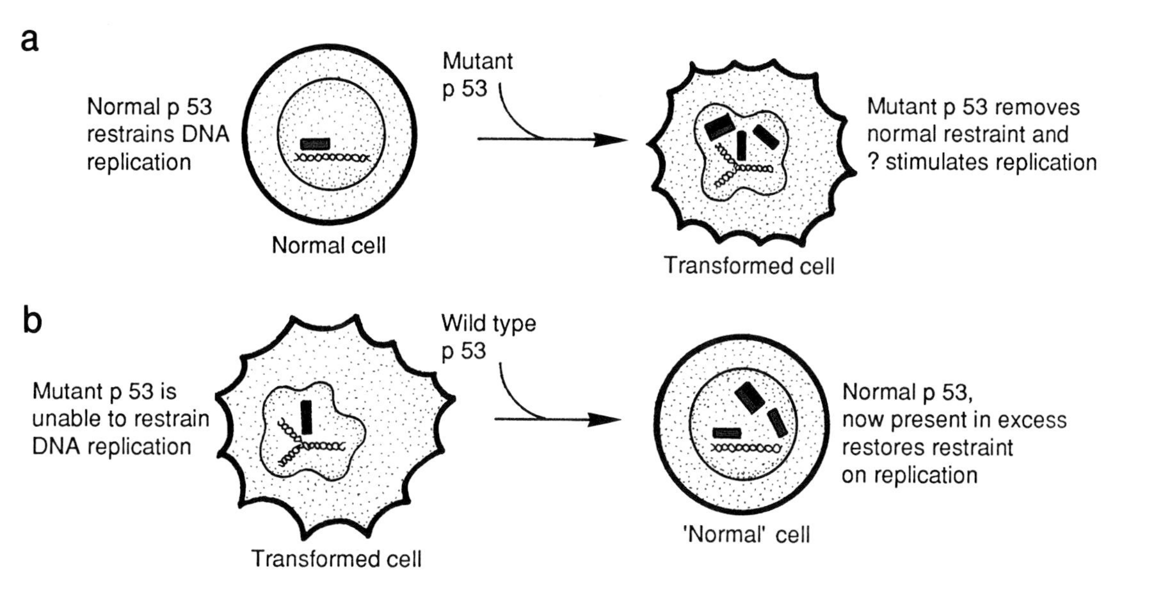

Fig. 10.29 p53 in carcinogenesis. Two experiments are represented. In **a**, mutant p53 transforms a cell of previously normal phenotype, when introduced *in vitro*. In **b** a cell of transformed phenotype, and with known mutation in its p53 gene, is treated so that normal p53 genes are introduced and integrate in the nucleus. The transformed phenotype is reversed.

recently, purified candidate chromosomes and genes have been tested for oncosuppressor activity by insertion into tumour cells *in vitro*. *RB-1*, wild-type p53, the oncosuppressor at 11p13 (defective in Wilms' tumour), and genes on chromosome 18q and 5q have all been shown to reverse aspects of the malignant phenotype of suitable target cells in culture.

The Functions of Cancer Genes

The products of proto-oncogenes form links in a signalling system that extend from the cell exterior to the heart of the nucleus (Table 10.8). Some oncogenes code for growth factors (e.g. c-*sis*, *int*-2). Others code for growth factor receptors (c-*fms*, c-*erb*-B1). These are transmembrane molecules with tyrosine kinase activity in their intracytoplasmic domains. Normally, the kinase is not activated unless the receptor is occupied by its ligand but activating mutations in c-*erb*-B1 free the kinase from dependence on ligand binding and render it continuously active.

Another large family of oncogenes (of which c-*src* is the prototype) codes for tyrosine kinases which have no extracellular domains themselves, and hence are called non-receptor tyrosine kinases. They do participate in signalling activities, however, for they are anchored into the plasma membrane in close proximity to a separate receptor protein. The natural substrates of these kinases include calpactin (a protein of the cytoskeletal network underlying the plasma membrane) and the integrins (which link ECM receptors to the proteins of adhesion plaques). Binding of mRNA to ribosomes depends upon an enzyme called S6 kinase which is also activated by tyrosine phosphorylation. Hence the proto-oncogenes in this class are key elements in the control of cell shape, adhesiveness and the rate of protein synthesis, all aspects of cell biology which are altered in neoplasia.

The products of the *ras* family are small, membrane-anchored GTP-binding proteins. In the

Table 10.8 Some cellular proto-oncogenes

Cell location	Family	Proto-oncogene	Notes on function
Exported protein	Growth factors	*sis*	PDGF B subunit
		int-2	FGF family
Cell membrane	'7-Span' transmembrane protein	*mas*	Angiotensin receptor
	Tyrosine-kinase-linked receptors	*erb*-B1	EGF receptor
		erb-B2 (*neu*)	
		fms	CSF-1 receptor
		kit	Receptor for haemopoietic stem cell factor
	'Non-receptor' tyrosine kinases	*src* }	Phosphorylate multiple substrates, including integrins, calpactin and other cytoskeletal proteins.
		fps }	
		yes }	
		lck	Transmits CD-4 linked signal in lymphocytes
	GTP-binding proteins	H-*ras* }	Calcium-mediated signal transduction
		Ki-*ras* }	Multiple cellular effects
		N-*ras* }	
Cytoplasm	Serine-threonine kinases	*raf*	
		pim-1	
		mos	p34 kinase activator; triggers mitosis
	Mitochondrial proteins	*bcl*-2	inhibits apoptosis in lymphocytes
Nucleus	Leucine zipper proteins	*fos* }	AP-1 transcription factor
		jun B }	
	Helix-loop-helix proteins	L-*myc* }	Maintain cells in cycle; multiple effects on transcription
		c-*myc* }	
		N-*myc* }	
	Steroid receptor superfamily	*erb*-A1	Thyroid hormone receptor
	Other DNA-binding proteins	*myb* }	Haemopoietic differentiation
		ets }	
	Tyrosine kinase	*abl* }	
	Other nuclear protein	*ski*	Muscle differentiation

PDGF, platelet derived growth factor; FGF, fibroblast growth factor; EGF, epidermal growth factor; CSF, colony stimulating factor.

presence of a second protein called GAP (*G*TPase *a*ctivating *p*rotein) the *ras*–GTP complex is a potent activator of many cell processes, but GAP also terminates this activity by stimulating the *ras* protein to hydrolyse GTP to GDP. Activating mutations in *ras* genes always affect the GTP-binding sites; they inhibit the GTPase activity and render the *ras*–GTP complex stable, even in the presence of GAP. The *ras* genes regulate cell proliferation, influence the expression of glycoconjugates on the cell surface, switch on and off developmental and differentiation programmes and inhibit cell death. However, their immediate substrates are not known.

Intracytoplasmic proto-oncogene products include serine-threonine kinases, one of which, c-*mos*, activates the cell cycle p34 kinase. The only known proto-oncogene whose product is localized to mitochondria is *bcl*-2, essential for cell survival during B-lymphocyte maturation. Finally, there are several proto-oncogenes whose products localize to the nucleus, bind to DNA, and presumably influence transcription: *fos* and *jun* (which dimerize to form the transcription factor AP-1), *erb*-A (a member of the gene superfamily which includes the thyroid hormone receptor and steroid receptors), *myc*, *myb*, *abl*, *ets* and *ski*.

Much less is known of the function of oncosuppressor genes, but their products also appear to be located at various points in an intracellular signalling system. The protein products of *RB-1* and p53 bind to the transforming proteins of DNA viruses (see Table 10.5) and presumably also to endogenous nuclear proteins of the replication fork. In suitable target cells p53 activates apoptosis. The 18q gene (*DCC*) has a nucleotide sequence which suggests it codes for a transmembrane adhesion protein. *NF-1* has a domain which is closely similar to the *ras* GAP. An animal oncosuppressor locus appears to code for proteins which (perhaps indirectly) inhibit angiogenesis.

There are many interactions amongst these proteins and between them and other components of the intracellular signalling systems. Thus, many growth factors cause increases in cytosolic calcium through activation of protein kinase C and diacylglycerol; *ras*-GTP has a similar effect although probably by a different route; increased cytosolic calcium induces transcription of *fos*, *jun*-B, *myc*, and other immediate early genes; and GAP is a potential substrate of the receptor kinases, perhaps explaining why the tyrosine kinases appear to require *ras* for their activity. In the opposite direction, TGFβ probably exerts its growth-suppressive effect by stimulating binding of the *RB-1* product in the nucleus, which in turn down-regulates *myc* and *fos* transcription.

Multistage Carcinogenesis, Tumour Progression and Cancer Genes

Oncogenes were first identified through their ability to transform cultured cells into which they had been introduced. In practice, transformation seldom occurs in experiments of this design, unless the recipient cells have already acquired some abnormal growth pattern, such as immortality. Diploid fibroblasts freshly cultured from rodent embryonic tissue do not transform in response to expression of single oncogenes. Addition of a second different oncogene, however, may allow transformation to full tumorigenicity. Only certain oncogene pairs cooperate well in this way. Often the products of two cooperating oncogenes are located at quite different points in the signalling system – e.g. oncogenes whose products are nuclear proteins tend to cooperate with those whose products are on the cell membrane.

Very similar conclusions are reached from experiments *in vivo*. Oncogenes were introduced into primitive rodent embryonic stem cells *in vitro*, and the stem cells were then returned to the blastocyst of early embryos. These embryos are capable of continuing development, and the resulting full grown mice are chimaeras, comprising cells with normal genomes admixed with cells bearing the 'transgene' – the experimentally introduced oncogene. Hence such mice are called **transgenic animals**. The transgene can be engineered to ensure that it is expressed only in certain tissues or circumstances. For example, when spliced to the insulin gene enhancer sequence, it was expressed preferentially in pancreatic β cells, whereas a transgene spliced to the immunoglobulin enhancer was selectively expressed in B lymphocytes (Fig. 10.30). Perhaps unexpectedly, animals bearing oncogenes introduced like this are often initially normal. With time, their islet cells or lymphocytes may show hyperplasia. When tumours develop, however, they are focal and monoclonal, and if multiple appear at different times. Since all cells in the tissue of choice (islet or B lymphocyte) expressed the oncogene, yet few gave rise to tumours, it appears that expression of a given oncogene alone is inadequate for tumorigenesis *in vivo* also. Some other event, or events, themselves inadequate without the oncogene, must cooperate with it.

It appears very likely that similar events occur during the development and progression of neoplasms in man. During the course of a lifetime,

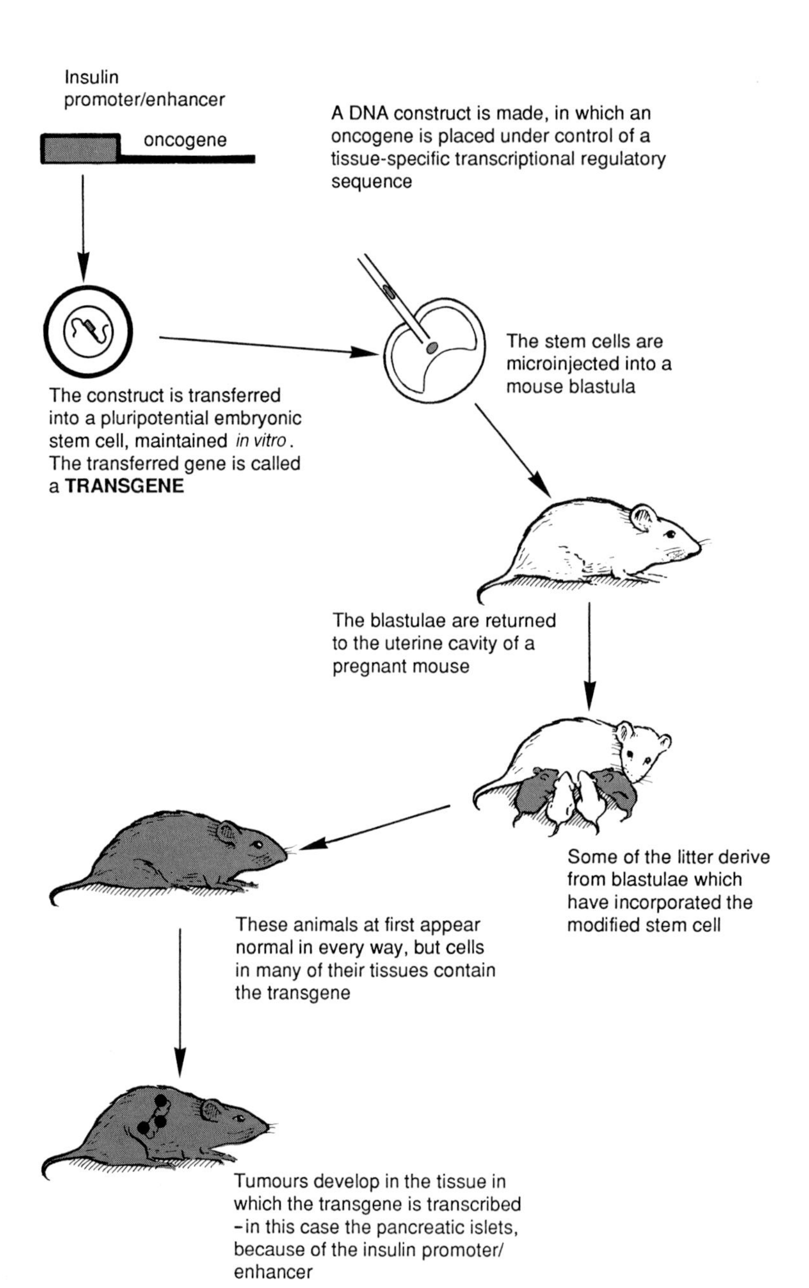

Fig. 10.30 Tissue specific oncogene-driven carcinogenesis in transgenic mice.

cells in many tissues may acquire activating mutations, or may lose the function of one allele of an oncosuppressor. These events do not affect cell phenotype or growth rate, however, until joined by others. At this stage a benign tumour, or intraepithelial neoplasia, may appear. Further addition of critical genetic lesions may produce stepwise increases in aggressiveness. Alternatively, the development of aneuploidy, by creating multiple synchronous allelic imbalances, may engender cells in which a new set of cancer genes are suddenly involved together (Fig. 10.31a).

This scenario raises another interesting issue. A single abnormal gene might be inherited and carried by many individuals, with no clinical effect save that fewer subsequent genetic events would

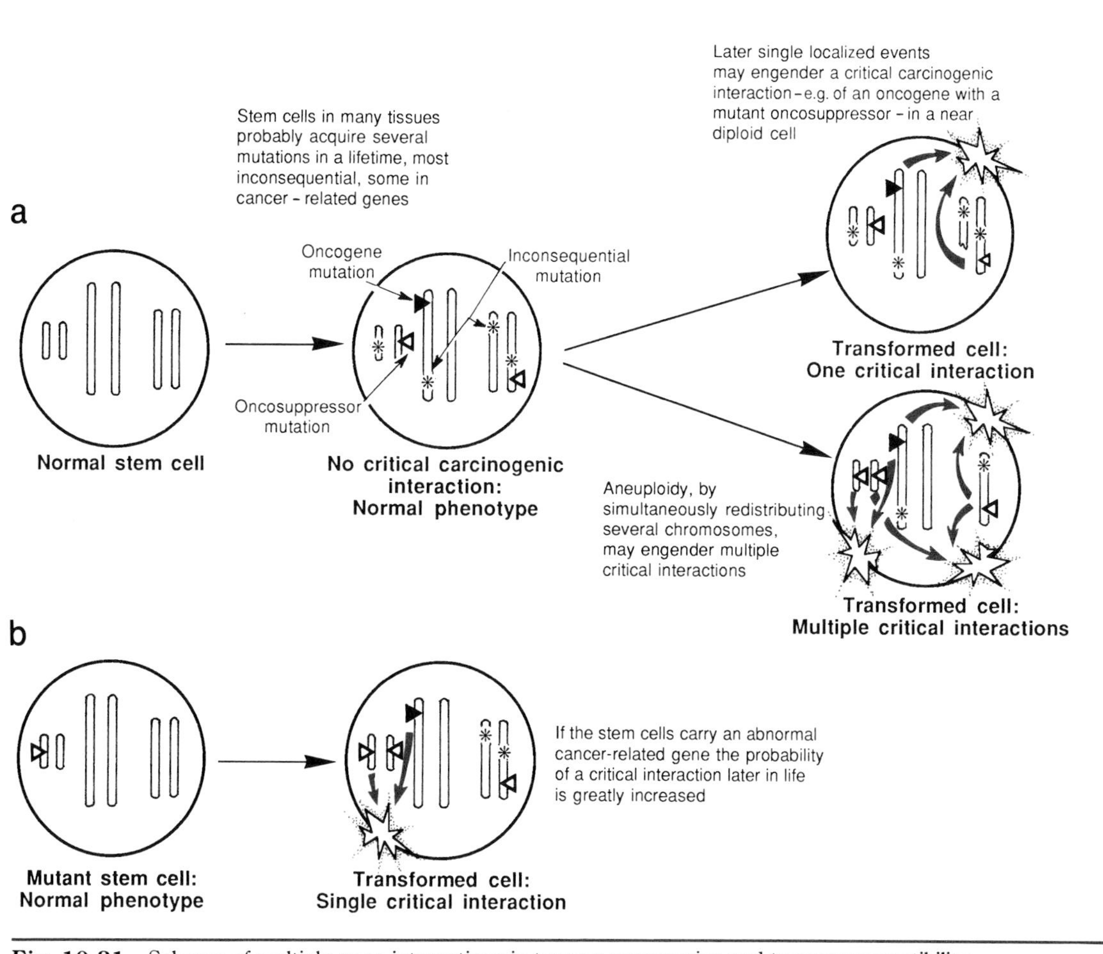

Fig. 10.31 Scheme of multiple gene interactions in tumour progression and tumour susceptibility.

be required for full tumorigenesis. Such individuals would not necessarily ever develop cancer, for they might escape the subsequent events, but if living in a suitably carcinogenic environment they would appear abnormally susceptible to tumour development (Fig. 10.31b). It seems very probable that such susceptibility genes will be identified in the near future, and could in theory help to focus cancer screening on persons most at risk. The application of genetic methods to identify cancer risk in whole populations, however, carries profound social implications.

Causation of Human Cancer

The preceding sections have reviewed the intracellular events which may be responsible for the transition from the normal to the neoplastic state. This section addresses the question of how and why these events accumulate in common human tumours.

The Role of Cancer Epidemiology

When cancer of a particular type appears at unexpectedly high frequency in well defined populations, analysis of the distinctive features of these populations can lead to recognition of a potential carcinogenic agent. Definitive proof of the agent's role in carcinogenesis then requires some kind of intervention: removal of the agent, or protection against its effects ought to lower cancer incidence. The history of cancer epidemiology contains outstanding examples of the success of this approach in circumstances when rare tumours cluster in distinctive communities. One of the earliest recognized instances of chemical carcinogenesis was the scrotal squamous carcinoma of the soot-begrimed chimney-sweeps of 18th century England. It is much more difficult to track down the carcinogens responsible for common human cancers because, by definition, the risk factors are more widely spread amongst life patterns perceived as entirely normal. None the less, epidemiology continues to provide major clues in the search for the agents that cause human cancer, and has also provided two important generalizations.

First, **environmental agents appear to be involved in the genesis of the great majority of human tumours**. The evidence comes from comparison of cancer incidence in different parts of the world. Few tumours show constant incidence, and complex differences emerge (Table 10.9 and see also Fig. 10.16). Thus, carcinoma of the upper gastrointestinal tract (stomach and oesophagus) is commoner in developing than in 'westernized' countries, whilst the opposite is true for carcinoma of colon and rectum. However, populations that become more 'westernized' in diet, even if remaining ethnically stable, tend to adopt 'Western' cancer patterns. Moreover, migrant populations often adopt the cancer incidence of their host country within a generation. These observations show that many of the differences in cancer incidence between countries must be due to environmental rather than inherited factors. It has been estimated that if the environment could be modified to incorporate the features affording the lowest cancer incidence for all tumours, world cancer incidence would fall by around 80%.

The second generalization is that **multiple independent events are involved in the genesis of all common human cancers**. This derives from the fact that incidence of all the common cancers of adult life rises increasingly steeply with patient age. Mathematical modelling of the age–incidence curves makes it extremely improbable that only a single carcinogenic event is involved per tumour stem cell; depending on the assumptions made, at least two and probably as many as five or six independent events may be involved. The rest of this section explores the nature and causes of these events in several common human tumours.

Table 10.9 Some examples of variation in cancer incidence between different communities

Cancer type	High incidence location	Low incidence location	Cumulative % incidence* in high incidence location	Ratio of high to low incidence
Skin	Australia	India	>20	>200:1
Oesophagus	NE Iran	Nigeria	20	300:1
Lung	UK	Nigeria	11	35:1
Stomach	Japan	Uganda	11	21:1
Liver	Mozambique	UK	8	100:1
Nasopharynx	Singapore (Chinese)	UK	2	40:1

*This is the percentage of the total population that will have experienced the cancer shown by the age of 75 years.

Colorectal Cancer

There is good reason to believe that many carcinomas of the colon and rectum evolve from adenomas. Thus, it is possible in this common human tumour to compare all stages in a presumed progression from normal through adenoma to carcinoma. More is known of the acquired genetic changes in colorectal carcinoma than any other human cancer. Ki-*ras* and p53 show activating mutations in around 50%, and alleles are consistently deleted which include the gene for p53 (around 70%), the *DCC* gene on chromosome 18q (70%) and the familial polyposis gene, *APC* on 5q (50%). A further presumptive oncosuppressor gene, *MCC* (for *m*utated in *c*olorectal *c*ancer) is located close to *APC* and is frequently included in the 5g21 allele deletions. Several other allele deletions are observed at consistent loci but lower frequency. In general, carcinomas show more genetic changes than adenomas, and the prognosis of carcinomas with multiple genetic changes is substantially worse than that of those with few.

The contents of the lumen of the large bowel include several substances that could cause these changes, although the role of none is proven. Fecapentaenes are products of digestion of food constituents by *Bacteroides* species. Butyric acid, another food constituent, is also potentially carcinogenic. Nitrosamines and nitrosamides are formed endogenously by bacterial metabolism, or can be present within foodstuffs. Benzopyrene and other polycyclic aromatic hydrocarbons are produced by high temperature cooking. The bowel mucosa contains the P450 enzyme system necessary to activate these molecules. Cooking also produces a range of 'pyrolysis products' (e.g. substituted pyridoindoles) which are carcinogenic in animals. Even water that has filtered through some peat-rich soils may contain trace quantities of polycyclic hydrocarbons.

Genetic susceptibility is also a factor in human colorectal carcinogenesis. In addition to familial polyposis coli, there are several less well defined but probably much commoner familial cancer syndromes. It has been estimated that as much as 10% of all colorectal cancer patients have some family history. Indeed, there is evidence to suggest that most patients with colorectal neoplasms (adenomas and carcinomas) carry a tumour susceptibility gene which is present in around 20% of the population.

Lung Cancer

It was in lung cancer that the first statistical evidence was produced to associate a common human cancer with an environmental agent, tobacco smoke. Consistently acquired genetic changes in lung cancer include mutation of p53 and Ki- and N-*ras*, and allele deletions involving the retinoblastoma oncosuppressor gene on chromosome 13q14, and as yet incompletely defined loci in 3p and 11p. There are no family syndromes involving lung cancer; presumably hereditary susceptibility is overshadowed at this site by environmental carcinogens. Foremost amongst these are constituents of tobacco smoke, including polycyclic hydrocarbons and nitrosamines. Epidemiological observations suggest that approximately 80% of lung cancer is smoking-related. Automobile exhaust fumes also contain known carcinogens and may contribute to lung cancer risk. Another potential candidate is the rare gas radon (^{222}Rn), a radioactive product released continuously, although at very low concentrations, from soil and responsible for about half of all background radiation in Britain. The cumulative exposure to radon is greater for people who live in ground floor houses and when air circulation is restricted. Exposure also varies with geographic location. There is evidence that lung cancer risk after adjustment for smoking habits, correlates with ^{222}Rn exposure. Industrial exposure to asbestos is another potent carcinogenic stimulus, and the risk is greatly amplified by smoking. The mechanism of carcinogenesis is not known. Asbestos is more closely associated with mesothelioma, a tumour of the pleura (p. 583).

Breast Cancer

At least a third of all breast cancers have mutations of the p53 gene, and in a similar proportion there is an allele deletion involving the p53 gene (and perhaps other loci) on 17p. There are also consistent deletions of alleles in 17q, the *RB-1* gene, and a locus at 11p13 which could include the Wilm's tumour oncosuppressor gene. Amplification of the c-*erb*-B2 locus occurs in 10–20% of tumours, and is an indicator of poor prognosis in tumours that have begun to involve lymph nodes. Genetic susceptibility to breast carcinoma is evident from the existence of many breast cancer families, in some of which there is also increased susceptibility to tumours at other sites.

Knowledge of the carcinogens responsible for these changes, however, is very rudimentary. One of the few strong leads from epidemiology highlights as a risk factor the number of menstrual cycles completed over the years. Thus nulliparous women constitute a high risk group. In each menstrual cycle breast ductular epithelium undergoes a phase of proliferation, which may have a promotional effect. About half of breast cancers possess oestrogen receptors and regress, at least temporarily, on treatment with anti-oestrogens such as tamoxifen. The nature of the carcinogens which are inducers for breast cancer, however, remains unknown.

Cervical Neoplasia

In terms of abnormality in DNA, the outstanding feature in infiltrative cervical carcinoma, and the intra-epithelial neoplasia that appears to precede it, is the intranuclear presence of human papilloma virus (HPV). When HPV colonizes squamous epithelial cells, it may replicate to high copy number, initiate synthesis of the late viral proteins that contribute to capsid formation, and assemble to reconstitute infectious virions. This **productive infection** is responsible for transfer of the virus by venereal contact. It may be subclinical, but it also causes a characteristic structural change (koilocytosis) in the keratinocytes of the upper layers of the epithelium, where most of the virus replication occurs (Fig. 10.32). The epithelium itself may also become focally hyperplastic, forming a lesion clinically recognized as a wart. These changes, however, are reversible and not neoplastic. Cells at the junction between the squamous epithelium of the ectocervix and the columnar, mucin-secreting epithelium of the endocervical canal appear to be particularly susceptible to infection. Here the virus DNA can persist at low copy number, expressing the transforming viral early genes E_6 and E_7. Cells in which this is going on tend to show neoplastic behaviour. The least degrees of structural disorganization (CIN 1) are associated with HPV types 6 or 11 and there is some doubt as to whether this constitutes a premalignant lesion. More severe changes (CIN 2 and 3, and infiltrative carcinoma) are associated with HPV types 16 or 18. In CIN 1 and 2, the viral DNA remains as a closed circle (i.e. an episome), but in many cases of CIN 3 and most of infiltrative car-

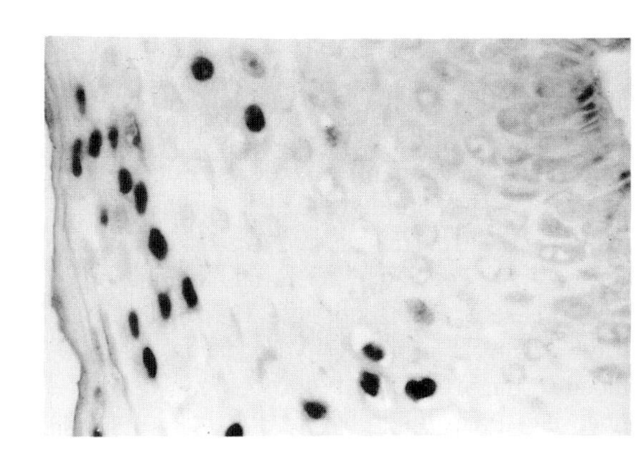

Fig. 10.32 HPV genomes revealed by *in situ* hybridization in cervical epithelium. This section was hybridized to a DNA probe consisting of sequences of HPV type 11. By means of a linked histochemical reaction, the sites to which the probe bound are revealed by deposition of a black dye. The photomicrograph shows how the labelled nuclei are restricted to the upper half of the epithelium (on left). This is the location of HPV viral replication. Although the basal cells are also infected with the virus, there is no viral replication, and the number of copies of viral genome per cell is below the level of detection.

cinoma it is usually integrated into the host cell genome. A consistent feature, however, is continued expression of the viral transforming genes E_6 and E_7.

There is much to encourage the view that HPV plays a causative role in cervical carcinoma. The disease shares the same epidemiological niche as the virus, with strong association with multiple sexual partners and early age of coitus. The neoplastic epithelium contains the virus in a high proportion of cases. There is a relationship between more aggressive cytological changes and HPV 16 and 18 in particular, which also engender more aggressive tumours in experimental systems than HPV 6 and 11. The critical transforming genes are consistently conserved and expressed. Despite this catalogue of information to incriminate HPV in cervical carcinogenesis, the human data prove nothing more than an association. Demonstration of causality cannot come from observations of this type: that must await a prophylactic vaccine.

There are other abnormalities in the DNA of cells from cervical neoplasia. Some carcinomas carry mutations of Ha-*ras* genes. This can be associated with allele loss involving parts of chromosome 11 that include the Ha-*ras* locus, a pattern suggesting that normal *ras* gene activity has been lost from these cells. Potential mutagens include tobacco carcinogens, as smoking is a risk factor for CIN, and tobacco metabolites have been found in the cervical mucus of smokers.

Hepatocellular Carcinoma

Because of its prevalence in the densely populated regions of China and central Africa, hepatocellular carcinoma is one of the commonest malignant tumours in the world, although it is relatively rare in Britain. There is a strong correlation with previous infection by hepatitis B virus (HBV). Thus, people with serum antibodies to the HBV surface antigen (a reliable guide to previous infection) have a 200-fold increased probability of contracting hepatocellular carcinoma, as compared to members of the same communities who are antibody negative. Chronic infection with hepatitis viruses is followed by hepatic carcinoma in animal and bird models. None the less, HBV does not contain a transforming gene, nor does it integrate in any consistent relation to hepatocyte genes. Indeed, it has sometimes proved impossible to recover HBV from the tumours at all. This has led to the view that the real role of HBV may be simply to engender chronic hepatocellular damage. Repair of this involves continuous recruitment of hepatocytes into the proliferation cycle, and this may serve as a promotor stimulus and render them particularly susceptible to mutagenic carcinogens.

Recently, however, an open reading frame (called X) in the HBV genome has been shown to be a transactivating gene, i.e. it codes for a product which alters the level of transcription of other genes, including those of the host hepatocyte. Moreover, transgenic animals which expressed the X gene in their livers (but did not contain other HBV genes) developed hepatocellular tumours in the absence of obvious hepatocellular damage. This suggests that one effect of HBV infection may be to switch on transcription of proto-oncogenes that are not normally expressed in hepatocytes. This in cooperation with other events, may effect carcinogenesis.

We know a little of what these other events may be. The regions of the world in which hepatocellular carcinoma is common are also places where exposure to the potent hepatocellular carcinogen aflatoxin B_1 is high. Aflatoxin is a product of the fungus *Aspergillus fumigatus*, which grows on mouldy foodstuffs, including grain and nuts. It interacts with DNA through an epoxide metabolite. Activating mutation in p53 and *ras* genes are observed occasionally in hepatocellular carcinomas and are of a type known to be caused by interaction with this epoxide.

Neoplasms associated with Epstein–Barr Virus

Burkitt's Lymphoma

This is a B-cell lymphoma which is the commonest childhood malignant tumour in parts of Africa and Papua New Guinea. It has a tendency to grow in soft tissues around the face and jaw. In the search for causative factors for this tropical neoplasm, four observations are of particular importance: (1) Epstein–Barr virus (EBV) genomes are present in almost all the tumours; (2) children with high titres of antibody to EBV capsid proteins are at greatly increased risk of contracting the lymphoma; (3) the tumour cells consistently have a chromosomal translocation, in which the c-*myc* proto-oncogene (on chromosome 8q24) is juxtaposed to one of the immunoglobulin splice sites (the heavy chain locus at 14q32, or less commonly the light chain loci for kappa at 2p12 or lambda at 22q11); and (4) the territory in which the lymphoma is found corresponds precisely to that of holo-endemic malaria.

As EBV has two known transforming genes (see Table 10.5) and can immortalize B cells *in vitro*, it is a strong candidate as a causative factor in lymphomas. A problem arises from the sheer universality of EBV infection, compared with the rarity of Burkitt's lymphoma. In all countries of the world, at least 85% of adults have antibody titres that show they have been exposed to the virus, although most will have had no symptoms, and the remainder will have experienced only the non-neoplastic febrile condition of infectious mononucleosis. The paradox is resolved by the observation that most individuals infected by EBV tend to retain the virus within nasopharyngeal B cells. Clones of cells expressing viral antigens are generated from time to time, but these are deleted by cytotoxic T cells. In Africa, however, the children may meet their first infection at an earlier age, and at a time when their T-cell reactions are severely constrained as a result of the prevailing massive exposure to malarial infection. Perhaps for this reason the transformed cells escape deletion. Amongst the EBV-transformed cells there are some in which imperfect splicing at the immunoglobulin loci has led to the translocation of c-*myc* into the midst of an actively transcribing immunoglobulin gene. The result is constitutive c-*myc* expression. This, together with the EBV transforming genes, appears to be a gene cooperation capable of sustaining growth of the lymphoma.

Outside of malarial regions, there is a B-cell lymphoma with the same histology, B-cell phenotype and c-*myc* translocation as Burkitt's, but without EBV. It tends to occur in older patients, and affect abdominal rather than facial lymphoid tissue. Presumably, in these lymphomas, another oncogene substitutes for EBV.

Nasopharyngeal Carcinoma

This is the most common carcinoma in southern China, but also occurs in parts of Africa and amongst Eskimos in the Arctic. It originates in the squamous epithelium that overlies the lymphoid tissue of the nasopharynx. All tumour cells bear multiple copies of the EBV genome. As with Burkitt's lymphoma, it is clear that the virus cannot be the only carcinogenic agent: only a small minority of infected people develop the tumour, and only after a latent period of 20–50 years. Since Chinese immigrants to other countries fail to lose their increased risk of nasopharyngeal carcinoma, inherited genetic factors may also be involved.

EBV DNA is also found in a proportion of other B- and T-cell lymphomas, including **Hodgkin's disease** (p. 657).

Adult T-cell Leukaemia/Lymphoma (ATLL)

This rare leukaemia is consistently associated with HTLV-1 (human T-cell leukaemia virus), a retrovirus related, but not identical to the human immunodeficiency virus responsible for AIDS. Although HTLV-1 infection is far commoner than the leukaemia, areas of the world with high incidence of infection coincide with areas where ATLL is also most frequent (e.g. southern Japan, southeast USA, S. America, and parts of Africa). Integrated proviral genomes are consistently present in the leukaemic cells, but not elsewhere. As with human tumours, all the virus-associated tumours except Burkitt's lymphoma, infection precedes development of leukaemia by decades, suggesting the existence of additional carcinogenic factors. HTLV-1 may exert its effect through its *tat* gene, a transactivating gene which initiates IL-2 receptor expression in infected T cells, and hence renders them liable to continuous growth stimulation from the IL-2 they secrete themselves. It is the only retrovirus known to be directly involved in carcinogenesis in man (HIV, by immunosuppression, may be involved indirectly).

Genetic Determinism in Human Tumours

The past few years have brought amazing new insights into molecular events that appear to underlie carcinogenesis and tumour progression. It is easy to get the impression that every human tumour type will ultimately be shown to have a unique genetic determinism: in other words, knowledge of changes in certain genes would accurately predict tumour behaviour and ultimately be the basis of specific corrective therapy. There are several reasons why the correctness of this proposition cannot yet be taken for granted.

First, we do not know how often single cells within normal tissues accumulate multiple genetic defects yet still remain phenotypically normal. The clonal expansion, within tumours, of cells bearing specific defects need imply only that the defects are permissive for such clonal growth.

Second, some of the available evidence for the role of gene changes in tumour pathology suggests that the number of accumulated defects is more important than the time sequence with which they occur. Thus, Ki-*ras* mutation can occur within colorectal adenomas (and apparently contribute to the clonal expansion of their cells) but may also appear for the first time in carcinomas that have evolved from adenomas without the Ki-*ras* mutation.

Third, none of the available methods of tumour analysis would detect 'hit and run' agents. Some herpes viruses appear to be carcinogenic in experimental systems, yet do not persist within the tumour cells. This result has been interpreted to mean that the virus induces critical carcinogenic events in the host cell genome (perhaps in a very specific way) but is then lost from the cell itself. If agents of this type are involved in human carcinogenesis, hints as to their nature might derive from epidemiological observations, but they would be very difficult to analyse directly in human tumours.

Fourth, we know surprisingly little about the interactions between specific, putatively carcinogenic gene changes and the state of the cell in which they occur. It is intuitively easy to accept the idea that cells within a tissue may undergo a set of gene changes which permits the development of a benign tumour, and subsequently evolve to a malignant one, through the accumulation of further events. Indeed, there is good evidence in the colorectal adenoma-carcinoma sequence that such processes do take place. Even amongst colorectal tumours, however, there is no proof that all carcinomas evolve through an adenoma phase, and it is certain that the majority of adenomas do not progress to carcinoma. The possibility remains open that subtle differences between the cells of tissues may influence the ways in which they respond to the same gene changes. Or there may be certain combinations of target cell and gene changes which permit the development of benign, non-progressive tumours, and others which encourage progression to malignancy.

Further Reading

Useful Short Articles

Arends, M. J. and Wyllie, A. H. (1991). Apoptosis: mechanisms and roles in pathology. *International Review of Experimental Pathology* **32**, 223–54.

Basset, P., Belloca, J. P., Wolf, C., et al. (1990). A novel metalloproteinase gene specifically expressed in stromal cells of breast carcinomas. *Nature* **348**, 699–704.

Birchmeier, W., Behrens, J., Weidner, K. M., Frixen, U. H. and Schipper, J. (1991). Dominant and recessive genes involved in tumor cell invasion. *Current Opinion in Cell Biology* **3**, 832–40.

Bruce, W. R. (1987). Recent hypotheses for the origin of colon cancer. *Cancer Research* **47**, 4237–42.

Dunlop, M. G. (1991). Allele losses and onco-suppressor genes. *Journal of Pathology* **163**, 1–5.

Folkman, J. and Klagsbrun, M. (1987). Angiogenic factors. *Science* **325**, 442–7.

Nicholson, G. L. (1988). Cancer metastasis: tumour cells and host organ properties important in metastasis to specific secondary sites. *Biochimica et Biophysica Acta* **948**, 175–224.

Onions, D. (1991). Integration of viruses into chromosomal DNA. *Journal of Pathology* **163**, 191–7.

Potten, C. S. and Loeffler, M. (1990). Stem cells: attributes, spirals, pitfalls and uncertainties. Lessons for and from the crypt. *Development* **110**, 1001–20.

Sobel, M. E. (1990). Metastasis suppressor genes. *Journal of the National Cancer Institute* **82**, 267–76.

Tiollais, P., Pourcel, C. and Dejean, A. (1985). The hepatitis B virus. *Nature* **317**, 489–95.

Wiedemann, L. M., McCarthy, K. P. and Chan, L. C. (1991). Chromosome rearrangement, oncogene activation, and other clonal events in cancer: their use in molecular diagnostics. *Journal of Pathology* **163**, 7–12.

Major Reviews and Books

Heim, S. and Mitelman, F. (1989). Primary chromosome abnormalities in human neoplasia. *Advances in Cancer Research* **52**, 1–43.

Klein, G. (1989). Tumorigenic DNA viruses. *Advances in Viral Oncology*, **8**. Raven Press, New York.

Levin, B. (1991). Driving the cell cycle: M phase kinase, its partners and substrates. *Cell* **61**, 743–52.

Levin, B. (ed.) (1991). Reviews on oncogenesis. *Cell* **64**, 235–336.

Lynch, H. T. and Hirayama, T. (1989). *Genetic Epidemiology of Cancer.* CRC Press, Florida.

Waterfield, H. D. (1989). Growth factors. *British Medical Bulletin* **45**.

11

Drug- and Radiation-induced Injury

As the impact of nutritional deficiency and infectious diseases has declined in the Western world, diseases due to other environmental factors – e.g. industrial pollution, cigarette smoking, stress and drugs – are placing an increasing burden on our medical resources. The diseases produced by pollutants, smoking and stress are discussed in the appropriate system chapters. However, some aspects of the pathology of adverse drug reactions (iatrogenic diseases), drug dependence and radiation-induced injury cannot be satisfactorily covered in this way. We have decided to review each of these topics separately in this chapter, but in some instances, drug-induced injury is dealt with in greater detail in the appropriate system chapter.

Adverse Drug Reactions

Adverse reactions to drugs are a common cause of morbidity and hospital referral. Less commonly they may be fatal. Drug-related injuries may be incidental and complicate therapeutic use of drugs, or they may be induced by self-poisoning or as a consequence of drug dependence. Study of the biochemical and molecular mechanisms of adverse reactions to drugs has increased our understanding not only of the basis of toxicity but also of wider pathophysiological mechanisms. For example, the importance of glucose-6-phosphate dehydrogenase (G-6-PD) in haematological diseases was revealed by the investigation of haemolytic anaemia induced by primaquine and other oxidizing drugs.

Adverse reactions are closely monitored and in the United Kingdom the system of reporting suspected cases by 'yellow card' to the Committee on Safety of Medicines, while not ideal, does allow for collection of information on a nationwide basis. If in doubt, doctors should report any adverse event, especially those involving new drugs.

Classification of Adverse Drug Reactions

There are several alternative approaches to the classification of adverse reactions to drugs (Table 11.1). A pragmatic classification might divide reactions into those which are life threatening and clinically serious and those which are less serious though troublesome to the patient. Alternatively, the reactions can be divided into those that are frequently observed (5–10% or more of patients) and those that are only seen rarely (less than 1%). Other more mechanistic classifications include reversible (functional) effects compared to irreversible reactions. Finally, adverse reactions can be divided into those where the mechanism is related directly or indirectly to the known properties of the drug – predictable or type A reactions – and those where the injury is unpredictable, type B. This classification fits best with the pathological aspects of drug-induced injury.

Table 11.1 Classifications of adverse drug reactions

Reversible (functional) reactions – self-limiting, full recovery expected. Includes actions of competitive agonists and antagonists at receptors, and inhibition of enzymes

Irreversible reactions – drug-induced injury to cells with cell death or permanent impairment of function. Recovery will only occur after formation of new enzyme or receptor, or from division or growth of undamaged cells

Type A: **predictable reactions** result from known pharmacological properties of drugs

(1) Primary – direct result of drug reaction
(2) Secondary – indirect consequence of drug action

Type B: **unpredictable reaction** – not expected from known pharmacological properties

(1) Toxic effects – high dose (or concentration) with tissue injury, due to physical or chemical properties but which cannot be predicted on the basis of pharmacological properties
(2) Idiosyncratic – therapeutic or low dose; often immunological or genetically determined mechanism of amplification

Type A Reactions

Type A reactions are common, predictable, dose dependent and have a low mortality. The effects are due to an exaggerated but otherwise known pharmacological action of the drug, in part dependent on the drug itself and in part on the patient's metabolic response to the drug. Similar adverse reactions may sometimes be produced in experimental animals and thus, the mechanism can be investigated; adverse reactions in preclinical trials are important in determining whether the drug is marketed. The dose and the therapeutic ratio are important factors in the development of type A reactions: the higher the ratio the less likely is an adverse drug reaction. The pharmacodynamic effect of a drug may be influenced by pharmacokinetic factors such as absorption, distribution and binding in the blood or tissues and the rates of metabolism and excretion. Many drugs exert their therapeutic effect after transformation to active metabolites. Thus, if the rate or extent of metabolism is potentiated by concurrent treatment with another drug, tissue injury may occur with smaller doses. Similarly, concurrent disease may enhance drug action, e.g. the depressant effect of morphine in patients with advanced liver disease.

Type B Reactions

Type B reactions are rare, unpredictable, usually not dose dependent and some have a relatively high mortality. The adverse reaction cannot be explained on the basis of the pharmacological properties of the drug. The mechanisms involved are not well understood, and the reactions are not reproducible in experimental animals. In type B reactions there is a qualitative abnormality in the response to a drug in susceptible individuals. This susceptibility may be due to a genetically determined enzyme deficiency, e.g. drug-induced haemolytic anaemia in G-6-PD deficiency (p. 602), and the development of a systemic lupus erythematosus (SLE)-like syndrome in patients who are slow acetylators (p. 417). There may be an abnormal immunological response, the drug (or its metabolites) acting as an allergen or hapten and triggering a hypersensitivity reaction, e.g. acute anaphylaxis (type I reaction) with penicillin, or immune-complex disease (type III reaction) with sulphonamides.

Systematic Review of Adverse Drug Reactions

Drug-induced injury to the liver is reviewed in greater detail here to illustrate how drug-induced diseases resemble, and may mimic, many non-iatrogenic illnesses. Diagnosis of drug toxicity thus requires considerable clinical awareness.

Liver

The liver is involved in about 8% of reports of adverse drug reactions. This is a reflection of its central role in the metabolism and excretion of many drugs. Virtually any type of liver disease may be caused by drugs (Table 11.2) and this differential diagnosis should be considered in most morphological abnormalities identified in the liver.

Table 11.2 Liver injury which may be drug induced

	Drug*
Acute hepatitis	Halothane
Massive/submassive necrosis	Paracetamol
Granulomatous hepatitis	Phenylbutazone
Chronic hepatitis	Methyldopa
Cirrhosis	Methotrexate
Cholestasis	
mixed hepatic/cholestatic	Chlorpromazine
cholestatic	Anabolic steroids
damage to intrahepatic bile ducts	Carbamazepine
chronic biliary disease	Chlorpromazine
Fatty change	
macrovesicular	Corticosteroids
microvesicular	Phenytoin
Non-alcoholic steatohepatitis (alcohol-like hepatitis)	Amiodarone
Lysosomal storage disorder (phospholipidosis)	Amiodarone
Vascular lesions	
veno-occlusive disease	Pyrrolizidine alkaloids
hepatic vein thrombosis	Contraceptive steroids
peliosis hepatis	Anabolic steroids
Tumours	
liver cell adenoma	Contraceptive steroids
angiosarcoma and cholangiocarcinoma	Thorotrast

*Only one example of each is given, but a number of drugs may be responsible for each type of injury.

Adaptive Changes

A number of drugs, e.g. barbiturates or phenytoin, when given over a long time, cause hypertrophy of the smooth endoplasmic reticulum (SER) which effects an induction or enhancement of the enzymes involved in the metabolism of these drugs. Enzymes are responsible for the biotransformation of drugs, i.e. the process by which drugs are transformed into more soluble metabolites or made more suitable for conjugation with endogenous substrates such as glucuronic acid, prior to excretion in the bile or in the urine. The induction of enzymes in response to one drug may result in the enhanced metabolism of a second drug, requiring the therapeutic dose of the second to be

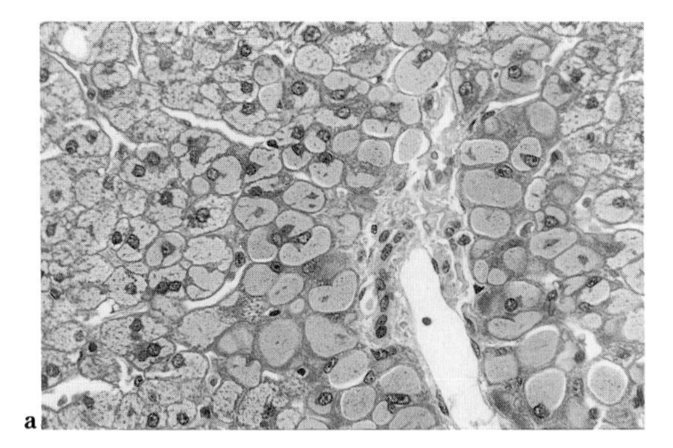

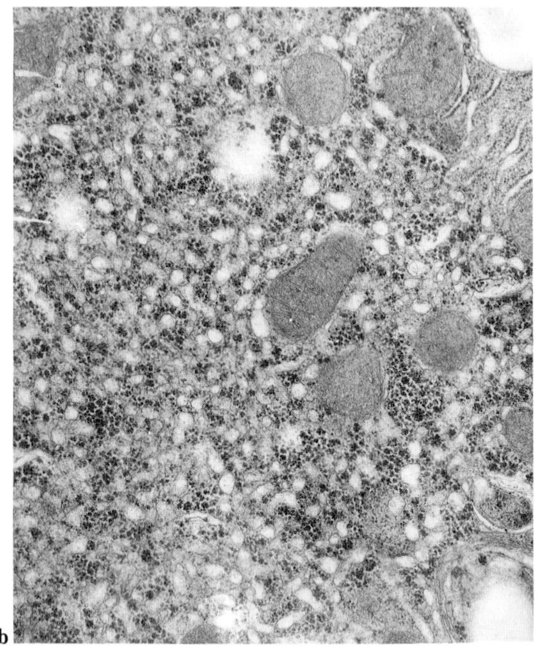

Fig. 11.1 **a** Induction effect on hepatocytes – human liver in a patient on Antabuse (disulfiram) for treatment of alcoholism: note the 'ground glass' inclusions in periportal hepatocytes; these are due in part to proliferation of the smooth endoplasmic reticulum. **b** Electron micrograph of rat liver showing phenobarbitone-induced hyperplasia of the smooth endoplasmic reticulum: a number of mitochondria are present and the dense particulate matter is glycogen. × 12000.

increased, or increasing its risk of producing an adverse reaction. 'Induced' hepatocytes are enlarged and their cytoplasm shows a granular 'ground glass' appearance (Fig. 11.1) which may mimic the ground glass hepatocytes seen in chronic hepatitis B infection.

The complexity of some drug interactions is illustrated if we consider the hepatotoxic effects of the broad spectrum antibiotic rifampicin. Factors which influence the likelihood of toxicity include combination with antituberculous drugs such as isoniazid. Isoniazid itself has been linked with liver damage, particularly as part of a drug-induced lupus erythematosus syndrome in patients with the slow acetylator phenotype. Slow acetylators rely more heavily than fast acetylators on the hydrolysis pathway for isoniazid inactivation. The hydrolysis pathway produces isonicotinic acid which is harmless, and hydrazine which may be a provoking agent for systemic lupus erythematosus. Rifampicin, which is a potent inducer of hepatic metabolizing enzymes, induces the enzyme which hydrolyses isoniazid. The combination of slow acetylator status and exposure to rifampicin will combine to increase the risk of hepatotoxicity with isoniazid. Rifampicin hepatotoxicity, however, also has a genetic component: patients who excrete only low concentrations of desacetyl-rifampicin in their urine have a lower risk of hepatotoxicity than other patients. Finally, poor nutritional status will also increase the likelihood of toxicity.

Hepatitis and Liver Cell Necrosis

Acute hepatitis may be produced by a wide range of drugs, e.g. halothane and phenothiazines. The histological appearances may be indistinguishable from those seen in acute viral hepatitis although unusual or unexpected features such as the location and severity of the injury or the presence of eosinophils may provide a hint of a drug-induced aetiology. Chronic hepatitis has been reported with methyldopa and nitrofurantoin; hepatitis characterized by granuloma formation may be caused by a variety of drugs of which the sulphonamides and phenylbutazone are good examples. Submassive or massive necrosis may occur with some drugs and is usually most marked in zone 1 of the acinus; causative drugs include paracetamol, halothane and allopurinol.

Paracetamol is a widely used analgesic which, in therapeutic doses (4 g per day), has a good safety record although overdosage with only 20 g may be fatal if not treated vigorously. Paracetamol is metabolized in the liver through two pathways. About 90% of the drug is normally conjugated with glucuronic acid or sulphate, resulting in water soluble products which are non-toxic and can be excreted easily by the kidney. The remainder is metabolized by an alternative pathway, the mixed function oxidase system, which produces an intermediate substrate which is highly reactive and potentially toxic to liver cells. Under normal circumstances this intermediate is conjugated with glutathione and thus detoxified. The capacity of the liver to conjugate drugs with glucuronic acid or sulphate is saturable and therefore, overdosage of paracetamol leads to a greater proportion being metabolized by the mixed function oxidase system. Supplies of glutathione within the liver are limited and, in overdosage, toxic metabolites of paracetamol are formed which cannot be inactivated sufficiently quickly to prevent hepatotoxicity. Enzyme inducers such as alcohol will increase the activity of the mixed function oxidase system and exacerbate the toxic effects of paracetamol.

Provided glutathione stores are not exhausted, paracetamol does not produce detectable damage. Sulphydryl containing compounds such as methionine (given orally) or *n*-acetylcysteine (administered intravenously) act as substitutes for glutathione and may prevent the development of fulminant hepatic failure. Nomograms are available which relate the plasma paracetamol level and time since ingestion to the risk of toxicity (Fig. 11.2). In cases of doubt, however, it is wiser to treat the patient with sulphydryl compounds.

Fatty Change and Non-alcoholic Steatohepatitis

Microvesicular fatty change, similar to that seen in acute fatty liver of pregnancy (p. 782), characterizes liver injury following intravenous tetracycline. A similar pattern of fat accumulation may be

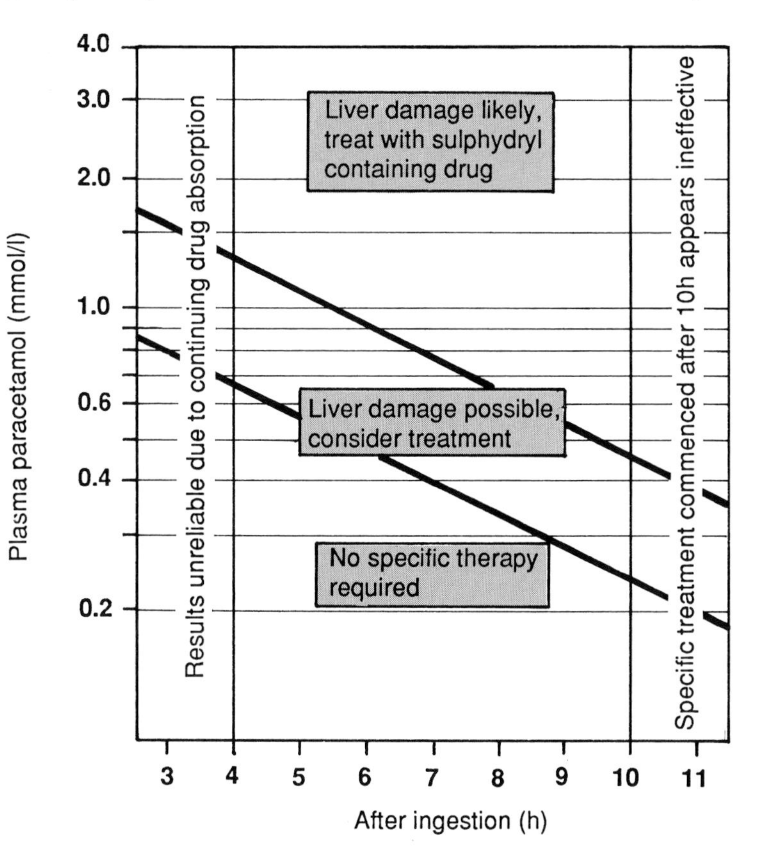

Fig. 11.2 Nomogram for the management of paracetamol poisoning. (Redrawn with permission from *Lecture Notes on Clinical Pharmacology*, eds J. L. Reid, P. C. Rubin and B. Whiting. Blackwell Scientific Publications, Oxford, 1989.)

caused by phenytoin and is seen in Reye's syndrome (p. 781) in which salicylates may have a contributory role. Macrovesicular fatty change may be caused by methotrexate and is one of the morphological lesions associated with alcohol abuse. All the features of alcoholic hepatitis (p. 761), including the formation of Mallory bodies, can be produced by amiodarone, a cardiac antidysrhythmic drug.

Fibrosis and Cirrhosis

Administration of methotrexate (e.g. in the treatment of severe psoriasis) is associated with fatty change, hepatic fibrosis and eventually cirrhosis. Liver function tests may remain normal and such patients should have a liver biopsy about once a year in order to monitor progressive fibrosis. Cirrhosis is a rare complication of drug therapy but it has been reported as a sequel to methyldopa or nitrofurantoin-induced chronic hepatitis. This has happened where the drugs have been administered over a prolonged period.

Tumours

Liver cell adenomas are a recognized complication of the use of contraceptive and anabolic steroids. A cause–effect relationship has been established on the basis of tumour regression following withdrawal of oral contraceptives. Thorotrast, an α-wave emitting radiological contrast medium which has now been withdrawn, was associated with the development of hepatic angiosarcomas and of hepatocellular and cholangiocarcinomas. Thorotrast, which has a half-life of many years, accumulated in Kupffer cells and other cells of the mononuclear phagocyte system. Tumours developed some 20 years after its administration.

Jaundice

The mechanisms of jaundice are discussed in detail in Chapter 17. Drugs may induce haemolytic jaundice. Clinical jaundice may develop in association with drug-induced hepatitis and may be a marked feature in so-called combined cytotoxic–cholestatic drug injury, e.g. isoniazid induced. In other patients, however, jaundice with intrahepatic cholestasis is the predominant feature, so-called cholestatic drug injury. Drugs may interfere at any point in the hepatic pathway of bilirubin secretion and excretion: its uptake by the liver cell, its conjugation, its secretion into the canaliculus, its transfer along the canaliculus and its excretion from the liver via the biliary system. Morphologically, there is hepatocellular bilirubin retention and bile concretions are present in canaliculi and may also be found in cholangioles and in bile ducts.

Cholestatis, as a complication of the use of phenothiazine drugs such as chlorpromazine, provides one of the best examples of a type B adverse drug reaction. Jaundice occurs in about 1% of all patients who receive the drug. It usually begins after 1–5 weeks of treatment, but in a few patients jaundice develops after a single dose, while in others it develops after many months of treatment. The onset is usually acute with fever, and a peripheral blood eosinophilia suggests a hypersensitivity reaction. In two-thirds of the patients prompt recovery follows within 6 weeks of withdrawal of the drug, but in others 3–12 months may be required and in a small number of patients a prolonged cholestatic syndrome resembling primary biliary cirrhosis (p. 767) has developed. A remission may occur despite continuation of therapy, an observation which would not favour a hypersensitivity reaction as the mechanism for the jaundice. A small proportion of patients develop hepatic necrosis and in some instances this has been fatal.

Haemopoietic System

Some drugs are designed to produce toxic effects on the haemopoietic system and marrow suppression by such cytotoxic agents is a typical example of a dose-related predictable reaction. Unpredictable drug-induced blood dyscrasias account for about 10% of reported drug reactions but they are responsible for about 50% of drug-related deaths. Various patterns of adverse reaction occur. Agranulocytosis is most common, followed by thrombocytopenia and haemolytic anaemia; aplastic anaemia is extremely rare.

Generalized marrow depression is common after chemotherapy for cancer and supportive measures and protection from infection may be required. Agranulocytosis, which may be immunologically mediated, occurs with antithyroid drugs, particularly carbimazole, with phenylbutazone and with antihistamines. The incidence with carbimazole has been reported to be 0.1% and is mainly restricted to women over the age of 40. It develops quickly, always within 3 months of instituting treatment, and withdrawal leads to recovery. Thrombocytopenia is usually due to immune destruction of platelets, the drug probably acting as a hapten (e.g. quinidine). Peripheral destruction of platelets may be induced by a direct toxic effect (e.g. by ristocetin). Thrombocytopenia due to hypoplasia of megakaryocytes may also occur (e.g. with phenylbutazone or gold salts). Drug-induced haemolytic anaemia (p. 610) and megaloblastosis with or without megaloblastic anaemia (p. 612) are discussed elsewhere.

Malignant haemopoietic neoplasms (especially acute non-lymphocytic leukaemia) may develop in patients who have been treated for lymphoma by combined chemotherapy and radiotherapy. There may be a delay of up to 15 years before the development of this complication.

Immune System

Corticosteroids and other immunosuppressants suppress T-cell immune responses. As a result, patients taking these medications are prone to reactivation of tuberculosis and opportunistic infections with *Pneumocystis carinii*, fungi or cytomegalovirus present particular problems. The increased incidence of malignant tumours in patients on immunosuppressive medication may be related to impaired immune surveillance.

Many of the side-effects of drugs are due to immunologically mediated hypersensitivity reactions. Drugs may also produce autoimmunity, the best known examples being drug-induced SLE and autoimmune haemolytic anaemia due to α-methyldopa. Hydralazine-induced SLE characteristically occurs in HLA-DR4 positive females who are slow acetylators and are taking high doses of the drug (>200 mg/day). Antibodies to nuclear constituents, particularly histones, are characteristic of drug-induced SLE. A list of drugs causing SLE is given in Table 11.3.

Table 11.3 Drugs associated with an SLE syndrome

Hydralazine	Ethosuximide
Procainamide	Propylthiouracil
Practolol	Methylthiouracil
D-Penicillamine	Trimethadione
Isoniazid	Diphenylhydantoin

Some drugs, particularly the anticonvulsants phenytoin and carbamazepine, the antirheumatic gold salts and penicillamine, produce IgA deficiency which may be accompanied by deficiencies of IgG_2 and IgG_4. Recurrent bacterial infections may become a problem, requiring gammaglobulin replacement therapy. The deficiency usually resolves slowly on withdrawal of the offending drug.

An infectious mononucleosis-like syndrome characterized by lymphadenopathy and fever is an occasional complication of anticonvulsant therapy, particularly phenytoin. Affected lymph nodes show perifollicular T-zone hyperplasia and the differential diagnosis from lymphoma may be difficult.

Cardiovascular System

Cardiac Arrhythmias

Paradoxically, the drugs which most commonly induce cardiac arrhythmias are those used for the treatment of arrhythmia. Life-threatening arrhythmias may occur in digitalis overdosage and this is potentiated by hypokalaemia.

Heart Failure

In patients whose myocardial function is maintained by a high level of adrenergic drive, e.g. after cardiac surgery, β-adrenergic blockers can precipitate cardiac failure combined with bradycardia and hypotension. Myocarditis may occur as an immunologically mediated phenomenon or as a toxic effect of drug therapy. Hypersensitivity myocarditis occurs with a variety of drugs including methyldopa and penicillin. Toxic myocarditis is associated with cytotoxic drugs, particularly adriamycin. Progression to interstitial fibrosis may occur even after withdrawal of the drug. Endocardial fibrosis may be a feature of drug-induced myocarditis or may be confined to the cardiac valves. The latter is a rare complication of methysergide therapy.

Drug-induced Effects on Blood Pressure

Hypertension. Most drugs which produce a chronic rise in blood pressure do so by causing salt and water retention. This occurs with corticosteroids and contraceptive steroids. Hypertension may be a direct feature of vasoconstrictor drugs such as ephedrine, a constituent of some nasal decongestants.

Hypotension may be an undesired effect of drugs with an α-adrenoreceptor blocking effect, particularly phenothiazines. Antihypertensive drugs, such as captopril, which act by inhibiting angiotensin converting enzyme (ACE), may produce profound hypotension. In volume depleted patients and those with heart failure this may occur with the first dose.

Damage to Blood Vessels

Vasculitis (p. 464) can be induced by numerous drugs, including ampicillin and chlorothiazide. The pathogenesis is probably related to the deposition of antigen–antibody complexes in vessel walls.

Peripheral arterial spasm, causing Raynaud's disease and occasionally gangrene, may be a consequence of the excessive use of ergot-containing drugs for the treatment of migraine.

Intravascular thrombosis. Oral contraceptive agents with a high oestrogen content are associated with a sixfold increase in the risk of venous thrombosis and are an important cause of stroke in young adult women. This hazard is much less with the low-oestrogen contraceptive preparations which are now widely used. Chemotherapeutic agents used in cancer, amiodarone or diazepam may cause thrombosis because of their irritant effect when administered intravenously. Any extravasation of irritant drug is likely to cause a severe local reaction or necrosis.

Respiratory System

Specific Pharmacological Effects

Opiates, barbiturates and other sedative drugs cause central depression of respiration and may cause ventilatory failure in patients with chronic bronchitis or emphysema. Oxygen therapy may have the same effect by reducing the hypoxic respiratory drive in patients with severe, chronic obstructive lung disease and respiratory failure. β-adrenoreceptor blocking agents, even those with relative β_1 selectivity, may provoke bronchospasm in asthmatic patients.

Allergic Reactions

Bronchial asthma and pulmonary eosinophilia may be caused by a variety of therapeutic agents. These include proteins such as antisera and vaccines and drugs of low molecular weight which act as haptens.

Diffuse Pulmonary Disease

Diffuse alveolar damage is a non-specific reaction to a wide range of insults, including drugs. There is widespread damage to alveolar lining cells, particularly type I pneumocytes, and capillary endothelial cells. When mild, this may lead only to proliferation of type II pneumocytes. More severe reactions are associated with an alveolar exudate and hyaline membrane formation. Organization may occur, producing pulmonary fibrosis. Drugs causing diffuse alveolar damage are numerous and include cytotoxic agents, e.g. bleomycin, chlorambucil, cyclophosphamide, gold salts, nitrofurantoin and penicillamine.

Gastrointestinal Tract

Ulceration

Ulceration in the gastrointestinal tract may be related to the direct effect of drugs in the mucosa, a systemic effect on the mucosa, abnormalities in epithelial turnover or opportunistic infection. Ulceration of any part of the gastrointestinal tract may be caused by cytotoxic agents or steroid therapy. Potassium chloride tablets and tetracyclines and their derivatives are recognized causes of oesophageal ulceration.

Non-steroidal anti-inflammatory drugs (NSAIDs) are common causes of gastric ulceration. They act by inhibiting the formation of prostaglandin which is required to maintain the physicochemical barrier of the gastric mucosa. Although direct injury from aspirin or indomethacin is known to occur, parenteral preparations can also lead to upper gastrointestinal ulceration. The ulceration is associated with chronic blood loss and this may be aggravated by NSAID-induced effects on platelet aggregation with an increased bleeding time. NSAID-induced iron-deficiency anaemia is probably the most common drug-induced haematological abnormality.

Most of the drugs that injure the stomach are able to cause similar, although less severe damage in the small intestine: thus, aspirin can cause erosions at the tips of villi, while indomethacin can cause inflammation and ulceration of the small intestine with subsequent stricture formation. Potassium chloride is an important cause of small intestinal ulceration, a hazard which is lessened by the use of slow release or enteric coated tablets.

Alterations in Gastrointestinal Flora

Broad spectrum antibiotics cause diarrhoea in up to 30% of patients. This is related, in the majority of cases, to an alteration in the bacterial flora of the colon. In some cases, however, there is a true colitis (pseudomembranous colitis) due to the overgrowth of a toxin-producing organism, *Clostridium difficile* (p. 709). Staphylococcal enterocolitis is a rare but severe complication of broad spectrum antibiotic therapy.

Alteration in Muscle Activity

Anticholinergic drugs may cause gastro-oesophageal reflux due to reduction in the tone of the lower oesophageal sphincter. A syndrome of pseudo-obstruction or even paralytic ileus may be induced by anticholinergic drugs, tricyclic antidepressants, phenothiazines and opiates. Laxative abuse, particularly with anthraquinone laxatives (senna, cascara), phenolphthalein and magnesium sulphate, may cause chronic diarrhoea. In the case of the anthraquinone laxatives there may be abnormal mucosal pigmentation – melanosis coli. Permanent damage to the myenteric plexus may result in persistent diarrhoea.

Malabsorption

Drugs may cause malabsorption by several mechanisms. Neomycin and cholestyramine bind bile acids leading to malabsorption of fat and fat soluble vitamins. Neomycin damages enterocytes with loss of disaccharidase activity, and may cause partial villous atrophy. Colchicine and antimitotic drugs cause partial villous atrophy by reducing cell turnover. Many drugs, including neomycin and para-amino salicylic acid, interfere with the absorption and transport of vitamin B_{12}, and may cause megaloblastic anaemia. Anaemia due to folate deficiency may result from long-term anticonvulsant therapy, especially with phenytoin.

Miscellaneous

Acute pancreatitis has resulted from exposure to pentamidine, used for the treatment of leishmaniasis and *Pneumocystis carinii* pneumonia in patients with the acquired immunodeficiency syndrome (AIDS).

Gingival hyperplasia is a well recognized complication of chronic phenytoin toxicity and less commonly with cyclosporin and some dihydropyridine calcium antagonists.

Kidney and Urinary Tract

Drug-induced renal disease is common and 20–30% of all cases of acute renal failure are drug induced. The kidney and the liver are the major excretory organs for drugs and their metabolites. Drugs or their metabolites may damage the urinary system during filtration, secretion, concentration or excretion. The renal pelvis, the ureters and bladder are also susceptible to toxic injury.

Although the kidneys account for only about 0.4% of body weight, they receive about one-quarter of the cardiac output, resulting in heavy exposure of the kidney to potentially nephrotoxic drugs. Excreted drugs and metabolites undergo glomerular filtration and some may be reabsorbed via the tubular epithelium. Some may be secreted directly into the tubules. In the distal nephron the concentrating ability of the medulla increases the interstitial concentration of drugs and their metabolites. Drugs which produce renal impairment may in turn reduce their own rate of clearance and, in the presence of impaired renal function from other causes, toxic serum concentrations of drugs and metabolites may result.

In common with the liver, most types of renal disease can be drug induced. They include glomerulonephritis, tubular and interstitial injury, renal papillary necrosis and lesions of the urothelium including tumours. These are dealt with in detail in Chapter 19.

Central Nervous System and the Special Senses

The blood–brain barrier to a large extent protects the brain from many drugs which cause damage elsewhere in the body. The posterior root ganglia, autonomic ganglia and peripheral nerves are not so protected, and peripheral neuropathy is a side-effect of many drugs. Brain damage can result from the circulatory effects of drugs. Hypotensive agents predispose to cerebral infarcts, while monoamine oxidase inhibitors can cause paroxysmal hypertension leading to cerebral haemorrhage. Prolonged hypoglycaemia may be an unpredictable effect of the sulphonylurea hypoglycaemic agents, resulting in confusion or dementia in the elderly.

Drugs may damage the central nervous system directly by affecting either neurons or glia. Neurotoxicity has been reported with a number of cytotoxic and immunosuppressive drugs. Cytarabine used in the treatment of leukaemia, is commonly associated with signs of cerebellar dysfunction. Cyclosporin has produced grand mal seizures, which may be dose-related. Oligodendrocyte damage due to intrathecal methotrexate therapy causes demyelination. Ataxia may be a feature of any drug with CNS depressant effects, but is most commonly recognized with anticonvulsants such as sodium valproate or phenytoin. Excessive doses of sedative drugs are associated with coma. This is seen with benzodiazepines or opiates. Provided supportive measures are undertaken, recovery from drug-induced coma is usually complete, but permanent damage may occur after serious metabolic disturbances such as cerebral anoxia or hypoglycaemia.

Epilepsy is characterized by a low threshold for seizures. In a patient with a low seizure threshold the risk of convulsions after drug treatment is increased. Apparently normal individuals with a low seizure threshold may have a convulsion in response to certain drugs including vaccines and high doses of theophylline. Overdosage of anticonvulsant drugs may itself be epileptogenic.

Acute dystonic reactions or extrapyramidal side-effects including parkinsonism are well recognized adverse effects of the phenothiazines, which have dopamine receptor antagonist properties. Metoclopramide may be associated with oculogyric crisis. Long-term treatment with phenothiazines may result in tardive dyskinesia.

The adverse effects of drugs on the special senses are summarized in Table 11.4.

Endocrine System

Suppression of the pituitary–adrenal axis occurs with exogenously administered glucocorticoids. Although short-term courses of high dose steroids cause minor disruption of the corticosteroid re-

Table 11.4 Common adverse effects of drugs on the special senses

	Drug
Deafness	Aminoglycosides, loop diuretics
Tinnitus	Aspirin toxicity, mefenamic acid
Taste disturbance (dysgeusia)	Captopril, penicillamine, antithyroid drugs
Blindness	Quinine, tobacco
Blurred vision	Anticholinergic drugs
Cataract	Corticosteroids (prolonged use), possibly isotretinoin
Disturbance of colour vision	Amiodarone
Glaucoma	Topical steroids, anticholinergic drugs
Optic neuritis	Almitrine, cimetidine
Retinopathy	Chloroquine, oral contraceptive drugs

sponse to stress, this effect lasts only a few days and does not appear to be a clinical problem. Long-term treatment with low doses of corticosteroids results in atrophy of the adrenal cortex. Withdrawal of long-term treatment must therefore be performed gradually and under supervision.

Drug-induced glucose tolerance and diabetes mellitus result from interference with the release of insulin (e.g. thiazide diuretics or diazoxide), or from anti-insulin effects (e.g. glucocorticoids), or from pancreatic damage (e.g. the cytotoxic agent streptozotocin).

Hypothyroidism and goitre have been associated with chronic lithium treatment. Iodine-containing drugs such as amiodarone produce a variety of disturbances of thyroid function and interfere with thyroid function tests.

Gynaecomastia is a feature of anti-androgen treatment (e.g. stilboestrol for the management of prostatic carcinoma), and may occur with other drugs, including spironolactone, cimetidine and occasionally digoxin.

Skin and Tegmenta

There are numerous clinical forms of cutaneous drug eruption and these may mimic natural disease. The histopathological changes are usually the same whether a disease is idiopathic or drug induced. An unusual but interesting skin reaction is the fixed drug eruption, in which blisters or erythematous areas develop at one or a few fixed sites on the skin. These eruptions resolve when the drug is withdrawn and reappear at the same sites if re-exposure occurs. Non-steroidal anti-inflammatory drugs and broad spectrum antibiotics are most often implicated.

Hair loss is commonly seen with cytotoxic drug treatment. Most cytotoxic drugs affect rapidly dividing cells including the hair bulb, producing alopecia. The antihistamine drug terfenadine has also been associated with alopecia. In contrast, minoxidil, a peripheral vasodilator used for treatment of severe hypertension, produces a striking and generalized increase in hair growth. This has militated against its use as an antihypertensive drug, particularly in women. More recently, however, local application of minoxidil has proved useful in the treatment of male baldness.

Drug-induced Damage to the Embryo or Fetus

Toxins may injure the developing organism at any phase in its prenatal development. The major organs are formed over a relatively short period of time (Fig. 11.3). The gestational age at exposure to the drug determines whether or not it exerts a teratogenic effect. A teratogenic effect results in a structural abnormality or deformity which may be sufficiently distinctive as to be diagnostic of drug exposure (Table 11.5). Phocomelia, the shortening of limbs which occurred with exposure to thalidomide in the late 1950s and early 1960s, is a good example. There is also considerable species variation, and absence of teratogenesis in preclinical toxicology testing is no guarantee of safety in human pregnancies.

In addition to major congenital abnormalities less severe changes may also occur. These include the fetal alcohol syndrome in which there are facial

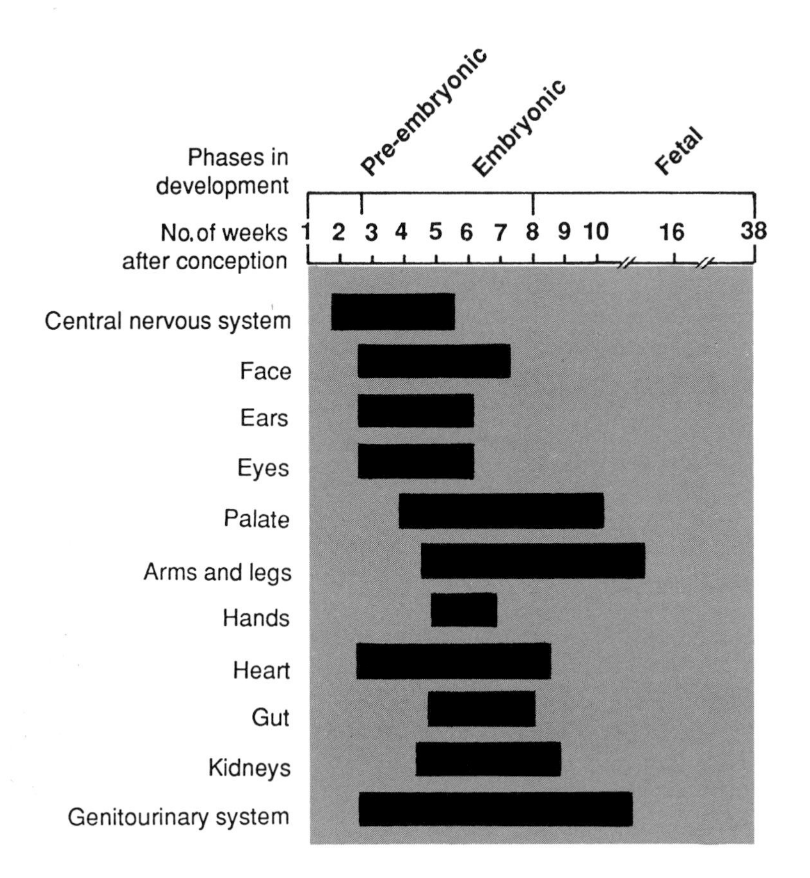

Fig. 11.3 Timing of embryonic and fetal development. (Redrawn with permission from Whittle, M. J. and Hanretty, K. P. (1987). Identifying abnormalities. Chapter 2. In *Prescribing in Pregnancy*, Ed. P. C. Rubin. BMJ Publications, London.)

Table 11.5 Teratogenic effects of drugs

	Effect	Incidence	Prenatal diagnosis
Lithium	Cardiac defects (Ebstein's complex)	10–12%	Feasible
Warfarin	Chondrodysplasia punctata/facial abnormalities;	5%	Unlikely
	central nervous system abnormalities	4%	Feasible
Phenytoin	Craniofacial defects; limb defects; reduced growth	30%	Feasible
Primidone and phenobarbitone	Facial clefting; cardiac defects	Unknown	Feasible
Sodium valproate	Central nervous system defects	2–3%	Feasible
Sex hormones	Cardiac defects; multiple anomalies	Unknown	Feasible

Reprinted with permission from Whittle, M. J. and Hanretty, K. P. (1987). Identifying abnormalities. Chapter 2. In *Prescribing in Pregnancy*, Ed. P. C. Rubin. BMJ Publications, London.

abnormalities and permanent impairment of physical and mental development. Tetracycline acts as a chelating agent and may interfere with bone growth in the fetus. It is deposited in bones and teeth, producing discoloration of the milk teeth.

Functional abnormalities may also occur, some of which only declare themselves postnatally. Sulphonamides, which are highly protein bound, will displace bilirubin from plasma binding sites. If the drug is used just prior to delivery the increased free concentration of bilirubin is not cleared by the placenta and crosses the poorly formed blood–brain barrier in the neonate: its deposition in the basal ganglia causes kernicterus. Aspirin may be used during pregnancy to prevent recurrent abortion or pre-eclampsia. Its use immediately prior to delivery increases the risk of maternal and neonatal bleeding complications. High doses of NSAIDs interfere with prostaglandin production and may cause premature closure of the ductus arteriosus with devastating haemodynamic effects.

Maternal exposure to opiates or sedative drugs during labour will lead to a sedated neonate which may have to be given antagonists. Chronic maternal exposure to opiates in drug abusers results in fetal tolerance and dependence. If this risk is not anticipated prior to delivery then the neonate will suffer a withdrawal syndrome.

Drug Resistance

The phenomenon of acquired resistance of bacteria to antibiotics is well recognized and has been discussed in Chapter 8. Recently, a special form of drug resistance occurring in tumours has been documented – multidrug resistance (MDR). Ths is characterized by cross-resistance to a wide variety of hydrophobic cytotoxic drugs including the vinca alkaloids (vincristine, vinblastine) and anthracyclines. Reduced intracellular accumulation of the drug is caused by increased expression of the MDR gene, *mdr-1*, which encodes a 170 kDa membrane protein, P-glycoprotein. This has significant homology with bacterial membrane transport proteins and is thought to act as an efflux pump, thus preventing drug access to intracellular sites. This protein is expressed normally in some human tissues, including epithelial cells of the gut and adrenal cortex. Tumours arising at these sites are known to be intrinsically resistant to these hydrophobic cytotoxic agents. In some tumours a subpopulation of cells express the MDR phenotype prior to treatment. These cells continue to proliferate when the majority of the tumour cells have been killed by the cytotoxic drugs, resulting in local 'recurrence' of tumour.

Drug Dependence

Drug dependence is a complex behavioural phenomenon caused by chronic administration of centrally acting drugs, such as morphine, barbiturates, alcohol (i.e. ethanol) or cocaine. Repeated administration of such drugs alters behaviour, which is characterized by an increasing urge to continue drug administration. This compulsion may be reinforced by the appearance of a physical abstinence syndrome that occurs when drug administration stops. Drug dependence can be divided into: (1) **psychological dependence**, which is the principal characteristic that defines drug dependence and is marked by an urge to continue drug administration and by anxiety if this is impossible; and (2) **physical dependence** which occurs only with some drugs, such as alcohol and morphine, and is marked by the appearance of a physical abstinence syndrome on drug withdrawal. The nature of the abstinence syndrome depends on the drug.

Dependence, like tolerance, is an adaptive response to repeated drug administration. Since tolerance and drug dependence develop in parallel, explanations of the origin of the former also seek to explain the latter in a unitary hypothesis. This is justifiable, since tolerance to the acute effects of dependence-producing drugs is primarily due to adaptation of the central mechanisms affected by the drug. Such pharmacodynamic tolerance may reflect the development of physical dependence. A second type of tolerance, which occurs in drug dependence, is caused by enhanced drug metabolism and excretion. This pharmacokinetic tolerance is less important and contributes only indirectly to dependence, by reducing the concentration of the drug at its site of action, thereby creating the need to increase the dose to obtain the desired effect.

The term drug dependence is used whether or not there is a physical withdrawal syndrome and applies equally to the inclination to use caffeine and to the compulsion to self-administer heroin. Since the consequences of taking drugs such as caffeine and heroin are so dissimilar, the term, drug dependence, is of limited value. It is therefore necessary to specify the type of dependence being considered – opiate dependence, alcohol dependence, etc. The use of these drugs during pregnancy can cause dependence and withdrawal symptoms in the newborn child.

Drug Misuse and Substance Abuse

Drug misuse and substance abuse can be considered together, since any substance that modifies a biological system, whether or not it is a therapeutic agent, can be defined as a drug. Obviously, what constitutes drug misuse depends on society and current attitudes prevailing within it. Since this is a sociological rather than a pharmacological problem, drug misuse will be considered here only insofar as it is associated with drug dependence.

Other Pathological Consequences of Drug Dependence

In addition to the effects outlined in the following paragraphs intravenous self-administration of drugs is associated with a high risk of local and systemic infection, notably hepatitis, HIV-1 transmission, infective endocarditis and with toxic effects related to the use of additives. Chronic alcohol intake is associated with injury to the liver, brain and cardiovascular systems and these are discussed in the appropriate system chapters.

Factors Affecting the Development of Dependence

There is little known about the nature of the adaptation underlying psychological dependence. In contrast, although the withdrawal syndrome can be readily analysed and quantified, the neurochemical changes underlying the development of physical dependence are only partially understood.

The Chemical Structure of the Drug

This is important, since it determines where and how the drug acts and what mechanisms it affects. Morphine has a characteristic molecular structure and acts on specific receptors on nerve terminals to inhibit transmitter release. In contrast, alcohol does not act on a particular receptor but enters biological membranes and alters their fluidity, so that its effects are less specific and more widespread. The adaptation of neuronal mechanisms to chronic administration of morphine is therefore likely to be different from that produced by alcohol. This difference is reflected in the dissimilar abstinence syndromes produced by their withdrawal.

The Dose, Frequency and Duration of Drug Administration

These determine whether, and to what extent, drug dependence develops. Continuous or frequent intermittent administration of a sufficiently high dose of many centrally acting drugs will produce dependence. In general, the higher the dose and frequency of drug administration and the longer the duration of drug treatment, the greater will be the dependence. The dependence can be quantified by measuring the severity of the abstinence syndome (Fig. 11.4).

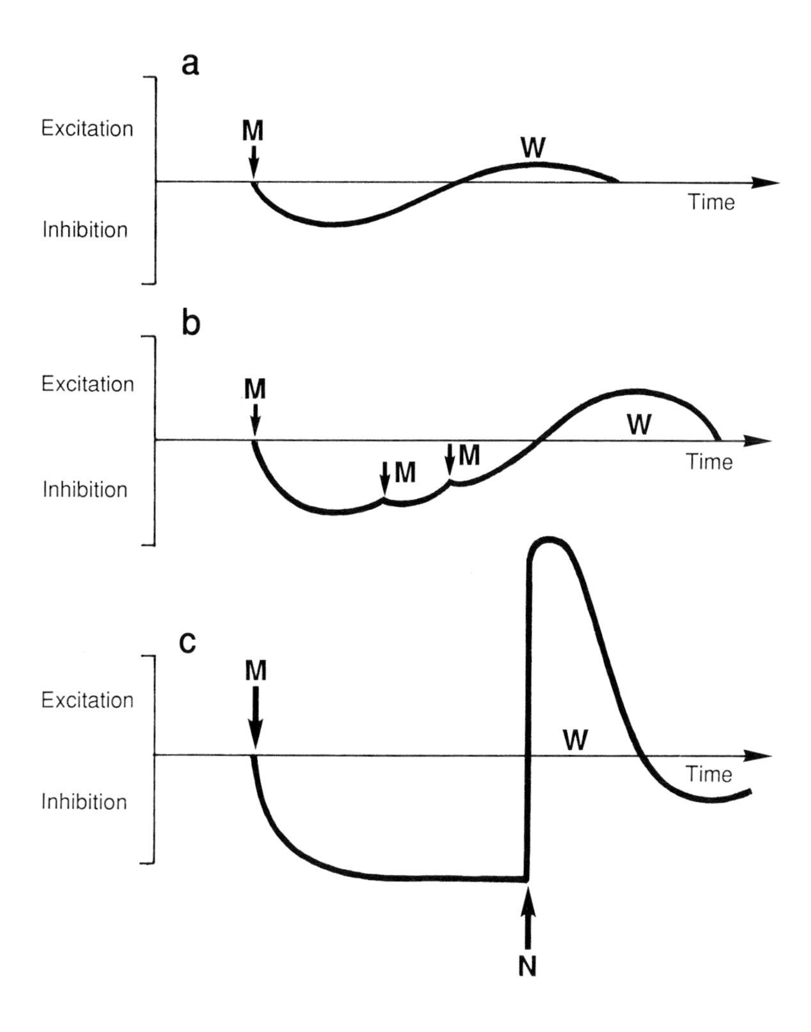

Fig. 11.4 Diagram to show the effects of administering a dependence-producing drug, morphine (M) in different ways. In the upper panel (**a**), a single dose of morphine administered at the arrow, depressed a hypothetical neuronal mechanism below the mean level of activity. The extent of inhibition is small and recovery occurs as the drug is metabolized and excreted. Recovery is also due to pharmacodynamic tolerance, caused by adaptation of the mechanism inhibited by morphine. The excitatory withdrawal phenomenon (W) is small since the inhibition was slight but if the dose had been large, so that the initial perturbation had been bigger, the withdrawal phenomenon would have been correspondingly bigger. In the middle panel (**b**), three similar doses of morphine were administered. Neither the second nor the third dose produced as big a response as the initial dose. In this situation, pharmacodynamic tolerance and dependence develop quickly. This is reflected in the larger excitatory withdrawal phenomenon. In the lower panel (**c**), an intravenous infusion of increasing concentration of morphine was commenced at the arrow. The increasing concentrations infused offset the effects of the rapidly developing pharmacodynamic tolerance. The infusion was stopped at the second arrow and a single large dose of the opiate antagonist, naloxone (N) was administered. This immediately precipitated a powerful excitatory withdrawal phenomenon, which was short-lived since the antagonist was more rapidly excreted than the morphine, which briefly reasserted its inhibitory effect. This panel illustrates the important point that as long as the dose is sufficient, the homeostatic adaptation responsible for dependence will remain latent. Its existence will only be revealed when plasma levels of the drug fall below a critical value or when the drug is displaced from its receptors by an antagonist.

The Route of Drug Administration

Dependence can be produced by administering drugs orally, intravenously or by inhalation. The rate of development of dependence is faster if the drug is given intravenously than when given orally. Intravenous administration or inhalation are popular routes for drug misuse because the acute effects they produce are more rapid in onset and more intense than those achieved by other routes.

The Simultaneous Administration of Other Drugs

When several drugs are administered together, complex interactions can occur. These not only influence the acute effects, which may be additive, opposed or synergistic, but also affect the capacity of a drug to cause dependence. Thus, the ability of morphine to produce dependence can be prevented by simultaneously administering the opiate antagonist, naloxone, which blocks opiate receptors and prevents morphine acting. This is a simple example with a predictable outcome. However, when drugs are abused for 'recreational purposes', complex mixtures of impure drugs may be used with unpredictable consequences.

Types of Dependence

The mechanisms of drug dependence, the clinical features and the withdrawal syndromes are different for each group of drugs. Features of dependency of some of the more important groups are discussed below, and their mechanisms of action and characteristics of their withdrawal syndromes are summarized in Table 11.6 and Fig. 11.5.

Opiate Dependence

Dependence is produced by morphine and other chemically related derivatives. Opiates act presynaptically on receptors for opiate peptides (endorphins) to inhibit transmitter (noradrenaline and dopamine) release at various central and peripheral synapses (Fig. 11.5). This effect is responsible for the ability of opiates to relieve anxiety and produce euphoria in some people,

Table 11.6 Features of some of the different types of drug dependence

	Examples of drugs in group	Withdrawal symptoms
Opiate	Morphine, heroin, pethidine, dipipanone, methadone	Anxiety; unproductive displacement activity; autonomic effects – yawning, lachrymation, rhinorrhoea, anorexia, nausea, vomiting, intestinal spasm, tachycardia, raised blood pressure, pupillary dilatation
Barbiturates*	Mainly short-acting barbiturates – amylobarbitone, quinalbarbitone	Irritability, insomnia, hallucinations, convulsions, death
Alcohol	Ethanol	As for barbiturates
Benzodiazepines	Diazepam; chlordiazepoxide; lorazepam, nitrazepam, and temazepam	Anxiety, irritability, 'rebound' insomnia; tremor, nausea, vomiting and convulsions
Cocaine	Cocaine	Depression, fatigue

*Non-barbiturate sedative hypnotics such as glutethimide and methaqualone produce a similar dependence.

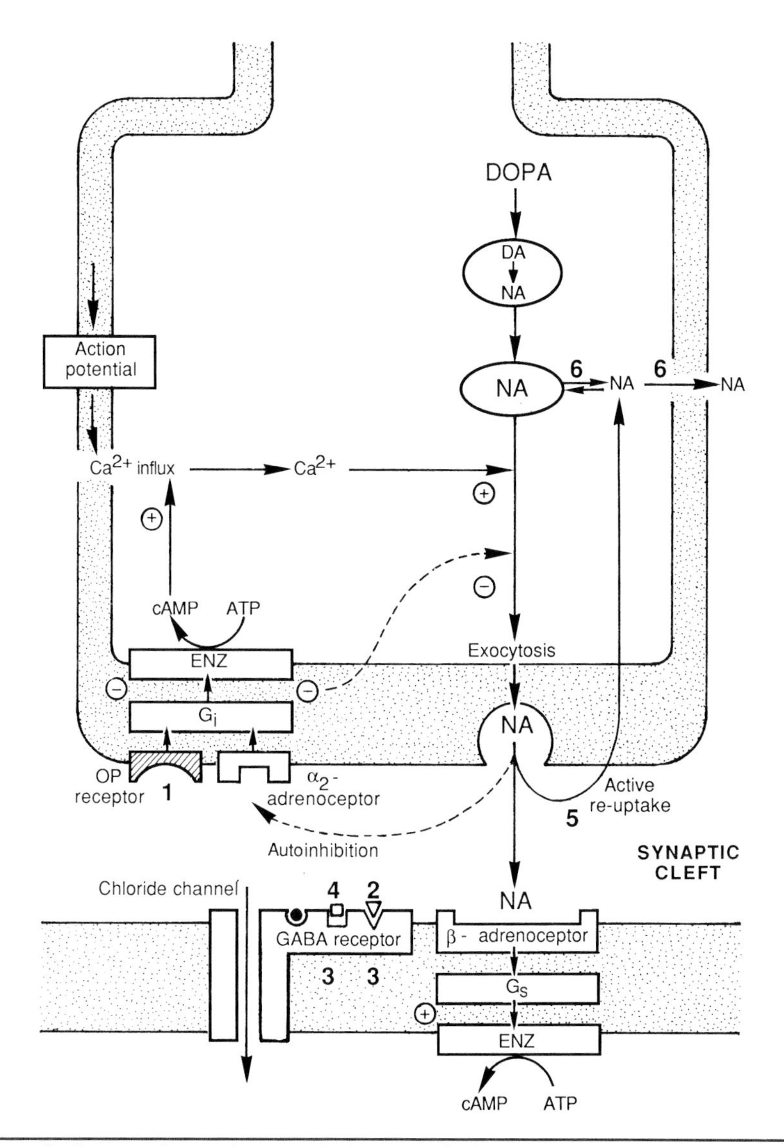

Fig. 11.5 Schematic diagram of synaptic transmission in the CNS showing the sites where dependence-producing drugs act. This diagram is speculative and is based on evidence from central and peripheral sites and model systems. The presynaptic neuron shown is noradrenergic but the information applies also to dopaminergic nerves. The synthesis of noradrenaline (NA) and dopamine (DA) from dihydroxyphenylalanine (DOPA) is shown. The mechanism by which α_2-adrenoceptor mediated autoinhibition and opioid peptide (OP) receptor mediated inhibition of transmitter release occurs via inhibition of adenylate cyclase and blockade of calcium entry is also shown. Both the presynaptic α_2-adrenoceptor and the OP receptor may be linked via the inhibitory GTP binding protein (G_i) to the enzyme, adenylate cyclase (ENZ). Also illustrated is the postsynaptic β-adrenoceptor, linked to the stimulatory GTP binding protein (G_s) and adenylate cyclase (ENZ). The sites and mechanisms affected by the major dependence-producing drugs are numbered. 1, **Opiates** act presynaptically on receptors for endogenous opioid peptides (OP) to inhibit transmitter release. This may involve inhibition of the calcium influx, required for transmitter release and probably also involves hyperpolarization of the nerve terminal and inhibition of adenylate cyclase. 2, **Barbiturates** act at a site (▽) adjacent to the GABA receptor, which operates the chloride channel. Barbiturates promote the action of GABA (●), which opens the chloride channel. 3, **Alcohol** and **solvents** distribute in the lipid membrane to increase its fluidity and alter the functioning of various receptors, including the GABA receptor. 4, **Benzodiazepines** act allosterically at a site (□) close to the GABA receptor to increase its affinity for GABA (●). 5, **Cocaine** inhibits the active re-uptake of noradrenaline, so that noradrenaline accumulates in the synaptic cleft. 6, **Amphetamines** are taken up by the active re-uptake mechanism and displace noradrenaline and/or dopamine from the storage vesicles and from the cytosol. Amphetamines also prevent the active re-uptake of noradrenaline.

providing a powerful motivation for the non-medical use of these drugs. The exogenous opiates may also inhibit the synthesis or release of endorphins.

Repeated administration of an opiate inevitably produces tolerance, especially to the euphoric effects. Where the intention is to elevate mood, increasing the dose is ineffective and this objective becomes progressively more elusive as dependence develops. The effect on synthesis and release of endorphins may be responsible for the withdrawal syndrome which is produced either by stopping drug administration or, more rapidly and with greater intensity, by giving an opiate antagonist, such as naloxone, which displaces the opiate from its receptor. From about 10 hours after administration of the last dose of the drug, the characteristic signs of the abstinence syndrome appear, are maximal after 48 hours and subside over the following week. However, some physiological and behavioural abnormalities may persist for up to 6 months.

Barbiturate–Alcohol Dependence

Since the barbiturates and alcohol produce similar types of dependence and since each can substitute for the other to prevent the appearance of the abstinence syndrome, barbiturate–alcohol dependence is usually considered as a single phenomenon, although the mechanisms by which these drugs act are dissimilar. Barbiturates act at a site adjacent to the γ-aminobutyric acid (GABA) receptor to enhance the ability of GABA to open the chloride channel and cause inhibition. Alcohol distributes in the lipid membrane and increases its fluidity and may alter the functioning of various receptors indirectly. Recent evidence suggests, however, that alcohol may have more specific effects. Various receptor-operated (GABA) ion channels are more sensitive to the acute effects of alcohol than the voltage-operated calcium channels. However, adaptation to the chronic administration of alcohol appears to be associated with increased numbers of voltage-operated receptors on neuronal cell bodies. In severe alcoholism, where malnutrition and cirrhosis develop, tolerance may diminish due to impaired capacity to metabolize alcohol. With the barbiturates, the effects of withdrawal gradually diminish within a week but with alcohol, when there is damage to the CNS, recovery will be slower and incomplete.

Benzodiazepine Dependence

The benzodiazepines are sedative hypnotics which also reduce muscle tone and coordination and have anticonvulsant activity. They act allosterically at a site close to the GABA receptor to increase its affinity for GABA and thus open the chloride channel. Tolerance to their effects develops rapidly. Psychological dependence develops during prolonged treatment with normal therapeutic doses, and barbiturates and alcohol increase the likelihood of dependence. Chronic treatment with high doses, especially of the short-acting benzodiazepines, lorazepam or temazepam, can produce physical dependence, in which there is a mild syndrome with tremor, nausea, vomiting and convulsions.

Cocaine Dependence

Cocaine, an alkaloid derived from the leaves of the coca plant, is a powerful local anaesthetic and central stimulant which can be inhaled, smoked, ingested or injected intravenously or subcutaneously. It inhibits the active re-uptake of noradrenaline or dopamine by the neuron so that these transmitters accumulate in the synaptic cleft.

Cocaine causes behavioural arousal, and feelings of euphoria, exhilaration, increased intellectual and physical capacity, and indifference to fatigue. With repeated administration, these feelings are replaced by agitation, insomnia and panic. Peak effects occur approximately 15–20 minutes after inhalation. Repeated doses of cocaine administered by this route at 30-minute intervals, over several hours, cause restlessness, hallucinations and paranoia. When the drug is excreted these effects are replaced by depression and fatigue, possibly due to down-regulation of receptors in the synaptic cleft. Cocaine produces powerful psychological dependence but does not cause physical dependence or tolerance. Dependence may be more likely to develop if the cocaine is 'freebased', as it is in 'crack'.

Amphetamine Dependence

Amphetamines are taken up by the neuronal uptake process in the same way as noradrenaline or dopamine. Once in the nerve terminal, amphetamines displace noradrenaline or dopamine from the storage vesicles or the cytoplasm so that these transmitters accumulate in the synaptic cleft, as in cocaine dependence. Down-regulation of aminergic receptors also occurs with prolonged amphetamine abuse.

Amphetamines are, like cocaine, psychomotor stimulants. They cause euphoria, increased peripheral sympathetic activity, locomotor activity and mental alertness. In high dosage and with repeated administration a stereotyped pattern of behaviour develops that resembles acute schizophrenia.

Nicotine Dependence

Nicotine has complex effects that are further complicated by the way it is administered. During smoking, blood levels rise and produce a discrete effect, but as soon as smoking stops the blood level and effects decline rapidly. Nicotine acts at acetylcholine receptors in sympathetic ganglia and in the adrenal medulla causing catecholamine release. Nicotine withdrawal syndrome may be suppressed by amphetamine, suggesting the control mechanism may be similar to that responsible for amphetamine dependence.

Other Causes of Drug Dependence

The following drugs are all capable of producing psychological dependence but physical dependence is unusual.

Cannabis causes psychological dependency by a mechanism that may depend on the lipid solubility of its principal constituent, tetrahydrocannabinol.

Hallucinogens include psilocin from the *Psilocybe* mushrooms, mescaline from a Mexican cactus and lysergic acid diethylamide (LSD) from ergot. They act centrally to distort perception of time and cause sensory confusion with frightening hallucinations and paranoid delusions. LSD acts at central 5-hydroxytryptamine (5-HT) receptors to mimic 5-HT.

Caffeine and the chemically related methylxanthine, theophylline, are central stimulants. They have complex actions, the most important being their ability to inhibit phosphodiesterase which breaks down intracellular cyclic adenosine monophosphate (cAMP).

Mechanisms of Physical Dependence

Various hypotheses have been postulated to explain the phenomenon of physical dependence. Since dependence-producing drugs are chemically and pharmacologically diverse, it seems likely that more than one mechanism is involved. A common theme in most hypotheses is that chronic treatment with such drugs produces a homoeostatic adaptation in the central mechanism affected by the drug. This adaptation would also be responsible for the pharmacodynamic tolerance, would be latent during drug administration and revealed on withdrawal. The magnitude of the adaptation and thus, the severity of the dependence, would reflect the extent to which the central mechanism had been perturbed by the drug. For example, prolonged inhibition of a central mechanism would produce a latent hyperexcitability, reflected in developing tolerance during treatment and in the magnitude of the abstinence syndrome. A number of hypotheses have been proposed to explain drug dependence and the abstinence syndrome.

(1) As morphine inhibits transmitter release, it is possible that prolonged inhibition might allow the transmitter to accumulate in the nerve terminals, so that when morphine blockade is removed, the large amount of transmitter released would produce withdrawal.

(2) Pharmacological (functional) 'denervation' produced by drugs that inhibit transmitter release, and surgical denervation, both deprive the postsynaptic membrane of the influence of the transmitter. Following surgical denervation, the sensitivity of the postsynaptic membrane to transmitter increases. Pharmacological 'denervation' may have a similar effect, so that when the drug is withdrawn and transmission is resumed, the transmitter is released on to a supersensitive postsynaptic membrane.

(3) In a biosynthetic pathway, the end product of the reaction may regulate the amount of enzyme available to catalyse an earlier reaction. Thus, if a drug inhibited an enzyme that catalysed a late reaction in the sequence, the reduction in end product would remove the inhibition on the production of the earlier enzyme. As a result, the amount of this enzyme would increase so that eventually more substrate would be available to compete with and overcome the effect of the drug. Such a mechanism, involving enzyme induction, might explain tolerance during drug administration and also withdrawal hyperexcitability.

(4) In cultured neuroblastoma-glioma cells, morphine acts on opiate receptors that are linked through an inhibitory GTP binding protein, G_i, which regulates adenylate cyclase. Normally, morphine inhibits adenylate cyclase and reduces cAMP levels in this model system. During chronic exposure to morphine, cAMP levels return to normal, even in the presence of the morphine. Whether this adaptation is due to induction of adenylate cyclase or to uncoupling of the opiate receptor from its regulatory G_i protein is unclear. Moreover, whether such a mechanism operates in the central nervous system and how it might affect neurotransmission, remains to be determined.

(5) Chronic treatment with morphine might interfere with the production of endogenous opioid peptides, so that their regulatory role is progressively supplanted by exogenous opiates. Drug withdrawal would result in a loss of homeostatic regulation, which would eventually be restored by recovery of endogenous production.

Most hypotheses seeking to explain drug dependence are highly speculative and none is successful in explaining even opiate dependence, about which most is known. It is unlikely that drug dependence will be explained by a single hypothesis, since it involves so many complex alterations in and interactions between neuronal and hormonal mechanisms.

Radiation-induced Tissue Injury

The discovery of radium in 1896 by Madame Curie was soon followed by its widespread use in the treatment of many and various diseases. Since it was used without clear understanding of its mode of action or knowledge of its potential for damage of normal tissues, disasters occurred – loss of fingers and serious skin and bone damage in patients. Röntgen's discovery around the same time of the properties of X-rays, generated by striking a metal target with a stream of electrons, led to the development of alternative machines for the treatment of many different diseases. X-rays were found to be particularly useful for skin disorders such as psoriasis and eczema, for fungating malignant tumours and for painful bones and joints. When treatment was given to the whole body, the lymphocyte count was reduced, and symptomatic improvement was produced in patients with leukaemia or lymphoma.

The amount of treatment which was given was

determined empirically on the basis of the reaction of the skin. Different levels of damage were recognized – erythema, dry desquamation and moist desquamation (superficial ulceration). It was soon recognized that, if ulceration developed, treatment could not be continued without risking permanent injury. It was not realized until many years later that late damage could occur which was not predictable from the acute effect of radiation on the skin, and that radiation, as well as curing cancer, could cause it.

Types of Ionizing Radiation

We are all subject to irradiation (Fig. 11.6) – cosmic radiation from deep space, natural radiation in the earth and air, background radiation from nuclear weapon fallout and, increasingly, from the use of radiation and radioactive materials in industry and in diagnostic and therapeutic medicine. To this is added accidental escape from nuclear energy sources such as at Chernobyl and Sellafield.

Ionizing radiation falls into three categories: electromagnetic radiation (X-rays and γ-rays), charged particles (electrons, protons and nuclei) and uncharged particles (neutrons). External sources for the therapeutic administration of ionizing radiation include X-ray machines, electron accelerators and γ-ray sources. Internal irradiation follows the ingestion or parenteral administration of many radioactive isotopes (radionuclides) used for diagnostic or therapeutic purposes.

The emission of radiation energy is measured in roentgens. Of greater importance clinically is the amount absorbed by the targeted tissue and this is measured in Grays (Gy). The dose of radioactivity released by an isotope is measured in becquerels (Bq). This radioactivity is measured over a defined period and is determined by the rate of decay of the isotope. The half-life of an isotope is the time over which half its atoms undergo disintegration.

Physical Properties of X-rays

A brief discussion of the physical properties of X-rays helps our understanding of the various types of damage which they may produce. The intensity (I) of electromagnetic radiation at a point reduces as the distance (d) from its source increases according to the inverse square law ($I \propto 1/d^2$). As radiation passes through a material its intensity is reduced by one of three types of interaction:

(1) **The photoelectric effect** occurs when a photon interacts with an orbital electron ejecting it from the nucleus and losing most of its own energy in the process. The vacancy in the atomic shell is then filled by an electron from an outer shell, producing so-called 'characteristic' radiation. This process of photoelectric absorption (PE) is strongly dependent on the atomic number (Z) of the element or the density of the material through which the X-rays pass (PE $\propto Z^3$); absorption will therefore be greater in bone than in other soft

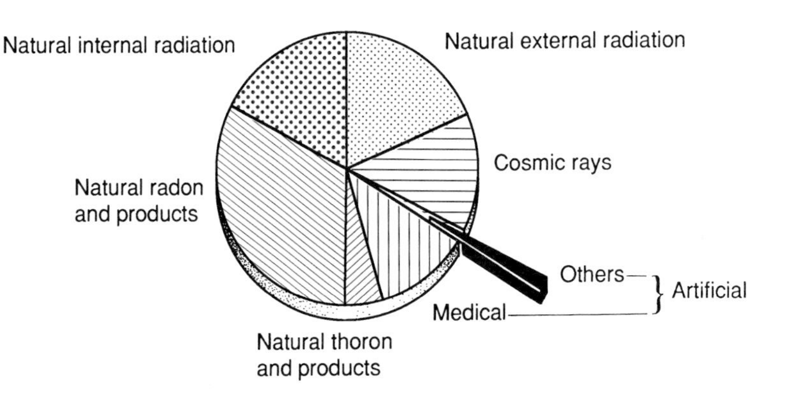

Fig. 11.6 Individuals are continuously exposed to radiation from different sources. This pie diagram shows the contributions made by each source.

tissues, a property which is exploited for X-ray diagnosis. This mode of interaction is predominant with low energy X-rays (up to 1 MeV – million electron-volts) known as superficial or orthovoltage radiation.

(2) **The Compton effect** refers to the release of loosely bound orbital electrons which leave the atoms with energy imparted from the incident photon, which then continues its passage with a reduced energy to interact with other electrons. This process is not dependent on atomic number but on electron density.

(3) At photon energies of greater than 1.02 MeV the process of **pair production** predominates, in which the incident photon disappears with the production of a positron and a negative electron which interact with surrounding cells.

Megavoltage radiation (energies higher than 1 MeV) produces its effects mainly by the process of Compton interaction. Because of its initial energy, megavoltage irradiation, unlike orthovoltage treatment, does not produce its maximum effect on the skin but at a depth where absorption interactions begin to be effective.

Until the 1960s therapeutic radiation used orthovoltage X-rays. Because of the long time scale to manifestation of late tissue injury, complications due to its increased absorption in bone and skin are still seen in clinical practice. The widespread use of megavoltage equipment coincided with the introduction of chemotherapeutic agents which may themselves modify the effect of radiation. All these factors must be considered in assessing the effects of radiation on tissues.

Biological Effects of Radiation

Mechanisms of Tissue Damage

Radiation causes cell and tissue damage by the transfer of its energy to these tissues as it passes through them. The damage may be either of excitation or ionization type. Ultraviolet-induced damage is an example of excitation type, but most irradiation-induced damage has both components. A potent *in vitro* effect of radiation is to inhibit the ability of the cells to multiply in appropriate tissue culture conditions. The percentage of cells which retain this ability, after a given dose of radiation, can easily be measured by counting the number of cellular clones in cultures of the irradiated cells. If the irradiated cells are allowed a period of 'recuperation' after the radiation insult and before cloning them, the percentage survival increases, indicating the cells' ability to repair radiation damage. The various types of radiation all give different shapes of survival curves when applied to the same tissue or cell. This is attributable to their varying abilities to transfer their energies to the tissue through which they are passing. The amount of energy transferred per micrometre of track of a particle or photon is referred to as the linear energy transfer (LET). Thus, slow moving, highly charged particles such as the α-particle produce much tissue ionization (high LET), whilst electrons move more rapidly through the tissues and give rise to more widely spaced ionization events (low LET) (Fig. 11.7). For an equal dose of

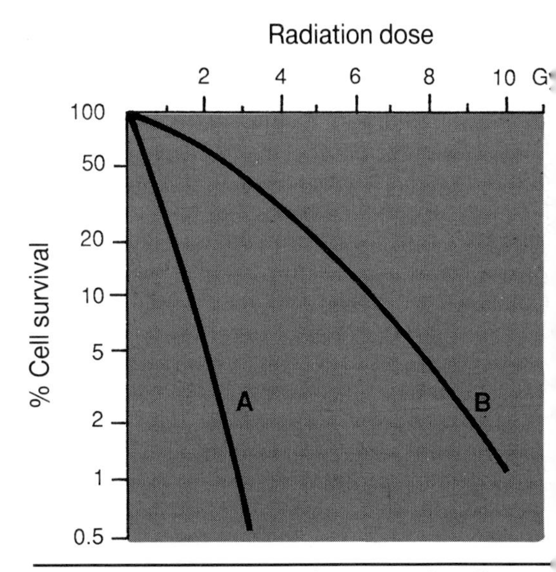

Fig. 11.7 The comparative cytotoxic effects of α-particles (A) and electrons (B).

adiation, high LET produces more biological damage than low LET.

Two theories, the target and the indirect, have been proposed to explain radiation-induced cell njury. The **target theory** proposes a direct effect, with damage to some specific sites or some specific molecules in the cells. The **indirect heory** suggests that ionization leads to the radiolysis of water with the generation of free hydroxyl adicals (OH•) which damage cell membranes, nucleic acids and cellular enzymes.

Factors Which Modify Tissue Damage

Any radiation absorbed by the body will cause damage to normal as well as abnormal cells but, in the latter, repair of damage may be less efficient and a satisfactory therapeutic ratio may be obtained. The therapeutic ratio will depend on the radiosensitivity of both the tumour being treated and the normal tissues which surround it. Thus, a lymphoma in a lymph node in the neck will require only a low dose of radiation to eradicate it and, because surrounding normal tissues can tolerate high doses, the therapeutic ratio is high. In contrast, a carcinoma of the cervix will only be eradicated by high doses of irradiation which may be poorly tolerated by the adjacent rectum.

In practice, therapeutic dosages are determined mainly by the tolerance of normal tissues (Table 11.7). This tolerance can be affected by a number of factors. Radiation damage is inversely proportional to age at treatment and special care has to be taken to minimize effects on normal tissues in children. In general, the smaller the volume of tissue being irradiated the higher the dose which can be given. If small daily fractions are used or treatment is given at a low dose rate, repair of radiation damage is possible in normal tissues and fewer acute and late side-effects will be seen. This is the rationale for radical treatment being fractionated over 6 or 7 weeks. Failure of these repair mechanisms may have serious consequences.

Higher energy X-rays will produce less skin and bone damage than orthovoltage beams. Diseases such as diabetes or atherosclerosis which impair blood supply to tissue will increase the likelihood of

Table 11.7 Critical radiation doses to different organs

	Dose (Gy) for permanent damage	Modifying factors	Effect
Bone	70	Chemotherapy	Necrosis
Epiphyses	13		Impaired growth
Soft tissues in children (breast, muscle)	20–30	Surgery	Hypoplasia
Brain	40–70	Age, treatment, volume, fraction, size, chemotherapy	Necrosis
Eye	6		Cataract
Lung	20–25	Fraction, size, chemotherapy	Pneumonitis
Kidney	12–15		Renal insufficiency, hypertension
Liver	30	Partial hepatectomy	Radiation hepatitis, veno-occlusive disease
Gonads	6–15	Chemotherapy, age	Delayed puberty, infertility
Pituitary	>40		Impairment of growth hormone production
Thyroid	>30		Hypothyroidism

Data reproduced from *Cancer in Children*, p. 41, by permission of Springer-Verlag.

overt radiation damage, as will previous surgery, because of altered blood supply. Drug–radiation interactions are of increasing importance although the late consequence of such interactions may not yet have been fully realized. Such interactions may be additive or potentiating. Examples of such interactions include adriamycin and actinomycin which affect the skin, cisplatin and bleomycin which affect the lung, and methotrexate which affects lung and gastrointestinal mucosa.

Effects of Radiation on Tissue and Cells

DNA is the cellular constituent most sensitive to radiation. Changes include the formation of pyrimidine dimers, cross-links and single- and double-stranded breaks. Repair is usually rapid but sometimes damage is irreparable and major chromosomal and chromatid alterations occur. The number of these mutations is related to the radiation dose (Fig. 11.8). These include deletions, translocations, fragmentation and adhesion breaks between chromosomes. Polyploidy and aneuploidy may be seen. Gross cytological abnormalities may be seen in biopsy material (Fig. 11.9). This radiation damage to DNA accounts for the inhibition of cell division, infertility, and somatic and germline mutations. There is increasing evidence that germline mutations may be transmitted to the children of irradiated parents and may explain the increased incidence of leukaemia in the offspring of workers in the nuclear energy industry. The problem of neoplastic transformation in irradiated cells is discussed later.

The effects produced in the body by ionizing radiation are classified as acute and late. Acute changes occur within hours or days of treatment, depending on how it is scheduled, whereas late changes occur after months or years. Acute effects are believed to be due to depletion of stem cells in an organ or tissue and will become clinically obvious when cell numbers are reduced below the levels at which regeneration can keep pace with cell death. If treatment is continued beyond this point, death of the tissue may occur and lead to

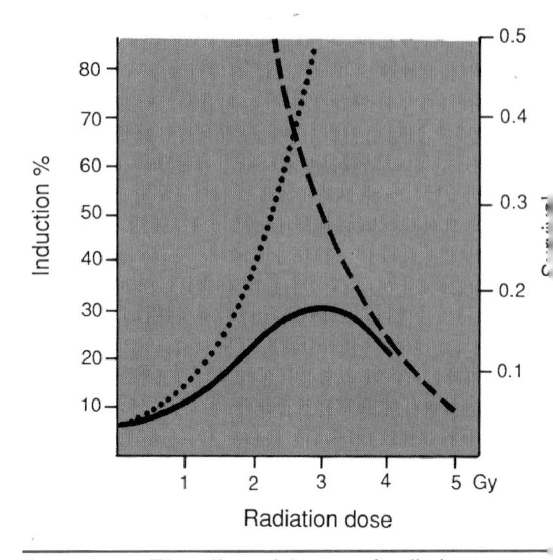

Fig. 11.8 The effect of dosage of radiation on mut tion rate in mice. As the dose is increased, the mutatio rate rises (....), but the survival rate diminishes (---- The incidence of mutation-dependent abnormalit (——), in this case leukaemia, is dependent on mutatic and survival rates.

irreversible damage. Tissues which are suscep ible to these acute effects include bone marrow skin and gastrointestinal mucosa, in which conti uous turnover of cells occurs. If time is allowed fc recovery of the tissue, further treatment can ofte be given without permanent damage.

In contrast lung, central nervous system, bone kidney and liver may show no evidence of damag by irradiation until long after the insult. Manifesta tion of the injury may be precipitated by othe factors. For example, interstitial pneumonitis a evidence of damage to the lungs by whole bod irradiation given before bone marrow transplanta tion may only be manifested when graft-versus host disease develops. Late damage in variou organs is thought largely to be related to endc thelial damage leading to intimal thickening an occlusion of blood vessels (Fig. 11.10), impair ment of blood supply and ischaemic fibrosis c necrosis. In the lung, damage to the endotheliu leads to proliferation of type II pneumocytes thickening of the basement membrane and conse quent impairment of gas exchange. Alternativ mechanisms for late damage have been propose for organs such as the liver where damage may nc

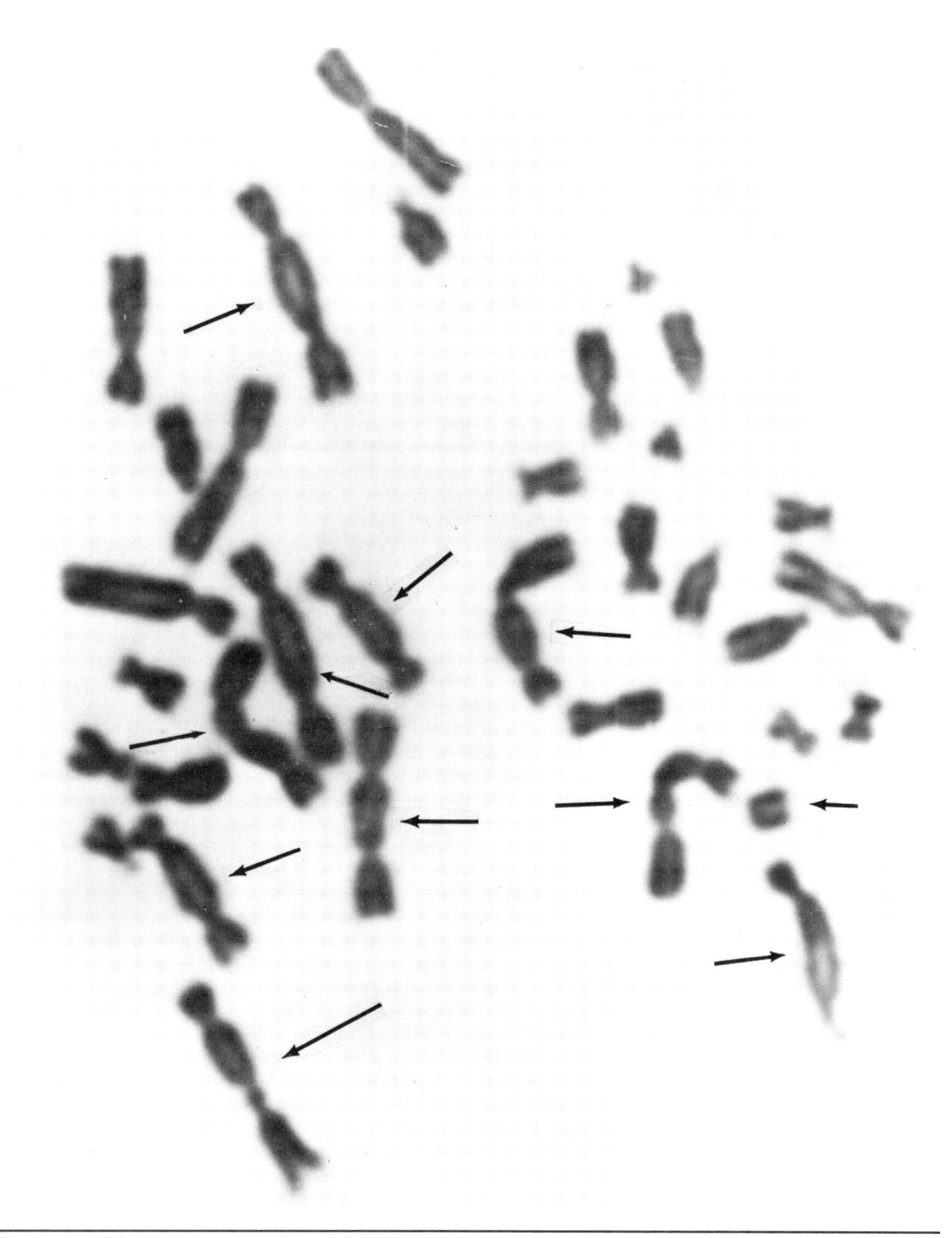

Fig. 11.9 Dividing lymphocyte in peripheral blood culture from a patient with bronchial carcinoma and spinal metastases, treated by 5 Gy of ^{60}Co radiation to the lumbar spine. This cell shows the result of extensive chromosome breakage due to radiation followed by random fusion of broken ends. There are nine dicentric chromosomes, one possible tricentric, one acricentric fragment and at least three other abnormal chromosomes. 44 centromeres can be counted, indicating elimination of two chromosomes. (Aceto-orcein stain × 200.) (Professor M. A. Ferguson Smith.)

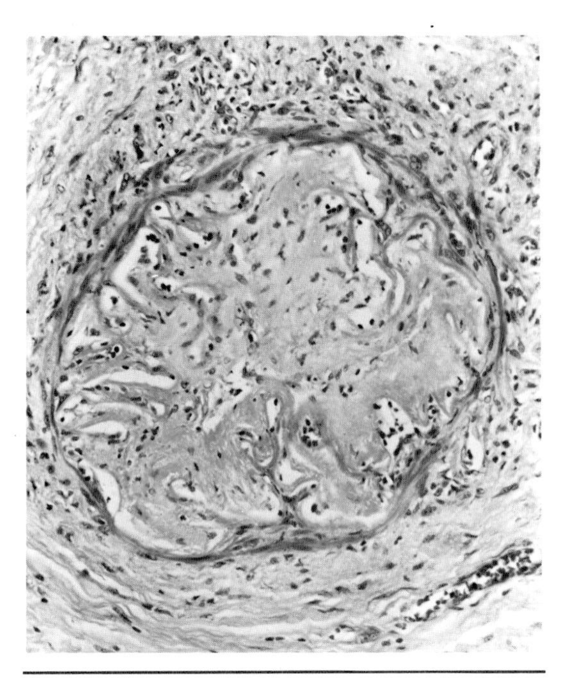

Fig. 11.10 A small artery occluded by hyaline fibrous tissue following radiotherapy. × 126.

be manifest until a stimulus to proliferation may reveal latent damage to presumed stem cells not previously required to function.

Effects of Local Irradiation

Skin and Tegmenta

Acute erythema occurs after irradiation of the skin by doses of more than 40 Gy. Occasionally, individuals may be more sensitive – those with the DNA repair defect of ataxia telangiectasia and those with fair skin and red hair, especially if of Celtic origin. *In vitro* irradiation of cultured fibroblasts from such individuals will demonstrate increased radiosensitivity. Continuation of treatment leading to superficial ulceration may delay healing for several weeks. Acute reactions may be followed after months or years by thinning and fibrosis of the skin and the development of telangiectasia, multiple tiny distorted vessels appearing in the skin. These skin reactions are not seen after megavoltage irradiation when the maximum energy deposition occurs beneath the skin.

Temporary epilation, because of damage to proliferating cells in the hair follicle, occurs after doses as low as 6 Gy but is reversible up to doses of approximately 40 Gy. Growing teeth may be damaged directly by irradiation, leading to abnormal shapes and fragile cusps. More damage occurs when the salivary glands have been irradiated: saliva secretion is reduced and is altered in quality to a viscous non-lubricating substance which promotes the development of caries.

Central Nervous System and Special Senses

In the central nervous system a transient demyelination occurs at 6–8 weeks after whole brain irradiation and gives rise to a syndrome of somnolence, while irradiation of the cervical cord gives rise to Lhermitte syndrome in which flexion of the neck produces paraesthesiae in the lower limbs. Most cases resolve spontaneously but in some, late damage may range from a poorly defined loss of intellectual function, especially in children, to transient myelitis or frank necrosis in the spinal cord. Necrosis in brain tissue is observed after high doses (in excess of 60 Gy) and after high dose/fraction treatments. It has been observed more frequently after neutron irradiation. Permanent damage to the spinal cord may be seen as transverse myelitis leading to paraplegia in severe cases. Pituitary damage may lead to endocrine hypofunction.

Radiation doses in excess of 6 Gy will produce cataract in varying percentages of patients according to its schedule of administration. It is due to damage to the proliferating cells at the margin of the lens which then fail to replace damaged cells within the lens. Radiation to the middle ear may produce deafness, perhaps because of impaired mobility and fibrosis of the ossicular bones.

Bones and Soft Tissues

Effects on these tissues are most marked after irradiation in childhood because of impaired growth. Irradiation before epiphyseal closure may lead to premature fusion and loss of growth potential so that spine or limbs are shortened. Asymmetrical irradiation may lead to failure of vertebral growth and development of scoliosis which will be worsened by the effects on surrounding muscles. Failure of muscle growth may be obvious after neck irradiation in childhood though no effect would be detectable after similar irradiation in adulthood.

After chemotherapy or irradiation of the hips, avascular necrosis may be seen, in some cases leading to pathological fracture. High doses of orthovoltage irradiation were associated with necrosis because of its preferential absorption in bone, but this is rarely seen with megavoltage treatment. Similarly, after high dose treatments, necrosis of cartilage may occur.

Damage to lymphatics produces lymphoedema with fibrosis. The most severe examples have been seen after orthovoltage irradiation to the axilla after mastectomy for carcinoma of the breast. The fibrosis may also involve the brachial plexus and lead to severe and intractable arm pain and eventually weakness. Clinically apparent damage does not occur after megavoltage irradiation unless doses of 60 Gy are exceeded.

Lungs

The lungs are very sensitive to radiation, with a tolerance dose of only 20 Gy when both lungs are treated with conventional fractionated irradiation. If single treatments are given (as during whole body irradiation for patients with leukaemia) the maximum tolerated dose is only 10 Gy. Concomitant administration of several cytotoxic drugs such as cyclophosphamide or bleomycin further diminishes tolerance. After treatment by tangential fields to the breast or direct fields to the supraclavicular fossa, radiological evidence of fibrosis is frequent though usually asymptomatic. Acute radiation pneumonitis may be seen at 1–6 weeks after treatment due to proliferation of type II pneumocytes; this can often be reversed by administration of steroids in high dosage. Later, development of fibrosis may lead to progressive impairment of gas exchange and restriction of exercise capacity.

Cardiovascular System

Acute changes to the heart are not seen after therapeutic irradiation. Late damage may be manifest by the premature development of arteriosclerosis 20–30 years after irradiation of the mediastinum, for example in patients with Hodgkin's disease.

Gastrointestinal Tract

Acute responses of the large and small bowel to radiation usually limit therapeutic doses. Diarrhoea, in severe cases with passage of blood and mucus, may necessitate discontinuing treatment after doses of 45–55 Gy. If this diarrhoea is ignored or controlled, continued irradiation will lead, in a proportion of patients, to persistent haemorrhage, diarrhoea or fistulae requiring resection of affected bowel. The severity of the acute response (diarrhoea) appears reliably to predict late damage. In some cases damage to the blood supply leads to strictures which cause obstruction. This problem may be difficult to resolve surgically since loops of bowel may be caught up in a densely fibrotic reaction throughout the abdomen or pelvis. Ulceration of the duodenum has recently been reported as a late effect of irradiation of the upper para-aortic lymph nodes.

Liver

Acute radiation damage from doses to the whole liver above 20 Gy may lead to liver cell necrosis with clinical jaundice. This may be fulminating, leading to death within 6–8 weeks or may resolve spontaneously. Veno-occlusive disease (p. 749) may occur as a late complication of smaller doses. This is seen most commonly when cytotoxic drugs such as methotrexate have been given at the same time as irradiation, and is characterized by intimal proliferation involving hepatic vein branches. It carries a mortality rate of approximately 50%.

Kidney

Functional impairment of the kidney is usually clinically important only when both kidneys are irradiated or when the remaining kidney is treated after nephrectomy. Raised amounts of β_2-microglobulin appear in the urine, indicating tubular damage, but reduced creatinine clearance is uncommon. Radiation nephritis mostly due to vascular injury occurs late, producing chronic renal failure and hypertension.

Gonads

Both male and female germ cells are sensitive to radiation injury and infertility is a frequent outcome. In the testis the interstitial cells and Sertoli cells are more radioresistant than the germ cells and survive. In the female the follicular granulosa cells are more sensitive than the germ cells.

Immune System

High dose local irradiation to the bone marrow may result in loss of activity for several months. Eventually repopulation occurs, presumably by migration of stem cells from other areas. Whole body irradiation may be given in doses of 10–15 Gy to ablate the bone marrow because rescue from the inevitable death can be obtained by infusion of harvested autologous or allogeneic marrow.

Whole body or total nodal irradiation has a profound effect on immune competence. Lymphocyte counts fall within 24 hours of irradiation and remain low for 18–24 months; macrophage populations are obliterated but recover after 6–8 weeks and immunoglobulin production is impaired for up to one year. Irradiation-induced lymphopenia is useful in preventing allograft rejection or graft-versus-host disease. It has also been used with limited success in the treatment of intractable rheumatoid arthritis and ankylosing spondylitis.

Other Organs

Damage to the **pancreas** is rare and produces malabsorption. The **thyroid** is very sensitive, and hypothyroidism is common after even low doses of radiation although increased pituitary activity (TSH) may compensate for this. Fibrosis in the **bladder** can seriously reduce its capacity, and telangiectasia results in troublesome haematuria.

Second Tumours

Ionizing radiation is a recognized cause of cancer (p. 405). Malignancy may develop in up to 3% of patients treated with radiation. The incidence is increased when chemotherapy is also given. The majority of tumours occur within the site of previous irradiation, i.e. cancer of the rectum after successful treatment of carcinoma of the cervix. In some instances, a pre-existing genetic abnormality predisposes to cancer induction and is associated with specific tumour types such as bone sarcomas. In other situations, familial clusters of cancers are found. Lymphoproliferative disorders are the commonest type of second tumour occurring in patients who have been immunosuppressed for long periods following systemic irradiation.

Total Body Radiation

Although relatively large doses of radiation (>40 Gy) can be used to treat local lesions, only 1–3 Gy whole body exposure produces acute radiation syndromes. In some cases the lethal dose of radiation may be as low as 2 Gy while in the absence of medical treatment doses of 7 Gy are uniformly fatal.

The features of the *haemopoietic syndrome* which occurs with doses between 2 and 5 Gy include lymphopenia, neutropenia and thrombocytopenia with anaemia occurring later. After exposure to doses of radiation between 5 and 10 Gy the *gastrointestinal syndrome* occurs with nausea, vomiting and diarrhoea leading to vascular collapse and death within 3 days. Sepsis is common. When exposed to doses of above 50 Gy listlessness, drowsiness, convulsions, coma and death occur within 1–2 hours – the *cerebral syndrome*. Survivors of whole body radiation exposure have a high incidence of leukaemias, lymphoma and solid tumours, particularly of thyroid, lung, breast and bone.

Further Reading

Adverse Drug Reactions

D'Arcy, P. F. and Griffin, J. P. (1986). *Iatrogenic Diseases*, 3rd edn. Oxford University Press, Oxford.

Davies, D. M. (1981). *Textbook of Adverse Drug Reactions*. Oxford University Press, Oxford.

Griffin, J. P. (1988). *Manual of Adverse Drug Interactions*, 3rd edn. J. Wright, Bristol.

Hayes, A. W. (1982). *Principles and Methods in Toxicology*. Raven Press, New York.

Meyler, L. (1988). *Side Effects of Drugs: Encyclopaedia of Adverse Reactions and Interactions*, ed. M. M. G. Dukes. Elsevier, Amsterdam.

Reid, J. L., Rubin, P. C. and Whiting, B. (1992). *Lecture Notes in Clinical Pharmacology*, 4th edn. Blackwell Scientific Publications, Oxford.

Riddell, R. H. (1982). *Pathology of Drug-induced and Toxic Disease*. Churchill Livingstone, Edinburgh, London, New York.

Stockley, I. H. (1982). *Drug Interactions*. Blackwell Scientific Publications, Oxford.

Drug Dependence

Bickel, W. K., Stitzer, M. L., Liebson, I. A. and Bigelow, G. E. (1988). Acute physical dependence in man: effects of naloxone after brief morphine exposure. *Journal of Pharmacology and Experimental Therapy*, **244**, 126–32.

Drug Abuse Briefing (1988). 3rd edition. Published by the Institute for the Study of Drug Dependence, 1 Hatton Place, London, EC1N 8ND.

Jaffe, J. H. (1985). In *Goodman and Gilman's The Pharmacological Basis of Therapeutics*, 7th edn, pp. 532–81, eds A. G. Gilman, L. S. Goodman and F. Murad. Macmillan, New York, London.

Laurence, D. R. and Bennett, P. N. (1987). *Clinical Pharmacology*, 6th edn, pp. 301–432. Churchill Livingstone, Edinburgh, London, New York.

Liskow, B. I. and Goodwin, D. W. (1987). Pharmacological treatment of alcohol intoxication, withdrawal and dependence: a critical review. *Journal of Studies in Alcoholism* **48**, 356–70.

Portnow, J. M. and Strassman, H. D. (1985). Medically induced drug addiction. *International Journal of Addiction* **20**, 605–11.

Radiation-induced Tissue Injury

Casarett, C. W. (1980). *Radiation Histopathology*. CRC Press Inc., Boca Raton, Florida.

Hall, E. (1972). *Radiobiology for the Radiobiologist*. Lippincott Publishers, Philadelphia.

Schwartz, E. E. (Ed.) (1983). *Biological Basis of Radiotherapy*. Elsevier Publications, Amsterdam.

Walter, J., Miller, H. and Bomford, C. K. (1976). *A Further Textbook of Radiotherapy*. Churchill Livingstone, Edinburgh, London, New York.

12

Cardiovascular System

Blood Vessels and Lymphatics

Arteries

Normal structure of arteries. The walls of arteries are composed of three coats (Fig. 12.1a): the innermost, or **intima**, consists of the endothelium separated by a thin layer of loose connective tissue from the internal elastic lamina – a thick fenestrated cylinder of elastic fibres which appears in histological sections as a wavy line but which is kept taut *in vivo* by the blood pressure. The **media** consists of a tight spiral of smooth muscle cells which lie in a meshwork of elastic and collagen fibres. The amount of stroma increases with vessel size: in the arterioles and smallest arteries it is very scanty, while in the aorta and larger arteries its volume exceeds that of the smooth musc... component. An external elastic lamina separates the media from the **adventitia**, a thin layer of loosely arranged collagen and elastic fibres, rich in lymphatics and traversed by the nerves which supply the medial smooth muscle.

All layers of the smallest arteries and arterioles are supplied with oxygen and nutrients, by diffusion from the lumen. Larger arteries have small

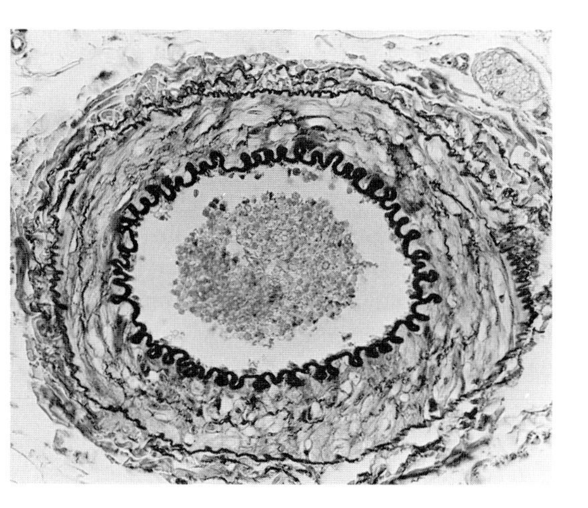

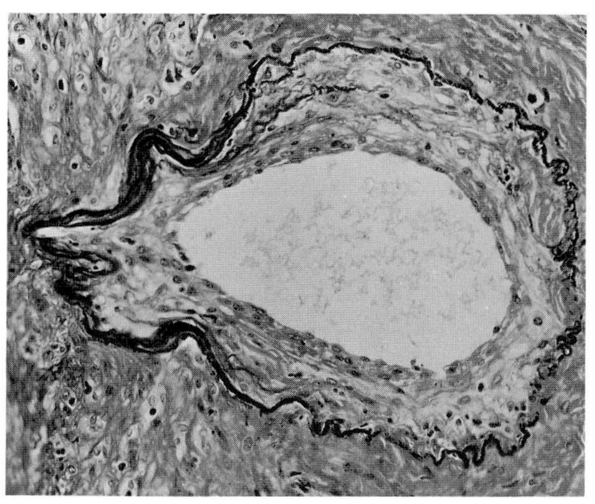

Fig. 12.1 **a** Normal medium sized artery in transverse section. The internal and external elastic laminae are seen as black wavy bands. ×10. **b** Endarteritis obliterans in a leg artery proximal to an old amputation. The internal elastic lamina marks the outer limit of the thickened fibrous intima. ×15.

vessels, the **vasa vasorum**, which supply the adventitia and outer part of the media, while the inner part of the wall depends on diffusion from the lumen for nourishment.

The differences in structure of the media of arteries of various sizes are reflected in their functions. The large elastic arteries absorb part of the force of left ventricular systole and their recoil helps to sustain the pressure for continued blood flow during diastole. The smaller arteries and arterioles (**resistance vessels**) regulate the overall arterial pressure and the blood flow to individual organs and tissues: these functions are reflected in the predominance of smooth muscle in the media. This smooth muscle has a rich autonomic innervation which, together with circulating levels of vasoactive hormones and factors produced by the endothelial cells, controls the calibre.

The smooth muscle cells of the media are not only contractile, they also synthesize the matrix proteins of the artery, the principal ones being collagen, elastin and proteoglycans. In disease states such as hypertension, atheroma and in response to injury, the smooth muscle cells undergo hypertrophy, divide and synthesize increased amounts of matrix. They also migrate through the fenestra of the internal elastic lamina into the intima where they may multiply and synthesize extracellular matrix proteins.

The endothelium is not a passive non-wettable lining (Fig. 12.2); it regulates the activity of platelets and has an important role in modulating both coagulation and fibrinolytic systems (p. 84). The endothelium also directly regulates vascular tone by secreting the vasodilator **endothelium derived relaxant factor** (EDRF), whose action is counterbalanced by the secretion of the vasoconstrictor peptide **endothelin**, currently the most potent vasoconstrictor known. The discovery that the endothelial cell may secrete at least 30 biologically active agents has stimulated a flood of research into its reactions in health and disease.

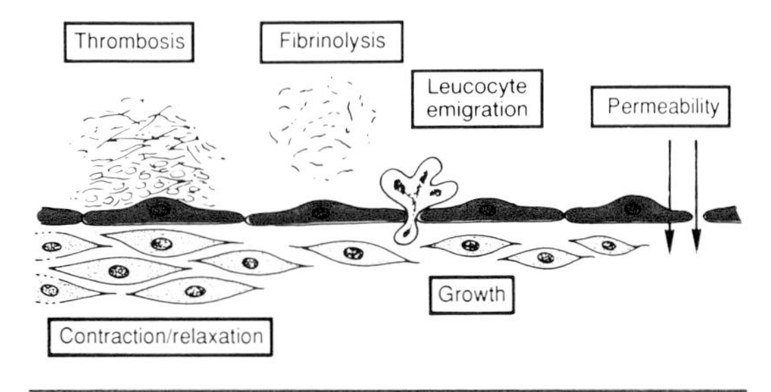

Fig. 12.2 A diagram showing some endothelial cell functions which are important in vascular physiology and in the reactions of blood vessels in disease. Subendothelial smooth muscle cells are also shown; their contraction/relaxation and growth may also be modified by endothelial cells (see text).

Effects of ageing. The structure of all arteries changes progressively with advancing age, changes which constitute **arteriosclerosis**. The intima becomes thickened and fibrosed, sometimes with reduplication of the internal elastic lamina. The smooth muscle and elastic fibres of the media are partly replaced by collagen. This results in increased rigidity and tortuosity of the walls, features well seen in the prominent temporal and brachial arteries of some elderly people. The increased rigidity contributes to the age-related increase in systolic and pulse pressures, but otherwise arteriosclerosis is of little clinical significance.

The walls of arterioles become thickened due to accumulation of plasma proteins in the vessel wall, so-called plasmatic vasculosis. This is followed by deposition of collagen. The histological appearance is termed **hyaline* arteriolosclerosis** and is particularly prominent in the arterioles of the spleen and the afferent arterioles of the glomeruli. If severe, it may result in narrowing of the lumen. Changes similar to those of ageing occur in the arteries and arterioles in persistent hypertension and in diabetes mellitus. However, in both conditions the changes develop earlier in life and progress more rapidly.

Compensatory changes. The muscular and elastic nature of the arterial wall readily allows it to adjust to variation in blood flow. This may be physiological, as in the increased blood flow in the uterine arteries during pregnancy. These vessels dilate, their wall becomes thickened with an increase in elastic fibres and an increase in the size and number of medial smooth muscle cells. Similar changes occur in the arterial wall in hypertension (p. 458).

Persistent reduction in blood flow results in a process of **involution**. Examples are found in the arteries in the stump following amputation of a limb. In the artery wall smooth muscle and elastic tissue are partially replaced by hyaline collagen. The lumen is further reduced by thickening of the intima, a process termed **endarteritis**: medial smooth muscle cells migrate into the intima and proliferate to form a thick concentric layer which gradually becomes fibrosed (Fig. 12.1b). Endarteritis also occurs in arteries exposed to chronic inflammation, for example in the base of a peptic ulcer, and this obliteration may prevent serious haemorrhage. However, the endarteritis of tuberculous meningitis (p. 826) or syphilis (p. 316), or following radiotherapy (p. 434) can cause serious effects due to ischaemia.

* (from the Greek 'hyalos' meaning glass; hyaline is applied to homogeneous, refractile (glassy), usually eosinophilic material on light microscopy).

Atheroma

In most developed countries atheroma is responsible for more deaths than any other disease. It causes narrowing of the lumens of arteries, is often complicated by occlusive thrombosis, and is the main cause of disability and death from heart disease, of cerebral infarction and of ischaemia of the lower limbs and gut. It is virtually always present in some degree in middle-aged and old people in most industrialized Western countries.

The lesions of atheroma consist of patches (**plaques**) of intimal thickening of arteries, due mainly to accumulation of lipids, proliferation of smooth muscle cells, and formation of fibrous tissue. The alternative term atherosclerosis is sometimes used because the lesion has a soft, lipid-rich part ('athere', porridge) and a hard (sclerotic) fibrous component. The shorter term **atheroma** has historical priority and is less easily confused with the quite separate process of arteriosclerosis.

Macroscopic Appearances

The earliest deposits of lipid in the intima of the aorta and large arteries occur predominantly in childhood and adolescence and are known as **fatty streaks**. They appear as yellow, slightly raised areas on the luminal surface, which enlarge and coalesce to form irregular yellow streaks. They consist of accumulations of lipid droplets beneath the endothelium, both free and as aggregates within macrophages (Fig. 12.3). Fatty streaks are almost invariably present at autopsy in the aortas of children and adolescents, and their presence and extent bear no relationship to the incidence of atheroma in older members of the community; some regress, but it is possible that some of them persist and progress to atheroma. By contrast, the incidence and extent of fatty streaks in the coronary arteries of young people correlate with the amount and severity of atheroma in the community and they may represent the early stage of this disease. Other lesions which may precede atheroma include foci of intimal oedema and increase in ground substance, termed **gelatinous patches**, and small intimal thickenings composed of smooth muscle cells, collagen and other extracellular matrix proteins (**intimal cushions**) which occur at the branching points of arteries.

In atheroma-prone communities, the earliest atheromatous lesions occur from young adulthood onwards. In large arteries they consist of small, disc-like, slightly raised patches of intimal thickening with a smooth glistening surface. The patches enlarge and thicken by further deposition of lipid deep in the intima and by fibrosis more superficially (i.e. adjacent to the lumen). When viewed from the intimal surface, these raised plaques may appear yellow or white, depending on the amount of white fibrous tissue overlaying the yellow lipid deposits. In any individual, the patches vary in size and thickness, reflecting their development and slow growth throughout adult life.

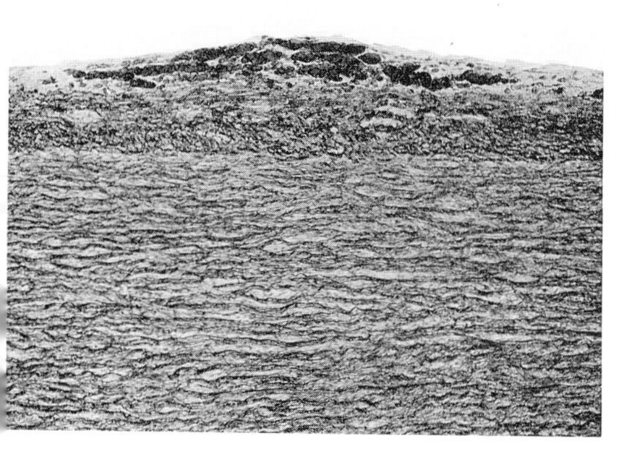

Fig. 12.3 Section of the aorta of a child showing a fatty streak. (Frozen section: lipid stained black.) ×20.

Aorta. Atheroma occurs mainly in the abdominal aorta, often developing first around the origins of the intercostal and lumbar branches (Fig. 12.4). Severe atheroma of the thoracic aorta is unusual except in diabetics in whom atheroma is often extensive and severe. The patches vary in size up to several centimetres in diameter and may become confluent (Fig. 12.5). If a large patch is cut across, lipid-rich, paste-like material can be expressed from its deeper part, and fibrous thickening is seen as a white layer overlying this. The proportions of lipid and fibrous tissue, however, vary considerably. The plaque may crack or ulcerate and thrombus is then deposited on the surface. Calcification may convert the plaque to a hard brittle plate. Plaques showing ulceration, calcification or thrombus deposition are referred to as **complicated atheroma**, and may produce great irregularity of the luminal surface of the aorta (Fig. 12.5). The plaques may erode into the media, causing weakening of the wall; an aneurysm may develop, with the danger of rupture. Plaques developing adjacent to the origin of the mesenteric, the renal or other arteries may seriously narrow the ostia of these vessels and cause ischaemia.

Other arteries. Atheroma occurs in arteries of all sizes down to approximately 2 mm diameter. The general features are similar to those in the aorta. However, in smaller vessels atheroma often involves the whole circumference of the artery, causing degrees of luminal narrowing down to virtual occlusion. The narrowing may be concentric or eccentric (Figs. 12.6, 12.7). Atheroma tends to affect especially the coronary and cerebral arteries and the arteries to the legs. There may be considerable variation in the distribution of atheroma; in some instances the aorta is mainly affected, in others the cerebral arteries and/or the coronary arteries. The coronary arteries are more

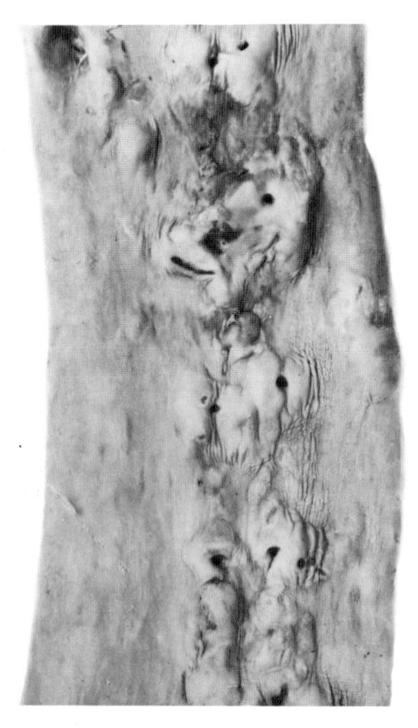

a

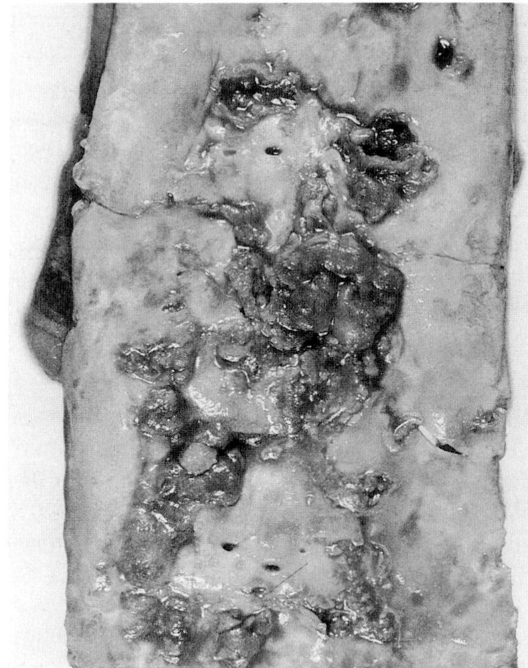

b

Fig. 12.4 **a** Mild atheroma of the abdominal aorta. The lesions are seen as raised patches and are located mainly around the origins of the arterial branches. ×0.8. **b** Complicated atheroma showing ulceration of plaques with superimposed thrombus formation.

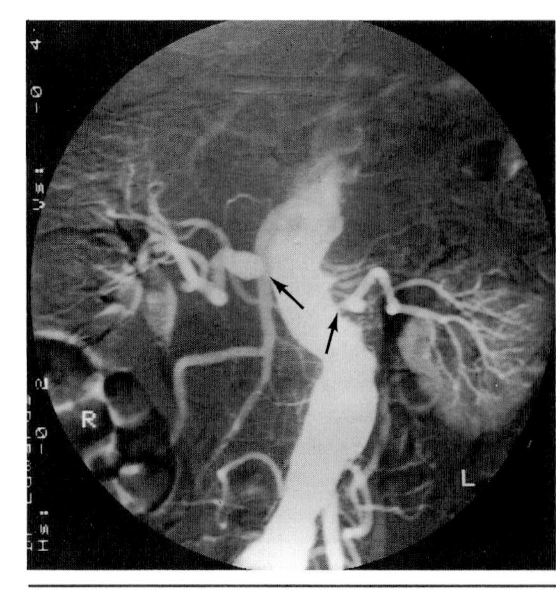

Fig. 12.5 Aortogram showing distortion of the abdominal aorta due to atheroma. In addition note that there is bilateral renal artery stenosis (arrows).

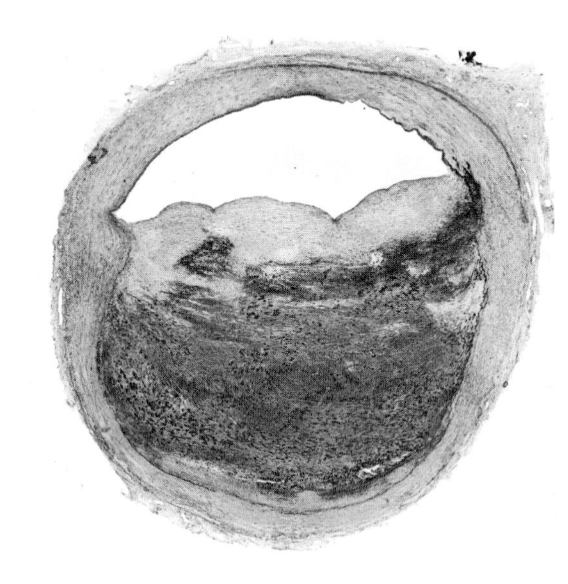

Fig. 12.6 Severe atheroma of the superior mesenteric artery causing eccentric narrowing of the lumen. The lipid in the plaque is stained dark.

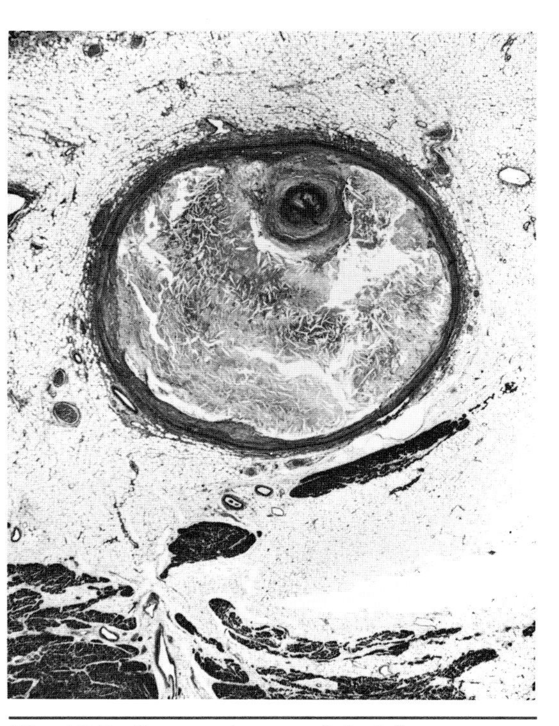

Fig. 12.7 Severe atheroma of the left coronary artery in a patient with myxoedema. The lumen has been greatly narrowed by atheroma and occluded by recent superadded thrombus, which appears dark. ×10.

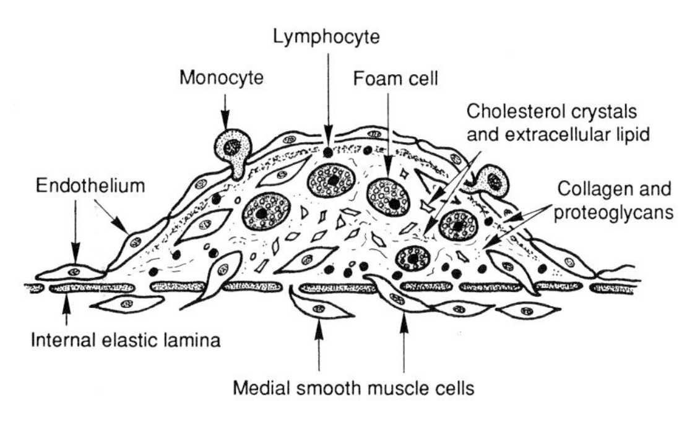

Fig. 12.8 A diagram of an early atheromatous plaque showing the constituent cells. The foam cells are derived from two sources: from smooth muscle cells which migrate into the intima from the media and from macrophages derived from circulating monocytes. The cellular interactions are indicated in Fig. 12.13.

often involved at an early age than any other vessels. Severe atheroma of the cerebral arteries is found chiefly in the elderly. Usually only the first few centimetres of the mesenteric arteries are affected, and the leg arteries are frequently severely affected.

Microscopic Appearances

The early changes are due to the proliferation of smooth muscle cells in the intima and the accumulation of lipids in 'foam cells'. These are of two lineages: some are macrophages derived from monocytes which adhere to and then penetrate the endothelium, and others are medial smooth muscle cells which proliferate and migrate into the intima (Fig. 12.8). The macrophages and the smooth muscle cells absorb lipid and their cytoplasm becomes swollen with lipid globules (Fig. 12.9a). Extracellular lipids also accumulate deep in the intima (i.e. close to the media) in relation to elastic fibres and the internal elastic lamina. As the patch develops, thin strands of connective tissue appear subendothelially and between the foam cells and form the fibrous part of the lesion. Areas of necrosis develop in the deeper part of the lesion, converting it to a structureless accumulation of extracellular lipids, cholesterol crystals and tissue debris. Infiltration by neutrophil polymorphs and other inflammatory cells is common (Fig. 12.9b).

The internal elastic lamina is eventually disrupted and lipid deposition, necrosis and fibrosis then erode into the adjacent media. As the plaque thickens, the underlying media becomes thin and atrophic. Small blood vessels grow into the atheromatous plaque from the vasa vasorum and also from the lumen and these vessels may haemorrhage, contributing altered blood constituents to the plaque contents. Some plaques may crack or rupture, causing haemorrhage into the plaque and leading to the formation of thrombus. This sequence of development is shown diagrammatically in Fig. 12.10 and in Fig. 12.44.

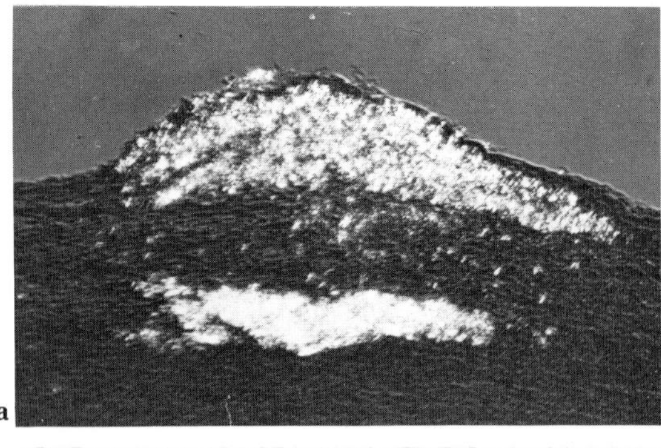

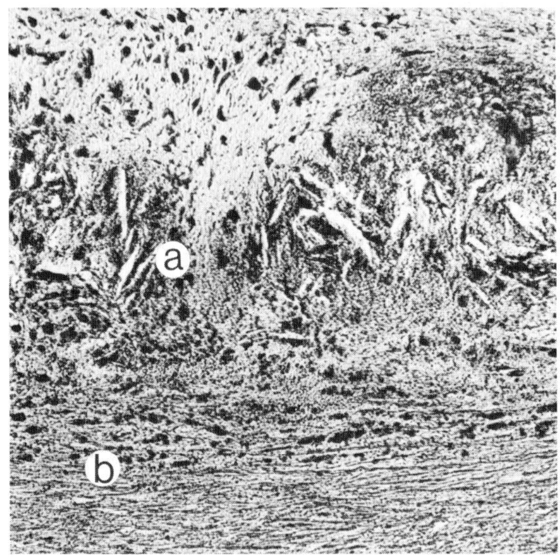

Fig. 12.9 **a** Doubly refractile intimal cholesterol and cholesterol esters in early atheroma of the aorta photographed by polarized light. **b** Section showing part of an atheromatous plaque of the aorta. In the deep part of the intima there is degenerate lipid-rich material (a), the spindle-shaped spaces being due to cholesterol crystals. Lipid accumulation stops fairly abruptly at the junction with the media (b). ×110.

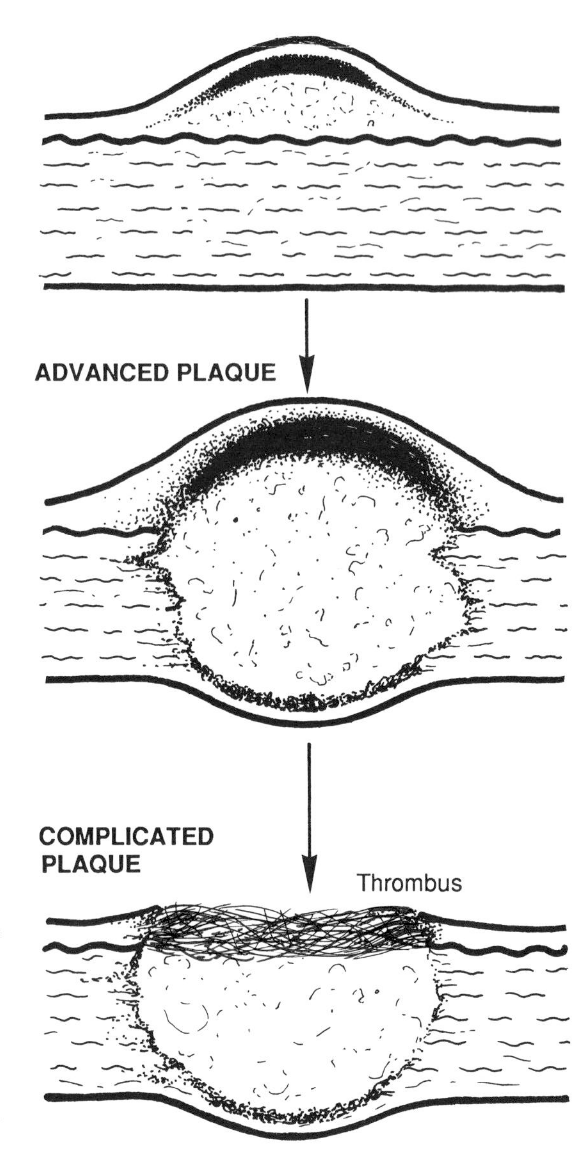

Fig. 12.10 The development of an atheromatous plaque. The early plaque is a slightly raised intimal lesion. The advanced lipid plaque erodes into the media, producing necrosis. The thickening of the wall causes atrophy of the remaining smooth muscle. If the fibrous cap ruptures, the plaque becomes a complicated plaque with superimposed thrombus (see Fig. 12.4).

Clinical Effects

The effects of atheroma are summarized in Table 12.1. They vary depending on the size of artery involved. Uncomplicated atheroma of large arteries usually has no clinical effects because it does not reduce the lumen significantly or seriously weaken the wall. In advanced cases, however, an **aneurysm** may form (p. 471). Mural thrombus seldom causes complete occlusion of the aorta except at or near its bifurcation, with resulting coldness and weakness of the legs, muscle wasting and sexual impotence (Leriche syndrome). Frag-

Table 12.1 Clinical complications of atheroma

Ischaemic heart disease (p. 488)
Sudden death
Angina pectoris
Myocardial infarction
Cardiac arrhythmias
Cardiac failure
Cerebral ischaemia (p. 817)
Transient cerebral ischaemic attacks
Dementia
Cerebral infarction
Mesenteric ischaemia (p. 720)
'Abdominal claudication'
Malabsorption syndrome
Bowel infarction
Peripheral vascular disease
Intermittent claudication
Gangrene
Renovascular hypertension (p. 464)
Renal artery stenosis
Aneurysms
Aorta (p. 471)
Iliac and popliteal arteries
Cerebral vessels (p. 823)

ments of thrombi and atheromatous debris from ulcerated plaques may, however, form emboli which lodge in arteries of the legs and abdominal organs such as the gut, kidneys and spleen.

The most important effects of atheroma are due to involvement of smaller arteries. The lumen may be progressively narrowed by an atheromatous plaque causing chronic ischaemia, or suddenly occluded by thrombosis which often causes infarction. In smaller arteries, thrombosis is often precipitated by a crack in the fibrous cap rather than complete ulceration of the plaque. Since the most important effect of this is coronary artery thrombosis this process is discussed in more detail on p. 489. Atheroma is the chief cause of **ischaemic heart disease**, the largest single cause of death in the developed countries. **Cerebrovascular disease** is also very common, the result of atheroma of the carotid, vertebral and intracerebral arteries (p. 818). Aneurysms are not a complication of atheroma of the smaller arteries, except occasionally in the arteries of the circle of Willis (p. 823).

The leg arteries are often severely atheromatous, especially in diabetics and in cigarette smokers, causing **peripheral vascular disease**. A collateral circulation initially develops but eventually this becomes inadequate: relative muscle ischaemia can then be induced by exercise producing severe pain in the leg, relieved by rest – **intermittent claudication**. In time, ischaemia may become so severe as to cause gangrene, which usually starts in the toes and spreads proximally. The arteries of the arm are seldom severely affected by atheroma; this may be due to their lower pulse pressure with a consequent reduction in haemodynamic stress.

Aetiology and Risk Factors

Atheroma has been the subject of an enormous amount of investigation. Approaches to elucidating its aetiology are difficult, for it has usually been present for many years before symptoms develop. Investigations have been mainly along three lines: (1) epidemiological studies have been used to detect risk factors, i.e. factors which are associated with an increase or decrease in the risk of developing atheroma; (2) intervention trials have been conducted to determine whether altering the risk factors, for example by modifying the diet, stopping cigarette smoking, or reducing cholesterol concentration with lipid-lowering drugs reduces the subsequent incidence of severe atheroma and its complications; and (3) biomedical laboratory research, including the experimental production of atheroma-like lesions in animals, and the study of cells *in vitro* have aimed at detecting the pathogenetic mechanisms involved in the development and growth of atheromatous plaques.

Epidemiological investigations require some grading of atheroma in communities and in individuals, but hitherto there have been no simple methods of detecting the disease unless it gives rise to symptoms. Recently, however, angiographic methods have been used to assess the results of intervention studies. Autopsy studies indicate a good general correlation between ischaemic heart disease (IHD), both fatal and non-fatal, and the severity of atheroma. It is customary, therefore, to regard IHD as an indicator of the extent of atheroma in a community and to search for risk factors associated with the age-adjusted mortality rates from IHD which are known for many countries. Risk factors are recognized by demonstrating a statistically significant association between exposure and disease. A list of some 240 risk factors for IHD have been compiled from numerous investigations but we will deal with only the major independent ones of which age, sex, hyperlipidaemia, hypertension, cigarette smoking and diabetes are the most important.

Age and Sex

Atheroma progresses slowly throughout adult life. It is not an inevitable accompaniment of ageing, but all the evidence suggests that the causal factors exert their effects over a long period, and that duration of exposure to them is of major importance. A lower incidence of IHD in women until after the menopause has been observed in all communities studied. It reflects the slower progress of atheroma in premenopausal women than in men, and is likely to have a hormonal basis, although this has not been identified.

Hyperlipidaemia

The presence of lipids and cholesterol in atheromatous plaques has already been described. Conditions which are associated with hyperlipidaemia often predispose to the development of atheroma which may be premature and of increased severity. Cholesterol and other lipids are relatively insoluble and circulate as lipoprotein particles. Each particle comprises a hydrophobic lipid core containing free and esterified cholesterol and triglyceride and an outer hydrophilic layer in which phospholipid and apolipoproteins are present. Apolipoproteins are ligands which bind to receptors on cells. They are divided into groups which are labelled alphabetically (Apo-A, B, C etc.) within which there are subclasses labelled numerically (Apo-A1, Apo-A2 etc). The major lipoproteins and some of their features are listed in Table 12.2 (also shown in Table 7.5). They show decreasing size and increasing density from the chylomicrons through very low density lipoproteins (VLDL) and low density lipoprotein (LDL) to high density lipoprotein (HDL); within each lipoprotein group the lipoprotein particles also vary in size. The cells have receptors for apolipoproteins; lipoproteins can be internalized by endocytosis and metabolized, or they can be modified by enzymes on the cell surface.

Lipid Metabolism

The two metabolic pathways involved in the transport and metabolism of cholesterol are outlined in Fig. 12.11. The exogenous pathway involves dietary fats and commences in the intestine while the endogenous pathway involves synthesis and processing in the liver and other tissues.

Table 12.2 Features of the various lipoproteins

Particle	Diameter (nm)	Approximate triglyceride/cholesterol ratio and cholesterol content (%)	Apolipoprotein
Chylomicron	80–1200	20:1 (<5%)	A-1, A-2, A-4, B-48 and C
Very low density lipoprotein (VLDL)	30–80	3:1 (25%)	B-48, C, E
Intermediate density lipoprotein (IDL)	25–35	2:3 (40%)	B-100, E
Low density, lipoprotein (LDL)	15–25	1:5 (65%)	B-100
High density lipoprotein (HDL)	5–15	1:4 (<20%)	A-1, A-2, C

Exogenous pathway. In the intestine, fatty acids and cholesterol are produced by digestion of food, and some cholesterol is derived from the bile (p. 786). These lipids are absorbed into the intestinal epithelial cells where they are re-esterified to form cholesterol esters and triglycerides and are packed into chylomicrons. The chylomicrons are carried in the lymph from the gut and enter the circulation via the thoracic duct. The enzyme lipoprotein lipase, on capillary endothelial cells, hydrolyses the triglycerides into glycerol and fatty acids. The fatty acids are taken up by adipose tissue and muscle while the cholesterol-containing remnants are ingested by hepatocytes via chylomicron remnant receptors, the number of which, unlike LDL receptors (Fig. 12.12), is not influenced by the amount of cholesterol in the hepatocyte. The apolipoproteins are catabolized and the cholesterol released. The outcome of this pathway is to deliver triglycerides derived from food to adipose tissue and to muscle and to supply cholesterol to the liver.

Endogenous pathways. The liver is the principal site of endogenous lipid synthesis. Hepatocytes synthesize triglycerides and cholesterol and, as we have seen, cholesterol is also derived from the metabolism of chylomicron remnants. Some of the cholesterol goes into the bile with bile acids and some is secreted with the blood as VLDL. In a way similar to chylomicron metabolism, the triglycerides of VLDL are removed by lipoprotein lipase in fat and muscle. The resulting residue ('VLDL remnant') contains both cholesterol and triglycerides and is known as intermediate density lipoprotein (IDL). Some IDL is rapidly taken up by the liver while the rest is converted to LDL by

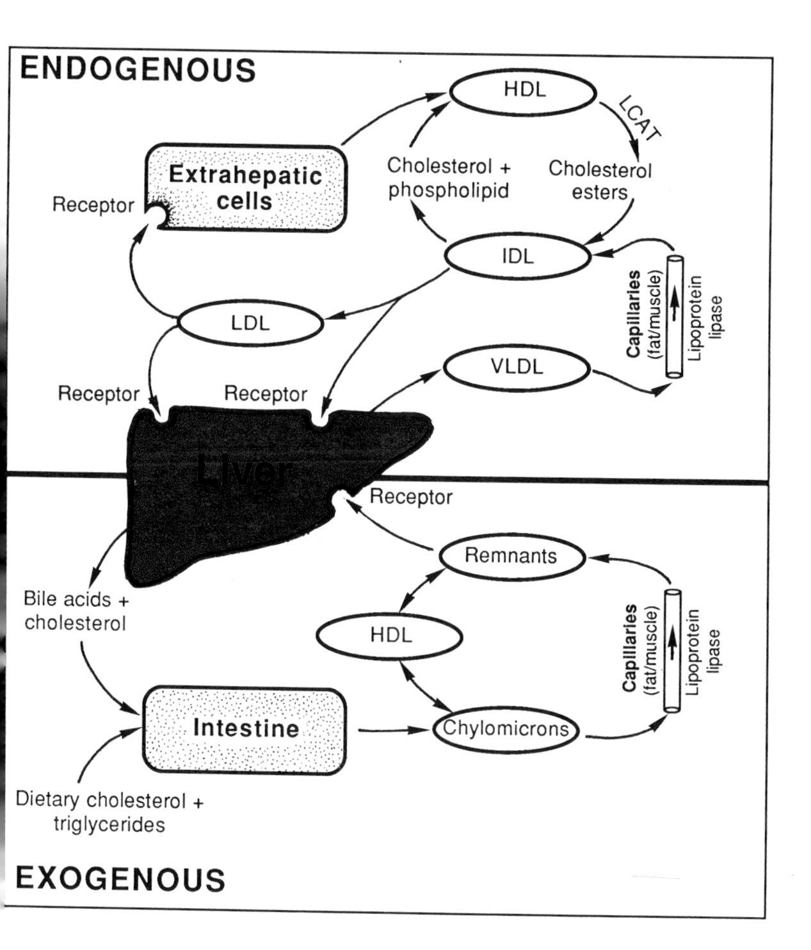

Fig. 12.11 Some of the exogenous and endogenous pathways for metabolism of lipoproteins. These are discussed at length in the text. The action of LCAT (lecithin cholesterol acetyltransferase) on HDL occurs in the plasma. VLDL – very low density lipoprotein; LDL – low density lipoprotein; IDL – intermediate density lipoprotein; HDL – high density lipoprotein.

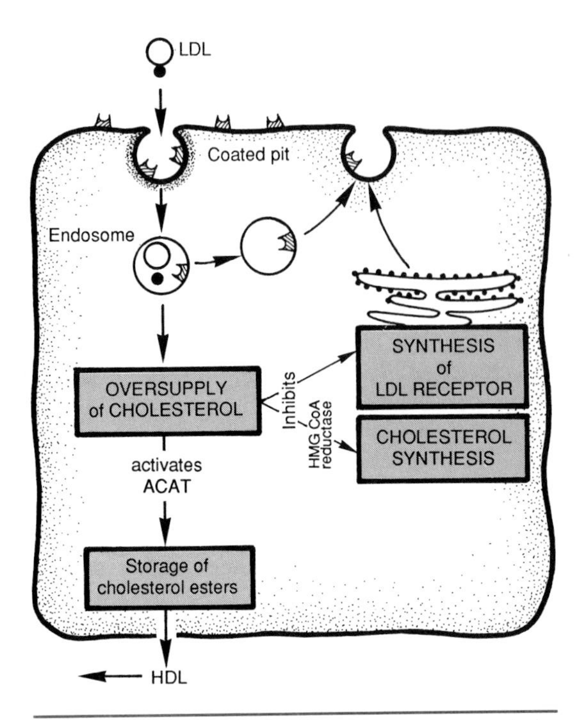

Fig. 12.12 Circulating LDL is internalized by receptor-mediated endocytosis into endosomes where the receptor dissociates and is recycled. Lysosomal enzymes then break down the apolipoprotein and unesterified cholesterol is released into the cytoplasm. Intracellular cholesterol level is controlled by three mechanisms: (1) inhibition of the enzyme HMG CoA reductase (3-hydroxy-3-methyl-glutamyl CoA reductase) which decreases cholesterol synthesis; (2) inhibition of LDL receptor synthesis; (3) activation of the enzyme ACAT (acyl cholesterol acetyltransferase) which esterifies cholesterol for intracellular storage and possibly subsequent removal from the cell.

removal of the remaining triglycerides and Apo-E at a site which remains to be determined.

The LDL is responsible for 70% of the measured levels of cholesterol in the blood. Most cells possess receptors for LDL which provides most of the cholesterol required for cell membrane and steroid synthesis. Receptor-mediated endocytosis and probably other pathways are involved in the cellular uptake of LDL. The liver possesses by far the greatest number of LDL receptors and 75% of plasma LDL is removed by hepatocytes. Thus, the level of cholesterol in the blood is largely controlled by its removal via LDL receptors in the liver.

The number of receptors on each hepatocyte is regulated by the cholesterol content of the cell (Fig. 12.12). Increasing the cholesterol content of hepatocytes switches off the synthesis of LDL receptors, thereby causing a rise in the plasma LDL levels. Conversely, low cholesterol absorption causes increase in hepatocyte LDL receptors and lowers the blood LDL levels. This can also be achieved by interrupting the enterohepatic circulation of bile acids (p. 786). When the reabsorption of bile acids from the bowel is prevented, the hepatocytes increase the conversion of cholesterol to bile acids, intracellular cholesterol falls and the synthesis of hepatocyte LDL receptors increases. This lowers blood cholesterol by increased hepatocyte LDL uptake. This knowledge is important in devising strategies to treat hyperlipidaemias.

HDL is synthesized mainly in the small intestine and in hepatocytes. HDL also takes up cholesterol from cells and other lipoproteins. In the blood, lecithin cholesterol acyl transferase (LCAT) esterifies the cholesterol. The cholesterol esters are then transferred by cholesterol ester transfer protein (CETP) to LDL and taken up by the liver. Thus, HDL is important in the transport of cholesterol from peripheral tissues to the liver.

A novel lipoprotein (a) which has similar electrophoretic mobility to LDL and contains a unique apolipoprotein (a) has recently been found to predict the risk of IHD. There are raised serum levels of lipoprotein (a) in familial hypercholesterolaemia. However, a raised plasma level of lipoprotein (a) confers a high risk of IHD, even when LDL and other lipids are normal. Lipoprotein (a) shows partial sequence homology with plasminogen. It has been suggested that lipoprotein (a) may bind to endothelial cells and possibly interfere with fibrinolytic mechanisms. It also binds to fibrin and extracellular matrix proteins and could therefore promote plaque formation.

Epidemiological studies of lipids as risk factors. Mean adult levels of total plasma cholesterol (TC) vary in different communities from about 3.9 mmol/l (150 mg/dl) to over 7 mmol/l (275 mg/dl).

In countries with a mean TC level around 4 mmol/1 IHD is rare, while those with means of 5.2 or more invariably have high rates of IHD. In prospective studies TC levels are predictive of the risk of developing IHD.

The levels of LDL relate closely to TC levels, and prospective studies have demonstrated that LDL levels are predictive of the risk of IHD. High VLDL levels might be of some predictive value, possibly because LDL is derived from the metabolism of VLDL in the plasma and there is a correlation between the levels of the two. By contrast, a number of prospective studies have demonstrated that plasma levels of HDL are related inversely to the risk of IHD; HDL levels may be of greater predictive value than TC or LDL levels within, but not between, communities. The way in which these lipids could interact with the vessel wall in atherogenesis is considered below.

Inherited abnormalities of lipid metabolism. Hyperlipidaemia may be inherited or may be secondary to another disorder. In the Friedrickson (WHO) classification (Table 12.3) the hyperlipidaemias are grouped according to the class of blood lipid which is in excess. An understanding of the precise biochemical defect responsible is leading to a logical classification of hyperlipidaemia based on abnormalities of apolipoproteins, of enzymes involved in lipid metabolism and of receptors for lipoproteins.

Table 12.3 The Friedrickson classification of the primary hyperlipidaemias

Type	Lipoprotein increased	Primary disorder
I	Chylomicrons	Lipoprotein lipase or apo-C11 deficiency
IIa	LDL	LDL receptor defect
IIb	LDL and VLDL	LDL receptor defect
III	IDL	Apo-E abnormalities
IV	VLDL	Unknown; ? hepatic lipase deficiency
V	Chylomicrons and VLDL	Lipoprotein lipase or apo C-11 deficiency

The best studied example is the monogenic form of familial hypercholesterolaemia. These patients have a predisposition to atheroma because of raised plasma LDL levels. This is due to deficiency of cellular LDL receptors caused by one of almost 30 known mutations of the LDL receptor gene (p. 268). Heterozygotes constitute 1/500 of live births and possess 50% of the normal number of LDL receptors. The reduced LDL uptake by the liver results in plasma levels which are two to four times higher than normal. There is at least an eight-fold increase in the risk of IHD, and this develops in early adulthood. Homozygotes constitute 1/1 000 000 of live births and usually die of vascular disease in childhood. In heterozygotes, plasma LDL can be lowered by a low cholesterol diet, by stimulating the synthesis of hepatic LDL receptors, by treatment with drugs which inhibit HMG CoA reductase and therefore cholesterol synthesis (Fig. 12.12) and by administration of cholestyramine which interferes with the enterohepatic circulation of bile acids.

Hypertension

In prospective studies increased blood pressure (both systolic and diastolic) has been consistently shown to be associated with a subsequent increased risk of IHD. In some community studies the risk in the 20% of the population with the highest pressures was four times that for the 20% with the lowest pressures. The relationship between blood pressure and IHD is not a simple linear one and there is considerable clinical debate as to the levels above which the risk is increased.

Cigarette Smoking

Smoking is one of the most powerful risk factors for IHD. The incidence of IHD is directly correlated with the number of cigarettes smoked per day, and prospective studies have shown that the relationship holds for individuals. On giving up smoking, the risk falls over several years to that of matched non-smokers. The mode of action of cigarette smoking remains uncertain but it seems likely that, in part, it acts via the coagulation system. Cigarette smoke has been shown to decrease endothelial PGI_2 synthesis, and to increase platelet aggregation *in vitro*; smokers have raised blood fibrinogen levels.

Diabetes Mellitus

Diabetes confers a two-fold increase in the risk of IHD. In addition, the rates of IHD are the same in diabetic men and women, the lower rate of IHD in premenopausal women being abolished. However, diabetics have a particular tendency to develop other complications of atheroma, especially cerebrovascular and peripheral vascular disease. The mechanisms involved in producing more severe atheroma in diabetics are complex. They are in part related to the hypertension and hyperlipidaemia which occur when there is carbohydrate intolerance. The hyperlipidaemia is due to overproduction and decreased metabolism of VLDL; there is hypertriglyceridaemia and also low HDL levels. There is as yet no good evidence that control of blood glucose levels lowers the risk of IHD.

Other Risk Factors

Diets rich in saturated fatty acids and cholesterol are associated with high mean plasma levels of TC, LDL and VLDL, while with diets containing a high content of unrefined carbohydrate and low in saturated fats and cholesterol these indices are low. Prospective studies in middle-aged men have demonstrated that the risk of IHD is related directly to: (1) the percentage of calories derived from saturated fats; (2) high ratios of saturated/polyunsaturated dietary fats; and (3) dietary intake of cholesterol. The risk of IHD has an inverse relationship to the amount of dietary vegetable fibre and to the amount of polyunsaturated fats in the diet. There is also some evidence that consumption of fish oils containing unsaturated fats may be protective.

Alcohol consumption of more than 5 units (50 mg) daily is associated with an increased risk of IHD. Alcohol consumption also carries associations with obesity, cigarette smoking and raised blood pressure, but even when allowance is made for this, alcohol consumption still appears to be an independent risk factor. The evidence that those who consume small amounts of alcohol (less than 2–3 units per day) have a lower risk of IHD than total abstainers is not strong and provides only a small grain of comfort!

Regular physical exercise has a protective effect on the risk of IHD. **Obesity** is regarded as an independent risk factor. However, it is additive when other risk factors are present.

The concentrations of **calcium in water supplies** bear an inverse relationship to mortality rates from IHD but the relationship is not strong. **Oral concentraceptives** are a risk factor, possibly by increasing the risk of thrombosis and by their effect on blood pressure and plasma lipids; the risk is slight but appears to be greatly increased by smoking. **Behavioural patterns and stress:** people classified as having type A behavioural pattern, who are ambitious, aggressive, bustling, impatient and short-tempered are particularly at risk.

The risk factors considered above are synergistic, each adding to the risk of developing IHD. They also contribute to the risk of cerebrovascular and peripheral vascular disease, both of which are also major complications of atheroma.

Genetic Predisposition

The various environmental risk factors which we have just considered are likely to account for most of the differences in the IHD rates between communities, but they do not predict accurately which individual members of a given community will develop IHD. There is a predisposition to IHD in some families with no known risk factors; a family history of early death from IHD in parents or grandparents is a recognized risk factor within such a family. The greater degree of concordance for IHD in monozygotic twins than in dizygotic twins of the same sex suggests that genetic factors are involved. It is possible that hitherto unrecognized, genetically determined variations in apolipoprotein metabolism and in their membrane receptors will prove relevant.

Intervention Trials

In order to promote a given risk factor from a statistical association with a disease to a causative relationship it is necessary to show that modification of the factor influences the incidence or the severity of the disease. Many intervention trials have been carried out, involving 'lifestyle' changes, attempts to reduce cholesterol levels, or both. However, these trials are difficult to design and are very costly. In addition, they may be carried out prospectively on patients in whom clinical signs or symptoms have developed. The results obtained have not been entirely conclusive, and, although reductions in ischaemic events have resulted from the use of drugs which lower serum cholesterol, no effect on total mortality has been found. However, for communities at high risk of IHD, reduction in fat intake, in blood cholesterol levels and in blood pressure, together with stopping smoking and regular physical exercise confer benefits.

Pathogenetic Mechanisms: Biomedical/ Laboratory Research

In 1852 Rokitansky suggested that atheromatous plaques resulted from repeated formation of mural thrombi which became covered by endothelium and were replaced by fibrous tissue to form a plaque of initmal thickening – the thrombogenic or encrustation theory. The lipid of the plaque was presumed to be derived from constituents of the thrombi. Four years later, Virchow proposed that atheroma was initiated by an 'irritation' (inflammatory lesion) of the arterial intima with insudation of plasma into the injured zone and subsequent fibrosis and 'fatty degeneration'. This insudation theory gained wide acceptance. In 1972 Ross and Glomset (see Ross, 1986) postulated that all of the features of an atheromatous plaque could be explained by endothelial injury and this response to injury hypothesis has recently attracted the most attention.

Thrombogenic Theory

In support of this theory, platelets and fibrin are commonly detectable by electron microscopy as a fine layer on the surface of the plaque and by immunohistological techniques in the plaque itself. Incorporation of thrombus could play a role in the growth of complicated plaques and this process has been intensively studied in the coronary arteries (p. 492). However, the amount of lipid in most plaques is greater than could be derived from such thrombi and there is good evidence that much of the accumulated lipid is derived by insudation of plasma lipoproteins into the intima. It is now widely accepted, therefore, that both mural thrombosis and insudation of plasma lipids are involved in atherogenesis. It is also believed that these processes and the proliferation of smooth muscle cells seen in the early lesion could be the result of endothelial injury or dysfunction.

Insudation of Lipid

The predominant lipid in atheromatous lesions is cholesterol and most of it is derived from the plasma. Studies in animals have shown that plasma proteins and some lipoproteins normally enter the intima. Such influx is greater in certain sites, notably around the ostia of branches of the aorta. Incubation of segments of aorta in culture fluid rich in lipoproteins show that LDL and HDL enter the intima. The LDL accumulates in the intima in much greater amounts than HDL and the net influx is proportional to its level in the plasma.

LDL metabolism in the artery wall. In the vessel wall LDL can be chemically modified by endothelial cells and macrophages and possibly by exposure to chemical factors generated by platelets and other leucocytes. These modifications include acetylation and oxidation, the latter of which can be effected by macrophage-derived free radicals. Macrophages in the vessel wall normally take up small amounts of native LDL by receptor-mediated endocytosis which is regulated by negative feedback. However, they take up modified LDL at a greatly increased rate by other means, the so-called scavenger pathway. This uptake of modified LDL is not regulated. The lipid accumulates in macrophages (and also in smooth muscle cells) as lipid droplets, producing so-called foam cells.

Oxidized LDL is antigenic and autoantibodies to oxidized LDL are common in patients with atheroma. Antigen—antibody complexes may be taken up by macrophages via Fc receptors. Oxidized LDL is chemotactic for monocytes and their recruitment in this way could contribute to plaque growth. Oxidized LDL is also toxic to endothelial cells and adversely affects their function. There is thus, increasing evidence that oxidized LDL generated in the vessel wall may be a means whereby raised blood LDL levels are associated with atheroma.

HDL can accept and incorporate free cholesterol from the surface of various cell types in culture, including smooth muscle cells. HDL may therefore provide a clearance system for cellular cholesterol, preventing its accumulation in the tissues. HDL may also prevent the chemical and physical changes such as oxidation and acetylation which promote the uptake of LDL by macrophages in the vessel wall. These observations would be in accord with the apparently beneficial effect of raised plasma levels of HDL.

Reaction to Injury Hypothesis

(Fig. 12.13)

Analysis of the possible interactions between cell types occurring in the atheromatous plaque led Ross and Glomset (1972) to suggest that atheromatous plaques may develop as a response to injury of the endothelium. Much of the evidence came from study of the arterial lesions of experimental hypercholesterolaemia in animals. The early changes involve retraction and loss of some endothelial cells, giving rise to small areas of denudation. This causes increased permeability to macromolecules and increased adhesion of platelets and monocytes. The monocytes penetrate into the intima, becoming macrophages; factors released by activated platelets, macrophages and the endothelium then initiate the smooth muscle proliferation and migration.

A transient injury would presumably cause no permanent lesion, while a chronic or long-standing insult would predispose to an atheromatous plaque. The increased permeability would be responsible for the accumulation of lipid; proliferation of modified smooth muscle cells which secrete extracellular matrix proteins would form the other extracellular components of the plaque.

Later, Ross (1986) suggested that more subtle

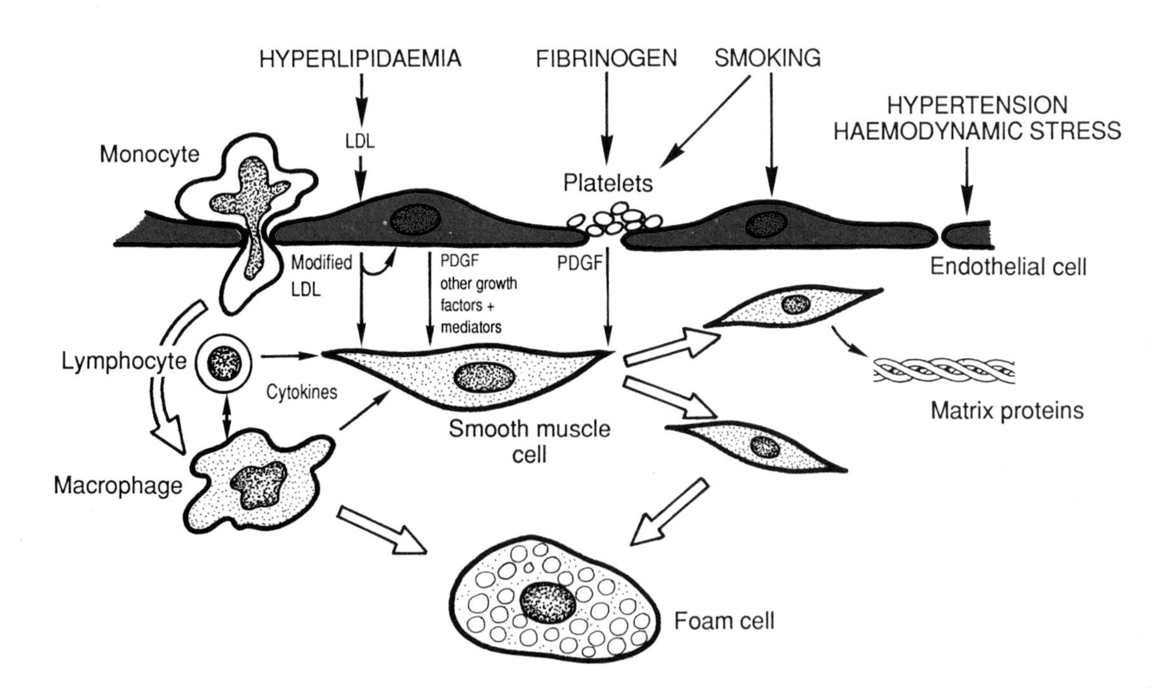

Fig. 12.13 A diagram showing how risk factors could interact with the cells which are involved in atherogenesis. The actions of chemical mediators are indicated by small arrows and the large arrows show cellular responses.

injury, without morphological evidence of cell damage, altered endothelial cell function and induced smooth muscle proliferation. Hyperlipidaemia may cause endothelial injury. This may be mediated by LDL which can be demonstrated in atheromatous plaques. The formation of oxidized LDL may also cause endothelial damage. This hypothesis of modified LDL-induced endothelial injury does not, however, explain the typical focal distribution of atheroma. This may be determined by superimposed haemodynamic factors, of which shear stress is thought to be the most important. Haemodynamic stress is greater at certain sites: the pulse pressure in the abdominal aorta, iliac arteries and leg arteries are much higher than in the brachial arteries. In man atheroma is more severe in chronic hypertension where *haemodynamic* stress is increased. The orifices of artery branches and vessel bifurcations are areas with low *shear stress* and there atheromatous plaques are common. Increased endothelial turnover and permeability at such sites has been demonstrated in experimental animals.

Endothelial cells have a critical role in haemostatic mechanisms (p. 84). Injury to the endothelium results in platelet and leucocyte adherence. Activation of these cell types could result in the release of growth factors and cytokines which affect the proliferative activities of subendothelial smooth muscle cells. Smooth muscle cells appear early in atheromatous lesions. The stimulus responsible for their proliferation

Table 12.4 Cell types involved in atheroma plaque formation and their possible roles

	Thrombus formation	Lipid accumulation	Production of matrix proteins	Effects on other cells
Endothelial cell	Key role in thrombus formation and fibrinolysis (see text)	Affect permeability to lipoproteins. Role in LDL metabolism	Secrete some collagen and extracellular matrix proteins	Stimulate migration and proliferation of smooth muscle cells
Platelets	Key role in thrombus formation	May modify LDL	—	Smooth muscle cell proliferation
Smooth muscle cells	—	Take up LDL and other lipids to become 'foam cells'	Synthesize most of the collagen and proteoglycans of the plaque	May stimulate or inhibit cell proliferation
Macrophages	Scavenger role	Oxidize and acetylate LDL. Take up lipids avidly to become foam cells. May inhibit lipoprotein lipase activity	Secrete proteases and other enzymes which may modify extracellular matrix	Smooth muscle cell proliferation and migration
Lymphocytes	—	TNF may inhibit lipoprotein lipase activity	—	Smooth muscle cell proliferation. Interaction with macrophages
Neutrophils	Scavenger/phagocytic activity	—	Secrete proteases and other enzymes producing continued injury and continued inflammation	—

was thought to be PDGF which is now known to be released not only by platelets but by other cell types involved in atherogenesis (Table 12.4), including smooth muscle cells. Fibroblast, epidermal and colony stimulating growth factors may also stimulate cellular proliferation. Conversely the release of growth inhibitory factors such as heparin, proteoglycan or transforming growth factor β (TGFβ) may inhibit cell proliferation.

Smooth muscle cells also elaborate extracellular matrix proteins such as proteoglycans, collagen and elastin and these contribute to the bulk of the plaque. It has been suggested that smooth muscle cell proliferation may be a primary event in atherogenesis. The proliferation of smooth muscle in any one plaque has been shown to be monoclonal or, at least oligoclonal. This led to the idea that smooth muscle proliferation may be initiated by mutagens such as viruses and anthracene derivatives, a hypothesis which has not, however, been confirmed.

In human atheroma there may be a prominent inflammatory response. Activated T lymphocytes and neutrophil polymorphs are plentiful; complement components can be demonstrated. A continuing inflammatory process may have a role in perpetuating the injury to the vessel wall and in some cases may result in fibrous thickening of the vessel wall and of the adjacent tissues.

In summary, the response to injury hypothesis encompasses the thrombogenic theory, the lipid insudation hypothesis and the effects of haemodynamic factors. While this concept is attractive, it remains highly speculative. Much of the evidence is derived from the study of atheroma in experimental animals and in addition, the behaviour of cells in tissue culture may not reflect *in vivo* activities. However, the response to injury hypothesis emphasizes that atherogenesis has much in common with the processes of chronic inflammation, healing and repair.

The role of oxidized LDL in initiating the earliest lesions is supported by experiments where the development of atheromatous lesions was inhibited by antioxidant drugs. There is little doubt but that a high level of plasma LDL is important in the development and progression of atheroma. Indirect evidence suggests that continuous or repeated endothelial cell injury over a long period is also a causal factor, increasing endothelial permeability to plasma lipoproteins and promoting platelet adhesion and thrombus formation. These elements contribute to the growth of the plaque both directly and also indirectly, by releasing growth factors which stimulate smooth muscle proliferation. The postulated endothelial cell injury seems likely to be due to a combination of haemodynamic stress aggravated by some of the known risk factors such as hypertension, high levels of LDL and possibly circulating chemicals such as those derived from cigarette smoking.

In populations who are most conscious of the known risk factors the incidence of IHD has fallen. Recent studies using quantitative coronary artery angiography have shown that changes in lifestyle with lowering of risk factors and drug-induced reduction of serum cholesterol levels can prevent progression and even induce regression of individual atheroma lesions.

Systemic Hypertension

The term hypertension, used without qualification, is synonymous with systemic arterial hypertension. However, hypertension, defined as raised pressure in a vascular bed, may affect the liver (portal hypertension, p. 772) and the lung (pulmonary hypertension, p. 542). Hypertension affects 15–20% of the population in many developed countries and is a major factor in their high mortality from cardiovascular disease.

Blood pressure rises through childhood and adolescence and reaches the plateau of normal adult levels in the third decade. However, mean blood pressure continues to increase with age but there is considerable individual variation in this increase. In any population, blood pressure has a distribution curve which is skewed to the right; any dividing line between normal and abnormal is arbitrary. There is good evidence, however, of an inverse relationship between the height of the blood pressure and life expectancy; this includes variation within the normal range. This applies to both the systolic and diastolic pressures. Rough working definitions of hypertension have been laid down by the World Health Organisation as follows:

hypertension: systolic pressure $\geq$ 160 mmHg and/or diastolic pressure $\geq$ 95 mmHg;

borderline hypertension: systolic pressure = 140–160 mmHg and/or diastolic pressure = 90–95 mmHg.

Normal blood pressure shows a circadian variation with low levels during sleep. Stimuli such as exercise, exposure to cold, emotion and change from a supine to a standing position cause an increase in blood pressure. In some individuals the blood pressure rise with such stimuli is excessive and the term 'labile hypertension' is then applied.

Classification and Causes of Hypertension (Table 12.5)

In about 95% of cases of hypertension the cause is not apparent and these patients are said to have **primary, essential** or **idiopathic** hypertension. In the remaining 5% hypertension is **secondary** to other disease processes: diseases of the kidneys are nearly always responsible (**'renal hypertension'**) but occasional cases result from functioning adrenal tumours or Cushing's syndrome. Hypertension may develop in pregnancy in so called pre-eclampsia. Coarctation of the aorta (p. 519) is accompanied by hypertension in the arteries arising proximal to the constriction. Regardless of the aetiology, hypertension may be divided into benign and malignant types sometimes also referred to as chronic or accelerated respectively.

Table 12.5 Classification of hypertension

Essential (95%)	Benign 90%
	Malignant 10%
Secondary (5%)	Benign 80%
	Malignant 20%
Renal diseases	
Renovascular diseases (p. 464)	
Renal parenchymal diseases (p. 895), e.g. chronic glomerulonephritis, chronic pyelonephritis and others – virtually any cause of chronic renal failure	
Adrenal diseases	
Conn's syndrome (primary hyperaldosteronism)	
Cushing's syndrome	
Phaeochromocytoma	
Congenital adrenal hyperplasia	
Other endocrine diseases	
Thyrotoxicosis	
Hypothyroidism	
Acromegaly	
Hyperparathyroidism	
Miscellaneous	
Pre-eclampsia	
Alcohol abuse	
Renin-secreting tumours	

In **benign hypertension** the rise of blood pressure is usually slow, progressing over many years, and the level is only moderately raised. Many patients with benign hypertension lead active lives for many years and die of some independent disease. Unless the blood pressure is controlled by antihypertensive drugs, however, it frequently causes disability and death from heart failure, and greatly increases the risk of myocardial infarction and cerebrovascular accidents.

Malignant hypertension is characterized by a very high blood pressure, by eye changes which include retinal haemorrhages and exudates and sometimes papilloedema, by rapidly progressive renal injury terminating in uraemia, and, rarely, by hypertensive encephalopathy. The pathological hallmark of this state is fibrinoid necrosis of arterioles. These special features are due to the rapid rise of blood pressure, often to very high levels. Unless treated, patients with malignant hypertension usually die within a year or so, but frequently the blood pressure can be reduced by antihypertensive drugs and the outlook is then greatly improved.

Benign and malignant hypertension should not be regarded as separate conditions. Malignant hypertension supervenes in a small proportion of cases of benign esential hypertension although more often it arises in hypertension secondary to renal disease. In many cases, malignant hypertension occurs apparently *de novo*, i.e. without evidence of preceding benign hypertension.

Changes in Blood Vessels

Benign hypertension causes changes in arteries of all sizes. In vessels from the aorta down to the smallest arteries, the changes are widespread and are termed **hypertensive arteriosclerosis**. Changes in the arterioles, **hyaline arteriolosclerosis**, tend to affect the viscera and, in particular, those of the kidneys. Malignant hypertension causes distinctive changes in the smaller vessels, particularly the arterioles, and these require separate description.

Large and medium-sized arteries. In the early stages the changes consist mainly of medial hypertrophy (Fig. 12.14) and an increase in elastic fibres. The increased smooth muscle mass in these small resistance vessels is responsible for increased responsiveness to pressor agonists. In long-standing hypertension the medial smooth muscle is replaced by collagen and other matrix proteins and proteoglycans. The arterial walls are thickened and rigid, the lumen is dilated and the vessels are often elongated and tortuous. There is loss of arterial compliance and this contributes to an increase in the systolic blood pressure. The dilatation is accompanied by thickening of the intima and, in medium-sized arteries, there is also reduplication of the internal elastic lamina (Fig. 12.15). An extreme increase in proteoglycans in the media of large arteries is known as 'myxoid degeneration' and explains why hypertension is the most important predisposing factor in aortic dissection (p. 474).

The arteriosclerotic changes described above are similar to those observed in normotensive elderly subjects. Atheroma is more severe in individuals with chronic hypertension, and there is no doubt that prolonged elevation of the blood pressure aggravates this condition.

Hypertension thus at first causes hypertrophy of the arterial walls, with increase in muscle and elastic fibres, followed by arteriosclerosis and a

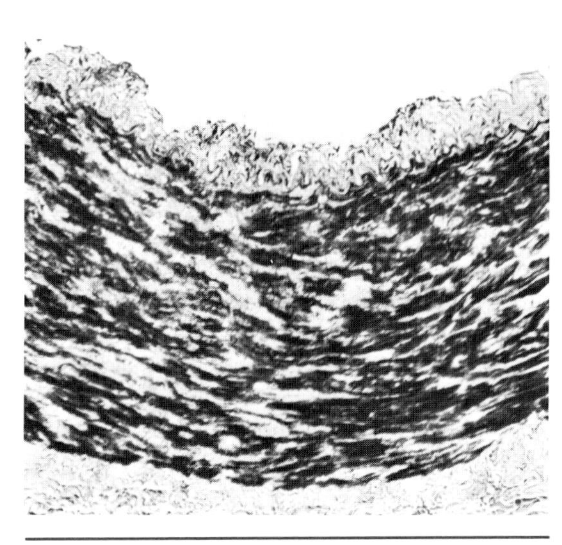

Fig. 12.14 Section of hypertrophied radial artery, from a case of systemic hypertension in a young subject, showing hypertrophy of the media. (Smooth muscle appears black.) ×140.

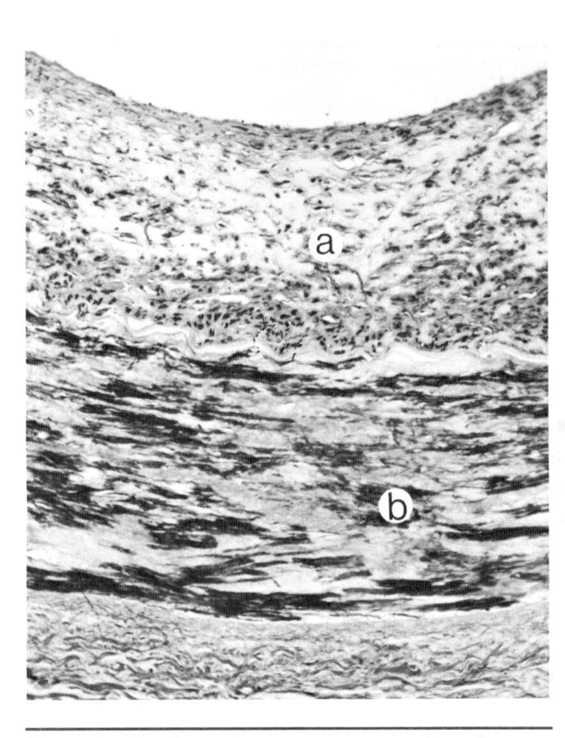

Fig. 12.15 Part of a transverse section of an arteriosclerotic artery. The intima **a** is thickened, while the muscle (shown as black) of the media **b** is partly replaced by fibrous tissue. (Compare with Fig. 12.14.) ×200.

tendency to severe atheroma. The early hypertrophic changes occur only in young subjects: in older patients with chronic hypertension, arteriosclerosis and atheroma predominate.

Small arteries and arterioles. In arteries of 1 mm diameter or less, and in the arterioles, the changes differ from those in the larger vessels, and they differ also in benign and malignant hypertension.

(1) **Benign hypertension.** The small arteries show a more pronounced degree of concentric intimal thickening: in the smallest arteries the intimal change predominates, and may result in atrophy of the media and narrowing of the lumen, in contrast to the dilatation seen in the larger arteries.

The arterioles undergo hyaline thickening of their walls (**hyaline arteriolosclerosis**), which consists at first of patchy deposits of hyaline material, initially beneath the endothelium and then involving the full thickness of the wall. The hyaline change gradually extends to involve the whole circumference, and when severe it replaces all the normal structures of the wall except the endothelium. This change also occurs in diabetes mellitus (p. 801) and in old age in the absence of hypertension. In both normotensive and hypertensive subjects hyaline arteriolosclerosis occurs most commonly in the spleen, then in the afferent glomerular arterioles of the kidneys (Fig. 12.16), and in the pancreas, liver and adrenal capsules. In all these sites, the change is appreciably commoner and more severe in hypertensives. Hyaline arteriolosclerosis is uncommon in the arterioles of the brain, gastrointestinal tract, pituitary, thyroid, heart, skin and skeletal muscles. The hyaline appearance is due in part to **plasmatic vasculosis**, the deposition in the vessel walls of proteins derived from the plasma. Some of the glycoproteins present may be due to excess synthesis of basement membrane material. The result is loss of medial smooth muscle cells, thickening of the wall and narrowing of the lumen.

In the kidney, hypertensive arteriolosclerosis is accompanied by sclerosis of glomeruli and consequent loss of nephrons. It causes renal impairment in the form of diminished functional

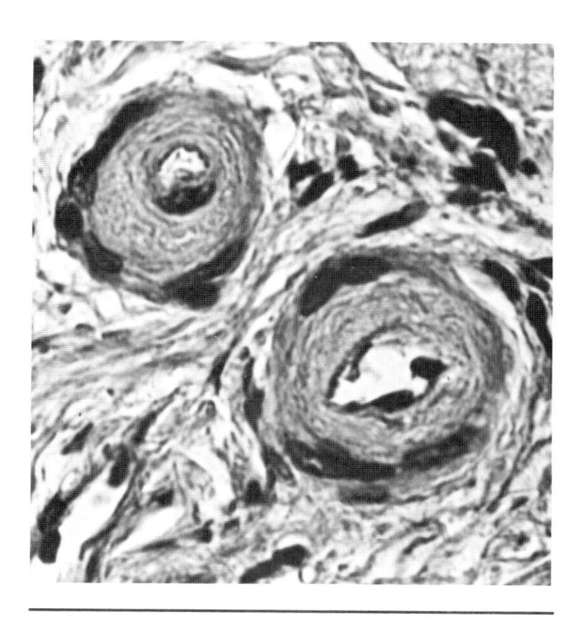

Fig. 12.16 Hyaline arteriolosclerosis in chronic systemic hypertension. The arteriole is not only thickened, but the smooth muscle cells of the media have been replaced by acellular hyaline material.

reserve. Unlike malignant hypertension, it only occasionally causes renal failure; no clinical effects have been defined in other affected organs.

In summary, benign hypertension causes medial hypertrophy in the resistance vessels. This causes increased vascular resistance in response to the prevailing pressor stimuli. In sustained hypertension, the hypertrophy is replaced by arteriosclerosis and arteriolosclerosis. Arteriosclerosis causes decreased compliance of the arterial tree, leading to raised systolic pressure, and arteriolosclerosis causes a long-standing increase in resistance, leading to permanent hypertension. In this way structural changes in the arterial tree will perpetuate hypertension regardless of its aetiology.

(2) **Malignant hypertension.** The histological hallmark of acute malignant hypertension is **fibrinoid necrosis** of small arteries and arterioles (Fig. 12.17). Fibrinoid necrosis consists of a focal area of plasma insudation into an artery, accompanied by cytological evidence of necrosis of the smooth muscle cells of the media. The presence of plasma proteins is confirmed by histologi-

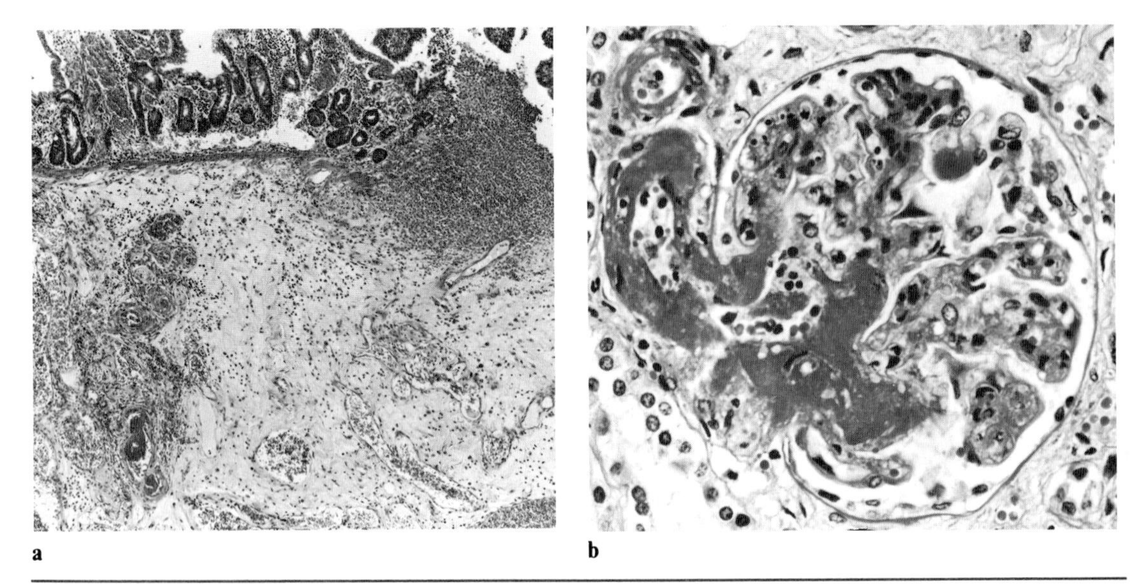
a b

Fig. 12.17 Arteriolar lesions in malignant hypertension. **a** Ulceration of the colonic mucosa due to fibrinoid necrosis and thrombosis of arterioles: one such vessel is seen (lower left) in the submucosa. **b** Fibrinoid necrosis of a glomerular afferent arteriole and part of the tuft.

cal staining reactions for fibrin or fibrinogen, hence the term fibrinoid. The lesions are often accompanied by extravasation of red blood corpuscles forming tiny haemorrhages, and by thrombosis of the lumen which may cause small infarcts. The kidney is the principal target organ. The most commonly affected vessels are the afferent glomerular arterioles and the distal interlobular arteries. When the afferent arteriole is affected, the fibrinoid necrosis may extend into the glomerulus (Fig. 12.17) and rupture of capillaries may cause haematuria and produces visible 'flea-bite' haemorrhages on the surface of the kidney.

The second arterial lesion in malignant hypertension is **proliferative** ('onion-skin') **endarteritis** found mainly in the renal interlobular arteries. The considerable thickening of the intima produces severe narrowing of the lumen (Fig. 12.18). The diffuse damage to the vascular tree may be accompanied by intravascular coagulation which accentuates the endothelial cell damage. The passage of blood at high pressure through a damaged vascular bed with intravascular coagulation causes red cell fragmentation – **microangiopathic haemolytic anaemia** (p. 610).

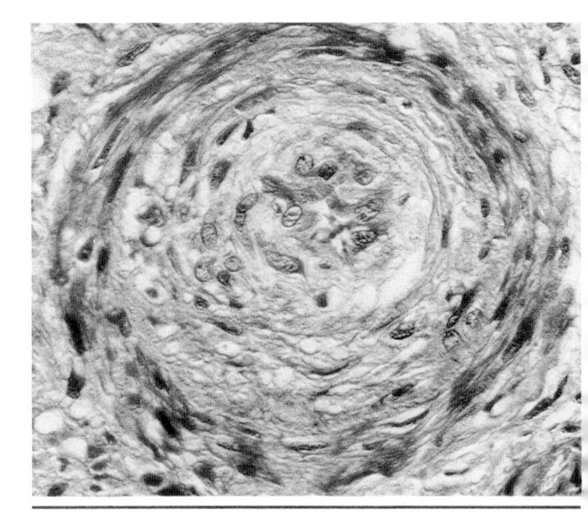

Fig. 12.18 A renal interlobular artery showing endarteritis. There is narrowing of the lumen due to intimal thickening. The media (dark) is atrophied. Interference contrast microscopy. ×290.

Pathogenesis of the Arterial Lesions

A rise in intraluminal pressure can overcome the normal reflex vasoconstriction of an artery. This is more likely to occur when the rate of rise is rapid. The failure to resist the pressure causes focal dilatation. There is increased permeability and plasmatic vasculosis; this is associated with histological evidence of smooth muscle cell necrosis resulting in fibrinoid necrosis. The proliferative endarteritis is best regarded as the healing stage of many types of arterial damage, all of which have in common endothelial cell injury. The cellular intimal thickening is caused by migration of smooth muscle cells through fenestra in the internal elastic lamina. Their proliferation and migration is probably stimulated by endothelial damage, platelet activation and the release of growth and chemotactic factors. The cells then orientate themselves circumferentially and secrete matrix proteins; the intima is initially oedematous and rich in proteoglycans, but later becomes collagenized.

In malignant hypertension the severe arterial damage causes renal ischaemia and stimulation of the renin–angiotensin system (p. 75). The high plasma levels of potent vasoconstrictors such as angiotensin II, noradrenaline and vasopressin can, in some cases, lead to the development of a vicious circle (Fig. 12.19). High levels of plasma aldosterone may result from renin release and the generation of angiotensin II – 'secondary hyperaldosteronism'.

Thus, in the early stages of malignant hypertension the arterial damage is caused by the failure of the vessel to resist the rise in pressure. The forced dilatation causes increased permeability and muscle cell necrosis. Intravascular coagulation then occurs and this may aggravate the vascular damage, cause renal ischaemia, widespread infarcts and microangiopathic haemolytic anaemia. The endarteritis is a healing response but is responsible for long-term renal ischaemia.

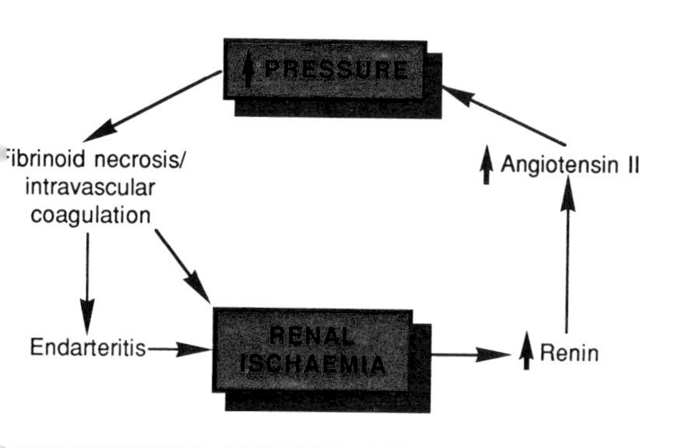

Fig. 12.19 The vicious circle of malignant hypertension. The vascular damage induced by hypertension causes renal ischaemia which leads to high plasma levels of vasoconstrictors such as angiotensin II, further increasing the blood pressure.

Course and Clinical Features

Benign (essential) hypertension. As already stated, this is much the commonest type of hypertension. The blood pressure rises very gradually over a period of years, in most cases to moderately high levels, e.g. 180/100 mmHg, but occasionally much higher. The increase nearly always starts between the ages of 45 and 55 years, and individuals with a resting blood pressure consistently below 140/85 at this age are unlikely to develop essential hypertension.

Benign hypertension is usually symptomless, and many cases come to light during routine medical examination for insurance or other purposes. Common symptoms include palpitations, audible pulsation in the head, headaches, attacks of dizziness particularly on stooping, and reduced exercise tolerance.

Without treatment, about 60% of patients with benign hypertension die of ischaemic heart disease or heart failure: this is due to the increased work load thrown on the left ventricle and to the commonly associated severe coronary artery atheroma. About 30% of patients die from cerebral haemorrhage or infarction, and 10% from various causes unrelated to the hypertension. Although changes occur in the kidneys, renal failure is uncommon. When heart failure develops, however, there is usually a moderate rise in the blood urea level. In those patients who progress from benign to malignant hypertension, renal failure inevitably supervenes.

Malignant hypertension. This develops in less than 10% of patients with benign essential hypertension. In those cases not preceded by chronic hypertension, the onset is often between 30 and 34 years of age. It can result in heart failure or cerebral haemorrhage, but without effective treatment renal injury is severe and usually causes death within a year.

Eye changes are an important diagnostic feature and lesions in the small arteries in the retina cause oedema, haemorrhages, infarcts and exudates, and blindness may ensue. Papilloedema, associated with cerebral oedema, is often present. Hypertensive encephalopathy, characterized by epileptiform fits and transient paralysis, is caused by cerebral oedema resulting from failure of the resistance vessels of the brain to withstand the increased blood pressure.

Modern antihypertensive drugs have revolutionized the prognosis. The vicious cycle of renal ischaemia and renin release can be interrupted by drugs which block angiotensin converting enzyme. Most patients who do not develop a cerebral haemorrhage or myocardial infarction in the acute phase, can be effectively treated. However, those who have sustained severe arterial damage often develop proliferative endarteritis which causes chronic renal failure due to ischaemia several years later.

Aetiology of Essential Hypertension

The blood pressure is a product of the cardiac output and the peripheral vascular resistance, and hypertension is attributable to an increase of one or both of these factors. The cardiac output is increased in the early stages of essential hypertension in some patients, and also in the early stages of experimental renal hypertension in rats. In established hypertension, however, cardiac output is normal, and maintenance of the high blood pressure is therefore attributable to increased peripheral resistance. In normal circumstances the peripheral resistance is controlled by the muscular tone in the arterioles throughout the body, and the major aetiological problem is the elucidation of the factors which, by increasing arteriolar tone, bring about the various types of hypertension. The structural changes in the resistance vessels are widely regarded as the result of hypertension, and not the cause. Vasoactive hormones such as angiotensin II and noradrenaline cause growth of smooth muscle cells *in vitro* and a similar effect *in vivo* could cause or augment the arterial hypertrophy. The hypertrophy of the resistance vessels could thus contribute to the hypertension by an increased response to pressor agents. The structural changes in the arterioles and small arteries (arteriolo- and arteriosclerosis) contribute to the maintenance of chronic hypertension once the vascular changes have become established.

Essential hypertension is a disease of middle and old age and is commoner in women. The mortality rates for men, however, are 1.5–2 times that for women with the same level of pressure. The possible ways by which essential hypertension could arise are numerous but, as yet, the reasons why the regulation of blood pressure is abnormal in this disease are not fully understood.

Genetic and Racial Factors

The distribution of blood pressure in human populations is unimodal, suggesting that, like height and other constitutional factors, the inheritance is polygenic. In essential hypertension familial aggregation of blood pressure levels also suggests a genetic component. This has been confirmed by studies in twins and by comparison between the adopted and natural children of the same parents.

Hypertension is twice as prevalent in black Americans as in the white population; and, furthermore, hypertensive black males have a death rate about six times that of white males with the same levels of blood pressure.

Environmental Factors

Stress. Urban populations have higher blood pressures than rural populations and the adverse effects of urban living are confirmed by the rise in blood pressure of rural populations migrating to the cities. These and similar studies suggest an effect of stress which could be mediated by the sympathetic nervous system.

Diet. Most Western populations who have a high incidence of hypertension have a high salt intake. The prevalence of hypertension in populations correlates with the salt intake. In animals, high salt intake also causes hypertension. However, there is a wide variation in susceptibility to salt which is genetically determined and probably operates early in life. Transplant experiments indicate that susceptibility to the hypertensive effect of salt is conferred by the kidney. In spite of the strong epidemiological and experimental evidence the role of high salt diet as a cause of hypertension in man remains controversial.

Diets which are high in sodium are usually low in potassium. Potassium supplements ameliorate the effects of experimental hypertension. Low potassium intake may therefore be a factor in the tendency to hypertension in man. Calcium and magnesium deficiency have also been implicated in the development of hypertension, but this evidence remains scanty.

Prenatal. Recent evidence sugests that the environment *in utero* may be important. Low birth weight predisposes to hypertension in adult life and there is experimental evidence that the renin–angiotensin system may be involved.

Cell Membrane Abnormalities

Multiple abnormalities of membrane cation transport systems have been described in patients with essential hypertension, e.g. sodium–potassium co-transport is reduced, and there is a small reduction in the activity of the ouabain-sensitive sodium pump. The handling of calcium by the cell membrane is also abnormal. Originally discovered in red and white blood cells, preliminary evidence suggests that these membrane abnormalities may also affect vascular smooth muscle cells. Their effect would be to lower resting membrane potential and increase contractility.

The cation transport systems of the cell membrane and the fluidity of the membrane itself are influenced by its lipid composition. Abnormalities of membrane lipids are now being described in the blood cells of hypertensive patients, and in vascular smooth musle cells in hypertensive animals. Epidemiological studies reveal relationships between blood lipids, blood pressure and membrane cation transport. An underlying defect in lipid metabolism may therefore be responsible for the abnormalities of membrane cation transport.

Nervous System

Resting vascular tone is controlled by the sympathetic nervous system and there is sympathetic overactivity in some cases of early essential hypertension and in some experimental models of hypertension. In hypertension the baroreceptor reflexes are set too high but this is likely to be a secondary defect.

Sympathetic nerves innervate the juxtaglomerular apparatus and their stimulation causes renin release mediated by a β-adrenergic receptor mechanism. Sympathetic nerves also contain a variety of neuropeptides, of which some such as neuropeptide-Y are potent vasoconstrictors. Neuropeptides are likely to prove important in the regulation of the cardiovascular system.

Circulating Pressor Agents

In essential hypertension plasma renin levels are normal in 60% of patients, high in 15% and low in 25%. There is no good evidence, however, that the renin-angiotensin system is directly involved in the pathogenesis of essential hypertension. Similarly, no important role for catecholamines, atrial natriuretic factor (ANP) and other hormones has been shown. Kinins and some of the prostaglandins are vasoactive and have local functions in the kidney contributing to the regulation of renal blood flow and electrolyte transport. There is no evidence, however, that altered activity of these systems is important in any type of human or experimental hypertension.

Secondary Hypertension

The causes of secondary hypertension are listed in Table 12.5. Of these, renal causes are ten times commoner than all the others. Renal hypertension may be due to renovascular disorders or diseases of the renal parenchyma.

Renovascular Hypertension

The commonest cause is renal artery stenosis usually caused by fibromuscular dysplasia or atheroma of the renal artery. Other diseases which affect the intrarenal arterial branches cause hypertension by similar mechanisms. In unilateral renal artery stenosis, the hypertension has three phases: (1) a rise in the circulating levels of renin and angiotensin II leading to a rise in blood pressure. If the renal artery constriction or the ischaemic kidney is removed, the blood pressure returns to normal; (2) after some days or weeks, in spite of lower renin and angiotensin levels hypertension persists; however, removal of the constriction or the affected kidney still restores blood pressure to normal; (3) in the third stage, after some months, plasma renin and angiotensin levels are normal but chronic hypertension is established. Hypertension persists when the ischaemic kidney is removed, but in some cases may be cured by removal of the contralateral kidney.

In the early and intermediate phases of renal artery stenosis the blood pressure is controlled by both the direct pressor action of plasma angiotensin II and a slow hypertensive effect of uncertain mechanism. In the third stage the hypertension is maintained because of damage to the contralateral kidney. Eventually the hypertension becomes permanent, as occurs in hypertension from any cause, the blood pressure being maintained by permanent changes in the vascular tree.

Renal Parenchymal Diseases

Hypertension is common in the early stages of many renal diseases such as glomerulonephritis and indeed may complicate virtually any renal disease. In some cases there is sodium and water retention and in others the renin–angiotensin system may be activated by a fall in renal perfusion. The mechanisms, however, are often more complex. In chronic renal failure, hypertension is invariable and may aggravate the renal damage. Blood pressure is lowered by dialysis, suggesting that the hypertension is largely due to sodium and water retention. A rise in body sodium and water should normally suppress the renin-angiotensin system. In chronic renal failure, however, plasma renin levels are usually normal, suggesting a failure of the suppression mechanisms, i.e. the 'normal levels' are inappropriately high.

Adrenal Causes of Hypertension

Phaeochromocytomas cause hypertension mainly because of the high levels of circulating catecholamines. The hypertension is episodic in 50% of cases and is often severe. In Conn's syndrome (primary aldosteronism) raised aldosterone levels stimulate sodium and water retention which causes mild hypertension. The syndrome should not be confused with secondary hyperaldosteronism which occurs in some cases of malignant hypertension with high levels of renin and angiotensin II, the latter stimulating aldosterone secretion by the adrenal cortex. In Cushing's syndrome both glucocorticoids and mineralocorticoids contribute to the hypertension and salt-retaining precursor steroids cause hypertension in cases of congenital adrenal hyperplasia (p. 1098).

Other Causes

The mechanisms of the hypertension in acromegaly, in thyroid hypo- and hyperfunction and in pre-eclampsia are not fully understood, nor are the mechanisms of hypertension in alcohol abuse. Renin secretion by tumours of the kidney – tumours of the juxtaglomerular apparatus, renal cell carcinomas and nephroblastomas – are rare causes of hypertension as is the 'inappropriate' secretion of renin by non-renal malignant tumours such as bronchial carcinoma. The high systolic pressure which occurs in the elderly is thought to be due largely to the decreased compliance of the aorta such that it cannot absorb the pressure rise of the pulse wave.

Vasculitis (Angiitis)

This term covers a heterogeneous group of conditions (Table 12.6) in which there is focal inflam-

Table 12.6 Vasculitis. (a) classification on a broad aetiological basis. (b) Classification according to the size of vessel involved

(a)

Non-infective systemic vasculitis
- Polyarteritis nodosa
  - Classical type
  - Microscopic polyarteritis (microangiopathic variant)
- Giant-cell arteritis
- Takayasu's disease
- Wegener's granulomatosis
- Buerger's disease (thromboangiitis obliterans)

Vasculitis in other diseases
- Associated with connective tissue disease
- Henoch–Schönlein purpura
- Serum sickness vasculitis
- Miscellaneous group
  - in association with drugs, malignancy, cryoglobulinaemia
- Churg–Strauss syndrome
- Kawasaki disease (mucocutaneous lymph node syndrome)

Infective systemic vasculitis
- Rickettsial, fungal and other causes
- Syphilis

(b)

Aorta and large arteries
- Giant-cell arteritis
- Takayasu's disease
- Aortitis: syphilitic and other types

Medium-sized and small arteries
- Polyarteritis nodosa
- Arteritis in connective tissue diseases
- Wegener's granulomatosis
- Churg–Strauss syndrome
- Kawasaki disease
- Giant-cell arteritis
- Buerger's disease
- Takayasu's disease
- Fungal vasculitis

Arterioles, capillaries and venules
- Henoch–Schönlein purpura
- Microscopic polyarteritis
- Wegener's granulomatosis
- Churg–Strauss syndrome
- Rickettsial vasculitis

mation of the walls of blood vessels, usually arteries or arterioles but veins and capillaries can also be affected. In severe arteritis there is necrosis of an artery wall, which may result in occlusive thrombosis, rupture or aneurysm formation. The healing phase often causes severe permanent narrowing of the lumen, resulting either from organization of thrombus or from endarteritis obliterans, and chronic ischaemia is likely to result.

Aetiology and Pathogenesis

In the vast majority of cases of vasculitis, the aetiology is unknown. In the vasculitis of serum sickness and in the vasculitis which occurs in systemic lupus erythematosus and rheumatoid arthritis there is immune-complex deposition and the mechanisms involved are discussed on p. 213. In a small proportion of cases of polyarteritis nodosa (less than 10%) the lesions are due to deposition of complexes containing hepatitis B surface antigens; other viruses and streptococci have also been implicated as antigens. Occasionally vasculitis develops following the administration of drugs; in these cases the drugs may act as an immunogen resulting in immune-complex deposition or there may be a local allergic or hypersensitivity reaction following binding of the drug to endothelial cells. Circulating anti-endothelial cell antibodies are present in some cases of vasculitis implying a type II hypersensitivity reaction. These autoantibodies may be useful in monitoring disease activity but their role in pathogenesis is dubious. In graft rejection, antibodies to major histocompatibility complex (MHC) antigens bind to endothelium and are implicated in the vascular damage which occurs (p. 225).

The diagnosis of vasculitis is established on the basis of the clinical and histological features, the distribution of the lesions and the presence of other diseases. The histological features show considerable variation but essentially comprise inflammation of the vessel wall which may be predominantly acute, a mixture of acute and chronic or may be granulomatous. Thus, neither a satisfactory aetiological nor morphological classification exists. Every effort should be made to try to identify and eliminate any possible cause. The pattern of vessel involvement is helpful in making a diagnosis and Table 12.6 combines both a list of the various vasculitis syndromes and also their distribution. There is often a good clinical response to immunosuppressive or cytotoxic drugs and so early treatment is indicated.

Polyarteritis Nodosa

In this disease multiple foci of necrosis, inflammation and usually thrombosis followed by healing, occurs in the walls of medium-sized and small arteries. Vessels in any part of the body may be affected, but the lesions are found predominantly in kidneys, heart, skeletal muscle, gastrointestinal tract and nervous system. The condition occurs over a wide age range, but mainly between 20 and 40 years and more often in men than in women.

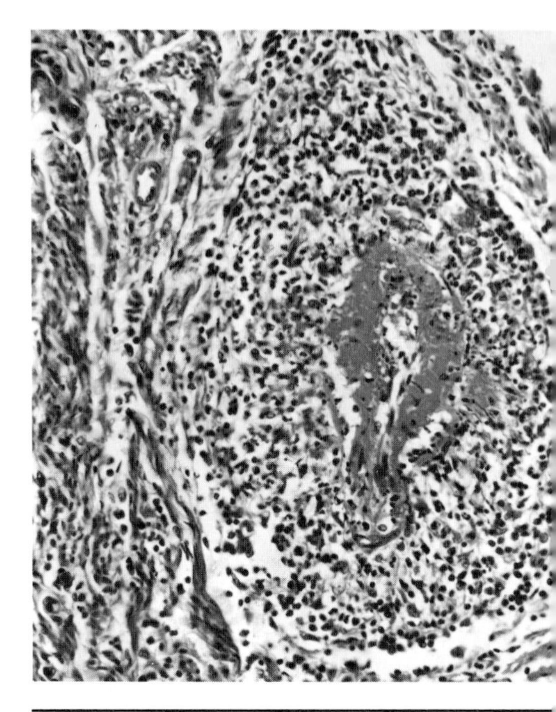

Fig. 12.20 An acute lesion of polyarteritis nodosa in a small artery in the kidney. There is fibrinoid necrosis and an intense inflammatory cell infiltrate in and around the wall of the artery. ×100.

Pathological Findings

The early lesion consists of fibrinoid necrosis of the media and intima of a small or medium-sized artery (up to about 3 mm diameter) or an arteriole. Necrosis is accompanied by acute inflammation with a neutrophil and eosinophil polymorph infiltration of the whole thickness of the vessel wall, particularly intense in the adventitia and surrounding tissue (Fig. 12.20). Lesions affect the whole circumference of smaller arteries, but often only a segment of the wall of the larger vessels (Fig. 12.21). Occlusive thrombosis is common in the acute stage, and in some cases the artery ruptures with severe haemorrhage. The acute changes progress to more chronic inflammation, with replacement of the necrotic vessel wall by fibrous tissue infiltrated with lymphocytes, plasma cells and macrophages, and the thrombus undergoes organization. The weakened wall may stretch to form an aneurysm, but even without this, the healed lesion may produce a nodular fibrotic thickening of the vessel wall.

Clinical Features

The disease may be severe and rapidly fatal. More often the course extends over some years, with periods of quiescence alternating with the recrudescence of new lesions. In most patients, however, death eventually results from lesions in the kidney, heart or other organs, and these are often accompanied by hypertension due to renal ischaemia. The clinical features show great variation. In severe cases there is fever, prostration, neutrophil (and sometimes eosinophil) leucocytosis and a very high ESR. Lesions in the small arteries of peripheral nerves result in paraesthesiae, and symptoms may arise from ischaemia

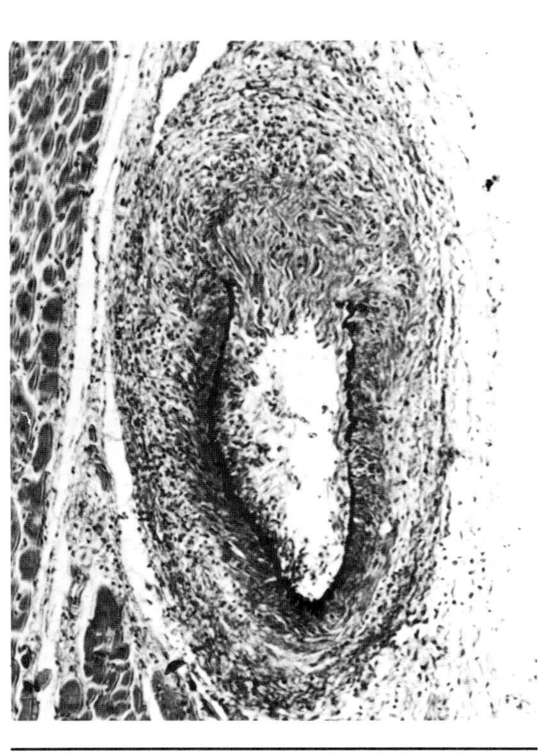

Fig. 12.21 Polyarteritis nodosa involving a coronary artery. The lesion is less acute than in the previous figure. Part of the circumference of the vessel wall (above) has been severely damaged, with interruption of the internal elastic lamina (stained black) and replacement of the inner part of the wall by fibrous tissue. There is more diffuse inflammatory cellular infiltrate. ×70.

of virtually any tissue. Angina, cardiac failure, renal failure and hypertension are among the commoner manifestations, but infarction of the gut or in the brain can also occur. In some cases angiography shows multiple aneurysms, or in others the vasculitis can be confirmed by skeletal muscle, renal or skin biopsy.

Microscopic (Microangiopathic) Polyarteritis

This form of vasculitis affects small arteries, arterioles and capillaries and the lesions are found predominantly in the skin, kidney, gut, skeletal muscles and heart. The lesions tend to develop simultaneously and thus show similar features in affected organs. In addition to the vessel involvement, rapidly progressive glomerulonephritis occurs in many cases (p. 901). Antineutrophil cytoplasmic antibodies are present in the sera of over 90% of patients.

Giant-cell (Temporal, Cranial) Arteritis

Giant-cell arteritis is commonest in the temporal arteries; however, since the temporal arteries are affected by other types of arteritis and giant-cell arteritis affects other vessels, the term temporal arteritis is best avoided. It occurs mostly in old people of both sexes. It is sometimes widespread and the aorta and its major branches may be involved.

There is inflammation of the whole thickness of the affected arteries, affecting either a continuous length of the vessel or appearing as multiple focal lesions along it. The vessel wall is involved in a granulomatous reaction, with accumulation of lymphocytes, macrophages and multinucleated cells of both Langhans' and 'foreign body' types which appear to develop around fragments of the internal elastic lamina. In the end-stage of the disease there is fibrous thickening of the intima and scarring of the media with thrombotic occlusion of the lumen (Fig. 12.22).

Clinically there may be localized reddening, tenderness, pain or nodularity of the arteries. There may be headache, facial pain, visual disturbances and sometimes blindness (from involvement of the retinal arteries) and cerebral infarction. In some instances, the disease occurs in association with polymyalgia rheumatica (p. 232). It is of unknown aetiology, and responds rapidly to corticosteroid treatment.

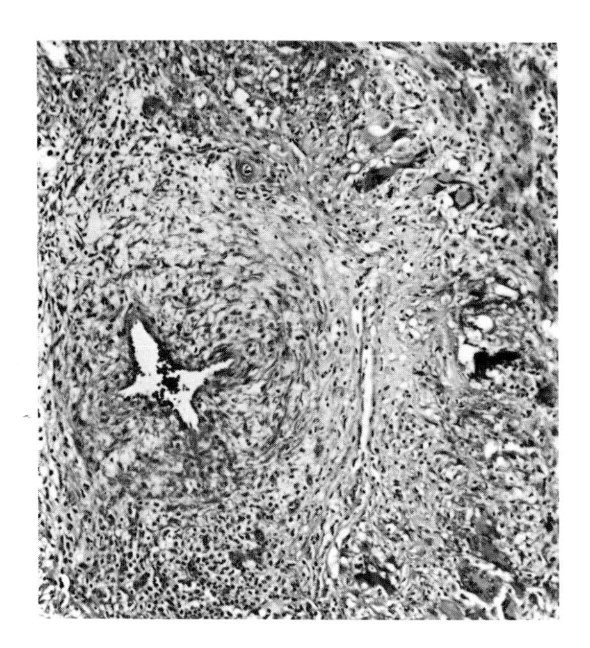

Fig. 12.22 Section of the temporal artery in giant-cell arteritis, showing multinucleated giant cells lying in relation to the internal elastic lamina (now disrupted and seen only as small fragments). There is gross intimal thickening and a very narrow lumen.

Other Miscellaneous Vasculitides

Takayasu's Disease

This is a rare condition, of unknown aetiology, affecting mainly young women (male: female ratio 1:4). It was first reported from Japan in 1928 but occurs world wide. The aorta and the large arteries arising from the aortic arch are affected by a granulomatous arteritis in which there are Langhans' giant cells and necrosis of the vessel wall. Medial and intimal fibrosis follow, sometimes with superadded thrombosis, thus producing narrowing or occlusion of the subclavian, carotid and innominate arteries (hence the term **pulseless disease**). There is ischaemia of the limbs accompanied by various visual and neurological defects which may extend to total blindness and hemiparesis. Involvement of the coronary, renal and other visceral arteries occasionally occurs with consequent ischaemic syndromes.

Wegener's Granulomatosis

In this disease there is vasculitis and necrotizing granulomatous inflammation involving the nose and upper respiratory tract, the lungs (p. 527) and kidneys (p. 902) in various combinations. Males are affected twice as commonly as females. There may be accompanying skin rashes, polyarthritis and polyneuritis. Cytotoxic drugs such as cyclophosphamide cure 90% of patients.

Buerger's Disease (Thromboangiitis Obliterans)

Buerger's disease is a vasculitis of medium-sized and small arteries and veins, with thrombosis, organization and recanalization of the affected vessels. It occurs predominantly in males, affects mainly the legs, but sometimes the arms, and gives rise to severe pain and progressive ischaemic changes which may progress to gangrene. Features which distinguish Buerger's disease from atheroma with superadded thrombosis are its early onset, its inflammatory nature, predilection for smaller vessels, and involvement of veins as well as arteries and of the arms as well as the legs.

Pathological findings. Short segments of the affected arteries and veins are occluded by thrombus and there is intense neutrophil infiltration of both the thrombus and the whole thickness of the vessel wall. These acute changes give way to chronic inflammation, and the thrombus is replaced by granulation tissue containing lymphocytes, macrophages and multinucleated giant cells (Fig. 12.23). The inflammatory changes eventually subside and fibrosis extends into the sur-

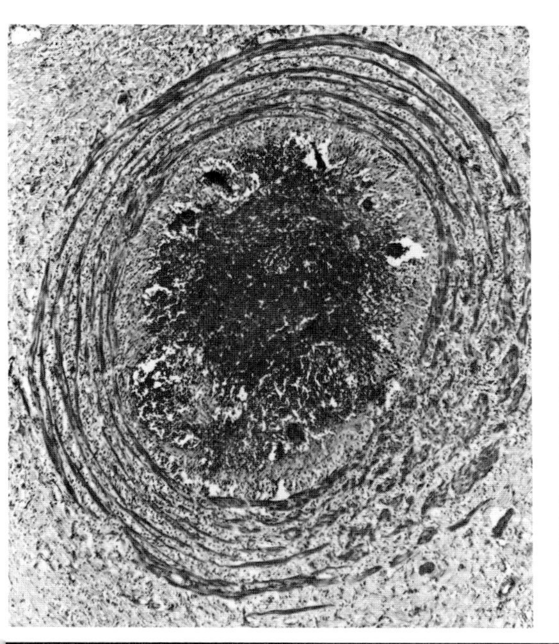

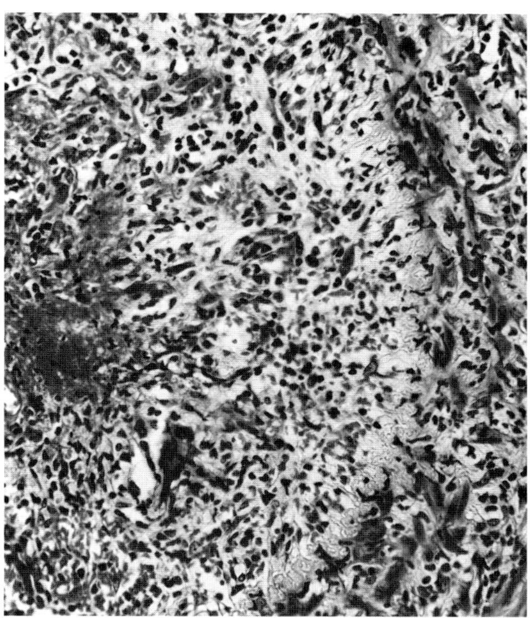

Fig. 12.23 Buerger's disease. Left, a superficial vein, showing inflammation of the wall, thrombosis and early organization. Several multinucleated giant cells lie in and adjacent to the thrombus. ×60. Right, an older lesion with more advanced organization of the thrombus: note the giant cell (below centre) and pleomorphic inflammatory infiltrate. ×250.

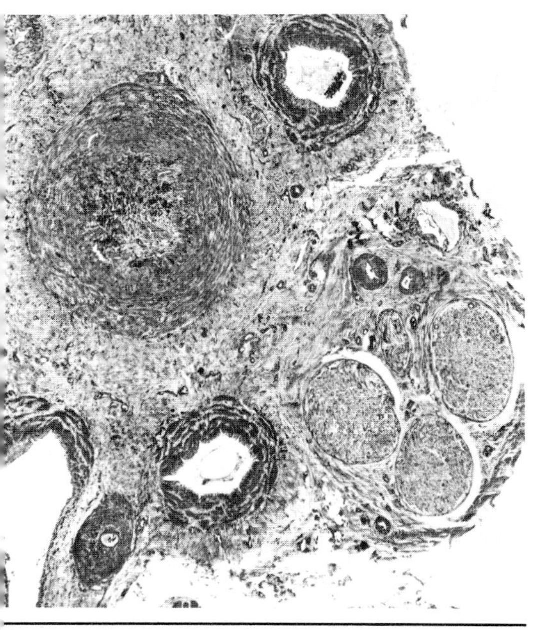

Fig. 12.24 Buerger's disease. Occlusion of the posterior tibial artery (upper left) and surrounding fibrosis extending around the adjacent veins and nerves. ×32.

rounding connective tissue and may involve the entire neurovascular bundle (Fig. 12.24).

There is an increased prevalence of HLA-A9 and B5 in patients with Buerger's disease, suggesting a genetic predisposition. The single known important predisposing factor is cigarette smoking. The disease is practically confined to heavy smokers; its progress is arrested or diminished by giving up smoking and resumption of smoking produces an exacerbation.

Infective Vasculitis

Arteries are relatively resistant to bacterial invasion and in acute infections the arteries in the inflamed tissues are usually spared unless suppuration or gangrene occur. Infected emboli, for example in infective endocarditis (p. 511) may cause an acute arteritis at the site of impaction: if severe, this may result in necrosis and rupture or the development of a so-called mycotic aneurysm. The purpuric rash of meningococcal septicaemia (p. 295) is caused by an acute meningococcal vasculitis affecting the cutaneous capillaries.

More widespread invasion of arterioles, capillaries and venules by micro-organisms can give rise to a vasculitis, causing necrosis and thrombosis of the vessels. This occurs in the **rickettsial diseases**, e.g. typhus and Rocky Mountain spotted fever (p. 329). A severe systemic vasculitis of this type may be caused by *Pseudomonas aeruginosa* which often infects patients with severe burns and those who are immunosuppressed. In immunosuppressed patients and drug addicts **fungal infections** such as aspergillosis and mucormycosis cause increased tissue destruction due to their ability to invade veins and arteries, causing thrombosis and infarction. **Tuberculosis** most often causes endarteritis of the arteries in an infected area, but occasionally necrosis of the wall may result in haemorrhage into a tuberculosis cavity in the lung and fatal haemoptysis.

The aorta (and indeed the coronary, renal and cerebral arteries) may be affected in rheumatic fever, **rheumatic arteritis**. The adventitia and outer media show non-specific chronic inflammation.

Syphilis causes lesions in the small vessels involved in primary, secondary and tertiary lesions, and also affects the aorta and rarely its larger branches. The lesions of small vessels consist of fibrous thickening of the intima and adventitia and perivascular infiltration of lymphocytes and plasma cells, endarteritis and periarteritis (Fig. 12.25). Their effect is to narrow the small vessels, causing local ischaemia. These changes occur in the vasa vasorum of the thoracic aorta, producing an irregular patchy loss of the musculoelastic laminae of the media and replacement by collagenous tissue, **syphilitic mesaortitis**. This is frequently accompanied by aneurysmal dilatation of the thoracic aorta and other complications.

Aortitis resembling syphilitic mesaortitis but of unknown aetiology occurs in some patients with **ankylosing spondylitis**, **Reiter's syndrome** and **psoriatic arthritis** (pp. 994–5). It affects mainly the root of the aorta and, as in syphilis, may cause aortic incompetence. However, in ankylosing spondylitis, unlike syphilis, there is often thickening of the valve cusps and even subaortic fibrosis. In other cases an aortitis of unknown aetiology occurs as an isolated disease.

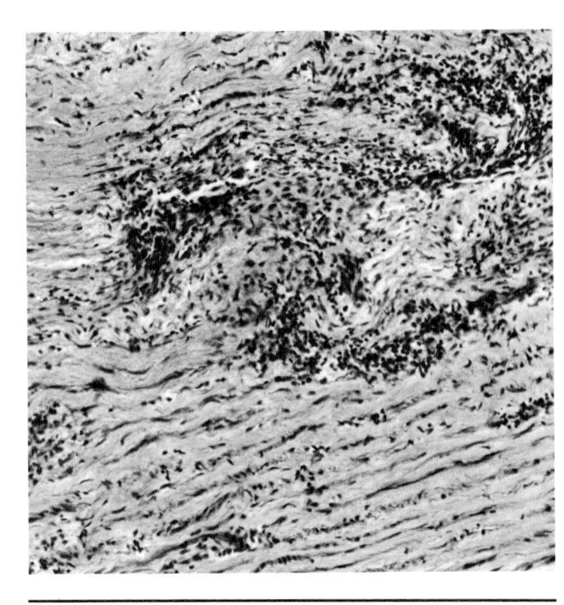

Fig. 12.25 Section of a syphilitic aorta, showing chronic inflammation around the small vessels in the media, with destruction of the musculo-elastic laminae. ×160.

Churg–Strauss Syndrome (Eosinophilic Granulomatous Vasculitis)

This is characterized by asthma, vasculitis of small arteries and veins and extravascular granulomatous inflammation with necrosis and intense eosinophil infiltration in the surrounding tissues. The lungs are most commonly affected although other organs such as spleen, skin and peripheral nerves may also be involved.

Kawasaki Disease (Mucocutaneous Lymph Node Syndrome)

This affects mainly children. It is a febrile illness characterized by skin rashes, inflammation of the conjunctival and buccal mucosae, generalized lymphadenopathy and sometimes arthritis. There is an arteritis resembling polyarteritis nodosa associated with circulating antibodies to endothelial cells. Unlike infantile polyarteritis nodosa there is spontaneous recovery in the large majority in 3–6 weeks; coronary arteritis develops in approximately 2% of cases sometimes with a fatal outcome.

Vasculitis in Other Diseases

Arteritis with lesions indistinguishable from polyarteritis nodosa occur in a number of diseases (Table 12.6). In **connective tissue diseases**, notably systemic lupus erythematosus and rheumatoid arthritis, the vasculitis is usually associated with circulating immune complexes and a reduction in the levels of some serum complement components. **Henoch–Schönlein purpura**, which may sometimes follow streptococcal or viral infections, affects the skin and gut and may cause glomerulonephritis (p. 902). **Malignancies** associated with vasculitis include lymphomas, hairy-cell leukaemia, myeloma and angioimmunoblastic lymphadenopathy. In **cryoglobulinaemia** (p. 640) palpable necrotizing skin lesions may be accompanied by arthritis, hepatosplenomegaly and a diffuse proliferative glomerulonephritis. Drugs which have been associated with vasculitis include penicillin, sulphonamides, gold salts and amphetamines.

Aneurysms

An ***aneurysm*** *is a localized vascular dilatation caused by stretching of the wall.* Symmetrical stretching of the whole circumference produces a fusiform aneurysm, while stretching of part of the circumference causes a saccular aneurysm, which bulges from one side of the artery. The term dissecting aneurysm is a misnomer for what is more correctly described as arterial dissection and is discussed separately. The term aneurysm is also loosely applied to conditions which include traumatic and false aneurysm, arteriovenous aneurysm and cirsoid or racemose aneurysm.

Pathogenesis. The force which expands an aneurysm is the blood pressure, but for an aneurysm to form there must be local weakening of the media which stretches. Stretching usually results in further weakening, so that once an aneurysm has formed it tends to expand, and then commonly ruptures. The weakness in the vessel wall may be congenital or may be acquired. The acquired lesions are most commonly atheroma, syphilitic mesaortitis, infection (mycotic aneurysm) and vasculitis.

Atheromatous Aneurysm

In Europe and North America, atheroma is the commonest cause of aortic aneurysm. Atheromatous aneurysms occur usually after the age of 60, are much commoner in males and 50% of patients are hypertensive. Atheromatous aneurysms are usually fusiform (Fig. 12.26). The aneurysm forms as a result of weakening of the media overlying atheromatous plaques due to extension of the plaque into the media. These aneurysms are a complication of severe atheroma and affect especially the abdominal aorta distal to the origin of the renal arteries. Atheromatous aneurysms occasionally occur in the thoracic

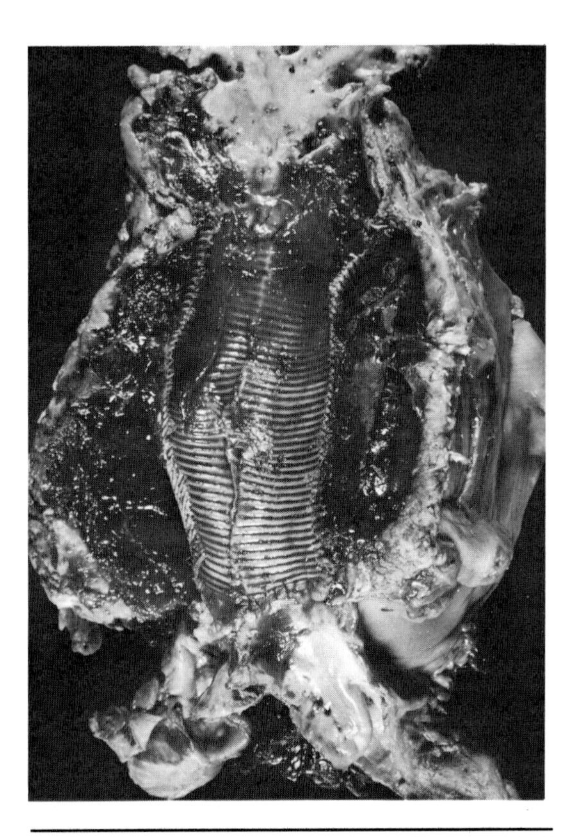

Fig. 12.26 Atheromatous aneurysm of the abdominal aorta arising below the origins of the renal arteries. The aneurysm, which is fusiform, had been repaired by a dacron tube.

aorta, but seldom in the ascending aorta. Atheroma also causes aneurysms in other arteries, most frequently in the common iliac arteries. Much less common are aneurysms of the popliteal artery and of the splenic, renal and other visceral arteries.

Effects. Pressure effects from abdominal aortic aneurysms are not conspicuous and the lesion is often diagnosed incidentally. Large aneurysms are liable to rupture, giving rise to massive retroperitoneal, and occasionally intraperitoneal haemorrhage, frequently with a fatal outcome. The larger the aneurysm, the greater the risk of rupture. Large expanding aneurysms should thus be bypassed by insertion of a prosthetic graft (Fig. 12.26). Mural thrombus frequently forms over the atheromatous plaques and may form thick layers filling the whole sac; embolism may occur and occlude the vessels of the legs. Extension of the aneurysm to involve the origins of the renal or mesenteric arteries produces ischaemic effects.

Syphilitic Aneurysm

Historically, syphilis was the commonest cause of large aneurysms of the thoracic aorta and occurred most frequently in the aortic arch, the abdominal aorta being rarely affected. Syphilitic aneurysms are now very rare.

The weakness in the aortic wall arises because of syphilitic mesaortitis which develops 20 or more years after contracting the disease. The primary lesion is in the vasa vasorum of the thoracic aorta leading to local ischaemia in the media with patchy loss of musculoelastic laminae. In places, the patches coalesce and involve the whole thickness of the media (Fig. 12.27). Dense fibrous intimal thickening develops, overlying the areas of medial stretching, and is seen on the intimal surface as

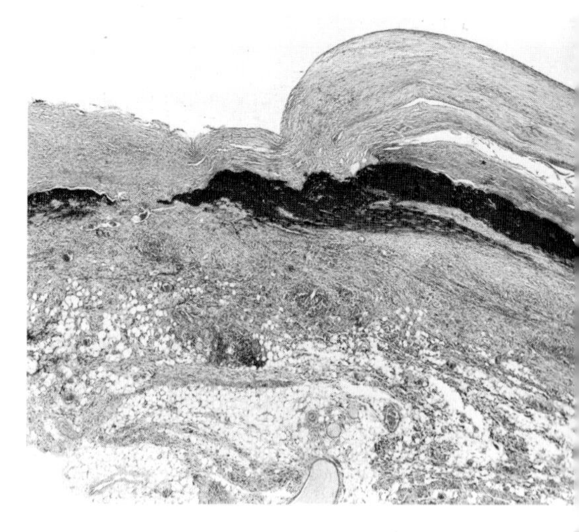

Fig. 12.27 Syphilitic aortitis; elastic tissue appears black. The section shows part of a thickened intimal plaque (upper right) and irregularity, thinning, and interruptions in the elastic tissue of the media, which has also lost most of its muscle and is grossly thinned: the paler tissue below is the adventitia and adjacent fatty tissue. ×10.

smooth grey-white areas, which extend and fuse, and become irregularly contracted to produce a wrinkled 'tree-bark' appearance (Fig. 12.28) and stellate scars. It is often associated with severe atheroma.

Effects. Pressure effects commonly occur leading to (1) superior mediastinal compression; (2) dysphagia; (3) bronchial obstruction with progression to pneumonia; (4) paralysis of the left recurrent laryngeal nerve; (5) painful vertebral erosion. Dilatation of the root of the aorta causes incompetence of the aortic valve leading to left ventricular hypertrophy and failure. Coronary artery narrowing due to involvement of their orifices by mesaortitis is now a rare cause of myocardial ischaemia. Rupture results in massive fatal haemorrhage with bleeding into the oesophagus, mediastinum or sometimes externally because of erosion through the sternum.

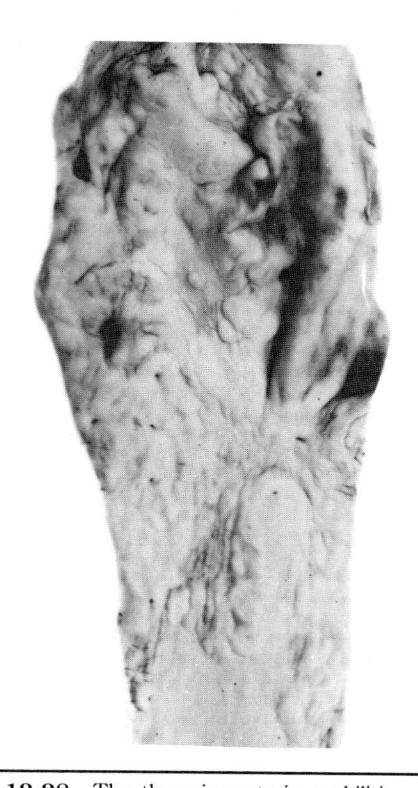

Fig. 12.28 The thoracic aorta in syphilitic aortitis. The arch of the aorta is stretched, with localized bulgings, thickened intimal patches and irregular wrinkling and scarring. In this example the changes stop abruptly below the arch. ×0.5.

Other Aneurysms

Infective (mycotic) aneurysms are the result of infection of the vessel wall either directly from an adjacent inflammatory process such as tuberculosis or due to the impaction of an infected embolus, e.g. in infective endocarditis.

Cerebral aneurysm. Saccular, 'berry' aneurysms on the circle of Willis usually arise because of congenital weakness in the arterial wall; some may be acquired as a result of atheroma. The sites of occurrence and the effects of rupture are discussed fully on p. 823. Microaneurysms of the deep penetrating branches of the cerebral arteries may occur in association with hypertension and are important causes of cerebral haemorrhage (p. 822).

Cardiac aneurysm is a complication of ischaemic heart disease (p. 496).

Capillary aneurysms are seen in the fundi in diabetic retinopathy (p. 884).

Arterial Trauma

Injury to the wall of an artery by a penetrating wound or blunt trauma may result in the development of a **traumatic aneurysm** due to a stretching of the fibrous scar. Complete penetration of an artery may give rise to a **false aneurysm** in which the sac is formed by fibrous tissue. Injury of an adjacent artery and vein may result in an arteriovenous fistula; in some instances the connection is by a channel with a fibrous wall, which may dilate to form an **arteriovenous aneurysm.**

A **cirsoid** or **racemose aneurysm** is a form of arteriovenous fistula which appears as a pulsatile swelling consisting of tortuous and dilated arteries and veins with multiple intercommunications. The commonest site is the scalp, and it may cause pressure atrophy of the underlying bone. The condition is sometimes congenital, probably due to birth injury but is more often the result of a blow on the head. Similarly, a **carotid-cavernous sinus aneurysm** resulting from a fracture base of the skull gives rise to great engorgement of the orbital veins and oedema of the orbit and conjunctiva.

Arterial Dissection

Dissection may affect many arteries but is commonest in the aorta. Aortic dissection is the commonest cause of rupture of the aorta. The initiating event is a tear in the intima of the aorta, through which blood enters and tracks between the inner two-thirds and outer third of the media, dissecting the wall into inner and outer layers. In most patients the blood bursts through the thinner outer layer of the wall usually within the first few days, and without surgical treatment the condition is usually fatal from massive haemorrhage. Dissection is spontaneous in the majority of cases but traumatic aortic dissection may be caused by blunt chest injury and may follow arterial catheterization and surgery.

The initial tear is usually transverse and, in 60% of cases, is in the ascending aorta (Fig. 12.29); in 30% of cases the tear is in the beginning of the descending aorta and at various sites in 10%. It is usually less than 3 cm in length but may involve the whole circumference. The extent of dissection varies greatly: in some patients the blood bursts out through the wall almost immediately with little dissection; the dissection may remain localized and thrombosis and organization of the blood in the media results in healing. Usually, however, blood tracks proximally and distally in the media. Most commonly it reaches the aortic ring and ruptures into the pericardial sac, causing death from cardiac tamponade or producing distortion of the valve ring and aortic incompetence. Therefore, dissections of the ascending aorta have a worse prognosis than those originating more distally. The dissection may also track distally along the arch and into the abdominal aorta, and then rupture into the mediastinum, pleura, retroperitoneal tissue or peritoneal cavity.

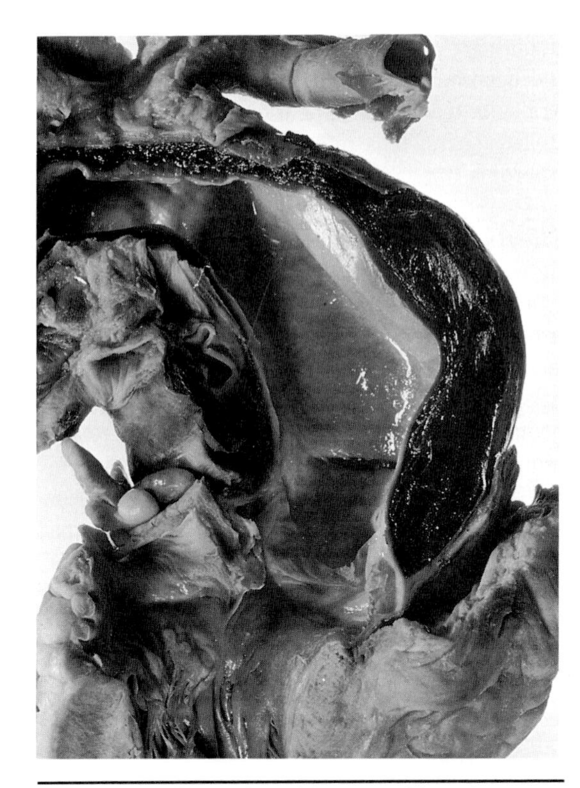

Fig. 12.29 Dissection of the aorta. There is a transverse tear of the inner part of the wall of the ascending aorta and blood has tracked proximally and distally within the media. Death was caused by haemopericardium. ×0.5.

The blood in the media can compress any of the branches of the aorta and can track along them, causing acute ischaemia: the coronary arteries are most often affected and myocardial infarction can result.

Occasionally, a second tear occurs on the inner aspect of the aortic wall, sometimes in an atheromatous patch in the abdominal aorta and the blood can flow through the second tear and re-enter the lumen. If the patient survives, the channel formed in the media becomes surrounded by fibrous tissue and lined by endothelium, giving a 'double-barrelled' aorta (Fig. 12.30).

Clinically, aortic dissection is three times commoner in males. The patient develops severe

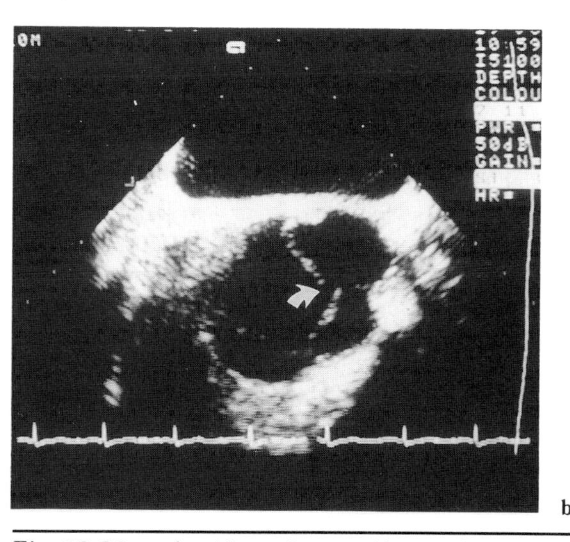

b

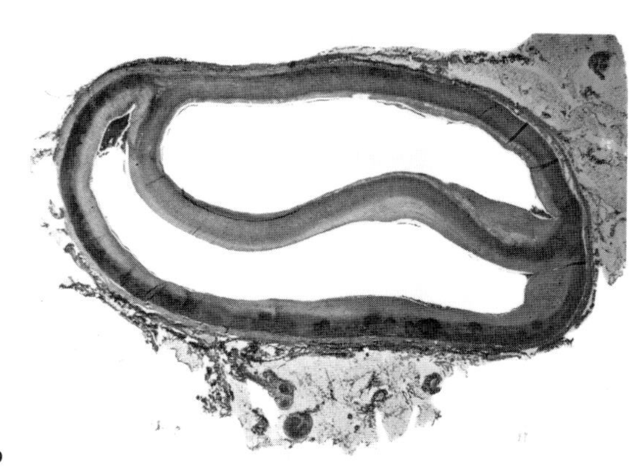

Fig. 12.30 **a** An oblique ultrasound image of the descending aorta showing an acute aortic dissection. There is a small tear (arrow) with a thin flap separating the true and false lumens. **b** A healed aortic dissection: in this case the dissection had burst back into the lumen through a second tear, giving rise to the 'double-barrelled' aorta seen here in cross-section.

tearing pain in the chest, becomes shocked and death may occur at any time from haemorrhage or from compression of the coronary arteries or other vessels. In 90% of cases there is a fatal outcome within a few days, but early diagnosis and prompt surgical treatment have improved the immediate prognosis.

Pathogenesis. The two important factors in aortic dissection are the blood pressure and weakness of the media. During ventricular systole the frictional force of the blood thrusts the intima in the direction of blood flow and when there is degeneration of the media this allows irregular increase in the sliding movement of the inner part of the wall and eventually results in a tear. Once this has happened the weakness in the media facilitates dissection by the escaping blood.

The weakness of the media is attributed to myxoid degeneration. This consists of patchy loss of elastic fibres and replacement of the musculoelastic tissue by accumulation of proteoglycan-rich extracellular matrix (Fig. 12.31). Areas of medial necrosis are found in 60% of cases at autopsy but this is probably secondary ischaemic damage due to shearing of the vasa vasorum. The cause of the myxoid degeneration is unknown. Similar changes can occur in hypertension and with increasing age. In pregnancy there is an increase in matrix proteoglycans in the arteries and this predisposes to dissection.

There is a high incidence of myxoid degeneration and aortic dissection in Marfan's syndrome, a hereditary disorder in which there is defective cross-linking of collagen. Aortic dissection can also occur in Ehlers – Danlos syndrome, in which there is a genetic defect in procollagen formation and in pseudoxanthoma elasticum in which there is a fragmentation of the medial elastic fibres. The experimental induction of defects in collagen cross-linking may result in arterial dissection. These experimental and clinical data suggest that in some instances the defect in the media in aortic dissection may have a metabolic basis.

Other Arterial Diseases

Raynaud's disease and Raynaud's phenomenon. This is an area in which there has been confusion in terminology. Raynaud's original description in 1862 was of a series of patients with

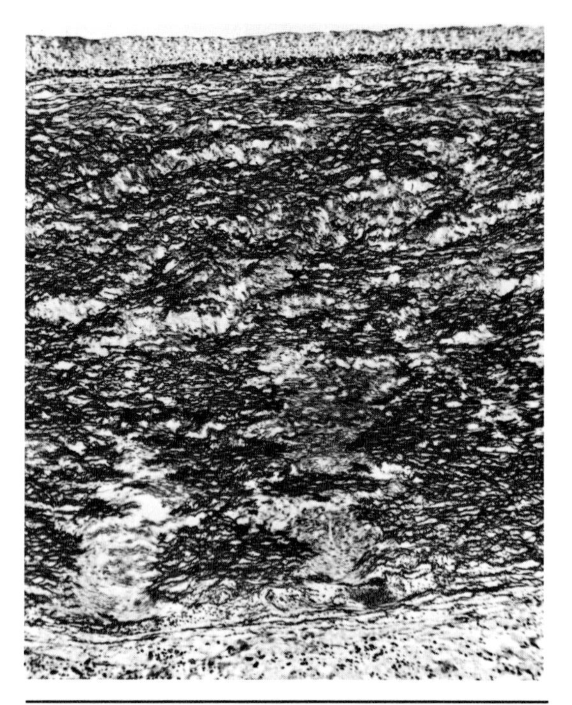

Fig. 12.31 Medial degeneration of the aorta. There are irregular pale gaps in the elastic tissue of the media. These represent the accumulations of proteoglycan-rich (myxoid) extracellular matrix. The patient was a woman of 24 who died of an aortic dissection. ×50.

intermittent abnormal impairment of the circulation through the extremities on exposure to cold. This is **Raynaud's disease**: it occurs mainly in young women, usually starting in adolescence and often continuing indefinitely. It usually affects the fingers of both hands symmetrically and occasionally the tip of the nose, ears and toes. On exposure to cold or in response to emotional stimuli the fingers become cold and white and may be numb or extremely painful. The circulation is restored by warmth, but trophic changes may eventually occur and whitlows are common: ulceration and gangrene seldom occur. There are no histological abnormalities in the vessels. The pallor of the skin suggests that in addition to arterial constriction there is also vasoconstriction of the capillary circulation. The mechanisms causing this vasoconstriction are not known. Recent studies have suggested that there might be a local dysfunction of peptidergic innervation of the digital vessels.

Raynaud's phenomenon consists of symptoms similar to those of Raynaud's disease but accompanying a number of other diseases or attributable to other mechanisms. These include: connective tissue diseases such as progressive systemic sclerosis and systemic lupus erythematosus; Buerger's disease; trauma from the use of vibratory power tools or pressure as in the thoracic outlet syndrome, drug or toxin induced (ergot, β-adrenergic blockers and polyvinyl chloride monomer); tumours secreting vasoactive peptides (carcinoids, phaeochromocytoma); and haematological diseases with impaired circulation in the extremities (cryoglobulinaemia and other hyperviscosity syndromes).

In Raynaud's phenomenon vessel involvement is not always symmetrical and trophic changes, ulceration and gangrene may occur. In cases where gangrene develops, thrombosis and recanalized vessels may be present. The mechanisms in Raynaud's phenomenon probably differ depending on the causal agent. In some instances there is probably a combination of local neurovascular dysfunction similar to that in Raynaud's disease but which is aggravated by a variety of factors. Raynaud's phenomenon may be an early manifestation of progressive systemic sclerosis (p. 231); the combination of **c**alcinosis, **R**aynaud's phenomenon, o**e**sophageal involvement, **s**clerodactyly and **t**elangiectasia constitutes the CREST syndrome.

Mönckeberg's sclerosis (calcification of the media). This disease, of uncertain cause, is characterized by dystrophic calcification in the media in the major arteries of the legs in elderly people. It probably represents an exaggeration of the normal increase of calcium salts in arteriosclerotic vessels. It may also affect the arteries of the arms and less commonly visceral arteries. The affected vessels are dilated and show transverse bars due to deposition of calcium in the circular medial muscle layer. Occasionally, true bone may be formed in an area of calcification, and may even contain red marrow. The radiological appearance is striking but since there is no arterial narrowing there are no significant clinical effects.

Fibromuscular dysplasia is a condition of unknown aetiology which affects medium-sized arteries mainly in females. There are various types but in all of them the structure of the artery wall is focally abnormal. Most often there is fibrous or fibromuscular thickening of the wall leading to stenosis. The renal arteries are most commonly affected causing renal artery stenosis. The carotid, vertebral and splanchnic arteries may also be involved. Alteration of the normal structure of the media gives rise to both true aneurysms and to dissection.

Veins

Compensatory enlargement of the veins takes place, as in the arterial system, when there is a sustained increase in blood flow – in the uterine veins during pregnancy and in the collateral veins following obstruction of a major vein. As in the case of arteries, dilatation is followed by hypertrophy of the various elements in the wall of the vessels with an increase in collagen and elastic tissue.

Thrombophlebitis and Phlebothrombosis

A distinction is sometimes made between **thrombophlebitis**, by which is meant a primary inflammatory condition of the vein, with secondary thrombosis, and **phlebothrombosis**, in which a thrombosis, of the vein occurs with, at most, mild accompanying inflammatory change. The presence of thrombus in the lumen of the vein sets up reactive changes so that differentiation between mild thrombophlebitis and phlebothrombosis may not be possible. Venous thrombosis and its consequences are discussed on p. 93.

Multiple venous thromboses occur in **thrombophlebitis migrans**. This usually affects superficial veins, but sometimes also deeper ones, in any part of the body. In some cases the cause is not apparent, in others it is a paraneoplastic syndrome associated with a carcinoma, most often of the pancreas but also of breast, stomach, bronchus or ovary. The thrombotic episodes may be the first clinical manifestation of the cancer.

Infective thrombophlebitis may occur in the veins of the diploë and dural sinuses in middle-ear infection, in the uterine veins in puerperal sepsis, in the veins of the bone marrow in suppurative osteomyelitis, and occasionally in the pulmonary veins in bronchiectasis. Veins involved in such lesions undergo thrombosis and the thrombus becomes infected by bacteria; fragments may break away and produce pyaemia. Portal pylephlebitis may complicate acute inflammation of abdominal organs (appendix, fallopian tube for example) or may follow umbilical catheterization in neonates; it may result in liver abscesses or portal vein thrombosis.

Chronic Phlebitis

Chronic inflammation causes reactive thickening of vein walls; the small veins are affected in this way in all chronic inflammatory conditions. The changes are analogous to endarteritis. Veno-occlusive disease of the liver giving rise to the Budd–Chiari syndrome is discussed on p. 749.

Venous spread of tumours occurs commonly, the best example being renal cell carcinoma. Such invasion is usually accompanied by thrombosis. Occlusion of a vein by tumour can result in retrograde flow with retrograde spread of tumour in a venous plexus, e.g. metastasis to the lumbar spine in prostatic carcinoma.

Varicose Veins

Dilatation and tortuosity of veins is termed **varicosity** and a dilated vein is a **varix**. Varices arise from increase in the blood pressure within veins, resulting either from (1) the effects of gravity, e.g. in the leg veins, sometimes aggravated by compression proximally, or (2) obstruction to flow of major veins leading to increased pressure in collateral veins.

'Gravitational' varicosity occurs in the saphenous system of the legs, notably the long saphenous vein. The condition is much commoner in women, and there is a distinct hereditary predisposition. Obesity, pregnancy and occupations involving prolonged standing are additional risk factors. Prolonged standing causes pressure and distension of the leg veins. Eventually the veins become permanently stretched, leading to incompetence of the valves. The venous stasis causes impaired nutrition of the tissues of the lower legs. This leads to eczema and pigmentation. Minor trauma may give rise to varicose ulcers which are susceptible to infection and heal with difficulty.

Haemorrhoids are varicosities of the haemorrhoidal venous plexuses, projecting from the surface just above or below the anorectal junction. Bleeding may cause iron deficiency and rupture causes painful swelling in the perianal subcutaneous tissue. They may also become thrombosed or prolapse through the anal sphincter and become strangulated.

Varicocele (p. 1065) is another 'gravitational' varicosity. It affects the pampiniform plexus of veins around the spermatic cord.

The most important 'obstructive' varicosity occurs in portal hypertension due most commonly to cirrhosis of the liver (p. 772). Anastomoses between the portal and systemic systems develop, producing **oesophageal varices**; bleeding from them is a common cause of death in cirrhosis.

Tumours and Malformations of Blood Vessels

Benign Vascular Tumours

Congenital malformation of blood vessels are common and many of the lesions called angiomas are not truly tumours but hamartomas. They are present at birth, their enlargement ceases with the growth of the patient and they comprise a mixture of vascular and other mesenchymal elements.

Haemangiomas

These comprise a mass of blood vessels atypical or irregular in arrangement and size.

Capillary haemangiomas consist of a dense network of vessels of capillary size (Fig. 12.32). They are commonest in the skin, where they form one of the two common types of naevus or birthmark, but also occur in the internal organs, the liver, spleen and kidney for example. Most are small, but larger lesions occur, e.g. the 'port-wine stains' of the face, which consist of capillary-like vessels with an abnormally large lumen. Capillary angiomas are usually well defined, deep red or purple. The vessels have a more prominent endothelial lining than normal capillaries and endothelial cells may be seen scattered or in clusters without formation of a lumen (Fig. 12.32). The stroma consists of a well formed collagen. There is no capsule, and at the margin the capillaries often give a false impression of invasion of the adjacent tissues.

The **juvenile capillary haemangioma** or 'strawberry naevus' is present in the skin at birth. They may grow rapidly for some months but then gradually shrink in the first few years of life before regressing completely, usually by the age of 5.

Cavernous haemangiomas are found in the skin, subcutaneous tissue, lips and tongue and also in the liver, pancreas and brain. They consist of relatively large, interconnecting, sinus-like vascular spaces (Fig. 12.33). In the liver they form deep purple, well defined masses, usually polygonal

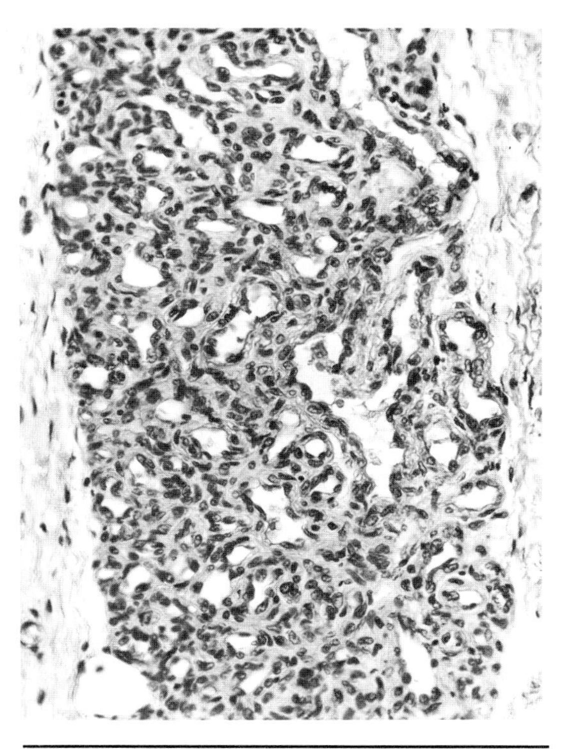

Fig. 12.32 Capillary angioma showing well formed capillaries with prominent endothelial cells. The solid areas between capillaries include many cells which appear to be endothelial cells not related to a lumen. ×200.

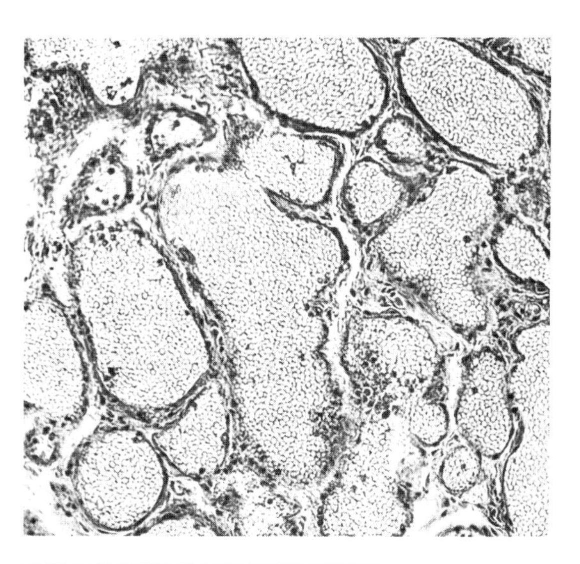

Fig. 12.33 Cavernous angioma of subcutaneous tissue, showing large intercommunicating spaces filled with blood. ×130.

rather than round and not raised above the surface.

Multiple angiomatosis syndromes. Angiomas are often multiple, and are also a component of several autosomal dominant diseases. These include: (1) hereditary haemorrhagic telangiectasia or **Osler–Weber–Rendu disease** in which there are multiple small angiomas in skin and mucosae and sometimes in liver and spleen. There is a strong tendency to haemorrhage but this can usually be controlled; (2) **von Hippel–Lindau disease** in which there are cerebellar and retinal angiomas with cysts of liver and pancreas; and (3) **Sturge–Weber syndrome** with facial and meningeal angiomas.

Epithelioid haemangioma (angiolymphoid hyperplasia, Kimura's disease) affects young and middle-aged adults, especially around the head and neck. The lesion consists of a cluster of vessels lined by large plump ('epithelioid') endothelial cells admixed with inflammatory cells in which eosinophils are often prominent. It is uncertain whether these lesions represent true tumours or an abnormal tissue response to trauma or infection. They may be multiple and can recur after excision, but never metastasize.

Glomangioma (Glomus Tumour)

This uncommon lesion arises from the glomus bodies, which control skin blood flow and temperature, particularly in the fingers and toes. In its most characteristic form, the glomangioma is a small bluish nodule, usually near the end of a finger or toe and extraordinarily tender to touch. The tumour consists of two kinds of tissue (Fig. 12.34): the first is angiomatous, with spaces containing blood, lined by endothelium, and separated by connective tissue containing varying amounts of smooth muscle; the other is cellular, with rounded or cuboidal glomus ('myoid') cells which show some of the ultrastructural features of smooth muscle cells. The tumour contains numerous

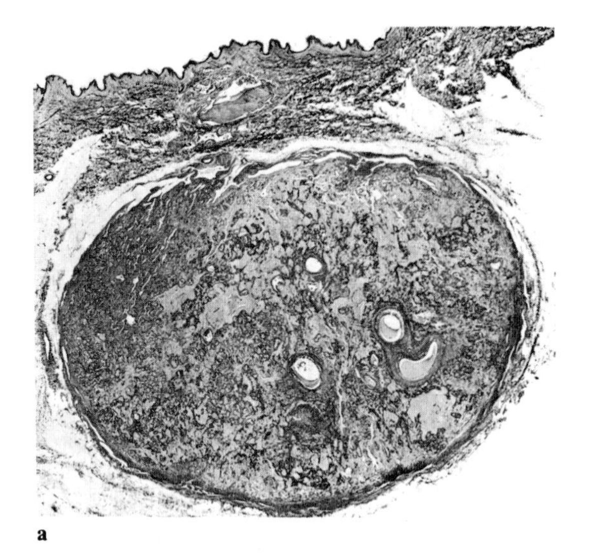

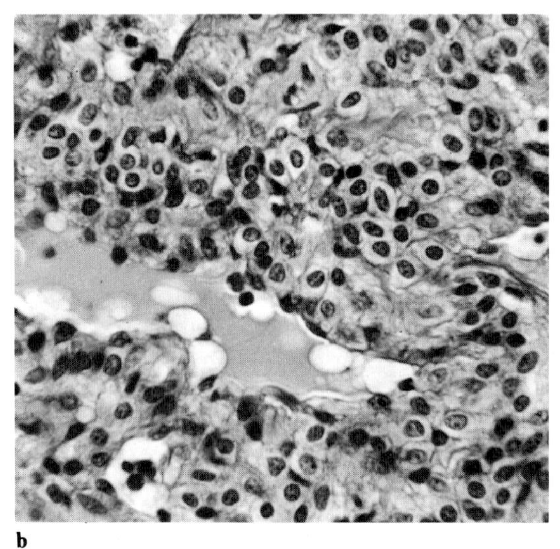

Fig. 12.34 **a** Glomangioma. Small subcutaneous encapsulated growth showing the coiled arteriole. ×8. **b** The clear myoid cells surrounding a vascular space. ×350.

myelinated and non-myelinated nerve fibres. Glomangiomas sometimes occur in deeper tissues, but the characteristic pain occurs only with those in the limbs.

Chemodectomas are rare tumours which arise from the glomus tissue derived from the branchial arches, viz. the carotid body, glomus jugulare and aorticopulmonary bodies. Chemodectomas occur also in other sites, including the organ of Zuckerkandl. They are sometimes incorrectly termed non-chromaffin paragangliomas, but do not produce any endocrine effect. They are nearly always benign but rare cases of malignancy with metastases have been reported. Their anatomical site may render complete removal difficult.

The commonest site is in the carotid body and these have an increased frequency in people (and their cattle) living at high altitudes, for example in the High Andes where carotid body hyperplasia due to long-standing hypoxaemia (p. 575) is a predisposing factor. Histologically, the tumour is composed of clusters of chief cells with clear cytoplasm and a round nucleus, enclosed in a framework of fibrous tissues which contains a rich sinusoidal blood supply. Chemodectomas at other sites have the same general features as those of the carotid bodies.

Glomus jugulare tumours are usually recurrent, bleeding aural polyps arising in the middle ear; they may also present intracranially.

Malignant Vascular Tumours

These are rare and show varying grades of malignancy ranging from indolent, slow-growing tumours, haemangioendotheliomas, to highly aggressive very poorly differentiated angiosarcomas. The endothelial cell nature of these tumours can often be confirmed by immunohistochemical techniques demonstrating the presence of factor VIII related antigen in the tumour cells or their ability to bind to the lectin *Ulex europaeus*. Electron microscopy will demonstrate the presence of Weibel–Palade bodies in the cells (p. 85).

Haemangioendotheliomas

Three subgroups of these are recognized.

Epithelioid haemangioendothelioma shows primitive vascular differentiation, usually confined to small intracellular lumina within individual cells. The tumours are usually associated with a large vessel, often a vein. They may occur in soft tissue sites, in the liver and in the lung. One-third metastasize to local lymph nodes.

Spindle-cell haemangioendothelioma occurs in young adult males, often in the hand. The histological appearances are a mixture of cavernous vascular spaces with intervening spindle-cell areas. Beginning as one nodule, they often become multifocal and occasionally metastasize.

Malignant endovascular papillary angioendothelioma is a rare low-grade angiosarcoma which occurs in the skin in childhood and may metastasize.

Angiosarcomas

These tumours show a wide range of differentiation. The commonest sites are the skin, breast, soft tissues and liver. Some of those in the skin arise in areas of chronic lymphoedema and there is some debate as to whether or not they are lymphangiosarcomas, an issue which can be avoided by using the non-committal term angiosarcoma. Angiosarcomas commonly show a disparity between their histological behaviour and the degree of malignancy; for example, angiosarcoma of the breast is commonly well differentiated histologically, yet it is the most malignant of all tumours of the breast. Angiosarcomas of the liver have attracted interest. Although very rare, they have been aetiologically associated with exposure to Thorotrast (a radioactive contrast medium used until the 1950s), arsenicals used in agriculture and most recently vinyl chloride monomer used in the plastics industry.

Kaposi's sarcoma is described on p. 1140 and its association with the acquired immunodeficiency syndrome is further discussed on p. 246.

Haemangiopericytoma

This tumour consists of short spindle cells arranged round many small vascular clefts. Silver stains and electron microscopy confirm that the tumour cells are outside the basement membrane of the vessels and that they are pericytes. They occur most commonly in the legs and in retroperitoneal tissues. Their behaviour can be difficult to predict but half of them will metastasize.

Lymphatic Vessels

Lymphatic vessels are thin-walled endothelial lined channels present in almost all tissues and as numerous as capillaries but not readily visualized histologically because they collapse. Terminal lymphatics drain into collecting lymphatics which progressively increase in size and finally drain into veins in the neck via the thoracic duct or the right lymphatic duct. Valves are present in collecting lymphatics to ensure unidirectional lymph flow. On route to the bloodstream lymph passes through a number of lymph nodes which act as filters along the lymphatic system (p. 650).

Electron microscopic studies show that lymphatic endothelium is thinner and more irregular than that of blood capillaries and its basement membrane is tenuous and incomplete. Junctions between endothelial cells are simpler in form and gaps are normally present between endothelial cells in some terminal lymphatics. Fine fibrils join the outer surface of the endothelial cells of terminal lymphatics to collagen fibres and other connective tissue structures. Collecting lymphatics have a more regular endothelium and smooth muscle cells are present in their walls.

Function of lymphatics. The role of plasma proteins in maintaining the normal oncotic pressure in the blood has already been discussed (p. 74). Many plasma proteins, however, carry out their functions in the extravascular spaces and in order to conserve these proteins they return to the circulation via the lymphatic channels. Electron microscopic studies show that large marker particles, and therefore presumably plasma proteins, enter terminal lymphatics via intercellular junctions or gaps. Flow of lymph along lymphatics is in part a passive process due to the valved structure and pressure from adjacent tissues and in part active due to contraction of smooth muscle cells in collecting lymphatics. The roles of lymphatics in inflammation and infection (p. 115) and in the spread of malignant tumours (p. 386) have already been discussed.

Lymphatic Obstruction: Lymphoedema

Chronic obstruction of lymphatics may give rise to interstitial accumulation of lymph (lymphoedema). When this is prolonged there is proliferation of connective tissue in the lymphoedematous area, resulting in a firm, non-pitting oedema. The most striking examples are seen in **filariasis**, in which obstruction of major lymphatics, together with recurrent inflammation in the affected region, may lead to gross thickening of the tissues known as **elephantiasis**: the legs and sometimes the male external genitalia may be involved (p. 1183). In non-tropical countries, extensive carcinomatous permeation of lymphatics is a more common cause of lymphoedema; this may follow surgical removal of lymphatics or destruction of lymphatics by radiotherapy. This was sometimes seen following radical mastectomy and radiotherapy of the axilla for breast cancer, where the arm, deprived of its lymphatic drainage, developed gross lymphoedema, in which angiosarcomas have occasionally developed.

Tumours and Malformations of Lymphatics

Lymphangioma. This may be composed of numerous lymphatic vessels – the plexiform lymphangioma – but more frequently it has a cavernous structure (Fig. 12.35). Dilatation and diffuse growth of vessels may give rise to enlargement of an organ, e.g. the tongue (macroglossia). Like haemangiomas, lymphangiomas are essentially hamartomas. The more diffuse lesions may be difficult to distinguish from the effects of lymphatic obstruction. Lymphangiomas, whether diffuse or compact, are commonest in the skin and subcutaneous tissue. Each forms a somewhat ill-defined, doughy or semi-fluctuant swelling, containing large, intercommunicating lymphatic spaces. Lymphangiomas of the neck, retroperitoneum or mesentery may undergo great dilatation, forming a large multilocular ramifying cystic mass – **cystic hygroma**. Occasionally a single cyst is formed which may be distinguished from other cysts by its endothelial lining.

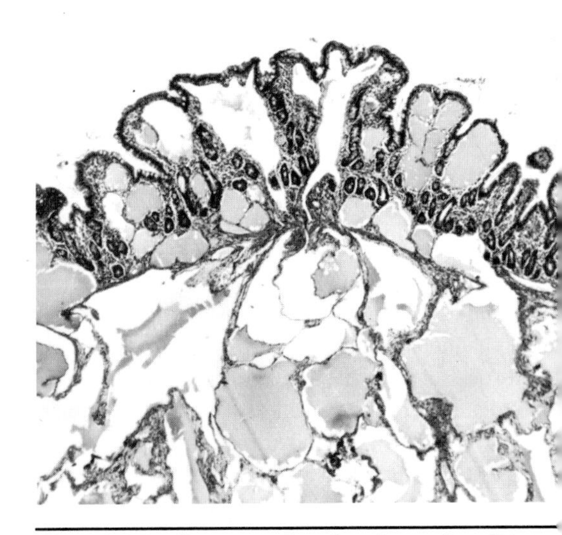

Fig. 12.35 Cavernous lymphangioma of small intestine. It is made up of large intercommunicating spaces filled with clear lymph (which has coagulated and then shrunk in processing the tissue). The lesion involves both mucosa and submucosa.

Lymphangioendothelioma (lymphangiosarcoma) is a doubtful entity and its association with chronic lymphoedema and haemangiosarcoma has been mentioned above.

The Heart

Diseases of the heart and circulation are the commonest causes of death in most industrial countries. About one-third of all deaths in the UK can be attributed to heart disease (Fig. 12.36), in the great majority due to ischaemic heart disease. In developing countries, ischaemic heart disease is less common but of increasing importance; the main causes of heart disease in these areas are rheumatic valvular disease and myocardial infection; for example Chagas' disease due to *Trypanosoma cruzi*, is a major form of heart disease in South America. The incidence of congenital heart disease has not changed but is assuming a greater importance because of major advances in cardiac surgery. The expanding scope of cardiac surgery also embraces correction of acquired valvular lesions, coronary artery bypass and cardiac transplantation, and this, as we shall see, has had implications for the pathologist.

The work of the heart. Assuming the resting stroke volume of the heart is 66 ml, at 72 beats per minute the left ventricle has a minute volume of about 5 litres, and a daily output of 7200 litres (about 7.5 tons). The normal heart has great reserve power, and this can be substantially increased by physical training. During exertion, there is a greater venous return with consequent increase in diastolic filling and stretching of the muscle fibres; the response is a more vigorous contraction (Starling's law) and a greatly increased stroke volume. The heart rate also increases during exertion and these two factors together can raise the minute volume to about seven times that of the resting state. This physiological performance can be maintained only if the myocardium is healthy, the valves function efficiently, the conducting system of the heart co-ordinates contraction of the chambers, and peripheral resistance to blood flow is not grossly abnormal. Disturbance of any of these requirements can cause cardiac failure.

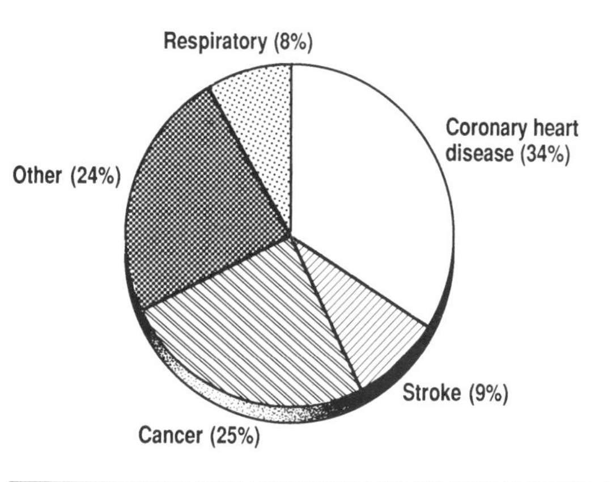

Fig. 12.36 Pie chart showing distribution of main causes of death in Scotland in 1987.

Cardiac Failure

The terms cardiac failure and heart failure are synonymous and refer to *that state in which impaired cardiac function fails to maintain a circulation adequate for the metabolic needs of the body despite an adequate blood volume.* Consequently there is inadequate perfusion of the tissues leading to a syndrome in which the most important features are fatigue, breathlessness and oedema. These result from a complex interaction of many factors: impaired cardiac output ('forward failure') and increased central venous pressure ('backward failure'); impaired gas exchange in the lungs; activation of neurohumoral mechanisms causing disturbances of salt and water balance; and changes in skeletal muscle function.

Heart failure is a clinical syndrome and not a single diagnosis or pathological entity. Furthermore, there is a spectrum of heart failure ranging from mild asymptomatic cardiac dysfunction, through more severe failure with reduced exercise tolerance but in which compensatory mechanisms (ventricular hypertrophy, peripheral vasoconstriction, salt and water retention) maintain tissue perfusion, and finally, to a stage in which compensatory mechanisms are exhausted and symptoms and signs of failure occur at rest.

The causes of heart failure are summarized in Table 12.7. Essentially, failure is due to an abnormal increase in the work required of the myocardium, weakness or inefficiency of the myocardial contraction, or a combination of both.

Table 12.7 Causes of heart failure

Right ventricle	Left ventricle
Increased workload	Increased workload
Pulmonary hypertension due to:	Systemic hypertension
left ventricular failure	Aortic and mitral valve disease
chronic lung disease	Coarctation of the aorta
left-to-right shunting with increased blood flow	Increased cardiac output:
Pulmonary embolism	anaemia
Pulmonary and tricuspid valve disease	thyrotoxicosis
Myocardial injury	Myocardial injury
Ischaemia/infarction	Ischaemia/infarction
Myocarditis	Myocarditis
Cardiomyopathy	Cardiomyopathy

Pathophysiological Concepts

The heart must not only expel enough blood during systole, it must also fill adequately during diastole. Heart failure most commonly results from impaired cardiac emptying, or 'systolic failure'; less commonly impaired filling leads to 'diastolic failure'. These simple concepts apply equally to both the right and left ventricles and their respective circulations. Although the pressure in the pulmonary circulation is much lower, the flow within it must equal that in the systemic circulation. Myocardial ischaemia produces a combination of both diastolic and systolic dysfunction since relaxation, like contraction, is an energy consuming process.

Systolic Failure – Inadequate Emptying

Impaired ventricular contraction. The normal left ventricle expels at least 50% of its contents during systole. This is known as the left ventricular ejection fraction (LVEF) and is the best clinical measure of ventricular systolic function. The weakened ventricle cannot achieve a normal LVEF and enlarges to accommodate the increased residual volume plus the blood which arrives from the atrium. This enlargement can be viewed as a compensation for impaired contraction (Fig. 12.37). The wall tension required to maintain pressure is proportional to the square of the radius of the heart (Laplace's law). Since wall tension is an important determinant of myocardial oxygen demand, maintenance of the stroke volume when the heart dilates incurs an increased metabolic cost. During exercise, the cardiac output cannot rise appropriately; this leads to the characteristic symptoms of tiredness and breathlessness. The tiredness is due to underperfusion of the exercising muscles. The breathlessness is due to the combination of (a) a rise in pressure and volume in the pulmonary circulation leading to decreased compliance in the lungs; and (b) increased anaerobic metabolism with accumulation of lactate causing acidosis and stimulating the respiratory centre.

Increased volume load. Incompetence of the heart valves leads to an increased volume load on the appropriate ventricle. In aortic or mitral incompetence, the left ventricle has to accommodate not only the volume of blood returning from the lungs but also the regurgitant volume from the left atrium in the case of mitral incompetence and from

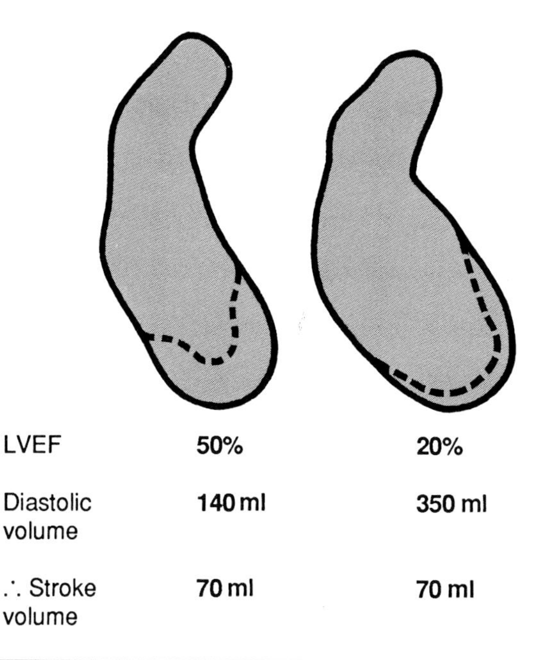

Fig. 12.37 Diagrammatic representation of a left ventriculogram. The dotted line outline shows the left ventricular (LV) chamber and proximal ascending aorta at end systole and the solid line shows the end diastolic outline. Enlargement of the left ventricle allows the maintenance of a normal stroke volume at rest, despite a severe impairment in contractility reflected in a reduction of the left ventricular ejection fraction from 50% to 20%.

the aorta in the case of aortic incompetence. This leads to dilatation accompanied by hypertrophy and, ultimately, to heart failure. Intracardiac shunts due, for example, to congenital heart disease also impose a volume load on the lower pressure chamber, i.e. right atrium and ventricle in atrial septal defect and right ventricle in ventricular septal defect.

Pressure overload is usually due to increased pressure in the systemic or pulmonary circulation (systemic or pulmonary hypertension) and stenosis of the aortic or pulmonary valves. These cause pressure overload in the left and right ventricle respectively. Myocardial hypertrophy increases the power of contraction and maintains the stroke volume for a time. Ultimately, dilatation and fibrosis occur, leading to impaired contractility and heart failure.

Diastolic Failure – Inadequate Filling

Pericardial diseases. Accumulation of fluid in the pericardium or the presence of pericardial thickening and calcification impedes the filling of all four cardiac chambers during their diastolic phases. This causes raised pressure in both systemic and pulmonary venous systems and clinically is first detected by distension of the jugular veins in the neck.

Stenosis of the tricuspid or mitral valve impairs filling of the right and left ventricle respectively. In mitral stenosis this causes raised pressure in the pulmonary circulation and later this is followed by right ventricular failure due to the increased load on the right ventricle. The peripheral venous pressure is raised, leading to oedema and hepatomegaly.

Atrial arrhythmias, especially atrial fibrillation, may precipitate heart failure because the tachycardia leaves less time for the heart to fill and, in addition, the final phase of ventricular filling due to normal atrial contraction is lost.

Decreased myocardial compliance also impairs ventricular filling. This occurs in severe left ventricular hypertrophy where there is also fibrosis, typically hypertrophic cardiomyopathy (p. 498) and, to a lesser extent, in all cases of severe hypertrophy. Decreased compliance also occurs in amyloid infiltration (p. 250).

Severe endocardial thickening as in endomyocardial fibrosis (p. 499) gives rise to diastolic dysfunction by restricting ventricular expansion in diastole.

Manifestations of Cardiac Failure

In mild degrees of cardiac failure the heart is no longer able to increase its output sufficiently to fulfil extreme metabolic demands, as in strenuous physical activity, but is still able to meet lesser demands. With increase in severity the cardiac reserve is further diminished, leading to decreasing exercise tolerance until, in severe failure, the circulation is inadequate even at rest.

Failure may be acute or chronic depending on whether the causal factors, impaired myocardial efficiency or increased workload, develop rapidly or slowly. The causal factors may affect predominantly either ventricle, giving rise to left or right ventricular failure, or both may be affected, with consequent total heart failure.

Acute heart failure occurs when the causal factors develop rapidly or suddenly. Examples include myocardial infarction, gross pulmonary embolism, arrhythmias, myocarditis, rheumatic fever and rupture of a valve cusp. In severe acute failure (most often due to myocardial infarction) the cardiac output falls drastically and there is peripheral vasoconstricion due to increased sympathetic activity. The term **cardiogenic shock** is then appropriate. The full picture of cardiogenic shock (p. 108) develops in only a small proportion of cases, but when it does the outlook is poor.

Chronic heart failure occurs when the causal factors develop slowly. The commonest causes are myocardial ischaemia, systemic arterial hypertension, chronic valvular dysfunction and diseases of the lungs with pulmonary hypertension. Chronic failure usually develops insidiously, but acute failure may progress to chronic failure. In chronic failure, cardiac output is diminished and tissue hypoxia results. Although two-thirds of cases die from progressive failure, the other third die suddenly, probably due to an arrhythmia. As with acute failure, the clinical and pathological changes depend on the nature of the causal factors and whether they affect mainly the left, right or both ventricles.

Left ventricular failure (LVF) The common causes of cardiac failure affect the left ventricle more than the right. However, LVF usually leads to right ventricular failure so that, in the later stages, the picture is that of chronic congestive failure. The commonest cause of LVF is ischaemic heart disease, particularly myocardial infarction. Other causes include systemic hypertension, aortic valve disease and mitral valve incompetence.

As failure develops, the left ventricle can no longer pass on all the blood it receives during diastole, causing dilatation which further impairs contraction. Eventually, the dilatation results in stretching of the mitral ring with consequent mitral valve incompetence, leading to venous congestion, pulmonary oedema (Fig. 12.38) and further reduction of left ventricular output.

The main clinical features of LVF are dyspnoea

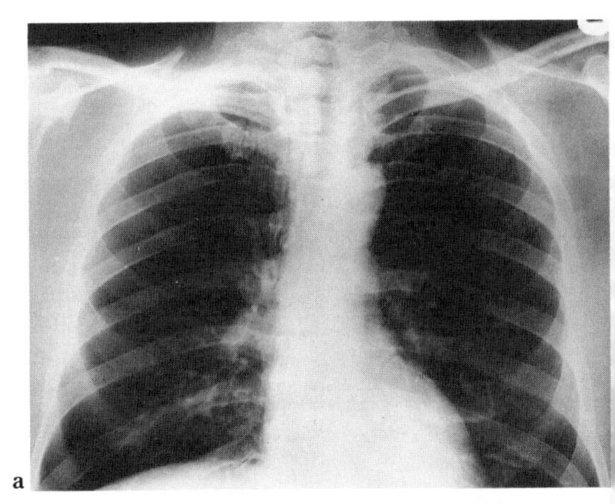

a

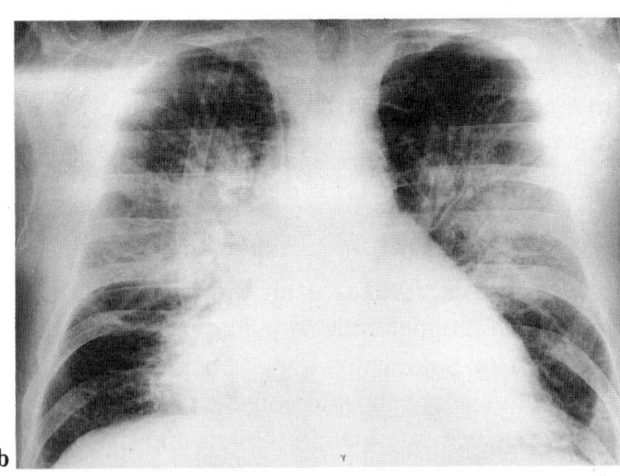

b

Fig. 12.38 **a** Chest radiograph showing a normal heart shape and size with clear lung fields. **b** Chest radiograph showing cardiac enlargement and unfolding of the aortic arch in a case of hypertension.

and cough due to pulmonary congestion and oedema. In acute failure, death may occur rapidly from acute pulmonary oedema and the picture is sometimes complicated by cardiogenic shock. During the early stage of chronic failure, the left ventricle fails to meet increased circulatory demands so that undue dyspnoea and cough are precipitated by physical activity. As failure increases, exercise tolerance diminishes until pulmonary congestion is present even at rest. Acute exacerbations of LVF commonly occur at night (**paroxysmal nocturnal dyspnoea**). Such attacks result from increased venous return in the recumbent position and from an increased blood volume following resorption of fluid from the extravascular space. The pulmonary congestion and oedema of LVF are most pronounced when there is severe imbalance between the functional capacities of the left and right ventricles.

Right ventricular failure (RVF) occurs most often as a consequence of pulmonary hypertension, and in most industrial countries the commonest cause of this is left ventricular failure due to ischaemic heart disease. When the left ventricle fails, pulmonary arteriolar vasoconstriction with a rise in pulmonary arterial pressure occurs in response to the increased pressure in the left atrium and pulmonary veins. The mechanisms of this are not fully understood. The most acute form of RVF is seen in pulmonary embolism. A massive embolus is usually fatal within minutes, but multiple large emboli can cause acute RVF and multiple embolism over a long period occasionally causes chronic RVF.

When the right ventricle fails, it becomes dilated as it is unable to eject all the blood which enters during diastole (Fig. 12.62). Stretching of the tricuspid ring results in incompetence. The right atrium dilates and there is a rise in central venous pressure which gives rise to the changes of **systemic venous congestion** and peripheral **'cardiac' oedema** (p. 76).

Congestive (biventricular) heart failure develops usually in cases of left ventricular failure, although both ventricles may fail simultaneously as a result of diffuse or extensive myocardial damage, e.g. extensive infarction, severe myocarditis, beriberi and congestive cardiomyopathy. Congestive failure can also result from conditions which increase the workload of both ventricles, for example lesions of the mitral and aortic valves and states in which there is a persistently raised cardiac output, such as thyrotoxicosis, anaemia and congenital abnormalities with left-to-right shunts. In these latter states, failure is associated with the usual fall in cardiac output, but the fall is relative to the previous abnormally high output so that, even in failure, the absolute output may be normal or even increased. The term '**high output failure**' is then applied.

Compensatory Mechanisms in Cardiac Diseases

Myocardial hypertrophy occurs in the walls of the affected chambers in response to increased pressure and increased volume load. In conditions of increased volume load, hypertrophy is accompanied by dilatation during diastole which stimulates increased systolic contraction (Starling's law). The atria also undergo compensatory changes when their workload is increased, but their capacity for hypertrophy is limited. The causes of left and right ventricular hypertrophy are those of right and left ventricular failure, with the important exception of myocarditis. Progressive left ventricular hypertrophy demands an increased blood supply; failure to meet this demand, as a result of coronary artery insufficiency, results in left ventricular failure.

Even in the presence of normal coronary arteries gross left ventricular hypertrophy results in relative ischaemia. It is associated with fibrosis of the myocardium, diastolic dysfunction (p. 485) and a tendency to sudden death due to ventricular arrhythmias.

Neuroendocrine factors in heart failure. Apart from the intrinsic compensatory mechanisms described above during heart failure stimulation of the sympathetic nervous system occurs and there is increased secretion of a number of vasoactive factors (Fig. 12.39). Sympathetic activation is stimulated via stretch receptors in the aorta, atria and pulmonary veins; those in the aorta respond to a fall in pressure, the others to a fall in volume. Increased sympathetic activity increases the heart rate (β_1 stimulation) and myocardial contractility (β_1 and α_1 stimulation) both of which help to maintain cardiac output and lead to vasoconstriction. Activation of the renin–angiotensin–aldosterone system (p. 75) with sodium and water retention which increase blood volume is due partly to increased sympathetic activity but mainly results from reduced renal perfusion. This effect may ultimately be detrimental, however, and aggravate the heart failure.

An understanding of these neuroendocrine mechanisms has suggested new therapeutic approaches to the clinical management of cardiac failure. Thus, angiotensin converting enzyme (ACE) inhibition may be used to counteract the effects of the renin–angiotensin system and more recently agents which stimulate atrial natriuretic peptide (ANP) secretion have been developed.

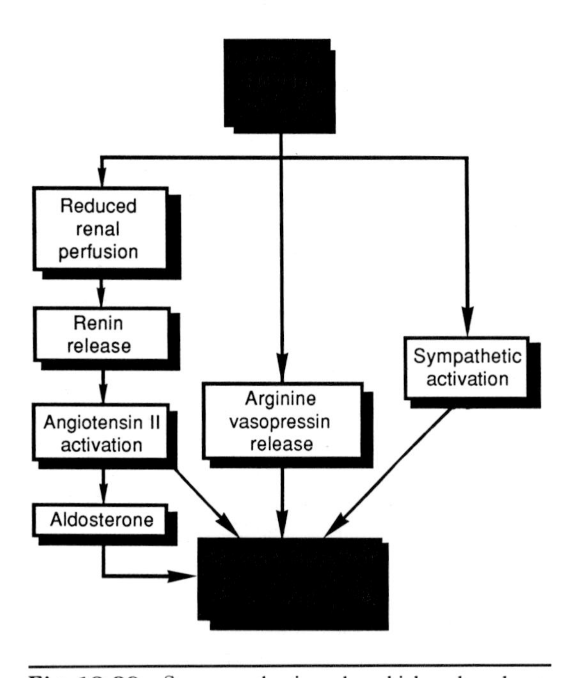

Fig. 12.39 Some mechanisms by which reduced cardiac output causes vasoconstriction and salt and water retention.

Ischaemic Heart Disease (IHD)

Ischaemic heart disease (IHD) is the leading cause of death in most industrialized countries. In the UK it accounts for 30% of male deaths and 20% of female deaths. There are marked geographical variations in the death rates from IHD. Finland, Scotland and Northern Ireland have the highest rates for males, closely followed by the USA, Australia and England and Wales. Lower rates are found in the Netherlands and Germany, still lower rates in Sweden and France; the outstanding exception to the relationship between industrialization and IHD deaths is provided by Japan, in which the rate is less than 10% of that in Finland. These striking epidemiological differences are attributed to differences in environment and in lifestyle. Migrants from a low risk country to a high risk country assume the risk of the latter.

In many industrialized countries death rates for IHD have fallen in both men and women over the past 20 years. The fall has been greatest (about 30%) in the USA but rates have also fallen in other countries such as Australia and Finland. The overall rates in the UK have begun to fall, especially in males less than 65 years old and in the higher socioeconomic groups and particularly in doctors, a group in which smoking has been reduced more than in most others. In contrast, death rates for IHD are rising in Eastern Europe.

Death rates for IHD increase with age and most deaths occur after the age of 40. Overall death rates are higher for men than for women, but IHD affects men earlier and for the age groups up to 65 the rates are very much higher for men. Some of the risk factors for IHD have been discussed earlier in the section on atheroma – diet, hyperlipidaemia, blood pressure, smoking, psychosocial factors, water hardness and alcohol consumption. This is because IHD is almost always due to narrowing of the lumen of one or more major coronary arteries by atheroma, often with complete occlusion by superadded thrombosis.

Atheroma of the Coronary Arteries

The general features of atheroma are described on p. 442. A small lesion may significantly narrow an artery the size of the coronary arteries. Stenoses producing a significant reduction in flow occlude the diameter of the vessel by at least 50%, which gives rise to a 75% reduction in cross-sectional area (Fig. 12.40). The pathology of the artery at the site of the stenosis will govern its ability to contract under vasomotor stimuli. Vessels with eccentric stenoses retain an arc of normal wall which remains responsive to vasomotor stimuli and these stenoses are regarded as potentially 'dynamic'. Concentric lesions produce atrophy of the medial muscle and are regarded as 'fixed'. The proportion of each type varies considerably in individual patients but in one series up to 56% of patients had at least one segment of dynamic high-grade stenosis with the potential for variation in calibre.

The atheromatous lesions may be largely fibrous (60%) or contain a large lipid pool which is semi-fluid at body temperature. In older subjects, the coronary arteries are commonly calcified and complete occlusion with variable degrees of re-canalization may be found at autopsy. In patients presenting with symptoms of IHD, coronary arteriography in life usually underestimates the extent of atheroma as found at autopsy. In populations with a high incidence of IHD asymptomatic coronary artery atheroma is found at autopsy in young persons dying from other causes.

A plaque may remain static, enlarge slowly and gradually obstruct the lumen, or rupture and occlude the lumen acutely, usually in association with thrombosis and/or spasm of the artery. Rupture of a plaque commonly causes unstable angina, sudden death or acute myocardial infarction. With slowly developing lesions which allow time for the development of a collateral circulation from another major artery (Fig. 12.41), subsequent occlu-

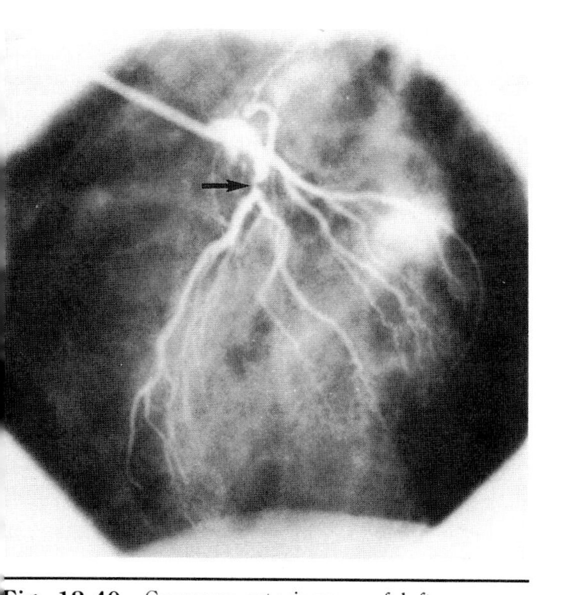

Fig. 12.40 Coronary arteriogram of left coronary artery. The arrow indicates severe atheromatous narrowing in the proximal portion of the left anterior descending artery (LAD), the major branch of the left coronary artery.

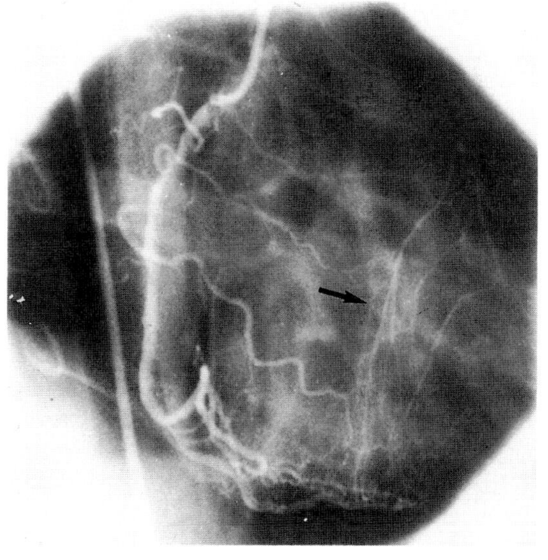

Fig. 12.41 Coronary arteriogram of the right coronary artery. The arrow indicates collateral vessels arising from the terminal portion of the right coronary artery and coursing vertically to anastomose with an occluded LAD.

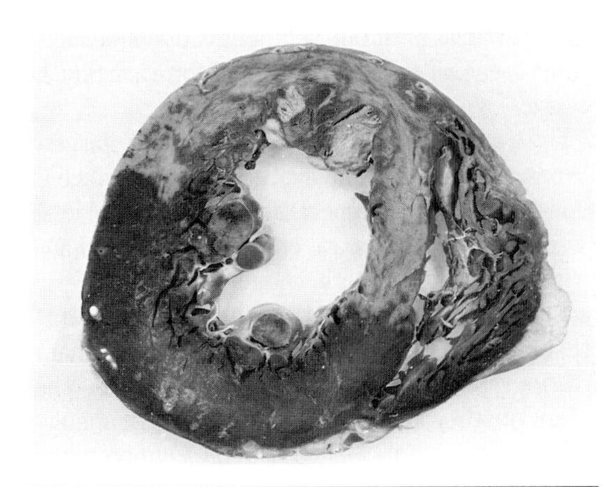

Fig. 12.42 Transmural myocardial infarction of several days' duration, due to occlusive thrombosis of the anterior descending coronary artery. The infarct appears pale and involves the anterior parts of both ventricles and of the septum. The coronary arteries have been injected for radiography (Professor M. J. Davies). ×0.5.

sion of the vessel may produce little disturbance in blood flow and few, if any, clinical symptoms.

Clinically, ischaemic heart disease may present as angina pectoris, myocardial infarction, chronic ischaemia with cardiac failure, or a sudden death which may occur without prior warning. There is overlap between these clinical syndromes.

Angina Pectoris

***Angina** is episodic chest pain of variable severity often described as 'gripping' or 'crushing'.* It is due to reversible myocardial ischaemia and is caused by an imbalance between myocardial oxygen supply and demand. The pain is usually retrosternal and may radiate to the neck and jaw or to the upper aspect of either or both arms and hands. Attacks are brought on by factors which increase the work of the heart and include physical activity, exposure to cold, emotional upset, or a heavy meal. An ECG at the time of the attack usually shows the changes of myocardial ischaemia and these regress with resolution of the attack. Ischaemia, however, does not always cause pain. Ambulatory ECGs in patients with angina show that up to 70% of ischaemic episodes are 'silent'; the frequency of chest pain therefore underestimates the true frequency of episodes of myocardial ischaemia in patients with angina pectoris.

Coronary arteriography delineates the number of vessels affected and this, together with other investigations of cardiac function, allow the clinician to classify patients into high or low risk groups. The most important variables in determining the prognosis are the severity of ischaemia induced by exercise testing, the state of left ventricular function and the number of vessels involved. Coronary artery bypass grafts or angioplasty (p. 522) may relieve symptoms and surgery also improves the prognosis in selected patients.

Angina occurs when increased myocardial workload occurs in the face of impaired perfusion. The myocardium extracts 80% of the oxygen from the blood passing through it. Thus, increased demand for oxygen must be supplied by increased blood flow. If the coronary arteries have fixed stenoses this is impossible and ischaemia results. Therefore, patients with angina pectoris usually have severe atheromatous narrowing and sometimes occlusion of one or more of their major coronary arteries and often one may be occluded. Arteriograms may demonstrate enlarged anastomotic channels which bypass or, more commonly, fill the occluded vessel by retrograde flow (Fig. 12.41). In most cases autopsy reveals myocardial scarring or more recent infarction. Myocardial infarction may either cause angina by diminishing the blood supply to surviving myocardium around the infarct or it may relieve angina by eliminating an area of myocardium with an inadequate blood supply.

Other causes of excessive oxygen demand include left ventricular hypertrophy secondary to hypertension or valvular disease, cardiomyopathies (p. 498) and hyperthyroidism (p. 1086). In aortic valvular disease the left ventricular workload is increased but coronary perfusion may be either relatively or absolutely reduced. Severe anaemia limits oxygen delivery and can predispose to angina. These diseases may therefore cause angina in the absence of significant coronary artery narrowing.

Stable angina. This is the commonest form of angina and many sufferers live for over 30 years. It is due to progressive stenosing coronary artery atheroma.

Variant angina (Prinzmetal's angina). In this form, the attacks of pain are not related to increase in workload and can occur at rest. They are caused by spasm of the large and medium-sized coronary arteries, often at a site of atheromatous narrowing. In 15% of cases, however, the coronary arteries appear normal. The mechanisms of the vasospasm are not known.

Unstable angina. This clinical pattern may supervene in previously stable angina or may commence *de novo*. There is a sudden increase in the severity and duration of episodes of chest pain, which begin to occur more frequently and often at rest. The pathogenesis is similar to that of acute myocardial infarction. In some patients, unstable angina may progress to myocardial infarction or sudden death.

Myocardial Infarction (MI)

The mortality of acute MI is approximately 30–35% with 50% of these deaths occurring within an hour of onset from ventricular fibrillation. The survivors suffer from variable degrees of impaired cardiac function. Younger patients generally pursue an uncomplicated course while older patients suffer heart failure and arrhythmias and thromboembolism more frequently.

Although atrial infarction also occurs in 20% of cases the ventricular myocardium is predominantly affected. There are two types of myocardial infarction: (1) 90% are **regional**, most of which are transmural and affect the myocardium lying within the region supplied by a major coronary artery which is almost always occluded by thrombus; (2) 10% are **subendocardial**, affecting the inner half or one-third of the ventricular wall throughout most or all of its circumference. In such cases the major coronary arteries are severely atheromatous but recent occlusion by thrombus is unusual.

Regional MI

Regional infarcts vary greatly in size but most are at least 2 cm across and many are much larger (Figs 12.42, 12.43). The frequency of involvement

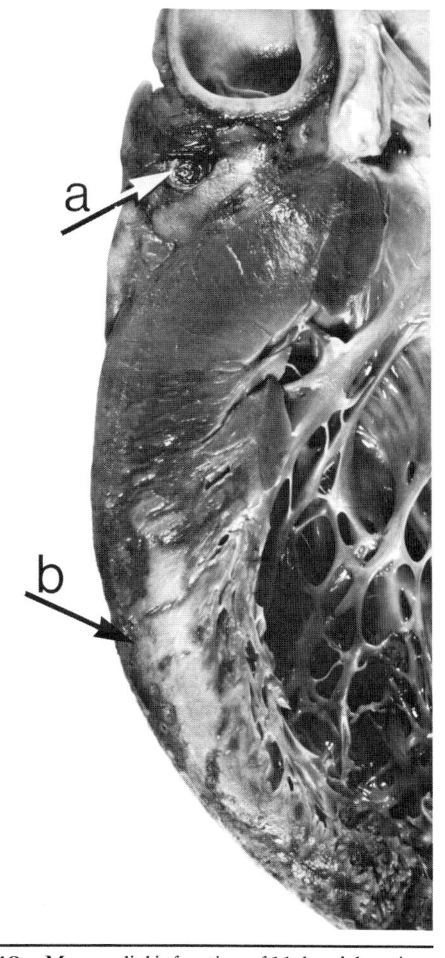

Fig. 12.43 Myocardial infarction of 11 days' duration. The anterior descending branch of the left coronary artery **a** is occluded by thrombus and the extensive infarction of the wall of the left ventricle is seen as areas of pallor and surrounding congestion. **b** Note also mural thrombus at the apex.

of the coronary arteries and the distribution of infarction are as follows:

(1) anterior descending branch of the left coronary artery (40–50% of cases). The infarct is anterior, extending from the apex, up the anterior wall of the left ventricle, often involving the anterior part of the interventricular septum and the adjacent anterior wall of the right ventricle.

(2) right coronary artery (30–40% of cases). The infarct is inferior (posterior), extending from the apex up the inferior wall of the left ventricle often involving the adjacent parts of the interventricular septum and of the inferior (posterior) wall of the right ventricle.

(3) circumflex branch of the left coronary artery (15% of cases). The infarct involves the lateral wall of the left ventricle.

Thrombosis of the left main coronary artery or of two major arteries occurs much less commonly, accounts for the remaining cases and is, of course, associated with more extensive infarction. The extent of infarction depends on the site of occlusion, (i.e. proximal or distal) within the artery, and on the presence of a collateral circulation. Gradual atheromatous narrowing of a major branch may result in opening up of collateral vessels (Fig. 12.41) so that when it is finally occluded by thrombus only a small infarct, at the most, is produced.

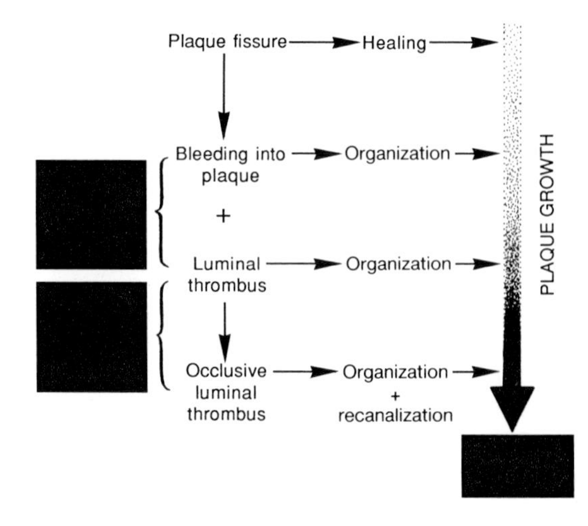

Fig. 12.44 The role of plaque fissure in the genesis of plaque growth is shown. The diagram also indicates the relationship between the consequences of plaque fissure and three major syndromes of IHD. (Modified from Davies, M. J. and Thomas, A. C. (1985). *British Heart Journal* **53**, 363–73.)

Pathogenesis

There is now convincing evidence that three of the acute clinical events in ischaemic heart disease – unstable angina, myocardial infarction and sudden death – usually result from cracking or ulceration of an underlying atheromatous plaque (Fig. 12.44). The sequence is thought to be:

(1) fissuring, cracking or rupturing of a plaque which has a lipid pool;
(2) penetration of blood into the plaque;
(3) acute enlargement of the plaque with thrombosis of the lumen;
(4) occlusion of the lumen.

The role of thrombotic occlusion of the coronary arteries has been confirmed by clinical angiography. This shows occlusion of the supplying artery in 90% of patients with an acute MI. Vasospasm may contribute to the occlusion, but the predominant cause is thrombus formation. Spontaneous relief of the vasospasm and activation of fibrinolytic mechanisms will relieve the occlusion so that at autopsy thrombotic occlusion is demonstrated in only a minority of cases with myocardial infarction. However, post-mortem angiography will confirm the presence of severe atheroma and the presence of plaque fissuring.

Thrombi may occur at areas of endothelial damage over a severe atheromatous stenosis. However, fissuring or ulceration of a plaque is thought to be the mechanism which initiates the sequence of events which have just been summarized. Fissuring and thrombosis are thought to be common events which often heal and may be a factor in the growth of a plaque (Figs 12.44, 12.45). The precipitating cause of severe fissuring leading to occlusion is unknown. Shear stress at the site of a plaque, surges in blood pressure, and local vasospasm have all been implicated. Once thrombus has formed the following sequences are possible: (1) spontaneous lysis; (2) platelet embol-

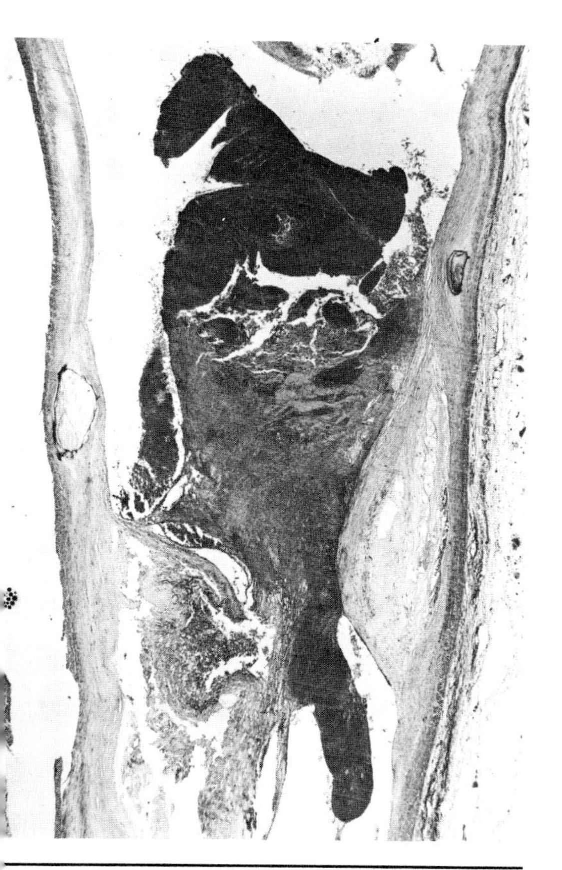

Fig. 12.45 Coronary artery in longitudinal section, showing an ulcerated atheromatous plaque (left, lower) with occlusion of lumen by thrombus. ×15.

zation which may aggravate the ischaemia distal to the occlusion; (3) continued thrombus formation progressing to local occlusion and propagation of the thrombus distally and proximally. Platelet activation at the site of thrombus formation will result in the release of vasoactive factors such as thromboxane (p. 140), possibly inducing vasospasm. The roles of endothelin and EDRF (p. 36) have still to be established. It should be clear therefore that coronary artery thrombosis is a dynamic and progressive process and the factors which determine the clinical syndromes and ultimate outcome are complex.

Morphological Features

Initially the necrotic muscle appears grossly and microscopically normal. Myocardial necrosis cannot be recognized in patients dying less than 6–8 hours after the onset. The first changes visible at autopsy are blotchy pallor and congestion followed in 24–48 hours by palpable softening. The colour gradually changes to grey-brown and then to yellow-grey, and there may be haemorrhages, particularly at the margin (Fig. 12.43). After a few days the infarct becomes more sharply defined by the development of a red zone of granulation tissue around its margin, and removal of the dead myocardium by organization proceeds gradually. There may be a fibrinous or haemorrhagic pericarditis which may be generalized or localized to the area of infarction. On the inner aspect of the infarct the endocardium and a thin layer of subendocardial myocardium remain viable, nourished by blood from the lumen; in patients surviving for several days mural thrombus is often formed on the endocardial surface. Microscopically, the infarcted muscle shows the changes of 'coagulative necrosis' (p. 25) after 8 or so hours: it is invaded by polymorphs and after a few days digestion by macrophages and organization can be seen at the margins (Fig. 12.46). The dead muscle is replaced

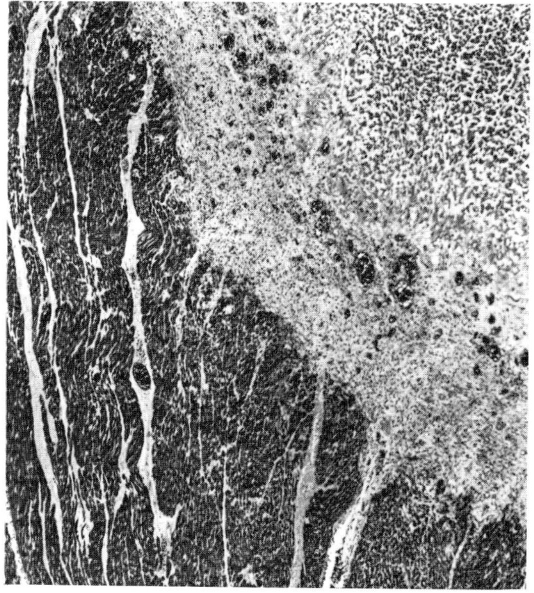

Fig. 12.46 Infarct of myocardium of 12 days' duration. The necrotic heart muscle (upper right) is separated from the surviving muscle by a zone of cellular and vascular granulation tissue. ×40.

by a fibrous scar over the next 6–8 weeks (Fig. 12.47a). Hypertrophy of the non-infarcted myocardium occurs and the chamber enlarges to compensate for the decrease in contractility caused by the infarct, thus maintaining the stroke volume (see Fig. 12.37). In 25–30% of transmural regional infarcts, stretching of the infarcted zone occurs. This may lead to aneurysm formation.

In patients dying from recent infarction regional scars which represent previous clinically silent infarcts are common. In some cases the areas o fibrosis are more diffuse with myocytes scattere among the fibrous tissue (Fig. 12.47b). Thes findings indicate chronic ischaemia with gradua loss of myocardial fibres and fibrous replacement

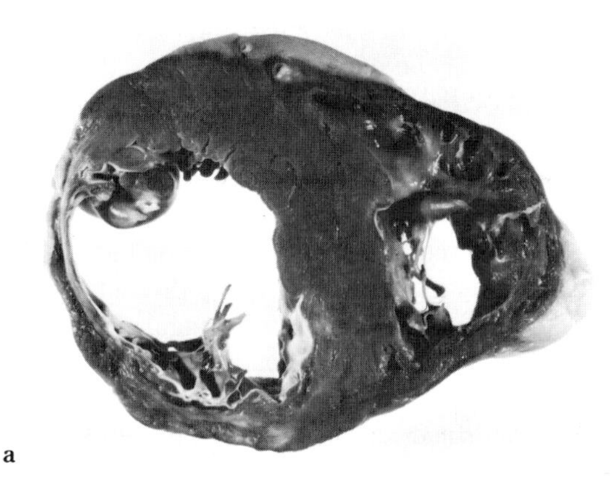

a

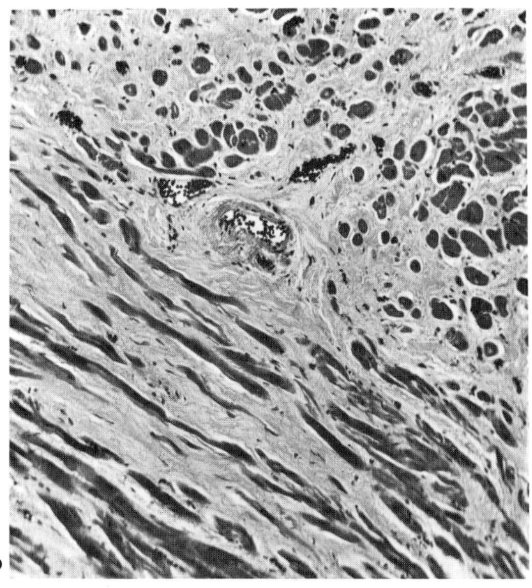

b

Fig. 12.47 **a** Old infarct represented by replacement of the lateral and posterior wall of the left ventricle by a relatively thin fibrous scar. **b** Part of an area of diffuse myocardial scarring throughout which some myocardial fibres have survived; this has probably resulted from chronic ischaemia.

Causal Factors

Factors carrying an increased risk of ischaemi heart disease, including MI, are discussed o p. 447. They include raised levels of blood chol esterol associated with a lipid-rich diet, cigarett smoking, hypertension, a sedentary lifestyle, ex cessive consumption of alcohol and genetic fac tors. These are all 'chronic' factors, and, whil they promote the development of atheroma, som of them may also predispose to superadded throm bosis. Precipitating factors are largely unknow but include sudden unaccustomed exercise, emo tional stress and cocaine abuse. Enhanced coag ulability is common in patients with ischaemi heart disease and plasma fibrinogen levels ar raised in some forms of hyperlipidaemia, notabl type II.

Unusual causes. Occlusion of a coronary arter by an embolus, with consequent regional infarc tion, is much less common than thrombosis; th embolus usually originates from intracardia thrombus and particularly from vegetations on th aortic valve. Rarer causes of occlusion includ polyarteritis nodosa, Buerger's disease, and in volvement of the ostia by aortic dissection or b the various forms of aortitis (p. 470).

Clinical Features and Course

The dominant symptom of MI is severe retro sternal pain. As in angina, it may radiate to th neck, jaw or arms, but it is not relieved by rest o vasodilator drugs and persists for at least one bu usually several hours and occasionally 1–2 days. I is generally accompanied by nausea, vomiting sweating, weakness and prostration. These earl features are usually dramatic, but there is a spec trum of severity of symptoms and in some case myocardial infarction is 'silent', with little or n pain or constitutional upset.

Within the first few hours there is usually mil

fever, a moderate neutrophil leucocytosis and characteristic electrocardiographic changes. Necrosis of myocardium is followed by release of cellular enzymes with consequent rise in the serum levels. Serum glutamic-oxalacetic aminotransferase rises in 6–8 hours, peaks at about 36 hours and returns to normal usually within a week. Lactic dehydrogenase (LDH) rises and peaks slightly later. These enzymes are released also by injury to other organs or skeletal muscle. However, a rise in serum LDH-1, an LDH isoenzyme, is more specific, while serum CPK-MB, a creatine phosphokinase isoenzyme, rises in 2–3 hours, peaks at about 36 hours, and is virtually diagnostic of myocardial necrosis. Acute myocardial infarction is confirmed clinically by pathological Q waves on the ECG together with appropriate enzyme changes.

Outcome of Myocardial Infarction

The mortality of acute MI is impossible to determine precisely because many patients who suffer sudden (instantaneous) cardiac death would not have developed infarction had they lived while others would. However the mortality of 'heart attacks' (sudden cardiac death and myocardial infarction) is 30–50% with 50% of all deaths occurring within the first hour. Overall, about 30–50% of patients with acute MI die, mainly from ventricular fibrillation, during the first week. The 'in hospital' mortality varies with the age of the patient and the size of the infarct but overall is approximately 15%. The subsequent mortality in the first year and succeeding years is 10% and 5% respectively.

The early mortality has been substantially reduced by the introduction of intravenous thrombolytic therapy with streptokinase and the administration of aspirin. The survival benefit is greatest in those treated earliest. In some series, the institution of fibrinolytic therapy within one hour of the onset of symptoms has reduced the mortality by 50%, which provides further evidence for the role of thrombosis in the acute event.

The most important single factor in determining outcome is the size of the infarct, although the extent and severity of atheroma in other coronary arteries are also important. In 'high risk' patients with post-infarction angina or with reversible ischaemic changes in the ECG during exercise testing, coronary angiography may be carried out with a view to performing angioplasty or coronary bypass surgery. In about one-third of patients subjected to angiography after MI the 'culprit artery' is not critically narrowed, suggesting that coronary spasm perhaps precipitated by fissuring of a plaque may have been responsible.

Cigarette smoking increases the risk of sudden death after MI. Treatment with beta blockers significantly reduces the risk of sudden death and re-infarction in the first year or two after MI; whether they confer improved long-term survival is less certain.

Complications of Myocardial Infarction

Arrhythmias. Ventricular fibrillation is by far the commonest cause of death in MI. Primary ventricular fibrillation occurs in the first 24 hours after infarction (usually within the first hour) and is thought to be responsible for most sudden deaths. Secondary ventricular fibrillation occurs some days later and is associated with extensive infarction and a significantly reduced short- and long-term prognosis. The occurrence of frequent premature ventricular beats after the first month or so indicates a particular liability to ventricular fibrillation. By involving the conducting system, MI may also cause various grades of heart block and other arrhythmias.

Cardiac failure. Extensive infarction of left ventricular muscle can cause acute heart failure. If this progresses to cardiogenic shock the mortality rate is 80%. Infarction also predisposes to heart failure which may develop at any time after infarction and indicates a poor prognosis.

Mural thrombosis. Following acute myocardial infarction, release of tissue thromboplastin from the damaged muscle, damage to the endocardium and localized eddying of blood predispose to mural thrombosis in the ventricles (Fig. 12.43 and Fig. 12.48). This is seen at autopsy in about 30% of cases who have had an MI; in patients who survive, the thrombus is eventually organized. Systemic emboli can result from mural thrombosis, but are less frequent than might be expected.

Venous thrombosis. Systemic venous thrombosis usually affecting the leg veins occurs in up to 30% of cases but fatal pulmonary embolism is an uncommon cause of death in myocardial infarction.

Rupture of infarcted myocardium occurs in about 5% of cases, at any time within the first 10 days. Most often the rupture occurs in the wall of the left ventricle and causes haemopericardium and death from cardiac tamponade.

Rupture of either the interventricular septum or of a mitral papillary muscle may also occur (Fig. 12.49), precipitating or aggravating acute heart failure. These complications can be confirmed and assessed using two-dimensional and Doppler echocardiography. Surgery is lifesaving in selected cases but the mortality rate is high.

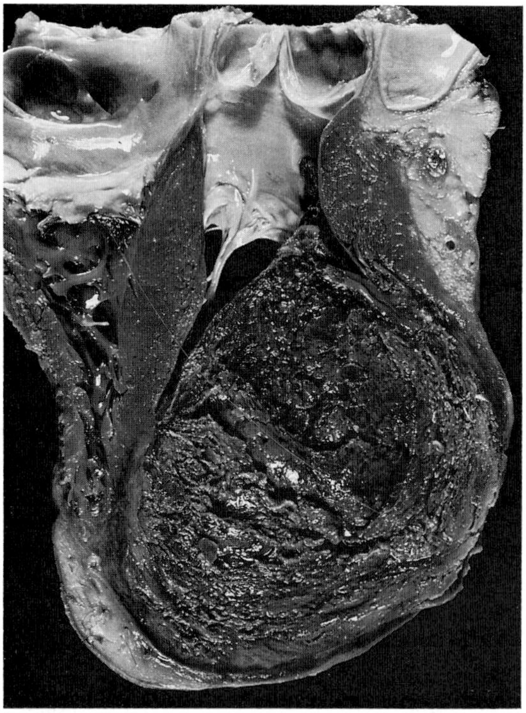

Fig. 12.48 Cardiac aneurysm following myocardial infarction. The wall of the left ventricle is stretched and thinned: thrombus has built up on it and now fills the aneurysm.

Cardiac aneurysm. The healing infarct of the left ventricle may stretch to form a cardiac aneurysm. This occurs in 12–15% of long-term survivors. Laminated thrombus tends to form in the cavity (Fig. 12.48) and may cause embolism. The aneurysm impairs ventricular function, causing cardiac failure which in some cases can be corrected by surgical excision of the aneurysm.

Angina pectoris. In some patients angina pectoris dates from a myocardial infarction because occlusion of a major coronary artery may render the surrounding areas of myocardium chronically ischaemic.

Recurrence of infarction. Individuals who have had a myocardial infarct are prone to re-infarction because of the underlying coronary artery disease.

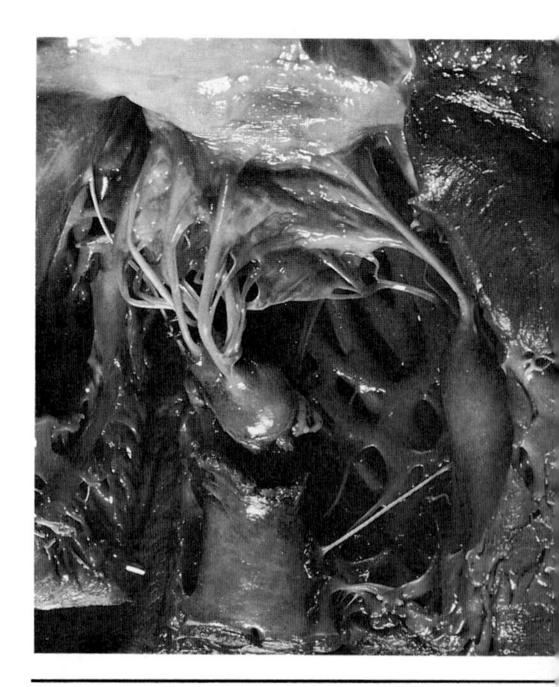

Fig. 12.49 Rupture of a necrotic papillary muscle in a patient with myocardial infarction.

Cigarette smoking greatly increases and beta blockers significantly reduce this risk.

Post-infarction (Dressler's) syndrome. Occasionally patients may develop pericardial and pleural effusions, a raised ESR, fever and leucocytosis up to 10 weeks following infarction. Raised titres of myocardial antibodies and resolution of the symptoms following corticosteroid therapy suggest an autoimmune response.

Subendocardial MI

Less than 10% of myocardial infarcts are subendocardial, affecting the inner part of the left ventricular myocardium. The infarct may be focal but when subendothelial infarction affects most or all of the circumference of the left ventricle it is sometimes called **global infarction** (Fig. 12.50). The major coronary arteries are usually severely narrowed by atheroma and at autopsy, in 75% of cases, there is no recent thrombotic occlusion. However, as with regional infarcts the true incidence of thrombosis may be greater. The immediate cause of infarction is failure of perfusion due to a fall in blood pressure. In some cases, the hypotension may be precipitated by a coronary artery occlusion and occasionally, combined transmural and subendocardial infarction can occur. In others, infarction may follow an episode of shock.

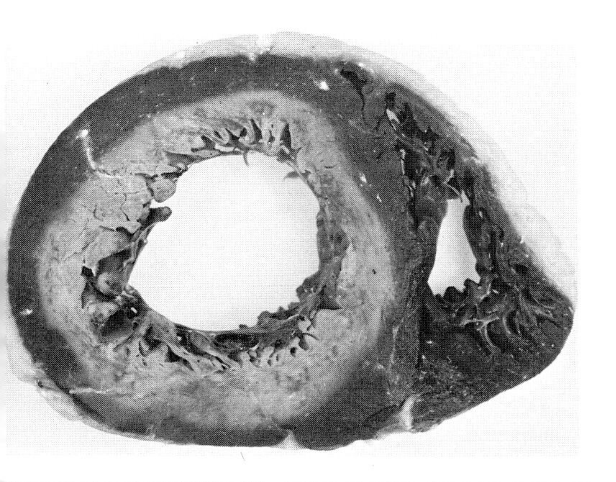

Fig. 12.50 Global subendocardial myocardial infarction of several days' duration. The infarcted myocardium is pale. Note also mural thrombi. The coronary arteries have been injected for radiography (Professor M. J. Davies).

The blood supply to the inner part of the ventricular myocardium is relatively precarious, and the combination of ventricular hypertrophy and coronary atheroma predisposes to diffuse subendocardial infarction, which is precipitated by a fall in coronary artery perfusion. In some instances, particularly when left ventricular hypertrophy is due to aortic valve disease, subendocardial MI occurs even without serious coronary artery disease.

Subendocardial MI is not complicated by pericarditis, nor by rupture of the ventricular wall or septum; otherwise its clinical features and complications resemble those of regional MI. In patients who recover, organization of the dead muscle leads to subendocardial scarring.

Other Effects of IHD

Sudden death. Ischaemic heart disease is the commonest cause of sudden cardiac death. There may be a history of angina, previous infarction, evidence of chronic heart failure, or chest pain immediately before death, but sometimes there are no warning symptoms. At autopsy there is usually severe coronary atheroma with or without old organized thrombotic occlusions. Recent occlusive coronary thrombosis is found in only about 30% of such cases and furthermore, the majority of patients resuscitated from what would undoubtedly have otherwise been sudden cardiac death do not develop a regional MI. Accordingly, while coronary thrombosis is an important cause of sudden death, coronary artery atheroma without recent superadded thrombosis is even more important. The role of coronary artery vasospasm remains uncertain.

Ischaemic heart disease is also the commonest cause of various grades of **heart block** and other arrhythmias and of chronic heart failure, whether or not there has been previous myocardial infarction.

The Cardiomyopathies

These comprise a heterogeneous group of conditions in which there is chronic myocardial dysfunction of uncertain cause. Thus, the diagnosis is based on exclusion of other identifiable causes of ventricular dysfunction. Endomyocardial biopsy is helpful in excluding specific heart muscle disorders and may reveal features typical of one or other form of cardiomyopathy. Cardiomyopathy is classified as hypertrophic, dilated or restrictive and may be further divided into primary types of unknown aetiology and secondary types which occur in association with some systemic disorder.

Hypertrophic cardiomyopathy (HCM) is characterized by variable but often massive hypertrophy of the left ventricle and especially of the interventricular septum, but with no dilatation. Function is affected by (1) decreased compliance of the left ventricle which interferes with diastolic filling; (2) the asymmetrical hypertrophy of the septum which may obstruct the outflow from the left ventricle; and (3) mitral regurgitation which is common and probably due to distortion of the ventricle by the asymmetrical hypertrophy.

Hypertrophic cardiomyopathy is an autosomal dominant disorder with a high degree of penetrance. Symptoms may occur at any age and sudden death is common. Microscopic examination shows gross hypertrophy of myocytes accompanied by interstitial fibrosis. There are areas of disarray in which there is a disordered, whorled arrangement of muscle fibres such that normal cellular orientation is lost. There is also disorganization of the myofibrillary architecture within cells which also contain increased glycogen. The diagnosis is usually made by echocardiography (Fig. 12.51).

Dilated (congestive) cardiomyopathy (DCM). These patients present with unexplained congestive heart failure. All four chambers are dilated (Figs 12.52, 12.53), the myocardium is pale and flabby, and there is often ventricular mural thrombus and endocardial thickening. The microscopic features are non-specific. Some myocardial

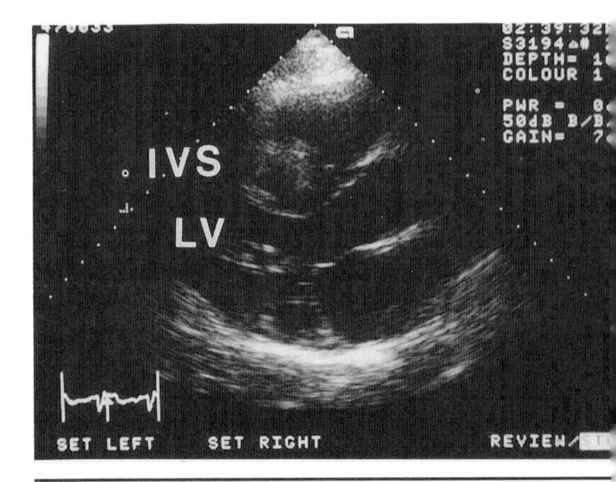

Fig. 12.51 Echocardiogram in hypertrophic cardic myopathy: the interventricular septum (IVS) is grossl thickened and the left ventricular chamber (LV) is smal

fibres may show gross hypertrophy while other appear thinned. There may be interstitial fibrosi with an increase in chronic inflammatory cells.

In rare instances dilated cardiomyopathy show familial aggregation. Some cases are associate with alcohol abuse. Many cases may represent th end-stage of a slowly progressive or relapsing vir myocarditis, an autoimmune reaction to myocar dial tissue initiated by some past injury, or injur from a number of potential toxins. Conditions i which congestive failure arises from an unusu

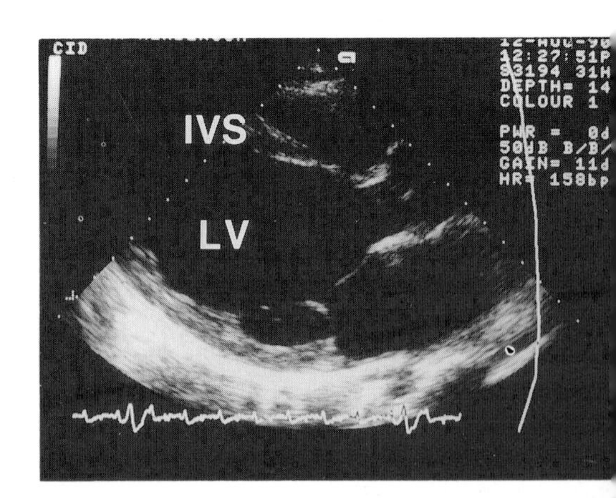

Fig. 12.52 Echocardiogram in congestive cardic myopathy: even at end systole, the left ventricle (LV) enlarged and the interventricular septum (IVS) thinned.

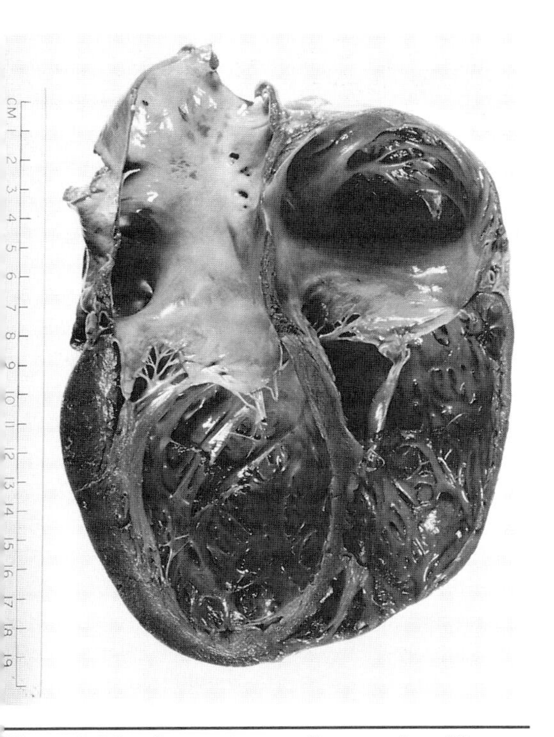

Fig. 12.53 Congestive cardiomyopathy. The anterior half of the heart is viewed from behind. The chambers are grossly dilated and there is some mural thrombus at the apex of the left ventricle.

cause may be misdiagnosed as DCM, e.g. beriberi (p. 348), haemochromatosis (p. 770), acromegaly (p. 1081) and Pompe's disease (p. 254).

Restrictive (obliterative) cardiomyopathy. This is the least common form of cardiomyopathy and includes two conditions – endomyocardial fibrosis and endocardial fibroelastosis. They are characterized by abnormal rigidity mainly due to gross endocardial thickening without myocardial disease. The rigidity interferes with the filling and emptying of the affected chambers so that progressive, diastolic heart failure results.

Endomyocardial fibrosis (EMF) is characterized by fibrosis of the endocardium and the immediate underlying myocardium of the inflow tracts of either or both ventricles. The fibrosis also involves the papillary muscles and chordae tendineae, causing incompetence of the mitral and/or tricuspid valves. The fibrous tissue restricts ventricular muscle contraction. Mural thrombosis and embolic phenomena may occur.

Endomyocardial fibrosis occurs sporadically world wide and is usually associated with marked eosinophilia. The condition is endemic in tropical Africa, Uganda and Nigeria in particular, in parts of southern India and, with a lower frequency, in Venezuela and Brazil. In these regions EMF occurs in children and young adults and is a significant cause of cardiac morbidity and mortality. The geographical distribution of tropical EMF remains unexplained. In both sporadic and endemic forms of the disease the initial endocardial damage is thought to be related to the eosinophilia and specifically to the toxic effects on the heart of eosinophil leucocyte major basic protein.

Endocardial fibroelastosis is an unusual cause of heart failure in infants and young children and is of unknown aetiology. A diffuse layer of dense, white avascular tissue, composed largely of elastic fibres, develops in the endocardium, usually of the left atrium and ventricle. It obscures the trabecular pattern of the endocardial surface and affects also the papillary muscles and chordae tendineae and sometimes produces thickening of the mitral and aortic valve cusps. The mechanical effects of the thickened endocardium and valve lesions lead to progressive heart failure.

Myocarditis

Myocarditis is inflammation of the myocardium which occurs as a result of (1) direct involvement by the causal agent; (2) toxin-mediated injury; (3) a local hypersensitivity reaction. The causes are numerous and are summarized in Table 12.8. The commonest causes are viral. Toxoplasmosis may affect the myocardium in neonates and in immunocompromised patients. *Trypanosoma cruzi* is endemic in South America, affecting 30% of the population and with a high mortality rate (p. 1154).

Table 12.8 Causes of myocarditis

Viral infection	Coxsackie A and B echoviruses, influenza virus, Epstein–Barr virus, herpesvirus and HIV
Rickettsiae	*Chlamydia* (psittacosis), *Coxiella* (Q fever), typhus fever
Bacteria	Suppurative myocarditis due to pyogenic infection Toxin mediated – diphtheria, typhoid fever
Other micro-organisms	*Trypanosoma cruzi* (Chagas' disease) Toxoplasmosis Weil's disease *Borrelia burgdorferi* (Lyme disease) *Trichinella* Various fungi
Hypersensitivity	Acute rheumatic fever Connective tissue diseases – rheumatoid arthritis and systemic lupus erythematosus Cardiac allograft rejection Drug-induced e.g. penicillin, streptomycin
Miscellaneous: uncertain aetiology	Giant-cell (Fiedler's) myocarditis Sarcoidosis

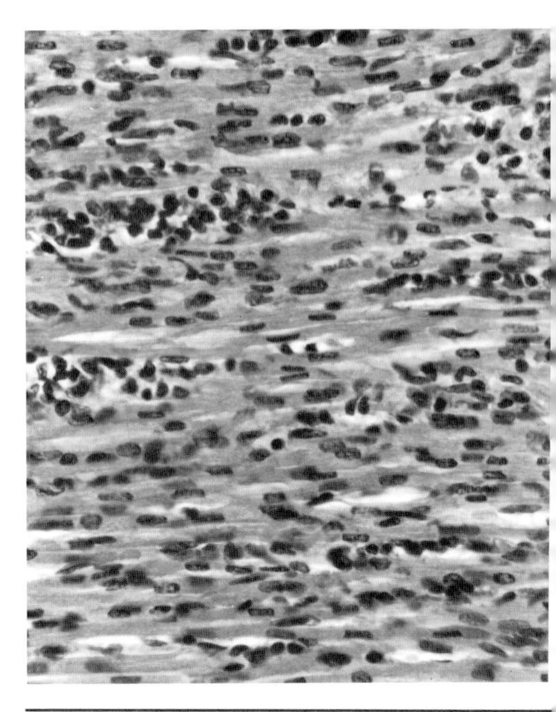

Fig. 12.54 Myocarditis due to coxsackie B virus from a child of 11 months. The field illustrates the extensive focal infiltration with macrophages and lymphocytes. ×320.

Viral myocarditis. Cases occur in infants but young adults, particularly male, are most often affected. The condition is usually mild and complete recovery is the rule. It may, however, be more severe with rapid and sometimes fatal cardiac failure. Asymptomatic cardiac involvement is believed to occur in many common viral illnesses – influenza, chickenpox, measles, mumps – and may be responsible for some of the sudden deaths during strenuous exercise in subjects suffering from apparently trivial upper respiratory infections. In some cases of congestive cardiomyopathy a previous history suggestive of viral myocarditis may be elicited. Myocarditis is a common feature of intrauterine rubella infection.

Histologically, there is interstitial oedema of the myocardium, infiltration by mononuclear cells, predominantly lymphocytes and macrophages, and sometimes plasma cells and eosinophils (Fig. 12.54). Necrosis of individual muscle fibres tends to be focal and may therefore not be seen in endomyocardial biopsies.

Suppurative myocarditis, caused by pyogenic bacteria, occurs in septicaemia and pyaemia, and also as a serious complication of acute infective endocarditis in which infection occurs by embolization of the coronary arteries or by direct spread from the valve lesions. As in other tissues, *Staphylococcus aureus* gives rise to localized abscesses while *Streptococcus pyogenes* causes a spreading infection with extensive necrosis and haemorrhage.

Toxic 'myocarditis' was a major feature of diphtheria, and similar appearances, presumed to be toxic in origin, may be seen in pneumococcal pneumonia, typhoid fever, septicaemia and other severe acute bacterial infections. Microscopically, there are numerous small foci of coagulative necrosis which are surrounded by an inflammatory nfiltrate consisting mostly of macrophages and ymphocytes, although polymorphs may be present also (Fig. 12.55). The necrotic muscle fibres subsequently undergo absorption and are replaced by small fibrous scars.

Hypersensitivity reactions. Myocarditis is one of the most serious features of acute rheumatic fever, and is dealt with in the next section. Myocarditis may also complicate rheumatoid arthritis and systemic lupus erythematosus but is among the less common and less serious lesions of hese conditions.

Granulomatous myocarditis. Granulomas are found in the myocardium at autopsy in 25% of cases with active sarcoidosis. Clinical evidence of cardiac involvement however, is very unusual.

In **Fiedler's giant-cell myocarditis** there is focal myocardial necrosis with a granulomatous reaction in which eosinophils are conspicuous and multinucleated giant cells, apparently derived from damaged muscle fibres, may be present.

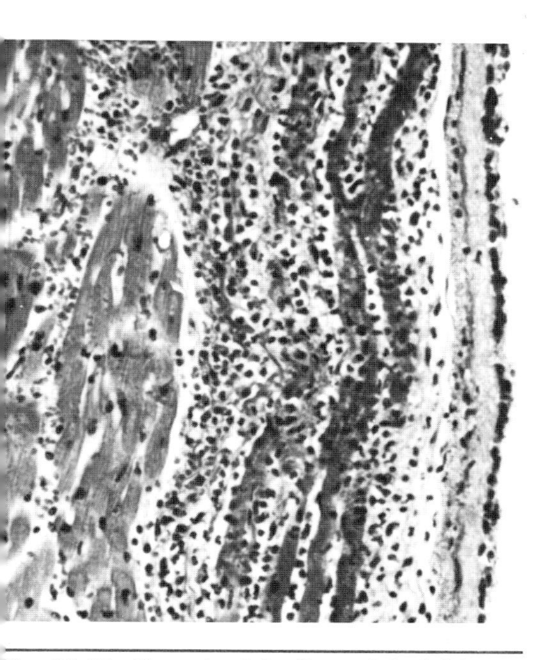

Fig. 12.55 Necrosis of the fibres of the left bundle branch, with an inflammatory reaction, in a fatal case of diphtheria. ×225.

Rheumatic Heart Disease

Acute Rheumatic Fever

This is an acute febrile illness in which lesions occur in the heart, the joints and the subcutaneous tissue. It follows an attack of streptococcal pharyngitis and occurs mainly in children and young adults, aged 5–20 years. Its incidence has fallen greatly in developed countries as a result of improved living conditions and the use of antibiotics but it is common in some parts of Africa, India, the Middle East and South America.

Heart failure due to diffuse myocardial injury may occur during the acute illness and is very occasionally fatal. In the large majority of cases myocardial function usually recovers completely. Subsequent disability is due to injury to the cardiac valves which results in permanent distortion, often leading to chronic heart failure. Rheumatic fever tends to recur after subsequent attacks of streptococcal pharyngitis and each recurrence increases the risk of serious valvular disease.

Changes in the Heart

Although all three layers of the heart are affected in acute rheumatic fever (**pancarditis**) the severity of their individual involvement varies greatly.

The pericarditis is exudative with effusion of serous fluid and deposition of fibrin on both pericardial surfaces, sometimes as a thick layer, giving them a rough, shaggy appearance which has been compared with that observed when two generously buttered pieces of bread are pressed together and then pulled apart. The fibrin is removed by organization and this may cause pericardial fibrosis and adhesions.

Myocarditis. In fatal acute cases, the myocardium is flabby and the ventricles, particularly the left, are dilated. Sometimes tiny pale foci may be just visible. These are the **Aschoff bodies**, pathognomonic of rheumatic carditis. They are scattered throughout the myocardium (Fig. 12.56), being particularly numerous in the left atrium and ventricle. The Aschoff bodies develop in the connective tissue septa of the myocardium. Microscopy reveals a focus of eosinophilic hyaline material which contains fibrin and indicates exudation of plasma proteins from small vessels. This is surrounded by an aggregate of lymphocytes, macrophages, occasional polymorphs and larger cells with two or three nuclei or a single convoluted nucleus (Fig. 12.57). In time the Aschoff bodies subside and healing occurs, leaving minute focal scars in the connective tissue of the myocardium.

Endocarditis. The endocardium shows diffuse inflammatory oedema and a light cellular infiltration. Aschoff bodies develop and are particularly numerous in the posterior wall of the left atrium just above the insertion of the posterior mitral cusp. Healing may result in thickening and irregularity of the endocardium in this area (McCallum's patch). In acute rheumatic fever, however, the most prominent endocardial lesion consists of small **thrombotic vegetations** forming a line of

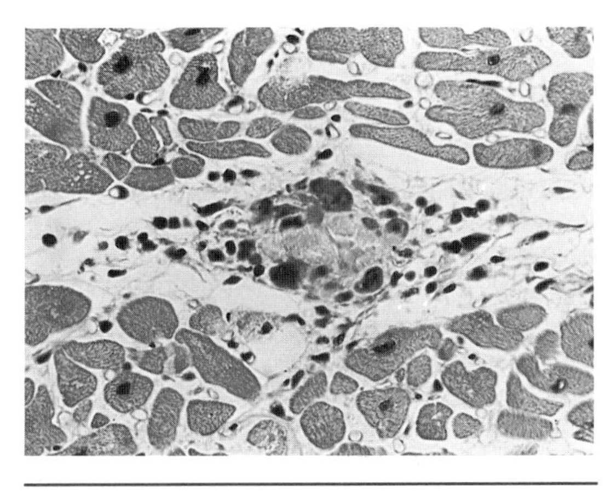

Fig. 12.56 Rheumatic myocarditis: Aschoff body in the myocardium of a child who died of heart failure. Central hyaline material is surrounded by macrophages, some with large or multiple nuclei, and by lymphocytes. ×310.

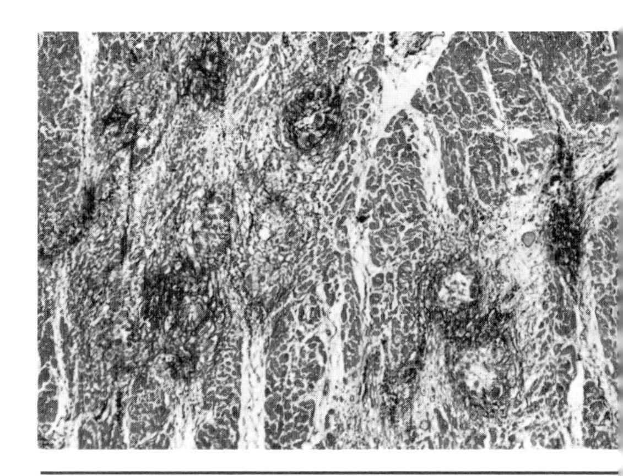

Fig. 12.57 Rheumatic myocarditis: healing stage showing fibrosis around Aschoff bodies (Masson's trichrome stain: collagen appears dark). ×48.

fine, grey-pink, firm nodular deposits on the surface of the valve cusps. They form mainly on the lines of contact between the cusps when the valves close (Fig. 12.58). Similar vegetations form on the chordae tendineae.

Microscopically, Aschoff bodies are seen on the valves but in addition, and more significantly, there is an acute inflammatory oedema, infiltration by neutrophil polymorphs, lymphocytes and macrophages and focal fibrinoid necrosis; focal ulceration occurs and acute thrombotic vegetations are formed in these areas (Fig. 12.59). There is an ingrowth of capillaries from the base of the valves and the acute changes are followed by organization of the vegetations and more diffuse fibrous thickening of the cusps. Organization of the vegetations on the cusps results in fibrous union between adjacent cusp margins. Organization of vegetations on the chordae tendineae lead to their becoming matted together as thick, fibrous bands, particularly at their valvular ends: this causes shortening of the chordae and distortion of the cusps. With recurrent acute attacks, the injury to the valve is more severe and further fibrous thickening and deformity result.

When patients die in the acute illness, all four valves are commonly inflamed, but residual effects with permanent distortion are usually confined to the mitral and aortic valves, probably because of their greater haemodynamic stresses. These late effects are described on p. 505.

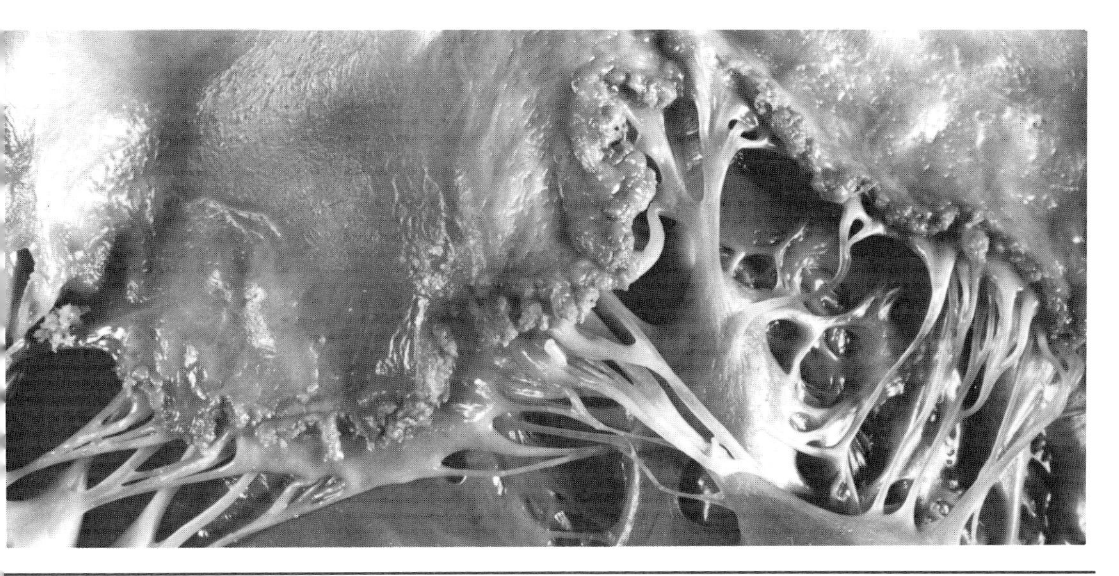

Fig. 12.58 Mitral valve in acute rheumatic endocarditis, showing the small vegetations which form along the line of opposition of the cusps. ×2.

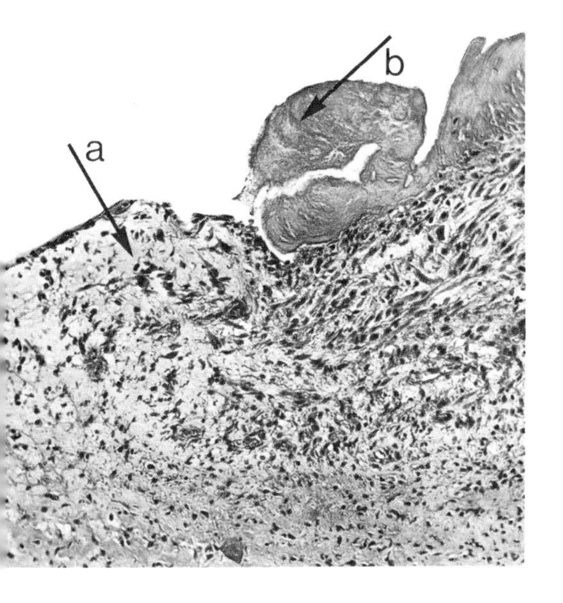

Fig. 12.59 Section of the mitral valve in acute rheumatic endocarditis. The cusp shows inflammatory oedema **a** and cellular infiltration, and appears to be vascularized. Where the cusps meet, the oedematous tissue has ulcerated and platelets have been deposited on the ulcerated surface to form the early vegetation **b**. ×80.

Changes in Other Tissues

The joints show mild inflammatory changes in the synovium sometimes accompanied by effusions; the tendons and their sheaths may show similar changes. **Subcutaneous nodules** may develop over bony prominences of the arms and legs, most commonly on the extensor surface of the elbow and overlying the ulna. The nodules are between 1 and 2 cm in diameter, painless and resemble enlarged Aschoff bodies. Various erythematous skin rashes may occur, the commonest being **erythema marginatum**, and in some cases there may be a mild **encephalitis** causing chorea.

Clinical Features

Rheumatic fever develops usually 2–4 weeks after a streptococcal sore throat. Symptoms may be mild but there is usually fever, tachycardia, malaise and arthralgia flitting from joint to joint: the affected joints are sometimes swollen. The most serious effect on the heart at this stage is the myocarditis which causes various degrees of acute heart failure. Signs of acute pericarditis usually appear later in the acute illness, and the valvular lesions are undetectable at this stage, although there may be evidence of secondary mitral incompetence due to dilatation of the left ventricle or valvular abnormalities resulting from previous attacks. Chorea may develop during or apart from the acute illness, as may the skin rashes and subcutaneous nodules. There is no specific test for rheumatic fever. A raised erythrocyte sedimentation rate, anaemia, slight leucocytosis and high titres of streptococcal antibodies such as antistreptolysin O (ASO) are usually present.

Aetiology and Pathogenesis of Acute Rheumatic Heart Disease

Rheumatic fever (RF) occurs as a sequel to pharyngeal infection with *Streptococcus pyogenes*, Lancefield group A. Approximately 3–5% of individuals develop rheumatic fever after streptococcal pharyngitis, and those who do are very liable to have recurrent attacks after further episodes of pharyngitis. There is thus strong individual predisposition. The serotypes of *Streptococcus pyogenes* are of importance, for some outbreaks of streptococcal pharyngitis are not associated with RF, even in subjects who have had previous attacks of RF. Treatment of streptococcal pharyngitis with antibiotics does not abolish the risk of subsequent RF, but long-term administration of penicillin prevents further attacks of streptococcal pharyngitis and of RF.

Streptococci are not found in the heart in fatal cases of RF nor is acute carditis caused directly by streptococcal toxins. It develops after recovery from the infection and is associated with unusually strong and persistent antibody responses to various streptococcal antigens, streptolysin and hyaluronate. Indeed, a high titre of antistreptolysin (ASO) is widely used as a diagnostic aid. The association of RF with a strong immune response suggests the possibility of a hypersensitivity reaction. Two mechanisms have been invoked: an autoimmune reaction triggered by the streptococcal infection, and an inappropriate immune response producing antibodies which cross-react with cardiac tissue antigens. Immunofluorescence studies on heart tissue from fatal cases of acute myocarditis show immunoglobulin and complement diffusely bound to the myocardial fibres and also to the cardiac valves. These antibodies can be absorbed both by normal myocardial antigens and by streptococcal antigens. Antisera to streptococcal antigen(s) react with human (and rabbit) sarcolemma. It is thus clear that *Streptococcus pyogenes* and myocardium share common antigens. However, similar antibodies occur after uncomplicated streptococcal infections and in patients who develop post-streptococcal glomerulonephritis but not rheumatic fever.

The cardiac lesions could also be due to a type 4 hypersensitivity reaction. In support of this are experiments in which animals immunized with streptococcal antigens produced lymphocytes cytotoxic to cardiac myocytes in tissue culture. Spleen cells but not antibodies caused cardiac damage when injected into normal animals.

In summary, therefore, rheumatic fever is preceded and accompanied by the development of antibodies cross-reacting with streptococcal components and myocardium and heart valves. The binding of antibody and complement to myocardial sarcolemma and cardiac valves in the acute phase suggests that these cross-reacting antibodies could be of pathogenic importance. However, type 4 (cell mediated) hypersensitivity could also be involved in causing tissue injury *in vivo*.

Chronic Rheumatic Heart Disease

Following recovery from rheumatic fever the function of the myocardium usually returns to normal, although minute fibrous scars mark the site of healed Aschoff bodies. Organization of fibrinous pericarditis commonly results in fibrous pericardial adhesions or even obliteration of the sac, but the fibrous tissue is seldom thick or rigid enough to impair cardiac function. By contrast, injury to the valves commonly causes permanent deformity resulting in stenosis or incompetence or a combination of both defects. In about 30% of patients with rheumatic fever these valve lesions eventually lead to heart failure. The risk of chronic endocarditis, however, depends on age, being higher following rheumatic fever in early childhood and in patients with repeated attacks. Sometimes the valvular changes progress rapidly, but more often there is an interval of 5–30 years of apparent good health before the clinical features of valvular disease develop. In patients treated surgically for post-rheumatic valvular disease, Aschoff bodies can often be detected in excised atrial tissue. This suggests that rheumatic heart disease can smoulder subclinically for many years, thus explaining the slow progression of the valvular disease.

In chronic rheumatic heart disease both the mitral and aortic valves are affected in about 50% of cases and the mitral valve alone in about 25%. The mitral, aortic and tricuspid valves are involved in about 15% of cases, while involvement of all four valves or of the aortic valve alone is rare. The susceptibility of the mitral and aortic valves to rheumatic injury is probably due to the degree of haemodynamic stress they must withstand. The valves on the right side of the heart are virtually never affected alone.

Disorders of the Heart Valves

Serious reduction in the size of the valve orifice (stenosis) will increase the pressure load in the preceding chamber, while failure to close completely (incompetence) will result in regurgitation of blood and thus increase the volume load on both sides of the valve. Either defect, if severe, is likely to result in cardiac failure.

Abnormalities of the cardiac valves may be congenital or acquired. In many parts of Africa, Asia and South and Central America, rheumatic fever remains the major cause of acquired valvular disease at all ages. In most industrialized countries rheumatic fever has virtually disappeared and chronic rheumatic valvular disease is now encountered mostly in middle and old age; thus valve lesions from other causes have increased in relative importance. Any abnormality of the cardiac valves increases the risk of infective endocarditis (p. 511).

Diagnosis and assessment of valvular lesions is mainly carried out by echocardiography supplemented in some cases by measurements of central pressures and of blood flow. Surgical repair of heart valves and replacement of severely damaged valves by prostheses produce good results in suitable patients while balloon valvuloplasty is also possible in a minority of stenoses, especially those affecting the mitral.

THE MITRAL VALVE

Normal functioning of the mitral valve depends on the mechanical efficiency of its cusps, chordae and papillary muscles, on the pliability and size of the fibrous valve ring or annulus, and on the adequacy of left ventricular contraction which normally halves the area of the orifice during systole. The circumference of the normal adult valve is approximately 8 cm and valves measuring less than 5 or more than 12 cm are likely to have been functionally defective.

Changes with age. In old people the mitral valve cusps are slightly thickened and the posterior cusp often becomes stretched and bulges towards the atrium. Yellow patches of thickening and degeneration similar in structure to atheroma are common and may be accompanied by fibrosis and calcification. These changes do not usually have serious effects on the functioning of the valve.

Mitral Stenosis

Rheumatic fever is the major cause of mitral stenosis. Women are affected more often than men, and in approximately two-thirds of cases the aortic valve is also involved. Valve lesions resembling those following rheumatic fever are seen occasionally in patients with SLE (p. 229). In rheumatoid arthritis minor distortion of the valve is common but seldom causes disability.

Each mitral cusp consists of a central fibrous plate (fibrosa) covered on either side by loose subendothelial connective tissue. The cusps are normally avascular but, in chronic rheumatic disease, they are thickened, and distorted, vascularized throughout, and consist of dense fibrous tissue which may be infiltrated with lymphocytes and plasma cells and, in some cases, may be irregularly calcified. The cusps are fused together along much of their free margins, thus forming a fibrous diaphragm with a central curved slit-shaped ('button hole') or oval orifice (Fig. 12.60), the area of which depends partly on the extent of fusion of the cusps and partly on their rigidity. Pure stenosis results when the diaphragm formed by the fused cusps is relatively thin and pliable. Greater thickening and rigidity usually results in a combination of stenosis and incompetence, particularly when the chordae become fused to form a rigid channel below the valve cusps, giving the valve a funnel-shape (Fig. 12.61).

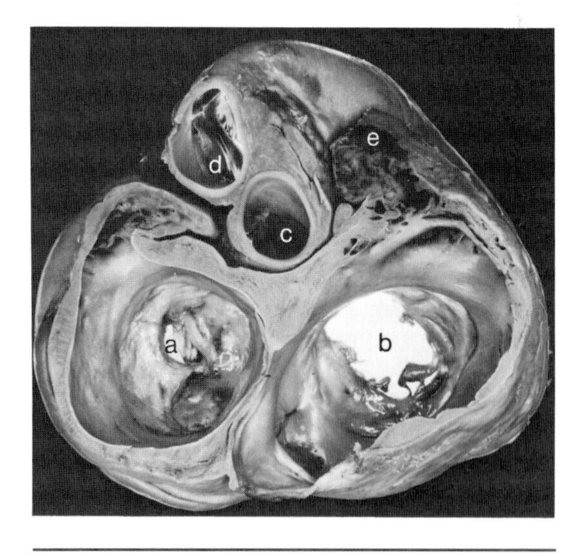

Fig. 12.60 Horizontal section through the atria in a case of mitral and tricuspid stenosis, as seen from above: **a** mitral valve, severely stenosed; **b** tricuspid valve, moderately stenosed; **c** aorta; **d** pulmonary artery; **e** right atrial appendage containing thrombus. ×0.6.

Effects

The capacity of the left atrial myocardium to undergo hypertrophy is very limited and mitral stenosis soon results in enlargement and dilatation (Fig. 12.61). Atrial fibrillation is common and almost always accompanies gross dilatation, but the cause–effect relationship is obscure. Thrombus formation is common in the left atrium, particularly in its appendage, and is almost always present in patients with atrial fibrillation. Systemic embolism may occur, the commonest serious effect being cerebral infarction.

Initially the raised left atrial pressure is sufficient to drive the normal volume of blood into the left ventricle, but, as mitral stenosis increases in severity, the requirement for increased blood flow during physical exercise cannot be met and, with severe stenosis, even the resting blood flow is reduced. Dyspnoea and persistent cough result from pulmonary congestion and oedema. Attacks of acute pulmonary oedema are brought on by exercise and paroxysmal nocturnal dyspnoea occurs during the night (p. 540). Mild haemoptysis may occur due to haemorrhage from engorged pulmonary capillaries.

Increased pulmonary venous pressure leads, by mechanisms which are not well understood, to increased tone and hypertrophy of the pulmonary arterial tree. This reduces the danger of pulmonary oedema, but restricts further the pulmonary blood flow and, by causing pulmonary hypertension leads to right ventricular hypertrophy (Fig. 12.62) and eventual failure with generalized oedema. In most cases the pulmonary hypertension will be relieved by surgical correction of the mitral stenosis.

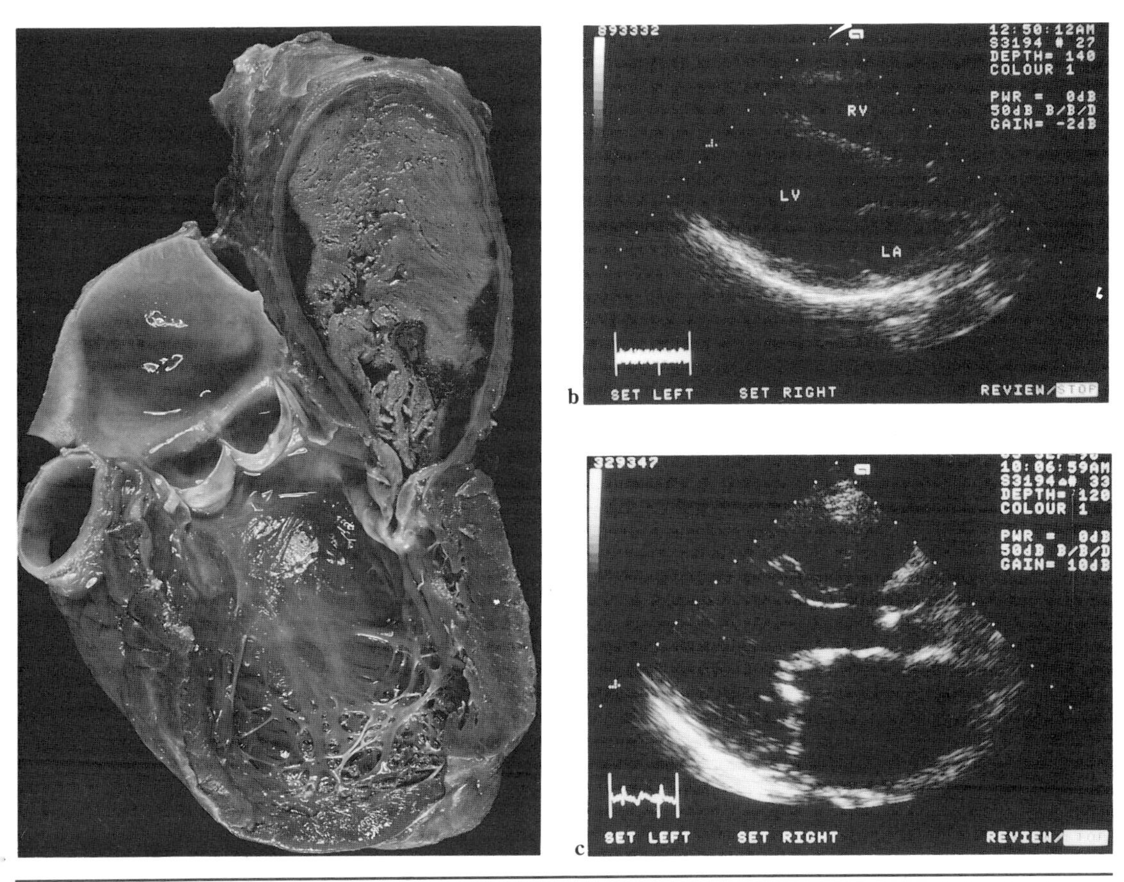

Fig. 12.61 **a** Severe post-rheumatic mitral stenosis. The cusps are grossly thickened and the chordae are thickened and fused, forming a narrow channel below the cusps. The left atrium is grossly distended and almost filled with thrombus. **b** & **c** Echocardiograms: parasternal long axis view of the heart. The left ventricle (LV) and mitral valve leaflets can be seen in diastole. In the normal **b** the mitral leaflets are thin and widely open and the left atrium is small. In the patient with mitral stenosis **c** the leaflets are thickened and open poorly in diastole and the left atrium is dilated.

Mitral Incompetence

There are a number of causes of mitral incompetence.

(1) Lesions of the valve cusps and chordae. Post-inflammatory scarring of the mitral valve may follow rheumatic or infective endocarditis. Fibrosis and contraction of the cusps, and thickening and rigidity of the chordae, if severe, may hold the cusps firmly in a partly open position. Increased rigidity of the cusps and fusion along part of their free margins often results in a combination of stenosis and incompetence; pu incompetence is unusual. Rapid or sudden mitral incompetence may develop in infective endocarditis as a result of perforation of cusps or rupture of affected chordae.

The **floppy mitral valve** or **mitral valve leaflet prolapse syndrome** is becoming a relatively important cause of mitral incompetence in countries where the incidence of rheumatic heart disease has declined. The valve cusps and chordae become stretched and the latter may rupture. This is due to degenerative changes in the zona fibrosa of the cusps. The zona fibrosa is focally replaced by loose fibrous tissue which contains abundant pro-

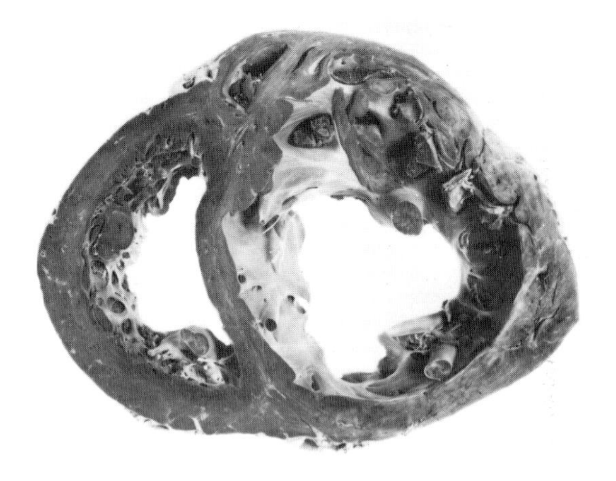

Fig. 12.62 Transverse section of the ventricles from a patient with mitral stenosis who died of right ventricular failure. The right ventricle (on the right) is hypertrophied and dilated, the left one relatively small. ×0.75.

teoglycans. During ventricular systole the slack in the valve cusps is taken up and the chordae are jerked taut, giving an audible systolic click. Part or all of one or both cusps bulge into the atrium (Fig. 12.63) and regurgitation may result, with a systolic murmur following the click.

Minor degrees of 'floppy valve' change occur in about 5% of people. The posterior cusp is usually more affected. Its segments or scallops become slightly thickened and at autopsy appear dome-shaped, bulging towards the atrium. The anterior cusp shows a single dome-shaped bulge. Incompetence is usually slight unless one or more of the chordae rupture. As in any abnormal valve, haemodynamic disturbance and mechanical trauma may lead to some thickening of the cusps. Thickening and occasionally fusion of the chordae may also develop, and the appearances can sometimes be confused with rheumatic lesions. A floppy mitral valve occurs in some cases of Marfan's syndrome, osteogenesis imperfecta or pseudoxanthoma elasticum. Changes in the valve leaflets are probably analogous to those which occur in the large arteries in these diseases (p. 475).

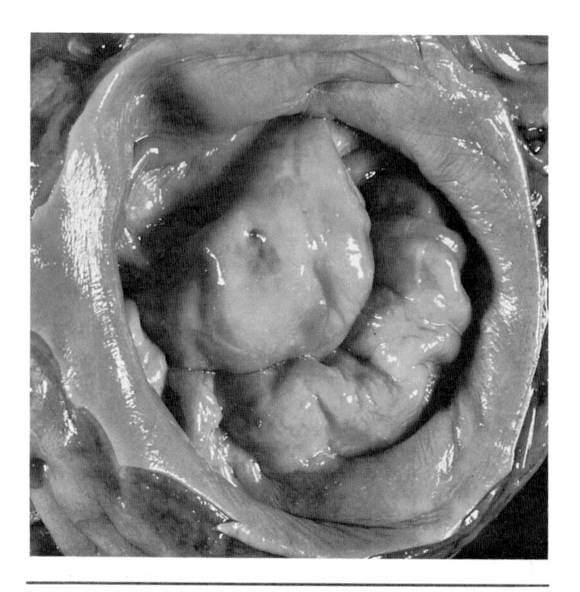

Fig. 12.63 Floppy mitral valve. The left atrium has been opened to show the thickened cusps bulging into it.

(2) Papillary muscle ischaemia. Loss of contractility of a papillary muscle as a result of ischaemic fibrosis may cause incompetence by allowing the related cusp to prolapse into the atrium. Rupture of an infarcted papillary muscle may complicate a myocardial infarct, causing sudden and severe regurgitation, and results in rapidly fatal left ventricular failure. Surgical repair is possible in some patients.

(3) Dilatation of the mitral ring is seen most frequently as a consequence of dilatation of a failing left ventricle, e.g. in ischaemic heart disease or systemic hypertension. It may occur rarely and as a primary event, in some cases of Marfan's syndrome, osteogenesis imperfecta and pseudoxanthoma elasticum. In these diseases there is mitral ring involvement as distinct from the floppy mitral valve.

Effects

Incompetence of the mitral valve allows regurgitation of blood into the left atrium during ventricular systole. The left atrium becomes distended but the additional volume of blood passes freely into the left ventricle during ventricular diastole, and stretching of the left ventricle by the extra volume load results in more forcible contraction. When mitral incompetence develops gradually, there is time for the left ventricle to undergo hypertrophy, and unless the leakage is severe this enables it to eject the normal amount of blood into the aorta in spite of the mitral leak. Although 'compensated', the left ventricle is nevertheless handicapped by the mitral leak. Its maximal effective stroke volume is reduced and accordingly, exercise tolerance is diminished and fatigue and weakness are often the presenting symptoms. Even during exercise, the pressure in the left atrium does not increase greatly during ventricular diastole, and attacks of acute pulmonary oedema with exertional and nocturnal dyspnoea are much less common than in mitral stenosis. Although atrial fibrillation commonly develops, left atrial thrombosis and embolic phenomena are observed less often than in mitral stenosis.

Eventually the increased volume load leads to left ventricular failure. As its contractions weaken and residual blood accumulates in it, the pressure in the left atrium rises also during ventricular diastole and pulmonary congestion and oedema develop. Death may result from left ventricular failure, but in some cases pulmonary congestion leads to pulmonary hypertension and right ventricular failure may supervene.

In **acute mitral incompetence**, the left ventricle is unable to compensate and fails rapidly. The left atrium cannot dilate rapidly to accommodate the additional volume of blood entering it and so the left atrial pressure rises rapidly, leading to severe pulmonary congestion and oedema.

In cases of **combined mitral stenosis and incompetence**, pulmonary congestion and oedema lead to pulmonary hypertension, right ventricular hypertrophy and eventual failure.

THE AORTIC VALVE

The fibrosa of the aortic cusps is continuous with the valve sleeve which consists of fibrous and elastic tissue. Proximally the sleeve is attached to the muscular interventricular septum and to the fibrous base of the anterior mitral cusp. Distally it continues into the aortic media at the level of attachment of the aortic cusp commissures. The sleeve thus supports the valve cusps and forms the sinuses of Valsalva.

Aortic Stenosis

In the UK rheumatic endocarditis accounts for about 20% of cases of aortic stenosis: about 65% of cases are due to calcific aortic stenosis, many of which are calcified bicuspid valves: 5% are due to other congenital abnormalities and in the remaining 10% the cause is uncertain.

In **post-rheumatic aortic valve disease** the cusps are thickened, vascularized, rigid and partly adherent and stenosis is usually combined with incompetence. In over 90% of cases the mitral valve is also affected. By contrast, **calcific aortic stenosis** is usually associated with a normal mitral valve and presents as stenosis, usually without serious incompetence. The changes in calcific aortic stenosis are an exaggeration of those seen commonly in old age: the cusps become thickened by fibrosis and irregular nodules of dystrophic calcification develop, usually starting at the base of the cusps and extending towards the free margin. The calcified nodules project from the aortic surface of the cusps, rigidity of which converts the orifice to a narrow slit (Fig. 12.64). Calcific aortic stenosis in a **congenitally bicuspid aortic valve** (Fig. 12.65) develops in a younger age group and becomes apparent between 40 and 60 years of age. In **congenital aortic valve stenosis** the cusps are usually fused to form a diaphragm with a central or eccentric orifice.

Effects

Reduction of the area of the valve orifice by over 50% increases significantly the resistance to ejection of blood into the aorta and there is left ventricular hypertrophy. In most patients this maintains an adequate cardiac output for many years. However, to achieve this compensated state, the left ventricle must generate a considerable pressure (sometimes over 250 mmHg) to overcome the resistance of the stenotic valve. Since the pressure in the aorta is not increased, and may fall below normal during ventricular di-

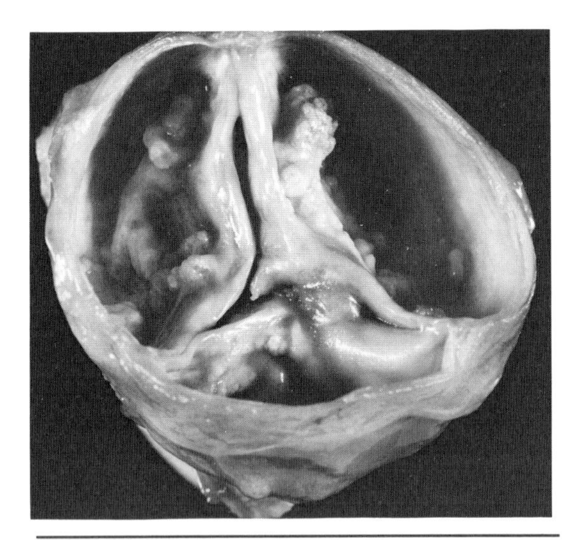

Fig. 12.64 Calcific stenosis in an aortic valve in an elderly patient.

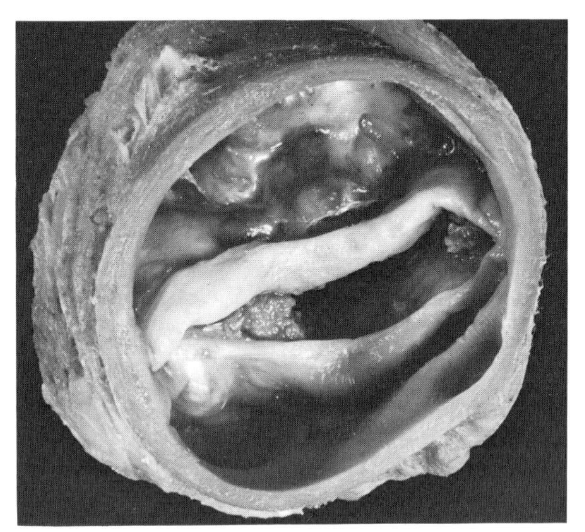

Fig. 12.65 Calcific aortic stenosis in a younger patient and superimposed on congenitally bicuspid valve.

astole, coronary perfusion pressure is diminished. These factors – increased pressure load and diminished coronary circulation – together with left ventricular hypertrophy, predispose to angina pectoris, which can sometimes occur in the absence of coronary atheroma. Fainting is a common symptom, perhaps due to transient arrhythmias triggered by the increased workload on the left ventricle, and some 15% of people with aortic stenosis die suddenly, presumably from ventricular fibrillation. Death may also result from left heart failure.

Aortic Incompetence

This increases the workload of the left ventricle which, at each contraction, must expel both the normal stroke volume and the amount of blood regurgitated during ventricular diastole.

Lesions of the valve cusps. Fibrous thickening and contraction of the cusps in **rheumatic heart disease** is still an important cause of aortic valve incompetence, but this is usually combined with stenosis and in most cases the mitral valve is also affected. Incompetence may also be associated with **calcific aortic valve stenosis**, while some bicuspid valves, particularly those with grossly unequal cusps, are incompetent at birth or become so in youth. In **infective endocarditis**, erosion or rupture of a cusp causes acute valve aortic incompetence.

Dilatation of the aortic valve sleeve, with consequent aortic incompetence, may be inflammatory or non-inflammatory. The inflammatory lesions include syphilitic aortitis and a similar form of aortitis which occurs occasionally in association with inflammatory joint diseases, e.g. in ankylosing spondylitis and rarely in Reiter's syndrome and rheumatoid arthritis.

Non-inflammatory stretching of the aortic valve sleeve is rare and usually of unknown cause. If an aortic dissection extends proximally to involve the aortic valve sleeve one or more cusps may be displaced because they lose their attachment. This causes acute aortic incompetence.

Effects

The increased volume of blood which has to be expelled by the left ventricle results in a raised systolic blood pressure, while during diastole the regurgitation of blood results in a rapid fall to abnormally low pressure. The pulse pressure is thus increased, giving a collapsing (water-hammer) or 'Corrigan's pulse. In response to the increased volume and pressure loads, the left ventricle hypertrophies and dilates and a state of compensation may last for many years. However, coronary blood flow, compromised by the reduced diastolic pressure, may not meet the demands of the hypertrophied left ventricle and so, as in aortic stenosis, angina pectoris is often a feature, but arrhythmias and sudden death are less common. Eventually the left vetricle fails with a fatal outcome.

THE TRICUSPID VALVE

The commonest cause of primary tricuspid valve disease is infective endocarditis due to intravenous drug abuse. In about 15% of cases of post-rheumatic valvular disease, the mitral, aortic and tricuspid valves are affected. The changes in the tricuspid are similar to those in the mitral valve, but usually less severe and give rise to tricuspid stenosis or a combination of stenosis and incompetence. The carcinoid syndrome also causes tricuspid stenosis, either pure or combined with incompetence, and stenosis also results from congenital malformations of the valve. Pure incompetence due to dilatation of the valve ring is a feature of right ventricular failure.

Tricuspid stenosis or incompetence or a combination of the two have similar effects. Pressure rises in the right atrium, which dilates, the central venous pressure increases and systemic venous congestion develops with 'cardiac' oedema. When associated with mitral stenosis or left ventricular failure, the tricuspid lesions tend to reduce the degree of pulmonary venous congestion and hypertension by limiting the volume of blood reaching the left side of the heart.

THE PULMONARY VALVE

Pulmonary stenosis is a feature of the carcinoid syndrome (p. 731) but occurs more commonly as a congenital malformation. It causes hypertrophy and eventual failure of the right ventricle.

Pulmonary incompetence may accompany stenosis in the carcinoid syndrome, but is more often secondary to pulmonary hypertension with dilatation of the pulmonary artery and valve ring. It occurs also as a congenital malformation and rarely in infective endocarditis. The mechanical effects are not serious unless there is pulmonary hypertension, and indeed the valve may be excised in patients with refractory infective endocarditis without greatly impairing cardiac function.

INFECTIVE ENDOCARDITIS

When micro-organisms gain entrance to the bloodstream, they are usually rapidly eliminated. In some circumstances, however, they may settle on the endocardial surface, usually of the valve cusps, with the formation of thrombi known as **vegetations**. This condition – infective endocarditis – is characterized by fever, toxaemia, embolic phenomena, heart failure and sometimes glomerulonephritis (p. 907). It is usually fatal unless the infection can be eliminated by antibiotic therapy. Traditionally, infective endocarditis is classified into acute and subacute types; the former affects a normal heart, and is rapidly fatal because it is due to bacteria of high virulence, the latter affects a damaged organ and gives rise to a more prolonged illness because it is due to less virulent organisms. The distinction is valuable but many patients present features intermediate between these two extremes and so it is best to regard infective endocarditis as a spectrum of diseases. The causal agents include a wide range of bacteria and fungi, *Coxiella burnetii*, *Chlamydia* and possibly viruses.

Predisposing Factors

The main factors which predispose to infective endocarditis are (1) conditions which cause bacteraemia, septicaemia or pyaemia; (2) abnormalities of the heart which favour the lodgement of micro-organisms on the endocardial surface, usually of the valves; (3) impairment of the host's defence mechanisms.

Bacteraemia, septicaemia and pyaemia. Everyone develops transient and clinically silent bacteraemia from time to time. Transient bacteraemia commonly follows tooth extractions, tonsillectomy and adenoidectomy, and even hard chewing or vigorous use of a toothbrush, particularly when there is periodontal infection (p. 676). Obvious infections, such as boils, carbuncles, bacterial pneumonias and infections of the urinary, gastrointestinal and biliary tracts are associated with bacteraemia and, much less often, septicaemia and pyaemia. Of increasing recent importance is intravenous drug abuse in which the tricuspid and pulmonary valves are commonly affected.

Surgery on the gut, biliary or genitourinary tracts, and even such minor procedures as urethral catheterization, cystoscopy and sigmoidoscopy cause transient bacteraemia. Such procedures do not carry a significant risk of infective endocarditis unless there is predisposing valvular disease or depression of defence mechanisms.

Abnormalities of the heart. Distortion of the heart valves predisposes to infective endocarditis. Chronic rheumatic valvular disease is still a most important underlying condition. In developed countries other valve lesions, calcific aortic stenosis, floppy mitral valve and congenital bicuspid aortic valve have increased in relative importance. Even the minor degenerative changes which occur in the valves with age predispose to infective endocarditis, and help to explain its occurrence in middle-aged and old people. In children, congenital heart lesions predispose to infection, e.g. Fallot's tetralogy, patent ductus arteriosus and interventricular septal defects. Valve prostheses, intracardiac catheters and pacemakers also predispose to infective 'endocarditis'.

Thrombus forms on distorted valves and at sites where turbulence and rapid jets of blood strike the endocardium. The thrombi which form are not usually visible macroscopically, but they provide shelter for entrapped micro-organisms and as these multiply they invade the underlying valve cusp and also promote the deposition of larger, readily visible vegetations which provide further protection from the host's defence mechanisms.

Impaired defence mechanisms. Immunodeficiency and impaired function of phagocytes, whether caused by natural disease or cytotoxic therapy, predispose to infective endocarditis. There is an increased liability to infection in this condition and in addition micro-organisms settling on the endocardium have a better chance of survival and multiplication.

Subacute Infective Endocarditis (SIE)

This is usually caused by bacteria of relatively low virulence. The most common is the 'viridans' group of α-haemolytic streptococci which form part of the normal flora of the mouth and pharynx and are important in periodontal infection, followed by *Streptococcus bovis*, a gut commensal and *Staphylococcus epidermidis*, a skin commensal which inevitably infects indwelling venous catheters and exteriorized pacemaker wires. Other commensals, such as diphtheroids, coliform bacilli, bacteroides and mycoplasmas are responsible for occasional cases. *Coxiella burnetii* accounts for about 3% of cases, occurring usually in young and middle-aged adults. Fungal endocarditis occurs in intravenous drug abuse from the use of dirty syringes and also occurs in immunosuppressed patients and following open heart surgery. The fungi most often involved are candida, aspergillus and, in some warm countries, histoplasma.

Pathological Features

The lesions consist of friable, soft, shaggy thrombi of variable size, projecting from the surface of the valve cusps (Fig. 12.66). They usually develop on the contact surface of a cusp, where they may be patchy or continuous, and also spread to the con-

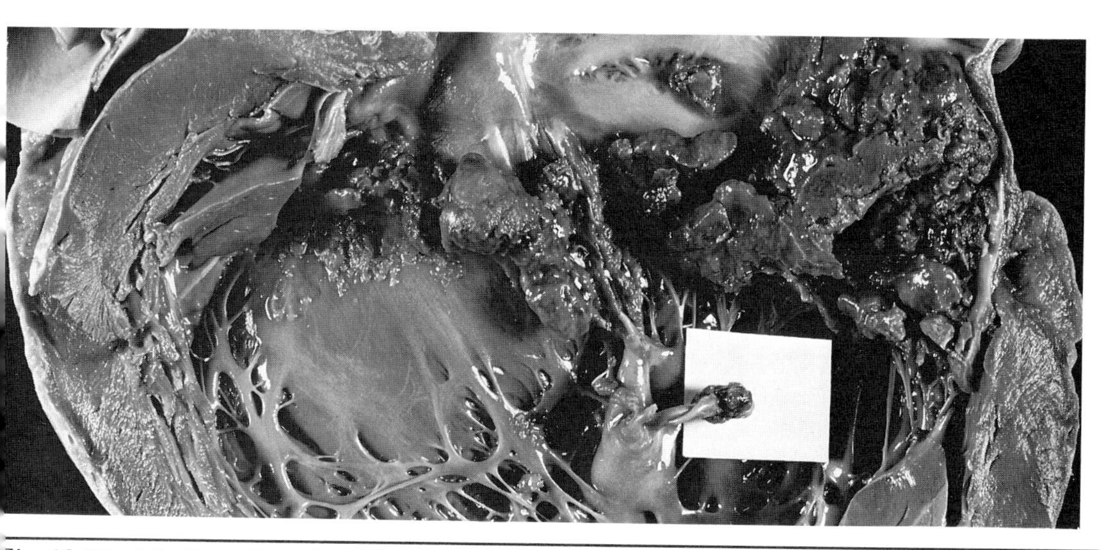

ig. 12.66 Infective endocarditis of the mitral valve. The vegetations have covered the cusps and extended on to he posterior wall of the left atrium. A ruptured chorda is displayed.

act surfaces of the adjacent cusp(s). Spread from he aortic valve to the anterior mitral cusp, and *vice ersa*, is common. The micro-organisms eventu-lly invade the cusp tissue and cause necrosis, which may lead to rupture of the cusp. They may lso extend along and cause rupture of the chor-lae, destructive changes which are more frequent nd severe in acute bacterial endocarditis. The esions may spread from the mitral valve to McCallum's patch in the left atrium, and from the ase of a valve cusp into the adjacent myocardium r into the root of the aorta.

Microscopically, the vegetations consist mostly f fibrin and platelets and contain colonies of micro-rganisms. Polymorphs are usually scanty. The nderlying cusp is vascularized, thickened and brosed and may have areas of necrosis. It is nfiltrated with polymorphs and macrophages and nay show invasion by bacteria.

Eradication of the infection by antibiotics is ollowed by gradual repair of the damaged cusps nd slow organization of the vegetations, resulting n gross and irregular scarring and distortion of the usps and fibrous thickening and matting of the hordae. The end result may be indistinguishable rom chronic rheumatic valvular disease, but sually the cusps are more irregularly thickened nd calcified.

Clinical Features and Course

Subacute infective endocarditis often starts insidiously with irregular fever, malaise and mild anaemia. Petechiae may appear, usually in small numbers, in the skin, mucous membranes and retina and 'splinter' haemorrhages are seen under the nails: these are probably embolic. The spleen is usually enlarged and palpable. Cardiac murmurs may be present from previous heart disease or may develop and change in quality as the infective lesions progress. Clinical features may arise from embolization of vegetations, causing infarction of the brain, myocardium, spleen and kidneys. Gross or microscopic haematuria results from renal infarction or glomerulonephritis. Heart failure eventually develops and is the commonest cause of death. It may be progressive due mainly to increasing valvular damage, but it may deteriorate suddenly due to rupture of a valve cusp or chordae or from myocardial infarction. The other major causes of death are embolic phenomena and renal failure.

Untreated SIE is invariably fatal, usually within a few months. With antimicrobial therapy the mortality is reduced to less than 50% and with early and adequate administration of an appropriate antibiotic the mortality may be reduced to less than 15%. Isolation of the micro-oganism is thus urgent and sometimes requires repeated blood cultures. In about 20% of cases no causal organism can be found. This may be due to recent administration of antibiotics, usually in amounts sufficient to sterilize the blood temporarily. In other instances, negative cultures occur because the causal organism does not grow in ordinary cultures, e.g. coxiella, mycoplasma or fungi. Occasionally an organism is cultured but is mistakenly regarded as a contaminant, e.g. diphtheroids or *Staph. epidermidis.* If blood cultures are negative, the decision to start therapy on suspicion is often difficult. Vegetations may be seen clearly on echocardiography which is a mandatory investigation when SIE is suspected; failure to visualize them does not, however, exclude their presence.

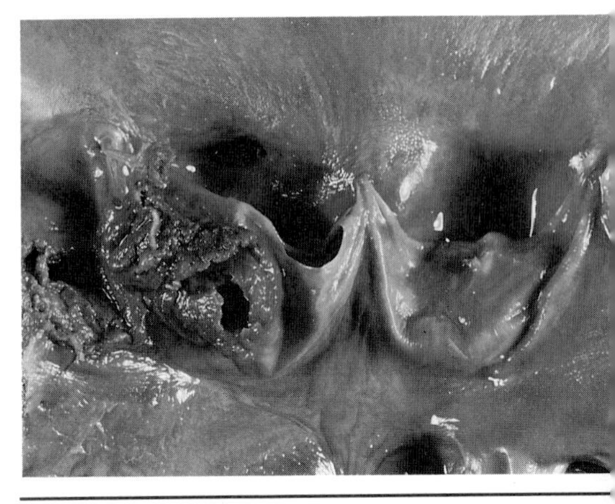

Fig. 12.67 Acute infective endocarditis of the aorti[c] valve. The lesion has involved the adjacent parts of tw[o] cusps, one of which (left) is largely destroyed and th[e] other (centre left) is perforated. There is an earl[y] vegetation on the remaining cusp.

Acute Infective Endocarditis

This is a much more severe infection than SIE and without effective treatment is fatal within a few days or weeks. The commonest causal organism is *Staphylococcus aureus* followed by *Streptococcus pyogenes* and enterococci. In immunodeficiency states less virulent bacteria, including those responsible for SIE, can cause acute endocarditis or conditions of intermediate severity.

Pathological Features

The vegetations resemble those of SIE, but tend to be larger and may be localized to one part of a valve (Fig. 12.67). They consist mainly of fibrin containing large clusters of bacteria surrounded by neutrophil polymorphs. The more virulent organisms rapidly invade the affected cusps, producing necrosis and suppuration, and often cause cusp 'aneurysms' or complete rupture (Fig. 12.67). The vegetations commonly extend to and cause rupture of the chordae tendineae. Spread of infection from the aortic valve to the adjacent aorta may cause a mycotic aneurysm or rupture. The organisms may also spread into the myocardium causing necrosis and abscesses. The mitral and aortic valves are more commonly involved; the tricuspid valve is often affected in intravenous drug addicts.

Clinical Features and Course

The clinical features are those of a severe acut[e] bacterial infection. Blood culture is nearly alway[s] positive. There are cardiac murmurs which ma[y] change rapidly as the valve cusps are destroyed[.] Septicaemia may develop and embolic fragment[s] produce septic infarcts in the brain, kidneys, lun[g] and spleen. In the absence of early and effectiv[e] antibiotic therapy, the condition is fatal within day[s] from overwhelming infection or within weeks fro[m] acute heart failure due to a combination [of] toxaemia, destruction of the affected valves an[d] septic myocarditis. Even with intensive treatmen[t] the mortality is over 50%, and following th[e] institution of antibiotic therapy early surgery i[s] now the preferred option.

Other Valvular Lesions

Non-infective thrombotic endocarditi[s] consists of the formation of sterile thromboti[c] vegetations on the heart valves, usually in a patch[y] fashion along the lines of closure of the cusps of th[e] mitral and aortic valves. The vegetations ar[e] smaller than those in infective endocarditis an[d]

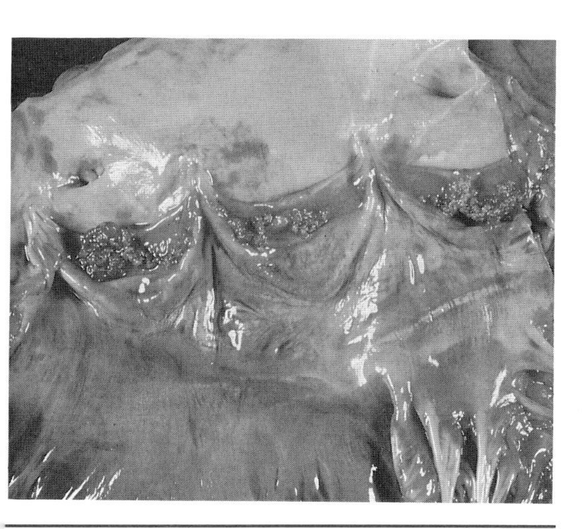

Fig. 12.68 Thrombotic vegetation of the aortic valve in a patient who died of cancer.

softer, larger and less regular than those in rheumatic endocarditis (Fig. 12.68). They are usually asymptomatic but both systemic embolism and secondary infection of the thrombi are complications. In most instances, the condition is discovered at autopsy in patients who have died of cancer or other wasting diseases, and it is sometimes called **marantic** or **terminal endocarditis**. It may be associated with the venous thrombosis which occurs in some patients with carcinoma of the pancreas or of other internal organs.

Libman–Sacks endocarditis develops in patients with systemic lupus erythematosus and usually involves the mitral and tricuspid valves. The vegetations are sterile and are softer, more friable and usually larger than those of rheumatic endocarditis; they are also more widely dispersed and may involve both sides of the valve cusps, extending onto the adjacent mural endocardium.

Disorders of the Conducting System

The conducting system consists of specialized cardiocytes (myocytes) which initiate the heartbeat in the sinoatrial node and conduct the impulse through the A–V node and then in turn through the common A–V bundle (bundle of His) and the left and right bundle branches to the apex of the ventricle, which is the first region to contract. Disturbances of cardiac rhythm complicate many types of heart disease: some of them are due to damage to the conducting system, the most vulnerable parts of which are the A–V bundle and its right and left branches; many of them, e.g. extrasystoles, paroxysmal tachycardia and atrial fibrillation, are due to 'spontaneous' impulses or irregularities arising in the myocardium.

Conducting system defects may be congenital or acquired. The latter include ischaemic or degenerative injury, inflammatory conditions such as myocarditis, sarcoidosis or connective tissue diseases (rheumatoid arthritis), infiltrative disorders such as amyloidosis or metastatic tumour, and finally, surgical trauma.

Ischaemia or infarction (Fig. 12.69) is the main cause of A–V nodal dysfunction. Prolongation of the PR interval of the ECG, intermittent dropping of beats due to failure of conduction or complete A–V dissociation leading to heart block are characteristic complications of acute myocardial infarction. Right bundle branch block is easily detectable on the ECG but in many cases no morphological cause can be established at autopsy. Left bundle branch block is more commonly associated with a morphologically detectable abnormality (Fig. 12.70).

Congenital Heart Disease

Little is known of the causation of congenital abnormalities of the heart. Rubella infection of the mother in the first 3 months of pregnancy is associated with serious abnormalities in 10–20% of infants of which heart disease constitutes about 50%.

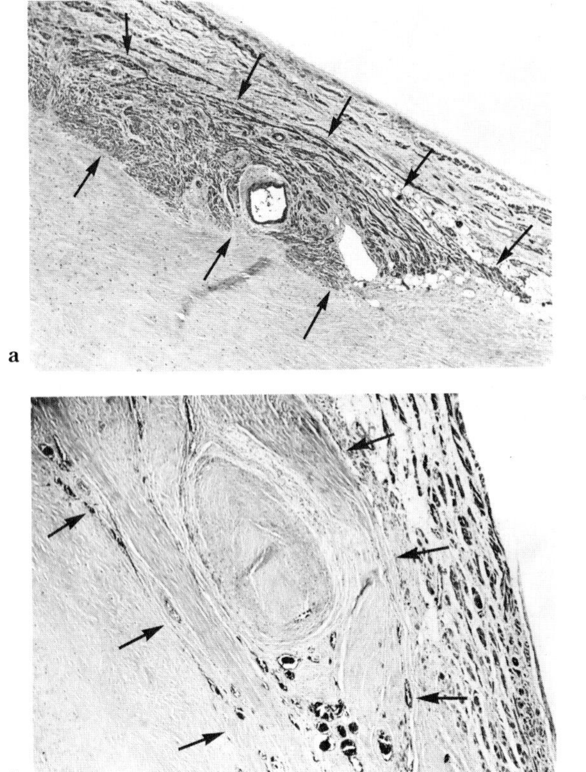

Fig. 12.69 Ischaemic fibrosis of A–V node. Above, normal A–V node (outlined by arrows), lying between the endocardium and central fibrous body. Below, ischaemic fibrosis of A–V node from a patient with heart block. (Professor M. J. Davies.)

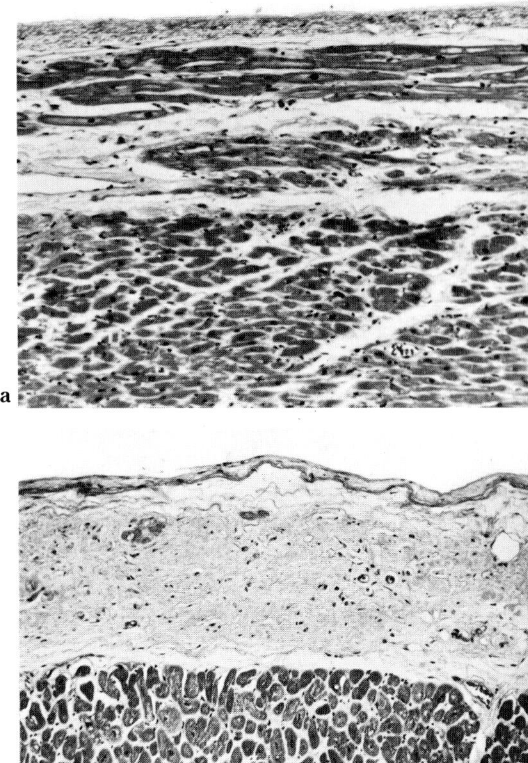

Fig. 12.70 'Idiopathic' bundle branch fibrosis. Above, normal left bundle branch from the heart of a young man, consisting of groups of fibres lying between the ventricular myocardium and endocardium surface. Below, almost complete loss of left bundle branch in a case of heart block. (Some loss of fibres occurs as a normal feature of ageing.) (Professor M. J. Davies.)

A high proportion of congenital abnormalities of the heart result from defects or variations in the formation of the septa in the developing heart. At an early stage of development the heart consists of three chambers or parts, an atrial, a ventricular and the aortic bulb; division of each of these into two takes place separately. Of special importance is the relation of the ventricular septum to the division of the distal portion of the bulb into the beginning of the aorta and of the pulmonary artery. The ventricular septum grows upwards from the apex, with a curved margin resulting from the growing folds on the anterior and posterior walls, until ultimately there is a relatively small aperture at the base. The aortic bulb undergoes division into two nearly equal parts with the formation and fusion of two longitudinal folds in its wall; the two vessels formed must rotate spirally in order to establish their normal continuity with the ventricles. The septum of the bulb ultimately fuses with the upgrowing ventricular septum, the last portion to close being represented by the membranous part of the septum.

Important abnormalities occur in connection with the growth of these two septa. The positions of the pulmonary and aortic valves do not correspond exactly with the junction of the primitive ventricle and the aortic bulb. This is especially the case on the right side, where the lower part of the bulb becomes the upper part of the right ventricle or conus, and, as we shall see, this part is sometimes abnormally narrow.

While some of the anomalies are incompatible with extrauterine life, in many, the circulatory dynamics allow survival for varying periods of time. Recent advances in diagnostic methodology, including cardiac catheterization and angiocardiography, allow the surgeon to establish the nature and extent of the defects and so cure or alleviation of many of the conditions can be effected.

It is convenient to divide the anomalies into those which produce cyanosis and those which do not. The cyanosis results from admixture of a relatively large volume of venous blood with the oxygenated blood leaving the heart, i.e. a venous–arterial shunt exists. The lowered O_2 tension in the arterial blood leads to a compensatory erythrocytosis and this makes cyanosis more prominent. The cyanosis may be further aggravated by impaired oxygenation of the blood by the lungs, in conditions where there is pulmonary involvement or when heart failure develops.

Cyanotic Group

Malformations of the aortic bulb – pulmonary and aortic stenosis. The commonest of these result from an unequal division of the bulb. Most frequently the septum is pushed to the right, so that the aorta is abnormally large and arises partly from the left and partly from the right ventricle (i.e. it is dextraposed); there is usually also a defect in the ventricular septum. The result is pulmonary stenosis or obstruction, but the site of the narrowing varies: sometimes the pulmonary artery is small, the division of the bulb being markedly unequal, and occasionally the small pulmonary artery is completely obliterated. In other cases the narrowing is mainly at the valve, the cusps being partly fused to form a thickened diaphragm with a reduced aperture. More rarely, there is a narrowing of the part of the right ventricle below the valve, that is, the part which is derived from the bulb. All these abnormalities interfere with the flow of blood into the pulmonary artery, and lead to varying degrees of right ventricular hypertrophy. Some of the blood from the right ventricle passes through the interventricular septum and into the aorta. The ductus arteriosus usually remains open after birth and the lungs receive part of their blood supply through it. The foramen ovale also remains open and may be very large.

The commonest anomaly of the cyanotic group and one which is amenable to surgery is the **tetralogy of Fallot**. In this there is **obstruction in the outflow tract of the right ventricle**, usually from stenosis of the pulmonary valve, though the obstruction may be in the infundibular part of the right ventricle. This results in **right ventricular hypertrophy** and the pressure in this chamber is raised so that some of the unoxygenated blood in the chamber is shunted into the aorta through a high **interventricular septal defect.** The **aorta partially over-rides the septal defect** and so, in addition to receiving oxygenated blood from the left ventricle, it also receives venous blood from the right ventricle. All degrees of severity exist in the stenosis of the right ventricular outflow, the size of the septal defect and the dextraposition of the aortic root. In extreme cases the pulmonary orifice and artery may be atretic and blood reaches the lungs from the aorta through a patent ductus arteriosus. In about 25% of cases of Fallot's tetralogy, there is a right aortic arch.

Eisenmenger's complex. The features resemble those in Fallot's tetralogy, but there is no obstruction to the outflow from the right ventricle. The pressure gradients across the high interventricular septal defect are such that little right-to-left shunting of blood and hence little cyanosis, occurs at first. Later, with the onset of pulmonary hypertension and changes in the pulmonary vessels, overt cyanosis occurs, partly from admixture cyanosis and partly from faulty oxygenation of the blood by the lungs.

Transposition of the great vessels. A curious anomaly results from failure of the proximal aorta and pulmonary artery to undergo the spiral rotation necessary for the establishment of their correct relationships with the ventricles. In consequence, the aorta arises from the right ventricle and the pulmonary artery from the left. While such a condition alone is incompatible with extrauterine life, it may sometimes be compensated, for a time, by persistence of the ductus arteriosus, a patent foramen ovale, or a defect of the interatrial or interventricular septum; often these defects are present in combination. In this condition the chief difficulty is the effectiveness of the mechanism allowing oxygenated blood to reach the systemic circulation. Therefore, the greater the volume of the shunt, the better the admixture of arterial blood to venous blood and the less marked is the cyanosis.

Truncus arteriosus. In this anomaly the aorta and the pulmonary arteries arise from a common stem vessel. The pulmonary arteries may be replaced by enlarged bronchial arteries. The truncus arises from both ventricles and over-rides a ventricular septal defect. Sometimes the septum fails to develop and a single ventricular cavity exists. Defects of the interatrial septum are also common.

Single ventricle with a rudimentary outlet chamber. A single ventricle provides blood to both the aorta and pulmonary artery, which may arise separately or from a rudimentary outlet chamber. The interatrial septum may or may not have developed normally, resulting in **cor binatrium triloculare** or **cor biloculare** respectively.

Tricuspid atresia is associated with defective development of the right ventricle which, in extreme cases, is virtually absent. Blood passes from the right to the left atrium through a defect in the interatrial septum. The pulmonary artery is small, arising from the underdeveloped right ventricle. In some cases the vessel is atretic or occupies an abnormal position. Blood usually reaches the lungs from the aorta via a patent ductus arteriosus.

In **aortic atresia**, a rare condition, the aortic orifice is hypoplastic, the ascending aorta hypoplastic or atretic, and the left ventricle poorly developed or absent. Circulation of blood is maintained by shunting of oxygenated blood from the left atrium into the right atrium and thence to the right ventricle and pulmonary artery. From this, the aorta is filled via a patent ductus arteriosus.

Pure congenital pulmonary stenosis. Here the course of the circulation is essentially normal but sometimes there is a patent interatrial septum. The lesion is a stenosis of either the pulmonary valve or the infundibulum of the right ventricle. The right ventricle is hypertrophied and forces the blood past the obstruction. If the interatrial septum is intact, cyanosis is not necessarily present; if there is interatrial communication a right-to-left shunt may be established with consequent cyanosis.

Anomalies of the venous return. These may involve the systemic or the pulmonary veins and vary greatly in detail. The superior and/or the inferior vena cava may open into the left atrium, thus shunting reduced systemic venous blood into the arterial side of the systemic circulation. In other cases, some of the pulmonary veins open into the right atrium: this results simply in an excessive amount of oxygenated blood being pumped around the pulmonary circulation and cyanosis will not occur.

Acyanotic Group

Aortic valve stenosis and subaortic stenosis may each occur as an isolated abnormality as may also a **bicuspid aortic valve**. The overall incidence of the latter is approximately 2% and it is usually symptomless in early life, but predisposes to the development of infective endocarditis and calcific aortic stenosis.

Patent ductus arteriosus may coexist with many other anomalies, but it may be the only abnormality present, in which case closure by surgery restores the circulation to normal. Failure to close the ductus leads eventually to hear ailure, and there is a risk of infective 'endocarditis' endarteritis) of the ductus. In a few cases there is issociated pulmonary hypertension and blood flow n the ductus may then be reversed so that un- oxygenated blood passes from the pulmonary artery into the aorta via the ductus, usually mmediately beyond the origin of the left subcla- vian artery. Such a patient may thus have a cyano- ic tinge in the nailbeds of the toes but not in those of the hands.

nteratrial septal defect. This is one of the commonest congenital malformations of the heart. Even when the defect is large, it appears to have ittle effect on the circulation. Rarely, a piece of letached thrombus, e.g. from the leg veins, basses from the right atrium through the defect to each the left atrium and causes crossed or para- loxical embolism. While probe patency of the oramen ovale may be demonstrable in up to 25% of normal hearts, the important malformations are of three main types: persistent ostium primum, ostium secundum and persistent atrioventricularis communis. In this last condition, there is often usion of the tricuspid and mitral valves to form a common atrioventricular valve. Lutembacher's lisease consists of an interatrial septal defect with nitral stenosis.

nterventricular septal defect. A high septal lefect is frequently part of another congenital anomaly such as Fallot's tetralogy. An isolated nigh interventricular septal defect (maladie de Roger) is not uncommon; the size and location of the aperture varies.

Anomalies of the aortic arch are commonly ssociated with Fallot's tetralogy, but as isolated nomalies they rarely cause symptoms. However, vhen a vascular ring is formed around the trachea nd oesophagus by a right aortic arch and left lescending aorta together with a persistent ductus rteriosus, ligamentum arteriosum or an anom- lous left subclavian artery, pressure effects, nainly on the trachea, may result. A double aortic rch may give similar symptoms.

oarctation (stenosis) of the aorta. Slight narrowing of the aorta between the left subclavian artery and the orifice of the ductus arteriosus, i.e. in the interval where the two main streams of the fetal circulation cross, is not very uncommon and occurs predominantly in males. The stenosis is rarely severe, but all degrees of narrowing up to complete atresia of the aorta have been recorded. With severe narrowing, an extensive collateral system from the carotid and subclavian arteries links the aorta above and below the narrowed segment. The pulses in the legs are poor compared with those of the arms. Hypertension develops and death is likely to ensue from cardiac failure, cerebral haemorrhage or, less commonly, from local complications associated with the site of coarctation, e.g. aneurysm or dissection. Coarctation of the aorta may be associated with other congenital abnormalities, but frequently it is the only abnormality present and, moreover, it is one that can be cured by surgery.

Other abnormalities of the valves. Sometimes there is excess or deficiency in the number of the cusps of the semilunar valves; occasionally there are four cusps, usually somewhat unequal in size, but, as a rule, there is no interference with the efficiency of the valve. There may, however, be only two cusps, usually in the aortic valve; one cusp is usually larger than the other. Bicuspid aortic valves predispose to calcific aortic stenosis and also bacterial endocarditis. Very rarely recorded.

In **Ebstein's disease** there is downward displacement of the tricuspid valve so that the upper part of the right ventricle comes to be a functional part of the right atrium. The course of the circulation is normal.

Diseases of the Pericardium

The pericardium is a fibrous sac which surrounds the heart and, like the peritoneum and pleura, it comprises visceral and parietal layers which line the cavities. Accumulation of fluid and blood can occur and it may be the site of acute and chronic inflammation. Multiple minute punctate haemorrhages occur on the visceral and parietal layers in various purpuric conditions (p. 640) and this may also be a prominent feature in cases of death by suffocation. The causes of pericardial disease are summarized in Table 12.9.

The pericardial sac can dilate to contain over a litre of fluid without rise in pressure, but only if the fluid accumulates slowly. If accumulation is rapid, even a small volume of fluid raises the pericardial pressure, interferes with cardiac filling and leads to **cardiac tamponade**, a form of cardiogenic shock with low cardiac output. There is severe hypotension with a low pulse pressure, particularly during inspiration (pulsus paradoxus) and death ensues. Cardiac tamponade is usually due to haemopericardium but may be caused by a tense effusion.

A pericardial effusion is a non-inflammatory accumulation of fluid in the pericardial sac. The commonest cause of this is metastatic carcinoma.

Table 12.9 Causes of pericarditis

- Infections
  - Viral – Coxsackie A, B, adenoviruses, influenza
  - Bacterial
    - Pyogenic organisms
    - Tuberculosis
  - Fungal
- Malignant disease
  - Direct spread from carcinoma of bronchus or oesophagus
  - Metastatic tumour
- Myocardial infarction
- Metabolic
  - Uraemia
  - Hypothyroidism
- Immunologically mediated
  - Rheumatic fever
  - Connective tissue diseases: rheumatoid arthritis, systemic lupus erythematosus and others
  - Post-cardiotomy or post-myocardial infarction (Dressler's syndrome)
- Iatrogenic
  - Post-radiation
  - Drug hypersensitivity reaction
- Idiopathic
  - Benign recurrent or relapsing

Effusions may also occur in cardiac failure, in association with other causes of oedema (renal, hepatic, gastrointestinal and nutritional) and in myxoedema.

Pericarditis

The clinical features of acute pericarditis include fever, tachycardia and usually chest pain, although the condition is sometimes clinically silent. If the volume of exudate in the sac is small, as in early or mild pericarditis, pain results from rubbing together of the inflamed, roughened pericardial surfaces, it is sharp and 'stabbing', and accompanied by an audible friction rub synchronous with the heart beat. If fluid is more abundant, it separates the pericardial layers and the heart sounds become muffled.

Morphologically, there are the usual features of acute inflammation of a serosal lining. Active hyperaemia, inflammatory oedema and emigration of leucocytes occur in the pericardial tissue, exudate accumulates in the pericardial sac and fibrin is deposited on its surface. Depending on the cause, these changes may be mild and brief, with accumulation of clear or slightly turbid fluid and dulling of the inflamed surfaces by a fine layer of fibrin, or they may be of greater severity, with turbid, blood-stained or purulent fluid and formation of a thick layer of fibrin on the surfaces. A fine deposit of fibrin on the pericardial surfaces undergoes lysis, but a thicker layer is removed by organization with consequent fibrous thickening and adhesion of the two layers of the pericardium and, if gross, fibrous thickening of the sac may lead to constrictive pericarditis.

Viral and idiopathic pericarditis. This is usually a mild pericarditis which occurs most often in young adults. It subsides within 2 weeks but in some 25–30% of cases there may be recurrences (benign recurrent viral pericarditis), the mechanisms of which are uncertain. In many cases of presumed viral pericarditis attempts to isolate a virus are unsuccessful.

Bacterial pericarditis may complicate septicaemia or pyaemia, bacterial pneumonia, empyema and an ulcerating carcinoma of the bronchus or oesophagus. The causal organisms are most often pyogenic cocci, notably *Staphylococcus aureus*, *Haemophilus influenzae* and streptococci.

Tuberculous pericarditis is common in chronic pulmonary tuberculosis. The route of infection is presumed to be by lymphatics or from an infected pleura. There is often an abundant exudate which is turbid or blood-stained and tubercles may be visible on the pericardial surfaces. The morphological features are typical and may progress to fibro-obliterative calcification of the pericardial sac.

Other causes of acute pericarditis. Mild pericarditis usually develops in the first week in patients with transmural **myocardial infarction**. A mild acute diffuse persistent pericarditis may occur as part of a post-infarction, post-cardiotomy, post-traumatic syndrome or sometimes non-cardiac thoracic surgery (Dressler's syndrome). In all these conditions the detection of antibody reactive with extracts of myocardial tissue has been reported, suggesting an autoimmune hypersensitivity reaction triggered by injury to the heart. Acute pericarditis occurs as an incidental feature in some cases of **systemic lupus erythematosus** and **rheumatoid arthritis**; in occasional cases in rheumatoid arthritis there may be progression to constrictive pericarditis. Fibrinous pericarditis is a feature of **uraemia** and is related to the level of the blood urea; it resolves spontaneously with dialysis.

Constrictive pericarditis. This is a rare condition characterized by obliteration of the pericardial sac by a thick layer of dense fibrous tissue which sometimes becomes calcified. It can result from prolonged pyogenic or from tuberculous pericarditis and also occurs as a complication of rheumatoid arthritis; in many cases it is of unknown aetiology.

The fibrous tissue interferes with the filling of the heart and this may be aggravated by constriction of the great veins as they enter the atria. The clinical picture is thus one of progressive congestive heart failure associated with a small heart, and a low stroke volume. If the heart can be freed by resection of the thickened pericardium the symptoms are relieved and for most patients the long-term outlook is good.

Tumours of the Heart and Pericardium

Primary tumours of the heart are very rare. **Fibroma**, **myxoma**, **lipoma**, **haemangioma** and **lymphangioma** are occasionally encountered, especially in the left atrium. The commonest is the **cardiac myxoma**, comprising a myxomatous mass up to several centimetres in diameter, projecting into the cavity from the margin of the foramen ovale, and which may create a ball-valve obstruction of the mitral valve and may mimic the clinical features of mitral stenosis. Microscopically they comprise polygonal or stellate cells in a loose myxoid matrix rich in proteoglycans. **Rhabdomyoma** of congenital origin occurs especially in the ventricles as multiple rounded nodules of pale, translucent tissue. It consists of large branching cells in which striped myofibrils are found; the cells have a vacuolated cytoplasm and contain much glycogen. In 30% of cases, the rhabdomyomas are associated with multiple discrete gliomatous growths in the cerebral hemispheres – tuberous sclerosis (p. 850); in some cases there are malformations of the kidneys and liver, and adenoma sebaceum on the face (Bourneville's disease).

Metastatic tumours in the heart and pericardium are common, occurring in about 10% of all fatal malignancies. Bronchial carcinoma, by direct spread, involves the heart more frequently than any other neoplasm (30% of cases). Melanoma metastasizes surprisingly often to the heart, and other primary sources include breast, gastro-intestinal tract and lymphomas.

The Pathology of Cardiac Surgery Procedures

The widespread application of curative or palliative surgical management for congenital and acquired heart disease has led to greatly improved quality of life and increased survival for many patients. These procedures, which include valve replacement with prostheses, coronary artery bypass grafts and cardiac transplantation have generated new and increasingly important aspects of cardiac pathology which are now briefly reviewed.

Valve Prosthesis – Complications

These are either mechanical or biological with animal (usually porcine) leaflets. The main complications are valve failure, thrombus formation, infective endocarditis, paravalvular leaks and haemolysis.

Valve failure. Degeneration and/or calcification of tissue valves usually occurs slowly, giving time for further surgery. Failure of one of the components of a mechanical valve is usually an emergency, especially if a moving part sticks or becomes disconnected with complete loss of valve function, and the possibility of embolism in the latter event.

Thrombus formation. Permanent anticoagulation is mandatory for patients with mechanical valves but is not routinely required for biological valves. The risk of systemic embolism is about 1.5% per patient year and is similar with either type of valve. Early, small emboli arising from thrombi on the sewing ring are as frequent with both types. Later, larger thrombi causing embolism or rarely valve dysfunction, are more common with mechanical valves.

Endocarditis is a serious complication with a high mortality rate (60%). It occurs with equal frequency on biological or mechanical valves at a rate of approximately 0.5–1% per patient year. *Staphylococcus epidermidis* is the commonest organism (30% all cases) followed by streptococci. Infection with yeasts or fungi is much rarer. Prompt recognition is vital and early valve replacement may improve the prognosis.

Haemolysis results from mechanical trauma due to contact between blood and the 'abnormal' surfaces of a valve prosthesis. Clinically important haemolysis rarely occurs with a normally functioning valve, though biochemical evidence of haemolysis can be demonstrated in many patients. Less than 5% of patients become anaemic. Paravalvular leak is thought to be the main reason for such significant haemolysis. Paravalvular leak may occur with any prosthesis and may be large enough to warrant repair or replacement.

Coronary Artery Bypass Grafts and Angioplasty

Vascular conduits are the standard method of coronary artery bypass grafts (CABG). The left internal mammary artery is the favoured conduit for the left anterior descending artery, supplemented by saphenous venous grafts for the circumflex and right coronary arteries. The major complication in CABGs is late narrowing or occlusion especially in saphenous vein grafts. The graft closure rate may be up to 15% in the first 6 months due to thrombosis, and 2–5% per annum thereafter due to atheroma/thrombosis. Patency rates of left internal mammary grafts may be as high as 90% at 10 years.

Coronary artery bypass is effective in relieving symptoms in most patients for up to 10 years. It significantly improves survival in high risk groups such as those with severe reversible ischaemia and associated impairment of left ventricular function, in disease of the left main stem artery, and in triple vessel disease.

Angioplasty

This is an alternative form of revascularization in which dilatation of vascular stenoses is achieved using a balloon catheter introduced into the coronary artery via a percutaneously inserted catheter. Percutaneous transluminal coronary angioplasty (PTCA) is the term applied to this technique. Rupture of the artery during the procedure is surprisingly uncommon, emergency surgery being required in only 3%. Immediate success rates are very high (80–90%). Subsequent abrupt closure is usually due to dissection, accompanied by spasm or thrombosis. Restenosis at 6–9 months is the commonest late problem and affects up to one-third of patients treated.

Cardiac Transplantation

Cardiac transplantation is a technically straightforward and logical operation for patients with intractable heart failure. The first cardiac transplant recipient lived for 18 days in 1967; his death was due to a combination of infection and acute rejection. Since then, improvements in immunosuppression have largely been responsible for greatly increased survival and the operation is carried out routinely in many large medical centres. If there is pulmonary hypertension, the lungs are also transplanted. The 5-year survival reaches 85%.

Endomyocardial biopsy has improved the management of rejection; the severity of the rejection is graded histologically and used to monitor the dosage of immunosuppressive drugs. Acute rejection occurs from 3–5 days postoperatively; later, it may be combined with chronic rejection, evidence of which may be found from about one month. There is a myocarditis and in addition, important changes occur in the arteries. The intima becomes infiltrated by inflammatory cells and becomes thickened due to cellular proliferation and lipid accumulation. The end result resembles atheroma and causes considerable narrowing of the lumen.

Further Reading

Braunwald, E., (ed.) (1991). *Heart Disease*, 4th edn. W. B. Saunders, Philadelphia.

Brown, M. S. and Goldstein, J. L. (1986). A receptor mediated pathway for cholesterol homeostasis. *Science* **232**, 34–47.

Camilleri, J.-P., Berry, C. L., Fiessinger, J.-N., and Bariety, J. (eds) (1989). *Diseases of the Arterial Wall*. Springer-Verlag, Berlin, Heidelberg.

Dalen, J. E. and Alpert, J. S. (eds) (1987). *Valvular Heart Disease*, 2nd edn. Little Brown & Co., Boston.

Kaplan, N. M., Brenner, B. M. and Laragh, J. H. (eds) (1987). *The Kidney in Hypertension*. Raven Press, New York.

Prevention of Coronary Heart Disease in Scotland. Report of the Working Group on Prevention and Health Promotion. Brief authoritative reviews of risk factors and intervention trials. HMSO, Edinburgh, 1990.

Ross, R. (1986). The pathogenesis of atherosclerosis – an update. *New England Journal of Medicine* **314**, 488–500.

Silver, M. D. (ed.) (1983). *Cardiovascular Pathology*. Churchill Livingstone, Edinburgh.

Thompson, W. D. and Smith, E. B. (1989). Atherosclerosis and the coagulation system. *Journal of Pathology* **159**, 97–106.

13 Respiratory System

The primary function of the respiratory system – oxygenation of the blood and removal of carbon dioxide – requires that air be brought into close approximation with blood. Accordingly, the respiratory tract is particularly exposed to infection, both by microbes in the inspired air and by spread downwards of the bacteria which commonly colonize the nose and throat. Another important hazard is presented by inhalation of pollutants found in the form of dusts, smokes and fumes, a particularly important example being cigarette smoke. These pollutants are responsible for the high incidence of chronic bronchitis, chronic lung disease and bronchial carcinoma in many parts of the world. The lungs are the only organs, apart from the heart, through which all the blood passes during each circulation: accordingly, cardiovascular diseases which disturb pulmonary haemodynamics are likely to have serious secondary effects on the lungs, e.g. pulmonary oedema, and conversely diseases of the lungs which interfere with pulmonary blood flow have important effects on the heart and systemic circulation. In short, ***normal cardiac and pulmonary function are closely interdependent***.

Respiratory Infections

The defences of the respiratory tract against infection include: the cough reflex, upward flow of the surface film of mucus which coats the air passages and is impelled by ciliated epithelium, the secretion of IgA antibodies, and the phagocytic activity of alveolar macrophages.

Bacterial infections of the respiratory tract may be primary, occurring in healthy individuals, or secondary to a large number of conditions which depress resistance. Primary infections have become much less common in many of the developed countries: they include laryngeal or nasal diphtheria, bacterial pneumonia due usually to *Streptococcus pneumoniae*, pulmonary tuberculosis, pneumonic plague and anthrax pneumonia. Primary pneumonia due to various pyogenic bacteria is, however, relatively common in infants and old people. Secondary bacterial infections occur especially when the local resistance of the respiratory mucosa is lowered by various virus infections, such as the common cold, influenza, or measles and when there are persistent abnormalities such as chronic bronchitis or bronchiectasis. In these conditions, bacteria growing in the nose and throat extend downwards, usually giving a mixed infection.

Virus infections. Most acute respiratory disease seen in general medical practice every winter is caused by viruses (Table 13.1). Acute viral pharyngitis (presenting as 'sore throat') and the common cold are frequent and comparatively trivial. Others, like bronchiolitis in infants due to respiratory syncytial virus, may be fatal. Measles, and to a lesser extent other xanthemas of childhood, may be followed by acute tracheobronchitis and pneumonia usually due to bacterial infection.

The clinical syndromes due to acute respiratory virus infections depend to some extent on the age of the patient and the extent to which the respiratory tract is invaded. These syndromes are not sharply defined and may be produced by many different viruses. Nevertheless, recognizable clinical syndromes produced by viruses in the respiratory tract are the common cold (coryza), viral sore throat, influenza, infantile croup, infantile acute bronchiolitis and 'atypical pneumonia'.

Table 13.1 The respiratory viruses

Virus group	No. of serotypes	Disease
Influenza virus	3	Influenza
Parainfluenza viruses	4	Croup, colds, lower respiratory infections in children
Respiratory syncytial virus	1	Bronchiolitis and pneumonia in infants, colds in older children
Rhinoviruses	> 100	Colds
Adenoviruses	33	Pharyngitis, conjunctivitis
Coronaviruses	3	Colds
Coxsackieviruses	Types A21, B3	Colds
Echoviruses	Types 11, 20	Colds
'Virus pneumonia agents' (not true viruses)	A heterogeneous group	Atypical pneumonia

The common cold occurs throughout the world, including tropical countries, and exposure to low temperature does not appear to be a predisposing factor. It is caused mainly by the *rhinoviruses* of which there are more than 100 serologically distinct types. There is no cross-immunity so that repeated infections are common. Rhinoviruses belong to the family of picornaviruses which also include enteroviruses. Other viruses which cause common colds are parainfluenza, respiratory syncytial, corona, and more rarely some coxsackie- and echoviruses.

Adenoviruses are the main cause of '**viral sore**

throat' in which the pharyngitis is sometimes accompanied by conjunctivitis. They cause epidemics of acute respiratory disease as well as endemic pharyngitis and follicular conjunctivitis. There are about 30 serological types of these DNA viruses.

The *parainfluenza viruses* cause a respiratory infection intermediate in severity between the common cold and influenza. They are the major cause of acute laryngo-tracheobronchitis (succinctly termed 'croup') in young children. There are four serological types of these large RNA viruses.

Respiratory syncytial virus infection is common in young children, generally giving rise to trivial signs and symptoms. However, it is highly virulent for children under 1 year of age, especially infants less than 6 months old, and is responsible for most hospitalized cases of acute bronchiolitis or pneumonia in young children.

The most serious virus infection of the respiratory tract is **influenza**. This mainly involves the upper respiratory tract and is a febrile illness often followed by lassitude and depression. Influenza virus is an RNA virus (Fig. 13.1) and three major antigenic types exist, A, B and C; there is considerable antigenic variation within them. Strains of the virus are further classified by two outer antigens – H, haemagglutinin and N, neuraminidase antigen, However, these antigens are not stable because the virus undergoes considerable genetic re-assortment (*antigenic shift*) and also minor but progressive change (*antigenic drift*). When the H antigen undergoes shift, a new strain may emerge to which there is no pre-existing immunity and a pandemic develops. This happened in 1918, 1957 (strain H2N2) and 1963 (strain H2N3). In such pandemics, rapidly fatal **influenza viral pneumonia** may occur in previously healthy young people. However, in most epidemics bacterial complications are the chief cause of pneumonia. During influenza epidemics it is important to protect those who are at special risk, such as chronic bronchitics.

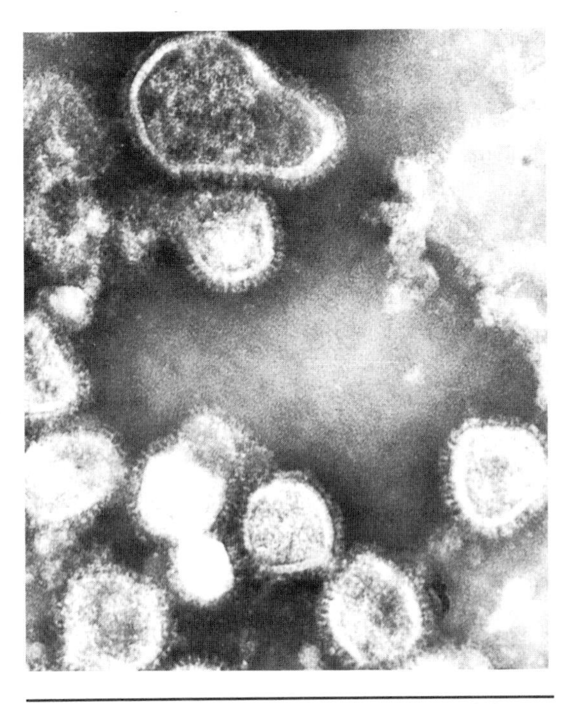

Fig. 13.1 Individual virus particles of the influenza H3N2 Hong Kong strain showing spikes of haemagglutinin by which the particle attaches itself to susceptible cells in the respiratory mucosa. Electron micrograph. ×128 000. (Dr D. Hobson.)

Nose, Nasal Sinuses and Nasopharynx

Inflammatory Conditions

Apart from the common cold, hay fever is the commonest cause of **acute rhinitis**. It is an acute allergic or atopic rhinitis, which occurs as a result of sensitization to certain pollens, such as that of Timothy grass or to house dust, animal dandruff, feathers or other specific antigens. Atopic hypersensitivity is also a factor in some cases of nasal polyps.

Acute sinusitis is generally a complication of acute infection of the nose, less commonly of dental sepsis. Gram +ve cocci such as *Streptococcus pyogenes, Streptococcus pneumoniae* or *Staphylococcus aureus* are the usual causal organisms.

Acute nasopharyngitis usually accompanies either acute rhinitis or acute tonsillitis in which *Streptococcus pyogenes* is the common pathogen.

The histopathology of acute inflammation of the nose, sinuses and nasopharynx is similar. There is hyperaemia and oedema of the mucosa, and the mucosal glands are hyperactive. In virus infections, neutrophil polymorphs are generally sparse in both the mucosa and the exudate until secondary bacterial infection supervenes, but thereafter increasing numbers of neutrophils migrate through the mucosa and the exudate becomes mucopurulent. There is a variable degree of loss of the superficial ciliated epithelium. In allergic states, oedema of the submucosa is a prominent feature, giving rise to polypoid thickening of the mucosa. The mucosal glands are often enlarged and distended and the oedematous stroma is characteristically infiltrated by numerous eosinophil polymorphs.

Chronic rhinitis, sinusitis and nasopharyngitis may follow an acute inflammatory episode which has failed to resolve. Inadequate drainage of the sinuses, nasal obstruction due to polyps, or enlargement of the nasopharyngeal lymphoid tissue (adenoids), may be underlying factors.

Nasal polyps. Chronic recurrent inflammation of the nose, particularly of an allergic aetiology, may lead to polypoid thickening of the mucosa. Polyps are rounded or elongated masses commonly arising from the region of the middle turbinate. They are often bilateral, a point of distinction from nasal tumours. Nasal polyps are usually gelatinous in consistency with a smooth, shiny surface. They consist of a core of loose oedematous connective tissue containing occasional mucous glands and covered by normal ciliated respiratory type of epithelium (Fig. 13.2), but squamous metaplasia is common. Lymphocytes, plasma cells and eosinophils infiltrate the submucosa to a variable degree.

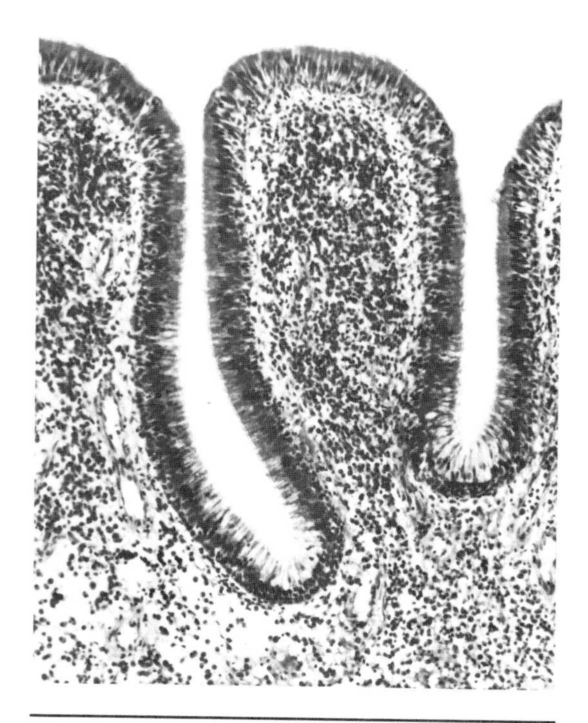

Fig. 13.2 Section through the surface of a nasal polyp showing the respiratory epithelium and the loose oedematous stroma infiltrated with chronic inflammatory cells. ×100.

Chronic granulomatous rhinitis. In contrast to acute infection, specific forms of chronic infection of the nose are rare in most communities. Chronic granulomas may be due to tuberculosis, tertiary syphilis, leprosy, scleroma or fungal infections such as aspergillosis or rhinosporidiosis.

Two rare forms of necrotizing granuloma of uncertain nature occur in the upper respiratory tract. In one form, **Wegener's granulomatosis**, a necrotizing vasculitis with giant cells develops, usually in the nose or the maxillary sinuses, followed by similar lesions in the lung and associated with disseminated lesions of polyarteritis particularly in the kidneys. **Malignant midline granuloma of the nose**, presents as an ulcerated lesion which spreads progressively to erode the soft tissues and bones around the nose.

Histologically, the lesion consists of proliferating lymphocytes and macrophages and it is now thought to be a T-cell lymphoma.

Benign Tumours

The commonest benign tumours of the nose are **haemangioma** of the septum and **squamous papilloma** of the vestibule. A much less common tumour is the **juvenile angiofibroma** which usually occurs in the nasopharynx. It appears in childhood, almost exclusively in boys, and tends to become quiescent by the end of the second decade. It is an enlarging vascular tumour which readily bleeds. It may cause bone erosion and destruction by pressure atrophy.

Malignant Tumours

Transitional-cell epithelial tumours are common in the nasal passages. Some of these do not recur and may be termed **transitional cell papillomas**: some recur in the same form, and some show a rapid change to **squamous cell carcinoma.** Squamous-cell carcinoma is common in the nose and nasal sinuses, but **anaplastic carcinoma** and **adenocarcinoma** also occur.

Nasopharyngeal carcinoma, usually squamous-cell, often poorly differentiated or of anaplastic type, is particularly common in China, Malaysia, Indonesia and East Africa. There is a prominent lymphocytic infiltrate in the tumour stroma and the lesion is also referred to as a lymphoepithelioma. This tumour is closely associated with the Epstein–Barr virus.

Larynx and Trachea

Inflammatory Conditions

Acute Inflammation

Mild **acute laryngitis and tracheitis** are commonplace where there is atmospheric pollution with any form of smoke. While these factors in themselves are rarely the cause of significant clinical laryngeal disease, they may be of importance in predisposing to viral and bacterial infections. The viruses concerned have been considered above. The bacteria commonly involved are *Streptococcus pneumoniae, Streptococcus pyogenes* and *Neisseria catarrhalis.* Once secondary bacterial invasion occurs it may progress to bronchitis. Acute laryngotracheitis commonly complicates acute febrile states such as measles, influenza and typhoid. It usually subsides but it may pass into the chronic stage.

Pseudomembranous inflammation is usually due to secondary infection by *Streptococcus pyogenes*, *Staphylococcus aureus* or *Streptococcus pneumoniae* following infection with parainfluenza virus. In a minority of cases *Haemophilus influenzae* is the secondary invader. Frequently such infections spread to involve the bronchial tree as **laryngo-tracheobronchitis**. In this condition there is necrosis of epithelium and the formation of an extensive fibrinous membrane on the trachea and main bronchi. There may be pronounced oedema of the subglottic area, resulting in stridor. In laryngo-tracheobronchitis the danger of laryngeal obstruction is, in general, greater than that of toxaemia or lung infection but bronchopneumonia and lung abscess are recognized complications. Pseudomembranous inflammation may result also from the action of corrosive substances or from the inhalation of irritating gases, notably ammonia.

Diphtheria produces a primary acute

oseudomembranous inflammation but this is now very rare in countries where prophylactic immunization is carried out. It usually affects the fauces, soft palate and tonsils but may also involve the nose, larynx, trachea and bronchi. The local lesions are characterized by the formation of a false membrane composed of fibrin, neutrophil polymorphs and necrotic epithelium and containing lumps of *Corynebacterium diphtheriae*. In the lower larynx and trachea the epithelium is columnar and the coagulated exudate rests on the basement membrane from which it separates easily and is coughed up. Over the vocal cords, where the mucosa consists of squamous epithelium, the membrane is firmly adherent. When it s coughed up from the trachea, it may remain attached to the vocal cords and may then impact in the larynx and cause suffocation. In nasal diphtheria the infection is often unilateral and the child may appear to have a cold with discharge from one nostril. This type may be overlooked until the appearance of palatal paralysis, myocardial failure or other toxic effects of diphtheria (p. 291).

Acute epiglottitis, which is caused by *Haemophilus influenzae* type B, is a disease of early childhood which may lead to death within a few hours of onset. Histological examination shows swelling of the tissues due to acute inflammatory oedema and infiltration by neutrophil polymorphs. There is no mucosal ulceration.

Sore throat, hoarseness, subglottic oedema and non-specific arytenoid granulomas may follow brief endotracheal intubation during general anaesthesia for a surgical operation. Endotracheal intubation exceeding 48 hours, using a tube with an inflatable cuff, may lead to pressure injury and abrasion of the trachea with production of large ulcers which expose the underlying cartilaginous rings. Such ulcers, which may be oval or linear transverse lesions, are often located on the anterolateral surface of the trachea: they may become infected by organisms such as *Pseudomonas aeruginosa* and *Candida albicans* and may be covered by a pseudomembrane. Occasionally, prolonged intubation is complicated by the development of tracheo-oesophageal fistula or tracheal stenosis.

Oedema of the glottis is an acute inflammatory oedema of the loose tissue of the upper part of the larynx and not of the vocal cords. The aryepiglottic folds and the tissues around the epiglottis become greatly swollen and tense. The false cords also are affected. This is an important lesion as the swelling may lead to obstruction and death by suffocation, particularly in children. Oedema of the glottis may occur in cardiac and renal diseases but rarely to such an extent as to cause serious results. Oedema of the glottis is also caused by the trauma following impaction of a foreign body in the larynx and may be produced by irritating gases or scalding fluids. It occurs in angio-oedema and in some cases this form has proved fatal.

Chronic Laryngitis

Chronic inflammation of the larynx and trachea is frequently associated with excessive smoking. The mucous glands are swollen and give the surface a granular aspect. Heavy smoking also leads to squamous metaplasia of the larynx which is common among city dwellers and chronic bronchitics. Among heavy smokers the entire larynx, including the subglottis and upper trachea, may become lined by squamous epithelium, thus interfering with clearance of mucus. Extensive squamous metaplasia is almost always present in patients who develop laryngeal carcinoma.

Tuberculous laryngitis occurs secondary to pulmonary tuberculosis, the tubercle bacilli being carried directly to the larynx in the sputum. Any part of the larynx or, less commonly the trachea, may be affected but the disease usually starts first, and is most pronounced, in the arytenoid region and on the vocal cords. Tuberculosis may spread deeply and involve the perichondrium of the arytenoid cartilages; there is chronic thickening, caseation and ulceration, and fragments of dead cartilage may be discharged. The lesion is often very painful; there may be considerable inflammatory swelling and oedema of the glottis may supervene.

Benign Tumours

Small **inflammatory polyps** also called singer's nodes are common and may contain fibrous tissue or amyloid and show myxoid degeneration. They may cause hoarseness and may become ulcerated and painful because of inflammation. **Squamous papilloma** is the commonest benign tumour of the larynx. It occurs usually on the vocal cords and especially at the commissure. In adults it is generally single, may recur after removal, but seldom becomes malignant. In children, usually under the age of 5 years they are mostly of viral aetiology (papilloma viruses), multiple, occur anywhere in the larynx, and regress spontaneously at puberty, sometimes with great rapidity. **Angioma, myxoma, lipoma** and **granular cell myoblastoma** sometimes arise in the larynx but are all very rare.

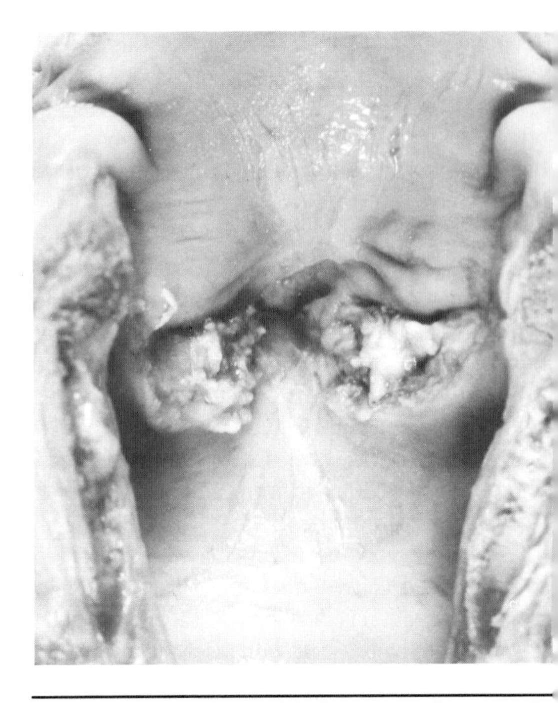

Fig. 13.3 Carcinoma of the larynx, causing extensive ulceration of the vocal cords. The false cords are intact ×2. (Dr J. Watt.)

Malignant Tumours

Squamous carcinoma is the commonest malignant tumour of the larynx, and occurs most often in men over 50 years old. There is an association with tobacco smoking and other inhaled pollutants. When the tumour is on the true or false vocal cords, it is usually less invasive and has a better prognosis than when it arises in the upper part of the larynx or in the subglottic region. Carcinoma of a vocal cord appears first as a small indurated patch, sometimes with a papillary surface, and subsequently ulcerates (Fig. 13.3). A carcinoma of the larynx infiltrates and destroys the surrounding tissue; ulceration may be accompanied by infection which may extend into the bronchi and lungs. Metastatic spread to local lymph nodes and distant sites may occur.

The trachea is a rare site of tumours.

The Bronchi

The ciliated and mucus-secreting cells of the bronchial epithelium are intimately concerned in the defence of the airways and lungs against bacteria and foreign material. Certain viruses may damage the ciliary mechanisms of the respiratory epithelium, thus facilitating invasion of the deeper parts of the bronchial tree and lung by bacteria. Chronic irritation of the bronchi by polluted air and particularly by cigarette smoke may lead to the hyperplasia and hypertrophy of goblet cells and mucous glands which is an important feature in chronic bronchitis.

Scattered among the ciliated respiratory epithelial cells in the bronchi and especially in the respiratory bronchioles are the non-ciliated *Clara cells*. These have all the features of apocrine secretory cells; the secretory product accumulates within smooth cisternae at the apex of the cell, and the apical region is then extruded into the bronchiolar lumen. They are thought to secrete a surfactant-like substance.

Pulmonary endocrine cells (Feyrter cells), arranged singly and in groups, are found throughout the bronchial epithelium. These clear cells are argyrophilic. They belong to the APUD system responsible for the secretion of polypeptide hormones. The peptides concerned are bombesin and calcitonin. Bombesin-containing cells become prominent in the early stages of plexogenic pulmonary arteriopathy (p. 543) when vascular smooth muscle cells are moving from the pulmonary arterial media into the lumen. Pulmonary endocrine cells, in this case containing calcitonin, become prominent in hypoxia, e.g. in subjects living at high altitude or suffering from chronic bronchitis and emphysema. Groups of pulmonary endocrine cells constitute the so-called neuroepithelial bodies which may be airway chemoreceptors. The increase in calcitonin-containing cells in the bronchioles in hypoxic conditions is enhanced in areas of bronchopneumonic consolidation, suggesting that infection may also affect them. The polypeptide hormones are stored in the cell cytoplasm in vesicles which ultrastructurally are electron dense, so-called dense-core vesicles. Dense-core vesicles are also seen in bronchial carcinoid tumours and in small cell bronchial carcinomas.

Acute Bronchitis

A distinction must be made between acute inflammation of the larger, extralobular bronchi (**acute bronchitis**) and of the small, intralobular bronchi and bronchioles (**acute bronchiolitis**). These different anatomical sites influence the likely consequences and hence seriousness of the inflammatory reaction. Acute bronchitis of the adult affects the large and medium-sized bronchi. It is usually mild but may be the cause of much disability when it aggravates an established chronic bronchitis, especially in aged or debilitated subjects. Except as a complication of influenza, acute bronchiolitis is rare in healthy adults, because bacteria do not readily become established so far down the bronchial tree. It does, however, occur in children, old people and in states of debility: it is a serious condition owing to the liability of the organisms to spread to the adjacent acini and cause bronchopneumonia.

Catarrhal bronchitis is characterized by excessive secretion of mucus together with inflammatory exudation. If the inflammatory stimulus (usually bacterial) persists, neutrophil polymorphs appear and the sputum changes from a mucoid secretion to yellow muco-pus. In very severe cases the superficial part of the bronchial wall may be shed with exposure of deeper tissues – so-called **ulcerative bronchitis**. Much acute bronchitis is probably initiated by viruses or mycoplasma which impair local defence mechanisms and allow secondary bacterial invasion of which *Haemophilus influenzae* and *Streptococcus pneumoniae* are the commonest. *Staphylococcus aureus* and *Streptococcus pyogenes* can produce a severe purulent bronchitis in infants. Inhalation of smoke or irritant gases such as sulphur dioxide or chlorine is a rare cause of acute bronchitis.

Chronic Bronchitis

In spite of its name, chronic bronchitis is not primarily an inflammatory disease but consists of metaplastic and other changes resulting from chronic irritation of the bronchial epithelium. The clinical entity is defined as a persistent cough with the production of sputum, on most days for a period of at least 3 months in at least 2 consecutive years. The two main irritants responsible are cigarette smoke and atmospheric pollution. The effects of atmospheric pollution may be aggravated by dampness and fog, when sulphur dioxide and other gases may accumulate and give rise to the lethal aerosol called smog. Chronic bronchitis is exceptionally common in heavy smokers and in industrialized areas. It is especially prone to occur in middle-aged men.

The chronic irritation of the bronchial epithelium leads to a pronounced hypertrophy and hyperplasia of mucous glands within the bronchial wall and an increase in the number and proportion of goblet cells, at the expense of ciliated cells, in the lining epithelium. Goblet cells appear also in the terminal bronchioles, where they are normally absent. The changes are persistent and lead to an excessive production of mucus. Areas of squamous metaplasia of the bronchial epithelium are common in chronic bronchitis, especially in heavy cigarette smokers.

Excessive production of mucus, combined with the loss of ciliated epithelium, results in its accumulation causing obstruction of bronchi and bronchioles. Secondary bacterial colonization of the retained secretion occurs, usually by *Haemophilus influenzae* and *Streptococcus pneumoniae*. Thus, in chronic bronchitis the lower respiratory tract, which is normally sterile, is very liable to be infected. A viral infection or irritation by inhaled pollutants may be sufficient to precipitate an acute exacerbation, with more extensive invasion by bacteria already present in the bronchial tree. When such secondary pyogenic infection occurs, the sputum changes from a glairy mucus to a frankly yellow pus. Bouts of acute infection of this type may occur several times during the course of a year, especially during winter.

It is important to distinguish between chronic bronchitis, which is based on a chronic irritation of the bronchial tree, and pulmonary emphysema, which is a destructive disease of the lung substance. The two conditions commonly exist together because of common aetiological factors but they are quite distinct. Clinicians and respiratory physiologists, however, are inclined to refer to chronic bronchitis and emphysema together as **chronic obstructive airways disease**. Organic obstruction to airways may, in fact, occur in cases of chronic bronchitis without emphysema. The episodes of mucopurulent inflammation may give rise to ulceration, scarring and destruction. This in turn, however, may lead to destruction of alveolar walls and emphysema may develop. Chronic bronchitis must also be distinguished from bronchial asthma.

Bronchial Asthma

In bronchial asthma there is widespread bronchial obstruction due to paroxysmal muscular spasm and plugging by thick mucus. Clinically, acute attacks are characterized by a feeling of tightness in the chest, difficulty in breathing, and particularly in exhaling, which is accompanied by loud wheezing and coughing which, during the attack, tends to be non-productive. In both types of asthma psychological factors are of importance and in many patients the attacks are more likely to occur during periods of anxiety or emotional disturbance. As the attack subsides, thick viscid sputum, which contains eosinophils, is coughed up. An attack may last from a few minutes to days and may vary in severity from mild dyspnoea to wheezing with severe respiratory distress. Attacks may occur almost continuously, so-called *status asthmaticus*. In a minority of cases right ventricular hypertrophy occurs as a response to pulmonary hypertension resulting from repeated episodes of alveolar hypoxia. Bronchial asthma may be classified into extrinsic and intrinsic types.

Extrinsic Asthma

This usually starts in childhood or early adult life and may be preceded by infantile eczema or hypersensitivity to foodstuffs. It is due mainly to atopic (type I) hypersensitivity (p. 205) to one or more extrinsic antigenic substances ('allergens'), inhalation of which brings on an attack within a few minutes. Such hypersensitivity occurs in individuals who have a genetically determined predisposition to develop reaginic antibodies of IgE class; skin or provocative inhalation tests with the allergen(s) responsible typically produce an immediate (type I) reaction. These allergens include various pollens, animal dandruff, house dust and various fungi. The most important allergen in house dust is provided by mites, notably *Dermatophagoides pteronyssinus* (Fig. 13.4) which infests mattresses and lives on human squames. Inhaled excreta or fragments of the mite produce an asthmatic reaction in sensitized individuals. *The*

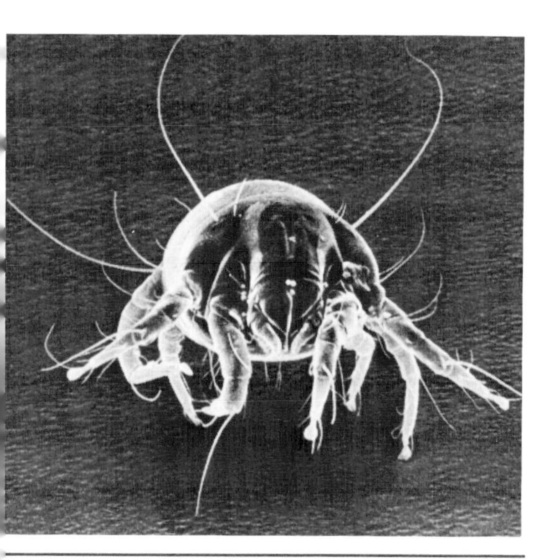

Fig. 13.4 The house-dust mite. *Dermatophagoides pteronyssinus*. ×300. (By courtesy of Bencard.)

prognosis in extrinsic asthma is good, although deaths may result from overmedication or from sudden withdrawal of corticosteroids.

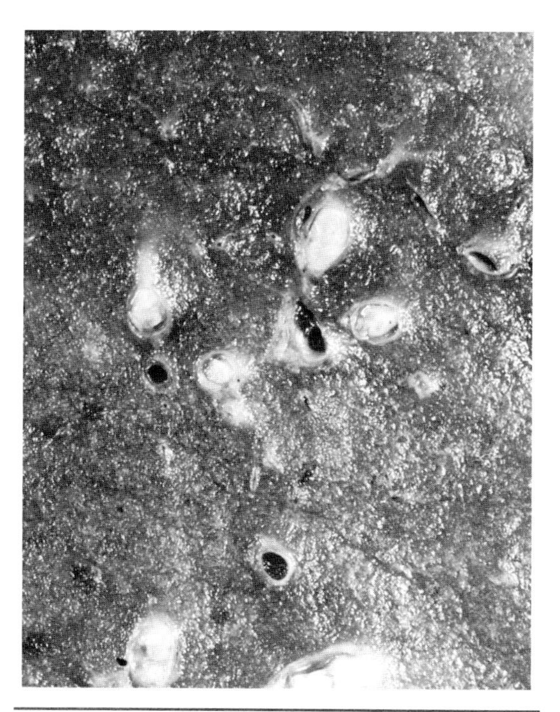

Fig. 13.5 The cut surface of a lung from a patient who died during an acute attack of bronchial asthma. The bronchi are distended by plugs of tough, white, mucoid material. ×2. (Dr P. S. Hasleton.)

Intrinsic Asthma

This usually develops later in adult life in subjects without an individual or family history of atopic diseases. Skin tests or provocative inhalation tests fail to reveal a responsible allergen. Nasal polypi are common. The prognosis is less good than in extrinsic asthma. Patients tend to develop drug hypersensitivities, particularly to aspirin and penicillin, and administration of these drugs may then be followed by a generalized atopic reaction which is sometimes fatal. *Intrinsic asthma is commonly associated with chronic bronchitis,* and atopic hypersensitivity to allergens provided by bacteria in the infected bronchi has been suggested, although this has seldom been established.

Pathology

When death has occurred during an acute attack the lungs, at autopsy, appear overdistended with air and fail to collapse. Their cut surfaces show occlusion of many segmental bronchi by plugs of tough mucous material (Fig. 13.5). Focal bronchiectasis may be present but chronic emphysema is slight or absent. Microscopic examination shows plugging of bronchi by mucinous material containing eosinophils and normal or degenerate columnar respiratory epithelial cells. The cellular elements tend to form twisted strips, known as Curschmann's spirals, which may be found in asthmatic sputum. There is hyaline thickening of the epithelial basement membrane. The submucosa shows vascular congestion, oedema and infiltration by eosinophils from which Charcot's crystals are formed. The number of mast cells may be increased. There is hypertrophy of the smooth muscle of the small bronchi and bronchioles, clearly associated with the repeated spasm of these airways (Fig. 13.6). In long-standing cases the changes of chronic bronchitis may also be present.

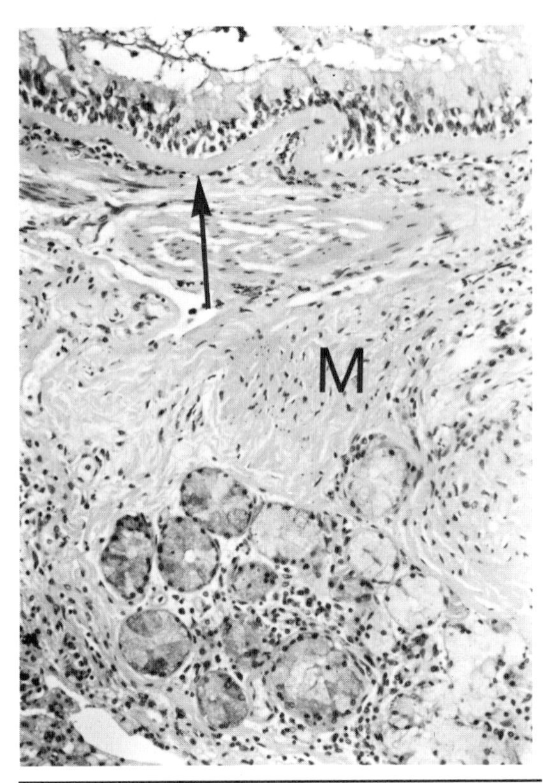

Fig. 13.6 Bronchial asthma. The bronchial lumen (top) contains mucinous material and is lined by intact respiratory epithelium. The basement membrane shows a characteristic hyaline thickening (arrow). The layer of bronchial smooth muscle (M) is hypertrophied and there is a proliferation of mucous glands (bottom). ×130.

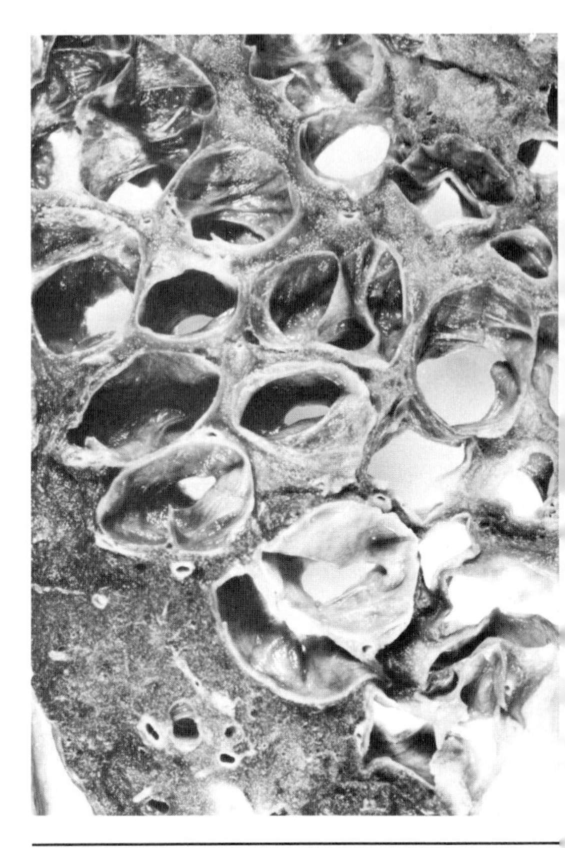

Fig. 13.7 Bronchiectasis. There is pronounced dilatation of bronchi which appear crowded together with obliteration of intervening lung substance. The dilated bronchi have thick white fibrous walls and their lumina are tortuous and lined by congested mucosa.

Bronchiectasis

Bronchiectasis is an abnormal and irreversible dilatation of the bronchi, which may be generalized or localized, and may result in the formation of multiple large spaces or cavities. It is the result of chronic necrotizing infection of bronchi and bronchioles. There is usually fibrosis of the surrounding lung tissue with obliteration and destruction of the smaller bronchi and bronchioles (Fig. 13.7). For a time the cavities are almost dry, but later secretion accumulates, becomes purulent, and ulceration of the wall occurs. Initially the bronchiectatic cavities may be wholly or partly lined by respiratory or simple columnar epithelium but later squamous metaplasia sometimes supervenes.

Without effective treatment, bronchiectatic cavities eventually become persistently infected with putrefying micro-organisms; purulent fluid accumulates in them and is decomposed, causing foul-smelling breath and sputum. Organisms may spread from the bronchiectatic cavities to the alveolar tissue, either by the air passages or by direct ulceration, and cause pneumonia or a lung abscess. In such conditions the wall of a vein may become involved, with the formation of septic emboli and the development of **secondary abscesses**, particularly in the brain. Severe **haemoptysis** may occur and **amyloidosis** may be a late complication.

In chronic bronchiectasis pulmonary haemodynamic changes may result from such factors as alveolar hypoxia and fibrous obliteration of pulmonary arteries. There is usually considerable enlargement of the bronchial arteries with the development of bronchopulmonary vascular anastomoses.

Aetiology

Three main factors are involved: there is loss of aerated lung substance so that the force of inspiratory expansion of the chest falls, in the affected part of the lung, on the bronchial walls alone; mechanical weakening of the supporting tissue of the bronchial wall is caused by inflammatory changes; and finally, there is contraction of fibrous bands connecting the bronchial wall with the fibrosed and adherent pleura. Any major degree of pulmonary collapse with negative intrapleural pressure is followed almost at once by dilatation of the bronchi supplying the collapsed zone; this dilatation may subsequently disappear when the lung becomes re-expanded. Permanent collapse is, however, followed by fibrosis and the bronchi remain dilated.

Bronchiectasis is usually a sequel of bronchiolitis and bronchopneumonia in childhood with partial collapse and imperfect resolution; it may also follow failure of a part of the lung to expand at birth (***atelectasis***). In children the bronchopneumonia may be primary or may complicate whooping cough or measles. In adults it is often secondary to influenza. In chronic pulmonary tuberculosis with fibrotic change, saccular bronchiectatic cavities are common in association with tuberculous cavities, and they also occur in silicosis and fibrotic conditions generally. In infants suffering from ***fibrocystic disease (cystic fibrosis) of the pancreas***, the trachea and bronchi contain tough mucoid secretion which soon becomes infected; bronchopneumonia follows and bronchiectasis is a common sequel. Other less common causes of bronchiectasis include ***Kartagener's syndrome***, in which there is an inherited immotility of cilia, and ***immunodeficiency syndromes***; in both of these, repeated bronchial infection may occur.

Bronchial Obstruction

Various degrees of obstruction may occur up to complete occlusion and either large or small bronchi may be affected. Progressive obstruction of a **large bronchus** is most frequently produced by a primary carcinoma infiltrating the wall and growing into the lumen, less commonly by pressure of massively enlarged lymph nodes and rarely by pressure of an aneurysm of the aortic arch. Sudden obstruction may be produced by an inhaled foreign body. This may obstruct the bronchus completely, the air in the related part of the lung is absorbed rapidly and pulmonary collapse follows. Usually, however, obstruction is partial at first, resulting in the accumulation of secretions and oedema fluid with some degree of bronchial dilatation. Bacterial infection follows, leading to a purulent bronchitis which, by further extension, may bring about suppurative bronchopneumonia. Occasionally, when infection is less severe, there may be considerable aggregation of lipid-rich macrophages – ***endogenous lipid pneumonia.***

Obstruction of individual small bronchi does not lead to collapse of the segment of lung supplied, because collateral ventilation from adjacent lobules through the pores of Kohn and canals of Lambert, connecting bronchioles to distal air passages, supplies enough air to expand the obstructed segment. In fact, it is more likely to become distended.

Obstruction of bronchioles is usually produced by a purulent or fibrinous inflammatory exudate, notably in bronchopneumonia. In bronchial asthma the obstruction is in part due to the spasmodic contraction of the walls of the bronchioles. If the obstruction is such that air can be sucked in and cannot be expelled then hyperinflation may occur in the area supplied by the obstructed bronchioles. Such hyperinflation is at first reversible when the obstruction is removed. However, if the obstruction is persistent, destruction of the wall may occur, leading to centrilobular emphysema.

The Lungs

The essential function of respiration is to provide oxygen for and to remove excess carbon dioxide from the cells of the body. This involves the controlled absorption of oxygen to oxygenate mixed venous blood and the elimination of carbon dioxide so that normal blood gas tensions are maintained. Respiration in its clinical sense is generally restricted to those aspects which concern the major airways and lungs. Respiration in its broader physiological context involves four processes. The first act of respiration is **ventilation** which is the exchange of gases between the alveolar spaces and external atmosphere. Then in the lungs the blood gases exchange with alveolar air by **diffusion** across the alveolar walls. The blood is used to **transport** gases to and from the tissues, and **exchange** between blood and tissue cells occurs in the systemic capillaries.

Although primarily involved in gas exchange, the lungs also have important non-respiratory functions: they act as a filter for the blood passing through them and are also concerned in the metabolism of certain vasoactive substances. This is facilitated by the fact that all the blood passes through the lungs in a single circulation. The pulmonary capillary bed is a huge network. The average diameter of the capillaries is about 8 μm. Particles ranging in diameter from 10 to 75 μm tend to be delayed in passing through the pulmonary circulation. Small emboli such as fibrin clots, bone marrow etc., are trapped in the lungs and may be cleared by the action of proteolytic enzymes and phagocytosis. Significant proportions of circulating 5-hydroxytryptamine, bradykinin, prostaglandins and noradrenaline may be removed from the blood during its passage through the lungs. The lung is probably the main site for the conversion of the relatively inactive decapeptide angiotensin I to the potent systemic vasoconstrictive octapeptide angiotensin II. The enzyme mechanisms responsible for the clearing and activation of these vasoactive substances are probably localized in the endothelium of the pulmonary vessels.

Respiratory Failure

The primary function of the lungs, as stated, is to add oxygen to and remove carbon dioxide from the circulating blood. Thus, ***respiratory failure is defined in terms of hypoxaemia, when the arterial oxygen tension has fallen below 60 mmHg (8.0 kPa) as a result of lung disease in a patient breathing air at sea level.*** In some forms of respiratory failure there is associated carbon dioxide retention so that arterial tension of this gas rises above 45 mmHg (6.0 kPa). Respiratory failure is said to be of type I when there is no associated carbon dioxide retention and of type II when there is.

Mechanisms of Arterial Hypoxaemia

A low inspired partial pressure of oxygen in the ambient air occurs at high altitude; a lowered oxygen tension in inspired air may also occur if a patient is accidentally ventilated at a low oxygen concentration, as from a faulty anaesthetic or inhalational therapy device. However, these are specifically excluded in the above definition of respiratory failure for there is no lung disease involved.

Mismatching of alveolar ventilation to perfusion is best illustrated by the extreme and theoretical situation where all the cardiac output goes to one lung and all the inspired air to the other, which is clearly incompatible with life. Ventilation–perfusion imbalance is the commonest cause of respiratory failure in clinical practice, and develops in most pathological processes which involve substantial parts of the lungs such as chronic bronchitis and emphysema, bronchial asthma and pulmonary oedema.

Alveolar hypoventilation causes hypoxaemia associated with a high arterial carbon dioxide tension.

An increase in shunt fraction is blood passing from the right heart to the systemic arterial circulation without being oxygenated in the lung. The shunt fraction is increased in congenital right-to-left cardiac shunts, and is also the commonest cause of hypoxaemia in pulmonary collapse. It also plays a role in the low arterial oxygen tension seen in both pneumonia and the adult respiratory distress syndrome.

The 'alveolar-capillary block syndrome' describes hypoxaemia brought about by interstitial lung disease due to thickening of the alveolar capillary membrane. In the normal lung, alveolar gas is separated from capillary blood by the alveolar-capillary membrane which is composed of three distinct anatomical layers: alveolar epithelium, a narrow interstitial zone, and capillary endothelium (Fig. 13.8a). It is now known that hypoxaemia in this syndrome arises from mismatch of alveolar ventilation to perfusion. It was thought that respiratory function tests designed to measure the diffusion of carbon monoxide across

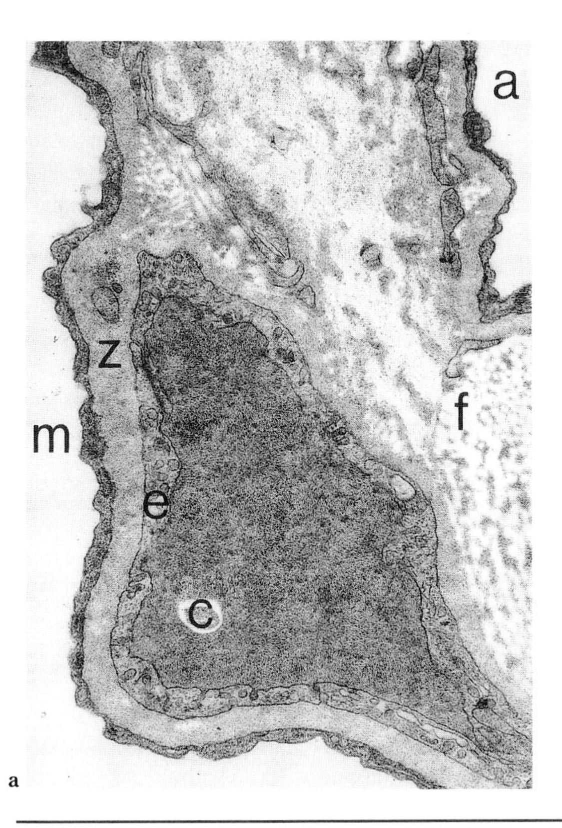

a

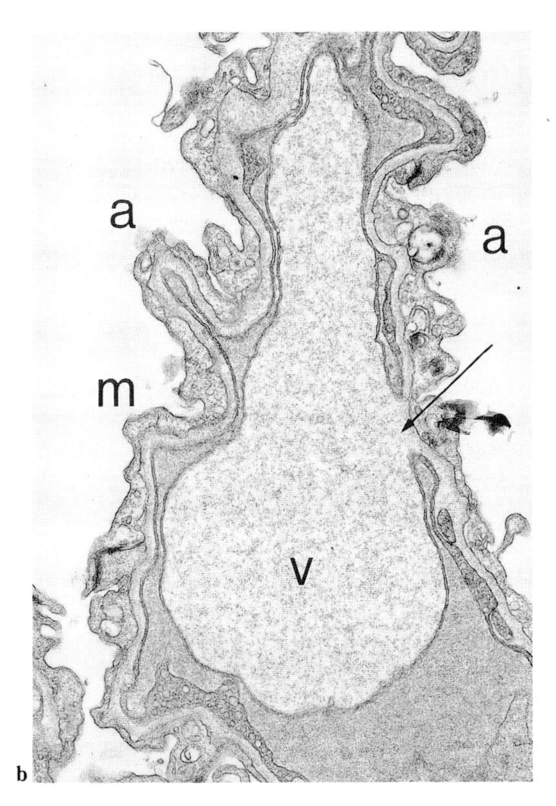

b

Fig. 13.8 **(a)** Electron micrograph of alveolar wall in normal human lung. The capillary lumen (c) is lined by endothelial cells (e). The alveolar spaces (a) are lined by membranous pneumonocytes (m). In the thinnest portion of the blood–air pathway the endothelial cell is separated from the membranous pneumonocyte by a granular amorphous zone (z) consisting of their fused basement membranes. Elsewhere, the endothelial and epithelial cells are separated by an interstitial space containing collagen (f). ×20 000. **(b)** Electron micrograph of a pulmonary capillary from a rat showing the features of pulmonary oedema caused by acute exposure to a simulated high altitude corresponding to the summit of Mount Everest (8850 m; atmospheric pressure 250 mmHg). The capillary contains an endothelial vesicle (v) which has been cut in longitudinal section and assumes the shape of the capillary. Its pedicle is indicated by an arrow. The alveolar spaces (a) are lined by membranous pneumonocytes (m). ×12 500.

the alveolar-capillary membrane specifically identified this syndrome. This, however, is not true because impaired diffusion of this gas also occurs where there is mismatching of alveolar ventilation to perfusion.

In clinical practice direct measurement of oxygen and carbon dioxide tension in arterial blood, with knowledge of the gas concentration being inspired at the same time, allows the difference between alveolar and arterial oxygen tension to be estimated with enough accuracy to separate these different mechanisms at the bedside.

The Clinical Recognition of Respiratory Failure

This depends on recognizing central cyanosis clinically. Most observers can detect this in daylight if the arterial oxygen saturation is below 90%. This is associated with 1.5 g of reduced haemoglobin/dl, if the total haemoglobin is 15 g/dl. Consciousness is lost when arterial oxygen tension is around 30 mmHg (4.0 kPa). Hypoxaemia also causes tachycardia, a raised cardiac output and eventually, systemic hypotension. In chronic hypoxaemia, as found in chronic bronchitis and emphysema, the patient becomes tolerant of hypoxia and a lower arterial oxygen tension can then be sustained. Thus, partial pressures of oxygen around 50 mmHg (6.65 kPa) and of carbon dioxide around 50 mmHg (6.65 kPa) are common in these patients when they are in a chronic stable state.

'Pink Puffers' and 'Blue Bloaters'

Patients with chronic bronchitis and emphysema tend to fall into two clinical patterns, although many show a spectrum between. Pink puffers are thin with marked chest hyperinflation and are often very breathless: they have **type I respiratory failure** with modest hypoxaemia with no carbon dioxide retention. Characteristically they do not develop pulmonary hypertension and right ventricular hypertrophy, nor do they develop secondary polycythaemia. In contrast, blue bloaters, with **type II respiratory failure**, have more marked central cyanosis, again with chest hyperinflation, but may not be so breathless. However, they may also have secondary polycythaemia, with a raised jugular venous pressure and ankle oedema. Only 30% of these patients survive 5 years, but long-term oxygen therapy given for more than 19 hours in the 24-hour day can prolong their life. This is a practical treatment given by an oxygen concentrator in the patient's home.

In **sleep hypoxaemia** arterial oxygen tension and saturation fall transiently, particularly during 'rapid eye movement' sleep. Hypoxaemia is aggravated in this type of sleep in patients with chronic bronchitis and emphysema. In the **sleep apnoea syndrome** the upper airway transiently obstructs for more than 10 seconds many times in each hour of sleep, airflow then ceasing at the nose and mouth, despite continued inspiratory efforts. The arterial oxygen saturation falls recurrently in each apnoeic episode. Obstructive sleep apnoea may affect 1–10% of the population, and must be suspected in snorers, either obese or of normal weight, who have daytime sleepiness. Excess nocturnal hypoxaemia sleep in blue bloaters further aggravates pulmonary hypertension and right ventricular hypertrophy.

Causes of Type I Respiratory Failure

Hypoxaemia without carbon dioxide retention is common in many types of extensive lung disease: acute attacks of bronchial asthma; pulmonary oedema; pneumonia of whatever aetiology; pulmonary collapse; pulmonary thromboembolism; and in extreme obesity, particularly when lying down. Interstitial lung diseases such as fibrosing alveolitis, sarcoidosis, allergic alveolitis, asbestosis and other pneumoconioses are also well recognized causes.

Arterial blood gas measurements define the status of gas exchange, but are not diagnostic of any specific pathology in the lung. The low arterial carbon dioxide tension associated with the hypoxaemia can cause respiratory alkalosis. A low carbon dioxide tension usually persists despite oxygen therapy; therefore, the alveolar hyperventilation causing this low carbon dioxide tension is not due to hypoxic stimulation of arterial chemoreceptors, but is most likely the result of the disease process stimulating intrapulmonary vagal afferent fibres, which then cause the hyperventilation, irrespective of the arterial oxygen tension.

Respiratory function tests may indicate the cause of respiratory failure. Thus, a variable peak expiratory flow rate (PEFR) or forced expiratory volume in one second (FEV_1) in bronchial asthma contrasts with the persistently low PEFR or FEV_1 in chronic bronchitis and emphysema. Lung volumes are increased in these conditions. In contrast, in interstitial lung disease all lung volumes are reduced, again with a low FEV_1 and PEFR, and a low capacity for diffusion of carbon monoxide across the alveolar-capillary wall. This is termed a restrictive pattern of respiratory function. In emphysema the low transfer factor for carbon monoxide is associated with a low FEV_1 and an increase in both total lung capacity and residual volume.

Causes of Type II Respiratory Failure

This implies alveolar hypoventilation, most commonly from chronic bronchitis and emphysema. This may occur in an acute exacerbation with a raised carbon dioxide tension and low pH. When it is chronic and the arterial oxygen tension lowered, say, to 50 mmHg (6.65 kPa) and arterial carbon dioxide raised to 50 mmHg (6.65 kPa) the pH may be normal, acidosis being corrected by reabsorption of bicarbonate in the renal tubules. The severity of an acute exacerbation is thus shown by disturbance of the arterial pH more than the level of the arterial carbon dioxide tension in these patients. Alveolar hypoventilation can also arise if *narcotic overdosage* depresses respiration in head injuries, with *thoracic and chest wall deformities* (e.g. kyphoscoliosis), or with *trauma* (e.g. crushed chest injury).

Treatment of Respiratory Failure

Type I respiratory failure requires oxygen inhalation, and as there is no carbon dioxide retention this can be given either as 2–3 litres of oxygen/min by nasal prongs, or if arterial hypoxaemia is more severe, by adding to this an oxygen mask delivering 6 litres/min of oxygen.

Type II respiratory failure is more difficult to treat. Correction of the low arterial oxygen tension by high concentrations of inspired oxygen carry a hazard, particularly in chronic bronchitis and emphysema. Many of these patients depend upon hypoxaemia to stimulate their breathing, for their high carbon dioxide tension fails to act as a ventilatory stimulant. Treatment thus depends upon providing enough oxygen to prevent death from hypoxaemia, but not too much so as to reduce ventilation and thereby aggravate carbon dioxide retention, leading to death from respiratory acidosis. Clinical experience has shown this can be achieved by giving enough oxygen (usually by 1–3 litres/min by nasal prongs) to provide an arterial oxygen tension over 50 mmHg (6.65 kPa) without causing the arterial pH to fall below 7.2. If controlled oxygen therapy fails to achieve these levels, ventilatory stimulant drugs and finally mechanical ventilation is needed. Mechanical intermittent positive pressure ventilation is essential in patients with type II respiratory failure from bronchial asthma, in the rare cases of type II failure in pulmonary oedema, and in patients with chest trauma.

Pulmonary Oedema

In pulmonary oedema there is an excessive extravascular accumulation of fluid in the lung. It can result from (1) an **imbalance of hydrodynamic**

forces across the alveolar-capillary wall which causes excess fluid to leave the capillaries and (2) **increased permeability** of the endothelial layer of the pulmonary capillaries.

The fine structure of the alveolar septum is shown in Fig. 13.8a. Capillary blood is separated from alveolar air by three distinct anatomical layers: capillary endothelium, a narrow interstitial zone and alveolar epithelium. The capillary endothelium is pitted by *caveolae intracellulares* whose nodular walls represent enzyme clusters. These globular particles, 6 nm in diameter, contain angiotensin-converting enzyme (ACE) which converts the inactive decapeptide angiotensin I to the active octapeptide angiotensin II. Normal alveolar capillary endothelial cells are joined by tight junctions containing narrow constrictions. Sandwiched between the capillary endothelium and alveolar epithelium is an interstitial zone of variable width (Fig. 13.8a). The alveolar septa are devoid of lymphatics, which first appear in the interstitial space surrounding terminal bronchioles, small arteries and veins. Over 95% of the area of the alveolar wall is lined by the thin, extensive *membranous pneumonocytes*. The margins of adjacent membranous or granular pneumonocytes abut bluntly or overlap with the formation of narrow clefts. These clefts are obliterated by fusion of opposing cell membranes.

Escape of fluid into the interstitial space is dependent, as elsewhere, on Starling's equation. Accumulation of fluid in the *alveolar* spaces is a late and not an inevitable manifestation of interstitial pulmonary oedema. The pulmonary lymphatics have a considerable reserve capacity but when this is exceeded, fluid begins to accumulate in the lung. It first accumulates in the loose, readily distensible connective tissues around the bronchi and larger vessels and next distends the thick, collagen-containing portions of the alveolar wall. Fluid-filled vesicles may form in the alveolar-capillary walls, lifting the pulmonary endothelium away from the basement membrane and projecting into the pulmonary capillaries (Fig. 13.8b). The final stage of pulmonary oedema is accumulation of fluid within the aveolar spaces. The route whereby fluid escapes from the interstitial tissues to the alveolar spaces is uncertain, although it is usually assumed that it is related to the opening, perhaps temporarily, of some of the intercellular junctions between membranous pneumonocytes.

Pulmonary oedema may occur in patients with **left ventricular failure** or **mitral stenosis** who develop elevation of the pulmonary venous pressure. Pulmonary oedema which follows **overloading of the circulation** with intravenous infusions is probably also due to failure of the left ventricle. The acute pulmonary oedema which may follow **sudden withdrawal of a pleural effusion** is generally attributed to a sudden increase in the negative intrathoracic pressure. Pulmonary oedema may occasionally occur in patients with **raised intracranial pressure** from whatever cause; the mechanism of production of this oedema is not clear. **High-altitude pulmonary oedema** is an uncommon complication following ascent to altitudes over 3000 metres. It is unusual in that it occurs in otherwise healthy individuals. Susceptibility to high-altitude pulmonary oedema is not limited to lowlanders, for if a high-altitude dweller spends even a few hours at sea level, he may develop pulmonary oedema soon after returning to the mountains. **Toxic gases and fumes** such as nitrogen dioxide, chlorine and phosgene may damage the alveolar wall and produce pulmonary oedema.

Other Conditions in which there is Pulmonary Oedema

Hyaline Membrane Disease and Infantile Respiratory Distress Syndrome

It has been known for many years that in infants who die in the neonatal period following a clinical diagnosis of a so-called respiratory distress syndrome, the lungs are airless, collapsed and firm, sometimes with microscopic 'hyaline membranes' lining the peripheral airways. The respiratory distress syndrome, which develops within a few minutes or hours of birth, is characterized by a rapid respiratory rate, increasing respiratory difficulty, cyanosis despite high concentrations of inspired oxygen and increasing pulmonary opacification on chest X-ray. The babies have severe functional right-to-left shunting and very low lung compliance. The mortality rate varies between 20 and 40%.

The respiratory distress syndrome is most common in premature infants and 10–15% of those with a birth weight of 2500 g or less develop the syndrome. The syndrome may also develop in infants born by Caesarean section, in infants born of diabetic mothers, in the second as compared with the first of twin pairs, and as a complication of birth asphyxia, intracranial haemorrhage, infections and various congenital abnormalities.

Microscopically, the alveoli are collapsed while the terminal and respiratory bronchioles are distended and lined by thick eosinophilic hyaline membranes of variable composition: they may contain fibrin, necrotic epithelial cell debris, and keratinized cells presumably derived from inhaled amniotic fluid. If the infants survive the first few days they seem to recover completely, although pulmonary fibrosis may ensue in a small minority.

It should be borne in mind that, in about 30% of cases with a clinical respiratory distress syndrome, hyaline membrane disease may not be found in the lung. The aetiology of hyaline membrane disease remains uncertain. Surfactant deficiency due to prematurity is the most frequent and important cause. Hyaline membranes are not seen in stillborn infants and their presence is related to breathing. Other factors include increased permeability of the alveolar capillaries, inhalation of amniotic fluid and exudation of blood contents.

Sometimes such infants develop massive pulmonary haemorrhage involving two or more lobes of the lung. Occasionally this is associated with bleeding into the subarachnoid space or cerebral ventricles. Such bleeding has been ascribed to oxygen toxicity or to the insertion of a catheter too far down the endotracheal tubes.

'Shock Lung' and Adult Respiratory Distress Syndrome

Respiratory failure is the cause of death in many patients who have suffered major trauma or haemorrhage causing shock. With improved techniques of resuscitation and blood transfusion, the syndrome of post-traumatic pulmonary insufficiency or 'shock lung' has emerged as one of the most frequent and life-threatening complications to occur in these patients.

Shock lung occurs within one or two days of the traumatic episode, following the initial resuscitation procedures. A similar clinical and pathological picture may occur in septic/endotoxic shock, oxygen toxicity, inhalation of toxic irritants, narcotic overdosage, following cardiac surgery with cardiac bypass and in aspiration pneumonia. The patient gradually becomes hypoxaemic with acidosis despite oxygen therapy, and mortality is high. Initially, the chest radiograph shows patchy opacities attributed to pulmonary oedema and collapse. This progresses to almost totally opaque lung fields in the severely affected patient and there is decreased lung compliance.

The factors involved in shock lung are complex and often multiple. Basically there is a variable combination of shock, sepsis, oxygen therapy and drug therapy. There may be fat embolism, pulmonary oedema, aspiration of gastric contents, oxygen toxicity, pulmonary microembolism and sometimes over-transfusion. The microemboli may comprise or arise in traumatized tissue. Disseminated intravascular coagulation and endotoxaemia occur in some patients. Diffuse damage to the alveolar walls results; there is endothelial and epithelial injury, oedema, sloughing of lining cells and atelectasis.

At autopsy, the lungs are heavy, beefy and oedematous. Microscopically, in early cases, there is intra-alveolar oedema with extravasation of erythrocytes. Intra-alveolar fibrinous exudate and hyaline membranes develop later. In long-standing cases, pulmonary fibrosis ensues, and the alveolar walls become lined by metaplastic cuboidal epithelium.

Uraemic Lung

This term is used to describe a chronic form of pulmonary oedema which, radiologically, produces a characteristic butterfly-shaped shadow that extends outwards from the hilum of both lungs. At autopsy, the lungs are voluminous and rubbery and, on squeezing, a frothy fluid exudes from the cut surface. Microscopically there is a fine fibrin network in the alveoli, and hyaline membranes may be formed. In long-standing cases focal organization of the exudate may be present.

Pulmonary Vascular Disease

Diseases of the heart affect the lungs and diseases of the lungs affect the heart. The anatomical basis of this inter-relationship is the pulmonary vasculature. Normally the blood pressure in the pulmonary arterial tree is only one-sixth of that in the systemic. The pulmonary arteries are thinner than the systemic arteries and consist of a layer of circularly orientated smooth muscle sandwiched between well formed elastic laminae. The pulmonary arterioles, unlike the systemic ones, do not have a muscular media, their walls consisting mainly of a single elastic lamina. Normal pulmonary arterioles are thus incapable of exerting significant resistance to the flow of blood through the lungs. The main way in which diseases of the heart and lung affect each other is through the production of pulmonary arterial hypertension and associated hypertensive pulmonary vascular disease.

The term '*cor pulmonale*' has been used in a general sense to mean involvement of the heart secondary to lung disease. Unfortunately it is also used to describe hypertrophy or failure of the right ventricle, brought about by involvement of the pulmonary circulation by lung disease. Since this term has no precise meaning its use is best avoided.

Pulmonary Hypertension

There are many diseases which will cause pulmonary arterial hypertension and associated pulmonary vascular disease. Pulmonary hypertension may be arbitrarily defined as a systolic blood pressure in the pulmonary circulation exceeding 30 mmHg (4.0 kPa). There are various forms of hypertensive pulmonary vascular disease, and one cannot predict what vascular lesions are present from a knowledge of the level of the pulmonary arterial pressure. Rather the form of the vascular changes depends upon the nature of the underlying disease process. This is of considerable practical importance, since the different forms of pulmonary vascular disease are reflected in different levels of pressure, flow and resistance in the pulmonary circulation, which, in turn, have an important effect on the clinical picture and course. The causes of pulmonary hypertension are summarized in Table 13.2 and the various forms of

Table 13.2 Causes of pulmonary hypertension

Secondary to cardiac conditions
*Congenital cardiac shunts
Increased left atrial pressure
Left ventricular failure
Secondary to hypoxia
Chronic obstructive lung disease
Native highlanders
Secondary to fibrosis
Pneumoconioses
Interstitial pulmonary fibrosis
Miscellaneous
Pulmonary thromboembolism
*Hepatic cirrhosis; portal vein thrombosis
Toxins and drugs
Idiopathic
*Primary pulmonary hypertension
Pulmonary veno-occlusive disease

*Only these conditions lead to plexogenic pulmonary arteriopathy.

hypertensive pulmonary vascular disease that they are associated with are as follows:

1. Congenital cardiac shunts. A large congenital cardiac defect between the right and left ventricles or between the aorta and the pulmonary trunk will lead to pulmonary arterial hypertension from birth, due to direct transmission of systemic arterial pressure and flow into the pulmonary circulation. Examples of such post-tricuspid shunts are ventricular septal defect, patent ductus arteriosus, persistent truncus arteriosus and aortopulmonary septal defect. Pre-tricuspid shunts, such as atrial septal defects, produce pulmonary hypertension in adolescence or adult life as a result of the effect of a prolonged excessive blood flow on the pulmonary vasculature.

Provided the defect is large enough, a characteristic form of pulmonary vascular disease occurs. Initially there is hypertrophy of the medial coat of the small pulmonary arteries, while pulmonary arterioles develop a distinct muscular media and resemble systemic arterioles. This is followed by migration of smooth muscle cells from the inner half of the media, to form a cellular intimal proliferation of myofibroblasts in the pulmonary arteries and arterioles. These cells produce matrix proteins and so the intimal thickening becomes fibrous and finally fibroelastic. These intimal changes lead to organic occlusion of pulmonary arteries. This is followed by dilatation of the pulmonary vasculature which may be generalized or localized.

Localized dilatation lesions are clusters of thin-walled branches of small pulmonary arteries arising proximal to the sites of occlusion. They form a collateral circulation to maintain a flow of blood to the pulmonary capillary bed, and are termed angiomatoid lesions. Sometimes a characteristic proliferation of myofibroblasts and mesenchymal cells takes place within them in a plexiform pattern to give the structure its name of plexiform lesion (Fig. 13.9). These thin-walled branches may rupture to give rise to pulmonary haemosiderosis. Finally, widespread fibrinoid necrosis of the small pulmonary arteries may occur if the pulmonary arterial pressure rises rapidly or severely.

This florid form of hypertensive pulmonary vascular disease, designated **plexogenic pulmonary arteriopathy**, is characteristic of pulmonary hypertension due to congenital cardiac shunts. However, it may also occur in other forms of pulmonary hypertension, e.g. in primary or idiopathic forms, and in the rare cases of pulmonary hypertension which may complicate hepatic cirrhosis or portal vein thrombosis.

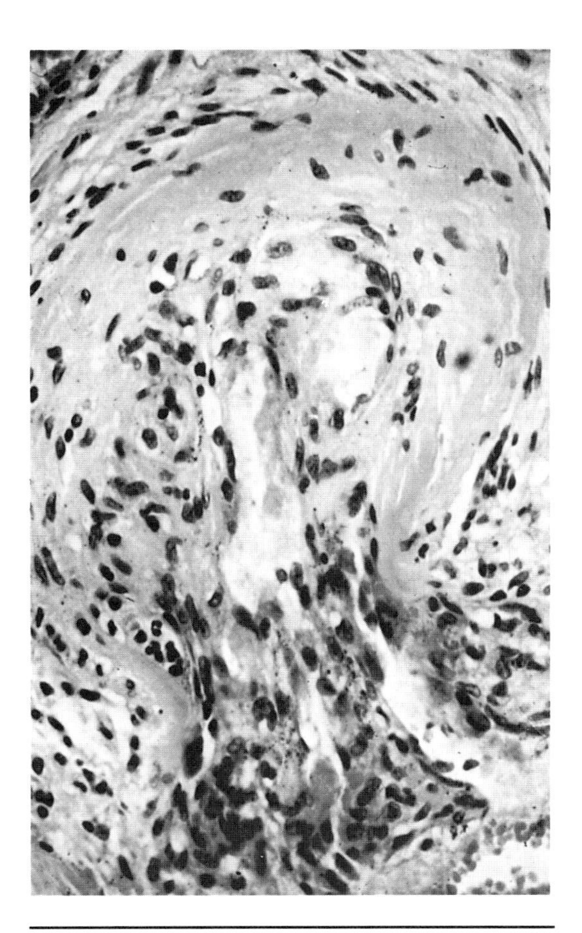

Fig. 13.9 Plexiform lesion from a girl of 12 years with a large ventricular septal defect. The parent muscular pulmonary artery shows fibrinoid necrosis. Its dilated sac contains a proliferation of myofibroblasts and fibrillary cells. ×150.

In the early stages of this form of pulmonary vascular disease the medial hypertrophy and intimal fibrosis are associated with pulmonary arterial hypertension with a high pulmonary flow, and a moderate increase in pulmonary vascular resistance which is largely reversible. The later dilatation lesions and necrotizing arteritis are associated with severe pulmonary hypertension, a reduced pulmonary blood flow, and a severely and irreversibly increased pulmonary vascular resistance. Hence, the early clinical picture of a large congenital cardiac shunt is dominated by signs of left ventricular hypertrophy, increased pulmonary blood flow, and left-to-right shunting of blood with no cyanosis. The later phase, however, is dominated by clinical signs of right ventricular hypertrophy, diminished pulmonary blood flow, and right-to-left shunting of blood with cyanosis. In the early stages surgical correction of septal defects is usually followed by the reversal of the associated pulmonary hypertension. In the later stages, however, the pulmonary hypertension is irreversible and this contraindicates attempts at corrective surgical treatment apart from heart/lung transplantations.

2. Hypoxia. Any state of chronic hypoxia will induce pulmonary arterial hypertension and associated changes in the pulmonary arteries. Thus, pulmonary hypertension occurs in anyone living at high altitude and is consistent with a healthy and active life. It also complicates chronic obstructive or interstitial lung diseases, *kyphoscoliosis, chronic mountain sickness* and the *Pickwickian syndrome.*

In this variety there is smooth muscle hypertrophy in the media of the terminal portions of the pulmonary arterial tree. This increases pulmonary vascular resistance. There is insignificant intimal fibrosis, however, and thus *the pulmonary hypertension and associated pulmonary vascular disease of chronic hypoxia are largely and rapidly reversible.* Another feature of hypoxia is the development of longitudinal muscle in the intima of pulmonary arteries and arterioles. Hyperplasia of the carotid bodies also occurs (p. 575).

3. Elevation of left atrial pressure. Any disease that brings about a sustained significant elevation of blood pressure in the left atrium is complicated by pulmonary venous and arterial hypertension and associated hypertensive pulmonary vascular disease. Conditions which lead to chronic left atrial hypertension include chronic left ventricular failure from any cause (p. 486), mitral stenosis or incompetence, and the rare myxoma of the left atrium. In its early stages there is medial hypertrophy and intimal fibrosis of pulmonary arteries and muscularization of pulmonary arterioles. Rarely in the later stages there is fibrinoid necrosis of pulmonary arteries. Plexiform and other dilatation lesions do not occur in this group. The pulmonary veins develop a distinct muscular media so that they may resemble small muscular pulmonary arteries. They also show intimal fibrosis.

Pulmonary venous hypertension with chronic congestion causes pulmonary oedema. Persistent pulmonary congestion and oedema are associated with a hyperplasia of granular pneumonocytes and the development of interstitial fibrosis of the lung. Red blood cells may be extruded from the distended pulmonary capillaries into the alveolar walls and spaces (Fig. 13.10). Their phagocytosis and destruction in macrophages results in collections of haemosiderin-laden macrophages within the alveoli – pulmonary haemosiderosis. The ferric iron may also be deposited on reticulin and elastic fibres in the walls of alveoli and in pulmonary arteries and veins where it may provoke a giant cell reaction. The combination of rusty discoloration of the lung due to this deposition of ferric salts, and firmness of the pulmonary parenchyma due to increase in fibrous tissue in the alveolar walls, accounts for the classical description of brown induration.

Other mineral deposits which may occur in chronic pulmonary venous hypertension include nodules of osseous metaplasia which present a characteristic radiological picture. A much rarer manifestation is microlithiasis, in which myriad laminated concretions of calcium phosphate bound within an organic envelope containing ferric salts, are deposited in the alveolar spaces.

4. Pulmonary fibrosis. Both massive and interstitial pulmonary fibrosis may become complicated by pulmonary hypertension and pulmonary vascular changes which are initially muscular in type and reversible. Later there is obliterative fibrosis of pulmonary arteries and arterioles with an irreversible increase in pulmonary vascular resistance.

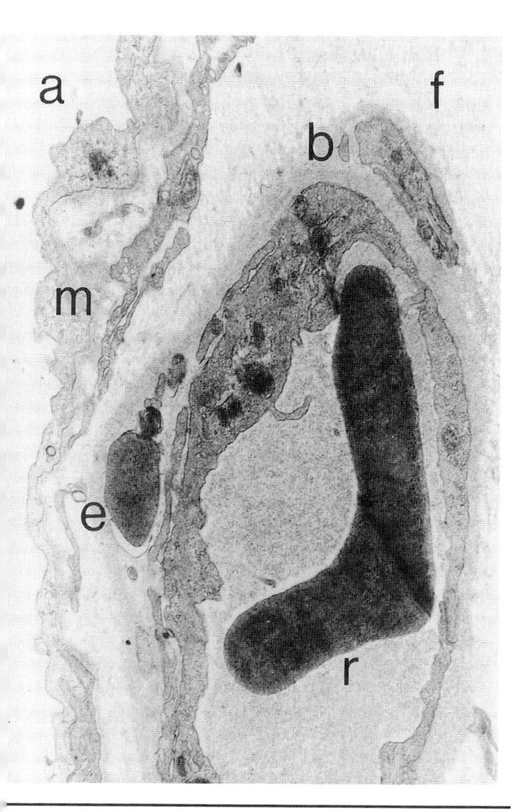

ig. 13.10 Alveolar wall in mitral stenosis. The al-
›olar capillary contains a red cell (r) and is surrounded
dense fibrous tissue (f) which displaces it inwards
om its normal superficial position beneath the mem-
anous pneumonocyte (m) lining the alveolar space (a).
he capillary basement membrane (b) is thickened and
ntains a disintegrating extravasated erythrocyte (e).
ectron micrograph. ×12 375.

xamples of pneumoconioses which may lead to ılmonary hypertension are silicosis and beryl-sis. In rheumatoid arthritis and some other con-ctive tissue diseases, pulmonary fibrosis, ›neycomb lung and a peculiar form of pulmonary ıscular disease occurs.

Miscellaneous. Primary or idiopathic pulmo-ry hypertension tends to occur in children under , in young women 20–30 years, and may be milial. It is now thought that local neurohumoral ctors are involved, producing vasoconstriction ıich leads to vascular changes in the pulmonary teries and arterioles. Pulmonary veno-occlusive disease is a distinct disease leading to pulmonary hypertension.

Recurrent pulmonary thromboembolism may give rise to significant pulmonary hypertension with associated pulmonary vascular disease characterized by organizing, organized and recanalized thrombus.

Toxins can produce pulmonary hypertension in animals, e.g. feeding with seeds or foliage of pyrrolizidine alkaloid-containing plant species like *Crotalaria* or *Senecio.* In man the toxic oil syndrome in Spain was thought to be due to ingestion of adulterated rape-seed oil, and there were reports of an epidemic of primary pulmonary hypertension thought to be due to the anorexigen *aminorex fumarate.*

Pulmonary Embolism

Thromboembolism

By far the commonest sites of origin of thrombi leading to pulmonary embolism are the deep veins of the legs, especially in the calf. Pulmonary thromboembolism is very rare in children but opinion is divided as to whether age or sex affects its incidence in adults. Predisposing factors are described on p. 97. There is no doubt that pulmonary thromboembolism is very common indeed. In one study, carried out in hospitals in Oxford, its incidence, as determined by examination of the left lung in a routine autopsy service, was 12%. A detailed histological examination of the right lung from the same cases revealed an incidence of 52%. It is likely that pulmonary thromboembolism is almost ubiquitous in hospital patients coming to autopsy.

The lungs have an astonishing capacity to dispose of thromboemboli. Even large fresh thrombi are absorbed by the lungs in dogs in 6 weeks and small ones much more rapidly. Two main groups of processes are involved, chemical and cellular. Chemical disposal is by fibrinolysis and predominates in the disposal of small thrombi. Lung tissue has a high content of fibrinolysins, present in the intima of both pulmonary and systemic arteries.

Cellular processes of organization and recanalization seem to be more important in the disposal of larger thromboemboli.

Massive pulmonary thromboembolism. Massive pulmonary embolism is a classical clinical emergency brought about by sudden occlusion of the pulmonary trunk or one of its main branches by a large embolus (Fig. 13.11). In the normal human lung, rather more than half the pulmonary arterial bed must be occluded before the clinical syndrome of fatal acute massive embolism will appear. In the presence of pre-existing pulmonary hypertension, however, occlusion of one primary branch of the pulmonary trunk has important haemodynamic effects. The increased pulmonary vascular resistance which occurs in pulmonary embolism in man is more likely a mechanical effect of blockage of pulmonary arteries rather than due to the effect of vasoactive substances liberated from pulmonary emboli.

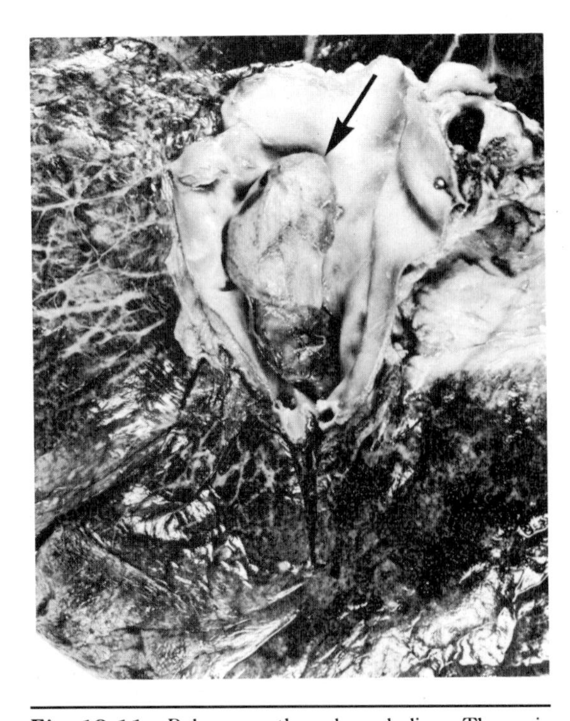

Fig. 13.11 Pulmonary thromboembolism. The main pulmonary artery at the hilum of the lung has been opened to reveal a pale thromboembolus (arrow) lying free in its lumen.

Pulmonary infarction. Pulmonary arterial oc clusion alone commonly fails to produce infarctio of the lung and an additional important requiremer appears to be an increased pulmonary venou pressure. Infarction is, therefore, common i patients with mitral stenosis and occurs mor often in the lower lobes, where the pulmonar venous pressure is likely to be higher. In additior the lung bases are more prone to be affected b bronchial occlusion, pleural effusion and infectior all factors shown experimentally to favou infarction.

Recurrent pulmonary embolism. In this cor dition there is a gradual occlusion of the pulmonar arterial bed over a period of time which ma extend to several years. Infarction is not a featur but there is a progressive increase in the pu monary vascular resistance, leading to sever pulmonary hypertension, right ventricular hype trophy and failure as previously described. I many patients with recurrent pulmonary throm boembolism the source of venous thrombi is no found. It may well be that chronic pulmonar thromboembolism is not caused by the productic of an excessive number of thromboemboli, but b the intrinsic inability of the pulmonary circulatic to deal with them, due possibly to an inadequa endothelial fibrinolytic system.

Non-thrombotic Pulmonary Embolism

The pulmonary capillary bed is a most effecti filter of particulate matter in the blood and manner of fragments may be found impacted in These may be of intrinsic origins or may be e trinsic, injected as part of a transfusion or dr injection.

Bone marrow embolism may follow bone fra tures, thoracic operations involving the sternu rib fractures due to external cardiac massage, spontaneous fracture due to tumour metastases bones. Masses of megakaryocytes may be fou impacted in the pulmonary capillaries, especia after surgical operations and in cases of pulmona thromboembolism.

Fat embolism commonly occurs after accidents involving fractures of bones or contusion of adipose tissue. Fat embolism in the lungs is very common: it rarely causes significant symptoms, unless very extensive, when it can be fatal.

Amniotic fluid embolism to the lung occurring in women during or shortly after childbirth, may be fatal. By contrast, small fragments of trophoblast are frequently found in the lungs of pregnant women dying from various causes, but rarely give rise to symptoms.

Tumour cells are trapped in the pulmonary capillary bed like other particulate matter: they may degenerate or grow to form metastases. Recurrent emboli from the right atrium in cases of cardiac myxoma may lead to pulmonary hypertension.

Air embolism may arise from many causes, including surgical and diagnostic procedures such as intravenous infusion, abortions, and the induction of a pneumothorax. If the volume of air is large, it may cause death by arresting the pulmonary circulation. At autopsy, the pulmonary trunk must be opened under water to reveal air embolism.

Pulmonary Emphysema

Pulmonary emphysema is a permanent enlargement of the air spaces distal to the terminal bronchiole, accompanied by destruction of their walls. The definition of emphysema must include the concept of permanent enlargement of air spaces, implying destructive changes, in contrast with their temporary overinflation as, for example, in bronchial asthma.

Microanatomy

In order to understand emphysema it is necessary to be familiar with the microanatomy of the terminal air passages. Large bronchi have cartilage plates of irregular shape in their walls and as they divide into small bronchi the amount of cartilage decreases. With further division in the airways increase in number and decrease in size, and the point at which the cartilage disappears is taken as the dividing line between the small bronchus and the bronchiole. The small bronchi have a few mucous glands in their walls, whereas in the bronchioles the only mucin-secreting cells are goblet cells in the lining epithelium. The bronchioles branch further and alveoli can arise directly from their walls. At this point the bronchioles are termed ***respiratory bronchioles*** while the ***terminal bronchiole*** is the last small bronchiole not to bear alveoli. The respiratory bronchioles may branch threee to five times. The first order of respiratory bronchioles have only a few alveoli, but these increase with each division. Eventually they form *alveolar ducts* whose walls are lined entirely by alveoli (Fig. 13.12a) The fundamental unit of the lung – the ***respiratory acinus*** – is the portion of lung tissue formed by the branching of a single terminal bronchiole as just described (Fig 13.12a).

The cut surface of a distended lung shows hexagonal areas of parenchyma, some 1–2 cm across, outlined by fibrous septa (Fig. 13.12b). Each hexagonal area is called a ***lung lobule***; it contains the lung tissue supplied by three to five terminal bronchioles which radiate from the centre, and therefore consists of three to five respiratory acini.

Classification of Emphysema

The classification of emphysema is based on its anatomical distribution within the lobule as this can be recognized by naked eye examination of slices of fixed, inflated lung. Many detailed classifications of emphysema exist, but here we will present a simplified version of the major types of emphysema which are of clinical importance.

Centrilobular Emphysema

In this type, the enlarged terminal airspaces are the respiratory bronchioles (Fig. 13.13a). In the

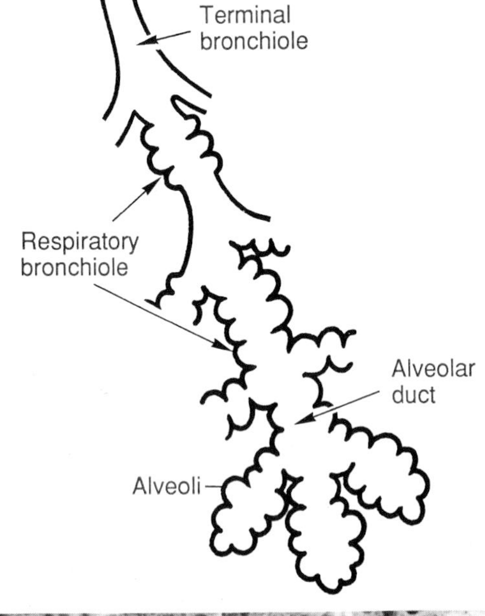

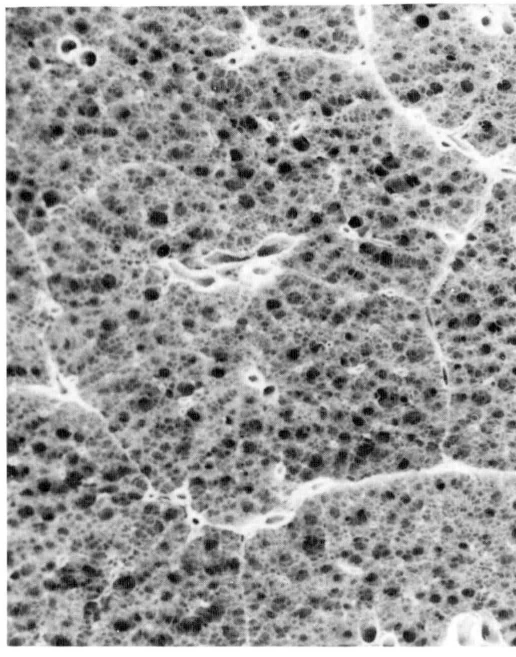

Fig. 13.12 **(a)** Model of normal respiratory acinus: each acinus is formed by branching of a single terminal bronchiole into a number of respiratory bronchioles which eventually form alveolar ducts whose walls are lined entirely by alveoli. **(b)** Normal adult lung. Note the hexagonal lobule in the centre of the field with the terminal bronchiole and accompanying pulmonary arteries in its centre. (Barium sulphate impregnation.) ×4. (Professor W. R. Lee.)

early stages of the disease the alveolar ducts and alveoli distal to the dilated bronchioles are normal. Thus in slices of fixed, inflated lung the enlarged air spaces are seen in clusters around the centre of the lobule, while the periphery of the lobule is spared – hence the description centrilobular (Fig. 13.13b).

Centrilobular emphysema occurs predominantly in male smokers and often in combination with chronic bronchitis. As described earlier these patients tend to have chronic hypoxia and a raised $P\text{ACO}_2$. This leads to pulmonary hypertension and right ventricular failure. Thus the patient will be cyanosed and have peripheral oedema – the 'blue bloater'.

The lesions of centrilobular emphysema are more common and more severe in the upper lobes and histologically there are dilated air spaces and chronic inflammation centred around bronchioles and bronchi.

A similar pattern of centrilobular emphysema is seen in coal workers and others exposed to carbon dust; this is termed ***focal dust emphysema*** (Fig. 13.13c). Because of its more focal nature and the absence of chronic bronchitis, this tends to be a milder disease and rarely causes right ventricular failure. Histologically the dilated respiratory bronchioles are surrounded by carbon pigment. The relationship of centrilobular emphysema to smoking and inhalation of coal dust suggests a role for these agents in the pathogenesis of the disease.

Panacinar Emphysema

In this type, there is permanent enlargement initially of alveolar ducts and alveoli, and later the disease progresses with destruction of respiratory bronchioles, thus involving the entire acinus – panacinar emphysema (Fig. 13.14a,b). In lung slices it is readily recognized by diffuse areas of abnormally large air spaces throughout the lobule (Fig. 13.14c).

Panacinar emphysema is the form of emphysema which occurs in α_1-antitrypsin deficiency. Although patients with panacinar emphysema usually do not have chronic bronchitis, it is a severe condition with overdistension of the chest and obvious radiological evidence of emphysema

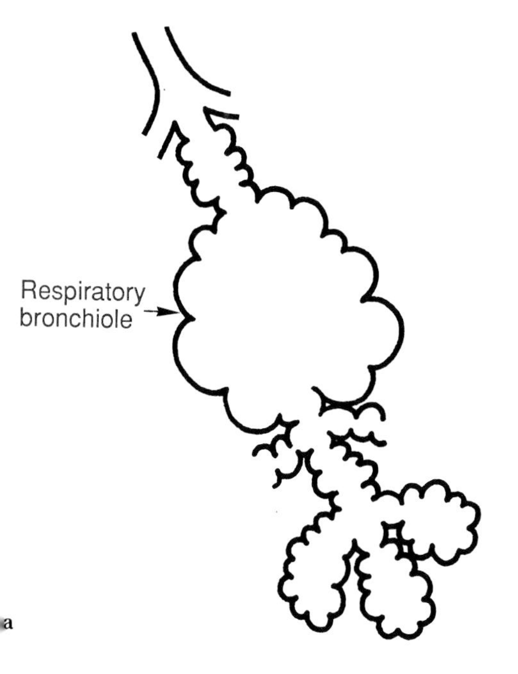

a

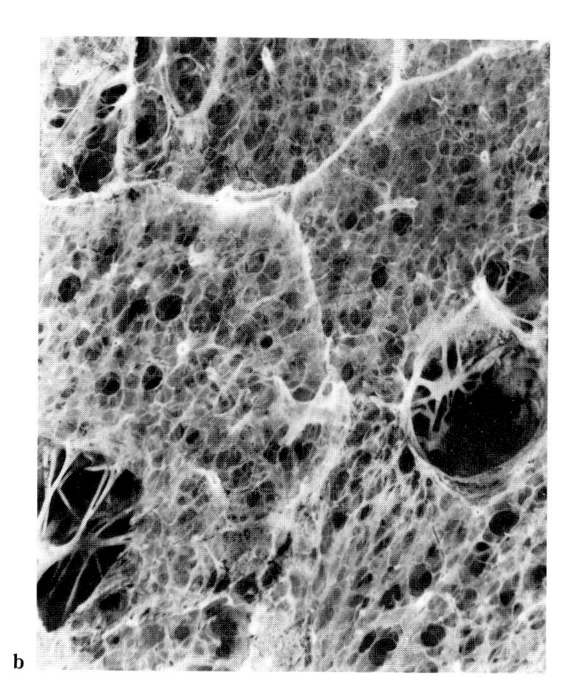

b

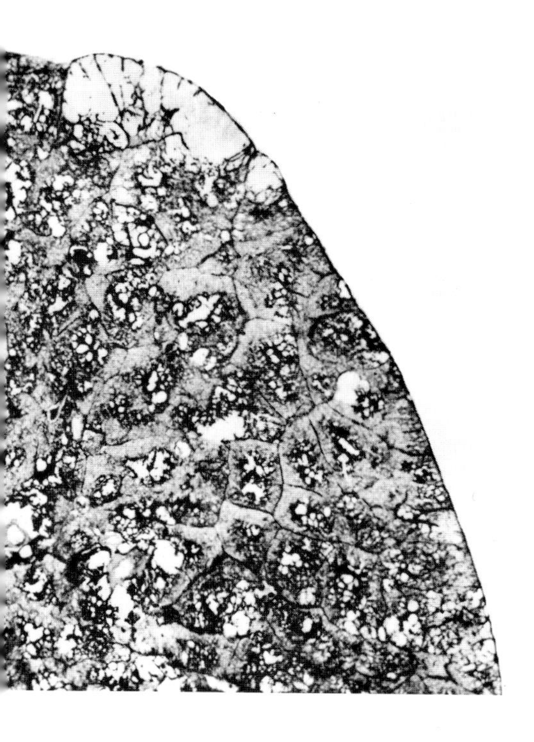

Fig. 13.13 **(a)** Centrilobular emphysema in which the dilatation of the air spaces affects the respiratory bronchioles; **(b)** Section of lung impregnated with barium sulphate, showing centrilobular emphysema. Note the punched out centrilobular spaces containing fibrous strands and blood vessels and the relatively normal parenchyma at the periphery of the lobules. ×7. (Professor W. R. Lee). **(c)** In focal dust emphysema it is again the respiratory bronchioles which become dilated; this is an example in coalminers' pneumoconiosis. Gelatin embedded lung section. ×1.

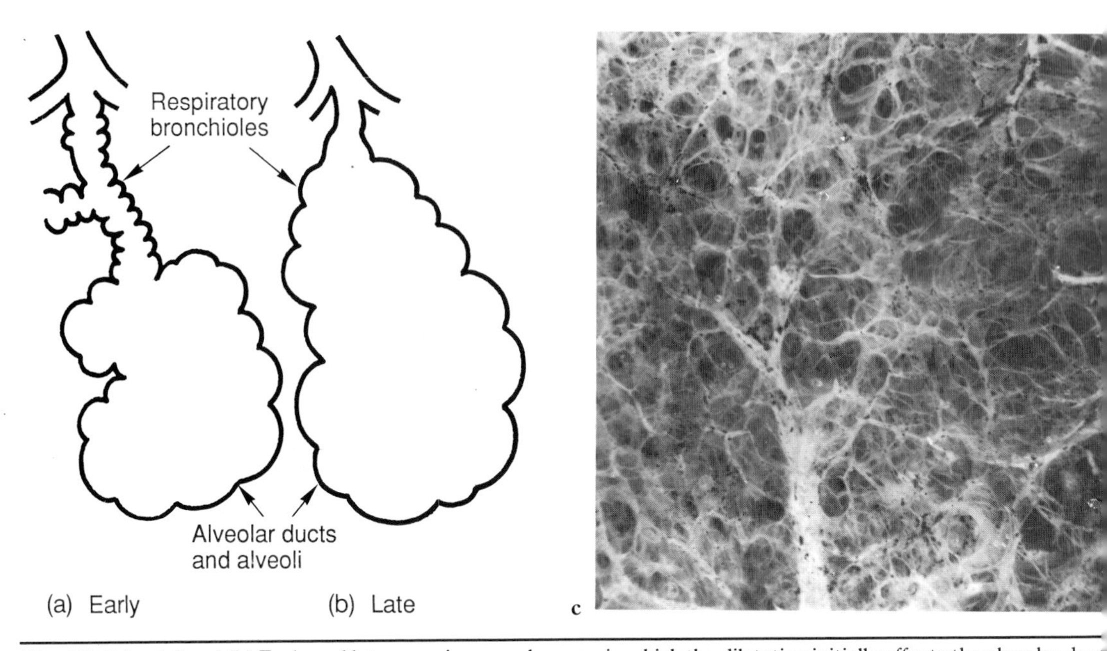

Fig. 13.14 **(a)** and **(b)** Early and late panacinar emphysema in which the dilatation initially affects the alveolar duc and alveoli and then extends to involve the respiratory bronchioles. **(c)** Severe panacinar emphysema. Parts of tw secondary lobules are shown, with a thickened interlobular septum (lower central). The alveolar walls throughout th lobules have been largely destroyed, with formation of emphysematous spaces. Atrophic lung tissue and som surviving small vessels are seen as fine strands. (Barium sulphate preparation.) ×8. (Professor W. R. Lee.)

There is a reduced diffusing capacity due to extensive lung destruction, but a normal $P\text{AO}_2$ and $P\text{ACO}_2$ can be maintained at rest by hyperventilation. The patient therefore is described as a *'pink puffer'* whose main disability is breathlessness rather than right ventricular failure.

The macroscopic appearances of panacinar emphysema are impressive. The lungs are voluminous, often obscuring the anterior surface of the heart, and the diaphragm is depressed. The emphysema is more pronounced along the anterior borders of the lungs, and when due to α_1-antitrypsin deficiency is most severe at the bases. The enlarged air spaces may become cystic and project from the pleural surface, forming bullae. It is worth noting that in some cases of severe centrilobular emphysema the dilatation of respiratory bronchioles may be so pronounced that it becomes impossible to distinguish them from cases of panacinar emphysema.

The Pathogenesis of Emphysema

Current evidence indicates that emphysema is du to an imbalance between protease and ant protease activities in the lung. Thus, in exper mental animals inhalation of papain, a proteolyt enzyme which degrades elastin, or of neutropl derived elastase produces emphysema. In adc tion, patients who have a homozygous defect f α_1-antitrypsin (α_1AT) have a high incidence severe panacinar emphysema developing befo the age of 40 years. Heterozygotes tend to b unaffected but damage induced by cigarette smo ing (usually centrilobular emphysema) procee more rapidly than in normal individuals.

α_1AT is synthesized in the liver and is present serum and tissue fluids where it acts as an inhibit of proteases, especially elastase. Its main functi appears to be the neutralization of elastase r leased by neutrophils during an inflammatory r sponse. As a result, in α_1AT deficiency, any stimulus which activates neutrophils in the lung nay result in uninhibited elastase-induced tissue lestruction.

The role of smoking in the pathogenesis of emphysema may also involve imbalance in protease–antiprotease activities (Fig. 13.15). Cigarette smoke causes the accumulation of neutrophils and macrophages around respiratory bronchioles and, by damaging lysosomes, induces hem to release elastase. Not only can macophage elastase not be inhibited by α_1AT but oxidants in cigarette smoke also inhibit the action of α_1AT. The net result is an increased elastase activity with decreased anti-elastase activity in the egion of the respiratory bronchioles, initiating issue destruction and hence centrilobular emphysema.

Once the initial damage to the lung tissue has occurred, the pressure of inspired air expands the damaged portion into an emphysematous space. As this enlarges, the pressure required to cause further distension decreases and a vicious circle of dilatation and destruction ensues. In chronic bronchitis this is further aggravated by the increased pressure associated with coughing.

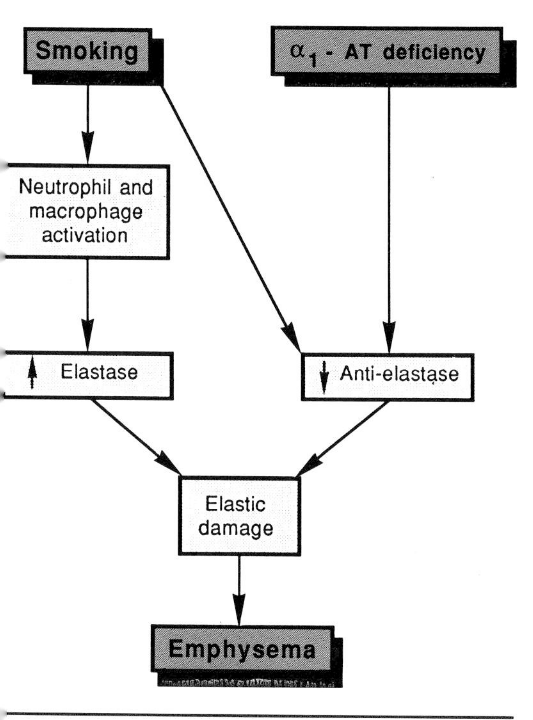

Fig. 13.15 Line drawing to show the possible mechanisms by which an imbalance between proteases/elastase and antiproteases/α_1-antitrypsin (α_1–AT) and anti-elastase may result in elastic damage.

Clinicopathological Correlations

The two main syndromes associated with what is clinically referred to as **chronic obstructive airways disease** have been discussed above and in the earlier section on respiratory failure (p. 538). The type I patient, in whom the emphysema is commonly but not invariably panacinar, is the 'pink puffer' who does not have significant hypoxia and whose main disability is breathlessness. There is radiological evidence of emphysema. At rest the partial pressures of O_2 and CO_2 are normal. The type II patient, in whom the emphysema is commonly centrilobular, is the 'blue bloater' who has significant hypoxia and is likely to develop peripheral oedema. The radiological evidence of emphysema is minimal. At rest the partial pressure of O_2 is low and that of CO_2 raised.

Adequate fixation is important for the demonstration of emphysema at autopsy. The whole lungs should be distended with formol saline through the trachea until the pleural surfaces are smooth and then left for 2–3 days before cutting. Barium sulphate may also be used to impregnate slices of fixed lungs (Figs 13.13b and 13.14c). Another technique is the preparation of sections 300 μm thick, of gelatin-embedded lungs (Fig. 13.13c). The application of morphometric techniques such as 'point-counting' sections of lung make it possible to determine the internal surface area and the number of surviving alveolar spaces. The normal total area of the exchange membrane is about that of a squash court (70 m^2). It is reduced in centrilobular emphysema and greatly diminished in severe panacinar emphysema. The number of alveolar spaces falls from 300 million to as low as 40 million in severe panacinar emphysema.

The classical concept that right ventricular hy-

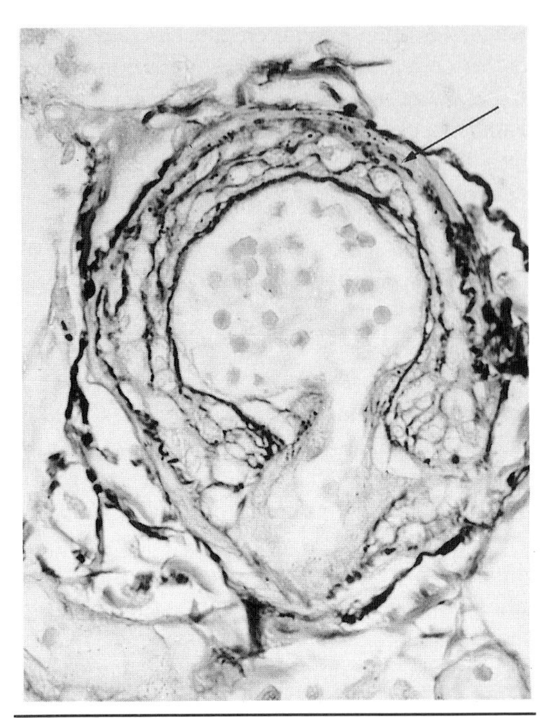

Fig 13.16 Transverse section of muscular pulmonary artery from a man of 64 years with centrilobular emphysema. The original media of circularly orientated smooth muscle (arrow) is thin. In the intima there is a thick layer of longitudinal muscle, many of the cells being separated by elastic fibrils (which appear dark). ×768.

pertrophy in emphysema in due to loss of pulmonary capillary bed is incorrect. In fact, right ventricular hypertrophy appears to be commoner in centrilobular emphysema in which the reduction in internal surface area, and so presumably in capillary bed is smaller. Chronic hypoxia causes pulmonary hypertension with hypertensive vascular disease (Fig. 13.16). The right ventricular hypertrophy reflects the degree of pulmonary hypertension which is present and this topic has been discussed earlier.

Other Types of Emphysema

In these, the term emphysema is used less strictly. **Compensatory emphysema** is a term used to describe the overdistension of alveoli which may occur around areas of collapsed lung tissue or during acute attacks of bronchial asthma, which may occur when a lung or lobe is removed surgically. It is more accurately described as 'overinflation' as no destruction of alveolar walls occurs.

Senile emphysema refers to the increase in size of alveolar spaces and decrease in the internal surface area of the lungs which occurs in some elderly people. Again it is due to overdistension rather than destruction and is of little clinical significance.

Localized emphysema may occur around scars or adjacent to interlobular septa or the pleura, or may only involve one lung (unilateral emphysema).

Interstitial emphysema follows laceration of the lung substance. This may be a traumatic laceration, for example due to a fractured rib or perforating wound, or it may be due to overdistension of the alveolar spaces with rupture of their walls. The latter is commoner in children and occurs in whooping cough, bronchiolitis and diphtheria. The alveolar walls rupture as a result of over-expansion during forced inspiration, and blebs of air extend along the junction of the interlobular septa with the pleura. When air is abundant it may extend to the tissues at the root of the neck giving rise to subcutaneous crepitant emphysema.

Collapse of Lung Tissue

The term **atelectasis** is derived from the Greek for 'imperfect expansion' and it should be restricted to denote failure of the lungs to expand properly at birth and distinguished from **acquired collapse** of a previously expanded lung. A lung may collapse because something presses on it from without (pressure collapse), or because there is obstruction of a bronchus with resulting absorption of air in the corresponding area of lung tissue (absorption collapse).

Pressure collapse. The lung may be compressed from without by a pleural effusion, haemothorax, empyema or pneumothorax. The absence of bronchial obstruction leaves the secretions from lung and bronchi free to drain up the bronchial tree and the collapsed lung tissue does not usually become seriously infected. The changes in it result from the haemodynamic alterations and associated vascular changes. Collapse due to empyema may be considerable so that the lung becomes very small and lies posteriorly against the side of the vertebral column. When the exudate on the visceral pleural surface becomes organized, pleural thickening results and prevents re-expansion of the lung even when the infection is overcome. Accordingly it is important to drain the pleural cavity and obtain re-expansion of the lung before this happens.

Absorption collapse. This is a commoner condition than pressure collapse and follows acute and complete obstruction of a large bronchus. Following such obstruction, collateral air ventilation may for a time keep the obstructed segment of lung filled with air provided the surrounding lung is normal. However, as the air gradually disappears it is largely replaced by secretion and oedema fluid so that the lung does not change much in size. Acute absorption collapse follows inhalation and impaction of foreign bodies; mucus plugging of bronchi during and after anaesthetics; after tracheostomy; in lung infections; or in terminal illnesses. Chronic bronchial obstruction may be caused by tumours, enlarged lymph nodes and aneurysms. In absorption collapse, bronchial secretions beyond the obstruction are very likely to become infected and suppurative. When the collapse has lasted for some time pulmonary fibrosis occurs and this is irreversible. The local pulmonary artery branches show narrowing of the lumen with intimal fibroelastosis.

Atelectasis, or incomplete expansion of the neonatal lung, may be caused by failure of the respiratory centre or, in premature infants, because the lung is insufficiently developed. It may follow hyaline membrane disease (p. 540) or may result from laryngeal dysfunction and obstruction of the air passages. These causes are, however, responsible for only a small proportion of atelectatic neonatal lungs. In many infants with severe atelectasis, no cause can be demonstrated at autopsy.

Acute Pulmonary Infections

Bacterial Pneumonias

The most common acute inflammatory disorders of the lung are the various types of pneumonia, which is defined as an inflammatory condition of the lung characterized by consolidation due to the presence of exudate in the alveolar spaces. The pneumonias may be classified anatomically into bronchopneumonia and lobar pneumonia.

Bronchopneumonia is an inflammatory condition of the lung that occurs when micro-organisms colonize the bronchioles and extend into the surrounding alveoli, leading to numerous discrete foci of consolidation (Fig. 13.17). The many causal organisms include *Streptococcus pneumoniae, Staphylococcus aureus, Streptococcus pyogenes, Klebsiella pneumoniae, Haemophilus influenzae, Pseudomonas aeruginosa* and *Legionella pneumophila.*

It occurs most commonly in infancy, in old age and in patients with some debilitating condition such as cancer, uraemia or a stroke. In debilitating conditions and whenever there is prolonged bed rest or interference with the respiratory muscles, retention of pulmonary secretions in dependent parts of the lungs may occur and then become secondarily infected – so-called ***hypostatic bronchopneumonia.*** Patients may also become infected in hospital, *nosocomial infections,* when bacteria may be spread from one patient to another and when the bacteria may have acquired resistance to antibiotics.

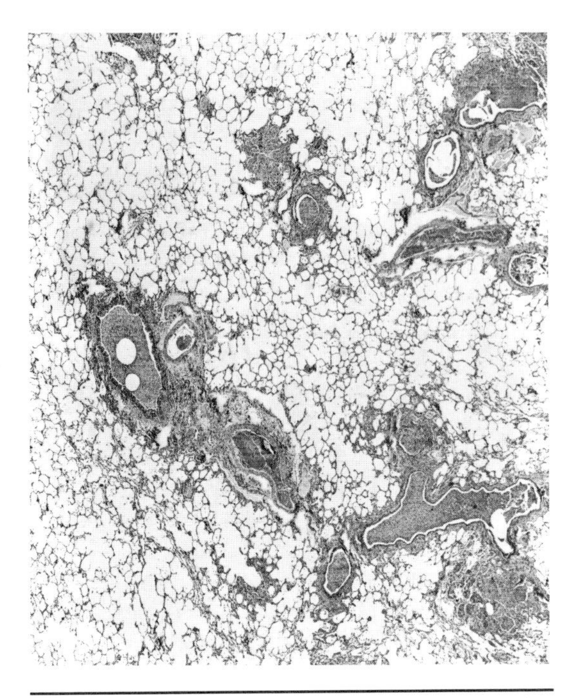

Fig. 13.17 Acute bronchiolitis and early broncho-pneumonia. The bronchioles are filled with exudate which is extending into the associated respiratory acini and peribronchiolar alveoli. ×10.

Acute respiratory virus infections, and chronic diseases such as chronic bronchitis, bronchiectasis and cystic fibrosis predispose to bronchopneumonia. It may develop in patients with congestive cardiac failure. It may follow general anaesthesia, due to the adverse effect of narcotic drugs on respiration and ciliary activity.

Bronchopneumonia occurs most often in the lower lobes of the lungs and at autopsy is seen as focal dark red or grey areas of about 1 cm diameter, which are firmer than the surrounding lung; each appears to be centred around a bronchiole from which a bead of pale yellow pus can be expressed. If progressive, the focal areas of consolidation become larger and eventually coalesce to produce lobular pneumonia, and with further extension it may simulate lobar pneumonia. The microscopic lesions of bronchopneumonia are an acute bronchiolitis with filling of the surrounding peribronchiolar alveoli by an inflammatory exudate rich in neutrophil polymorphs. Complete resolution is uncommon, except in mild cases, because there is usually a variable amount of damage to, and destruction of, the walls of bronchioles with consequent small foci of fibrosis. If fibrosis of the lung is extensive, bronchiectasis may develop.

The clinical features depend on the extent of the lung involvement and the virulence of the causal agent. The patients are usually pyrexial; there is a productive cough and clinical signs of consolidation. Radiological examination will define the extent of this. The complications of bronchopneumonia include lung abscesses, pleural infection with empyema, pericardial infection with suppurative pericarditis and bacteraemia with distant metastatic abscesses in other organs, e.g. brain.

Lobar pneumonia. In this condition infection leads to a watery inflammatory exudate in the alveoli. This flows directly into bronchioles and related alveoli, filling them and spilling over into adjacent lobules and segments of the lung. Damage to the bronchiolar walls, although present, is relatively unimportant. The exudate and bacteria spread through the lumens rather than the walls of the terminal airways. The consolidation is sharply confined to the affected lobe, which is diffusely affected (Fig. 13.18).

Since the widespread use of antibiotics the fully developed picture of classical lobar pneumonia is not often seen in Britain. However, it is still a common disease in many developing countries and fatal untreated cases may also be encountered in those who lie neglected at home or who decline medical aid, in vagrants, and in alcoholics who become exposed to cold. The disease predominates in males and may occur at all ages. However, it is uncommon below the age of one year and is most often seen in adults between the ages of 30 and 50 years.

The anatomical type of pneumonia (bronchopneumonia, lobar) and the complications which may develop, depend on the aetiological agent. Thus, it is more appropriate to classify the bacterial pneumonias on the basis of the causal organisms.

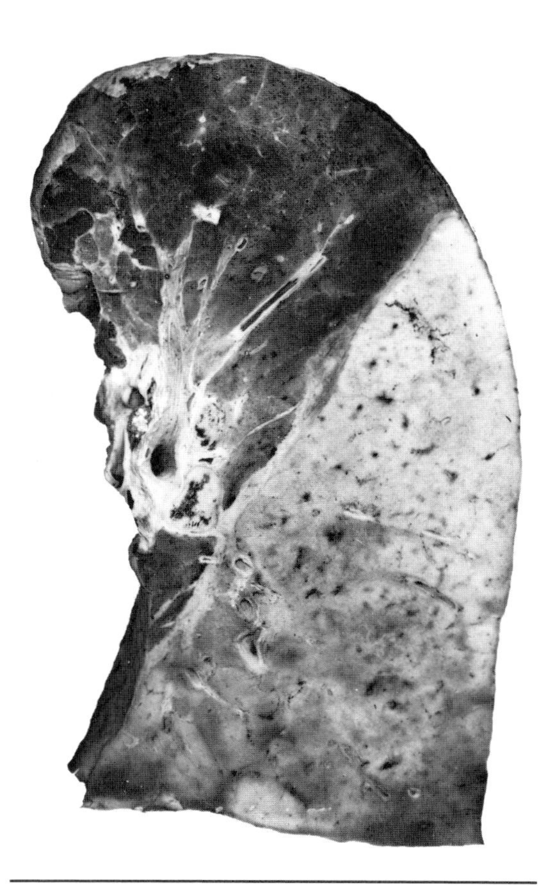

Fig. 13.18 Acute lobar pneumonia with grey hepatization in lower lobe and red hepatization in part of upper lobe. ×⅓.

Pneumococcal Lobar Pneumonia

The causative agent is *Streptococcus pneumoniae*, a Gram +ve diplococcus which can be serologically typed according to the antigenic properties of its polysaccharide capsule. The capsule prevents effective phagocytosis by polymorphs and macrophages unless type-specific antibody is present. Pneumococci with large capsules (e.g. type III) tend to be more virulent than those with small capsules.

Structural changes. It has been customary to recognize the following four stages in the progress of untreated pneumococcal lobar pneumonia; it must be emphasized that these stages occur in untreated cases in adults and the use of antibiotics profoundly alters the classical clinical and pathological picture.

1. *Acute congestion*, the initial phase, lasts for one or two days and is one of acute congestion and oedema. Macroscopically the affected lobe is heavy, dark red and firm: abundant frothy red fluid can be squeezed from it. Large numbers of pneumococci are seen in stained smears prepared from the cut surface. Microscopically, the alveolar capillaries are engorged with erythrocytes. The alveolar spaces are filled with eosinophilic oedema fluid containing many Gram +ve diplococci and neutrophil polymorphs.

2. *Red hepatization.* This phase lasts from the second to the fourth days of the disease. The pleural surface of the affected lobe is covered by greyish-white friable tags of fibrin. The cut surface appears dry, firm, red and granular and feels like liver. Affected lung tissue is airless and sinks in water. Microscopically, the capillary engorgement persists, but the exudate in the alveolar spaces now contains a fine network of fibrin, large numbers of extravasated red cells and numerous neutrophil polymorphs.

3. *Grey hepatization.* In this stage of late consolidation (4–8 days) the affected lung may weigh up to 1500 g. Fibrinous pleurisy is present and the cut surface is dry, granular and grey (Fig. 13.18). The affected lobe feels firm. Microscopically, the alveolar spaces are distended and filled by a dense network of inspissated fibrin containing neutrophil polymorphs, many of which are dead and disintegrating (Fig. 13.19) and occasional degenerating erythrocytes.

4. *Resolution* begins on the eighth day with the migration of macrophages from the alveolar septa into the exudate, which is gradually liquefied by fibrinolytic enzymes and absorbed or coughed up. Complete resolution and re-aeration take from 1 to 3 weeks. Since there is minimal tissue destruction in lobar pneumonia, the lung parenchyma returns to normal but the pleural exudate is commonly organized with the formation of fibrous adhesions between the two surfaces.

Clinical features. The onset is sudden and the

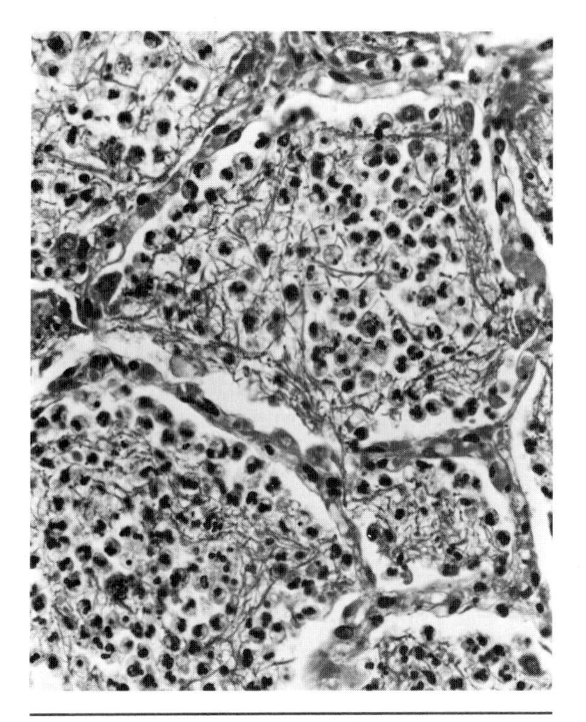

Fig. 13.19 Lobar pneumonia. The alveolar spaces are filled with exudate containing a fibrin network and many neutrophil polymorphs. ×235.

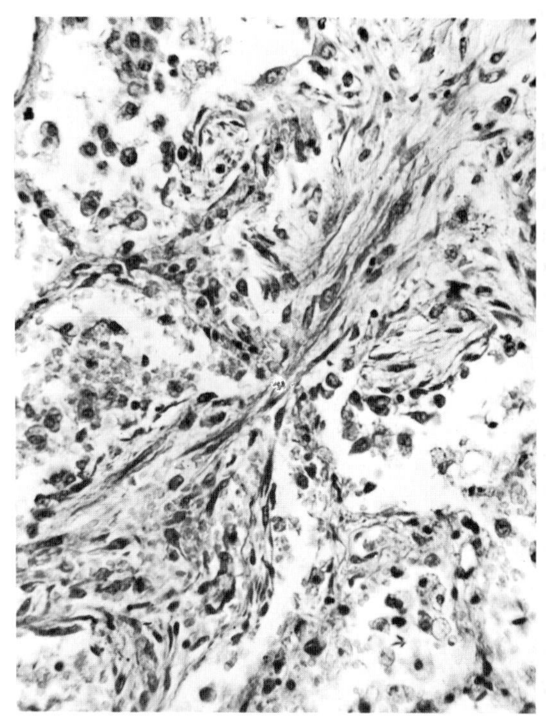

Fig. 13.20 Organization of alveolar exudate in the lung. The inflammatory exudate has been replaced by cellular fibrous tissue which can be seen passing from one alveolus to another through the pore of Kohn in the centre of the picture. ×390.

patient has a fever with rigors and sharp pleuritic pain on respiration. When a lower lobe is involved, diaphragmatic pleural pain may be referred to the tip of the shoulder. Partly because of the pain, breathing is shallow and rapid, and there is usually a cough productive of brown or blood-stained sputum. There is a neutrophil polymorphonuclear leucocytosis from an early stage. Bacteraemia may occur, blood cultures being positive in about 30% of cases. Antibodies to pneumococci appear at the stage of grey hepatization; the organisms are rapidly eliminated and the fever subsides by crisis.

The principal complications of pneumococcal lobar pneumonia are as follows:

1. *Organization of exudate.* In about 3% of cases resolution does not occur and the fibrinous exudate occupying the alveoli becomes organized (Fig. 13.20). Fibroblasts grow in from the alveolar septa, and the tissue becomes fibrosed.

2. *Pleural effusion* occurs in about 5% of treated cases and empyema in less than 1% of treated cases.

3. *Lung abscess* is a complication which has practically disappeared since the introduction of antibiotics.

4. Bacteraemic spread may result in endocarditis, meningitis, arthritis and otitis media.

Staphylococcal Pneumonia

Staphylococcus aureus is usually a secondary infection in patients with chronic lung disease such as cystic fibrosis. Its incidence rises sharply during epidemics of influenza, measles and pertussis, when it may be responsible for an acute, lethal haemorrhagic bronchopneumonia in affected children and adults. In this severe form, staphylococci invade the lungs about 36 hours after the onset of nfluenza. At autopsy, the lungs appear purple and ıre heavy due to haemorrhagic pulmonary)edema.

In patients who survive this acute phase, multi-)le foci of greyish-white bronchopneumonic con-solidation develop and suppurate, forming abscess :avities. There is much lung destruction and the)leura at this stage is thickly coated with fibrinous)r fibrinopurulent exudate. Empyema and pneu-nothorax may occur from rupture of pulmonary ıbscess into the pleural cavity. In children, a valvular obstruction may occur at the junction of an ıbscess cavity and bronchus to produce a rapidly :xpanding air-filled **tension cyst** or **pneu-natocele**. The cyst, which can be several cen-imetres in diameter, may rupture into the pleural :avity to produce a **tension pneumothorax**. Jsually the air is absorbed after the infection is)vercome.

Klebsiellar Pneumonia

Klebsiella pneumoniae (Friedlander's bacillus) is a Gram −ve bacillus with a very thick mucoid cap-ule that inhibits phagocytosis. It is an infrequent :ause of pneumonia but important because the nfection is destructive, with a high mortality rate ınd a high incidence of complications. It tends to ccur especially in men over the age of 50 years vho are chronic alcoholics, diabetics, or have oral epsis. Most infections commence in the right ıng, usually in the posterior segment of the upper obe.

Streptococcal Pneumonia

Pneumonia due to *Streptococcus pyogenes* is rare nd usually secondary to influenza or measles. In evere cases death occurs within 36–72 hours and he lungs appear purple with a fibrinous pleurisy.

Pseudomonas Pneumonia

Following the introduction and combined use of ntibiotic and corticosteroid drugs, Gram −ve rganisms in general, and *Pseudomonas eruginosa* in particular, have become of greater nportance as causes of bacterial pneumonia. This nay also complicate tracheostomy and mechanical entilation apparatus commonly becomes colon-ized by *Pseudomonas aeruginosa*. It is most important to sterilize respiratory equipment properly after use to prevent the spread of infection.

Unfortunately, *Pseudomonas aeruginosa* may survive and proliferate in water, soap solutions, stored blood, infusion fluids and in some antiseptics. A characteristic feature of pseudomonas pneumonia is bacterial invasion of pulmonary arteries, leading to necrosis of the vessel with subsequent haemorrhage or thrombosis and then pulmonary infarction.

Haemophilus Pneumonia

This is most often seen in young children after a viral infection or in adults with chronic bronchitis and emphysema.

Legionnaire's Disease

An outbreak of severe pneumonia affected 180 of about 4400 persons attending the Annual Convention of American Legionnaires in Philadelphia, USA during July 1976, causing 29 deaths. Investigation revealed that the pneumonia was caused by a hitherto unknown Gram −ve coccobacillus which has been named *Legionella pneumophila*. One proven source of infection is the water in air-conditioning systems. The lungs show either a lobar or a bronchopneumonia (Fig. 13.21). The intra-alveolar exudate contains abundant fibrin and variable numbers of macrophages and neutrophil polymorphs. Unlike many bacterial pneumonias, macrophages may predominate. Acute vasculitis and focal necrosis of alveolar septa occur in about one-third of cases. *Legionella pneumophila* can be demonstrated histologically using the Dieterle's silver staining method and also by immunofluorescence microscopy. Culture is extremely difficult. Since the original description of the disease, numerous cases have been reported in North America and Europe and several other species of legionella are now known to cause pneumonia.

Aspiration Pneumonia

This results from the inhalation of food, gastric contents, or infected material from the

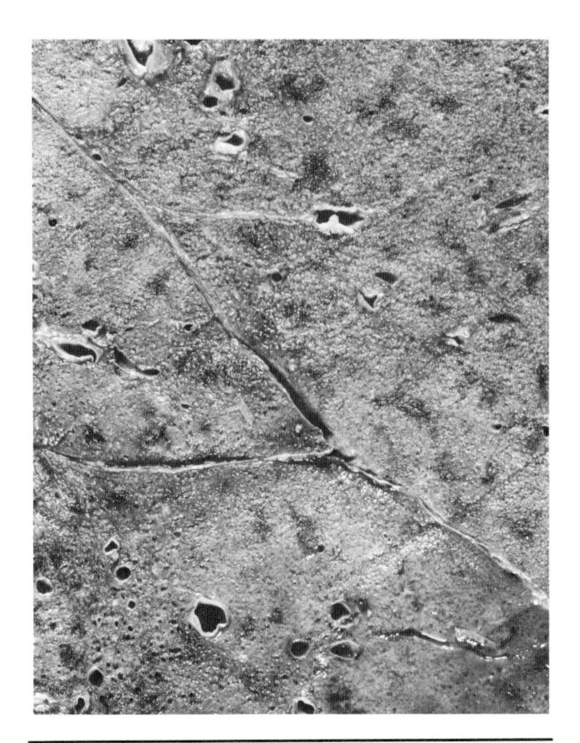

Fig. 13.21 The cut surface of the right lung in Legionnaire's disease, showing the adjacent parts of upper, middle and lower lobes, all of which are diffusely consolidated by inflammatory exudate. ×0.7. (Dr J. F. Boyd.)

oropharyngeal region. The likelihood of this happening is increased in unconscious patients, drunkenness, epilepsy and neurological disorders affecting swallowing. It may follow anaesthesia, and it may result from partial drowning, particularly in dirty water.

Massive inhalation of gastric contents may lead to rapid death from asphyxia. The aspiration of smaller amounts of sterile acid gastric contents produces pulmonary oedema due to chemical irritation of the alveolar walls: a few hours after aspiration the patient dramatically develops cyanosis, dyspnoea and shock, and cough with blood-stained sputum. If the acute episode is survived secondary bacterial infection is likely to follow. Non-sterile aspirate rapidly causes widespread bronchopneumonia, which becomes confluent with multiple areas of necrosis. A granulomatous reaction with foreign-body giant cells may be seen surrounding vegetable matter from food.

Viral and Other Uncommon Forms of Pneumonia

In viral respiratory infections there may be proliferation of bronchial, bronchiolar and alveolar epithelium, sometimes with formation of multinucleated giant cells, followed by necrosis. The bronchial, bronchiolar and alveolar walls are infiltrated by lymphocytes and mononuclear cells. Neutrophil polymorphs are few or absent in the inflammatory cell infiltrate, which is mainly interstitial except in influenza. Inclusion bodies may be demonstrated in lung tissue and secretions in infections with *Chlamydia trachomatis* or cytomegalovirus but otherwise the viral nature of a pneumonia can often only be inferred from the above histological features. The nature of a viral pneumonia can be confirmed by isolation of the virus or by demonstrating a rising or high titre of specific antibodies in the patient's serum. In spite of their varied pathogenesis, viral pneumonias mostly present a broadly similar clinical picture which is commonly referred to as **atypical pneumonia**.

As noted earlier, viral infections of the lung, and especially influenza, predispose the respiratory tissues to secondary bacterial invasion and when this occurs the distinctive histological appearances of viral pneumonia are often obscured.

Viral Pneumonias

Influenza occurs endemically in most countries but about every 3 years it causes an epidemic. Every 40 years or so a major epidemic or worldwide pandemic appears, as in 1918 when a large percentage of the world's population was affected. Recent pandemics have all been caused by type A virus and the subtypes causing successive pandemics have differed markedly in their important outer (H and N) antigens. Infection is spread by inhalation of droplets of infected secretions.

Influenza virus colonizes and causes necrosis of the columnar epithelium of the respiratory tract. At this stage the tracheobronchial mucosa is lined by basal or reserve cells and the submucosa is acutely inflamed but infiltrated mainly with lymphocytes. In mild cases these changes are probably restricted to the trachea and larger bronchi, but in severe cases they extend down to involve the terminal bronchioles. In patients who recover from the initial infection, the epithelium regenerates: at first it is of simple squamous type and devoid of cilia. During this phase the lung defence mechanisms are impaired and there is a considerable risk of secondary bacterial infection (Fig. 13.22). Differentiation to pseudostratified ciliated columnar epithelium occurs in about 3 weeks.

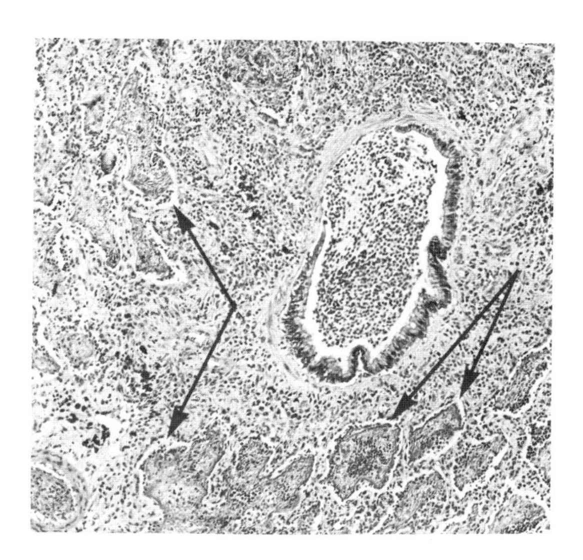

Fig. 13.22 Influenza with secondary bacterial bronchopneumonia. There is an acute inflammatory exudate in the bronchiole and in the surrounding alveolar spaces (arrows): the exudate in the alveoli is rich in fibrin and appears dark. ×60.

Primary influenzal pneumonia is almost always fatal. The alveoli become filled with a mixture of oedema fluid, fibrin, red blood cells and mononuclear cells (lymphocytes and macrophages). These changes are accompanied by an interstitial mononuclear cell infiltrate in half the cases. In the most severely affected parts of the lung there may be focal necrosis of the alveolar walls, which are lined by hyaline membranes.

Cytomegalovirus causes opportunistic infections in man, notably in the fetus, in premature infants and in subjects with primary or secondary immunodeficiency diseases. Patients treated by bone marrow transplantation are particularly susceptible. In adults the lungs may be involved as part of a serious widespread infection, the salivary glands and kidney being affected more frequently than the lungs. The changes occur in both bronchiolar and alveolar epithelium. Cells enlarge so that they are five to six times the size of their uninvolved neighbours.

Giant-cell pneumonia. In patients with measles dying early in the disease, notably in children with a deficiency in cell-mediated immunity, the epithelium of the bronchioles may be hyperplastic. Numerous giant cells may develop by fusion of alveolar lining epithelial cells and may contain inclusion bodies.

Other Uncommon Forms of Pneumonia

Psittacosis (ornithosis). Infection with various species of *Chlamydia* (p. 329) is very common in birds. Infection in man is acquired by inhalation of the excreta of infected birds. Cross-infection from human patients to healthy attendants may occur by droplet spread. The infection should be suspected in any patient who presents with atypical pneumonia where there is a history of contact with birds, especially parrots, budgerigars and pigeons. Infection produces a bronchopneumonia in which the alveoli are filled with exudate containing mainly macrophages, fibrin and often red cells. Very few polymorphs are present. The disease is occasionally fatal.

Q fever. This condition is caused by *Coxiella burnetii* which primarily infects cattle, sheep and goats. Man is usually infected by handling infected carcasses, by inhaling dust from infected barns and straw, or by drinking raw milk containing the organisms. Stockyard workers, farmers, shepherds and medical laboratory staff may be exposed to infection during the course of their work. The disease most commonly presents as an atypical pneumonia, with headache and muscle pains as prominent symptoms. The course of the illness is usually short (up to 8 days) and benign, but chronic infection can occur. Endocarditis is a rare complication and is frequently fatal.

Mycoplasma pneumoniae (p. 320) causes a low-grade bronchopneumonia in which the walls of the bronchioles are thickened by an interstitial mononuclear cell infiltration, while the lumina contain mucopurulent material. In some alveoli there is fibrinous exudate tending to undergo organization, in others oedema and haemorrhage. The onset is usually gradual and the mortality is low but resolution is often somewhat delayed.

Pneumocystis carinii (p. 1161) is an opportunistic infection which may frequently occur together with cytomegalovirus. It is a common cause of pneumonia in immunodeficiency states (p. 237).

Lymphoid interstitial pneumonia which is of unknown cause, affects persons of all ages, including infants. It is a slowly progressive condition and the diagnosis is usually made following lung biopsy. Histologically, the alveolar septa are distended with masses of mature lymphocytes intermingled with large pale macrophages and plasma cells. Large lymphoid follicles may be present. Differentiation from a malignant lymphoma may be difficult.

Eosinophilic pneumonia may occur in acute and chronic forms, both of which may be accompanied by peripheral blood eosinophilia. Acute eosinophilic pneumonia is a brief, mild, self-limiting illness commonly referred to as *Löffler's syndrome*. In chronic eosinophilic pneumonia, which may last for several months or years, the alveolar spaces contain proteinaceous exudate mixed with eosinophils and mononuclear cells. The alveolar septa and pulmonary interstitial tissues are heavily infiltrated with plasma cells, lymphocytes, eosinophils and macrophages. Most cases of eosinophilic pneumonia are of unknown cause but some are related to adverse drug reactions, or infection by *Aspergillus*, *Filaria* and *Dirofilaria*.

Pulmonary alveolar proteinosis is a rare chronic disease of unknown cause, which can affect persons of all ages. It is manifested clinically by dyspnoea, a cough often productive of yellow sputum, increasing fatigue and loss of weight. Some patients recover spontaneously but the disease is fatal in about one-third of cases. Histologically, the alveolar spaces are distended by granular eosinophilic PAS positive material, and lined by prominent granular pneumonocytes. The alveolar septa are devoid of inflammatory cells and fibrosis is usually absent. The nature of pulmonary alveolar proteinosis is obscure. It may represent a stereotyped reaction of the lung to different types of injury, rather than being a single disease entity.

Pulmonary granulomatosis. The lungs are sometimes the principal site of involvement by a number of distinctive types of focal, destructive and infiltrative vascular disease and granulomatosis not produced by known infectious agents, nor associated with rheumatoid arthritis. There is tissue necrosis accompanied by a chronic, cellular inflammatory reaction, which is not the result of occlusive lesions of the blood vessels. The necrotic lesions are surrounded by chronically inflamed granulation tissue with multinuclear giant cells. Several forms of granulomatosis have been identified and classified according to their histological picture, location within the lung and behaviour. They include ***Wegener's granulomatosis*** (p. 527), ***allergic granulomatosis, bronchocentric granulomatosis*** **and** ***necrotizing sarcoidosis***.

Exogenous lipid pneumonia follows the inhalation of oily material into the lungs. This is associated with the long-term use of oily drops or sprays taken for rhinitis, or the accidental aspiration of any mineral oils. The patients are often symptomless and the lung lesion is usually revealed by chance during radiographic examination or at necropsy. Microscopically the oil may be seen lying free or in foamy macrophages, and there are multinucleate giant cells with accompanying lymphocytic infiltration and fibrosis.

Endogenous lipid pneumonia is seen distal to obstruction of a major airway, most often due to a tumour. Macrophages with foamy cytoplasm accumulate within alveolar spaces. They may degenerate with the liberation of cholesterol and other lipids and the formation of cholesterol clefts.

Lung Abscess

Lung abscess presents clinical and radiological features which must be distinguished from those of necrosis in a malignant tumour or cavitation due to tuberculosis; these two diagnoses must be considered automatically whenever there is a clinical suspicion of lung abscess.

Causes. The commonest cause of a lung abscess is inhalation of infected material during unconsciousness and sleep. An abscess may form beyond an *obstructed bronchus* and this may be the first sign of a bronchial carcinoma or impacted foreign body. Pyogenic infection of *bronchiectatic* or *tuberculous cavities* results in abscess formation, and another important group of lung abscesses may complicate pneumonia caused by type III *Streptococcus pneumoniae, Klebsiella pneumoniae, Staphylococcus aureus* or *Streptococcus pyogenes.* Less common causes of lung abscess include infection of a pulmonary infarct, septic emboli in the lung as in pyaemia due to acute osteomyelitis or acute infective endocarditis, amoebic abscesses due to *Entamoeba histolytica,* trauma to the lung, or direct extension from a suppurating focus in the oesophagus, mediastinum, subphrenic area or vertebral column.

Localization. Abscesses due to inhalation of infected foreign material are likely to be located in the lower part of the right upper lobe or at the apex of the right lower lobe. The right bronchus is more in line with the trachea than the left and is thus more likely to receive aspirated foreign material. Small foreign particles are able to travel further into the lung and may produce a subpleural abscess. An abscess arising as a result of bronchiectasis tends to be centred around the affected bronchus, while an abscess complicating pneumonia has no primary relationship to a major bronchus. Pyaemic abscesses, which are usually staphylococcal or streptococcal, are scattered widely throughout the lungs, although they are likely to be small and mainly subpleural.

Complications. It is possible for a small lung abscess to heal completely, leaving a fibrous scar with a small central sterile cavity. An abscess near the pleura induces a fibrinous or purulent pleurisy which may progress to *empyema.* An abscess communicating with a bronchus may rupture into the pleural cavity to give a *bronchopleural fistula* and *pyopneumothorax.* Abscess formation in staphylococcal pneumonia may result in *tension cysts* or *pneumatoceles.* Serious *haemorrhage* may occur if an abscess erodes a pulmonary or bronchial artery. *Meningitis* or *cerebral abscess* may develop from bloodstream spread of the infection.

Chronic Pulmonary Infections

Pulmonary Tuberculosis

A general account of tuberculosis is provided on p. 300 and the basic information contained in it is essential to the understanding of this account of pulmonary tuberculosis. Tuberculosis affects the lungs more often than any other organ, partly because inhalation is now the commonest mode of infection, but also because lung tissue provides a favourable environment for the growth of the organism. The pattern of tuberculosis varies greatly in different populations. In those with a high prevalence of the infection, there is a high rate of primary infection in childhood, and survivors may remain free of further clinical evidence of infection or may subsequently develop secondary (chronic or reactivation) pulmonary tuberculosis. This is the traditional pattern and gave rise to the terms 'childhood' (i.e. primary) and 'adult' (i.e. secondary) tuberculosis. The pattern has however, changed in many of the developed countries where improved living standards, population screening, immunization and effective drug therapy have very greatly reduced the prevalence of all forms of tuberculosis. The result is that tuberculosis in childhood has become increasingly rare; primary tuberculosis is seldom seen because of a high level of immunization and most new cases are now in the middle-aged or elderly and represent recrudescence from a healed primary or secondary lesion which has remained latent for many years. Such old latent lesions are liable to be activated by any chronic debilitating disease, by corticosteroid or other immunosuppressive therapy, by chronic alcoholism, the development of diabetes mellitus, following partial gastrectomy and in workers with silicosis.

Primary Pulmonary Tuberculosis

In patients who have not previously had tuberculosis, inhalation of tubercle bacilli causes a **primary lesion**, also termed the **Ghon focus**. This is usually single, 1–2 cm in diameter, and situated just beneath the pleura, usually in the midzone of either lung. Microscopic examination shows central caseation and peripheral tubercles; the lesion enlarges by spread of mycobacteria, which are taken up and carried by macrophages, so that tubercles form in the adjacent lung tissue, replacing alveolar walls and filling air spaces, and as they enlarge these peripheral tubercles become incorporated in the central caseous area.

Lymphatic spread of *Mycobacterium tuberculosis* occurs in the primary infection; tubercles are often seen along the line of the lymphatics between the Ghon focus and the hilar lymph nodes, and both the tracheobronchial and adjacent mediastinal nodes often become extensively involved, greatly enlarged and caseous. The combination of the Ghon focus and tuberculous lymphadenitis is termed the **primary complex** (Fig. 13.23). In children, the affected hilar and tracheobronchial lymph nodes form a caseous mass which is much larger than the peripheral Ghon focus. In some adults with a primary infection, the reverse is the case.

In most instances, the Ghon focus undergoes healing: if small, by fibrous tissue; if larger, the caseous centre usually persists and is converted into a hard calcified nodule, often partly ossified and enclosed in fibrous tissue. Such a healed lesion is readily visible in chest radiographs. The affected hilar and tracheobronchial lymph nodes usually heal and may become heavily calcified.

The primary complex is symptomless in 90% of cases, but the pleura may be infected directly from the Ghon focus, causing a pleural effusion or rarely *tuberculous empyema*. In some cases the Ghon focus or hilar lymph nodes may involve and ulcerate into a bronchus, with consequent aspiration and tuberculous bronchopneumonia or dissemination may occur by the bloodstream resulting in either generalized miliary tuberculosis or one or more metastatic lesions, e.g. in the kidneys or joints. These serious complications are particularly liable to develop in very young, malnourished or debilitated children.

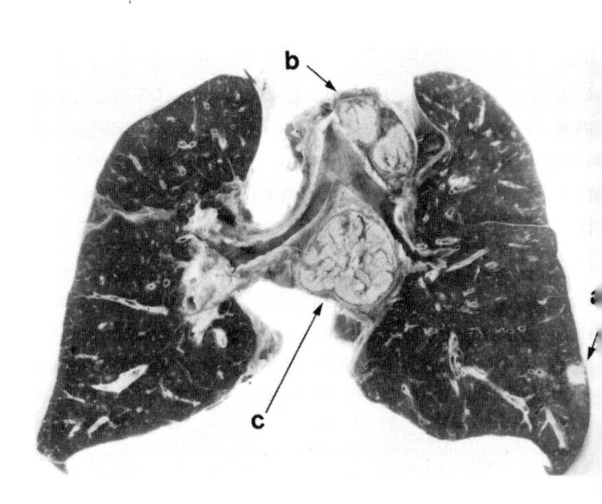

Fig. 13.23 Primary pulmonary tuberculous complex. Lung of child with primary lesion (a) in right lower lobe and enlarged tracheobronchial lymph nodes (b and c).

Acute tuberculous bronchopneumonia can develop from the primary infection by aspiration of infected caseous material throughout the bronchial tree either from the Ghon focus, or more commonly, from caseous lymph nodes at the hilum. The resulting tuberculous bronchopneumonia is relatively acute, and usually affects both lungs, although one is often involved more extensively than the other. The lung tissue is studded with numerous small pneumonic patches (Fig. 8.16) which are arranged in groups or clusters around the terminal bronchi. The microscopic features are quite atypical for tuberculosis. Acute tuberculous bronchopneumonia can occur also in patients with reactivation pulmonary tuberculosis.

Secondary (Reactivation or Chronic) Pulmonary Tuberculosis

During the primary tuberculous infection, or following BCG immunization, the patient develops cell-mediated immunity to antigens of the tubercle bacillus; this is demonstrable by a positive tuberculin skin test (a delayed hypersensitivity reaction to tuberculoprotein) which is associated with increased resistance to subsequent infection.

Post-primary infection can be endogenous, resulting from reactivation of a dormant primary or post-primary lesion, or it may be exogenous, i.e. caused by organisms in inhaled dust, etc. Some of the causes of reactivation of a dormant primary lesion have already been mentioned, but in many instances, none of these factors is responsible.

The common sites for post-primary pulmonary tuberculosis are the posterior or apical segment of the upper lobe and the superior segment of the lower lobe. The anatomical location of the lesion is attributed to the good ventilation but relatively low blood flow in these areas. The re-infection lesion results from proliferation of *Mycobacterium tuberculosis* in the wall of a bronchiole or alveolus. Tubercle follicles develop and the lesion enlarges by formation of new tubercles at the margin and in the adjacent lung tissue. The infection spreads by the lymphatics, but, because of the immune state, it induces a delayed hypersensitivity reaction from the onset, lymphatic spread is strictly localized, and the hilar lymph nodes are not usually affected. The early reactivation lesion thus comes to consist of a cluster of follicles which, as they enlarge and caseate, become confluent, producing one or more larger lesions which contain yellowish caseous material. Because of the partial state of immunity which exists, progress of the lesion is slow, the tubercles are well developed and there is conspicuous formation of fibrous tissue at their periphery. If healing does not now occur, some of the nodules will spread to involve the wall of a bronchus and blockage of the lumen follows. The lesion may become encapsulated by fibrous tissue or the caseous material may be gradually discharged along the bronchus, leaving a small cavity. Bronchial spread to the upper parts of other lobes and to the other lung may occur, and chronic pulmonary tuberculosis is frequently bilateral.

The cavities may coalesce and can become very large (Fig. 13.24). Even with cavitation, enlargement of the tuberculous lesions is usually slow: there is considerable overgrowth of fibrous tissue, not only around the cavities, but also in a diffusely spreading manner. In this way the lung shrinks and bronchiectasis may be superadded. Pulmonary and bronchial blood vessels involved in the wall of a cavity usually become occluded by endarteritis obliterans (p. 442). Sometimes, however, the wall of an artery may be weakened and rupture; this may be preceded by aneurysm formation. Serious and sometimes fatal haemorrhage results. This is to be distinguished from the coughing up of blood-stained sputum, or the slight bleeding which commonly occurs from small vessels in the wall of a cavity.

If at any time there is rapid spread of large numbers of bacilli by the air passages, as may happen when a caseous focus suddenly discharges into a bronchus, the patient's resistance may be overcome and tuberculous bronchopneumonia supervenes. It is not uncommon to find the latter in the lower parts of the lungs, while chronic cavity formation is present in the upper lobes (Fig. 13.24). In patients dying from chronic pulmonary tuberculosis, and particularly when there has been breakdown of resistance and extensive bronchopneumonia, blood dissemination with acute miliary tuberculosis may occur. Tuberculous ulcers may

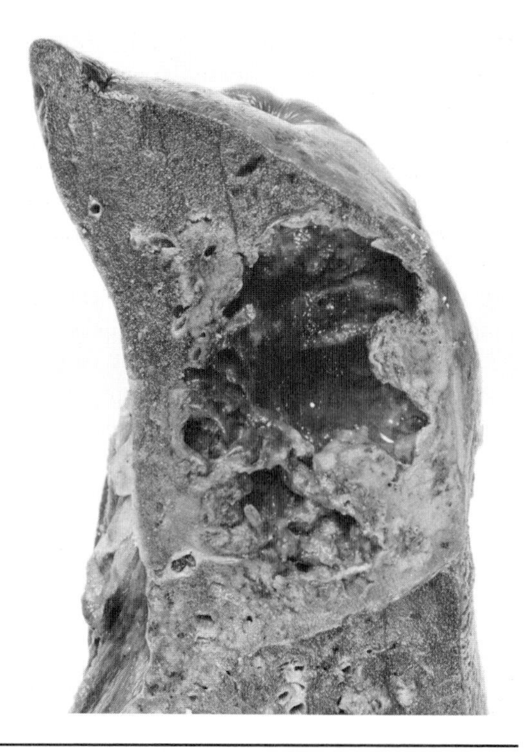

Fig. 13.24 Cavitating chronic pulmonary tuberculosis. Much of the upper lobe is occupied by a large irregular cavity with a necrotic lining and a fibrous wall in which paler caseous patches are seen. Fibrosis is most extensive below and lateral to the cavity, where it extends to the pleura. Irregularity of the cavity is due to persistence of fibrosed remnants of bronchi and blood vessels involved in the lesion.

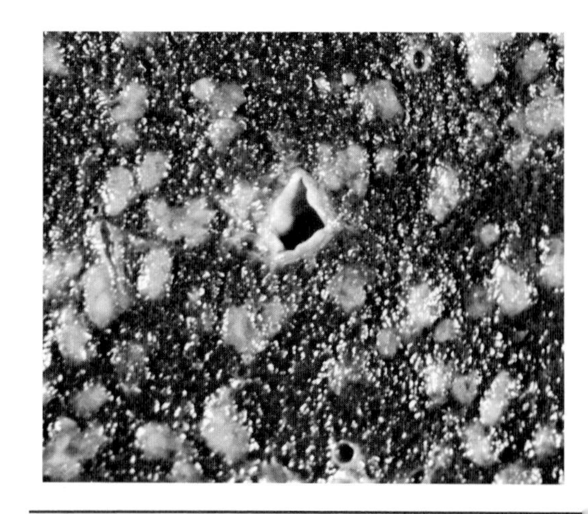

Fig. 13.25 Acute miliary tuberculosis. The cut surface of the lung shows numerous discrete grey tubercles. ×5.

develop in the larynx or in the intestine from direct infection by bacilli in sputum. *Secondary amyloidosis* is a common complication of chronic tuberculosis.

Generalized Miliary Tuberculosis

In developed countries where the prevalence of tuberculosis is low, miliary tuberculosis occurs most commonly in the elderly. In contrast, where the prevalence of tuberculosis is high, it occurs most frequently in childhood. The pulmonary lesions are part of an acute generalized tuberculosis, which occurs when a large number of mycobacteria gain entrance to the bloodstream. In miliary tuberculosis, lesions are usually more numerous in the lungs than in any other organ. They consist of grey tubercles which may be too small to be visible by the naked eye or up to 3 mm in diameter (Fig. 13.25).

The Effects of Specific Chemotherapy

If adequately carried out in the early stages of the apical lesion, chemotherapy leads to rapid healing with minimal fibrosis. In excavated lesions, whether chronic or bronchopneumonic, the caseous lining disappears and is replaced by a layer of vascular granulation tissue which, in turn, is converted to a thin smooth fibrous layer, over which an epithelial lining may eventually grow, leaving a persistent cavity which may or may not communicate with a bronchus.

Sarcoidosis

Sarcoidosis is a systemic disease of unknown aetiology in which non-caseating epithelioid cell granulomas are scattered throughout several organs. The general features of the condition are described on p. 313.

The lungs are involved more frequently than any other organ. In Europe and North America the commonest presentation of the disease is an abnormal routine chest radiograph. The following patterns of radiological abnormality can be distinguished: (1) hilar node enlargement with normal lung fields (38%); (2) hilar node enlargement with pulmonary infiltration (50%); (3) pulmonary infiltration without hilar node enlargement (7%); and (4) pulmonary fibrosis with honeycomb lung (5%).

Most patients have no physical disability and the radiological changes regress within 2–3 years. About 10–20% of patients develop chronic progressive pulmonary sarcoidosis, which is frequently associated with crippling dyspnoea, respiratory failure and pulmonary hypertension. About 5% of patients with chronic progressive pulmonary sarcoidosis die within 10–15 years of the disease being recognized.

Pathological examination of the lungs at an early stage of the disease reveals typical, non-caseating, epithelioid-cell granulomas distributed along the lymphatics in the pleura and septa and along pulmonary arteries, veins and bronchi. They usually heal with minimal fibrosis. In chronic progressive sarcoidosis an interstitial fibrosis develops which leads eventually to honeycomb change (p. 567): in this late stage, no trace of the original sarcoid granulomas can usually be found.

Actinomycosis and Nocardiosis

Actinomycosis is caused by *Actinomyces israelii* (p. 320) which produces a chronic granulomatous reaction with pus formation. About 20% of actinomycotic infections involve the lungs and thorax. Pulmonary actinomycosis may be primary or secondary, the latter usually resulting from spread of disease from below the diaphragm, particularly from the liver. About 75% of pulmonary cases are primary and the disease commonly occurs in the lower lobes, where it forms a dense fibrotic lesion honeycombed with small abscess cavities. The pus contains 'sulphur granules' which are colonies of *Actinomyces israelii.*

Nocardiosis is due to infection by *Nocardia asteroides*, an aerobic organism which usually enters the body through the lungs. It produces abscesses which may be large and cavitating or small and multiple. Infection is usually associated with immunodeficiency states. The organism does not form colonies, but occurs as branching filaments which are Ziehl–Neelsen +ve and Gram +ve and appear black using the methenamine silver stain.

Fungal Infections (Mycoses)

Most pulmonary fungal infections are **opportunistic**, arising as a result of breakdown in cellular and humoral defence mechanisms, and from the sustained use of antibiotics, which may so alter the normal human bacterial flora that fungi which are normally non-pathogenic may grow and invade the tissues. Until recent years, many of the pulmonary fungal diseases (mycoses) were little known and constituted an unimportant group of conditions. However, since the introduction of therapeutic immunosuppressive agents and antibiotics, the importance of fungal diseases has changed dramatically. The pulmonary mycoses usually encountered in Britain are aspergillosis, candidiasis and cryptococcosis; occasionally histoplasmosis (p. 332), coccidioidomycosis and blastomycosis may be acquired from overseas travel.

Aspergillosis, the commonest pulmonary mycosis in the British Isles, is usually due to infection by *Aspergillus fumigatus.* The hyphae are 3–4 μm in diameter, show frequent tranverse septa, and exhibit dichotomous branching at acute angles (Fig. 13.26). Four types of lung disease may occur: (1) atopic subjects may develop reaginic antibodies to constituents of aspergillus, and suffer episodes of bronchial asthma following heavy exposure to the spores; (2) some patients develop precipitating antibodies and on further exposure to the spores may have attacks of extrinsic allergic alveolitis; (3) aspergillus can colonize tuberculous

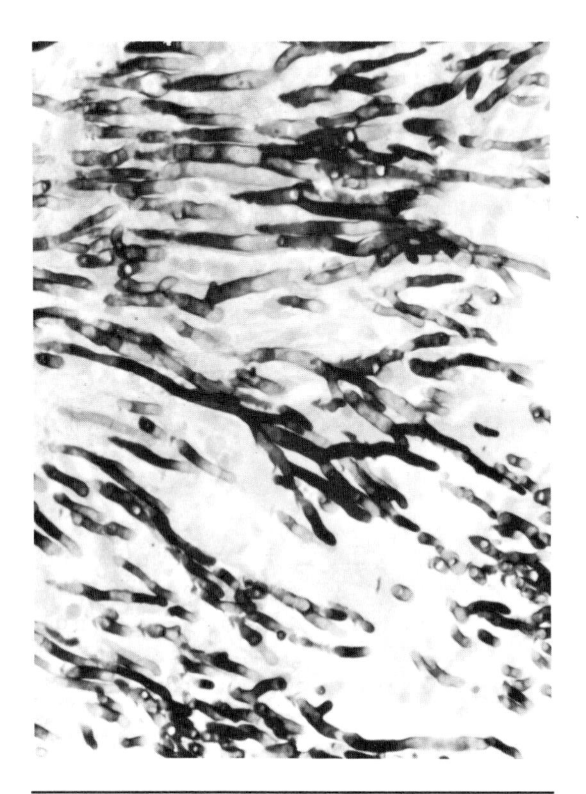

Fig. 13.26 Invasive pulmonary aspergillosis. The hyphae of *Aspergillus fumigatus* show frequent transverse septa and exhibit dichotomous branching at acute angles. From a patient who received cytotoxic therapy for Hodgkin's disease. Methenamine silver stain. ×375.

or bronchiectatic cavities in the lung, producing a rounded mass of fungus (mycetoma). The chest radiograph shows an opaque spherical mass which almost completely fills the cavity, leaving a crescentic 'halo' of air between the mycelial mass and the cavity wall; (4) in immunosuppressed patients, infection may produce diffuse nodules of haemorrhagic consolidation and necrosis. Such consolidated areas contain ramifying hyphae of *Aspergillus fumigatus* which may invade pulmonary arteries and veins, leading to thrombosis and metastatic foci in other organs.

Candidiasis. *Candida albicans* (p. 332) is a normal commensal in the pharynx, where it can give rise to the lesion of *thrush*. Bronchopulmonary infection is rare, occurring as a result of severe underlying disease, immunological deficiency states or because of long-term treatment with antibiotic or corticosteroid drugs. Sometimes the trachea and bronchi are lined by the fungus and hyphae extend into the mucosa; the lungs may show pneumonic consolidation with areas of necrosis and infiltration by neutrophil polymorphs.

Cryptococcosis (torulosis). The most usual presentation due to infection by *Cryptococcus neoformans* (p. 333) is a meningoencephalitis, but respiratory tract infection can occur with the production of granulomas containing numerous yeasts with a mucinous capsule which stains red with mucicarmine.

Pulmonary Complications of the Acquired Immunodeficiency Syndrome (AIDS)

Patients with AIDS frequently present with pulmonary complications which are associated with a high mortality rate. The most commonly recognized pathogen is *Pneumocystis carinii* which causes pneumonia at least once in 50–90% of all patients. Other opportunistic infections include *cytomegalovirus pneumonia, atypical mycobacterial disease,* invasive *candidiasis, toxoplasmosis, cryptococcosis, histoplasmosis* and *aspergillosis.* More than one pathogen may frequently be involved. Non-infective complications include *Kaposi's sarcoma, lymphoid interstitial pneumonia* and *malignant lymphoma.*

Pulmonary Fibrosis (Diffuse Interstitial Disease of the Lung)

Pulmonary fibrosis is a result or complication of many of the diseases described in this chapter (Table 13.3). Localized fibrosis may result from organization of acute pneumonias and pulmonary infarcts or from tuberculosis. Chronic diffuse pulmonary damage proceeding to interstitial fibrosis may be caused by inhalation of inorganic mineral dusts (the pneumoconioses), biological organic dusts (extrinsic allergic alveolitis), or by inhalation of fumes. It may also result from ionizing radiation and as an adverse reaction to a number of drugs and toxins. It may complicate sarcoidosis and certain systemic connective tissue and vasculitic diseases. In many cases, however, no cause can be established and this includes a group of unusual diseases (idiopathic pulmonary fibrosis) characterized by inflammation of the lower respiratory tract or alveolitis with diffuse alveolar damage and then progression to alveolar and interstitial fibrosis.

Table 13.3 Pulmonary fibrosis: causes and associated conditions*

Occupational and environmental dusts
- Mineral/inorganic dusts – coal, silica, asbestos etc.
- Biological/organic dusts – thermophilic actinomyces, (farmer's lung), avian protein (bird fancier's disease, pigeon breeders' lung) etc. These dusts are also associated with extrinsic allergic alveolitis
- Inhalants – oxygen, sulphur dioxide, nitrogen dioxide, mercury vapour

Infections
- Post-pneumonic – bacterial, viral, fungal and protozoal
- 'Shock' lung – adult respiratory distress syndrome

Drugs and toxin
- Cytotoxic agents – busulphan, cyclophosphamide, azathioprine
- Non-cytotoxic drugs – nitrofurantoin, penicillamine, gold
- Toxins – Paraquat

Ionizing radiation

Miscellaneous
- Sarcoidosis
- In association with systemic connective tissue or vasculitic diseases, e.g. rheumatoid arthritis, systemic lupus erythematosus, systemic sclerosis

*In the majority of cases no cause can be established – see section on primary (idiopathic) pulmonary fibrosis.

Clinically, patients with diffuse interstitial lung disease present with progressive breathlessness, a dry unproductive cough and irregular patchy infiltrative opacities mainly in the basal areas on chest radiography. The functional changes in the lungs are of a restrictive rather than obstructive nature with reduction in lung compliance, lung volume and oxygen diffusion capacity. Type I respiratory failure and right ventricular failure supervene in many cases.

Morphologically the end stage of many of these disorders is **honeycomb lung**. Honeycomb lung describes a non-specific acquired condition in which cystic spaces develop in fibrotic lungs. The term honeycomb lung refers to the naked eye appearance of the lung at autopsy. Small cystic spaces, up to 1 or 2 cm in diameter, develop in the fibrotic lung. The cysts have smooth grey-white walls, and the surrounding lung is pale, firm and fibrous (Fig. 13.27). The presence of cysts beneath the visceral pleura gives the external surface of the lungs a nodular appearance which simulates that of the liver in macronodular cirrhosis. The essential change in honeycomb lung is obliteration by fibrosis or granulomas of some of the bronchioles and alveolar spaces with compensatory dilatation of unaffected neighbouring bronchioles.

Pneumoconiosis and Industrial Lung Diseases

Pneumoconiosis is a comprehensive term covering a group of lung diseases resulting from the inhalation of dust. The group can be subdivided according to whether the inhaled dusts are in-

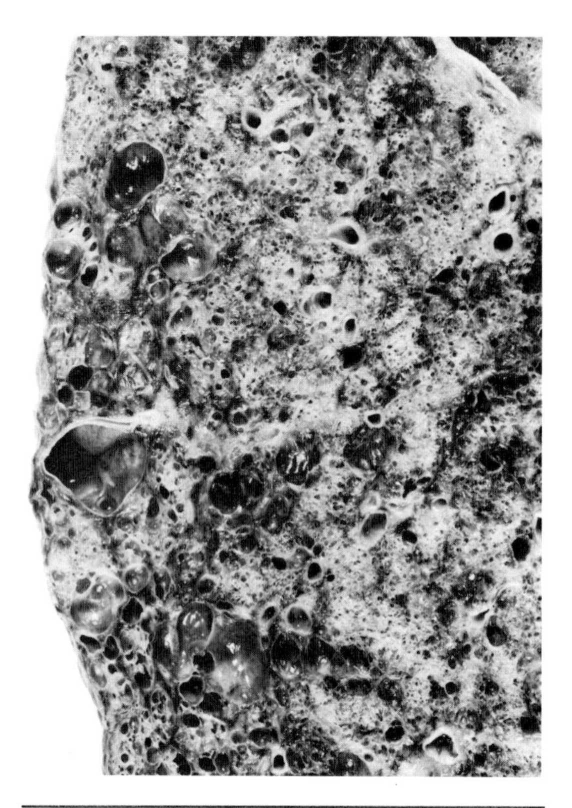

Fig. 13.27 Honeycomb lung showing cystic spaces, predominantly subpleural (left) and which represent dilated terminal bronchioles surrounded by dense fibrous tissue.

organic or organic. Their number continues to increase as new industrial hazards are created. The type of lung disease varies according to the nature of the inhaled dust. Some dusts are apparently inert and cause little or no damage, whereas others may cause widespread lung destruction and fibrosis. Certain dusts are antigenic and cause damage through immunological reactions, while others may predispose to tuberculosis or to neoplasia. The factors which determine the extent of damage caused by an inhaled dust include its physical state, its chemical composition, its concentration, the duration of exposure, and the coexistence of other lung diseases.

The size of the inhaled dust particles determines which will reach the alveoli and whether dust will penetrate the thin alveolar epithelium or remain within the alveolar lumen. Practically all inhaled particles of more than 5 μm diameter are trapped in the nasopharynx, trachea and major bronchi, from where they are swept upwards, entangled in mucus, by the action of cilia. Particles less than 1 μm are probably exhaled. Particles between 1 and 5 μm in diameter are most likely to reach the alveoli. Shape of particles is important; long and thin asbestos fibres, up to 300 μm in length and less than 0.1 μm diameter, may reach the alveoli. Submicronic particles, <0.02 μm, may penetrate type I epithelial cells and enter the interstitium. Larger particles are incorporated into the alveolar walls.

Mineral (Inorganic) Dusts

Anthracosis. This is caused by the inhalation of atmospheric soot particles; it is found in some degree in all adults, and it is more marked in those who live in the highly polluted atmosphere of industrial areas; it produces the blackening seen in the adult lung at autopsy. Some of the inhaled particles are engulfed by macrophages and retained within alveoli adjacent to bronchioles, in blood vessels and fibrous septa, beneath the pleura and at the edges of lung scars. Some particles are carried to the hilar lymph nodes.

Coal-workers' Pneumoconiosis

This is due to the inhalation of coal dust particles and occurs in persons who handle soft bituminous coal with a low silica content. It occurs in two stages, simple coal-workers' pneumoconiosis and progressive massive fibrosis (complicated pneumoconiosis).

Simple pneumoconiosis of coal workers. The intra-alveolar coal dust particles are fairly evenly distributed within the lungs but maximal changes occur in the upper two-thirds of each lung. The particles are ingested by macrophages and are retained in relatively immobile alveoli, including those adjacent to the respiratory bronchioles. The dust accumulation provokes a local fibrotic reaction and after several years there is obliteration

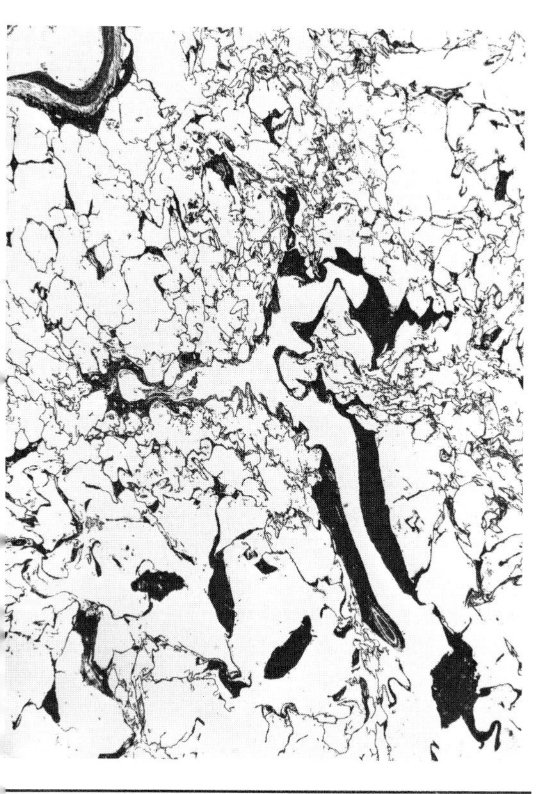

Fig. 13.28 Simple pneumoconiosis of coal-workers with focal dust emphysema, showing localization of dust accumulation in the walls of the second order of respiratory bronchioles. ×7.

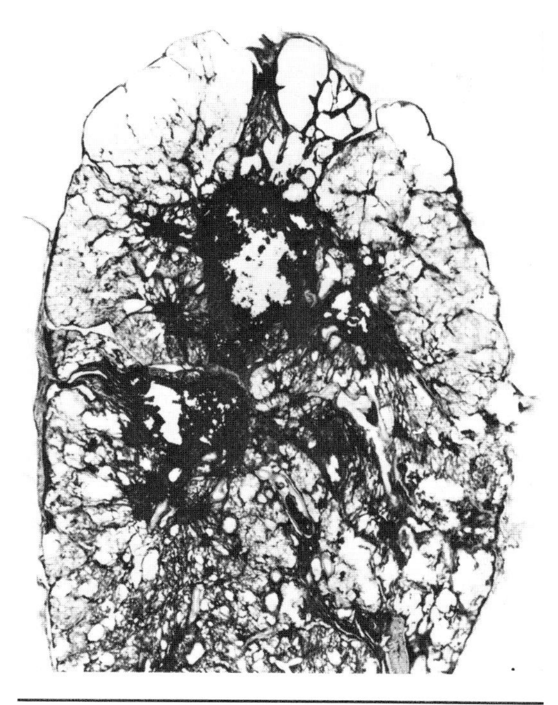

Fig. 13.29 Thick section of the lung of a coalminer, showing very severe emphysema and two foci of progressive massive fibrosis, seen as solid black areas with, in this instance, central cavitation. ×0.5

of the peribronchiolar alveoli and atrophy of bronchiolar smooth muscle. The respiratory bronchioles dilate to produce *focal dust emphysema,* characterized by abnormal clusters of dust-blackened centrilobular air spaces (Figs 13.13c and 13.28). Simple pneumoconiosis may be seen in the chest radiographs of coal workers who are free from symptoms. It appears to have no adverse effect on pulmonary function and does not significantly alter life expectancy.

Progressive massive fibrosis. After 10–20 years at the coal face a small proportion of workers with simple pneumoconiosis develop massive confluent areas of fibrosis in the upper lobes (Fig. 13.29). These irregular masses of black fibrous tissue may break down centrally and may become infected by tuberculosis. Progressive massive fibrosis is a serious and incapacitating disease; death results from respiratory failure, tuberculosis or right heart failure.

There has been considerable debate about the cause of progressive massive fibrosis. Concomitant tuberculosis may play a role, as careful examination of these lungs at autopsy has found tuberculous infection in 40% of cases. The initial tissue breakdown may be ischaemic in origin due to obliteration of pulmonary artery branches. Immunological mechanisms may also be involved, as some patients' serum contains antinuclear antibodies and rheumatoid factors.

Silicosis. Wherever rock is cut, as in granite, sandstone and slate quarries or in coal, gold, tin or copper mining, silica dust fills the air. Stonemasons, sandblasters, boiler scalers and those

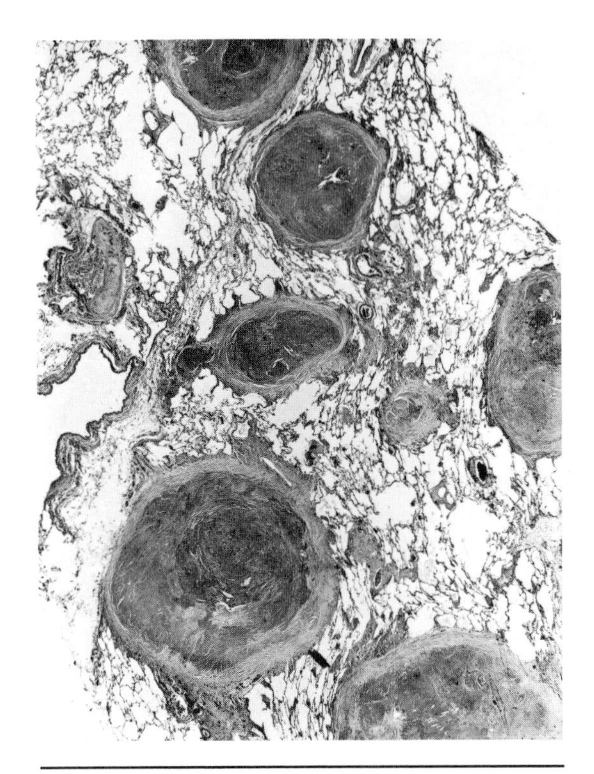

Fig. 13.30 Silicosis. The lung contains multiple nodules consisting of laminated fibrous tissue. There is no inflammatory cellular infiltrate. ×7.

involved in glass and pottery manufacture may also be exposed. The inhaled particles, less than 5 μm in diameter, are deposited in immobile air spaces as in anthracosis, but in contrast with soot deposition, silica induces a dense fibrous reaction, forming *silicotic nodules* (Fig. 13.30). These contain particles of birefringent silica surrounded by concentric rings of fibrous tissue. The fibrosis obliterates the lumen of bronchioles and pulmonary blood vessels and pleural adhesions may form over nodules. At autopsy the pleura is thickened and adherent, and the lungs contain multiple, discrete, greyish-black nodules which may coalesce to form large confluent masses of fibrous tissue.

The cause of pulmonary fibrosis in silicosis is uncertain. Two possibilities are that silica is antigenic and provokes fibrosis by an immunological mechanism, or that collagen formation is stimulated by the release of lysosomal enzymes by macrophages which have ingested silica particles. Silicosis leads to progressive respiratory impairment and death may be due to respiratory failure or right ventricular failure secondary to pulmonary hypertension. There is also an increased susceptibility to tuberculosis.

Asbestosis

In addition to fibrosis of the lungs, asbestos exposure can also cause pleural fibrous plaques and mesothelioma. Asbestos is a general term embracing a number of fibrous silicates of magnesium. The three types of asbestos which are most important commercially are *chrysotile* (white asbestos), *crocidolite* (blue asbestos) and *amosite* (brown asbestos). They are used for their fire-resistant properties, and as thermal and acoustic insulators. Thus, the widest exposure has occurred in shipyards and in the building industry and in engine and motor manufacturing.

Chrysotile fibres are soft and are more likely to be retained in the proximal small airways, while the rigid fibres of crocidolite and amosite travel readily in the airstream and so reach the periphery of the lung. These properties may explain why chrysotile causes lesions in the lung but rarely pleural mesothelioma. The most important factor in the development of asbestosis is the amount of dust inhaled; heavy exposure for a few years or exposure to low levels over many years are equally likely to result in asbestosis.

Inhaled asbestos fibres (50 μm long and 0.5 μm diameter) are mostly retained in the respiratory bronchioles of the lower lobes. In time they pass into the alveolar ducts and spaces where fragments are engulfed by macrophages. Complete fibres are surrounded by macrophages and become coated with iron and protein, producing the characteristic drumstick shaped asbestos body (Fig. 13.31). It should be emphasized that the finding of asbestos bodies in the sputum or lung is only an indication of past exposure to asbestos and is not proof of the presence of disease due to asbestos.

Fibrosis is first evident around respiratory bronchioles and then spreads to involve alveolar ducts and alveoli which are progressively obliterated.

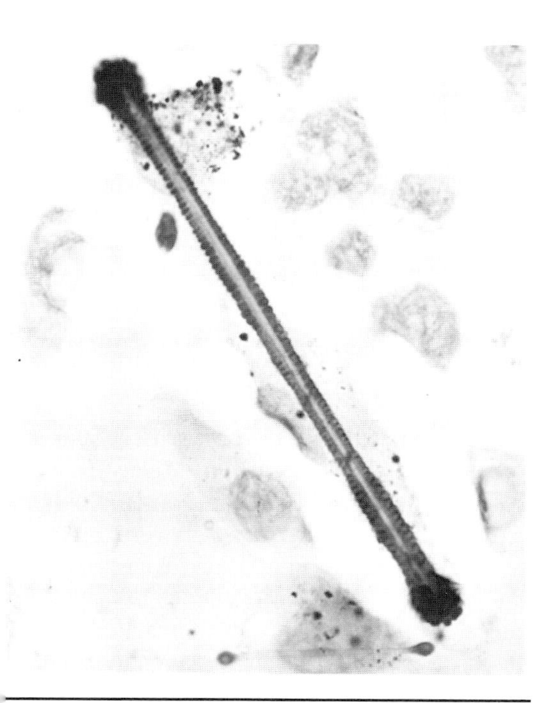

Fig. 13.31 An asbestos body in the lung. The needle-like asbestos fibre is enclosed in a crenellated protein deposit with club-shaped ends. The body is partly enveloped by two macrophages (which also contain dust pigment), and a smaller asbestos body (below) is almost completely engulfed within a macrophage. ×900.

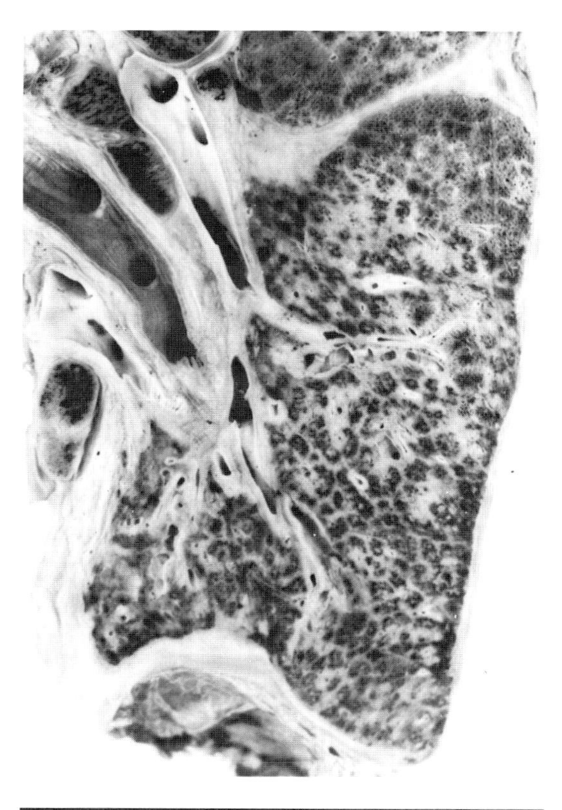

Fig. 13.32 Pulmonary asbestosis showing pronounced fibrosis and shrinkage of the lower lobe and gross pleural thickening. ×¾.

Unaffected bronchioles undergo compensatory dilatation and the disease may progress to honeycomb lung. The disease commences in the subpleural region of the lower lobes and causes thickening of the visceral pleura. (Fig. 13.32). Fibrosis progresses upwards and inwards so that eventually the middle lobes and lower parts of the upper lobes may be affected. The mechanism by which asbestos causes pulmonary fibrosis is not understood. It has been suggested that, like silica, asbestos stimulates macrophages to secrete fibrogenic lysosomal enzymes or immunological factors may play a role.

Asbestosis causes respiratory failure due to destruction of lung tissue. This may be accompanied by pulmonary hypertension with right ventricular hypertrophy and failure. Asbestosis does not predispose to pulmonary tuberculosis, but it is the only form of pneumoconiosis with a high risk of carcinoma of the lung. Approximately half of British male asbestos workers with asbestosis die of lung carcinoma, which arises in the vicinity of the fibrosis, usually in the lower lobe. The neoplasm may be of any cell type but is usually an adenocarcinoma. Surveys of the smoking habits of asbestos workers have shown only a slight increase in the prevalence of lung cancer among non-smokers. However, heavy smokers (more than 20 cigarettes a day) have an 80–90-fold greater predisposition to lung cancer. The combined effects of asbestos and smoking therefore appear to be synergistic rather than additive.

Caplan's Syndrome

This is characterized by the presence of nodules, up to 5 cm in diameter, scattered fairly evenly throughout the lungs of workers who are exposed to inhaled dusts, including coal dust, silica and asbestos. Rheumatoid arthritis is usually present but occasionally the nodules develop several years before the arthritic manifestations. Rheumatoid factor is present in the blood. Cavitation and calcification of the nodules is common. Not all patients with rheumatoid disease and pneumoconiosis develop Caplan's syndrome. The central parts of the nodules show concentric black and pale yellow rings, the pale zones frequently being liquefied. Histologically, the lesions are modified rheumatoid nodules with a central zone of dust-laden fibrinoid necrosis.

Biological (Organic) Dusts

Inhaled organic dusts may affect the bronchi, as in the case of byssinosis, or may produce an extrinsic allergic alveolitis.

Byssinosis

This is an occupational disease which develops after many years of exposure to dust in the cotton, flax and hemp industries. It is thought to be due to bronchoconstriction induced by cotton dust or associated bacteria from the cotton bales. The pathological changes are indistinguishable from those of chronic bronchitis.

Extrinsic Allergic Alveolitis

In addition to their causal role in asthma, inhaled organic dusts can induce an Arthus (type III) reaction (p. 213) in the alveoli in which circulating precipitating antibodies react with inhaled antigen. The clinical syndromes produced by this latter reaction are known collectively as extrinsic allergic alveolitis. Their symptoms and pathological manifestations are similar but their origins diverse. The individual diseases are generally recognized by names descriptive of their occupation or the nature of the antigenic dust (Table 13.3).

The most acute and severe is **farmer's lung** (which also occurs in cows!). The clinical features consist of acute episodes of fever, headache and malaise with cough, dyspnoea and basal pulmonary crepitations, arising 4–5 hours after exposure to the dust and persisting for 24 hours. Histologically the alveolar walls are thickened by an infiltrate of lymphocytes, plasma cells, mononuclear cells and occasional eosinophils. Sarcoid-like granulomas occur in relation to respiratory bronchioles in about 70% of cases. Repeated exposure as commonly occurs with bird fanciers leads to the development of a diffuse interstitial fibrosis which may progress to honeycomb lung.

Other occupational diseases. Beryllium provokes granulomatous lesions in the lung which may be indistinguishable from sarcoidosis. This may proceed to fibrosis – *berylliosis*. Severe, acute and chronic damage affecting both the upper and lower respiratory airways may occur due to toxic metal fumes, e.g. aluminium and cadmium and toxic gases, e.g. chlorine, ammonia and oxides of nitrogen.

Idiopathic Pulmonary Fibrosis (Fibrosing Alveolitis)

In this group of conditions the cause of the lung damage is unknown. Similar clinical and histological features may occur in association with systemic connective tissue or vasculitic diseases. The diagnosis is one of exclusion and a lung biopsy (open or transbronchial) is required to exclude recognized causes of pulmonary fibrosis such as extrinsic allergic alveolitis or pneumoconiosis. Aetiological theories have included some form of autoimmunity in that serum autoantibodies may occur in some patients.

The basic pathogenesis appears to be diffuse alveolar wall damage similar to that seen in adult respiratory distress syndrome but occurring and progressing less rapidly. Histologically, there is often overlapping between the various stages and components of the alveolar injury but broadly these comprise: (1) an alveolar exudate in which there is oedema, hyaline membrane formation and inflammatory cells. Many of the alveolar walls are lined by type II, granular pneumonocytes which have proliferated and replaced necrotic membranous pneumonocytes. Many alveolar spaces contain pulmonary macrophages; (2) an interstitial inflammatory cell infiltrate consisting of lymphocytes, plasma cells and polymorphs; (3) fibroblastic proliferation which is mainly interstitial (in the alveolar walls) but may be intra-alveolar; and (4) progressive obliterative fibrosis producing severe architectural disturbance. Two separate entities have been defined and it is of some clinical importance to recognize these in that their respective prognosis is different.

In **usual interstitial pneumonia (UIP)** the distribution is patchy and the alveolar walls are thickened due to a combination of fibrosis and infiltration by lymphocytes, plasma cells and occasional polymorphs (Fig. 13.33). There is progressive fibrosis and the patients die from respiratory failure after several years.

Desquamative interstitial pneumonia (DIP) is more diffuse; the alveoli are filled with macrophages and the alveolar walls show only minimal fibrosis (Fig. 13.34). The name, however, is a misnomer because the intra-alveolar cells are true macrophages and are not derived from desquamated alveolar wall lining cells. The prognosis is usually good and the patients respond to corticosteroid therapy.

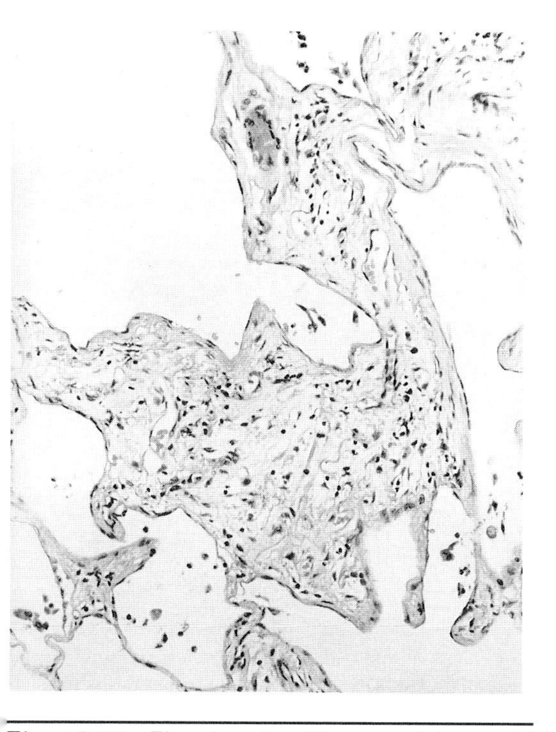

Fig. 13.33 Fibrosing alveolitis – usual interstitial pneumonia (UIP). The alveolar walls are thickened due to a combination of fibrosis and infiltration by lymphocytes and plasma cells with smaller numbers of eosinophils and neutrophil polymorphs. Many of the alveolar walls are lined by cuboidal epithelial cells. Scanty mononuclear cells are present in the alveolar spaces. ×120.

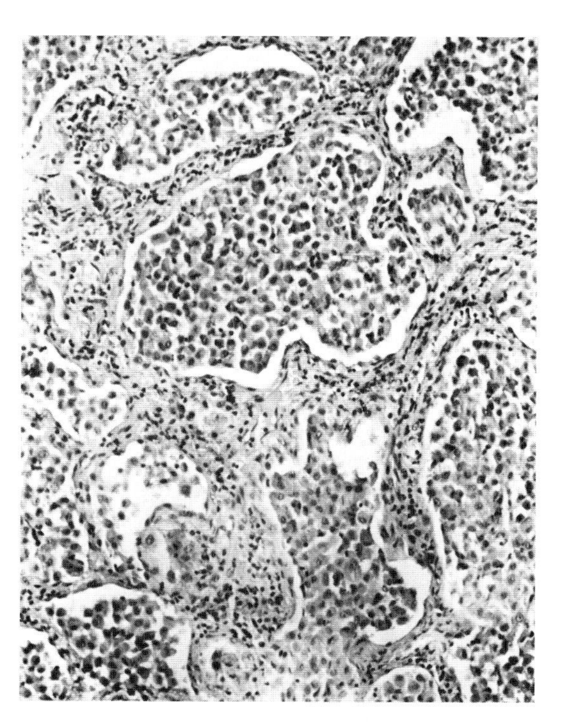

Fig. 13.34 Desquamative interstitial pneumonia (DIP). The alveolar spaces are filled with macrophages. There is only slight fibrous thickening of the alveolar walls. ×130. (Professor D. B. Brewer.)

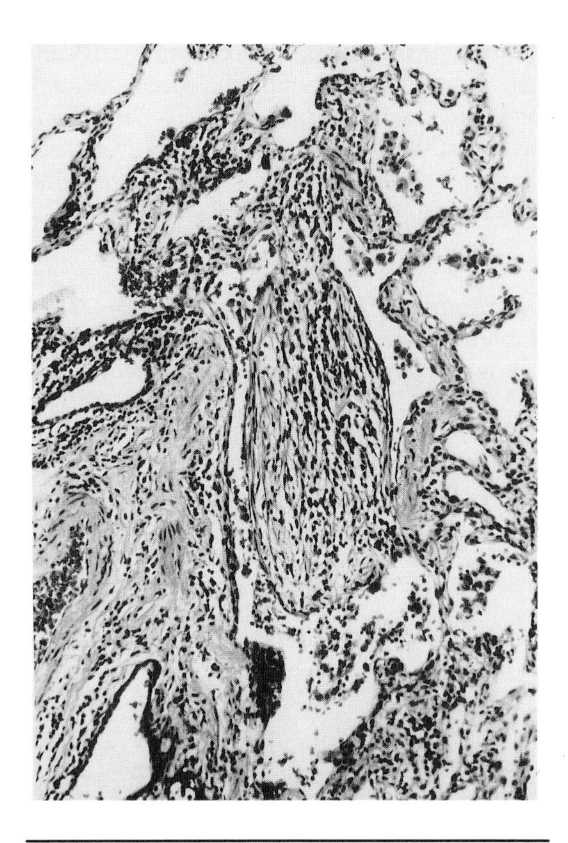

Fig. 13.35 Bronchiolitis obliterans organizing pneumonia (BOOP). The lumen of a longitudinally sectioned respiratory bronchiole is occupied by an oval plug of cellular fibrous tissue. The adjacent alveolar walls are thickened and infiltrated by chronic inflammatory cells. ×120.

Table 13.4 Drug and toxin induced lung injury

Lung disease	Examples of drugs/toxins which may cause these
Pulmonary hypertension	Pyrrolizidine alkaloids; aminorex fumarate (an anorexigen); denatured rape-seed oil ('toxic oil syndrome')
Bronchial asthma	Aspirin, penicillin and many others
Eosinophilic pneumonia	Nitrofurantoin
Adult respiratory distress syndrome	Busulphan; cyclophosphamide; prolonged oxygen administration
Pulmonary fibrosis	Nitrofurantoin, cyclophosphamide; pencillamine; Paraquat

Bronchiolitis Obliterans Organizing Pneumonia (BOOP)

This is another idiopathic condition which must be distinguished from fibrosing alveolitis. It is characterized by whorls of fibrous tissue within the alveoli (Fig. 13.35). These balls of fibrous tissue are also present in the lumens of distal bronchioles (bronchiolitis obliterans). This disease is very sensitive to corticosteroid therapy and indeed many cases appear to resolve spontaneously. The aetiology is not known but there is evidence that some cases may have an infective cause or be drug induced and indeed BOOP is probably best considered to be a non-specific form of lung injury rather than a specific disease.

Drug and Toxin Induced Lung Injury

Many drugs and chemical substances may give rise to clinical signs and symptoms which may mimic naturally occurring diseases (p. 418). Some of these agents produce morphological changes in the lung (Fig. 13.36). However, none of the lesions associated with drugs is unique; they correspond to lesions which have already been described and the associations are briefly summarized in Table 13.4: it is emphasized that the list of drugs is by no means complete and indeed that only examples are given.

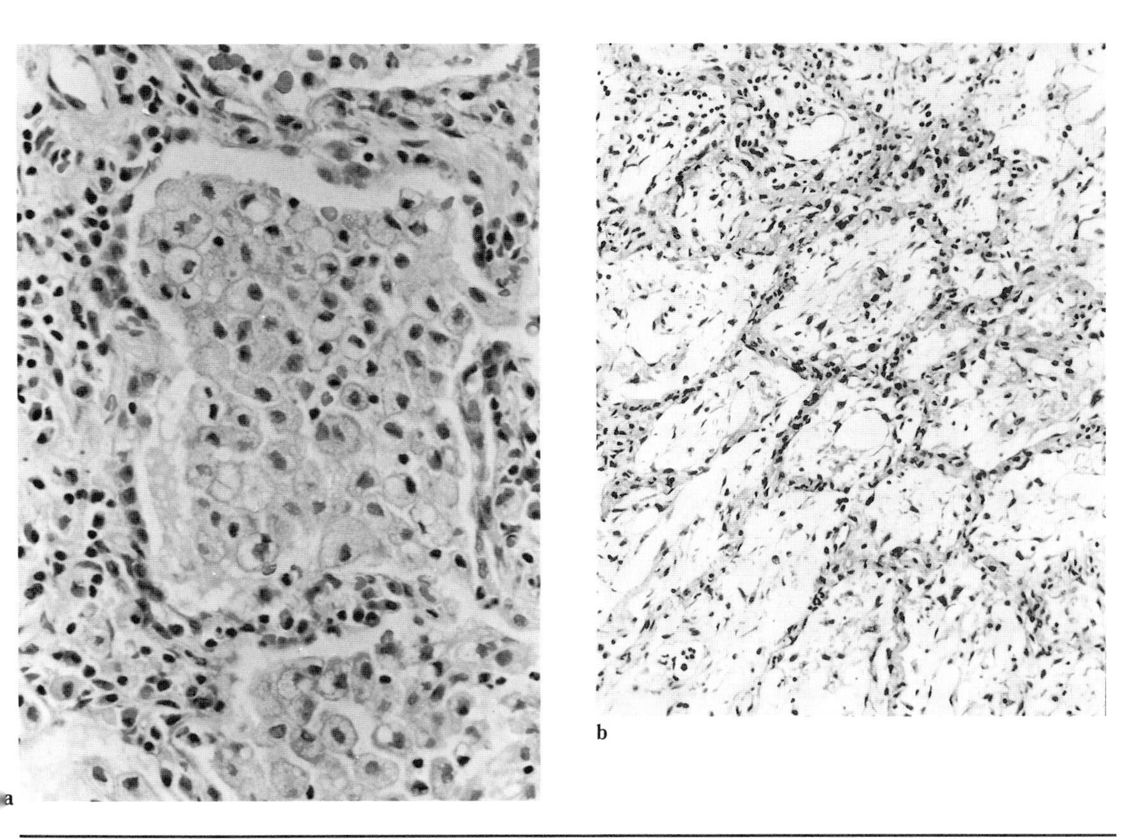

Fig. 13.36 Drug and toxin induced lung injury. **(a)** Amiodarone lung toxicity. The alveolar spaces contain large macrophages with abundant pale foamy cytoplasm. The alveolar walls are thickened and infiltrated by plasma cells, lymphocytes and scanty neutrophils. There is patchy cuboidal cell metaplasia of the alveolar epithelium. ×300. **(b)** Paraquat lung. The alveolar spaces are occupied by loose-textured cellular fibrous tissue; from a 31-year-old man who underwent lung transplantation 16 days after exposure to paraquat. ×120. (Section donated by Dr D. W. Chamberlain.)

The Carotid Bodies

These are small nodules of tissue, a few millimetres across, lying in the bifurcation of the common carotid artery. They receive their blood supply through the glomic arteries which usually arise from the bifurcation but sometimes from the internal or external carotid arteries. The carotid bodies are usually ovoid but may be double, bilobed or leaf-shaped. They comprise clusters of chief (type I) cells which contain dense-core granules in which are found the vasoactive peptides: leu- and met-enkephalins, substance P and vasoactive intestinal peptide (VIP). In contradistinction, bombesin is found around the glomic arteries. Biogenic amines such as dopamine, adrenaline and serotonin are also present. The clusters are surrounded by elongated (type II) cells which resemble Schwann cells.

Under certain circumstances such as chronic hypoxia in high-altitude natives, in chronic bronchitis and emphysema, in intracardiac shunts with reversal of flow, and in systemic hypertension, the carotid bodies enlarge so that their combined weight exceeds 30 mg (Fig. 13.37). With increasing age, in systemic hypertension and most not-

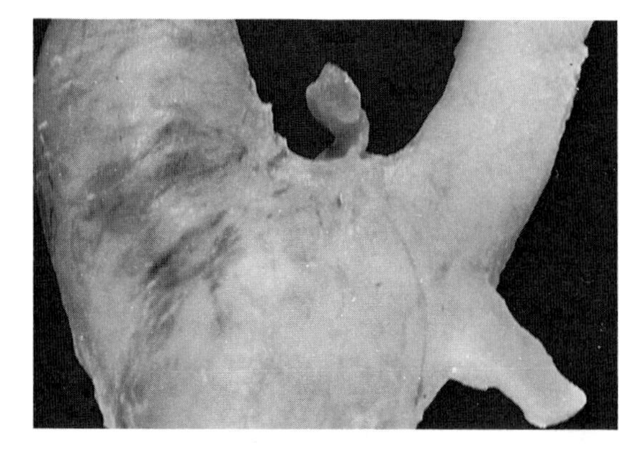

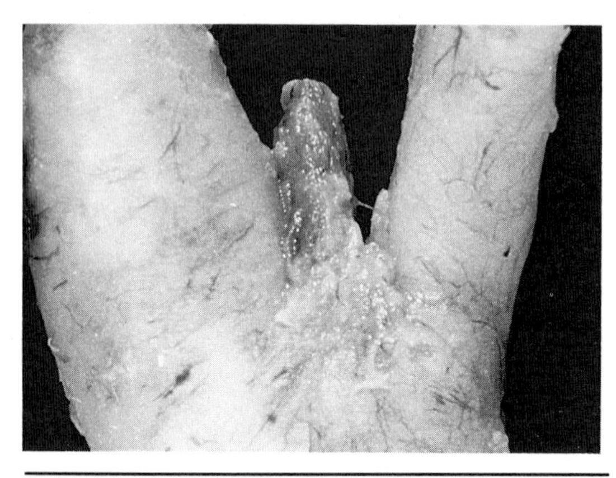

Fig. 13.37 The carotid body. Upper, the normal appearance (weight 10 mg). Lower, hyperplastic (weight 35 mg). From a 74-year-old man who died from chronic bronchitis and panacinar emphysema. Both ×3.

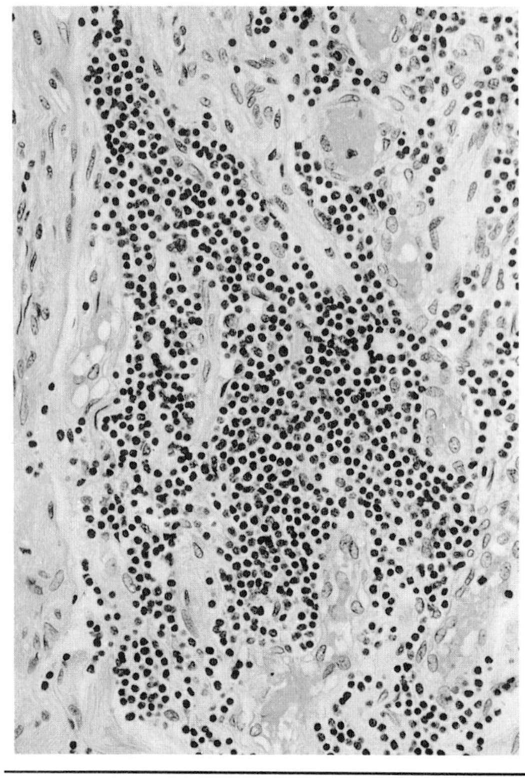

Fig. 13.38 Chronic carotid glomitis, comprising large focal aggregates of lymphocytes amongst the glomic tissue. From a 53-year-old man dying from a myocardial infarct. ×321. (Dr Q. Khan.)

ably in coarctation of the aorta there is proliferation of type II cells.

Over the age of 50 years a diffuse infiltrate of lymphocytes – chronic carotid glomitis – appears in the carotid bodies (Fig. 13.38), and is thought to be an autoimmune reaction to senescent nerve fibrils.

Chemodectoma of the carotid bodies is described on p. 480.

The Pleura

Pleural Effusion

Pleural effusions can be caused by diseases which interfere with the mechanisms that maintain the normal balance of entry and removal of water, electrolytes and protein into and out of the pleural cavity. The following are the more important causes.

1. *Increased intracapillary pressure* due to either left or right ventricular heart failure or an increased blood volume.

2. *Increased capillary permeability* due to pleural inflammation which in turn may be due to pneumonia, pulmonary tuberculosis, pulmonary infarction, connective tissue diseases, bronchial carcinoma, mesothelioma, subphrenic abscess and acute pancreatitis.

3. *Hypoproteinaemia* in patients with the nephrotic syndrome or cirrhosis of the liver.

4. *Impaired lymphatic drainage of the lung* in carcinomatous permeation of lymphatics and in neoplasms involving the hilum of the lung.

As with oedema fluid in general, pleural effusions may be rich in plasma proteins when they are due to increased capillary permeability, i.e. **inflammatory exudates**, or of low protein content when due to haemodynamic or osmotic disturbances or lymphatic obstruction, i.e. **transudates**. As elsewhere, inflammatory exudates may be serous, serofibrinous, purulent or haemorrhagic. The number and types of cell present will depend on the cause of the inflammation. A haemorrhagic exudate should always raise the suspicion of neoplastic infiltration, pulmonary infarction or tuberculosis.

Empyema or pyothorax is a collection of purulent exudate or pus in a pleural cavity. It may be due to infection of the pleura from the lung or occasionally from penetrating injuries of the chest wall. Less commonly infection of the pleura may arise from the bloodstream or through the diaphragm from abdominal disease such as a subphrenic abscess. In lung abscess, bronchiectasis and bronchial carcinoma, infection may extend into the pleural cavity and cause empyema. A post-pneumonic lung abscess may discharge simultaneously both into a bronchus and into the pleural cavity, resulting in a ***bronchopleural fistula*** and ***pyopneumothorax.*** Empyema may also result from perforation of the oesophagus and mediastinitis, and as a complication of thoracic surgery.

Haemothorax is a collection of blood in a pleural cavity. It may be due to trauma to the chest wall and lung, or result from rupture of an aortic aneurysm.

Chylothorax is the accumulation of an opalescent creamy fluid in the pleural cavity due to obstruction of, or injury to, the thoracic duct. Obstruction is commonly due to pressure exerted by enlarged mediastinal lymph nodes, while trauma may be accidental or a complication of thoracic surgery.

Pneumothorax

Pneumothorax is the presence of air in a pleural cavity. It causes the lung on that side to collapse to an extent depending on the volume of air admitted. Therapeutic pneumothorax was, at one time, used to deflate the lung in order to accelerate healing of pulmonary tuberculosis. Pneumothorax may be traumatic, or it may arise spontaneously due to the escape of air from the lung through a hole in the visceral pleura. Traumatic pneumothorax may be due to a penetrating injury of the chest wall or it may occur accidentally during the withdrawal of pleural fluid.

Primary or spontaneous pneumothorax occurs in the absence of any clinical evidence of underlying disease, most commonly in young males between the ages of 20 and 40 years. In some cases it is recurrent and rarely bilateral. Occasionally thoracotomy has revealed a tear in the visceral pleura at the site of attachment of a fibrous adhesion.

Secondary spontaneous pneumothorax occurs in patients who have evidence of underlying lung disease – most commonly emphysema, asthma or active pulmonary tuberculosis.

Once rupture of the lung surface has occurred, air continues to escape into the pleural cavity until the pressure gradient reaches zero or until the aperture is sealed by collapsing lung tissue. Occasionally, a valve-like mechanism occurs so that air enters the pleural cavity during inspiration but cannot escape during expiration: the pressure within the affected pleural cavity then steadily increases to produce a **tension pneumothorax** leading to mediastinal shift and compression of the opposite lung. In uncomplicated cases the pleura seals spontaneously and the air is gradually absorbed in a few weeks. Complications include pleural effusion, haemorrhage and infection.

Tumours of the Bronchi, Lungs and Pleura

Benign Tumours

The so-called **chondroma** or **adenochondroma** of the lung forms an ovoid, largely cartilaginous mass. It is usually discovered by chance on radiological examination. There is a discrete, rounded, mass-shadow which requires surgical intervention to exclude a bronchial carcinoma. These tumours consist of mature cartilage with clefts lined by flattened or respiratory type epithelium and with collections of adipose and fibrous tissue (Fig. 13.39). They are best regarded as hamartomas. **Fibromas** and **lipomas** rarely occur.

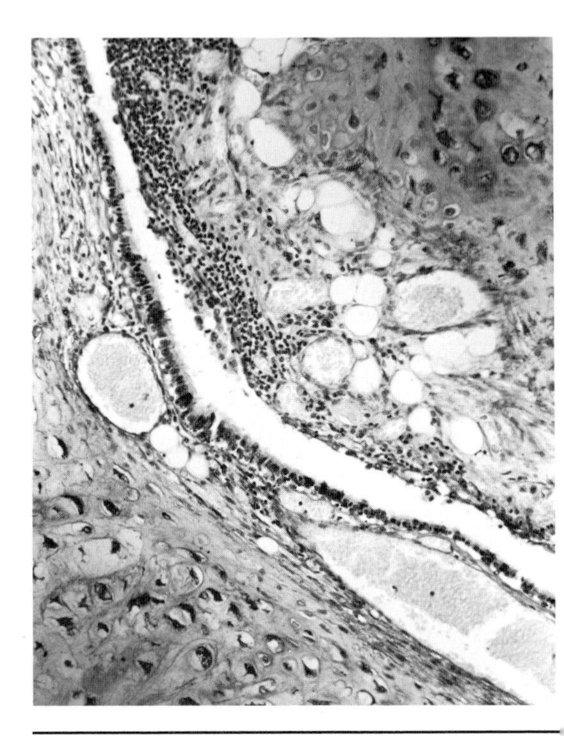

Fig. 13.39 Section of a cartilaginous hamartoma ('adenochondroma') of lung. This field shows an epithelial-lined space with cartilage on either side, some adipose tissue and blood vessels. ×50.

Malignant Tumours

Bronchial Carcinoma

This is the commonest primary tumour of the lung. It is now the commonest fatal cancer in men in many countries and in women is second only to cancer of the breast. Like other carcinomas, the incidence increases with age; it is most common between 40 and 70 years but some 2–3% of cases occur in younger patients.

Aetiology

The most important factor in the dramatic rise in the incidence of bronchial carcinoma is the habit of smoking, particularly cigarettes. The statistical risk of cancer increases proportionately to the number of cigarettes smoked. The smoking of cigars appears to be safer and the smoking of pipes safer still. In the UK, the habitual smoking of 25 cigarettes or more a day has been shown to be associated with a 12% risk of dying from bronchial carcinoma. In ex-cigarette smokers the risk gradually diminishes and after 10 years of abstinence it is not much greater than in non-smokers. The mode of action of cigarette smoke is uncertain. Analysis of the 'tar' from cigarette smoke reveals at least 18 hydrocarbons, 10 of which can induce carcinomas when applied to the shaven skin of small experimental animals. There is as yet no clear relationship between atmospheric pollution and the development of bronchial carcinoma, although the incidence is higher in non-smokers who live in cities, in which the atmosphere is polluted by carcinogens, than in those living in rural areas. Recent reports suggest that the incidence is also increased in the non-smoking spouses of cigarette smokers, i.e. due to 'passive smoking'.

There are other rarer but established causes of

bronchial carcinoma. These include work in the chromate industry, in haematite mining and with asbestos. Asbestos exposure is also associated with malignant mesothelioma; in contrast to mesothelioma, the risk of bronchial carcinoma is considerably increased in the asbestos worker who is a smoker, the two factors appearing to act synergistically.

Pathological Features

Macroscopically, bronchial carcinoma presents a variety of appearances depending upon the site of origin, the extent of local spread, and the degree of bronchial obstruction produced.

Usually the tumour forms a mass surrounding the main bronchus to the lung or to one lobe (Fig. 13.40 – *hilar type*. The bronchial mucosa may be ulcerated or may be merely roughened and nodular. Lymphatic spread often produces further nodules in the mucosa towards the bifurcation of the trachea. The carcinoma narrows the lumen of the affected bronchus, causing obstruction. Retention of secretions then occurs and is followed by infection with consequent bronchopneumonia and abscess formation. The tumour spreads by the lymphatics, giving rise to massive metastases in the mediastinal nodes, which are often enveloped in the tumour mass and cannot easily be distinguished. Extension to the lymph nodes of the neck is frequent. Retrograde spread occurs along the peribronchial and perivascular lymphatics so that even the smaller bronchi and vessels may be ensheathed by tumour. Permeation of lymphatics just beneath the visceral pleura produces a delicate white lacework pattern, visible on the external surface of the lung – *lymphangitis carcinomatosa*. Direct invasion of the pericardial sac may occur and the carcinoma may compress and occlude the superior vena cava, causing marked cyanosis. Infiltration of the heart is sometimes obvious on gross examination, and on careful histological examination of autopsy material it is found to be frequent.

Less frequently the tumour originates from a peripheral bronchus – *peripheral type*. Sometimes the exact site of origin is uncertain. These tumours are more likely to be adenocarcinomas, are less commonly associated with smoking, and are sometimes associated with areas of scarring (scar cancers).

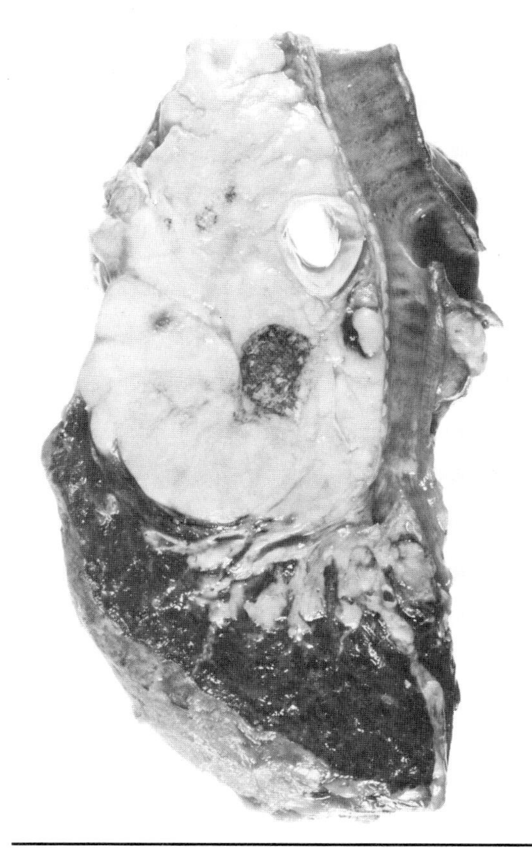

Fig. 13.40 Bronchial carcinoma. The main mass of tumour is at the hilum and has compressed and displaced the lung tissue. An enlarged lymph node, showing dust pigmentation and white flecks of tumour, lies within the mass. The major bronchi and pulmonary vessels are extensively infiltrated by tumour and appear thickened.

The Spread of Lung Cancer

Invasion of the lymphatics has been emphasized and this may involve the pleura, forming a thick ensheathment of the surfaces or as multiple discrete nodules. A haemorrhagic pleural effusion is common. When the tumour is at the apex of the lung, extension to the adjacent thoracic cage may involve the lower cords of the brachial plexus and the sympathetic chain, so that pain and sensory disturbances occur (*Pancoast's syndrome*).

Metastases may be widespread and may involve virtually any organ in the body. Spread may occur to the lymph nodes of the neck, axilla or groin, before the primary tumour presents localizing signs. Ipsilateral lymphatic spread to the adrenals is common.

There is a special tendency particularly of small cell types to metastasize in the brain, and this may overshadow the primary bronchial tumour clinically. Surgical exploration for a cerebral neoplasm should always be preceded by a careful survey of the lungs to exclude primary bronchial carcinoma. Metastases in liver and in the bones are common, the thoracic vertebrae being especially frequently involved, possibly by the retrograde venous route. It should be kept in mind that widespread metastasis may occur from a small and clinically silent bronchial carcinoma. Even at autopsy the primary tumour may be very difficult to find.

Associated Phenomena

Bronchial carcinoma may be associated with a number of paraneoplastic syndromes. *Neuropathy* and *myopathy* are mediated by humoral factors from the tumour. *Cushing's syndrome* with adrenal cortical hyperplasia is due to secretion of an ACTH-like hormone by tumours of small cell type. Other rare systemic effects of bronchial carcinoma are the *carcinoid syndrome, hypercalcaemia, hyponatraemia, encephalopathies, neuropathies, hypertrophic osteoarthropathy* and *gynaecomastia. Migrating phlebitis* and *gross lymphoedema* may also occur and may be the presenting symptoms.

Histological Types

Lung tumours are usually classified according to the criteria recommended by the World Health Organisation (1982). Histological classification is important because it has prognostic and therapeutic implications. There are four major histological types: squamous-cell carcinoma, (approximately 35–50% overall); small-cell carcinoma (20–30%); adenocarcinoma (15–30%); and large-cell carcinoma (10–15%). Sometimes a tumour may have a mixed histological pattern, e.g. squamous combined with small-cell, or adenocarcinoma. Squamous-cell carcinomas, adenocarcinomas and large-cell carcinomas are treated by surgical resection whenever there is a reasonable chance of complete removal; small-cell carcinomas are treated by radiotherapy and chemotherapy because metastases are almost always present by the time the diagnosis is made.

Squamous-cell carcinoma (Fig. 13.41) usually arises in a large bronchus near the hilum. These tumours are prone to massive necrosis and cavitation, especially after radiotherapy, and cause severe or fatal haemorrhage more frequently than any other lung cancer. They probably arise from bronchial epithelium which has undergone squamous metaplasia, areas of which are frequently seen in the bronchial mucosa of cigarette smokers and patients with chronic bronchitis. In about two-thirds of cases exfoliated malignant squamous cells can be identified in the sputum.

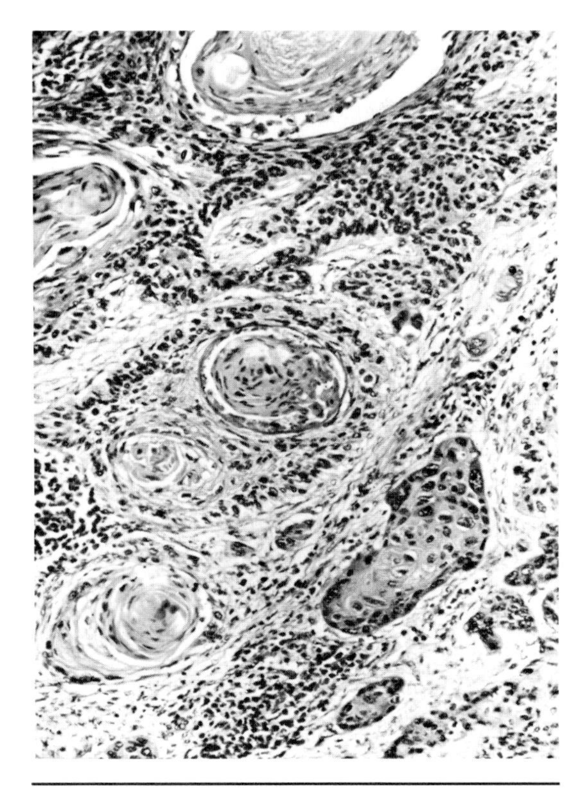

Fig. 13.41 Keratinizing squamous-cell carcinoma of bronchus with well developed cell nests. ×130. (From a section kindly loaned by Dr Whitwell.)

Small-cell carcinoma also commonly arises from a main bronchus in the hilum and malignant cells can be identified in the sputum in about two-thirds of cases. Small-cell carcinomas are derived from the pulmonary endocrine cells and this explains the endocrine syndromes commonly associated with them. Dense-core neuroendocrine granules can be seen in the tumour cells on electron microscopy. Three varieties of small-cell carcinoma are recognized but their biological behaviour and response to therapy are the same. All three types are highly cellular and stroma is usually scanty. The oat-cell carcinoma is composed of uniform small cells, generally larger than lymphocytes, with dense round or oval nuclei, diffuse chromatin, inconspicuous nucleoli, and very sparse cytoplasm (Fig. 13.42). Small-cell carcinoma, intermediate-cell type, is composed of small cells with nuclear characteristics similar to the oat cell but with more abundant cytoplasm. Combined oat-cell carcinoma is a tumour in which there is a definite component of oat-cell carcinoma with squamous cell and/or adenocarcinoma.

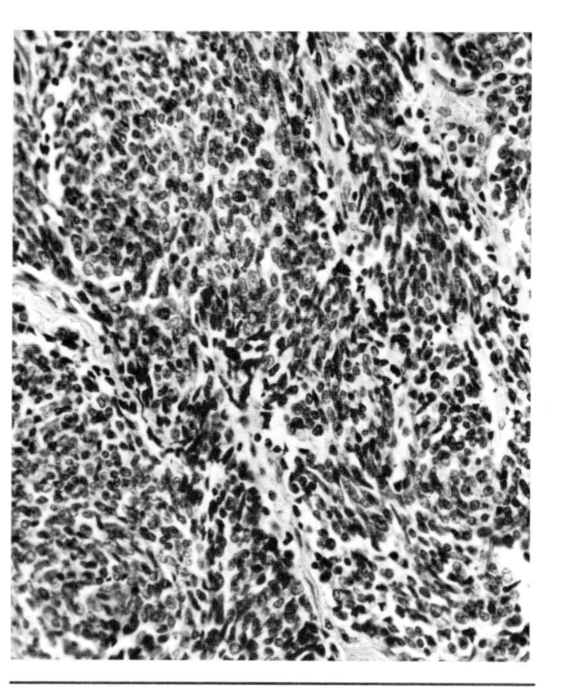

Fig. 13.42 Oat-cell carcinoma of bronchus. This neoplasm is composed of small, uniform, darkly staining ovoid cells, with scanty supporting stroma. ×115.

Adenocarcinoma. More than half of these tumours arise at peripheral sites within the lung, and malignant cells are detectable in the sputum in only about half the cases. They may be subclassified into acinar adenocarcinoma, papillary adenocarcinoma, bronchioloalveolar carcinoma and solid carcinoma with mucus formation. Bronchioloalveolar carcinoma is a type of mucus-secreting tumour in which cylindrical tumour cells grow along the walls of pre-existing alveoli (Fig. 13.43); they may produce a grey pneumonic mucoid appearance in the lung. Solid carcinoma is a poorly differentiated adenocarcinoma lacking structural differentiation, but with mucin-containing vacuoles in many of the cells. In reaching a diagnosis, special care must be taken to exclude metastasis from an adenocarcinoma in the gastrointestinal tract, pancreas or ovaries. Glandular variants which may include *cribriform (adenoid cystic)* and *mucoepidermoid* carcinomas

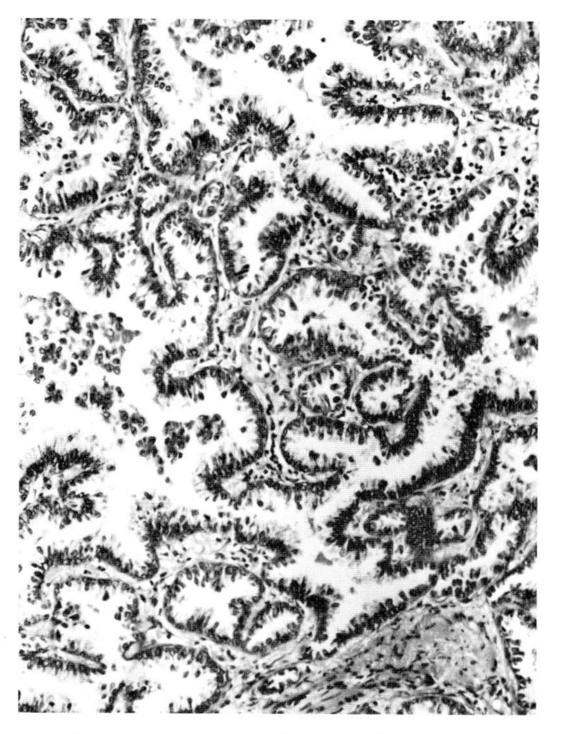

Fig. 13.43 Bronchioloalveolar carcinoma. The alveolar walls are lined by tall columnar neoplastic cells. ×125. (Section loaned by Dr F. Whitwell.)

are thought to arise from bronchial submucosal glands.

Large-cell carcinoma. This neoplasm is composed of cells with large nuclei, prominent nucleoli, abundant cytoplasm and usually well defined cell borders, without the characteristic features of squamous-cell, small-cell or adenocarcinomas. On electron microscopic examination they usually turn out to be poorly differentiated variants of squamous and adenocarcinoma.

Bronchial Carcinoids

The term 'bronchial adenoma' has, in the past, been erroneously applied to these tumours. They are slowly growing malignant tumours of which less than 10% may metastasize to local lymph nodes and to other organs such as liver. It is not possible to predict their prognosis on the basis of their histological appearance, but the 5-year survival is usually more than 80%. They comprise about 1% of tumours of the lung and they occur most commonly in people under the age of 40 years and with equal frequency in the sexes. Macroscopically, the tumour forms a 'dumb-bell' lesion, intraluminal growth being connected by a relatively narrow neck to invasive growth in the adjacent lung tissue. Endoscopic resection is therefore not practicable. The tumour sometimes causes haemoptysis and usually partial bronchial obstruction with bronchiectasis beyond. Histologically, they resemble the carcinoid tumours of the alimentary canal. About 50% show the argyrophil reaction and 20% show the argentaffin reaction (p. 729). They occasionally give rise to the carcinoid syndrome (p. 731). On electron microscopy, they show characteristic intracytoplasmic neurosecretory granules (Fig. 13.44). Bronchial carcinoids that show histological evidence of malignancy are classified as atypical. These atypical carcinoids comprise 10% of all bronchial carcinoids and metastasis may occur in over 70% of cases.

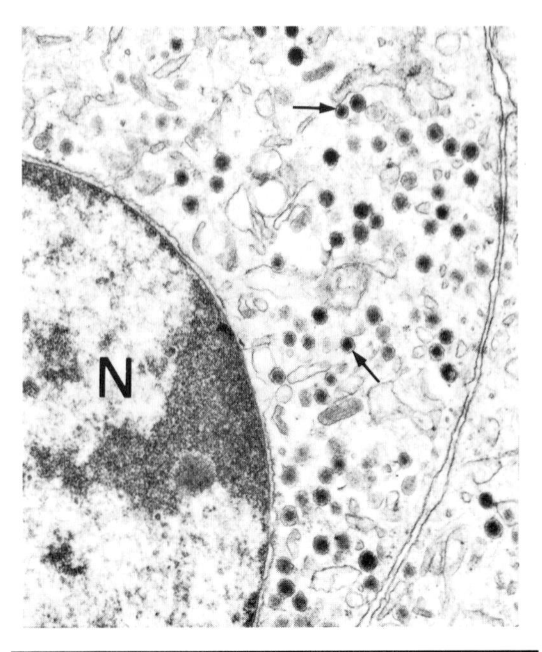

Fig. 13.44 Bronchial carcinoid tumour. Part of a neoplastic cell containing a nucleus (N) and numerous small electron-dense neurosecretory granules (arrows). ×18 750. (Dr W. Taylor.)

Secondary Tumours in the Lung

The lung is the great filter of the bloodstream so it is not surprising that a wide variety of tumours may give rise to pulmonary metastases. *Sarcomas* of all types commonly metastasize to the lung by the bloodstream. Spread of carcinoma to the lungs is also common both by the lymphatics and by the bloodstream. Spread by lymphatics is common in *breast carcinoma*, the tumour cells of which may spread to the pleural lymphatics and thence to the lungs. *Abdominal carcinomas* may spread to hilar lymph nodes and thus extend into the lung. When the lymphatics of the lung are involved, extensive cuffing of blood vessels and bronchi may result – *lymphangitis carcinomatosa.* Other metastatic tumours include *renal cell carcinoma, testicular tumours* and *lymphomas*.

Pleural Mesothelioma

Benign mesotheliomas are rare tumours, often called pleural fibromas, and they may attain a large size. There is no relationship to asbestos exposure. In contrast, in 1960 malignant mesothelioma was noted to be associated with occupational and environmental exposure to asbestos in South Africa. Only about 10–15% of the cases recorded in the UK appear to be unrelated to asbestos. On the other hand, the incidence of the tumour in people with industrial exposure to asbestos is very low. In cases of pleural mesothelioma, the duration of exposure to asbestos varies from as little as 3 months to 60 years. The degree of exposure is, however, likely to have been intense for at least part of the time. The latent period between exposure and the development of mesothelioma is very long, usually more than 20 years and sometimes more than 40. In asbestos workers who are also smokers, the tabacco smoking does not influence the risk of mesothelioma. The fibre type which has been most associated with mesothelioma is *crocidolite*. The source of exposure has usually been occupational but cases have occurred in people exposed to air pollution in the vicinity of asbestos mines and factories.

The tumour affects both the visceral and parietal layers of the pleura, leading to the formation of a layer of grey-white tissue 0.5–3 cm in the thickness, which obliterates the pleural cavity, ensheaths and compresses the lung, and extends into the interlobar fissures (Fig. 13.45). The histological picture presents a variable pattern with either carcinomatous or sarcomatous features or a mixture of the two. The carcinomatous pattern usually consists of tubular and papillary structures in a loose stroma. The sarcomatous pattern consists of spindle cells. Asbestos bodies are seen in the lungs but not in the tumour. Metastasis to hilar and abdominal lymph nodes is fairly common. Secondary deposits can also arise in the other lung, the liver, thyroid, adrenals, bone, skeletal muscle and brain.

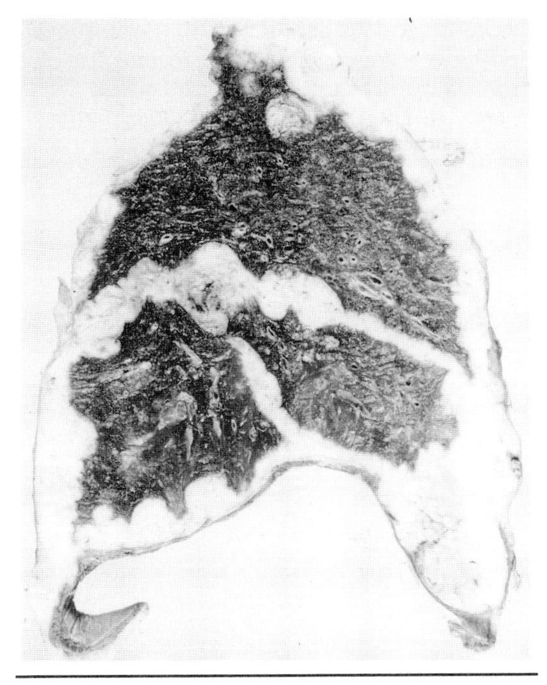

Fig. 13.45 Mesothelioma: note how the tumour (white) encases the lung tissue extending around the lobes and into the interlobar fissures.

Further Reading

Dail, D. H. and Hammar, S. P. (eds) (1988). *Pulmonary Pathology*, pp. 1200. Springer Verlag, New York.

Harris, P. and Heath, D. (1986). *The Human Pulmonary Circulation*, 3rd edn, pp. 702. Churchill Livingstone, Edinburgh.

Heath, D. and Smith, P. (1991). *Diseases of the Human Carotid Body*. Springer-Verlag, London.

Heath, D. and Williams, D. R. (1989). *High-altitude Medicine and Pathology*, pp. 352. Butterworths, London.

Katzenstein, A.-L. A. and Askin, F. B. (1990). *Surgical Pathology of Non-neoplastic Lung Disease*, 2nd edn, pp. 603, W. B. Saunders Company, London.

Spencer, H. (1984). *Pathology of the Lung*, 4th edn, pp. 1200. Pergamon Press, Oxford.

Thurlbeck, W. M. (ed.) (1988). *Pathology of the Lung*, pp. 832. Thieme Medical Publishers Inc., New York.

Wagenvoort, C. A. and Wagenvoort, N. (1977). *Pathology of Pulmonary Hypertension*, pp. 345. John Wiley & Sons, London.

14

The Blood and Bone Marrow

Introduction

This chapter is devoted to abnormalities of the red cells, leucocytes and platelets of the blood and to disorders in the production of the elements of the blood in the bone marrow. Lymphocytes are a component of the blood leucocytes; however, apart from the lymphocytic leukaemias, their disorders are considered in Chapter 6; the lymphomas which overlap in some aspects with the lymphocytic leukaemias are discussed in Chapter 15, which deals with diseases of the lymphoreticular system. These subdivisions are arbitrary and convenient, but the student should appreciate the considerable overlap which exists between disorders of the haemopoietic and lymphoid systems.

Haematological abnormalities are commonly encountered in medical practice. They may be primary, indicating disease in the blood-forming organs, or secondary, reflecting disease in another system. The latter occur more frequently. The ready accessibility of biopsy material, either venous blood or bone marrow, makes preliminary investigation of haematological disorders a straightforward exercise. As with other medical laboratory specialties, haematologists have taken advantage of developments in engineering and electronics to automate labour-intensive routine procedures; they have harnessed the data processing and communication capabilities of the computer. Furthermore, they are now capitalizing on the many recent developments in molecular biology.

Physical Features of Blood

Blood volume. The circulating blood volume in adult males is 5 litres, slightly less in females, and is related to lean body mass. Centrifugation of a column of venous blood in a narrow-bore glass tube shows that about 45% consists of cells (packed cell volume – PCV or venous haematocrit) and 55% of plasma. Accurate measurement of blood volume requires radioisotope dilution methods. Increase in the PCV results from a rise in the red cell mass (erythrocytosis) or a fall in plasma volume (haemoconcentration). Conversely, a decrease in PCV follows reduction in red cell mass (anaemia) or a rise in plasma volume (haemodilution).

Blood viscosity depends on the concentration of red cells and the protein content of the plasma. Increased blood viscosity, due to an increased PCV (e.g. polycythaemia), an increase in protein concentration (e.g. paraproteinaemia), a reduction in deformability of red cells (e.g. sickle cell disorders) or an increase in leucocytes (various leukaemias) may slow the blood flow and lead to thrombotic episodes.

Development of Blood Cells

Haemopoiesis first appears in the embryonic yolk sac at about 3 weeks. From about 6 weeks the liver becomes a haemopoietic organ and by 12 weeks is the major site, spleen, lymph nodes and thymus making minor contributions. Haemopoiesis starts in the marrow at 16–20 weeks and this becomes the main contributor by 30–36 weeks. Haemopoiesis in the liver diminishes, a few foci persisting until 1–2 weeks after birth; hepatic haemopoiesis is more prominent in premature infants and will persist in neonatal anaemic states, e.g. haemolytic disease of the newborn.

During childhood the marrow is normally the only source of new blood cells and all marrow is haemopoietic. Progressive replacement of haemopoietic (red) marrow by fatty (yellow) marrow occurs in late childhood, and by early adult life (16–18 years) red marrow is confined to the proximal ends of long bones, to vertebrae, ribs, sternum, pelvis and skull. With the exception of the skull these are the sites at which marrow aspiration or biopsy can be performed in adults. The tibial tubercle is the site of choice in infants.

Fatty marrow may revert to red marrow, an adaptive response to a need for increased production, e.g. compensatory erythroid hyperplasia in chronic haemolytic anaemia. The liver and spleen may also resume their fetal haemopoietic function in children with severe sustained anaemia such as the thalassaemias or in adults with myelofibrosis: this is termed extramedullary haemopoiesis.

Haemopoietic microenvironment. Haemopoiesis occurs in extravascular spaces within the marrow cavity but the mechanisms by which the mature cells enter the blood vessels are unclear. Granulocytes are motile and can probably migrate through the sinusoidal wall; megakaryocyte cytoplasmic processes project between endothelial cells, allowing release of platelets: but the mode of entry of the non-motile red cells is not known. The destruction of the sinusoidal architecture in myelofibrosis or following invasion by metastatic carcinoma cells may explain the frequent occurrence of circulating immature blood cells in these conditions, the leucoerythroblastic reaction.

The microenvironment in the bone marrow permits the proliferation and maturation of blood cell precursors and in this the marrow stroma is essential. The structural arrangements of the cells which constitute the marrow stroma – sinusoidal lining cells, fat cells and fibroblasts – are poorly understood. It is clear that the stroma produces haemopoietic stimulating growth factors which do not circulate. They act in a paracrine system for local effect and cannot be detected in the circulation. Erythropoietin may be detected in blood but is produced in the kidney. When marrow is ectopically transplanted, haemopoiesis is reconstituted only after the stroma has developed.

Haemopoietic Differentiation

All blood cells arise from a pluripotent stem cell. Haemopoietic stem cell proliferation maintains the stem cell pool (self-renewal) and provides precursors for all blood cells (differentiation). This is outlined in Fig. 14.1. The lymphopoietic stem cell gives rise to mature T and B lymphocytes which are capable of polyclonal expansion as part of an immune response (Chapter 3). The multipotent haemopoietic stem cell gives rise to erythroid, megakaryocytic and myelomonocytic committed stem cells whose progeny differentiate to produce the functional end cells, the erythrocytes, platelets, monocytes and granulocytes. Stem cells are capable of self-renewal but with lineage-specific commitment self-renewal becomes limited. The cells undergo differentiation and further proliferation leads to the production of functional end cells. They are end cells in that they have a finite lifespan. Therefore, normal or increased numbers of end cells arise by continuous replication of stem cells and their entry into the committed precursor cell pool. These functional roles, however, are extremely varied and in the inflammatory response, for example, the neutrophil function is regulated and can be modified by a number of factors.

Stem cells cannot be identified morphologically in the bone marrow. Their pluripotential nature was first demonstrated by experiments in which marrow cells from a normal mouse were injected intravenously into a mouse whose own haemopoietic cells had been destroyed by whole-body X-irradiation. The injected cells produced colonies of cells in the bone marrow and spleen and each colony was shown to arise from a single stem cell. If the cells of a single colony were injected into a second irradiated mouse they could also produce colonies indicating that they also contained stem cells. This technique provided a method of assay for pluripotent and multipotent stem cells expressed as colony forming units – spleen (CFU-S). Colony forming cells can also be obtained from human marrow and they have been investigated using *in vitro* gel cultures and long-term bone marrow culture techniques. As shown in Fig. 14.1 erythrocytes and megakaryocytes have a common stem cell (CFU-E/Mega) and similarly granulocytes and monocytes (CFU-G/M).

Haemopoietic cell differentiation is governed by programmes encoded in genomic DNA, triggered by signals transmitted to the nucleus via cell surface receptors for growth factors. A number of haemopoietic growth factors have been identified and it seems that these act in concert to control production of specific cell lines. Three broad groups exist: (1) multipotent factors, e.g. interleukin 3 (IL-3) which stimulates proliferation and differentiation of stem cells. Granulocyte macrophage colony stimulating factor (GM-CSF) is somewhat more restricted and promotes growth of macrophage, neutrophil and eosinophil precursors; (2) lineage restricted factors, e.g. granulocyte- and monocyte-colony stimulating factors (G-CSF and M-CSF respectively), which affect cells committed to a specific line of differentiation; and (3) lineage – promiscuous factors (e.g. various interleukins and transforming growth factor β) which act on relatively mature cells of one or more line. T lymphocytes and monocytes have a primary role in growth factor production as have stromal cells. Various interleukins can affect myeloid cell production. Erythropoietin is somewhat different to these growth factors as it is produced in the kidney and transported humorally to the marrow to stimulate terminal differentiation of erythroid precursor cells.

These growth factors have therapeutic application in restoring depressed haemopoietic activity. cDNAs of several factors have now been cloned and recombinant factors produced. The anaemia of renal failure has been corrected by recombinant erythropoietin and acceleration of bone marrow recovery following high-dose chemotherapy and autologous bone marrow transplantation has been produced by GM-CSF. Clinical trials suggest that

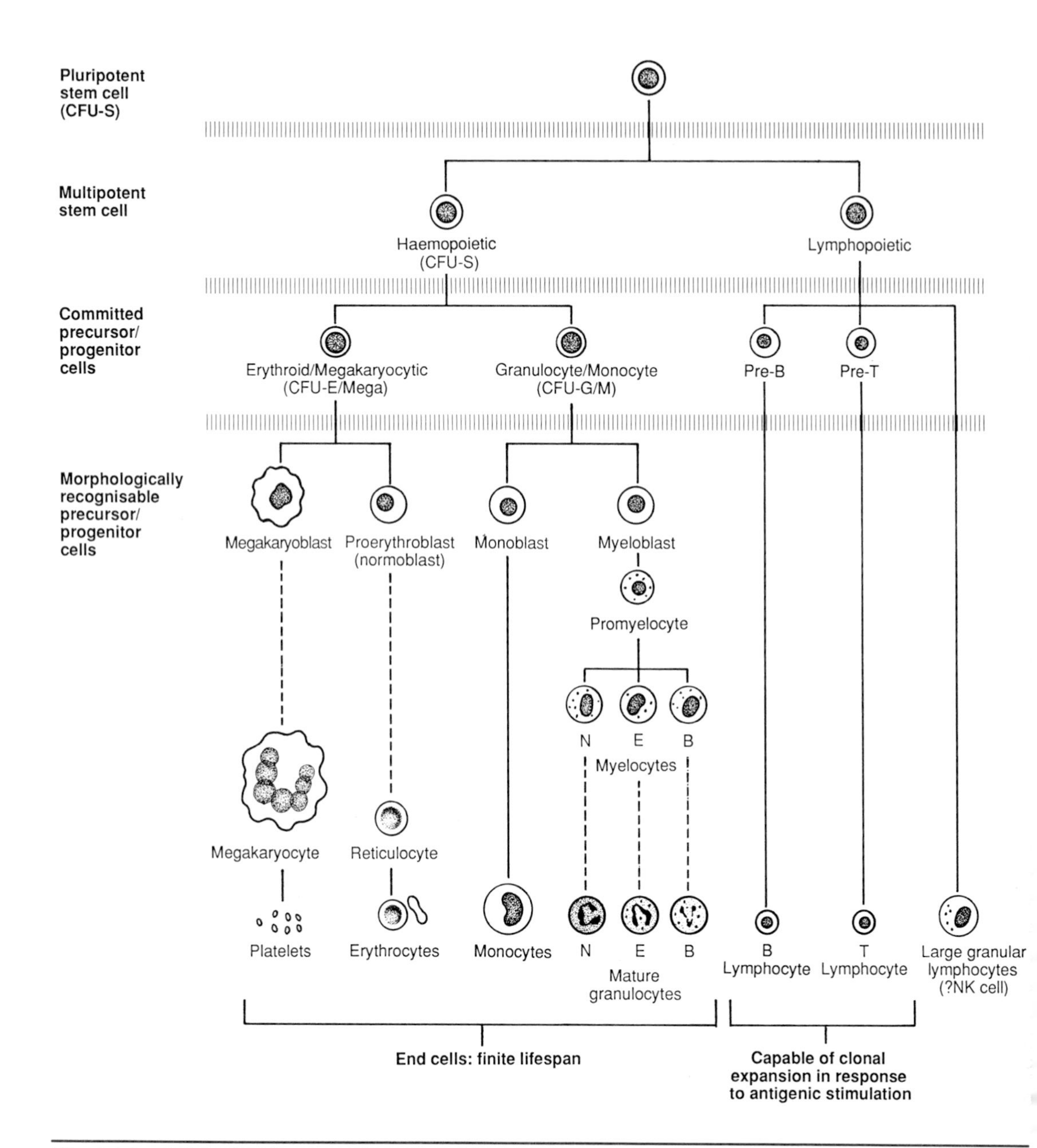

Fig. 14.1 This is a highly schematic outline of normal haemopoiesis. The maturation of the lymphopoietic cells is discussed in Chapter 5.

The haemopoietic system shows the early precursor cells and the mature (end) cells; the intervening cell types, showing the progressive maturation of the individual cell lines, is omitted. The pluripotent and multipotent cells can divide and produce colony forming units (CFU) in the spleen (S) or in long-term marrow cultures. The committed precursor/progenitor cells may also proliferate as colony forming units – erythroid/megakaryocytic (E/Mega) and granulocyte/monocyte (G/M). These cells also respond to growth factors (see text), colony stimulating factors (CSF), e.g. CSF-GM; erythropoietin is a key factor in the maturation of the erythrocyte series. The haemopoietic end cells have a finite lifespan but they are far from being end cells in terms of the functions they subserve. The lymphoid series are capable of clonal expansion and undergo further maturation before undertaking their functional roles; they also produce long-lived ('memory') cells.

GM-CSF or G-CSF may benefit patients with myelodysplastic syndromes (MDS) and aplastic anaemia. Thrombocytopenia may respond to IL-3. In relation to the use of growth factors in MDS it is interesting to note that the genes coding for IL-3, GM-CSF and M-CSF are all located on the long arm of chromosome 5 which in turn is the chromosome most frequently found to be abnormal in MDS. The role of growth factors in the myeloid leukaemias is still uncertain, as myeloid leukaemia cells also express receptors for growth factors which in theory may enhance leukaemic growth. Similar concerns relate to MDS cells and to the role of autocrine growth factor production by myeloid leukaemia cells to stimulate their own growth.

Bone Marrow Biopsy

The diagnosis of many blood disorders depends on microscopic examination of aspiration or trephine marrow biopsies. The overall marrow cellularity and the presence of specific blood cell precursors can be assessed. The ratio of haemopoietic cells to fat cells is normally 1:1; in marrow hypoplasia the proportion of fat cells is increased while increased haemopoietic cellularity characterizes the dyserythropoietic anaemias and the leukaemias. The normal ratio of myeloid to erythroid precursors ranges from 2.5:1 to 12:1 but this is almost invariably disturbed in the various anaemias and leukaemias. The normal marrow contains less than 3% plasma cells and less than 10% lymphocytes. Silver stains normally show only a few delicate reticulin fibres, but these increase dramatically in myelofibrosis. Evaluation of marrow iron is done using the Prussian blue reaction (Perls' stain): some 40% of normoblasts contain haemosiderin granules, so-called sideroblasts. Increased numbers of sideroblasts occur whenever haem or globin synthesis is depressed and progressive increase in iron within mitochondria produces ring sideroblasts (p. 619). Absence of stainable iron in the marrow indicates iron deficiency.

The proportion of cells in mitosis, normally 1–2%, gives an indication of overall haemopoietic activity. Radioisotopically labelled compounds can be used for detailed evaluation of marrow function: tritium-labelled thymidine for overall activity, ^{52}Fe or ^{59}Fe for assessment of erythropoiesis and ^{99m}Tc-labelled colloid for monocyte-macrophage function.

Erythrocytes

Erythropoiesis

Normal red cell maturation (normoblastic erythropoiesis) involves (1) diminution of cell size, (2) reduction in nuclear size, condensation of chromatin and eventual extrusion, (3) loss of cytoplasmic RNA and (4) concurrent production of haemoglobin (Fig. 14.2). Three mitotic divisions occur between the pro-normoblast and late normoblast, each intermitotic interval lasting 16 hours. Shortening of the intermitotic interval with normal maturation produces increased numbers of red cells, e.g. after haemorrhage or in haemolytic anaemia. Reduction in the number of mitoses results in red cells which are larger than normal (macrocytes), e.g. in megaloblastic anaemia, whilst increase in the number results in smaller red cells (microcytes), e.g. in iron deficiency anaemia.

The **reticulocyte** is the immature red cell following extrusion of the nucleus. Maturation to an erythrocyte takes 48–72 hours, the final 24 hours being in the peripheral circulation. Reticulocytes contain polyribosomes, RNA and mitochondria and can synthesize haemoglobin. This explains the diffuse basophilia (polychromasia) with Romanowsky staining. Reticulocytes can be counted after staining with supravital dyes such as azure B or cresyl blue (Fig. 14.3). However, this method is being replaced by flow cytometry techniques using RNA stains coupled to fluorophores. The reticulocyte count is usually expressed as a percentage of the total red cell count (adult reference range 0.5–2.0%), but the absolute count is more informative (adult reference range 25–75 × 10^9/l). The reticulocyte

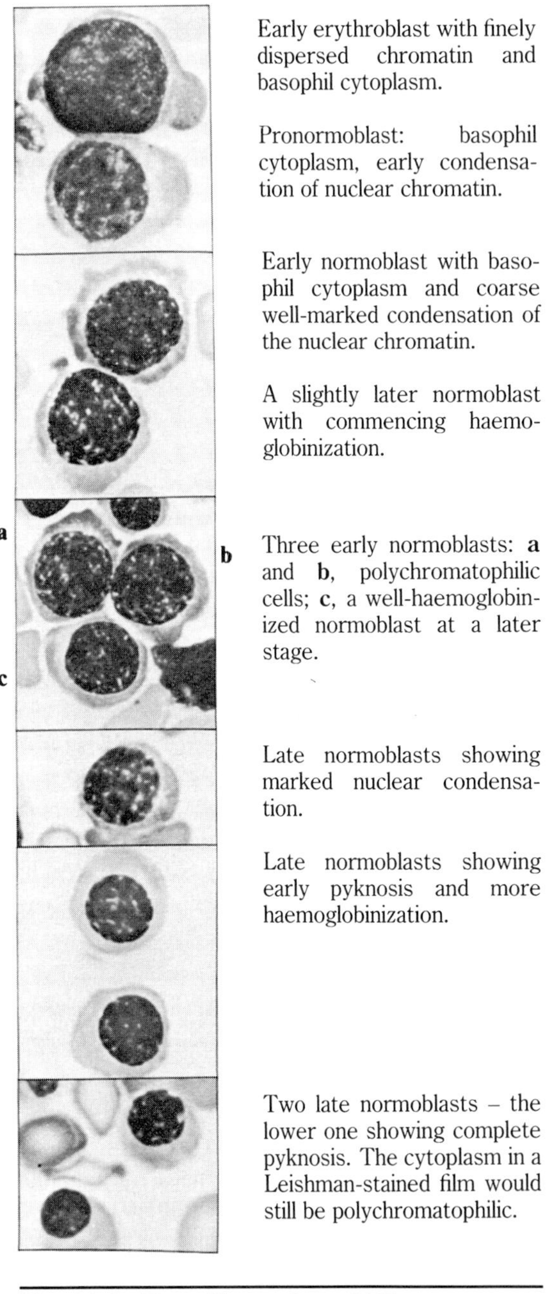

Fig. 14.2 Normoblast series. ×1000.

count is a useful measure of erythropoietic activity. It rises following haemorrhage, during haemolysis and in response to haematinic therapy.

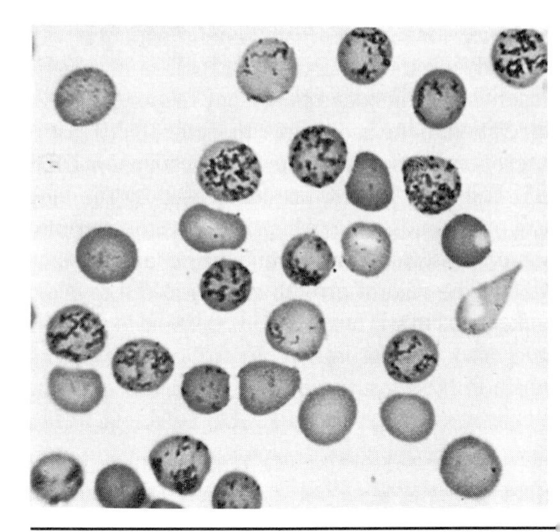

Fig. 14.3 Blood smear in haemolytic anaemia, showing numerous reticulocytes containing varying amounts of reticulum. Supravital staining with cresyl blue. ×100.

The count is reduced when there is marrow failure or ineffective erythropoiesis; the reappearance of reticulocytes is an indicator of marrow recovery.

The growth factors which affect erythropoiesis have already been mentioned. **Erythropoietin** is responsible for the fine control of erythropoiesis and determines the rate at which the erythroid precursor cell (CFU-E) gives rise to normoblasts. It is produced in the kidney in response to hypoxia: small amounts are also produced by the liver and spleen. It controls the rate at which normoblasts are produced and also influences the rate of cell maturation, haemoglobin synthesis and the release of red cells into the circulation. Thyroxine, growth hormone and androgens stimulate red cell production by increasing erythropoietin production.

In addition to the reticulocyte count, an estimate of the myeloid: erythroid ratio in a marrow biopsy gives an assessment of erythropoietic activity. However, in order to assess the effectiveness of marrow function, ferrokinetic studies following an injected dose of radioactive iron are required. From the plasma iron clearance (i.e. the rate of clearance of transferrin-bound iron from the

Table 14.1 Normal adult red cell values expressed as mean ± two standard deviations

	RBC ($\times 10^{12}$/l)	PCV (l/l)	Hb (g/dl)*
Male	5.5 ± 1.0	0.47 ± 0.07	15.5 ± 2.5
Female	4.8 ± 1.0	0.42 ± 0.05	14.0 ± 2.5

*WHO recommends expression of haemoglobin concentration in g/l.

plasma) and the plasma iron content, it is possible to calculate the plasma iron turnover (normally 72–144 μmol/l/day). Plasma iron turnover reflects the total amount of erythropoietic tissue, both effective and ineffective. Reappearance of radioactive iron in circulating red cells is an indicator of effective erythropoiesis. Normally 70–80% of administered iron is so used and can be detected 7–9 days after injection. The sites of erythropoiesis may be demonstrated by surface counting radioactivity over the spleen, liver and sacrum.

Features of the Red Cells

The primary red cell measurements include the *red cell count (RBC), packed cell volume (PCV)* and *haemoglobin concentration (Hb).* The reference range for each measurement is given in Table 14.1. For any individual, fluctuations occur within these ranges. The ranges vary with age and sex and are affected by atmospheric pressure, increasing with height above sea level.

A quantitative assessment of red cell size and haemoglobin content can be made using the primary red cell measurements to obtain estimates of average volume of red cells (*mean cell volume – MCV)*; average weight of haemoglobin in each cell (*mean cell haemoglobin – MCH)*, and average concentration of haemoglobin in each cell (*mean cell haemoglobin concentration – MCHC)*. MCV is calculated by dividing PCV (l/l) by RBC ($\times 10^{12}$/l), and is expressed in femtolitres (fl). MCH is derived by dividing Hb in g/l by RBC ($\times 10^{12}$/l), and is expressed in picograms (pg). MCHC is obtained by dividing Hb (g/dl) by PCV (l/l) and is expressed in g/dl. The adult reference ranges are shown in Table 14.2. These red cell indices are not influenced by age, sex or altitude. They are now all measured using automated electronic counters. The degree of accuracy of red cell counting makes the MCV and MCH prime diagnostic measurements in the morphological classification of anaemia (Table 14.3). With automated analysis the range of MCHC narrows to 30–36 g/dl and this limits its diagnostic usefulness.

Table 14.2 Red cell indices: reference range for healthy adults

Mean cell volume (MCV)	80–100 fl
Mean cell haemoglobin (MCH)	27–32 pg
Mean cell haemoglobin concentration (MCHC)	30–36 g/dl

Red cells in an individual are not uniform in volume, but exhibit a range. The determination of 'average' volume (MCV) gives useful information in cases of major abnormality, but it is insensitive to minor variations at extremes of the range and it is incapable of detecting more than one population of cells. Using automated cell counters volume distribution may be displayed graphically or numerically (standard deviation or coefficient of variation). The *red cell distribution width (RDW)*, reflects the variation in cell volume and is a measure of anisocytosis: it is increased in iron deficiency and megaloblastic anaemias (Fig. 14.4).

Table 14.3 Morphological classification of anaemia

	Red cell indices	
	MCV	MCH
Normochromic/normocytic	Normal	Normal
Hypochromic/microcytic	Low	Low
Normochromic/macrocytic	High	Normal

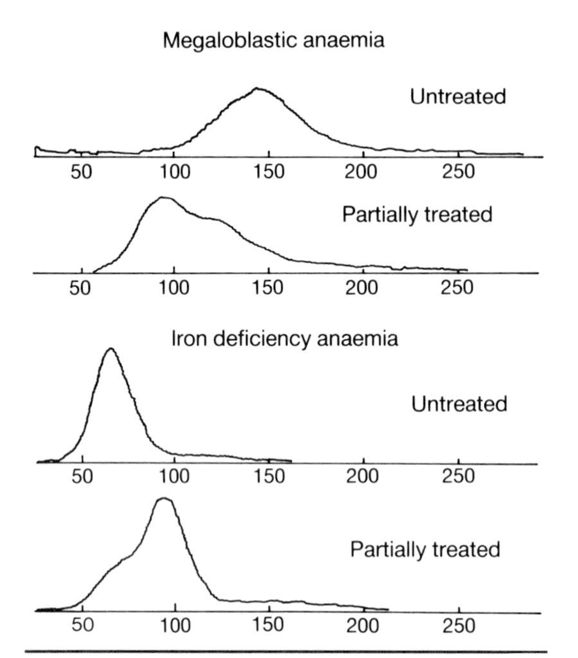

Fig. 14.4 Red cell volume (fl) distributions in untreated and partly treated megaloblastic anaemia (above) and untreated and partly treated iron deficiency anaemia (below).

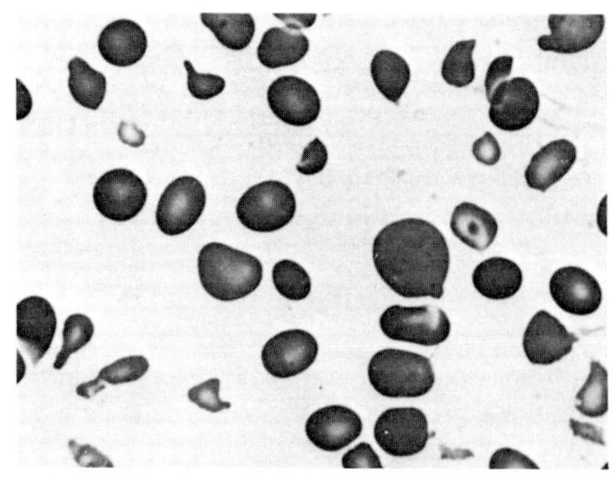

Fig. 14.5 Red cells in pernicious anaemia, prepared from below the buffy coat, showing gross aniso-poikilocytosis. ×650.

Morphological Changes in Red Cells

In health, red cells vary little in size and shape. They are biconcave discs with an average diameter of 7.0 μm (range 6.0–8.5 μm). The diameter of the small lymphatic nucleus serves as a gauge on microscopy. Because of the bioconcavity, red cells stain more heavily at the periphery. Central pallor should not exceed one-third of the red cell area (normochromia).

Changes in size and shape. Anaemia is often associated with variation in erythrocyte size (anisocytosis) and irregularities in shape (poikilocytosis). Abnormally large cells, macrocytes, are numerous in megaloblastic anaemia, aplastic anaemia and liver disease. Small red cells occur typically in iron-deficiency anaemia and thalassaemia – microcytic anaemia. Poikilocytes occur in any severe anaemia (Fig. 14.5) but are prominent in megaloblastic anaemia. Mechanical injury to red cells in microangiopathic haemolytic anaemia results in red cell fragmentation (Fig. 14.6). In spherocytosis red cells assume a globular shape, are reduced in diameter and are uniformly densely stained. Other shape changes include sickle cells associated with haemoglobin S (p. 605), rod cells (p. 618) found in iron deficiency,

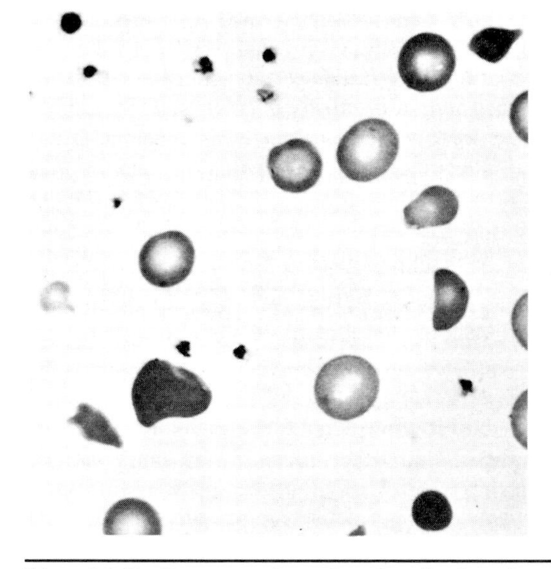

Fig. 14.6 Fragmentation of red cells in microangiopathic haemolytic anaemia. ×1000.

thalassaemia and liver disease and oval cells in hereditary elliptocytosis (p. 602).

In hypochromia or 'ring-staining' (see Fig. 14.26) the red cells show staining only at their periphery. Iron deficiency is the most common cause but this may also occur in sideroblastic anaemia, anaemias of chronic infection and in thalassaemia (defective globin synthesis). Red cell dimorphism describes a mixture of normochromic and hypochromic red cells and is seen in iron deficiency anaemia responding to treatment, following transfusion of normal cells to a patient with a hypochromic anaemia, and in sideroblastic anaemia.

Red cell inclusion bodies. Some are vestiges of cell elements normally lost during maturation and others are due to pathological change. Macrophages in the spleen normally remove inclusions without destroying the red cells, a process which takes place in the red pulp and is referred to as pitting. If the spleen has been removed or is atrophic, cells with inclusions circulate in large numbers. *Pappeneheimer bodies* are small (1 μm diameter) deeply basophilic granules giving a Prussian blue reaction for ferric iron and correspond to the iron granules seen in marrow sideroblasts. *Howell–Jolly bodies* are granules of nuclear chromatin, 1–2 μm or more in diameter (see Fig. 14.22) and occur most commonly in megaloblastic and haemolytic anaemias. *Heinz bodies* are demonstrated by supravital staining (see Fig. 14.14). They consist of denatured globin, and occur in the haemoglobinopathies and in chemically induced haemolytic anaemia. A few Heinz bodies are seen following splenectomy. *Punctate basophilia* describes clumps of RNA seen as minute blue granules on Romanowsky staining (Fig. 14.7) and occurs in infection, chronic lead poisoning, drug and chemical induced haemolytic anaemia, and myelodysplastic syndromes.

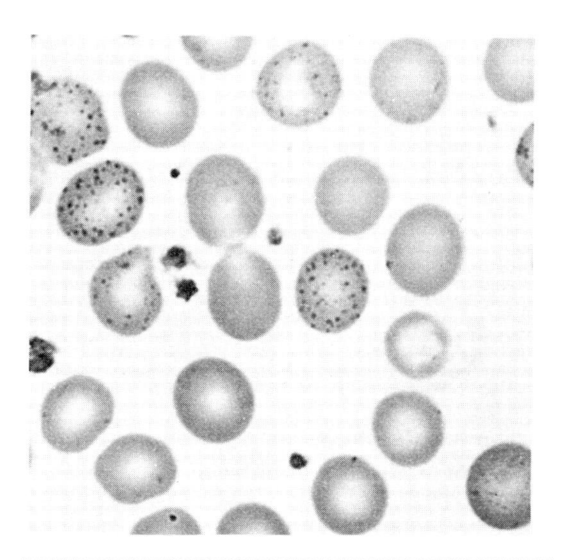

Fig. 14.7 Blood smear showing punctate basophilia ×1250.

Erythrocytosis

Chronic hypoxia (e.g. chronic respiratory or cardiac failure, congenital heart disease, living at high altitude) stimulates erythropoietin production with consequent elevation of RBC (erythrocytosis). This is often inappropriately called secondary 'polycythaemia', which implies increase in all formed elements. Only red cells are increased in erythrocytosis and when due to hypoxia it is compensatory. Rarely, erythrocytosis results from increased formation of erythropoietin by certain tumours, most commonly renal carcinoma, or by cystic lesions or ischaemia of the kidney.

Leucocytes

The three main classes of leucocyte in the blood, granulocytes, monocytes and lymphocytes, differ in lineage, morphology and function. Increase or decrease of leucocytes in disease can affect any or all of the different types. Increase in total number above 11 × 10^9/l is leucocytosis while diminution below 4 × 10^9/l is leucopenia. The differential leucocyte count on stained blood films is a useful diagnostic procedure. Reference ranges in adults are shown in Table 14.4. The advantage of deter-

Table 14.4 Reference range for white cell count (WBC) and differential in healthy adults ($\times 10^9$/l)

White cell count (WBC)	4.0–11.0
Granulocytes	
Neutrophils	2.5–7.5
Eosinophils	0.04–0.44
Basophils	0–0.1
Lymphocytes	1.5–3.5
Monocytes	0.2–0.8

mining the absolute rather than the proportional number for each class must be stressed.

Neutrophil Granulocytes

Neutrophil Leucocytosis

The commonest cause of neutrophil leucocytosis is bacterial infection, usually in the range of 15–25 $\times 10^9$/l, but occasionally up to 50 $\times 10^9$/l. Moderate increase may also occur in connective tissue diseases and accompany tissue necrosis, e.g. in myocardial infarction, burns and with rapidly growing tumours undergoing ischaemic necrosis. Transient neutrophil leucocytosis develops within a few hours of major haemorrhage and in acute haemolysis. In very severe infection and toxic states, the neutrophil nuclei may fail to segment and the cytoplasm may contain deeply staining coarse azurophilic granules of variable size (toxic granulations).

In bacterial infection immature forms, metamyelocytes or myelocytes may be found in the circulation. An exaggerated form of this with circulating myeloblasts, a **leukaemoid reaction**, may mimic leukaemia. A leukaemoid reaction may also occur with severe haemolysis and as a paraneoplastic reaction to some tumours. The neutrophil alkaline phosphatase score is high, however, in contrast to chronic granulocytic leukaemia.

A leucoerythroblastic reaction comprises circulating immature granulocytes accompanied by nucleated red cells, erythroblasts. It may occur in patients with massive haemorrhage, severe haemolysis, acute hypoxia or severe infection, but also occurs where there is bone marrow replacement, e.g. by metastatic tumour or in myelofibrosis.

Neutrophil Leucopenia (Neutropenia)

This occurs as an isolated event or with reduction of all cell types (pancytopenia). Neutropenia results from failure of marrow production or from excessive peripheral destruction or consumption; the causes are summarized in Table 14.5. The term **agranulocytosis** refers to severe neutropenia which predisposes to infections with pathogenic or commensal organisms. These infections frequently involve the mouth and oropharynx producing widespread necrotizing ulceration. Cutaneous, perianal and vaginal lesions may also occur. It is most commonly seen in drug-induced neutropenia.

A large number of drugs cause neutropenia, and this may be the result of depressed granulopoiesis or accelerated granulocytic destruction. Some drugs, e.g. cytotoxic drugs used to treat malignant disease, cause predictable marrow depression

Table 14.5 Causes of neutropenia

Depression of granulopoiesis
- Marrow hypoplasia/aplasia (p. 619)
  - Idiopathic
  - Acquired, e.g. irradiation, drugs
- Marrow replacement syndromes
- Megaloblastic anaemia (p. 612)
- Overwhelming infection, e.g. septicaemia, miliary tuberculosis

Accelerated or excessive destruction of neutrophils
- Immunologically mediated
  - Drug induced
  - Autoimmune neutropenia
- Hypersplenism

Miscellaneous
- Some infections, e.g. typhoid fever; infectious mononucleosis, HIV and other viruses
- Connective tissue diseases, e.g. systemic lupus erythematosus
- Genetic: congenital agranulocytosis, cyclical neutropenia

With others the reaction is idiosyncratic; the most important include, for example, phenylbutazone, chlorpromazine and other phenothiazines, sulphonamides, frusemide and antithyroid drugs. These may cause marrow depression or may act as haptens, attach to neutrophil membranes and provoke an immunological reaction. In autoimmune neutropenia circulating antibodies to granulocytes are present.

Functional Disorders of Neutrophils

The capacity of the neutrophil to combat infection depends on its response to chemotactic stimuli, its ability to recognize and phagocytose microorganisms and its ability to destroy these organisms intracellularly. Neutrophils use a number of compounds generated by the partial reduction of oxygen to achieve bacterial killing. The metabolic pathway that forms these compounds is known as 'respiratory burst' which leads to increased oxygen uptake, superoxide (O_2^-) production, H_2O_2 formation and hexose monophosphate shunt activity. The potency of H_2O_2 to effect bacterial killing is augmented by the enzyme myeloperoxidase together with halide (Cl^-) ions.

The aetiologies of functional disorders of neutrophils are summarized in Table 14.6. Defects in each of these and their aetiology are summarized in Table 14.6. Defects of chemotaxis and opsonization are discussed in relation to the acute inflammatory response (Chapter 4). Glucocorticoid therapy impairs neutrophil locomotion and ingestion and is one of the common causes of neutrophil dysfunction.

The Chediak–Higashi syndrome is a rare autosomal recessive disorder characterized by defective skin pigmentation, neuropathy, frequent bacterial infections and an increased risk of developing lymphomas. The neutrophil count is low and they contain giant lysosomes. There are a number of defects of neutrophil function including impaired chemotactic responsiveness, phagocytosis and bacterial killing.

Chronic granulomatous disease of childhood. The more common mode of inheritance is X-linked. It may also occur as an autosomal recessive; approximately 20% of patients are female. Affected individuals suffer from recurrent protracted infections in skin, bones, liver and many viscera with extensive granuloma formation; death occurs at an early age. There is deficient hydrogen peroxide (H_2O_2) formation with an inability to destroy catalase producing organisms such as *Staphylococcus aureus*. The defect can be demonstrated *in vitro* by the failure of neutrophils to reduce nitroblue tetrazolium (NBT) dye.

Table 14.6 Functional disorders of neutrophils

Predominant abnormal function*	Causes
Locomotor	Lazy leucocyte syndrome Diabetes mellitus, corticosteroids, renal failure, alcoholism Chediak–Higashi syndrome
Recognition and phagocytosis	Complement and antibody deficiency states; severe malnutrition; immune complex diseases, e.g. rheumatoid arthritis; glomerulonephritis
Bacterial killing	Chronic granulomatous disease Iron deficiency

*There may be some overlap between the functional loss due to these causes.

Miscellaneous Morphological Abnormalities of Neutrophils

The presence of toxic granulations in severe infections has already been mentioned. *Döhle bodies* are intracytoplasmic inclusions in mature neutrophils thought to be ribosome-containing remnants of promyelocyte cytoplasm. These are found in pregnancy and in association with severe infection, burns and tumours. They also occur in the May–Hegglin anomaly in which there are giant platelets and a mild functional bleeding disorder.

Hypersegmented neutrophils, *macropolycytes*, sometimes with more than five lobes, occur in megaloblastic anaemia and in uraemia. The *Pelger-Huët* anomaly is a rare inherited, clinically silent defect, characterized by failure of nuclear segmentation: in heterozygous individuals most mature neutrophils are bilobed. An acquired similar disorder known as the pseudo-Pelger change occurs in myelodysplastic syndromes and various infections.

Eosinophil Granulocytes

Increased numbers of eosinophils (eosinophilia) occurs: (1) in parasitic infections where the level may exceed $3 \times 10^9/l$; (2) in association with a number of type I hypersensitivity reactions, e.g. asthma, skin diseases, drug-induced: (3) in the hypereosinophilic syndromes, e.g. Loeffler's syndrome (p. 560); (4) in association with malignancy, e.g. in granulocytic leukaemias and Hodgkin's disease. A fall in the eosinophil count occurs in response to excess circulating glucocorticoids.

Basophil Granulocytes

Increased numbers of basophils may occur in chronic granulocytic leukaemia and the chronic myeloproliferative syndromes and this may be of diagnostic value. A basophilia may rarely be found in myxoedema and even less frequently in chickenpox or chronic ulcerative colitis.

Lymphocytes

Lymphopoiesis and the immunological functions of lymphocytes are described in Chapter 3. Lymphocytes account for a higher proportion of total leucocytes in young children than in adults. The number is highest after birth, due to increasing antigenic experience at this time, and gradually falls in subsequent years. Lymphocytosis occurs in whooping cough, and may rise to $100 \times 10^9/l$. Lymphocytosis also occurs in virus infections, particularly infectious mononucleosis in which the cells are large and of abnormal appearance. Although B (and not T) lymphocytes carry the receptor for Epstein–Barr virus the atypical lymphocytosis in infectious mononucleosis has been identified as a reactive T (CD8+) response. Other infections characterized by lymphocytosis include typhoid and paratyphoid fevers, brucellosis, influenza, secondary syphilis, toxoplasmosis and cytomegalovirus infections. High lymphocyte counts are also seen in acute infective lymphocytosis of young children. The major cause of gross lymphocytosis is chronic lymphocytic leukaemia.

Lymphopenia is normal in the elderly and is often a feature in connective tissue diseases, in marrow hypoplasia and rarely in acute infections. In infancy, reduced B cell and/or T cell counts are features of some of the immunological deficiency syndromes (p. 237) and a selective CD4 + T cell lymphopenia characterizes HIV infection (p. 243). Severe lymphopenia results also from irradiation and the use of cytotoxic drugs, including glucocorticoids.

Monocytes

Monocytes (Fig. 14.8) are circulating cells of the mononuclear-phagocyte system. When stimulated, they enlarge, show increased motility and metabolic activity and become macrophages.

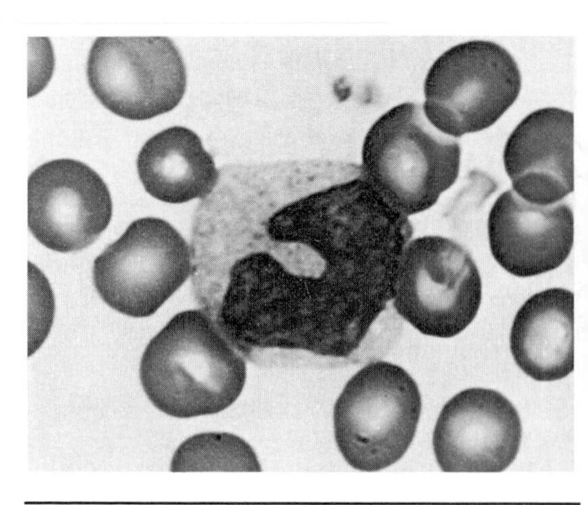

Fig. 14.8 Monocyte in a blood smear. ×1250.

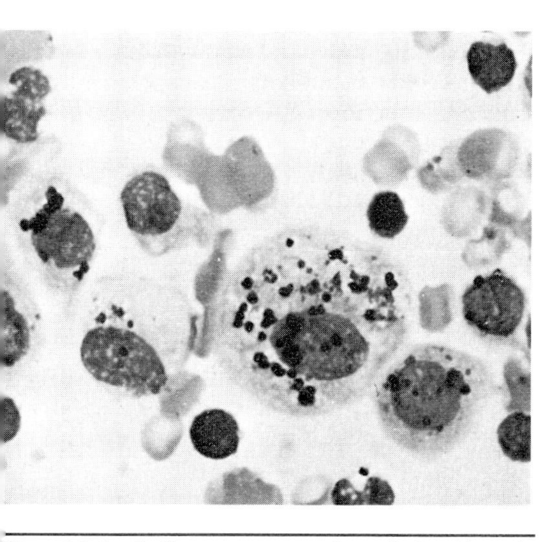

Fig. 14.9 Buffy coat preparation of the blood in malaria, showing monocytes containing pigment. ×680.

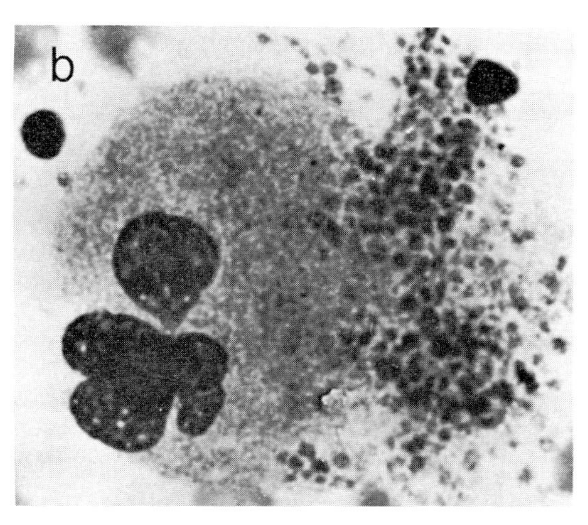

Fig. 14.10 Megakaryocyte cell showing partial conversion of the cytoplasm to platelets. ×600.

Their roles in the inflammatory response (Chapter 5) and in the immune response (Chapter 3) have already been discussed. A peripheral blood monocytosis occurs in subacute infective endocarditis, in brucellosis, tuberculosis, typhus and other rickettsial diseases, and in certain protozoal infections – malaria, trypanosomiasis and kala-azar. In chronic malaria, the monocytosis is often marked and some cells contain pigment granules (Fig. 14.9). The possibility of monocytic or myelomonocytic leukaemia must always be considered in patients with a persistent monocytosis.

The Platelets

Platelets are anucleate fragments of megakaryocyte cytoplasm (Fig. 14.10) and although not cells in the true sense, they possess a complex structure of organelles and tubular systems. The normal platelet count is 150–450 × 10^9/l. Platelets can adhere to the walls of damaged blood vessels and to each other, forming aggregates. They secrete a number of chemical mediators, the most important of which is thromboxane A_2 (TxA_2), the most potent aggregating agent known. They are weakly phagocytic. Platelets perform a number of important functions: (1) maintaining the integrity of vascular endothelium (p. 86); (2) forming the primary haemostatic plug following vessel injury (p. 89); (3) activation of the blood coagulation system (p. 80); (4) producing mediators involved in vessel wall repair, regulation of vascular tonicity and in inflammatory reactions (p. 139); and (5) producing growth factors (p. 156).

Platelet disorders (p. 640) may be grouped into three broad categories: (1) increase in platelet numbers which may be reactive (thrombocytosis) or neoplastic (thrombocythaemia); (2) reduction in platelet numbers (thrombocytopenia); (3) defective platelet function (qualitative disorders).

The Anaemias

Definition and Types of Anaemia

Anaemia is defined as a reduction in the haemoglobin concentration below the reference range, usually, but not invariably, accompanied by a reduction in red cell mass. Anaemia develops when the rate of marrow red cell production fails to keep pace with destruction or loss of cells. The anaemias are classified as follows:

1. Excess loss or destruction
   (a) loss – post-haemorrhagic
   (b) destruction – haemolytic
2. Failure of production
   (a) diminished production with marrow hyperplasia – dyserythropoietic
   (b) diminished production with marrow hypoplasia – hypoplastic or aplastic

In haemolytic and post-haemorrhagic anaemias, there is increased output of red cells, *effective erythropoiesis.* In dyserythropoietic states, however, although hyperplasia occurs, cell maturation is slow; some red cell precursors are destroyed in the marrow and production is not increased, *ineffective erythropoiesis.* In aplastic or hypoplastic anaemias compensatory hyperplasia does not occur despite stimulation by erythropoietin.

Effects of Anaemia

The main effect of anaemia is a reduction in the oxygen-carrying capacity of blood resulting in tissue hypoxia. The patient complains of tiredness, dizziness, paraesthesiae of the extremities, and exertional dyspnoea. Certain compensatory adjustments occur leading to an increase in cardiac output, a fall in circulation time and increase in tissue perfusion. These changes lead to a bounding pulse with high pulse pressure, palpitation, cardiac enlargement and haemic murmurs; if the anaemia worsens, high output cardiac failure is a risk, especially if the load is further increased by injudicious blood transfusion. If anaemia develops rapidly, symptoms are severe, whereas remarkable tolerance is seen when the haemoglobin level falls slowly. Pallor, mild pyrexia and slight splenomegaly may result from anaemia *per se.* Fatty change, especially in the liver and heart, is the most constant finding in patients dying with severe anaemia.

Anaemias of Blood Loss or Red Cell Destruction

Post-haemorrhagic Anaemia

Restoration of plasma volume after acute haemorrhage causes temporary dilution of blood with a fall in red cell count. The first evidence of regeneration of red cells after haemorrhage is a reticulocytosis, the degree of which is an indicator of haemopoietic activity. Occasionally, nucleated red cells may be present. As regeneration is completed, the reticulocyte count gradually returns to normal. These changes result from erythroblast proliferation in the bone marrow (Fig. 14.11). Neutrophil leucocytosis and thrombocytosis, of moderate degree, appear within hours of haemorrhage but decline in 2 or 3 days unless haemorrhage recurs. Chronic blood loss is the most common cause of iron-deficiency anaemia.

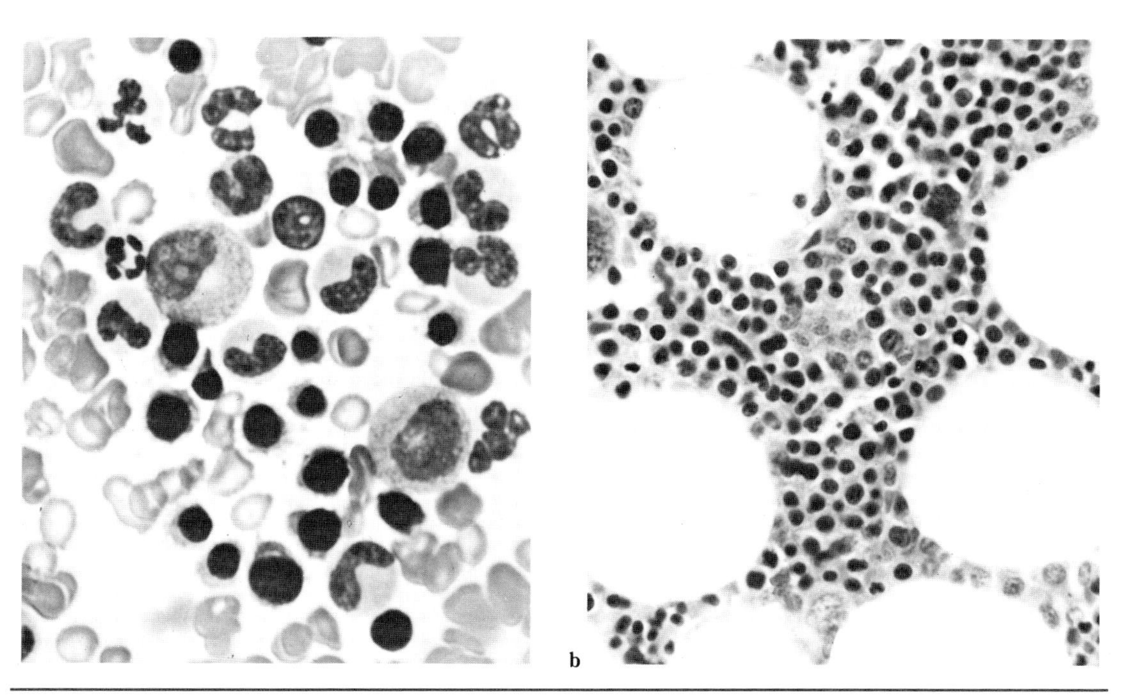

Fig. 14.11 The haemopoietic marrow, showing an erythroblastic reaction following haemorrhage. **(a)** Marrow smear: there is an increased proportion of normoblasts, at various stages of maturity, as compared with myelocytes. ×850. **(b)** Marrow section: the cellular haemopoietic tissue has increased at the expense of the fat cells. ×500.

Haemolytic Anaemias

Classification of Haemolytic Disorders

Shortening of red cell survival is the essential diagnostic feature of haemolytic disease. Important points in the classification of haemolytic disorders are: (1) the site of haemolysis (extravascular or intravascular); (2) intrinsic defect of the red cells ('intracorpuscular defect') or extrinsic agent acting on normal red cells ('extracorpuscular defect'); (3) hereditary or acquired (Table 14.7).

Measurement of Red Cell Lifespan

A sample of the patient's red cells are labelled *in vitro* with radiochromium (^{51}Cr) and re-injected. The rate of disappearance of radioactivity is estimated from serial blood samples and is proportional to the rate of red cell destruction. It is customary to calculate the time taken for the concentration of ^{51}Cr to decay to 50% ($T_{1/2}$) of its initial value. Provided haemorrhage can be excluded, red cell survival is estimated from these data. In addition, by placing an external scintillation counter over the liver and spleen, sites of red cell sequestration and destruction can be ascertained. This information can predict the potential benefit of splenectomy on red cell survival.

General Features

The haemolytic disorders are characterized by increased destruction of red cells and shortening of their lifespan. There is compensatory increase in erythropoiesis but anaemia develops when the rate of destruction exceeds that of production.

Table 14.7 Classification of haemolytic anaemia

Hereditary
- Red cell membrane defects
  - Hereditary spherocytosis
  - Hereditary elliptocytosis
- Red cell enzyme defects
  - Glucose-6-phosphate dehydrogenase deficiency (hexose monophosphate shunt defect)
  - Pyruvate kinase deficiency (Embden–Meyerhof pathway defect)
- Haemoglobinopathies
  - Abnormal globin chains (haemoglobin variants)
  - Decreased globin chain synthesis (thalassaemias)

Acquired
- Autoimmune haemolytic anaemias
  - Warm antibody types
  - Cold antibody types
- Isoimmune haemolytic anaemia
  - Haemolytic disease of the newborn
  - Haemolytic transfusion reaction
- Drug-induced immune haemolytic anaemia
  - Haemolysis due to toxins and chemicals
  - Mechanical damage to red cells (red cell fragmentation syndromes)
- Miscellaneous
  - Hypersplenism
  - Parasitic invasion of red cells
  - Paroxysmal nocturnal haemoglobinuria
  - Secondary: liver disease, dyserythropoietic anaemias

The absence of anaemia does not exclude haemolytic disease. In all haemolytic disorders, irrespective of cause, there are increased rates both of haemoglobin catabolism and of erythropoiesis; this combination provides the laboratory basis for diagnosis.

In most haemolytic disorders red cells are destroyed by macrophages in the spleen, liver and bone marrow, **extravascular haemolysis.** Moderately damaged cells are phagocytosed in the spleen whereas more severely damaged cells undergo phagocytosis in any tissues containing vascular channels lined by macrophages (liver, spleen and bone marrow). **Intravascular haemolysis** with escape of haemoglobin into the circulation is due to severe red cell membrane damage by antibody and complement, toxic chemicals or mechanical trauma.

Changes Resulting from Increased Destruction of Red Cells

Following red cell phagocytosis, haemoglobin is degraded to haem and globin. Haem iron is released and transported to the marrow and the residual porphyrin rings are broken down to bilirubin; the peptide chains of globin are hydrolysed to their constituent amino acids and re-enter the general metabolic pool. Production of bilirubin exceeds the liver's capacity to remove it, and the plasma level rises; clinical jaundice occurs with levels >50 μmol/l. The bilirubin is unconjugated but bound to albumin and therefore does not enter the urine (acholuric jaundice). Increased excretion of conjugated bilirubin by the liver leads to excess stercobilinogen in the gut. Increased absorption of stercobilinogen from the gut cannot all be dealt with by the liver and appears in the urine as urobilinogen. The high bilirubin content of bile predisposes to the formation of pigment gallstones, most often in the inherited haemolytic anaemias. High levels of plasma bilirubin in haemolytic disease of the newborn may cause toxic damage to the brain, kernicterus (p. 840).

Intravascular haemolysis results in free haemoglobin appearing in the plasma (normally less than 1 mg/dl); a proportion becomes bound to haptoglobin to form a complex of molecular weight 150 000 and therefore too large to pass into the urine. This complex is removed by hepatocytes. If intravascular haemolysis is severe, haptoglobin disappears completely from plasma. Reduction in the levels of haptoglobin also occurs when haemolysis is extravascular. When the haptoglobin-binding capacity becomes saturated, free haemoglobin circulates. Some is removed by hepatocytes but two other degradation pathways exist: (1) it may be dissociated into half-molecules (α β dimers of molecular weight 32 000), which pass into the glomerular filtrate. Haemosiderin granules in exfoliated epithelial cells in the urine are a sensitive indicator of intravascular haemolysis; (2) it may be oxidized to methaemoglobin from which the haem becomes dissociated and either complexes with haemopexin and passes into hepatocytes, or combines first with albumin to form methaemalbumin which subsequently transfers haem to haemopexin as the latter becomes available. Elevation of plasma methaemalbumin is a useful indicator of intravascular haemolysis (Schumm's test).

Changes Associated with Compensatory Erythropoiesis

In haemolytic states, the marrow is capable of increasing red cell production to a maximum of six times normal. The reticulocyte count is always increased. It is often assumed that the magnitude of reticulocytosis reflects the degree of shortening of red cell lifespan, but the relationship is inexact. Anaemia in haemolytic disease is usually normocytic but there may be a slight macrocytosis. The marrow shows erythroblastic hyperplasia, haemopoietic tissue extending down the shafts of long bones. Eventually the medullary cavity becomes widened with loss of bony trabeculae and thinning of cortical bone. Megaloblastic change due to folic acid deficiency may develop. In severe, chronic cases, extramedullary haemopoiesis may occur. In addition haemosiderin accumulates in Kupffer cells and splenic macrophages.

Hereditary Red Cell Membrane Defects

The red cell membrane consists of a lipid bilayer. Membrane lipids are in equilibrium with plasma lipids and therefore may be altered by diet or disease. The ratio of cholesterol to phospholipid influences the deformability of the red cell membrane, increase in cholesterol tending to make the cell less deformable. The physical properties of the membrane are largely due to a submembrane protein meshwork which functions as a cytoskeleton. Like all cells, the red cell regulates its volume and water content primarily through control of sodium and potassium ions. This depends on both an intact cell membrane and a supply of energy in the form of ATP.

The surface-to-volume ratio of red cells can alter considerably in disease. Red cells become spherocytic as surface-to-volume ratios decline and this can arise because of loss of membrane surface (microspherocytes) or by gain in cell volume (macrospherocytes). The cell becomes less deformable as it becomes more spheroidal. The **osmotic fragility test** is a useful indirect measurement of this surface-to-volume ratio. When red cells are placed in hypotonic salt solution they swell, rupture and haemoglobin escapes. With normal red cells, the first trace of lysis is usually seen in 0.42% saline; initial lysis occurring below 0.4% or above 0.5% is abnormal, indicating diminished or increased fragility respectively.

Hereditary Spherocytosis

This chronic haemolytic disease which occurs worldwide, is inherited as autosomal dominant with incomplete penetrance. In about 25% of patients there is no family history, the defect arising by spontaneous genetic mutation. The cytoskeleton of the red cell membrane consists of a number of proteins, spectrin, ankyrin, actin, anion exchange protein, and various glycophorins. These form an interlocking structure underlying and attached to the red cell membrane. In hereditary spherocytosis there is a qualitative or quantitative defect in the spectrin molecule which results in membrane instability, the red cells having a spheroidal shape and reduced plasticity.

The microspherocytes become trapped in the red pulp of the spleen because they lack the deformability necessary to enable them to pass through the clefts between endothelial cells in the venous sinusoids in order to return to the circulation. The spleen therefore occupies a central role in this disorder. Following splenectomy survival of red cells returns to normal. Transfused cells survive normally in patients with hereditary spherocytosis.

Clinically, the disease is characterized by fluctuating acholuric jaundice dating from early childhood. Anaemia may be insignificant but acute episodes of severe anaemia occur. These crises result from (1) increase in the rate of red cell destruction (haemolytic crisis), caused by infection or pregnancy or (2) reduced marrow erythropoietic activity due to folic acid deficiency or parvovirus B19 infection ('hypoplastic crisis').

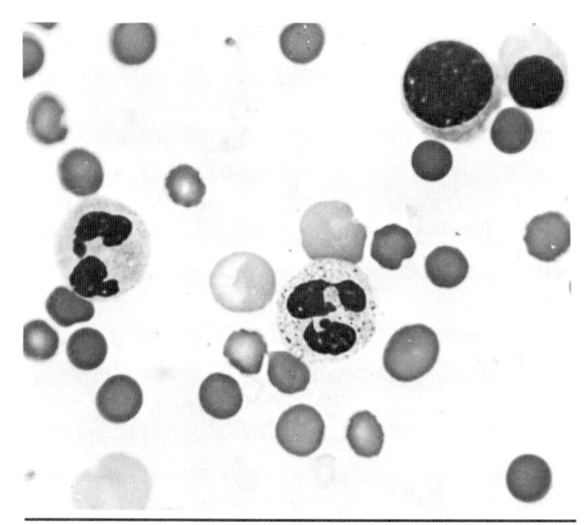

Fig. 14.12 Blood smear in hereditary spherocytosis. Note the small, densely staining spherocytes. ×780.

Splenomegaly (500 g or more) is invariable. Most untreated patients develop pigment gallstones and some develop chronic leg ulcers. The diagnosis is suggested when haemolysis is associated with microspherocytes in the peripheral blood (Fig. 14.12) and is confirmed by an increased osmotic fragility of the red cells. Although splenectomy prevents haemolysis, the microspherocytosis and increased osmotic fragility of the cells persist.

Hereditary Elliptocytosis

This is an inherited disorder characterized by elongated red cells in the peripheral blood. Two variants are recognized, both of which have autosomal dominant inheritance. In one the abnormal gene is linked to the Rh blood-group genes. The disorder is more common than hereditary spherocytosis and is a milder disease. It may also involve spectrin. Clinically, red cell production keeps pace with destruction in 90% of cases, and anaemia becomes overt in the other 10% in whom splenectomy may be required.

Hereditary Red Cell Enzyme Defects

Normal red cell survival is dependent on the integrity of two enzyme systems concerned in glucose metabolism, (1) the hexose monophosphate shunt and (2) the Embden–Meyerhoff anaerobic glycolytic pathway (Fig. 14.13).

The *hexose monophosphate shunt* produces NADPH. This NADPH contributes additional reducing power and mediates the production of reduced glutathione. Reduced glutathione is an important intracellular buffer as it protects against exogenous and endogenous oxidants which would threaten to oxidize haemoglobin to methaemoglobin by loss of single electrons from the four haem ion atoms. Conversion of glucose to pyruvate in the *Embden–Meyerhoff pathway* results in production of 2 moles of ATP for each mole of glucose catabolized. In addition, NAD is reduced to NADH. ATP maintains the internal membrane flexibility and red cell shape. Lack of ATP reduces red cell survival leading to extravascular haemolysis. The NADH produced by this pathway is also necessary to maintain haem iron in the ferrous state.

Glucose-6-phosphate Dehydrogenase (G-6-PD) Deficiency

Deficiency of G-6-PD is among the commonest inherited diseases in the world, affecting up to 40% of persons of Mediterranean, South East Asian and Negro ancestry. By contrast, the incidence is low in Northern Europeans and Japanese. Inheritance is X-linked. Clinical disease may occur very occasionally in females when the random inactivation (lyonization) of the X-chromosome results in a predominance of affected red cells. The deficiency is most common in areas where malaria is endemic, reflecting the protection which deficient cells afford against falciparum malaria. The principal effect is a fall in NADPH production with a decrease in reduced glutathione. Haemoglobin is readily oxidized to methaemoglobin, which precipitates as Heinz bodies (Fig. 14.14).

More than 150 isoenzymes of G-6-PD are recognized. They show variation in geographical distribution and in turn there is a wide clinical spectrum of disease depending on the isoenzyme involved. The two main variants associated with clinical disease are: (1) G-6-PD A^- which affects

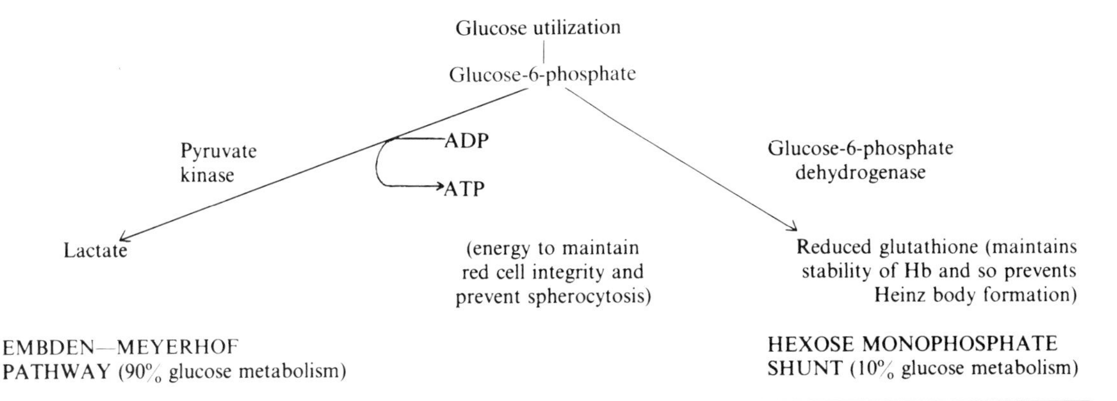

Fig. 14.13 Two enzyme systems of importance in determining the lifespan of the red cells.

Negroes and in which normal amounts of enzyme are produced, but it is unstable so that decreasing amounts are found in ageing red cells; and (2) G-6-PD Mediterranean-Oriental in which the enzyme activity is relatively reduced in all red cells.

The commonest clinical presentation is an acute haemolytic episode in response to oxidant stress, e.g. acute infection, drugs or diabetic ketoacidosis. The drugs which can act as oxidants include antimalarials, sulphonamides, nitrofurantoin, aspirin and vitamin K. In some cases, usually in Mediterranean regions, haemolysis may follow ingestion of the fava bean – favism. In G-6-PD A$^-$ deficiency, the haemolytic episode is self-limiting as young red cells have a higher concentration of G-6-PD. Spontaneous haemolysis occurs in 5% of affected neonates in Mediterranean countries and the Far East and the main danger is kernicterus (p. 840). If this can be prevented, prognosis is good, haemolysis ceasing spontaneously in 2–3 months. Northern Europeans with G-6-PD deficiency often exhibit chronic low grade haemolysis which is exacerbated by infection.

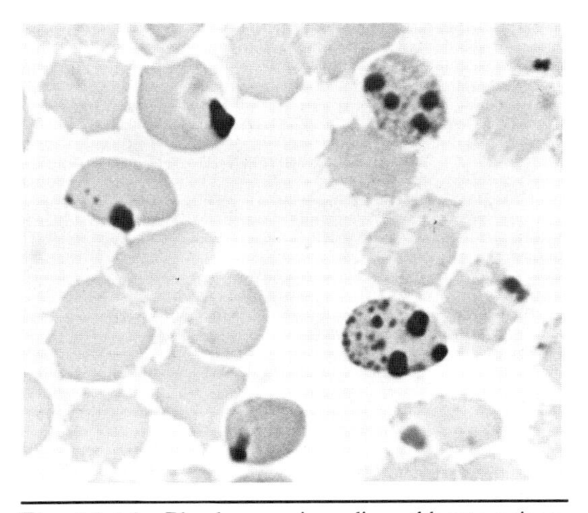

Fig. 14.14 Blood smear in sodium chlorate poisoning, stained with methyl violet to show Heinz bodies. ×1400.

The diagnosis of G-6-PD deficiency is suggested by contracted and fragmented cells in the blood film and by the demonstration of Heinz bodies. Reticulocytes have higher levels of G-6-PD than mature cells and enzyme assay results can be misleading during a haemolytic episode; thus it should be performed later.

Pyruvate Kinase (PK) Deficiency

This is much less common than G-6-PD deficiency and is inherited as autosomal recessive. Haemolysis occurs only in the homozygous state. The anaemia, which may be moderate to severe, causes relatively mild symptoms as there is a shift to the right in the O_2 dissociation curve due to a rise in intracellular 2,3-diphosphoglycerate. Pyruvate kinase deficiency presents in childhood with mild jaundice. Reticulocyte counts can be very high. Paradoxically, osmotic fragility may be decreased due to the presence of osmotically resistant reticulocytes. The diagnosis is made by measuring erythrocyte pyruvate kinase activity.

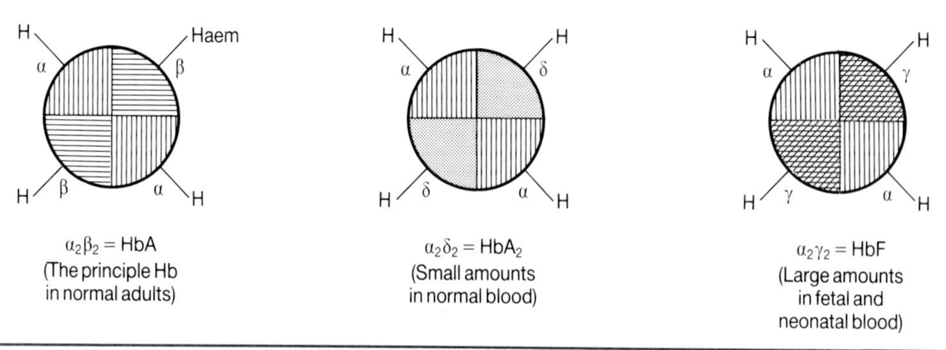

Fig. 14.15 The structure of the normal haemoglobins.

Haemoglobinopathies

Haemoglobin is a globular protein (molecular weight 65 000) consisting of two pairs of polypeptide chains and four haem groups, one being attached to each chain. The haem groups transport oxygen. The haemoglobin type is determined by the amino-acid sequence in the polypeptide chains. Four chains occur normally in adults, α, β, γ and δ. Normal haemoglobins consist of two α chains linked to two β (HbA) or δ chains (HbA$_2$) (Fig. 14.15). Alpha chains contain 141 amino acids, the others 146. Globin chains have a spiral configuration and the constituent amino acids are located both internally (non-polar, non-charged) or externally (polar, charged); the non-polar internal amino acids form a scaffold which preserves the rigidity and configuration of the globin chain. Haemoglobins differ in their electrophoretic mobility (Fig. 14.16), solubility and resistance to alkali denaturation. These features, together with their chromatographic properties, are used for their identification.

Replacement of fetal haemoglobin (HbF) by HbA starts before birth; HbA accounts for 96% and HbA$_2$ for 3% of the haemoglobin normally present by one year. Haemoglobinopathies result from abnormalities in the synthesis of the globin chains, the haem groups being normal. Two main varieties occur: (1) in which a gene mutation or deletion results in the production of abnormal globin chains – the haemoglobin variants; and (2) in which complex genetic defects result in lack of or decreased synthesis of globin chains – the thalassaemia syndromes. The presence of a haemoglobinopathy results in both impairment of red cell production and a reduced survival time in the circulation. The anaemia is, therefore, partly dyserythropoietic and partly haemolytic.

Haemoglobin Variants

The haemoglobin variants, in 90% of cases, occur because of substitution of a single amino acid. Over 300 variants are recognized but only a few produce clinical manifestations, the most common being haemoglobins S, C, D and E. Haemoglobin variants resulting from substitution of external (polar) amino acids produce clinical disease only in the homozygous state; the commonest and most important is sickle cell anaemia. The internal (non-polar) amino-acid variants produce disease in the heterozygous state; homozygotes are non-viable.

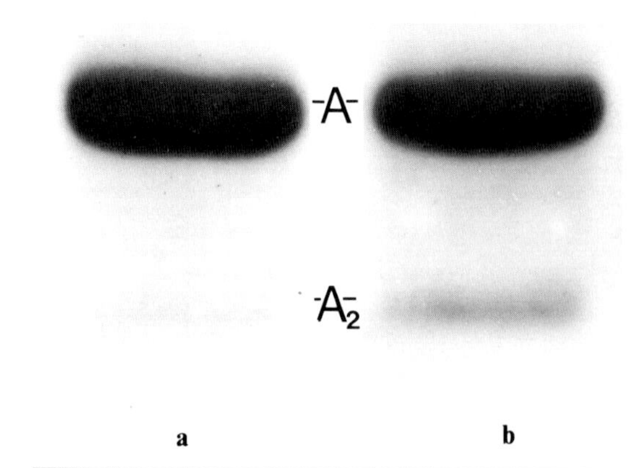

Fig. 14.16 Starch-gel electrophoresis of haemoglobins. **(a)** Normal. **(b)** Thalassaemia minor, showing increase in HbA$_2$.

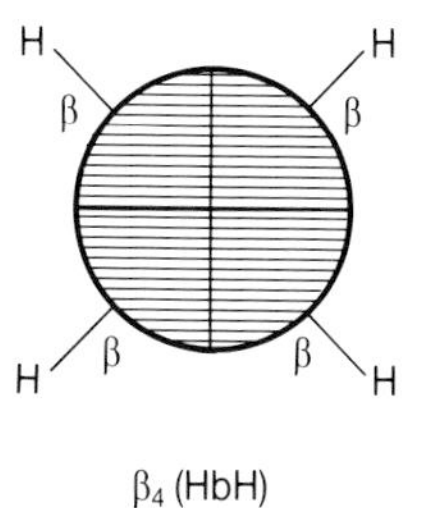

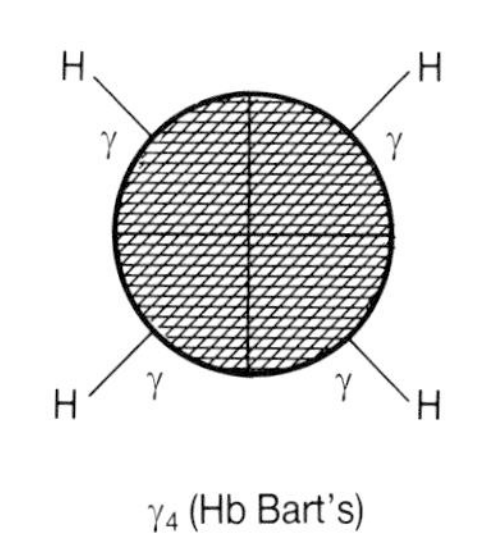

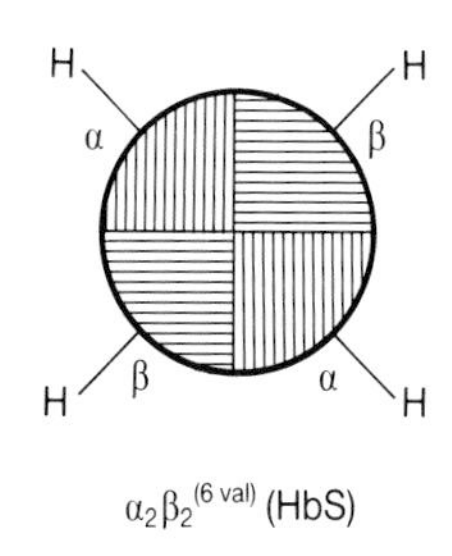

Fig. 14.17 The structure of some abnormal haemoglobins.

Sickle cell disease

Haemoglobin S ($\alpha_2\ \beta_2\ 6^{val}$) differs from HbA in the substitution of valine for glutamic acid in the sixth position of the β chain amino-acid sequence (Fig. 14.17). Homozygotes (HbSS), in whom all the haemoglobin is HbS, always manifest features of sickle cell disease and this may be fatal in childhood. Heterozygotes (HbAS) have about 40–50% HbS and are usually asymptomatic as they only manifest symptoms under severe anoxic conditions – the sickle cell trait. The abnormal gene follows the same geographical distribution as falciparum malaria; people who carry the sickle cell gene are protected against malaria.

Sickling of red cells occurs as a result of polymerization of deoxygenated HbS molecules so that they become stacked linearly. Initially the process is reversible when the haemoglobin is reoxygenated, but eventually membrane damage occurs with permanent sickling. Sickling is demonstrable *in vitro* by adding a reducing agent to blood (Fig. 14.18).

Clinical symptoms occur in homozygotes and develop at about 6 months old. There is a chronic haemolytic anaemia and recurrent painful vaso-occlusive crises occur due to sickled erythrocytes blocking small blood vessels. This leads to tissue ischaemia and infarction, most commonly affecting bones, liver, spleen, lungs, brain and retina; leg ulceration is common and priapism may occur in the male. These crises may be precipitated by minor infections, severe cold, exercise, dehydration and pregnancy. Although splenomegaly occurs in young children, repeated crises with splenic infarction result in splenic atrophy (autosplenectomy). Patients are prone to serious bacterial infections, particularly pulmonary infection, septicaemia, meningitis, osteitis and osteomyelitis (the latter frequently due to salmonella infection). Severe infection may also precipitate bone marrow hypoplasia (aplastic crisis) as can parvovirus B19 infection or folate deficiency.

In **sickle cell trait** (HbA/S), symptoms are absent or mild, but sickling is demonstrable *in vitro*. It is, however, important to establish the diagnosis because sickling occurs during severe or prolonged hypoxia. Thus Negroes, in whom the trait may occur in 10–20%, should be screened on admission to hospital.

Combination of HbS with other variants is not uncommon. The most frequent, HbS/C, is clinically similar to HbSS but less severe. HbF reduces the risk of sickling; this explains why

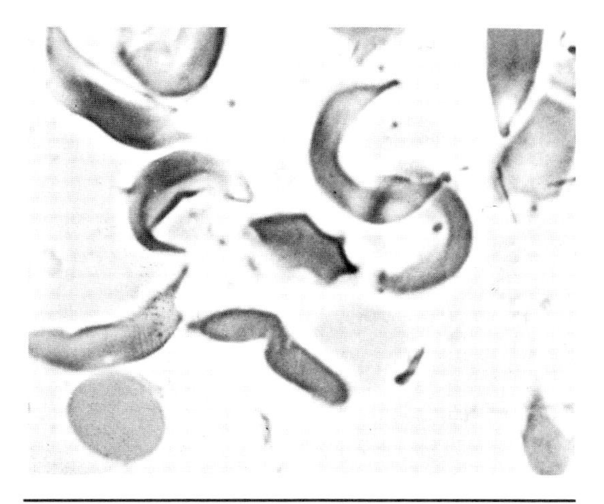

Fig. 14.18 Blood from a subject with sickle cell trait showing the characteristic distorted shapes assumed when the red cells are subjected to a low oxygen tension. ×1000.

clinical symptoms therefore do not develop before the age of 6 months. When there is persistence of HbF, sickle cell disease is often a benign disorder. The combination of HbS/thalassaemia is described later.

Variants with internal amino-acid substitutions

Three categories exist. The largest comprises the **unstable haemoglobin variants.** The amino-acid substitutions affect the attachment site of haem. Even heterozygous individuals (Hb Koln is the commonest), suffer from non-spherocytic haemolytic anaemia. Since unstable haemoglobins readily become denatured, Heinz body formation is a typical feature and this can be demonstrated when the cells are incubated *in vitro*. The second group, the HbM variants, produce a type of **congenital methaemoglobinaemia** characterized clinically by cyanosis due to the failure of methaemoglobin to bind oxygen. **Altered affinity haemoglobins** constitute the third group; most bind oxygen strongly, with consequent tissue hypoxia and erythrocytosis but some bind oxygen weakly and present with cyanosis.

The Thalassaemia Syndromes

The thalassaemias are inherited disorders in which there is diminished production of normal globin chains, most often the α or β chain. Thalassaemia genes occur in all races but α thalassaemias are found mainly in the Middle and Far East and in Africa whereas β thalassaemias are most prevalent in Mediterranean countries.

Thalassaemias are inherited as autosomal codominant and each disorder may occur in a homozygous or heterozygous form. Because the synthesis of one globin chain is reduced, there is a relative excess of other globin chains. However, the red cells are still deficient in haemoglobin and thus are hypochromic and microcytic. Excess globin chains may precipitate in the cell causing haemolysis.

Alpha (α) thalassaemia

The α chains are coded for by two duplicated genes on chromosome 16; thus, deletion of all four genes is required to suppress α chain synthesis completely. Varying abnormalities are produced when fewer genes are deleted and these, together with the clinical features, are summarized in Table 14.8. Diagnosis is made by demonstrating a reduced α/β chain ratio.

Beta (β) thalassaemia

The β chains are coded for by a single gene on chromosome 11. Mutations in this gene result either in a failure to synthesize β chains (β^0) or in reduced synthesis of β chains (β^+). Numerous mutations, usually single base changes, have been described and these can (1) cause decreased or absent transcription of the gene; (2) prevent RNA splicing so that mRNA is structurally abnormal; (3) result in the formation of a 'stop' codon so that

Table 14.8 Classification and clinical features of α-thalassaemias

	Genotype	Clinical and laboratory features	Comments
One gene deletion	–α/αα	Silent α-thalassaemia;	–
Two gene deletions	– –/αα or α–/α–	α thalassaemia trait; mild anaemia and hypochromia	–
Three gene deletions	– –/–α	HbH disease; haemolytic anaemia (Hb 7–9 g/dl); red cells severely hypochromic with HbH inclusions; may become folate deficient	Excess of β chains combine to form an unstable tetramer HbH (β4) (Fig. 14.17)
Four gene deletions	– –/– –	Lethal *in utero* with hydrops fetalis	Excess of γ chains combine to form tetrameric Hb Barts (γ4) (Fig. 14.17)

Table 14.9 Classification and clinical features of β thalassaemias

Genotype	Clinical and laboratory features	Comments
β^0/β^0 β^+/β^+	Severe hypochromic microcytic anaemia; increased reticulocytes; target cells and basophilic stippling: increased iron stores	Thalassaemia major; transfusion dependent; absent HbA, excess α chains form aggregates in red cells and red cell precursors
β^0/β β^+/β	Mild to moderate hypochromic microcytic anaemia	Thalassaemia minor; raised HbA_2

there is interruption of mRNA translation. In the absence of β chains the excess of α chains precipitate in red cells and lead to haemolysis. A brief classification of the β thalasssaemias is given in Table 14.9.

Clinical and pathological features. The β thalassaemias can be classified as major, minor or intermedia. Homozygous β^0 thalassaemia (β^0/β^0) always results in thalassaemia major. There is absence of HbA, and 98% of the haemoglobin is HbF. Patients are severely anaemic and depend on blood transfusion. Homozygous β^+ thalassaemia (β^+/β^+) presents a range of severity and is classed as thalassaemia major when anaemia is severe or intermedia when it is moderate. Both heterozygous β^0 and β^+ thalassaemia (β^0/β and β^+/β) are graded thalassaemia minor. These cause mild anaemia, elevation of HbA_2 and, in some forms, also elevation of HbF.

In *thalassaemia major,* severe anaemia develops within a few weeks of birth. Splenomegaly is prominent due to red cell haemolysis and extramedullary haemopoiesis. The peripheral blood shows reticulocytosis, nucleated red cells, and target cells (Fig. 14.19). Many patients die in infancy or childhood, while those surviving longer develop severe haemosiderosis, cardiac failure being a common cause of death. Prolonged marrow hyperplasia causes thickening of the calvarium, giving mongoloid facies and a 'hair on end' appearance to the skull X-ray. **Thalassaemia intermedia** is less severe, whereas **thalassaemia minor** usually presents in adult life as mild hypochromic microcytic anaemia.

The diagnosis rests initially on the discovery of anaemia, hypochromia, microcytosis and target cells and changes in the proportions of HbF and HbA_2 (Fig. 14.16). Confirmation of the diagnosis is by measurement of the α/β globin chain synthesis ratio (normally 1:1). Prenatal diagnosis is possible by globin chain analysis on fetal blood in the second trimester or by chorionic villus biopsy in the first trimester. This can normally provide 100 μg of pure fetal DNA and permit detailed gene studies.

A rare form of thalassaemia is δ/β *thalassaemia.*

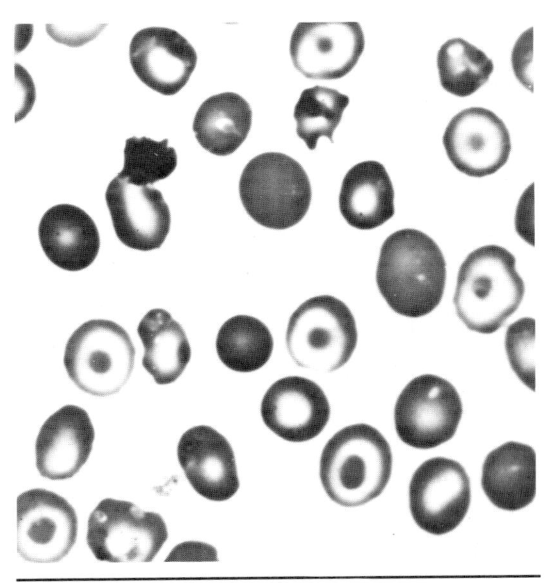

Fig. 14.19 Target cells in a case of thalassaemia. ×1000.

This occurs when there is deficient production of both δ and β chains. When homozygous, the symptoms are those of thalassaemia major. β thalassaemia can also coexist with α thalassaemia. In this case the α/β globin chain synthesis ratio is balanced, haemolysis is reduced, and clinically there is thalassaemia intermedia.

Thalassaemia can occur in combination with the haemoglobin variants in areas where there is a high frequency of both gene defects. In α thalassaemia the severity of sickle cell disease may be reduced because the HbS levels in red cells is slightly decreased. HbS/β^- thalassaemia can produce a spectrum of clinical severity: with β thalassaemia, HbS levels are increased and thus β^+ may result in clinical symptoms in patients with sickle cell trait while β^0 may result in a severe sickle cell syndrome. β thalassaemia in association with HbC or HbD is mild, not requiring treatment. HbE/β thalassaemia is severe.

Autoimmune Haemolytic Anaemias

A common cause of acquired haemolytic anaemia is the development of an autoantibody capable of binding to, and damaging red cells. Autoimmune haemolytic anaemia occurs in two forms which differ in the thermal range of reactivity of the antibody, namely warm and cold antibody types.

Warm Antibody Type

In this form an IgG class autoantibody binds strongly to red cells at 37°C. In some cases, the antibody is Rh antigen specific and, like Rh isoantibodies is 'incomplete', i.e. it does not cause agglutination of red cells suspended in saline. *In vivo* the red cells become microspherocytic and are destroyed prematurely in spleen, liver and marrow, i.e. extravascular haemolysis.

This chronic haemolytic anaemia occurs at any age and in both sexes, but is commonest in women over 40 years. In 50% of cases it is idiopathic while the others complicate autoimmune disorders such as systemic lupus erythematosus or rheumatoid arthritis. It may also occur in patients with leukaemias or lymphomas. Acute self-limiting forms occur in children following various infections and in adults following drug therapy, most often α-methyldopa. In the chronic form there is fluctuating haemolytic anaemia with splenomegaly. Microspherocytosis and increased osmotic fragility are usual. Antibody bound to red cells is detectable by the direct antiglobulin test with anti-IgG (Coombs' test); antibody can be eluted from the cells and is sometimes detectable in low titre in the serum.

Cold Antibody Type

These are due to autoantibodies usually of IgM class which have enhanced activity at 4°C. The antibody produces two effects: (1) autoagglutination of red cells and (2) sensitization of red cells to complement activation with consequent intravascular haemolysis.

Cold Agglutinin Disease

This may occur in a chronic idiopathic form in the elderly or may be associated with lymphoma or connective tissue disease; the antibody is usually monoclonal. Anaemia is mild to moderate but may become severe in cold weather. An acute mild form may follow infection by *Mycoplasma pneumoniae* or Epstein–Barr virus, and is self-limiting after a few weeks. The antibody response is polyclonal.

Episodes of haemolysis occur on exposure to the cold; acrocyanosis (Raynaud's phenomenon) is prominent and must be distinguished from Raynaud's disease (p. 475). The direct antiglobulin test is usually positive using antibody to complement components. In all forms, red cell agglutination occurs on the peripheral blood film and when blood counts are performed on automated equipment erroneous results occur.

Paroxysmal Cold Haemoglobinuria

Originally described in syphilis, this very rare form of cold antibody haemolysis is now seen as a transient complication of virus infections such as mumps or infectious mononucleosis (where it is often accompanied by a false-positive Wassermann reaction) or as an autoimmune disorder in adults. The cold antibody is of IgG class and reacts with antigens of the P system. On exposure to cold the antibody binds; it is then capable of strong complement fixation and causes intravascular haemolysis. The mechanism of haemolysis was elucidated by Donath and Landsteiner who demonstrated haemolysis *in vitro* by first chilling the blood to allow the cold antibody to react with the red cells, followed by warming to allow complement activity. This test is still used.

Isoimmune Haemolytic Anaemias

Haemolytic Disease of the Newborn

Fetal red cells enter the maternal circulation during labour, in the course of obstetric manipulations and during abortion. They may provoke maternal antibody formation to blood-group antigens foreign to the mother and derived from the father. Such isoantibodies are of IgM class in the primary response but switch to become IgG class. These can cross the placenta in subsequent pregnancies and cause haemolytic anaemia in the fetus. Some degree of fetal/maternal incompatibility is inevitable, but the Rh system, particularly the D antigen, is responsible for most severe cases of haemolytic disease of the newborn. This occurs in only a small proportion of pregnancies at risk (i.e. those with a Rh negative mother and a Rh positive father) because: (1) the first-born child is not affected unless the mother has been previously immunized by blood transfusion or abortion; (2) the father is sometimes heterozygous (Dd), in which case the fetus has a 50% chance of being Rh negative; (3) ABO incompatibility between mother and fetus prevents immunization of the mother by the fetal D antigen; incompatible fetal red cells (say Group A) entering the maternal circulation are destroyed by the mother's natural (anti-A) isoantibody before they can stimulate production of Rh antibodies. ABO incompatibility itself rarely causes severe haemoglobin disease of the newborn because natural isoantibodies are usually of IgM class and incapable of crossing the placenta.

Haemolytic disease of the newborn varies in severity. In mild forms there may be transient jaundice and anaemia – *congenital haemolytic anaemia*; treatment may be unnecessary or consists only of blood transfusion. A more severe form, *icterus gravis neonatorum*, requires urgent treatment. Jaundice develops shortly after birth and if the level of unconjugated serum bilirubin exceeds 250 μmol/l there is risk of permanent brain damage – kernicterus. The neonate is anaemic, with reticulocytosis and nucleated red cells in the blood (*erythroblastosis fetalis*). There is hepatosplenomegaly and extramedullary haemopoiesis is seen in the spleen, liver, kidneys, adrenals and other viscera. Very severe anaemia causes intrauterine or neonatal death with marked oedema and congestive cardiac failure – *hydrops fetalis*.

All women are screened for isoimmune red cell antibodies during pregnancy. Where there is materno-fetal incompatibility, the mother's serum should be examined at regular intervals during the pregnancy. Haemolytic disease in the fetus can be confirmed by finding raised bilirubin levels in the amniotic fluid. Early delivery may save some infants, but with others intrauterine fetal transfusion with Rh negative blood is indicated. At birth, diagnosis can be confirmed by a positive direct antiglobulin test on fetal neonatal red cells and exchange transfusion may be necessary.

Isoimmunization may be prevented by maternal intravenous injection of anti-D within 3 days of delivery. The anti-D coats fetal Rh positive cells causing their rapid clearance from the circulation before an immune response can be initiated. Prophylaxis is also appropriate for all Rh negative women with Rh positive husbands following abortion, amniocentesis or other obstetric manipulation. Incompatibilities in other blood group systems, e.g. Kell and Duffy, occasionally cause haemolytic disease of the newborn. In a small proportion of group O mothers natural IgG isoantibodies to A or B antigens may exist and can cause mild haemolytic disease in the fetus.

Miscellaneous Types of Haemolytic Anaemia

Drug-induced Immune Haemolysis

Various drugs are capable of inducing immune destruction of red cells. They may be mediated in one of two ways:

Antibody directed against drugs. There are two mechanisms. First, the drug e.g. penicillin or cephalosporin, binds firmly to red cell membranes and antibody develops against the hapten-cell/membrane complex. Haemolysis is seldom severe and ceases on discontinuing the drug. The second occurs via a drug induced immune complex mechanism when antibody is formed against a drug/plasma-protein complex; the reaction of antibody and complement with the bound complex releases activated complement fragments to attack 'innocent bystander' red cells and cause lysis. Moderate haemolytic anaemia develops accompanied by haemoglobinuria. Drugs causing this reaction include quinidine, phenacetin, digoxin, sulphonamides and chlorpropamide.

Antibody directed against normal red cells. The drug appears to induce autoantibody formation against normal red cells by mechanisms which are not understood. The most common is the antihypertensive drug α-methyldopa. The Coombs' test becomes positive in 10% of patients some months after starting therapy and may remain positive for many months after stopping therapy. Only a small proportion develop anaemia.

Haemolytic Toxins and Chemicals

Infection with bacteria which secrete haemolytic toxins (e.g. phospholipases) can produce severe acute intravascular haemolysis. Examples are *Clostridium welchii* and *Streptococcus pyogenes*.

Haemolytic chemicals include phenylhydrazine, compounds of lead, arsenic and copper, saponin and potassium chlorate. In chronic lead poisoning red cells develop increased mechanical but diminished osmotic fragility; red cells tend to microcytosis and hypochromia although the patient is not iron deficient; such cells are short-lived, and mild anaemia results. Lead also precipitates reticulocyte RNA producing punctate basophilia (see Fig. 14.7). Lead interferes with haemoglobin synthesis, particularly iron utilization, and ring sideroblasts occur in the marrow.

Mechanical Damage to Red Cells (Red Cell Fragmentation Syndromes)

Red cell fragmentation occurs in March haemoglobinuria, in microangiopathic haemolytic anaemia, in patients with prosthetic heart valves and in patients with severe burns.

March haemoglobinuria consists of acute haemoglobinuria, occurring after long marches or running on hard surfaces and results from mechanical injury to red cells in the soft tissues of the plantar aspect of the feet.

Microangiopathic haemolytic anaemia is characterized by red cell fragmentation (see Fig. 14.6) and thrombocytopenia. It is observed in toxaemia of pregnancy, in malignant hypertension, thrombotic thrombocytopenic purpura, the haemolytic-uraemic syndrome of childhood, with metastatic mucin secreting carcinoma and in septic shock. The common factor is widespread fibrin deposition in small blood vessels due to either vascular damage (microangiopathy) or to disseminated intravascular coagulation (DIC).

Paroxysmal Nocturnal Haemoglobinuria

In this rare disorder an abnormal stem cell clone lacks the cell membrane glycoprotein decay accelerating factor (DAF). This protein restricts activation of complement by the alternate pathway accelerating the inactivation of C3 convertase (p. 142). The red cell, white cell and platelet progeny of the clone are all abnormal. In addition to chronic haemolysis, there is mild thrombocytopenia and leucopenia, repeated thrombotic episodes, mainly venous (portal and cerebral veins) and increased liability to infection. There is a high incidence of aplastic anaemia and acute leukaemia, supporting the suggestion that the syndrome is the result of proliferation of an abnormal multipotent cell. However, in some patients, there is a progressive diminution of the number of abnormal cells and apparent spontaneous remission may occur.

The increased sensitivity of red cells to complement-mediated lysis provides the basis for diagnosis. In Ham's test the increased complement activity of acidified serum (pH 6.4) is sufficient to lyse the deficient red cells but not normal cells. The slight fall in plasma pH during sleep enhances haemolysis and produces the nocturnal haemoglobinuria characterizing this condition. Haemosiderin granules accumulate in the kidney (Fig. 14.20) and are usually detectable in the urine. Patients are often iron deficient due to the urinary iron loss. However, iron administration may cause a reticulocytosis with exacerbation of haemolysis. Blood transfusion is dangerous unless washed or reconstituted frozen cells are used; even small volumes of plasma cause haemolysis due to the presence of activated complement components.

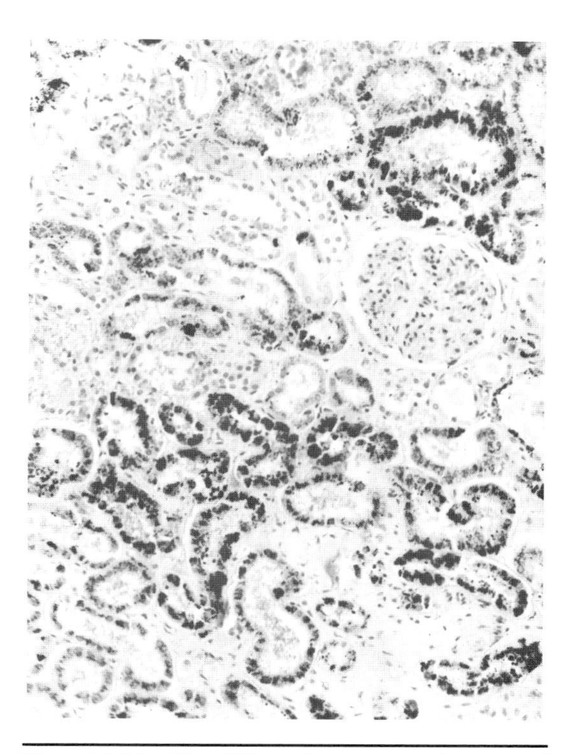

Fig. 14.20 The kidney in paroxysmal nocturnal haemoglobinuria stained by the Prussian blue reaction, showing accumulation of haemosiderin in the tubular epithelium due to prolonged haemoglobinuria. ×100.

Haemolytic Disease Caused by Parasitic Invasion of Red Cells

This occurs in malaria and Oroya fever. In the former, haemolysis can be intravascular and extravascular. In black water fever, a condition which occurred mainly in Europeans with falciparum malaria, there was severe and often fatal intravascular haemolysis.

Hypersplenism

The hypersplenism syndrome comprises splenic enlargement, reduction in one or more of the peripheral blood formed elements, normal or hyperplastic haemopoietic marrow, and, most importantly, cure by splenectomy. By convention the syndrome does not include conditions in which splenomegaly results from haemolytic anaemia or thrombocytopenia. The anaemia of hypersplenism results from increased destruction of pooled red cells in the spleen and an expansion of plasma volume with consequent dilution of the red cell mass.

Dyserythropoietic Anaemias

While the marrow is of normal or increased cellularity in these conditions, red cell production is diminished (dyserythropoiesis or ineffective erythropoiesis) and anaemia results. Of the various types (Table 14.10) the most important are the megaloblastic and iron deficiency anaemias. The congenital forms are rare, of recessive inheritance and show varying degrees of anaemia associated with ineffective erythropoiesis.

Table 14.10 Causes of dyserythropoietic anaemia

Primary	
Hereditary	
Acquired (myelodysplastic syndromes)	
Secondary	
Impaired DNA synthesis	
Vitamin B_{12} deficiency	megaloblastic anaemias
Folic acid deficiency	megaloblastic anaemias
Impaired haem synthesis	
Iron deficiency	
Defective iron utilization	
Impaired globin synthesis	
Haemoglobinopathies	

The Megaloblastic Anaemias

These anaemias are characterized by a distinct abnormality of haemopoiesis known as megaloblastic change (Fig. 14.21) which affects production of granulocytes and platelets as well as red cells; the effect on erythropoiesis is most conspicuous. The commonest cause of megaloblastic anaemia is deficiency of either Vitamin B_{12} or folic acid; less often it follows cytotoxic drug therapy which inhibits DNA synthesis (e.g. cytosine arabinoside, hydroxyurea, 6-mercaptopurine and methotrexate). Megaloblastic anaemia is characterized by an increase in mean cell volume (MCV) of the red cells and is a common cause of macrocytic anaemia. However, other forms of anaemia can be macrocytic in the absence of megaloblastic change, e.g. anaemia following severe haemorrhage, haemolysis, or in extramedullary haemopoiesis because of a high reticulocyte count, in alcohol abuse, chronic liver disease and myxoedema, and rarely in some forms of aplastic or refractory anaemia.

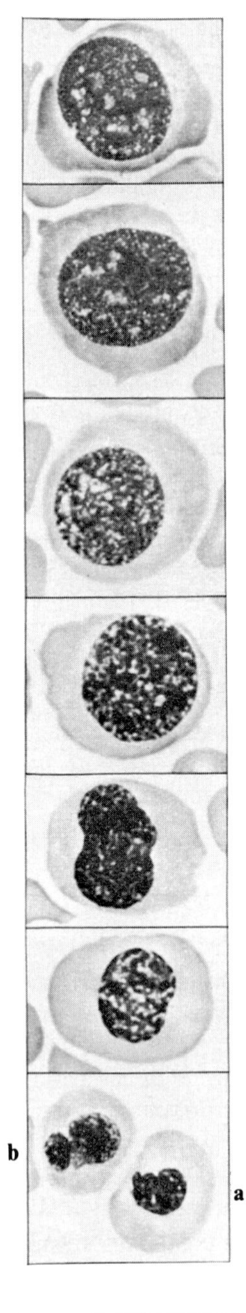

Early erythroblast: note the basophil cytoplasm and evenly dispersed nuclear chromatin containing several nucleoli.

Promegaloblast: nucleoli persist, nuclear chromatin shows commencing fine reticular condensation, cytoplasm basophilic. Note contrast to the coarse aggregation of nuclear chromatin in the normoblast series.

Early megaloblast: nuclear chromatin is finely reticulate, cytoplasm shows diminished basophilia and early haemoglobinization.

Polychromatophilic megaloblast with haemoglobinization in advance of nuclear maturation.

Later polychromatophilic megaloblast.

Late megaloblast with some nuclear condensation.

Two late megaloblasts, one showing nuclear pyknosis (**a**) and the other nuclear fragmentation (**b**).

Fig. 14.21 Megaloblastic series. ×1000.

The Physiological Actions of Vitamin B_{12} and Folic Acid

These substances, which act as coenzymes, are important for normal cell function, particularly cell division. The main action of folic acid is the transfer of single carbon units during methionine, DNA and RNA synthesis and during the breakdown of homocysteine. Only the polyglutamate form of folic acid is active biologically. Vitamin B_{12} (hydroxocobalamin) contains two major components: a corrin (porphyrin-like) ring and a nucleotide group consisting of a base and phosphorylated ribose. Hydroxocobalamin is biologically inert and requires enzymatic conversion to the active forms adenosylcobalamin and methylcobalamin. Vitamin B_{12} is required for the intracellular conversion of the transport form of folic acid, 5-methyltetrahydrofolate, to the active polyglutamate. This explains why vitamin B_{12} deficiency leads to megaloblastic haemopoiesis, largely due to failure of DNA synthesis and accounts for tests of folic acid deficiency being positive in vitamin B_{12} deficiency.

Blood Picture

In both vitamin B_{12} and folic acid deficiency red cells, granulocytes and platelets are reduced in number, i.e. pancytopenia. The red cells show an increased MCV, often preceding anaemia. As anaemia develops the red cells show increasing anisocytosis and macrocytosis and in advanced cases they may be abnormal in shape (poikilocytes), or may be nucleated with megaloblastic features (Fig. 14.22). The reticulocyte count is reduced. Neutropenia is associated with the early appearance of large hypersegmented neutrophils with six or more lobes (macropolycytes). Platelets are moderately reduced but severe thrombocytopenia resulting in purpura may occasionally occur.

Bone Marrow Features

Even when anaemia is minimal there is marked expansion of haemopoietic tissue throughout the long bones (Fig. 14.23) and the marrow itself shows hypercellularity with loss of fat spaces. All haemopoietic elements are affected to some degree, but erythroid hyperplasia is most marked with the erythroid to myeloid ratio approaching 1:1. Erythropoiesis undergoes megaloblastic change, the essential feature of which is a delay in nuclear maturation with the accumulation of many cells in an early stage of development, i.e. maturation arrest. These cells have an increased nuclear size and a delicate chromatin pattern (Fig. 14.24). A variety of other dyserythropoietic abnormalities occur, including nuclear polyploidy and fragmentation, with formation of Howell–Jolly bodies (Fig. 14.22). The formation of haemoglobin in developing erythroblasts is less affected and this asynchrony between nuclear and cytoplasmic maturation is one of the most distinctive features of megaloblastic erythropoiesis. Interference with granulocyte development is identified by abnormal (giant) metamyelocytes. Megakaryocytes are often reduced in number.

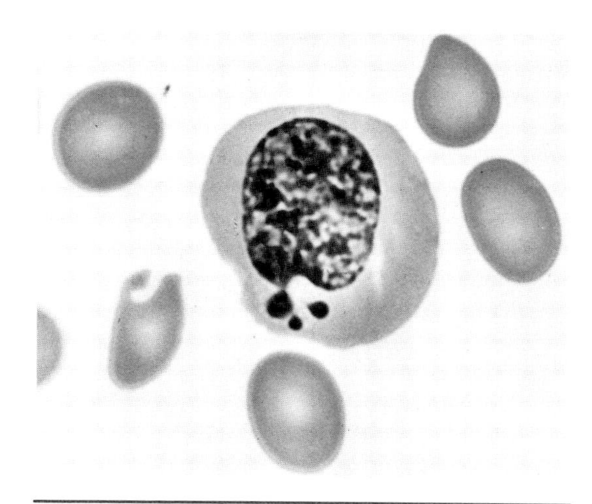

Fig. 14.22 Blood smear in pernicious anaemia showing a megaloblast with Howell–Jolly bodies. ×1300.

Neurological Changes

These are conspicuous only in vitamin B_{12} deficiency and may develop before anaemia becomes apparent. The principal lesion is subacute combined degeneration, characterized by discontinuous demyelination of the long pyramidal tracts and posterior columns of the mid-thoracic region of

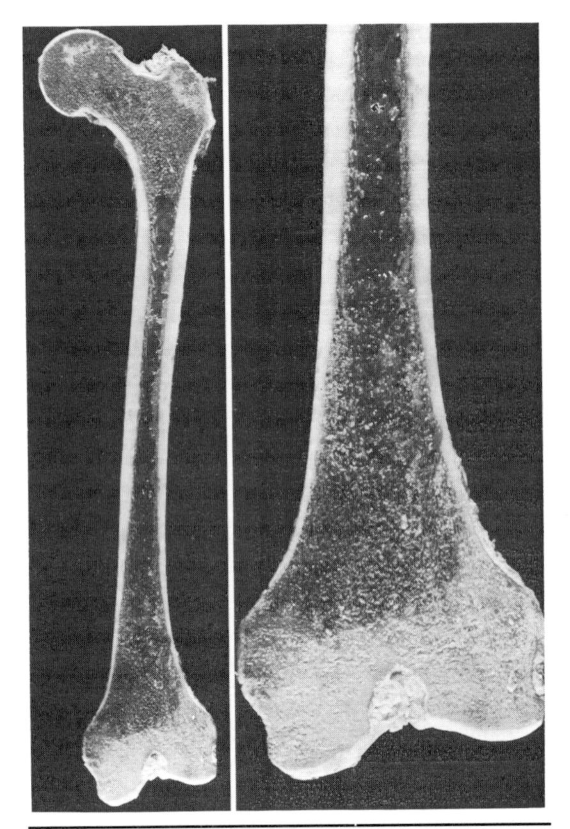

Fig. 14.23 *Left*, Section of femur in pernicious anaemia, showing the dark red marrow throughout the shaft. *Right*, lower end.

the spinal cord (p. 842). There may be patchy demyelination in large peripheral nerves and in the cerebral hemispheres. Psychiatric disturbances are not uncommon in vitamin B_{12} deficiency ('megaloblastic madness').

Early recognition of the neurological effects is mandatory because, although they can be arrested by treatment, they may not be completely reversible. The administration of folic acid alone can exacerbate the condition. Should urgent treatment of a megaloblastic anaemia be required before the cause is established, both vitamin B_{12} and folic acid must be given.

Effects on Other Tissues

Atrophic glossitis and oral ulceration are common features of vitamin B_{12} deficiency. In both vitamin B_{12} and folic acid deficiency, mild villous atrophy

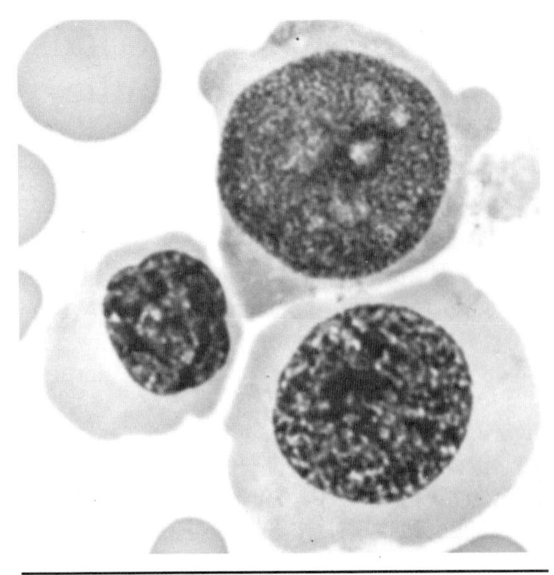

Fig. 14.24 Smear of bone marrow in pernicious anaemia, showing a promegaloblast (*above*) and two typical haemoglobinized megaloblasts. ×1700.

occurs in the small intestine. Sterility due to disturbed germ cell maturation is described in both sexes in vitamin B_{12} deficiency and is reversed by therapy. Slight to moderate splenic enlargement, due to increased red cell destruction or to extramedullary haemopoiesis, is often present.

Causes of Vitamin B_{12} Deficiency

These are summarized in Table 14.11. The most important is malabsorption due to intrinsic factor (IF) deficiency – pernicious anaemia – and this is discussed in greater detail separately.

The sole source of vitamin B_{12} is food of animal origin – meat, fish, eggs and dairy produce – and the minimal daily requirement is 1 μg. Normally liver stores will provide the total needs for 3–5 years. Thus inadequate dietary intake must occur over years; this may happen in underdeveloped parts of the world or in strict vegans.

As vitamin B_{12} is absorbed in the distal ileum, extensive disease in this area will interfere with its absorption – Crohn's disease, ileal resection, tropical sprue and lymphoma. Competitive loss of

Table 14.11 Causes of vitamin B_{12} deficiency

Decreased intake	Vegans; nutritional deficiency (rare)
Malabsorption	Gastric causes; atrophic gastritis, post-gastrectomy, congenital intrinsic factor deficiency
	Ileal causes: blind-loop syndrome with bacterial overgrowth, Crohn's disease and ileal resection, tropical sprue, infestation with *Diphyllobothrium latum*, chronic pancreatitis, drugs
Increased requirements	Pregnancy, haemolytic anaemia, disseminated malignancies

vitamin B_{12} occurs in states of intestinal stasis with bacterial overgrowth – blind loops, diverticulae and in intestinal infestation with the fish tape worm *Diphyllobothrium latum* (p. 1173). In chronic pancreatitis the fall in pH may reduce absorption. A number of drugs, e.g. biguanides, may also inhibit absorption. Vitamin B_{12} levels fall during pregnancy.

Pernicious Anaemia

Pernicious anaemia results from chronic atrophic autoimmune type A gastritis. In so-called juvenile pernicious anaemia there is a congenital intrinsic factor deficiency or production of defective intrinsic factor. Intrinsic factor deficiencies also result following gastrectomy.

Classical pernicious anaemia is most prevalent in North Europeans but can occur in all races. It occurs mainly in the elderly, and there is a strong familial tendency. There is convincing evidence that the chronic atrophic type A gastritis belongs to the group of organ-specific autoimmune diseases and patients and their relatives have a high incidence of autoimmune thryoiditis (p. 1089). The autoantibodies which are found in association with chronic atrophic gastritis are: (1) *antibody to parietal cells*, reactive with the microvilli of the canalicular system and present in the serum of 90% of patients; (2) antibody to the vitamin B_{12} binding site of intrinsic factor – *blocking antibody* – present in the serum and gastric juice of 60% of patients; (3) antibody reacting with IF and vitamin B_{12}–IF complexes – *binding antibody* present in the serum and gastric juices of 50% of patients and always in the presence of blocking antibody. The role of autoimmunity in the atrophic gastritis responsible for pernicious anaemia is discussed on p. 693. However, it should be borne in mind that some patients have no autoantibodies and conversely that parietal cell antibodies can occur in a significant proportion of elderly people with chronic gastritis and no evidence of pernicious anaemia. The intrinsic factor antibodies are much more specific for pernicious anaemia.

The histological changes in the stomach are described elsewhere (p. 694). Symptoms due to the gastritis are seldom significant. There is, however, an increased risk of gastric carcinoma, and this may supervene in some 5–10% of patients with pernicious anaemia.

The Diagnosis of Vitamin B_{12} Deficiency States

Once megaloblastic anaemia has been diagnosed by marrow examination, it is necessary to establish whether it is due to vitamin B_{12} or to folic acid deficiency. Vitamin B_{12} deficiency is established by the demonstration of a reduced level of the vitamin in the serum, measured by radio immunoassay. There is a wide range of normality (100–1200 μg/l) and each laboratory has its own standards. The cause of vitamin B_{12} deficiency can usually be determined by the Schilling test: a small dose of vitamin B_{12} labelled with ^{58}Co is administered orally, together with a parenteral 'loading dose' of 1000 μg unlabelled vitamin B_{12} to minimize utilization of the labelled B_{12} absorbed from the gut. The quantity absorbed is assessed by measuring urinary excretion of labelled vitamin B_{12} over 24 hours. With normal absorption more than 10% of the labelled dose appears in the urine. When there is intrinsic factor deficiency absorption is subnormal. A second stage of the test can then be carried out: intrinsic factor deficiency is indicated if the vitamin B_{12} is absorbed normally when given with oral intrinsic factor. Although demonstration of intrinsic factor deficiency is necessary for the definitive diagnosis of pernicious anaemia, the presence of histamine-fast achlorhydria in patients with megaloblastic anaemia establishes the diagnosis beyond reasonable doubt.

Causes of Folic Acid Deficiency

Dietary sources of folic acid include green vegetables, cereals, meat, fish and eggs. The average Western diet contains 650 μg folic acid daily, but up to 90% may be destroyed by cooking. The minimum daily requirement is 50 μg. Storage capacity provides for 80–100 days, the principal site being the liver. The absorption of folic acid occurs in the jejunum. The causes of folic acid deficiencies are listed in Table 14.12.

Inadequate dietary intake occurs in milk-fed babies (especially if premature), in the elderly and in chronic alcoholics. Coeliac disease and tropical sprue cause malabsorption of folic acid; malabsorption may also occur post-gastrectomy, in extensive Crohn's disease, in diffuse lymphomatous involvement of the small bowel and during phenytoin therapy. A rare cause is an inherited defect in the mucosal transport of folate.

Folic acid requirements are increased in pregnancy, in diseases producing increased haemopoietic activity, e.g. chronic haemolytic states, and in widespread malignancy when increased DNA synthesis requires additional folic acid. A number of drugs act as folic acid antagonists. Some inhibit dihydrofolate reductase (methotrexate, trimethoprim, pyrimethamine and triampterine); some may interfere with both intestinal absorption and intracellular folate metabolism (sulphasalazine); and some act by a mechanism not yet defined (alcohol, cycloserine and oral contraceptives).

Table 14.12 Causes of folic acid deficiency

Decreased intake	Nutritional deficiency, alcoholism
Malabsorption	Coeliac disease, tropical sprue, extensive Crohn's disease, gastrectomy, drugs
Increased requirements	Physiological: pregnancy, prematurity and infancy
	Pathological: chronic haemolytic anaemias, myeloproliferative disorders, disseminated malignancy, chronic inflammatory disease (e.g. rheumatoid arthritis), haemodialysis
Impaired utilization	Drugs, folic acid antagonists, e.g. methotrexate
	Liver diseases

The Diagnosis of Folic Acid Deficiency

Anaemia with megaloblastic haemopoiesis in the absence of vitamin B_{12} deficiency suggests deficiency of folic acid. Serum folate level may be measured by radioimmunoassay and the reference range is 3–15 μg/l. All folate-deficient patients show a low serum folate level but low serum levels may occur during immediate dietary deficiency in the absence of genuine deficiency. The red cell folate level is a measure of body folate stores (adult reference range is 160–640 μg/l packed red cells); however, a haematological response to folic acid remains the most convincing evidence of deficiency.

Iron Deficiency Anaemia

There is no regulatory mechanism for iron excretion and body iron content is controlled by absorption from the gut. About 70% of the 3–4 g of iron in the body is incorporated in the haem of haemoglobin: 5% is in myoglobin, and small but important amounts are incorporated in cellular cytochromes, other haem containing enzymes such as catalase and peroxidase and non-haem iron enzymes such as xanthine oxidase and ribonucleotide reductase. The remainder (0.3–1.4 g) is mostly in storage form in macrophages of the spleen, bone marrow, and liver and in various tissue cells, particularly hepatocytes.

Normal Iron Metabolism

Iron absorption occurs mainly in the duodenum and proximal jejunum. Dietary iron consists of haem, which is absorbed as metalloporphyrin, and non-haem iron which is absorbed mainly as ferrous salts, ferric salts being very poorly absorbed. The precise mechanism of iron uptake by the mucosal epithelium is not clear. The amounts taken up bear an inverse relationship to the total storage iron in the body (Fig. 14.25) and, within limits, varies directly with the amount available in the diet. Absorption of *non-haem iron* is aided by an acid pH; alcoholic drinks increase iron uptake by stimulating gastric acid secretion and also because some drinks contain iron. Gastric achlorhydria and the presence in the diet of compounds such as phytates from cereals, tannates and other food preservatives results in the formation of non-absorbable polymers. *Haem* is an important source of dietary iron because the proportion absorbed is relatively high. Overall, normal individuals absorb about 10% of the iron in a good mixed diet.

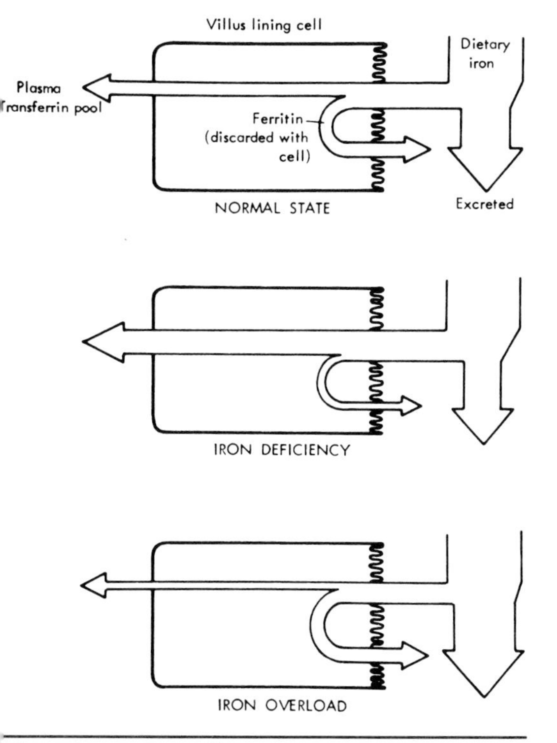

Fig. 14.25 The effect of the total iron store on absorption of dietary iron by intestinal epithelium. Only a fraction of the available dietary iron is normally taken up by the epithelium (*upper*): the fraction taken up is increased when total storage iron is depleted (*middle*) and decreased when the iron store is increased (*lower*). Of the iron taken up by the epithelium, the proportion transferred to the plasma transferrin pool is similarly affected by the total iron store.

Iron loss. In children and adult males, less than 1 mg of iron is lost passively from the body daily and this is replaced by absorption of iron from a balanced diet. In females, the average daily loss is increased by menstruation to about 1.6 mg and in the second and third trimesters of pregnancy to 3 mg due to fetal requirements. Therefore iron balance can be precarious in women of reproductive age where iron deficiency is common. Negative balance results from excessive loss and/or from impaired intake or absorption relative to requirements. Negative balance is compensated initially by mobilization of iron stores and by enhanced absorption, but eventually stores are depleted and the characteristic changes of iron deficiency appear in the blood.

Plasma iron. The normal average level is 13–32 μmol/l, 95% of which is in the form of transferrin. Transferrin possesses two binding sites for iron and is normally only about 30% saturated in the plasma. Transferrin is the form in which iron is transferred between the intestinal mucosa, red cell precursors in the marrow and liver cells. The macrophages of the spleen, marrow and liver do not have transferrin receptors and acquire iron by the breakdown of senescent red cells. Plasma iron status is now assessed on the basis of serum ferritin estimation (v.i.).

Storage iron. Iron is stored in macrophages in the spleen, marrow and liver. Hepatocytes also contain storage iron and for practical purposes these two cell types represent the main store. The iron is stored in two forms: (1) ferritin, which consists of micelles of ferric oxide and phosphate enclosed in protein molecules, and which is water soluble and present in the cytosol; and (2) haemosiderin, present in lysosomes and in which the protein of ferritin has been degraded; it is insoluble, is seen as golden-yellow intracytoplasmic granules and gives the Prussian blue (Perls') reaction on treatment with hydrochloric acid and potassium ferrocyanide, the intense blue colour being due to formation of ferri-ferrocyanide. In states of negative iron balance iron is transferred from the intracellular ferritin and haemosiderin of macrophages and hepatocytes to the plasma transferrin pool and anaemia does not develop until after the stores are depleted.

Causes of Iron Deficiency Anaemia

Chronic blood loss is the only way large quantities of iron are lost from the body. The loss of 10–15 ml blood daily (5–7 mg iron) is equivalent to the maximum amount of iron absorbed from a normal diet. Heavy menstrual bleeding and occult bleeding from unsuspected lesions of the gastrointestinal tract, especially peptic ulceration or ulcerated tumours, commonly present with iron deficiency anaemia. Infestation by hookworm (ancylostomiasis) causes considerable gastrointestinal bleeding and is probably the most important cause of iron deficiency worldwide (p. 1179).

Malabsorption of iron. Iron is absorbed mainly in the duodenum and disease there causes iron deficiency, e.g. coeliac disease. Normal gastric acid secretion is necessary for iron absorption and gastrectomy or achlorhydria predispose to iron deficiency.

Low dietary intake is important in infants before weaning, especially in developing countries. Dietary deficiency is, however, seldom the sole cause of anaemia.

Changes in the Blood and Bone Marrow

When iron stores are totally depleted no Prussian blue stainable iron is present in the bone marrow. There is erythroid hyperplasia and the late erythroblasts show defective haemoglobinization. The red cells become hypochromic and microcytic; poikilocytosis is present and in severe deficiency ring staining and narrow elliptocytes (rod cells) may be seen (Fig. 14.26).

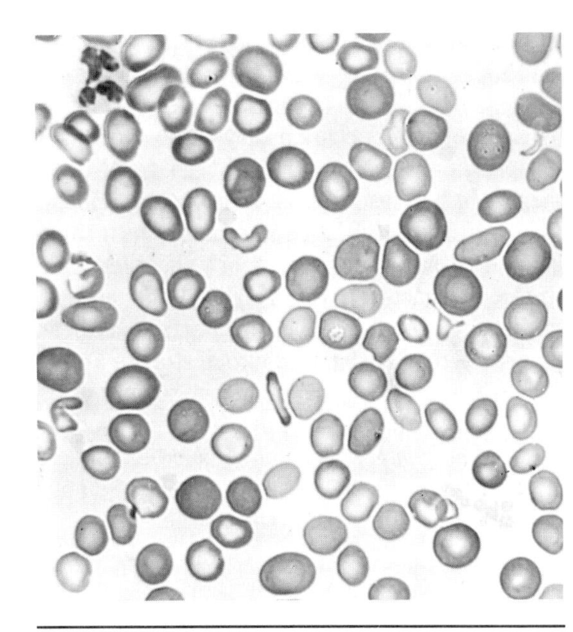

Fig. 14.26 Blood smear in iron deficiency anaemia, showing some variation in the size of red cells and some rod cells: note also ring staining which is, however, not diagnostic. ×800.

In latent iron deficiency the blood picture may be normal but serum iron levels are low, transferrin saturation is less than 15% (normal 30%) and serum ferritin levels less than 14 μg/l (normal range 20–100 μg/l). With increasing iron deficiency, serum total iron binding capacity rises due to increased hepatic synthesis of transferrin and the saturation levels fall to less than 10%.

Changes in Other Tissues

These occur because of depletion of iron-containing enzymes in the tissues. The nails become striated and brittle and may eventually become spoon-shaped (koilonychia). Atrophic glossitis, fissuring of the angles of the mouth and dysphagia due to folding of lax mucosa in the upper oesophagus (oesophageal web) may occur. The latter, the Brown–Paterson–Kelly or Plummer–Vinson syndrome, may predispose to post-cricoid oesophageal carcinoma. Atrophic gastritis may result in achlorhydria and this will aggravate iron deficiency. The oral and nail changes usually respond to iron, but achlorhydria may be permanent.

Iron deficiency is the commonest cause of hypochromic microcytic anaemia, but any failure of haemoglobin synthesis will have the same effect. In some patients the fault lies in globin chain synthesis (thalassaemia) while in others haem synthesis is inadequate (sideroblastic anaemias).

Anaemias Due to Disorders of Iron Metabolism

Anaemias of Chronic Disease

In chronic infection, rheumatoid arthritis, systemic lupus erythematosus, disseminated carcinoma and other wasting diseases, there is a mild microcytic anaemia due to a block in iron release from macrophages: plasma iron is low but total iron-binding capacity is also reduced, therefore iron saturation is not as low as in iron deficiency. The result, however, is adequate marrow iron that cannot be utilized and erythroblast maturation is delayed. Serum ferritin is normal or raised. There is reduced erythropoietic activity in the marrow and often a mild reduction in red cell lifespan. So long as the causal condition persists, so does the anaemia.

Sideroblastic Anaemias

These are characterized by the presence of Prussian blue staining iron granules arranged around the nuclei of erythroblasts in a ring fashion (ring sideroblasts). The appearance is due to impairment of iron utilization within the cell, producing mitochondria laden with iron. A rare inherited form of this disorder is X-linked, occurring in males in childhood or adolescence. The more common form, **primary acquired sideroblastic anaemia**, occurs in middle-aged or elderly subjects who present with symptoms of mild anaemia. Such patients may eventually develop acute non-lymphoblastic leukaemia. **Secondary sideroblastic anaemia** is caused by specific toxins such as alcohol, antituberculous drugs, chloramphenicol and lead, or may be associated with leukaemias and other myeloproliferative disorders, carcinomatosis and erythropoietic porphyria.

Aplastic and Hypoplastic Anaemias

Anaemia is termed aplastic when little or no cellular marrow exists and hypoplastic when marrow is merely of reduced cellularity. Aplasia restricted to red cell precursors (*pure red cell aplasia*) may be congenital (*Blackfan–Diamond anaemia* or *erythrogenesis imperfecta*) or acquired, usually in adults and often associated with a *benign thymoma* (p. 646). It is, however, more usual for all cell lines to be involved, resulting in pancytopenia. Rarely this may be congenital (*Fanconi anaemia*, usually associated with other abnormalities, e.g. skeletal malformations and congenital heart disease) but is more commonly acquired.

Acquired Aplastic Anaemia

Marrow aplasia may occur predictably in individuals given cytotoxic drugs or irradiation as treatment for malignant disease and its development is dose dependent. It is usually possible to avoid serious marrow damage by careful monitoring of the peripheral blood and adjustment of treatment. This form of aplasia is not included under the heading of 'acquired aplastic anaemia'.

However, marrow aplasia may result from an

idiosyncratic reaction to drugs and this is a dose-independent reaction. This and the other types of acquired aplastic anaemia are comparatively rare, and in 50% of cases the disease is idiopathic (Table 14.13). The incidence of aplastic anaemia in Caucasians is approximately 3–4 per million population per year, but is higher in the Far East. There is a male preponderance and there are two peaks in age distribution – one in an under 20 age group and a second in older persons. In drug-associated cases there is usually a delay of 1–6 months between exposure and the onset of pancytopenia.

In viral hepatitis the aplastic anaemia usually develops after infection in the non-A, non-B variety but in others it may occur simultaneously with the hepatitis. Parvovirus infection may cause an aplastic crisis in sickle cell disease and in other haemolytic states such as hereditary spherocytosis. Although a rare condition, interest in aplastic anaemia has been stimulated by improved methods of support and treatment, particularly by the introduction of allogeneic bone marrow transplantation. A functional definition of aplastic anaemia is failure of haemopoietic stem cells to proliferate and differentiate in the absence of any predictable cause. Aplastic anaemia associated with viral hepatitis and Epstein–Barr virus carries a poor prognosis. Short-term marrow cultures from patients with aplastic anaemia show reduction in all types of committed precursor cells but whether the stem cell failure results from an intrinsic defect or because of damage to the haemopoietic microenvironment is not known. The ability of bone marrow transplants to cure some cases of aplastic anaemia favours the former although there is some evidence that T cell derived factors from patients with aplastic anaemia will depress *in vitro* marrow cultures from normal individuals. Acute leukaemia may supervene in patients with aplastic anaemia, suggesting that the marrow hypoplasia is a preleukaemic state.

Clinically, patients present with symptoms related to the anaemia, with minor persistent infections or with a bleeding tendency. The peripheral blood shows pancytopenia and the reticulocyte count is reduced. The red cells are normochromic and normocytic and the lymphocyte count may be normal. The marrow is hypocellular and fatty (Fig. 14.27) though islands of haemopoietic tissue persist. Both marrow aspirate and trephine biopsy are essential for diagnosis. The main differential diagnoses to be excluded are preleukaemia and a

Table 14.13 Aetiology of acquired aplastic anaemia

Idiopathic
Drugs*
  Idiosyncratic reaction, e.g. chloramphenicol, phenylbutazone, indomethacin, gold
Chemicals
  Benzene, insecticides, analine dyes
Infections
  Viral hepatitis, Epstein–Barr, cytomegalo- and parvoviruses
Associated with
  Autoimmune disease, paroxysmal nocturnal haemoglobinuria

*Irradiation and drugs which on a dose-dependent basis predictably cause marrow aplasia are excluded.

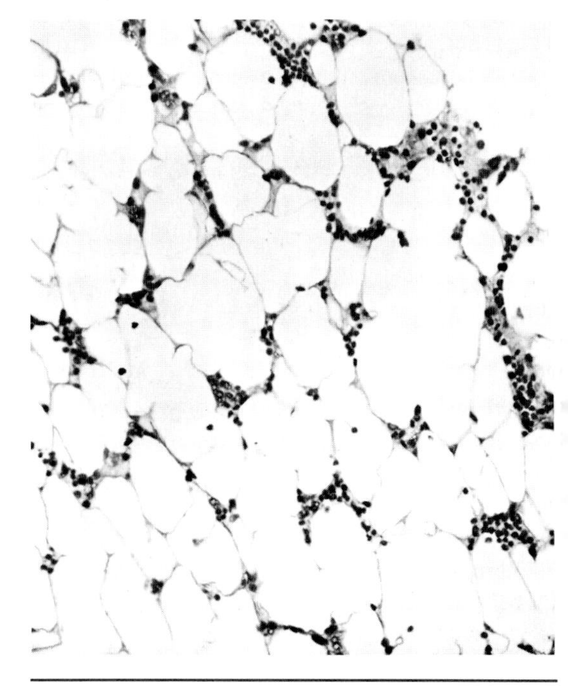

Fig. 14.27 Sternal marrow biopsy in aplastic anaemia due to chloramphenicol. There is great reduction in the numbers of cell types. ×250.

myelodysplastic syndrome. The treatment initially comprises supportive therapy with prophylactic antibiotics and red cell and platelet transfusion. Androgen therapy (oxymetholone) may be of value. Immunosuppression with corticosteroids and antilymphocyte globulin is the next line of treatment. In patients under 40 years allogeneic bone marrow transplantation may be attempted, haematological remission occurring in 50–60% of patients.

Other Conditions Associated with Anaemia

Pregnancy. The haemoglobin level falls during normal pregnancy due to an increase in plasma volume – physiological anaemia. There are, however, increased demands for iron and folic acid. Good antenatal care requires careful haematological assessment and supplementation of the diet with both iron and folic acid.

Liver diseases. The mild anaemia of acute and chronic liver disease is often characterized by the presence of target cells and there may be mild haemolysis. Folic acid deficiency may sometimes occur, in part due to impaired storage. Zieve's syndrome with frank haemolysis and hyperlipidaemia may complicate alcohol-induced cirrhosis. Gastrointestinal bleeding and hypersplenism will aggravate any anaemic state.

Renal diseases. Anaemia is often severe in chronic renal failure. The major cause is decreased erythropoietin production by the kidneys. Recombinant erythropoietin is now used with considerable benefit.

Malignant disease. Anaemia may occur as a non-metastatic effect of many malignant diseases. There may be disordered iron metabolism, and folic acid deficiency due to increased utilization by tumour cells or as a result of chemotherapy. Bone marrow replacement by metastases will also cause anaemia with a leucoerythroblastic reaction, particularly when metastases are numerous or when they stimulate an osteosclerotic reaction, a common feature with prostatic cancer.

Neoplasias of the Haemopoietic Tissues

The commonest of these are the leukaemias, usually myeloid (granulocytic) or lymphoid, in which neoplastic cells circulate in the blood. The myelodysplastic syndromes, which are not initially neoplastic, often progress to leukaemia and include many of the disorders classified as preleukaemias. The chronic myeloproliferative disorders form another group consisting of (1) polycythaemia rubra vera, a proliferation mainly of the erythroid series, (2) myelofibrosis, a related condition in which there is also fibrosis of the marrow, and (3) essential thrombocythaemia, in which megakaryocytic proliferation predominates. These last three conditions have overlapping features and intermediate forms are observed, reflecting an origin from a pluripotent haemopoietic stem cell. Neoplasia of lymphoid cells include lymphoid leukaemias and plasma-cell tumours, most of which originate in the marrow, and also the lymphomas, nodal and extranodal, which are discussed in Chapter 15.

General features. Although haemopoietic neoplasias are classified by the predominant cell type, there may be proliferation of two or more cell lines. Megakaryocytic proliferation and thrombocytosis are common features of chronic granulocytic leukaemia, while erythroid, myeloid and megakaryocytic cells all proliferate in polycythaemia rubra vera. Most forms of haemopoietic neoplasia differ from carcinomas and sarcomas in that they usually infiltrate the marrow and other tissues diffusely, rather than forming distinct tumour masses. They suppress and replace the normal haemopoietic elements, with consequent reduction in the production of red cells, white cells and platelets. A high degree of cell differentiation, i.e. maturation, is usually associated with a chronic course, and impaired differentiation with more aggressive behaviour, but virtually all forms are malignant and likely to be fatal in the untreated patient.

The Leukaemias

Leukaemia is a primary neoplastic clonal disorder of the bone marrow. The neoplastic cells escape into the blood where they may be present in large numbers, hence leukaemia. Leukaemias are divided into two forms, acute and chronic. Acute leukaemias involve proliferation of immature cells while the chronic forms involve maturing cells. Untreated patients with acute leukaemia follow a relentless, downhill course to death in weeks, whereas those with the chronic forms survive longer. With more effective therapy, however, this is changing radically.

The two main acute leukaemias are acute lymphoblastic (ALL) and acute non-lymphoblastic (ANLL): the latter can show myeloid, monocytic, erythroid or megakaryocytic differentiation. The two main chronic types are chronic lymphocytic leukaemia (CLL) and chronic granulocytic leukaemia (CGL).

The annual incidence of leukaemia (all types) in the general population is about 9 per 100 000; this increases to 69 per 100 000 in the over 65 age group. With the exception of ALL over 50% of leukaemias occur in the elderly.

The Acute Leukaemias

Acute leukaemias may be divided by age into those of childhood, 80% of which are ALL and those in adults (>15 years), 85% of which are ANLL. The characteristic cell in acute leukaemia is a poorly differentiated immature 'blast' cell which fails to differentiate. Acute leukaemia cells in culture can be induced to differentiate by the addition of certain agents, including corticosteroids, haemopoietic growth factors and some chemicals. However, treatment of acute leukaemia still depends mainly on destruction of the leukaemic cells rather than modification of their behaviour.

Clinical features. The clinical features of acute leukaemia are attributable mainly to failure of normal haemopoiesis. This leads to the triad of *anaemia, recurrent infection* due to reduction in normal leucocytes, and *bleeding* due to thrombocytopenia. In children the disease appears abruptly, with fever, weakness, pallor, bleeding from the gums and petechial haemorrhages into the skin. Intercurrent infection is common and without treatment the course from onset to death may be only a few weeks. In adults, the disease may be more insidious, but the clinical features are similar.

Blood picture. The leucocyte count is raised in about 50% of cases but may be normal or low in others. The diagnostic feature is that most of the cells are blasts, with nucleoli and a high nuclear/cytoplasmic ratio. Anaemia and thrombocytopenia are invariable.

Bone marrow. Marrow aspirate shows a marked increase in cellularity, most of the cells being primitive blasts (Fig. 14.28). Normal haemopoietic elements, especially neutrophils and megakaryocytes, are sparse. There is extension of leukaemic marrow along the shafts of long bones.

Other tissues. Extensive diffuse tissue infiltration occurs during the course of acute leukaemia, and almost any organ can be affected. Splenic enlargement is common but seldom gross. Lymph node enlargement is frequently seen in ALL but is unusual in ANLL. In some instances of childhood ALL, a thymic lymphoid tumour (Sternberg's

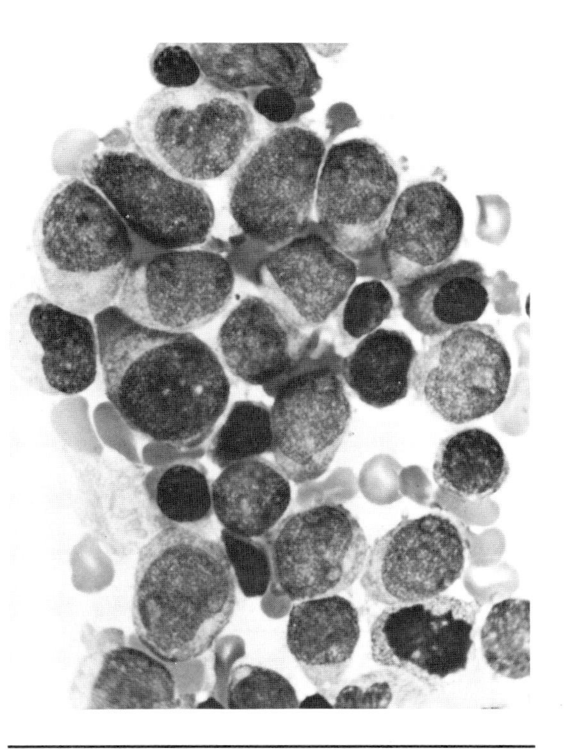

Fig. 14.28 Smear of sternal marrow in acute leukaemia. Nearly all the cells are primitive 'blasts' with a large nucleus containing one or more nucleoli, and with scanty basophilic cytoplasm. ×750.

tumour) precedes the onset of T cell ALL. Leukaemic cells in ALL are often deposited in the subarachnoid space and may escape destruction during treatment because, with the exception of methotrexate in high dosage, cytotoxic drugs do not reach an effective concentration in the cerebrospinal fluid. Such cells provide a nidus from which relapse may occur. Similarly, ALL cells which have infiltrated the gonads, especially the testes, may be a source of relapse. Meningeal and testicular involvement is rare in ANLL.

Diagnosis of Acute Leukaemia

The diagnosis of acute leukaemia is based on the clinical features, the blood picture, and the morphology of the bone marrow. To assess prognosis and select appropriate treatment it is necessary to distinguish between ANLL and ALL (Table 14.14) and to identify their subtypes. Leukaemia subclassification follows the protocols of the French–American–British (FAB) co-operative group based on the morphology of leukaemic cells stained by Romanowsky methods (Tables 14.15

Table 14.14 Differential diagnosis of acute lymphoblastic leukaemia (ALL) and acute non-lymphoblastic leukaemia (ANLL)

	ALL	ANLL
Morphological		
Cell size	Small/moderate	Moderate/large
Nuclei	Usually 1 or 2 nucleoli	Frequently more than 2 nucleoli
Cytoplasm	Scanty/moderate; homogeneous	Moderate/abundant; granular, sometimes with Auer rods
Cytochemical		
Peroxidase/Sudan black B	Negative	Positive
Acid phosphatase	Positive	Usually negative
Nuclear terminal deoxynucleotidyl transferase (Tdt)	Positive	Occasionally positive
CD 19 (pan B)	Positive (common and null ALL)	Negative
CD 7 (pan T)	Positive (T cell)	Negative
CD 13 and CD 33	Negative	Positive

Table 14.15 The French–American–British (FAB) morphological classification of acute lymphoblastic leukaemia (ALL) with the corresponding immunophenotype and incidence

FAB classification; morphological features	Immunophenotype	Membrane markers	Approximate incidence	
			Children	Adults
L1 Small; homogeneous cell population L2 Large; heterogeneous cell population; one or two nucleoli	Early B cell: null (n) cell ALL†	CD19	10%	35%
	Pre B cell: common (c) ALL††	CD19 and CD10*	75%	50%
	T cell ALL	CD2 and CD7	10%	10%
L3 Large; vacuolated cytoplasm; heterogeneous cell population; nucleoli prominent	Mature B cell: ALL†††	CD19 and sIg	<1%	2%

† Ig heavy chain rearrangement.
†† Ig heavy ± light chain rearrangement.
††† Ig heavy and light chain rearrangement.
* Also intracytoplasmic μ chain.
sIg, surface immunoglobulins.

Table 14.16 The French–American–British (FAB) morphological classification of acute non-lymphoblastic leukaemia (ANLL)

	FAB classification	Comments
M0	Undifferentiated myeloblastic	No cytochemical markers can be defined
M1	Acute myelocytic leukaemia without differentiation	
M2	Acute myelocytic leukaemia with differentiation	Also on M2-baso: basophil myeloblasts present
M3	Acute promyelocytic leukaemia	Hypergranular promyelocytes M3-variant: hypogranular promyelocytes
M4	Acute myelomonocytic leukaemia	Myeloid elements resemble M2; peripheral blood monocytosis
M5	Acute monocytic leukaemia	
M6	Acute erythroleukaemia	
M7	Acute megakaryocytic leukaemia	Myelofibrosis may also occur

and 14.16). This can be augmented by cytochemistry and immunophenotyping markers and by cytogenetic studies. Only 2% of adult and less than 1% of childhood acute leukaemias fail to be categorized using these methods.

Immunophenotyping or cell marker analysis has been facilitated by the development of monoclonal antibodies and this has defined many clusters of differentiation (CD) antigens. Thus, the blast cells in common ALL express CD antigens which may also be found on normal bone marrow precursors while those in T cell ALL express the antigens of thymic cells. Leukaemic cells therefore express normal differentiation antigens, but sometimes hese appear in abnormal combinations which are not seen in their normal counterparts. No leukaemic specific surface marker has yet been found. mmunophenotyping, in addition to its use in diagnosis, has contributed to our understanding of eukaemogenesis, is of value in determining prognosis and possible lines of treatment and is of value n the follow-up of patients after chemotherapy or one marrow transplantation. The techniques of igh resolution chromosome banding (p. 50) vith the demonstration of chromosomal abnormalities have been of similar diagnostic and prognostic usefulness. These techniques are still at a levelopmental stage but may ultimately replace norphological criteria for classification of the leukaemias (and other myeloproliferative disorders).

Acute Lymphoblastic Leukaemia (ALL)

Childhood. This is the common acute leukaemia of childhood, but, rarely, can occur in adults. About 80% of childhood acute leukaemias are ymphoblastic and the highest incidence is in the irst 5 years of life. The morphological and mmunophenotypic features are outlined in Table 14.15. About one-third of the common ALL cases ave cytoplasmic μ chains and are thus derived rom pre-B cells (p. 169). About 75% of childhood ALL express the common ALL antigen (CD10) vhile the percentage is lower in adults. The emonstration of the nuclear enzyme DNA polymerase terminyl transferase (TdT) is an important ool in ifferentiating ALL from ANNL. TdT is seldom resent in ANNL but present in most cases of ALL.

Chromosomal abnormalities are often found in ALL. Hyperploidy with chromosome numbers beween 50 and 60 may occur and is associated with a ood prognosis. Translocations also occur: the hiladelphia (Ph) chromosome t(9;22) is present in % of cases and t(4;11) is found in 5% of cases oth adults and children) and in 75% of cases aged ess than 6 months. In B cell ALL a t(8;14) is ound, a translocation also seen in Burkitt's lymphoma (p. 670); in T cell ALL t(9;22) and t(4;11) have been reported. These abnormalities, especially if they persist after treatment, are all associated with a poor prognosis.

Also of clinical significance is the morphological/immunological subclassification. Common ALL is usually of L1 type and occurs more frequently in girls, with a peak incidence between 3 and 7 years. The white cell count is usually between 5 and 15 × 10^9/l and the response to treatment is good. Null ALL, also of L1 morphology, has a worse prognosis than common ALL. T-ALL tends to occur in older children, particularly boys, where it can be associated with the presence of a thymic tumour; the leukaemic cells express intrathymic T cell markers and are thus immature. It is characterized by a high WCC (>40 × 10^9/l). Response to treatment is poor and relapse from surviving cells in the meninges is common. In general, males, a high WCC at presentation, age less than 2 or more than 10, chromosomal abnormalities, apart from hyperploidy and L3 morphology are bad prognostic signs. Null, B- and T-ALL all do worse than cALL.

Adults. The distribution of the various subtypes is different from that in children, null cell ALL being more common (Table 14.15). About 20% have the Ph chromosome. The prognosis in general is worse than in children, but remission lasting 5 years or more can now be achieved in about 25% of cases.

Acute Non-lymphoblastic Leukaemias (ANLL)

The acute non-lymphoblastic leukaemias occur in all age groups and include eight subtypes (M0 and M1–7) in the FAB classification as listed in Table 14.16. These emphasize the considerable heterogeneity which exists within this group and justifies the use of the term acute non-lymphoblastic rather than acute myeloblastic leukaemia. Division into further subtypes has resulted from cell-marker and cytogenetic studies.

The FAB *type MO* is undifferentiated myeloblastic leukaemia which does not stain with any of the cytochemical markers listed in Table 14.14.

Types M1–3 are all leukaemias of the myeloblast series but differ in the degree of differentiation. In *M1*, less than 10% of the cells differentiate sufficiently to produce azurophil granules or give a positive peroxidase or Sudan black B reaction. Most cells have large rounded nuclei and up to four prominent nucleoli. In *M2* the cells have bilobed or reniform nuclei, usually an Auer rod, azurophil granules, and are peroxidase and Sudan black B positive; variable numbers of cells differentiate into abnormal promyelocytes, myelocytes and even granulocytes. In *M3*, most of the cells are rich in peroxidase-positive azurophil granules; some contain bundles of Auer rods and resemble promyelocytes. Two populations of cells are present in *M4*, myeloblasts and monoblasts. These may be distinguished by non-specific esterase activity; both cell types are positive but pretreatment with sodium fluoride inhibits the reaction of monoblasts. In *M5*, most of the leukaemic cells are monoblasts. *M6* is characterized by the presence of both myeloblasts and primitive erythroblasts; some of the latter have multiple or lobed nuclei and account for 30% of nucleated cells in the marrow. Type *M7* is megakaryocytic leukaemia.

Over 50% of ANLL are M1 or M2; about 30% are M4, and M3, 5, 6 and 7 are uncommon. With intensive chemotherapy, M3 has the longest survival, while M6 has a poor prognosis. The remaining types show considerable individual variation in response to treatment.

Chromosomal abnormalities are found in over 80% of cases of ANLL, the commonest abnormality being trisomy 8. Some translocations are associated with specific subtypes; t(15;17) is unique to the M3 type and t(8;21) is found in about 25% of M2 cases, usually young males. Inversion of 16 or deletion of 16q occurs in about 25% of M4 cases and is associated with eosinophilia. Chromosomal abnormalities may also influence prognosis; t(8;21) and inv.16 indicate a favourable prognosis, t(15;17) and del Y are of intermediate prognosis and others carry a poor prognosis. In cases of secondary leukaemia following cytotoxic therapy or environmental exposure to carcinogens, chromosomal abnormalities, for example monosomy 7 or 5, are extremely common (>90%).

The Chronic Leukaemias

Chronic lymphocytic leukaemia (CLL) is rare below 40 years of age, the median age of onset being 50–60 years. It accounts for almost 50% of leukaemias occurring after the age of 60 years. The median age of onset of chronic granulocytic leukaemia is 30–40 years, but it occurs over a wide age range and can occur in children. In both diseases, large numbers of leucocytes circulate in the blood and eventually infiltrate various tissues. In most cases the initial leukaemic proliferation is readily controlled by drugs, but many patients with CLL remain well without treatment. In contrast, in CGL the prognosis is poor due to the occurrence of an acute phase (blast transformation) characterized by decreasing cell maturity and greater resistance to therapy.

Chronic Lymphocytic Leukaemia (CLL)

Blood picture. The outstanding feature is a marked increase in leucocytes, often 100 × 10^9/l or higher; nearly all are mature small lymphocytes (Fig. 14.29). Although the disease appears to originate in the marrow, pancytopenia is a late feature. However, autoimmune haemolytic anaemia and thrombocytopenia occur as early complications in about 10% of cases. There is often a reduction in normal serum immunoglobulin levels and paraproteinaemia, usually IgM, occurs in 5% of cases. In CLL 95% of cases are of B cell and 5% of T cell lineage. The leukaemic B cells possess surface immunoglobulin (sIg) and show light chain restriction, express CD19 and CD20 antigens and do not contain TdT. They are long lived with low proliferative activity. Chromosomal changes are found in half the cases, trisomy 12 being the most common.

Bone marrow. From an early stage the bone

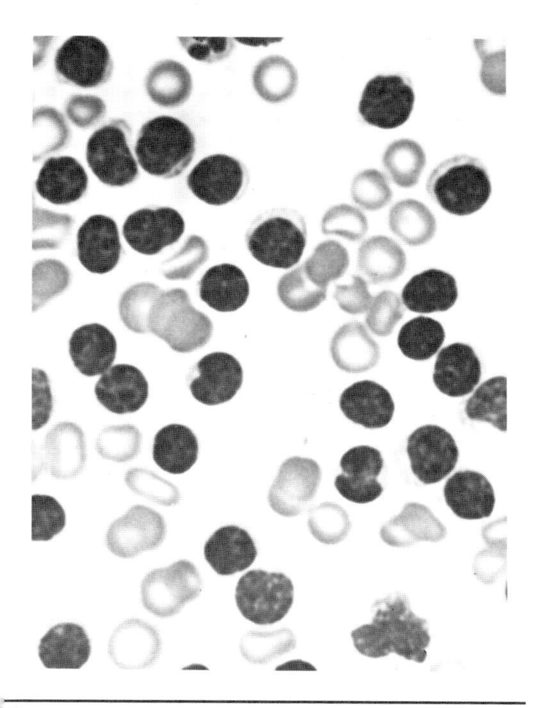

Fig. 14.29 Blood smear in chronic lymphocytic leukaemia. Most of the leukaemic cells have the appearances of normal small lymphocytes, a narrow ring of pale cytoplasm enclosing a round, dense nucleus of about the diameter of a red cell. ×750.

marrow shows excess lymphocytes initially focal but later diffusely replacing normal haemopoietic cells and extending into the fatty marrow.

Other tissues. Generalized lymph node enlargement is often the presenting sign. The nodes are soft and rubbery and appear homogeneous, pinkish-grey on section. Microscopically, nodal architecture is lost and replaced by a diffuse lymphocytic infiltrate. The spleen may be enlarged, due to extensive infiltration by lymphocytes filling the red pulp and obscuring the Malpighian bodies. Similarly the liver may be enlarged.

Staging of CLL based on physical examination and blood picture, is performed to assess the extent of disease and indicate prognosis. Two staging systems in common use are shown in Table 14.17. Both are of prognostic value and are of help in determining appropriate therapy. Poor prognostic features at presentation are large numbers of circulating prolymphocytes, massive splenomegaly and evidence of marrow failure.

Diagnosis and course. Minimum diagnostic criteria are: (1) a persistent circulating lymphocyte count of $>5 \times 10^9$/l, and (2) bone marrow lymphocytosis >30%. The clinical course is extremely variable: it may be rapidly progressive with a fatal outcome in 1–2 years or it may be static over decades. There is an increased susceptibility to bacterial infection and bronchopneumonia is often the immediate cause of death.

Variants of Chronic Lymphocytic Leukaemia

Prolymphocytic leukaemia. This may be B cell (80%) or T cell (20%) and largely comprises prolymphocytes. Typically the white cell count is high, splenomegaly is pronounced with little lymphadenopathy and the disease progresses more rapidly than typical CLL.

Hairy-cell leukaemia. This is of B cell lineage, the descriptive term deriving from the presence of circulating malignant cells which have multiple fine hair-like cytoplasmic projections. Pancytopenia is usually present. The diagnosis is confirmed by the cytochemical demonstration of cytoplasmic tartrate-resistant acid phosphatase in the hairy cells. The disease occurs mainly in elderly males who present with general ill-health. Lymph node enlargement is uncommon but massive splenomegaly with hypersplenism occurs as the disease progresses and with severe neutropenia the patients may benefit from splenectomy. Marrow fibrosis also occurs. There are recent reports of a clinical response to interferon-γ. Median survival is about 5 years.

T cell CLL. These, as already indicated, are rare but CD4 positive and CD8 positive subtypes are now recognized. The CD4 positive cases pursue an aggressive clinical course while the CD8 positive cases have a better prognosis. In the latter the cells show abundant granular cytoplasm; severe erythroid and myeloid hypoplasia may occur.

Table 14.17 Clinical staging of chronic lymphocytic leukaemia

Rai *et al.* (1975)	
Stage 0	Lymphocytosis of blood and marrow only
Stage I	Lymphocytosis and enlarged lymph nodes
Stage II	Lymphocytosis and enlarged liver or spleen or both, with or without enlarged nodes
Stage III	As with O, I and II but Hb < 11 g/dl
Stage IV	As with O, I, II or III but platelet count < 100 × 10^9/l
Binet *et al.* (1981)	
Group A (good prognosis) – more than 10 years	HB > 10g/dl: platelet count > 100 × 10^9/l; fewer than three sites of palpable organ involvement
Group B (intermediate)	Hb and platelet count as for A *but* 3 or more sites of palpable organ involvement
Group C (poor prognosis) – less than 2 years	Hb < 10 g/dl; platelet count < 100 × 10^9/l

Chronic Granulocytic Leukaemia (CGL)

While commonest in adults of 30–40 years, this disease can occur at any age. The clinical picture is usually dominated by gross hepatic and splenic enlargement. Signs of impaired marrow function, such as anaemia or thrombocytopenia, are inconspicuous until late in the disease. After a variable period, usually several years, ANLL or common ALL supervene.

It is generally accepted that CGL arises as a result of a mutation or series of mutations in a single pluripotential haemopoietic stem cell. Evidence for this comes from studies on CGL patients heterozygous for glucose-6-phosphate dehydrogenase (G-6-PD) isoenzymes, which have revealed that all the leukaemic cells express the same isoenzyme. Confirmatory evidence for the monoclonal origin of CGL comes from the distribution of the Philadelphia (Ph') chromosome in haemopoietic precursors of CGL patients: it is found in cells of granulocytic, erythroid, megakaryocytic and even B-lymphoid origin. Acute transformation in CGL may affect any or several of these lineages.

The Philadelphia (Ph') chromosome (p. 72) is a reciprocal translocation of parts of the long arms of chromosomes 9 and 22 – t(9;22)(q34;q11). In approximately 90% of CGL patients the Ph chromosome can be identified in marrow cell metaphases, and they have a median survival of 42 months whereas the remainder are Ph negative and have only a 15-month median survival. In occasional patients the Ph positive stem cells do not dominate haemopoiesis completely and both Ph +ve and Ph −ve metaphases are found: this is associated with a relatively long survival. It has recently been found that treatment with alpha interferon can increase the percentage of normal metaphases and can rarely even lead to loss of the Philadelphia chromosome. The development of additional chromosome changes during the chronic phase of CGL is, however, a grave prognostic sign and indicates incipient acute transformation; additional chromosomal changes are present in over 80% of cases with acute transformation and some of these have been described earlier. It is worth reiterating that a few cases of ALL and ANLL are also Ph chromosome positive.

Blood picture. The outstanding feature is the gross circulating leucocytosis, sometimes exceeding 300 × 10^9/l. While many are mature neutrophil granulocytes (Fig. 14.30), metamyelocytes and myelocytes are always present and in rapidly progressing cases myelocytes may predominate (Fig. 14.31). Occasionally eosinophils are numerous and a significant increase in basophils is a useful diagnostic feature. Anaemia is generally moderate, but

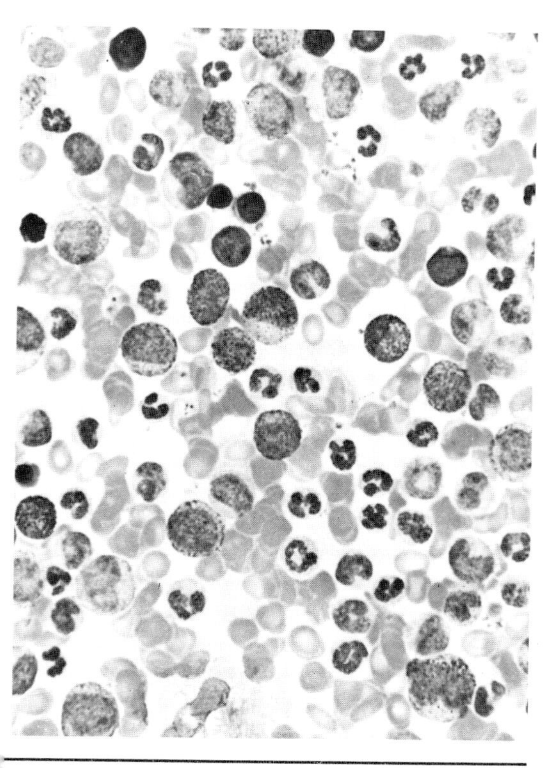

Fig. 14.30 Blood smear in chronic granulocytic leukaemia, showing myelocytes, neutrophil granulocytes and intermediate forms; two erythroblasts are seen above centre of field. ×500.

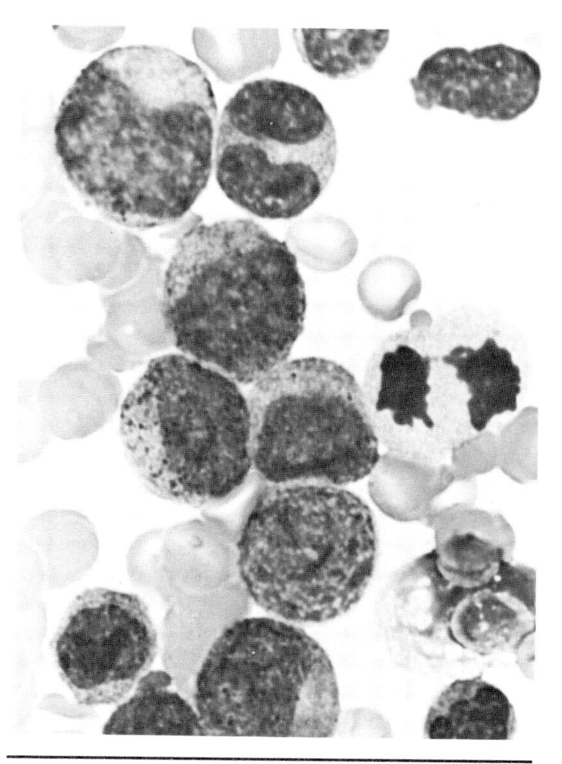

Fig. 14.31 Blood smear in chronic granulocytic leukaemia, showing a finely granular myelocytes and neutrophil granulocytes. One cell is in mitosis. ×1000.

increasing anaemia and other features of marrow failure may indicate transformation to an acute phase. In 75% of patients acute transformation is myeloblastic, whereas in the remaining 25%, transformation is lymphoblastic, usually of common ALL type. Occasionally blast cells are of more than one lineage, e.g. myeloblasts and lymphoblasts. Most patients in blast-cell crisis die within 6 months despite treatment.

The diagnosis of CGL is usually easy, but a pronounced reactive leucocytosis (leukaemoid reaction) can closely mimic CGL. Features which confirm the diagnosis of CGL include: (1) a high proportion of myelocytes; (2) an absolute increase in proliferating marrow cells; (4) low levels of alkaline phosphatase in leukaemic neutrophils in contrast to reactive leucocytosis; and (5) elevation of serum vitamin B_{12}, probably due to an increase in plasma vitamin B_{12}-binding protein.

Bone marrow. Haemopoietic marrow is replaced by soft pale pink or greenish tissue extending into the long bones (Fig. 14.32). The marrow cellularity is greatly increased due to granulocyte precursors, mainly myelocytes, and megakaryocytes.

Other organs. There is massive enlargement of the spleen which may exceed 3 kg, often causing discomfort or leading to spontaneous rupture. It is firm and the cut surface has a mottled appearance with areas of infarction. The red pulp is packed with leukaemic cells, but much of the splenic enlargement is due to extramedullary haemopoiesis. The Malpighian bodies are obscured by the massive cellular infiltration. The lymph nodes are not usually involved until a late stage of the disease. The liver may show extensive sinusoidal infiltration by leukaemic cells. Dif-

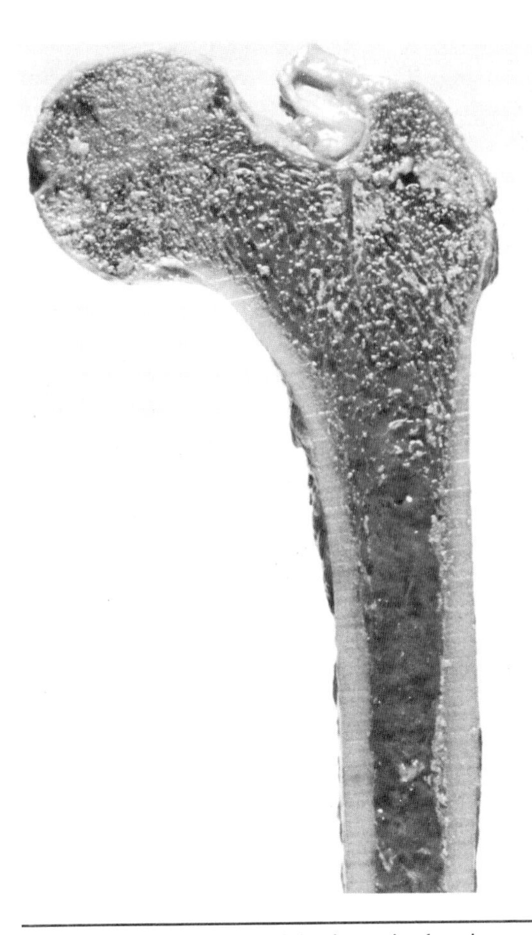

Fig. 14.32 Upper end of the femur in chronic granulocytic leukaemia. Pale marrow occupies the whole shaft. The marrow cavity is also widened by resorption of bone trabeculae.

fuse infiltration of other organs, including central nervous system, may occur.

Other features include fatty change of organs secondary to anaemia and widespread petechial haemorrhages due to thrombocytopenia or defective platelet function. Occasionally more extensive haemorrhage occurs, especially in the brain, and haemorrhagic infarcts may occur as a result of diffuse microvascular occlusion by leukaemic cell aggregates. The serum uric acid level is usually elevated, especially during cytotoxic drug therapy. Unless prevented by appropriate treatment this may lead to secondary gout with impaired renal function due to urate crystal deposition in the tubules.

Variants of Chronic Granulocytic Leukaemia

It is apparent from recent advances in characterization of leukaemic cells that CGL may comprise a number of entities. The major categories of Ph positive and Ph negative CGL have already been described. *Juvenile CGL* is a rare disorder occurring under the age of 5 years but with a very characteristic clinical and haematological picture. The leukaemic cells are Ph negative and originate from a fetal stem cell; a high level of HbF is found in the red cells. In a further type of juvenile CGL monosomy 7 occurs in the leukaemic cells and HbF levels are not increased. In both types the response to treatment is poor.

Aetiology of the Leukaemias

The cellular changes involved in carcinogenesis and the factors inducing them are discussed in Chapter 10. This should be read before the following account, which is restricted to leukaemogenesis.

Hereditary Factors

There is no strong evidence that heredity plays any significant role. A high incidence of CLL has been reported in some families and the concordance rate of ALL in monozygotic twins has been estimated to be over 20%, but this may be due to environmental factors.

Ionizing Radiation

The leukaemogenic effect of irradiation has been established by observing an incidence of leukaemia at least ten times that expected in the following situations: (1) patients treated for ankylosing spondylitis by irradiation of the spine (AML and CGL), (2) radiologists practising in the 1930s–40s (usually CGL), and (3) survivors of the atom bomb explosions in Japan in 1945 (mostly ALL in children and CGL in adults; less often ANLL). In each group, the incidence of leukaemia peaked between 4 and 8 years after exposure. The clinical and pathological features of post-irradiation leukaemias are the same as those of 'spontaneous' leukaemias. The incidence of leukaemia bears a close, but not linear relationship to irradiation dose. There is less certainty about the possible leukaemogenic effects of fetal exposure to diagnostic X-ray examination in pregnancy or of radioactive phosphorus given to patients with polycythaemia rubra vera.

Chemicals and Drugs

The only industrial chemical known with certainty to be leukaemogenic is benzene, prolonged exposure to which increases the risk of developing ANLL and possibly CGL and CLL. The leukaemia is preceded by marrow hypoplasia, often for several years. There is also firm evidence that cytotoxic and immunosuppressive drugs, particularly alkylating agents, used to treat various neoplastic and non-neoplastic diseases increase the risk of ANLL. Leukaemia develops a few years after the start of treatment and is preceded by a variable period of dyserythropoiesis.

Chromosomal Abnormalities

As noted earlier, chromosomal abnormalities of different types may occur in all forms of leukaemia and some have prognostic significance. The causal role of such abnormalities is strongly suggested by (1) the association of particular chromosomal changes with particular types of leukaemia, e.g. the Ph' chromosome with CGL; (2) the increased incidence of leukaemia in individuals with syndromes attributable to congenital chromosome abnormalities, e.g. ALL or ANLL in trisomy 21 (Down's syndrome); and (3) the fact that irradiation and leukaemogenic drugs damage DNA and cause chromosomal abnormalities. However, it is also possible that the chromosomal changes occur as a secondary effect in genetically unstable leukaemic cells.

Leukaemogenic Viruses

The implication of oncogenic retroviruses in the leukaemias of domestic fowls and in a range of leukaemias and lymphomas in cats, rodents, cattle and non-human primates, has led to a search for leukaemogenic viruses in man.

Retrovirus-like particles and viruses resembling retroviruses associated with leukaemia in non-human primates have been isolated from human leukaemias and lymphomas, but a causal relationship has not been established. The exception is human T-cell leukaemia virus (HTLV-1) a retrovirus which causes a form of adult T-cell leukaemia/lymphoma endogenous in parts of Japan (p. 408).

A Unifying Concept of Leukaemogenesis

Most studies on leukaemogenesis indicate the importance of chromosome abnormalities, whether occurring spontaneously or induced by irradiation, chemicals or by integration of a retrovirus. The many possible ways in which chromosomal rearrangements may effect transformation to a neoplastic cell are illustrated by the leukaemias. The translocations observed in leukaemia affect regions rich in cellular oncogenes and the sites of the immunoglobulin genes. Some translocations observed in various leukaemias involve chromosomes carrying the genes for immunoglobulins (2, 22 and 14) and may activate cellular oncogenes (c-*oncs*) by bringing them into proximity with Ig promotor genes.

In CGL the Ph' chromosome, a small chromosome 22, results from a translocation t(9;22)(q34;q11). The breakage point of chromosome 22 recurs within a short sequence region (5.8 kb) termed the breakpoint cluster region (*bcr*). This translocation leads to the insertion of the c-*abl* oncogene from chromosome 9 into the *bcr* which is part of the BCR gene on the Philadelphia chromosome. The essential result is the formation of a *bcr–abl* fusion gene which is transcribed using the BCR promoter to produce a chimeric *bcr–abl* mRNA. Translation of the mRNA results in the synthesis of a hybrid protein which exhibits *in vitro* tyrosine kinase activity and which is considered to be probably responsible for the malignant transformation. Even in some cases of Ph' CGL the C-**abl** gene can be detected in the *bcr*.

Translocations most often related to B-cell ALL are t(8;14) in 80% of cases, t(2;8) and t(8;22), each of which may transfer the cellular oncogene c-*myc* on chromosome 8 to the vicinity of the Ig genes and their promoters. Chromosomes 14, 2 and 22 carry genes coding for immunoglobin heavy chains and kappa and lambda light chains respectively. Part of chromosome 22 transferred to chromosome 9 in Ph' +ve CGL contains c-*sis*, which may be a structural gene for platelet-derived growth factor which possesses mitogenic activity.

Activation of cellular oncogenes by integrated proviruses of leukaemogenic retroviruses, which do not themselves possess a viral oncogene, depends on chance insertion of the provirus at a particular site in cellular DNA. Apart from Burkitt's lymphoma there is no strong evidence that DNA viruses are involved in human leukaemia or lymphoma.

The latent period of some years between exposure to irradiation or leukaemogenic chemicals and the development of leukaemia suggests that, like carcinogenesis in general, the development of leukaemia is a multi-step process. Chromosome abnormalities increase the likelihood of further abnormalities by rendering the affected cells genetically unstable or conferring on them a growth advantage. This is seen in individuals with Ph' +ve CGL in whom Ph' +ve stem cells gradually dominate haemopoiesis: blast-cell crisis is attributable to an additional chromosome abnormality which may occur in either a stem cell of the CGL clone or in a pluripotent Ph'+ve stem cell which is not yet neoplastic. The development of resistance to cytotoxic drugs in leukaemia is also explicable by an additional chromosome abnormality in a leukaemic stem cell.

Finally, two further aspects of leukaemogenesis deserve comment. One is the suppressive effect of leukaemic proliferation on the haemopoietic activity of normal stem cells. This occurs in most forms of leukaemia. It may result from insensitivity of leukaemic cells to a factor termed leukaemia-associated inhibitory activity (LIA) which is an acidic isoferritin produced by monocytes and macrophages. LIA inhibits normal cells in the S-phase of mitosis but fails to inhibit proliferation of leukaemic cells. The second is the possible role of immunosuppression in leukaemogenesis. Radiation and leukaemogenic drugs are immunosuppressant and so are the leukaemogenic retroviruses of animals. There is, moreover, an increased incidence of leukaemia in some of the congenital immune deficiency states, e.g. ataxia telangiectasia and the Wiskott–Aldrich syndrome.

Bone Marrow Transplantation

Bone marrow transplantation is now an accepted treatment modality in a number of conditions. Since bone marrow contains progenitors of lymphoid and haemopoietic cells it has the potential (1) to provide the means for marrow recovery after high dose chemotherapy or total body irradiation for haematological (and possibly other) malignancies; (2) to produce a new haemopoietic system in aplastic anaemia; (3) to replace defective lymphoid stem cells in various immune deficiency syndromes; and (4) to replace defective cell lines in inherited disorders such as the haemoglobinopathies or enzyme deficiency syndromes, e.g. the mucopolysaccharidoses.

Currently most transplants are performed with donor/recipient pairs fully HLA compatible. Unlike other organ transplants allograft rejection rarely occurs as patients are severely immunocompromised. In addition, however, because the donor marrow contains immunocompetent T cells which can react against the HLA antigens of the recipient, a graft-versus-host (GVH) reaction can occur with consequent GVH disease (p. 225). Prevention of this is theoretically possible if the T cells can be removed, e.g. by using monoclonal anti-T cell antibodies. However, it seems that reduction in T cells in the graft may also render it more susceptible to graft failure. Autologous marrow transplantation or 'rescue' employs the recipient's own cells in cases of haematological malignancy and following attempts to remove or 'purge' malignant cells before re-infusion. Effective conditioning regimens are required to eradicate leukaemic cells (e.g. in the meninges) or to destroy genetically defective progenitor cells in inherited disorders, otherwise the risk of disease recurrence is high. Such regimens utilize high dose chemotherapy and radiotherapy; their long-term oncogenic risks are unknown.

The marrow graft is obtained from the donor's iliac crests. A single cell suspension is produced and injected intravenously. The marrow infusion is usually well tolerated and after 14 days discrete aggregates of haemopoietic cells, usually of one cell type, are detectable in the marrow. Marrow cellularity then increases rapidly, a rise in the number of normal blood cells signals graft productivity and successful engraftment.

Other Neoplastic Disorders

The Myeloproliferative Disorders

This is a group of disorders characterized by abnormal, excessive and sustained proliferation of erythropoietic, granulopoietic and megakaryocytic components of the bone marrow, often accompanied by fibrosis (myelofibrosis) and extramedullary haemopoiesis. Three diseases are included – polycythaemia rubra vera (primary polycythaemia), myelofibrosis and essential thrombocythaemia. This grouping is justified because of occurrence of cases with intermediate features, frequent evolution of one entity into another within the group, e.g. polycythaemia rubra vera into myelofibrosis, and invariable involvement of more than one haemopoietic cell line in the neoplastic process. These features suggest that myeloproliferative disorders originate from a stem-cell abnormality. Their neoplastic nature is suggested by the absence of any known physiological stimulating factors and by the demonstration of glucose-6-phosphate dehydrogenase isoenzyme homeogeneity in the haemopoietic cells of heterozygotes. This last observation suggests a monoclonal proliferation of stem cells and all may terminate as ANLL. Although chromosome abnormalities occur, they are neither consistent nor specific. Many of the morphological abnormalities are common to the group and differ only in degree: they include (1) haemopoietic hyperplasia, (2) an increase in reticulin or in some cases collagen deposition in the marrow, (3) an increase in morphologically abnormal megakaryocytes which are often present in clusters, and (4) the presence of extramedullary haemopoiesis.

Polycythaemia Rubra Vera (Primary Polycythaemia)

This is distinguished from secondary polycythaemia (erythrocytosis), which is usually the result of raised erythropoietin levels and may occur in hypoxic states or as a paraneoplastic effect, for example in hepatocellular and renal carcinoma. In contrast, serum erythropoietin levels are usually reduced in the primary type.

In polycythaemia rubra vera erythroid precursors predominate in the marrow but, in common with all these disorders, myeloid and megakaryocytic elements also proliferate. It occurs in 1 per 100 000 of the population, usually after 40 years of age, and with a male preponderance.

Laboratory features The outstanding feature is a marked increase in red cell mass; the red cell count usually exceeds 7×10^{12}/l, and the haemoglobin concentration may exceed 18.0 g/dl. A packed cell volume of 0.6 l/l at sea level is virtually diagnostic. The red cell mass, however, should be estimated, both to confirm the diagnosis and to ascertain the severity of the disease, particularly as peripheral blood cell values do not correlate closely with red cell mass. The increase in red cell mass may deplete iron stores and the red cells may become microcytic. About 50% of patients show elevation of the total white cell count involving neutrophils, eosinophils and basophils and two-thirds have an elevated platelet count. The neutrophil alkaline phosphatase score is usually increased, often to very high levels.

The clinical features are caused by the increase in red cell mass and consequently in blood volume and viscosity, and by the hypermetabolic state associated with myeloproliferation. Patients complain of various non-specific symptoms of which headaches, blurring of vision and generalized pruritus, particularly after a hot bath, are common. The hypervolaemia results in engorgement of the microcirculation which, together with erythrocytosis and peripheral vascular stasis produces a plethoric appearance to the face. The elevated blood viscosity leads to hypertension and a thrombotic tendency which may result in myocardial and cerebral ischaemia. Platelets may be functionally deficient, in spite of their increased number, and spontaneous haemorrhage may occur, particularly into the gastrointestinal tract. There is an unexplained increased incidence of peptic ulceration. The spleen is usually enlarged and firm. Increased haemopoietic cell turnover may be reflected by elevation of serum uric acid levels and secondary gout with renal impairment develops in 10% of cases.

Treatment is directed mainly at reducing the red cell mass and thus the blood viscosity. This may be achieved by repeated venesection or by administration of radioactive phosphorus or myelosuppressive drugs. The disease is often advanced when first detected but may run a prolonged course. Death usually results from the effects of hypertension or from thrombotic episodes, but with improved control a long survival (a median of 13 years) may be achieved. Approximately 15% develop myelofibrosis and a further 10% ANLL or ALL. The incidence of leukaemic transformation is increased in patients treated with radioactive phosphorus or myelosuppressive drugs. This may be due to treatment but could also represent the natural progression of the disease.

Myelofibrosis

This usually develops in the over 50 age group. There is increased fibroblast activity in the haemopoietic marrow, resulting in a great increase in reticulin and collagen fibres (Fig. 14.33). The fibroblast proliferation, however, appears to be reactive to an underlying myeloproliferative disorder rather than part of a neoplastic process itself, as it is not monoclonal. It has been suggested

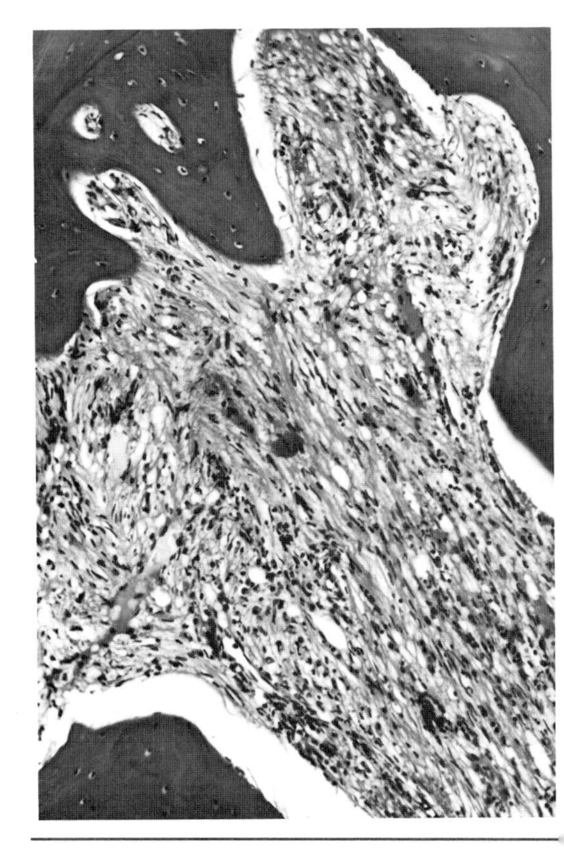

Fig. 14.33 Myelofibrosis. Section of bone showing replacement of the haemopoietic marrow by fibrous tissue.

that the fibroblast proliferation occurs in response to the release of growth factors by proliferating, presumably abnormal megakaryocytes/platelets. While myelofibrosis may be a primary disorder it has already been noted that CGL and polycythaemia rubra vera may transform to a myelofibrotic state. The marrow component is invariably accompanied by extramedullary haemopoiesis in the spleen and liver. No chromosomal changes have as yet been identified.

Clinical and laboratory features. The onset is usually insidious, symptoms being due to either anaemia or splenomegaly. The spleen is greatly enlarged, up to 4 kg or more, and abdominal pain due to splenic infarction is not uncommon. The liver may also be enlarged. Both organs show extensive extramedullary haemopoiesis.

Needle aspiration of the marrow is often unsuccessful ('dry tap') and trephine or open biopsy may be necessary for diagnosis. The diagnostic feature is diffuse fibrosis with disappearance of haemopoietic elements. In some cases there is an increase in bony trabeculae (osteosclerosis). The haemopoietic elements in the marrow may be focally or diffusely increased and abnormal megakaryocytes are seen. The blood picture shows anaemia with marked polychromasia, anisocytosis and poikilocytosis with 'tear-drop' red cells and a leucoerythroblastic reaction. Some patients become folate deficient, with a raised MCV. The number of granulocytes is variable but the platelet count is usually increased. The neutrophil alkaline phosphatase score is very high, and the serum uric acid raised.

As the disease progresses, all formed elements tend to decrease due primarily to impaired haemopoiesis, but this may be aggravated by hypersplenism. The median survival from the time of diagnosis is about 3 years. Most patients die from myocardial infarction or cerebrovascular accidents, but some from marrow failure with severe haemorrhage or infection. About 10% develop ANLL.

Essential Thrombocythaemia

In this very rare disorder megakaryocytic hyperplasia and excessive platelet production predominate. The platelet count often exceeds $1000 \times 10^9/l$, but many are functionally defective and haemorrhage from the gastrointestinal tract is common, leading to iron deficiency. There may be a moderate neutrophil leucocytosis and the neutrophil alkaline phosphatase score is high. Thrombotic episodes with infarction of internal organs are common; thus, the spleen, which may be enlarged initially may reduce in size because of repeated infarction. There is a high mortality from haemorrhage and/or thrombosis but many patients may survive for up to 10 years. A proportion progress to myelofibrosis and less frequently to ANLL.

Myelodysplastic Syndromes (MDS)

These are primary stem cell disorders occurring spontaneously in the elderly, or in younger patients who have received protracted treatment with cytotoxic drugs and/or radiotherapy. The group has in common morphological abnormalities in the bone marrow with maturation defects resulting in ineffective haematopoiesis. There is variable but, in certain types, predictable progression to ANLL. The term preleukaemia has been applied to these syndromes but is inappropriate in that only in retrospect can it be established with certainty. In addition to detection of the peripheral blood and bone marrow abnormalities, accurate diagnosis may require cell kinetic, cytogenetic and marrow culture studies. Five categories have been defined by the French–American–British (FAB) group (Table 14.18).

The categories are identified by the percentage of blast cells seen in the peripheral blood and in the bone marrow, the morphological abnormalities in all cell lines (reflecting ineffective haematopoiesis)

Table 14.18 French–American–British (FAB) group classification of the myelodysplastic syndromes

Refractory anaemia and/or pancytopenia (RA)	Patient usually under 50; 'Micromegakaryocytes' present in marrow; some transform to ANLL
Primary acquired sideroblastic anaemia (RA-S)	See p. 619: with ringed sideroblasts
Refractory anaemia with excess of blasts (RAEB)	Patients usually over 50; 30% develop ANLL
Refractory anaemia with excess of blasts in transformation (RAEB-t)	
Chronic myelomonocytic leukaemia (CMML)	Patient over 50; this is an absolute peripheral monocytosis ($>2 \times 10^9$/l) with abnormal forms; 40–50% develop ANLL

and the frequency with which ANLL develops. Chromosomal abnormalities are seen in 70% of primary cases and in over 90% of secondary cases, the most commonly found being trisomy 8, loss of 5, 7 or Y and deletion of parts of 5 or 20. The most common single abnormality is $5q^-$ which is associated with the $5q^-$ syndrome, namely refractory anaemia in elderly females associated with a good prognosis. Multiple chromosomal abnormalities carry a worse prognosis.

Plasma Cell Neoplasms

These comprise a group of disorders in which there is a monoclonal neoplastic proliferation of plasma cells resulting in multiple tumour deposits within the marrow (multiple myeloma), a single tumour mass which is often extramedullary (plasmacytoma), or diffuse infiltration of marrow, lymph nodes, spleen and liver by malignant cells (Waldenström's macroglobulinaemia and other syndromes). These tumour cells secrete immunoglobulins or components of the immunoglobulin molecule and some of the clinical and pathological features are due to the excessive production of these proteins. The term gammopathy is sometimes applied to this situation, reflecting the previous classification of immunoglobulins as gamma-globulins.

Plasma cells are derived from B lymphocytes and are normally responsible for the synthesis and secretion of immunoglobulins. Plasma cell tumours arise from B cells in a late stage of differentiation. There is proliferation of a single clone of cells producing a monoclonal immunoglobulin of a single heavy chain class, one type of light chain and identical sequences of amino acids in the variable region of each chain. These monoclonal proteins are usually detected in the blood and are paraproteins or myeloma (M) proteins. The further along the differentiation pathway (i.e. towards plasma cells) the malignant transformation occurs the more likely is the secretion of a paraprotein. Monoclonal immunoglobulins may be of any isotype although IgG is the commonest followed by IgA and IgM; IgD and IgE are rare.

In some instances excess light or heavy chains are synthesized and occasionally only light chains (light chain disease) or heavy chains (heavy chain disease) are produced and in the absence of complete Ig molecules. Because of their low molecular weight (25 kDa) light chains are excreted in the urine as monomers or dimers and are detected as Bence Jones protein.

Detection and Characterization of Paraproteins

Paraproteins are detected by electrophoresis of serum or urine on cellulose acetate strips or in agarose gel, and usually appear as discrete dense bands in the globulin region (Fig. 14.34a). They can be definitely characterized by immunoelectrophoresis (Fig. 14.34b), although isoelectric focusing (Fig. 14.34c) is now more frequently used on account of its greater sensitivity. Bence Jones protein is best detected by electrophoresis of

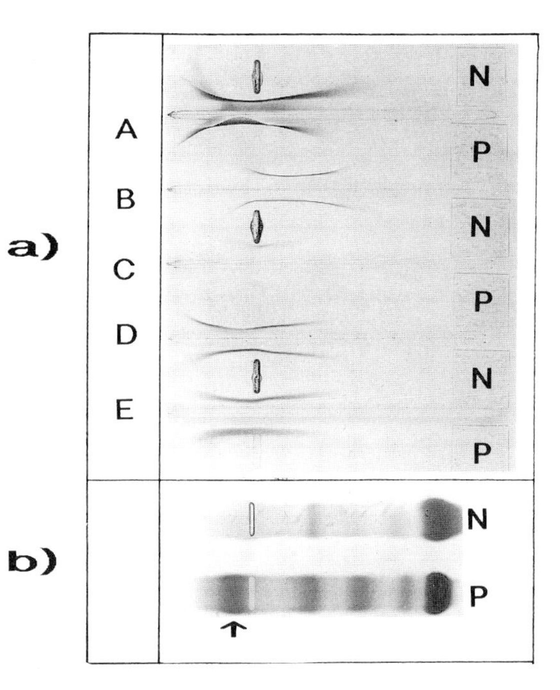

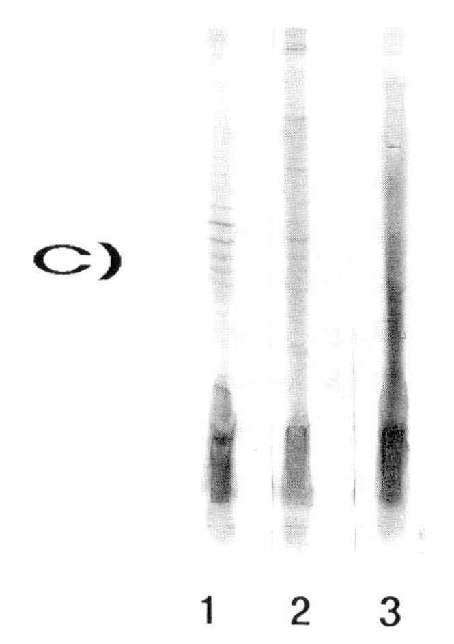

Fig. 14.34 (**a**) Immunoelectrophoresis (anode to the right) of normal serum in wells 1, 3, 5 and myeloma serum in wells 2, 4, 6. Antisera in the troughs are as follows: A, anti-IgG; B, anti-IgA; C, anti-IgM; D, anti-light chain; E, anti-light chain. Note the abnormal precipitin arc between the patient's serum and anti-IgG and anti-antisera. Diagnosis, IgG paraprotein. (**b**) Zonal electrophoresis (anode to the right) of normal serum (upper track) and myeloma serum (lower track). Note the extremely dense band (arrowed) to the cathodal side of the origin in the patient's serum. (c) Isoelectric focusing of IgG-myeloma serum (1), serum containing oligoclonal bands (2) and normal serum (3). This very sensitive technique reveals a series of clear but closely associated bands in track 1, which is typical of a monoclonal IgG antibody. The greater number of less dense bands shown in track 2 is described as oligoclonal and is produced by proliferation of a small number of clones. In this case the patient was HIV positive. Normal serum (track 3) does not show any clear bands due to the great heterogeneity of antibodies in normal individuals.

urine followed by immunofixation or by immunoelectrophoresis. However, Bence Jones protein is also readily detected by adjusting a urine sample to pH 4–6; heating results in precipitation of the light chain at 50°C but they become soluble again at 80°C.

Monoclonal Gammopathy of Undetermined Significance (Benign Monoclonal Gammopathy)

Monoclonal proteins sometimes occur in apparently healthy individuals, the incidence increasing with age, from 1.5% of individuals over 50 years of age to 3% over 70 years. A Swedish study has shown a population prevalence of paraproteins of 0.5% and only 1% of these had myeloma. In contrast, in general hospital practice 75% of patients incidentally found to have paraproteins will have some form of malignant disease (of these 85% will have myeloma and the remainder some other malignancy of the lymphoreticular system). Of the remaining 25% which are classified as benign, 60% will have no apparent underlying pathology, 20% will have a connective tissue disease (Chapter 6) and 20% will be associated with other underlying chronic diseases.

Benign paraproteins may be transient or persistent. In the former case, B cells are producing a monoclonal protein in response to an antigenic stimulus, but are under normal homeostatic controls. In the latter, it is probable that some normal regulatory process has broken down. All patients who have paraproteinaemia should be investigated to exclude underlying malignancy. Those found to be normal should be monitored regularly, however, as a proportion of them will develop a B cell malignancy or multiple myeloma.

Multiple Myeloma

In multiple myeloma neoplastic proliferation of plasma cells or their precursors is usually confined to the bone marrow but may spread to other sites. The disease occurs in elderly patients, mean age of presentation 60 years, is rare before 40 years of age and has an annual incidence of 2–3 per 100 000. The diagnosis is usually not difficult and depends on the presence of osteolytic lesions on X-ray, the demonstration of a monoclonal protein in the serum and/or urine and the typical cellular changes in the bone marrow. Monoclonal IgG is the most frequent paraprotein in myeloma (50%). IgA is found in 25% of cases and only light chains (Bence Jones myeloma) in 20%. In Bence Jones myeloma the light chains are filtered by the kidneys and the paraprotein can only be found in the urine and not in serum.

The aetiology and pathogenesis are not known. Prolonged antigenic stimulation may produce plasma cell tumours in experimental animals but there is no evidence for this in humans. In some 10% of cases a serum paraprotein may precede signs of tumour by many years. Some Japanese atomic bomb survivors developed multiple myeloma. The disease is commoner in blacks than whites and there are some reports of multiple familial cases. Chromosomal abnormalities have been identified on 14 band q32 but of a different pattern to that seen in Burkitt's lymphoma and other B cell tumours.

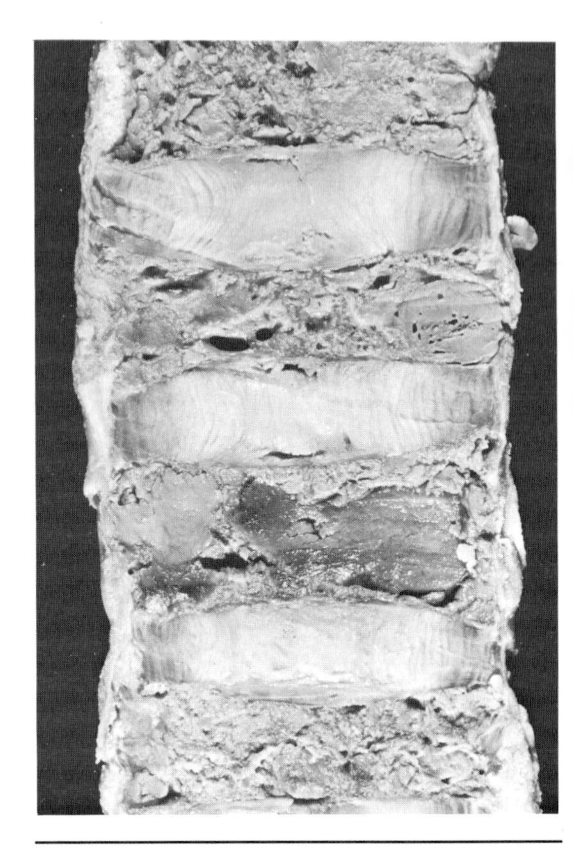

Fig. 14.35 Multiple nodules of myeloma in vertebral column. The vertebral bodies show compression collapse.

Pathological features. There are multiple 'punched out' lesions in bones affecting the vertebral column (Fig. 14.35), ribs, skull, femur, pelvis and other flat bones. Vertebral collapse and pathological fractures occur. The tumours arise in the medullary cavity and extend to the cortex; bone resorption is due to tumour secretion of osteoclast activating factors. Widespread proliferation in the marrow may produce diffuse osteoporosis. Extramedullary extension to involve spleen, liver, lymph nodes and other organs may occur late in the disease and, very rarely, plasma cell leukaemia may be found.

The cytological features are variable. Many are recognizable as mature plasma cells (Fig. 14.36) but more primitive cells – plasmablasts and cells intermediate in appearance between lymphocytes and plasma cells – may occasionally predominate. Bi- and trinucleate cells and intracytoplasmic protein aggregates (Russell bodies) are often seen, but are not of diagnostic significance. Plasma cells are present in normal marrow, and their number is increased in chronic inflammatory conditions but seldom to more than 10% of all cells.

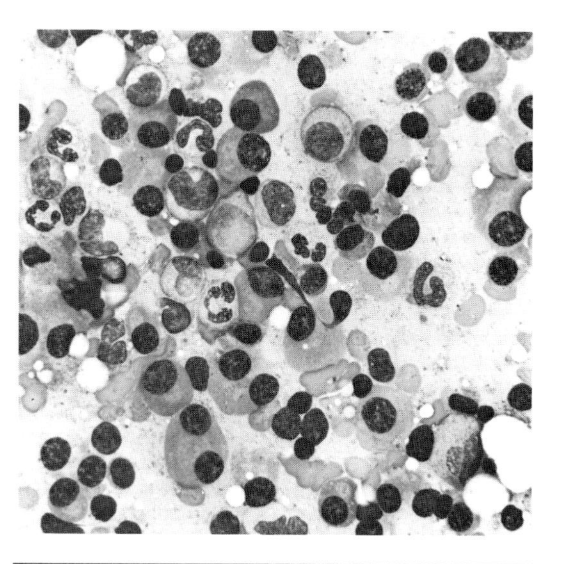

Fig. 14.36 Smear of sternal marrow aspirate in multiple myeloma, showing large numbers of plasma cells. ×600.

Clinical features. Bone pain and pathological fractures are common presenting features. Marrow replacement by the tumour and marow depression by tumour cell secretions result in a normochromic normocytic anaemia, neutropenia and thrombocytopenia. Red cell haemolysis and quantitative platelet dysfunction with a bleeding tendency may be caused by the paraproteins. Neutropenia and immunoglobulin deficiency lead to increased susceptibility to infection, the commonest cause of death. A hyperviscosity syndrome similar to that seen in Waldenström's macroglobulinaemia also occurs, particularly with IgA which may polymerize. The paraprotein causes marked rouleaux formation, sludging of red cells and a very high ESR; the ESR in light chain myeloma may not be elevated. Hypercalcaemia due to the increased bone resorption is present in 30% of cases and may be sufficiently severe to cause constipation, abdominal pains and mental confusion; polyuria with hypercalciuria develops and nephrocalcinosis may contribute to renal failure. Renal failure is a very common cause of death due to myeloma nephropathy or amyloidosis (p. 924).

The disease varies in clinical aggressiveness. Some patients with indolent forms live for many years while in others death may occur in 2–3 months. With chemotherapy and other therapeutic measures an increasing number of patients now survive for 5 years or more. The use of alpha interferon for maintenance treatment is currently under investigation.

Plasmacytoma

Localized plasmacytomas are far less common than multiple myeloma. These occur as a single deposit in the bone marrow or more commonly, in extramedullary sites (extramedullary plasmacytoma) such as the lungs and the upper respiratory tract. Morphologically they resemble the lesions seen in multiple myeloma. At presentation, paraproteins are present in the sera of approximately 25% of these patients. Up to 60% of patients with an osseous lesion will go on to develop multiple myeloma. Extramedullary lesions may be cured by resection or with combined radiotherapy and chemotherapy.

Waldenström's Macroglobulinaemia

This is an uncommon condition constituting about 5% of the plasma cell dyscrasias. It develops in the over 50 age group and there is a male preponderance. There is marrow, lymph node, spleen and liver infiltration, the tumour cells comprising lymphocytes and plasmacytoid cells (intermediate between lymphocytes and plasma cells) which may contain PAS positive nuclear inclusions. The hallmark of the disease is the production of large amounts of IgM. The serum IgM is between 25 and 80 g/l; it is insoluble and precipitates on dilution in water – the Sia test.

The clinical features are largely attributable to the hyperviscosity syndrome which results from the IgM paraproteinaemia. The increased blood viscosity impedes circulation through the capillary beds, and this is aggravated by red cell aggregation and sludging of the blood. Patients develop neurological symptoms, with dizziness, pareses and visual impairment. Mucosal haemorrhage may occur, due in part to impaired blood flow and in part to impaired platelet function. In contrast to myeloma, lytic lesions in bone do not develop. The symptoms are relieved by plasmapheresis and cytotoxic chemotherapy induces temporary remission. The median survival is about 5 years.

Heavy Chain Disease

These are extremely rare neoplastic conditions in which lymphoid proliferation in the tissues is associated with the presence in the serum of immunoglobulin heavy chains and which are usually incomplete.

Alpha chain disease is the commonest and affects the small intestinal mucosa particularly the ileum. It occurs in young adults, mainly in the Mediterranean region, Asia and South America. There is abdominal pain and severe malabsorption. Mucosal biopsy shows an infiltrate of polyclonal plasma cells and lymphocytes, and this has given rise to the term immune proliferative small intestinal disease (IPSID). In the early stage a clinical response to antibiotics may occur, suggesting that the proliferation is a response to some micro-organisms. Many cases, however, progress to an invasive immunoblastic B-cell lymphoma with a poor prognosis.

Gamma chain disease and *μ chain disease* (the rarest) present with features of lymphoma or chronic lymphocytic leukaemia and the paraprotein abnormality is detected on immunoelectrophoresis. Both carry a poor prognosis.

Cryoglobulinaemia

Cryoglobulins are immunoglobulins which precipitate on cooling and may be polyclonal or monoclonal. The latter usually indicate lymphoreticular neoplasia, and a mixed pattern occurs (essential mixed cryoglobulinaemia) with some autoimmune diseases (Chapter 6). The clinical features are a combination of ischaemia – Raynaud's disease and inflammation due to complement activation – vasculitis and glomerulonephritis.

Platelet Disorders

As has been previously described platelets have important functions in normal haemostasis and in the acute inflammatory response. There are a number of primary platelet disorders, quantitative and qualitative, which are now briefly discussed.

Thrombocytopenia

The causes are summarized in Table 14.19. Thrombocytopenia exists when the platelet count is less than 150×10^9/l. Sponaneous haemorrhage does not usually occur with counts above 20×10^9/l unless infection is present. Detection of the cause of thrombocytopenia is often difficult and a diagnosis of 'idiopathic' thrombocytopenic purpura should not be made too readily.

Decreased Production of Platelets

Acquired causes are by far the commonest. Depressed platelet production, recognized by a paucity of megakaryocytes in the marrow, is seen in the aplastic/hypoplastic anaemias, in the megaloblastic anaemias and when there is marrow replacement due to leukaemia or metastatic tumour. A number of drugs/toxins can cause

Table 14.19 Causes of thrombocytopenia

Decreased production of platelets
- Acquired
  - Marrow disorders
  - Aplastic and hypoplastic anaemias
  - Marrow replacement syndromes: leukaemia, carcinomatosis
  - Megaloblastic anaemias
- Specific impaired platelet production
  - Drugs and toxins: alcohol, cytotoxic drugs, phenylbutazone, gold
  - Viral infections: EBV
- Hereditary
  - Wiskott–Aldrich syndrome

Immunologically mediated destruction of platelets
- Autoimmune thrombocytopenia purpura
- Isoimmune neonatal and post-transfusion
- Drug hypersensitivity reactions
- Viral infections: EBV, HIV

Increased consumption of platelets
- Disseminated intravascular coagulation
- Thrombotic thrombocytopenic purpura
- Microangiopathic disorders: haemolytic uraemic syndrome
- Sequestration:
  - Spleen: hypersplenism
  - Vascular tumours – giant haemagiomas

Miscellaneous
- Severe sepsis
- Massive transfusion

thrombocytopenia in occasional recipients, possibly by selective suppression of megakaryocytes. These include chronic alcohol ingestion, cytotoxic drugs and thiazide diuretics. Rubella infection may be associated with thrombocytopenia in children. Thrombocytopenia also occurs in the rare Wiskott–Aldrich syndrome (p. 240) in which there is immunodeficiency with recurrent infection and eczema. In myelodysplastic syndromes thrombocytopenia is frequently associated with the presence of abnormal or micromegakaryocytes.

Immunologically Mediated Destruction of Platelets

Autoimmune Thrombocytopenic Purpura

This disorder occurs chiefly in children and young adults. In children the onset is acute, often preceded by a viral respiratory infection, and in most cases the disorder is self-limiting, lasting only 2–4 weeks. Platelet destruction is thought to be due to autoantibodies against platelets or to virus-associated immune complexes which are adsorbed onto platelets. The adult type, occurring mainly in females aged 20–40 years, develops insidiously and usually persists for months or years. The antibody is usually of IgG_3 class. It can cross the placenta and thus neonatal thrombocytopenia may occur, even when splenectomy has been carried out in the mother (see below).

Autoimmune thrombocytopenia may also occur in association with other autoimmune disorders, e.g. systemic lupus erythematosus or myasthenia gravis, and may occasionally accompany autoimmune haemolytic anaemia. It may also complicate lymphoma and chronic lymphocytic leukaemia, although in these marrow replacement may also be a factor.

The clinical pattern of bleeding varies from mild cutaneous purpura to gross uterine or gastrointestinal haemorrhage. In severe cases intracerebral bleeding is a particular danger. Many patients respond to immunosuppressive drugs and splenectomy is beneficial in a proportion, simply by removing the site of platelet destruction; circulating levels of platelet associated antibodies do not fall; however, following splenectomy there may be a remarkable transient overswing in platelet count, which can exceed 1000×10^9/l. In some patients, platelets which are very heavily coated by antibody are removed mainly by the Kupffer cells and these patients are unlikely to benefit from splenectomy.

Isoimmune Neonatal and Post-transfusion Thrombocytopenia

Platelets, like other haemopoietic cells, have specific isoantigens. Of these, platelet A1 antigen (PLA-1) is present in 98% of adults. However, PLA-1 negative patients who receive PLA-1 positive platelets in blood transfusions develop isoantibodies. During pregnancy PLA-1 negative mothers may become immunized to their PLA-1 positive babies, producing neonatal thrombocytopenia, a situation comparable to that which occurs in isoimmune haemolytic anaemia (p. 609).

Other Acquired Causes

Drug-induced hypersensitivity reactions may cause thrombocytopenia by mechanisms similar to that which occur in drug-induced haemolytic anaemia (p. 610). Drugs which have this side-effect include quinidine and sulphonamides. Viral infections associated with thrombocytopenia include Epstein–Barr virus and cytomegalovirus. Thrombocytopenia may occur also with HIV infection, and indeed is the commonest haematological disorder in AIDS.

Increased Consumption of Platelets

The features of disseminated intravascular coagulation (DIC) are discussed elsewhere (p. 91); widespread sequestration of platelets takes place within intravascular thrombi. Platelets, in common with red cells, may be mechanically destroyed in all the microangiopathic haemolytic anaemia syndromes (p. 610) and in thrombotic thrombocytopenic purpura (p. 90). Massive splenomegaly from a variety of causes may result in increased sequestration of platelets and other blood cells, and thrombocytopenia may be a manifestation of hypersplenism (p. 648). Sequestration of platelets may also occur in vascular tumours.

Thrombotic Thrombocytopenic Purpura

This is a rare disorder of young adults (20–40 years), more common in females and characterized by thrombocytopenia, haemolytic anaemia, fever, neurological signs and renal failure. In contrast to DIC there is no clotting deficiency. Widespread intravascular, platelet-rich microthrombi develop and this affords an explanation for the thrombocytopenia. The haemolysis is of mechanical aetiology comparable to that seen in various microangiopathies and the microthrombi cause widespread organ ischaemia. There is some evidence that decreased endothelial synthesis of PGI_2 is the primary defect, allowing inappropriate platelet aggregation in blood vessels.

Thrombocytosis

Very marked elevation of the platelet count may occur in the myeloproliferative disorders. Secondary thrombocytosis may occur post-splenectomy, postoperatively, in haemorrhage or haemolysis, after extreme exercise and in collagen vascular diseases, in disseminated malignancy and in some chronic inflammatory diseases such as ulcerative colitis. Postoperative thrombocytosis is a contributory factor in deep venous thrombosis (p. 93).

Qualitative Platelet Abnormalities

A variety of haemorrhagic defects, both hereditary and acquired, exist, characterized by a normal platelet count but abnormal platelet function. Defects are recognized in all steps leading to formation of the haemostatic platelet plug, including adhesion, release and aggregation.

These hereditary disorders are rare, but the investigation of them has contributed enormously to the understanding of normal platelet function. The major types are summarized in Table 14.20.

Table 14.20 Some hereditary causes of qualitative platelet dysfunction

Membrane glycoprotein disorder	
Glanzmann's disease (thrombasthenia)	Absent aggregation; defective fibrinogen binding: lifelong haemorrhagic tendency; autosomal recessive
Bernard–Soulier syndrome	Large platelets; reduced adhesion; autosomal recessive
Defects in platelet secretion	
Storage pool disease	Absent dense granules; defective release of ADP; autosomal recessive
Grey platelet disease	Absent α granules; defective release
Thromboxane synthetase deficiency	Defective release of ADP

The severity of the bleeding is mild to moderate in the membrane glycoprotein disorder and is extremely variable in the others. Impaired platelet adhesion is also seen in Ehlers–Danlos syndrome due to the collagen abnormality. In von Willebrand's disease (p. 90) impaired platelet adhesion is due to deficiency of von Willebrand's factor.

Acquired forms of platelet dysfunction are more common and occur in uraemia, liver failure, the myeloproliferative disorders and paraproteinaemias. Many drugs and toxins interfere with platelet function, including aspirin and alcohol. Aspirin irreversibly blocks platelet cyclooxygenase resulting in impaired prostaglandin and thromboxane (TxA_2) synthesis. Aspirin is now used prophylactically to prevent arterial vascular thrombosis.

Further Reading

Adamson, J. W. (1989). The promise of recombinant human erythropoietin. *Seminars in Haematology* **26**, No. 2, Suppl. 2, 5–8.

Binet, J. L., Auquier, A., Dighiero, G., Chastang, C., Piguer, H., Goasguen, J. *et al.* (1981). A new prognostic classification of chronic lymphocyte leukaemia derived from a multivariate survival analysis. *Cancer* **48**, 198–206.

Campana, D., Coustan-Smith, E. and Janossy, G. (1990). Immunophenotyping in haematological diagnosis. In: Cavill, I. (ed.). *Baillière's Clinical Haematology* **4**, 889–919.

Catovsky, D., Melo, J. V. M. and Matutes, E. (1985). Biological markers in lymphoproliferative disorders. In: Bloomfield, C. J. (ed.). *Chronic and acute leukaemias in Adults*, pp. 69–112. Nijhoff Martinus, Boston.

Cook, J. D. (1982). Clinical evaluation of iron deficiency. *Seminars in Haematology* **19**, 6–18.

Dacie, J. V. (1988). *The Haemolytic Anaemias*, vol. 2; *The Hereditary Haemolytic Anaemias*, Part 2, 3rd edn. Churchill Livingstone, Edinburgh.

Gale, R. P. and Hoffbrand, A. V. (eds) (1986). Acute leukaemia. *Clinics in Haematology* **15**(3), 569–904.

Goldman, J. (ed.) (1987). Chronic myeloid leukaemia. *Baillière's Clinical Haematology* **1**, 869–1076.

Gordon-Smith, E. C. (ed.) (1989). Aplastic anaemia. *Baillière's Clinical Haematology* **2**, 1–190.

Hamblin, T. J. (1987). Chronic lymphocytic leukaemia. *Baillière's Clinical Haematology* **1**, 449–92.

Heim, S. (1990). Cytogenetics in the investigation of haematological disorders. In: Cavill, I. (ed.) *Baillière's Clinical Haematology* **4**, 921–48.

Hoffbrand, A. V. and Wickremasinghe, R. C. (1982). Megaloblastic anaemia. In: Hoffbrand, A. V. (ed.). *Recent Advances in Haematology*, Vol. 3, pp. 25–44. Churchill Livingstone, Edinburgh.

Jacobs, A. (1985). Iron deficiency and iron overload. *CRC Critical Reviews in Oncology/Hematology* **3**, 143–86.

Jones, A. L. and Millar, J. L. (1989). Growth factors in haemopoiesis. *Baillière's Clinical Haematology* **2**, 83–112.

Kyle, R. A. (1987). Monoclonal gammopathy and multiple myeloma in the elderly. *Baillière's Clinical Haematology* **1**, 533–56.

Lee, G. R. (1983). The anaemia of chronic disease. *Seminars in Haematology* **20**, 61–80.

Lewis, S. M. and Bayly, R. J. (eds) (1985). Radionuclides in haematology. *Methods in Haematology* **12**, 1–262.

Luzzatto, L. (1989). Inherited haemolytic anaemias. In: Hoffbrand, A. V. and Lewis, S. M. (eds.) *Postgraduate Haematology*, 3rd edn, pp. 167–82. Heinemann Professional Publishing, Oxford.

Oscier, D. G. (1987). Myelodysplastic syndromes. *Baillière's Clinical Haematology* **1**, 389–426.

Palck, J. (1987). Hereditary elliptocytosis, spherocytosis and related disorders: consequences of a deficiency or a mutation of membrane skeletal proteins. *Blood Reviews* **1**, 147–68.

Pearson, T. C. and Messinezy, M. (1987). Polycythaemia and thrombocythaemia in the elderly. *Baillière's Clinical Haematology* **1**, 355–88.

Petz, L. D. (1980). Drug induced immune haemolytic anaemia. *Clinics in Haematology* **9**(3), 455–82.

Prentice, H. G. and Brenner, M. K. (1988). Recent advances in bone marrow transplantation in the treatment of leukaemia. In: Hoffbrand, A. V. (ed.). *Recent Advances in Haematology*, vol. 5, pp. 153–78. Churchill Livingstone, Edinburgh.

Rai, K. R., Sawitsky, A., Cronkite, E. P., Charona, A. D., Levy, R. N. and Pasternak, B. S. (1975). Clinical staging of chronic lymphocytic lukaemia. *Blood* **46**, 219–84.

Reis, M. D., Griesser, H. and Mak, T. W. (1988). Gene rearrangements in leukaemias and lymphomas. In: Hoffbrand, A. V. (ed.). *Recent Advances in Haematology*, Vol. 5, pp. 99–120. Churchill Livingstone, Edinburgh.

15

The Lymphoreticular System

The lymphoreticular system encompasses all those tissues and cellular elements which subserve the immunological process, the microanatomical and physiological aspects of which are described in detail in Chapter 5. In order to understand the clinical and pathological features of lymphoreticular disease, however, it is worthwhile to summarize here some of the general aspects of the system. Application of the term lymphoreticular is a kind of historical compromise, yet serves to emphasize the close functional relationship that exists between lymphocytes and cells of the mononuclear phagocyte system – formerly referred to as the 'reticuloendothelial' system. A notable feature of the lymphoreticular system is its wide dispersal throughout the body: lymphoreticular elements may be encountered in almost any tissue at one time or another. Even so, these elements do form discrete aggregates which are divided into two main categories. First, there are the **primary** or central lymphoid organs such as the bone marrow and thymus gland which provide the microenvironment necessary for the production of lymphocyte precursors and for their initial antigen independent phase of development. The immunocompetent cells which subsequently emerge are then despatched, for the most part, to a **secondary** group of lymphoid organs which are strategically located to confront antigenic material either at its point of entry into the body or following penetration of the tissue spaces or vascular channels. These organs include the lymph nodes, spleen and mucosa-associated lymphoid tissues (MALT). Other organs, such as liver, skin and again the bone marrow might also be included since they contain specialized elements of the mononuclear phagocyte system. It needs to be re-emphasized that, in order to maintain the comprehensive integrity of the immunological defence mechanism, lymphocytes continuously recirculate and that many of the lymphoid elements in the secondary organs are only temporary residents (p. 172). The widespread distribution and continuous recirculation of the cellular elements accounts for many of the important features of lymphoreticular disease, such as the common development of generalized lymphadenopathy, hepatosplenomegaly and alterations in the peripheral blood lymphocyte population.

Thymus

This organ is located in the superior part of the anterior mediastinum, overlying the pericardium. It is basically an epithelial structure, the cortical part of which is derived from ectoderm whereas the medullary component is an endodermal outgrowth of the third and fourth branchial pouches. Within the micro-environment provided by the epithelium in the outer cortical part of the thymus, T-lymphocyte precursors, originally derived from the bone marrow, undergo an initial phase of antigen independent proliferation and development (see p. 200). This process is maximal during childhood, the thymus enlarging from infancy to reach its greatest size (30–40 g) at about puberty. Thereafter, the gland gradually decreases in bulk and weighs only about 15 g in late adult life. Failure of the epithelial component of the thymus to develop results in severe immunological deficiency (p. 239).

Thymic Enlargement

The main causes of this are outlined in Table 15.1. True hyperplasia is rare. Most cases of non-neoplastic enlargement are due to the presence in the medulla of fully developed lymphoid follicles with germinal centres. Some B lymphocytes are present in the thymus, but lymphoid follicles are seldom found normally and their presence can usually be regarded as pathological – '**thymitis**'. The commonest disease associated with this type of reaction is myasthenia gravis, an autoimmune disorder in which the development of antibodies to the acetylcholine receptors on the motor end plates of striated muscle leads to undue and occasionally life threatening muscular fatigue on exertion (p. 879). Removal of the hyperplastic thymus usually, but not invariably, induces remission of the disease. Thymitis may also be found in other autoimmune diseases both of organ-specific and non-organ-specific type (Table 15.1).

Table 15.1 Causes of thymic enlargement

Causes
True hyperplasia
Follicular hyperplasia (thymitis)
in association with myasthenia gravis, systemic lupus erythematosus, rheumatoid arthritis and other autoimmune diseases
Tumours
thymoma
carcinoid
lymphoma (Hodgkin's disease, T-lymphoblastic, mediastinal B-cell)
germ-cell tumours (seminoma, teratoma)

Tumours

Most distinctive, although rare, is the thymoma. This is an epithelial tumour which generally behaves like a low-grade carcinoma, invading structures in the local vicinity (pleura, pericardium) yet seldom metastasizing (<10%). Histologically, the tumour cells may exhibit a spindle or round cell morphology and may show squamous differentiation: in most cases they are interspersed with normal cortical and medullary thymocytes and, on occasion, this may be so pronounced as to lead to misdiagnosis of lymphoma. While often found incidentally (e.g. on routine chest radiography) thymoma has some interesting clinical associations. It is found in 10–20% of cases of myasthenia gravis but only in a quarter of these does removal of the tumour induce remission. Other disturbances associated with this tumour include red cell aplasia (p. 619), hypogammaglobulinaemia and autoimmune disorders such as polymyositis and systemic lupus erythematosus (SLE).

Neuroendocrine or carcinoid tumours occur but are uncommon. They may secrete ACTH and produce Cushing's syndrome (p. 1098). Occasionally, highly malignant 'oat-cell' carcinoid variants are encountered.

Several types of lymphoid neoplasia may arise in and primarily affect the thymus. These include (as one might expect) a tumour of T-lymphocyte precursor cells (lymphoblastic lymphoma) which commonly evolves into acute leukaemia. Hodgkin's disease, usually of the nodular sclerosis type, may also arise in the thymus, particularly in young women. More recently, a B-cell lymphoma, of large cell type, has been described. This tumour also exhibits sclerosis and tends to affect young adults. Lastly, the thymus is one of the favoured sites for the development of germ cell tumours; both teratomas and tumours resembling seminomas are well recognized.

Spleen

In normal adult life the spleen weighs between 100 and 200 g and receives 200–800 ml of blood per minute. It represents the only lymphatic tissue specialized to filter the blood. The function of the spleen is intimately related to its structure and in particular to its vascular arrangements (Fig. 15.1). Blood flows through the spleen by two main routes. More important is the slow transit mode (30–60 minutes) by which blood from the arterioles opens into a meshwork of vascular channels (the red pulp) and subsequently flows into the sinusoids which represent expanded radicles of the portal venous system. The red pulp is richly endowed with cells of the mononuclear phagocyte system which tend to be concentrated in the adventitia of the sinusoids. The latter channels are lined by transversely disposed endothelial cells separated by slit-like spaces approximately 3 μm in diameter and which have to be negotiated by red cells before they can re-enter the venous circulation. The slow pathway through this meshwork of vessels results in blood becoming concentrated to a haematocrit of approximately 80%, placing the red cells under considerable metabolic stress. There is also a rapid transit mode for blood flow through the spleen (2 minutes) with blood passing directly from the arterioles to the venous sinsuoids, and the greater proportion of the blood follows this route. The spleen contains abundant lymphoid tissue. This mainly takes the form of a sheath around the trabecular arterioles (the Malpighian bodies) and includes both T- and B-cell areas.

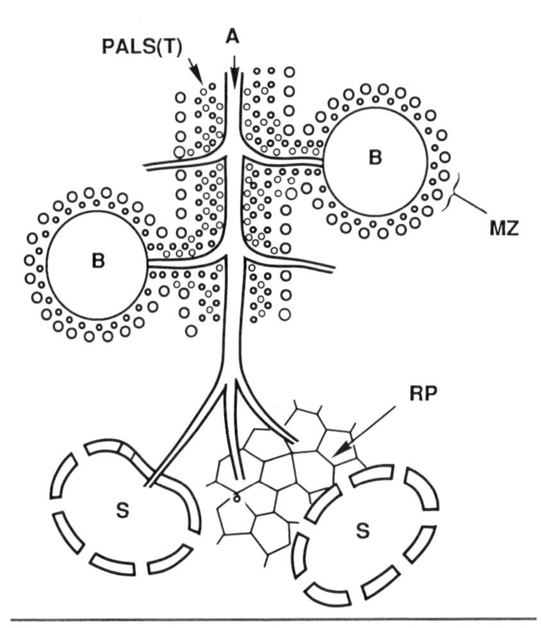

Fig. 15.1 A diagrammatic representation of splenic structure. Note that the arterial radicles either pass directly into the venous sinusoids (S) or, more often, enter the red pulp (RP). The periarteriolar lymphoid sheath (PALS) has distinct T- and B-cell areas. The marginal zone (MZ) may represent a site of lymphocyte entry into the spleen.

The spleen has a number of major functions. The first of these is phagocytic. The spleen monitors the bloodstream, its abundant phagocytes removing unwanted waste products and, more importantly, foreign materials and microorganisms of all kinds. More specifically, the spleen, by virtue of its vascular arrangements in particular in the slow transit mode, represents a testing ground for red cells. It disposes of time-expired red cells and abnormal red cell forms (**culling function**). It also removes certain intracellular inclusion bodies consisting, for example, of residual DNA (Howell–Jolly bodies), denatured haemoglobin (Heinz bodies) or haemosiderin (Pappenheimer bodies) from red cells. This remarkable so-called **pitting function** is also undertaken by macrophages and without damaging the red cell membrane. The spleen also has important immunological functions. It has a major role in counteracting blood infection, largely by producing IgM immunoglobulin. Removal of the spleen, especially in the first 2 years of life but also in adult life, unquestionably predisposes to severe and sometimes fatal blood infections, especially with pneumococci.

Hypersplenism

Most pathological processes involving the spleen result in its enlargement. This not only renders the organ palpable (a useful clinical sign) but may cause quite serious abdominal discomfort. More importantly, however, splenomegaly usually leads to expansion of the red pulp with increased sequestration and, when pronounced (splenic weight in excess of 1 kg), to premature destruction of the formed elements of the blood. The result is known as hypersplenism, a state of pancytopenia which is associated with compensatory bone marrow hyperplasia. The diagnosis of hypersplenism is seldom easy, haematological improvement following splenectomy being the only wholly convincing criterion.

Hyposplenism

This is not very common. Occasionally the spleen is absent at birth (usually in association with cardiac anomalies such as dextrocardia) and of course the spleen may be removed surgically, sometimes for haematological states such as hereditary spherocytosis or autoimmune thrombocytopenic purpura, but more often as a result of trauma or in the course of other surgical procedures (e.g. gastrectomy). Some diseases are associated with atrophy of the spleen. Coeliac disease is the best example of this, the reduction in spleen size being associated with a generalized state of immunodeficiency. Other causes include sickle cell disease (p. 605) and essential thrombocythaemia (p. 635) in both of which splenic atrophy is due to progressive microvascular occlusion.

Splenic hypofunction is usually evident from examination of the peripheral blood in which there is an accumulation of abnormal red cells (schistocytes, target cells) and red cells which retain the inclusions normally removed by the pitting mechanism, e.g. Howell–Jolly bodies (p. 593). It has already been noted that removal of the spleen may predispose to recurrent bacterial infections and splenic atrophy may have similar consequences.

Splenic Enlargement

The main causes of this are listed in Table 15.2. Some of these, however, deserve special mention.

Table 15.2 Important causes of splenomegaly

Inflammatory and immunological states
- Bacterial
  - typhoid fever, tuberculosis, brucellosis, subacute bacterial endocarditis
- Viral
  - infectious mononucleosis; cytomegalovirus
- Protozoal and metazoal
  - malaria, leishmaniasis, trypanosomiasis, toxoplasmosis, echinococcosis
- Sarcoidosis
- Rheumatoid arthritis, Felty's syndrome, systemic lupus erythematosus
- Amyloidosis

Congestive states
- Hepatic cirrhosis
- Schistosomiasis
- Portal vein thrombosis
- Budd–Chiari syndrome

Haematological disorders
- Haemolytic anaemias
- Autoimmune thrombocytopenic purpura
- Extramedullary haemopoiesis

Storage diseases
- Gaucher's disease
- Niemann–Pick disease
- Mucopolysaccharidoses

Neoplastic states
- Hodgkin's disease
- Non-Hodgkin's lymphoma
- Chronic leukaemias: myeloid and lymphocytic
- Acute leukaemias (uncommon)
- Myeloproliferative syndromes
- Primary vascular tumours
- Metastatic tumours (uncommon)

Inflammatory and Immunological Diseases

Splenic enlargement commonly takes place when pathogenic micro-organisms – bacterial, viral, fungal or protozoal – have been present in the bloodstream for prolonged periods. The protozoal infections provide some of the most striking examples of massive splenic enlargement. The so-called big spleen disease, a form of hypersplenism prevalent in equatorial Africa, is due to persistent malaria of the quartan variety (p. 1144). Massive splenomegaly is also an important feature of visceral leishmaniasis (p. 1151). Infections of the spleen carry the risk of splenic rupture: the hazard appears to be especially great in infectious mononucleosis (p. 652). Of the other inflammatory conditions, mention must be made of Felty's syndrome, an expression of long-standing rheumatoid arthritis (p. 992) in which the spleen is greatly enlarged, due to marked follicular hyperplasia, and causes hypersplenism with an increased susceptibility to recurrent bacterial infections; nodular regenerative hyperplasia of the liver (p. 750) is also an associated feature.

Portal Hypertension

This is the mechanism which leads to splenic enlargement in association with hepatic disturbances such as cirrhosis, the Budd–Chiari syndrome and schistosomiasis. In all these conditions there is congestion of the red pulp and the histological changes are distinctive: there is marked dilatation of the sinusoids and their walls become thickened. There may also be periarteriolar haemorrhages which subsequently become converted into fibrous nodules heavily encrusted with haemosiderin and calcium salts (so-called Gamna–Gandy bodies).

Haematological States

Certain abnormalities of red cells lead to impairment of their elasticity or deformability with consequent entrapment in the red pulp of the spleen. Spherocytosis and various other haemolytic anaemias (p. 601) provide the best examples of this phenomenon. In these conditions the spleen is invariably enlarged; histologically, the accumulation of red cells in the red pulp is evident and leads to compression of the sinusoids. In hereditary spherocytosis splenectomy cures the disease without rectifying the red cell defect. Splenectomy may also be of benefit in some cases of autoimmune thrombocytopenic purpura in which platelets tend to be sequestered in the red pulp (p. 640). The spleen is seldom much enlarged in this disease. Histologically, the most distinctive feature is the presence in the red pulp of histiocytes, with a foamy appearance attributable to the presence of ingested platelets.

Metabolic Diseases

Inherited defects of lysosomal enzymes concerned with the disposal of cellular breakdown products leads to the massive accumulation of these products, usually within the mononuclear phagocyte system (p. 258). Splenomegaly, sometimes accompanied by hypersplenism, is usually a prominent feature in such circumstances. The most striking example of this is the adult form of Gaucher's disease in which there is infiltration of the red pulp by histiocytes with a distinctive bloated appearance caused by the accumulation of glucocerebroside. Due to the presence of this material these cells are strongly positive with the PAS reaction. A similar situation arises in Niemann–Pick disease, the material accumulating in the spleen and elsewhere in the mononuclear phagocytic system being mainly sphingomyelin.

Neoplastic States

Splenomegaly is a major feature of haematological tumours. This is especially true of the chronic leukaemias, either granulocytic (myeloid) or lymphocytic type, in which the spleen becomes massively infiltrated by leukaemic cells. In myelosclerosis, splenic enlargement is due mainly to extramedullary haemopoiesis (p. 634). Malignant lymphomas of either Hodgkin's or non-Hodgkin's type commonly involve the spleen: by contrast carcinomas only very rarely do so. It should also be noted that primary tumours of the spleen are uncommon. It is possible, however, that some lymphomas, e.g. hairy cell leukaemia, are of splenic origin and occasional vascular tumours have been described.

Lymph Nodes

Under normal conditions lymph nodes are small, bean-shaped structures which, even in their major peripheral locations (e.g. cervical, axillary or inguinal) are seldom palpable. Their primary function is to entrap and, if need be, to mount an immune response to foreign agents or unwanted materials which have gained access to the tissue spaces. To bring this about lymph nodes are surrounded by a peripheral sinus which receives the afferent lymphatics emerging from the tissue spaces (p. 481). From this peripheral basin a second series of sinuses traverse the node and

Table 15.3 Important causes of lymphadenopathy

REACTIVE STATES

Acute lymphadenitis
  Pyogenic infections
 	
Follicular hyperplasia
  HIV infection and AIDS
  Rheumatoid arthritis, systemic lupus erythematosus and other connective tissue and autoimmune diseases
 	
Paracortical reactions
  Drug hypersensitivity (e.g. anticonvulsants)
  Viral infection
    Epstein–Barr, cytomegalovirus, herpes simplex
 	
Sinus reactions
  Sinus histiocytosis with massive lymphadenopathy
  Sinus B-cell reactions
 	
Histiocytic reactions
  Anthracosis, post-lymphangiography and other foreign materials
  Dermatopathic lymphadenopathy
 	
Miscellaneous
  Histiocytosis X
  Angiofollicular lymph node hyperplasia
	Granulomatous reactions
	  Infective
	    tuberculosis
	    syphilis
	    toxoplasmosis
	    chlamydial
	    fungal
	    leishmaniasis
	    acute mesenteric lymphadenitis
	  Miscellaneous (uncertain aetiology)
	    cat scratch disease
	    necrotizing histiocytic lymphadenitis
	    sarcoidosis
	    Crohn's disease
	
	Whipple's disease
	
	Vasculitis

NEOPLASTIC STATES

Metastatic tumour
Hodgkin's disease
Non-Hodgkin's lymphomas, including leukaemias

merge to form a single efferent lymphatic which subsequently conveys lymph back to the venous system. The sinuses are richly endowed with cellular representatives of the mononuclear phagocyte system which line the sinus wall and sometimes appear to be suspended within the lumen by cytoplasmic strands. These cells take up antigen and present it by way of intermediary antigen presenting cells to the lymphoid elements which lie within the connective tissue framework between the sinuses, the B-cell areas being located in the outer cortex, while the T-cell areas mainly occupy the deeper cortical zones (paracortical zones). The medullary region around the radicles of the efferent lymphatic is the preferential location for plasma cells.

When lymph nodes are affected by disease they usually become enlarged and palpable. The main causes of this are listed in Table 15.3. In broad terms they can be divided into reactive and neoplastic states. In view of the extended accounts which are subsequently given of the primary neoplastic conditions which affect lymph nodes the student should bear in mind that numerically they constitute a minor, albeit an important component of diseases which affect lymph nodes (Table 15.4).

Table 15.4 Lymph node biopsies examined at the Western Infirmary Glasgow in 1989

	No.	%
Non-malignant conditions		
Reactive changes	106	47
Tuberculosis	4	2
Sarcoidosis	1	0.4
Toxoplasmosis	1	0.4
Malignant disease		
Metastatic tumour	69	30
Non-Hodgkin's lymphoma	36	16
Hodgkin's disease	10	4.4

Overall (227 specimens): non-malignant (49%); metastatic tumours (30%); primary lymphoid neoplasms (21%)

This places in perspective the relative incidence of the various lymph node diseases.

Reactive Lymphadenopathy

Lymph nodes are commonly enlarged due to transient and sometimes severe acute inflammatory changes taking place during the course of pyogenic or other rapidly developing infections involving the tissue spaces (acute lymphadenititis). Lymphadenopathy may also arise as a consequence of chronic inflammation. Sometimes this presents distinctive changes, e.g. granuloma formation, but more often is caused by proliferation of the main lymphoid and histiocytic elements. It is convenient to classify these chronic reactions (which may or may not be infective in origin) according to the predominant reactive element (Table 15.3) although it has to be appreciated that it is by no means uncommon for all the cellular elements to be affected in some degree.

Acute Lymphadenitis

During any acute infection involving the subcutaneous tissues organisms may gain entry into lymphatics and reach the draining lymph nodes. Here the organisms initially encounter (and may be phagocytosed by) sinus histiocytes which become swollen and eventually constitute an effective, though by no means infallible, barrier to further spread of the infection. The typical features of acute inflammation such as vascular congestion and neutrophil emigration may develop in and around the sinuses and may extend into the perinodal tissues (periadenitis) or into the cortical parenchyma. Sometimes suppuration follows. This type of lesion is especially well exemplified in the cervical nodes in acute streptococcal tonsillitis.

Follicular Hyperplasia

Germinal centre (or secondary follicle) formation within the cortical B-cell zones of a lymph node is regarded as a marker of antigen exposure and it is thus not surprising that this phenomenon may become pronounced in many reactive states. In diagnostic terms, follicular hyperplasia is a nonspecific change and may be seen in draining lymph nodes in relation to such diverse conditions as peptic ulcer, chronic inflammatory bowel disease and syphilis.

In human immunodeficiency virus (HIV) infection persistent lymphadenopathy may be an important feature which precedes the onset of AIDS (p. 243). Follicular hyperplasia is the most striking histological feature observed initially. Even at an early stage the follicle mantles appear to be deficient: later the germinal centres themselves tend to break down (folliculolysis). The paracortical T zones may also be expanded at first, but as the condition advances, they also become progressively depleted, mainly due to destruction of virally infected T-helper cells.

In rheumatoid arthritis lymphadenopathy and splenomegaly are by no means uncommon. Histologically, the lymph nodes may show well marked follicular hyperplasia (Fig. 15.2) usually accompanied by an increase in medullary plasma cells. The spleen may show similar expansion of the B-cell zones. The disease may be complicated by a malignant lymphoma but curiously, this tends to be of T-cell type.

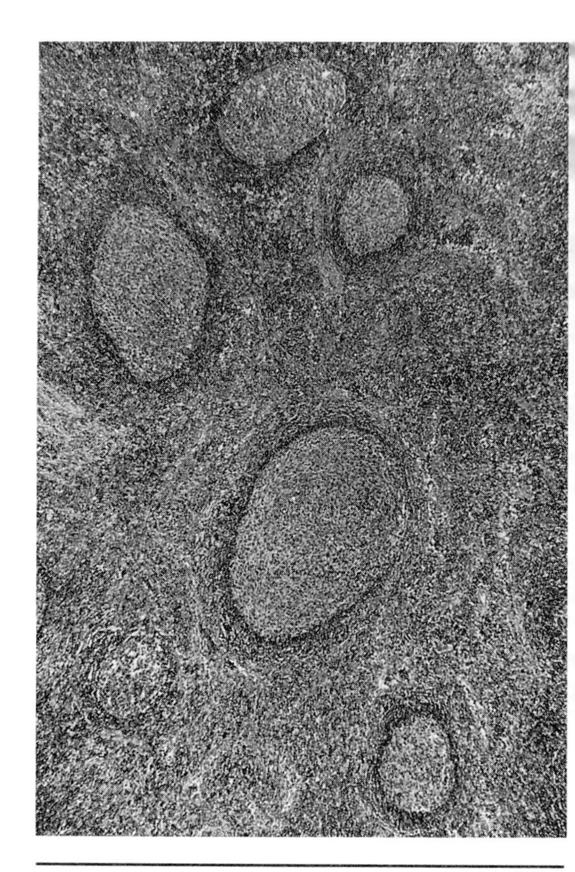

Fig. 15.2 Lymph node in rheumatoid arthritis, showing follicular hyperplasia with conspicuous germinal centres. ×50.

Paracortical (T-cell) Hyperplasia

The normal T zone in a lymph node occupies the deep cortex (paracortical zone) and consists mainly of small lymphocytes interspersed with antigen presenting cells (interdigitating reticulum cells) and post-capillary venules with their tall plump endothelial cells through which lymphocytes gain entry into the node. Transformed or activated lymphocytes (immunoblasts) are usually sparse but in T-cell reactions become much more numerous and lead to paracortical expansion. While reactions of this kind are by no means uncommon they tend to be especially pronounced in drug hypersensitivity reactions and in association with certain viral infections. **Infectious mononucleosis** due to the Epstein–Barr (EB) virus provides the most striking example in the latter category. The EB virus grows mainly in B cells and may cause extensive damage to the B-cell areas in lymph nodes. This is invariably accompanied by a striking paracortical T-cell reaction with pronounced immunoblastic proliferation (Fig. 15.3). This combination of changes can be alarming and is sometimes mistaken for a lymphomatous (neoplastic) process. The basic nodal architecture and, in particular, the sinus network are preserved and, characteristically, transformed lymphocytes are found within the sinuses. The atypical mononuclear cells which can invariably be found in the peripheral blood may also represent transformed lymphocytes, probably of T-cell type.

Sinus Histiocytosis

This term refers to the proliferation of the histiocytic cells which normally occupy the sinus

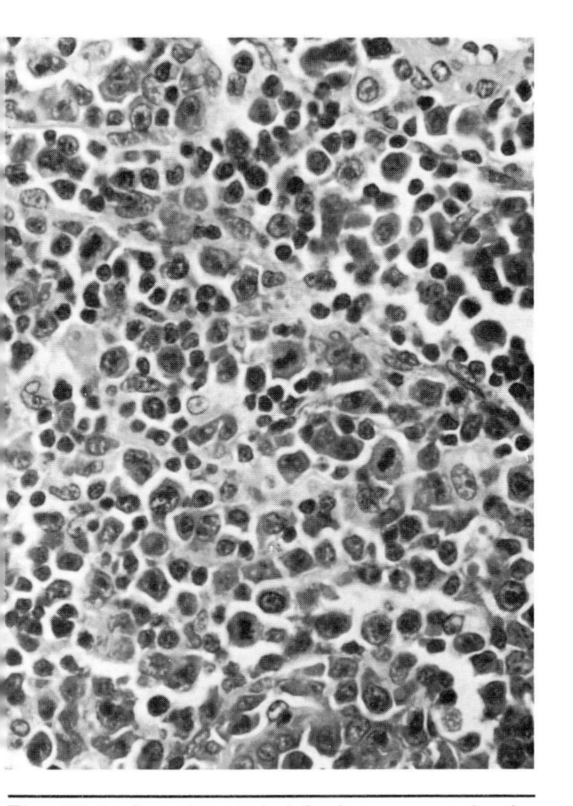

Fig. 15.3 Lymph node in infectious mononucleosis, showing large numbers of lymphoblasts in the paracortex. Mitoses are conspicuous and a sinus (upper right) also contains blast cells. ×520.

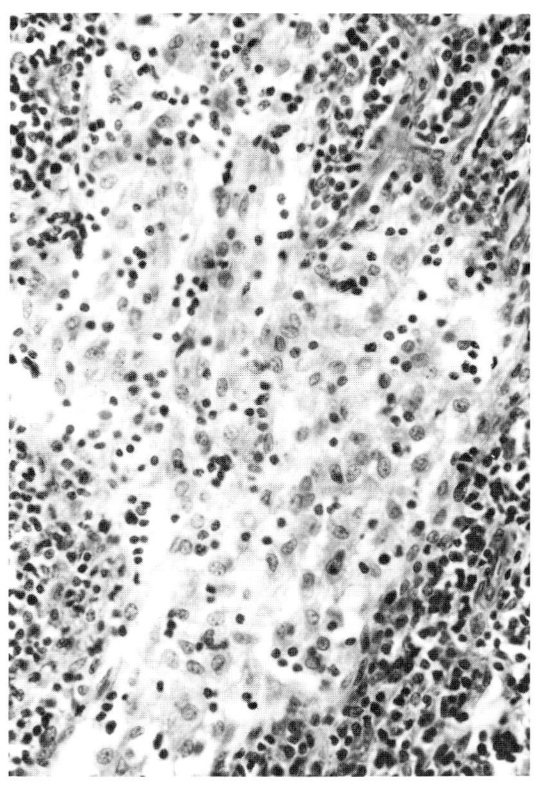

Fig. 15.4 Lymph node showing reactive sinus hyperplasia: an enlarged sinus containing increased numbers of macrophages. ×120.

network (Fig. 15.4) and is seen in many inflammatory and reactive states. It may be prominent in lymph nodes draining carcinomas without there being metastatic spread. In some rare diseases, however, sinus histiocytosis is a predominant feature.

In sinus histiocytosis with massive lymphadenopathy (Rosai–Dorfman disease), a self-limiting condition, which usually affects black children or young adults, there is striking nodal enlargement (usually cervical) due to the proliferation of histiocytes within the sinuses and sometimes in the nodal parenchyma. The histiocytes are markedly swollen and contain numerous phagocytosed cells, especially lymphocytes. The cause is unknown.

Sinus B-cell Reactions

In certain infections such as toxoplasmosis, EB virus infection and HIV infection there may be a proliferation of B cells with monocytoid (monocyte-like) features within sinuses. This has to be distinguished from true sinus histiocytosis.

Parenchymal Histiocytic Reactions

Foreign substances and cellular debris from endogenous sources are commonly found in lymph nodes. These materials either arrive at the lymph nodes within histiocytes or are taken up by sinus histiocytes: in either event the affected cells migrate into the paracortical zones where, failing rapid disposal of the offending material, they tend to accumulate. This phenomenon is most readily seen in the hilar or peribronchial lymph nodes which, in city dwellers at least, invariably show some paracortical infiltration by histiocytes stuffed with anthracotic carbon pigment derived from the inhalation of soot. Other materials which produce histiocytic nodal reactions include silicon elastomers (used in the structuring of synthetic joints) and the radiological contrast medium Lipiodol (used during lymphangiographic procedures).

Dermatopathic lymphadenopathy. This is the best example of a nodal reaction caused by endogenous factors. During certain skin diseases, especially lichenoid conditions and mycosis fungoides, the breakdown of epidermal cells releases cellular debris, particularly cell wall lipid and melanin pigment, into the tissue spaces. Much of this material reaches lymph nodes where it is taken up by histiocytes, mainly in the paracortical zones and can lead to pronounced lymph node enlargement.

Granulomatous Reactions

Epithelioid granuloma formation is a common and important histological finding in a lymph node. As is evident from Table 15.3 the aetiology is diverse. Even now tuberculosis must head the list especially if the granulomas show central necrosis, whether or not this has the classical features of caseation.

Sarcoidosis is an important cause of lymphadenopathy. The granulomas rarely show central necrosis but may undergo progressive hyalinization as the disease evolves. It is important to note that sarcoid-like granulomas may be found in lymph nodes draining malignant tumours (e.g. carcinoma of breast), and some malignant lymphomas (especially of T-cell type) may be accompanied by granuloma formation. This is also true of Hodgkin's disease; indeed, granulomas may be found in sites such as spleen, bone marrow and liver even in the absence of direct tumour involvement. The reasons for granuloma formation in these circumstances are not fully understood but may relate to some immunological response to tumour antigens.

Toxoplasmosis is due to infection by the protozoon *Toxoplasma gondii* and is probably contracted through contact with domestic animals, notably cats (p. 1158). Whereas in neonates the disease can result in severe neurological disturbances in adult life lymphadenopathy is the most prominent clinical finding, systemic symptoms often being vague or mild.

Histologically, the lymph nodes show pronounced follicular hyperplasia and there may also be a prominent B-cell reaction in the sinuses. Even more distinctive is the presence of small epithelioid granulomas which tend to impinge upon reactive germinal centres (Fig. 15.5). Organisms can seldom be detected histologically: reliance has to be placed upon serology to confirm the diagnosis.

Cat scratch disease, another hazard of cat ownership, is almost certainly infective although the organism responsible has not yet been convincingly identified. Lymphadenopathy is the main clinical feature.

Histologically, the affected nodes exhibit a characteristic type of granulomatous lesion. It tends to have an irregular Y shaped or serpiginous structure and consists of epithelioid histiocytes which are disposed in a palisaded fashion around areas of central necrosis or suppuration (Fig.

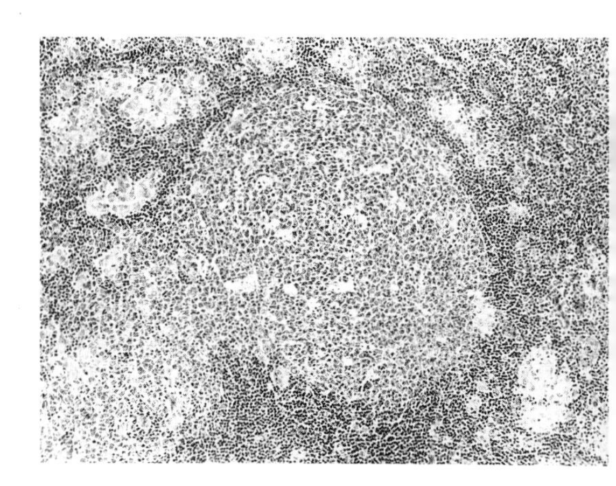

Fig. 15.5 Toxoplasmosis. There is a pronounced B-cell reaction with enlarged germinal centres. Small epithelioid cell granulomas, often impinging upon the germinal centres are also present. H & E ×70.

15.6). An almost identical type of nodal appearance may be seen in chlamydial infections such as lymphogranuloma inguinale and also in the childhood condition, acute mesenteric lymphadenitis, which is due to infection by *Yersinia pseudotuberculosis*.

Necrotizing histiocytic lymphadenitis (Kikuchi's disease) mainly affects young Japanese women and has only occasionally been seen elsewhere. It resolves spontaneously in a few months. Histologically, the lymph nodes show foci of cortical and paracortical necrosis which are surrounded by histiocytes but these are of the phagocytic and not the epithelioid variety and are often associated with a marked immunoblastic reaction. A notable feature is the absence of neutrophil polymorphs. The cause is uncertain: a yersinial infection has, however, been suspected in some cases.

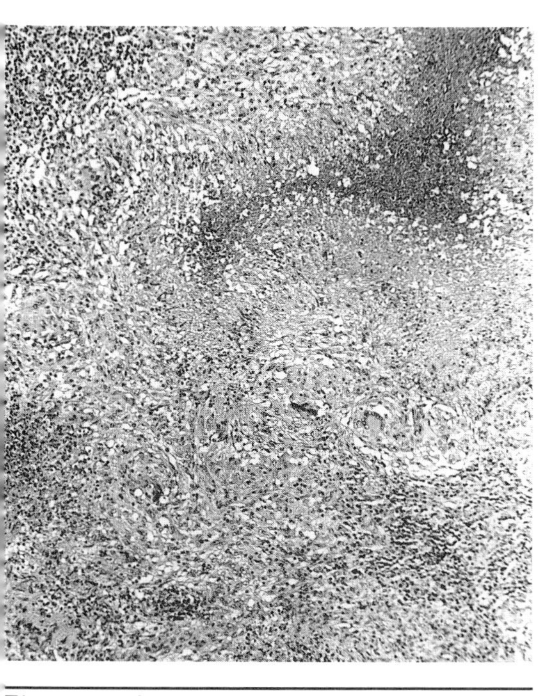

Fig. 15.6 Cat scratch disease. The affected lymph nodes contain irregularly shaped granulomatous lesion with areas of central necrosis surrounded by palisaded epithelioid cells and giant cells. H & E × 60.

Miscellaneous Lymph Node Lesions

Most of these listed in Table 15.3 are part of systematized diseases discussed elsewhere. Worthy of special mention, however, are two other conditions, histocytosis X, a proliferative lesion of Langerhans cells, and the enigmatic condition known as angiofollicular lymph node hyperplasia or Castleman's disease.

Histiocytosis X. This term applies to a group of conditions characterized by the proliferation of a particular type of histiocyte known as the Langerhans cell, probably an antigen presenting cell. This cell, which is normally found within the epidermis and sometimes in other epithelial surfaces (p. 1109) has a curious lobulated nuclear morphology and S-100 protein can be demonstrated by immunohistochemical methods in the cytoplasm. Electron microscopy reveals an even more distinctive cytoplasmic feature, namely the presence of tiny structures resembling tennis rackets in shape (Birbeck granules). In the granuloma-like lesions of histiocytosis X, Langerhans cells are almost always accompanied by eosinophils, sometimes in large numbers. The disease varies in severity. **Letterer–Siwe** disease which affects children below the age of 4 years is the most severe form and involves mainly the lymphoreticular system, skin and lungs; it is invariably fatal. In the less aggressive form, **Hand–Schüller–Christian disease**, the lesions are similarly distributed; hepatosplenomegaly and lymphadenopathy are prominent and bony involvement (especially of the skull) is usual. The least serious form is the solitary lesion known as **eosinophil granuloma**. While this usually affects bone (p. 983) it may involve a lymph node. Here the Langerhans cell proliferation takes place mainly within sinuses although it may extend into the parenchyma. Eosinophils may be so numerous as to produce solid masses which may show central breakdown (so-called eosinophilic abscesses).

Angiofollicular lymph node hyperplasia (Castleman's disease). Usually this takes the form of a symptomless mediastinal mass consisting of abnormal lymphoid tissue which shows a paucity of sinusoids yet exhibits numerous follicular structures histologically. These lack true germinal centres which are replaced by groups of large cells (probably dendritic reticulum cells) enclosing a prominent blood vessel with thick hyalinized walls and surrounded by concentric rings of mantle zone lymphocytes (hyaline-vascular type) – Fig. 15.7. There is also a less common form in which there are multiple lesions mainly affecting peripheral lymph nodes: histologically, the nodes may have normal looking germinal centres but there is massive interfollicular plasma cell infiltration (plasma cell type). This type may be accompanied by systemic symptoms such as fever and weight loss. The cause of angiofollicular lymph node hyperplasia is not known. Some regard it as essentially hamartomatous, but it sometimes appears to arise in relationship to immunodeficiency states such as AIDS and can occasionally be followed by the development of a lymphoma.

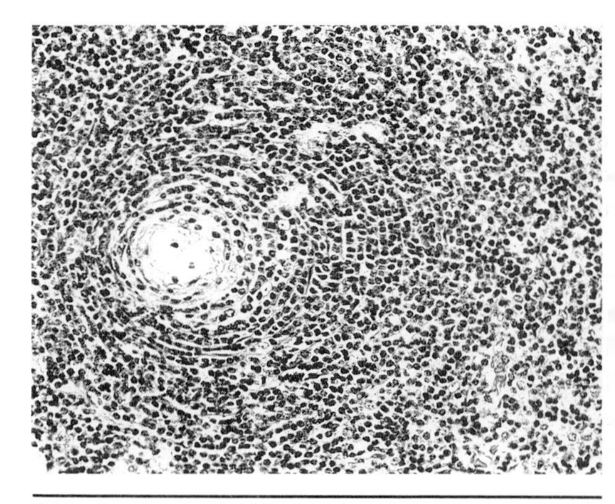

Fig. 15.7 Angiofollicular lymph node hyperplasia (Castleman's disease). Abnormal follicles with a central hyalinised blood vessel, surrounded by rings of lymphocytes are typical of the 'hyaline-vascular' form. H & E ×175.

Neoplastic Diseases of Lymph Nodes

It cannot be overemphasized that the tumours most often encountered in lymph nodes are metastatic rather than primary. With the exception of rodent ulcer (basal cell carcinoma) all carcinomas (and melanomas) have the capacity to metastasize by way of the lymphatic system. Whilst carcinomas constitute by far the commonest metastatic tumour in lymph nodes, some sarcomas (e.g. malignant fibrous histiocytoma and synovial sarcoma) also have the capacity to spread by this route, although more commonly they metastasize by the bloodstream. The most common primary tumours are the malignant lymphomas which are discussed below. The only other primary tumour at all common in lymph nodes is Kaposi's sarcoma (p. 1140), especially the form which complicates AIDS in male homosexuals.

Malignant lymphoma is now widely preferred as the term to describe primary tumours of the lymphoreticular system and gains justification from the increasing likelihood that most of these tumours arise from lymphocytes. It should also be noted that all lymphomas are regarded as malignant in the sense that they all exhibit the ability to disseminate or metastasize and most, if left untreated, will limit the lifespan of the affected individual. In terms of natural history, however, lymphomas vary greatly in behaviour: some are capable of bringing about a fatal outcome in a few weeks or months (high-grade) whereas others may take many years to do so (low-grade).

As might be expected from the widespread distribution of the lymphoreticular system malignant lymphomas may arise from almost any organ. However, most originate in the primary or secondary lymphoid organs, especially the lymph nodes. Moreover, when lymphomas metastasize they tend to mimic the recirculating behaviour of normal lymphocytes and spread, initially at any rate, to other parts of the lymphoreticular system through either lymphatics or blood vessels. Widespread lymphadenopathy and splenomegaly are thus common features. Tumour cells are also commonly found in the blood (leukaemic phase) and bone marrow.

It is customary to separate Hodgkin's disease from the other types (not surprisingly referred to as the non-Hodgkin's lymphomas) by virtue of its distinctive histological appearance and continuing debate regarding its histogenesis. This distinction is to some extent arbitrary and may ultimately prove to be unnecessary.

Hodgkin's Disease

This was probably the first lymphoma to be described (in 1832) and is still one of the most common, accounting for about 30% of all malignant lymphoma cases. It was pathologically characterized at the turn of the century following descriptions of the histological marker cell by Sternberg (1898) and Reed (1901) and which now bears their names – the Reed–Sternberg (RS) cell. It has a biphasic age incidence with peaks in early adult life (about 30 years of age or, in so-called third world countries, late childhood) and again in late middle age. Although the cause is unknown there is some epidemiological evidence to suggest a possible link with viral infection: certainly the incidence of the disease parallels that of ubiquitous viral diseases such as Epstein–Barr virus infection; but other factors (possibly genetic in origin) may also be involved.

Clinical Features

Lymph node enlargement, involving the neck or mediastinum, is by far the most common presenting feature. Only rarely does the disease arise in an extranodal site (e.g. skin or bone marrow). In some cases there are systemic symptoms such as low-grade intermittent pyrexia, sweating, pruritus and weight loss; the presence or otherwise of these symptoms is a further subdivision of the clinical stages (Table 15.5). Occasionally the enlarged nodes are painful, especially after alcohol ingestion. There may be anaemia, usually of the secondary type and this can be accompanied by peripheral blood neutrophilia or eosinophilia. Deficiencies of cell mediated immunity may be troublesome even at an early stage and can lead to opportunistic infections, e.g. herpes zoster, tuberculosis or fungal infection.

The disease is seldom confined for long to the lymph node groups primarily involved. There may, of course, be local invasion of adjacent organs, but the most striking form of initial spread is by way of the lymphatics to adjacent nodal groups and subsequently to distant nodes. The spleen too may be involved at a relatively early stage. Only later are extranodal sites such as bone marrow and liver affected, probably as a result of blood spread. Eventually, metastases may appear in many organs outwith the lymphoreticular system. This pattern of spread forms the basis of the clinical staging system outlined in Table 15.5. Clinical staging is important since it not only helps to assess the prognosis but also to determine the kind of treatment that is given. Staging involves careful clinical examination, X-ray examination, lymphangiography, bone marrow biopsy and computerized tomography to assess liver and splenic

Table 15.5 Hodgkin's disease: clinical staging system* (Ann Arbor)

Stage	Description
I	Disease confined to one lymph node group or involvement of a single extranodal site (I_E)
II	Disease confined to several lymph node groups on the same side of the diaphragm†, or with minimal involvement of adjacent extranodal site (II_E)
III	Disease present in lymph node groups on both sides of diaphragm with minimal involvement of adjacent extranodal site (III_E)
IV	Diffuse involvement of one or more extranodal tissues, e.g. bone marrow or liver

*Each stage is further subdivided according to whether there are systemic symptoms (A) or not (B).
†Spleen regarded as lymph node for staging purposes.

involvement. Liver biopsy and splenectomy may also be carried out.

Pathological Features

Macroscopically, lymph nodes affected by Hodgkin's disease vary in appearance (Fig. 15.8). In some cases they are discrete and rubbery in consistency, the cut surface being featureless and greyish-pink in colour. In other cases the lymph nodes are more fibrous and less well defined and may show yellow areas of necrosis.

Histologically, the disease has two distinctive features. First is the RS cell regarded as the neoplastic component of the cellular infiltrate, recognition of which is essential for diagnostic purposes. The RS cell is a large cell with either two nuclei or a bilobed nucleus. Each nuclear component has a large central eosinophilic nucleolus surrounded by a clear zone, the heterochromatin being condensed at the periphery (Fig. 15.9a). The cytoplasm is quite abundant and usually amphophilic (i.e. purple with H & E stains) and pyroninophilic (i.e. stains with pyronin dyes due to a high RNA content). Pleomorphic and mononuclear forms of the RS cell may also be conspicuous: the latter are known as Hodgkin cells and are especially helpful in identifying metastatic lesions (e.g. in liver or bone marrow) when the typical RS cells are sparse. Other variants of the RS cell are: (1) the lacunar cells which show peripheral cytoplasmic vacuolation so that they appear to lie in clear spaces (Fig. 15.9b); (2) the so-called lymphocytic-histiocytic (L and H) type (or popcorn cell) with a multilobated or convoluted nucleus and relatively small nucleoli (Fig. 15.9c).

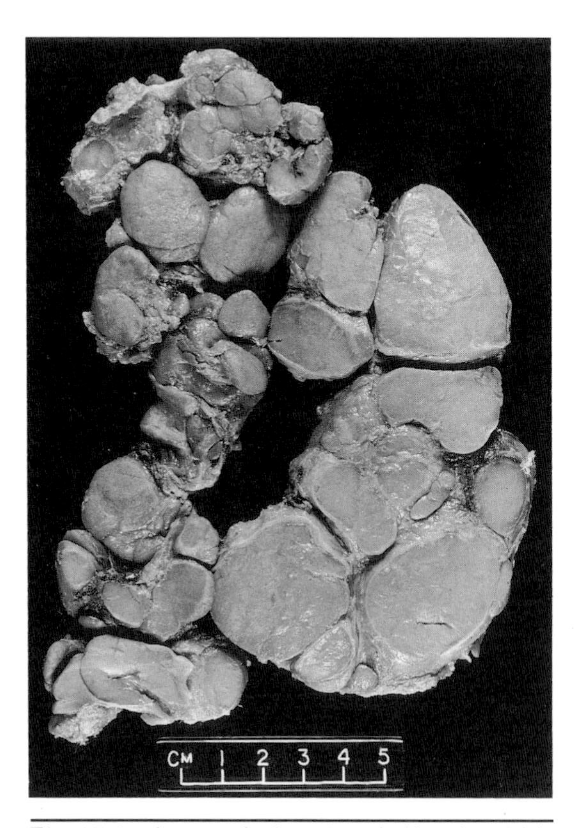

Fig. 15.8 A group of enlarged cervical lymph nodes in Hodgkin's disease. The largest nodes are becoming matted together.

The second important feature of Hodgkin's disease is that the RS cells evoke a striking cellular response which progressively ablates lymph node architecture. This response involves not only leucocytes such as lymphocytes, plasma cells, histiocytes, neutrophils and eosinophils in variable proportion, but may include a fibroblastic reaction.

It has long been recognized that Hodgkin's disease varies greatly in terms of its clinical aggressiveness and that behaviour can, to some extent, be linked to the histological features. The Rye histological classification system recognizes this principle and subdivides Hodgkin's disease into four main subtypes (Table 15.6), the essential basis for the classification being the frequency of the RS cell and its variants and the patterns of the accompanying cellular response.

Table 15.6 Hodgkin's disease: histological subtypes (Rye classification)

Lymphocyte predominance
Nodular sclerosis
type I
type II
Mixed cellularity
Lymphocyte depletion

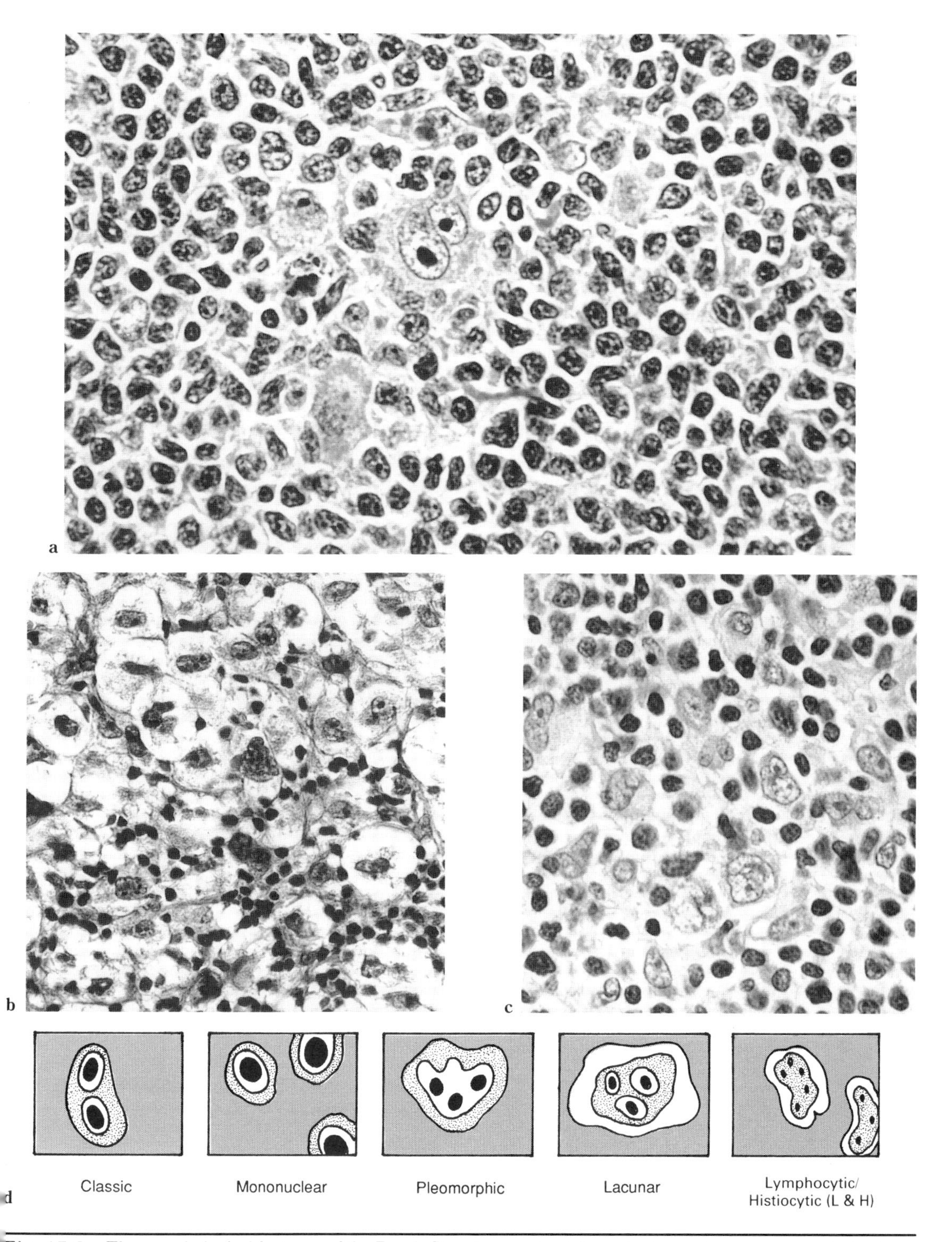

Fig. 15.9 The morphological features of the Reed–Sternberg cell and its variants are shown in these photomicrographs and in addition are illustrated diagrammatically in **d**. **a** Classic Reed–Sternberg cell, binucleate or with a mirror-image nucleus, vesicular chromatin and a prominent eosinophilic nucleolus; the number of nuclei and of nucleoli may vary as shown in the diagram (see also Fig. 15.11). **b** Lacunar variant: the cell appears as if to lie within a vacuole. **c** Lymphocytic–histiocytic – L and H variant; the nucleus is multilobated or convoluted creating a popcorn-like appearance; hence the term 'popcorn cells'.

Lymphocyte predominace. This subtype accounts for about 10% of Hodgkin's disease cases and is mainly found in young adult males. Histologically, there are two main features: first, classic RS cells are very sparse, the main neoplastic element being the L & H (popcorn) cell and secondly, the cellular response consists almost exclusively of lymphocytes and histiocytes, the latter sometimes forming small granulomas. Currently there is some debate that this subtype may in reality be a B cell lymphoma.

Nodular sclerosis. This is the most common subtype, accounting for 60–70% of cases in Europe and North America, rather less in tropical countries. It mainly affects young adults, especially females. Histologically, diagnosis depends upon recognition that the neoplastic infiltrate is disposed in a series of nodules, each surrounded by thick bands of birefringent collagen (Fig. 15.10). Classic RS cells are found in the lesions but lacunar cells are more characteristic. The cellular response within the nodules varies: usually it consists mainly of lymphocytes or shows a mixed cellularity pattern as described below (**nodular sclerosis type 1**): sometimes, however, there is pronounced lymphocyte depletion in most of the nodules, or the RS cells are unusually pleomorphic (**nodular sclerosis type 2**). In either type there may be granuloma formation or foci of necrosis.

Mixed cellularity. This might be regarded as the archetypal form of Hodgkin's disease and is common in the third world. It only accounts, at most, for about 20% of cases in Europe and North America, and tends to affect adults in later life. Histologically, most of the tumour cells are either classic RS or mononuclear (Hodgkin) cells (Fig. 15.11) and the cellular response consists not only of lymphocytes but includes plasma cells, neutrophils and eosinophils. Histiocytes are often prominent and there may be epithelioid granulomas. A sclerotic reaction in the form of a tangled network of reticulin fibres (not a banded pattern as in nodular sclerosis) is usual. Necrosis is common.

Lymphocyte depletion. Fortunately this subtype accounts for less than 5% of cases in most series. Older adults are usually affected. In histological terms (Fig. 15.12) the appearances differ from mixed cellularity in that either the cellular response is severely deficient in lymphocytes (this often being associated with diffuse sclerosis) or the neoplastic cell population includes not only classic RS cells but many pleomorphic forms, sometimes with giant nucleoli.

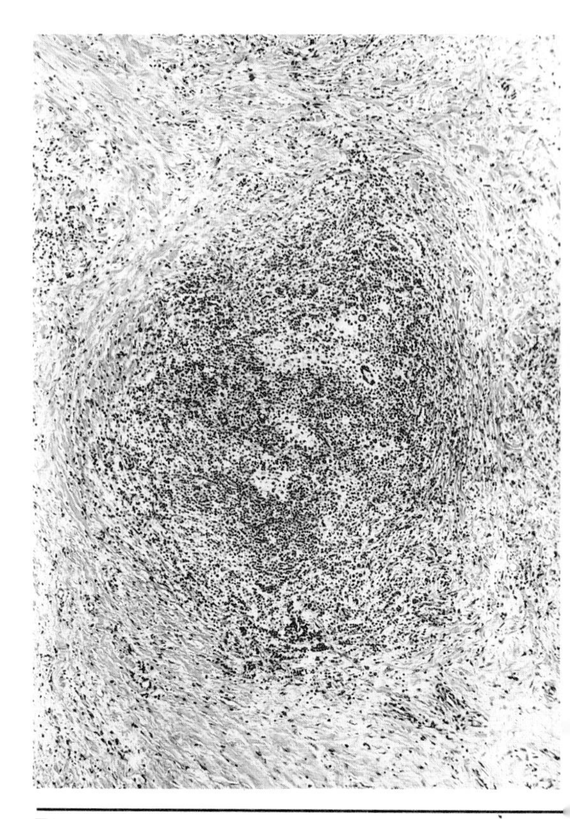

Fig. 15.10 Hodgkin's disease, nodular sclerosis. There is a nodule of tumour growth encased by thick bands of collagen. H & E ×60.

The Significance of the Subtypes

Long-term survival in Hodgkin's disease is usually associated with the lymphocyte predominance or nodular sclerosis type 1, the presence of numerous lymphocytes or banded sclerosis in the lesions presumably representing a good response to the tumour. Mixed cellularity indicates a dimin-

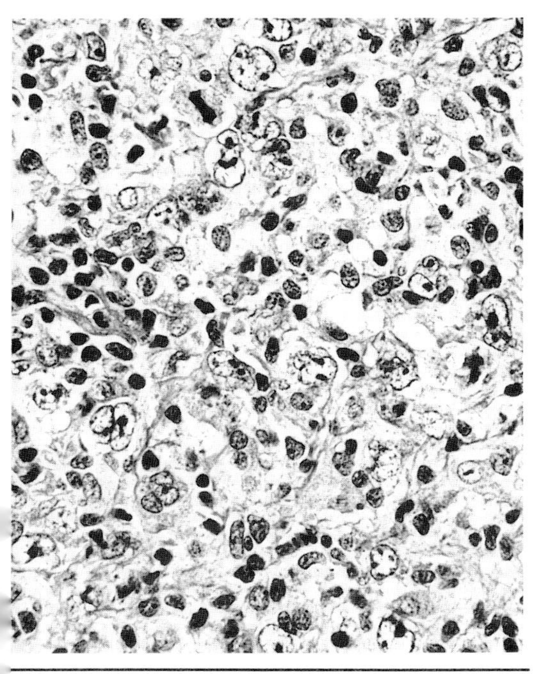

Fig. 15.11 Hodgkin's disease, mixed cellularity. There are numerous Reed–Sternberg cells relative to the reactive lymphocytic and plasma cell populations. H & E × 454.

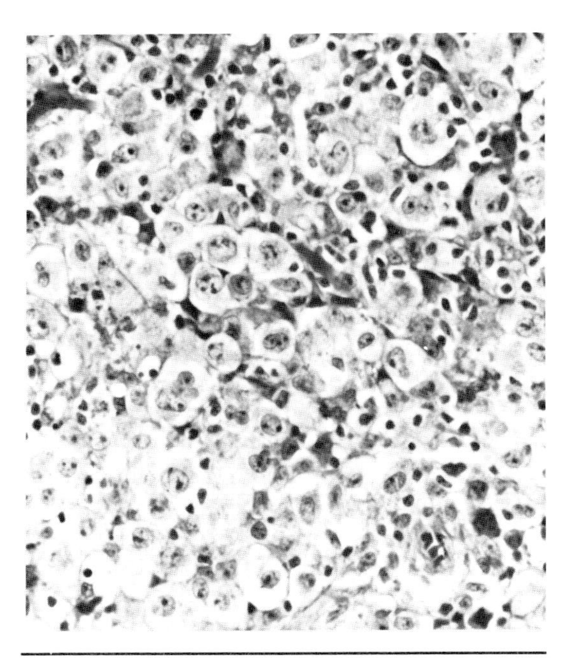

Fig. 15.12 Lymphocyte-depleted Hodgkin's disease. Most of the cells are neoplastic showing mononuclear and pleomorphic variants; lymphocytes are few. ×520.

ishing response and is associated with a poorer prognosis. In both the nodular sclerosis type 2 and the lymphocyte depletion subtype it is apparent that the response has failed and the disease is correspondingly highly aggressive. In some cases there may be a transition from lymphocyte predominance to mixed cellularity or even lymphocyte depletion, indicating progressive response failure. It should also be noted that the nodular sclerosis type 1 and the lymphocyte predominance subtype are often in clinical stage 1 or 2 at presentation, whereas the others are more likely to have advanced to stages 3 and 4.

The Nature of Hodgkin's Disease

While it has long been accepted that the RS cells and their variants, including the mononuclear Hodgkin cell, are the neoplastic elements, they have so far eluded exact histogenetic identification, with the exception of the RS variant seen in lymphocyte predominance which seems to be of B-cell origin. Reed–Sternberg cells do not consistently demonstrate any of the usual lymphocyte or histiocyte lineage markers. Similarly, no consistent clonal rearrangement of either the Ig or T-cell receptor (TCR) genes has been shown. Rather perversely, however, they express the granulocyte antigen identified by CD15 antibody (p. 188) although plainly they are not of granulocytic origin. There is nevertheless, accumulating evidence to suggest that the RS cell arises from lymphocytes probably of B-cell origin. It often expresses lymphocyte activation antigens such as the MHC class 2 marker HLA-DR, interleukin-2 receptor (CD25) and CD30, a property shared with a group of anaplastic large cell non-Hodgkin lymphomas. It may well be the case that Hodgkin's disease only differs from these in that it derives from a lymphoid cell which, during activation, has lost its lineage identification antigens, yet through the production of lymphokines elicits the pronounced cellular response so typical of the disease. The agent responsible for activation has not been defined but, as has already been mentioned, some epidemiological studies support an infective aetiology, and in this respect the Epstein–Barr virus remains a strong contender.

The Non-Hodgkin's Lymphomas (NHL)

These tumours exhibit considerable diversity with regard both to morphology and behaviour. It is now recognized that the morphological variation is due to the fact that even though most NHL are of lymphoid derivation they may arise from either B- or T-cell subpopulations and, to some extent, recapitulate the different phases of the maturation and post-maturation life cycle of lymphocytes (p. 169). Contrary to what was thought prior to 1970 it is now apparent that few, if any, NHL take origin from cells of the mononuclear phagocyte system. It is also to be realized that while most NHL seem to develop in lymph nodes, at least 30% arise in extranodal sites, especially bone marrow, thymus, skin, gastrointestinal tract, respiratory tract, gonads and CNS, and that this may influence their behaviour.

If left untreated almost all NHL will ultimately lead to a fatal outcome. Some do so quickly (i.e. within 1 year) and are referred to as **high-grade** in terms of aggression. Such tumours tend to behave very much like carcinomas, i.e. there is usually an identifiable primary site of origin which may be locally destructive, with subsequent spread occurring in a relatively predictable fashion either by lymphatics or eventually via the bloodstream. They can thus be staged in much the same way as Hodgkin's disease. The only exceptions to this rule are the lymphoblastic lymphomas which mostly evolve into acute leukaemia. The **low-grade** NHL generally pursue a more indolent clinical course. Paradoxically, however, many become widely disseminated at an early stage. This is not so much an expression of metastatic potential as a reflection of the circulatory behaviour of lymphocytes. All the same, this roving tendency makes these tumours difficult to treat and eradicate.

The great majority of low-grade NHL arise in later adult life and approximately 80% of these (in Western countries at any rate) are of B-cell type. On the other hand, high-grade NHL can arise at almost any age although lymphoblastic types are mainly encountered in early life. Whilst the causation is far from clear, some form of immunological perturbation appears to have an aetiological role in at least some instances. Non-Hodgkin's lymphomas may, for example, complicate immunodeficiency states; and Burkitt's lymphoma affects young children whose immune responses have been depressed by endemic malaria, creating an environment in which B cells infected by EB virus are allowed to persist and eventually undergo malignant transformation. In adult life, drug-induced immunosuppression and AIDS may predispose to similar tumours, some of which are EB virus related. High-grade T-cell tumours are unusually common in the Orient, especially Japan. Here too, a virus may be implicated, in this instance a retrovirus (HTLV-1), which is endemic in some of the southern islands of the Japanese archipelago and predisposes to a distinctive leukaemia–lymphoma syndrome.

Typing and Classification of the Non-Hodgkin's Lymphomas

Whilst the majority of cases of NHL can be identified on morphological features in appropriately stained histological sections, a significant proportion present notoriously difficult diagnostic problems which can only be resolved (and sometimes not even then) by specialized techniques involving the use of immunohistochemistry (see Fig. 15.16) and cytogenetics (see Figs 15.17 and 15.23). One major difficulty encountered is the distinction between neoplastic and reactive lymphoid proliferations. The fact that all cells in a lymphoma are derived from a single cell, i.e. are monoclonal, whereas a reactive process originates from many cells, i.e. is polyclonal, is crucially important in this regard. Thus, all cells in a B-cell lymphoma will produce immunoglobulin with the same light chain (this is termed light chain restriction) which can be recognized in tissue sections using antibodies to κ or λ light chains linked to a suitable chromogen. Likewise, all tumour cells in a B-cell lymphoma will show the same (clonal) rearrangement of the immunoglobulin genes, which can be demonstrated by the Southern blotting technique (p. 57; Fig. 15.13). T-cell tumours can be identified using similar forms of DNA analysis, this time to show clonal rearrangement of the T-cell antigen receptor genes (p. 189). Indeed at present, this is the only reliable way of identifying T-cell neoplasia with certainty. Such techniques may be employed to subtype lymphomas, and in particular to distinguish between B- and T-cell variants.

The accurate classification of NHL is important, not only to assess prognosis, but in the refinement of therapeutic regimens which can only take place if like is compared with like. There are several ways in which NHL can be classified. The Kiel system outlined in Table 15.7 is now widely used in Europe and the UK. In its most recent form the NHL are subdivided into B- and T-cell types as well as low- and high-grade categories. In general, low-grade tumours tend to consist mainly of small cells (with the suffix -cytic) and affect adults in later life whilst high-grade tumours usually consist of large cells (suffix -blastic) and can be found at almost any age. Within the B-cell group the various subcategories can be linked to phases in the B-lymphocyte life cycle. This is less easily achieved with T-cell tumours, although thymic or precursor phase and post-thymic or peripheral forms are recognized.

Clinicians involved in the treatment of NHL do not necessarily require such detailed classification at present and may prefer to use the National Cancer Institute (USA) International Working Formulation, which was designed principally for clinical usage and related to survival. This system divides NHL into three grades – low, intermediate and high – without subdivision into B- and T-cell types. The correspondence between the Working Formulation and the Kiel classification is outlined in Table 15.7 and, as can be seen, there is some overlap between the grades in the two systems. This causes little difficulty in clinical practice so long as one system is consistently applied. Some of the morphological features on which the Kiel and Working Formulation are based are shown diagrammatically in Fig. 15.14; in addition some of the terminology is defined in the footnotes.

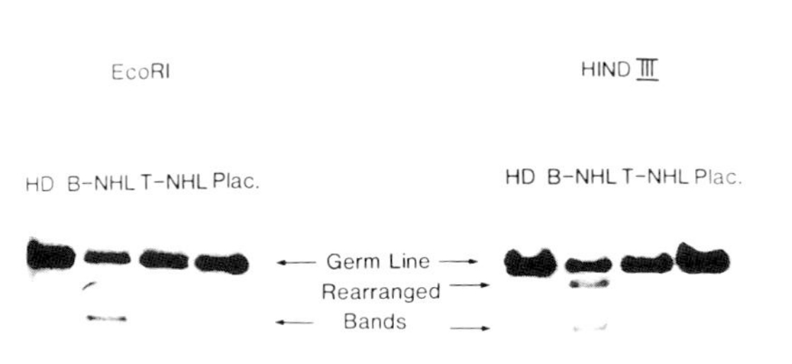

Fig. 15.13 Southern blot analysis of extracted DNA following digestion with the restriction enzymes EcoR1 and Hind III and hybridization with a J-region Ig heavy chain probe. The DNA from Hodgkin's disease (HD), T-cell non-Hodgkin's lymphoma (T-NHL) and normal human placental tissue show only the germline configuration of the gene. By contrast, DNA extracted from a B-cell non-Hodgkin's lymphoma (B-NHL) shows the presence of clonal gene rearrangements consistent with a neoplastic proliferation of B lymphocytes.

Low-grade B-cell Lymphomas

In Western countries the majority of cases (approximately 50%) of NHL fall into this group. Lymphadenopathy is the mode of clinical presentation in most cases. Macroscopically, the lymph nodes tend to be discrete and rubbery in consistency, and the cut surface shows a uniform smooth greyish-pink appearance.

Lymphocytic type. One of the commonest types of lymphoma, this tumour usually arises in the bone marrow and leads to chronic lymphocytic leukaemia—CLL (p. 626). Elderly people are

Table 15.7 Kiel classification of B-cell and T-cell lymphoma shown in relation to the International Working Formulation designed principally for clinical usage

	B-cell lymphomas		Working Formulation	T-cell lymphomas	
			LOW-GRADE		
Low-grade	Lymphocytic: chronic lymphocytic and hairy cell leukaemia ←→	A	Small lymphocytic: chronic lymphocytic leukaemia ←→	Lymphocytic: chronic lymphocytic leukaemia; Small cerebriform cell: mycosis fungoides and Sézary syndrome	Low-grade
Low-grade	Lymphoplasmacytoid ←→		Plasmacytoid		Low-grade
Low-grade	Plasmacytic: multiple myeloma	B	Follicular: predominantly small cleaved cell		Low-grade
Low-grade	Centroblastic/centrocytic follicular ←→	C	Follicular: mixed small cleaved and large cell		Low-grade
			INTERMEDIATE GRADE		
Low-grade	Centroblastic/centrocytic diffuse	D	Follicular: predominantly large cell		Low-grade
Low-grade	Centrocytic ←→	E	Diffuse: small cleaved cell		Low-grade
		F	Diffuse: small and large cell ←→	Angioimmunoblastic lymphadenopathy; Lymphoepithelioid; T zone lymphocytic; Pleomorphic, small cell	Low-grade
High-grade	Centroblastic ←→	G	Diffuse: large cell		
			HIGH-GRADE		
High-grade	Immunoblastic ←→; Anaplastic	H	Large cell: immunoblastic, plasmacytoid, clear cell, polymorphous ←→	Immunoblastic; Pleomorphic, medium or large cell (HTLV-1); Anaplastic	High-grade
High-grade	Lymphoblastic ←→	I	Lymphoblastic: convoluted: non-convoluted ←→	Lymphoblastic	High-grade
High-grade	Burkitt's lymphoma	J	Small non-cleaved cell: Burkitt's lymphoma		High-grade

Diagonal interrupted lines link: Plasmacytic: multiple myeloma ↔ Centroblastic/centrocytic follicular ↔ B; Centroblastic/centrocytic diffuse ↔ F; Centroblastic ↔ D.

The interrupted lines ←→ indicate approximate correlations in terms of cell size.

Fig. 15.14 Schematic outline of the cell types on which the morphological classification of the non-Hodgkin's lymphomas is based. The B lymphocytes undergo maturation in lymphoid follicles and, in the germinal centres, centrocytes and centroblasts are recognized; there is uncertainty as to the pathways which the maturing B cell follows in the germinal centres and this is indicated by the discontinuous lines. Both B cells and T cells become immunoblasts which then further mature to produce plasma cells and activated T cells respectively.

The student **must not** assume that the various subtypes of non-Hodgkin's malignant lymphoma (ML) as classified in Table 15.7 arise from the individual cell types shown in this diagram. The morphological classification is based on the predominant cell type present in the tumour and, as for the leukaemias, the tumours are the result both of proliferation and variable degrees of maturation or differentiation. *Immunoblasts*: these are large cells, about four times the size of lymphocytes, and which have a vesicular nucleus with a prominent central nucleolus (usually basophilic) and abundant pyroninophilic cytoplasm. They are B or T lymphocytes which have been transformed in response to antigenic stimulations and may arise from 'virgin' cells or from memory cells (shown by double lines ⇌). *Centroblasts*: these are a particular type of transformed B cell normally confined to germinal centres. They may be up to four times the size of lymphocytes and have a round vesicular nucleus with multiple nucleoli located peripherally. *Centrocytes*: these are also confined to germinal centres and distinguished from centroblasts by virtue of their nuclei, which are hyperchromatic and appear notched or cleaved. *Lymphoblasts*: these are putative lymphocyte precursor cells up to twice the size of lymphocytes, have a high nuclear to cytoplasmic ratio and the nuclei have a fine stippled chromatin pattern with 2–5 small nucleoli.

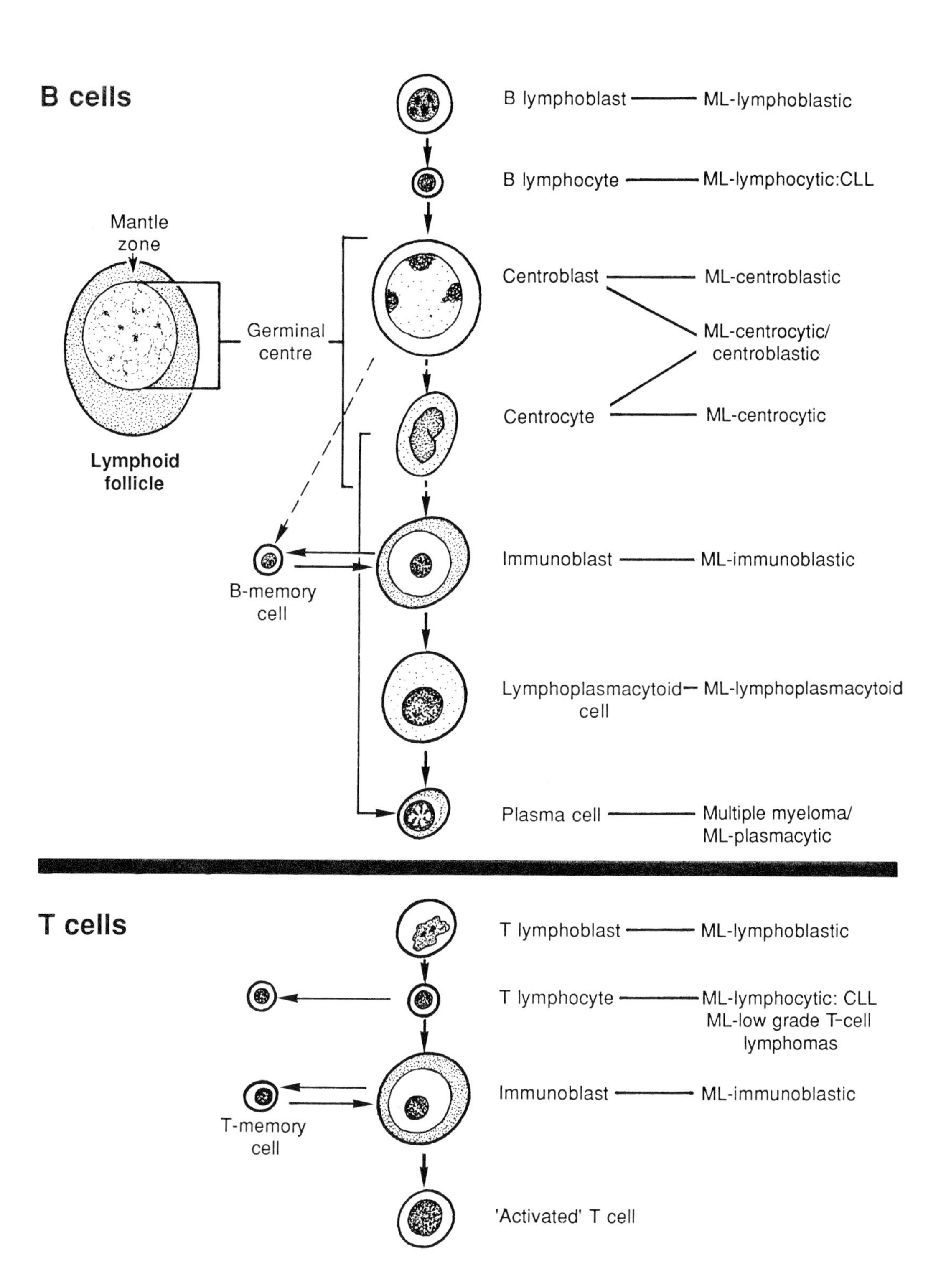
B cells
B lymphoblast
ML-lymphoblastic
B lymphocyte
ML-lymphocytic:CLL
Mantle zone
Germinal centre
Lymphoid follicle
Centroblast
ML-centroblastic
ML-centrocytic/ centroblastic
Centrocyte
ML-centrocytic
B-memory cell
Immunoblast
ML-immunoblastic
Lymphoplasmacytoid cell
ML-lymphoplasmacytoid
Plasma cell
Multiple myeloma/ ML-plasmacytic
T cells
T lymphoblast
ML-lymphoblastic
T lymphocyte
ML-lymphocytic: CLL
ML-low grade T-cell lymphomas
Immunoblast
ML-immunoblastic
T-memory cell
'Activated' T cell

usually affected. Lymph node and splenic enlargement, however, become common as the disease progresses and ultimately many tissues may become involved. Histologically, the neoplastic infiltrate consists for the most part of small lymphocytes, not readily distinguished from normal forms (Fig. 15.15). In lymph nodes the normal architecture becomes ablated by this infiltrate which invariably includes groups of larger nucleolated cells, some resembling immunoblasts (proliferation foci). With treatment, many patients survive for 5 years or more; death is commonly due to infection (e.g. bronchopneumonia), precipitated by the hypogammaglobulinaemia which is an important complication of the disease process.

Lymphoplasmacytoid type. By no means rare, this tumour resembles lymphocytic types in that it mainly affects the elderly and commonly involves bone marrow, lymph nodes, spleen and liver. Occasionally it arises in extranodal sites, e.g. the subcutaneous tissues. The distinctive histological feature of the tumour infiltrate is that, in addition to lymphocytes (the predominant tumour cell), plasmacytoid lymphocytes and/or plasma cells are readily detected. Sometimes immunoglobulin (staining with PAS) can be seen in the perinuclear space of the lymphoid cells (Dutcher bodies). Not surprisingly, the tumour often produces immunoglobulin, usually IgM, in large quantities; the associated clinical entity is Waldenström's macroglobulinaemia (p. 639).

Plasmacytic type. For reasons as yet obscure, most tumours of plasma cells arise in the bone marrow to produce the condition known as multiple myeloma (p. 637). Only occasionally do they develop primarily in extramedullary sites such as lymph node or gastrointestinal tract.

Centroblastic/centrocytic type (follicular lymphoma). This is by far the commonest type of NHL, accounting for about 40% of all cases. It is mainly a disease of adult life, only rarely arising before the age of 30 years and affecting males and females in equal numbers. Lymph nodes are primarily affected, but the disease is often widespread with splenic and bone marrow involvement at the time of clinical presentation. Histologically, the tumour may exhibit a follicular or diffuse (or both) architecture (Fig. 15.16) and consists of germinal centre cells, centrocytes and centroblasts, in variable proportion. Sometimes in follicular forms the distinction from reactive follicles is difficult and requires demonstration that the immunoglobulin present on the surface of tumour cells shows light chain restriction (Fig. 15.16b,c). Cytogenetically, these tumours also frequently show a chromosomal translocation, t(14;18), involving the immunoglobulin heavy chain genes in the tumour cells (Fig. 15.17). The breakpoint region on chromosome 18 affected by this translocation is the site of a possible oncogene known as *bcl2*. The usual centrocyte-predominant form is compatible with a median survival of about 7 years and sometimes much longer. In a substan-

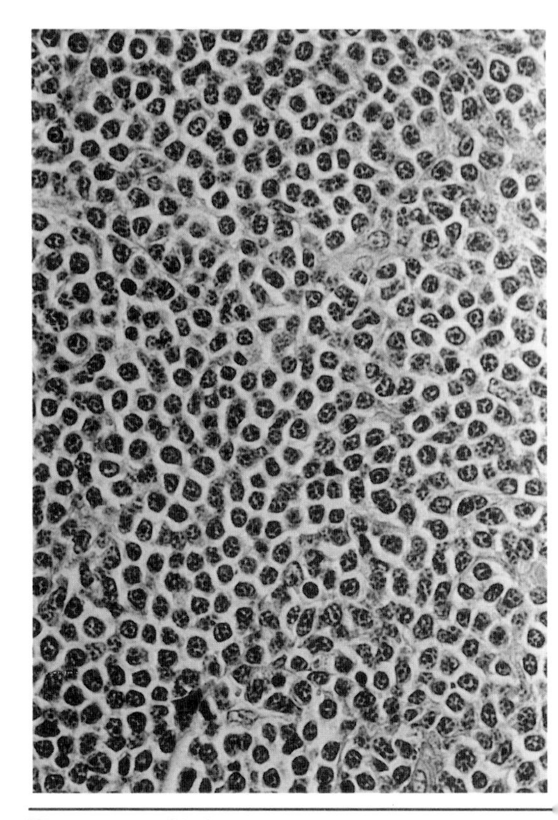

Fig. 15.15 Malignant lymphoma, lymphocytic. The tumour consists mainly of small lymphocytes. H & E × 520.

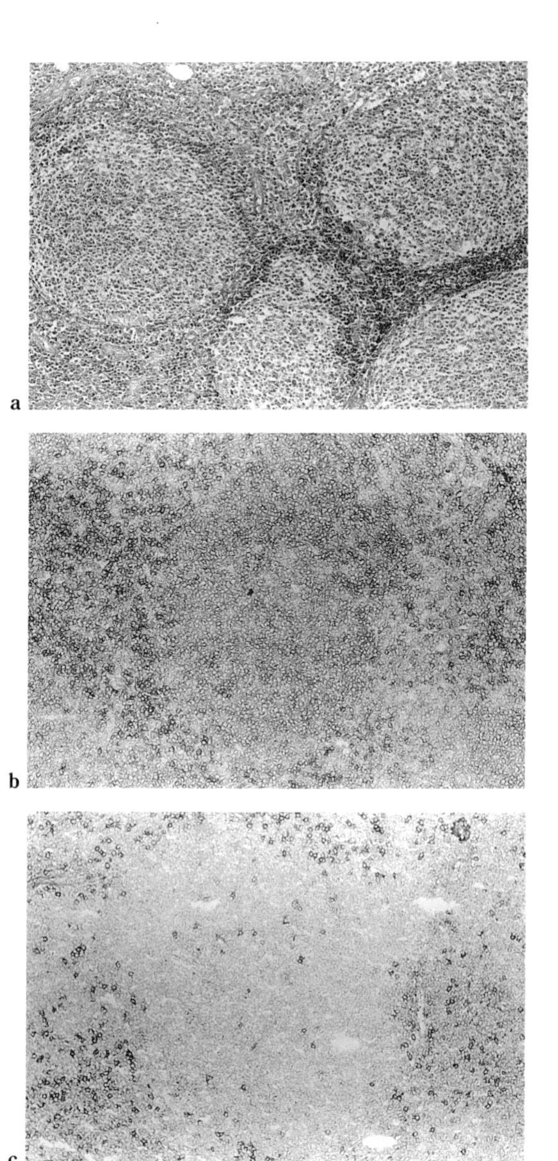

Fig. 15.16 Malignant lymphoma, follicular. The tumour nodules resemble germinal centres, but have a more ill-defined outline and lack tingible body macrophages (**a**; H & E ×180). Immunoperoxidase stains reveal that the tumour cells exhibit 'light chain restriction', i.e. the presence of ϰ chain at the cell surface (**b**), but not λ chain (**c**).

tial proportion of cases, however, the tumour transforms into a much more aggressive lymphoma, usually of centroblastic type with a survival time of a few months.

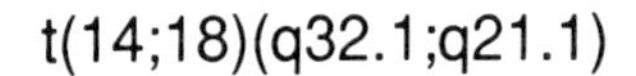

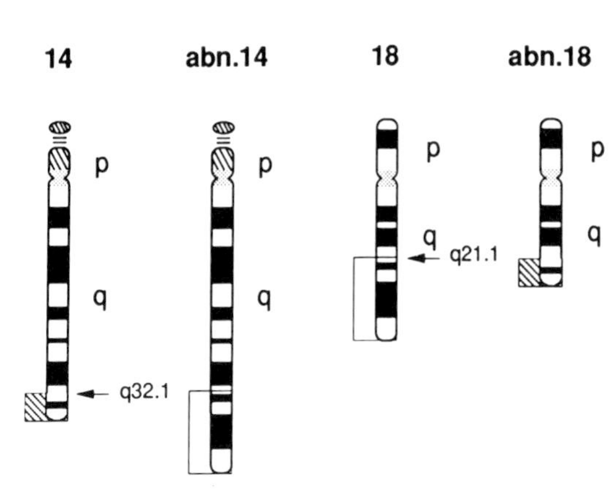

Fig. 15.17 The t(14:18) translocation characteristic of follicular non-Hodgkin's lymphoma. The 14q32 break is in the Ig heavy (IgH) chain gene complex and the break at 18q21 is immediately upstream of the *bcl-2* gene such that the translocation brings an intact *bcl-2* under the regulatory control of IgH-flanking sequences.

Centrocytic type. The most aggressive member of the low-grade B-cell lymphomas, the tumour consists exclusively of centrocytes (Fig. 15.18) and is usually diffuse, lacking a true follicular architecture. There is some doubt as to whether it actually arises from true germinal centre cells and could originate from mantle zone cells (see Fig. 15.14). In contrast to the follicular lymphomas they are more common in males and the median survival is about 3 years.

Low-grade T-cell Lymphomas

Most of these tumours (in Western countries accounting for less than 10% of all cases of NHL) derive from peripheral or post-thymic lymphocytes and usually affect adults. Some present, as expected, with lymphadenopathy but they have varied manifestations ranging from leukaemic change to extranodal lesions, mainly in the skin.

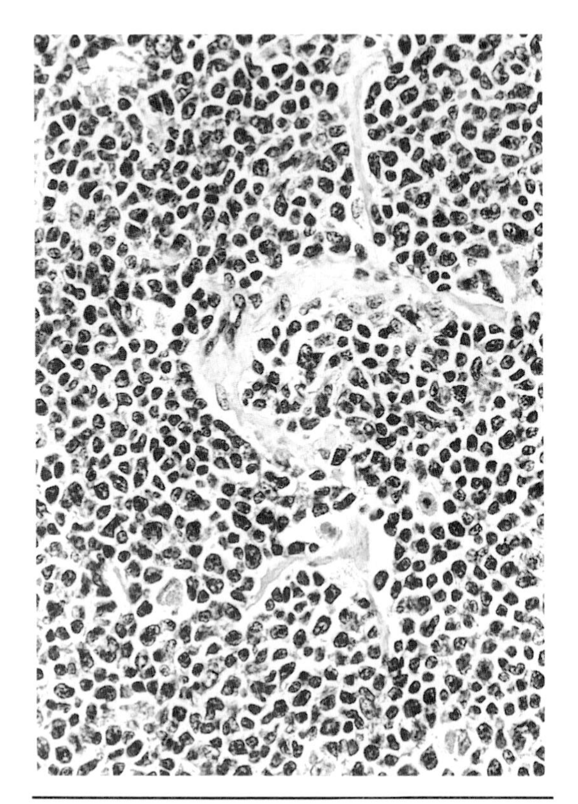

Fig. 15.18 Malignant lymphoma, centrocytic. The tumour consists exclusively of small cells with irregularly-shaped nuclei. Note the thickened hyalinized blood vessels. H & E ×365.

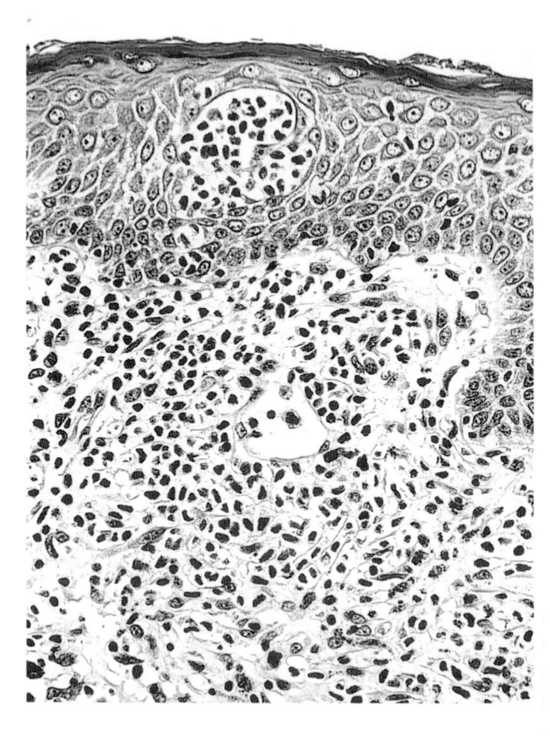

Fig. 15.19 Mycosis fungoides. In this type of lymphoma the skin is heavily infiltrated with small lymphoid cells with irregularly shaped nuclei. Note the presence of tumour cells lying in nests within the epidermis ('Pautrier micro-abscesses'). H & E ×350.

Lymphocytic type. Several variants of this tumour have been described. Most present as forms of chronic lymphocytic leukaemia and all are rare. The T-helper (CD4) cell form is the commoner and is much more aggressive than B-cell leukaemias. Histologically the tumour cells, as seen in lymph nodes or bone marrow, have a distinctly irregular, rough, knobby nuclear shape, a common feature of T cells. The T-suppressor (CD8) cell form also known as T-gamma-lymphocytosis, is much more indolent, yet produces curious effects, such as suppression of normal haemopoiesis and neutropenia in particular. The tumour cells, as seen in the peripheral blood, may resemble large granular lymphocytes (p. 197).

Small cerebriform cell type. The tumour cells derive their name from their curious serpiginous nuclear structure, best seen in electron micrographs. This tumour usually presents initially in the skin (Fig. 15.19) as **mycosis fungoides** (p. 1136). When an erythrodermatous variant of this is associated with lymphadenopathy and the presence of similar tumour cells in the blood the condition is referred to as the **Sézary syndrome.** The predominant tumour cells are CD4 positive. The clinical behaviour is indolent with a median survival of 7–8 years.

Angioimmunoblastic lymphadenopathy (AILD). Clinically, this tumour affects adults in later life and presents with generalized lymphadenopathy, often associated with systemic disturbances such as fever, skin rash, haemolytic anaemia and polyclonal hypergammaglobulinaemia. Histologically, the lymph node architecture is completely disrupted by a proliferation of neoplastic T cells which take the form of small lymphocytes (often with clear cytoplasm) and immunoblasts. These T cells, predominantly CD4 positive, elicit a series of complex responses, including the infiltration of plasma cells, eosinophils, histiocytes sometimes forming small granulomas, and dendritic reticulum cells, with the proliferation of thick-walled branching (arborizing) blood vessels resembling post-capillary venules (Fig. 15.20). The disease runs a rapid course relative to other low-grade non-Hodgkin's lymphomas and is difficult to control even with chemotherapy. Sometimes it evolves into a high-grade immunoblastic lymphoma.

Lymphoepithelioid type (Lennert's lymphoma). This too is a quite aggressive disease, only marginally worthy of inclusion in the low-grade category. It presents with generalized lymphadenopathy, sometimes with involvement of pharyngeal lymphoid tissue, but systemic symptoms are seldom prominent. Histologically, lymph nodes show loss of structure due to a proliferation of T cells and immunoblasts, which are associated with the presence of conspicuous epithelioid histiocytes, forming small granulomas. Like AILD, this disease may transform into a high-grade immunoblastic lymphoma.

T-zone lymphocytic type. This lymph node tumour represents the obverse of follicular (centroblastic/centrocytic) lymphoma, in that the neoplastic infiltrate specifically expands the paracortical areas of lymph nodes and recapitulates the structure of the normal T zone (including post-capillary venules and interdigitating reticulum cells). Often the normal B-cell areas survive and indeed may show marked germinal centre formation, presumably a response to the proliferation of neoplastic T cells which are usually CD4 positive.

Pleomorphic small cell type. As already mentioned, irregularity of their nuclear outline is a notable feature of T-cell tumours and this is most marked in those associated with HTLV-1 infection. The term pleomorphic as used here refers primarily to the nuclear irregularity. Many such tumours are highly aggressive, but those in which small cells (i.e. comparable in size to mature lymphocytes) predominate, tend to progress more slowly and are low-grade. Most of these tumours arise in lymph nodes but they may become leukaemic.

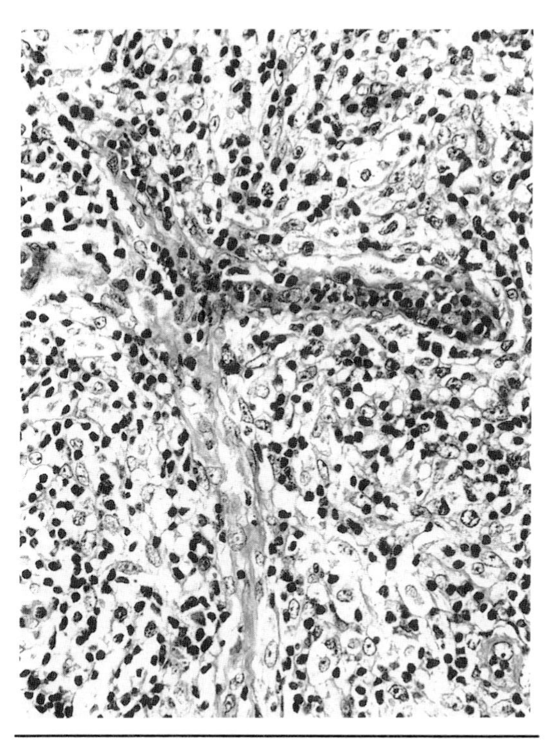

Fig. 15.20 Malignant lymphoma T-cell type. This tumour presents the features of 'angioimmunoblastic lymphadenopathy'. Note the 'arborizing' blood vessels and the small lymphoid tumour cells with 'clear' cytoplasm. H & E ×286.

High-grade B-cell Lymphomas

Approximately 30% of all non-Hodgkin's lymphomas fall into this category. Apart from Burkitt's lymphoma, most consist of large lymphoid cells with a nuclear diameter about four times larger than that of a normal lymphocyte. While most arise in lymph nodes an origin from extranodal locations (e.g. gastrointestinal tract or Waldeyer ring) is by no means rare.

Centroblastic type. This usually involves lymph nodes and affects adults in later life. As its name implies, the tumour cell is of germinal centre derivation; some evolve from follicular (centroblastic/centrocytic) lymphomas, others arise *de novo*. Histologically, the infiltrative pattern may be nodular or diffuse and the infiltrate consists almost exlusively of large cells, the nuclei of which include two or more peripherally located nucleoli (Fig. 15.21a). The nucleus is usually spheroidal, but irregularly shaped or multilobated forms have been described. Untreated, this tumour usually pursues a rapid course with extensive dissemination in the final stages.

Immunoblastic type. Also commonly involving lymph nodes, this highly aggressive neoplasm may arise either *de novo* (especially in the elderly) or from low-grade B-cell neoplasms such as chronic lymphocytic leukaemia or lymphoplasmacytoid tumours. It may also complicate immunodeficiency states. Histologically, the cells are disposed in a diffuse pattern, are large and possess nuclei with prominent central nucleoli (Fig. 15.21b). They may have an overtly lymphoplasmacytoid appearance with abundant purple cytoplasm due to a high RNA content, and are sometimes accompanied by plasma cells.

Burkitt's lymphoma. This interesting tumour is found mainly, but not exclusively, in tropical countries (especially East Africa) and its relationship to holo-endemic malaria and Epstein–Barr virus infection is discussed earlier (p. 408). It mainly affects young children and has a distinctive and largely extranodal pattern of growth. In males, the jaw bones are most often the site of primary involvement, whereas in females the ovaries are commonly affected. Peripheral lymph nodes are rarely involved and the disease seldom becomes leukaemic.

Histologically, the tumour cells exhibit a diffuse, almost coherent pattern, are a little larger than small lymphocytes and have a high nuclear/cytoplasmic ratio. The rapid growth of the tumour is reflected by the high mitotic rate and the presence of numerous histiocytes containing nuclear

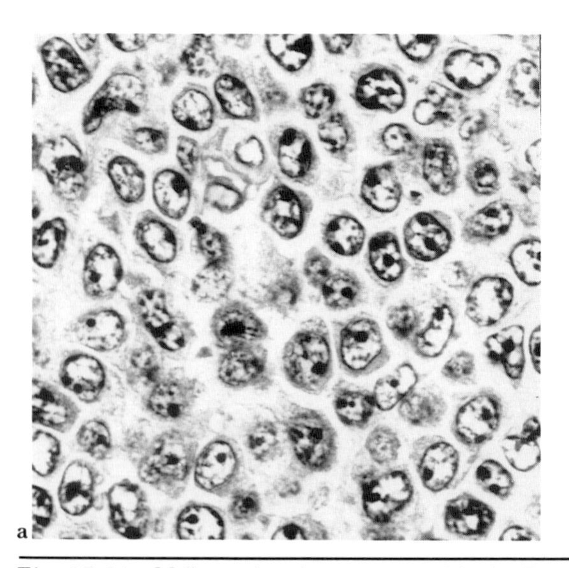

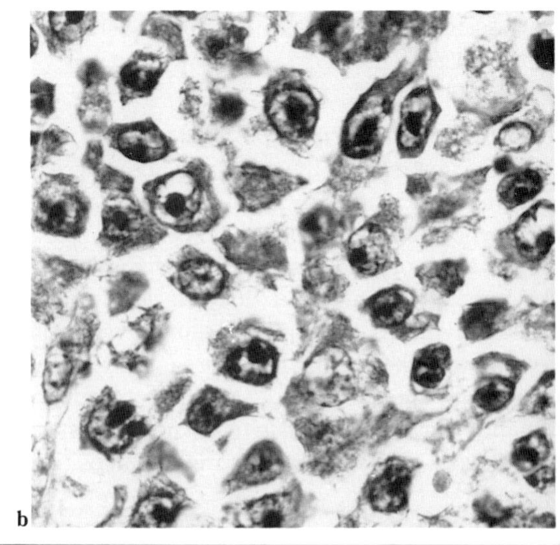

Fig. 15.21 Malignant lymphoma: **a** centroblastic. The tumour is composed of large lymphoid cells, the nuclei of which include prominent nucleoli, often peripherally located. H & E ×850; **b** immunoblastic. The cells in this tumour are also large but the nuclei possess prominent central nucleoli. H & E ×850.

debris (from apoptotic cells), which is responsible for the typical 'starry-sky' histological appearance (Fig. 15.22). Paradoxically, the extraordinary high rate of cell replication renders the tumour very responsive to chemotherapy and a favourable outcome can now be expected in the majority of cases. Like follicular lymphomas, a chromosomal alteration is usually present (Fig. 15.23), in this case commonly a translocation t(8;14), less often t(8;2) or t(8;22). The occurrence of this change within a population of EBV-infected B cells may result in proliferative advantage due to activation of the *c-myc* oncogene and may be the final step in neoplastic transformation (p. 394).

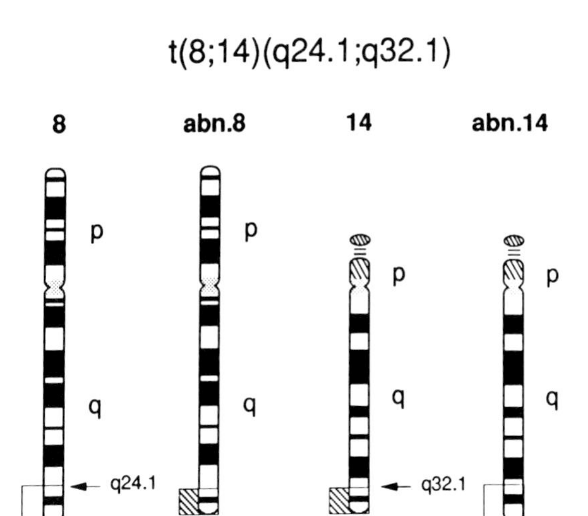

Fig. 15.23 The t(8:14) translocation characteristic of Burkitt's lymphoma (both 'endemic' and non-EB virus-associated). The same translocation is found in some other high-grade B-cell tumours. The 8q24 breakpoint passes through the *c-myc* gene and the 14q32 breakpoint through the Ig heavy chain gene complex.

High-grade T-cell Lymphomas

These are not very common in Europe and America, but in epidemiological terms are much more important in oriental countries such as Japan. The histological appearances are very variable.

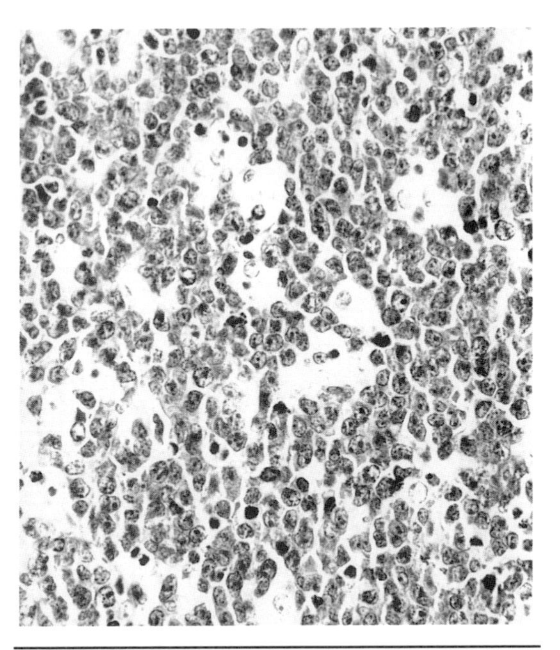

Fig. 15.22 Burkitt's lymphoma. The tumour cells are closely packed and have a high nuclear-cytoplasmic ratio. The high mitotic rate and the numerous 'starry sky' histiocytes reflect the rapid proliferation rate of the cells. H & E ×545.

Pleomorphic medium or large cell type. These are the tumours characteristically found in the Far East and may or may not be associated with HTLV-1 infection: when they are, they not only involve the lymph nodes and spleen but commonly affect the skin, and are often associated with leukaemic change (leukaemia/lymphoma syndrome, p. 408). Hypercalcaemia is another notable feature. Histologically, the cells are CD4 positive and may be slightly larger than lymphocytes or of large size and show pronounced irregularity of nuclear outline. Often the cells show variation in size and there may be some giant cells, the presence of which is regarded as a marker of viral aetiology.

Immunoblastic type. In both clinical and pathological terms these are very similar to the B-cell types, and are equally common even in Western countries. They may evolve out of low-grade tumours such as AILD and may be associated in some instances with HTLV-1 infection. Histologically, the tumour cells may be indistinguishable from the B-cell form, but may show clearing of the cytoplasm and are more often associated with T lymphocytes than plasma cells. The prognosis is grave once the disease has spread from its initial site.

Lymphoblastic type. These tumours appear to arise from T-cell precursors and are found mainly in adolescent males (2:1 compared with females). The thymus is primarily involved in more than 50% of cases and the patient may present with the effects of a mediastinal mass. The haematological features of acute lymphoblastic leukaemia may be present at the outset or develop after a discrete tumour has been detected. Phenotypically, the tumour cells may express the markers of intrathymic lymphocytes (CD2, CD5 and CD3) or occasionally may co-express CD4 and CD8. Histologically, the cells grow in a diffuse, closely packed manner, are slightly larger than small lymphocytes and have a high nuclear/cytoplasmic ratio. The nuclei usually have a twisted or convoluted shape, and possess a fine chromatin pattern with only small, inconspicuous nucleoli (Fig. 15.24). Untreated the disease pursues an aggressive course with widespread dissemination and death within a short time.

Fig. 15.24 Lymphoblastic lymphoma, T-cell type. The cells have a high cytoplasmic ratio and often exhibit a convoluted nuclear morphology. H & E × 826.

Large cell anaplastic type. This recently delineated group of tumours brings together lymphomas which may be of T- or B-cell lineage (but most commonly T-cell) composed of large pleomorphic cells lacking distinctive morphological characteristics (Fig. 15.25), yet expressing lymphocyte activation antigens, notably CD30. .In lymph nodes, these tumours produce focal ex-

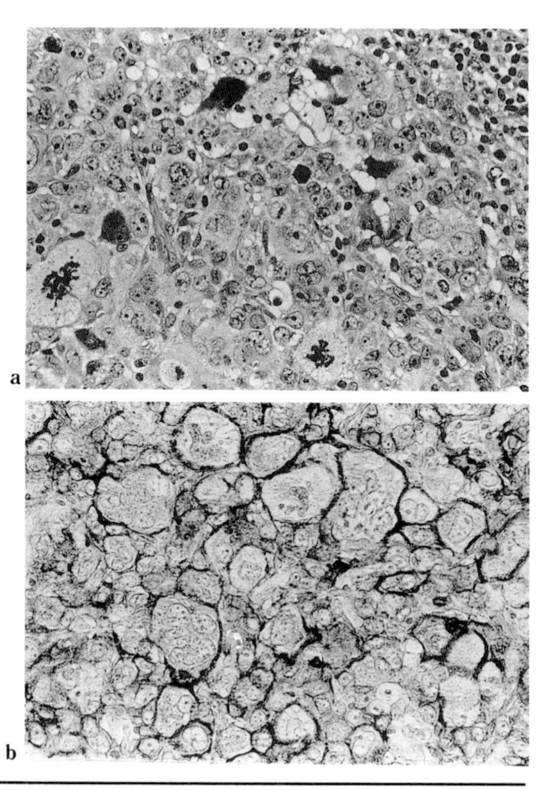

Fig. 15.25 **a** Malignant lymphoma, large cell anaplastic type. The tumour cells show marked pleomorphism with many binucleate and giant forms, and there are several grossly abnormal mitoses (H & E ×210). **b** The cells also exhibit CD30 positivity an indication of 'activation' (Immunoperoxidase staining).

panding aggregates or involve the sinusoids, resembling the condition formerly known as malignant histiocytosis, and they have sometimes been misdiagnosed as metastatic carcinoma or sarcoma. Young adults are commonly affected and the tumours are considered high-grade in terms of behaviour, although following treatment they are not as aggressive as might be expected. One feature of considerable current interest lies in their morphological resemblance, in some parts, to Hodgkin's disease, even to the extent of producing 'RS-like' giant cells with CD15 positivity. It may well be that Hodgkin's disease will come to be regarded as a variant of this tumour category.

Further Reading

Lauder, I. (1991). T cell malignant lymphomas. In *Recent Advances in Histopathology*, No. 15, pp. 93–112, eds P. P. Anthony and R. N. M. MacSween. Churchill Livingstone, Edinburgh.

Lennert, K. (1978). *Malignant Lymphomas other than Hodgkin's Disease*. Springer-Verlag, Berlin.

Lukes, R. J. (1971). Criteria for involvement of lymph node, bone marrow spleen and liver in Hodgkin's disease. *Cancer Research* **31**, 1755–67.

Stansfeld, A. G. (1985). *Lymph Node Interpretation*. Churchill Livingstone, Edinburgh.

Stansfeld, A. G. *et al.* (1988). Updated Kiel classification. *Lancet* **1**, 292 (also *Lancet* **1**, 603).

Stein, H., Mason, D. Y., Gerdes, J. *et al.* (1985). The expression of the Hodgkin's disease associated antigen Ki-I in active and neoplastic lymphoid tissue: evidence that Reed–Sternberg cells and histiocytic malignancies are derived from active lymphoid cells. *Blood* **66**, 848–58.

Sucki, T., Lennert, K., Tu, L-Y., Kijuaki, M., Sato, E., Stansfeld, A. G., Feller, A. C. (1987). Histopathology and immunohistochemistry of peripheral T-cell lymphomas: a proposal for their classification. *Journal of Clinical Pathology* **40**, 995–1015.

The non-Hodgkin's lymphoma pathologic classification project. (1982). National Cancer Institute sponsored study of classifications of non-Hodgkin's lymphoma. *Cancer* **49**, 2112–35.

16

Alimentary Tract

The Oral Cavity, Salivary Glands and Oropharynx

The Oral Cavity

In general, the tissues of the mouth are subject to the same types of lesion found in other sites but often show distinctive features peculiar to the mouth. In addition there are a number of specific lesions related to the teeth and their supporting structures.

The most frequent diseases in the mouth are dental caries and non-specific chronic inflammation of the soft tissues immediately related to the teeth. The principal aetiological agents in both of these diseases are oral bacteria. Bacteria in the mouth are found in saliva, adherent to the epithelium and in adherent deposits on tooth surfaces. These deposits are **dental plaque** consisting of bacteria in an organic matrix of bacterial and salivary origin. Calcium salts may be deposited in dental plaque to form **dental calculus**.

The Teeth

Teeth consist of three specialized calcified tissues (Fig. 16.1): the **dentine** is a thick layer of calcified collagenous tissue surrounding the soft tissues of the pulp, the **enamel**, which forms the hard outer layer of the crown, and is non-cellular, consisting largely of calcium apatite crystals in a delicate organic matrix, and the **cementum**, which overlies the dentine of the root(s). At the apex of each root is an apical foramen through which vessels and nerves enter the pulp.

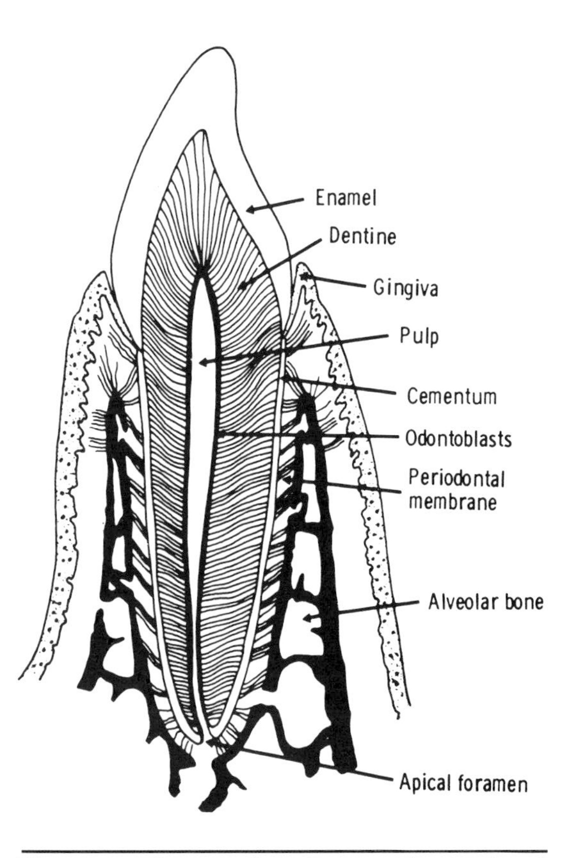

Fig. 16.1 Cross-section of an anterior tooth and related tissues.

Developmental abnormalities. Tooth development and eruption of the first dentition followed by the second dentition begin at about 3 months of intrauterine life and continue until the early 20s. During this period many developmental abnormalities can occur in the number of teeth, in their form and colour, in the structure of individual tooth elements and the times of eruption and shedding of teeth. These abnormalities result from various factors, both genetic and environmental. An example of iatrogenic disease is the permanent staining of the calcified dental tissues caused by administration of some tetracyclines during tooth development.

Dental caries is the progressive destruction, by bacteria and their products, of the calcified tissues of the teeth exposed to the oral environment. Caries itself, and consequent inflammation of the tooth pulp, are the commonest causes of tooth loss up to middle age.

Dental caries usually starts in two principal areas of the tooth: the fissures on the occlusal or biting surfaces of posterior teeth and the areas between teeth (**proximal caries**). Both of these are areas of relative stagnation in which plaque is likely to accumulate. The bacteria within the plaque produce various organic acids, the resulting pH depending on factors such as the thickness of the plaque and the concentration of dietary sugars. The initial attack upon enamel (Fig. 16.2) is by the acid, which produces decalcification. At first this is a painless process, but, as the lesion extends through the enamel, dentine is involved and toothache starts. Bacteria do not enter the enamel until decalcification has so weakened the structure that breakdown has occurred to form a cavity. At this stage the acid conditions within the cavity particularly favour the growth of **lactobacilli**, which appear to be the main organisms involved in dentine caries. The organisms initially penetrate the dentinal tubules, but then cause softening and distortion of the dentine by a combination of de-

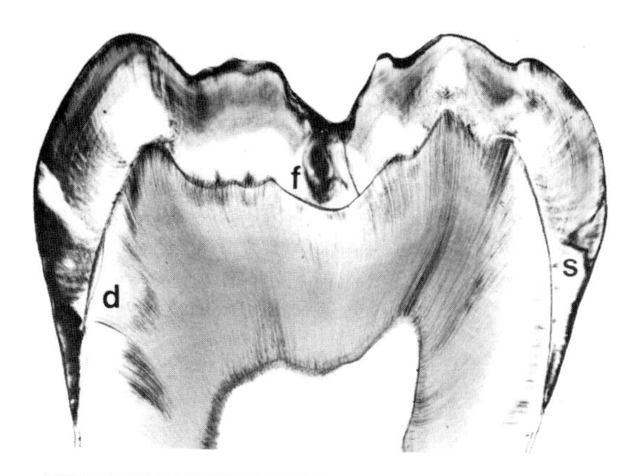

Fig. 16.2 Ground section of a molar tooth crown showing early smooth surface enamel caries (s), fissure caries (f) and early dentine caries deep to enamel caries (d). ×6.

calcification and proteolytic breakdown of the collagen matrix. The carious dentine becomes yellow by absorption of pigment from bacterial metabolic products and from the mouth; the process then extends through the dentine towards the dental pulp.

Dental caries may also start at the neck of the tooth either by involving the cementum and then the dentine, or, if cementum is deficient, by directly attacking the dentine. This form of caries is more common in older patients in whom recession of the gingiva is common.

In the very early stages of enamel caries, the damage is reversible, but thereafter caries of enamel and dentine is progressive except in unusual circumstances where the area becomes self-cleaning and the lesions may be arrested.

Lesions of the dental pulp. The dental pulp is a vascular connective tissue confined within the rigid pulp chamber and root canals in the dentine. The most frequent and clinically significant lesions of the pulp are inflammatory lesions (**pulpitis**) due to the extension of the carious process into dentine and then to the pulp. Physical injury, e.g. heat and chemical irritation from filling materials, may also give rise to pulpitis.

Pulpitis may be acute or chronic. Because the changes are occurring within the rigid confines of the pulp chamber there is increase in pressure due to inflammatory exudate. Consequently acute pulpitis is very painful and may proceed quickly to necrosis of the pulp. If the insult to the pulp is less severe, chronic pulpitis may result with loss of specialized cells such as odontoblasts. The pulp may eventually undergo necrosis, which is often symptomless.

Clinically the non-vital tooth lacks lustre and may be discoloured by the leaching of products of the necrotic pulp into the dentine. In children, a large carious cavity penetrating quickly to the pulp may result in a large opening into the pulp chamber, leading to open pulpitis from which exudate can drain and a mass of granulation tissue may extend as a **pulp polyp**, into the carious cavity.

Periodontal Disease

Acute inflammation of the gingiva can arise from various physical, chemical and infective causes. **Acute ulceromembranous gingivitis (Vincent's infection)** is a distinctive condition in which there is necrosis of the interdental papillae with variable spread to other parts of the gingiva. There is overgrowth of two commensal organisms, *Fusobacterium fusiforme* and *Borrelia vincenti* but the exact relationship of these to the disease is not clear. A similar but more destructive type of gingivitis is seen in AIDS.

Chronic inflammation is very common in the periodontal tissues and is the most frequent cause of tooth loss in older individuals. A number of local and systemic factors are involved, but of these the most important is the bacterial plaque around the neck of the tooth.

For clinical convenience the lesions are divided into **chronic gingivitis** where the disease is confined to the gingiva and **chronic periodontitis** where the process involves the deeper tissues, causing retraction towards the root apex of the part of the gingiva attached to the tooth. Many mechanisms of tissue destruction have been described involving polymorphonuclear leucocytes, macrophages and both humoral and cell mediated immune mechanisms. It is probable that all of these are operative in different situations. The later stages of the disease involve the alveolar bone supporting the teeth. Osteoclastic resorption occurs and progresses to the formation of areas of deepening of the gingival sulcus, termed periodontal pockets. Infrequently there is an acute exacerbation of infection in such pockets and a periodontal abscess can arise.

Periapical Lesions

A variety of lesions can occur in the tissues related to the root apices of teeth. The most frequent of these arise from spread of infection from pulpitis, through the apical foramina of the tooth, to reach the periodontal membrane. This can result in an acute periapical abscess, a very painful condition which may be accompanied by cervical lymphadenopathy and generalized fever and malaise. Pus tracks through the adjacent bone and, after the periosteum is breached, a soft tissue abscess – a gumboil – develops and later discharges.

More frequently following low-grade pulpitis a periapical granuloma develops. This consists of a mass of granulation tissue heavily infiltrated with chronic inflammatory cells. There is resorption of surrounding bone, seen radiographically as a periapical radiolucency (Fig. 16.3). Acute exacerbation may result in an acute periapical abscess and conversely, a periapical granuloma can develop after an acute periapical abscess has pointed and drained.

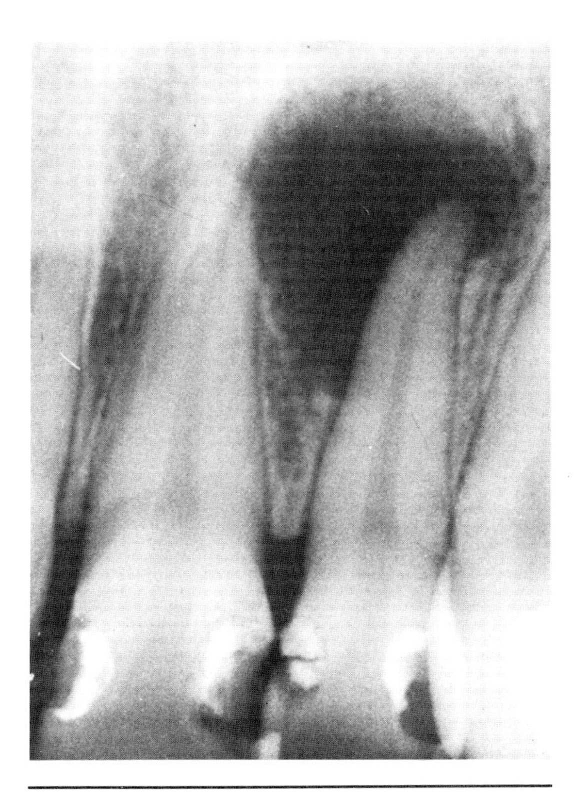

Fig. 16.3 Radiograph of upper anterior teeth with large restorations. The upper lateral incisor is non-vital and a radiolucency is present in the bone around the apex of the tooth.

Epithelial-lined Cysts of the Jaws

A number of different types occurs; they can be classified into odontogenic cysts, in which the epithelium is derived from the dental epithelial tissues, and fissural cysts which arise in areas of fusion of embryonic processes.

Odontogenic Cysts

These may be further subdivided into **inflammatory** and **developmental cysts** and categorized by their position in relation to the teeth. The commonest is the **dental cyst** (synonyms, **radicular** or **periapical cyst**) which is an inflammatory cyst developing from a periapical granuloma. Epithelial remnants related to the root are stimulated to grow and cyst formation occurs. If the affected tooth is extracted, the cyst may be left in the bone and remain as a **residual cyst**. The most frequent of the developmental odontogenic cysts is the **dentigerous cyst** which arises in the reduced enamel epithelium around the crown of a tooth which has failed to erupt. Closely related is the **eruption cyst** which presents as a bluish fluctuant swelling overlying the crown of an erupting tooth.

The odontogenic cysts described above are lined by non-keratinized stratified squamous epithelium which may include a few mucus-secreting cells. These cysts are usually symptomless unless infected and can grow to several centimetres with considerable bone destruction. They must be differentiated from the **odontogenic keratocyst** (synonym, **primordial cyst**) which has a distinctive keratinized stratified squamous epithelial lining. Its relationship to the teeth is variable and it occurs anywhere in the jaws, the most common site being in the mandibular molar area, often extending up into the vertical ramus of the mandible. The importance of this cyst lies in the frequency with which it recurs after attempted surgical removal, because of the friable nature of the lining and the presence of related small daughter cysts.

Fissural Cysts

The **nasopalatine cyst** arises in the nasopalatine canal in the midline of the anterior part of the hard palate. It may be entirely within the bone or present as a palatal swelling. A similar type, the **nasolabial cyst**, occurs in the upper lip below the ala of the nose, but this is within the soft tissues. The fissural cysts are usually lined by epithelium with numerous mucus secreting cells, but areas of non-keratinized stratified squamous epithelium may also be present.

Oral Mucosa

The oral mucosa is subjected to numerous physical insults and is exposed to vast numbers of microorganisms, and to food and other material introduced into the mouth. Oral epithelium has a high rate of cell turnover. In almost all lesions of oral mucosa, physical trauma and infection will play a role, and this may be superimposed upon a previously normal or abnormal mucosa. It is not surprising that these circumstances produce complex changes in disease which are not yet fully documented or understood.

Developmental abnormalities of oral epithelium. Apart from Fordyce's disease – the presence of pale yellowish sebaceous glands in the lining mucosa, especially of the cheeks – developmental abnormalities of oral mucosa are rare.

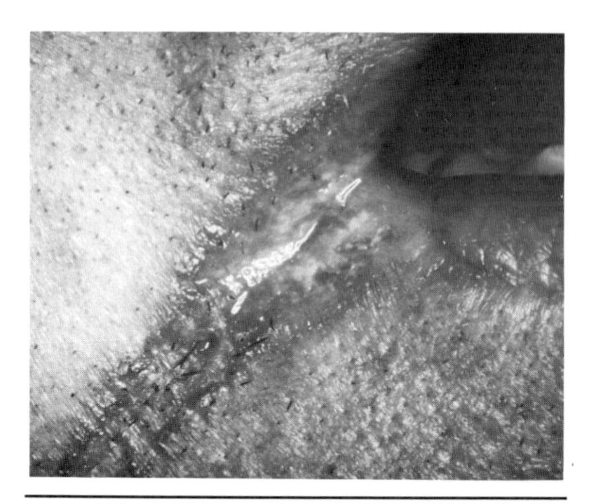

Fig. 16.4 Angular cheilitis showing typical moist skin fissuring.

Oral Candidiasis (Thrush)

Candida sp. are part of the oral flora of over half the population. *Candida albicans* is the most frequent of these. Thrush is an acute condition found most often in young children or debilitated adults and is characterized by detachable white fungal plaques on the epithelium. Chronic atrophic candidiasis is found under upper dentures, and is an inflammatory reaction to fungi which are mainly in the interstices of the fitting surface of the denture. Candidal hyphae may also be found in adherent hyperkeratotic lesions as chronic hyperplastic candidiasis (candidal leukoplakia). Persistent oral candidal infections are a frequent problem in patients with AIDS.

Angular Cheilitis (Fig. 16.4)

Angular cheilitis is a painful cracking at the angles of the mouth often of multifactorial aetiology. Infection with *Candida albicans* and *Staphylococcus aureus* is frequent. Underlying nutritional deficiencies, notably of the B group of vitamins and of iron, can predispose to the condition.

Virus Infections

The most frequent viral infection of oral epithelium is caused by herpes simplex virus types I and II. Acute herpetic gingivostomatitis is characterized by extensive painful ulceration and occasionally generalized upset. Secondary or recurrent herpetic lesions are more frequent, especially at mucocutaneous junctions round the lips and nose, where the initially vesicular phase is followed by ulceration and crusting.

Recurrent Oral Ulceration (Aphthous Ulceration)

Recurrent painful fibrin-covered ulcers, either singly or in crops, are a common and troublesome problem, particularly in childhood and adolescence and in the elderly. It may be associated with vitamin B group deficiencies, iron deficiency, or various food allergies.

Dermatoses

A number of diseases can involve the skin and mucosae. The skin manifestations of these are discussed in Chapter 24. The oral mucosal features are similar, but frequently not so clear cut, making diagnosis more difficult. Lichen planus (Fig. 16.5) is the most frequent of the dermatoses which affect the mouth. Other examples include pemphigus, benign mucous membrane pemphigoid, erythema multiforme and lupus erythematosus.

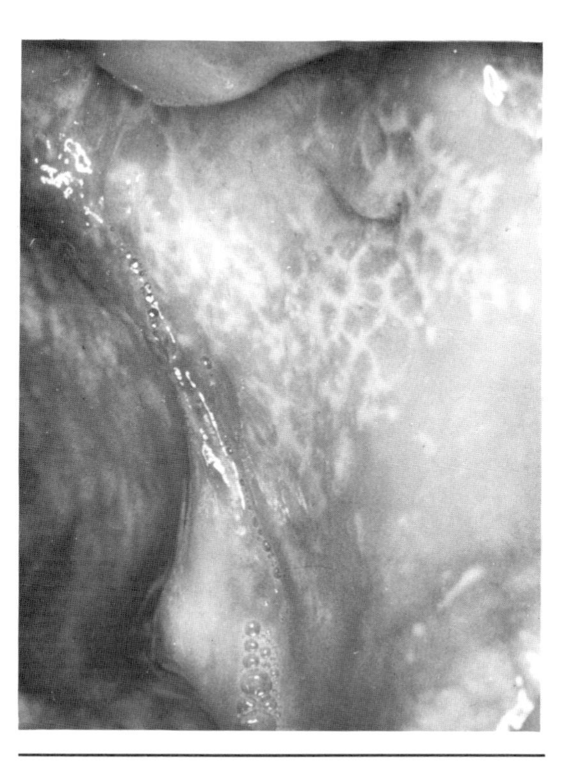

Fig. 16.5 Lichen planus of the cheek mucosa showing a reticular pattern of keratinized striae.

Leukoplakia. Leukoplakia is a clinical descriptive term commonly used to describe a white patch on the oral mucosa which cannot be attributed to a specific disease. It is not a pathological entity. The term covers a variety of histological changes. It is, however, commonly due to keratinization of a normally unkeratinized site or hyperkeratosis of a site where keratin is normally present. In many cases the aetiology is quite unknown, although chronic irritation from smoking, particularly pipe smoking, is a contributory cause in some.

Histologically the epithelium may show acanthosis or atrophy and a variable inflammatory infiltrate is present. A small proportion show dysplasia and are regarded as possibly premalignant. Progression of leukoplakia to squamous cell carcinoma occurs but is infrequent (<5% in 20 years). On the floor of the mouth and the ventral surface and lateral margins of the tongue leukoplakia is more prone to become malignant, particularly in elderly people. Leukoplakia arising on an atrophic epithelium or showing as areas of white upon an erythematous background (speckled leukoplakia) is also more likely to proceed to carcinoma. Speckled leukoplakias often appear to be associated with superficial infestation by *Candida albicans.*

Pigmentation. Melanin pigmentation, especially of the gingiva, is frequent in coloured races but is infrequent in whites. Melanin pigmentation of the lips and buccal mucosa occurs in Addison's disease. Perioral melanin pigmentation is a feature of the rare Peutz–Jeghers syndrome (p. 731).

Ingestion of various heavy metals can give rise to dark blue or black pigmented lines around the gum margins, where the pigment is deposited in soft tissues as sulphides following reaction with bacterial products from the dental plaque.

Soft Tissue Swellings

Fibrous overgrowths of the oral mucosa are a common response to chronic irritation. These may occur on labial or buccal mucosa as fibroepithelial polyps or in relation to the margins of old and ill-fitting dentures where the term denture-induced hyperplasia is used.

An epulis is a localized swelling on the gingiva. The common type is a reaction to chronic irritation, e.g. from dental calculus or the rough margin of a carious cavity or filling; it consists of a mass of cellular fibrous tissue frequently with metaplastic bone formation. Less commonly, such lesions consist of highly vascular granulation tissue and are then described as pyogenic granulomas: this may occur during pregnancy – pregnancy epulis.

Giant cell epulis is a distinctive lesion consisting of numerous multinucleated giant cells in a vascular stroma. The giant cell epulis is a superficial lesion with minimal bone involvement, but intraosseus lesions, such as central giant cell granuloma or osteitis fibrosa cystica may mimic a giant cell epulis if they extend to involve the gingival soft tissues.

Tumours of the Oral Mucosa

Squamous papilloma may occur at any site on the oral mucosa. *Haemangiomas* and less frequently *lymphangiomas* can arise in the oral mucosa and submucosa.

Squamous carcinoma accounts for more than 90% of oral malignancies. Despite the fact that early recognition should be possible, many oral cancers have a bad prognosis because the tumours are not recognized and treated when small. Although squamous carcinoma can occur at any oral site, more than half the lesions involve either the lower lip (Fig. 16.6) or the lateral border of the tongue (Fig. 16.7). Squamous carcinoma of the lower lip is much more frequent in males and exposure to sunlight appears to be an important causal factor. The lesion is most often seen as an ulcer which fails to heal. The tumour shows slow local spread and involves lymph nodes relatively late.

Intra-oral carcinomas as a generalization have a poorer prognosis the further posteriorly in the mouth they arise. Although some appear to develop from recognized premalignant lesions, over three-quarters of carcinomas develop in clinically normal mucosa. The earliest lesions are red rather than white and are symptomless. As successful treatment is dependent upon early diagnosis, it is important that lesions of the oral mucosa which do not relate to obvious causes, or which fail to respond to the removal of obvious causes, be biopsied.

Odontogenic tumours. The lesions designated odontogenic tumours are a group of rare lesions, of widely differing pathology, derived from the dental soft and hard tissues. Some of these lesions are neoplasms but several are hamartomas. The most important is the **ameloblastoma** which is an

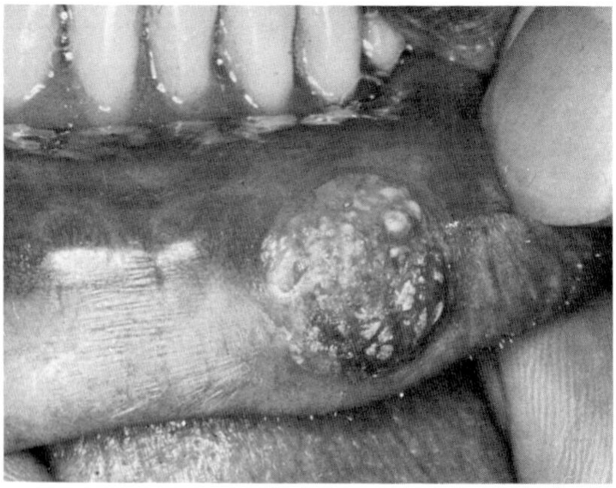

Fig. 16.6 Small exophytic squamous carcinoma of the lower lip.

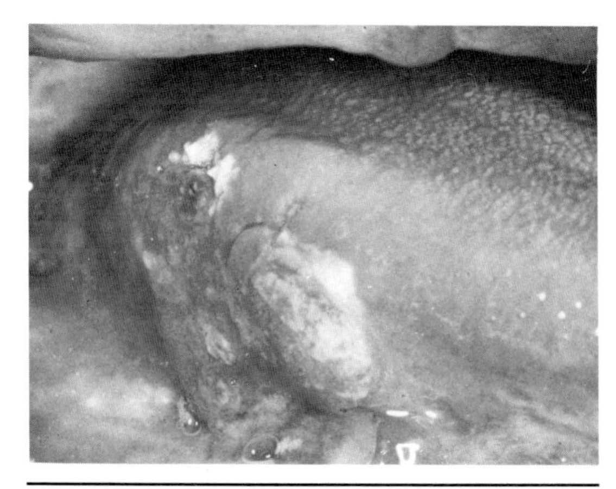

Fig. 16.7 Squamous carcinoma of the lateral margin of the tongue and lingual sulcus.

epithelial neoplasm of distinctive appearance (Fig. 16.8). Ameloblastomas are most frequent in the molar region of the mandible and are locally aggressive, often producing extensive bone destruction. When the tumour mass contains enamel and dentine the term **odontome** is used. A complex odontome consists of a disorganized mass of dental tissues, whereas a compound odontome consists of numerous small teeth.

The Salivary Glands

These include the three pairs of major glands – parotid, submandibular and sublingual – and numerous intra-oral minor salivary glands. The most frequent lesion of minor salivary glands is a **mucocele**. This is seen, especially, in the lower lip and presents as a bluish, slowly enlarging swelling due to leakage of mucus from a damaged duct. Histologically, there is pooling of mucus in soft tissues, surrounded by granulation tissue. A larger variant of this lesion occurs in the floor of the mouth involving sublingual glands and is known as a **ranula**.

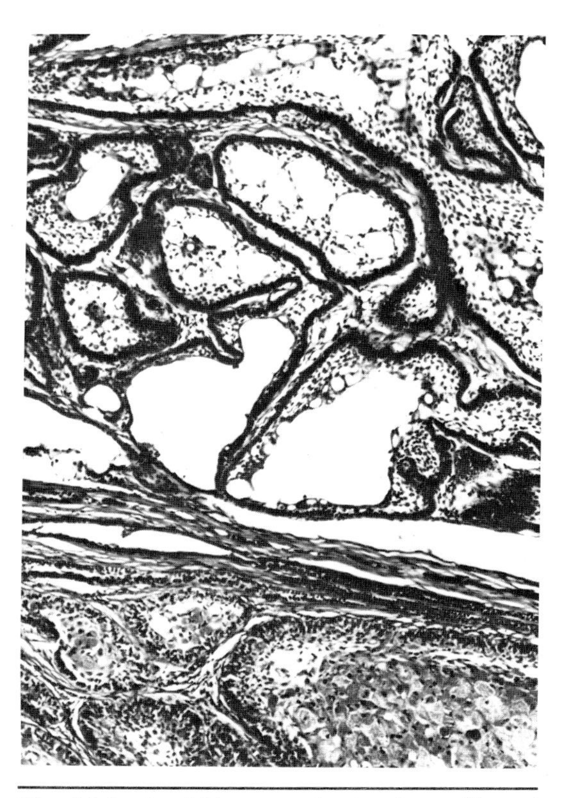

Fig. 16.8 Ameloblastoma, showing the proliferated epithelium in spaces enclosed in a well defined stroma. In places, the epithelium forms a loose network. The appearances resemble the enamel organ. The lower part of the field shows a histological variant of an ameloblastoma in which granular cells are present.

Inflammatory Lesions

Mumps is the commonest acute inflammatory lesion of the salivary glands. This viral infection has an incubation period of 3 weeks and infected individuals secrete the virus in their saliva for about a week before the main symptom of painful salivary gland swelling is evident and for just over a week thereafter. Both parotid glands are usually involved and sometimes also the submandibular. The salivary enlargement usually subsides without permanent damage to the glands. Mumps may be accompanied by orchitis or pancreatitis. Mumps virus is also a relatively frequent cause of aseptic meningitis.

Suppurative parotitis is due to infection by pyogenic cocci and occurs as a postoperative complication in dehydrated patients. It may also occur in elderly debilitated patients, sometimes as a sequel to septicaemia.

Chronic sialadenitis can occur in either the parotid or submandibular glands. In the latter it is often associated with salivary calculi. Duct obstruction leads to atrophy with marked acinar loss and interstitial fibrosis.

Autoimmune Sialadenitis

Sjögren's syndrome is an autoimmune condition involving salivary and lacrimal glands and seen mainly in older women. They complain of dryness of the mouth (xerostomia) and eyes (keratoconjuctivitis sicca). This may occur in isolation (sicca

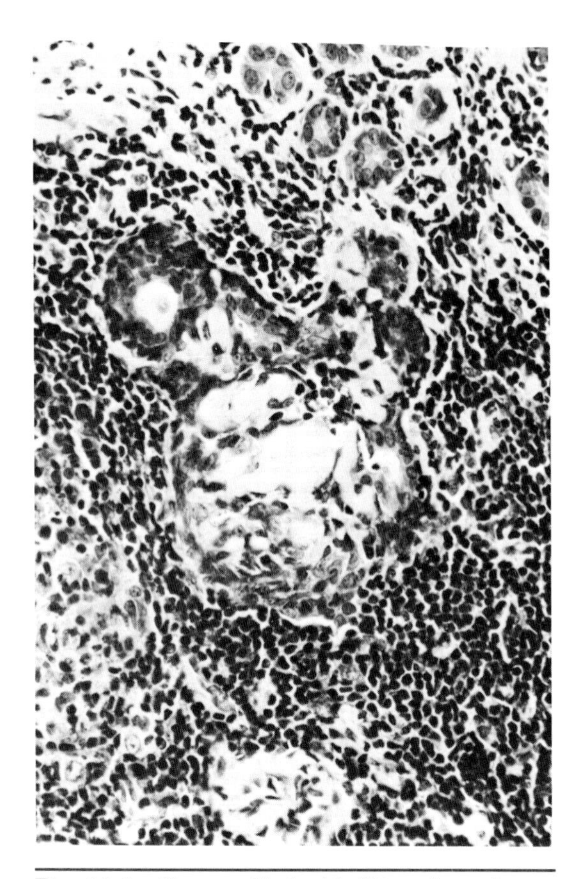

Fig. 16.9 The parotid gland in Sjögren's syndrome, showing heavy infiltration with lymphocytes, loss of glandular tissue and proliferation of duct epithelium to form a cellular mass containing foci of pale-staining hyaline material. ×320.

syndrome or primary Sjögren's syndrome) or as secondary Sjögren's syndrome associated with a non-organ specific autoimmune condition, most frequently rheumatoid arthritis. Microscopically, there is acinar loss and extensive infiltration of lymphocytes (Fig. 16.9). This may give obvious parotid swelling. In a small proportion of cases malignant lymphomas develop, usually at extra-glandular sites but sometimes in the salivary glands.

Salivary Gland Tumours

These tumours are uncommon and comprise approximately 2% of all tumours in man. Approximately 80% occur in the parotid gland, 10% each in the submandibular and minor salivary glands, and they very rarely involve the sublingual gland. Approximately 80% of salivary gland tumours are benign but again there are differences between the salivary glands, 85% of parotid ones being benign and only 60% of those in the other glands. The tumours show considerable and complex morphological variations but the reasons suggested for this histological diversity are numerous and none satisfactory. These tumours are difficult to treat and their clinical behaviour is often unpredictable. Similar tumours may occur in the lacrimal, nasal and sweat glands. A simple classification is shown in Table 16.1.

Table 16.1 Salivary gland tumours

Benign tumours
Pleomorphic salivary adenoma (PSA)
Adenolymphoma
Oxyphil or cystic adenoma
Soft tissue tumours: lipoma, haemangioma
Malignant tumours
Adenoid cystic carcinoma
Mucoepidermoid carcinoma*
Acinic cell carcinoma*
Adenocarcinoma
Carcinoma arising in a pleomorphic salivary adenoma
Non-Hodgkin's lymphoma (in association with autoimmune sialadenitis)

*Clinical behaviour unpredictable.

Pleomorphic Salivary Adenoma (PSA)

Over two-thirds of salivary gland tumours are of this type. They form slow-growing nodules, apparently well defined. The composition of individual tumours is very varied with solid, glandular and myxomatous areas representing varying combinations of glandular and myoepithelial cells (Fig. 16.10). The latter produce connective tissue mucins and may show metaplasia to cartilage. The

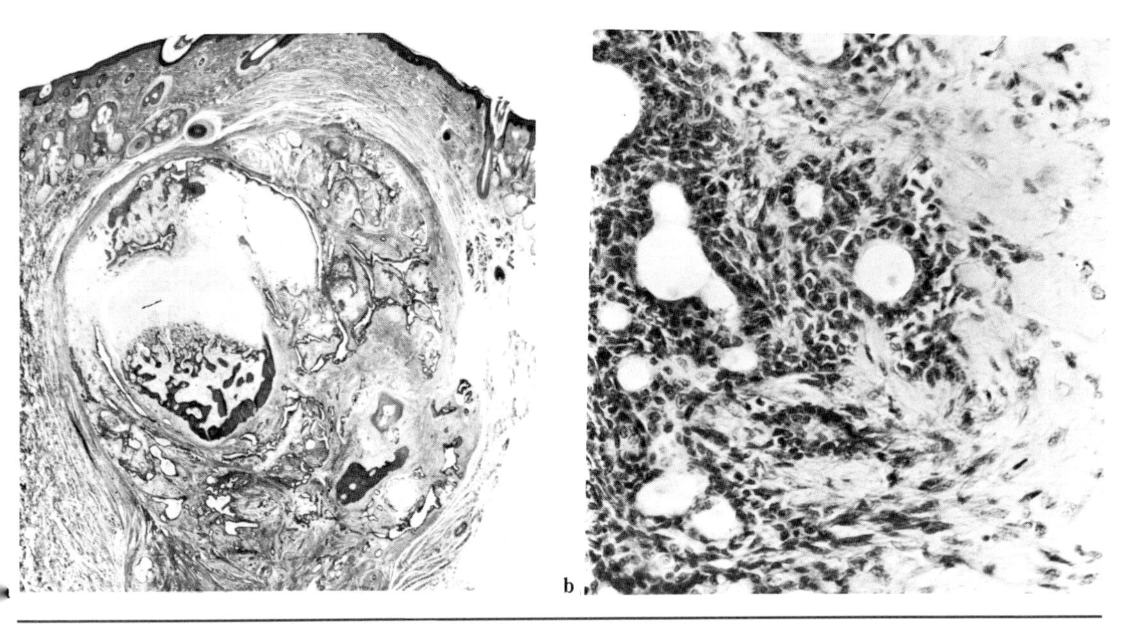

Fig. 16.10 **a** A small pleomorphic salivary adenoma of the lower lip. The tumour is roughly rounded and sharply defined. The pale part of the mushroom-shaped area within it is cartilage, which shows formation of bone trabeculae, seen as dark areas. ×7. **b** Pleomorphic salivary adenoma, showing gland-like epithelial structures, from which cells appear to be streaming off into the connective tissue stroma. ×200.

variable histological patterns account for the previous name 'mixed salivary tumour'. These tumours are benign and do not metastasize, but they often recur (sometimes after decades). This is largely due to the fact that small outgrowths of the tumour often protrude through the capsule and are left behind if close excision is done, while wide excision is made difficult by the facial nerve and other important structures. Carcinoma occasionally arises in a pre-existing PSA, and may show any of the histological variants discussed below.

Adenolymphoma

Adenolymphoma (Fig. 16.11), the second commonest tumour, is basically a papillary cystadenoma, with a characteristic two-layered epithelium of tall pink-staining mitochondrion-rich (oncocytic) cells and with abundant lymphoid tissue filling the stroma. In distinction from all other tumours of these glands, they occur chiefly in older men, are almost entirely limited to the

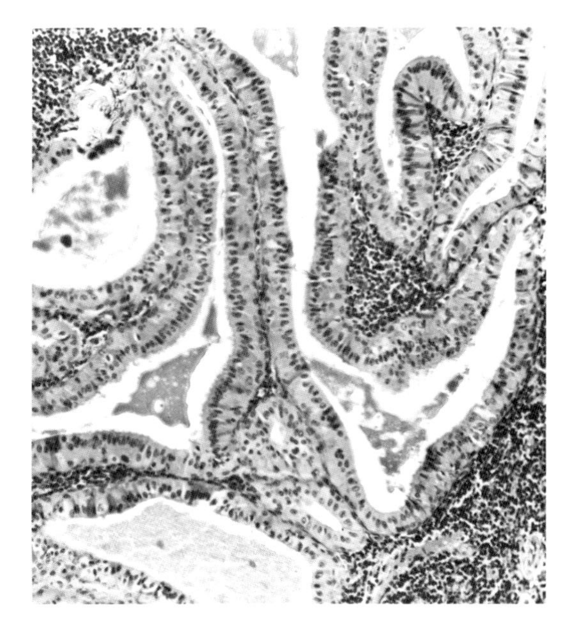

Fig. 16.11 Adenolymphoma of the parotid gland, showing the papillary architecture, with lymphoid stroma. ×130.

parotids and may be multiple and bilateral. They are benign.

Adenoid Cystic Carcinoma

Adenoid cystic carcinoma is the commonest malignant tumour and, though slow-growing and slower to metastasize, is often widely infiltrative and difficult to eradicate. It consists of masses of small, dark-staining cells which show a characteristic sieve-like or 'cribriform' pattern (Fig. 16.12) and has a particularly striking tendency to infiltrate along nerves.

Mucoepidermoid Carcinoma

These tumours comprise an admixture of squamous cell and mucus-secreting cells, and which may apparently blend within one another. They may be either benign or malignant. The degree of differentiation is some guide to likely behaviour but even well differentiated examples may metastasize to local lymph nodes or to distant sites, e.g. lung and bone.

Acinic Cell Carcinomas

These are usually well circumscribed slow-growing tumours of acinar cells, which can behave unpredictably; they tend to invade locally.

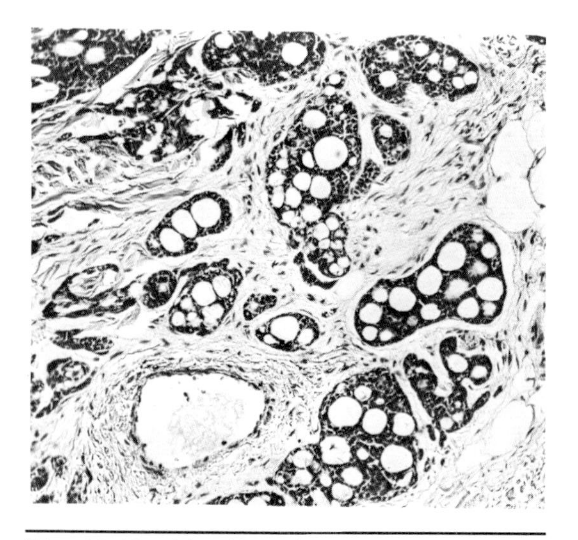

Fig. 16.12 Adenoid cystic carcinoma showing the characteristic architecture. ×90.

Other malignant neoplasms besides the varieties already mentioned, include ordinary adenocarcinomas and even squamous-cell carcinomas occur, and malignant lymphomas (sometimes apparently arising in Sjögren's lesions of long standing) may occur.

The Oropharynx

Tonsillitis. Acute tonsillitis is a common cause of sore throat. Haemolytic streptococci are the commonest infecting agents and give rise to acute inflammatory swelling with purulent exudate in the tonsillar crypts – follicular tonsillitis. The infection occasionally extends more deeply and involves the whole tonsil and adjacent tissues with frank suppuration; this is known as quinsy. From such a lesion streptococcal cellulitis may spread widely into the neck – Ludwig's angina – or even into the mediastinum or may give rise to a retropharyngeal abscess.

Acute streptococcal tonsillitis occurring alone or in scarlet fever is the usual antecedent infection in rheumatic fever and post-streptococcal glomerulonephritis. Chronic enlargement of the tonsils and adjacent lymphoid tissue commonly results from colonization by one or other of the many adenoviruses.

Vincent's angina is a painful necrotic ulcerating lesion on the fauces similar in every way to Vincent's infection of the gingiva.

Blood dyscrasias. Swelling, haemorrhage and ulceration of the gingivae occurs in agranulocytosis.

Diphtheria is an acute inflammation which affects most frequently the fauces, soft palate and tonsils, but may also attack the nose, or the larynx and trachea; it occurs chiefly in young children, but may also affect adults. Immunization programmes are largely responsible for the present very low incidence of diphtheria in many parts of the world.

The causal organism, *Corynebacterium dipth-*

theriae, exists in three main forms, *mitis*, *intermedius* and *gravis*, and infections with the last type tend to be more severely toxic and also to show greater local inflammatory reaction. The organisms remain strictly localized at the site of infection and the systemic effects are due to the formation and absorption of a powerful exotoxin which may cause myocardial damage with fatty change, fatty change in the liver and kidney, and polyneuropathy. The mechanisms of cellular injury are outlined on p. 291.

The local lesions are characterized by the formation on the affected surfaces of a false membrane composed of fibrin and leucocytes. In the fauces, palate and tonsils the stratified squamous epithelium becomes permeated by exudate which forms a fibrinous coagulum in which the epithelium is incorporated; it then undergoes extensive necrosis, producing a dull greyish-yellow pseudomembrane which can be detached only with difficulty owing to the attachment of the dead epithelium to the underlying tissues. When it is removed a bleeding connective tissue surface is laid bare. In *gravis* infections, membrane formation may be less obvious but inflammatory congestion and swelling are more marked and the cervical lymph nodes may be much swollen.

Diphtheria of the nasopharynx and of the larynx is described on p. 528.

Tumours of the Oropharynx

Benign tumours. The commonest is squamous papilloma which occasionally recurs after removal but rarely progresses to malignancy. Lymphangiomas occur, usually in the tonsillar region.

Malignant tumours. Squamous carcinoma and lymphomas occur in approximately equal numbers and together account for about one-third of extracranial malignant tumours of the head and neck (excluding skin tumours). Squamous carcinoma develops most often in the tonsillar region in elderly men. It usually ulcerates and becomes infected and death often results from aspiration bronchopneumonia. Lymphomas are of various types and arise in the lymphoid tissue of Waldeyer's ring.

Tumours of the nasopharynx are described on p. 528.

The Oesophagus

The oesophagus has a structure well adapted to its primary function in actively transporting ingested material of variable composition, texture and temperature from the oral cavity to the stomach. The mucosal surface is lined throughout by non-keratinized squamous epithelium overlying a lamina propria which includes blood vessels, lymphatics and nerves and is supported by a thin muscular layer, the lamina muscularis mucosae. The submucosa contains occasional racemose mucous glands. In the upper part of the oesophagus the muscularis propria includes striated muscle which reflects the initial voluntary phase of swallowing: more distally this layer consists exclusively of smooth muscle under autonomic control and is responsible for the peristaltic activity involved in the later phases of swallowing, culminating in relaxation of the cardiac sphincter and entry of ingested material into the stomach.

The distal oesophagus is an important site of anastomoses between the systemic and the portal venous systems. An increase in portal venous pressure causes dilatation of veins on either side of the gastro-oesophageal junction. On the oesophageal side these enlarged veins, known as **oesophageal varices**, are mainly located in the lamina propria and are readily eroded, causing haemorrhage. The dilated gastric veins may also rupture and cause severe bleeding. The most common causes of portal hypertension producing these effects are hepatic cirrhosis and schistosomiasis (p. 772). Oesophageal haemorrhage may also occur in peptic oesophagitis, mucosal laceration during vomiting (Mallory–Weiss syndrome) and from an ulcerated carcinoma.

Inflammatory Disease

Micro-organisms are not commonly involved in producing oesophageal inflammation unless there is some defect in mucosal resistance due for example to immunodeficiency states such as AIDS, cytotoxic drug treatment or diabetes mellitus. Two opportunistic organisms which exploit these defects deserve mention. **Herpes simplex** virus can cause ulcerative lesions at either end of the oesophagus, the proximal forms often being precipitated by intubation. The histological presence of pale, haematoxyphilic inclusions in the nuclei of epithelial cells (often multinucleated) at ulcer margins is characteristic. *Candida albicans* can also produce extensive oesophageal ulceration (often in continuity with oropharyngeal lesions) under similar circumstances. The ulcers tend to be white in colour and have congested margins, hence the alternative term **thrush**; using special histological stains such as the PAS reaction fungal hyphae can be readily seen penetrating the oesophageal epithelium.

Acute oesophagitis may also result from the ingestion of alcohol and hot fluids, corrosive agents, drugs (e.g. antibiotics), is commonly associated with cigarette smoking, and may complicate skin diseases (e.g. pemphigus) and the uraemia of chronic renal failure. It also occurs in graft-versus-host disease and Behçet's syndrome.

Reflux or Peptic Oesophagitis

This, the most common form of oesophageal inflammation is due to the persistent regurgitation of gastric juice into the lower oeosophagus. This phenomenon is normally prevented by the tonal activity of the cardiac sphincter, possibly supported by the constrictive action of the diaphragmatic muscle surrounding the oesophageal hiatus and the acuteness of the cardio-oesophageal angle. Any increase in intra-abdominal pressure (due for example to obesity or pregnancy, or simply by bending from an upright position) may compromise this anti-reflux mechanism. The herniation of the fundal portion of the stomach into the thorax, **hiatus hernia**, especially if this results in widening of the cardio-oesophageal angle, may have a similar effect (Fig. 16.13).

The effect of subsequent reflux may be compounded if there are high levels of gastric acid which not only enhances damage to the oesophageal mucosa but, by depressing serum gastrin levels, may reduce the tone of the cardiac sphincter and exacerbate reflux. The usual effects of gastric juice upon the squamous epithelium of the lower oesophagus is to produce superficial ulceration which is preceded by punctate erosion of the elongated papillae of lamina propria within the epithelial surface (Fig. 16.14). This produces

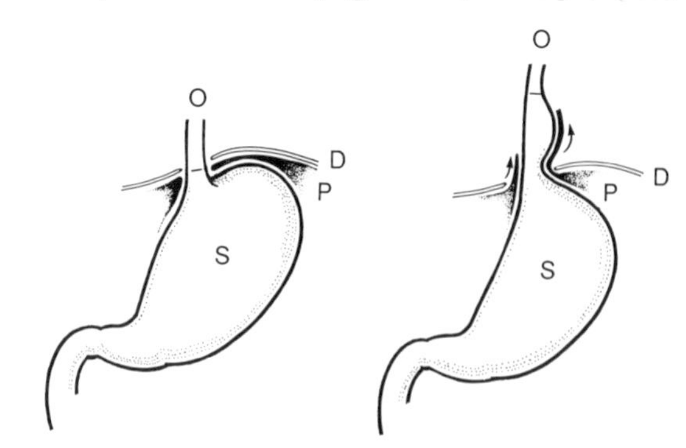

Fig. 16.13 Hiatus hernia 'sliding' type. Note the upward displacement of the cardia with loss of the cardio-oesophageal angle and 'pinchcock' action of diaphragm. O, oesophagus; S, stomach; D, diaphragm; P, peritoneal cavity (outlined in black).

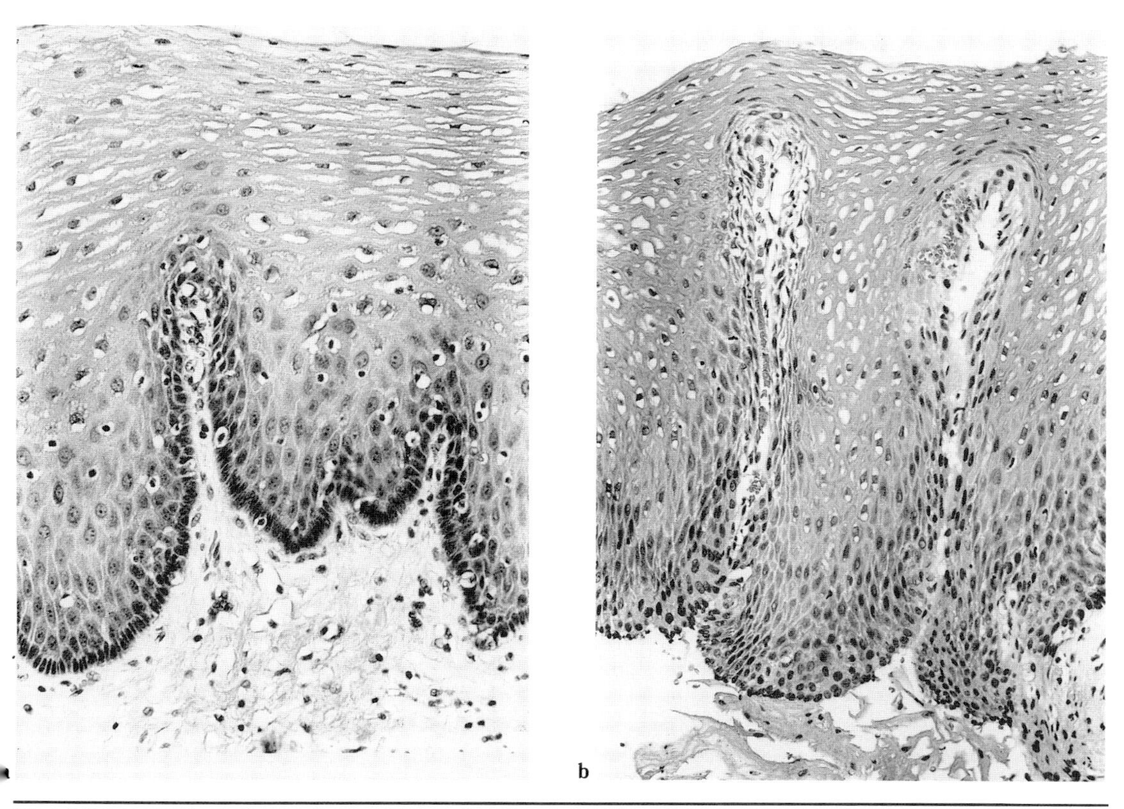

Fig. 16.14 **a** Normal oesophagus. Connective tissue papillae of the lamina propria extend upwards into the epithelium, but to a height less than half of the epithelial thickness. H & E × 179. **b** Reflux oesophagitis. The connective tissue papillae reach almost to the luminal surface of the epithelium. H & E ×150.

oesophageal pain and sometimes blood loss of sufficient severity to produce anaemia. The formation of granulation tissue beneath the ulcers may eventually lead to fibrosis and stricture formation.

Another important consequence of persistent reflux is the development of metaplasia in the oeosophageal mucosa, the squamous epithelium being replaced by columnar epithelium, so called **Barrett's oesophagus**. Usually this epithelium is of gastric type but at its advancing proximal edge it tends to exhibit an intestinal pattern, albeit of incomplete type (p. 700). Metaplasia has two potentially serious complications. First, it may predispose to true chronic peptic ulceration penetrating the entire thickness of the oesophageal wall, with the hazard of perforation or erosion of a major artery; secondly, it may evolve into dysplasia (i.e. intra-epithelial neoplasia) and in 10–15% of cases into invasive adenocarcinoma. Barrett's oesophagus is thus a premalignant conditions carrying a 30-fold increased risk of developing an adenocarcinoma when compared with the normal population.

Chronic Inflammatory Disturbances

These are rare. Involvement of the lower oesophagus in **Crohn's disease** (p. 713) is, however, becoming increasingly recognized and may occasionally cause oesophageal obstruction. Occasionally the diagnostic epithelioid granulomas can be detected in an oesophageal biopsy.

Miscellaneous Conditions

Oesophageal Diverticula

A diverticulum is a blind-ended protrusion of the lumen of an epithelial lined cavity beyond its natural border. Two types of diverticulum may arise in the oesophagus: traction diverticula and pulsion diverticula. A traction diverticulum is formed when the outer part of the oesophagus becomes involved in a sclerosing inflammatory process usually involving the mediastinal lymph node, e.g. tuberculosis. A pulsion diverticulum develops due to luminal pressure exploiting a weakness in the oesophageal wall. It usually occurs proximally, due to a weakness in the inferior constrictor muscle of the pharynx and generally presents posteriorly but sometimes anteriorly. They are properly referred to as pharyngeal pouches. They cause increasing oesophageal obstruction as they enlarge due to the accumulation of ingested material.

Inflammation and ulceration of diverticular mucosa occurs and may lead to perforation and mediastinitis.

Oesophageal Obstruction

This is the commonest cause of the distressing symptom **dysphagia**, defined as difficulty in swallowing. It not only causes progressive inanition but presents the hazard of regurgitation and inhalation of ingested material with subsequent pneumonitis, which is often fatal. The main causes of oesophageal obstruction are listed in Table 16.2 and are divided into four broad categories.

Table 16.2 Common causes of oesophageal obstruction

External compression
Mediastinal tumours (e.g. bronchial carcinoma)
Mediastinal lymphadenopathy (e.g. tuberculosis, primary and secondary malignancies)
Enlargement of the left atrium (as in mitral stenosis)
Vascular disorders (e.g. aneurysm of the aorta)
Pharyngeal pouch
Intrinsic lesions (strictures)
Carcinoma
Reflux oesophagitis
Corrosive liquids (e.g. 'lye' strictures)
Crohn's disease
Oesophageal occlusion
Foreign material
Polypoid tumours
Functional obstruction
Achalasia
Chagas' disease
Progressive systemic sclerosis
Kelly–Paterson (Plummer–Vinson) syndrome

External compression. This is most often the result of expanding lesions in the mediastinum, especially bronchial carcinomas arising close to the carina or lymph nodes in the same location enlarged as a result of metastatic carcinoma, lymphoma or infective processes such as tuberculosis. Occasionally the oesophagus is compressed by a dilated left atrium (following mitral stenosis) or by an aneurysm of the thoracic aorta. Pharyngeal pouches when distended with food may kink and obstruct the upper oesophagus.

Intrinsic lesions. Many oesophageal diseases lead eventually to narrowing of the lumen, i.e. to stricture formation. The most serious and important condition in this category is carcinoma of the oesophagus. Simple strictures are, however, by no means rare. The most common cause is reflux oesophagitis with or without hiatus hernia. Scarring and stricture formation may also follow the ingestion of corrosive liquids such as lye, an alkaline fluid used for cleaning purposes. Occasionally Crohn's disease may produce constriction of the oesophagus especially at the lower end.

Luminal occlusion. Foreign material, especially inadequately masticated masses of food, quite often bring this about. The effects are usually transient but can prove fatal. Occasionally a polypoid tumour may have similar consequences.

Functional obstruction. Disturbances of innervation or muscular activity may cause serious dysphagia even in the absence of any organic obstruction of the oesophagus. Of particular importance is **achalasia** of the oesophagus. In this disease, which usually affects young women, the normal wave of peristaltic activity initiated by swallowing dies out before it reaches the cardiac spincter which thus fails to relax, hence the alternative term cardiospasm. It has been shown histologically that there is a deficiency of ganglion cells in the distal oesophagus, the reason for this being unknown. As a consequence the proximal oesophagus becomes grossly distended (mega-oesophagus) by ingested material which may only succeed in entering the stomach by gravitational force. There is a serious risk of regurgitation and aspiration pneumonitis. There is also a slightly increased risk of oesophageal carcinoma. Incision through the muscle of the cardiac sphincter (Heller's operation) may alleviate the symptoms.

A very similar phenomenon may arise in **Chagas' disease**, caused by the protozoon *Trypanosoma cruzi* and which occurs almost exclusively in South America (p. 1154). This organism has a predilection for the muscle coats of tubular organs and in the chronic stage it causes widespread damage to the myenteric plexus. In the oesophagus damage to the myenteric plexus leads, as in achalasia, to defective peristalsis and mega-oesophagus.

The non-organ specific autoimmune disease **progressive systemic sclerosis** (p. 231) is a well recognized cause of damage to the oesophageal musculature and its replacement by fibrous tissue, possibly due to an ischaemic phenomenon mediated by vasculitis. The subsequent impairment of peristaltic activity may produce severe dysphagia, sometimes compounded by shortening of the oesophagus and reflux oesophagitis.

The dysphagia associated with iron deficiency anaemia and glossitis (the **Kelly–Paterson** or **Plummer–Vinson syndrome**) is probably related to spasm of the hypopharyngeal muscles mediating swallowing and is thus essentially functional. Occasionally, however, an oesophageal web or diaphragm has been demonstrated in such cases.

Oesophageal Rupture

In most instances this is brought about either by the ingestion of foreign bodies or by instrumentation involving the oesophagus, e.g. bouginage or endoscopy. It may, however, arise spontaneously as a result of violent vomiting (often alcohol related) with sudden distension of the lower oesophagus. The usual site of rupture is the posterior wall of the oesophagus just above the cardiac sphincter. In addition to the severe pain and the shock-like state which may be generated, the entry of regurgitated gastric contents into the mediastinum or sometimes the pleural cavity inevitably leads to severe infection which may be difficult to control. Explosive vomiting may also on occasion produce a mucosal tear which is localized either in the lower oesophagus or gastric fundus and may precipitate brisk haemorrhage, the so-called **Mallory–Weiss** syndrome.

Congenital Lesions

Most of these are due to disturbance in the structuring of the upper part of the endodermal tube and its respiratory and alimentary components. In many instances the middle part of the oesophagus fails to become cannulated (oesophageal atresia) and either blind end may communicate with the trachea (tracheo-oesophageal fistula). Sometimes such a fistula is the only abnormality. Such disorders are usually surgically remediable but congenital abnormalities of other organs often coexist.

Tumours

Carcinoma of the Oesophagus

This is by far the commonest oesophageal tumour. There are, however, enormous variations in its incidence throughout the world. In Scotland it accounts for only 2–3% of all malignant tumours but in parts of southern USSR, Iran, China and South Africa (especially the Transkei) it is the commonest form of cancer. Usually it occurs in the fifth decade and is three to four times more common in males. The tumour carries a grim prognosis: scarcely more than 10% of its victims survive for 5 years.

The aetiology of oesophageal carcinoma is far from clear. It is likely that diets including potentiating carcinogenic agents such as nitrosamines are responsible. Alcoholic beverages, tobacco or food contaminated by fungal toxins or silica may be implicated and nutritional defiency could be a contributory factor. In the lower oesophagus reflux oesophagitis associated with columnar cell metaplasia (Barrett's oesophagus), achalasia and longstanding strictures are recognized premalignant lesions. In the upper oesophagus, or more correctly the hypopharynx, there is some evidence (not too convincing) that iron deficiency may predispose to carcinoma, especially in women.

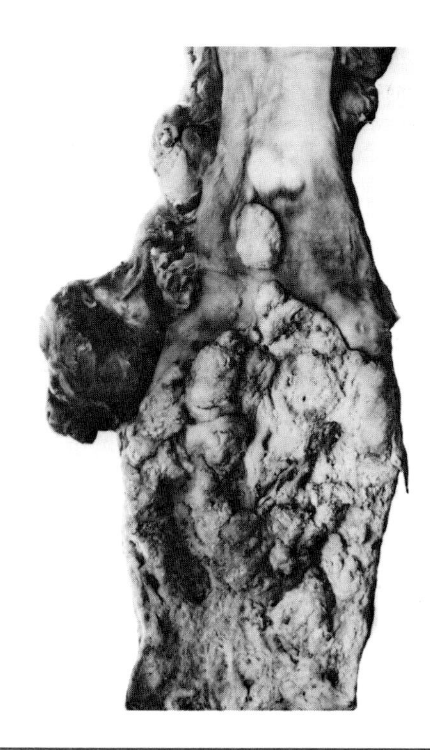

Fig. 16.15 Extensive ulcerating carcinoma in middle part of oesophagus.

Pathological Features

Most carcinomas arise in the middle third of the oesophagus. Distally located tumours are less common even though most adenocarcinomas fall into this category. The proximal oesophagus has the lowest incidence except possibly in iron-deficient women. Usually the tumour takes the form of an ulcer with raised margins: in most cases, however, infiltration of the oesophageal wall with thickening and stenosis is evident at the time of diagnosis. In some cases a polypoid fungating lesion may extend into and partially obstruct the lumen (Fig. 16.15). Superficial spread may lead to the appearance of nodules in the mucosa at some distance from the putative primary locus.

In most instances the tumour is a keratinizing squamous carcinoma sometimes associated with adjacent intraepithelial neoplasia (i.e. *in situ* carcinoma). A substantial proportion of malignant tumours in the distal oesophagus are adenocarcinomas, usually arising in Barrett's oesophagus. These have to be distinguished from adenocarcinomas arising in the stomach and spreading into the lower oesophagus.

The spread of oesophageal carcinoma may be less conspicuous than in other neoplasms since death commonly results from the effects of oesophageal obstruction notably inanition and aspiration pneumonitis, before extensive spread has taken place. There may be local spread to adjacent structures such as the mediastinum or pleural cavity. Lymphatic spread is also important and permeation of lymphatics in the lamina propria mucosae may lead to the appearance of tumour nodules at some distance from the primary site. Metastases to the local para-oesophageal lymph nodes is more common and occasionally blood spread to, for example, lung, brain or bone marrow is observed.

Other Oesophageal Tumours

Mesenchymal tumours are uncommon apart from leiomyomas. Occasionally these are malignant (leiomyosarcomas). Other rare but well recognized malignant tumours include carcinosarcomas (which usually present as a polypoid tumour causing oesophageal occlusion) and small cell carcinomas probably arising in neuroendocrine cells (p. 729). Tumours occasionally arise in the submucosal oesophageal glands: most resemble the mucoepidermoid tumours found in the salivary glands and may exhibit low-grade malignant behaviour.

The Stomach

While not essential to life, the stomach, by virtue of its role in the early phase of the digestive process, is important to the well-being of the individual as is evident from some of the serious nutritional disturbances which may be observed following gastric surgery. Unfortunately the stomach is afflicted by some of the most common and serious diseases encountered in clinical practice and surgery of some kind all too often becomes a necessity. The diagnosis of gastric disease has been significantly improved in recent years by the widespread use of fibreoptic endoscopy allowing biopsy of unsuspected lesions under direct vision.

The interpretation of these biopsies and an understanding of the lesions revealed require some knowledge of gastric structure especially at the mucosal level. Histologically, the gastric mucosa has two main compartments. Adjacent to the lumen is the foveolar area which includes the surface epithelium and gastric pits (tubular indentations) both of which are lined by columnar epithelium secreting neutral mucins. More deeply placed is a zone of glandular structures which open into the bases of the gastric pits. The stem cell population from which the surface and glandular epithelium is derived and replenished is located in the glandular neck region which often includes some mucous cells.

In terms of mucosal appearance, however, the stomach has three distinct zones (Fig. 16.16). In the **cardiac area** (seldom more than 1 cm in length) immediately distal to the oesophagogastric junction the glands secrete mucin and have a racemose structure but tend to be small and somewhat irregular in distribution. In the **body or fundus**, which occupies most of the stomach, the glandular compartment is much larger than the foveolar zone and consists of long tubular glands lined mainly by specialized cells most notably parietal cells (producing acid and intrinsic factor) and chief or zymogenic cells (producing pepsin). Conversely in the **pyloric antrum** (immediately proximal to the pylorus) the foveolar zone occupies most of the mucosa. The less prominent glandular compartment consists of racemose glands lined by mucin secreting cells and mixed with occasional parietal cells; neuroendocrine cells, most notably gastrin secreting G cells, are also present.

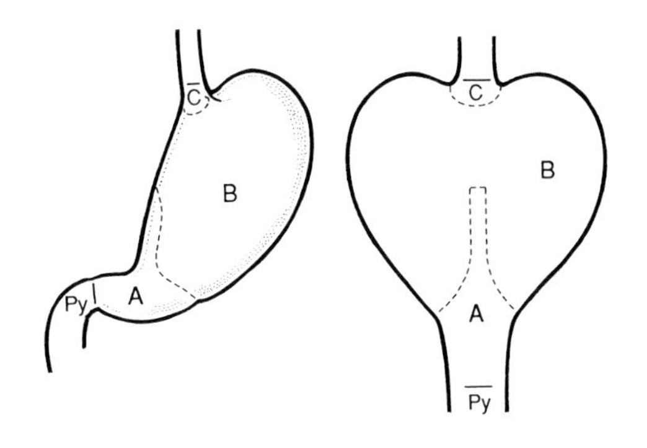

Fig. 16.16 Stomach: the three major zones as seen in lateral view (left) and on opening along the greater curvature (right). Note that the antrum (A) extends to a variable extent along the lesser curvature. B, body; C, cardiac region; Py, pylorus.

Vascular Disturbances

Gastric haemorrhage which is severe results in the vomiting either of fresh blood (haematemesis) or altered blood (coffee ground vomit) and is always a clinical emergency. The causes are listed in Table 16.3. In hepatic cirrhosis, quite apart from the variceal lesions in portal hypertension, foci of vascular ectasia have been observed to cause bleeding from the gastric fundus. In elderly individuals a similar form of ectasia may affect the antrum often producing red linear streaks in the mucosa (gastric antral vascular ectasia or so-called watermelon stomach). Severe iron-deficiency anaemia may be caused by recurrent haemorrhage from these lesions. Histologically, mucosal biopsies have shown dilated vascular channels (often with organizing luminal thrombus) associated with fibromuscular thickening of the lamina propria. The cause is unknown. Occasionally the protrusion of a large submucosal artery through a small mucosal erosion may also cause severe gastric haemorrhage (Dieulafoy lesions).

Gastritis

Considering the vast range of potentially damaging agents to which the stomach is exposed (either accidentally or deliberately) it is hardly surprising that inflammatory changes of one kind or another are extremely common and become increasingly so with advancing age. Until quite recently, however, remarkably little was known about the exact mechanisms involved and which agents could be incriminated with confidence. This is especially true of the more acute forms of gastric inflammation which often take the form of erosive lesions, but the common types of chronic gastritis have also proved difficult to explain and remain a source of controversy. At the time of writing, a new classification method (the Sydney system) has just been published. In this the histological features and the endoscopic features are combined. The endoscopic features include topography – gastritis of the body, gastritis of the antrum and pangastritis (antrum predominant, body predominant) – together with other visible characteristics such as oedema, erythema etc., which we need not detail here. The classification presented in Table 16.4 must at this stage be regarded as provisional but it is in part based on the Sydney system while also including the older or former terminologies.

Table 16.3 The common causes of gastric haemorrhage

Acute erosion (due e.g. to analgesics)
Acute peptic ulcer (stress-related)
Chronic peptic ulcer
Carcinoma of the stomach
Gastric varices (due to hepatic cirrhosis)
Gastric antral vascular ectasia

Acute Gastritis

This term is often applied to the acute gastric symptoms which arise during the course of infective fevers following dietary indiscretion or stress or the ingestion of agents such as alcohol, acids or alkalis. Histologically, the gastric biopsy shows acute superficial inflammation without glandular loss or atrophy. The pathological lesions responsible for the acute gastric symptoms seen in 'food poisoning' and associated with staphylococcal exotoxins, Salmonellae and *Yersinia* infections have not been clearly defined. Acute damage to the gastric mucosa due, for example, to alcohol or certain analgesic drugs may take the form of acute mucosal erosion associated with intense mucosal congestion, acute haemorrhagic gastritis. Similar changes may also be found in uraemia and in shock-like states.

Acute Gastric Erosions

The term erosion is applied to an ulcerative lesion which remains confined to the mucosa and does

Table 16.4 Classification of gastritis

Acute gastritis
Drug associated or other known gastric irritants with erosions
Infective (excluding *Helicobacter pylori*) – bacterial, viral, fungal, parasitic
Chronic gastritis
Autoimmune associated with severe atrophy (formerly type A gastritis)
Helicobacter pylori associated (formerly type B gastritis)
Idiopathic
Special forms of gastritis
Lymphocytic
Eosinophilic
Granulomatous (Crohn's associated, sarcoidosis, idiopathic)
Reflux
Post-gastrectomy associated
Radiation associated

In the Sydney system the topography of the gastritis as seen on endoscopy is included (antral, body, pangastritis) together with the macroscopic appearances (oedema, haemorrhagic, flat, raised, rugal appearances etc.). In addition, some of the histological and macroscopic features may be graded in terms of severity – mild, moderate or severe.

not transgress the lamina muscularis. Such lesions are a manifestation of acute mucosal damage and may produce gastric haemorrhage. They are often multiple and widely distributed in the stomach (Fig. 16.17). When located proximally in the body or fundus they can often be attributed to the ingestion of alcohol or drugs, especially aspirin, less frequently other non-steroidal anti-inflammatory drugs (NSAIDs). Such drugs may also produce more deeply penetrating ulcers sometimes causing haematemesis or even gastric perforation. The more common erosions located in the distal stomach or antrum may be infective in origin. Occasionally, erosions complicate hepatic cirrhosis, purpuric disorders or systemic infections, and sometimes cytomegalovirus is responsible, especially in immunocompromised individuals.

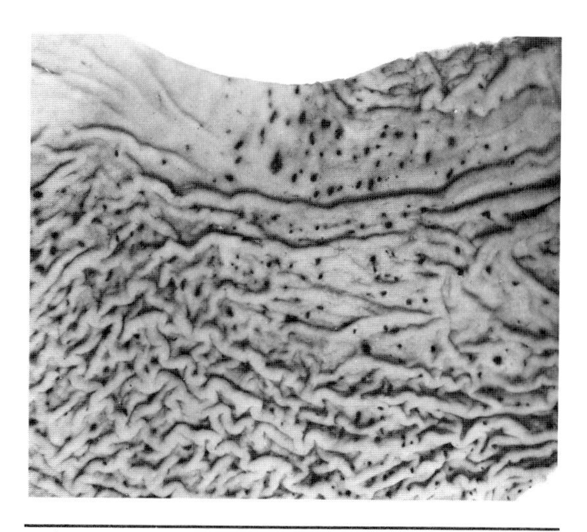

Fig. 16.17 Multiple minute haemorrhagic erosions of the gastric mucosa.

Chronic Gastritis

Autoimmune-associated Gastritis (Type A Chronic Gastritis)

In this condition of late adult life the fundus of the stomach is predominantly if not exclusively affected and severe mucosal atrophy is the usual end result. Gastric biopsies reveal that initially there is infiltration of the mucosa especially in the foveolar area by plasma cells and lymphocytes (chronic superficial gastritis). This is followed by gradual loss of the specialized cells in the glandular zone which becomes reduced in thickness (chronic atrophic gastritis; Fig. 16.18). Eventually complete gastric atrophy develops. Commonly, the specialized glands are replaced by mucin secreting glands (pseudopyloric metaplasia) or intestinal epithelium (intestinal metaplasia). These alterations result in progressive reduction in the secretion of acid, pepsin and intrinsic factor, eventually producing complete achlorhydria.

The condition seldom causes recognizable gastric symptoms, the major problem being vitamin B_{12} malabsorption and the development of megaloblastic anaemia (*pernicious anaemia*) (p. 615).

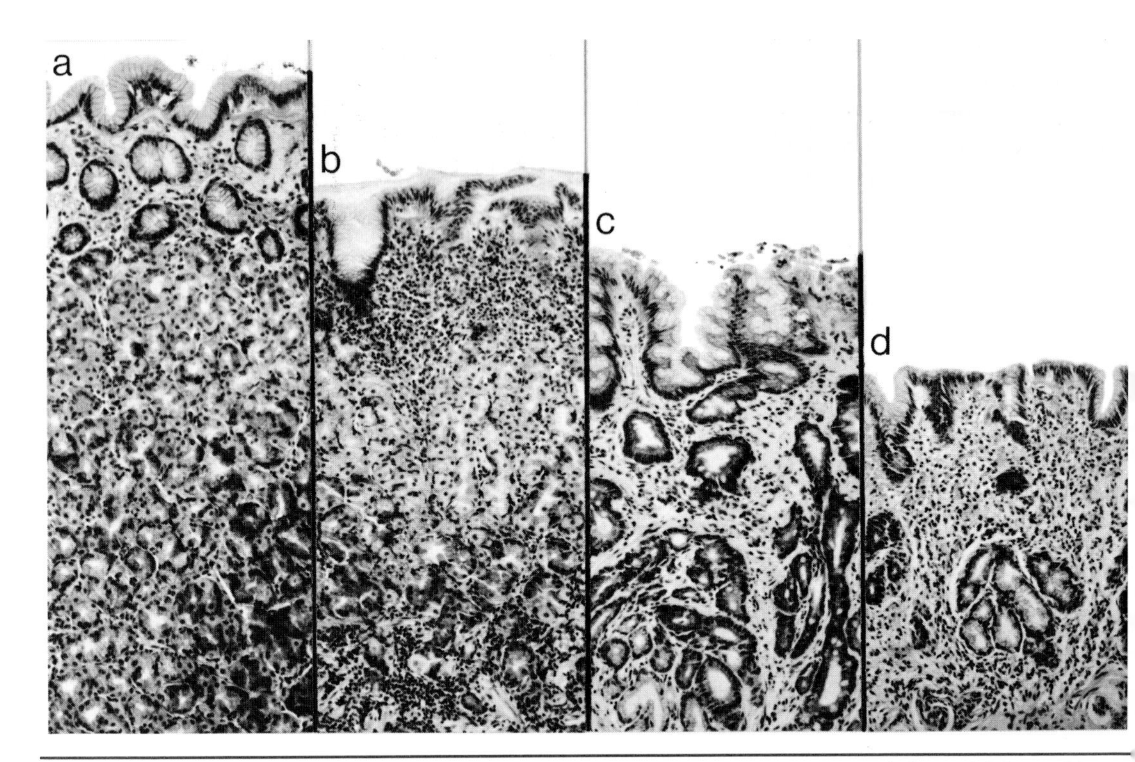

Fig. 16.18 Evolution of autoimmune chronic gastritis (type A). **a** Normal mucosa. **b** Superficial gastritis and atrophic gastritis affecting the deep part of the mucosa. **c** Complete loss of parietal and chief cells with intestinal metaplasia. **d** Complete atrophic gastritis. The remaining glands are of simple mucus-secreting type. In **b**, **c** and **d**, the full thickness of the mucosa is shown.

That the mucosal changes are mediated by autoimmune mechanisms is reflected by the presence in the serum of antibodies to parietal cells (in 90% of cases) and to intrinsic factor itself in 50% of cases. Antibodies of the latter type (often blocking the vitamin B_{12} binding site) may also be present in the gastric juice and are probably responsible for finally ablating vitamin B_{12} absorption. It should also be noted that this type of chronic gastritis is sometimes associated with other autoimmune diseases such as chronic thyroiditis and diabetes mellitus. Another important aspect of the disease is that it is associated with an increased risk of gastric carcinoma; it may also be complicated by the development of carcinoid tumours (p. 729) and occasionally, malignant lymphoma of the stomach.

Helicobacter *Associated Gastritis (Type B Chronic Gastritis)*

This, perhaps the commonest type of gastritis, tends to increase in prevalence with advancing years even though it can arise at any age. While any part of the stomach may be affected, the lesions are usually more pronounced in the antrum or junctional zone. Histologically, the predominant change is an intense plasma cell infiltration of the foveolar zone of the mucosa with variable involvement of the glandular zone. Some glandular atrophy and intestinal metaplasia may be observed on occasion and there may be hypochlorhydria of variable degree. More noticeable, however, is the almost invariable presence of neutrophils in the lamina propria or superficial epithelium (Fig

16.19) which often shows signs of mucin depletion or degradation (active gastritis).

In most cases minute curved bacillary organisms can be found in close apposition to the surface epithelium and can be visualized even in sections stained with H & E, although their identification is facilitated by special stains such as a modified Giemsa. The pathogenetic role of this bacterium, now referred to as *Helicobacter pylori*, is becoming increasingly accepted. They are present in over 80% of active chronic gastritis and are selective in that they inhabit exclusively gastric-type epithelium. The prevalence of *H. pylori* increases also with age. Serological testing for *H. pylori* specific antibodies suggest that the infection is generally acquired in early adulthood. However, *H. pylori* gastritis can also occur in children.

These observations are of considerable importance since this type of chronic gastritis is not only thought to be responsible for dyspeptic symptoms but may be involved in the pathogenesis of peptic ulcer and possibly gastric carcinoma.

Eosinophilic Gastritis

This may occur on its own or as a component of eosinophilic gastroenteritis, the features of which are discussed on p. 718.

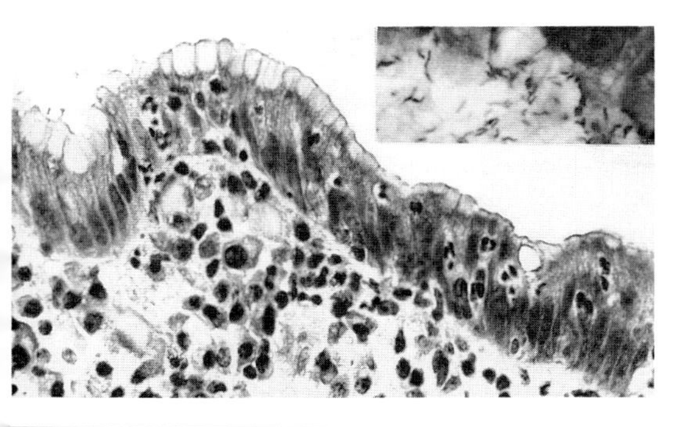

Fig. 16.19 *Helicobacter pylori* associated chronic gastritis (type B). The foveolar epithelium in acutely inflamed and in the underlying lamina propria there is a mixed acute and chronic inflammatory cell reaction: the causal organisms can just be visualized on the surface but are shown at a higher power in the inset.

Lymphocytic Gastritis

In this recently described entity the body of the stomach is usually involved and may be afflicted by persistent multiple mucosal erosions often surrounded by heaped up mucosa (varioliform gastritis). Histologically, the distinctive feature is the presence of an intense lymphocytic infiltrate within the surface and foveolar epithelium. These can be shown to be T cells. Some cases may represent a chronic reaction to *Helicobacter* infection, but the possibility of an unusual response to some local antigen has to be considered.

Granulomatous Gastritis

The presence of epithelioid cell granulomas in the stomach is now rarely attributable to tuberculosis or syphilis but may be associated with sarcoidosis, fungal infection and occasionally with peptic ulceration or carcinoma. The appearance of granulomas located mainly in the glandular zone of an otherwise normal gastric mucosa is also by no means rare in Crohn's disease. Granulomatous gastritis may also be encountered as an apparently isolated lesion: whether or not this represents a limited form of Crohn's disease remains to be determined.

Reflux Gastritis

Reflux of duodenal contents (including bile) into the stomach produces a histologically distinctive form of distal gastritis characterized less by the infiltration of inflammatory cells than by oedema and congestion of lamina propria mucosa and elongation and tortuosity of the gastric pits – foveolar hyperplasia. The role of this lesion in the aetiology of dyspepsia remains, however, controversial. A similar form of foveolar hyperplasia, associated with cystic dilatation of gastric glands and thickening of the lamina propria may be found in the vicinity of gastrojejunostomy stomas.

Peptic Ulcer

This common and important lesion is a distinctive form of ulceration which only develops in sites exposed to the action of gastric secretions. Most important of these is the stomach itself, the duodenum, the jejunum (following gastrojejunostomy or in Zollinger–Ellison syndrome), the distal oesophagus and Meckel's diverticulum in which there is heterotopic gastric mucosa (p. 719). Peptic ulcers exist in two main forms: the acute peptic ulcer which penetrates the lamina muscularis mucosae but does not extend more deeply than the submucosa, and the chronic peptic ulcer which penetrates the full thickness of the muscularis propria and has its base in the serosal layer of the organ involved or outwith the gut altogether.

Acute Peptic Ulcer

This can arise at any age and is usually related to stress in the form, for example, of severe burns (Curling's ulcer) or brain damage (Cushing's ulcer). Analgesic drugs such as aspirin may be implicated in some cases. Gastric haemorrhage is the usual form of clinical presentation and may be severe if a large submucosal artery becomes eroded. The lesions, usually 1–2 cm in diameter (seldom more) are commonly multiple and usually located either in the first part of the duodenum or in any part of the stomach. Should the lesions heal scarring is seldom evident.

Chronic Peptic Ulcer

The incidence of this lesion in its most common sites, viz. the stomach and duodenum, has shown substantial variation over the last 100 years, at least in Western countries. Both gastric and duodenal ulcers became extremely common in the early decades of the century, ultimately affecting almost 20% of all adult males in the UK at one time or another. The incidence has decreased considerably in recent years. The disease affects adults at any age but gastric ulcers are now particularly common in the older age groups especially in females. In general, however, duodenal ulcer is still more common and predominantly affects males. In uncomplicated cases post-prandial epigastric pain (dyspepsia) is the usual presenting symptom of peptic ulcer disease.

Macroscopic Features

The location of chronic peptic ulcers is decidedly restricted. In the stomach most are found at the junctional zone between antrum and body on the lesser curvature. In women this zone may extend so far proximally as to reach almost the cardia and ulcers correspondingly tend to be found high on the lesser curvature. In males, however, this zone is located more distally and many ulcers arise much nearer to the pylorus (prepyloric ulcers). The duodenum, however, is more often affected in males, much less so in females, but only the first 2.5 cm (the duodenal bulb) is involved as a rule. Chronic peptic ulcer is usually a solitary lesion. Sometimes there are two, seldom more. In the duodenum there may be ulcers on both the anterior and posterior walls ('kissing ulcers'). Occasionally a duodenal ulcer may be associated with a gastric ulcer, the distal lesion usually coming first. Most chronic ulcers measure between 1 and 3 cm in diameter but some are very much larger. They are usually circular or ovoid in shape and have a punched out appearance, the gastric rugae often appearing to converge upon the ulcer margin (Fig. 16.20). The walls of the ulcer crater usually shelve steeply but some show more shallow extensions if there has been recent ulcerative activity. The ulcer base may lie in the gastric or duodenal serosa but in many instances the ulcer erodes into the adjacent structures such as pancreas or liver.

Microscopic Features

Histologically, peptic ulcers have a distinctive appearance (Fig. 16.21). On the surface is a layer formed by neutrophils and structureless haematoxyphilic bodies which probably represent dead neutrophils. This overlies a zone of fibrinoid necrosis which, at a deeper level, becomes organized by granulation tissue. This in turn becomes

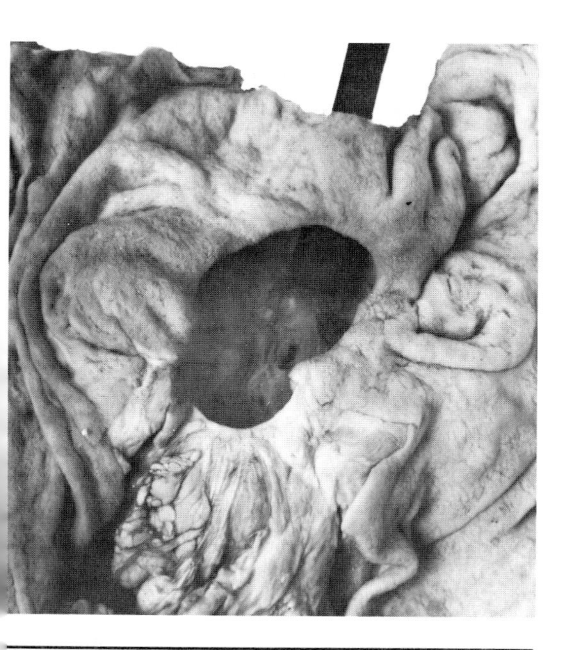

Fig. 16.20 Large chronic ulcer of duodenum just beyond the pylorus. The ulcer had perforated at the margin, as indicated by the pointer.

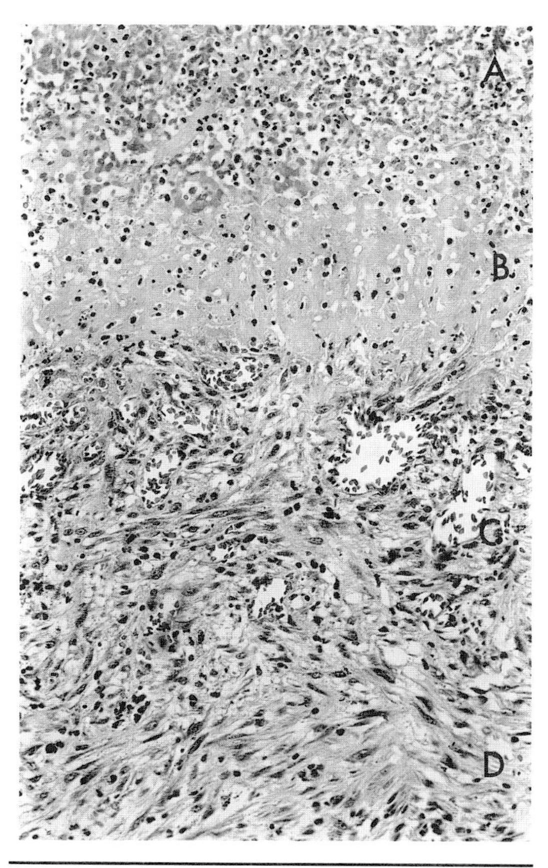

Fig. 16.21 Peptic ulcer. The base of the ulcer consists, from the lumen outwards, of a neutrophil layer, including many dead cells (A), a zone of fibrinoid necrosis (B), a layer of granulation tissue (C) and an outer layer of fibrous tissue (D). H & E ×153.

converted to fibrous scar tissue which extends into surrounding structures. As previously mentioned, in a chronic ulcer the muscularis propria of the organ involved is completely penetrated and its severed edge is to be found in the lateral wall of the ulcer. Sometimes this edge fuses with the lamina muscularis. There may be surprisingly little inflammatory reaction around peptic ulcers although some lymphocytes, plasma cells and eosinophils are usually found. Arteries in the base of the ulcer commonly show endarteritis obliterans. In the mucosa surrounding gastric ulcers, however, there is invariably evidence of chronic type B gastritis often accompanied by active gastritis and intestinal metaplasia. There may also be active mucosal inflammation around duodenal ulcers (duodenitis). At the edge of ulcers there is often evidence of mucosal regeneration and commencing re-epithelialization of the ulcerating surface. Healing of a chronic peptic ulcer will restore mucosal continuity but some scarring of the underlying submucosa and muscularis mucosa invariably persists.

Complications of Chronic Peptic Ulceration

Healing and scarring. Healing will restore mucosal continuity but some scarring of the underlying submucosa and muscularis mucosa invariably results. Contraction of the fibrous tissue may have serious effects. Most important of these is **pyloric stenosis** which may follow ulceration in the duodenal bulb or the prepyloric area and may provoke recurrent vomiting with dehydration and chloride depletion which is compensated by a rise in plasma bicarbonate. Extracellular potassium loss may be superadded so that biochemically there is hypokalaemic alkalosis. Narrowing may also take place at a higher level in the stomach in association with more proximally located gastric ulcers producing an 'hour-glass deformity' best seen on radiological examination.

Haemorrhage of some degree is an almost inevitable consequence of peptic ulceration; that it does not take place in overt form more often is due to the development of endarteritic changes in advance of the ulcerative process. The erosion of small blood vessels in the granulation tissue zone surrounding an ulcer frequently leads to the development of iron-deficiency anaemia (p. 616) and involvement of a larger submucosal artery (Fig. 16.22) in a rapidly advancing ulcerative process may cause more clinically evident bleeding as revealed by melaena or haematemesis. The most serious, and often life threatening type of haemorrhage takes place when a major artery becomes eroded. In the case of gastric ulcers on the lesser curvature, for example, the left gastric artery may be affected whilst with posteriorly located ulcers in the duodenal bulb it is the gastroduodenal artery which is at hazard. Haemorrhage from such a source is unlikely to cease naturally since the vessel is often embedded in the fibrous tissue reaction and is unable to contract properly. It is true that thrombus may form in the vessel lumen especially if there is a fall in blood pressure but when this is rectified by blood transfusion the thrombus is likely to become displaced and bleeding will recommence. Recourse to surgery is inescapable in such circumstances.

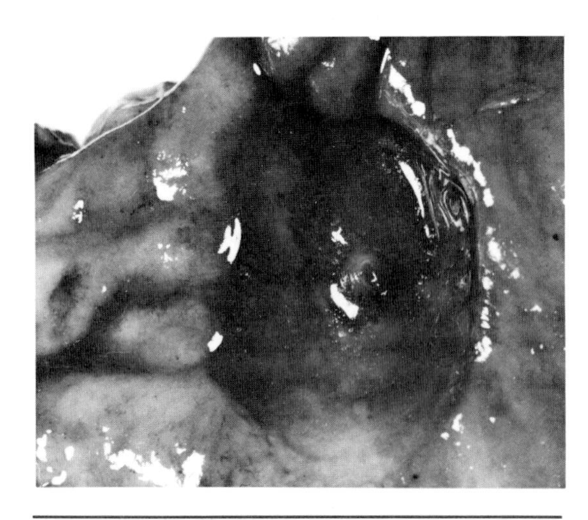

Fig. 16.22 A chronic gastric ulcer, showing an eroded artery from which fatal haemorrhage occurred.

Perforation. Perhaps the most clinically dramatic consequence of chronic peptic ulceration is perforation of the affected viscus with the escape of the gut contents into the peritoneal cavity. This is especially likely to happen with anteriorly located ulcers in the duodenal bulb but it may also complicate gastric ulcers. Perforation is most likely to take place if the ulcerative process advances rapidly and there is little time for a protective fibrous tissue mantle to develop in the serosal layers of gut. The material entering the peritoneal cavity is usually acidic and acts as a peritoneal irritant evoking severe abdominal pain; it is also potentially infective and acute peritonitis inevitably follows. Should such material enter the lesser sac (as may be the case with lesser curve gastric ulcers) it tends to track upwards behind the liver and may ultimately result in the development of a subphrenic abscess. It should also be noted that the presence of escaped gas under the diaphragm is an important radiological sign of perforation.

Development of carcinoma. Whilst the development of carcinoma in the regenerating epithelium at the margin of a chronic gastric ulcer is a well documented phenomenon it is probably an uncommon event, complicating less than 1% of such ulcers. It seems likely that the lesions which precede chronic peptic ulcer (? chronic gastritis) may also predispose to carcinoma and their concurrence on occasion is thus not surprising. Carcinoma never develops in a chronic duodenal ulcer.

The Aetiology and Pathogenesis of Chronic Peptic Ulcer

These are still far from clear. It seems improbable that the cause of chronic ulcers is the same as that of stress related acute peptic ulcers. However, the striking variations in chronic peptic ulcer incidence observed during this century suggest that environmental influences must be operating and psychological stress could well be one of these. Moreover, cigarette smoking and analgesic ingestion are widely regarded as at least contributory factors. Genetic factors might also be implicated. There is a relatively high incidence of duodenal ulceration in individuals who do not secrete blood group substances into their gastric juice and belong to blood group O. Chronic duodenal ulcer may be familial and there is a higher concordance in monozygotic as compared with dizygotic twins. The possibility that gastric ulcer and duodenal ulcer might have different causes is suggested by the fact that these diseases may segregate separately in families.

In pathogenetic terms, chronic peptic ulcer represents a disturbance of the normal balance between the potentially erosive effect of acid gastric juice and the resistance of the mucosal surface to this effect. In gastric ulceration gastric acid production is usually normal and may even be reduced and impaired mucosal resistance would appear to be the main problem. The cause of this is uncertain but chronic type B gastritis, possibly related to *H. pylori* infection and which is present in 70% of cases, may well be implicated. With regard to duodenal ulcer there is evidence that persistently high gastric acid levels, especially during the night, may be a major factor. In some instances there would appear to be failure of the normal feedback control of gastric acid secretion. A possible reason for this is that duodenal ulcer is invariably associated with chronic antral gastritis. Here again *H. pylori* infection may be involved since it is present in 90% of cases of duodenal ulcer. Furthermore, duodenal ulceration is commonly associated with the presence in the duodenum of metaplastic gastric epithelium, possibly an effect of acid hypersecretion, and this may be colonized by *H. pylori* with deleterious effects on mucosal resistance.

There is thus a possibility that *Helicobacter*-induced chronic antral or type B gastritis may be a crucial factor common to the development of both gastric and duodenal ulcers. In view of what was mentioned earlier, however, it is likely that additional factors determine where and when peptic ulcers might develop. The existence of such additional factors is suggested by the fulminating ulcer diathesis that may be produced by gastrinomas (the Zollinger–Ellison syndrome) and possibly other endocrine tumours which stimulate gastric acid secretion (p. 802). In this syndrome peptic ulcers occur not only in the common sites but also in unusual areas, e.g. the greater curvature of the stomach, the distal duodenum and the jejunum.

Tumours of the Stomach

Benign Tumours

The only benign connective tissue tumour at all common in the stomach is the **leiomyoma** which may arise either from the muscle coat or from blood vessels. Should such a tumour protrude into the gastric lumen it may become eroded and cause bleeding.

Benign epithelial **adenomas** usually take the form of sessile or pedunculated polyps and may give rise to gastric haemorrhage. Histologically, these tumours consist of abnormal glandular or papillary structures lined by epithelium, often of intestinal type and showing various degrees of dysplasia as revealed by nuclear crowding, hyperchromatism or loss of polarity. They have undoubted malignant potential (especially if they exceed 1 cm in diameter) but are decidedly rare. Most epithelial polyps in the stomach are non-neoplastic and show either foveolar or glandular hyperplasia (often both) accompanied by fibromuscular proliferation in the lamina propria – hyperplastic or regenerative polyps. Both neoplastic and regenerative polyps tend to be especially associated with chronic autoimmune (type A) gastritis.

It should also be noted that **inflammatory fibroid polyps**, lesions characterized histologically by the proliferation of fibrous tissue and blood vessels often associated with a pronounced eosinophilic infiltration, are almost certainly reactive rather than neoplastic. This lesion usually arises in the gastric submucosa and in its antral location may cause obstruction of the pyloric canal. Despite the eosinophilic infiltrate it does not appear to be associated with atopic allergy.

Gastric Carcinoma

Regrettably this is the most common gastric tumour. It carries a bad prognosis, less than 10% of patients surviving for more than 5 years after diagnosis, regardless of treatment. In global terms it is perhaps the most common fatal neoplasm but fortunately, it has been falling in incidence both in the UK and in the USA. In eastern Asia, especially Japan, in certain parts of South America especially Chile and other Andean countries, and in eastern and northern Europe including Iceland, gastric cancer still presents a formidable problem. The cause is unknown but dietary or other environmental factors operating from an early stage in life are currently thought to be important. A high incidence of gastric cancer has been associated with the consumption of salty or smoked foods or diets rich in fibre. Exposure of the stomach to large quantities of nitrates or nitrite is thought deleterious (due to the potential for the formation of nitrosamines) as are diets deficient in animal fat or meat. Dietary deficiencies may explain why the tumour also tends to be especially common in individuals of low socioeconomic status. Males are more often affected than females in the ratio of 3:2 and the disease usually arises in middle age or later adult life.

Premalignant Lesions

Certain gastric lesions appear to enhance the risk that carcinoma may develop. Mention has already been made of adenomas, and chronic type A autoimmune gastritis. Chronic type B gastritis may also be precancerous and could account for the occasional association between carcinoma and peptic ulcer already mentioned. An important feature of both main types of chronic gastritis is the appearance of intestinal metaplasia. Incomplete forms of this, in which goblet cells are found in association with atypical mucin secreting epithelium (Fig. 16.23) rather than enterocytes is thought by many to be especially associated with the development of carcinoma. Ménétrier's disease and gastric remnants remaining after gastric operations also appear to carry an enhanced risk of neoplasia. Recognition of such high risk conditions is important since it may be possible to detect the tumour at an early stage by regular endoscopic examination.

The early detection of gastric cancer. In the UK unselected population screening is probably not practicable but the delineation and regular endoscopic surveillance of high risk groups (e.g. post-gastrectomy states, chronic autoimmune gastritis) may be justified. Endoscopists are becoming more skilled in the recognition of suspicious lesions and the identification by histological and cytological means of dysplastic change or early carcinoma (i.e. tumours which have not invaded more deeply than the submucosa) may improve the outlook of the disease, as has happened in some parts of Japan.

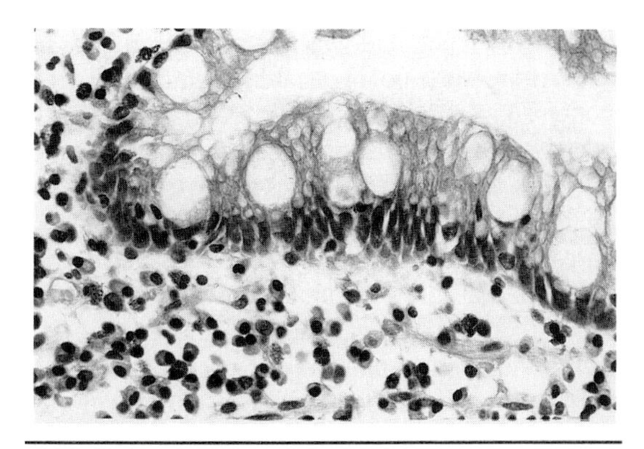

Fig. 16.23 Intestinal metaplasia, incomplete. Goblet cells are found in an epithelium consisting mainly of atypical mucoid cells. H & E × 300.

Clinical Features

The initial symptoms of gastric carcinoma tend to be ill-defined: there is often little more than vague malaise, anorexia or weight loss. Symptoms due directly to tumour growth such as those caused by pyloric or oesophageal obstruction or frank haematemesis may only occur late in the course of the disease. This explains why the tumour has usually reached an advanced stage before the diagnosis is made. Indeed the appearance of metastasis (as revealed for example by enlargement of peripheral lymph nodes) may be the first indication of the disease. Anaemia may also be a presenting feature: this may be of iron-deficiency type (due to gastric blood loss), megaloblastic type (due to coexistent pernicious anaemia), leuco-erythroblastic type (due to bone marrow metastasis) or haemolytic (due to low grade disseminated intravascular coagulation provoked by mucin released by tumour cells in the vicinity of blood vessels).

Pathological Features

Carcinoma may arise in any part of the stomach but most tumours appear to primarily involve the antrum. In a substantial and increasing number of cases the cardiac region is the site of origin. Most tumours of the intestinal type are exophytic in that their growth is directed mainly towards the lumen with the eventual formation of large fungating masses which are usually ulcerated (Fig. 16.24). The more diffuse histological types, on the other hand, tend to be endophytic with growth penetrating deeply into the stomach wall and often showing pronounced lateral spread, producing marked and extensive thickening of the gastric wall (leather bottle stomach or linitis plastica); there may or may not be ulceration in such cases (Fig. 16.25).

Histologically, the tumour almost always presents the features of a mucin secreting adenocarcinoma, but the appearances are very variable even in individual cases. There appears to be two

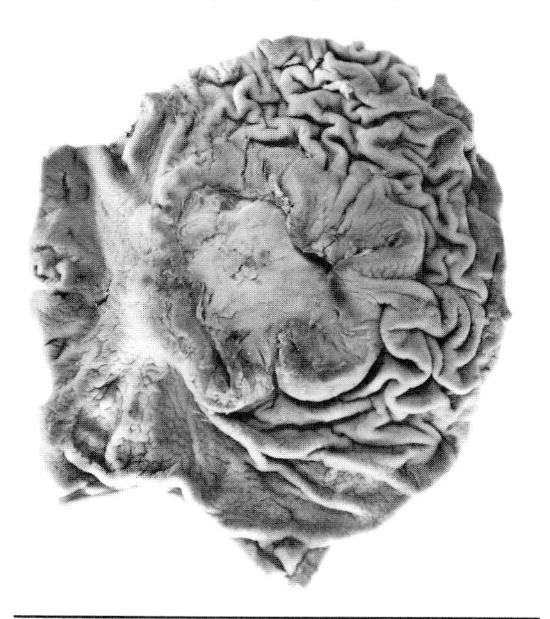

Fig. 16.24 Ulcerating scirrhous carcinoma of stomach, with thickened, raised margin and ulcerated base.

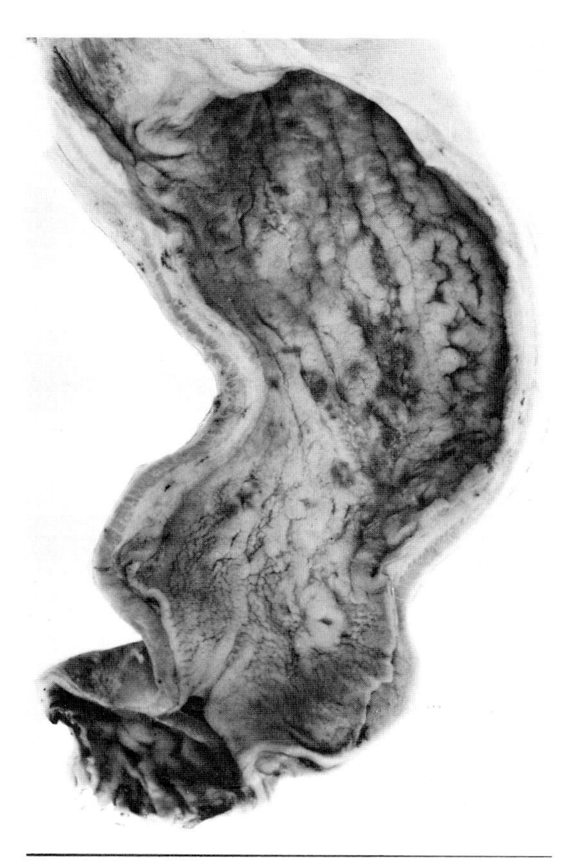

Fig. 16.25 Diffuse carcinoma of stomach. Note the general thickening of the wall without a localized tumour mass and with little ulceration.

main types, which form the basis of the Lauren classification. In the first the formation of glandular structures is the predominant feature, the appearances resembling colonic adenocarcinoma (Fig. 16.26). This type is associated with the presence of metaplastic intestinal epithelium and is the predominant type in areas with a high incidence of gastric carcinoma. In the second type the tumour exhibits a more diffuse infiltrative pattern: gland formation is often minimal and the neoplastic infiltrate takes the form of sheets of cells lying singly or in small groups. The cells may be distended with mucin with compression of the nucleus (**signet-ring cells**, Fig. 16.27). Both types may be preceded by a phase of intraepithelial or intramucosal neoplasia (often referred to as dysplasia) which is characterized by distortion of the normal mucosal gland pattern and varying degrees of epithelial atypia as revealed by impaired differentiation, nuclear crowding, nuclear hyperchromatism, loss of polarity and abnormal mitotic activity.

Spread of the tumour. Gastric carcinoma tends to spread rapidly and by a number of different routes. Local spread to adjacent organs, for example the greater or lesser omentum, duodenum or lower oesophagus, is often conspicuous. Especially with diffuse carcinomas there may be extensive spread within the peritoneal cavity, and in females (usually in the reproductive era) the ovaries may be conspicuously affected (so-called Krukenberg tumours (p. 1034). Whether or not this kind of spread is due to the exfoliation of cells into the peritoneal cavity (transcoelomic spread)

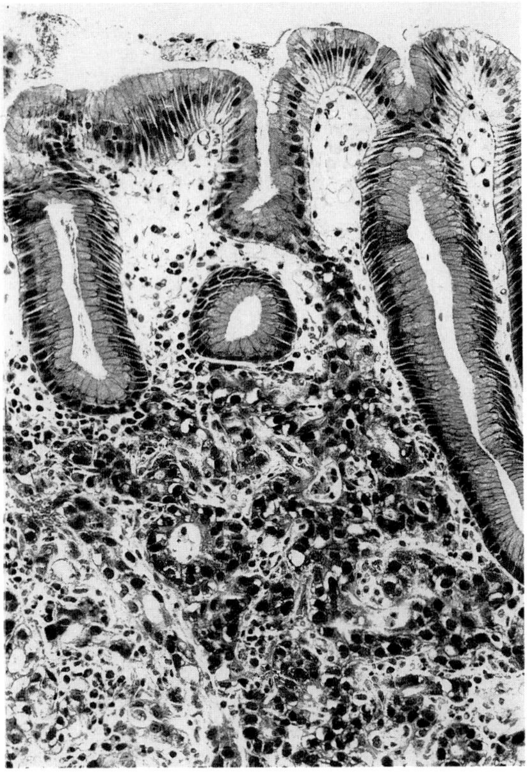

Fig. 16.26 Stomach. The mucosa is infiltrated by an adenocarcinoma showing considerable glandular differentiation ('intestinal' type). H & E ×150.

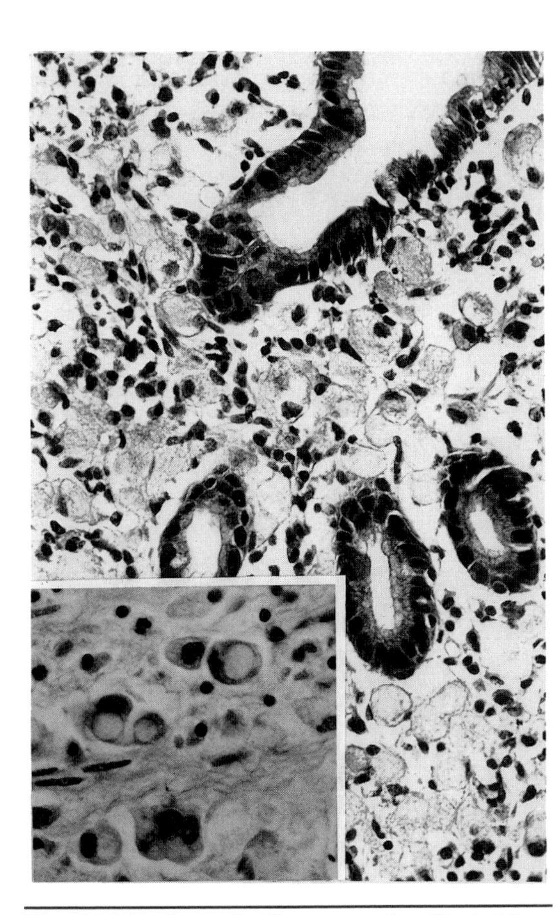

Fig. 16.27 Stomach. The mucosa is infiltrated by a carcinoma with extensive signet-ring cell differentiation ('diffuse' type). H & E ×150.

or lymphatic permeation by tumour cells is debatable. Local lymph nodes, especially in the lesser omentum, are often involved at an early stage and commonly there is spread to more distant nodes, for example the supraclavicular group. Lastly, spread by the bloodstream to such sites as liver, lung, brain and bone marrow is all too often observed and may indeed be the initial sign of the disease.

Other Malignant Tumours of the Stomach

Malignant Lymphoma

Of all parts of the alimentary tract the stomach is the commonest site of primary, as opposed to metastatic lymphoma. The more aggressive variants produce large lobulated intraluminal masses sometimes preceded by rugal enlargement. Almost all are of B-cell origin and many belong to the so-called mucosa associated lymphoid tissue (MALT) group (p. 172). Histologically, these are characterized by a predominance of small lymphoid cells (centrocyte-like cells) which seem to take origin from the outer marginal zone of lymphoid follicles and subsequently invade and destroy the gastric epithelium to produce what are referred to as lymphoepithelial lesions (Fig. 16.28). It is important to recognize this neoplasm since it is a very indolent tumour and amenable to local surgical excision: only at a late stage does it become systematized.

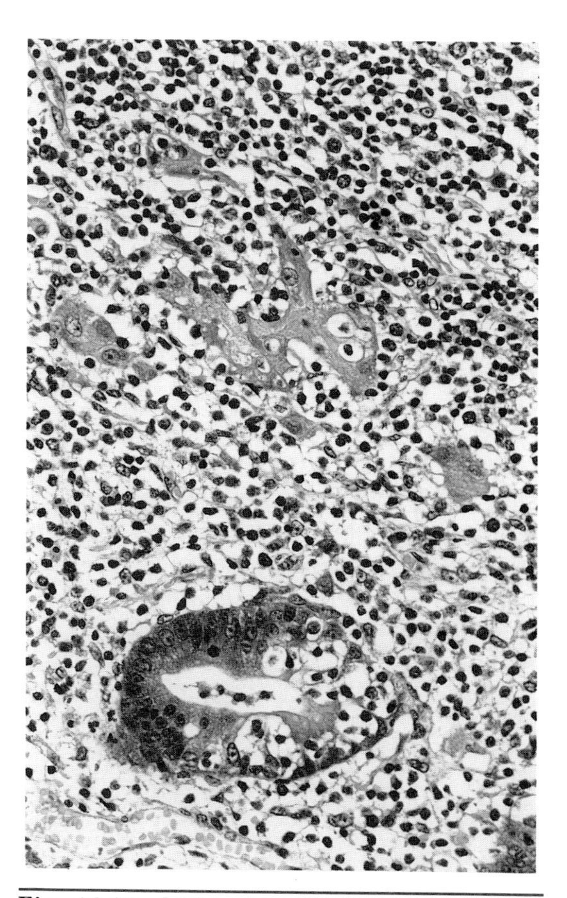

Fig. 16.28 Malignant lymphoma of stomach. The mucosa is overrun by lymphoid cells which are infiltrating and destroying the gastric epithelium ('lymphoepithelial' lesion). H & E ×257.

Carcinoid Tumours

Gastrointestinal carcinoid tumours are discussed in greater detail later. Gastric carcinoids may form globular tumours which tend to project into the gastric lumen and undergo ulceration. They may exhibit low-grade malignancy and metastasize to the liver. Histologically, they usually consist of packets or ribbon-like columns of uniform cells showing little mitotic activity. Some may secrete histamine and 5-hydroxytryptophane but endocrine effects are seldom evident clinically. Curiously, tumours of the gastric secreting G cells which are normally found in the gastric antrum are rare and most gastrinomas arise in the duodenum or pancreas. Multiple carcinoid tumours, sometimes showing low-grade malignancy, may complicate chronic autoimmune gastritis.

Leiomyosarcoma

Smooth muscle tumours in the stomach are usually benign but some show atypical histological features such as the presence of sheets or cords of cells with round nuclei and abundant clear cytoplasm (epithelioid leiomyomas) or large pleomorphic cells (bizarre leiomyomas). These are not necessarily more aggressive than ordinary simple leiomyomas but if they show more than the occasional mitotic figure they should be regarded with suspicion. Any smooth muscle tumour with more than five mitoses per 10 high power fields should be regarded as a leiomyosarcoma with the implication that it may metastasize either to the liver or to the lung. Histologically, such tumours will usually be highly cellular and show marked nuclear pleomorphism and hyperchromatism.

Miscellaneous Conditions

Congenital Abnormalities

Best known of these is **hypertrophic pyloric stenosis**, a condition which shows a marked male preponderance. It may well have a hereditary basis since the siblings and descendants of affected children often develop the disease and there is a high rate of concordance in monozygotic twins. It is characterized by pronounced circumferential thickening of the circular muscle of pylorus (Fig. 16.29), leading to recurrent vomiting, fluid depletion and failure to thrive. Surgical incision of the affected muscle (Ramstedt's operation) is usually effective in relieving the obstruction. Occasionally adults show a similar condition with only partial thickening of the pyloric muscle. In most cases pyloric stenosis in adults follows peptic ulceration. **Diverticula** occur in the pyloric and fundal region but are rare. Congenital **'hour-glass' contraction** may occur, but this lesion is more often the result of scarring around a chronic gastric ulcer.

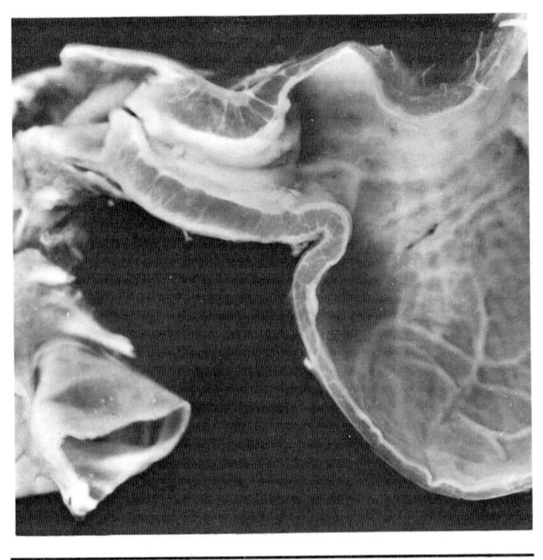

Fig. 16.29 Congenital stenosis of pylorus. The anterior wall at the pylorus has been cut away to show the greatly hypertrophied muscle at the pyloric antrum.

Hyperplastic Gastropathy

This term is applied to certain rare conditions of unknown aetiology in which there is localized or diffuse enlargement of the gastric rugae due to expansion of the foveolar or glandular zones of the gastric mucosa, sometimes both. This may or may not be associated with hypersecretory phenomena, and there is usually minimal inflammation so that the term gastritis is really inappropriate. Best known of these states is **Ménétrier's disease**, histologically characterized by diffuse foveolar hyperplasia and cystic change in the glandular zone which otherwise appears somewhat atrophic. Hypoalbuminaemia due to loss of protein into the gastric lumen is a notable feature of this disease and there is some evidence to suggest that there is an increased risk of gastric carcinoma. Gastric gland hyperplasia also occurs in patients with gastrinomas and the Zollinger–Ellison syndrome (p. 802).

The Intestines

The intestinal tract from the pylorus to the pectinate line in the anal canal has the same basic structure. The mucosal surface throughout is lined by columnar epithelium supported by a lamina propria which includes scattered leucocytic elements (mainly plasma cells) together with focal lymphoid aggregates (Peyer's patches) always most prominent in the distal part of the ileum. Between the mucosa and the submucosa is a thin layer of muscle, the lamina muscularis mucosae. The submucosa is free of epithelial elements, except for the mucus secreting Brunner's glands which are only found in the duodenum. The muscularis propria has an inner layer of circular muscle which is more or less continuous, and an outer layer of longitudinal muscle which, in the large intestine, is discontinuous and consists of three principal bands known as taenia coli.

The mucosa of the small intestine has a structure which reflects its vitally important function as the channel through which all nutrients finally gain entry into the body. It has two main compartments. The villus compartment includes virtually all the main functional elements, viz. the absorptive epithelial cells or enterocytes the population of which is reflected by the dimensions of the villi (Fig. 16.30). The basal compartment includes the crypts of Lieberkühn which are populated mainly by enterocyte precursor cells or stem cells from which the enterocyte population is continuously replenished in its entirety every 3 days or so. The crypts also include Paneth cells which produce lysosyme and may help to maintain the virtual sterility of the small bowel lumen. Even more important in this regard, however, is the rapid transit of material through the small bowel and which is dependent on the integrity of the musculature and its innervation. The large bowel has a more simple mucosal structure with a smaller enterocyte population reflecting its limited absorptive capacity (Fig. 16.31). On the other hand, mucin secreting goblet cells are much more nu-

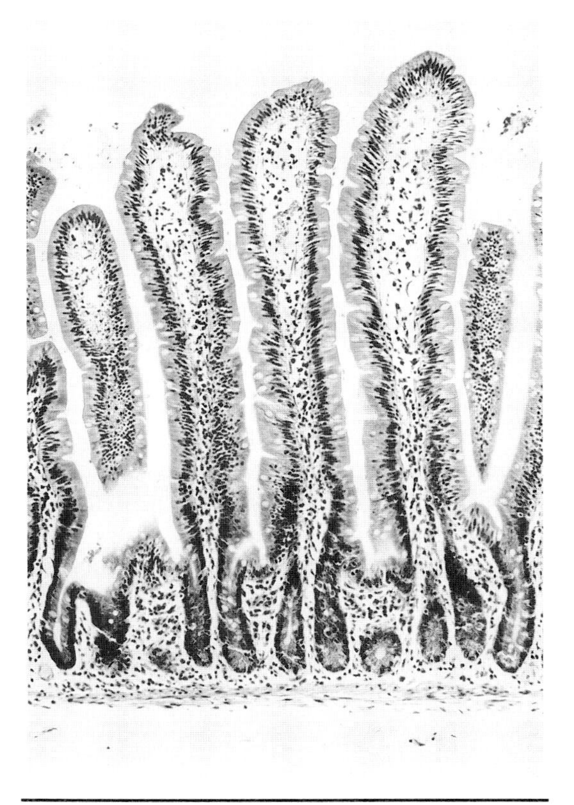

Fig. 16.30 Normal jejunal mucosa. Note that the finger-like villi are much longer than the crypts. H & E ×115.

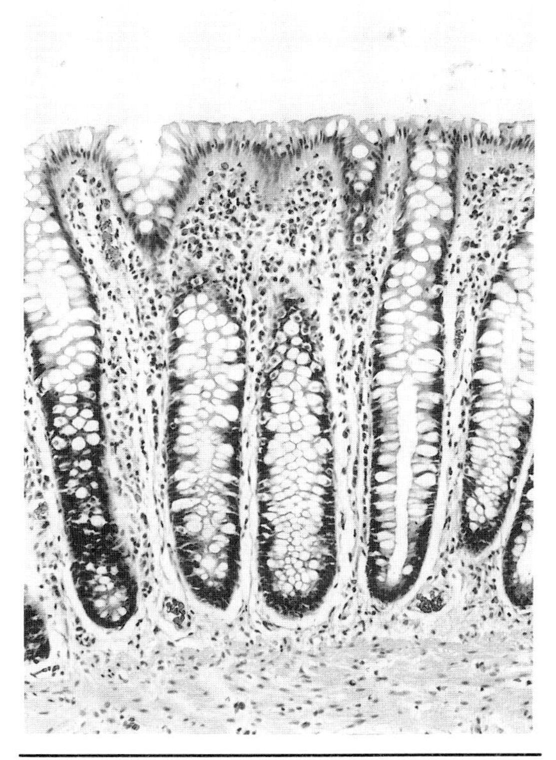

Fig. 16.31 Normal colonic mucosa. Inflammatory cells are found only in the upper part of the mucosa. H & E ×144.

merous, indicating the greater need for lubrication of the mucosal surface. Mucin may also exert a protective function: the colonic lumen of course sustains a large population of micro-organisms, many of which are potentially pathogenic.

Infective Diseases

In view of its exposed position it is hardly surprising that the intestine frequently shows inflammatory disturbance. Quite apart from the numerous primary infections which have ravaged mankind over the centuries it is to be noted that almost any kind of damage to the intestinal surface is likely to be exploited by the micro-organisms which normally inhabit the intestinal lumen.

Infective diseases, thus, constitute a common and important cause of morbidity in many communities, especially in the third world: even in industrialized societies, however, constant vigilance is required to keep these diseases under control. In pathological terms some produce highly distinctive changes (e.g. mycobacterial disease, typhoid fever) and occasionally the offending organism can be identified histologically (e.g. amoebiasis) or even with the naked eye (e.g. ascariasis). With most bacterial infections, however, the diagnosis is made using bacterial or immunological techniques. None the less, the presence of such infections may be suspected from the histological appearances of colorectal mucosal biopsies in particular. Typically these show acute reactive changes with oedema, congestion, haemorrhage and neutrophil infiltration in the lamina propria. Neutrophils may also traverse the epithelial lining of the crypts, sometimes forming small superficial crypt abscesses. As a rule plasma cells only become increased at a later stage in the process. There is seldom much distortion of the mucosal architecture and the changes tend to be self-limiting. Persistent changes should always raise the suspicion of chronic inflammatory bowel disease. It should be noted that not all infections are discussed here; some are more properly considered in the section on malabsorption. Parasitic diseases, including schistosomiasis, amoebiasis and other infestations are discussed in Chapter 25.

Salmonellosis

Organisms of salmonella species can produce lesions of varying severity in either the small or large intestine, sometimes both.

Typhoid Fever

This is undoubtedly the most dangerous form of salmonellosis. Human carriers provide the source of infection, there being no animal reservoir. Following the ingestion of food or water contaminated from such sources the offending organism, *Salmonella typhi*, a Gram-negative bacillus, penetrates the intestinal mucosa to gain entry into the lymphatics and the bloodstream and produce an initial bacteraemic phase in the disease process. This phase, during which systemic symptoms such as fever (with a progressive 'staircase rise'), a skin rash (rose spots) and sometimes lesions such as periostitis, perichondritis (involving the costal and laryngeal cartilage) or meningitis appear, lasts for about a week and over this period its true nature can only be diagnosed by blood culture. There is usually a leucopenia with a white cell count below 4 $\times 10^9$/l and the spleen is enlarged. The organism then reappears in the alimentary tract, possibly via bile excretion, its most favoured sites of settlement being the mucosal lymphoid aggregates in the distal small intestine, although solitary lymphoid follicles more proximally and distally are also affected. These then undergo explosive inflammatory swelling with the formation of ulcers which, being coterminous with the lymphoid tissue, tend to be round or ovoid in shape with their long axis parallel to the direction of intestinal flow (Fig. 16.32). Histologically, the lesions show intense congestion and infiltration with lymphocytes and plasma cells; neutrophils are virtually absent. Necrosis frequently takes place, the cell debris as well as extravasated red cells being taken up by histiocytes with abundant eosinophilic cytoplasm which form aggregates, so-called typhoid nodules. These inflammatory changes may extend deeply

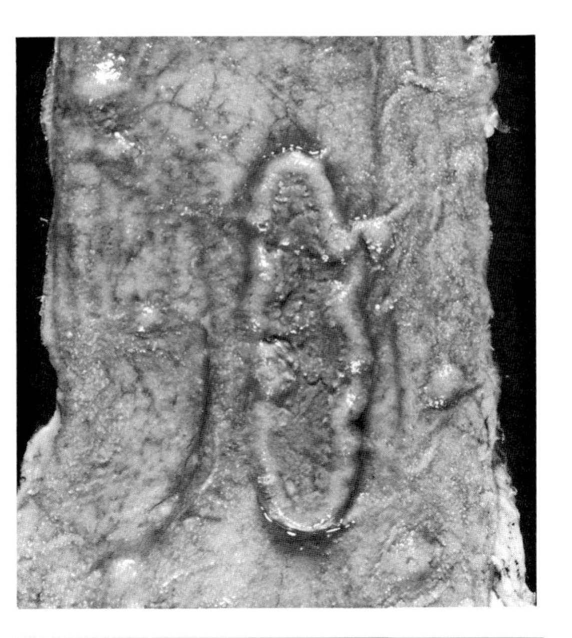

Fig. 16.32 The lower ileum in typhoid fever, showing necrosis and ulceration of the Peyer's patches and solitary lymphoid follicles.

into the intestinal submucosa and even into the muscularis propria: they may also be found in the mesenteric lymph nodes.

Such extensive lesions explain the most serious complications of the disease. These include severe intestinal haemorrhage due to erosion of a large submucosal blood vessel and perforation of the intestine or capsule of a lymph node with subsequent peritonitis, which despite its serious and often fatal consequences may produce few obvious symptoms. Intestinal stenosis rarely follows typhoid fever and with recovery mucosal healing is complete. During the intestinal phase (in which diarrhoeal symptoms become evident) the diagnosis can be readily made by stool culture and the serological Widal reaction (produced by antibodies capable of agglutinating the organisms in liquid suspension) becomes demonstrable. It is likely that the explosive nature of the intestinal lesions during this period represents a further expression of the immune response to the organism. Despite recovery from the acute phase of the disease, however, some individuals continue to excrete the organism in the faeces or less often in the urine. In most cases this carrier state is due to persistence of gallbladder infection (typhoid cholecystitis) probably initiated during the bacteraemic phase, and represents the reservoir from which all cases are directly or indirectly acquired.

Paratyphoid Infections

This disease, caused by one or other of the subtypes of *S. paratyphi*, is also an exclusively human affliction and its clinical and pathological features are very similar to those of typhoid albeit, in most cases, milder in degree and largely confined to the distal ileum. Here, too, the carrier state provides the reservoir of infection.

Salmonella Food Infection

This term is applied to a group of conditions with similar clinical features (usually including the acute onset of fever, abdominal pain and diarrhoea) caused by one or other of the numerous salmonella species, subtypes *S. typhimurium* and *S. enteriditis* being the best known, and which are derived from animal sources gaining access to food products. Whilst it is likely that both the small and large intestine become infected the lesions are best documented in the large bowel ('salmonella colitis') mucosal biopsies from which show the acute reactive features mentioned above. Despite the severe clinical effects and occasional systemic infective lesions these conditions are usually self-limiting: they may, however, be dangerous and even fatal in the elderly.

Cholera

This is a severe diarrhoeal disease caused by the curved Gram-negative bacillus *Vibrio cholerae*. Contamination of water supplies by this organism is usually involved and has led to explosive epidemics (even pandemics) in the past. The threat of this remains since the disease is still prevalent in several third world countries. The organism exerts its effects mainly upon the small bowel, where it may be present in massive numbers. They do not invade the bowel wall and obvious mucosal lesions are seldom conspicuous except possibly at the ultrastructural level. However, they produce a powerful endotoxin derived from the cell wall and which contains A and B subunits. The A subunit enters the enterocytes and acts as a powerful stimulus to adenyl cyclase activity. This enhances cyclic AMP formation and results in secretion of water and electrolytes into the intestinal lumen. This produces a colourless diarrhoea – 'rice-water' stool. Fluid depletion rapidly develops with hypervolaemic shock which, if not quickly corrected, leads to peripheral circulatory failure and death. While the organisms seldom seem to penetrate the intestinal mucosa they may persist in the gall-bladder and lead to a carrier state which provides the sole reservoir of this uniquely human disease.

Infantile Gastroenteritis

Severe diarrhoea with or without vomiting is particularly dangerous in infants and young children who can become rapidly dehydrated. In Western countries infections with strains of *Escherichia coli* have been shown to be responsible for many gastrointestinal illnesses of this kind. As with cholera the clinical effects of the infection with such organisms may be due to toxins but severe haemorrhagic inflammation, especially in the colon, has become increasingly recognized. Occasionally small bowel disease can lead to transient malabsorption due to a degree of villous atrophy. In older children infection with certain viruses, notably **rotaviruses** and **Norwalk viruses** may also lead to severe diarrhoeal illness followed by transient malabsorption.

Shigellosis

In global and historic terms bacillary dysentery, the disease caused by rod-shaped Gram-negative organisms of the *Shigella* species (*Shigella sonnei, Shigella flexneri* and *Shigella shigae*) is amongst the most common of all intestinal infections. The disease is transmitted by the faecal–oral, route the offending organism exerting its effects mainly in the large intestine. In children, however, the terminal ileum may be involved (ileocolitis). The typical dysenteric symptoms include debilitating diarrhoea, tenesmus (painful straining at defaecation) and the presence of blood or pus in the stools. Sigmoidoscopically, the large bowel shows pronounced mucosal congestion sometimes with focal erosions, but in severe cases there may be irregular and ragged ulceration. Histologically, the mucosa shows an acute inflammation sometimes with prominent crypt abscesses. Occasionally, colonic stricture follows severe or relapsing infection and a carrier state may also ensue.

Tuberculosis

Intestinal lesions in this disease are now rare in Western countries except in third world immigrants. Classically three main forms are recognized.

The primary complex (p. 303) was quite often located in the intestinal tract following the ingestion of milk contaminated with bovine tubercle bacilli. As in other sites, the primary lesion in the intestinal mucosa is inconspicuous, but there is pronounced enlargement of the mesenteric lymph nodes (**tabes mesenterica**) and in rapidly progressive cases spread to the peritoneal cavity. Pasteurization of milk and other measures have now virtually eliminated this process but enlarged calcified mesenteric nodes, indicative of a healed primary complex, are still seen in older adults.

Secondary tuberculosis. Ulceration may develop in the intestine, especially the ileum, if infected sputum from cavitating pulmonary lesions is swallowed, usually at an advanced stage of the disease. The lesions, exhibiting histologically the typical caseating epithelioid cell granulomas, may be localized initially in the lymphoid aggregates but later extend laterally to produce ragged undermined transversely disposed ulcers sometimes with nodular margins. Small nodules (tubercles) may be found on the serosal surface of the intestine and fistulous tracts may develop between intestinal loops producing short-circuiting of bowel contents and malabsorption.

Hyperplastic ileocaecal tuberculosis. As the name implies this form of the disease is characterized by pronounced inflammatory thickening producing obstruction in the vicinity of the ileocaecal valve. Pulmonary tuberculosis sometimes coexists and it is likely that this lesion represents a somewhat indolent version of the classic secondary form just described. It is still quite common in the Indian subcontinent, but now increasingly rare in UK natives. It should not be confused with Crohn's disease which may produce very similar ileocaecal lesions. A similar picture may also be produced in actinomycosis.

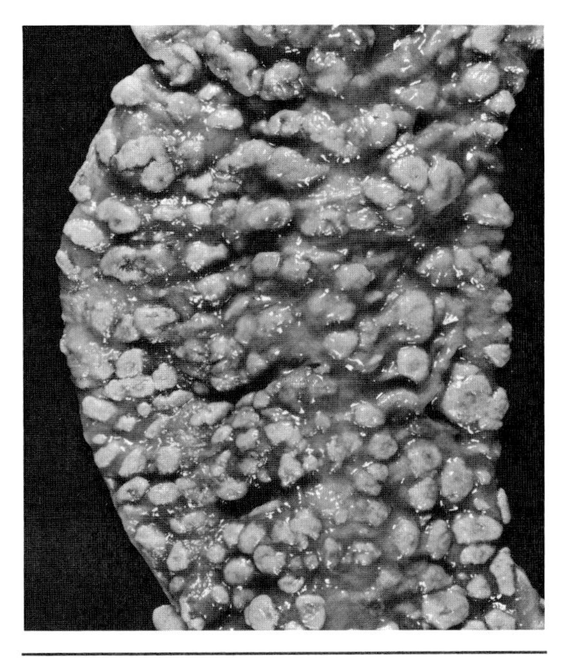

Fig. 16.33 Pseudomembranous colitis, showing the typical discrete raised patches of pseudomembrane and normal intervening mucosa.

Clostridial Disease

Anaerobic Gram-positive spore-forming bacilli belonging to *Clostridium* species (especially *Cl. perfringens*) may form part of the normal gut flora, but certain subtypes can cause severe necrotizing lesions in the ileum especially in states of privation. The ingestion of heavily infected porcine offal during wedding feasts in New Guinea causes the disease known as pig-bel. It is also possible that some cases of **neonatal necrotizing enterocolitis**, especially in premature infants, are due to an exploitation of intestinal hypoxic states by clostridia.

Pseudomembranous Colitis

In this disease foci of acute mucosal inflammation appear in the colon and sometimes in the distal ileum and can be identified sigmoidoscopally by the presence of discrete yellow plaques known as pseudomembranes (Fig. 16.33). While this phenomenon may be seen in a number of colitic diseases including shigellosis and ischaemic disease, it is usually due to the action of an exotoxin produced by *Clostridium difficile* in the gut lumen. Toxin formation by this organism, an occasional gut commensal, is promoted by the administration of certain antibiotics, e.g. lincomycin and ampicillin. The condition is thus, in most cases, an unusually severe expression of antibiotic-associated colitis. In elderly individuals the diarrhoea symptoms may be accompanied by a shock-like state which is often fatal. Histologically, the disease is initiated by damage to the colonic surface epithelium associated with neutrophil infiltration and an intense subepithelial fibrinous exudate which subsequently erupts through the mucosa to produce a fountain-like mass consisting of strands of fibrin enmeshed neutrophils. Often the crypts become occluded by exudate and become markedly dilated (Fig. 16.34). At a later phase toxin-mediated epithelial damage may extend to involve the full mucosal thickness.

Yersiniosis

Organisms of the species *Yersinia* are capable of producing a variety of clinical disturbances related

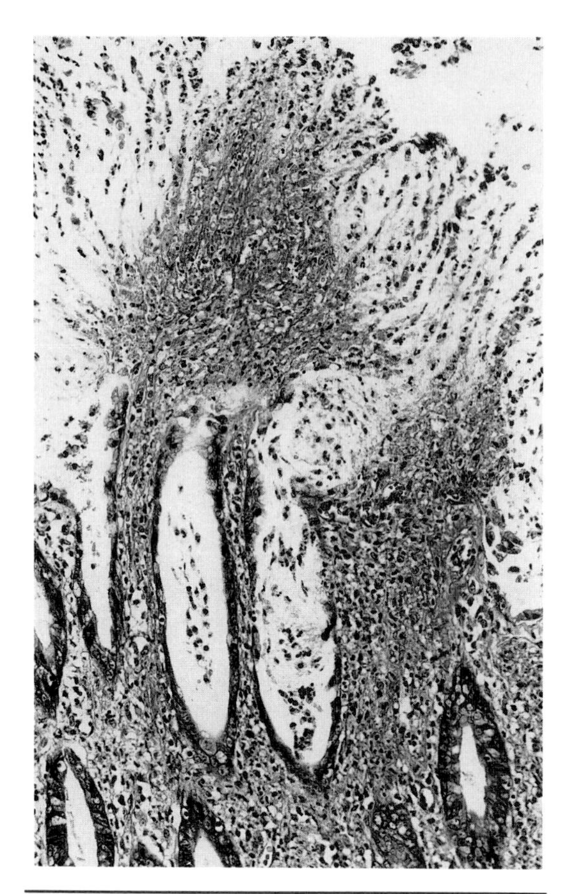

Fig. 16.34 Pseudomembranous colitis. The fountain-like purulent exudate arising from necrotic surface epithelium is characteristic. Note the crypt dilatation. H & E×153.

to the alimentary system. Best known of these is an appendicitis-like syndrome which may be due to acute inflammation of the appendix itself, acute terminal ileitis, or acute mesenteric adenitis. The last of these is usually caused by *Y. pseudotuberculosis* and is histologically characterized by irregular areas of suppuration surrounded by a palisaded, epithelioid, histiocytic reaction in which Langhans type giant cells may be present.

Actinomycosis

As a path of entry for the branching, colony-forming Gram-positive bacterium *Actinomyces israelii*, the intestine comes next to the mouth in order of frequency. The lesions consist of suppuration and ulceration of the wall of the gut, with a tendency to spread to involve the peritoneum or adjacent loops of gut, abdominal wall, etc. with formation of sinuses and fistulae. The wall of the appendix seems to be the most common portal of entry and spread to the wall of the caecum may occur. In the peritoneum, loculated abscesses between the coils of intestine may discharge into the bowel. Diagnosis can usually be made by finding colonies of *Actinomyces* on microscopic examination. Secondary actinomycotic abscesses may occur in the liver.

Campylobacter Infections

These are now well recognized as a cause of acute diarrhoeal illness, often associated with quite severe abdominal pain resembling appendicitis. In the UK, domestic animals (e.g. chickens) are thought to provide the reservoir for the infection. Initially it was thought that the small bowel was predominantly affected but an acute colitis is a commoner finding and mucosal biopsies reveal a typical acute inflammatory reactive pattern.

Sexually Transmitted Disease

Recent years have witnessed a striking increase in intestinal and especially colorectal infection transmitted as a result of anal intercourse in male homosexuals. Many of the above infections (salmonellosis, shigellosis, campylobacter) can be transmitted in this way as well as giardiasis (p. 1158) and viral infections such as herpes simplex. Proctitis caused by classic venereal diseases such as syphilis, gonorrhoea and lymphogranuloma venereum is also well recognized in homosexuals and should always be considered in the differential diagnosis of inflammatory bowel disease.

Idiopathic Inflammatory Bowel Disease

Sometimes simply referred to as inflammatory bowel disease (IBD) this term includes two major entities, ulcerative colitis and Crohn's disease. These are probably distinct conditions and will be discussed separately although some authorities believe that they represent differing expression of the same basic entity.

Ulcerative Colitis

This disease emerged as an entity during the latter part of the last century when it became apparent that there were serious forms of colitis which could not be attributed to a specific micro-organism. Ulcerative colitis is a chronic inflammatory process which, in definitive terms, is confined to the large intestine. Proctocolectomy effectively cures the disease. Individuals of any age from childhood onwards may be affected but the disease shows a predilection for young adults of either sex. Clinically, the main feature is diarrhoea associated at various times with the presence of blood, mucus or pus in the stools. The natural history of the disease is variable. Usually it pursues an intermittent course with exacerbations and remissions over many years but the symptoms may be continuous or unremitting from the outset. Some cases are mild and self-limiting. On occasion the disease can be acute and fulminating and sometimes rapidly fatal, even with the first attack of the disease. The aetiology is unknown. It seems improbable that a specific organism will be demonstrated. Some kind of autoimmune mechanism seems more likely although the evidence at present is tenuous: one possibility is that the disease arises in individuals who develop antibodies directed primarily towards enteric organisms but capable of cross-reacting with colonic epithelium. Corticosteroids administered systemically or locally can be effective in bringing about remission in many cases.

Pathological Features

Macroscopically, the disease primarily affects the rectum or sigmoid colon with variable extension proximally in a continuous fashion. The entire colon, including the appendix, is involved in 40% of cases. In some instances there may also be inflammation in the distal ileum, but this is thought to be of a reflux nature (backwash ileitis). Initially the diseased mucosa appears swollen and congested and bleeds readily when touched. Punctate erosions then appear and later give way to more extensive, irregularly disposed ulceration. Occasionally, ulceration is most prominent over the taeniae coli. In severe cases only a few islands of mucosa may survive, the ulcer bases consisting of a thin layer of granulation tissue overlying the circular muscle coat. Regenerative activity in surviving islands of mucosa, often accompanied by exuberant granulation tissue formation, may produce numerous intraluminal excrescences – pseudopolyps (Fig. 16.35).

Histologically, ulcerative colitis is primarily a disease of the colonic epithelium. The mucosa, during phases of disease activity, is congested and densely infiltrated with leucocytes. There is invariably evidence of recurrent epithelial damage and attempts at regeneration (Fig. 16.36a) as revealed by goblet cell depletion, irregularity of the crypts and crypt abscess formation (Fig. 16.36b). These abscesses are initiated by a focus of epithelial damage in the crypt lining through which neutrophils emigrate into the lumen and accumulate to such an extent as to produce crypt dilatation. Rupture of a crypt on to the luminal surface produces the erosions observed by the naked eye and is the herald of more extensive ulceration. The lamina propria mucosa shows intense plasma cell infiltration, associated with an increase in lymphoid aggregates in cases of long standing. Neutrophils may be observed marginating congested blood vessels and in the lamina propria. Sometimes eosinophils are also prominent. A common phenomenon is the herniation of inflamed mucosa into the underlying submucosa. Should a crypt abscess rupture in this location it may lead to extensive submucosal suppuration (lacunar abscess formation) with undermining of

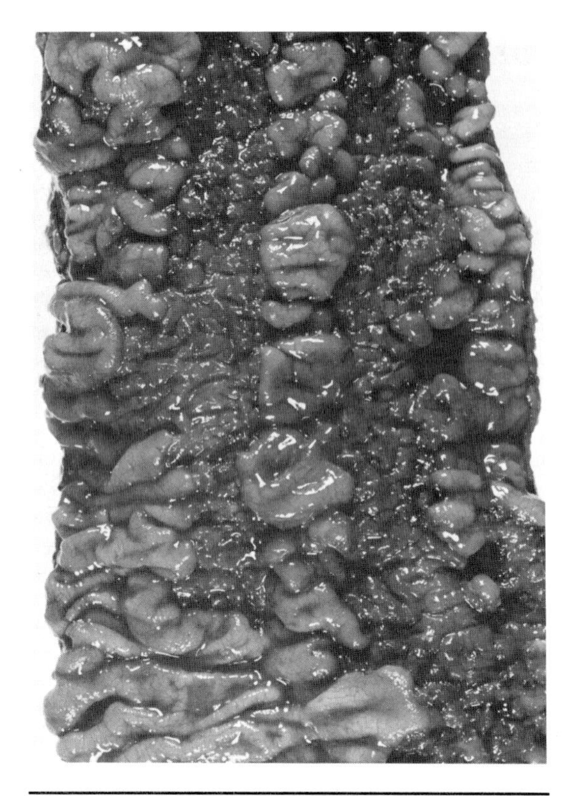

Fig. 16.35 The colon in chronic ulcerative colitis. The mucosa is extensively ulcerated and the surviving portions are swollen and hyperplastic with many undermined bridges of mucosa.

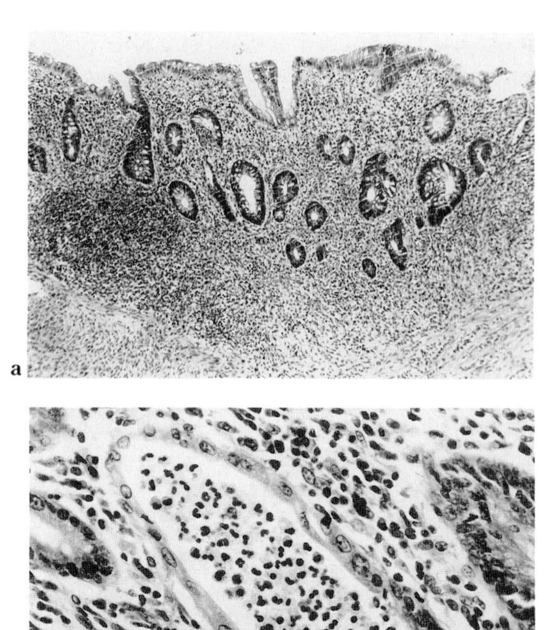

Fig. 16.36 **a** Ulcerative colitis. The colonic mucosa shows intense mucosal inflammation and there is goblet-cell depletion in the crypts which are irregular in disposition and widely separated from the lamina muscularis. H & E × 82. **b** Ulcerative colitis: crypt abscess. Note the dilatation of the crypt. H & E ×195.

the mucosa which may give way to produce extensive areas of ulceration. Another important change is Paneth cell metaplasia which, even if the disease goes into remission, remains as a marker of previous epithelial damage.

Complications

The most serious development is **toxic megacolon** during which the colon enters an atonic mode and becomes markedly thin and dilated. Perforation of the colon frequently follows and is often fatal. This change is associated with involvement of the muscularis propria in the deeply penetrating ulceration that may follow extensive lacunar abscess formation, and may be precipitated by antispasmodic drugs or secondary infection possibly provoked by steroid therapy. Simple stricture formation is surprisingly uncommon. On the other hand, **carcinoma** is a dangerous long-term complication especially when the disease involves the entire colon, appears early in life and has been present for 10 years or more. The cumulative hazard of carcinoma is 15% after the disease has been present for 30 years. Carcinoma may be preceded by a phase of intramucosal neoplasia (dysplasia) often arising in a flat (as opposed to a polypoid) mucosa and characterized by architectural and cytological epithelial atypia with nuclear pleomorphism, hyperchromatism, loss of polarity and increased mitotic activity. Detection of this change by regular endoscopy and biopsy is an indication for proctocolectomy before carcinoma develops.

There may be important **systemic complica-**

tions in addition to the anaemia and hypoproteinaemia which may follow persistent diarrhoea and blood loss. These include liver disease (e.g. primary sclerosing cholangitis and cholangiocarcinoma, p. 768), skin disease (e.g. pyoderma gangrenosum), arthritis including ankylosing spondylitis (p. 994), and iridocyclitis (p. 883). Some of these remit with remission of ulcerative colitis but others such as primary sclerosing cholangitis may progress independently of the colonic disease.

Crohn's Disease

The idea that there might be a chronic granulomatous disease of the intestine not attributable to tuberculosis only became accepted in the early 1930s but had been postulated long before that (Dalziel 1912). Initially it was thought that only the distal ileum was affected by the disease, hence the term regional ileitis as applied by Crohn *et al.* (1932). However, it is now realized that any part of the gut from the oral cavity to the anus and even sometimes extra-alimentary sites may be involved. Like ulcerative colitis the disease may arise at any age but young adults of either sex are predominantly affected. Clinically, however, the features are somewhat different. Obstructive symptoms (e.g. abdominal pain) tend to predominate and may be associated with pyrexia and a history of anorexia and weight loss, sometimes attributable to malabsorption. There may be diarrhoea if the colon is primarily afflicted. In contrast to ulcerative colitis surgical extirpation of the disease seldom if ever effects cure since the process has an unpleasant tendency to recur in 50% of patients.

The aetiology is unknown. The close resemblance to tuberculosis has sustained interest in the idea of a primary infective agent; recent studies suggest that this might well be so and that an atypical mycobacterium could be implicated. It remains possible, however, that patients with the disease have some kind of immunological deficit or abnormality which renders the gut unduly susceptible to organisms of low pathogenicity. In some instances this is a granulomatous vasculitis and thus the lesions could be ischaemic in nature.

Pathological Features

Macroscopically, what might be called the definitive lesions are discontinuous or patchy in distribution, the intervening gut seemingly being normal. Typically there is pronounced thickening of the gut wall with marked narrowing of the lumen and proximal gut distension due to obstruction (Fig. 16.37). The affected mucosa usually shows linear or laciform ulceration with intervening mucosal swelling producing a cobblestone appearance (Fig. 16.38). With small intestinal disease the mesentery may also be markedly swollen and the mesenteric lymph nodes enlarged. The site most commonly involved is the terminal ileum, often with extension to the ileocaecal valve and caecum. The colon may, however, be primarily affected as may on occasion other localities such as the oral cavity, oesophagus or upper small bowel.

Histologically, the inflammatory process typically involves all layers of the gut wall (i.e. it is

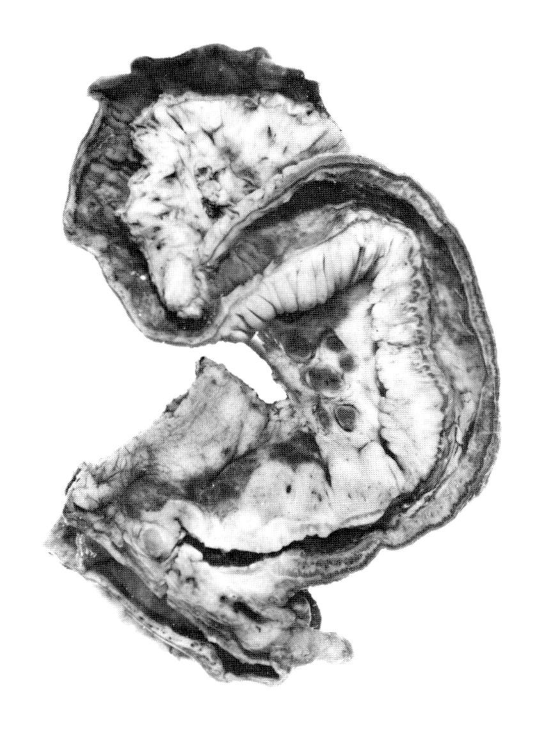

Fig. 16.37 Crohn's disease, showing diffuse thickening of the wall of the lower part of the ileum, with narrowing of its lumen.

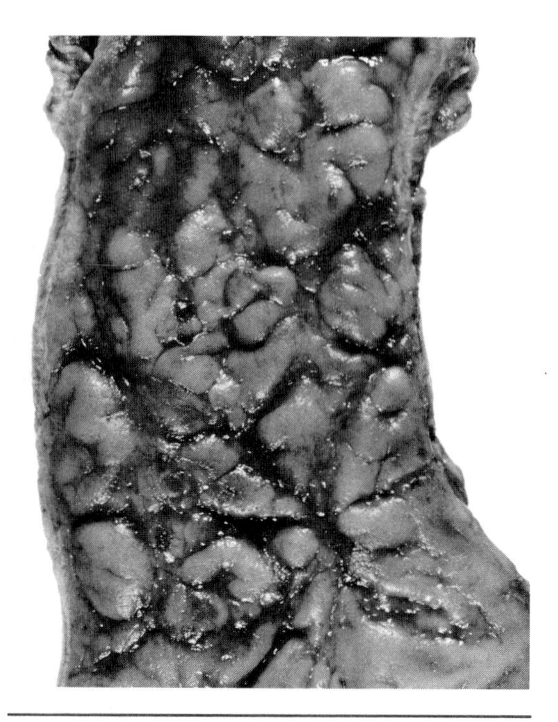

Fig. 16.38 The ileum in Crohn's disease, showing the 'cobblestone' appearance of the fissured, oedematous mucosa.

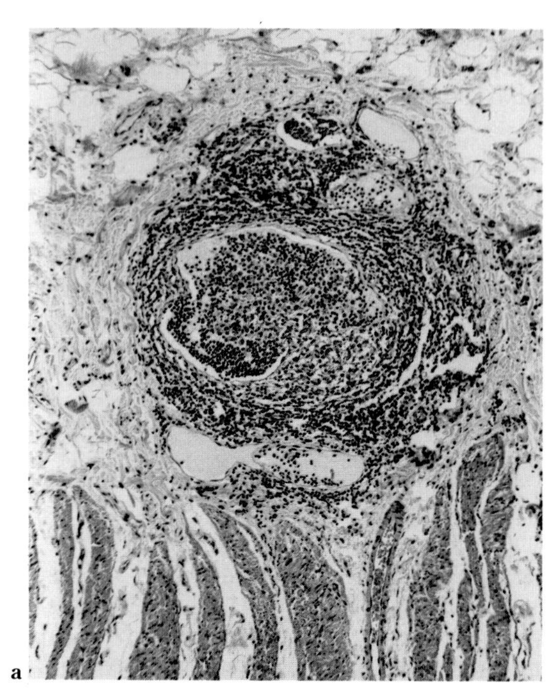

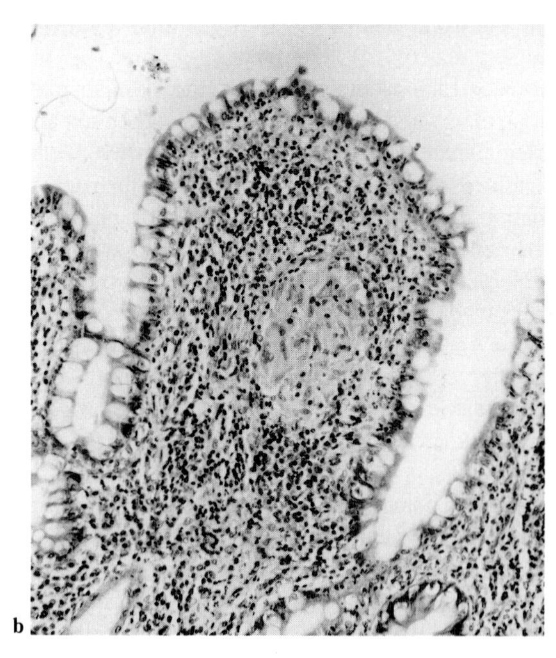

Fig. 16.39 **a** Crohn's disease. Lymphoid infiltration with early granuloma formation related to a lymphatic channel in the ileal submucosa. H & E × 71. **b** Crohn's disease. An epithelioid-cell granuloma is present in the ileal mucosa. H & E ×142.

transmural) and may extend into the mesentery. Focal lymphocytic infiltration is its most constant feature (Fig. 16.39a) but the formation of non-caseating epithelioid cell granulomas (Fig. 16.39b) is the diagnostic touchstone and may be seen, not just in the gut and mesentery, but also in the mesenteric lymph nodes. Both these phenomena are frequently related to lymphatics and may lead to lymphatic obstruction and dilatation. This is the likely explanation of the pronounced usually submucosal oedema which is mainly responsible, at least at first, for the thickening of the gut wall (Fig. 16.40). Later, fibrosis and more diffuse submucosal inflammation may be implicated. The involved mucosa usually shows a marked chronic inflammatory cell reaction, sometimes with crypt abscess formation and there may be superficial ulceration with the formation of intensely vascular granulation tissue. In many cases ulceration is associated with metaplasia of gastric type. Another important feature is the formation of deep fissures traversing the gut wall and sometimes

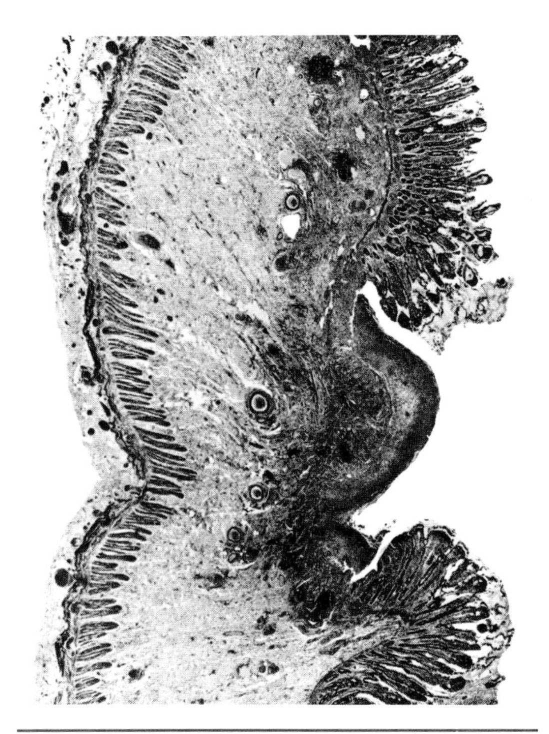

Fig. 16.40 Crohn's disease showing oedematous thickening, especially of the submucosa, with focal inflammatory infiltration and ulceration. ×10.

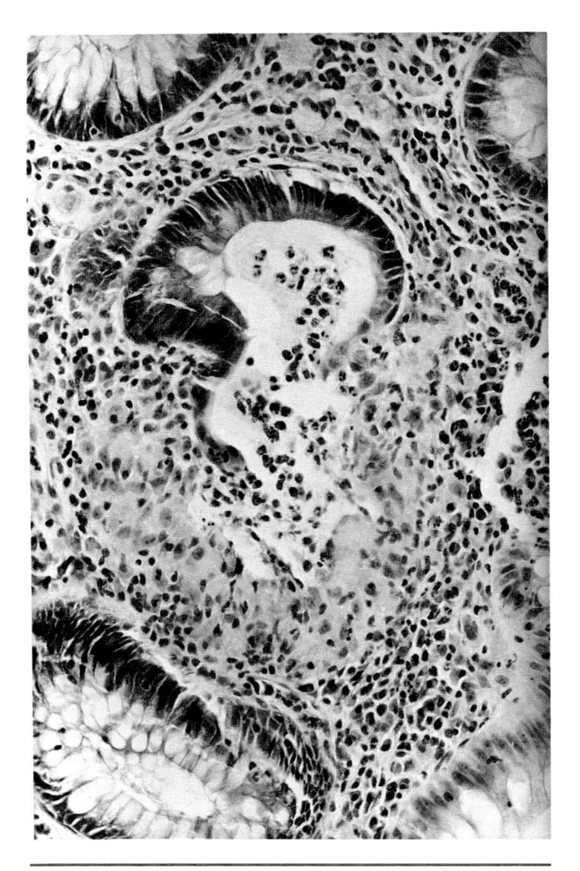

Fig. 16.41 Crohn's disease showing disruption of a crypt of the colonic mucosa and an associated epithelioid-cell granuloma. ×200.

giving rise to peri-intestinal abscesses; they may also be responsible for the development of fistulae. In some forms of the disease, especially in the colon, the mucosa may be predominantly and diffusely affected.

Characteristically in these cases there is a patchy non-specific chronic inflammatory reaction often without serious epithelial disturbance although granulomas may be detected and sometimes lead to crypt destruction (Fig. 16.41).

Complications

Reference has already been made to intestinal obstruction which, if not responding to conservative measures, may require surgical intervention. The development of fistulae especially between intestinal lesions and adjacent structures (including the skin surface) is unfortunately common, perianal fistulae which often accompany colonic Crohn's disease being particularly troublesome. Extensive disease of the terminal ileum may lead to bile salt depletion, causing steatorrhoea and predisposing to gallstones, or to impaired vitamin B_{12} absorption leading to megaloblastic anaemia (p. 612). Anaemia may also result from blood loss from ulcers or from impaired folic acid absorption. More serious nutritional problems may arise if extensive upper small bowel disease results in a generalized state of malabsorption. It is now recognized that Crohn's disease may predispose to the development of carcinoma in both the small and large bowel and, as in ulcerative colitis, may be preceded by dysplastic epithelial changes (Fig. 16.42). Systemic symptoms such as arthritis, skin disease, iridocyclitis and primary sclerosing cholangitis are also occasionally observed in Crohn's disease.

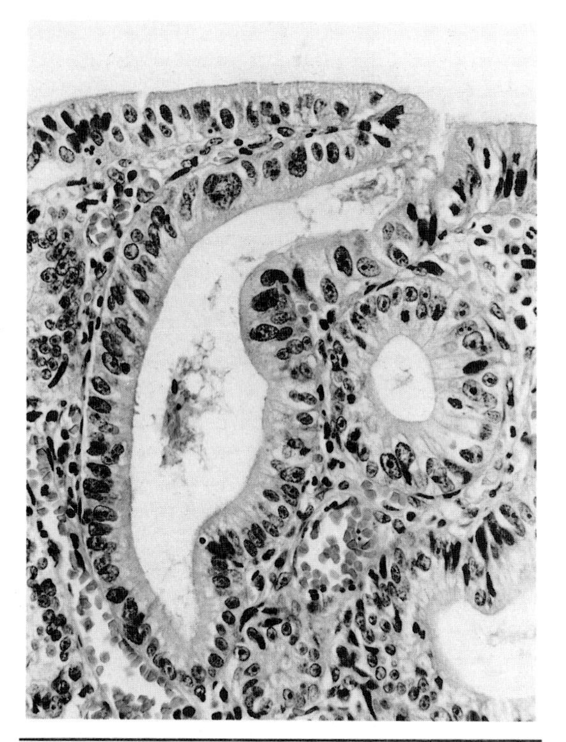

Fig. 16.42 Crohn's disease. There is a dysplastic change in the surface epithelium of the ileal mucosa. H & E ×326.

Appendicitis

The appendix may be involved in some of the diseases which afflict other parts of the large intestine including infections such as yersiniosis, tuberculosis and inflammatory bowel disease. The term acute appendicitis, however, is applied to the distinct entity characterized by acute transmural inflammation with peritonitis, and clinically by the acute onset of abdominal pain, initially periumbilical, but later shifting to the right iliac fossa where it is accompanied by the classic sign of 'rebound' tenderness.

The causation of this condition is far from clear. It is not primarily infective in origin. Many investigators would take the view that the initial event in most cases is outflow obstruction at or near the appendicular orifice. If, in a blind-ended structure like the appendix, this is sustained for any length of time there will inevitably be a rise in intraluminal pressure which could lead to mucosal ischaemia and eventual breakdown, with entry into the deeper structures of the potentially pathogenic organisms normally found in the colonic lumen. It is not hard to imagine that if an organism such as *Streptococcus faecalis* were to be given this opportunity, rapidly spreading cellulitis with peritoneal involvement might follow. Several other organisms, for example *E. coli*, and *Bacterioides* species may, however, be implicated. The cause of the initial episode of obstruction is uncertain. In some cases hard or calcified faecal matter (faecoliths) can be incriminated but other factors such as swelling of the mucosal lymphoid tissue due to viral infection, or infestation by *Oxyuris vermicularis* may be involved. It is also possible that, as in diverticular disease, dietary factors and in particular deficiency of dietary fibre could be of importance. Appendicitis has a high incidence in Western countries, children and young adults being especially affected, but it is still relatively uncommon in most tropical countries.

Pathological Features

Macroscopically (Fig. 16.43a), an acutely inflamed appendix is markedly swollen and intensely congested: the peritoneal surface is invariably roughened and may be covered by yellow plaques of fibrinous exudate. In unusually severe cases the appendix may be green or black in colour – gangrenous appendicitis.

Histologically, there is mucosal ulceration (Fig. 16.43b) with focal or extensive neutrophil infiltration in all the main layers of the appendicular wall (transmural inflammation) and including the serosa. There is often frank abscess formation. Not uncommonly, acute inflammation is found to be limited either to the mucosa or the serosal coat of the appendix. Limited mucosal inflammation is of doubtful clinical significance since it may be found incidentally (e.g. in appendices removed prophylactically during cholecystectomy). However, limited serosal inflammation invariably indicates the presence of acute inflammation elsewhere in the abdominal cavity.

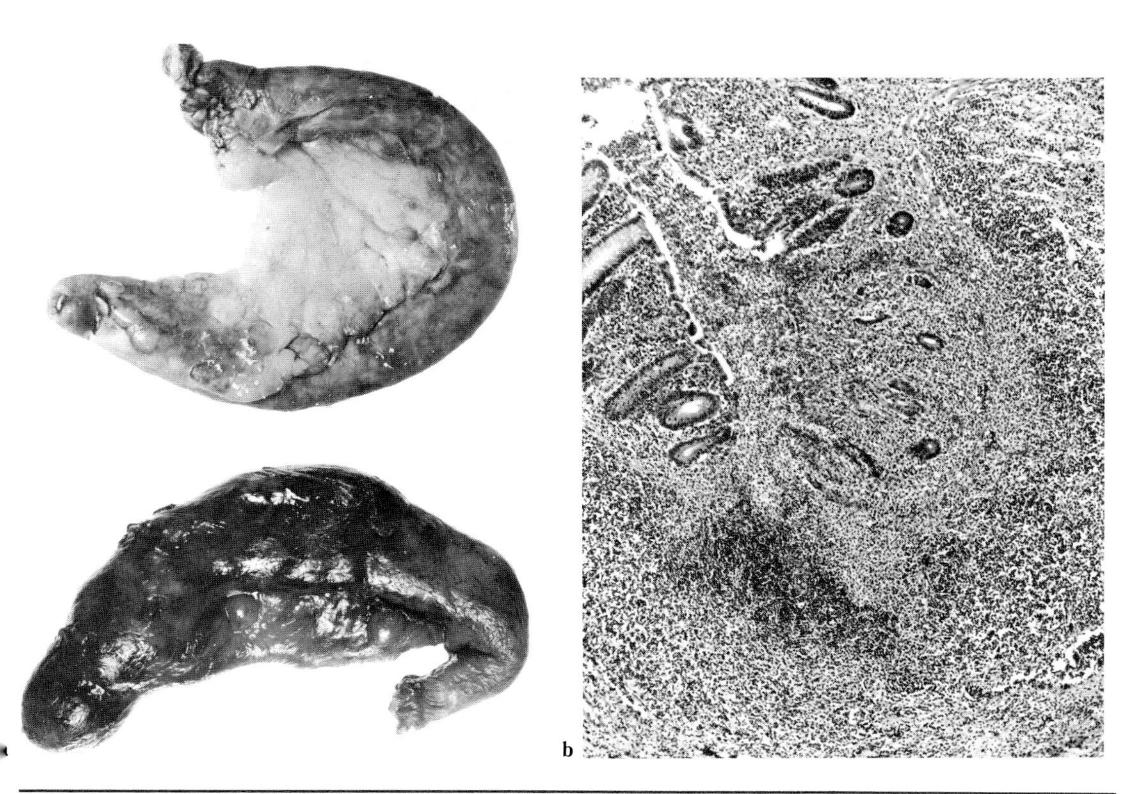

Fig. 16.43 **a** Acute appendicitis. Above, showing swelling and congestion and dulling of the serosal surface by fibrin. Below, gangrenous appendicitis, showing swelling, haemorrhage and fibrin deposition. **b** Acute appendicitis, showing a local ulcerative lesion in the mucosa with commencing abscess formation beneath. ×60.

Complications

Most serious is rupture of the appendix which may lead to **acute generalized peritonitis** or to **periappendicular abscess formation** if the site of rupture becomes sealed off by the blanketing action of the omentum. Thrombosis of the mesoappendicular vessels involved in the inflammatory process may lead to **gangrenous appendicitis**, and occasionally to embolic blood-borne spread of infection to the liver (portal pyaemia) or a spreading thrombosis with secondary suppuration extending up the portal vein (**portal pylephlebitis**). Should acute lesions resolve, some fibrous thickening of the appendix, especially in the submucosa, may lead to luminal stenosis and mucin accumulation, one form of **mucocele** of the appendix. Rupture of such a mucocele may take place and produce local periappendicular mucin accumulation and inflammation. The condition known as 'pseudomyxoma peritonei' (p. 739) in which there is extensive intraperitoneal mucin accumulation is probably not post-inflammatory and is much more likely to be related to the presence of a mucin secreting appendicular tumour. Sometimes a diverticulum may arise following acute appendicitis and can become a further source of acute inflammation. It is unlikely, however, that acute appendicitis ever becomes chronic: the condition known as 'grumbling appendix' is probably due to repeated acute episodes.

Other Inflammatory Diseases

Drug-induced Intestinal Disease

Mention has already been made of the role of antibiotics in the pathogenesis of pseudomembranous colitis. Other drugs may affect the intestine more directly, most notably the non-steroidal anti-inflammatory agents (NSAIDs). Mefenamic acid, for example, may cause a pronounced colitis and sometimes malabsorption accompanied by partial villous atrophy of the small bowel mucosa. Indomethacin administration especially in suppository form may result in acute proctitis. It is also suspected that NSAID can produce ileal ulceration and diaphragm formation (causing obstruction) as well as more extensive forms of mucosal necrosis. Enteric coated potassium tablets have for long been known to cause ileal ulceration. Cytotoxic drugs used in the treatment of leukaemia or intestinal carcinoma may cause severe mucosal damage in the intestinal tract.

Eosinophilic Gastroenteritis

Eosinophils are encountered histologically in a wide variety of inflammatory states in the intestine including vasculitis, parasitic infections, Crohn's disease and the hypereosinophilic syndromes (p. 560). In one group of conditions, however, these cells are the predominant element. The best known member of this group is eosinophilic gastroenteritis which is characterized by episodic segmental swelling of the small intestine associated clinically with abdominal pain and symptoms of obstruction. Histologically, this swelling is due to intense submucosal oedema accompanied by pronounced eosinophilic infiltration, often extending into the muscularis propria. The aetiology of this is seldom obvious; certain food products have, however, been incriminated and fish parasites may be responsible in some cases. There is often a history of atopic allergy and the intestinal disease may be accompanied by peripheral blood eosinophilia.

Eosinophils are also conspicuous in the so-called **inflammatory fibroid polyp** the gastric type of which is described on p. 700. The intestinal version has similar histological features. As the name implies, the lesion protrudes into the intestinal lumen and may cause intussusception). There is, however, usually no atopic history or peripheral blood eosinophilia.

Radiation Enteritis

Exposure of the intestine to ionizing radiation is usually an unwanted side-effect in the treatment of intra-abdominal or cervical cancer. The initial effect is damage to the epithelial stem cells in the crypts of Lieberkühn with a subsequent reduction in the functional enterocyte population. Clinically, this may lead to diarrhoea and, if the small bowel is mainly affected, to malabsorption. These effects are usually transient but there may be delayed consequences which become evident for many months or even years. These are due to progressive occlusion of blood vessels damaged during the initial phase of exposure, and are essentially ischaemic in nature. Ulceration and stricture formation occur. In the small bowel this may lead to intestinal stasis and malabsorption and in the large bowel to rectal bleeding or frank obstruction. Histologically, rectal biopsies show mucosal atrophy with epithelial damage, vascular hyalinization and sometimes atypical mesenchymal cells.

The Solitary Ulcer Syndrome

This troublesome condition may affect young adults, especially females, and is characterized by the presence in the distal rectum of recurrent ulceration (not always solitary) for which an infective cause cannot be demonstrated. It is probably caused by spasm of perirectal muscles and undue straining at defaecation with distal displacement of the mucosal lining of the rectum (mucosal prolapse). The shearing stress applied to the mucosa produces a characteristic histological appearance with surface epithelial damage, fibromuscular thickening of the lamina propria and sometimes displacement of crypts into the rectal submucosa. Similar changes may be found in other types of mucosal prolapse, e.g. in colostomy stomas.

Colitis cystica profunda This rare and usually incidental condition is caused by displacement of epithelium into the colonic submucosa with subsequent cyst formation. It is commonly the result of mucosal inflammation and may be seen in the vicinity of solitary ulcers.

Diverticular Disease

A diverticulum is an out-pouching of an epithelium lined cavity beyond its normal boundaries. It may either be a congenital structure, in which case it has a complete muscular coat, or acquired and lacking in a muscular coat, the wall comprising mucosa, lamina muscularis and an attenuated mantle of submucosal fibrous tissue. Three main varieties are recognized.

Meckel's diverticulum. This, the classic congenital diverticulum, represents the vestige of the embryonic vitello-intestinal duct, the distal part of which may be absent or represented by a fibrous cord attached to the umbilicus. Because of its origin a Meckel's diverticulum has an antimesenteric location in the distal ileum, in adults about 90 cm from the ileocaecal valve. It is found in 10% of people and is asymptomatic in about 80% of cases. In the others a variety of clinical disturbances may be observed. The diverticulum may become acutely inflamed, producing an appendicitis-like syndrome, or it can lead to obstruction as a result either of eversion and subsequent intussusception or of twisting of the bowel around the cord linking the diverticulum to the umbilicus. Sometimes the diverticulum contains heterotopic gastric mucosa, acid secretion from which causes peptic ulceration in the adjacent intestinal mucosa with the associated risks of haemorrhage or perforation of the intestine.

Acquired small bowel diverticula. These rare lesions of unknown aetiology are usually found in the duodenum or jejunum, in the latter location protruding into the mesenteric attachment alongside blood vessels. They may be associated with similar lesions in the colon. Usually multiple, they may enlarge to 3–4 cm in diameter in later adult life. They are often asymptomatic and seldom cause acute abdominal disturbances. Nevertheless, they tend to be repositories of abnormal bacterial proliferation in the small bowel which otherwise is almost sterile. This bacterial overgrowth may lead to malabsorption (p. 723).

Colonic diverticula. In contrast to the small bowel the colon is frequently beset by diverticula, the sigmoid colon being the most favoured site. In the UK, 10–15% of all adults over the age of 40 years are affected, but symptoms occur in only about 20% of cases. Clinical disturbances are, as a rule, produced by inflammatory change in the diverticula (diverticulitis). This may produce an appendicitis-like syndrome with pain tending to localize in the left iliac fossa. Rupture of a diverticulum may lead to pericolic abscess formation or sometimes to generalized acute peritonitis. Should the inflammation involve an adjacent organ a fistula may develop, colovesical fistula being the best recognized example of this. Persistent diverticular inflammation may ultimately lead to pericolic fibrosis with subsequent colonic obstruction. Occasionally a blood vessel running alongside the diverticular wall may rupture and produce brisk haemorrhage.

The aetiology of colonic diverticula is not known. The high incidence of diverticula in urbanized western society when compared with tropical areas suggests that dietary habits may be important. It has been postulated that low intake of dietary fibre leads to disturbed colonic motility with the generation of high intraluminal pressure pockets by unusually brisk segmental muscular contraction. This might lead to protrusion of the mucosa through points of weakness in the colonic wall located at sites of entry of blood vessels (Fig. 16.44). It is significant that diverticula often lie in two longitudinal rows between the taeniae coli, and the pronounced thickening of the muscular coat observed in many cases may be a further reflection of the disordered muscular activity thought to be responsible for the condition.

Vascular Disease

Ischaemic disease of the intestine is by no means uncommon and both clinically and pathologically exists in several forms. Most dramatic is haemorrhagic intestinal **infarction** which is due to occlusion of a major vessel such as the superior mesenteric artery. This may be due either to thrombosis, almost always related to an ather-

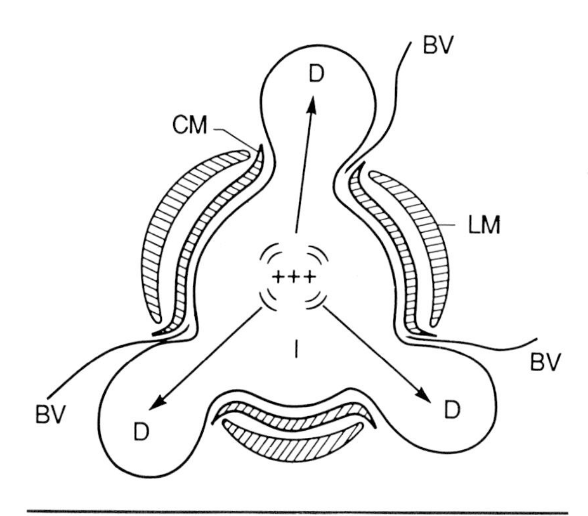

Fig. 16.44 Diverticulum formation in colon. The diverticula (D) arise when increased intraluminal pressure (+++) forces the mucosa through the circular component of the muscularis propria (CM) at points of weakness associated with the entry of blood vessels (BV) between the longitudinal muscle of the taeniae coli (LM).

omatous plaque close to the origin of the vessel, or embolism, usually from the left ventricle in cases of myocardial infarction or the left atrial appendage in mitral valve disease or other diseases associated with atrial fibrillation. The infarct is usually coterminous with the area supplied by the vessel (in the case of the superior mesenteric artery most of the small bowel and proximal colon) but is much less than that if there is good anastomotic support from adjacent vessels (p. 101). Severe narrowing of the superior mesenteric artery does not as a rule lead to infarction but if associated with similar stenosis of the coeliac axis may cause a syndrome of **abdominal angina**, which is characterized by post-prandial pain, sometimes malabsorption and weight loss.

The term **ischaemic enterocolitis** is applied to multiple, randomly distributed, focal ischaemic necrosis involving both small and large bowel and occurring in shock, congestive cardiac failure and uraemia. Hypotension and/or disseminated intravascular coagulation are involved in these cases. The splenic flexure of the colon is particularly susceptible to even lesser degrees of perfusion failure. The inferior mesenteric artery normally supplies this area but its origin is frequently narrowed in the elderly due to aortic atheroma or may be involved by an aortic aneurysm. This may be of little consequence if a proximal branch of the superior haemorrhoidal artery can take over the function of the inferior mesenteric artery; even so the blood supply at this 'watershed' site is always at best marginal and is readily compromised should there be a sustained fall in blood pressure. This may cause little more than a transient episode of rectal bleeding due to mucosal necrosis but can result in stricture formation (**ischaemic colitis**). Vasculitis due, for example, to polyarteritis nodosa, rheumatoid arthritis, systemic lupus erythematosus or possibly Henoch–Schönlein purpura may cause focal ischaemic damage. Ischaemic damage may develop in the large bowel proximal to an obstructive lesion. Increased intraluminal pressure interferes with mucosal perfusion and **'stercoral' ulceration** results.

Angiodysplasia of the colon. Severe haemorrhage from the large bowel may be caused by many diseases, most notably carcinoma, inflammatory bowel disease, ischaemia and diverticular disease. In elderly individuals, usually over 60, the importance of small vascular ectasias in the mucosa and submucosa especially of the caecum and ascending colon as a cause of severe and often multiple bleeding episodes is now well recognized. The cause of this condition, usually known as angiodysplasia, is, however, unknown. The diagnosis, when suspected, is usually established by selective mesenteric arteriography of the intestines.

Functional Disturbances of the Intestines

The Malabsorption Syndrome

The defective absorption of ingested nutrients is an important consequence of disease in the small intestine, especially if prolonged and extensive. Several different mechanisms (and sometimes more than one) may be implicated. These are summarized in Table 16.5. In some of the diseases listed only certain nutrients are affected. Disease of the distal ileum, for example, specifically interferes with the absorption of vitamin B_{12} and the reabsorption of bile salts (enterohepatic circulation, p. 785) with resultant bile salt depletion and fat malabsorption. It should also be appreciated that malabsorption is not always due to small bowel disease. In many tropical countries, for example, chronic pancreatitis is more important in this respect.

Table 16.5 The main causes of malabsorption

Cause	Examples
Inadequate digestion	Pancreatic insufficiency; hepatobiliary disease; post-gastrectomy
Intestinal damage	Coeliac disease; tropical sprue; post-infective malabsorption; Crohn's disease; parasitic disease; drugs; radiation enteritis; Whipple's disease; lymphoma; immunodeficiency; amyloidosis
Altered intestinal flora (bacterial overgrowth)	Jejunal diverticulosis; blind loops
Biochemical abnormality	Abetalipoproteinaemia; disaccharidase deficiency; specific amino-acid malabsorption, e.g. Hartnup disease; bile acid deficiencies
Lymphatic obstruction	Intestinal lymphangiectasia (congenital or acquired)
Inadequate absorptive surface	Intestinal resection or bypass
Endocrine disturbances	Carcinoid syndrome; Verner–Morrison syndrome (vipoma); diabetes mellitus; hypothyroidism
Circulatory disturbance	Mesenteric vascular insufficiency

Malabsorption may become manifest clinically in a wide, and somewhat bewildering variety of ways. The classic symptom, the passage of stools that are pale, bulky and offensive (due to **steatorrhoea**), is by no means invariable. Indeed the initial clinical features may not be directly related to the intestine at all. In infants and children malabsorption may be revealed by a failure to thrive or by disturbance of growth. Hypoproteinaemia, associated with oedema, may be the result not only of impaired amino-acid absorption but also of protein leakage into the lumen (**protein-losing enteropathy**), a feature of many gastrointestinal diseases. Isolated nutritional disturbances such as rickets or osteomalacia (due to vitamin D deficiency), anaemia (due to iron, folic acid or vitamin B_{12} deficiency – sometimes all three) or scurvy (due to vitamin C deficiency) may be the first indication of a malabsorptive state.

Peroral Intestinal Biopsy

This is of great importance in the investigation of malabsorption. Endoscopic biopsies can be taken under direct vision in the distal duodenum but not as yet beyond this point. To sample the jejunum or ileum the biopsy capsule is still required but has the disadvantage of taking random samples which are possibly unrepresentative of the intestinal mucosa as a whole. Either type of biopsy is capable of detecting histological abnormalities in two main categories. The first of these is variation in the functional enterocyte population as revealed by changes in villous architecture, usually taking the form of villous atrophy; such changes are found in several important diseases, notably coeliac disease and tropical sprue (Table 16.6). Secondly, biopsies may show pathological abnormalities not necessarily related to villous disturbance such as the presence of pathogenic organisms, amyloidosis, granulomas and other distinctive inflammatory changes.

Villous Atrophy

Under the dissecting microscope, the normal jejunal mucosa has tall, slender finger-shaped villi interspersed with occasional broader leaf-shaped villi, which are more conspicuous in the duodenum. The villi measure about 400 μm in height and usually account for about 70% of the total mucosal thickness. In tropical residents, however, and for reasons which are not clear, the villi are more often leaf-shaped and may even fuse to form short ridges.

In **partial villous atrophy** (Fig. 16.45) the villi show extensive fusion with the formation of long ridges or convolutions; histologically they appear shorter and broader than normal, although the crypts are enlarged and hyperplastic. The villous epithelium often shows degenerative change, and there is little doubt that the fundamental disturbance is a shortening of the lifespan of these cells with compensatory hyperplasia of the generative crypt cells. In the more severe **subtotal villous atrophy** (Fig. 16.46) villous fusion is more advanced and the mucosa appears completely flat both under the dissecting microscope and histologically. Epithelial degenerative changes are also more prominent. The term subtotal is sometimes confusing to the student; while the mucosa appears flat, the upper part still includes functional enterocytes, hence the use of the term subtotal.

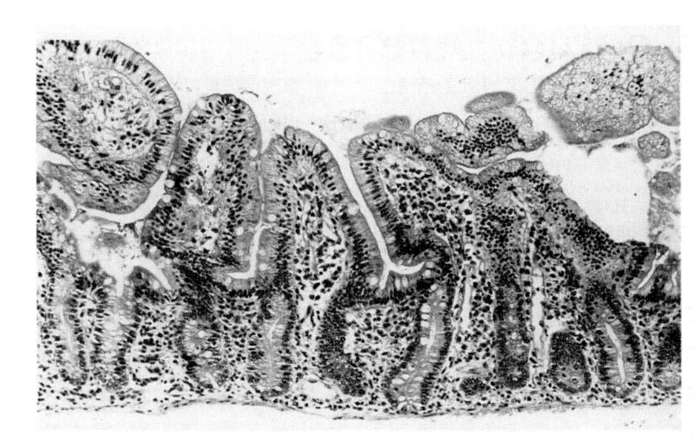

Fig. 16.45 Partial villous atrophy of the jejunal mucosa, crypt hyperplastic type; due to mefenamic acid hypersensitivity. Note that the crypts and villi are of equal height (cf. Fig. 16.30). H & E.

Table 16.6 The main causes of villous atrophy

Coeliac disease
Tropical sprue
Post-infective malabsorption
Crohn's disease
Immunodefiency (e.g. AIDS)
Drugs (e.g. mefenamic acid)

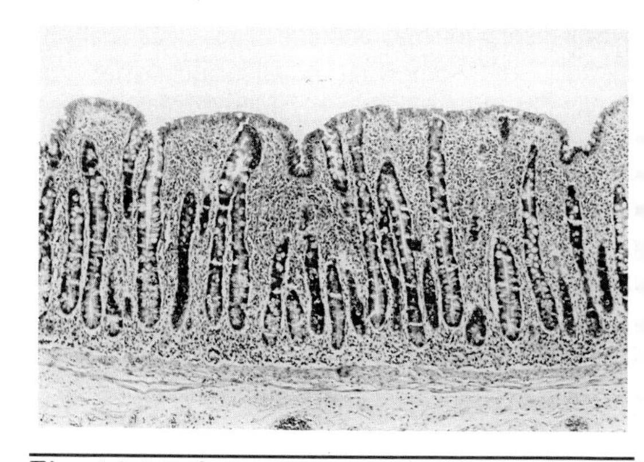

Fig. 16.46 Subtotal villous atrophy of the jejunal mucosa, crypt hyperplastic type, due to coeliac disease. Note the marked inflammatory reaction in the lamina propria. H & E.

Coeliac Disease

This is probably the most common intestinal cause of malabsorption, certainly in temperate climates. It frequently presents in infancy or early childhood not long after weaning has been established, but it may only become manifest in adult life. The current view is that the disease is caused by a genetically determined, abnormal, cell mediated immune response to the wheat protein gluten or a peptide derivative thereof, gliadin. There is a strong familial tendency and an association with the HLA-B8, DW3 and possibly other histocompatibility antigens.

The main pathological effect is damage to the mature enterocytes in the small bowel and depletion of the enterocyte population as revealed by severe villous atrophy, this usually being associated with pronounced plasma cell infiltration in the lamina propria and an apparent increase in intra-epithelial T lymphocytes, probably reflecting the immune mechanism responsible for the disease. Villous atrophy takes place despite the increased output of epithelial cells from the crypts which become markedly hyperplastic (Fig. 16.46). These changes are always maximal in the proximal small bowel. The diagnosis is established by demonstrating that withdrawal of gluten from the diet results in improvement in the villous architecture, reflecting restoration of the functional enterocyte population; hence the term gluten-sensitive enteropathy.

Apart from the nutritional or developmental consequences of malabsorption the most serious complication of coeliac disease is an increased risk of malignancy, usually a malignant T-cell lymphoma or less often a carcinoma in the small intestine. There also appears to be a greater predisposition to develop certain extraintestinal tumours, e.g. oesophageal carcinoma. Splenic atrophy is commonly observed in adult patients. Many, if not most patients with dermatitis herpetiformis (p. 1120) also have coeliac disease, although the intestinal lesions are usually mild; the bullous skin lesions are associated with IgA deposits on the basement membrane, and it has been suggested that the antibody is of gastrointestinal origin.

Tropical Sprue

As the name implies this malabsorptive disease is related to exposure to a tropical environment especially in central America and south east Asia. Both residents and visitors into the areas may be affected. Anaemia due either to folic acid or vitamin B_{12} deficiency (or both) is a common presenting feature, although there may be other severe nutritional effects. While the aetiology is not entirely clear it has been postulated that the disease is caused by persistent colonization of small bowel by aerobic enteric bacteria, this phenomenon possibly being initiated by an acute infection. In any event the small bowel mucosa shows villous atrophy, often of the partial type and which may respond to the administration of broad spectrum antibiotics.

Protozoal Diseases

The most important and ubiquitous disease in this category is *giardiasis* (p. 1158) usually contracted following ingestion of water containing the encysted form of *Giardia lamblia*. This may cause an acute diarrhoeal disturbance or it can produce more chronic effects including quite severe malabsorption. The diagnosis is usually made by histological examination of an intestinal biopsy which reveals the organism in its trophozoite phase in the gut lumen. Curiously, the intestinal mucosa may show little inflammatory reaction but there may be villous atrophy of some degree especially in immunodeficiency states which are often complicated by giardiasis.

Altered Intestinal Flora

Bacterial overgrowth in the small intestinal lumen occurs when there is stasis, e.g. in diverticula or blind loops following operative bypass procedures or acquired as a result of fistula formation or strictures. The mechanisms of the malabsorption in these patients is complex. The organisms may compete for nutrients such as vitamin B_{12}; they may interfere with bile salts causing fat malabsorption; or they may inactivate mucosal enzymes. The patients respond to antibiotic therapy and surgical management can be curative.

Whipple's Disease

In this rare, multisystem disorder intestinal disturbance associated with malabsorption is often the predominant feature. Other organs which may be involved include lymph nodes, joints, heart valves and lung and the central nervous system. Patients may first present because of this and it is of interest that the first patient described by Whipple presented with joint symptoms. Males in middle age or beyond are mainly affected. The intestinal biopsy findings are diagnostic (Fig. 16.47): the mucosa is diffusely infiltrated by histiocytes with abundant, finely granular and basophilic cytoplasm which stains strongly positive with the periodic-acid Schiff method. Similar cells are found in other affected organs. Electron microscopy reveals the presence, in these cells, of numerous secondary lysosomes containing rod-shaped bacteria in varying states of degradation.

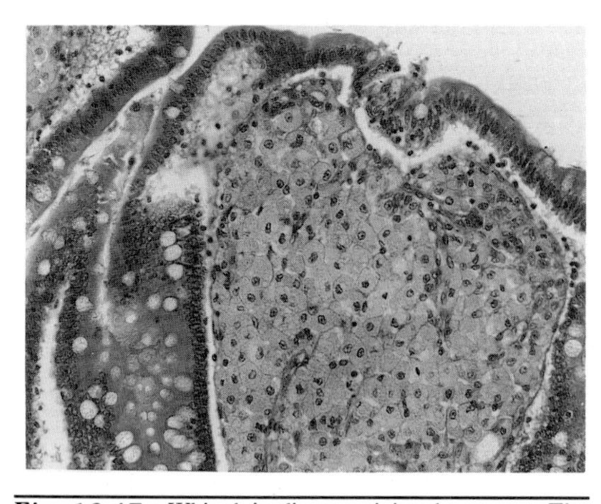

Fig. 16.47 Whipple's disease, jejunal mucosa. The lamina propria infiltrated by histiocytes showing abundant granular cytoplasm. H & E ×500.

Bacillary bodies may also be seen free in the lamina propria mucosae. The identity of these organisms has yet to be established, but they may be related to certain groups of streptococci. Nevertheless, it would appear that Whipple's disease is an infective process, a view supported by the favourable response to oral broad spectrum antibiotics. The curious epidemiology of the disease, however, suggests that the affected individuals might have some immunological deficit but evidence for this is not wholly convincing.

Abetalipoproteinaemia

In this rare condition, inherited as autosomal recessive, the proteins required for transport of triglycerides to the villus lymphatics from the enterocyte (where they have been resynthesized following absorption of monoglycerides and fatty acids) is apparently deficient. Triglyceride thus remains within the enterocyte (Fig. 16.48) and is lost when the cell is shed into the lumen, effectively resulting in fat malabsorption. Patients with this disorder often have retinal abnormalities and cerebellar dysfunction. A lipid defect in the membrane produces a curious spiny alteration on the red cell surface – acanthocytosis.

Disaccharidase Deficiency

The disaccharidase enzymes are found in the cell membrane on the apices of enterocytes. Lactase deficiency may occur in a congenital or acquired form and undigested lactose exerts an osmotic effect in the gut, producing diarrhoea and malabsorption. The diagnosis can be established by a lactose tolerance test or by measuring the lactase content of a mucosal biopsy.

Intestinal Lymphangiectasis

Obstruction of lymphatic flow from the intestine is an uncommon but well recognized cause of malab-

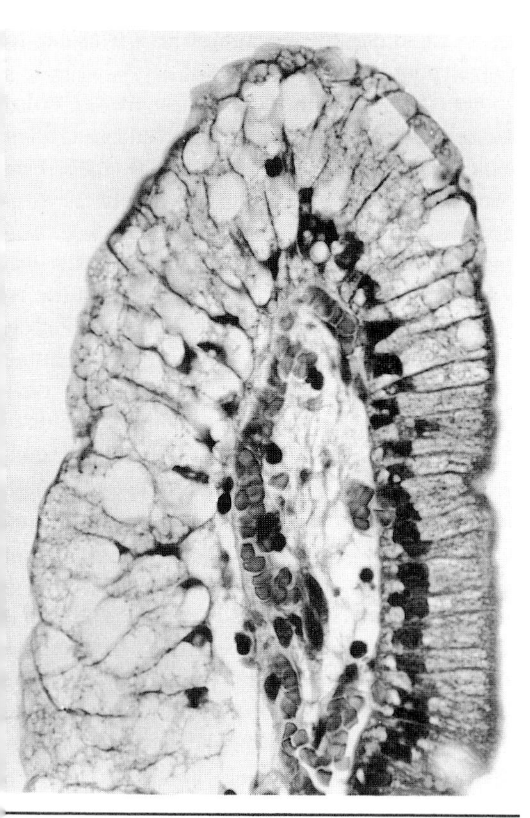

'ig. 16.48 Abetalipoproteinaemia. The enterocytes ‹ the tip of a jejunal villus are distended with lipid. H & E ‹570.

orption of fat and fat-related vitamins. Sometimes ıis is due to acquired disease of the mesenteric ·mph nodes (e.g. tuberculosis, lymphoma) but it ıay be a congenital disturbance often associated ·ith malformation of lymphatics elsewhere in the ody. In the congenital forms not only is fat lost ·om the body but lymphocytes as well and a state f immunodeficiency may arise. There may also be ubstantial loss of protein into the gut lumen – rotein-losing enteropathy.

mmunodeficiency States

lalabsorption is a well recognized feature of con- enital and acquired forms of immunodeficiency. In ıe latter category two disorders are of particular importance. In **nodular lymphoid hyperplasia** of the small intestine there is severe combined deficiency of IgA and IgM and to a lesser extent, IgG, possibly due to an acquired disturbance of B-cell maturation which is reflected by the presence of large, abnormal germinal centres and an absence of plasma cells in the intestinal mucosa. This defect is almost always complicated by severe giardiasis, in this instance accompanied by partial villous atrophy of the mucosa and malabsorption.

Severe malabsorption and nutritional disturbance may be a feature of AIDS especially in Africa (hence the term 'slim disease'). In some cases these effects may be due to opportunistic intestinal infection, especially those due to coccidial protozoa or *Mycobacterium avium intracellulare*. In the latter instance the intestinal mucosa is infiltrated by globoid, foamy histiocytes containing numerous alcohol acid-fast bacilli. In some cases of AIDS, however, malabsorption can be attributed to partial villous atrophy of the intestinal mucosa arising without obvious cause.

Intestinal Obstruction

While this is a potentially serious complication of many intestinal diseases it is important to realize that different mechanisms may be involved in its causation and that not all of the causative factors originate in the intestine itself. The mechanisms involved can be divided into four broad categories. The first of these and probably the most common is external compression which is of particular importance with regard to the small intestine. Secondly, there are disease processes of the intestinal wall capable of producing narrowing of the lumen (i.e. stricture formation). Third is luminal occlusion which *per se* is uncommon as a cause of obstruction. Lastly, there are functional disorders producing derangement of intestinal motility. The most important causes of intestinal obstruction are listed in Table 16.7.

Table 16.7 Main causes of intestinal obstruction

Cause	Examples
External constriction	Hernia; volvulus; intussusception; adhesions (postoperative); large intra-abdominal tumours
Intrinsic lesions	Malignant tumours (especially carcinoma); Crohn's disease; ulcerative colitis; diverticular disease; radiation damage; congenital strictures and atresias; acquired stricture – post-inflammatory, ischaemic, radiation damage
Luminal occlusion	Foreign material; polypoid tumours; gallstone ileus; meconium in cystic fibrosis
Functional obstruction	Bowel infarction; Paralytic ileus; Hirschsprung's disease

The Effects of Intestinal Obstruction

These are related not only to the underlying cause and its remediability but also to its location, the completeness of obstruction and the presence or absence of additional factors most notably interference with the intestinal blood supply.

In general terms obstruction taking place in the **proximal small intestine**, where the contents of the lumen are largely liquid, needs to be complete for the effects to become manifest but these develop quickly and are usually severe in degree. With obstruction distal to the ampulla of Vater there is rapid accumulation within the lumen, not only of ingested material and gas but also of the copious secretions (approximately 8 litres per day) from the biliary system, pancreas, stomach and intestine itself. With little capacity for reabsorption most of this largely liquid material pools in the obstructed bowel which, after an initial phase of enhanced propulsive activity, may become atonic and markedly dilated. Much of this material is subsequently lost by vomiting. Unless treatment is expedited the patient becomes rapidly depleted of fluid and electrolytes (especially sodium, potassium and chloride) with the hazard of peripheral circulatory collapse (p. 106). With more distal small bowel obstruction the onset of fluid depletion is less rapid due to the greater area available for reabsorption.

Obstruction taking place in the **distal colon** creates additional problems. Fluid and electrolyte depletion, while slow in onset, will ultimately develop, often being associated with the regurgitation of intestinal contents ('stercoral vomit'). Potassium depletion is especially dangerous since it may not be immediately apparent from the results of serum analysis and can lead to serious impairment of intestinal motility. The more immediate danger, however, is the pronounced rise in pressure which may take place in the colonic lumen especially if the ileocaecal valve retains competence ('closed loop obstruction' phenomenon). This pressure rise may seriously threaten mucosal viability and, by permiting the entry of enteric bacteria or their breakdown products precipitate endotoxic shock (p. 108). Frank ulceration may also develop in the obstructed bowel, especially in the vicinity of the caecum (stercoral ulcer) and there is a serious risk of perforation at this site. Obstruction of the colon (and occasionally at a higher level, e.g. terminal ileum) is often incomplete and sometimes transit of faecal material can be sustained by enhanced peristaltic activity in the obstructed segment which, as a result, becomes markedly hypertrophied as well as dilated.

Strangulation. This term is used when obstruction becomes complicated by interference with the blood supply to the bowel. This most often takes place when both the intestine and its vascular pedicle become subjected to external constriction and is seen with hernias, volvulus and intussusception (Fig. 16.49).

Hernias

This term, when unqualified, usually refers to protrusion of the peritoneal cavity beyond its natural boundaries, producing a hernial sac. A hernia develops when a local weakness in the abdominal wall is exploited by increased intra-abdominal pressure. The local weakness may be congenital, for example, at the umbilicus or the inguinal canal

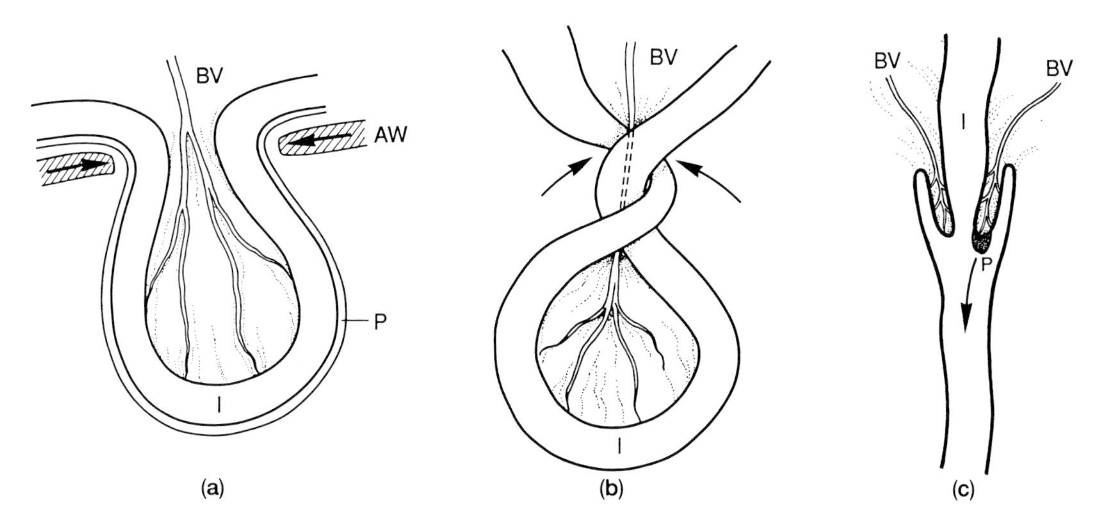

Fig. 16.49 **a** Hernia. A loop of intestine (I) has entered a hernial sac formed by protrusion of the peritoneal cavity (P) through a gap in the anterior abdominal wall (AW). Note the potential for constriction at the neck of the sac (arrows). BV, blood vessel. **b** Volvulus. A loop of bowel (I) has twisted leading to constriction of its lumen and compression of the vascular pedicle, BV, blood vessel. **c** Intussusception. A segment of bowel (I) has become invaginated due to the presence of a polypoid mucosal lesion (P). Note the potential for constriction of the bowel and its blood supply (BV) at the site of invagination (arrows).

or acquired as a result of surgical scars. The increase in intra-abdominal pressure may be due to factors such as muscular exertion, coughing or straining at defaecation. The commonest types of hernia are external, i.e. are visible on the surface of the body and include the inguinal, femoral, umbilical and postoperative (i.e. incisional) varieties. Inguinal hernias may be either **indirect** in which the protrusion passes lateral to the inferior epigastric artery and may, following the path of the gubernaculum and processus vaginalis, enter the scrotum; or **direct** when the protrusion passes medial to the artery and projects through the external abdominal ring. A femoral hernia passes under the inguinal ligament medial to the femoral vessels and is especially common in females. Hernias may also be internal, passing, for example, through the oesophageal hiatus (p. 686) or through the obturator foramen. Quite often a loop of bowel enters a hernial sac; usually it is reducible and readily replaced into the peritoneal cavity. It may, however, become impacted due to the formation of adhesions or due to the bulk of the bowel contents. There is then a hazard that the intestinal loop will become obstructed by external constriction at the neck of the sac; the vascular supply, especially the venous drainage, is compromised with resulting ischaemic damage and gangrene.

Volvulus

A loop of bowel may become strangulated when it twists or rotates through an angle in excess of 180° with the result that the lumen is obstructed and the vascular supply compromised simultaneously. This phenomenon most often takes place in the sigmoid colon when it possesses an unusually long mesocolon and becomes overloaded with faeces. Occasionally a volvulus develops in the small intestine when, especially in childhood, it becomes twisted around a congenital fibrous band (e.g. the remnant of the vitello-intestinal duct. In adult life adhesions developing between adjacent loops of bowel as a result of peritonitis or intra-abdominal surgery may have a similar affect.

Intussusception

This develops when a segment of bowel becomes invaginated into an adjacent segment usually lying distally. In most instances the result of this is strangulation of the invaginated segment or intussusceptum due to obstruction of its lumen and its blood supply at the initial point of invagination (Fig. 16.50). Intussusception is especially common in early childhood and is usually located in the distal ileum, the usual explanation for this being that the lymphoid tissue in this site and at this age may be unusually swollen possibly as a result of viral infection and, being mistaken as it were for a bolus of food, may be propelled distally by peristaltic activity.

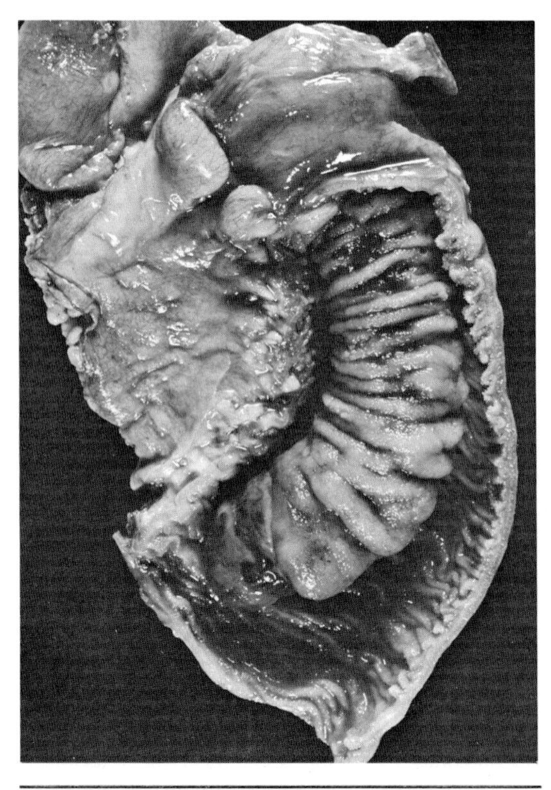

Fig. 16.50 Intussusception of the small intestine. The ensheathing section of gut has been cut open to show the invaginated loop, which is passing downward. The invaginated loop shows early haemorrhagic necrosis at the apex (near lower margin of excision) and near the entrance (at the top of the photograph).

Haemorrhage into the mucosa in Henoch–Schönlein purpura (p. 471) may have a similar effect. In adolescence or adult life polypoid small bowel lesions such as Peutz–Jeghers polyps, inflammatory fibroid polyps or polypoid tumours are usually responsible. Occasionally, infection of a Peyer's patch, e.g. by tuberculosis, may be implicated in adults. Polypoid lesions may also cause colonic intussusception but this is comparatively uncommon.

Functional Obstruction

Obstructive effects caused by interference with neuromuscular activity or co-ordination in the intestine are by no means uncommon. Pseudo-obstruction of this kind, sometimes of a chronic nature, may be due to metabolic disturbances such as diabetes mellitus or hormonal disorders, most notably hypothyroidism. The connective tissue disease progressive systemic sclerosis (p. 231) may, by damaging the intestinal musculature, have similar effects. In Chagas' disease (p. 1154) the myenteric plexus in the colon may be affected.

Undoubtedly the most serious acute condition in this category is **paralytic ileus** which is a feared complication of abdominal operations (often of a trivial nature) or which may arise as a result of intestinal infection, peritonitis or toxaemic states. There is serious impairment of intestinal motor activity with subsequent gross distension of the intestinal lumen. The fluid accumulating in distended bowel loops is effectively lost to the circulation and may lead to peripheral circulatory collapse. The cause of paralytic ileus is still uncertain; sympathetic overactivity may be implicated and this can certainly be aggravated by potassium depletion. Restoration of fluid and electrolyte balance is thus essential, and intubation with drainage of the distended bowel may be required before gut contractility returns.

Hirschsprung's Disease

A variety of congenital disorders involving the intestinal musculature and its innervation may also cause intestinal obstruction. Most important of these is Hirschsprung's disease, in which both the submucosal and myenteric plexuses over a variable part of the large bowel are found to be devoid of parasympathetic ganglia. This is the result of failure of the migration of neuroblasts during embryogenesis, innervation of the bowel taking place in a cephalocaudad direction in the first trimester of pregnancy. The aganglionic segment does not transmit peristaltic activity and appears collapsed. In contrast the proximal colon, being in effect obstructed, may become grossly distended with faeces and often markedly hypertrophied. This may involve the entire colon and caecum and sometimes the appendix (megacolon). The enhanced pressure in the lumen of the obstructed colon may lead to ischaemic or necrotizing colitis and sometimes perforation.

The aganglionic segment may be of variable length. In 85% of cases it is a short segment and does not extend beyond the sigmoid colon; long segment disease extends beyond the sigmoid and may reach the caecum (10%); total colonic aganglionosis in which variable lengths of small bowel are involved and finally ultra-short segment disease confined to the anorectal region comprise the remainder. In some cases of ultra-short segment disease the obstruction may be due to a disorder (achalasia) of the internal anal sphincter. The disease, which more often affects males in the ratio of 3:1 usually declares itself in the neonatal period with a failure to pass meconium. The disease, however, may be first diagnosed in infancy, childhood or even adulthood and the length of segment is not necessarily related to the clinical symptoms.

The diagnosis is established on suction biopsy of the rectal mucosa. The absence of ganglion cells or the presence of abnormal ganglia in the submucosa can be demonstrated on H & E stained sections, but the immunohistochemical demonstration of increased acetylcholinesterase activity in nerve fibres is more reliable. Excision of the aganglionic segment of gut usually restores normal function.

Tumours of the Intestine

Small Intestine

Tumours of any kind are surprisingly uncommon in this site: less than 1% of carcinomas arising in the gastrointestinal tract take origin in the small bowel. Even so, such tumours as are encountered here form an interesting group.

Mesenchymal Tumours

Connective tissue tumours such as lymphangioma, haemangioma and leiomyoma are all well recognized. The last may on occasion give rise to intestinal blood loss or predispose to intussusception. As in the stomach, bizarre or epithelioid variants as well as frankly malignant forms (leiomyosarcoma) may be encountered.

Carcinoid Tumours

This term is applied to a group of tumours which take origin from endocrine cells of varying type located within the epithelial lining of endoderm-derived structures, notably the gastrointestinal and respiratory tracts. These cells are part of the diffuse endocrine system (p. 1075). They comprise cells which are of neural crest origin but the majority are derived from epithelium differentiating from progenitor cells in the crypt zones. There are thus neuroendocrine and enteroendocrine (enterochromaffin) cells which subserve endocrine, neuroendocrine (neuropeptide) and paracrine functions. The cells have the capacity to take up silver stains, hence the term argentaffin cells; some require treatment with a reducing agent to take up the stains and are referred to as argyrophil cells. In addition they may be identified by immunohistochemical methods to demonstrate 'pan-endocrine markers', including neuron-specific enolase and chromogranin, or to demonstrate their specific secretory products. Some 40 different endocrine cell types are now recognized in the gastrointestinal tract and they secrete a large array of hormones some of whose functions are not clear. Serotonin-secreting enterochromaffin cells are the predominant cell type; D cells secreting somatostatin are also widely distributed. G cells secreting gastrin are numerous in the stomach; the others constitute minor populations variously distributed throughout the gastrointestinal tract.

Carcinoid (carcinoma-like) tumours may arise in the oesophagus, stomach and duodenum (foregut), in the jejunum, ileum, appendix and colon to the mid-transverse colon (mid-gut) and in the distal colon and rectum (hindgut). They constitute approximately 2% of all gastrointestinal tract neoplasms: some 75% arise in the mid-gut (50% in the appendix), 15–20% in the hindgut (mainly rectum) and the remainder in the foregut. The tumours may predominantly secrete one hormone and may be clinically identified on that basis – gastrinoma, glucagonoma etc. The majority of them secrete a number of hormones, but in many instances these are apparently non-functional and no distinctive syndromes result.

In the **appendix** carcinoid tumours are usually found incidentally and may be associated with acute appendicitis. They appear as small yellowish-brown nodules usually located towards the distal extremity. Histologically, they consist of packets of uniform polyhedral cells which in H & E sections may possess fine brick red granules. They exhibit the classic argentaffin reaction. The tumour seldom if ever metastasizes. In some carcinoids the cells secrete mucin in addition to 5-HT ('goblet cell carcinoids'). These forms often exhibit frankly malignant behaviour.

Ileal carcinoids show histological features virtually identical to the appendicular form (Fig. 16.51) but are often multiple, tend to be larger and frequently metastasize both to local mesenteric lymph nodes and the liver. The tumour also elicits

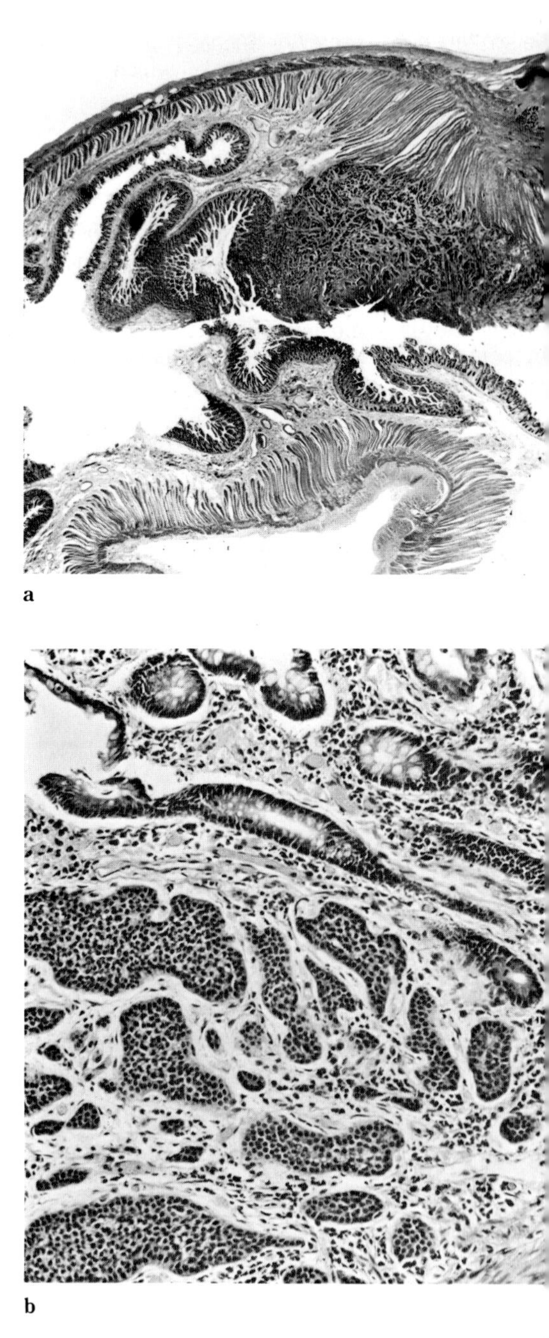

Fig. 16.51 **a** Carcinoid tumour of ileum, seen as the darkly stained tissue invading the circular muscle coat, which is greatly hypertrophied, and causing stenosis. There were hepatic metastases and the carcinoid syndrome developed. ×2.5 **b** Histologically, the tumour comprises clumps of small polygonal epithelial cells infiltrating the mucosa. ×125.

a striking fibrotic reaction and may cause intestinal obstruction. As long as the tumour is confined to the intestine the secretion of 5-HT scarcely matters in functional terms. With massive liver metastases, however, 5-HT and other secretory products such as kallikrein may be released into the systemic circulation producing the **carcinoid syndrome**. This comprises of flushing attacks which are often precipitated by alcohol consumption and are probably due to the secretion of kallikrein rather than 5-HT. The latter, however, being a potent stimulator of smooth muscle, is probably responsible for the diarrhoea and bronchospasm also observed and almost certainly for the subendocardial fibrosis which develops in the right side of the heart and may lead to pulmonary stenosis. The left side of the heart is less often affected since 5-HT is destroyed in the lungs. Clinically, the syndrome can be diagnosed by quantitative estimation in the urine of 5-hydroxyindole acetic acid (5-HIAA), the breakdown product generated by the action of amine oxidase on 5-HT in the liver and, to a lesser extent, in the lungs.

Adenomas and Carcinoma

Adenomas are rare. The duodenum is the most common site. They are sometimes multiple and may be associated with familial adenomatous polyposis. Like adenomas of the colon they are premalignant lesions and most carcinomas of the duodenum and ampulla arise from them; priampullary carcinomas, indeed may develop in 5% of cases of familial adenomatous polyposis.

Carcinoma. This tumour is decidedly rare (with only one-eightieth of the incidence of colorectal carcinoma) despite the fact that it may arise as a complication of both Crohn's disease and coeliac disease. Carcinoma has also a tendency to develop in blind loops. The tumour is an adenocarcinoma closely resembling the colonic type and tends to have a poor prognosis since by the time it produces symptoms (usually as a result of obstruction) spread to the mesenteric lymph nodes and even to the liver has often taken place.

Peutz–Jeghers syndrome. This condition which is inherited as autosomal dominant is characterized by abnormal pigmentation usually around the mouth and more persistently within the oral cavity, and the development of multiple polyps, mainly in the small intestine. These polyps are not true tumours but are best regarded as hamartomas, since histologically they often include all the epithelial components found normally in the intestinal mucosa together with a branching muscular stroma derived from the muscularis mucosae. They seem to arise mainly during adolescence and may cause intestinal bleeding or, more dramatically, recurrent intussusception. Only rarely if at all does a Peutz–Jeghers polyp undergo malignant transformation; however, there are reports of colorectal carcinomas arising in association with the Peutz–Jeghers syndrome.

Malignant Lymphoma

Malignant lymphoma arising primarily in the small intestine is by no means rare; indeed the gastrointestinal tract is the commonest site for extranodal lymphomas. Hodgkin's disease, however, does not arise in the bowel. In some parts of the world, including the UK, the incidence of lymphomas exceeds that of small bowel carcinoma. It exists in three main forms. First, are B-cell tumours similar to those arising in lymph nodes. A variant of this is a centrocytic B-cell tumour which may colonize all the lymphoid aggregates in the gastrointestinal tract to produce the dramatic condition known as **multiple lymphomatous polyposis**. This is an aggressive neoplasm which tends to systematize widely, may become leukaemic and carries a relatively poor prognosis. In adolescence and young adults a lymphoblastic type of B-cell lymphoma resembling Burkitt's lymphoma may arise, usually in the terminal ileum, and is often rapidly fatal.

Secondly, there is the condition referred to as **immunoproliferative small intestinal disease (IPSID)** in which the intestinal mucosa is diffusely infiltrated with plasma cells sometimes producing the heavy chain of IgA (alpha chain disease, p. 639). This disease is found mainly in the Middle East and around the south and east Mediterranean, hence the other name, 'Mediterranean lymphoma'. It may be associated with malabsorption. Infection may be a factor contributing to the functional disturbance. Indeed broad spectrum antibiotics may effect a remission in the early stages of the disease. IPSID is thought to be a neoplastic disorder of the MALT and a frank lymphoma of centrocyte-like cells may ultimately develop in many cases. The lymphoma resembles gastric lymphomas which also arise from the MALT.

Thirdly, a distinctive type of lymphoma may complicate coeliac disease. It is now thought to be a tumour of the intraepithelial T lymphocytes, hence the term **enteropathy-associated T-cell lymphoma**. This tumour usually declares its presence either by producing obstruction or by causing intestinal perforation. They may occur as a single ulcerating mass or as multiple tumours throughout the small intestine. There is often evidence of recurrent ulceration – ulcerative jejunitis – prior to these events. The development of lymphoma, usually in late middle age, may be the first indication of coeliac disease. The prognosis is generally, but not invariably, poor since the tumour rapidly spreads to lymph nodes, liver and bone marrow.

Large Intestine

In contrast to the small bowel, epithelial tumours, both simple and malignant, are all too common in the large intestine. Connective tissue tumours are rare; only leiomyoma and its malignant counterpart deserve mention. Malignant lymphoma is also uncommon but may on occasion complicate ulcerative colitis.

Adenomas (Benign Adenomatous Polyps)

Adenomas arise from the colorectal epithelium and invariably become elevated above the mucosal surface, i.e. they form polyps. These lesions may either be sessile (i.e. flat elevations) or pedunculated (i.e. possess a stalk). Histologically, adenomas exhibit varying degrees of epithelial dysplasia as revealed by nuclear crowding, hyperchromatism, loss of polarity or abnormal mitotic activity. They can be divided into two main types.

Tubular Adenomas

Tubular adenomas (65% of cases) are smooth with a lobulated surface and often pedunculated and consist mostly of glandular structures (Fig. 16.52) resembling colonic mucosa. They usually show little evidence of mucin secretion.

Villous Adenomas

Villous adenomas (10% of cases), on the other hand, generally exhibit a frond-like surface, are almost always sessile and consist of long papillary processes covered by epithelium often showing considerable mucin secretion (Fig. 16.53). Indeed the secretory activity may be such as to lead to

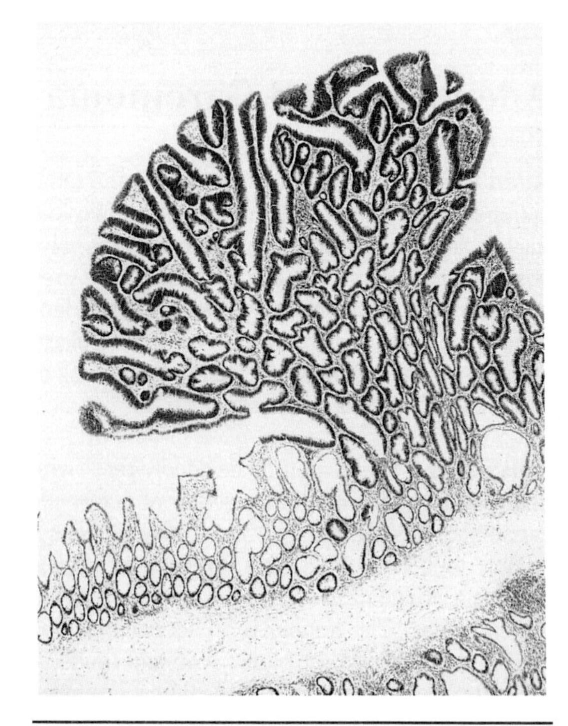

Fig. 16.52 Adenoma of colon, tubular type. Note the polypoid structure and smooth surface. H & E.

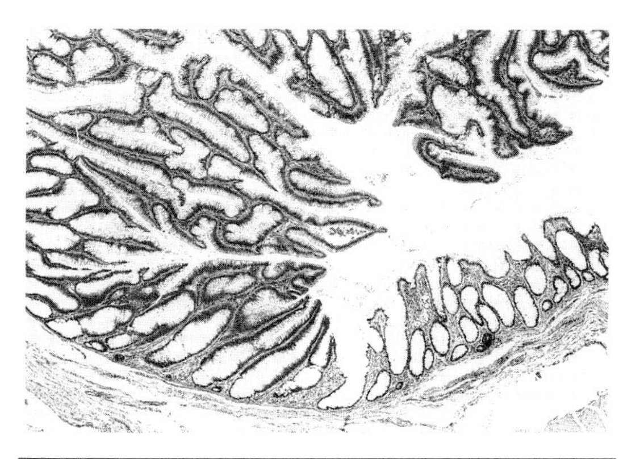

Fig. 16.53 Adenoma of colon, villous type. The lesion has a frond-like structure and shows marked mucin secretion. H & E.

potassium depletion. Some adenomas (25%) show mixed features and are referred to as **tubulovillous adenomas**.

Adenomas should be regarded as foci of intraepithelial neoplasia with the potential to evolve into invasive carcinoma. It is likely that, with the exception of those occurring in ulcerative colitis, most if not all colorectal carcinomas arise in this way. These lesions therefore require careful histological examination and examination of the excision margins, particularly with the sessile growths. The risk that an adenoma will undergo malignant transformation varies considerably and depends upon several factors.

Size. With adenomas less than 1 cm across the hazard is low. Such small adenomas are more evenly distributed throughout the large bowel and are even found in geographical areas with a low cancer incidence. Above 1 cm the hazard is greater and with adenomas larger than 4 cm and which have been removed incidentally a carcinoma will be present in approximately 50%. Over 50% of the larger adenomas are found in the rectum and sigmoid colon (the commonest sites for carcinoma) and in addition are most common in those parts of the world with a high cancer incidence.

Type. Size for size, villous adenomas carry a 10-fold higher risk than purely tubular types. In addition they are often larger at clinical presentation and this further increases the likelihood that they are already malignant.

Degree of dysplasia. Dysplasia may be graded as mild, moderate or severe. Severe dysplasia with pronounced architectural disturbance of gland formation and cytological abnormalities implies that mucosal invasion is imminent. This advanced form of dysplasia is sometimes referred to as **carcinoma *in situ*.**

Number. Obviously the presence of multiple adenomas will enhance the risk of colorectal malignancy in any individual case. This is particularly evident in adenomatous polyposis.

Polyposis Syndromes

The term polyposis embraces a group of conditions characterized by multiple polyps in the gut, some of which are inherited, some of which are acquired and some of which are neoplastic. These are listed in Table 16.8 and some of them have been discussed elsewhere.

Familial adenomatous polyposis (so-called polyposis coli) is inherited as autosomal dominant and the gene is on chromosome 5 in the q21–22 region. In affected individuals there is a progressive development of irreversible mainly tubular adenomas of the colon (Fig. 16.54). In addition adenomas may also occur in the upper gastrointestinal tract; in the duodenum in over 50% of cases, sometimes in the jejunum and ileum and in the stomach polyps occur.

Cytogenetic studies suggest that the adenomas are monoclonal. The tumours usually appear in late childhood, are more frequent in the rectosigmoid region and by adulthood there is diffuse involvement of the entire colon. Since each adenoma carries a risk of malignant transformation the development of carcinoma is inevitable by the third or fourth decade unless total colectomy is undertaken. Carcinoma may also arise in the duodenal adenomas.

In **Gardner's syndrome**, also autosomal dominant, the polyposis affects stomach and also duodenum in addition to the colon, and is accompanied

Table 16.8 Gastrointestinal polyposis syndromes

Syndrome	Mode of inheritance	Extra-intestinal lesions
Familial adenomatous polyposis	Autosomal dominant	
Gardner's syndrome	Autosomal dominant	Osteoma; lipoma; fibroma; thyroid and adrenal tumours
Turcot's syndrome	Autosomal recessive	Tumours in the central nervous system
Juvenile polyposis	Autosomal dominant in most cases	Occasional cases with congenital defects e.g. cleft palate
Cowden's syndrome	Autosomal dominant	Carcinoma of breast and thyroid
Peutz–Jegher's syndrome	Autosomal dominant	Buccal pigmentation; colorectal carcinoma
Cronkhite–Canada syndrome	Not inherited	Alopecia, atrophy of nails, hyperpigmentation of skin
Lymphoid polyposis	May be familial	

by a variety of other neoplastic lesions, e.g. osteomas and soft tissue tumours of the skin.

Turcot's syndrome comprises familial adenomatous polyposis in which there are also malignant tumours in the central nervous system.

Juvenile polyposis. The juvenile polyp as the name suggests is usually found in childhood. It is a globoid lesion which sometimes ulcerates and may measure up to 2 cm in diameter. They may sometimes be multiple (juvenile polyposis coli), with or without a family history. Histologically, the lesion consists of expanded and inflamed lamina propria associated with crypt dilatation and appears to be hamartomatous in nature. Only rarely does it exhibit dysplastic features and the risk of malignancy is very low (probably less than 10%).

Cronkhite–Canada syndrome. In this rare and usually fatal condition, diffuse gastrointestinal polyposis is associated with skin pigmentation, alopecia and atrophy of the nails. It is not related to any other forms of intestinal polyposis. There may be vomiting and severe diarrhoea with protein loss, the symptoms resembling ulcerative colitis. The polyps resemble juvenile polyps. A notable feature is the presence of microscopic mucus retention cysts in the intestinal mucosa.

Other Polypoid Lesions

Metaplastic polyps occur in adult life often in the elderly and are visible to the naked eye as a small, pale grey sessile nodule never more than a few millimetres across and histologically shows crypt elongation and a curious feathery mucoid change in the surface epithelium (Fig. 16.55). It lacks dysplastic features and does not apparently have malignant potential.

Lymphoid polyposis. Occasionally the lymphoid aggregates in the rectum undergo reactive hyperplasia and present a polypoid appearance (**benign lymphoid polyposis**). This harmless condition is found mainly in young women and may be the result of viral infection. It also occurs in immunodeficiency states.

Inflammatory polyps have been described in the section on inflammatory bowel disease (p. 711).

Carcinoma

This is amongst the most common of all lethal malignant tumours in urbanized western society. Large bowel carcinoma is, however, mainly a

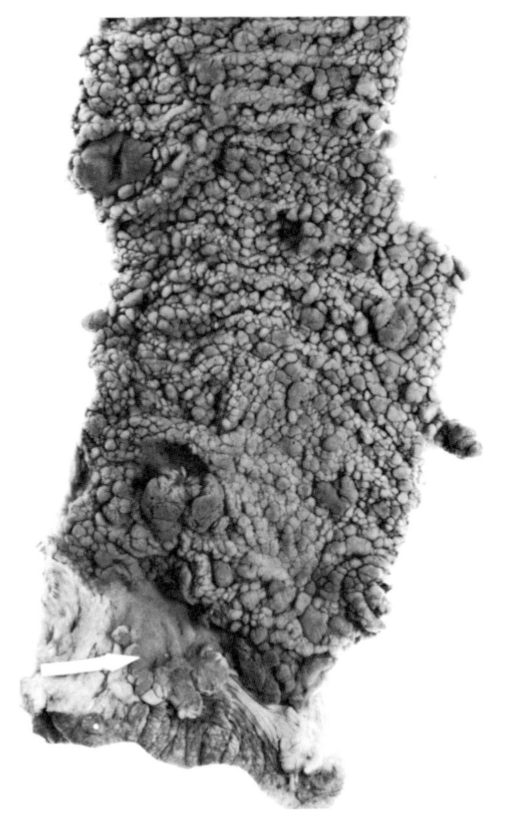

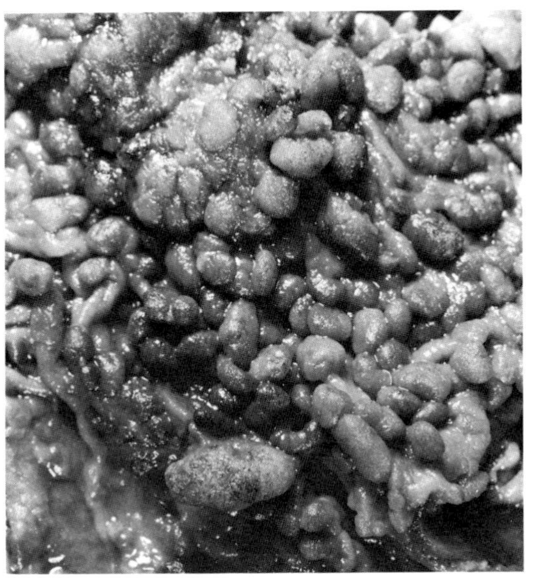

Fig. 16.54 Polyposis coli. Above, innumerable small polyps and several larger ones are present. Two small cancers have developed just above the anal margin. Below, showing the appearance of the individual polyps.

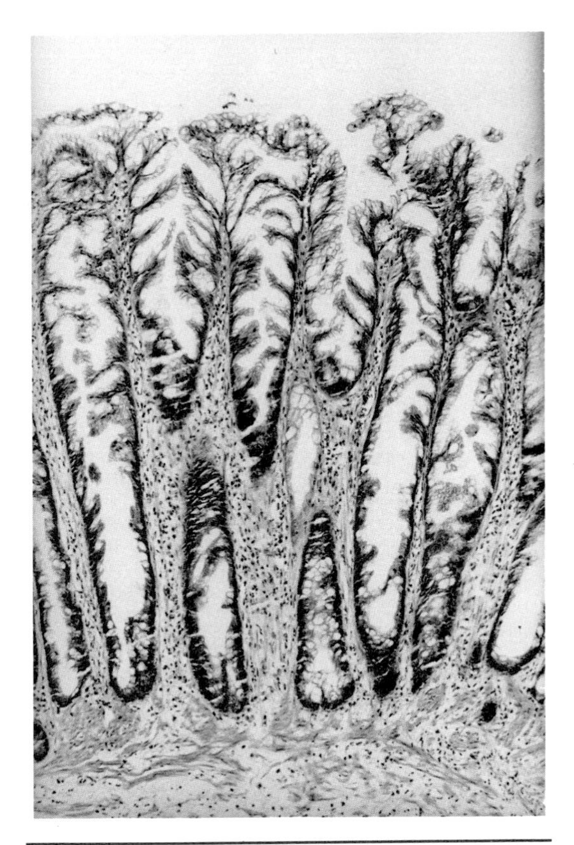

Fig. 16.55 Metaplastic polyp of colon. The surface epithelium has a characteristic 'feathery' mucoid appearance. H & E.

tumour of late adult life. It affects males and females in equal numbers.

Aetiology

Environmental factors are plainly involved. There is a marked geographical variation in incidence, the highest risk being in western urbanized communities. Low incidence areas include India, Africa and South America. Diets deficient in fibre with a high carbohydrate and fat content, leading to delay in the transit of faecal matter along the large bowel, may well be important since this would allow time for bacteria, especially anaerobes within the colonic lumen, to degrade substances such as bile acids with the possible generation of carcinogenic agents. The geographical incidence parallels that of diverticular disease in which dietary fibre has also been thought to be important

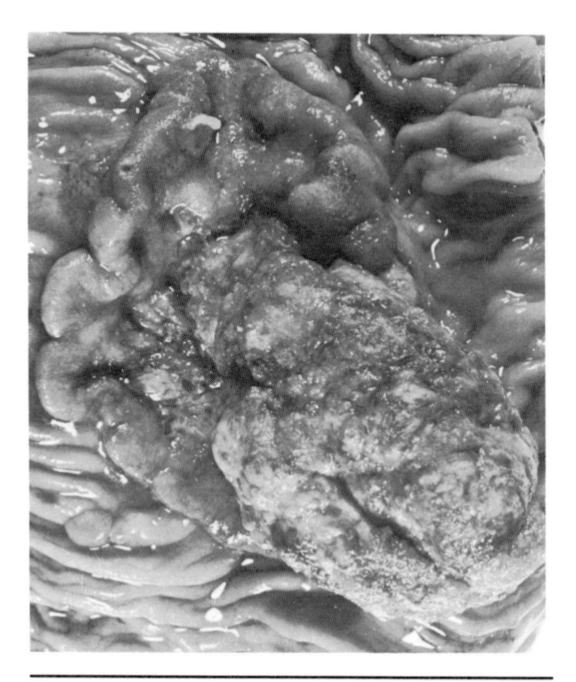

Fig. 16.56 Fungating carcinoma of the colon showing ulceration. Note the raised margin of the ulcer.

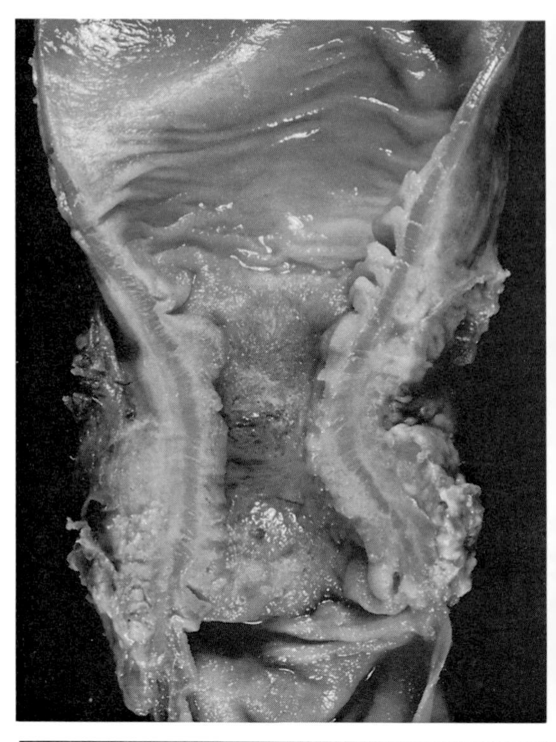

Fig. 16.57 Carcinoma of the descending colon. The tumour has ulcerated and caused obstruction, with consequent dilatation of the colon proximally and hypertrophy of the muscle coat.

aetiologically. The peak incidence is in the over 60 age group and the tumour is only rarely found in patients younger than 45 and this usually in association with adenomatosis coli or inflammatory bowel disease.

Precancerous lesions. Undoubtedly the most important of these are **adenomas** which we have just discussed. In terms of environmental factors it is noteworthy that the incidence of adenomatous polyps also parallels the incidence of carcinoma: in high incidence areas for carcinoma polyps are more common in the distal large bowel while in low incidence areas polyps are more common in the caecum and ascending colon where carcinoma also tends to occur. It now seems likely that the majority of carcinomas take origin from these lesions. In familial adenomatous polyposis the development of carcinoma is invariable if the condition is not treated and may take place at a relatively early age. The latter is also true of **inflammatory bowel disease** whose role in the pathogenesis of carcinoma has been discussed previously.

Clinicopathological Features

In males carcinomas develop most often in the rectum whereas in women the sigmoid colon is the more favoured site. In both sexes the caecum and ascending colon come next in terms of incidence. While carcinomas may initially appear polypoid (possibly reflecting their origin from adenomas) they later evolve into ulcerating lesions with elevated or rolled margins (Fig. 16.56). Often they encircle the gut (Fig. 16.57) and produce marked narrowing of the lumen (ring stricture formation) with eventual obstruction and all its subsequent effects, sometimes including ischaemic damage to the mucosa and stercoral ulceration (p. 720). In distal lesions these ulcerative and obstructive changes account for the early symptoms of rectal bleeding and alteration in bowel habit. In the caecum the tumours may attain a larger size before detection and may evolve into fungating masses prone to infection and ulceration. This accounts for the appearance of clinical disturbances such as fever (often accompanied by neutrophilia) and iron-deficiency anaemia prior to the onset of more obvious colonic symptoms.

Histologically, the tumour is almost always a mucin secreting adenocarcinoma, usually well or moderately well differentiated. Anaplastic signet-ring cell types are unusual. Occasionally the tumour presents the features of a mucoid carcinoma in which the tumour cells lie in lakes of extracellular mucin.

Spread and Prognosis

These tumours commonly penetrate the entire thickness of the intestinal wall to involve the serosa and sometimes extensive spread occurs within the peritoneal cavity. Involvement of adjacent structures such as bladder or pelvic wall may also take place. Lymphatic spread, initially to the paracolic lymph nodes, regrettably occurs at an early stage whilst blood spread to the liver is a relatively late phenomenon. The extent of spread can be used to assess the prognosis on any individual case. Using Duke's staging system it is notable that when the tumour is confined to the intestinal wall (stage A) the cure rate approaches 100% but when the tumour has penetrated the whole thickness of the wall (stage B) the cure rate falls to 70%. Lymph node metastases (stage C) reduce the cure rate to approximately 30%. Recent studies further suggest that the presence of a conspicuous lymphocytic infiltrate around the tumour, and an expanding as opposed to an infiltrative invasive margin represent favourable prognostic indicators.

Other Tumours

Carcinoids. These are relatively uncommon, comprising <1% of all colonic tumours. The general features have been discussed on p. 729. Hindgut carcinoids are largely confined to the rectum. They tend to present unusual histological patterns, the cells forming ribbons or trabeculae rather than packets as in the mid-gut. Small cell undifferentiated types also occur; they often produce multiple hormones. Rectal carcinoids are rarely argentaffin positive.

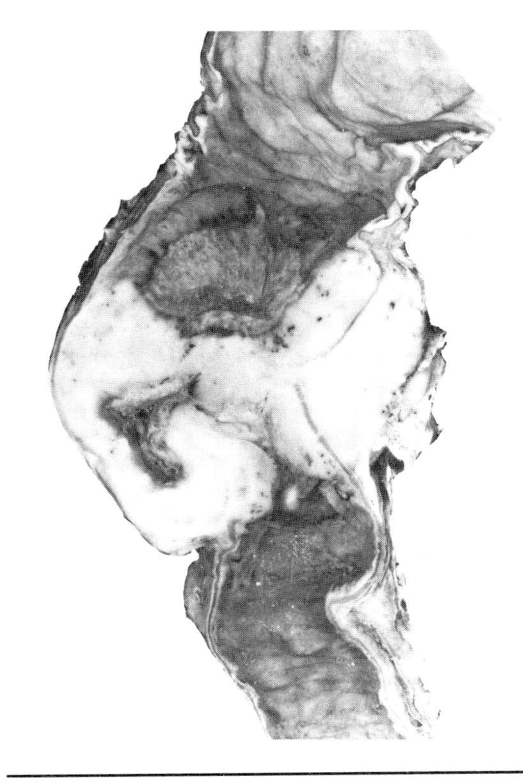

Fig. 16.58 Malignant lymphoma of the ileocaecal region.

Malignant lymphomas of the large bowel comprise 10% of all gastrointestinal lymphomas and probably less than 1% of malignancies in the colorectum. They are more common in the caecum and frequently extend to involve the ileum (Fig. 16.58). They may be associated with ulcerative colitis and usually arise in the rectum; as a complication of ulcerative colitis lymphoma is one-tenth as common as carcinoma.

Tumours of the Anal Canal

Malignant tumours are uncommon. Most are **squamous carcinomas**, but some exhibit a basaloid pattern resembling rodent ulcer (so-called cloacogenic carcinomas). Some tumours also show an admixture of mucin secreting and squamous elements (mucoepidermoid carcinomas). **Malignant melanomas** also occur in the anal canal. All these tumours tend to metastasize to both pelvic and inguinal lymph nodes and carry a poor prognosis.

The Peritoneum

Peritonitis

Acute peritonitis is nearly always due to spread of infection from an inflamed abdominal viscus. This may occur with appendicitis, cholecystitis, diverticulitis of the colon, infarction or strangulation of a segment of bowel and, in the female, salpingitis when the inflammation may remain confined to the pelvis – pelvic inflammatory disease. When there is perforation of a viscus then the peritonitis may be in part due to chemical irritation: the causes of perforation include peptic ulcer, typhoid ulcer, ulcerative colitis, stercoral ulceration and an ulcerated tumour, particularly a lymphoma. In acute haemorrhagic pancreatitis the escape of pancreatic enzymes provokes an intense chemical peritonitis in which fat necrosis is a prominent feature (p. 793). Acute spontaneous peritonitis (usually pneumococcal) may occur in children with the nephrotic syndrome and in adults may complicate hepatic cirrhosis when *E. coli* is the causal organism.

Peritonitis secondary to haematogenous spread is relatively uncommon. Patients treated by chronic ambulatory peritoneal dialysis may get peritonitis and in some instances there may be a low-grade inflammatory reaction to some chemicals in the dialysate. The causal organisms are extremely variable. *E. coli* infection is the most common either alone or in combination with other bacteria: other organisms include streptococci, staphylococci and anaerobes including clostridia, bacteroides and various Gram-negative bacteria.

In generalized peritonitis the surfaces are inflamed and a variable fluid exudate is present in the peritoneum. The exudate may become turbid or frankly purulent and there is usually a fibrinous deposit on the serosal surface. When the peritonitis has resulted from perforation of a viscus the reaction is usually more intense and haemorrhagic. The inflammation may sometimes be localized by the omentum and this may result in the formation of a periappendicular or peridiverticular abscess. Following resolution of the peritonitis residual foci of infection may occur, forming subphrenic, subhepatic or pelvic abscesses.

Acute generalized peritonitis is a serious condition *per se* which may, in addition, be accompanied by paralytic ileus, severe toxaemia, dehydration and electrolyte disturbances and a combination of septic and hypovolaemic shock. Recovery may be complicated by residual abscesses as already mentioned or by organization of the exudate to form fibrous adhesions between loops of bowel (Fig. 16.59). These may later cause intestinal obstruction due to kinking of the bowel, internal hernias or volvulus formation.

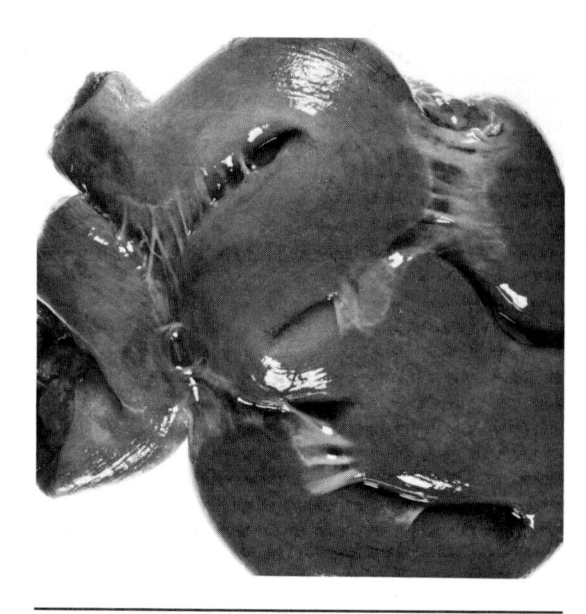

Fig. 16.59 Fibrous adhesion between loops of small intestine, resulting from organization of fibrin deposited during acute peritonitis.

Chronic peritonitis. Abscess formation secondary to acute peritonitis has already been mentioned. Tuberculous peritonitis is now uncommon. It may be localized or generalized and in the latter is usually the result of spread from a mesenteric lymph node or the fallopian tube. There is usually a peritoneal exudate and minute grey tubercles are scattered over the peritoneum and in the omentum. Surgically introduced foreign materials such as talc may produce a localized granulomatous reaction.

Miscellaneous Conditions

Mesenteric and omental cysts are of lymphatic origin and present in children either as painless masses or acutely as a result of rupture, torsion or intestinal obstruction.

Tumours

Primary tumours of the peritoneum are rare. Benign soft tissue tumours may arise in the retroperitoneal area and these include **lipomas, fibromas, neurofibromas** and **lymphangiomas. Mesothelioma** of the peritoneum presents features like those of mesothelioma of the pleura but is less frequent; in 85% of cases it is associated with exposure to asbestos.

Secondary tumours may appear as multiple 'seedling' deposits on the peritoneum and in the omentum sometimes with diffuse lymphatic permeation on the serosal aspect (Fig. 16.60) of the intestines or as larger discrete aggregates. The ovary, gastrointestinal tract and the pancreas are the origin of most primaries.

In mucoid carcinomas the peritoneum is filled with extensive soft translucent tumour deposits, a condition to which the term **pseudomyxoma peritonei** has been applied. Mucinous carcinomas of the ovary or appendix are the commonest primary sites, but the condition has also been associated with primaries in the gallbladder and pancreas.

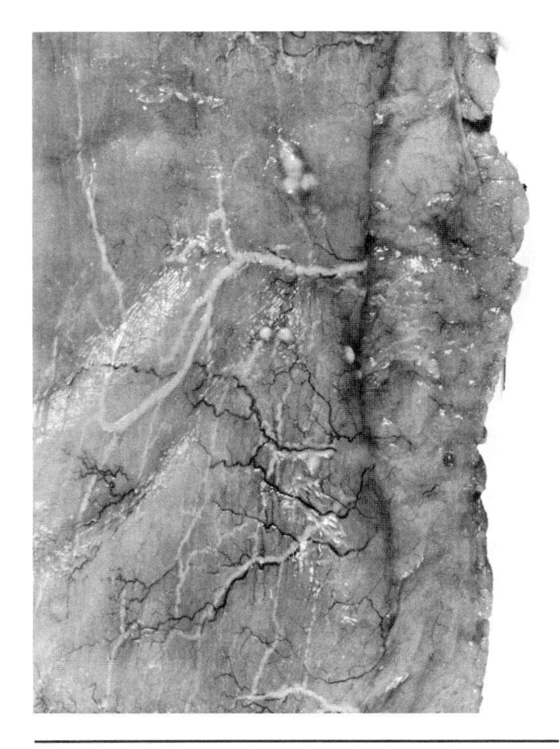

Fig. 16.60 Permeation of lymphatics in the serosa of the small intestine by gastric carcinoma cells.

Secondary sarcoma is rare but spread from leiomyosarcomas of the gastrointestinal tract or uterus may occur.

Retroperitoneal Fibrosis

Extensive formation of dense fibrous tissue in which there is an admixture of chronic inflammatory cells occurs retroperitoneally and sometimes extends into the mesentery. Retroperitoneal fibrosis may cause ureteric obstruction with hydronephrosis and pyelonephritis (p. 937). The aetiology is unknown but it may be a reaction to drugs, e.g. methysergide. It may be associated with Riedel's thyroiditis (p. 1093), sclerosing mediastinitis and primary sclerosing cholangitis (p. 768).

Further Reading

Appelman, H. D. (1984). *Pathology of the Oesophagus, Stomach and Duodenum.* Churchill Livingstone, Edinburgh.

Crohn, B. B., Ginzburg, L. and Oppenheimer, G. D. (1932). Regional ileitis; a pathological and clinical entity. *Journal of the American Medical Association* **99**, 1323–9.

Dalziel, T. K. (1913). Chronic interstitial enteritis. *British Medical Journal* **2**, 1068.

Filipe, M. I. and Jass, J. R. (1986). *Gastric Carcinoma.* Churchill Livingstone, Edinburgh.

Isaacson, P. G. and Spencer, J. (1987). Malignant lymphoma of mucosa-associated lymphoid tissue. *Histopathology* **11**, 445–62.

Jass, J. R., Love, S. B. and Northover, J. M. A. (1987). A new prognostic classification of rectal cancer. *Lancet* **1**, 1303–6.

Symmers, W. St. C. (1987). Alimentary system. In: Morson, B. C., ed. *Systematic Pathology*, 3rd edn, Vol. 3, Churchill Livingstone, Edinburgh.

Whitehead, R. (1989). *Gastrointestinal and Oesophageal Pathology.* Churchill Livingstone, Edinburgh.

Wyatt, J. I. and Dixon, M. F. (1988). Chronic gastritis – a pathogenetic approach. *Journal of Pathology* **154**, 113–24.

17

Liver, Biliary Tract and Pancreas

The Liver

The Anatomical Unit

The structural unit of the liver has long been considered to be the lobule arranged around a central hepatic venule and with portal tracts at its periphery (Fig. 17.1). In fact, the lobule forms a unit only in so far as blood from it drains into one central venule. It receives portal venous and hepatic arterial blood from several portal tracts, and its bile drains into several small bile ducts. On the basis of elegant microcirculatory studies, Rappaport and his colleagues (1954) have defined an alternative basic structural unit, the **acinus** (Fig. 17.2a); this is the parenchyma receiving blood from a single terminal portal venule and hepatic arteriole (termed together the **axial vessels**) and passing its bile into a single small duct in the same portal tract. The simple acinus lies between two hepatic venules into which its blood drains.

The simple acinus is subdivided into three zones (Fig. 17.2). The hepatocytes in zone 1 (**periportal zone**) are those nearest to the axial vessels; they receive blood rich in nutrients and oxygen and are metabolically more active than cells in the other zones. Zones 2 (**mid-zone**) and 3 (**perivenular zone**) are more peripheral to the axial blood supply; the cells of zone 3 are at the microcirculatory periphery of the acinus and are thus the most susceptible to hypoxic damage. Functional heterogeneity of hepatocytes is also reflected across the acinar unit with zonal variation in both enzyme distribution and bilirubin secretion.

Although the three zones of the simple acinus correspond loosely to the peripheral, mid-zonal and centrilobular zones of the traditional lobule, a comparison of Figs 17.1 and 17.2 shows that the correspondence is inexact. As differences in metabolic activities of hepatocytes generally depend on their relationship to the axial blood flow, and as this also influences patterns of pathological damage, these are best understood and described on the basis of the acinar concept. Thus, we shall refer in this chapter to the acinus as the basic anatomical and functional unit.

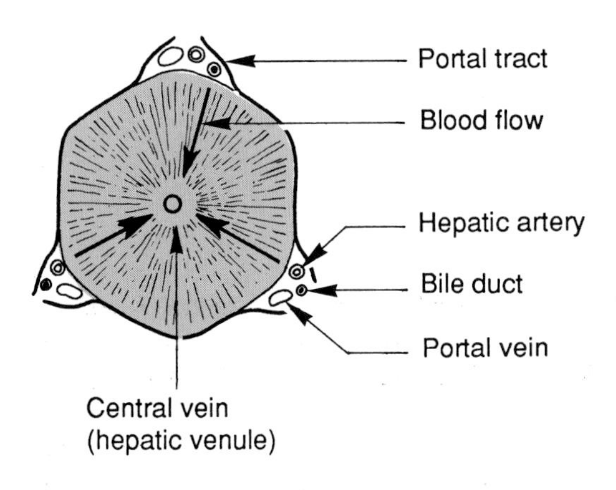

Fig. 17.1 Diagrammatic illustration of the hepatic lobule arranged round a single central (hepatic) vein into which blood flows.

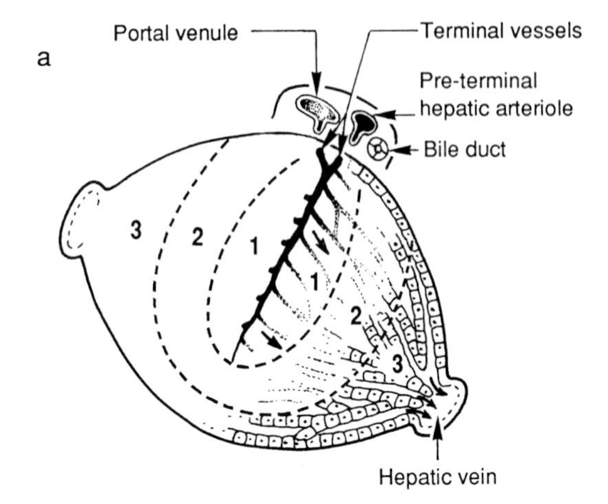

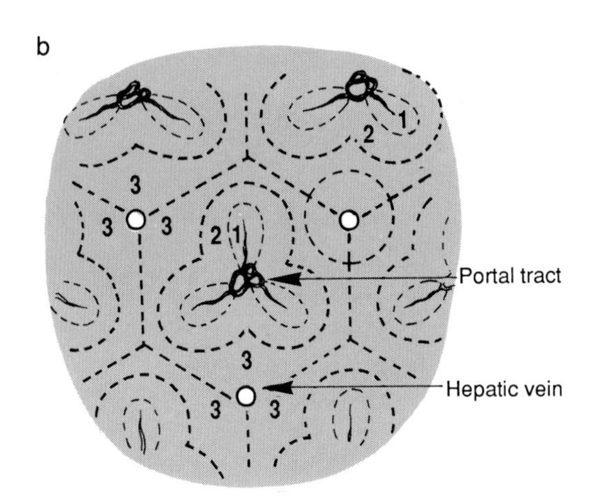

Fig. 17.2 **a** Diagrammatic illustration of the simple acinus arranged around the terminal branches of the hepatic artery, showing its blood draining into two hepatic vein branches. **b** Diagrammatic illustration showing the relationship between adjacent acini and how there is continuity between zones 3, i.e. the microcirculatory periphery of the acini.

Pathophysiology of Liver Disease

The liver has a very large number of important physiological functions. It is involved in the intermediary metabolism of proteins, carbohydrates and fats, in the synthesis of a number of plasma proteins such as albumin and fibrinogen, the production of various enzymes and the formation and secretion of bile. It is also responsible for the detoxification of endogenously produced waste products or exogenous toxins and drugs, and in the storage of proteins, glycogen, various vitamins and metals. Accordingly, the liver is liable to injury from a variety of causes, and injury to it may have profound metabolic effects.

Major Causes of Liver Disease

Certain virus infections damage the liver severely, causing acute hepatitis with extensive necrosis of liver cells. These include hepatitis A, hepatitis B, the non-A: non-B group and many others. Progression to chronic hepatitis is a complication of type B and some of the non-A: non-B group.

Injury from drugs and toxins. The liver cell is especially liable to injury because of its function of taking up and dealing with many metabolites, drugs and toxic substances. The vast number of chemicals used industrially and pharmacologically provide an ever-increasing hazard to the liver, particularly as certain chemicals which are harmless to most individuals can cause extensive liver damage in individuals with a special susceptibility, as yet unpredictable. A wide spectrum of hepatotoxic effects may be produced by the numerous drugs in clinical use (p. 413). The liver also receives blood draining the gastrointestinal tract, and is exposed to poisons and toxins absorbed from the gut.

Lesions of the biliary tract affect the liver in two ways. Biliary obstruction, if sufficiently prolonged, results in biliary cirrhosis, and the bile ducts are also a route of bacterial infection of the liver.

Injury from metabolic disturbances. In experimental animals specific dietary deficiencies can produce fatty liver and liver cell necrosis. Similarly, in man protein malnutrition can produce marked fatty change and there is evidence that malnutrition may considerably exacerbate other forms of injury. Specific enzyme deficiencies may cause various hepatic storage diseases (p. 746) or failure of bile excretion (p. 784).

Hypoxia. Owing to their active and complex metabolism, liver cells are readily injured by hypoxia, as in shock, venous congestion or anaemia. However, the dual blood supply to the liver affords some protection against hypoxic injury.

Tumours. Primary tumours of the liver are relatively uncommon in Britain though of great frequency in parts of Africa and the Far East: they are associated with cirrhosis. The liver is a very common site of metastatic carcinoma, particularly from primary tumours of the gastrointestinal tract.

Clinical Features of Disturbed Hepatic Function

Disturbances of function resulting from lesions of the liver and biliary tract are varied and complex. They may be considered under the headings hepatocellular failure and portal hypertension. These are described more fully later.

Hepatocellular failure arises when total liver cell function falls below the minimum required to maintain a physiological state. It results from loss of a large number of liver cells, and from impaired function of liver cells, attributable to interference with hepatic blood flow or interference with intracellular metabolic functions. Hepatic failure may be acute, as in massive liver cell necrosis due to hepatitis or drugs, or it may be chronic, for example in cirrhosis. The more important effects include:

(1) *changes in nitrogen metabolism* with a rise in the blood level of toxic nitrogenous compounds produced by bacteria in the gut and normally metabolized by the liver cells. These compounds are

particularly harmful to the central nervous system, causing hepatic encephalopathy;

(2) *jaundice* because of failure to remove bilirubin from the blood, to conjugate it and to excrete it in the bile;

(3) *failure to produce plasma proteins* in normal amounts, particularly albumin and clotting factors;

(4) *hormonal disturbances* attributable to interference with hepatic metabolism of various steroid and other hormones;

(5) *circulatory disturbances* with cyanosis and a hypervolaemic hyperkinetic circulation;

(6) *functional renal failure* (the hepatorenal syndrome).

Portal hypertension. This is caused by obstruction to the blood flow through the liver. As a result, veins which provide an anastomosis between the portal and systemic systems enlarge and some of the portal blood is shunted directly into the systemic circulation instead of passing through the liver. This increases the blood level of toxic compounds absorbed from the gut, thus aggravating the effect of hepatocellular failure on the central nervous system and other organs.

Biochemical Features of Disturbed Hepatic Function

The Liver Function Tests

Biochemical investigations are commonly used to assess the structural integrity of the liver, its ability to transport material from the blood into bile and its ability to synthesize and secrete substances into the blood. In clinical practice a group of tests is usually performed. These include the serum total bilirubin concentration as a measure of hepatic transport function and the severity of jaundice, the serum transaminase (aminotransferase) activity as a measure of the integrity of the liver cells, the serum alkaline phosphatase activity as an index of cholestasis, and the serum albumin concentration and the prothrombin time as an index of hepatic synthetic function.

The ability of the liver to metabolize various drugs, such as caffeine, and antipyrene, has also been used by some to assess the severity of liver disease, but these methods are rarely used in routine practice.

Bilirubin. Normal bilirubin metabolism is outlined on p. 783. Bilirubin in normal plasma is almost entirely unconjugated; both conjugated and unconjugated forms may accumulate during hepatobiliary disorders. Normally, the total serum bilirubin is less than 20 μmol/l, but in jaundiced adults the level exceeds 35–50 μmol/l. A small proportion of the normal population (2–5%) transport and conjugate bilirubin less effectively than the majority and these individuals may have minor increases in serum bilirubin concentration without other evidence of liver disease (Gilbert's syndrome). The causes of jaundice (clinical hyperbilirubinaemia) and the investigation of jaundiced patients are considered more fully on p. 783.

Transaminases. The activities in serum of two transaminases – aspartate aminotransferase (AST) and alanine aminotransferase (ALT) – have become widely used in the diagnosis of liver disease. AST is present mainly in the liver and the heart, although small amounts are present in several other tissues. ALT is also widely distributed, but its measurement in liver disease is rather more specific as its activity is relatively low in tissues other than the liver. The normal serum level for each is less than 40 iu/l.

Increased serum aminotransferase activity is a sensitive index of hepatocyte damage, but it has limited prognostic value. The increased activity results principally from the release of these enzymes from damaged hepatocytes. Acute liver damage, irrespective of the cause, usually increases the activity in serum more than tenfold but these values may be much higher in acute viral hepatitis and drug-induced hepatitis when there is widespread hepatic necrosis. In viral hepatitis the aminotransferase activity may be raised for as long as 2 weeks before the appearance of clinical jaundice. Aminotransferase activity may be raised also in chronic liver disease.

Alkaline phosphatase. The alkaline phosphatases are a family of isoenzymes that are widely distributed; they are found in particular in liver, bone, small intestine, placenta and kidney. Thus they are frequently elevated in patients with liver or bone disease, in the last trimester of pregnancy and in adolescents when bone turnover is maximal. The various isoenzymes can be estimated by biochemical techniques and the source of the elevated enzyme activity can be established.

In the liver alkaline phosphatase is found at the sinusoidal and canalicular borders of the hepatocytes. Therefore it is elevated in cholestatic liver disease; the higher the level of alkaline phosphatase, the more likely is extrahepatic cholestasis. The normal serum level is 20–85 iu/l.

Albumin. Albumin is the major secretory protein synthesized by the liver (some 8–14 g daily). The total exchangeable pool of albumin in the body is 280–350 g. About one-third of this is in the plasma, and two-thirds in the extravascular, extracellular space. It is important to remember that the concentration of albumin in the plasma (40–50 g/l) is much higher than in the extracellular space and that it is this concentration difference that accounts for its important role activity in determining the distribution of water in the body.

Hypoalbuminaemia is a feature of advanced chronic liver disease: it occurs in acute liver disease only if it is severe and of several weeks' duration. Hypoalbuminaemia in chronic liver disease is often taken as an indication of reduced hepatic albumin synthesis. However, in some cases albumin synthesis may be normal while the distribution or redistribution of albumin in the body is altered.

Other Biochemical Investigations

While the above group of biochemical investigations has proved to be of considerable help in the investigation of patients with liver disease other measurements may also be of value. Examples of these are:

(1) the serum immunoglobulins, the concentration of which are raised in most patients with chronic liver disease, e.g. IgG predominantly in chronic active hepatitis, IgA in alcoholic liver disease and IgM in primary biliary cirrhosis; and

(2) ceruloplasmin, the concentration of which rises in cholestasis and falls in the large majority of patients with Wilson's disease.

Coagulation factors. The liver is responsible for the synthesis of fibrinogen, prothrombin (factor II) and factors V, VII, IX and X. Failure of synthesis occurs in both acute and chronic failure, while, in the latter, vitamin K malabsorption due to cholestasis may also play a role. Assessment of these factors is made by measuring the **prothrombin time**. The extent of prolongation of the prothrombin time is roughly proportional to the severity of the hepatocellular injury and indeed, it is this index which is the most accurate predictor of outcome in acute hepatic failure.

Liver Cell Necrosis and Liver Cell Regeneration

Many of the causes of liver disease discussed above result in liver cell necrosis which, in turn, stimulates regeneration, and it is appropriate to discuss these before describing the specific types of disease.

Liver Cell Necrosis

This may be of variable extent:

(1) single scattered liver cells which die one by one (**apoptosis**) (p. 28). These cells become eosinophilic with a pyknotic nucleus which is eventually extruded leaving the **acidophilic** or **'Councilman' body**;

(2) small groups of hepatocytes – **focal necrosis** in relation to which macrophages and lymphocytes may accumulate. Focal necrosis occurs in acute viral and drug-induced hepatitis and as a non-specific reactive change in many systemic disorders;

(3) large groups of hepatocytes – **confluent necrosis**. This occurs in severe viral and drug-induced hepatitis and in acute ischaemic liver in-

jury. Confluent necrosis may extend between contiguous hepatic venules (central – central) or between hepatic venules and portal tracts (central – portal) – **confluent bridging necrosis**;

(4) extensive areas of the liver – **massive hepatic necrosis**, which represents a more severe degree of confluent necrosis and may be a sequel to viral hepatitis or drug injury. Clinically, it results in fulminant acute hepatocellular failure.

In chronic liver disease **piecemeal necrosis** occurs and is defined as destruction of liver cells at an interface between parenchyma and fibrous tissue, together with a predominantly lymphocytic or plasma cell infiltrate.

The factors which determine the topographical distribution of hepatic necrosis are not known but presumably these include zonal differences in enzyme distribution, cell metabolism and quality of blood supply. Ischaemic injury affects the perivenular zone of the acinus as do many drugs and toxins, for example alcohol and paracetamol. Less commonly, some agents, for example phosphorus, produce periportal injury, while yellow fever characteristically affects zone 2 of the acinus, producing a 'mid-zonal' pattern of necrosis.

Liver Cell Regeneration

Hyperplasia and hypertrophy of liver cells occur commonly as compensatory processes; indeed the liver is remarkable in its ability to regenerate in response to liver cell loss from whatever cause. Even when as much as two-thirds of the liver is removed, the weight of the organ is restored within a few weeks. The regenerative response is predictable and reproducible. In experimental animals the initial response, lasting for 24 hours, is one of liver cell hypertrophy; diffuse hyperplasia follows, initially commencing in periportal areas and peaking at about 30 hours. The proliferative response subsides when the original mass of the liver is restored. A similar response may follow a second or successive partial hepatectomies.

The factors responsible for the initiation and control of the regenerative response are not known, although local and circulating growth factors are important. The ability of the liver to regenerate allows it to recover from a variety of injuries and permits extensive surgical resection in the treatment of tumours. On the other hand, it may result in nodular regeneration, which occurs both as a recognized entity – nodular regenerative hyperplasia (pp. 111, 750) or as an essential component of cirrhosis (p. 764).

Metabolic Disorders and the Liver

Fatty Change

Lipid metabolism is outlined in Chapter 12. Because of their central role in fat metabolism, the liver cells are particularly prone to undergo fatty change, i.e. to accumulate in their cytoplasm droplets consisting mainly of neutral fat, and in adults a minor degree of fatty change is probably within physiological limits. In pathological obesity (p. 353) severe fatty change occurs in the liver, the accumulation of fat beginning and being greatest in periportal hepatocytes.

In addition to the causes of generalized fatty change – hypoxia, starvation or wasting disease, and numerous chemical and bacterial toxins – fatty change in the liver may also result from chronic malnutrition, alcohol abuse (p. 760) and in the rare conditions of acute fatty liver of pregnancy (p. 782) and Reye's syndrome (p. 781).

Fatty change in chronic malnutrition is a controversial topic of some importance because of the prevalence of malnutrition in many parts of the world. Severe malnutrition gives rise to a syndrome termed kwashiorkor, which affects infants and young children (p. 342). The syndrome is a complex one, attributable to a diet severely deficient in high-grade protein, but less deficient in total calories. The plasma albumin is low, there is nutritional oedema and features due to vitamin deficiency. The liver is severely fatty and may show mild fibrosis (Fig. 17.3); progression to cirrhosis does not occur.

Lipid Storage Diseases

In these conditions (p. 259) abnormal amounts of lipids (other than triglycerides) accumulate, mainly

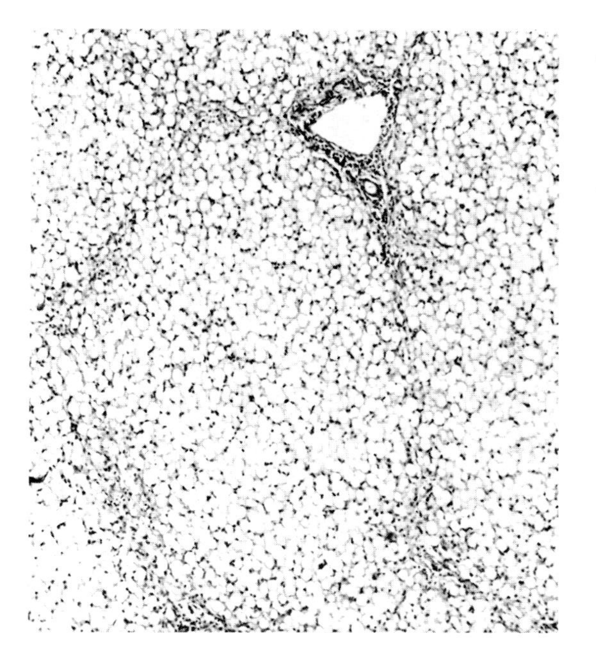

Fig. 17.3 Fatty liver in kwashiorkor. In addition to vacuolation of each liver cell by a large globule of fat, there is an apparent increase in fibrous tissue, seen as fine strands running through the parenchyma. ×40.

in cells of the mononuclear-phagocyte system, the Kupffer cells being consistently involved in Gaucher's disease (cerebroside accumulation) and Neimann-Pick disease (sphingomyelin). Hypercholesterolaemic lipid storage diseases rarely affect the liver.

Glycogen Storage Diseases

Glycogen storage diseases (p. 254) result from many different enzyme defects and the ultimate diagnosis depends on the demonstration of the specific defect. The liver cells are involved in types I, II, III, IV, VI and VIII, and the intracellular site of glycogen storage varies in the different types: electron microscopy may reveal diagnostically useful changes. Hepatocellular adenomas may develop in type I and cirrhosis in type IV. Excess of glycogen accumulates also in other metabolic disturbances, for example in diabetes mellitus.

Amyloidosis

The liver is involved in approximately 50% of cases of primary and secondary amyloidosis, but is less frequently involved in myeloma-associated amyloid. The SAA protein (p. 246) is synthesized by liver cells. The amyloid deposits accumulate in hepatic artery branches and in the perisinusoidal space, producing compression atrophy of the liver cell plates (Fig. 17.4). Amyloidosis only rarely causes hepatocellular dysfunction.

Other Metabolic Disorders

In a number of other metabolic disorders which affect the liver cirrhosis may result, e.g. haemochromatosis, Wilson's disease, alpha-1-antitrypsin deficiency, galactosaemia (p. 258).

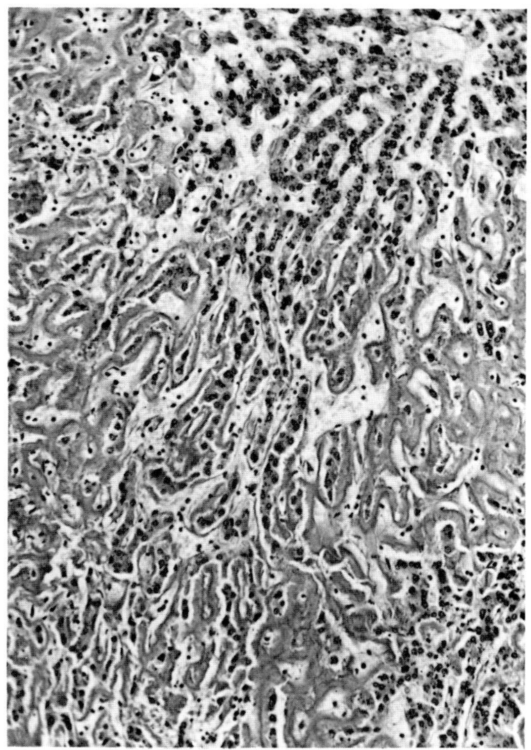

Fig. 17.4 Amyloidosis of the liver. The pale homogeneous amyloid has been deposited around the walls of the sinusoids, enclosing the column of liver cells, which are undergoing atrophy. The zone around the hepatic vein (*top right*) is least affected. ×115.

Circulatory Disturbances

The total hepatic blood flow is approximately 1.5 litres per minute, three-quarters of the blood being supplied by the portal vein and one-quarter by the hepatic artery. Thus, although hepatic arterial blood has a higher oxygen saturation (95%) than portal vein blood (85%), the latter normally provides approximately 70% of the hepatic oxygen requirement. Mixing of the two blood supplies takes place in the liver sinusoids, blood flow being controlled by sphincters at the portal and venular ends. Thus flow of arterial blood into the sinusoids may be intermittent, with consequent variations in the proportion of arterial and portal venous blood.

Hepatic Arterial Obstruction

The hepatic artery is rarely obstructed by disease. Fatal infarction can follow ligation of the main trunk, but adequate collateral circulation may prevent this. For this reason obstruction of smaller intrahepatic branches is usually without effect. However, local infarction may occur in polyarteritis nodosa and in acute bacterial endocarditis.

Portal Venous Obstruction

The normal portal venous pressure is 7 mmHg (0.9 kPa) and the most important effect of portal venous obstruction, whatever the site or cause, is portal hypertension. Impairment of the portal venous blood flow can arise from obstruction of the hepatic veins, the hepatic sinusoids, intrahepatic portal vein branches, or of the portal vein itself. The commonest and most important cause of obstruction is hepatic cirrhosis. Other intrahepatic causes include schistosomiasis (p. 1163), congenital hepatic fibrosis (p. 781) and metastatic or primary carcinoma of the liver. The portal venous pressure may also rise transiently in acute hepatitis – viral and alcoholic – due to sinusoidal compression by swollen liver cells.

Obstruction of the portal vein itself is uncommon. It can result from thrombosis, which may occur spontaneously or may complicate (1) umbilical sepsis in the neonatal period, (2) intra-abdominal sepsis, (3) direct invasion by tumour, (4) myeloproliferative disorders, (5) splenectomy, and (6) portal hypertension. Obstruction of the portal vein without thrombosis may result from pressure by tumours in or around the porta hepatis.

The effects of complete portal vein obstruction depend on the site. If it is in the portal vein alone nothing dramatic happens, but when it extends to occlude the ostium of the splenic vein, then the blood cannot drain via the splenic and gastro-oesophageal anastomoses and venous infarction of the bowel follows. Occlusion of a branch of the portal vein may sometimes be followed by 'red infarction' of the liver (Fig. 17.5), especially when venous congestion is also present. Such lesions, however, are not complete infarcts but are due to sinusoidal engorgement and atrophy of liver cells.

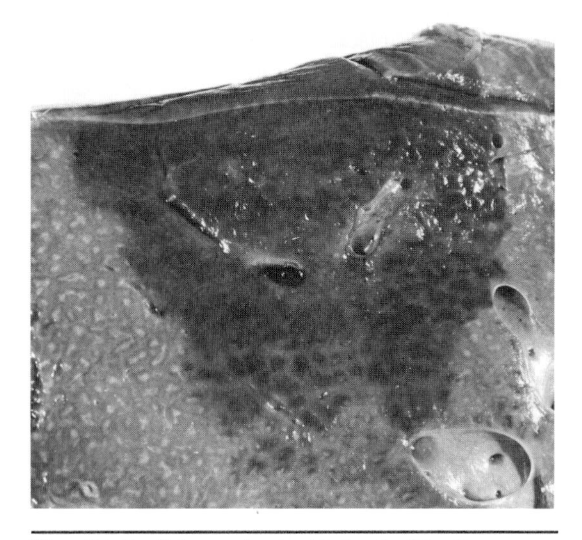

Fig. 17.5 Subcapsular 'red infarct' of the liver.

Hepatic Venous Obstruction

Obstruction of the major hepatic veins, clinically producing the Budd–Chiari syndrome, is rare. Spontaneous thrombosis of these vessels may occur in myeloproliferative disorders, in particular polycythaemia rubra vera (p. 633) and in thrombophlebitis migrans. It may also occur in pregnancy, in the post-partum period, or may be associated with the use of contraceptive steroids. In many instances the obstruction is due to endophlebitis, the aetiology being unknown. Compression by tumour masses or direct spread of tumour, for example hepatocellular carcinoma, in the major hepatic veins or the terminal inferior vena cava predisposes to thrombotic venous occlusion.

Intense engorgement of the liver results, with sinusoidal dilatation, perivenular congestion and haemorrhage, and there is atrophy and necrosis of liver cells. Abdominal pain and liver tenderness occur and ascites is usually severe. Death from hepatocellular failure results unless a porto-systemic venous shunt is carried out.

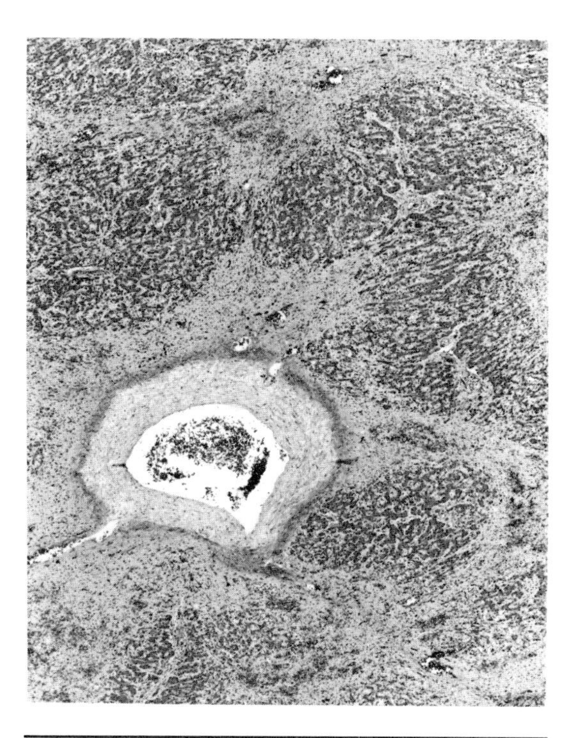

Fig. 17.6 Liver in veno-occlusive disease. There is extensive perivenular hepatocyte loss with replacement fibrosis and marked intimal fibrosis of the hepatic vein branch. ×28.

Veno-occlusive disease of the liver occurs in Jamaica and certain other tropical countries, probably as a result of drinking various plant or herbal medicines – 'bush teas'. The active agents are alkaloids of the pyrrolizidine group present in plants of the genera *Senecio* (ragwort), *Crotalaria* and *Heliotropium*. Changes are seen first around the hepatic venules which become obliterated by fibrosis (Fig. 17.6). Death may result from liver failure in acute cases, but a chronic stage may develop with progression to cirrhosis. Veno-occlusive disease may also result from irradiation of the liver, and has been associated with the use of immunosuppressants, oral contraceptive steroids and antineoplastic drugs.

Circulatory Disturbances due to Systemic Disease

Acute circulatory failure and shock. Impaired hepatic perfusion results from a fall in both hepatic arterial and portal venous blood flow as part of general circulatory failure. Initially the microcirculatory periphery (zone 3) of the acinus is injured, but involvement of zones 2 and 1 may occur in prolonged shock. Liver cell necrosis (Fig. 17.7) results, provoking an acute inflammatory reaction with infiltration of polymorphs. Biochemically, these changes are reflected by elevation of serum aminotransferases, which are sometimes as high as in acute viral hepatitis, and by variable increases in serum bilirubin levels.

Venous congestion. In the systematic venous congestion of acute cardiac failure the liver is enlarged, often tender, and microscopy shows sinusoidal dilatation and congestion in the perivenular areas. In chronic cardiac failure the changes are more marked (p. 111), with liver cell loss resulting from the continued effects of hypoxia and compression by the dilated sinusoids. Clinically, there may be mild jaundice, moderate or

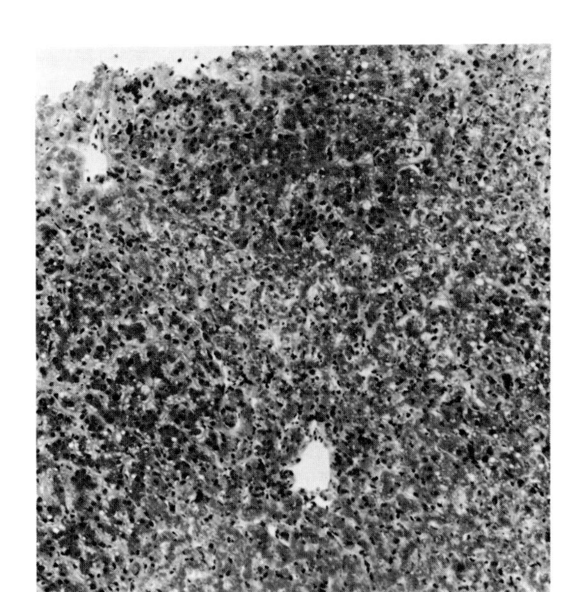

Fig. 17.7 Liver in acute circulatory failure: note the perivenular necrosis of hepatocytes producing bridging necrosis between adjacent branches of hepatic veins. ×80.

sometimes marked elevation of the serum aminotransferase levels and also a reduced rate of hepatic inactivation of various drugs. In very prolonged venous congestion, perivenular hepatocyte loss may be extensive. In some instances compensatory liver cell hyperplasia may occur with nodule formation and only minimal fibrosis – **nodular regenerative hyperplasia.** Sometimes replacement fibrosis takes place and fibrous septa link adjacent hepatic venous branches, resulting in architectural disorganization (Fig. 17.8); a true cirrhosis seldom, if ever, occurs.

Hepatitis

Hepatitis literally means any inflammatory lesion of the liver. In practice the term is not used for focal lesions, such as an abscess, but only when there is diffuse involvement of the liver. Hepatitis may be classified on an aetiological basis, and some types are best dealt with under the separate headings of alcoholic hepatitis and drug-induced hepatitis. Cirrhosis represents a late, irreversible and progressive stage of chronic hepatitis and is also discussed separately.

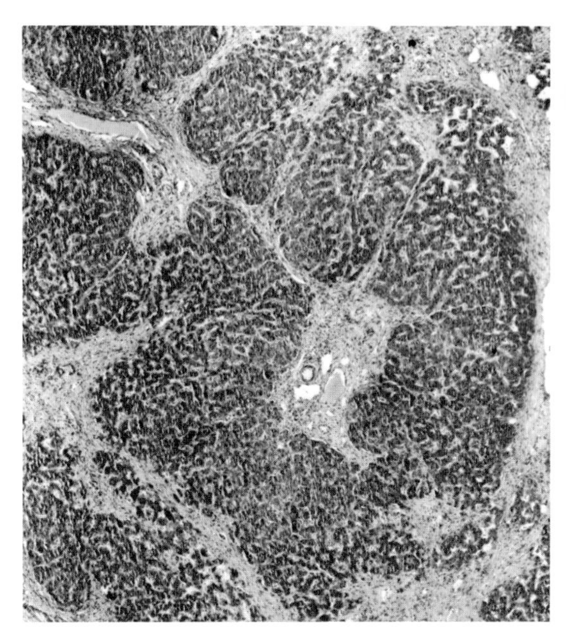

Fig. 17.8 Liver in chronic venous congestion: perivenular fibrosis has occurred with septate linkage between hepatic vein branches. Note the large portal tract (*central*) surrounded by surviving hepatic parenchyma. ×40.

In this section we deal with (1) acute viral hepatitis and with (2) chronic hepatitis, sometimes a sequel to acute viral hepatitis but often of unknown cause.

Acute Viral Hepatitis

This is an acute infection characterized by diffuse hepatitis with widespread liver cell necrosis. There are three well characterized viral types – hepatitis A (HAV), hepatitis B (HBV) and hepatitis D (HDV), and a less well characterized non-A: non-B group which includes a number of different viral infections. The features of these viruses are summarized and compared in Table 17.1.

Hepatitis A

Hepatitis A has an incubation period of 15–40 days, is transmitted by the faecal–oral route and

Table 17.1 Comparison of some of the features of acute viral hepatitis

	Type A (HAV)	Type B (HBV)	Types non-A: non-B	
			HCV	HEV
Incubation period	15–40 d	50–180 d	42–90 d	30–50 d
Patients	Children, young adults	Any age	Any age	Children, young adults
Transmission	Faecal–oral	Parenteral, perinatal, sexual	Parenteral and possibly faecal–oral	Faecal–oral; lower infectivity than HAV
Severity	Usually mild	Occasionally	Usually mild; relapse common	Usually mild; cholestasis
Mortality	1%	Variable, up to 10%	Not known, but fulminant hepatitis does occur	0.5–3%; 20% in pregnant women
Chronicity	Very rare	Common	Very common	Not known
Geographical distribution	World wide – occurs in epidemics	World wide – marked variation in incidence	Probably world wide	Asia and Africa but may be world wide
Virus and type	RNA picornavirus, 27 nm	DNA hepadna virus	RNA flavivirus or pestivirus, 40–50 nm	RNA virus, calcivirus, 32–34 nm

occurs both endemically and as epidemics. The infective agent is a picornavirus and associated 27 nm particles occur in the blood and faeces 3–4 weeks after exposure to the virus and can be demonstrated in the liver cell cytoplasm by immunocytochemical methods. Infection is commonest in children under 15, with a higher frequency in the lower socioeconomic classes. It is estimated that, during epidemics, up to 75% of the community may be infected, but in most the infection is anicteric and often subclinical. Acute infection can be diagnosed by the demonstration of anti-HAV IgM class antibody in the serum, while previous infection is characterized by the presence of IgG antibody which is protective. No carrier state exists. Passive immunization with pooled human IgG can prevent clinical disease.

Hepatitis B

Hepatitis B has an incubation period of 50–180 days; it is most frequently transmitted by blood and blood products. Whereas transmission was at one time a hazard of blood transfusion, the screening of blood donors for serum markers of HBV has virtually eliminated this. The virus may also be present in body fluids, saliva, semen and vaginal secretions and may also be transmitted by intimate physical contact including from mother to child and sexually. It is a particular hazard among active male homosexuals and intravenous drug abusers. The disease occurs in any age group. It is more severe than hepatitis A, with a higher mortality, and infection may result in the development of a carrier state or in progression to chronic liver disease.

Hepatitis B virus is a DNA virus, and is a member of the hepadna group, i.e. hepatic (hepa) DNA viruses. The complete infective virion (Dane particle) is a 42 nm particle consisting of a core of circular double-stranded DNA, a specific DNA polymerase and structural proteins, surrounded by an outer envelope of surface protein which is recognized serologically as hepatitis B surface antigen (HBsAg). The nucleocapsid contains two serologically distinct antigens, the core antigen (HBcAg) and 'e' antigen (HBeAg). Viral replication occurs in liver cell nuclei and HBcAg is released from the nucleus into the cytoplasm where infective viral particles are assembled. HBeAg is thought to be involved in this assembly process. The presence of HBeAg, HBV-DNA and viral DNA polymerase in the serum indicates active

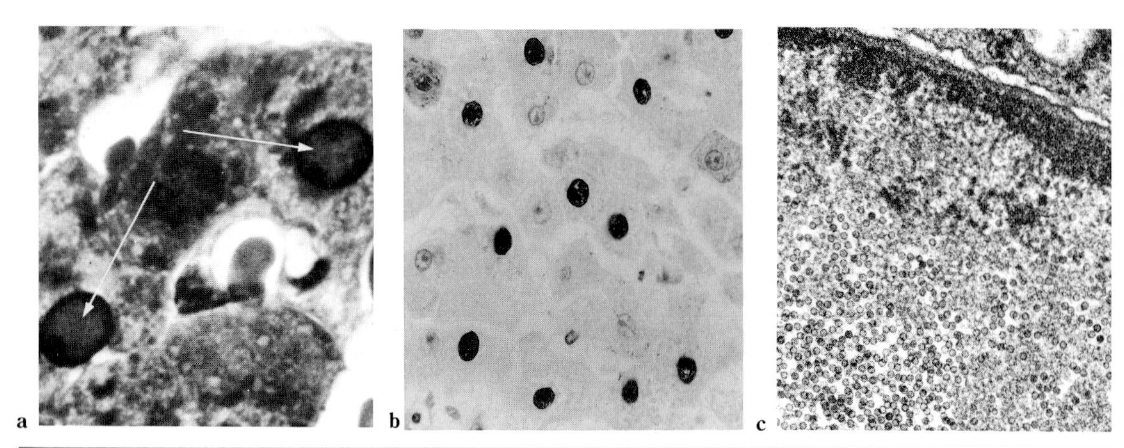

Fig. 17.9 Hepatitis B core antigen. **a** Nuclear excess of antigen producing 'sanded nuclei' (arrows). ×150. **b** Core antigens demonstrated by an immunoperoxidase technique: some nuclei are negative. **c** Intranuclear core particles demonstrated by electron microscopy: the nuclear membrane runs transversely across the upper part of the illustration. ×43 000. (Professor L. Bianchi, University of Basel, Switzerland.)

viral replication and correlates with infectivity of the blood.

Using immunocytochemistry, HBcAg is localized predominantly in the hepatocyte nucleus (Fig. 17.9), whereas HBsAg is found in the liver cell cytoplasm (Fig. 17.10). HBsAg, for reasons which are not understood, is produced in considerable excess and may accumulate in smooth endoplasmic reticulum producing the characteristic 'ground glass' hepatocytes (Fig. 17.10). Excess HBsAg also appears in the serum, and electron microscopy shows it to form small spheres and tubular structures 20 nm in diameter (Fig. 17.11). Four distinct antigenic subtypes of HBsAg exist; these are useful in epidemiological studies.

The patterns of antigen and antibody response

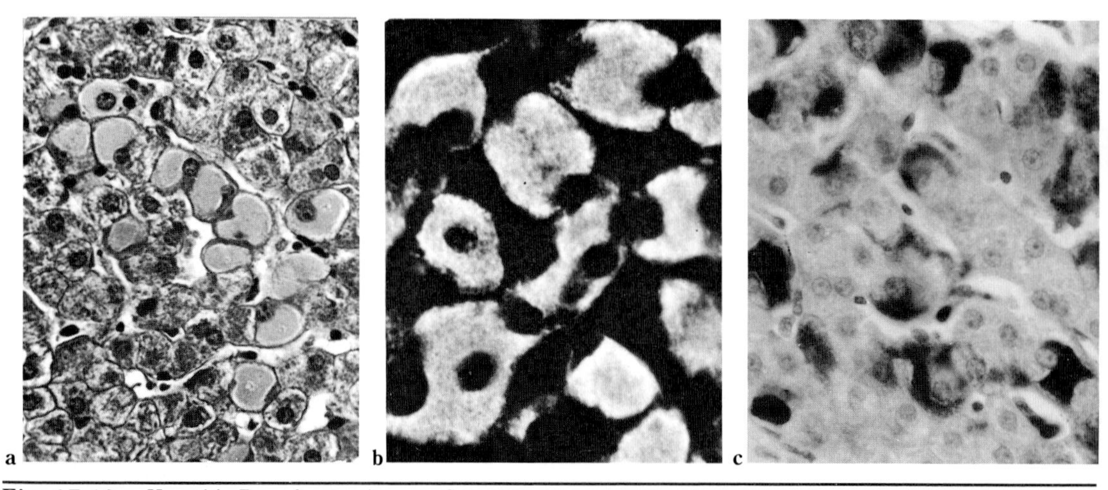

Fig. 17.10. Hepatitis B surface antigen. **a** Cytoplasmic excess of antigen producing 'ground glass hepatocytes' with an intracytoplasmic homogeneous inclusion. Masson's trichrome. ×250. **b** Specific immunofluorescence for surface antigen showing uniform cytoplasmic staining: the nuclei are negative. (Professor L. Bianchi, University of Basel, Switzerland.) **c** Surface antigen demonstrated by an immunoperoxidase technique: there are different patterns of expression by the liver cells.

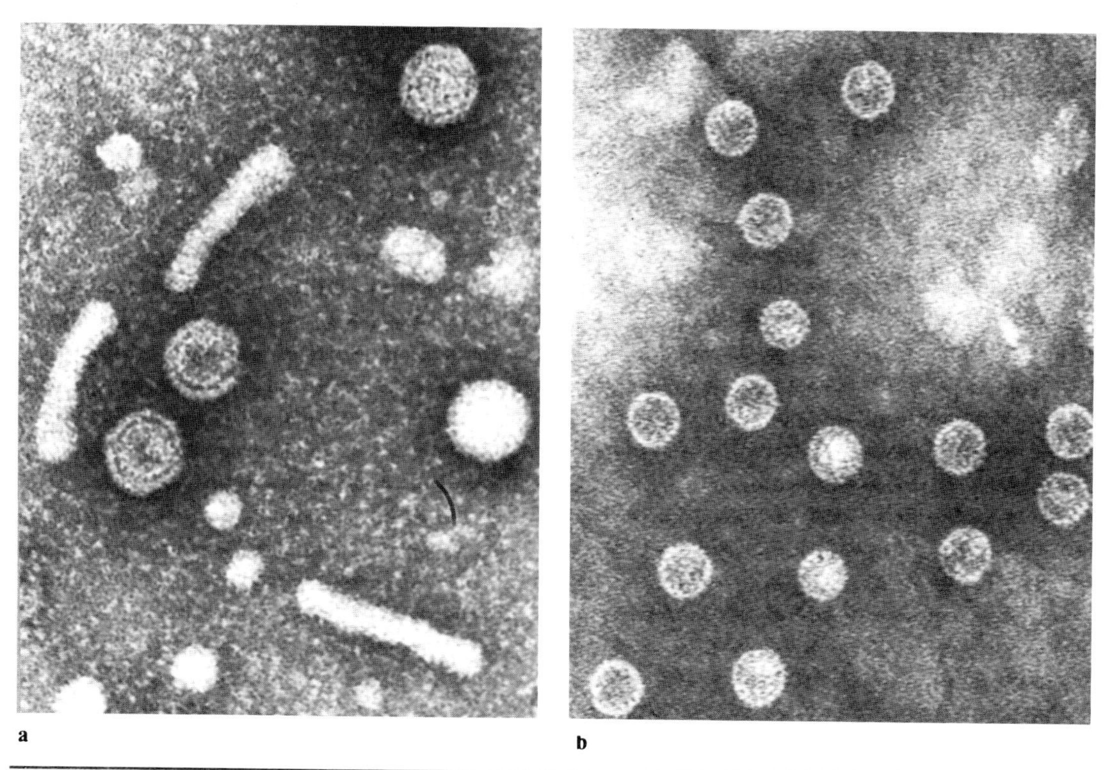

Fig. 17.11 Electron micrographs showing the morphological forms of the HBsAg. **a** This shows the small spheres and tubular structures (20 nm diameter) together with the larger double-shelled Dane particles (42 nm diameter). The small spheres, tubules and outer coat of the Dane particle comprise HBsAg. The inner part of the Dane particle is HBcAg. ×300 000. **b** A preparation of purified core particles – HBcAg. ×300 000. (Dr June Almeida.)

in the acute attack, with elimination of the virus and full clinical recovery, are shown in Fig. 17.12a. The development of antibody to HBsAg (HBsAb) occurs several months after infection. It is regarded as the protective antibody. While recovery with elimination of the virus is the outcome in most adult patients, about 5% develop chronic hepatitis and progress to cirrhosis and about 5% become chronic carriers; the pattern of antigen and antibody responses in these patients is shown in Fig. 17.12b. Chronic active hepatitis is associated with failure to produce HBsAb and persistence of HBeAg. In contrast, the chronic carrier produces HBeAb, but there is persistent production of HBsAg and a failure to produce HBsAb; such a carrier state may develop after a period of chronic active liver disease (Fig. 17.12b) with seroconversion to HBeAb positivity and cessation of viral replication.

The host factors which result in a failure of complete viral elimination are not fully understood, but viral persistence is more likely to occur in males and the incidence of carriers in the community shows marked geographic variation. In Britain it is in the order of 0.1%, whereas in parts of Africa and South-east Asia it is as high as 20%. Vertical perinatal transmission from mother to child is the most important mode of infection in countries with high carrier rates. The virus is transferred from mother to child as a result of close contact. In 5% of cases viral elimination occurs but, in contrast to adults, a carrier state arises in 95% of cases. This is thought to be due to the blocking effect of HBcAb acquired transplacentally. Active immunization against HBV infection is now available. A genetically engineered subunit vaccine which induces HBsAb protects against the virus.

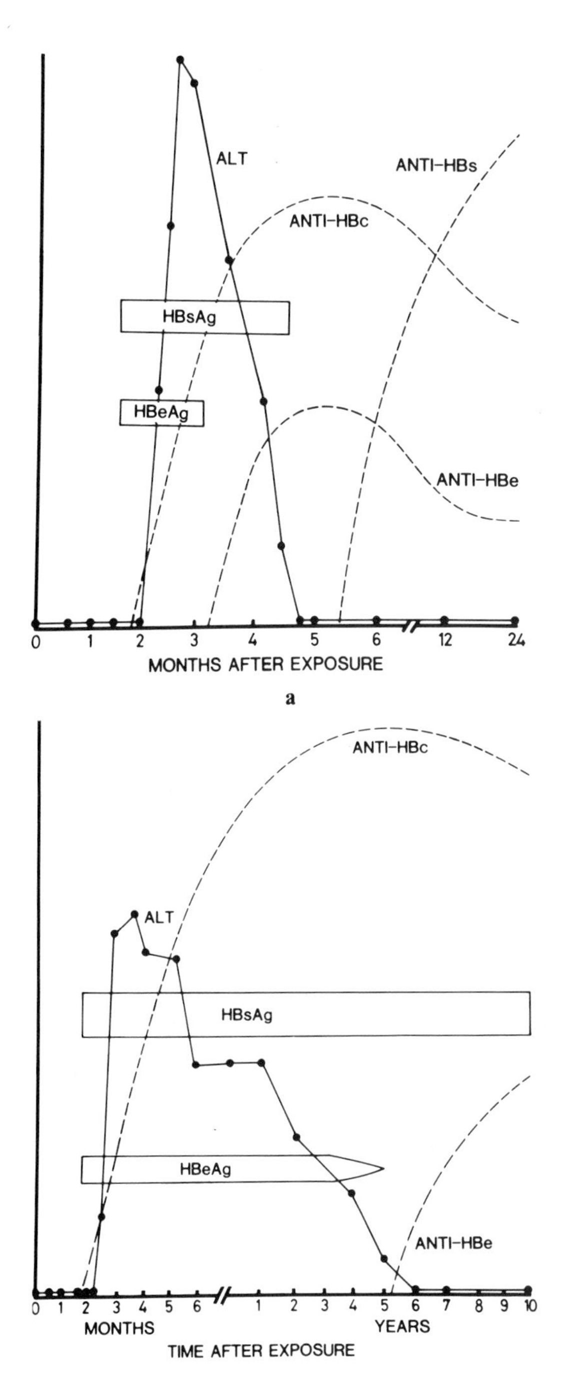

Fig. 17.12 Humoral responses in hepatitis B infections (see text). **a** With clinical recovery and viral elimination, **b** Chronic infection with continued viral replications. ALT, alanine aminotransferase. Units on the vertical axis are arbitrary.

Hepatitis D

Previously known as the delta agent, this is a defective RNA virus which usually requires HBV for its replication. The infective particle contains HDV RNA coated with HBsAg. Antigen can be detected in liver cell nuclei by immunohistochemistry. HDV, which occurs on a worldwide basis, modifies both acute and chronic HBV infections. It can be acquired simultaneously with HBV (co-infection) or it may secondarily infect chronic HBV carriers (super-infection). In both cases the clinical illness is more severe and the liver injury more extensive than infection with HBV alone.

Non-A: Non-B Hepatitis

The term non-A: non-B hepatitis was used to describe clinical cases of viral hepatitis in which the aetiological agent could not be defined. Most of these occurred after blood transfusion and a high proportion led to chronic hepatitis. At the time of writing two agents have been partially characterized; one associated with the transfusion of blood and blood products – parenteral non-A: non-B due to hepatitis C virus (HCV) – and another responsible for epidemic outbreaks and thought to be enterically transmitted – enteric non-A: non-B due to hepatitis E virus (HEV).

Hepatitis C

This has an incubation period of 42–90 days, is transmitted by blood and blood products and is now the most important cause of post-transfusion hepatitis. It is prevalent among intravenous drug addicts and co-infection with HBV can occur.

The causative agent has recently been identified by molecular cloning techniques and is thought to be a 10 000 nucleotide single stranded RNA virus which shares homology with the pestiviruses and flaviviruses. Although the viral particle itself has not been isolated, several serological assays are now available to measure anti-HCV antibody and HCV RNA can be measured in serum using the polymerase chain reaction. Clinically, antibody to HCV appears between 1 and 6 months after the acute illness.

Infection with this virus is an important cause of

chronic liver disease. It is estimated that 30–60% of post-transfusion HCV hepatitis patients develop chronic liver disease, characterized by an indolent course with recurring episodes of relapse and remission progressing to cirrhosis. The only treatment of proven value is alpha-interferon. Clearly an asymptomatic carrier state must exist and in Britain the prevalence among blood donors is 0.3–0.6%.

Hepatitis E

This has an incubation period of 35–40 days, is transmitted by the faecal–oral route and occurs epidemically in Asia and Africa. It causes an illness similar to hepatitis A. The causative agent is a single-stranded RNA virus, 32–34 nm, similar to the calciviruses. It mainly affects young adults in whom it causes a mild illness with jaundice; however, there is a high fatality rate in pregnant women. Progression to chronicity does not seem to occur. There is, as yet, no effective immunoprophylaxis.

Clinical and Biochemical Features

The early clinical features of acute hepatitis are severe nausea, anorexia, intolerance of fat, vomiting and fever. A 'serum-sickness-like' syndrome may be seen, with arthralgia and skin rashes. There is often epigastric pain and the liver is enlarged and tender. Jaundice develops 3–9 days after this prodromal illness and reaches a peak by 10 days, during which period the stools are pale and the urine dark. These features subside in 2–6 weeks but full clinical recovery may take longer. The serum bilirubin level is raised (80–250 μmol/1) and is mainly in the conjugated form. The serum enzymes AST and ALT may reach levels greatly in excess of 1000 iu/l early in the disease and then fall rapidly with the onset of jaundice. The one-stage prothrombin time is usually prolonged, and this provides the best single indication of the severity of the hepatitis.

Most patients recover completely from an attack. Mortality rates vary depending on the type of virus (Table 17.1). In very severe cases, death results acutely from fulminant liver failure due to massive hepatic necrosis. In some cases jaundice is deeper and persists for weeks or even months – **cholestatic hepatitis** – but eventually there is complete recovery. The development of chronic carrier states and of chronic active hepatitis and cirrhosis are discussed later. The **post-hepatitis syndrome** with vague features – undue fatigue, dyspepsia and hepatic pain – occurs in a small number of patients.

Pathological Features

Classical Acute Hepatitis

The morphological features of all types of acute viral hepatitis are virtually the same. There is diffuse hepatic involvement (Fig. 17.13) with more severe changes in the perivenular areas (acinar zone 3). The most striking feature is focal necrosis of hepatocytes. Many liver cells are swollen with a vacuolated hydropic cytoplasm. Some liver cells become eosinophilic and eventually the nucleus is extruded forming an acidophil or Councilman body. Associated with the necrosis there is a mononuclear inflammatory cell infiltrate, predominantly lymphocytic and there is reactive hyperplasia of Kupffer cells. A lymphocytic infiltrate is also seen in the portal tracts, but in hepatitis A plasma cells may be numerous. Mild cholestasis is also seen.

The liver quickly recovers from the acute injury, and, before the clinical attack has subsided, hypertrophy and hyperplasia are seen among surviving hepatocytes. As necrosis diminishes and resolution occurs, Kupffer cell activity becomes more prominent and aggregates of ceroid-laden macrophages are seen. Eventually the liver returns to normal.

The mechanisms of the liver cell injury are not fully understood but are probably immunological. Swelling of hepatocytes followed by lysis probably occurs, but this seems unlikely to be a direct effect of the virus since in chronic hepatitis virally infected cells may appear morphologically normal.

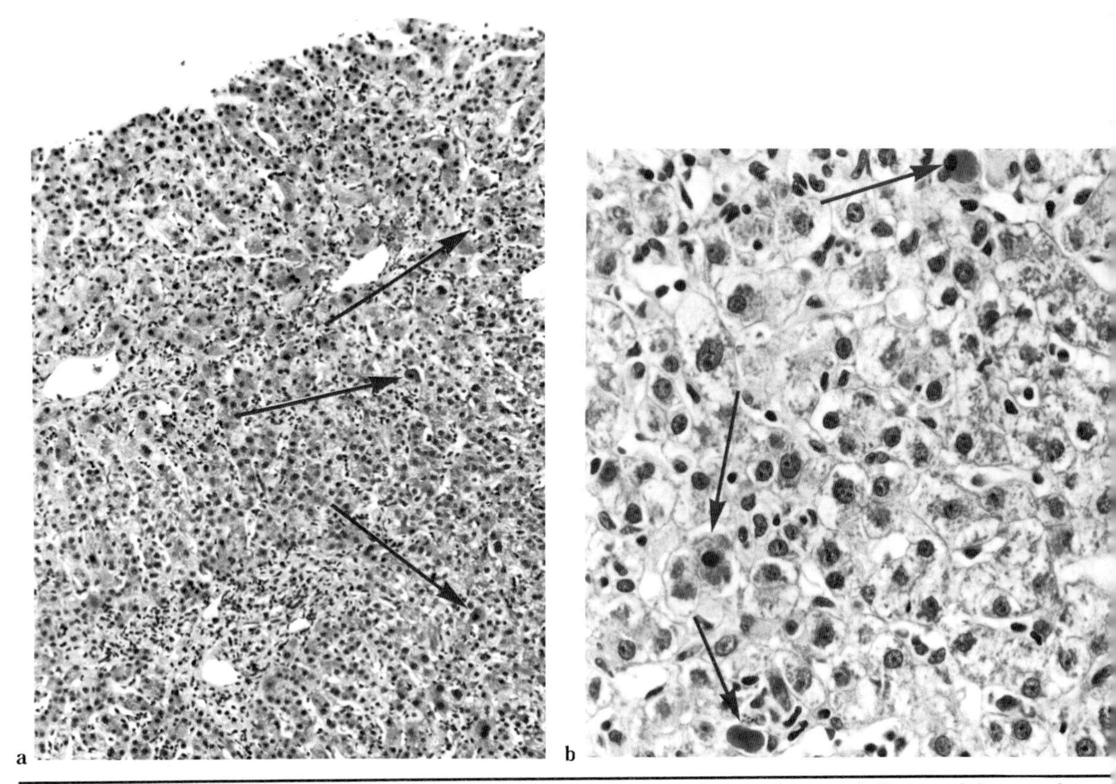

Fig. 17.13 **a** Liver in viral hepatitis. There is a moderately intense mononuclear cell infiltrate of the portal tract (*lower centre*), and a more intense diffuse parenchymal cell infiltrate with liver cell degeneration and a number of acidophil bodies (arrowed). ×120. **b** Perivenular area showing a number of ballooned hepatocytes, a diffuse mononuclear infiltrate, and a number of acidophil (Councilman) bodies (arrowed). ×360.

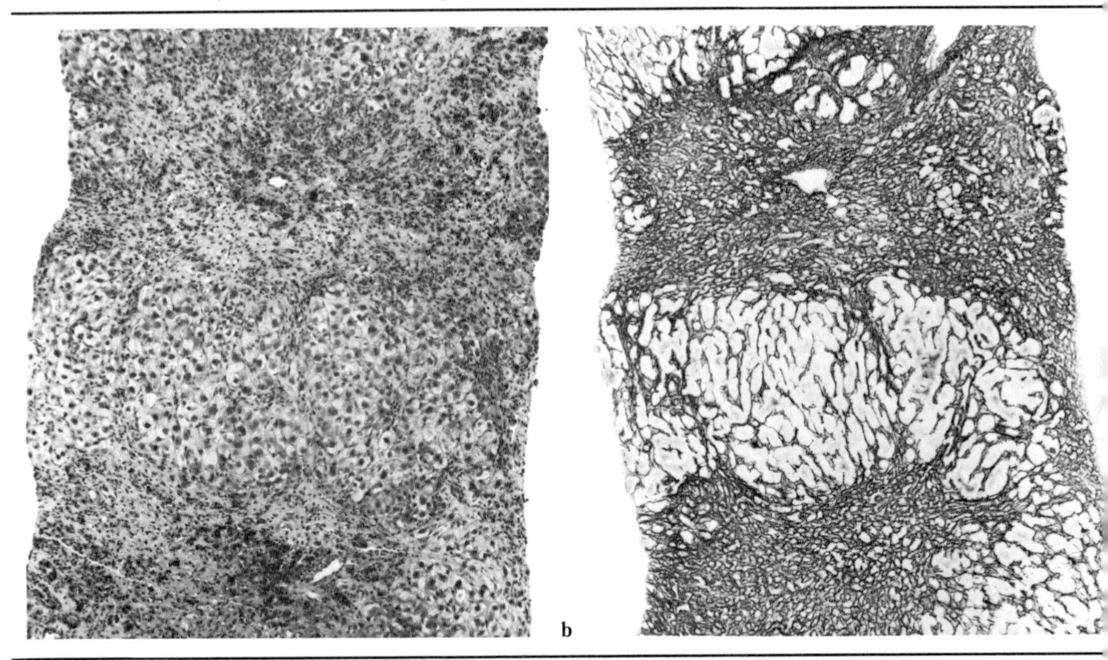

Fig. 17.14 Liver in viral hepatitis with bridging necrosis. Note the extensive confluent necrosis of liver cells, producing collapse of the reticulin framework. Full uneventful recovery occurred in this patient. **a** H & E ×60. **b** Gordon and Sweets' reticulin ×60.

Acute Hepatitis with Bridging Necrosis

In these cases there is more extensive loss of liver cells particularly in zone 3 (Fig. 17.14). There is lytic necrosis of hepatocytes, an intense inflammatory infiltrate and condensation of the reticulin framework. The areas of necrosis coalesce to form central–central and central–portal linkages as already described. Survival depends on the regenerative power of the spared parenchyma, and with survival there is usually a restoration of normal architecture.

Acute Hepatitis with Massive (Panacinar) Necrosis

There is confluent necrosis of all or nearly all the hepatocytes in large areas of the liver. It is in these patients that fulminant hepatic failure and death occurs in the acute attack, although it is not clear why this should happen in some cases of viral hepatitis. When death occurs early in the illness, the liver is approximately normal in size and is strikingly yellow due to bile-staining. In those who survive for some time, the dead cells disappear and the affected parts of the liver become shrunken, soft and red due to congestion and haemorrhage. If the patient survives longer, proliferation of the surviving liver cells produces pale regenerative nodules of varying size, and scarring occurs in the area of liver cell loss (Fig. 17.15), producing a shrunken nodular liver – **post-necrotic scarring.**

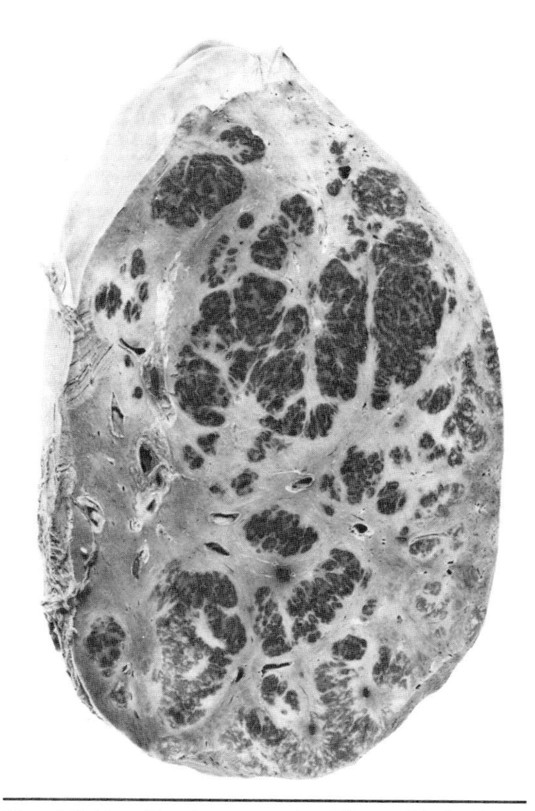

Fig. 17.15 Massive necrosis of liver with fatal outcome. The pale areas consist of fibrous tissue, the liver cells having undergone necrosis in the initial attack with subsequent autolysis. The dark nodular areas consist of tissue in which the liver cells survived the initial attack, but were destroyed in a fatal recurrence.

Hepatitis Due to Other Viruses

Yellow fever, caused by a group B arbovirus, occurs sporadically and in epidemics in certain parts of Africa and tropical America. The disease occurs in monkeys and is transmitted to man by the bite of *Aedes aegyptii* and certain other mosquitoes. It varies in severity from a mild febrile illness to fatal fulminant hepatic failure, acute renal failure and marrow depression. The hepatic lesion consists of mid-zonal necrosis in which acidophil bodies are prominent. (It was in yellow fever that Councilman first described these bodies.)

Acute hepatitis may occur as an unusual complication of infection by a number of non-hepatotropic viruses. These include **rubella** and **herpes simplex** in infancy and childhood, but rarely in adults. In **infectious mononucleosis** due to the Epstein–Barr virus, abnormal lymphoid cells may accumulate in the portal tracts and sinusoids, and a mild form of clinical hepatitis often occurs. **Cytomegalovirus** hepatitis in older children and adults causes a hepatitis which resembles closely acute viral hepatitis A or B.

Chronic Hepatitis

Chronic hepatitis is defined as inflammation of the liver continuing without improvement for at least 6 months. Chronic inflammation is also a feature of alcohol-induced liver injury, long-standing biliary obstruction, Wilson's disease and other metabolic disorders. While these conditions may also be associated with morphological features similar to those about to be described, and also run a chronic course, they are not strictly included under the heading chronic hepatitis and are classified on an aetiological basis.

Chronic hepatitis has traditionally been subdivided into a relatively benign form, chronic persistent hepatitis, in which the inflammation is largely confined to the portal areas, and a more aggressive form, chronic active hepatitis, in which there is portal, periportal and acinar involvement with progressive fibrosis ending in cirrhosis. It is perhaps best to regard chronic persistent hepatitis as the mildest form in the spectrum of chronic hepatitis. Such a pattern of liver injury may be seen in patients with chronic active hepatitis who go into remission, either spontaneously or due to immunosuppressant therapy (Fig. 17.17).

Chronic Active Hepatitis

Chronic active hepatitis (Table 17.2) may be classified as being of viral, autoimmune, drug-induced or unknown aetiology. About 10% of patients with acute hepatitis B fail to eliminate the virus and, of these, 5% progress to chronic active hepatitis with persistence of HBeAg and HBsAg in the serum and continued expression of both core and surface antigen in the liver. A chronic course occurs also in cases of parenteral (HCV) non-A: non-B hepatitis; serological identification of other viruses in this group may shed light on some of the cases currently of unknown aetiology. In autoimmune chronic active hepatitis antinuclear factors and smooth muscle antibodies occur: rheumatoid factor and microsomal antibody are less frequent. None of these antibodies is specific for chronic active hepatitis, and there is no evidence that they are of aetiological significance. Additional features in the autoimmune type of chronic active hepatitis include arthralgia, skin rashes, pleural effusions, thrombocytopenia, leucopenia and proteinuria attributable to glomerular lesions. Some patients also may have chronic inflammatory bowel disease, Sjögren's syndrome and other diseases of possible autoimmune aetiology.

Chronic active hepatitis may present acutely and be indistinguishable from an acute viral hepatitis, or it may be insidious with non-specfic symptoms of anorexia, tiredness, vague upper abdominal pain and often amenorrhoea. There is hepatomegaly, and a reactive splenomegaly which precedes the development of any portal hypertension. There may be hepatocellular failure, but the disease tends to fluctuate in severity. Biochemical tests show mild elevations of aminotransferase levels, but the occurrence and degree of jaundice varies. In the later stages more advanced changes of hepatocellular dysfunction occur. Without treatment chronic active hepatitis usually progresses to cirrhosis, although some cases may subside spontaneously.

Pathological Features

Chronic active hepatitis is manifest by continuing progressive inflammation with liver cell degeneration and bridging necrosis. The diagnostic histological lesion is **piecemeal necrosis**. This may be periportal (Fig. 17.16) or may be periseptal (Fig. 17.18) in areas of bridging hepatic necrosis. Continued inflammatory activity with fibrosis and septum formation between adjacent hepatic veins and between portal tracts and hepatic veins results in severe architectural distortion. Continuing injury produces a macronodular cirrhosis.

The features of acute hepatitis may be superimposed. In some instances, this may be the dominant feature – **chronic lobular hepatitis.** When chronic active hepatitis is a sequel to hepatitis B infection, 'ground glass' hepatocytes containing HBsAg can be identified (see Fig. 17.10). Core antigen can be demonstrated in liver cell nuclei (see Fig. 17.11) as can hepatitis D antigen when this virus is implicated.

Table 17.2 Aetiological types of chronic active hepatitis

	Clinical features	Serological markers
Autoimmune	Female predominance; HLA-B8, DR3 associated; peak incidence in teenage and perimenopausally. Extrahepatic features, e.g. arthralgia. Associated with other autoimmune diseases. Good response to immunosuppressants	High-titre non-specific autoantibodies: antinuclear, anti-smooth muscle and antimicrosomal
Viral hepatitis B	Male predominance. Wide age distribution. May be complicated by HDV infection. Poor response to immunosuppression but possible benefit from interferon-γ. Spontaneous remissions occur	HBV markers in serum (see Fig. 17.11). HBsAg, HBeAg, HBcAg
Viral hepatitis C	Commonest cause of post-transfusion hepatitis. Relapse and remission pattern characteristic	Anti-HCV and HCV RNA
Drug-induced	Idiosyncratic drug reactions, e.g. α-methyldopa, isoniazid, nitrofurantoin. Resembles autoimmune type	Low titre antinuclear and anti-smooth muscle antibodies present

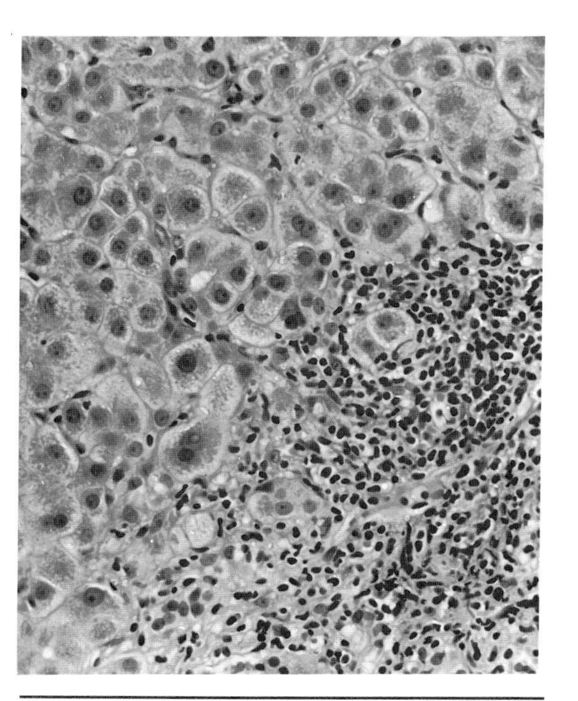

Fig. 17.16 Chronic active hepatitis with piecemeal necrosis. Note the irregular margin (limiting plate) between the portal tract fibrous tissue (lower right) and periportal liver cells, some of which are swollen and vacuolated and are entrapped and surrounded by chronic inflammatory cells. ×340.

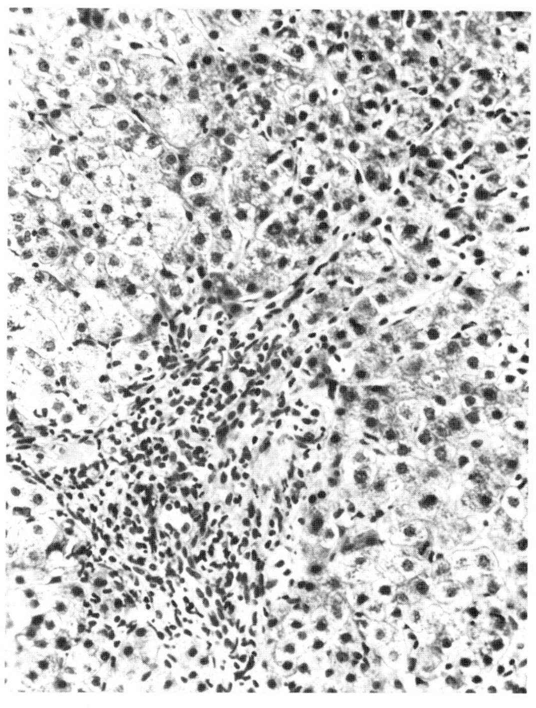

Fig. 17.17 Chronic active hepatitis in remission. There is a mononuclear cell infiltrate confined to the portal tract in the lower left quadrant with little or no involvement of the hepatic parenchyma. ×205.

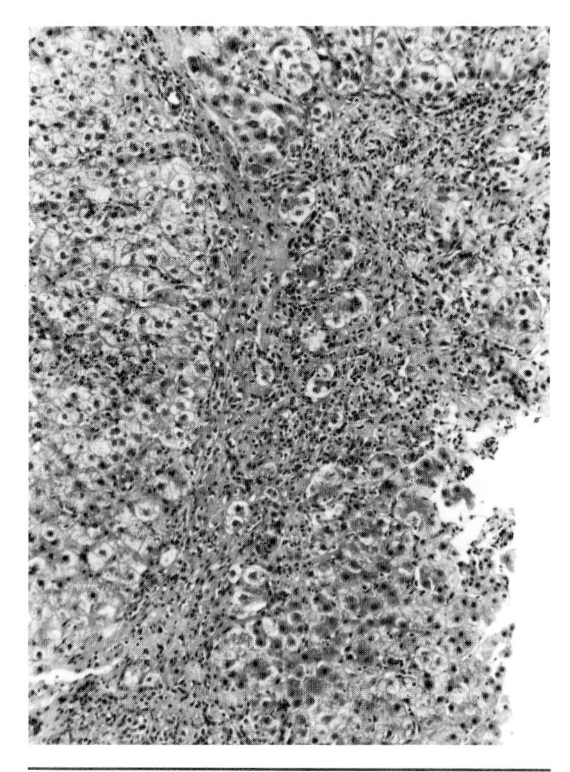

Fig. 17.18 Chronic active hepatitis with bridging septa causing architectural distortion; there is well marked piecemeal necrosis at the fibrous/parenchymal interface. ×120.

Alcoholic Liver Disease

The changes in the liver brought about by high alcohol consumption include fatty liver, alcoholic hepatitis, hepatic fibrosis and cirrhosis. Fatty change alone is a reversible disorder, while alcoholic hepatitis is considered to be the precursor of cirrhosis. Excess alcohol consumption alone has been shown to produce these hepatic lesions in man without any other obvious nutritional abnormality, and their degree and severity are related to the amount and duration of alcohol abuse. However, dietary imbalance and nutritional deficiencies, particularly of protein, may accompany alcohol abuse, and may aggravate the hepatotoxic effects of alcohol.

Alcoholic Fatty Liver

Under controlled conditions alcohol administration has been shown to produce hepatic fatty change regularly in man. After a single dose of alcohol the fatty acids which accumulate in the liver are derived from fat depots, whereas with chronic alcohol intake they are predominantly of dietary origin.

The relationships between alcohol metabolism and accumulation of fat in the hepatocyte are outlined in Fig. 17.19. Alcohol is broken down mainly by oxidation by alcohol dehydrogenase (ADH) in the cytoplasm. This results in the generation of hydrogen ions, and is reflected by an increase in the reduced: non-reduced nicotinamide adenine dinucleotide ratio (NADH:NAD), with a resultant change in reduction–oxidation (redox) potential. Some alcohol is also metabolized by microsomal enzymes in the smooth endoplasmic reticulum, this pathway being known as the microsomal ethanol oxidizing system (MEOS); it is dependent on the reduced form of NAD phosphate (NADPH). Normally the ADH:MEOS ratio for alcohol metabolism is approximately 3:1, but in chronic alcohol abuse, with an increase in smooth endoplasmic reticulum, a greater amount may be metabolized via the MEOS.

This increase in endoplasmic reticulum is a well recognized feature of alcoholic liver damage, and it seems likely that induction of a number of microsomal enzyme systems may accompany this increase and contribute to some of the other effects of alcohol on hepatocyte fat metabolism. In addition, the mitochondria are damaged by alcohol; they become swollen, sometimes markedly so, producing giant forms (Fig. 17.20d).

The cumulative effects of these changes on hepatocyte fat metabolism are as follows:

(1) accumulation of fatty acids, mainly because the NADH:NAD redox changes inhibit their oxidation via the citric acid cycle; this is aggravated by the direct damage to mitochondria. In addition there is an increase in the concentration of α – glycerophosphate and this results in trapping of fatty acids in the hepatocytes. These fatty acids are then esterified in the endoplasmic reticulum to

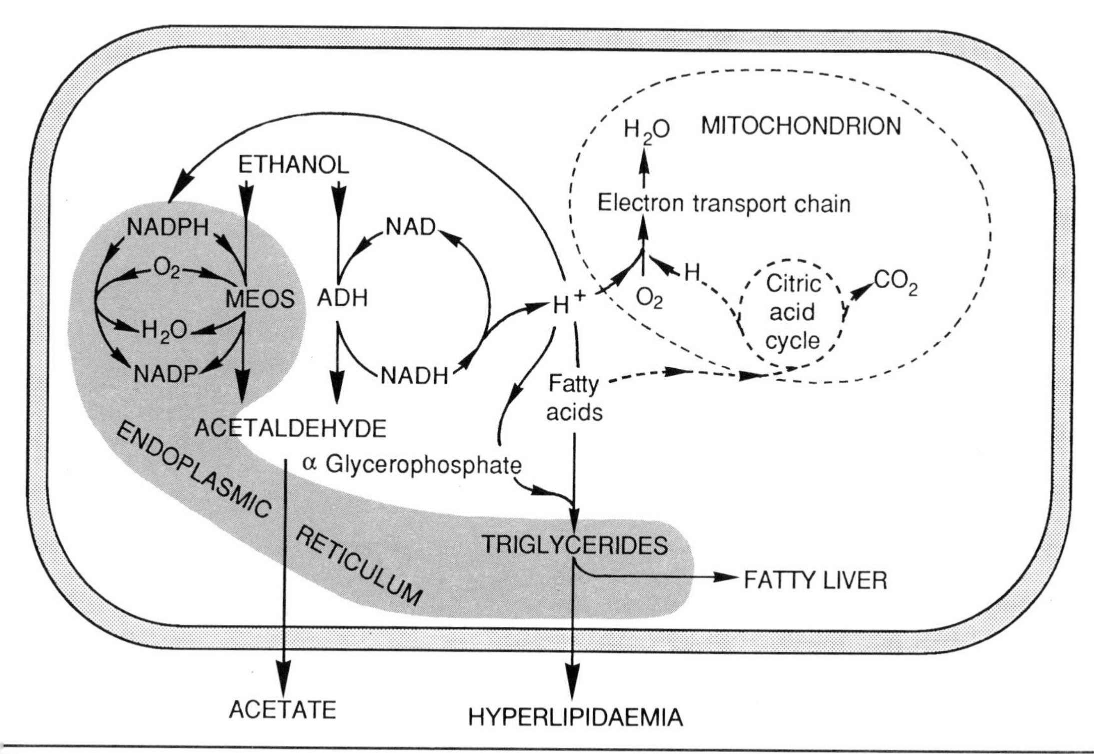

Fig. 17.19 Alcohol metabolism and fatty change in the liver cell, schematic representation. ADH, alcohol dehydrogenase; MEOS, microsomal ethanol oxidizing system. Pathways that are decreased by alcohol are represented by interrupted lines. (Modified after and printed with permission from Professor C. S. Lieber.)

triglycerides, some of which accumulate in the hepatocytes. In addition, however, increased lipoprotein synthesis occurs in the SER and some of these triglycerides are transported into the circulation, producing hyperlipidaemia;

(2) cholesterol esters also accumulate, and this is partly due to increased cholesterol production in the SER and partly to a reduced cholesterol catabolic rate.

These mechanisms combine to produce fatty change, which can be detected after only 2 days of excess alcohol. Conversely, stopping alcohol results in a rapid mobilization of the fat from hepatocytes. When the fatty change is severe, cholestasis and hepatocellular failure may develop.

Alcoholic Hepatitis and Cirrhosis

In contrast to our understanding of alcohol-induced fatty liver, the metabolic events that lead to the development of alcoholic hepatitis and cirrhosis are still not understood. Both the volume of alcohol and the duration of alcohol abuse are related to the development of these lesions. Estimates suggest that a daily consumption of more than 100g of alcohol (5 large whiskies, 5 pints of beer or 1 bottle of wine) represents a hepatotoxic level of alcohol intake. However, there are undefined host factors which determine susceptibility. Clinical evidence suggests that alcoholic hepatitis develops after 3–5 years of sustained alcohol abuse but this occurs in only about 35% of chronic alcoholics; in turn only one-third of these (i.e. 12% of alcoholics) progress to cirrhosis. Females, however, are at greater

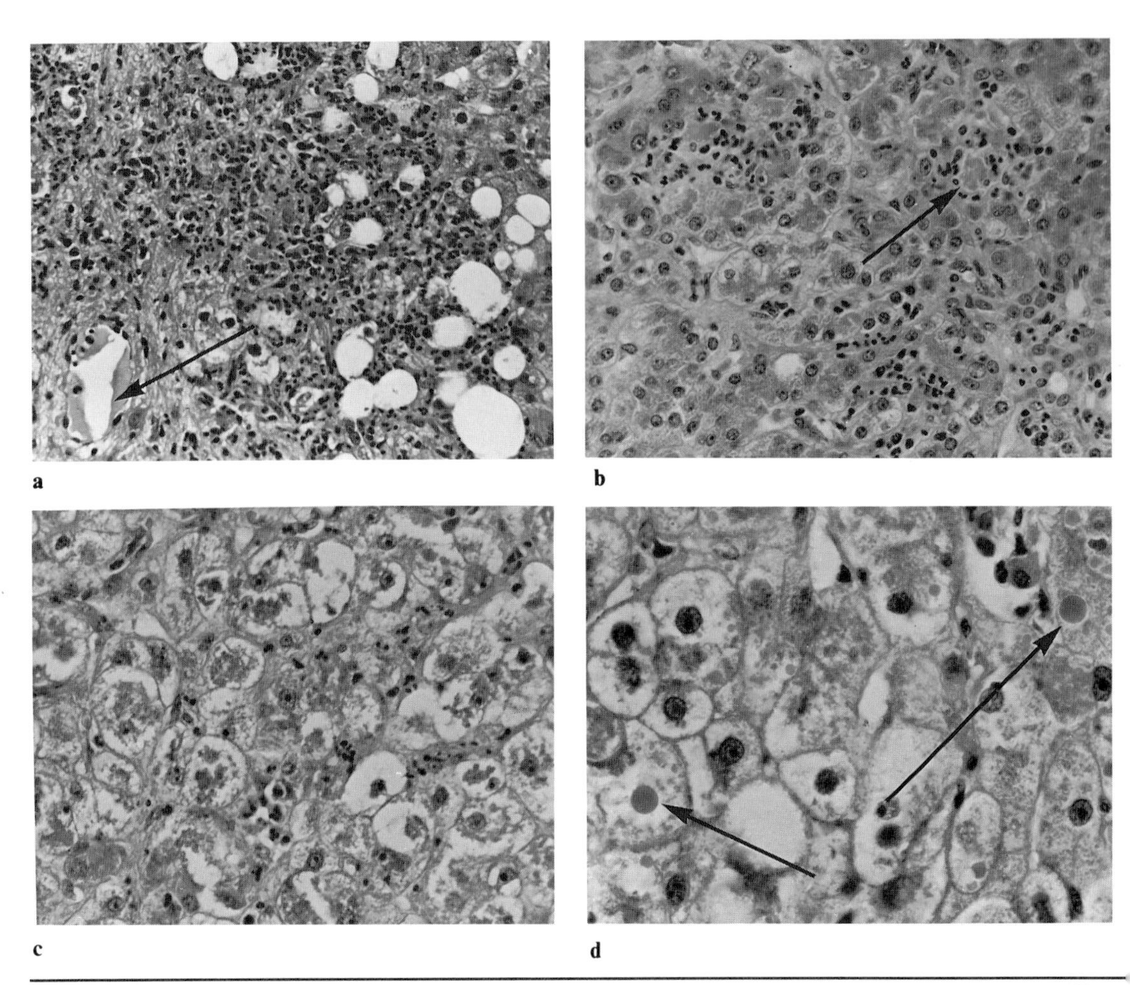

Fig. 17.20 Alcoholic hepatitis. **a** The perivenular distribution of the lesion is evident (hepatic vein arrowed). There is extensive liver cell necrosis with an inflammatory cell infiltrate. ×150. **b** Foci of liver cell necrosis with a neutrophil polymorph infiltrate, these cells in some areas (arrow) arranging themselves around Mallory body containing liver cells. ×270. **c** Mallory bodies are present (arrow) and a few neutrophil polymorphs are also seen. ×270. **d** Giant mitochondria (arrowed) within liver cells. ×350.

risk, developing alcoholic hepatitis with smaller daily amounts and over a shorter period of abuse.

In alcoholic hepatitis, which is usually superimposed on a fatty liver, there is ballooning and necrosis of hepatocytes, associated with a neutrophil polymorph reaction (Fig. 17.20b). The hepatitis develops around hepatic vein branches (Fig. 17.20a). Amorphous irregular eosinophilic aggregates of **Mallory's hyalin (Mallory bodies** – Fig. 17.20c) are seen within the cytoplasm of some hepatocytes; it has a fibrillar pattern on electron microscopy and represents an accumulation of intermediate filaments in the damaged cells. Giant mitochondria may also be noted (Fig. 17.20d). Fibrosis is an early feature, showing a pericellular distribution, and with continued liver cell loss, fibrous septa are formed. In some instances the hepatitis is severe with diffuse parenchymal involvement leading to liver failure.

Continuing alcoholic hepatitis results in progressive fibrosis and scarring; fibrous septa extend and form links between contiguous perivenular areas and between hepatic veins and portal tracts. The liver architecture is increasingly distorted and

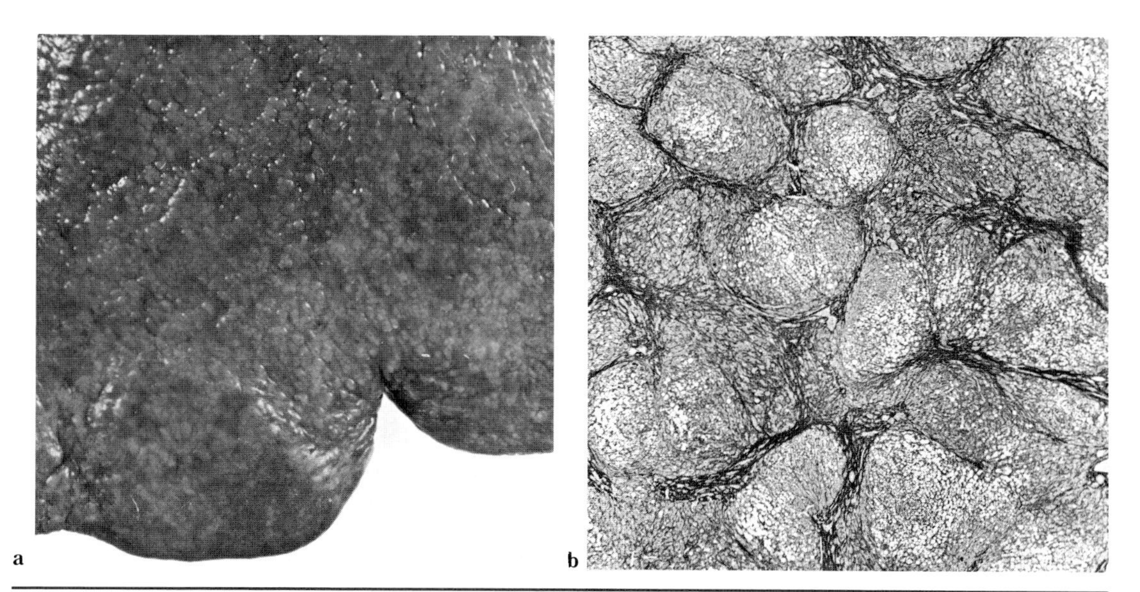

Fig. 17.21 Micronodular cirrhosis. *Left,* showing the fine uniform nodularity of the liver surface. ×0.75. *Right,* microscopy shows regular nodular regeneration: the hepatocytes in many of the nodules show marked fatty change. (Gordon and Sweets' reticulin) ×20.

eventually a micronodular cirrhosis is established (see Fig. 17.21). If there is still further parenchymal cell loss and fibrosis, with accompanying nodular regeneration, the end-stage liver may show a mixed or a macronodular cirrhosis.

In some cases alcohol may produce perivenular and pericellular fibrosis without an accompanying hepatitis. This lesion may also progress to cirrhosis. It is important to recognize alcoholic cirrhosis because it progresses more slowly than most other types, and may be limited by abstinence from alcohol. In addition to the features associated with cirrhosis of any aetiology the abuse of alcohol may also be associated with systematic effects: muscle wasting, cardiomyopathy, vitamin B and C deficiency, polyneuropathy, alcoholic gastritis and peptic ulceration, chronic pancreatitis, Dupuytren's contracture and changes within the central nervous system.

Pathogenesis of Alcoholic Hepatitis and Cirrhosis

The mechanisms whereby alcohol causes hepatitis and fibrosis are poorly understood. Free radical formation, lipid peroxidation, plasma membrane or organelle injury and immunological mechanisms have all been invoked, but none proven. However, many of the individual morphological features can be explained.

The ballooning of liver cells is due to retention of secretory proteins accompanied by water, the retention resulting from injury to secretory organelles. Mallory bodies are known to be composed of intermediate (pre-keratin) filaments; alcohol or acetaldehyde may cause disorganization of the cytoskeleton, resulting in aggregation of filaments or in a failure to disperse them. Finally, the Ito or perisinusoidal cell, is reponsible for the production of collagen within the liver. Proliferation of these cells may result from stimulation either by alcohol or its metabolites or by products of liver cell injury, producing the pericellular fibrosis characteristic of alcoholic liver disease.

Cirrhosis

Definition. *Cirrhosis is a condition involving the entire liver in which the parenchyma is changed into a large number of nodules separated from one another by irregular branching and anastomosing sheets of fibrous tissue.* It results from long-continued loss of liver cells, with a persistent inflammatory reaction accompanied by fibrosis and compensatory hyperplasia. The progressive loss and regeneration of liver cells occurs focally and leads to disruption of the normal architecture, so that the portal tracts and hepatic veins are spaced irregularly in the nodules of surviving parenchyma and in the fibrous septa. The condition is irreversible and the fibrosis and architectural distortion interfere with the flow of blood through the liver, with the result that loss of liver cells may continue even in the absence of the original cytotoxic agent (e.g. alcohol). Death usually results from hepatocellular failure, portal hypertension, or a combination of both.

It is important to emphasize that the changes of cirrhosis affect the whole liver. Localized scarring, for example post-hepatitic or focal nodular hyperplasia (p. 782), is not included within the term cirrhosis; nor are mild degrees of more generalized hepatic fibrosis unaccompanied by loss of normal architecture as seen in schistosomiasis (p. 1167).

Pathological Features of Cirrhosis

The liver may be of normal size or enlarged if there is fatty change or excessive development of hyperplastic regenerating nodules. Usually, however, it shrinks as the disease progresses, due to loss of liver cells exceeding regeneration, and terminally may weigh less than 1 kg. The surface is diffusely nodular and on section the parenchyma is divided up into rounded nodules separated by bands of fibrous tissue (Figs 17.21, 17.22). The colour varies considerably, being pale if there is fatty change, bile stained if there is cholestasis, and red if there is congestion.

Histologically, the liver shows loss of normal architecture. Fibrous septa dissect the parenchyma and the portal tracts and hepatic veins lose their regular spacing. These septa form links between portal tracts, between portal tracts and hepatic veins or between adjacent hepatic veins, and enclose regenerative liver cell nodules. Within the nodules, liver cells show focal hypertrophy and hyperplasia; this may compress adjacent liver cells which atrophy. Thus in some parts of the nodules the cells are enlarged, while in others they are small (Fig. 17.23). Some nodules may be partially divided by irregular septa extending into them. Small groups of liver cells may be entrapped in the fibrous septa and increased numbers of small bile ductular elements are also present – ductular proliferation. Cholestasis is not usually marked (except in biliary cirrhosis) but may develop terminally in hepatocellular failure.

Lymphocytes, and less commonly plasma cells are often present in fibrous septa and in portal tracts, the intensity varying considerably. Degeneration of liver cells may be observed, especially at the margins of the nodules and this, particularly if associated with heavy lymphocytic infiltration, is an indication that the disease process is progressing actively.

Classification of Cirrhosis

The differentiation of cirrhosis into various types has some clinical significance. Elucidation of the causes of cirrhosis and thus, eventually, its prevention, are dependent on distinguishing between various types. Cirrhosis may be classified on an aetiological basis or on the morphological appearances of the liver.

The morphological divisions are into a **micronodular** cirrhosis in which the nodules are approximately the same size, i.e. up to 3 mm in diameter, a **macronodular** cirrhosis in which the nodules are of variable size and may range up to 1 cm in diameter, and a **mixed** type in which both small and large nodules are present (Figs 17.21,

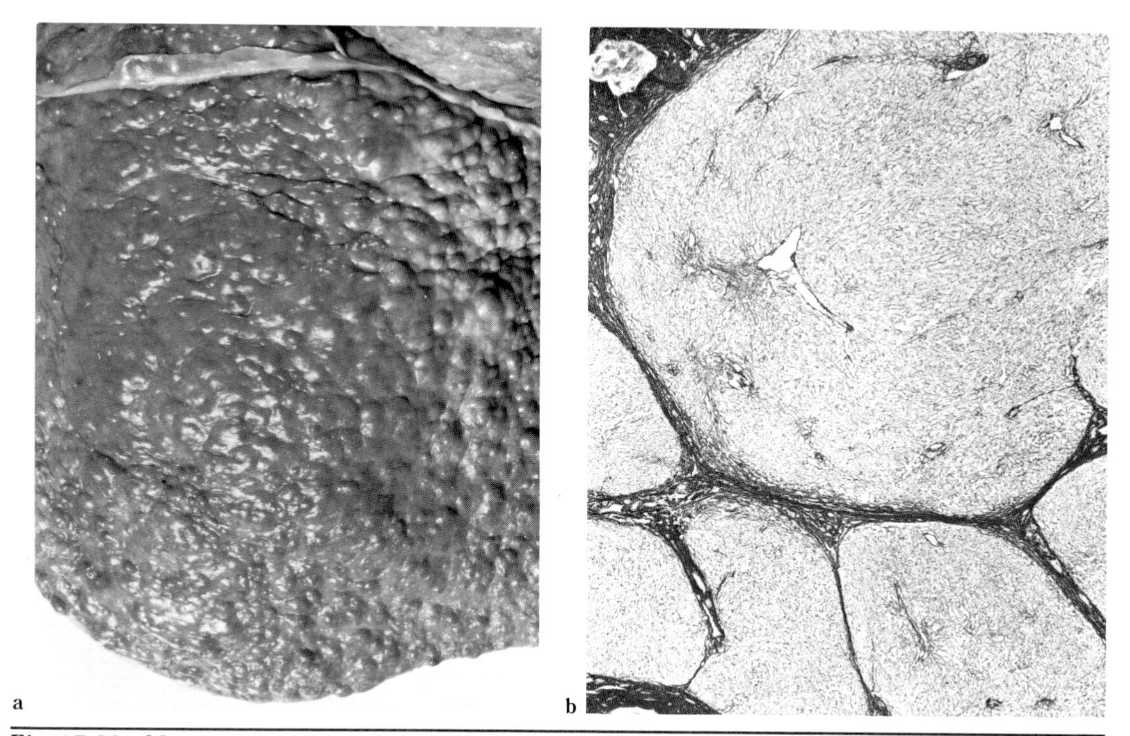

Fig. 17.22 Macronodular cirrhosis. *Left*, surface view, showing the coarse irregularity, with considerable variation of nodular size. ×0.75. *Right*, microscopy shows the variation in nodular size. (Gordon and Sweets' reticulin) ×20.

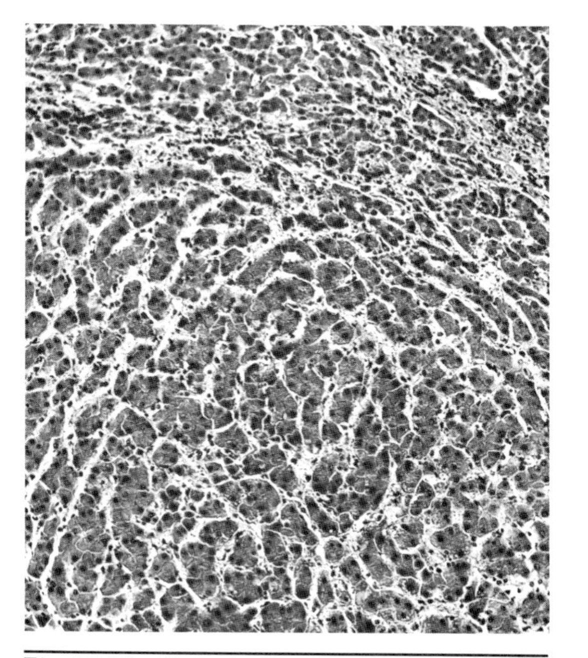

Fig. 17.23 Cirrhosis of liver, showing hypertrophy of the liver cells in a nodule, with stretching and atrophy of the adjacent cells in the upper part of field. ×90.

17.22). The value of this classification is doubtful as the correlation between aetiological factors and the morphology of the cirrhosis is poor. A mixed pattern is most frequently seen in end-stage cirrhosis and reflects the balance between continuing liver injury and the regenerative capacity of the liver. An aetiological classification of cirrhosis is given in Table 17.3.

In our experience, alcoholic cirrhosis comprises 30–35% of all cases, post-viral 15–20%, 40–50% are cryptogenic and the remainder form a miscellaneous group. The features of some of these will now be outlined briefly.

Pathogenesis of Cirrhosis

Cirrhosis results from long-continued loss of liver cells, accompanied by compensatory liver cell hyperplasia and nodule formation, and by chronic inflammation and progressive replacement fibrosis, i.e. chronic hepatitis. It is thus the

Table 17.3 Classification of cirrhosis

Acquired
- Alcoholic
- Post-hepatitic or post-viral
- Of unknown aetiology
  - cryptogenic
  - Indian childhood cirrhosis
- Biliary cirrhosis
  - primary
  - secondary (due to bile duct obstruction)

Inherited
- Inborn errors of metabolism
  - haemochromatosis
  - thalassaemia
  - Wilson's disease
  - alpha-1-antitrypsin deficiency
  - galactosaemia
  - type IV glycogen storage disease
  - tyrosinosis
  - fructose intolerance

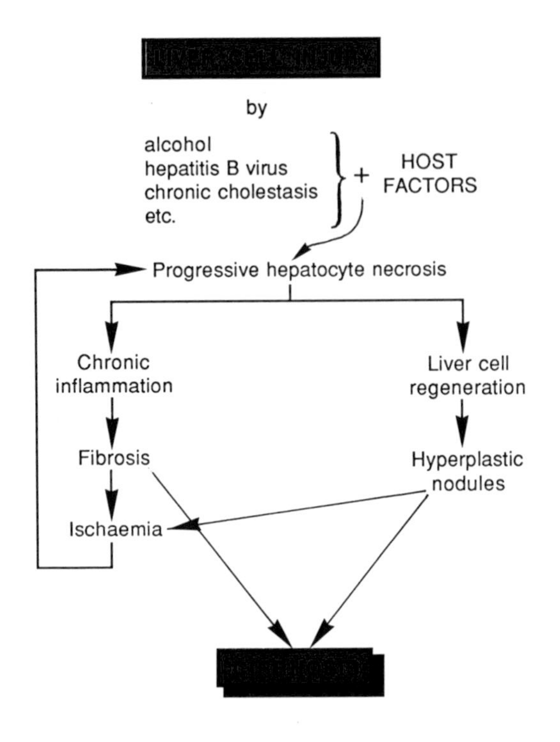

Fig. 17.24 The pathogenesis of cirrhosis.

outcome of prolonged hepatocellular necrosis. Eventually the irregular liver cell hyperplasia and fibrosis interfere with blood flow to such an extent that, whatever the initial cause of the injury, hepatocyte loss continues as a result of ischaemia and the changes become progressive, leading to death from hepatocellular failure and/or portal hypertension (Fig. 17.24).

The possible aetiological factors in human cirrhosis have already been enumerated. It is important to emphasize that cirrhosis is not a predictable outcome in many cases: the host factors which influence progression following viral hepatitis and in alcohol abuse are not known, although persistence of the original inflammatory stimulus may play a role. For example persistence of virus may explain the progression from an acute to chronic hepatitis in cases of type B and type C viral hepatitis. In other cases, an immunological reaction may occur, as has been postulated in some forms of chronic acute hepatitis. In the various forms of biliary cirrhosis, progression can be explained in part on the basis of chronic bile retention. The factors responsible for initiating hepatic fibrosis also remain obscure, but the importance of the fibrosis in the progression to the cirrhosis and in the development of the secondary effects of cirrhosis is not in doubt.

Complications of Cirrhosis

These include portal hypertension and hepatocellular failure which are described below. It is the major cause of these two conditions, particularly when they occur together. Liver cell carcinoma arises in 10–15% of all cirrhotic patients, but the incidence varies depending on the aetiology of the cirrhosis.

Alcoholic Cirrhosis

The pathological features have already been described (p. 764). Alcoholic cirrhosis is commoner in men than in women, and develops mainly between 40 and 70 years of age. Reduction in size of the liver is usually slight, and the early pattern of the cirrhosis is micronodular. Fatty change persists, thus the nodules appear pale and yellow. Later there may be a mixed or predominantly macronodular appearance and the degree of fatty change tends to diminish. The margins between nodules and fibrous septa are regular, the septa are narrow, bile duct proliferation is slight, and lymphocytic infiltration is usually not heavy. The presence of Mallory's hyalin is a useful diagnostic marker; it is, however, seen also in Wilson's disease, Indian childhood cirrhosis and in biliary cirrhosis.

Post-viral (Post-hepatitic) Cirrhosis

The liver is usually smaller than in alcoholic cirrhosis, fatty infiltration is slight or absent and the pattern of cirrhosis is usually macronodular (Fig. 17.22). The normal architecture is not completely lost, and can be detected in some of the nodules. The liver cells may vary considerably in size. Where there is piecemeal necrosis and the septa are heavily infiltrated with lymphocytes this indicates continuing activity of the hepatitis.

Post-hepatitic cirrhosis tends to occur usually at a younger age than alcoholic cirrhosis, although the range is wide. The disease has a poor prognosis, progressive portal hypertension and hepatocellular failure being more rapid than in alcoholic cirrhosis. There is also a higher incidence of liver cell carcinoma, especially where the cirrhosis is due to hepatitis B infection.

Cryptogenic Cirrhosis

In these patients the aetiology of the cirrhosis cannot be established either clinically or morphologically. The presumption is that the majority follow an episode of subclinical hepatitis. Most cases show a macronodular pattern.

Biliary Cirrhosis

Long-continued cholestasis, whether of extra- or intrahepatic origin, can lead to cirrhosis because of the harmful effect of retained bile on hepatocytes, often aggravated, in patients with major duct obstruction, by cholangitis. Two varieties are recognized:

(1) **primary biliary diseases** in which there is progressive destruction and loss of bile ducts, the mjaor types being primary biliary cirrhosis and primary sclerosing cholangitis; and

(2) **secondary biliary cirrhosis** resulting from prolonged mechanical obstruction of the larger biliary passages.

Primary Biliary Cirrhosis

This is an uncommon condition, occurring predominantly in middle-aged women, the female preponderance being 9:1. Clinically, the onset is insidious, frequently with pruritus, hyperpigmentation of the skin and a period of vague ill-health before jaundice appears. There is usually a marked degree of hepatomegaly. The level of jaundice may fluctuate and is initially mild. The serum alkaline phosphatase level is disproportionately high when compared with the increase in conjugated bilirubin. Serum aminotransferase levels are mildly raised and cholesterol levels may be markedly elevated. After a duration varying from months to many years, death results from liver failure or the complications of portal hypertension. In long-standing cases malabsorption develops, and there may be osteomalacia and osteoporosis (hepatic osteodystrophy).

Although the clinical and biochemical features are those of obstructive jaundice, the large intrahepatic and extrahepatic bile ducts are patent. The most conspicuous change is an infiltrate of lymphocytes and plasma cells in and around the epithelium of the smaller intrahepatic bile ducts of 50 μm or less in diameter. The epithelium shows degenerative changes (Fig. 17.25), and there is gradual destruction and loss of these smaller bile ducts. Epithelioid granulomas are found in about one-

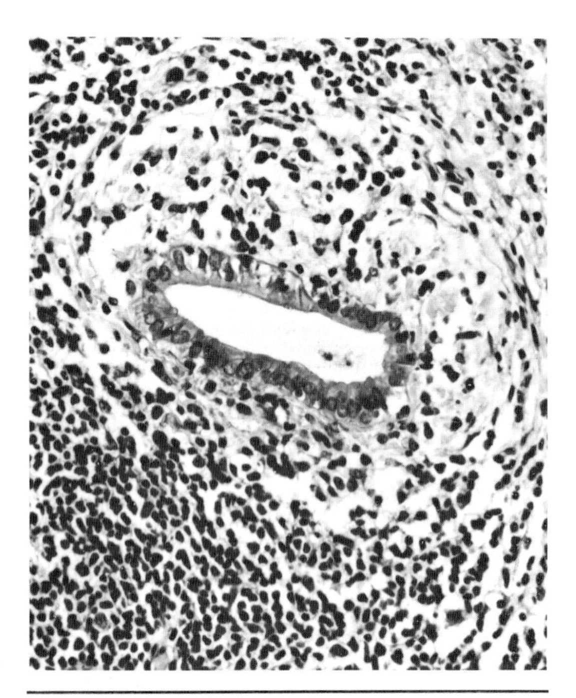

Fig. 17.25 Primary biliary cirrhosis, showing an intrahepatic bile duct with surrounding inflammatory reaction. The duct epithelium is unduly basophilic with vacuolation of the cells lining the upper margin. ×350.

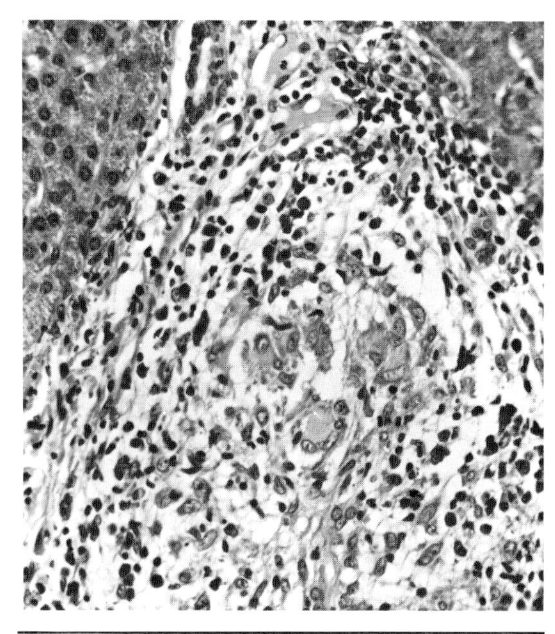

Fig. 17.26 Primary biliary cirrhosis, showing a granuloma with giant cells, lying in a portal area which is heavily infiltrated with lymphoid cells. ×350.

third of the cases and may be intimately related to bile ducts (Fig. 17.26). There is also a chronic inflammatory cell infiltrate in the portal tracts and this extends progressively to involve the periportal parenchyma and is accompanied by portal fibrosis. There is cholestasis, most marked in the periportal areas, and later, protein-bound copper accumulates in the periportal liver cells due to impaired excretion of copper in the bile. Mallory's hyalin is also seen in these hepatocytes. Eventually progressive fibrosis with portal–portal septum formation, continued loss and nodular regeneration of liver cells complete the evolution of cirrhosis, usually of a micronodular pattern.

Aetiology and pathogenesis. In this disease the initial lesion is a chronic non-suppurative granulomatous destruction of small bile ducts. Later, liver cell necrosis is superadded, probably due to cholestasis, and there is progression to cirrhosis. In virtually 100% of patients the serum contains, in high titre, an antibody which reacts with a non-organ specific mitochondrial antigen, and this is a valuable confirmatory serological test.

Primary biliary cirrhosis is thought to be an autoimmune disease, but the aetiology is not known. Familial cases may occur but no genetic factors have been identified. Many immunological abnormalities occur and other autoimmune diseases may coexist including Sjögren's syndrome and scleroderma. The invariable presence of anti-mitochondrial antibody titres is highly significant but does not explain the bile duct specificity of the disease.

Primary Sclerosing Cholangitis

This is also uncommon, shows a male preponderance of 4:1 and in 70% of patients is associated with chronic inflammatory bowel disease, especially ulcerative colitis. Clinically, patients present with obstructive jaundice. The disease is characterized by a chronic non-suppurative fibro-obliterative destruction of bile ducts in which there

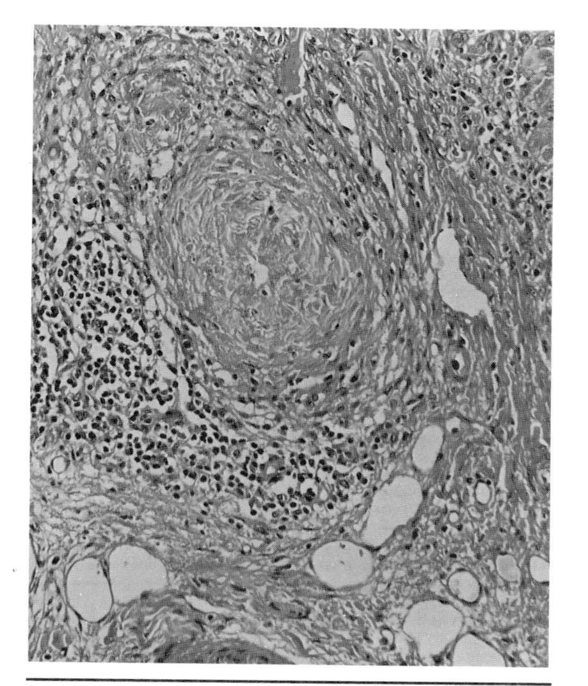

Fig. 17.27 Primary sclerosing cholangitis. In this portal tract the bile duct has been replaced by a dense whorl of fibrous tissue. ×210.

is progressive periductal fibrosis and eventual obliteration of bile ducts (Fig. 17.27). This can affect both intrahepatic and extrahepatic bile ducts. Diagnosis is made on cholangiography which shows irregular strictures and beading of the ducts (Fig. 17.28).

There is progression to cirrhosis, the pattern resembling that seen in primary biliary cirrhosis, but with a tendency to develop more rapidly. The aetiology of this disease is also not known and the association with chronic inflammatory bowel disease is obscure. There is a well recognized risk of these patients developing a cholangiocarcinoma (p. 780).

Secondary (Obstructive) Biliary Cirrhosis

Unrelieved obstruction to the outflow of bile from the liver from any cause, for example traumatic or malignant strictures of the common bile duct and biliary atresia, results in secondary biliary cirrhosis. The rate of development of cirrhosis is

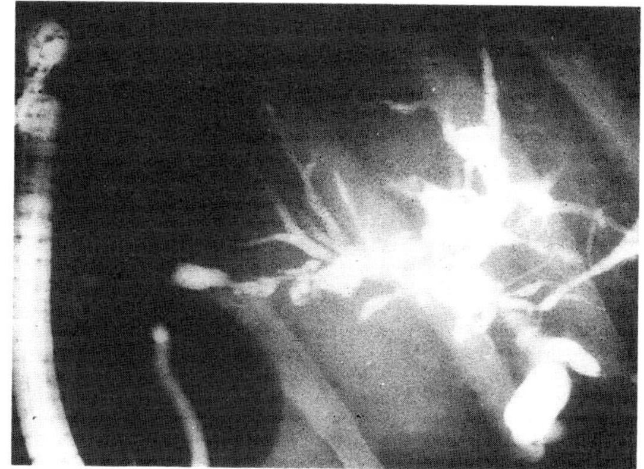

Fig. 17.28 Cholangiogram showing ectasia of intrahepatic ducts and abrupt 'cut off' of ducts in primary sclerosing cholangitis.

extremely variable, and depends partly on the degree of obstruction. In some cases, and particularly when obstruction is due to gallstones, an ascending bacterial cholangitis is superadded and may lead to abscess formation (Fig. 17.29). In obstruction due to neoplasms, e.g. carcinoma of the head of the pancreas, death usually results before cirrhosis has developed.

The early changes following biliary obstruction

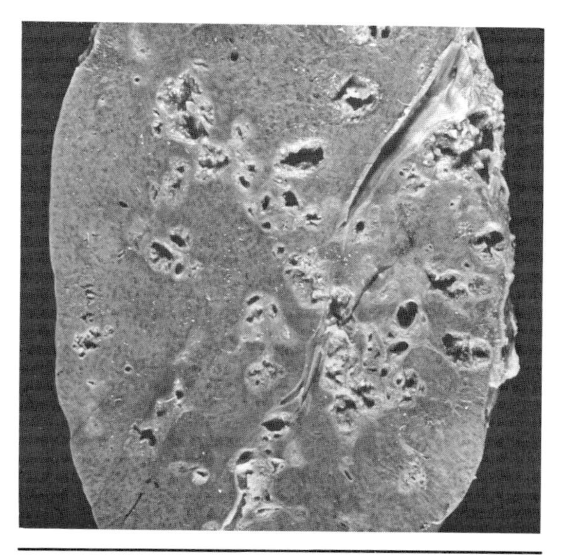

Fig. 17.29 Liver slice from a case of large duct obstruction and ascending cholangitis: numerous abscesses are present in the parenchyma.

consist of cholestasis. First, bile accumulates in hepatocytes, bile canaliculi and Kupffer cells, particularly in the perivenular zones and in small bile ducts. Subsequently the larger bile ducts become dilated and filled with bile. Extravasation of bile may occur producing bile lakes: this may be associated with focal necrosis of liver cells – bile infarcts. The retention of bile provokes an inflammatory reaction. This particularly involves the portal tracts, which become oedematous and infiltrated with lymphocytes, plasma cells and, most significantly, neutrophil polymorphs in and around the bile ducts – cholangitis (Fig. 17.30). There is periductal fibrosis, bile duct proliferation occurs and fibrous septa form, linking portal tracts. Loss of liver cells and fibrosis result in disturbance of architecture and, together with the development of regenerating nodules, progress to a micronodular cirrhosis. Grossly the liver is firm, enlarged and deeply jaundiced with a finely nodular surface. Portal hypertension may eventually supervene, but death results more often from liver failure or intercurrent infection.

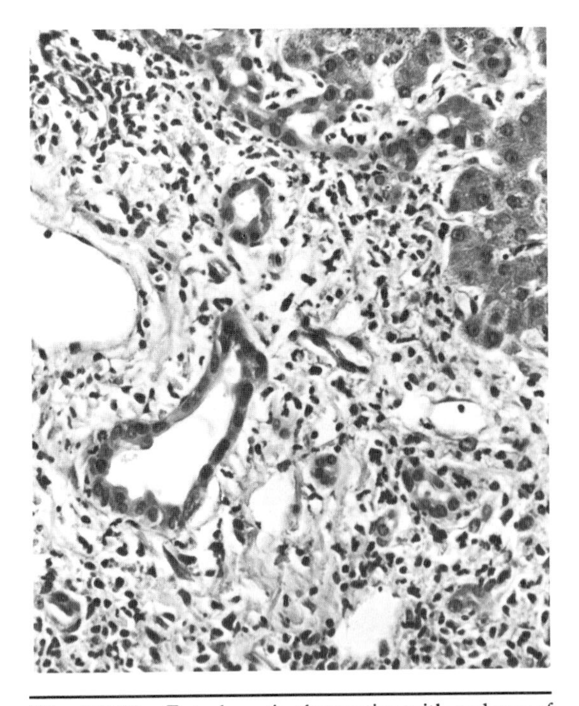

Fig. 17.30 Extrahepatic obstruction with oedema of the portal area, a prominent neutrophil infiltrate, some of which is closely related to the bile ducts, and early bile duct proliferation. ×250.

The best example of pure obstructive biliary cirrhosis without infection is seen in congenital atresia of the bile ducts. This may involve either the extrahepatic or intrahepatic biliary tree. In the extrahepatic variety there is marked jaundice and death occurs within a few months of birth. Patchy atresia of smaller intrahepatic bile ducts sometimes has a more prolonged course with survival into early adult life: secondary biliary cirrhosis develops, as described above.

Cirrhosis Due to Metabolic Disorders

Many of the metabolic abnormalities listed in Table 17.3 can cause cirrhosis in childhood. Other causes of cirrhosis in childhood include:

(1) **Indian childhood cirrhosis** which is common in 1–3 year olds in that country, is of unknown aetiology, but involves gross accumulation of copper in the liver cells;
(2) biliary cirrhosis due to atresia (see above); and
(3) cystic fibrosis (p. 272).

Haemochromatosis

The normal adult liver contains approximately 0.3 g of iron, more than half in the form of ferritin and the remainder as haemosiderin. The normal metabolism of iron and the consequences of iron deficiency are discussed on p. 617. Iron balance depends largely on the control of iron absorption from the gut; iron loss is normally small and can only be increased significantly by haemorrhage or venesection. Iron overload, haemochromatosis, can result from absorption of excessive amounts of iron, from parenteral administration of iron or a combination of these. We distinguish between primary or idiopathic haemochromatosis and secondary haemochromatosis the causes of which are summarized in Table 17.4. In primary haemochromatosis the excess iron deposits involve predominantly the hepatocytes and later the

Table 17.4 Causes of haemochromatosis

- Primary (idiopathic) haemochromatosis
- Secondary haemochromatosis
  - Increased iron intake
    - multiple transfusions
    - increased dietary iron: medicinal or iron-containing food and beverages
  - Ineffective erythropoiesis with marrow hyperplasia
    - thalassaemia
    - sideroblastic anaemia
  - Miscellaneous causes
    - alcoholic cirrhosis; porphyria; congenital absence of transferrin

Kupffer cells whereas in the secondary forms the converse is true. The haemosiderin deposits appear as brownish-yellow intracellular granules (haemosiderin) and are stained by the Prussian blue reaction (Perls' stain).

Primary haemochromatosis is characterized by excessive absorption of dietary iron from birth onwards and body stores may exceed 30 g instead of the normal 3–5 g. The disease has a frequency of 2 per 1000 and shows a 4:1 male preponderance, in part due to the protective effect of menstrual blood loss. It is inherited as an autosomal recessive trait. The disease-susceptibility gene is located on chromosome 6 and there is a significant linkage with HLA-A3 and a weak linkage with HLA-A14 and B7.

The nature of the metabolic defect responsible for the excessive iron absorption is not known. The proportion of dietary iron absorbed is abnormally high and as noted by Bothwell *et al.* (1979) the 'absorbostat' is set too high. This could be due to mucosal cell abnormalities, to a defect in post-absorptive secretion or in a macrophage defect resulting in uptake of excess iron by parenchymal cells. The plasma transferrin level is not increased but is usually more than 75% saturated (normal 30%).

Excess parenchymal cell accumulation occurs in liver, pancreas, endocrine cells and cardiac myocytes. The patient may present with features of cirrhosis or diabetes or show focal hyperpigmentation of the skin – **bronzed diabetes**. Other features may include pseudo-gout (p. 997), hypogonadism probably due to pituitary failure and congestive cardiomyopathy (p. 498).

In the liver excess iron deposits are present predominantly in hepatocytes, the most intense deposit occurring in zone 1 (periportal) (Fig. 17.31). Bile duct epithelium, Kupffer cells and portal tract macrophages are also involved especially in advanced disease. Hepatic fibrosis develops initially in the portal areas and in the later stage a macronodular cirrhosis becomes established. Although the development of cirrhosis and the intensity of iron deposition are not closely correlated, the iron is considered to be fibrogenic. Treatment is by repeated venesection and with iron removal some reduction of fibrosis occurs. Cirrhosis, however, cannot be reversed. In those in whom cirrhosis has developed, both treated and untreated, there is an increased incidence of primary carcinoma of the liver.

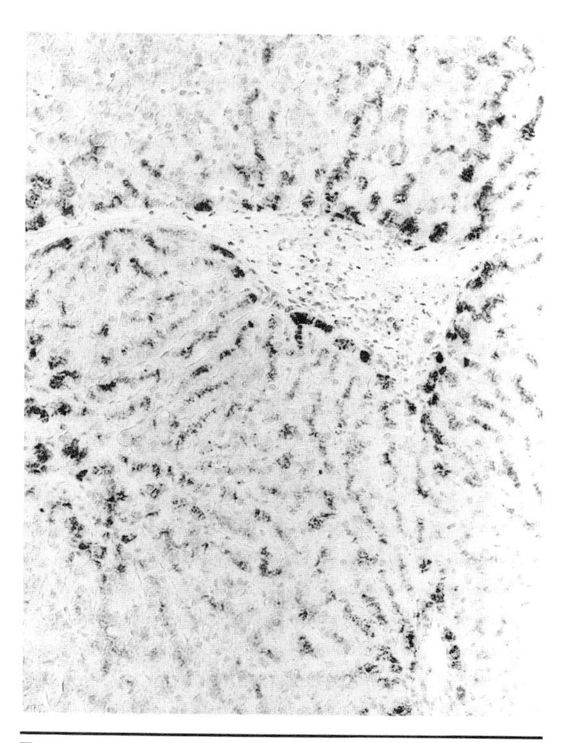

Fig. 17.31 Liver biopsy in haemochromatosis. The excess iron is stored mainly as haemosiderin in the hepatocytes, and is seen as dark granules. Perls'. ×150.

Secondary haemochromatosis. Many of the diseases associated with this are dealt with elsewhere. In contrast to the primary form, the iron accumulates initially and predominantly in macrophages. Subsequently parenchymal cell deposits develop and may produce fibrosis which occasionally results in cirrhosis. The best example of iron overload resulting from dietary factors was seen in South Africans of the Bantu tribe in whom the increased intake was due to the use of iron pots for cooking and for brewing beer. Increased iron absorption is promoted by alcohol; in alcoholic cirrhosis stainable iron deposits are frequently seen in liver biopsies.

Wilson's Disease (Hepatolenticular Degeneration)

This is a disorder of copper metabolism determined by a pair of autosomal recessive genes, on chromosome 13 and with a prevalence of 1 per 200 000 of the population. Increasing amounts of copper accumulate in and damage the liver, the lenticular nuclei, the kidneys and the eyes.

The biochemical abnormality in Wilson's disease is in the liver and a successful hepatic allograft is curative. The precise nature of the abnormality is uncertain. However, there is an increase in the hepatic lysosomal copper concentration presumed to be due to defective excretion of copper via the bile. Liver copper levels may be up to 20 times the upper limit of normal. There is also reduced hepatic synthesis of the serum copper glycoprotein, ceruloplasmin (the gene for which is on chromosome 3). Low serum levels of ceruloplasmin occur in the large majority of patients with Wilson's disease but is not diagnostic of the disease. The accumulation of copper in the liver begins in infancy and in time excess amounts diffuse from liver to blood and accumulate in and damage other organs.

The patient may present with an acute hepatitis, with fulminant hepatic failure, with chronic active hepatitis or with cirrhosis. This may occur from the age of 5 years onwards and Wilson's disease should always be considered in a young person with chronic liver disease. The histological features comprise fatty change, liver cell necrosis, chronic active hepatitis and progressive fibrosis resulting in a macronodular cirrhosis.

There is excess urinary copper excretion, and damage to tubular cells leads to aminoaciduria. In the eyes, deposits of copper in Descemet's membrane of the cornea produce the diagnostic Kayser–Fleischer rings. Treatment with D-penicillamine increases urinary excretion and depletes copper stores. This may prevent progression of the disease.

α_1-Antitrypsin Deficiency

The acute phase protein α_1-antitrypsin is a protease inhibitor produced by hepatocytes and macrophages and as many as 30 polymorphic variants are now known. The inheritance is autosomal codominant. The normal phenotype is MM and the normal serum levels are 2–4 g/l. The most important clinical variant is termed Z, and ZZ homozygotes have serum levels less than 50% of normal. The abnormal protein, showing a single amino-acid substitution (^{342}Glu→Lys) is synthesized but cannot be secreted by the liver cell and accumulates as PAS-positive globules predominantly in periportal hepatocytes (Fig. 17.32).

α_1-Antitrypsin deficiency is associated with panacinar emphysema and liver disease. In the liver it may cause neonatal hepatitis or the patient may present in later childhood or adulthood with cirrhosis. The mechanisms responsible for the cirrhosis are not known.

Portal Hypertension and Hepatocellular Failure

Portal Hypertension

The normal portal venous pressure is 7 mmHg (0.9 kPa). Portal hypertension occurs when there is obstruction to the blood flow within the liver or obstruction of the portal vein itself. The obstruc-

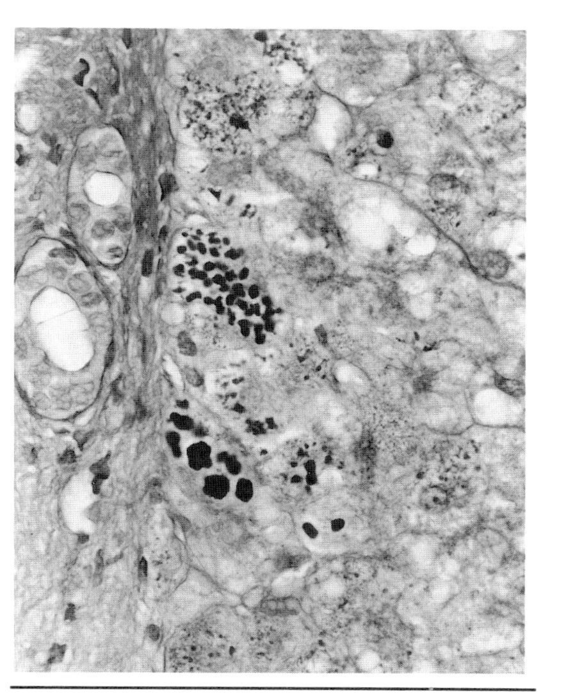

Fig. 17.32 α_1-Antitrypsin deficiency: PAS positive, diastase resistant globules are seen at the margins of cirrhotic nodules. ×385.

tion may be post-sinusoidal as in cirrhosis, veno-occlusive disease, hepatic vein obstruction, alcoholic hepatitis and congestive cardiac failure, or pre-sinusoidal as in schistosomiasis, congenital hepatic fibrosis and portal vein occlusion. Massive splenomegaly with increased splenic blood flow can also cause portal hypertension in the absence of obstruction. The effects of portal hypertension result from some of the portal blood bypassing the liver and entering the systemic veins at sites of portal-systemic anastomosis.

Portal-systemic anastomoses with varicosity of the veins occur in:

(1) the lower oesophagus and upper gastric fundus, between the left gastric vein (portal) and the azygos minor vein (systemic);
(2) the lower rectum and anus, between the superior haemorrhoidal (portal) and the middle and inferior haemorrhoidal veins (systemic);
(3) the falciform ligament between the left branch of the portal vein and the superficial veins of the anterior abdominal wall, via the paraumbilical veins, producing the clinical appearance of **caput medusae**; and
(4) at points of contact between abdominal viscera and the posterior abdominal wall.

The most important anastomoses are those at the gastro-oesophageal junction, where spontaneous rupture of large submucosal varices results in bleeding which may be fatal and also contributes to the development of hepatocellular failure.

Portal hypertension results in splenomegaly, primarily due to passive congestion, but often with lymphoid hyperplasia. **Hypersplenism** (p. 648) may result in anaemia, thrombocytopenia and granulocytopenia. Portal hypertension is also a major factor in the production of ascites. Surgical shunt procedures may be carried out to reduce the hypertension and thus the risk of bleeding from oesophageal varices, but this may increase the risk of hepatic encephalopathy.

Hepatocellular Failure (Liver Failure)

Although the liver has a large functional reserve and a high regenerative capacity when injured, liver insufficiency, manifest by failure of the liver cells to perform adequately their various functions, occurs both in patients with severe acute liver injury and in advanced cases of chronic liver disease.

Acute liver failure occurs in severe acute hepatitis of viral aetiology or as an adverse reaction to certain drugs, as a result of drug overdose or poisoning by certain hepatotoxic chemicals, in massive liver cell necrosis of unknown cause, and occasionally in severe fatty infiltration of the liver, particularly microvesicular steatosis. Hepatic failure results directly from the parenchymal cell injury and is a reflection of the degree of hepatocellular damage.

Chronic liver failure is most often due to cirrhosis. It may occur even in patients with a relatively large amount of surviving liver tissue and is attributable in part to the interference with hepatic blood flow which results from the disturbed liver architecture. Acute on chronic hepatic failure may be precipitated by factors such as gastrointestinal bleeding, the use of diuretic or narcotic drugs, bacterial infection, paracentesis, portacaval shunt and other surgical operations.

Because of the multiple functions of the liver, hepatic insufficiency gives rise to a complex syndrome, which includes neurological disturbances, jaundice, defects of blood coagulation and renal failure. Additional features include ascites and oedema and endocrine and circulatory disturbances, but these occur mainly in chronic failure. The mechanisms involved in these manifestations of liver failure are discussed below.

Hepatic encephalopathy. This comprises mental confusion with apathy, disorientation or excitement, a coarse flapping tremor and muscular rigidity, and finally hepatic coma. These are accompanied by characteristic changes in the electroencephalogram. All these features are reversible, and the only morphological changes which have been observed are in the astrocytes, the nuclei of which are enlarged. In occasional cases, however, progressive brain damage may occur. In acute liver failure, cerebral oedema is often a significant contributory cause of death.

The neurological disorder is due to metabolic disturbances and is potentially reversible. While the precise mechanism is not known, it is almost certainly of multifactorial aetiology and, in individual cases, the following factors may be involved in various combinations:

(1) failure of the liver to remove potentially toxic agents. In particular, nitrogenous bacterial metabolites absorbed from the gut may avoid detoxification in the liver, due to liver cell loss and/or portosystemic bypass of the liver. An increased nitrogen load from a high protein intake or in haemorrhage from oesophageal varices often precipitates hepatic encephalopathy. In most cases there is an increased level of ammonia in the blood, but the levels correlate only approximately with the depth of coma; moreover, the clinical features of ammonia toxicity as seen in urea-cycle enzyme deficiencies are different from those of hepatic encephalopathy. Other metabolic products of intestinal origin have also been implicated. False neurotransmitters, such as octopamine, may replace true transmitters in the brain. Gamma-aminobutyric acid (GABA), an inhibitory neurotransmitter, has produced many of the features of hepatic encephalopathy in experimental animals. It may also have a role in humans, by facilitating the activity of other neurodepressants.

(2) lack of factors normally produced by liver cells and which may be essential for normal neuronal function.

(3) increased cerebral sensitivity to a variety of agents, possibly due to interference with oxidative metabolism via the citric acid cycle and consequent ATP depletion.

(4) disturbances of amino-acid metabolism. These include an increase in serum aromatic amino acids and/or a decrease in branched-chain amino acids; increase in serum short-chain fatty acids and mercaptans may be important.

(5) changes in vascular permeability, particularly affecting the blood–brain barrier.

(6) hypotension, ammonia and electrolyte disturbances which accompany hepatic failure.

Jaundice is usual in acute hepatocellular failure, its severity reflecting the degree of hepatocellular damage. In very severe acute cases, however, death may result before jaundice has become conspicuous. In chronic failure the degree and type of jaundice depends upon the nature of the liver disease. In secondary biliary cirrhosis jaundice accompanies the development of hepatic dysfunction. In other cirrhoses, jaundice is a late but bad prognostic sign, usually mild, and due to failure of the hepatocytes to excrete bile.

Coagulative defects result primarily from defective synthesis of a number of coagulation factors by the liver. There may also be thrombocytopenia, anaemia and leucopenia due to hypersplenism, and, particularly in acute failure, disseminated intravascular coagulation with consumption of clotting factors.

Renal failure may develop in both acute and chronic hepatic failure. In the **hepato-renal syn-**

drome there is impairment of renal function without morphological damage. It is characterized by a reduced glomerular filtration rate and progressive oliguria, but without a fall in urine osmolarity. The mechanisms are unknown but the renal failure is reversible with improvement in hepatic function. Acute renal failure may also result from hypotension due to bleeding from oesophageal varices or as an additional complication when the liver failure is of a drug-induced aetiology. In these cases the kidneys show the features of acute tubular necrosis (p. 921).

Ascites and oedema. Ascites does not result from hepatocellular failure unless there is also portal hypertension. In chronic liver failure there is diminished production of plasma albumin, with a consequent fall in plasma oncotic pressure. The portal hypertension increases the intravascular hydrostatic pressure in the microvasculature in the abdomen, and, in addition, there is leakage of hepatic lymph because of obstruction to its outflow from the liver. Secondary hyperaldosteronism (p. 75) occurs inducing sodium retention, thus aggravating the oedema and ascites. The mechanism of secondary hyperaldosteronism in this situation is not clear. Peripheral oedema is due mainly to the fall in plasma oncotic pressure.

Endocrine disturbances. In chronic liver failure there is, in both sexes, a tendency to depression of libido, sterility and loss of body hair. In men the testes are frequently atrophic, and there may be gynaecomastia. These effects result from failure of hepatic inactivation of oestrogens, which have a stimulating effect upon the breast and may also suppress the production of pituitary gonadotrophin, thus explaining the testicular atrophy. In women menstrual irregularities, secondary amenorrhoea and breast atrophy occur. Two well known vascular changes in liver failure are, exaggerated mottling of the skin of the palms – 'liver palms' – and the development in the superior vena caval drainage area of small leashes of dilated vessels in the superficial dermis, radiating out from a central arteriole – 'spider naevi'. Both these features may occur in normal pregnancy and probably have a hormonal basis.

Circulatory disturbances. A hyperkinetic circulation, characterized by peripheral vasodilation and increased cardiac output and blood volume, may occur. This may be due to circulating vasoactive substances or impaired sympathetic responsiveness. Cyanosis with arterial hypoxia (the result of pulmonary arteriovenous shunting, p. 542) and finger clubbing develop in a small percentage of patients.

Infection. Bacteraemia, particularly with coliform organisms, can occur spontaneously when there is ascites.

Other features. In hepatocellular failure the breath has a peculiar sweetish smell termed 'foetor hepaticus', possibly due to failure of the liver to detoxify substances absorbed from the gut. Fever is common in acute failure, but profound hypothermia has been described in chronic failure. General ill-health with anorexia, wasting and vomiting is common.

Non-viral Infections of the Liver

Bacteria and Spirochaetes

Pyogenic infections. Because of improvements in diagnostic facilities and the earlier use of antibiotics, pyogenic infection of the liver is less common than it used to be. When it does occur, it is usually due to extension of bacteria within the biliary duct system – **ascending cholangitis**. *Escherichia coli*, either alone, or with other coliforms, is the commonest causal organism. Bile duct obstruction is the most important predisposing cause. The process extends into the liver tissue, giving rise to suppurative cholangitis in which the pus is characteristically bile-stained.

Multiple abscess formation in the liver also results from suppurative phlebitis affecting the veins around a septic focus in the abdomen or pelvis, for example in acute appendicitis, diverticulitis of the colon, or infected haemorrhoids. The infection may reach the liver by septic emboli or by portal pyelophlebitis. Umbilical sepsis in the neonate sometimes spreads to the intrahepatic portal vein radicles via the umbilical vein. Abscesses may also develop in the liver in septicaemia or pyaemia, but these are less frequent and less important than in other organs.

Leptospirosis. The spirochaete *Leptospira icterohaemorrhagiae* causes endemic chronic renal infection in rats, and can survive in water or damp conditions for some time after excretion in rat urine. It can penetrate the intact human skin or may gain entry via the respiratory or oral routes, and, after an incubation period of 10–15 days, causes an intense febrile illness (**Weil's disease**) with conjunctivitis, renal tubular damage, a haemorrhagic tendency, jaundice, focal myocardial and skeletal muscle necrosis and often a mild lymphocytic meningitis. The disease occurs chiefly in sewage workers, agricultural workers and fish handlers. Various other leptospira, including *L. canicola* from dogs, can cause a similar but usually milder disease in man.

Liver biopsy shows liver cell degeneration, prominent mitotic activity of the hepatocytes and sometimes focal necrosis, cholestasis and haemorrhage. In some cases, however, the changes are slight. After death, the liver cells are often rounded and separated from one another (Fig. 17.33).

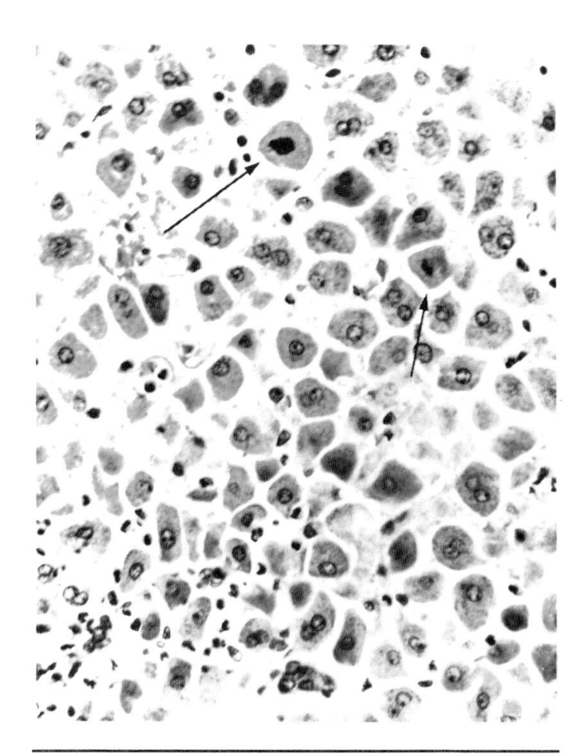

Fig. 17.33 Liver in Weil's disease: post-mortem liver showing separation and rounding of hepatocytes, proliferative activity (arrows) and focal liver cell necrosis with a related inflammatory cell infiltrate (lower left). ×400.

The mortality rate is about 15%. Death may occur in the first week, when haemorrhagic consolidation of the lungs is the principal finding. Later, death is usually due to renal failure and is almost always accompanied by hepatic involvement.

Tuberculosis. Tuberculous lesions are less common in the liver than in most other organs. In generalized tuberculosis miliary tubercles occur and are distributed irregularly in the parenchyma; rarely, a few large caseous lesions result from blood spread.

Syphilis. The liver is frequently affected in both congenital and acquired syphilis. In congenital syphilis the commonest lesion is diffuse interstitial pericellular fibrosis and spirochaetes are abundant. In acquired syphilis miliary granulomas may occur in the secondary stage. Hepatic gummas are a common feature of tertiary syphilis and, when healing occurs, scarring is extensive, producing gross distortion – *hepar lobatum*.

Parasitic Infestations

These are discussed in detail in Chapter 25 and only the major ones affecting the liver are mentioned here.

Schistosomiasis. Infestation by *Schistosoma mansonii* and *Schistosoma japonicum* produces hepatic fibrosis. It is the most important cause of portal hypertension in endemic areas and, indeed, is the commonest cause on a worldwide basis.

Amoebic abscess due to *Entamoeba histolytica* may complicate amoebic dysentery or may occur as an isolated lesion after the colonic disease has subsided.

Malarial parasites initially develop within hepatocytes and sometimes persist there for many years. In the erythrocytic phase colonized red cells are phagocytosed by Kupffer cells, which show marked hypertrophy and hyperplasia, and contain abundant dark brown granules of malarial pigment (haemozoin).

Opisthorchiasis results from invasion of the biliary tree by the larvae of the Chinese liver fluke (*Opisthorchis sinensis*). Secondary pyogenic infection may occur and adenomatous hyperplasia of bile duct epithelium, a precursor lesion of cholangiocarcinoma, is common in endemic areas.

Ascariasis is due to intestinal infestation by the roundworm *Ascaris lumbricoides*. It is prevalent in children in Africa and the Far East and in over a third of cases direct invasion of the common bile duct produces obstruction and cholangitis.

Other Causes of Hepatic Granulomas

Non-caseating granulomas frequently occur in the liver in a wide variety of disorders. Some are primary diseases of the liver, such as primary biliary cirrhosis and hepatic schistosomiasis, but most granulomas occur as part of a generalized disease process. These include sarcoidosis (in which the liver is involved in most cases), various fungal, rickettsial and parasitic diseases, allergic granulomatous diseases and drug-induced injury.

Tumours of the Liver

Benign Tumours

Benign tumours of the liver are rare, comprising approximately 5% of all hepatic neoplasms.

Liver cell adenomas bear a close microscopic resemblance to normal liver tissue, the cells forming regular trabeculae two or three cells thick. Bile canaliculi are present but bile ducts are absent. These tumours are usually very vascular, are often immediately subcapsular, and may present with intra-abdominal haemorrhage. They are well demarcated but not always encapsulated. An increased incidence has been found in women using the oral contraceptive pill and a causal association is now accepted.

Bile duct adenomas are very rare and are usually an incidental finding. They are composed of small bile duct elements in a fibrous stroma.

Haemangiomas, usually cavernous, dark purple and sharply demarcated from the surrounding hepatic tissue, are common. Most are less than 2 cm in diameter, but some are larger. They are usually superficial and may be mistaken for infarcts.

Liver Cell (Hepatocellular) Carcinoma

Liver cell carcinomas account for approximately 85% of primary malignant tumours of the liver, bile duct carcinomas for approximately 5–10% and the remainder are relatively rare tumours including haemangiosarcoma, hepatoblastoma, and mesenchymal tumours.

Hepatocellular carcinoma shows marked geographic variation in incidence. In this country it develops in approximately 1–3 per 100 000 of the population, whereas in parts of Africa and Far East Asia the incidence rises to 10–15 per 100 000. In all areas 80–90% of cases occur in males and the tumour supervenes on cirrhosis (predominantly of macronodular type) in 70–80% of cases. In cases without pre-existing cirrhosis, the male:female ratio is 2:1.

In low-incidence areas the tumour arises usually after the age of 50, and the proportion of cases of cirrhosis in which malignancy supervenes is low, estimates varying from 5 to 15%. By contrast, in high-incidence areas the tumour arises in the 20–40 age group. In such areas there is a much greater risk of tumours supervening in cirrhosis, some estimates being as high as 50% and clinical features of the tumour and of cirrhosis often present simultaneously. The tumour cells secrete α-fetoprotein and levels in excess of 10 ng/ml are found in the serum in 85% of cases.

Aetiological Factors

The precise relationship between cirrhosis and liver cell carcinoma is uncertain. While it is possible that cirrhosis is a premalignant lesion, neoplasia supervening on the long-standing and continued hyperplasia of the cirrhotic liver, two other possibilities must be considered. These are (1) that both the cirrhosis and the tumour are caused by one agent, and (2) that a liver which is cirrhotic is peculiarly predisposed to the carcinogenic effects of a variety of microbiological and/or chemical agents.

There is convincing evidence of an association between HBV infection and liver cell carcinoma:

(1) there is a close correlation between the hepatitis B carrier incidence and liver cell carcinoma;

(2) serological markers of hepatitis B infection (e.g. HBsAg or HBcAb) are found in 80–90% of patients with tumours even in some areas with a low overall incidence of liver cell carcinoma;

(3) liver cell carcinoma occurs much more frequently in HB-associated cirrhosis;

(4) prospective studies of chronic hepatitis B carriers have shown the relative risk of tumour to be 300 times greater than in non-carriers. In high carrier-rate areas prenatal transmission of HBV occurs and such early infection could be a factor in the early development of liver cell cancer;

(5) integrated DNA sequences of HBV have been shown in tumour cells and in liver cancer cell lines;

(6) in animal models of hepadna virus infection such as woodchucks and Pekin ducks, both chronic hepatitis and liver cell carcinomas occur. Thus, the evidence for an association between virus and tumour is strong. However, a direct oncogenic role for HBV is not established.

Experimentally, liver cell carcinoma has been produced in rats by feeding with aflatoxins, in particular aflatoxin B_1, a product of the fungus *Aspergillus flavus*. These and other mycotoxins and plant toxins may contaminate stored foods and cereals which are the staple diet in high incidence areas. This may explain in part the geographical variation in incidence in man.

Clinical and Pathological Features

Clinically, the features are usually those of the associated cirrhosis. Sudden clinical deterioration, right upper quadrant pain or the appearance of a hepatic mass may be noted. In 85% of cases the serum levels of α-fetoprotein are in excess of 10 ng/ml. The prognosis is dismal and 90% of patients are dead within 6 months.

Microscopically the tumour may form a single large mass (Fig. 17.34a), with central necrosis, haemorrhage and bile-staining, or may be multicentric (Fig. 17.34b). Extensive permeation of intrahepatic portal vein branches is a common feature. Extrahepatic metastases occur in less than half the cases, mainly in the lungs and lymph nodes. Microscopically the tumour cells closely resemble hepatocytes, their arrangement being more of less trabecular, with intervening sinusoids (Fig. 17.35). Bile canaliculi and intracytoplasmic inclusions such as Mallory bodies and α_1-antitrypsin granules may be seen. In other cases the tumour may be very poorly differentiated with tumour giant cells. A fibrolamellar variant, in which fibrous tissue separates the tumour cells, occurs in non-cirrhotic livers in younger people and is worth recognizing as it has a better prognosis.

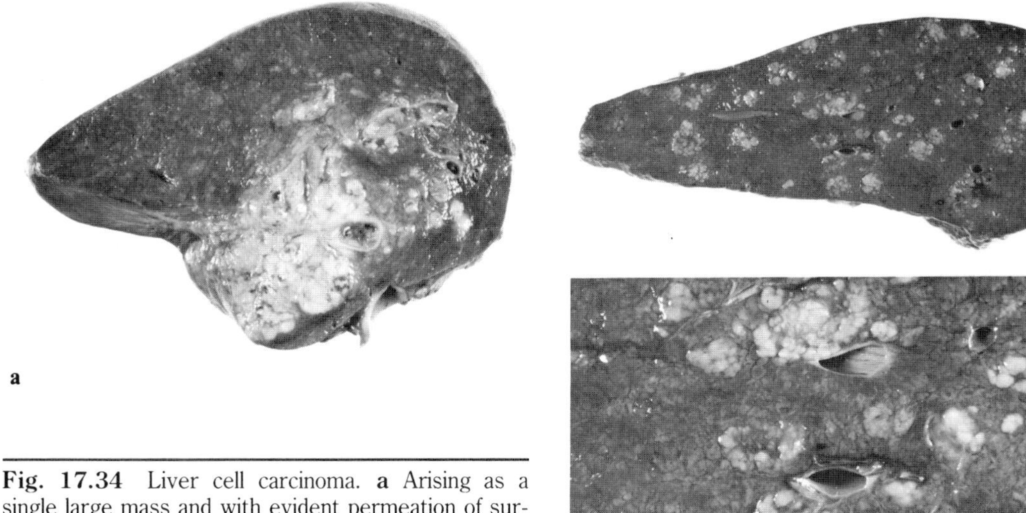

a

b

Fig. 17.34 Liver cell carcinoma. **a** Arising as a single large mass and with evident permeation of surrounding portal vein branches. **b** Arising as multicentric foci throughout the liver (shown also at higher magnification).

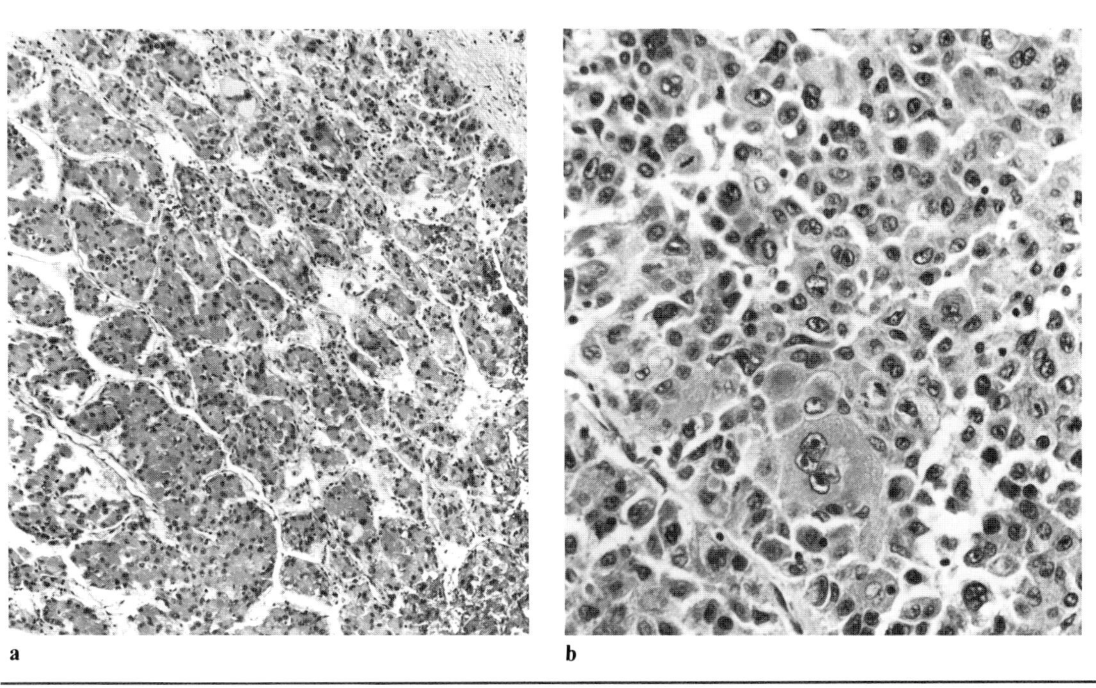

a

b

Fig. 17.35 Liver cell carcinoma. **a** Trabecular arrangement with endothelial-lined sinusoids separating the aggregates of tumour cells. ×75. **b** Individual tumour cells resembling hepatocytes with some binucleate and giant cell forms. ×250.

Bile Duct Carcinoma (Cholangiocarcinoma)

Primary tumours composed of cells resembling biliary epithelium (Fig. 17.36) are much less common than liver cell tumours. They are not associated with cirrhosis although there is an increased incidence in primary sclerosing cholangitis. There is no difference in sex incidence. In the Far East, where these are relatively frequent, about 65% of cases are associated with infestation by the liver fluke *Opisthorchis sinensis*.

Hepatoblastoma and Haemangiosarcoma

These are both very rare. Hepatoblastomas are congenital tumours of childhood and are composed of a mixture of epithelial and mesenchymal elements. Haemangiosarcomas are angioformative tumours. They have been associated with exposure to thorotrast and to arsenic, and more recently the tumour has been shown to be causally related to vinyl chloride monomer exposure.

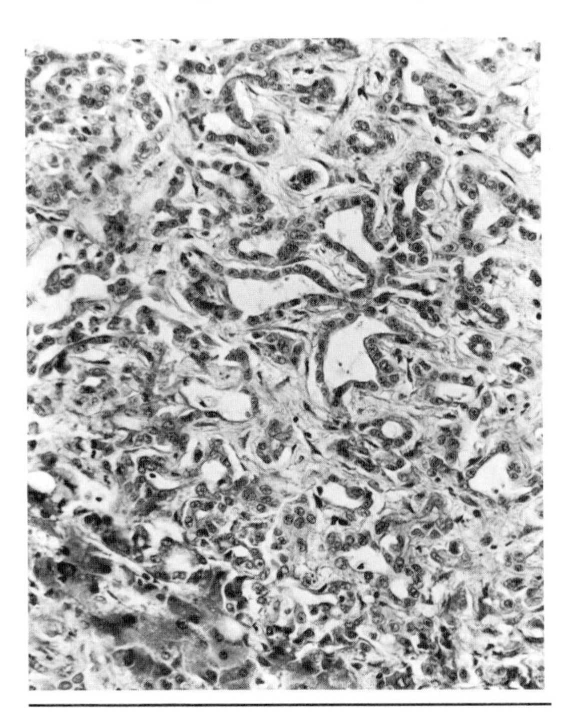

Fig. 17.36 Bile duct adenocarcinoma. There is a related fibrous (scirrhous) reaction. ×200.

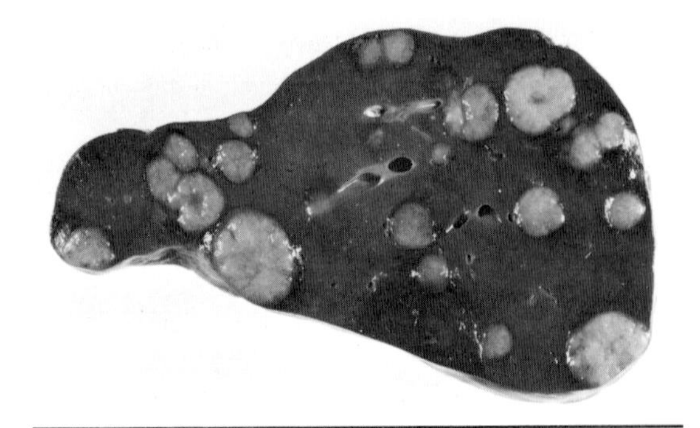

Fig. 17.37 Multiple secondary deposits in liver from a primary carcinoma of oesophagus.

Secondary Tumours

The liver is one of the commonest sites of secondary carcinomas of all kinds, notably from the gastrointestinal tract, lung and breast (Fig. 17.37). The liver becomes enlarged and its surface is beset with nodular elevations, some of which may show umbilication due to central necrosis. The organ may weigh 5 kg or more. Intrahepatic cholestasis and jaundice may develop from pressure on bile duct radicles. Leukaemic infiltration and involvement by malignant lymphomas is also common.

Other Disorders of the Liver

Drug and toxin-induced liver injury are discussed in Chapter 11.

Liver Diseases in Childhood

Many of the forms of liver disease which can occur in childhood are dealt with elsewhere. They include various metabolic disorders, biliary cirrhosis due to bile duct atresia or as a complication of fibrocystic disease of the pancreas, Indian childhood cirrhosis and congenital syphilis. There remain a few miscellaneous conditions which merit a brief description.

Neonatal hepatitis. This is now recognized to be due to a variety of causes. It may be the result of viral infections. HAV, HBV, cytomegalovirus, herpes simplex and rubella can all cause neonatal hepatitis. Metabolic disorders, e.g. galactosaemia, tyrosinaemia, total parenteral nutrition and α_1-antitrypsin deficiency may produce a similar histological picture as can biliary atresia. A number of cases are idiopathic. A striking feature is diffuse giant cell transformation of liver cells, some having 30–40 nuclei (Fig. 17.38). The precise aetiological diagnosis of neonatal hepatitis is both clinically and pathologically difficult.

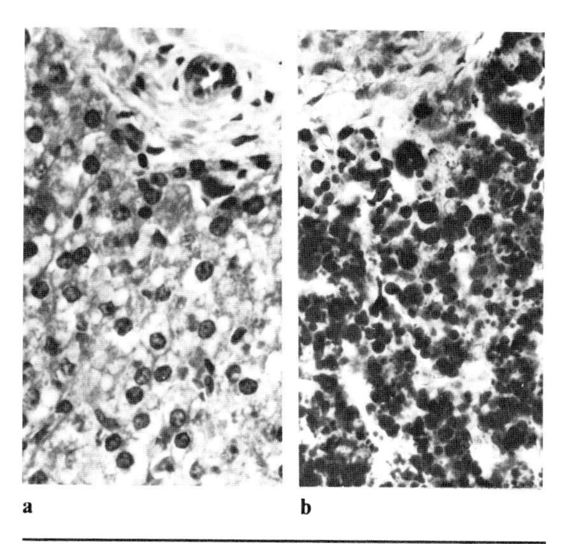

Fig. 17.39 Liver in Reye's syndrome: there is a severe degree of microvesicular fatty change. **a** H & E ×250. **b** Oil Red O ×250.

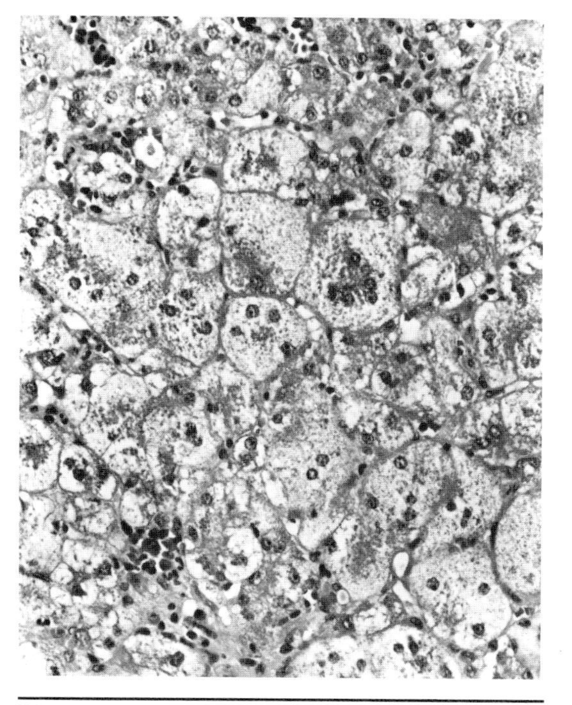

Fig. 17.38 Neonatal giant cell hepatitis: many of the liver cells are enlarged and multinucleate forms are evident. ×190.

Reye's syndrome affects children up to 10 years old. A mild upper respiratory infection is followed by convulsions, vomiting, fever, coma and death in up to 25% of cases. There may be hypoglycaemia and raised serum ammonia levels. The aetiology is uncertain and, while viral infection was suspected, there is now strong circumstantial evidence of an association with the use of aspirin. The liver is usually enlarged and shows very severe microvesicular fatty change (Fig. 17.39), which is seen also in the brain and myocardium.

Congenital Malformations

Cystic disease of the liver. Congenital cysts in the liver are rare and are usually associated with cystic disease of the kidneys; the latter condition, however, occurs much more commonly alone. The cysts vary greatly in size and number.

Congenital hepatic fibrosis. This is regarded as a form of cystic disease of the liver. It may be familial and is sometimes accompanied by cystic disease of the kidneys. Bands of dense fibrous tissue containing mature bile duct elements extend irregularly throughout the liver (Fig. 17.40), but the normal architecture is preserved between these. Affected individuals present in childhood or early adult life with portal hypertension, and when this is relieved surgically the prognosis is usually good because hepatocellular function is normal (*cf.* cirrhosis). However, there is an increased susceptibility to cholangitis.

Focal nodular hyperplasia. This is a benign circumscribed hamartomatous lesion in which there is a focal aggregation of hyperplastic liver cell nodules separated by fibrous septa. It is usually found incidentally and may be mistaken for tumour.

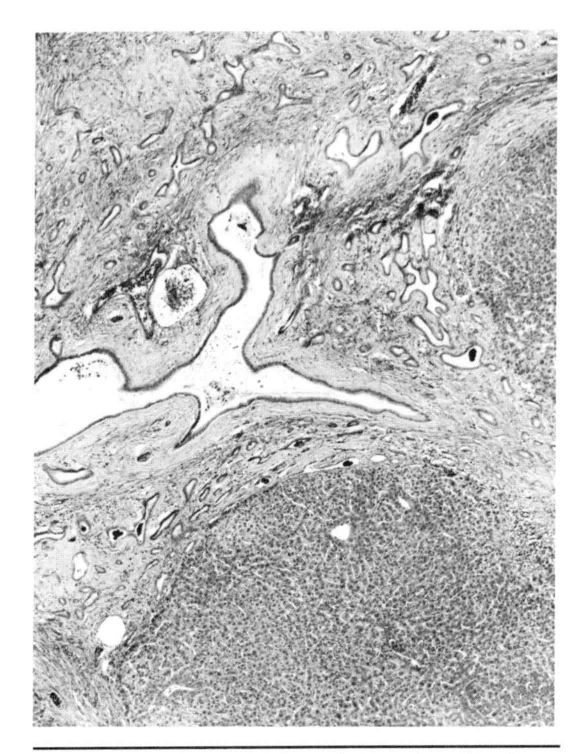

Fig. 17.40 Congenital hepatic fibrosis: wide fibrous septum within which are numerous mature bile duct elements, some of which contain inspissated bile. ×30.

Liver Disease in Pregnancy

Enterically transmitted non-A:non-B hepatitis – HEV – is associated with a high mortality in pregnancy.

A benign form of **intrahepatic cholestasis** may recur with each pregnancy and is probably due to increased levels of steroid hormones.

Acute fatty liver of pregnancy usually occurs in the last trimester and results in fatal hepatocellular failure in a proportion of cases. There is widespread fatty accumulation in hepatocytes, but of an unusual microvesicular appearance (Fig. 17.41). A similar appearance may occur with tetracycline toxicity. The lesion is thought to result from depressed hepatocyte protein synthesis with resultant accumulation of fat.

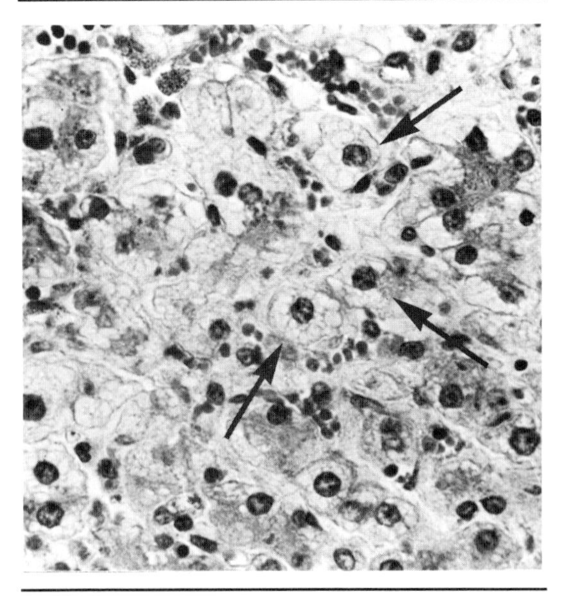

Fig. 17.41 Acute fatty liver of pregnancy: the hepatocytes are enlarged and contain multilocular droplets of fat arranged circumferentially round the nucleus (arrows). ×400.

Toxaemia of pregnancy. The liver is not usually injured but in fatal cases there are often foci of periportal necrosis and haemorrhage with fibrin thrombi. This is probably ischaemic, due to hepatic involvement in the disseminated intravascular coagulation now regarded as the pathogenetic mechanism in toxaemia of pregnancy.

Jaundice

Many of the hepatic causes of jaundice have been discussed above. In addition jaundice may develop as a complication of diseases of the gallbladder and pancreas. Jaundice is a clinical sign which is the result of yellow discoloration of the tissues with bilirubin. It is important to appreciate that jaundice and cholestasis are not synonymous terms as patients with jaundice may not be cholestatic and cholestatic patients may not be jaundiced. Jaundice generally appears first in the sclerae and when the serum bilirubin concentration reaches values of 35–50 μmol/l generalized jaundice appears. Hyperbilirubinaemia may result from excessive bilirubin production, a failure of bilirubin transport across the liver, or biliary obstruction. Cholestasis, on the other hand, is a failure of normal bile flow which gives rise to a typical clinical and biochemical syndrome. The two conditions meet in the biliary canaliculus where bilirubin is excreted into bile and bile flow is generated.

According to the duration and severity of the hyperbilirubaemia, the skin and sclerae show various degrees of yellow discoloration up to a deep orange colour, and occasionally, in chronic cases, the tissues may be olive-green owing to the formation of biliverdin, the oxidation product of bilirubin. The internal organs also are pigmented with the exception of the brain and spinal cord. However, even the brain does not escape in **icterus gravis neonatorum**, a condition associated with localized discoloration of the basal nuclei of the grey matter, kernicterus (p. 840). In patients with hyperbilirubinaemia conjugated bilirubin may also be excreted into the urine (only when the bilirubin is conjugated) and in the sweat; tears, saliva and gastric juice are not discoloured.

When the cause of the jaundice has been removed, the skin discoloration recedes rapidly. However, in more chronic cases of jaundice, both the hyperbilirubinaemia and the skin discoloration may recede much more slowly than expected. This is usually due to protein binding of the retained bilirubin to elastic tissue of the skin and, in the case of the blood, to albumin. The bound bilirubin has a biological half-life of about 23 days, explaining the slow resolution of the jaundice in these cases.

Bilirubin Metabolism by the Liver

Bilirubin is a tetrapyrrole derived from haem, principally found in haemoglobin: it is also present in myoglobin, catalase, peroxidase and the cytochromes. About 75% of the total production of bilirubin by the body is derived from haemoglobin, the remainder being produced by the liver from the catabolism of these other haem-containing proteins, from free haem and from ineffective erythropoiesis. Many tetrapyrroles are known to be water soluble but hydrogen bonding within the bilirubin molecule produces a structure in which the polar groups are no longer available to interact with water. Thus, bilirubin is highly insoluble in water.

Unconjugated bilirubin is transported in the blood almost totally bound to albumin. This binding process is reversible and has a high capacity, the upper limit being about 400 μmol of bilirubin per litre of plasma. While the reversible nature of the binding enables the uptake of bilirubin by the liver from the plasma, it also permits other substances, such as thyroxine and sulphonamides, in the plasma to compete with albumin for bilirubin binding. This may have clinical importance, particularly in neonates, in whom bilirubin displaced by these substances may enter the brain and cause kernicterus.

Bilirubin is taken up from the plasma almost exclusively by the liver. This process is facilitated by the size of the liver, by the fenestrated sinusoidal endothelium which allows easy access of plasma to the hepatocyte membrane and, possibly, by the presence of a bilirubin receptor on the membrane: the latter is controversial.

Once internalized within hepatocytes the

Table 17.5 Causes of hyperbilirubinaemia

	Comments
Predominantly unconjugated	
Increased bilirubin production	
ineffective erythropoiesis (dyserythropoiesis)	p. 611
haemolysis	p. 599
primary shunt hyperbilirubinaemia	Familial disease: premature destruction of red cells in marrow but normal red cell survival
Failure of bilirubin uptake	
Gilbert's syndrome	
Failure of bilirubin conjugation	
neonatal (physiological) jaundice	Relative deficiency of glucuronyl transferase in neonatal or premature babies: improves 2–3 weeks *post partum*
Criggler–Najjar syndrome	
type I	Absence of glucuronyl transferase, early death from kernicterus
type II	Partial deficiency of glucuronyl transferase; normal survival in many cases
Uncertain causation	
thyrotoxicosis	
Predominantly conjugated	
Failure of bilirubin excretion by hepatocytes	
Dubin–Johnson syndrome	Bilirubin fails to be secreted but not the other bile contents; brown granules accumulate in hepatocytes and give the liver a brown/green colour
Rotor syndrome	Similar to Dubin–Johnson: no pigment in hepatocytes
Byler disease	Recessive inheritance: cirrhosis and death in early infancy
Biliary flow obstruction	
Intrahepatic	
benign recurrent intrahepatic cholestasis	Possibly due to impaired canalicular bile flow
benign intrahepatic cholestasis of pregnancy	
chronic cholestatic syndrome – PBC; PSC	
cholestatic viral hepatitis	
intrahepatic biliary atresia	
Extrahepatic	
gallstones	
by extrinsic pressure on bile ducts; tumours primary or secondary	
biliary stricture	
pancreatitis	
extrahepatic biliary atresia	
Hepatocellular damage	
Acute hepatitis	
Alcohol-induced liver damage	
Chronic hepatitis	
Cirrhosis	
Tumours: primary and secondary	

bilirubin is bound to intracellular proteins in readiness for conjugation, principally with glucuronic acid, a reaction catalysed by the enzyme uridine diphosphate glucuronyl transferase. This leads to the formation of **conjugated bilirubin** comprising both mono- and diglucuronides which have a relatively high water solubility.

Little is known of the mechanism that leads to the excretion of the conjugated bilirubin into canalicular bile. Both mono- and diglucuronides are present in normal human bile in a ratio of about 1:4. It is appropriate to describe this last process as excretion because the bilirubin that is carried to the small intestine as bile is not subjected to reabsorption. There is therefore no established enterohepatic circulation of bilirubin in contradistinction to the active enterohepatic circulation of the bile acids.

Hyperbilirubinaemia

Bilirubin in normal plasma is almost entirely unconjugated: both conjugated and unconjugated forms may accumulate in hepatobiliary disorders. Hyperbilirubinaemia may therefore be classified as predominantly unconjugated or as predominantly conjugated. The causes of these types of hyperbilirubinaemia are set out in Table 17.5.

The student should bear in mind the fact that in many instances the mechanisms producing the hyperbilirubinaemia are complex and may be due to both hepatocellular injury and interference with bile flow. Drugs are a common cause of hyperbilirubinaemia and may interfere with bilirubin uptake, bilirubin conjugation, canalicular bile flow, and may cause bile duct injury.

The Gallbladder and Bile Ducts

Function of the Gallbladder

The relatively watery bile from the liver is stored in the gallbladder, concentrated by the absorption of water and electrolytes, and rendered more alkaline by the secretion of bicarbonate. Accordingly, with the addition of mucus from the mucosa, gallbladder bile becomes thick and mucoid. The normal structure of the mucosa is well suited to this absorptive function (Fig. 17.42). This concentrating ability of the gallbladder facilitates its radiological examination, in that certain iodine-containing compounds taken orally or administered intravenously are excreted and concentrated in the bile and, being radio-opaque, allow the gallbladder and the extrahepatic biliary system to be visualized. The discharge of gallbladder bile is stimulated by the entry of food into the duodenum, particularly fatty foods. This involves contraction of the gallbladder accompanied by relaxation of the sphincter of Oddi, a response mediated by cholecystokinin. Initially the gallbladder discharges only a proportion of its contents,

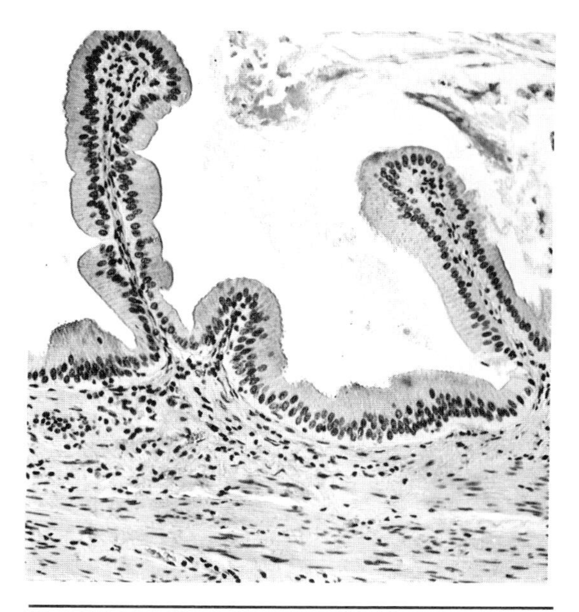

Fig. 17.42 Normal human gallbladder, showing delicate villous folds of mucosa covered by tall columnar epithelium. ×180.

and thereafter small quantities are passed at intervals; there is always some bile retained in the gallbladder. Between these periods of discharge the hepatic bile flows steadily into the gallbladder where it is concentrated, although a small amount bypasses the cystic duct and flows directly into the small intestine. Thus, small quantities of hepatic bile reach the duodenum even during periods of fasting.

Gallstones (Cholelithiasis)

Gallstones are formed from constituents of the bile – cholesterol, bile pigments and calcium salts – in various proportions, along with other organic material. They form usually in the gallbladder, but may also develop in the extrahepatic biliary tree and occasionally within intrahepatic ducts.

There is marked geographic variation in incidence, cholesterol stones being uncommon in developing countries. There is a very high incidence in North American Indians. Gallstones are commonest in late adult life, in women, especially multiparous, and in association with diabetes and obesity; the use of oral contraceptives may accelerate the development of gallstones. In patients who have undergone ileal resection there is an increased tendency for stone formation due to a decrease in the bile-acid pool.

Pathogenesis

The exact mechanisms of stone formation remain debatable, and it seems likely that changes in the composition of the bile, local factors in the gallbladder and biliary tract infection are predisposing causes.

Composition of the bile. Cholesterol is an important constituent of most gallstones. It is synthesized in the liver and excreted in the bile. Although extremely insoluble in water, it is kept in solution by the actions of phospholipids and bile salts, which together form molecular aggregates (mixed micelles) which are stable in the aqueous environment of the bile. The phospholipids are mainly (96%) lecithins with small amounts of lysolecithin and phosphatidyl ethanolamine. In water the phospholipids are dispersed as liquid crystals and these too interact with cholesterol, as a secondary solubilizing system, into bile. The ratio of cholesterol to bile acid conjugates and phospholipids in bile determines whether mixed micelles or phospholipid/cholesterol aggregates form: this in turn determines the overall solubility of the cholesterol in bile.

The primary bile acids are synthesized in the liver from cholesterol, the most important ones being cholic acid and chenodeoxycholic acid. They are secreted in the bile as conjugates with the amino acids glycine and taurine, the glycine/taurine conjugate ratio being 3:1. In the colon the primary bile acids undergo bacterial dehydroxylation to form the secondary bile acids, deoxycholic and lithocholic acid. These major bile acids, together with other minor forms, constitute the bile-acid pool; more than 85% of this is reabsorbed daily from the distal small intestine and colon and recycled (the enterohepatic circulation). It is the detergent-like properties of bile acids which promote the formation of micelles.

Gallstones tend to form when there is a relative excess of cholesterol to bile acids and phospholipids – '**lithogenic bile**'. This may result either from an increase in bile cholesterol or a decrease in the bile-acid pool: these changes are commonly found in patients with gallstones, but are unexplained. It is important to appreciate that the presence of lithogenic bile *per se* is not sufficient to explain the formation of gallstones in individual patients. Indeed, lithogenic bile can be found in both patients with and without gallstones. However, it is curious that cholesterol will form tiny microcrystals in bile from patients with gallstones much more rapidly in spite of the similarities in lithogenicity. It appears, therefore, that there are other, as yet undefined, factors that lead to the nidation of these microcrystals; further growth of microcrystals is taken to be the mechanism for the formation of gallstones.

Local factors in the gallbladder. It seems likely that these have some part to play in the formation of stones. The parts played in stone formation by the gallbladder mucosa, the mucus and glycoprotein which it secretes and the effects of local stasis are not known. There may also be a feedback effect on bile composition from the gallbladder and lithogenic bile shows a return to more normal composition following cholecystectomy.

Infections. It is doubtful whether infection is involved in the formation of cholesterol or pigment stones. The bile is sterile in most patients with such stones. Infection may, however, enhance the effects of local factors already mentioned and thus contribute to increase in size of stones and the formation of additional stones and mixed ones.

Types of Stone

Stones containing predominantly cholesterol are by far the commonest. It should be appreciated, however, that all cholesterol gallstones also contain calcium salts and a mucinous 'skeleton'. Indeed, the chemical composition of gallstones can be considered as a continuum consisting of varying proportions of cholesterol with calcium salts. Pigment and calcium carbonate stones are rare.

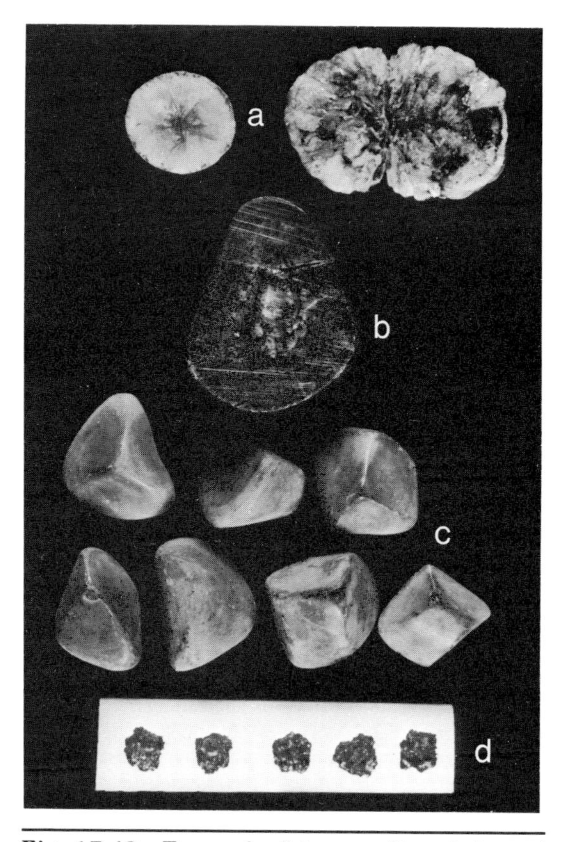

Fig. 17.43 Types of gallstones. **a** Two cholesterol stones; **b** combination stone: a cholesterol core coated by laminated surface deposits of mixed composition; **c** multiple faceted mixed stones; **d** bile-pigment stones.

Cholesterol Stones

These can be classified as mixed or laminated, pure and combination or compound cholesterol stones (Fig. 17.43).

Mixed or laminated gallstones. These, the commonest type, are always multiple and often very numerous (Fig. 17.43). They vary greatly in size from 1 cm or more in diameter to the size of sand grains, are irregular in shape and often faceted. On section they have a distinctly laminated structure, dark brown and paler layers alternating. These layers consist chiefly of cholesterol and bile pigment respectively, both containing also an admixture of calcium salts and organic material. They may lie free in the bile, or they may be tightly packed together within a contracted gallbladder with a thickened wall (see Fig. 17.45).

The pure cholesterol stone is usually solitary, oval, and may reach over 3 cm in length. It is pale yellow, soapy to the touch and floats in water. When broken across, the stone shows a crystalline structure composed of sheaves of cholesterol crystals which radiate outwards from the centre and there is no trace of lamination. Some solitary cholesterol stones, however, have a laminated cortex (Fig. 17.43) due to the secondary deposition of bile pigment and calcium salts, which occurs when the gallbladder becomes inflamed by superadded bacterial infection. These are called **combination** or **compound cholesterol stones**. They constitute the largest gallstones.

Bile Pigment Stones

Such stones are usually multiple, black, irregular in form or occasionally somewhat stellate (Fig.

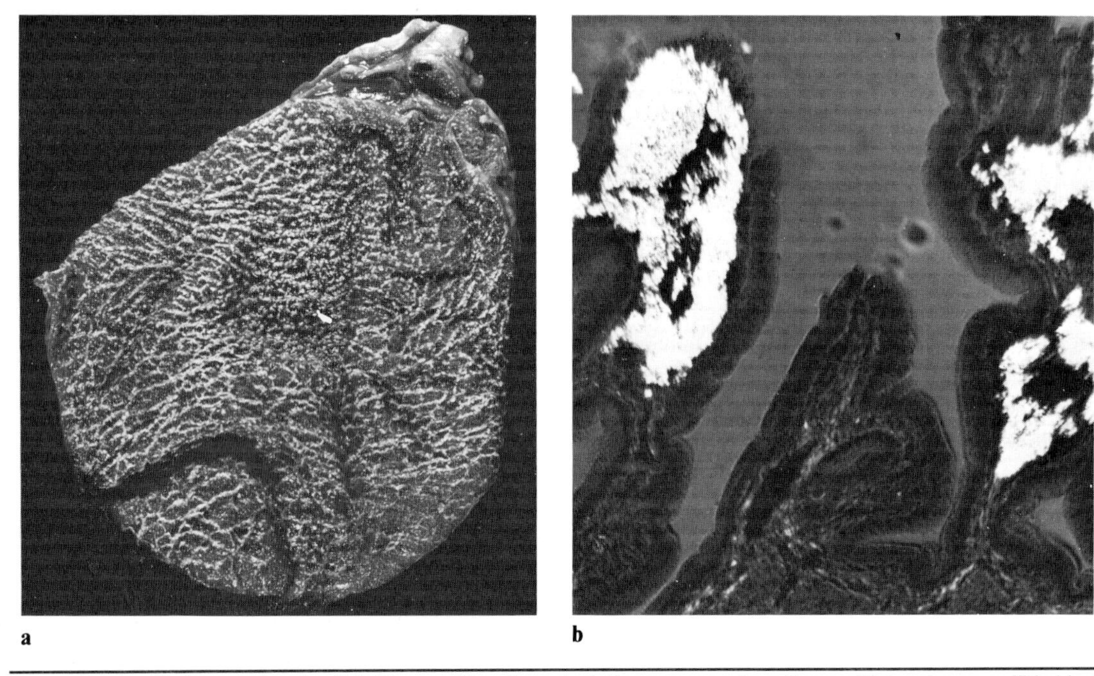

Fig. 17.44 Cholesterosis of gallbladder. **a** The characteristic macroscopic pattern of 'strawberry gallbladder'. **b** Deposits of cholesterol esters in papillae, viewed by polarized light. ×90.

17.43). They are composed chiefly of bile pigment and may be friable or hard. They are often present in chronic haemolytic anaemias and are usually due to excess of bile pigment in the bile. They may also be associated with parasitic infestations, e.g. malaria. The gallbladder usually appears normal.

Calcium Carbonate Stones

These are rare. They are multiple, small, pale yellowish and fairly hard.

Cholesterosis of the Gallbladder

This unimportant condition results from the patchy deposition of doubly refractile cholesterol esters within mucosal macrophages. This produces distinct yellowish flecking of the mucosa giving the appearance of so-called 'strawberry gallbladder' (Fig. 17.44). The lipid deposits may increase in size to form polypoidal nodules. It is associated with cholesterol stones in one-third of cases.

Cholecystitis

Inflammation of the gallbladder is one of the commonest causes of abdominal pain, and frequently necessitates cholecystectomy.

Acute Cholecystitis

Acute cholecystitis is nearly always associated with the presence of stones. In the early stages of acute cholecystitis bacteria cannot usually be cultured from the gallbladder. Therefore it is thought that the initial inflammation is chemically induced. Obstruction to the outflow of bile by a stone results in the bile becoming overconcentrated and this produces an irritant effect with consequent inflammation. Secondary bacterial infection may then occur, aggravating the inflammatory reaction. The organisms, which are thought to reach the gallbladder via the lymphatics are most commonly *Escherichia coli* or *Streptococcus faecalis*. Acute cholecystitis rarely occurs in the absence of stones, and is then usually associated with a source of infection elsewhere.

Pathologically, acute cholecystitis consists of varying degrees of oedema, fibrinous exudate and neutrophil infiltration, and there may be mucosal ulceration and haemorrhage. More severe changes occur when there is continued obstruction of the cystic duct, either by stone or by inflammatory oedema and exudate. The lumen may then become filled with pus – **empyema of the gallbladder**. Abscesses may also form in the wall, or there may even be necrosis of the wall with rupture into the peritoneal cavity. In acute cholecystitis, fibrin deposition on the serosal surface may undergo organization resulting in fibrosis and adhesions. The condition is often recurrent and may become chronic.

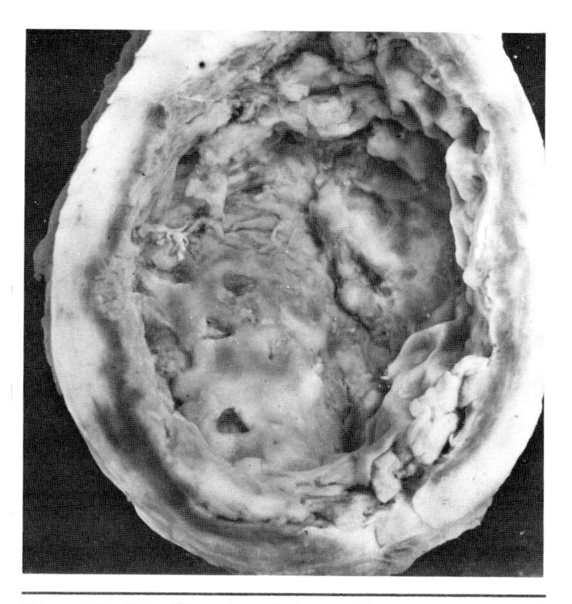

Fig. 17.45 Chronic cholecystitis, showing great thickening of wall. The gallbladder was packed with small rounded stones.

Chronic Cholecystitis

This may result from repeated attacks of acute cholecystitis. In many patients, however, the disease is one of insidious onset, accompanied by dyspeptic symptoms or biliary colic. Gallstones are almost always present. The gallbladder wall is shrunken and shows marked fibrous thickening (Fig. 17.45). The gallbladder becomes shrunken with a thickened fibrous wall whose lining is irregular. The microscopic appearances are variable. The muscle bundles within the wall are thickened and epithelial downgrowths through the muscle become more marked, forming gland-like structures known as **Rokitansky–Aschoff sinuses** (Fig. 17.46). Bile may rupture from these and elicit a granulomatous reaction and there may be a chronic inflammatory infiltrate in the submucosa or elsewhere in the wall with fibrosis.

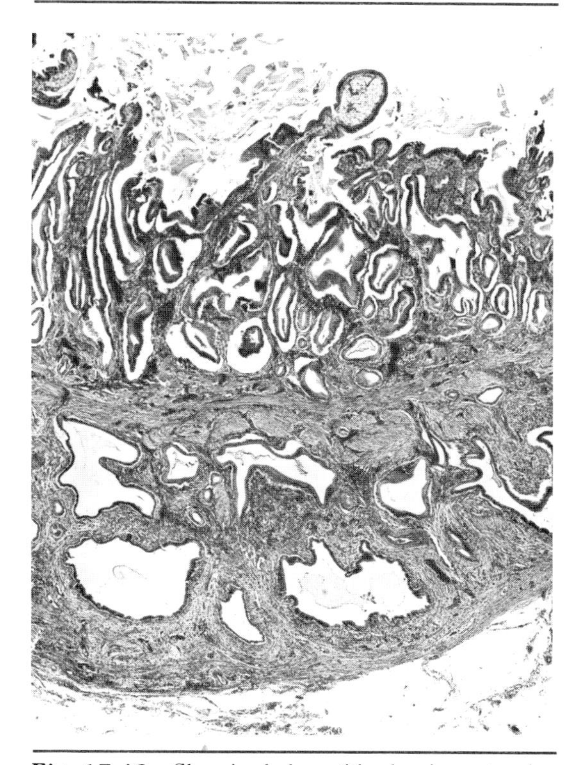

Fig. 17.46 Chronic cholecystitis showing extensive penetration of fundus of gallbladder by epithelial lined spaces lying between muscle and serosa (Rokitansky–Aschoff sinuses). ×20.

Complications of Cholelithiasis and Cholecystitis

Gallstones and infections of the gallbladder are so intimately related that the complications associated with them are best considered together. Some of these have been referred to already.

Gallstones, single or multiple, may be symptomless – silent stones. When a stone becomes impacted in Hartmann's pouch or in the cystic duct, marked distension of the gallbladder results; the bile pigments are absorbed and the contents become clear and mucoid – **mucocele** of the gallbladder (Fig. 17.47). In the presence of infection, however, the contents become turbid or purulent – **empyema** of the gallbladder. Inflammation of the wall may progress to necrosis, with escape of the contents into the peritoneal cavity producing localized or generalized peritonitis.

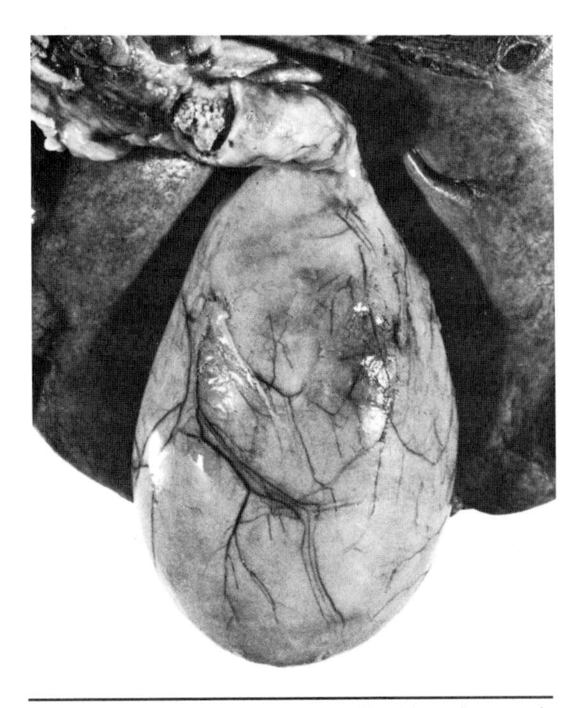

Fig. 17.47 Mucocele of the gallbladder. A stone is impacted in the cystic duct producing distension of the gallbladder, the contents of which have become clear and mucoid. Note how this accentuates the vascular markings on the serosa.

Stones may also obstruct the common bile duct, producing biliary colic, extrahepatic obstruction and jaundice. If the stone remains loose in the duct, the jaundice may be intermittent. Secondary bacterial infection is common, resulting in ascending cholangitis. In only a small proportion of cases does obstruction of the bile duct by stones lead to secondary biliary cirrhosis.

In chronic cholecystitis the wall becomes thickened and contracted over a mass of closely packed stones. There are often adhesions around the gallbladder and a stone or stones may ulcerate in one of several directions. A large stone of the compound cholesterol type may, for example, ulcerate through into the duodenum or less frequently into the colon. It may pass along the bowel or may become arrested to the small intestine, chiefly by contraction of the muscular coat, where it produces acute intestinal obstruction, termed **gallstones ileus**. Ulceration into the portal vein resulting in portal pyaemia has also been reported. Lastly, the irritation produced by gallstones may lead to carcinoma of the gallbladder or, more rarely, of the large ducts.

Tumours of the Biliary Tract

Benign tumours, such as fibroma, lipoma and papilloma, are all very rare.

Carcinoma of the gallbladder is uncommon and gallstones are an important factor in its causation, being present in 80% of cases. The commonest site is the fundus and next is the neck of the gallbladder. It is usually of a slowly growing, infiltrating type. Occasionally the gallbladder may be completely destroyed, only identifiable by the presence of a small cavity containing gallstones. Tumour may directly invade the liver (Fig. 17.48) or may metastasize to it, and to porta hepatis lymph nodes. In most cases the tumour is an adenocarcinoma, but squamous-cell carcinoma,

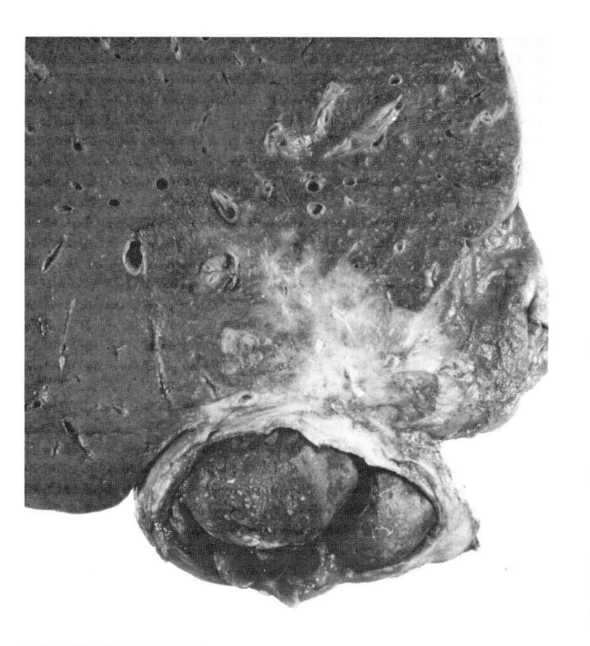

Fig. 17.48 Carcinoma of the gallbladder spreading directly into the overlying liver.

arising secondarily to metaplasia of the lining epithelium, also occurs.

Carcinoma occurs also in the **large bile ducts** and is usually a small and slowly growing tumour presenting with obstructive jaundice. The two commonest sites are the lower end of the common bile duct and the junction of the cystic and hepatic ducts, the latter being more frequent.

Of the very many individuals who develop gallstones, less than 2% develop carcinoma of the gallbladder; the incidence of bile-duct carcinoma is also low, although it is often not possible to determine whether a tumour around the ampulla has originated from bile duct or pancreas.

Congenital Anomalies

A large number of abnormalities of the gallbladder have been described and may affect its size, shape, position, relation to the liver, etc. Gallstones may occur more frequently at a younger age in association with these anomalies.

Varying degrees of extrahepatic **biliary atresia** may occur and may result in biliary cirrhosis. The rare **choledochal cyst** comprises a sac-like dilatation of part or all of the biliary tract, and is associated with jaundice and cholangitis.

The Pancreas

The pancreas is often thought of as two separate organs – an exocrine one concerned with digestion, and an endocrine one concerned with the metabolism of carbohydrate, fat and protein. Their association within one gland is simply regarded as fortuitous. However, knowledge of the embryology, anatomy, physiology and pathology of the pancreas militates against this simplistic approach.

Embryology. Dorsal and ventral pancreatic buds develop independently from the foregut. They fuse to give a single organ in which there is usually union of the duct systems of the two buds. The ventral bud eventually forms about one-tenth of the pancreas, identifiable as a 'lobe' in the posteroinferior part of the pancreatic head. In early fetal life the pancreas comprises a series of branching ductules from which are derived both acinar tissue and islet cells. Thus, the whole pancreas, exocrine and endocrine, is derived from foregut endoderm.

Structure. Connective tissue septa divide the pancreas into lobules. Within the lobule the secretory unit is the acinus, the cells of which have abundant cytoplasmic zymogen granules – membrane-bound sacs containing digestive enzymes. The secretory products pass into the acinar lumen and drain via intralobular and interlobular ducts to the main pancreatic duct. In 85% of cases the pancreatic duct joins the common bile duct to form the ampulla of Vater which then enters the duodenum. In 15% of cases the two ducts do not join to form an ampulla and they enter the duodenum separately.

The anatomy of the pancreatic blood supply is significant. Most lobules receive a single arterial branch and, within lobules, much of the circulation passes by arterioles to the islets, the exocrine tissue being supplied by a portal system of capillaries which drains the blood from the sinusoids of the islets (Fig. 17.49). The pancreatic acini around islets are thus exposed to very high levels of islet hormones – possibly several hundred times higher than the levels in the systemic circulation. Most of the endocrine cells are grouped together into islets, although individual endocrine cells can be found in duct epithelium and among acini. In the adult pancreas, islets in that part derived from the dorsal bud (superior anterior part of head, body and tail of the pancreas), consist of approximately 80% insulin-secreting (B) cells, 15% glucagon-secreting (A) cells, 4% somatostatin-secreting (D) cells and 1% pancreatic polypeptide-secreting (PP) cells. By contrast, in the part derived from the ventral bud, islets are composed of 18% B cells, 1% A cells, 2% D cells and 79% PP cells. Not surprisingly, this part of the pancreas is termed the PP-rich lobe and the remainder is called the PP-poor lobe. Because of the greater density of islets in the former, PP cells constitute 36% of all the endocrine cells in the pancreas.

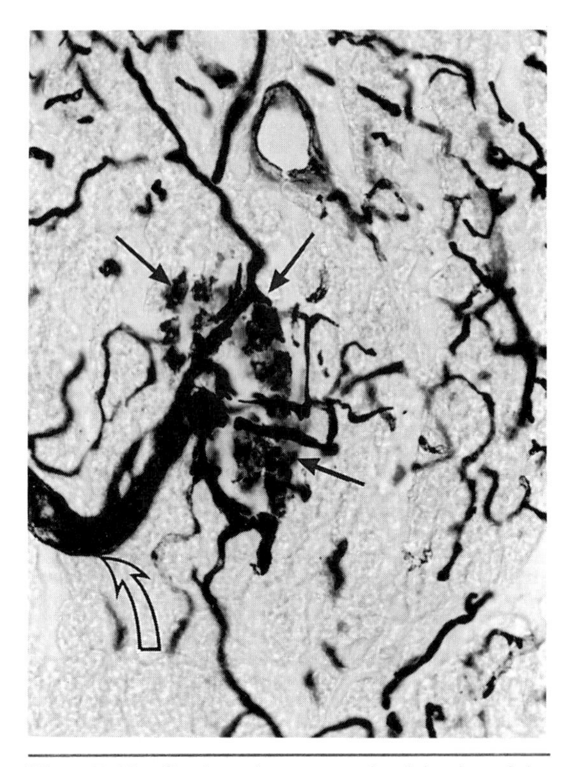

Fig. 17.49 Section of pancreas after injection of the blood vessels with India ink. The B cells of the islets have been stained black by the immunoperoxidase technique. The periphery of an islet is marked by straight arrows. An arteriole (curved arrow) breaks up into sinusoids which supply the islet and drain into capillaries which supply the surrounding exocrine tissue. ×120.

Functional aspects. The exocrine pancreas secretes about 1–2 litres per day of an alkaline fluid containing some 20 enzymes. Bicarbonate is secreted by the duct epithelium. The enzymes include proteases – trypsin and chymotrypsin – lipases, phospholipases, elastase and amylase. Protease inhibitors are also present within acinar cells and in the pancreatic secretion. Most enzymes are secreted in precursor forms which are activated in the duodenum, a process in which trypsin has a key role.

In addition to its systemic effects insulin is a major trophic hormone for the exocrine pancreas, increasing the rate of DNA and protein synthesis in acinar tissue. Weight for weight the exocrine pancreas synthesizes considerably more protein (mainly enzymes) than any other tissue in the body (eight times more than the liver, for example). Since one of the main actions of insulin in all cells of the body is to stimulate protein synthesis, it is interesting to speculate that the islets, with their distinctive blood supply, which ensures very high levels of insulin in the exocrine capillaries, have evolved to aid the massive protein-synthesizing requirements of the exocrine pancreas. Thus the pancreas, in some respects, functions as a single organ.

Pancreatitis

Pancreatitis is classified clinically and pathologically into acute and chronic forms.

Acute Pancreatitis

This is defined as an acute inflammatory process within the pancreas usually associated with necrosis of intrapancreatic acini and adipose tissue. If there is macroscopic haemorrhage the term **acute haemorrhagic pancreatitis** is used, but this probably simply represents the most severe form of acute pancreatitis.

Clinical features. The onset is sudden with abdominal pain, vomiting and collapse and may easily be confused clinically with perforation of a peptic ulcer. The diagnosis is confirmed by demonstrating a serum amylase level greater than 1200 iu/l. Two-thirds of patients admitted to hospital have a mild illness which settles readily with nasogastric suction and intravenous fluids. Severe pancreatitis, characterized by shock, hypocalcaemia, hypoxaemia and hyperglycaemia, is less common and carries a 50% mortality rate.

Macroscopic changes. The abdominal findings in severe cases are acute peritonitis with blood-stained ascitic fluid and white flecks of fat necrosis on the omentum (Fig. 17.50) and surface of the pancreas. The cut surface of the pancreas usually shows further flecks of necrosis, possibly in combination with haemorrhage, which may be confluent, resulting in a firm black necrotic mass (Fig. 17.51).

Microscopic changes. There appears to be at least two different anatomical sites where the initial damage may start (Foulis, 1984). In some cases, necrosis and an acute inflammatory infiltrate appear first within and around excretory ducts (**periductal necrosis** – Fig. 17.52). In others, necrosis develops at the periphery of pancreatic lobules (**perilobular necrosis** – Fig. 17.53). These two patterns can be correlated with aetiology.

Aetiology and Pathogenesis

In Western countries over 80% of clinically observed cases of acute pancreatitis are associated either with the presence of **biliary calculi** or

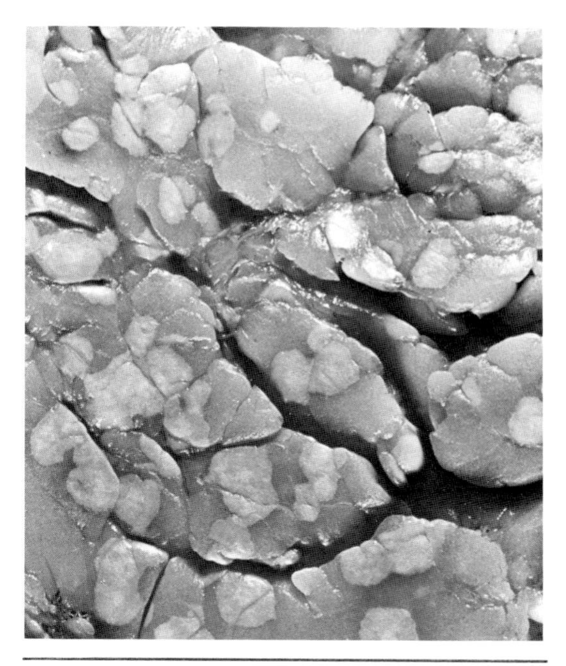

Fig. 17.50 Part of the greater omentum from a case of acute pancreatitis showing pale patches of fat necrosis. ×1.7.

alcohol abuse. These agents appear to initiate pancreatic necrosis by damaging pancreatic excretory ducts, since both are associated microscopically with duct inflammation and **periductal necrosis**. In 'gallstone pancreatitis', the initiating event appears to be the passage of a gallstone into the common bile duct, resulting in temporary obstruction of the pancreatic duct at the ampulla of Vater. If such patients are treated surgically within 48 hours, impacted gallstones are found at the ampulla in over 70% of cases. It has also been

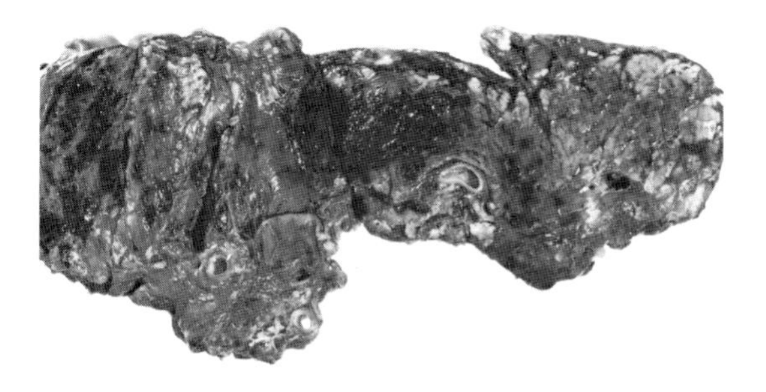

Fig. 17.51 Acute haemorrhagic pancreatitis. ×0.6.

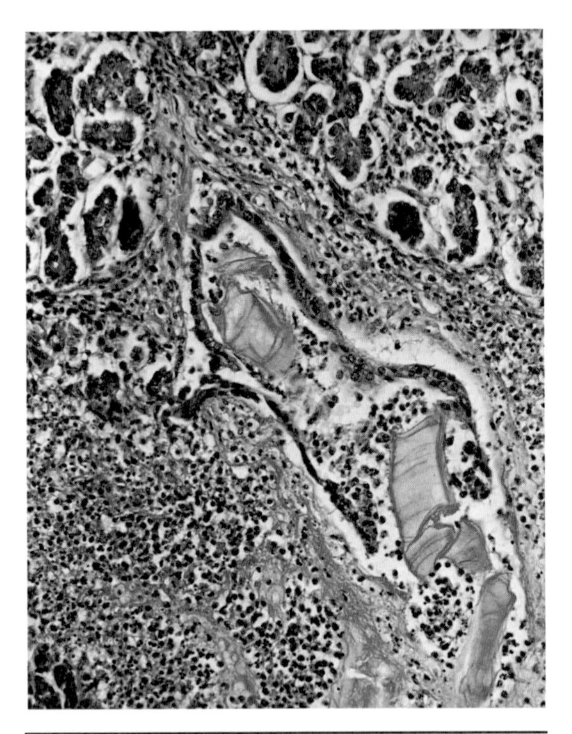

Fig. 17.52 Acute pancreatitis, showing periductal necrosis. An interlobular duct is dilated by protein-rich concretions. The surrounding acini are necrotic and there is an acute inflammatory infiltrate in and around the ducts. ×180.

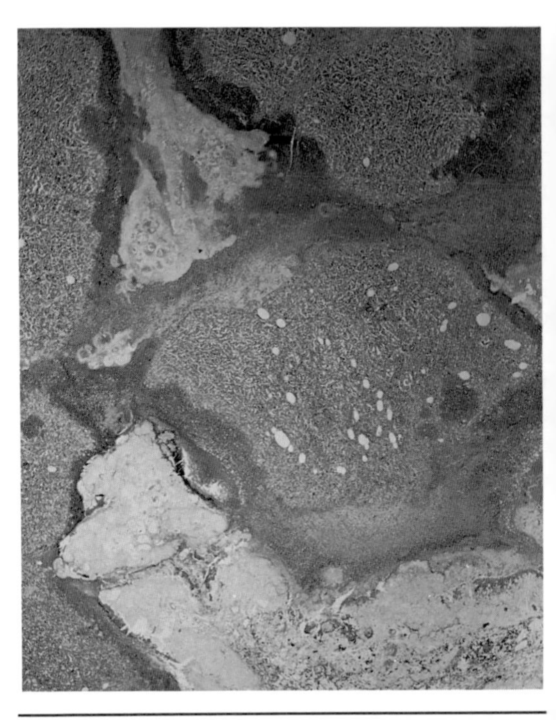

Fig. 17.53 Acute pancreatitis, showing necrosis of the peripheral parts of the lobules. (The necrotic tissue is mostly darker staining than the surviving tissue.) ×20.

shown by operative cholangiography that there is reflux of contrast material from the bile duct into the pancreatic duct, signifying a common exit channel, in 66% of patients with gallstone pancreatitis, but in only 20% of patients with gallstones but without pancreatitis. Thus reflux of bile into an obstructed pancreatic duct is the likely initial event. Normal bile alone does not damage the pancreatic duct, but infected bile or bile preincubated with trypsin causes ductal inflammation and necrosis when infused into the pancreatic duct at physiological pressure. Both infection and trypsin convert primary bile salts into secondary bile salts which are toxic to pancreatic duct epithelium. Bile is infected in at least 40% of cases of gallstone pancreatitis and, in the presence of an obstructing stone, bile which has refluxed into the pancreas can be altered by pancreatic trypsin.

Although in alcohol-associated acute pancreatitis the pancreatic ducts are also thought to be the initial site of damage, the mechanism causing this is not known, and is likely to be different from that involved in gallstone pancreatitis.

Acute pancreatitis can complicate **shock** from any cause and **hypothermia**. In these situations **perilobular necrosis** is found microscopically within the pancreas and the cause of the pancreatitis appears to be hypoperfusion. Pancreatic lobules are supplied by a single arterial branch and thus during prolonged hypotension the periphery of the lobule is prone to ischaemic damage. Hypothermia is associated with diminished prostacyclin synthesis resulting in an increased thrombotic tendency and this, in combination with hypotension, may precipitate thrombosis and perilobular necrosis in the pancreas.

Rarer causes of acute pancreatitis include direct pancreatic trauma, Pólya type gastrectomy, endoscopic exploration or radiography of the common bile duct and pancreatic duct, viral (notably

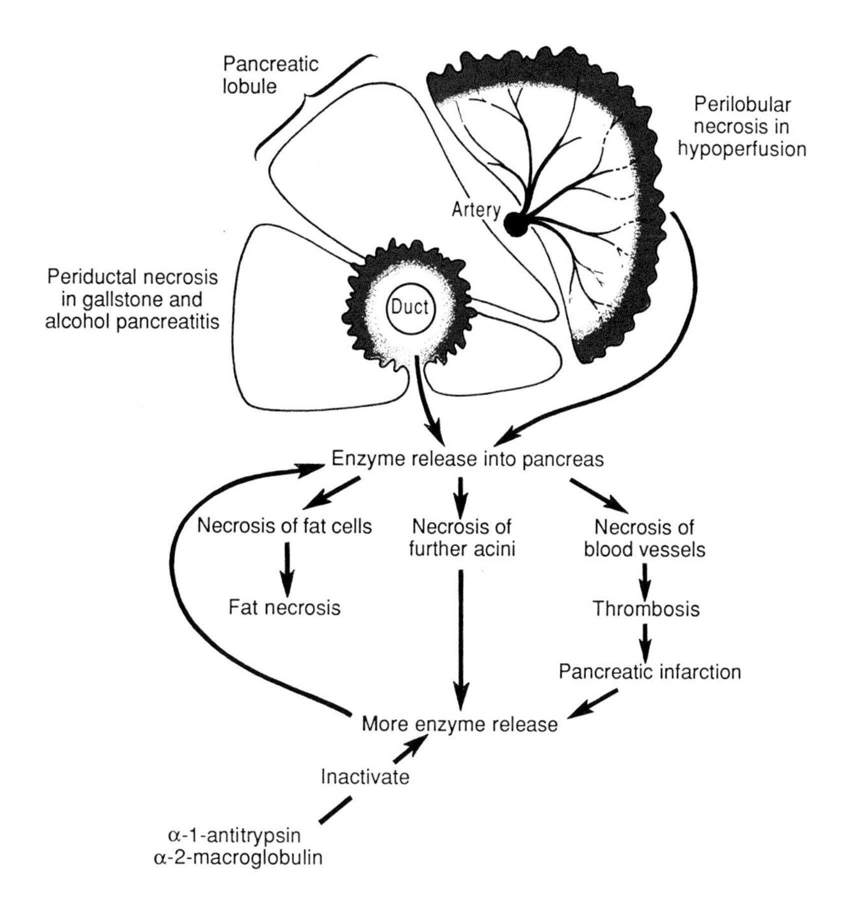

Fig. 17.54
Diagrammatic outline to show the mechanisms by which acute pancreatitis develops.

mumps) infection and drugs (azathioprine, valproic acid, diuretics and oral contraceptives). The incidence is also increased in hyperparathyroidism and in diabetes mellitus. Lack of pathological material in these conditions has precluded study of the pathogenetic mechanisms involved.

Wherever the process starts necrosis causes release of digestive enzymes into the substance of the pancreas. These enzymes are thought to damage further pancreatic parenchymal cells and blood vessels by a process of **autodigestion** (Fig. 17.54). Necrotic blood vessels, particularly veins, are liable to thrombose causing ischaemic damage to further areas of pancreas, thus initiating a vicious cycle of further enzyme release which may result in extensive coagulative necrosis of entire lobules and intervening ducts and blood vessels (**panlobular necrosis**) – this corresponds to the macroscopic appearance of acute haemorrhagic pancreatitis.

Defence Mechanisms

Plasma contains the antiproteolytic enzymes α_1-antitrypsin and α_2-macroglobulin and pancreatic juice contains pancreatic secretory trypsin inhibitor. These combine with active proteolytic enzymes such as trypsin to inactivate them. Release and activation of these antiproteolytic enzymes in the inflammatory exudate in acute pancreatitis may help inhibit the autodigestive process.

Complications of Acute Pancreatitis

Systemic. Severe acute pancreatitis is complicated by chemical peritonitis which, even in the absence of superadded bacterial peritonitis, can cause death from endotoxic shock due to escape of intestinal endotoxin into the circulation. Release of pancreatic enzymes into the blood may also contribute to the shock syndrome complex, in which adult respiratory distress syndrome (p. 541) and acute renal failure are serious, life threatening, additional complications.

Local. Sepsis in a necrotic pancreas may result in widespread suppuration or a **pancreatic abscess**. The causal organisms are *E. coli* and other gut commensals. Another local effect is the formation of a **pseudocyst** – a localized collection of pancreatic juice and necrotic debris resulting from disruption of the pancreatic ductal drainage. It is lined by granulation tissue and commonly forms in the lesser sac.

Chronic Pancreatitis

In this disease there is continuing pancreatic inflammation.

Clinical features. Most patients present with episodes of severe, erratic abdominal pain which may persist for years and lead to analgesic addiction. The pain may be exacerbated by food and thus weight loss may ensue. Some patients develop intermittent jaundice due to involvement of the common bile duct. Steatorrhoea and diabetes (exocrine and endocrine pancreatic failure) are usually later manifestations but may be the presenting features in the few patients in whom the disease process has been painless. Plain abdominal radiographs may show diffuse pancreatic calcification and endoscopic retrograde pancreatography will usually show strictures and distortions of the pancreatic ducts and pancreatic calculi in the ducts.

Macroscopically the pancreas is firm and the cut surface shows a smooth grey appearance with loss of normal lobulation. This change is the result of diffuse fibrosis. The main ducts are often focally dilated, sometimes forming cysts which contain calcified stones.

Microscopically, early lesions consist of ductal strictures and the presence of protein precipitates and inflammation in the ducts. The protein precipitates calcify and enlarge to form stones which obstruct branches of the ducts, leading to atrophy and eventual disappearance of acini drained by the ducts. In the late stage there is much periductal fibrosis and exocrine pancreatic atrophy but there is preservation of islets, which do not disappear as a result of duct obstruction (Fig. 17.55). They may, however, become embedded in fibrous tissue leading to relative ischaemia, dysfunction and resultant diabetes mellitus.

Aetiology and Pathogenesis

Most cases of chronic pancreatitis occur in patients who abuse alcohol. The disease is not associated with gallstones. Epidemiologically, it is common in wine drinking countries where a high alcohol intake is accompanied also by a diet rich in

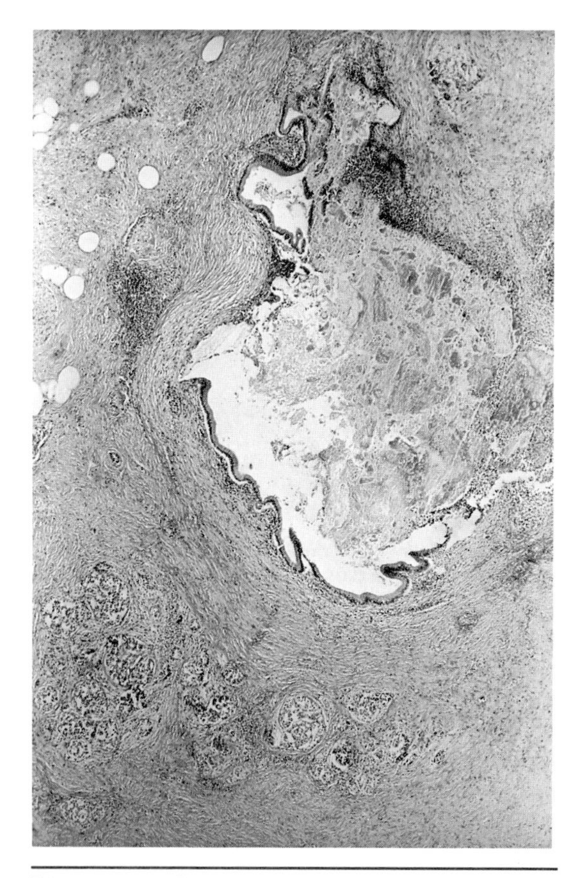

Fig. 17.55 Chronic pancreatitis showing ulceration and dilatation of a duct and periductal fibrosis. Note the loss of acini but preservation of islets. ×25.

protein. Alcohol increases the protein concentration in pancreatic juice with subsequent precipitation of concretions in the ducts: these form stones which ulcerate the ductal epithelium leading to periductal inflammation and fibrosis. This scar tissue contracts and causes ductal strictures with secondary dilatation of the duct behind the stricture and acinar atrophy.

It will be appreciated that the site of initial damage in the pancreas in both alcohol related acute pancreatitis and chronic pancreatitis is the pancreatic duct. Not surprisingly therefore, there is some overlap clinically and pathologically between these two conditions in affected alcoholics. Thus, a patient may present with typical acute pancreatitis and this may be the prelude to continuing chronic pain and the development of chronic pancreatitis. In turn patients with chronic pancreatitis may have particularly severe episodes of pain which clinically and biochemically are indistinguishable from an attack of acute pancreatitis.

Tumours of the Exocrine Pancreas

Apart from carcinoma, pancreatic tumours are rare.

Cystadenomas of the pancreas are often large and multiloculated. When they are lined by a non-mucin-secreting epithelium which contains glycogen they are benign. Some of the mucin-secreting multicystic tumours may be malignant, and are termed cystadenocarcinomas.

Carcinoma

Carcinoma of the pancreas has doubled in incidence in the UK during the last 50 years. The increase in the USA has been even higher and there it now ranks second only to colorectal carcinoma among alimentary tract cancers. It is commoner in males than females and increases progressively in incidence after the age of 50 years. Epidemiologically, it has been linked to smoking, a high-fat/high-protein diet, and possibly diabetes. There is no association with chronic pancreatitis or alcohol abuse. Sixty-five per cent of tumours are situated in the head of the pancreas where they usually obstruct the common bile duct, causing obstructive jaundice, sometimes before spread has occurred. By contrast, carcinoma arising in the body or tail of the pancreas is usually clinically silent until there are multiple metastases. Pancreatic cancer may also present with bizarre clinical effects due to unexplained venous thrombosis (migrating thrombophlebitis), peripheral neuropathy or myopathy.

Histologically, the tumour is an adenocarcinoma and usually provokes a scirrhous reaction (Fig. 17.56). It frequently obstructs the main pancreatic duct, and exocrine pancreatic tissue distal to the obstruction becomes atrophic with some associ-

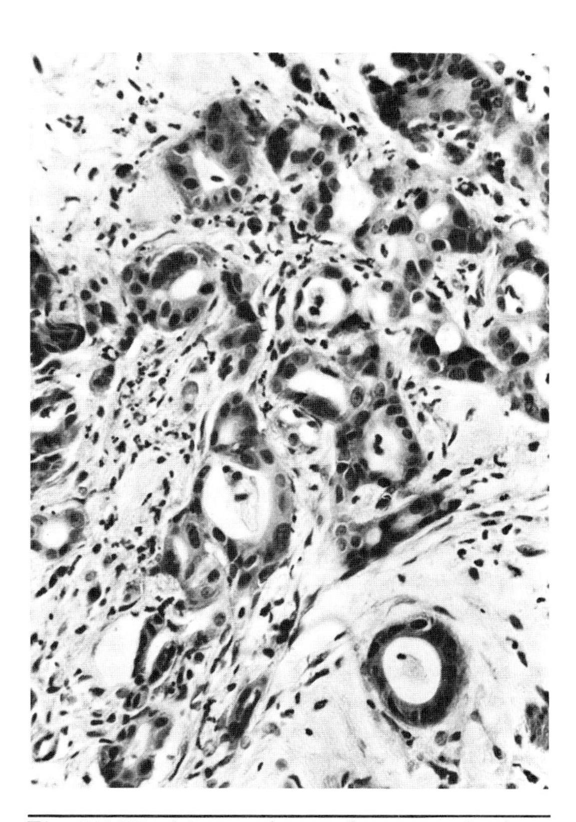

Fig. 17.56 Adenocarcinoma of pancreas showing a regular acinar pattern and with a related scirrhous reaction. ×250.

ated chronic inflammation. Biopsy of such tissue adjacent to the tumour may suggest an erroneous diagnosis of chronic pancreatitis. The tumour itself, with its small acini in a fibrous stroma, may in turn be difficult to distinguish from chronic pancreatitis. The presence of perineural tumour invasion, which is common in pancreatic carcinoma, is, however, diagnostic of malignancy. Percutaneous fine needle aspiration cytology under ultrasound guidance now offers an alternative means to making a definitive diagnosis.

The prognosis in carcinoma of the pancreas is extremely bad, 90% of patients not surviving 6 months. Resectional surgery is best confined to the rare low-grade cystadenocarcinomas and small tumours arising at the ampulla of Vater.

Cystic fibrosis. This disease is due to a generalized abnormality of exocrine gland secretion also involving bowel, bronchi, biliary tree and sweat glands as is discussed in detail on p. 272. The pancreas is always involved and microscopic changes can be seen even in fetal life. Inter- and intralobular ducts are dilated and filled with proteinaceous concretions and there is secondary acinar atrophy (Fig. 17.57). These changes occur diffusely throughout the pancreas and eventually result in almost total loss of exocrine pancreatic tissue with subsequent steatorrhoea clinically. Although islets are not destroyed in this obstructive process diabetes may eventually occur. The mechanism for this is not fully understood.

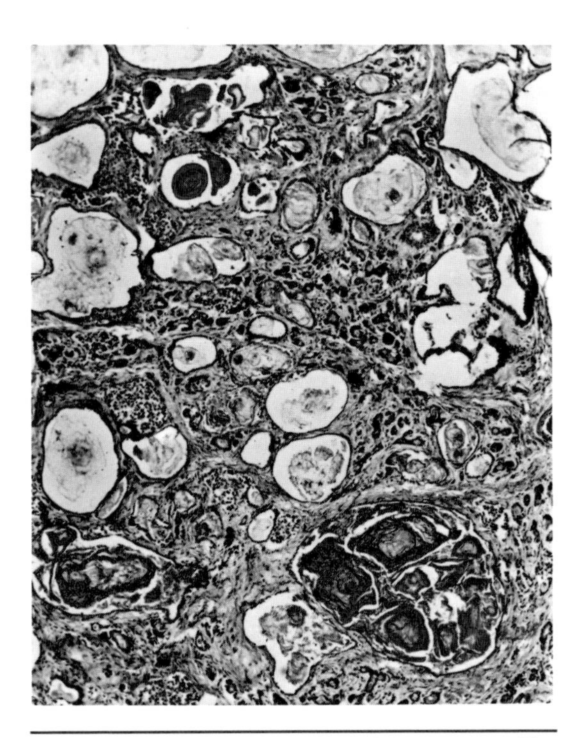

Fig. 17.57 Fibrocystic disease of the pancreas. The ducts and acini are filled with eosinophilic laminated secretion; the acini are either markedly atrophied or much dilated. ×50.

Congenital anomalies. These are of little significance. Annular pancreas, in which pancreatic tissue completely surrounds the duodenum, may present with neonatal duodenal obstruction. Ectopic pancreas may occur in the stomach, duodenum, jejunum, ileum and Meckel's diverticulum.

Diabetes Mellitus

Diabetes is not a single disease but the pathological and metabolic state caused by inadequate insulin action: a feature common to all types is glucose intolerance. It is defined clinically as either a fasting plasma glucose level greater than 7.8 mmol/1 (140 mg/dl) or a 2-hour post-prandial plasma glucose greater than 11 mmol/1 (200 mg/dl).

Insulin is a major anabolic hormone. It promotes the uptake of glucose by cells and the formation of intracellular glycogen from glucose. It stimulates cells to utilize amino acids for protein synthesis rather than for gluconeogenesis, and it promotes the uptake of free fatty acids by adipose tissue. Insulin lack therefore, results in a general catabolic state with loss of weight, hyperglycaemia, diminished protein synthesis, increased gluconeogenesis, and hyperlipidaemia due to lipolysis in adipose tissue. Although the renal threshold is usually raised, there is heavy glycosuria which results in an osmotic diuresis causing dehydration and thirst. In the liver, excess free fatty acids are converted via acetyl-CoA into ketone bodies which, in the absence of available glucose, are metabolized for cellular energy. The ketone bodies (acetoacetic acid, β-hydroxybutyric acid and acetone) dissociate to produce hydrogen ions, with a resulting metabolic acidosis (ketoacidosis). This complex of metabolic disturbances produces hyperosmolarity, hypovolaemia, acidosis and electrolyte imbalance, which have serious effects on the functions of neurons and result in one form of diabetic coma – ketoacidotic coma. The other major form, hyperosmolar non-ketotic coma, results from massive dehydration and profound hyperglycaemia in the absence of ketoacidosis. Relative or absolute overdosage with insulin causes hypoglycaemic effects, including coma which, unless treated, may be fatal.

Classification of Diabetes

Over 99% of cases of diabetes are caused by two diseases – types 1 and 2 diabetes; type 2 diabetes is ten times more common than type 1. The principal differences between the two are given in Table 17.6. Specific diseases in which diabetes occurs as a secondary event include chronic pancreatitis, haemochromatosis, cystic fibrosis, acromegaly, Cushing's syndrome and non-insulin secreting islet cell tumours. In haemochromatosis excess iron is taken up by B cells, but not by other islet endocrine cells, resulting in inhibition of insulin synthesis.

Table 17.6 Classification of diabetes

Type 1 diabetes	Type 2 diabetes
Onset under 40 years	Onset over 40 years
Thin patient	Obese patient
Affects 1 in 400 of population	Affects 1 in 40 of population
Liable to ketoacidotic coma	Liable to hyperosmolar non-ketotic coma
Requires insulin for therapy	Does not require insulin for therapy
Concordance rate for monozygotic twins 40%	Concordance rate for monozygotic twins 100%
Genetic link with class II MHC antigens	No genetic link with class II MHC antigens
Islet cell antibody present	Islet cell antibody absent
Insulitis present	Insulitis absent
B cells destroyed in pancreas	B cells not destroyed in pancreas
Islet amyloid absent	Islet amyloid present

Type 1 Diabetes (Insulin-dependent Diabetes)

In this disease insulin secreting B cells are selectively destroyed in the islets but A, D and PP cells are preserved. The process of B-cell destruction appears to take many years and the patient presents clinically with diabetes when about 80% of B cells are lost. Islets in which there is active B-cell destruction are inflamed – insulitis (Fig. 17.58). The infiltrate consists mainly of lymphocytes with a few macrophages.

Aetiology and Pathogenesis

There is evidence that genetic factors, autoimmunity and possibly viral infection may all be involved.

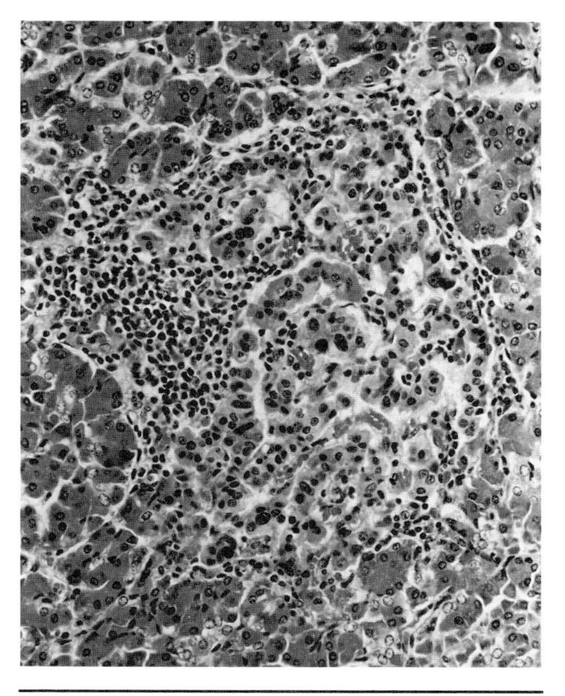

Fig. 17.58 Insulitis in an early case of type 1 diabetes. There is a lymphocytic infiltrate affecting this insulin-secreting islet. The polypoid endocrine cells are B cells. ×210.

Genetic factors. There is a significant link between type 1 diabetes and the class II major histocompatibility complex (MHC) genes – DP, DQ and DR in man. Persons carrying the DR3 allele have a relative risk ×5 of developing type 1 diabetes. The figure for DR4 is ×7 and that for DR3/DR4 heterozygotes is ×14. There is an even stronger association with the DQ gene. However, the concordance rate between identical twins is only 40%, indicating the involvement of non-genetic factors in the pathogenesis of the disease.

Immunological features. There is evidence for both humoral (islet cell antibodies) and cell mediated immunity directed against B cells. At presentation, at least 80% of patients have circulating cytoplasmic islet cell antibodies. Type 1 diabetes thus joins the group of organ specific autoimmune disease. Indeed, 15% of patients with type 1 diabetes also develop other organ specific autoimmune diseases such as thyroiditis, pernicious anaemia, and autoimmune Addison's disease.

Viral infection. Up to 30% of patients presenting with type 1 diabetes have serological evidence of recent or continuing coxsackie B infection. This virus is known to be trophic for the endocrine pancreas. Other viruses which have been implicated are mumps and rubella virus.

The evidence to date suggests that as yet unidentified environmental factors (possibly viruses) act on a particular genetic subpopulation to stimulate autoimmunity directed against the B cell. One finding that may be of relevance to this process is that B cells in type 1 diabetes, but in no other pancreatic disease, express the protein products of the class II MHC genes. Such class II MHC molecules are necessary for antigen presentation to helper T lymphocytes, the cells which initiate the immune response. Thus, the islet B cells in type 1 diabetes may become antigen presenting cells, presenting cell specific antigens to which there is no tolerance. This may stimulate autoimmunity. Whether a viral infection of B cells could lead to this abnormal expression of class II MHC products is not yet known.

Type 2 Diabetes (Non-insulin-dependent Diabetes)

The pancreas at clinical presentation of this disease does not show the same dramatic loss of B cells as that seen in type 1 diabetes. However, in about 70% of cases amyloid is present within islets (Fig. 17.59). The chemical nature of the amyloid protein has now been determined. It consists of a 37-amino-acid peptide known variously as islet amyloid polypeptide, amylin or diabetes associated peptide. There is strong circumstantial evidence that this protein is produced by B cells in both normal and diabetic subjects.

Aetiology and Pathogenesis

Patients with type 2 diabetes, obese people and 25% of the normal population show resistance to the action of insulin. These people thus have to hypersecrete insulin to achieve metabolic

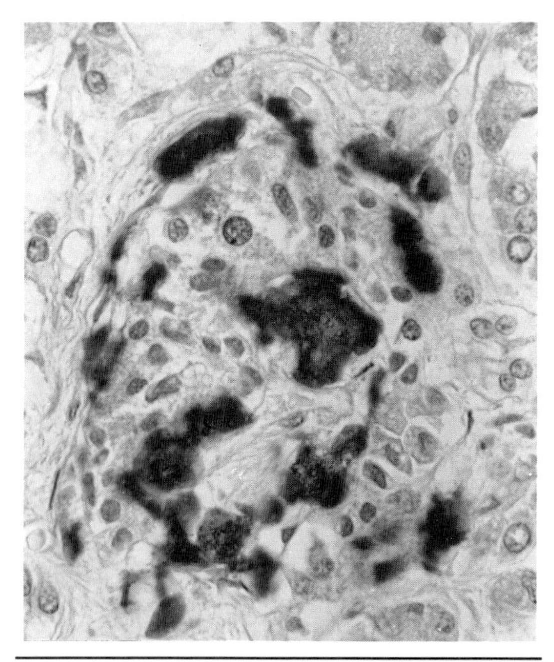

Fig. 17.59 Amyloid in an islet from a patient with type 2 diabetes. The islet amyloid polypeptide (amylin) is stained black using an indirect immunoperoxidase technique. ×500. (In conjunction with Dr Anne Clark.)

homeostasis. While in many normal people this, possibly genetic, disorder may cause no illness, it is proposed that in a minority there is eventual B-cell exhaustion with falling insulin secretion and hence the development of type 2 diabetes (Editorial, 1989). Thus, there may be both a qualitative and quantitative insulin insufficiency. The concordance rate for type 2 diabetes among monozygotic twins is 100%, suggesting that the failure of B cells to cope with prolonged insulin resistance may also be genetic. By the time the patient presents with type 2 diabetes there is a marked reduction in insulin response to a glucose load. Oral hypoglycaemic drugs, which are used to treat patients with this disease, increase the insulin output of B cells. The accumulation of amyloid in the islets may reflect long-standing B-cell hyperfunction where the islet amyloid polypeptide has been hypersecreted in parallel with insulin. It is interesting in this regard that amyloid of the same composition is also found in some insulinomas (Fig. 17.60).

Complications of Diabetes

Coma due to lack of diabetic control is now a relatively rare cause of death, and the mortality and morbidity of diabetes are due to the following complications.

Cardiovascular complications. It is customary to speak of diabetic macroangiopathy, most commonly affecting large muscular arteries, and diabetic microangiopathy, affecting arterioles and capillaries. The former is simply atheroma, which tends to develop early and become severe in diabetics of either sex. This, plus the fact that 50% of patients with type 2 diabetes have hypertension, results in 80% of adult diabetic deaths being due to cardiovascular, cerebrovascular, or peripheral vascular diseases. In diabetic patients with peripheral vascular disease, the small muscular arteries of the lower leg and foot are commonly affected. Thus, a toe may be gangrenous in the presence of normal femoral and popliteal pulses due to the fact that relatively small vessels are narrowed by atheroma.

In **diabetic microangiopathy** two types of lesion have been described: (1) a thickening of the basement membrane or an accumulation of basement membrane-like material in capillaries; and (2) endothelial cell proliferation together with basement membrane thickening. The cause of the microangiopathy is uncertain but it affects diabetics of all types, appears to be related to the duration of the disease and is probably aggravated by poor diabetic control. It is responsible for diabetic retinopathy (p. 884) and diabetic nephropathy (p. 913). Diabetic retinopathy is the commonest cause of blindness under the age of 65 years in developed countries.

Infections. There is an increased susceptibility to bacterial and fungal infections. Boils, carbuncles and urinary tract infections, sometimes complicated by pyelonephritis and renal papillary necrosis, are of frequent occurrence and may precipitate diabetic coma. Diabetics have an increased risk of tuberculosis, especially of the lungs, and unless treated, the disease tends to progress rapidly.

Other pathological effects. Trophic disturbances, such as ulceration of the fingers or toes and neuropathic arthropathy, may develop as complications of diabetic peripheral neuropathy. It is noteworthy that atheroma, diabetic microangiopathy, peripheral neuropathy and susceptibility to infections all tend to promote gangrene of the extremities in diabetes.

Pregnancy in diabetics used to be associated with a high incidence of toxaemia and congenital abnormalities in the fetus. Now, with aggressive diabetic management aimed at achieving as good metabolic control as possible, the risks to mother and child have been considerably reduced.

Tumours of the Endocrine Pancreas

An islet cell tumour is usually a solitary discrete nodule embedded in the pancreas. Microscopically, the tumour cells closely resemble normal islet cells, and form cords or clusters separated by fibrous stroma (Fig. 17.60). Distinction between benign and malignant tumours on a morphological basis is often difficult. For practical purposes, the tumours are most appropriately described in relation to the principal hormone which they produce.

Insulinoma. This is the commonest islet cell tumour and is associated clinically with recurrent attacks of hypoglycaemia, which may result in confusion, mania, dizziness or coma. These effects are reversed by taking glucose or by excision of the tumour. Insulinomas are rarely malignant.

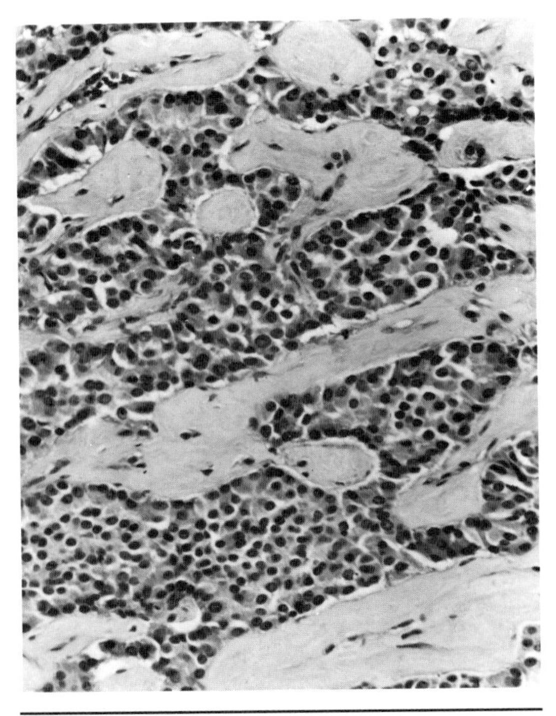

Fig. 17.60 A pancreatic islet cell tumour showing the cords and clusters of tumour cells. The stroma contains amyloid material. ×230.

Rarely, hyperplasia of the islets may produce clinical effects, e.g. idiopathic hypoglycaemia in infants.

Gastrinoma. Gastrin is normally produced only by G cells in the stomach and duodenum. A gastrin-producing cell has not been identified in the normal pancreas. However, two thirds of gastrinomas are found in the pancreas. Gastrinomas are associated with the **Zollinger–Ellison (Z–E) syndrome** in which persistent hypersecretion of acid gastric juice causes duodenal and even jejunal peptic ulceration which is difficult to control medically. In the multiple endocrine neoplasia type 1 **(MEN 1)** syndrome, adenomas of the parathyroids, pituitary, adrenal cortex and pancreas may be present in association with peptic ulceration. The latter is due to a duodenal or pancreatic gastrinoma. Over 60% of gastrinomas are malignant and while they metastasize, death due to dissemination of tumour is relatively unusual.

Other islet cell tumors are much less common, and may produce one of the following hormones or sometimes more than one (multihormonal tumours):

(1) **glucagon**; resulting in diabetes accompanied by peculiar skin manifestation;
(2) **somatostatin**, which inhibits both endocrine and exocrine pancreatic function leading to diabetes and steatorrhoea;
(3) **vasoactive intestinal peptide (VIP)**, causing watery diarrhoea, hypokalaemia and achlorhydria – **'WDHA' or the Verner–Morrison syndrome**;
(4) **pancreatic polypeptide hormone** which may produce no clinical symptoms; and
(5) **inappropriate (ectopic) hormones** resulting, for example, in the carcinoid syndrome or Cushing's syndrome.

Further Reading

Liver and Biliary Tract

Anthony, P. P. (1989). Liver tumours: an update. In *Recent Advances in Histopathology*, No. 14, Anthony, P. P. and MacSween, R. N. M. (eds), pp. 185–203. Churchill Livingstone, Edinburgh.

Desmet, V. J. (1984). Aspects of liver disease: cholestasis. In *Recent Advances in Histopathology*, No. 12, Anthony, P. P. and MacSween, R. N. M. (eds), pp. 146–58. Churchill Livingstone, Edinmburgh.

Farber, J. L. (1987). Xenobiotics, drug, metabolism, and liver injury. In *Pathogenesis of Liver Diseases*. IAP Monograph, Farber, E., Phillips, M. J. and Kaufman, N. (eds), pp. 43–53. Williams & Wilkins, Baltimore.

MacSween, R. N. M. and Burt, A. D. (1989). Pathology of the intrahepatic bile ducts. In *Recent Advances in Histopathology*, No. 14, Anthony, P. P. & MacSween, R. N. M. (eds), pp. 161–83. Churchill Livingstone, Edinburgh.

MacSween, R. N. M., Anthony, P. P. and Scheuer, P. J. (1987). *Pathology of the Liver*, 2nd edn. Churchill Livingstone, Edinburgh.

Portman, B. C. (1989). Liver biopsy in the diagnosis of inherited metabolic disorders. In *Recent Advances in Histopathology*, No. 14, Anthony, P. P. and MacSween, R. N. M. (eds), pp. 139–59. Churchill Livingstone, Edinburgh.

Scheuer, P. J. (1984). Aspects of liver disease: viral hepatitis. In *Recent Advances in Histopathology*, No. 12. Anthony, P. P. and MacSween, R. N. M. (eds), pp. 129–37. Churchill Livingstone, Edinburgh.

Scheuer, P. J. (1987). Viral hepatitis. In *Pathology of the Liver*, 2nd edn, MacSween, R. N. M., Anthony, P. P. and Scheuer, P. J. (eds), pp. 202–23. Churchill Livingstone, Edinburgh.

Shafritz, D. A. and Hadziyannis, S. J. (1987). Molecular pathophysiology of persistent hepatitis B virus infection in relation to chronic liver disease and primary hepatocellular carcinoma. In *Pathogenesis of Liver Diseases*. IAP Monograph, Farber, E., Phillips, M. J. and Kaufman, N. (eds), pp. 136–52. Williams & Wilkins, Baltimore.

Pancreas

Foulis, A. K. (1984), Acute pancreatitis. In *Recent Advances in Histopathology*, No. 12, Anthony, P. P. and MacSween, R. N. M. (eds), pp. 188–96. Churchill Livingstone, Edinburgh.

Foulis, A. K. (1989). R. D. Lawrence lecture: In type 1 diabetes, does a non-cytopathic viral infection of insulin-secreting beta cells initiate the disease process leading to their autoimmune destruction? *Diabetic Medicine* **6**, 666–74.

Editorial (1987). Pancreatic abnormalities in type 2 diabetes mellitus. *Lancet* 2, 1497–8.

Editorial (1989). Type 2 diabetes or NIDDM: looking for a better name. *Lancet* 1, 589–91.

18

The Nervous Systems: Voluntary Muscles: The Eye

The Central Nervous System

The central nervous system (CNS), i.e. the brain and the spinal cord, is composed of two types of tissue, both of which are involved in varying degree in disease processes. The first consists of the highly specialized **nerve cells (neurons)** with their processes and the **neuroglial cells**, all of which are of **neuroepithelial** origin. The second comprises the **meninges**, the **blood vessels** and their supporting connective tissue and the **microglia** (phagocytic cells) all derived from **mesoderm**.

The Meninges

The **dura mater** acts as a periosteum to the cranial bones but it can be stripped from the skull, e.g. by haemorrhage into the potential extradural space between the dura and the skull. Extensions of the dura – the **falx cerebri** and the **tentorium cerebelli** – subdivide the cranial cavity into three spaces, two supratentorial and one infratentorial (Fig. 18.1). The infratentorial space is more usually referred to as the posterior fossa. The subdural space lies between the dura and the outer surface of the arachnoid, and blood or pus can spread widely throughout it. The **arachnoid** is a continuous sheet in contact with the dura, while the **pia** is closely attached to the surface of the brain. The space between the pia and the arachnoid, known as the subarachnoid space, is traversed by delicate trabeculae of connective tissue into a series of intercommunicating spaces filled with **cerebrospinal fluid** (CSF). The subarachnoid space is widest in the cisterns at the base of the brain and within sulci. The major **cerebral arteries** and **veins** run in the subarachnoid space and from the arteries small **nutrient arteries** pass into the cortex. The nutrient arteries to the deeper structures of the brain are branches of the major arteries at the base of the brain (see Fig. 18.14).

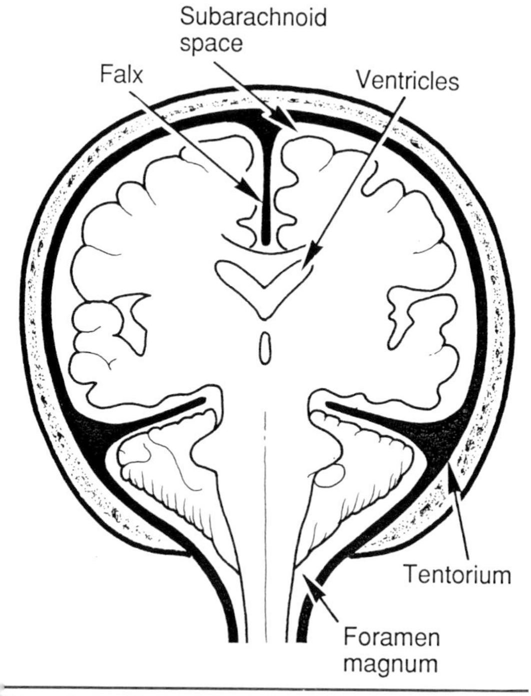

Fig. 18.1 The intracranial compartments; see text. (From Adams and Graham, 1988.)

The Source and Circulation of Cerebrospinal Fluid

The main source of CSF is the choroid plexuses in the ventricles. Its total volume is about 120–150 ml and it is renewed several times per day. The CSF produced in the lateral ventricles passes by the foramina of Monro into the third ventricle (Fig. 18.2), and then by the aqueduct of Sylvius to the fourth ventricle. Further CSF is formed in the third and fourth ventricles. It then passes through the exit foramina of Luschka and Magendie in the lateral recesses and roof respectively of the fourth ventricle to reach the subarachnoid space. There-

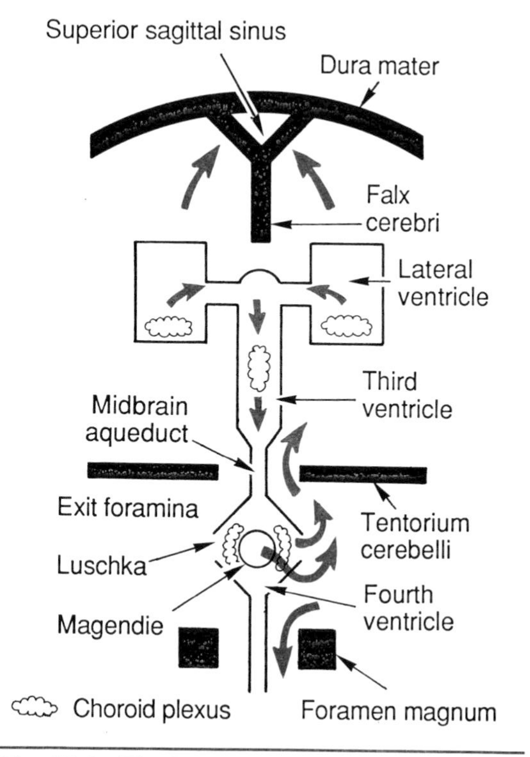

Fig. 18.2. The formation and circulation of CSF: see text. (From Adams and Graham 1988.)

after, it spreads through the subarachnoid space over the surface of the brain and spinal cord and is absorbed into the blood through arachnoidal granulations which project into dural venous sinuses.

Normal CSF is clear and colourless, does not coagulate and has a specific gravity of 1.006. It contains 0.15–0.45 g/l protein, 2.8–4.4 mmol/1 glucose, and approximately 128 mmol/1 sodium and 128 mmol/l chloride. A few lymphocytes may be found in normal CSF but rarely more than 4 per ml. Examination of the CSF often provides valuable information about diseases of the nervous system. Specimens are ordinarily obtained by lumbar puncture but ventricular or cisternal puncture may sometimes be indicated. The pressure of the CSF should always be measured as either an increase or decrease may be of diagnostic value. Microbiological, serological, cytological and biochemical investigations of the CSF are routine procedures in investigating diseases of the nervous system.

Cells of Neuroepithelial Origin

The **neuron** is one of the most complex cells in the body, and since it is incapable of dividing after the first few days of life, loss of neurons is irreversible. Immunocytochemistry for neurotransmitters has defined various functional types but all have a perikaryon or cell body, dendrites and an axon. A conspicuous feature in the perikaryon of large neurons is Nissl granules which are rich in RNA and are composed of stacks of rough endoplasmic reticulum and intervening groups of free ribosomes. Neurons also contain microtubules, neurofilaments, mitochondria and lysozomes. A feature of large neurons is the presence of lipofuscin (Fig. 18.3) which tends to increase in amount with age.

The remaining cells of neuroepithelial origin are the **neuroglia** – astrocytes, oligodendrocytes and ependymal cells. **Astrocytes** are stellate cells with branching processes which contain intracellular 10 nm fibres, a major component of which is glial fibrillary acidic protein. Astrocytes are attached to the walls of blood vessels by one or more swellings – the so-called foot processes. **Oligodendrocytes** are small cells with short processes and are intimately associated with the formation and maintenance of myelin. **Ependymal cells** form a single layer of cells lining the ventricular system and the central canal of the spinal cord.

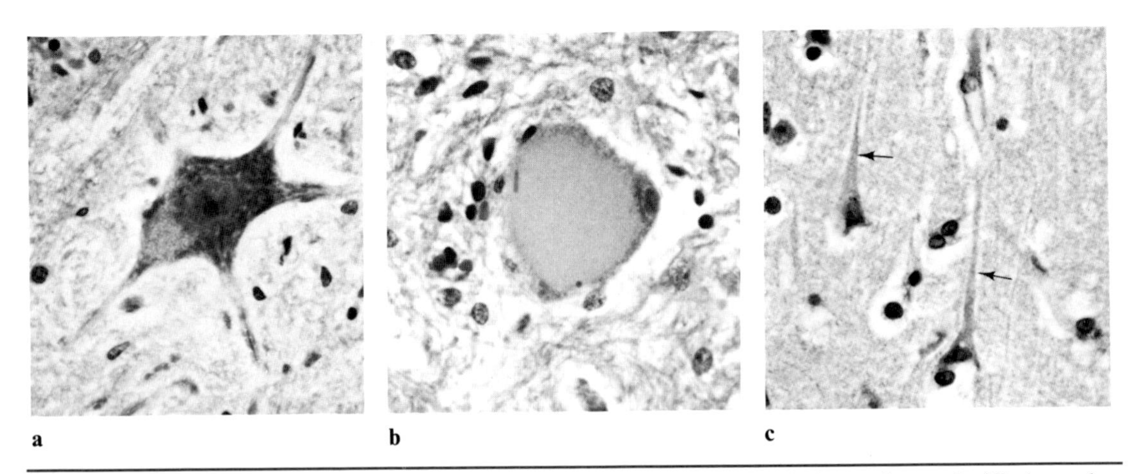

Fig. 18.3 Neurons. **a** Normal motor neuron in ventral horn of spinal cord. The dark granules are the Nissl granules. The pale area is the region occupied by lipofuscin. **b** Similar neuron showing the features of central chromatolysis. Note the pale homogeneous cytoplasm and the eccentric nucleus. **c** Neurons showing the features of ischaemic cell change. They are shrunken and contain dark hyperchromatic nuclei. All ×400.

The Reactions of the Nervous System to Disease

Neurons

Reactions of the neuron to disease take several forms.

Structural Changes Resulting from Hypoxia

Neurons require a constant supply of oxygen and glucose, and if this is inadequate they undergo a series of changes termed the ischaemic cell process. The earliest histological feature is **microvacuolation** due to swelling of mitochondria in an otherwise normal neuron. If the neuron is irreversibly damaged, then there is a gradual transition from the stage of microvacuolation to that of **ischaemic cell change**, in which the cell body shrinks and becomes triangular in shape: Nissl granules disappear, the cytoplasm becomes intensely eosinophilic and the nucleus triangular and pyknotic (Fig. 18.3). In the next stage incrustations appear – small dense granules lying on or close to the surface of the neuron. Finally, the neuron undergoes homogenizing change when the cytoplasm becomes progressively pale and homogeneous and the nucleus smaller. This type of damage is most commonly seen in the Purkinje cells of the cerebellum. Dead neurons are engulfed and then digested by microglia.

Changes in the neuroglia and blood vessels resulting from hypoxic damage are proportional to the severity of neuronal destruction. Mild to moderate selective neuronal loss is very difficult to recognize histologically unless there are also reactive changes in the neuroglia and microglia.

Reactions to Axonal Transection

Following axonal transection, changes take place proximally in the cell body – chromatolysis – and distally in the peripheral axon – Wallerian degeneration.

Central chromatolysis describes a process that occurs in the cell body between 5 and 8 days after transection. It can also occur as a response to certain virus infections and in some deficiencies of the vitamin B group. It is characterized by swelling of the cell body which becomes spherical, displacement of the nucleus to the periphery of the cell, and dispersion of the Nissl substance – chromatolysis – a change that is particularly marked in the centre of the cell body (Fig. 18.3). The cytoplasm becomes pale and homogeneous.

The chromatolytic reaction occurs in both central and peripheral neurons but particularly the latter, e.g. neurons in the motor nuclei of the brain stem and in the ventral horns of the spinal cord. This may be followed by recovery with or without axonal regeneration, or may proceed to degeneration and ultimate death of the neuron. Recent studies have shown that this response to injury is accompanied by an increase in protein synthesis and is therefore considered to be a regenerative phenomenon. Effective regeneration is, however, limited to the peripheral nervous system. In contrast, those neurons whose projections lie entirely within the CNS undergo ***retrograde degeneration*** and die.

Wallerian degeneration describes the series of changes that take place in the axon following transection. Both the proximal and distal ends of the severed axon swell to form axonal bulbs: they are thought to be due to a continuance of axoplasmic flow in both directions. They are most frequently seen adjacent to infarcts or in certain types of head injury as eosinophilic bodies and are most easily seen in sections stained for axons by silver impregnation. It is from the proximal swelling that growth of new fibres occurs in the peripheral nervous system – **regeneration**. In contrast, the distal axon and myelin sheath break down by the process of Wallerian degeneration. The axon becomes irregular and then breaks up into fragments and at the same time the myelin sheath is broken down into simpler lipids and ultimately neutral fat. Within the peripheral nervous system most of the breakdown products of myelin are removed by macrophages within weeks and the Schwann cells proliferate to form cords of cells within endoneural tubes, a necessary prerequisite for re-innervation. In contrast, the process within the CNS is very much slower, demonstrable microglia (macrophages) remaining within the affected tissue for many months or even years. Once myelin debris has been phagocytosed, its staining properties change largely due to the production of cholesterol esters which stain red with Sudan dyes and black with osmium in the Marchi technique. Wallerian degeneration of the long tracts in the spinal cord is dealt with in more detail on p. 851.

After damage to neurons, there may be some recovery of function which may be ascribed to plasticity, surviving neurons forming new contacts with neurons which have lost their afferent connections.

Other Alterations in Neurons

These are numerous and some are characteristic of specific diseases.

Alzheimer's neurofibrillary degeneration may be seen in occasional neurons in the cerebral cortex in normal old age but they are numerous in dementia of Alzheimer type (see p. 843) and in cases of Down's syndrome (see p. 847) surviving into adulthood.

Granulovacuolar degeneration which refers to one or more vacuoles in the cytoplasm of neurons is a degenerative change uncommon before the age of 65 years but thereafter increases in frequency in the pyramidal cells of the hippocampus. It is particularly apparent in dementia of Alzheimer type.

Lewy bodies are hyaline eosinophilic concentrically laminated inclusions, often with a central core and a surrounding pale peripheral rim, that occur characteristically in the substantia nigra and locus ceruleus in patients with idiopathic Parkinsonism (see p. 845).

Transneuronal degeneration occurs when the principal afferent connections to a neuron have been destroyed, e.g. in the external geniculate body after the loss of an eye.

Neuroglia

Astrocytes

Damage to the CNS is invariably accompanied by hypertrophy and hyperplasia of astrocytes, processes that are referred to as **gliosis** or **astrocytosis**, and are characterized by the formation of large amounts of intracellular 10 nm glial fibres. Usually the glial fibres are laid down in an irregular manner but occasionally they assume a regular and parallel arrangement – **isomorphic gliosis**.

Rosenthal fibres are homogeneous, hyaline, eosinophilic structures that are found in the perikaryon and processes of astrocytes. They are found in a variety of circumstances which include any long-standing gliosis and within some slowly growing glial tumours.

Oligodendrocytes

Very little is known about the causes or significance of reactive changes in oliogodendrocytes. Acute swelling occurs in many toxic processes and proliferation of perineuronal oligodendrocytes (**satellitosis**) occurs around degenerating neurons and is a normal occurrence with ageing.

Ependymal Cells

These show few reactive changes. Thus, when the ventricles enlarge as in hydrocephalus, the ependyma is stretched and then broken but the ependymal cells do not proliferate to fill the defects. A common but non-specific reaction to chronic irritation is the appearance of numerous small excrescences on the ventricular surface – **granular ependymitis**. They consist of focal proliferations of subependymal astrocytes.

Microglia

These belong to the mononuclear phagocyte system and, as in other organs, are seen in the CNS where there is tissue destruction.. In some conditions, microglia increase in length and become slightly thicker than normal and are known as **rod cells** (Fig. 18.4). When neurons are killed selectively, they become surrounded by macrophages and sometimes neutrophil polymorphs and undergo phagocytosis, a process known as **neuronophagia.** When brain tissue is destroyed the microglia act as macrophages: the cells become enlarged, rounded and laden with myelin breakdown products to appear as **lipid phagocytes** (Fig. 18.4).

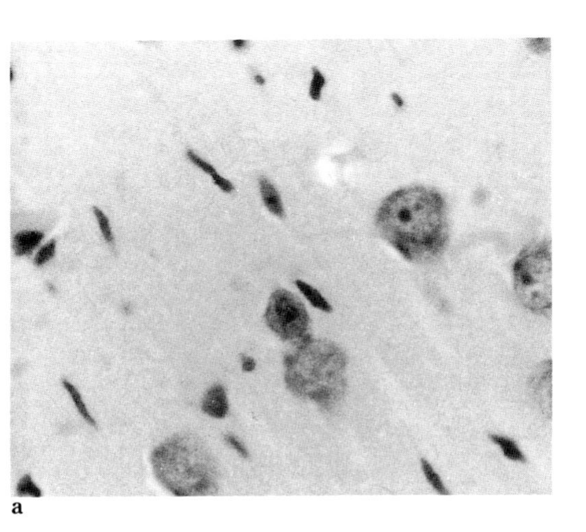

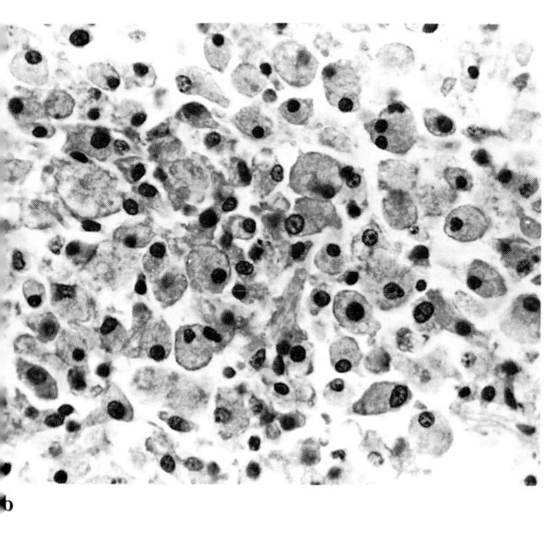

Fig. 18.4 Microglia. a The dark elongated nuclei represent rod cells among residual neurons. ×400. b Lipid-laden phagocytes in a cerebral infarct. ×510.

Blood Vessels

Whilst gliosis readily occurs when there is any damage to the brain, production of fibrous tissue is seen only when the injury is severe enough to damage blood vessels. For instance, when suppuration occurs within the brain there is usually a combined glial and fibroblastic response, often called a **gliomesodermal reaction.** Proliferation of capillaries is the rule around infarcts and abscesses, and in relation to rapidly growing cerebral tumours.

Intracranial Expanding Lesions

Once the fontanelles have closed in late infancy, the intracranial contents consisting of the brain (about 70% of the intracranial volume), CSF (about 15%) and blood (about 15%) are enclosed in a rigid bony container. Any increase in the volume of one of these components will, unless compensated for by a corresponding reduction of the others, lead to an increase in intracranial pressure. Thus, various pathological processes within the brain or on its surface such as tumour, haematoma or a massive recent cerebral infarct which lead to an increase in the volume of the intracranial contents will ultimately cause an increase in intracranial pressure. There is, however, a period of **spatial compensation** during which the intracranial pressure remains within normal limits. This compensation is brought about principally by a reduction in the volume of CSF, both within the ventricles and the subarachnoid space, and by a reduction in the volume of blood within the intracranial veins. Occasionally there is some loss of brain tissue adjacent to a slow growing tumour such as a meningioma. When all the available space has been utilized there is a critical point at which a further slight increase in the volume of the intracranial contents will cause an abrupt increase of intracranial pressure and rapid deterioration in the patient's condition. Near this critical point, arteriolar vasodilatation due to even a short period of increased arterial $P\text{CO}_2$, or the use of certain volatile anaesthetic agents, may be sufficient to produce this effect. The compensatory mechanisms fail more rapidly when the lesion is expanding rapidly than with one of similar size that has developed slowly. Intracranial expanding lesions also cause distortion of the brain and it has to be emphasized that distortion and displacement of the brain and the associated increase in intracranial pressure are often of greater significance with regard to the immediate survival of the patient than the nature of the lesion itself.

The clinical features of high intracranial pressure include headache, vomiting, a raised systolic blood pressure with a slow pulse and diminished consciousness passing into coma. Ophthalmoscopy will often reveal papilloedema, caused by both a reduction in anterograde axoplasmic flow in axons in the optic nerve and compression of the retinal vein where it traverses the subarachnoid space in the optic nerve sheath.

A **supratentorial intracerebral expanding lesion** produces a fairly standard sequence of changes (Fig. 18.5). As the lesion expands, so also does the hemisphere. CSF in the subarachnoid space is displaced and the convolutions become flattened against the dura; the sulci are progressively narrowed and at autopsy the surface of the brain looks dry. CSF is also displaced from the ventricular system with the result that the ipsilateral ventricle becomes smaller, whilst the contralateral ventricle may become larger. Further expansion of the lesion leads to distortion of the brain and a **lateral shift** of the midline structures, viz. the interventricular septum, the anterior cerebral arteries and the third ventricle (Fig. 18.5). Internal herniae then develop. The cingulate gyrus herniates under the free edge of the falx cerebri above the corpus callosum – the so-called **supracallosal** or **subfalcine** hernia. The most important hernia associated with an expanding lesion of this type is a **tentorial hernia** when the medial part of the ipsilateral temporal lobe is squeezed through the tentorial opening (Fig. 18.6). The herniated brain tissue compresses and

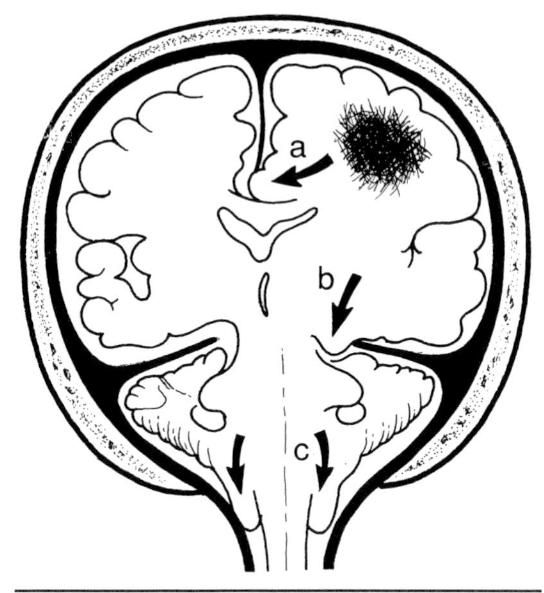

Fig. 18.5 Raised intracranial pressure. The effects of an intracranial expanding lesion. The subarachnoid space on the surface of the hemisphere is narrow, there is a shift of the midline structures, and internal herniae have developed. **a** = supracallosal hernia; **b** = tentorial hernia; **c** = tonsillar hernia, see Fig. 18.1. (From Adams & Graham 1988.)

displaces the midbrain which is pushed against the contralateral rigid edge of the tentorium. This pressure is often sufficient to produce a distinct groove on the surface of the midbrain. As a result of the inevitable plugging of the tentorial opening and the continuous production of CSF, a pressure gradient develops, the supratentorial intracranial pressure exceeding the infratentorial pressure, and this is associated with a rapid deterioration in the patient's conscious level.

Other structural abnormalities are caudal displacement of the brain stem, compression of the third and sixth cranial nerves with resultant disturbances of eye movement and pupillary reflexes and, less commonly, infarction of the ipsilateral medial occipital cortex brought about by compression of the posterior cerebral artery where it crosses the tentorium. A common terminal event in patients with supratentorial expanding lesions is haemorrhage into the midbrain and pons (Fig. 18.6), usually involving the tegmentum adjacent to the midline and thought to be due to a combination

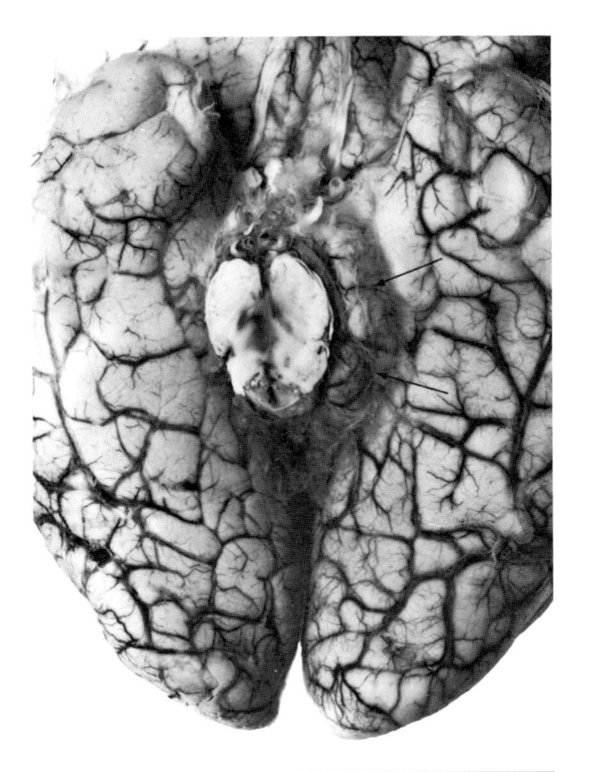

Fig. 18.6 Raised intracranial pressure. The medial part of the temporal lobe has pushed medially and downwards to form a tentorial hernia. The deep groove (arrows) indicates the position of the edge of the tentorium. There is also secondary haemorrhage into the brain stem.

of downward displacement of the brain stem, obstruction to venous drainage and stretching of arteries.

A supratentorial expanding lesion may also cause a **tonsillar hernia (cerebellar cone)**, i.e. impaction of the cerebellar tonsils in the foramen magnum (Fig. 18.5), but this type of lesion is more common with **infratentorial expanding lesions.** The tonsils compress the medulla and produce apnoea by distorting the respiratory centre. By obstructing the flow of CSF through the fourth ventricle, such herniation may further increase the intracranial pressure so that a vicious circle is set up.

In a patient with an intracranial expanding lesion lumbar puncture can precipitate internal herniation with serious consequences. Even if only a small amount of CSF is withdrawn, more may leak into the spinal extradural space via the puncture wound in the meninges. Lumbar puncture is therefore contraindicated in a patient thought to have a high intracranial pressure until the presence of an intracranial expanding lesion has been excluded by CT or MRI scanning.

Brain Swelling

This term is applied to an increase in the volume of the brain due to oedema or an increase in cerebral blood volume. Such an increase often makes an important contribution to an increased intracranial pressure. Vasodilatation leading to an increase in cerebral blood volume may occur in states of hypoxia or hypercapnia, or as a result of loss of vasomotor tone which may complicate acute brain damage. Brain swelling due to vasodilatation is a major factor contributing to an increased intracranial pressure in acute head injury.

Cerebral oedema is classified as vasogenic or cytotoxic. The **vasogenic type** corresponds to oedema elsewhere in the body resulting from an increased filtration pressure and/or increased permeability of the capillaries and venules. It is often prominent in the tissue around cerebral contusions, recent infarcts, a brain abscess and, very frequently, in association with a brain tumour. The oedema fluid is mainly interstitial and the cut surface of the brain appears pale and swollen. Microscopy shows separation of tissue elements by oedema fluid, and astrocytes may be swollen.

In **cytotoxic oedema**, which is less common, the fluid is intracellular. It occurs in some metabolic derangements and can be produced experimentally by several noxious agents. This is basically a disturbance of cellular osmoregulation, the blood–brain barrier to proteins remaining intact.

Hydrocephalus

The term hydrocephalus means an increased volume of CSF within the cranial cavity. In **internal** hydrocephalus the increased volume of CSF is within the ventricular system which thus becomes enlarged. In general the term hydrocephalus is used to denote this type. In **external** hydrocephalus the excess CSF is in the subarachnoid space. The hydrocephalus is said to be **communicating** if CSF can flow freely from the ventricular system to the subarachnoid space: if it cannot, it is **non-communicating**. **Compensatory** hydrocephalus (sometimes referred to as *ex vacuo*) occurs when the increased volume of CSF is compensatory to loss of brain tissue.

Pathogenesis

The commonest cause of hydrocephalus is ventricular enlargement secondary to cerebral atrophy (see p. 843): in these circumstances intracranial pressure is not increased. Hydrocephalus of acute onset with an increased intracranial pressure is most often due to **obstruction to the free flow of CSF**. Because of the ventricular enlargement there is a reduction in the bulk of the white matter in the cerebral hemispheres (Figs 18.7 and 18.8). In obstructive hydrocephalus it is the site of the lesion rather than its nature which is of importance. Thus, even a small lesion in a critical site adjacent to an interventricular foramen of Monro or the aqueduct in the midbrain (see Fig. 18.2) will rapidly produce hydrocephalus. The abnormality, however, need not be adjacent to the ventricular system since any process such as previous meningitis or subarachnoid haemorrhage that results in partial obliteration of the subarachnoid space, particularly at the level of the tentorial incisura (see Fig. 18.2), will also obstruct the flow of CSF. Hydrocephalus is also rapidly produced by a lesion in the posterior fossa of the skull. This may be a conventional expanding lesion but several of the obstructive lesions causing hydrocephalus are congenital, e.g. the Chiari malformations and the Dandy Walker syndrome (see p. 849). A rare cause of hydrocephalus is **gliosis of the aqueduct** in late adolescent or early adult life. This appears to be produced by a proliferation of periaqueductal astrocytes leading to progressive stenosis of the aqueduct.

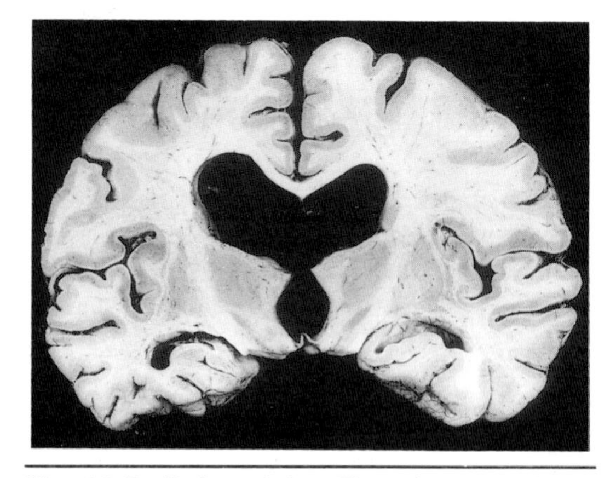

Fig. 18.7 Hydrocephalus. There is great enlargement of the lateral and third ventricles resulting from an expanding lesion in the posterior fossa.

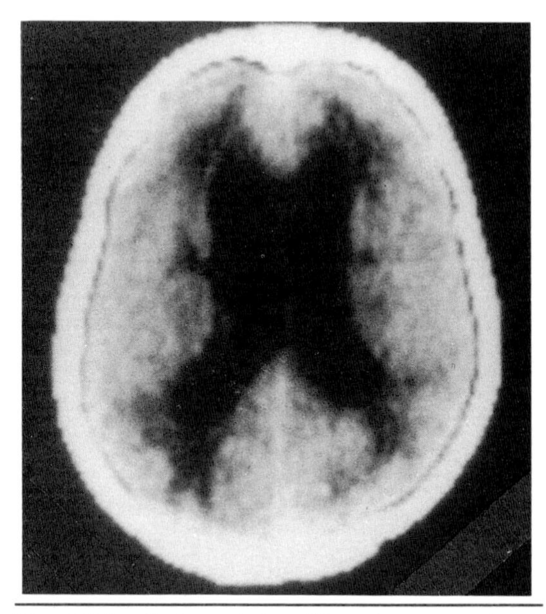

Fig. 18.8 Hydrocephalus. There is great enlargement of the lateral ventricles in a CT scan. (From Adams and Graham, 1988.)

If the obstruction to the flow of CSF is at a foramen of Monro, one lateral ventricle enlarges: if it is in the third ventricle or the aqueduct, both lateral ventricles enlarge; if it is at the exit foramina of the fourth ventricle, the entire ventricular system enlarges; if the obstruction is in the subarachnoid space, the entire ventricular system again enlarges but on this occasion the hydrocephalus is communicating in type because CSF can flow out of the exit foramina in the fourth ventricle into the subarachnoid space.

Other possible causes of hydrocephalus are **increased production of CSF** or **decreased absorption**. The former may occur in patients with a papillary tumour of the choroid plexus (p. 857). Decreased absorption of CSF may be a sequel to subarachnoid haemorrhage; it is suggested that the arachnoidal granulations may be partly obliterated by macrophages containing haemosiderin.

Normal Pressure Hydrocephalus

This syndrome has attracted considerable attention in recent years and is characterized by ventricular enlargement and a clinical syndrome consisting of progressive dementia, disturbance of gait and urinary incontinence or urgency. A routine measurement of the CSF pressure may show it to be normal but if patients thought to have this syndrome are subjected to continuous monitoring of intracranial pressure, episodes of moderate intracranial hypertension can often be demonstrated. For this reason it has been suggested that a more appropriate descriptive term might be **intermittent hydrocephalus**. The condition of patients with normal pressure hydrocephalus may be improved by surgical measures to reduce hydrocephalus such as a ventriculoperitoneal shunt. In the majority of cases the cause is not known, but in a proportion there may be a history of previous subarachnoid haemorrhage resulting from a head injury or a previous haemorrhagic stroke, leading to partial obliteration of the subarachnoid space.

Head Injury

In the United Kingdom trauma is responsible for more deaths in all age groups under 45 than any other single cause, and brain damage resulting from a head injury is the most important factor contributing to death or serious incapacity due to trauma. There are two principal types of head injury – missile and non-missile – and the mechanisms of brain damage are different in the two types.

In **non-missile** head injury there is sudden deceleration or acceleration of the head, as a result of which the brain moves within the cranial cavity engendering various shear strains within the brain. These strains are particularly severe when there is a rotational element in the acceleration/deceleration. It has now been established that all of the major types of brain damage seen in man as a result of a non-missile head injury can be reproduced experimentally by non-impact controlled, angular acceleration of the head. Thus, there need not be a direct blow to the head to produce brain damage in head injury – what matters is the acceleration/deceleration conditions that exist at the moment of injury. The causes of, and the incidence of structural abnormalities brought about by, non-missile head injury are given in Table 18.1.

Missile head injuries are produced by various types of object which fall or are propelled through the air. The object often enters the cranial cavity producing focal brain damage.

Fracture of the Skull

Many patients with a fracture suffer no significant brain damage whilst about 25% of fatal head injuries do not have a fracture: in patients with a fracture, however, there is a much higher incidence of secondary damage in the form of an intracranial haematoma. The fracture may be depressed, causing local pressure on the brain, and if there is also laceration of the scalp, the fracture is compound and a potential source of intracranial sepsis. Any fracture of the base of the skull provides a potential source of infection from the nasal passages, the paranasal sinuses or the middle ear. With such fractures there may be CSF rhinorrhoea or otorrhoea. Other complications of a fracture are tearing of a meningeal artery with the production of an extradural haematoma, or injury to the carotid artery within the cavernous sinus giving rise to a caroticocavernous fistula.

Table 18.1 Data from a consecutive series of 635 fatal non-missile head injuries on whom post-mortem examinations were undertaken in the Institute of Neurological Sciences, Glasgow

Sex	497 M (78%): 138 F (22%)
Type of injury	
Road traffic accidents	335 (53%)
Falls	222 (35%)
Assaults	31 (5%)
Other	47 (7%)
Incidence of	
Fracture of the skull	75%
Surface contusions	94% (mild in 6%, moderate in 78%, severe in 10%)
Gliding contusions	31%
Intracranial haematoma*	60%
Extradural	10%
Subdural	18%
Intracerebral	16%
'Burst lobe'	23%
Diffuse axonal injury	28%
Brain stem damage secondary to a raised intracranial pressure	53%
Hypoxic brain damage	55%
Brain swelling	53% (34% unilateral: 19% bilateral)
Intracranial infection	4%

For definition of types of damage, see text.
*Some patients had more than one haematoma.

Brain Damage in Head Injury

Primary brain damage such as surface contusions and diffuse damage to nerve fibres occurs at the moment of injury. Secondary brain damage such as intracranial haematoma and high intracranial pressure occur some time after the injury. One of the most important factors in the management of a head-injured patient is the early recognition of these complications.

Primary Brain Damage

Cerebral contusions. Surface contusions are the commonest form of brain damage directly attributable to injury. They may occur at the site of contact particularly if there is a depressed fracture of the skull, but in any non-missile head injury they tend to involve the frontal poles, the orbital gyri, the temporal poles and the inferior and lateral surfaces of the anterior halves of the temporal lobes (Fig. 18.9). These regions are vulnerable because movement of the brain within the skull brings them into forcible contact with bony protuberances of the base of the skull. Contusions are usually asymmetrical and they may be more severe on the side opposite the point of injury (**'contrecoup' injury**): thus, severe frontal contusions may occur in association with an impact in the occipital region but the reverse is not the case because the inner surface of the occipital bone is smooth. Contusions affect the crests of gyri but, if more severe, they may extend through the full thickness of the cortex into the adjacent white matter and be associated with some intracerebral haemorrhage and swelling. Old healed contusions are represented by golden brown shrunken areas of gliosis which have such a characteristic distribution and appearance that the post-mortem diagnosis of a previous head injury can be made with certainty.

The term **gliding contusion** is used to describe parasagittal foci of haemorrhage affecting the cortex and the adjacent white matter (Fig. 18.10).

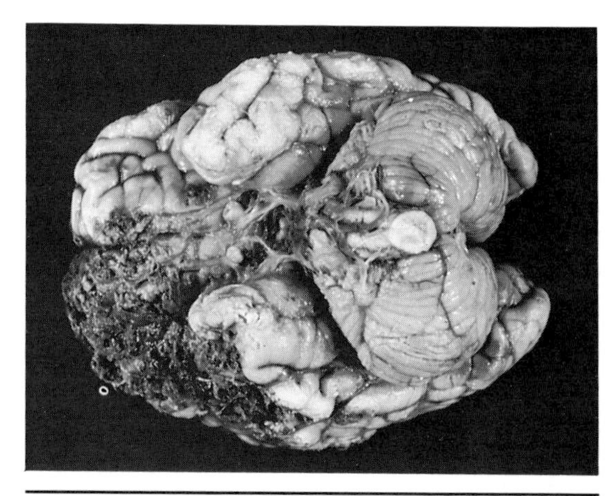

Fig. 18.9 Cerebral contusions. The right frontal lobe and the temporal pole are affected by haemorrhagic contusions.

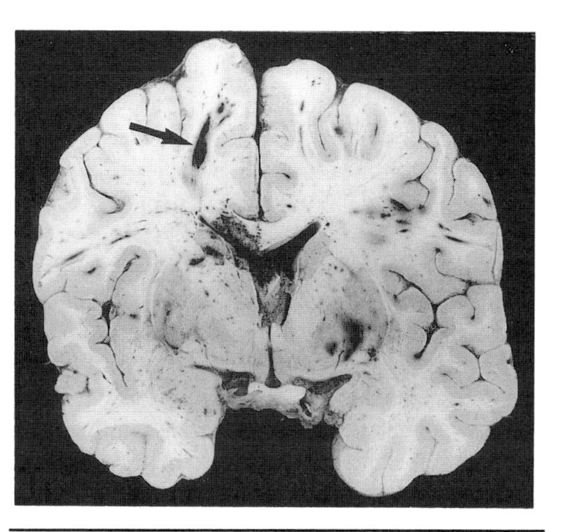

Fig. 18.10 Diffuse axonal injury. There is a haemorrhagic lesion in the corpus callosum to the left of the midline. There is also a gliding contusion (arrow) and a small haematoma in the right basal ganglia. (From Adams and Graham, 1988.)

Diffuse axonal injury. Nerve fibres are torn at the moment of injury as a result of shear strains produced by acceleration/deceleration forces, particularly rotational. This type of brain damage may occur in the absence of surface contusions and the only abnormalities observed at autopsy may be haemorrhagic lesions in the corpus callosum (Fig. 18.10) and in the dorsolateral quadrant or quadrants of the rostral brain stem. On other occasions the diagnosis can only be made as a result of histological examination. The striking abnormality is the presence of **axonal bulbs**, i.e. extruded axoplasm at the point of injury, in all regions of the brain (Fig. 18.11). In patients who survive for weeks or months – always in a severely disabled or vegetative state – there is enlargement of the ventricular system due to a reduction in the bulk of the white matter. There are often also small, shrunken, cystic lesions in the corpus callosum and in the rostral brain stem. Microscopy at this stage shows Wallerian degeneration in the cerebral and cerebellar hemispheres, the brain stem and the spinal cord secondary to the axonal disruption that occurred at the moment of injury.

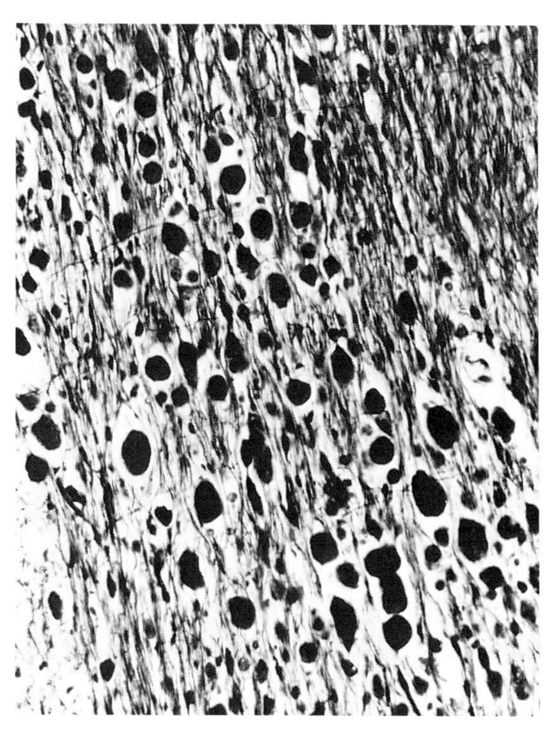

Fig. 18.11 Diffuse axonal injury. There are numerous axonal bulbs in the pons. (Palmgren silver stain.) ×320.

Secondary Brain Damage

Intracranial haemorrhage. This is a frequent complication of a head injury and is the commonest cause of deterioration and death in patients who have been conscious immediately after their injury. The incidence of haematoma is much higher in patients with a fracture of the skull. Traumatic intracranial haematomas may be extradural, subdural or intracerebral.

Extradural haematoma results from haemorrhage from a meningeal blood vessel, usually the middle meningeal artery. As the haematoma develops it gradually strips the dura from the skull to form a large ovoid mass (Fig. 18.12) that progressively compresses the adjacent brain. Only occasionally does an extradural haematoma occur in the absence of a fracture and then virtually only in young children. The initial injury may be apparently mild when the patient experiences a lucid

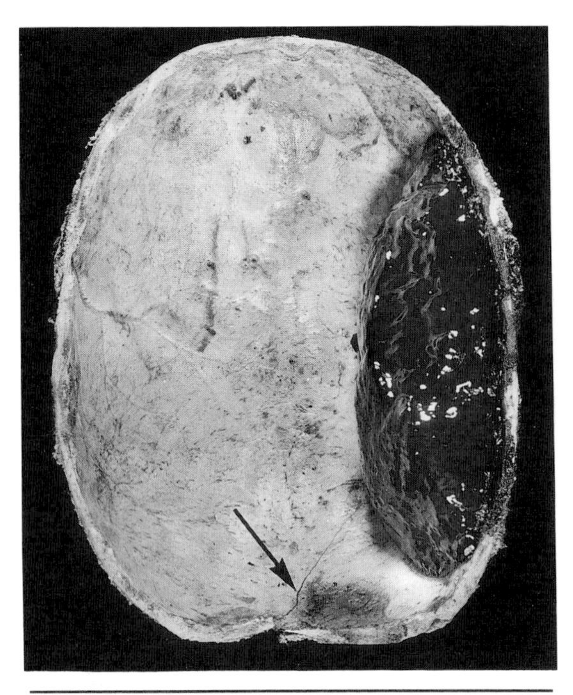

Fig. 18.12 Extradural haematoma. A large mass of blood clot has formed between the skull and the dura. There is also a fracture of the skull (arrow).

interval of some hours before developing headache and becoming drowsy. As the haematoma enlarges, the intracranial pressure (ICP) increases and the patient lapses into coma and may die unless the haematoma is evacuated. Extradural haematomas occasionally occur in the frontal and parietal regions or within the posterior fossa.

Subdural haematoma results from rupture of bridging veins which run into the superior sagittal sinus, or from haemorrhage into the subdural space from severe surface contusions. The blood spreads diffusely throughout the subdural space.

Acute subdural haematoma is a common autopsy finding if death has occurred soon after the injury. The haematoma may be large and act as an acute intracranial expanding lesion, or it may only be a thin film of blood. Even in these circumstances the ICP often increases because of associated swelling of the subjacent cerebral hemisphere. Some patients with acute subdural haematoma experience a lucid interval similar to that classically associated with extradural haematoma.

Chronic subdural haematoma presents weeks or months after an apparently trivial head injury. Indeed some patients deny any history of injury. The haematoma is gradually organized and becomes encapsulated in a fibrous membrane. Because chronic subdural haematoma is particularly common in old people who already have some cerebral atrophy and because the haematoma expands very slowly, probably as the result of repeated small haemorrhages into it, they may become quite large before symptoms appear. In untreated cases, however, death is usually attributable to brain damage secondary to a high intracranial pressure. Chronic subdural haematoma is frequently bilateral.

Intracerebral haematoma tends to be associated with contusions and occurs principally in the frontal or the temporal lobe. The term *burst lobe* is used to describe the combination of an intracerebral haematoma in continuity with a subdural haematoma through surface contusions (Fig. 18.13). Small, deeply seated intracerebral haematomas – often referred to as *basal ganglia haematomas* (see Fig. 18.10) – also occur and have

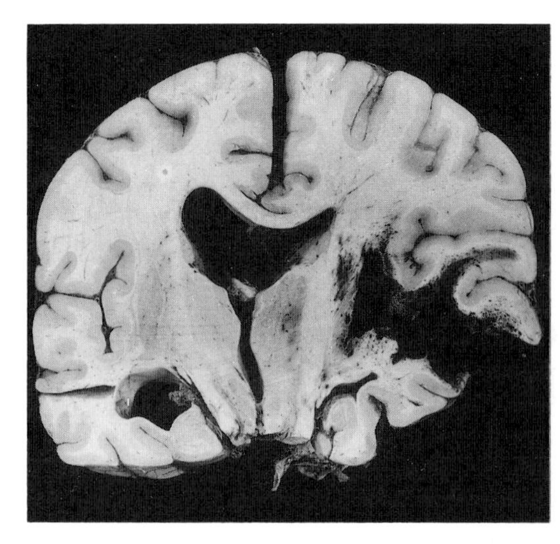

Fig. 18.13 A burst lobe. The large haematoma in the right temporal lobe was in continuity with an acute subdural haematoma.

a higher incidence in patients with diffuse axonal injury.

Raised Intracranial Pressure

It will be clear from the foregoing that secondary brain damage resulting from a head injury often causes an increase in intracranial pressure and hence distortion and herniation of the brain. The increase of intracranial pressure is often contributed to by brain swelling. There is always some swelling around contusions, swelling of the ipsilateral hemisphere is seen frequently in association with a subdural haematoma, and particularly in children there may be acute swelling of both hemispheres soon after injury.

Ischaemic Brain Damage

This occurs in about 90% of fatal head injuries. The pathogenesis of the ischaemic damage is not understood but it is probably attributable to some acute haemodynamic crisis soon after injury or shift and distortion due to raised intracranial pressure. In some cases, however, it may result from cardiorespiratory arrest or status epilepticus.

Infection

This is brought about by bacteria entering the skull through a compound fracture of the vault or through a fracture of the base of the skull. It usually presents as **meningitis** and its onset is not restricted to the early post-traumatic period because a small traumatic fistula from the subarachnoid space to one of the major air sinuses in the base of the skull may persist. **Intracranial abscess** is a rarer complication and is usually secondary to a penetrating injury.

Clinical Aspects of Head Injuries

The pathogenesis of brain damage due to a head injury is complex and the primary damage may be the beginning of an evolving process which may range from progressive improvement – as in most patients with so-called **concussion** – to death. There is an increasing tendency to think of brain damage in head injury as being focal or diffuse. Focal brain damage such as contusions and haematomas are easy to recognize neuroradiologically but this is not so with diffuse brain damage such as axonal injury and ischaemia whose presence may not be known until histological studies have been undertaken. Diffuse brain damage is probably the more important with regard to the clinical outcome since, unlike intracranial haematoma, much of it is not amenable to treatment.

The period of disturbed consciousness and the interval between the injury and return of continuous memory – **post-traumatic amnesia** – are probably more related to diffuse brain damage. Nevertheless, the management of head-injured patients has to be based on the knowledge that complications occur only too frequently and their development must be diagnosed as soon as possible. Thus, some extradural and acute subdural haematomas may occur in individuals with no other, or just trivial, brain damage.

Head injury is an important cause of **epilepsy**. About 10% of patients admitted to hospital with such an injury develop fits. These tend to occur in the first week after injury (early epilepsy) or are delayed for 2–3 months (late epilepsy). Factors predisposing to late epilepsy include a depressed fracture of the skull and an intracranial haematoma. Fits are less liable to recur in patients with early epilepsy than in those who develop late epilepsy. With penetrating head injuries the incidence of epilepsy is about 45%.

Circulatory Disturbances

Cerebrovascular disease in the form of a **stroke** – a sudden disturbance of cerebral function of vascular origin – accounts for about 10% of all deaths, and of those who survive some 15% remain severely disabled. The incidence rises with age, about 80% occurring in patients over 65. Data from retrospective epidemiological studies suggest that some 84% are due to infarction (53%

thrombotic, 31% embolic), leaving some 16% due to haemorrhage (10% with spontaneous intracerebral haemorrhage, 6% from a ruptured intracranial aneurysm).

A distinction is made between **transient ischaemic attacks** – a fully reversible neurological deficit often lasting for no more than a few minutes but occasionally up to 24 hours, in which it is assumed that no structural brain damage has occurred – and a **completed stroke** where permanent brain damage of varying severity has occurred. There are numerous risk factors associated with strokes. Atheroma and hypertension play dominant roles in the genesis of cerebral infarction but other important factors include abnormalities in serum lipids, diabetes mellitus, coronary artery disease, cardiac failure and atrial fibrillation. Additional factors are cigarette smoking, diet, obesity and alcohol consumption. Factors that predispose to spontaneous intracranial haemorrhage are hypertension, congenital anomalies, vascular malformations, arteritis and bleeding diatheses.

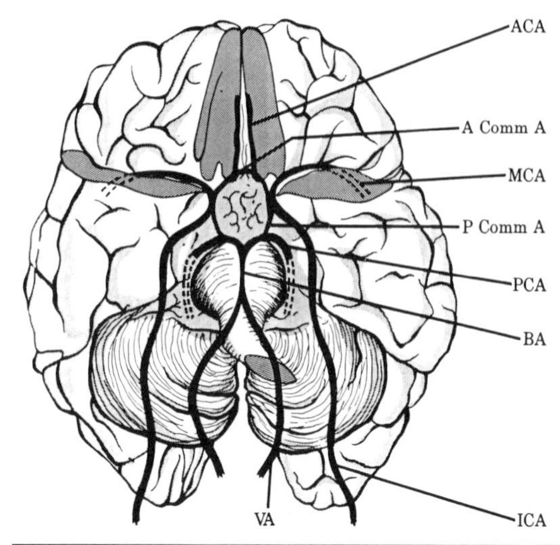

Fig. 18.14 Schematic diagram of the major arteries at the base of the brain. ACA, anterior cerebral artery; A Comm A, anterior communicating artery; MCA, middle cerebral artery; P Comm A, posterior communicating artery; PCA, posterior cerebral artery; BA, basilar artery; ICA, internal carotid artery; VA, vertebral artery.

Blood Supply of the Central Nervous System

The arterial supply to the cerebral hemispheres (Fig. 18.14) is derived from branches of the circle of Willis. The circle of Willis is an anastomotic channel between the major cerebral arteries at the base of the brain. Anastomoses between the external and internal carotid arterial systems are of the greatest importance if the blood flow through the internal carotid or vertebral arteries is compromised in any way. Thus, there is an increased incidence of cerebral infarction if these anastomoses are deficient as a result of some anomaly in the circle of Willis or acquired arterial disease such as atheromatous stenosis. The nutrient arteries which penetrate the brain substance are end arteries.

The blood supply to the spinal cord is derived from the spinal branches of the vertebral, deep cervical, intercostal and lumbar arteries which arise from the aorta in a segmental manner. These feed into an anterior spinal artery, which supplies the anterior two-thirds of the spinal cord and two smaller posterior spinal arteries (see Fig. 18.44).

Structural damage resulting from ischaemia usually takes the form of a cerebral infarct when there is necrosis of all tissue elements, viz. neurons, neuroglia and blood vessels. In less severe ischaemia only the most susceptible cells, viz. neurons, undergo necrosis. This is known as selective neuronal necrosis. In both situations neurons undergo the structural sequence of ischaemic cell change.

Cerebral Infarction

This results from a local arrest or reduction of cerebral blood flow and consists of an area of tissue within which all the cellular elements have undergone necrosis. An infarct may range from a small discrete lesion to necrosis of a large part of the brain: it may occur in any part of the brain but the commonest site is in the distribution of the middle cerebral artery. The entire arterial territory may be affected or only part of it (Fig. 18.15).

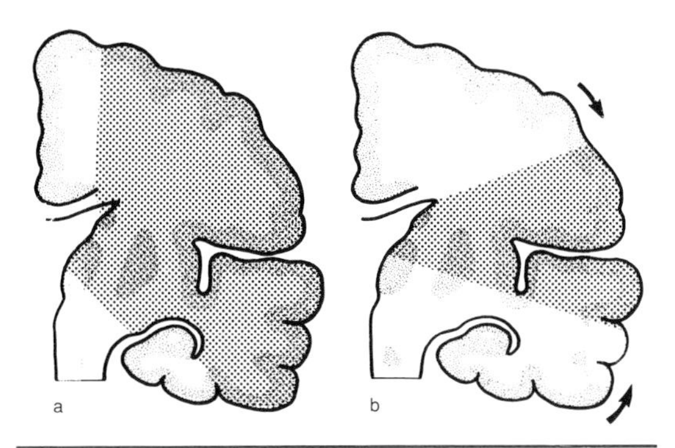

Fig. 18.15 Diagrammatic representation of infarcts in the territory supplied by a middle cerebral artery. **a** Infarct involving the entire territory. **b** Infarct restricted to the central territory. Arrows in **b** indicate collateral flow from the anterior and posterior cerebral arteries. (From Adams and Graham, 1988.)

The structural changes in a cerebral infarct depend upon the size of the lesion and the survival time. A cerebral infarct may be haemorrhagic or pale. An intensely haemorrhagic infarct may resemble a haematoma, but the distinctive feature is the preservation of the intrinsic architecture of the infarcted tissue (Fig. 18.16). A pale infarct less than 24 hours old may be difficult to identify macroscopically, but thereafter the dead tissue becomes soft and swollen and there is a loss of the normal sharp definition between the grey and white matter. At this stage histological examination will show ischaemic necrosis of neurons, pallor of myelin staining and, sometimes, polymorphs around the necrotic walls of vessels. If the infarct is large, swelling of the necrotic tissue and oedema of the surrounding brain may lead to its acting as an acute expanding intracranial lesion with raised intracranial pressure. Within a few days the infarct becomes distinctly soft and the dead tissue disintegrates (Fig. 18.17). Histological examination at this stage will show macrophages filled with globules of lipid (lipid phagocytes) produced by the breakdown of myelin (see Fig. 18.4), and, around the dead tissue, enlarged astrocytes and early capillary proliferation. During the following weeks the dead tissue is removed and there is a

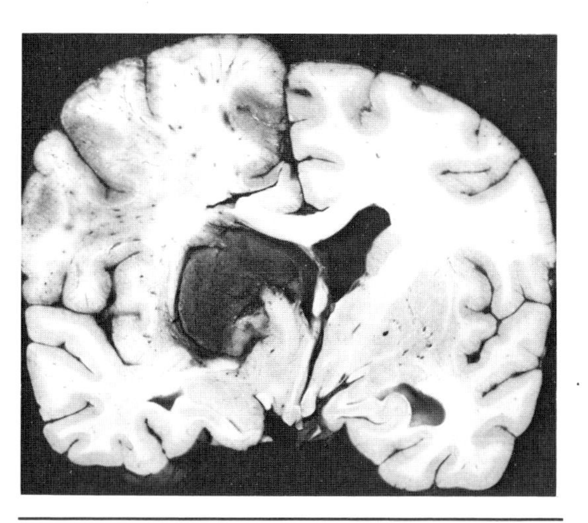

Fig. 18.16 Recent infarct in left cerebral hemisphere. The basal ganglia show the features of haemorrhagic infarction; the posterior part of the frontal lobe above the Sylvian fissure shows those of pale infarction. Note that the affected hemisphere is swollen and that there is displacement of the midline structures to the right.

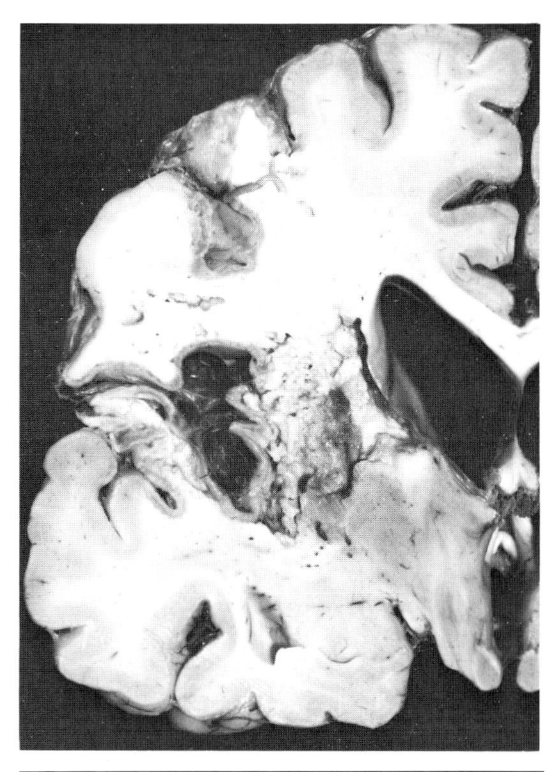

Fig. 18.17 Infarct of a week's duration in the left cerebral hemisphere. The dead tissue is disintegrating and there is already some shrinkage of the affected cortex.

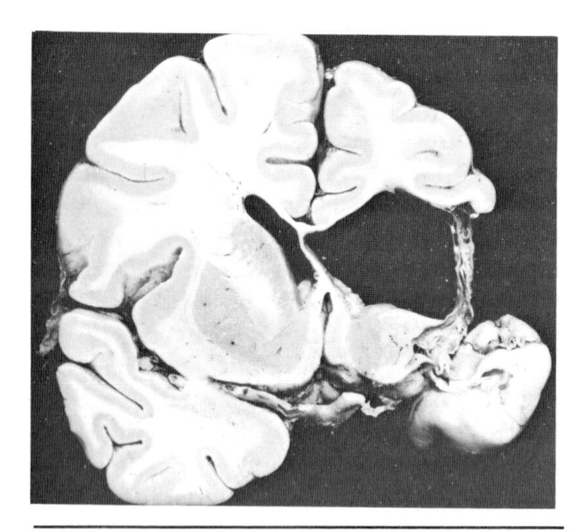

Fig. 18.18 Infarct of several years' duration in the right cerebral hemisphere. The dead tissue has been removed and the lateral ventricle is separated from the surface of the brain by a narrow web of tissue composed of meninges, ependyma and a few astrocytic fibres.

gliosis. The lesion ultimately becomes shrunken and cystic (Fig. 18.18), and the cyst is often traversed by small blood vessels and glial fibrils. If the infarct has been haemorrhagic, some of the macrophages will contain haemosiderin and the cyst wall will appear brown. Shrinkage of an infarct in the cerebral hemisphere is usually accompanied by enlargement of the adjacent lateral ventricle (Fig. 18.18). A consequence of infarction is Wallerian degeneration of the nerve fibres that have been interrupted. Thus, if the infarct involves the internal capsule, there is progressive degeneration and shrinkage of the corresponding pyramidal tract in the brain stem and spinal cord (see Fig. 18.49).

Pathogenesis of Cerebral Infarction

Embolism. Cerebral emboli may arise from vegetations of infective endocarditis, from mural thrombus in patients with arrhythmias or a myocardial infarct, and from non-bacterial thrombotic endocarditis in association with cachexia of advanced chronic disease. Brain damage due to embolism may also complicate open heart surgery, and more recently coronary artery surgery using cardiopulmonary bypass. Thrombus formation on ulcerated atheromatous lesions in the aorta and in the neck arteries is also another source of embolism.

Thrombus and atheroma. In addition to the intracranial arteries, the internal carotid and vertebral arteries in the neck are often affected. Atheroma of the cerebral arteries is usually associated with atheroma in other parts of the body, including the arteries to the limbs. Atheromatous stenosis does not necessarily lead to cerebral infarction because at normal blood pressure the internal cross-sectional area of an artery must be reduced by up to 90% before blood flow is impaired. In many cases, however, cerebral infarction results from a combination of systemic circulatory insufficiency and stenosis of the cervical and/or cerebral arteries by atheroma.

Infarction may also result from occlusion of arteries within the skull or in the neck. The commonest intracranial site of thrombotic occlusion is the middle cerebral artery. Atheromatous narrowings or occlusions may occur in any part of the carotid or vertebral arteries. The commonest site is at the origin of an internal carotid artery, but infarction results only if the collateral circulation is, or becomes, inadequate. In some cases, thrombosis extends along the internal carotid artery into the middle and anterior cerebral arteries to produce infarction of a large part of the cerebral hemisphere. When the vertebral arteries are more severely atheromatous or are occluded, ischaemic damage occurs characteristically in the brain stem, the cerebellum and the occipital lobes.

Miscellaneous causes of cerebral infarction. Types of vasculitis that cause infarction include **arteritis** due to micro-organisms and collagen diseases such as **polyarteritis nodosa, systemic lupus erythematosus** and **giant cell arteritis**. Cerebrovascular accidents may complicate various disorders including **polycythaemia rubra vera** and **sickle cell disease**, and may occur in **pregnancy and the puerperium**, and in women taking **oral contraceptives** and in cases of **drug addiction** due to heroin and lysergic acid diethylamide (LSD).

Selective Neuronal Necrosis

Neurons are dependent on a continuous adequate supply of oxygen and glucose. The supply of oxygen depends upon pulmonary function and on the cerebral blood flow which, in turn, depends upon the cerebral perfusion pressure which is the difference between the systemic arterial pressure and the cerebral venous pressure. Cerebral blood flow is controlled by an autoregulatory mechanism which maintains a relatively constant blood flow in spite of changes in perfusion pressure. In consequence, blood flow is maintained within normal limits even when systemic arterial pressure falls as low as 50 mmHg (6.65 kPa) provided the subject is in the prone position. At arterial pressures lower than this, the cerebral blood flow falls rapidly. Reduced cerebral blood flow can be brought about by cardiac arrest or an episode of hypotension. The former produces diffuse brain damage, the latter focal damage. Autoregulation may be impaired in chronic hypertension, in hypoxic or hypercapnic states, or in a wide range of acute conditions producing brain damage, e.g. head injury and strokes.

Brain Damage due to Cardiac Arrest

Many patients who suffer severe diffuse brain damage as a result of a cardiac arrest die within a few days. The brain damage is usually restricted to selective neuronal necrosis rather than frank infarction. Provided the patient has survived for more than about 12 hours, microscopic examination will disclose widespread and severe neuronal necrosis. Because of the selective vulnerability of groups of neurons to hypoxia, the necrosis is most prominent in the Ammon's horn (hippocampus), in the third, fifth and sixth layers of the cerebral cortex (particularly within the sulci of the posterior halves of the cerebral hemispheres), in certain of the basal nuclei and in the Purkinje cells of the cerebellum. After a few days the dead neurons disappear and reactive changes in astrocytes, microglia and capillaries become intense.

An essentially similar pattern of damage occurs in **carbon monoxide intoxication, status epilepticus** and **severe hypoglycaemia**.

Brain Damage due to Hypotension

This type of damage is concentrated in the **boundary zones** (watersheds) between the main cerebral and cerebellar arterial territories (Fig. 18.19). The infarcts tend to be largest in the parieto-occipital regions where the territories of the anterior, middle and posterior cerebral arteries meet. There is variable involvement of the basal nuclei, particularly the head of the caudate nucleus and the upper third of the putamen. The hippocampi, despite their extreme vulnerability to cardiac arrest, are usually not involved.

This type of brain damage appears to be caused by a major and abrupt episode of hypotension followed by a rapid return to normal arterial pressure. Because of the precipitous decrease in arterial pressure, autoregulation fails and the regions most remote from the parent arteries, i.e. the boundary zones, are subjected to the greatest reduction in cerebral blood flow. Many examples of this pattern of brain damage have been de-

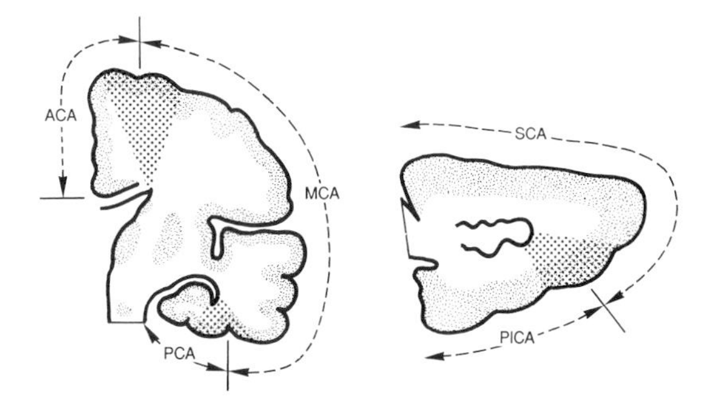

Fig. 18.19 Diagram to show arterial boundary zones (heavy stippling) in the cerebral and cerebellar hemispheres. They lie between the territories supplied by the major arteries. ACA, anterior cerebral artery; MCA, middle cerebral artery; PCA, posterior cerebral artery; SCA, superior cerebellar artery; PICA, posterior inferior cerebellar artery.

scribed in association with major operations under general anaesthesia, myocardial infarcts, or severe haemorrhage.

Spontaneous Intracranial Haemorrhage

The commonest causes are intracerebral haemorrhage secondary to hypertension, and subarachnoid haemorrhage resulting from a ruptured aneurysm.

Intracerebral Haemorrhage

The great majority of intracerebral haematomas develop in late middle age in individuals with **hypertension** due to rupture of one of the numerous **microaneurysms** found in the brain tissue of most people with hypertension.

The commonest site of hypertensive intracerebral haemorrhage is in the region of the basal ganglia and the internal capsule (Fig. 18.20): other sites are the pons and the cerebellum. The haematoma usually increases in size rapidly and produces a sudden rise in intracranial pressure and rapid distortion and herniation of the brain. The blood may rupture into the ventricles or through the surface of the brain directly into the subarachnoid space. The clinical onset is usually sudden, and patients with large intracerebral haematomas rarely survive for more than a day or two.

The appearance of the haematoma at autopsy varies with its duration. A recent haematoma is composed of dark red clot. If the haematoma is not large enough to be rapidly fatal, the periphery has a brownish colour after about a week and there are early reactive changes in capillaries and astrocytes in the adjacent brain. Gliosis leads eventually to the formation of a poorly defined capsule and if the patient survives, the clot is ultimately completely removed by macrophages and replaced by yellow fluid to form a so-called apoplectic cyst (Fig. 18.21).

Another common cause of spontaneous intracranial haemorrhage is rupture of a **vascular**

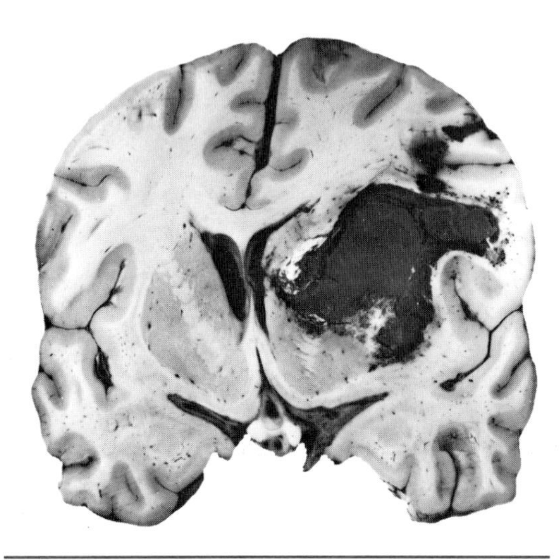

Fig. 18.20 Intracerebral haemorrhage. There is a large haematoma in the basal ganglia resulting from chronic hypertension.

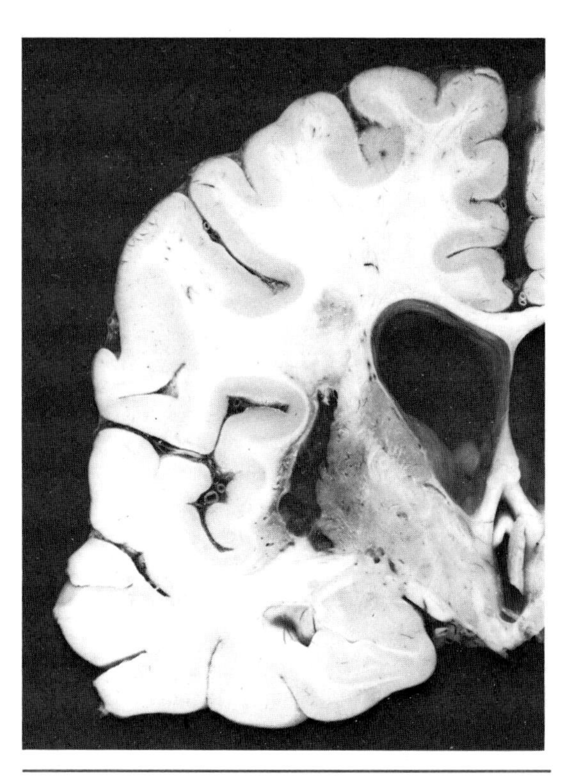

Fig. 18.21 Apoplectic cyst in the left hemisphere. The cyst is centred on the external capsule and the outer part of the lentiform nucleus.

malformation which may range in size from a small capillary angioma to a massive lesion composed of large, often thick walled vascular channels (Fig. 18.22). Many of these lesions are compatible with long survival, sometimes punctuated by episodes of subarachnoid haemorrhage. Other causes of spontaneous intracranial haemorrhage are **haemorrhage into tumours** and **blood dyscrasias**, e.g. acute leukaemia.

Subarachnoid Haemorrhage

Sixty-five per cent of patients presenting clinically with spontaneous (non-traumatic) subarachnoid haemorrhage have rupture of a saccular (berry) aneurysm on one of the major cerebral arteries. In about 5% the subarachnoid haemorrhage is due to rupture of a vascular malformation and in a further 5% it is due to some other disease, such as a blood dyscrasia or extension of either intracerebral or intraventricular haemorrhage into the subarachnoid space. In up to 25% of patients the cause is not found even after complete cerebral angiography.

Saccular aneurysms occur on the arteries of the base of the brain in about 1–2% of the adult population, most often at the bifurcation of a middle cerebral artery within a Sylvian fissure, the junction of the anterior communicating artery with an anterior cerebral artery, or at the junction of a posterior communicating artery with an internal carotid artery. They may also occur on the basilar artery and its branches. About 10–15% of patients who present with symptoms due to an aneurysm are found to have multiple (usually two or three) aneurysms.

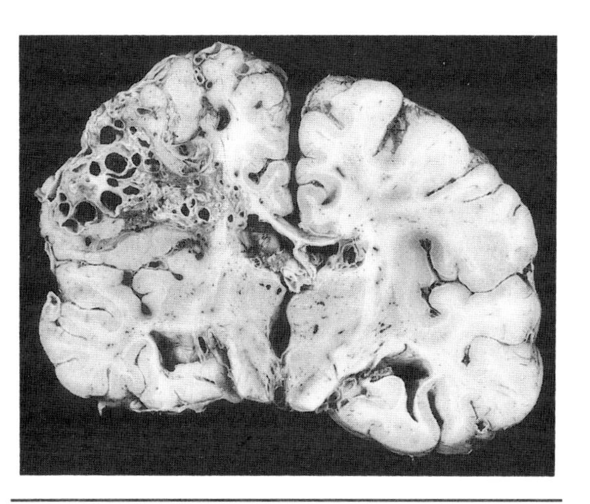

Fig. 18.22 Arteriovenous malformation. There is a large plexus of vascular channels of varying size in the upper part of the left cerebral hemisphere. (From Adams and Graham, 1988.)

They occur more commonly in women than in men and they are often referred to as congenital aneurysms; the developmental abnormality, however, is not the aneurysm itself but a defect in the medial coat of the artery at a bifurcation. Subsequent degeneration of the internal elastic lamina, probably brought about by early atheroma and hypertension, may be a prerequisite to the development of the aneurysm. Most aneurysms that rupture measure 5–10 mm in diameter. Some 10% of patients die during the first bleed, and a further 30% from its after effects within the next few days. A further 35% rebleed and die within the first year, most of these within the first 2 weeks.

When a saccular aneurysm ruptures, the haemorrhage may be limited to the immediate vicinity of the aneurysm, but more often it spreads extensively through the subarachnoid space. Blood may also track into the brain to produce an intracerebral haematoma, and if the aneurysm is embedded in brain tissue, intracerebral haemorrhage may occur without any subarachnoid haemorrhage. Anterior communicating artery aneurysms tend to burst into the frontal lobe, while posterior communicating aneurysms commonly rupture into the temporal lobe. Thus patients with ruptured intracranial aneurysms may have the clinical and pathological features of an acute expanding lesion in addition to subarachnoid haemorrhage. Such intracerebral haematomas often rupture into the ventricles.

Late intracranial complications include infarction which is most common in the region of the brain supplied by the affected artery. This is probably partly attributable to arterial spasm. Another complication is hydrocephalus.

Other types of aneurysm. Atheroma may be the cause of fusiform enlargement of a major cerebral artery but such aneurysms rarely rupture. **Mycotic aneurysms** produced by infected emboli may also occur on the cerebral arteries and may rupture to cause haemorrhage. An aortic dissection (p. 474) may extend into the carotid arteries thus restricting cerebral blood flow.

Thrombosis of the Veins and Venous Sinuses

This may be primary (non-infectious or marantic), or secondary to pyogenic infection (septic thrombosis).

Primary thrombosis is most frequent in poorly nourished and dehydrated children during the course of acute infections. It may occur in adults where predisposing factors include congestive cardiac failure, pregnancy and the puerperium, the use of oral contraceptives and various haematological disorders. If several cortical veins or the sagittal sinus are occluded venous infarction may occur.

Secondary thrombosis of the superior sagittal sinus may be due to spread of infection from the frontal sinus or a compound fracture of the skull. Middle ear infections may involve the lateral sinus.

Infections of the Central Nervous System

Protozoal and helminthic infections are discussed in Chapter 25.

Pyogenic Infections

The brain and spinal cord are relatively well protected from bacteria, but once micro-organisms have gained access the infection may spread rapidly by way of the CSF pathways. Furthermore, many micro-organisms which are relatively non-pathogenic elsewhere in the body can cause serious and often fatal infections of the nervous system. Inflammation of the meninges, **meningitis**, and inflammation of the brain, **encephalitis**, will be considered separately.

Meningitis

Meningitis may involve the dura – pachymeningitis – or the pia/arachnoid – leptomeningitis. The latter is by far the commoner and is generally simply referred to as meningitis.

Leptomeningitis. **Acute pyogenic meningitis** is caused by infection of the subarachnoid space. The causal organisms are many and varied, the commonest being *Neisseria meningitidis, Streptococcus pneumoniae* and the *Haemophilus group*. *Escherichia coli* is common in infants.

Most cases of meningitis are of haematogenous origin. In meningococcal meningitis the infection is spread by droplet infection from nasopharyngeal carriers, this being favoured by poor hygienic conditions. As a result, meningococcal meningitis may occur as an epidemic. The meningococci pass to the meninges by the bloodstream. During epidemics, cases of fatal meningococcal septicaemia can occur without there being time for meningitis to develop; other features in such cases include a haemorrhagic rash and spontaneous haemorrhage into the adrenal glands – the Waterhouse-Friderichsen syndrome. Meningitis may also be brought about by local spread from infection in the bones of the skull or after a compound fracture of the skull. Iatrogenic infection occasionally occurs from the introduction of micro-organisms at operation or during lumbar puncture.

The principal structural change is the presence of pus in the intracranial and spinal subarachnoid spaces. It is thickest within sulci (Fig. 18.23) and in the cisterns at the base of the brain. In rapidly fatal cases there may be no more than an excess of turbid fluid in the sulci, and histological examination is required to confirm the presence of acute inflammation. There is remarkably little involvement of the underlying cortex. The ventricles may contain turbid CSF and there may be fibrin or pus on the ventricular walls and on the choroid plex-

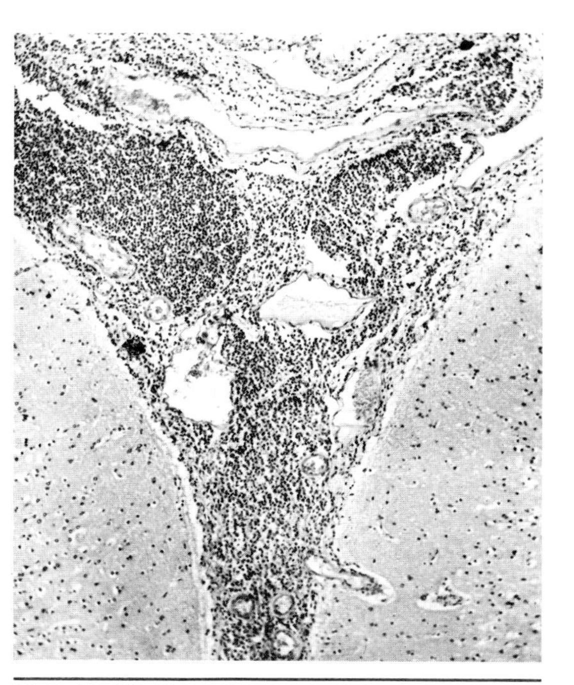

Fig. 18.23 Acute pneumococcal meningitis. The subarachnoid space is filled with purulent exudate.

uses. Mild hydrocephalus is common because the exudate interferes with the flow of CSF.

The precise diagnosis depends on examination of the CSF and this must be done as soon as possible whenever meningitis is suspected, even if there is a suspicion of a high intracranial pressure because this is the only means by which the precise diagnosis can be established. The CSF is turbid or distinctly purulent. There is a high cell count of neutrophil polymorphs. The protein content is raised and the sugar reduced or absent. The causal organisms are often apparent in stained films but sometimes they can be detected only by culture.

Vigorous early treatment with the appropriate antibiotic usually results in resolution of the exudate. If, however, treatment is delayed or inadequate, the exudate does not resolve and the meninges become thickened and oedematous. Organization of the exudate leads to obliteration of the foramina in the roof of the fourth ventricle and/or the subarachnoid space leading to hydrocephalus. Involvement of cranial nerves in the same process may result in partial paralyses. This process is now uncommon but was referred to as posterior basal meningitis.

Pachymeningitis

Acute inflammation of the dura is practically always due to extension of inflammation from the bones of the skull, resulting for example from chronic suppurative otitis media or a compound fracture of the skull. Suppuration occurs between the bone and the dura, resulting in the formation of an **extradural abscess**. The infection may spread through the dura when pus can spread widely over the cerebral hemisphere to form a **subdural abscess.**

Brain Abscess

The causative organisms include the common pyogenic cocci and many others – anaerobic streptococci, bacterioides, diphtheroids, coliforms, yeasts and fungi.

As with meningitis, the organisms may gain access to the brain by haematogenous dissemination. Such abscesses are often multiple and occur most frequently in the parietal lobes and in the cerebellum. The source of the infection may be anywhere in the body, but the primary site is often in the lung. In the past there was a close association between brain abscess and suppurative bronchiectasis but the latter disease can now be adequately controlled by antibiotics. For reasons that are not apparent, individuals with congenital cyanotic heart disease are particularly susceptible to brain abscess. Multiple small acute abscesses occur in pyaemia, whilst in a patient dying with infective endocarditis, numerous small perivascular inflammatory foci are found in the brain.

A commoner cause of brain abscess is direct spread of bacteria from the adjacent bone. The most important are chronic suppurative otitis media or mastoiditis. The bone is eroded by a chronic osteitis with the production of extradural and subdural abscesses. The bacteria then spread into the brain, diffuse bacterial meningitis being prevented by local adhesions in the subarachnoid space. If the source of infection is the middle ear, infection spreads upwards through the tegmen

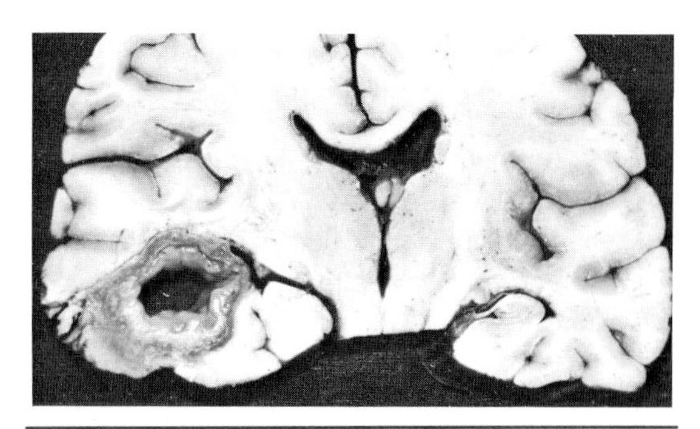

Fig. 18.24 Cerebral abscess. There is an encapsulated abscess in the left temporal lobe secondary to chronic suppurative otitis media.

tympani to the temporal lobe (Fig. 18.24). If the spread is from the mastoid antrum, the abscess occurs in the cerebellum. Occasionally, abscesses may be found both in the temporal lobe and in the cerebellum.

As in other tissues, the abscess becomes limited by a pyogenic membrane which, unless the infection is very severe and extends very rapidly through brain tissue and into the ventricles, soon becomes a well-defined capsule composed of connective tissue, new capillaries, enlarged astrocytes and macrophages. In the adjacent brain tissue there may be some oedema, gliosis and infiltration by macrophages and plasma cells. The symptoms of an abscess are often vague, and by the time the diagnosis is made it may contain thick, greenish-yellow pus, commonly with a foul odour because of the mixed bacterial flora. An abscess may remain latent for some months but it usually enlarges resulting in a high intracranial pressure. The abscess may become multilocular and may finally rupture into a ventricle or into the subarachnoid space.

Non-pyogenic Infections

Tuberculosis

Infection of the CNS by *Mycobacterium tuberculosis* is always secondary to disease elsewhere in the body and its frequency is therefore related to the incidence of tuberculosis in a given population. The infection takes two principal forms – tuberculous meningitis and tuberculomas.

Tuberculous meningitis. The bacilli almost always reach the subarachnoid space by the bloodstream, either as a component of miliary tuberculosis or spread from a tuberculous focus elsewhere in the body. Occasionally infection spreads to the subarachnoid space from tuberculosis of a vertebral body.

Tuberculous meningitis presents clinically as a subacute meningitis; the exudate is gelatinous or caseous and most abundant in the basal cisterns (Fig. 18.25), within sulci and around the spinal cord. Small tubercles measuring 1–2 mm in diameter may be seen in the pia-arachnoid adjacent to cortical blood vessels. The exudate obstructs the flow of CSF with the result that there is almost

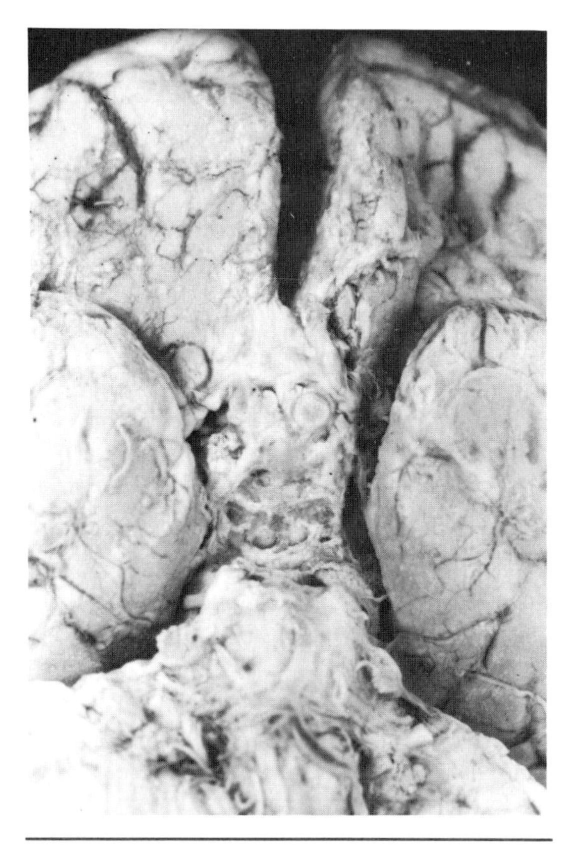

Fig. 18.25 Tuberculous meningitis. There is thick exudate at the base of the brain.

invariably a degree of hydrocephalus. On histological examination the exudate is fibrinocaseous in type, diffusely permeated by lymphocytes, plasma cells and macrophages. Langhans' type giant cells are only occasionally encountered. Obliterative endarteritis resulting in a great reduction in the lumina of affected arteries is the rule (Fig. 18.26). As a result of this there are often small infarcts in the brain or in the cranial nerve roots, leading to focal neurological signs.

The CSF is under increased pressure. It may be clear, but more often has an opalescent appearance. A fine fibrin web often appears on standing. Cells – lymphocytes and macrophages – are increased as is the protein. The glucose is reduced. In a suspected case of tuberculous meningitis the centrifuged deposit must be examined very carefully for acid-alcohol fast bacilli because of the time it takes for their culture. Thus, appropriate antibiotics should be administered to all suspected cases, even when tubercle bacilli cannot be found right away in the CSF.

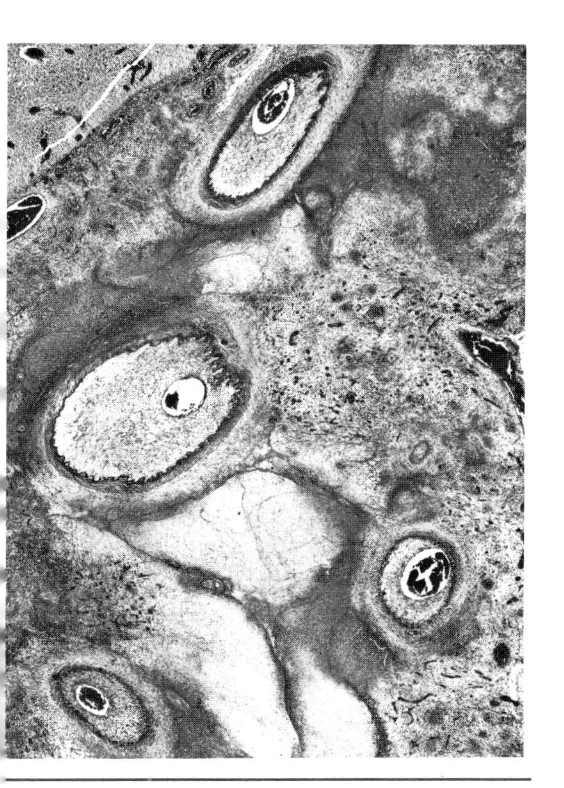

Fig. 18.26 Tuberculous meningitis. There is a severe obliterative endarteritis of arteries in the subarachnoid space.

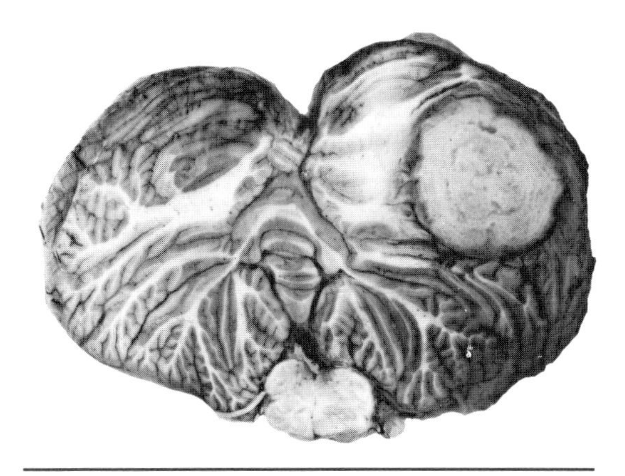

Fig. 18.27 Tuberculoma. There is a sharply defined caseous mass in a cerebellar hemisphere.

Tuberculoma. This takes the form of an encapsulated caseous mass (Fig. 18.27), and in countries where tuberculosis is rife they are a common cause of intracranial expanding lesions. In adults they usually occur in a cerebral hemisphere but in children they have a particular predilection for the cerebellum. They are composed of a core of caseous material surrounded by a broad band within which conventional tubercles and Langhans' type giant cells are conspicuous.

Syphilis

The spirochete, *Treponema pallidum*, gains access to the CNS early in the secondary stage of the disease as shown by some increase in cells and protein in the CSF, but only rarely does the patient exhibit the clinical features of a transient meningoencephalitis. Neurosyphilis presents in two principal forms – tertiary neurosyphilis and parenchymatous (quaternary) neurosyphilis.

Tertiary neurosyphilis. This may take the form of a subacute meningitis with lymphocytes and plasma cells in the subarachnoid space and a periarteritis – **meningovascular syphilis**. There may also be an obliterative endarteritis (Fig. 18.28), leading to focal ischaemic lesions in the brain and in cranial and spinal nerve roots. The rare **hypertrophic cervical pachymeningitis** is mainly produced by syphilis: the dura and arachnoid are thickened and adherent, gliosis occurs in the spinal cord and the nerve roots may be compressed. **Gummas** occur in the meninges, particularly over the convexity of the cerebral hemispheres or over the cerebellum. Within the abnormal tissue there is necrosis, a periarteritis and infiltration by lymphocytes and plasma cells.

Parenchymatous neurosyphilis. The pathogenesis of this type of syphilis remains unknown but the onset of the disease processes may be delayed for as long as 20 years after the primary infection. **General paralysis of the insane (GPI)** is a subacute encephalitis characterized clinically by a progressive dementia. The principal abnormalities are perivascular cuffing of vessels within the CNS by lymphocytes and plasma cells, and a similar inflammatory response in the subarachnoid space. If untreated, there is progressive cerebral atrophy as shown by the presence of small, rounded gyri and widened sulci. The ventricles are enlarged and there is often a granular ependymitis.

Tabes dorsalis is the result of selective degeneration of the posterior spinal nerve roots immediately proximal to the posterior root ganglia, there being selective involvement of the fibres responsible for pain, temperature and proprioception. The posterior nerve roots become grey and shrunken and the spinal cord also becomes reduced in size, particularly in its anteroposterior diameter, because of demyelination and shrinkage of the posterior columns due to Wallerian degeneration (Fig. 18.29). Tabes dorsalis most frequently affects the lumbosacral nerve roots but occasionally cervical nerve roots are the most severely affected, this being referred to as cervical tabes.

In both these conditions the CSF is abnormal. There is an increase in cells – mainly lymphocytes – and of protein. IgG is usually raised and of oligoclonal origin. The Wassermann reaction is usually positive.

Fungal Infections

Fungal infections of the CNS are invariably secondary to infection elsewhere in the body, but lesions at the portal of entry, e.g. in the lung, may

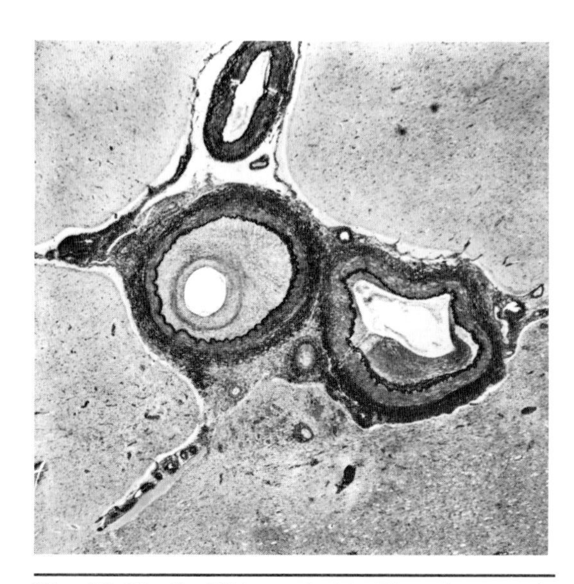

Fig. 18.28 Syphilitic meningitis. There is an established obliterative endarteritis in arteries in the subarachnoid space.

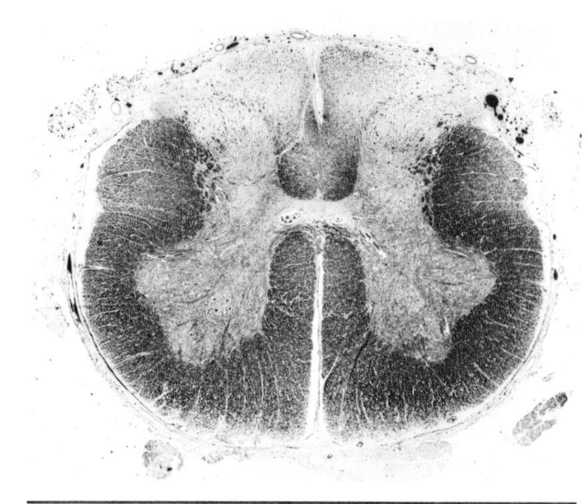

Fig. 18.29 Tabes dorsalis. There is degeneration of posterior nerve roots and the posterior columns in the lumbar spinal cord.

be small and readily overlooked. The brain therefore may appear to be the only organ involved. In other cases, however, infection of the CNS may simply be one of the manifestations of a generalized infection. Some fungi, e.g. *Cryptococcus neoformans*, may produce disease in man in the absence of predisposing factors, but opportunistic fungal infections are being increasingly observed in patients who are immunocompromised.

Cryptococcosis presents usually as a subacute meningitis. The exudate in the subarachnoid space is gelatinous and contains masses of encapsulated crytptococci. Flask-shaped cysts filled with cryptococci are frequently found in the superficial layers of the cortex.

Opportunistic fungal infections are caused mainly by *Candida albicans, Aspergillus fumigatus* and *Nocardia asteroides*. They generally produce multiple brain abscesses of various sizes. In the acute stages the abscesses resemble haemorrhagic infarcts, but later they may become encapsulated. Histological examination usually discloses abundant fungus, particularly at the edges of the abscesses, and a necrotizing vasculitis. Accurate identification depends on culture. Mucormycosis is a rarer opportunistic infection. It has a particular predilection for poorly controlled diabetic patients. The infection commences in the paranasal regions and spreads directly into the anterior fossa of the skull to produce selective involvement of frontal lobes.

Viral Infections

Patients with acute viral infections of the CNS present as aseptic meningitis or viral encephalitis. Most viruses reach the nervous system by way of the bloodstream, i.e. there is a viraemia, often after primary replication of the virus in lymphoid tissue. The viruses may enter the body by various routes, e.g. infections of the skin or mucous membranes (herpes simplex virus), by the alimentary tract (enteroviruses) or by the bites of an arthropod (arboviruses). A few viruses reach the nervous system by travelling along peripheral nerves (rabies virus).

Only a small proportion of individuals infected by potentially neurotropic viruses (i.e. viruses with a predilection for the nervous system) develop clinical evidence of neurological disease. Symptoms frequently occur late, when viraemia is subsiding and circulating antibody increasing, suggesting that at least a proportion of the brain damage is brought about by immunological reactions to antigens in the nervous system.

The CSF pressure may be slightly raised but the fluid is usually of normal appearance. There is an increased cell count – mainly lymphocytes and monocytes – with occasional plasma cells, and the protein is raised slightly. The glucose level is normal.

Aseptic meningitis is usually not a severe illness but it is a common acute infection of the CNS, particularly in children. It is most frequently caused by one of the many enteroviruses or by the mumps virus. Since aseptic meningitis is rarely fatal, little is known about its pathology which probably amounts to no more than infiltration of the subarachnoid space by lymphocytes, plasma cells and macrophages.

Acute viral encephalitis. There are several histological features common to all types of acute viral encephalitis. The most striking is the presence of lymphocytes and plasma cells in the subarachnoid space and as cuffs around blood vessels within the brain (Fig. 18.30). There is also diffuse hyperplasia of microglia with the formation of rod cells and small clusters of microglia. In regions where there is destruction of tissue, there is an astrocytosis and lipid-containing macrophages appear. Central chromatolysis, necrosis of neurons and neuronophagia (Fig. 18.31) are other features. In some forms of encephalitis inclusion bodies (Fig. 18.32) may be found in neurons, astrocytes and oligodendroglia. Necrosis may also occur, ranging from selective neuronal necrosis as in poliomyelitis, to frank infarction of grey and white matter as in herpes simplex encephalitis. The causal virus can usually be isolated from brain

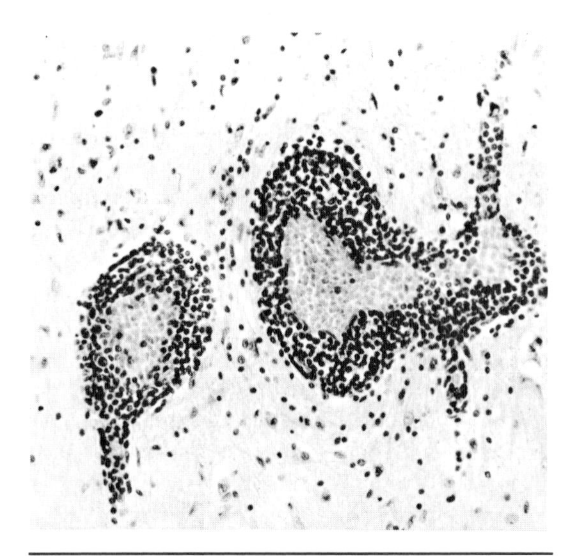

Fig. 18.30 Acute viral meningitis. These small blood vessels within the brain are cuffed by lymphocytes and plasma cells.

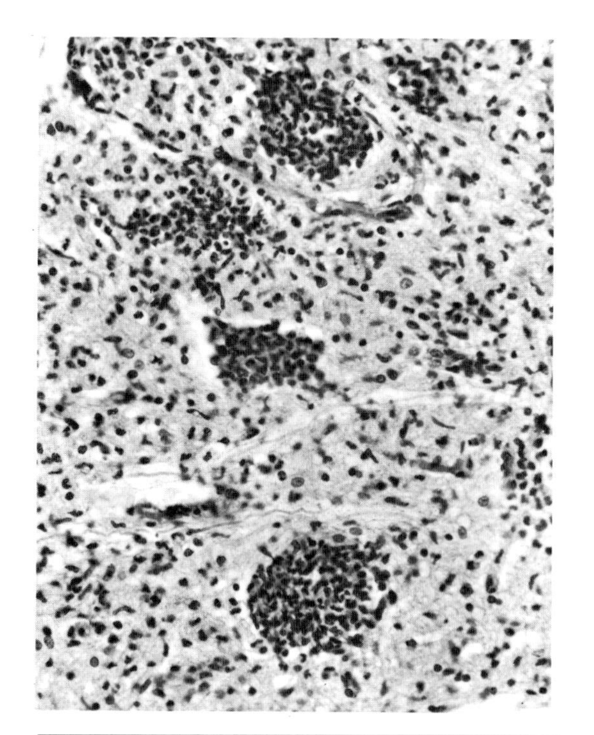

Fig. 18.31 Acute viral meningitis. The densely cellular aggregates are microglia engulfing dead neurons (neuronophagia).

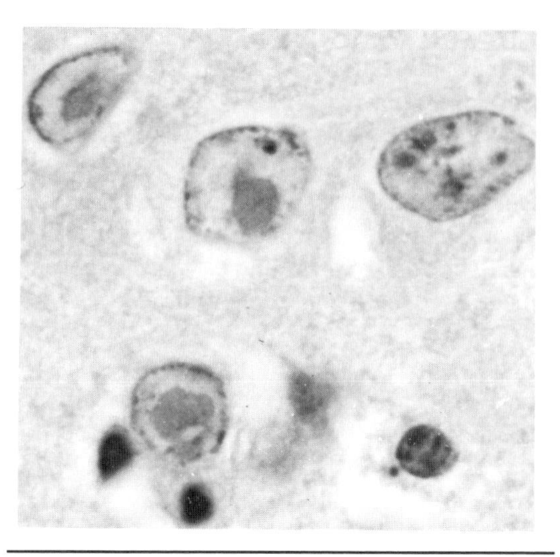

Fig. 18.32 Acute viral encephalitis. Three nuclei contain inclusion bodies.

tissue (biopsy or autopsy) but rarely from the CSF.

Infections with Herpes Viruses

The human herpes viruses that affect the CNS are herpes simplex virus (types 1 and 2), varicella zoster and cytomegalovirus. All are DNA viruses of similar morphology.

Herpes simplex virus (HSV) affects the CNS in one of three ways, the most important of which is an acute necrotizing encephalitis which is the commonest virus encephalitis encountered in western Europe. Other diseases produced by HSV are an aseptic meningitis, and a fulminating disseminated infection that may occur in infants and in immunocompromised individuals.

Herpes simplex encephalitis is a fulminating and often rapidly fatal disease, the distinctive feature being extensive and asymmetrical necrosis in the temporal lobes, the insulae and the cingulate gyri. Swelling of the more severely affected temporal lobe is often sufficient to produce a shift of the midline structures and a tentorial hernia (Fig. 18.33). The necrotic tissue may be focally haemorrhagic. If the patient survives the acute stage, the

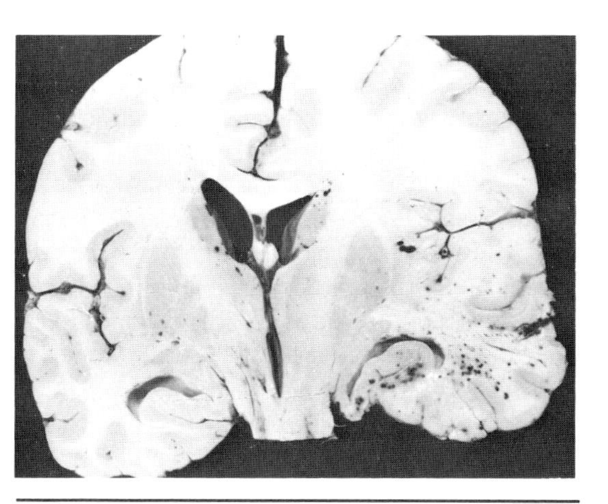

Fig. 18.33 Encephalitis due to herpes simplex virus. Within the swollen right temporal lobe there are many small haemorrhagic foci. There is also a shift of the midline structures to the left.

necrotic tissue becomes shrunken and cystic (Fig. 18.34). Although the necrosis has a selective distribution, histological examination will reveal a diffuse meningoencephalitis.

As a result of the development of appropriate antiviral agents, treatment should be commenced as soon as the diagnosis is considered. This may be confirmed by a brain biopsy. An acute inflammatory process will be seen in smears and sections, HSV antigen can often be identified by immunofluorescence and virus can usually also be isolated from the biopsy.

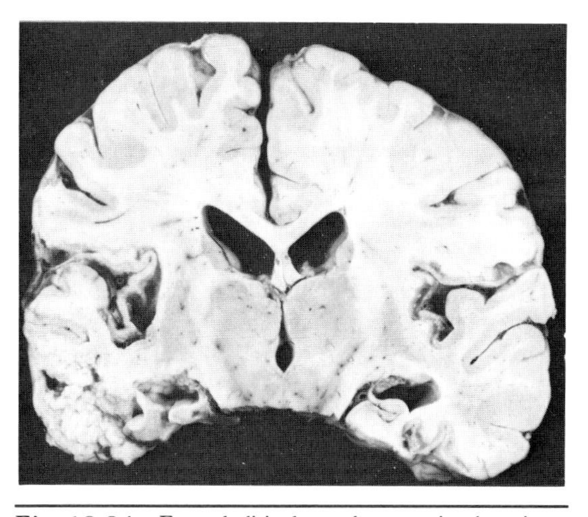

Fig. 18.34 Encephalitis due to herpes simplex virus. This patient survived for several weeks, severely brain damaged. The affected regions are now shrunken and focally cystic. The left temporal lobe is more severely affected than the right one.

Varicella Zoster (VZ). Primary infection with VZ virus produces varicella (chicken pox). During the period of the cutaneous eruption, the virus travels centrifugally along sensory nerves where it remains latent in sensory cranial and posterior root ganglia. When the virus reactivates it produces an acute necrotizing inflammatory response in the affected ganglion and travels down the nerve, producing a characteristic vesicular rash when it reaches the skin, the disease being known as herpes zoster (shingles). In its commonest form herpes zoster occurs in a dermatome supplied by one posterior root ganglion, most often in the thoracic region. The second commonest nerve involved is the ophthalmic division of the trigeminal nerve.

In the acute stage the affected ganglion is swollen and may be haemorrhagic. On microscopic examination there is an intense lymphocytic infiltration both within and around the ganglion (Fig. 18.35). There is usually necrosis of individual neurons and occasionally extensive necrosis throughout the ganglion. The inflammatory process often extends into the posterior nerve root and the ipsilateral dorsal quadrant of the spinal cord. As the inflammatory reaction diminishes, fibrosis occurs within the ganglion. The death of neurons leads to Wallerian degeneration in the nerve fibres in the ascending columns of the spinal cord.

What produces reactivation of the latent virus is not clear but in a small proportion of cases some precipitating factor such as physical trauma to the affected region has been identified. Immunological disturbances may also be important since zoster is common in patients with lymphoma. In patients undergoing treatment with cytotoxic drugs and corticosteroids, herpes zoster may become disseminated and lead to a generalized varicelliform rash and a fatal multifocal necrotizing encephalomyelitis.

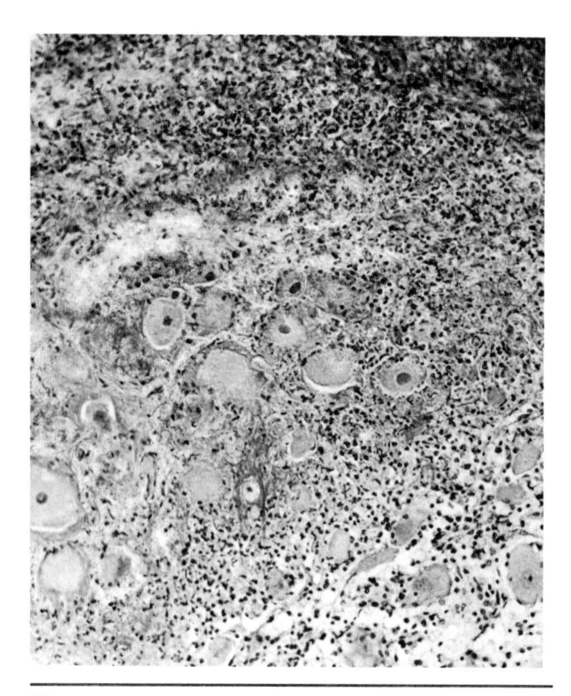

Fig. 18.35 Herpes zoster. This posterior root ganglion is heavily infiltrated by inflammatory cells.

Cytomegalovirus (CMV). Involvement of the CNS by cytomegalovirus is mainly due to infections acquired *in utero*. In the neonate it presents as an acute disseminated necrotizing encephalomyelitis with selective involvement of periventricular tissue. Cytomegalic inclusions may be found in various types of cell. Survivors are almost always mentally retarded, the principal abnormalities in the brain being hydrocephalus and periventricular calcification. Infection early in pregnancy may lead to malformations such as microgyria.

Infections with enteroviruses

The most important enteroviruses are the polioviruses, Coxsackie and ECHO viruses. All are small RNA viruses that are frequent causes of aseptic meningitis. They may also cause paralytic disease, i.e. acute anterior poliomyelitis, which is classically associated with the polioviruses but is caused occasionally by other enteroviruses. Overt paralysis occurs in probably no more than about 1% of individuals infected with the most pathogenic poliovirus – type I.

Enterovirus infections are usually contracted by ingestion of the virus which then multiplies in the pharynx and in the cells lining the gastrointestinal tract. Within a few days virus is present in adjacent lymphoid tissue and, if the antibody response is inadequate, virus reaches the CNS by the bloodstream. Faecal excretion of virus continues long after the acute infection.

Acute anterior poliomyelitis. The virus selectively attacks neurons in the ventral horns of the spinal cord, particularly in the lumbar and cervical enlargements, leading to paralysis of the limb muscles. The motor nuclei in the brain stem are also often affected – **bulbar polio** – when there may be early involvement of the respiratory centre. In a patient dying in the acute stage, the CNS is often of entirely normal appearance macroscopically but there may occasionally be foci of haemorrhage in the ventral horns in the spinal cord or in the brain stem.

Microscopic examination discloses the typical features of a generalized acute viral encephalitis with selectively severe involvement of the spinal cord or the brain stem. Neuronophagia (see Fig. 18.31) is conspicuous in the affected nuclei and central chromatolysis is often seen in neurons that have not been destroyed. With time the inflammatory changes subside and at least some of the paralysis may improve. This is not due to regeneration but to recovery of function in neurons that have been transiently affected by the inflammatory process.

In patients with residual paralysis who die long after the acute stage of the disease, there is loss of motor neurons in the affected ventral horns and atrophy of the related nerve roots. There is neurogenic atrophy of the affected muscles (see p. 871).

Infections with Arboviruses

Arboviruses are RNA viruses that are transmitted from host to host by bloodsucking insects. They multiply in both vertebrate and invertebrate hosts. Man is not a natural host for any arbovirus but during periods of epizootic spread among the natural hosts (usually wild birds and small mammals) he may become affected.

Several arboviruses can cause severe encephalitis in man, e.g. **St Louis encephalitis, eastern and western equine encephalitis** and **Japanese B encephalitis**, all of which are mosquito-borne. The structural changes are those of a disseminated encephalomyelitis, sometimes with focal necrosis. Tick-borne arboviruses are responsible for **Russian spring–summer encephalitis** and **louping ill.**

Rabies

Rabies remains a major problem in many countries of the world. The great majority of human cases can be traced to the bite of a rabid dog. The virus (a rhabdovirus) enters the body via the saliva contaminating the bite and reaches the CNS by travelling along peripheral nerves. The major reservoirs of the virus are the fox, the skunk and the jackal. The incubation of the disease varies greatly, its duration being related to the distance of the bite from the CNS. Sometimes it is as short as 2 weeks but, more commonly, it is 1–3 months or even longer. As the old name of hydrophobia implies, spasm of the muscles of deglutition on attempting to drink water may be the first or at least an early symptom.

In a fatal case the brain may appear normal macroscopically or perhaps slightly congested. Microscopic examination shows the features of a diffuse virus encephalitis, predominantly affecting grey matter. The pathognomonic histological feature are the Negri bodies. They appear as sharply defined rounded or oval acidophilic intracytoplasmic inclusions varying in size from 1 μm to 7 μm across. They may lie anywhere in the cytoplasm of the cell body or its dendrites, and two or more may be seen in one cell. Virus can be identified within the Negri body using immunofluorescent techniques or electron microscopy.

Persistent Virus Infections

The two infections of the nervous system which can most appropriately be classified as persistent virus infections are subacute sclerosing panencephalitis and progressive multifocal leucoencephalopathy.

Subacute sclerosing panencephalitis is caused by the measles virus. It is a rare form of subacute encephalitis occurring mainly between the ages of 4 and 20 years and usually fatal in 6 weeks to 6 months. It occurs some years after an apparently uncomplicated attack of measles. Its pathogenesis is not understood but it appears to be due to reactivation of measles virus which has remained latent in the brain since the time of the primary infection. There are high levels of both IgM and IgG oligoclonal antibodies in the blood and CSF. At autopsy the brain appears superficially normal but the white matter is often abnormally firm. Microscopic examination shows the features of a meningoencephalitis with widespread cuffing of blood vessels throughout the brain by lymphocytes and plasma cells. Neuronophagia is common, and varying numbers of residual neurons may contain intranuclear and/or cytoplasmic inclusion bodies. There is also considerable gliosis in the white matter. A similar disease process may occasionally result from infection by rubella.

Progressive multifocal leucoencephalopathy is caused by viruses which belong to the polyoma subgroup of papovaviruses. It is virtually restricted to immunocompromised patients. In the brain there are multiple small grey foci distributed widely throughout the white matter. These foci can coalesce to form large grey areas which may become cystic. Histological examination shows multiple foci of demyelination accompanied by macrophages, abnormal oligodendrocytes with large hyperchromatic nuclei containing ill-defined inclusion bodies, and large bizarre astrocytes. With electron microscopy, pseudocrystalline arrays of virions are present in oligodendrocytes.

Slow Virus Infections

There are at least two so-called slow virus infections of the CNS in man – kuru and Creutzfeldt–Jakob disease. Similar diseases occur in animals – scrapie in sheep, mink encephalopathy and bovine spongiform encephalopathy. All these conditions have a long incubation period, and an unremitting, and fatal, progressive course. This group of diseases is now classified as the **spongiform encephalopathies**. The transmissible agents have so far not been identified nor has their true nature been established. Experimental evidence suggests that they may be unique and not contain nucleic acid. The term prion has been introduced to describe such a proteinaceous infection particle and there is currently intense research to identify such highly unconventional infectious agents.

Kuru. The elucidation of this disease has been one of the most dramatic occurrences in the entire field of diseases of the nervous system in the past three decades. It is a subacute disease characterized by microcystic degeneration in the grey matter, referred to as status spongiosus, associated with loss of neurons and a great excess of hypertrophied astrocytes. Its peculiar importance is that it was the first progressive degenerative disease of the nervous system in man to be transmitted to another animal, first the chimpanzee but later other species, by injecting extracts of brain tissue from patients with the disease. The agent which is filterable and capable of replicating, has not been identified. Ritual cannibalism in the eastern highlands of New Guinea was the primary mode of transmission and the incidence of the disease has subsided since this practice ceased.

Creutzfeldt–Jakob disease is a progressive dementia of worldwide distribution, again characterized by status spongiosus and gliosis. It has been shown to be transmissible to other species. It has also been transmitted, accidentally, to man by implantation of contaminated electrodes in the brain, corneal grafting, by growth hormone extracted from pituitary glands from affected patients and dural grafts.

Human Immunodeficiency Viruses (HIV)

The brain is affected in more than 50% of individuals with AIDS. The commonest diseases are opportunistic infections such as toxoplasmosis, cryptococcosis, cytomegalovirus encephalitis and fungal infections. There is also an ill-understood AIDS dementia where the principal structural features seem to be microglial hyperplasia and the presence of multinucleated macrophage-type cells in which some HIV antigens have been demonstrated.

Demyelinating Diseases

These disorders of the CNS are characterized by **periaxial demyelination** in which there is destruction of myelin **with relative preservation of axons** (Table 18.2). They are distinct from genetic disorders of myelin formation – dysmyelination (leucodystrophy) – and from diseases causing breakdown of myelin secondary to neuronal destruction – Wallerian degeneration (see p. 807). The group includes chronic disorders in which there is conspicuous gliosis in the demyelinated areas, the most important being multiple (disseminated) sclerosis, and acute conditions associated with considerable inflammatory exudation such as acute disseminated (perivenous) encephalomyelitis and acute haemorrhagic leucoencephalitis.

Table 18.2 Diseases characterized by periaxial demyelination

Multiple sclerosis
Diffuse sclerosis
Neuromyelitis optica

Acute disseminated encephalomyelitis
Acute haemorrhagic leucoencephalitis

Progressive multifocal leucoencephalopathy
Central pontine myelinolysis
Subacute sclerosing panencephalitis
Carbon monoxide poisoning

Multiple (Disseminated) Sclerosis

This is the most common of the demyelinating diseases and is characterized by patchy demyelination and gliosis in the brain and spinal cord. It usually starts before 50 years of age and most often in adolescents and young adults. It is a chronic disease characterized clinically by relapses and remissions and resulting in increasing disability. The intervening periods of remission may extend over years, and the rate of progress and severity vary considerably. In some cases, the disease becomes relentlessly progressive in the later stages, but occasionally it is steadily progressive from the start leading to **ataxic paraplegia**. A common early symptom is an acute unilateral **optic neuritis** due to a focus of demyelination in the optic nerve. The clinical features of multiple sclerosis – often referred to as MS – are caused by foci of demyelination, known as plaques, irregularly distributed in the brain and spinal cord. Acute lesions are yellowish and soft; chronic lesions are firm, grey and slightly translucent.

In acute lesions there is periaxial demyelination with infiltration by lipid containing macrophages and perivascular cuffing by lymphocytes and plasma cells. As the plaque ages, the cellular infiltration decreases and vascular thickening and gliosis occur, but without much contraction or distortion. Partial clinical recovery from the disabling effects of the acute lesions is attributed to subsidence of inflammatory oedema in and around the acute lesions since the demyelinated axons may persist and function for a long time. Many of the axons, however, ultimately undergo Wallerian degeneration. The neurons in a plaque usually show little or no abnormality. Old plaques are readily identifiable as conspicuous pale areas in which there is complete loss of myelin and a fairly sharp line of demarcation from the adjacent normal tissue. Smaller plaques, up to a few millimetres across, are usually round or oval; larger ones are irregular, and may result from the confluence of smaller plaques. Typically, most of the lesions seen at autopsy are old; they vary greatly in number, size and distribution but are usually most

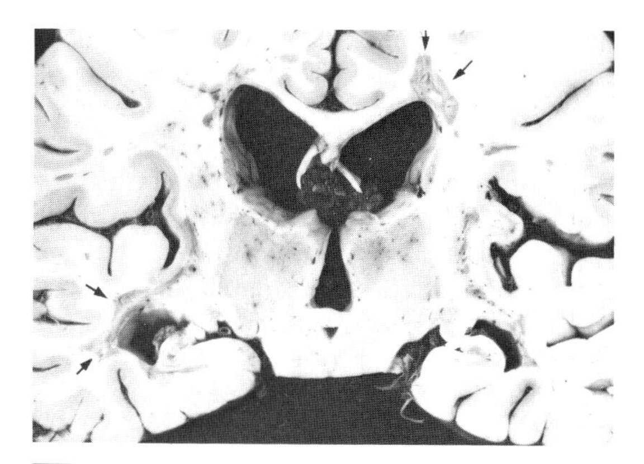

Fig. 18.36 Multiple sclerosis. There is a large grey plaque (arrows) of demyelination at the angle of a lateral ventricle.

easily seen in the white matter of the cerebrum, particularly at the edges of the lateral ventricles (Fig. 18.36) and at the junction of the cortex and white matter. Plaques do, however, occur in the cortex and central grey matter. They are common in the brain stem (Fig. 18.37), particularly around the aqueduct and fourth ventricle, and in the spinal cord. If there was a history of visual disturbances, a plaque can usually be found in the optic nerve.

There is, unfortunately, no test by which a definitive diagnosis can be established. By combin-

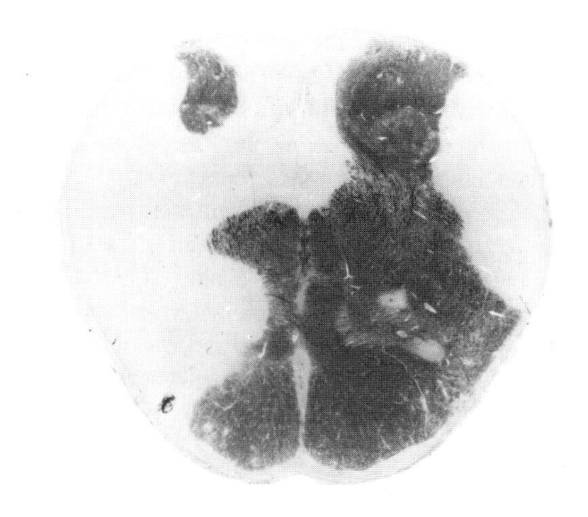

Fig. 18.37 Multiple sclerosis. Demyelinated plaques in the lower medulla are the pale areas. (Weigert–Pal method).

ing the clinical features, various electrophysiological studies and examination of the CSF, a diagnosis of multiple sclerosis can be achieved with varying degrees of certainty. High resolution CT scanning and MR imaging of the brain and spinal cord may help in the identification of plaques. The CSF in multiple sclerosis may contain more than five lymphocytes per ml, particularly during an acute episode, and in the majority of patients there is an increase in the immunoglobulin/albumin ratio with oligoclonal bands of IgG present. Whilst such bands are not specific, they are present in 85–95% of patients with definite multiple sclerosis.

Variants of Multiple Sclerosis

These include **neuromyelitis optica**, a disease of adults in which there is rapid loss of vision and the development of paraplegia due to extensive plaque formation in the brain, optic nerves and spinal cord; and **sudanophilic diffuse sclerosis**, a disease of childhood, usually acutely progressive, affecting the cerebral white matter, notably the occipital lobes, and in which prominent macrophage aggregates are seen in the lesions together with some axon loss.

Aetiology

Genetic and environmental factors both appear to be of importance. Genetic factors are suggested by an increased incidence of HLA-A3, B7, DR2 and DW2 in patients. Epidemiological studies point to an environmental factor being of importance in childhood, for there are considerable differences in the incidence of multiple sclerosis in various parts of the world, and people who migrate from one area to another after the age of about 14 retain the incidence of their childhood locality. There is an increased incidence of multiple sclerosis amongst siblings (particularly twins) and parents of patients with the disease, but it is not known whether this is attributable to genetic or environmental factors or to a combination of both. Whilst these studies might suggest an infective aetiology, there is no convincing evidence yet for this theory.

There is evidence of an immune reaction in multiple sclerosis, with an increase of lymphocytes in the CSF, and of T lymphocytes, both T4 and T8, and plasma cells in acute lesions. Oligoclonal bands of IgG are present in the CSF. These immunological factors could be interpreted as indicating either a response to a neurotropic virus or an autoimmune response to a neural tissue component as in experimental autoallergic encephalomyelitis. In support of a viral aetiology, the titres of antibody to measles virus are relatively high in both the serum and CSF, and antibodies to some other viruses are also raised. Isolation of various viruses from multiple sclerosis tissue has been reported and virus-like particles have been detected by electron microscopy, but the findings are conflicting and no consistent pattern has emerged. In support of an autoimmune aetiology, antibodies which together with complement cause demyelination of cultures of neural tissue have been detected in the serum of patients with multiple sclerosis. The evidence, however, is inconclusive as they also occur in various non-demyelinating diseases. Also, the acute demyelination complicating rabies prophylaxis in man and occurring in experimental allergic encephalomyelitis (both disorders which appear to have an autoimmune pathogenesis) occurs as a single acute episode and is perivenular, in contrast to the recurrent episodes of multiple sclerosis in which plaques are much larger and show no obvious relationship to small vessels.

Experimental autoallergic encephalomyelitis (EAE). This can be produced in various species of animal by the injection of brain extract or myelin basic protein of the same or different species emulsified in Freund's adjuvant. Whilst the role of the antibodies is unclear, there is good evidence that the lesions result from a delayed autohypersensitivity reaction in which sensitized lymphocytes and possibly macrophages react directly against the antigenic component of myelin. In some species the pathological changes are similar to those of acute disseminated perivenous encephalomyelitis in man, and may be caused by a similar immunological reaction. Acute perivenous encephalomyelitis and EAE are monophasic illnesses whereas multiple sclerosis is essentially a chronic relapsing condition. Nevertheless the analogy between EAE and MS has become closer with the development of chronic models of EAE in certain strains of guinea-pigs and mice.

Acute Disseminated (Perivenous) Encephalomyelitis

This monophasic and generally self-limiting disease occurs in older children and young adults and develops as an unusual sequel to (1) various acute virus diseases such as mumps, measles, chicken pox or rubella (post-infectious encephalitis); (2) respiratory infections presumed to be viral; and (3) primary vaccination against smallpox (post-vaccinal encephalitis) and anti-rabies inoculation. It is often of rapid onset, occurring between 5 and 14 days after the onset of the initial infection or immunization.

The lesions are diffusely distributed throughout the brain and spinal cord and are characterized histologically by perivenular demyelination associated with inflammatory oedema and infiltration mainly by neutrophil polymorphs in the acute state and later by lymphocytes and macrophages. As the condition complicates so many different acute infections, vaccination and immunization procedures, it is thought to be due to autoallergy in which a host-mediated response is directed against antigens such as myelin basic protein in the CNS; the possibility of an immune reaction against virus or virus-infected cells cannot, however, be excluded. Further evidence in favour of an immune reaction is provided experimentally in that the disease may be transferred to healthy animals by the injection of sensitized lymphocytes from an affected animal.

Acute Haemorrhagic Leucoencephalitis

This uncommon disease is characterized by a rapid and dramatic onset, a short clinical course and usually a fatal outcome. It may also occur as a sequel to viral infections, usually respiratory, and may also complicate septic shock, treatment with various drugs, and various other diseases assumed to be hypersensitivity reactions, e.g. thrombotic thrombocytopenic purpura.

At autopsy the brain is swollen and there are numerous petechial haemorrhages, particularly in the white matter. Microscopic examination shows focal necrosis of the walls of venules and arterioles, perivascular 'ball' and 'ring' haemorrhages and perivascular demyelination, often with infiltration first by neutrophil polymorphs and later by lymphocytes and macrophages. There is also oedema and an inflammatory exudate in the meninges. Although the aetiology is unknown, the condition is thought to be a hyperacute variant of acute disseminated perivenous encephalomyelitis and to be caused by the deposition of immune complexes and the activation of complement.

Other Forms of Periaxial Demyelination

There are a number of systemic conditions and intoxications that produce demyelination with the relative preservation of axons and neurons.

Central pontine myelinolysis is a condition that usually occurs in middle-aged patients who are alcoholic, chronically debilitated or malnourished. It is characterized by symmetrical demyelination in the central portion of the pons. It is thought to be related to a metabolic disturbance involving a fluid electrolyte imbalance and may be caused by the too rapid therapeutic correction of a low plasma sodium to normal levels.

Toxic demyelination with relative preservation of axons may be produced by various agents such as hexachlorophane and tin, and in association with carbon monoxide poisoning.

Viral diseases include progressive multifocal leucoencephalopathy and subacute sclerosing panencephalitis (see p. 833).

Metabolic Disorders

Although uncommon, primary (inherited) metabolic disorders make a considerable contribution to morbidity and mortality in children. Many are inherited as autosomal recessive diseases, although in a few there is X-linked recessive inheritance. Inherited metabolic defects involve many substances, e.g. lipids, carbohydrates, mucopolysaccharides, amino acids and trace metals. Many of the metabolic disorders have been discussed in Chapter 7. Depending on the particular disease, structural changes may or may not be present in the CNS. In some, however, the disease primarily affects the CNS whilst in others the primary disease involves other systems but is accompanied by impaired neuronal metabolism. Although the onset of clinical symptoms may not become apparent until adult life, the majority appear during childhood and frequently in the first few days of life.

The metabolic complexity of the CNS makes it dependent upon the functional integrity of other systems in the body. It is therefore not surprising that secondary metabolic effects on the CNS are often a manifestation of systemic disease. In many instances the clinical features are reversible and there are minimal morphological changes. It is only when the metabolic disorder has been profound and prolonged that structural changes occur.

Also discussed here are the non-metastatic (remote) effects of tumours on the CNS, and unusual clinical syndromes which may, in part, be metabolic in aetiology.

Primary (Inherited) Metabolic Diseases

Many of these disorders are due to deficiencies of particular lysosomal enzymes which play an essential role in the degradation of various normal metabolites or the breakdown products of cells. As a result the undegraded material accumulates in, and causes enlargement of, the lysosomes of certain cells, the distribution depending on the particular enzyme deficiency. Some of these disorders affect neurons which become enlarged with a ballooned appearance. Stored material can be detected histochemically, and electron microscopy demonstrates grossly enlarged lysosomes containing unmetabolized material. Diagnosis by assay of the relevant lysosomal enzymes in blood, urine, leucocytes or cultured fibroblasts is now often possible and has reduced the need for diagnostic biopsy of the CNS. The lysosomal storage disorders can be divided into two main groups: those that affect neurons – neuronal storage disorders – and those that affect the white matter – leucodystrophies. This classification is convenient, if somewhat artificial, as both neurons and white matter may be affected in many of the disorders.

Neuronal Storage Disorders

Principal amongst these are the **sphingolipidoses** and the **mucopolysaccharidoses**, the main types of which are listed in Table 18.3. The sphingolipidoses are probably the most important group of inherited metabolic disorders that affect the nervous system. The sphingolipids include gangliosides, cerebrosides, sulphatides and sphingomyelins, all of which are important constituents of the normal cell. One of the commonest storage disorders especially affecting neurons is **Tay–Sachs disease**, the classical infantile type of amaurotic familial idiocy. A particularly characteristic sign of the disease (but not restricted to it) is the cherry red spot at the macula due to retinal involvement. Typically, the cell bodies of affected neurons are greatly distended by an accumulation of stored material in enlarged lysosomes, some of which have distinctive electron microscopic appearances.

The Leucodystrophies

These are a complex group of uncommon disorders having in common diffuse symmetrical demyelination and gliosis of the white matter of the cerebral hemispheres, and sometimes also of the cerebellum, the brain stem and the spinal cord. Clinically they are characterized by various combinations of mental deterioration, motor impairment and sometimes a peripheral neuropathy.

Table 18.3 Principal neuronal storage disorders

Disorder	Enzyme affected	Substances stored
Disorders of lipid metabolism		
Sphingolipidoses		
GM_1-gangliosidosis (two types)	β-Galactosidase	GM_1-ganglioside, oligosaccharides, ceramide tetrahexoside
GM_2-gangliosidosis (several types including Tay–Sachs and Sandhoff)	Hexosaminidases	GM_2-ganglioside, ceramide trihexoside
Cerebrosidosis (Gaucher's disease, 3 types)	β-Glucocerebrosidase	Glucocerebroside
Sphingomyelinosis (Niemann–Pick's, 2 groups)	Sphingomyelinase	Sphingomyelin, cholesterol
Batten's disease (neuronal ceroid lipofuscinosis)	Not known	Lipofuscin-like substances
Disorders of glycosaminoglycan metabolism		
Mucopolysaccharidoses (MPS)		
Type I–II (Hurler's)	α-L-iduronidase	Acid mucopolysaccharides (heparan sulphate, dermatan sulphate, keratan sulphate and several gangliosides)
Type II (Hunter's)	Sulphoiduronate Sulphamidase	
Type III (Sanfilippo's – 4 subtypes)	Various	
Type IV (Morquio's – 2 subtypes)	Various	

There are several different types of leucodystrophy (Table 18.4), most of which are genetically determined and occur in childhood. They are therefore regarded as **dysmyelinating diseases** in the belief that the myelin is biochemically abnormal before it degenerates, in contrast to the primary demyelinating disorders in which myelination is thought to be normal prior to the onset of the demyelination. At autopsy the brain feels unusually firm and the white matter may be somewhat greyer and more translucent than normal. Histologically, there is widespread loss of myelin and in **metachromatic leucodystrophy** there is an accumulation of metachromatic material within neurons. Some cases of **sudanophilic leucodystrophy** in males are associated with adrenal

Table 18.4 Principal types of leucodystrophy

Disorder	Enzyme affected	Substances stored
Metachromatic	Arylsulphatase A	Sulphatides
Krabbe's	Galactocerebroside β-galactosidase	Galactocerebroside
Adrenoleucodystrophy	Not known	Very long chain fatty acid esters

In addition there are a number in which the enzyme defect has not been defined. These include spongiform, Alexander's (in which fibrillar material – Rosenthal fibres – are stored in astrocytes), Pelizaeus–Merzbacher and Cockaynes' leucodystrophy insufficiency which may precede or accompany the onset of neurological illness, or may remain subclinical. It has been suggested that the majority of males with sudanophilic leucodystrophy are cases of **adrenoleucodystrophy**, a characteristic feature of which is the presence of ballooned vacuolated adrenal cortical cells containing linear lamellar bodies with distinctive fine structural features.

Other Inborn Errors of Metabolism with CNS Involvement

Neonatal hypothyroidism, phenylketonuria and galactosaemia are the most important of these because they can be detected by screening tests in infants, and brain damage can be prevented or reduced either by replacement therapy or by exclusion of the precursor substances from the diet.

Hepatolenticular degeneration (Wilson's disease) (p. 772) is an autosomal recessive disorder of copper metabolism in which there is accumulation of copper in the liver (producing cirrhosis) and in the brain. The copper accumulates mainly in the putamen and caudate nucleus, which become soft, shrunken and ultimately cystic. Clinically the patients develop muscular tremors and spasticity. The CNS involvement tends to develop later than the hepatic cirrhosis, but is also preventable by treatment with penicillamine.

Subacute necrotizing encephalomyelopathy (Leigh's syndrome) is a recessive disorder that is more common in males, usually presenting in infancy but with some cases occurring in juveniles and adults. Clinically, there is ataxia, muscle weakness, visual disturbance and intellectual deterioration. The pathological findings are similar to Wernicke's disease. The metabolic error affects mitochondria with deficiency of a number of enzymes in brain and muscles.

Secondary Metabolic Disorders

Metabolic encephalopathies may occur as a result of hepatic failure, uraemia, renal dialysis and transplantation, diabetes mellitus (hyper- and hypoglycaemia), hyper- and hypothyroidism, acidosis and alkalosis, hypoxia, carbon dioxide narcosis and carbon monoxide poisoning. Another example is central pontine myelinolysis. With many of these there are often only minor morphological changes in the brain emphasizing the predominantly biochemical nature of the encephalopathy.

Hepatic Encephalopathy

This invariably accompanies severe liver failure. Cases of massive hepatic necrosis accompanied by an acute hepatic encephalopathy are characterized by rapidly developing coma. On the other hand, in cases of liver disease with cirrhosis, particularly when there is portal systemic shunting of blood, chronic hepatic encephalopathy develops. There may be no histological abnormalities in the CNS in cases of acute fulminant hepatic encephalopathy, but in some, Alzheimer astrocytes may be present. These large astrocytes with strikingly vesicular swollen nuclei are a prominent feature of chronic hepatic encephalopathy and may be widely distributed throughout the grey matter. Hepatic encephalopathy is due to an accumulation of neurotoxic substances in the blood as a result of liver failure. The possible nature and effects of these substances are discussed more fully on p. 774.

Kernicterus

This is a metabolic disorder in the perinatal period also known as bilirubin encephalopathy. In the fetus, bilirubin is excreted by the placenta, so jaundice becomes severe only after birth. Severe jaundice in infancy carries the risk of brain damage. Necrosis of neurons and bile staining are seen particularly in the hippocampus and basal nuclei. If not fatal, the damage is likely to cause choreoathetosis, spasticity and often mental deficiency. The condition is particularly likely to occur when the plasma level of unconjugated bilirubin exceeds 250 μmol/l. By far the commonest cause of this in full-term Caucasian infants is haemolytic anaemia due to fetal–maternal Rh incompatibility. In some other ethnic groups, haemolysis due to G-6-PD deficiency is an important cause (p. 602). Other causal factors include functional immaturity of the liver in premature infants, liver injury of various kinds and genetically determined defects in bilirubin conjugation. Hypoxia during labour or at birth, or due to severe anaemia, may be contributory factors and the administration of excess vitamin K analogues tends to aggravate haemolysis and so may increase the jaundice.

Non-metastatic (Remote) Effects of Malignant Tumours

Many tumours metastasize to the brain and the spinal cord. Others, however, particularly carcinoma of the bronchus and lymphoma, may have an indirect effect on the nervous system, at different levels, singly or in combination. Various neurological syndromes develop in about 6% of all patients with carcinoma: there is no constant relationship between the course of the neurological disorders and that of the carcinoma. They may develop concurrently or the neurological disorder may antedate evidence of tumour. The commonest disorder is a **peripheral neuropathy** (p. 863) which may be predominantly motor or sensory, or of mixed type. Other conditions in this group are a **myasthenic syndrome** (p. 879), a **diffuse encephalomyelitis** characterized histologically by perivascular cuffing with lymphocytes and affecting particularly the medial parts of the temporal lobes – **limbic encephalitis**, and **subacute cerebellar atrophy** characterized by a severe loss of Purkinje cells and degeneration of the long motor and sensory tracts in the spinal cord.

The aetiology of these disorders is uncertain. Many suggestions have been put forward and they include toxins, infections, autoimmune processes, and metabolic and endocrine disorders. The presence of inflammatory lesions in the nervous system, similar to those seen in virus infections, certainly suggests the possibility that a neurotropic virus is the cause of encephalomyelitis. An alternative explanation is that of an antigen–antibody reaction since specific circulating antibodies against neural tissue have been described in some cases. Infections occur commonly in patients with lymphoma, and are usually due to loss of immunocompetence.

Deficiency Disorders and Intoxications

Deficiencies of vitamins and protein are responsible for various neurological disorders. In the developed countries of Europe and North America many cases of vitamin deficiency are due to alcoholism, less commonly to malabsorption from gastrointestinal tract disease and rarely to food fads. In contrast, the deficiency syndromes that are common in certain underdeveloped countries are usually due to an inadequate food supply. Malnutrition may cause irreparable brain damage at certain critical periods of both prenatal and postnatal development.

Interest in the effect of toxins on the nervous system has been growing rapidly. Some toxic disorders may occur as a result of exposure to a host of substances that include drugs (e.g. phenytoin, chemotherapeutic agents), pest control products, industrial chemicals (e.g. carbon disulphate and solvents), chemical warfare agents, food additives, heavy metals (e.g. lead and mercury), the products or components of living organisms, and other substances that include, for example, alcohol, inhalants or narcotics.

Deficiency Disorders

Vitamin B_1 (Thiamine)

In addition to causing beriberi and a peripheral neuropathy, vitamin B_1 deficiency sometimes presents as a **Wernicke–Korsakoff syndrome**

(Wernicke's encephalopathy). The deficiency may be chronic as in alcoholism, prolonged malnutrition and malabsorption, or it may be acute, e.g. as a complication of persistent vomiting. Chronic alcoholism remains the commonest underlying cause in a well nourished community. The disorder was common among prisoners in the Far East during the Second World War and was attributed to an acute dietary deficiency.

The clinical features include disturbances of consciousness, ophthalmoplegia, nystagmus, and ataxia with, if untreated, terminal coma. The blood pyruvate level is raised and if the deficiency state is chronic there is usually also a peripheral neuropathy. Improvement following the administration of vitamin B may be dramatic. Some patients die in the acute phase of the disease. There are petechial haemorrhages in the mamillary bodies, in the floor and walls of the third ventricle, around the aqueduct in the midbrain and in the floor of the fourth ventricle. In patients who have survived an acute attack the macroscopic abnormalities may be restricted to slight granularity in the affected areas and the mamillary bodies are small. In chronic cases who develop a persistent psychosis the mamillary bodies are structurally damaged. They become shrunken, there is loss of myelin and they often have a brownish discoloration on section, due to deposition of haemosiderin, evidence of previous haemorrhage.

Vitamin B_{12} (Cyanocobalamin)

Deficiency of vitamin B_{12} affects the haemopoietic system (p. 612), epithelial surfaces and the nervous system, and within the latter structural abnormalities are found in the spinal cord and in the optic and peripheral nerves. The best known is **subacute combined degeneration of the spinal cord**, where there are degenerative changes in the lateral and posterior columns, particularly in the thoracic region (Fig. 18.38). In early cases there is focal swelling and ballooning of myelin sheaths; these lesions progressively enlarge, thereby imparting a characteristic spongy appearance to the affected white matter. Eventually there is loss of myelin, degeneration of axons and phagocytosis of the debris by macrophages. Similar histological appearances are occasionally seen in the white matter of the cerebral hemispheres and, more rarely, in the optic nerves.

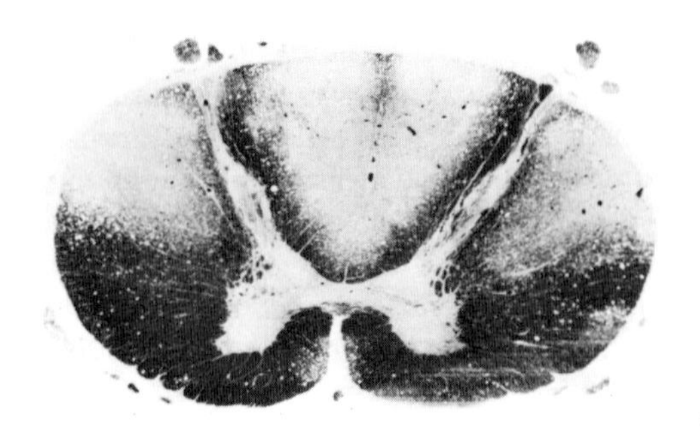

Fig. 18.38 Subacute combined degeneration. There is conspicuous demyelination in the posterior and lateral columns.

The biochemical basis for the various deleterious effects of this particular deficiency upon the nervous system is not known. Lesions in the spinal cord similar to those found in human B_{12} deficiency have been produced in monkeys exposed to nitrous oxide which is thought to inactivate one of the vitamin B_{12} dependent enzymes, thereby causing a depletion of methionine and a deficiency of the methyl group. Since highly effective purified preparations of vitamin B_{12} have been available for treatment of pernicious anaemia, this complication is now uncommon. Similar lesions have been found even more rarely in some other chronic diseases, e.g. malabsorption syndromes, leukaemia, diabetes and carcinoma. Subacute combined degeneration may develop in the pre-anaemic stage of pernicious anaemia. The administration of vitamin B_{12} in adequate doses is completely effective in preventing the development of neural lesions.

Ageing and the Dementias

The adult brain weighs between 1200 g and 1600 g and remains fairly constant throughout middle age;

after about the age of 65 years it becomes smaller as a result of atrophy, and the cerebral hemispheres shrink away from the skull. At autopsy the meninges, especially over the vertex, may become thickened and opalescent. Atrophy of the brain is shown by the presence of firm, rather narrowed gyri and widened sulci, particularly at the frontal and temporal poles, in contrast to the cerebellum which tends to be well preserved. On section there is thinning of the cortex, a reduction in the amount of white matter and compensatory enlargement of the ventricular system. Microscopical changes include some loss of neurons, and the presence of a few senile plaques in grey matter, and occasional examples of granulovacuolar and neurofibrillary degeneration.

The Dementias

Dementia is a generalized disturbance of higher mental functions in an otherwise alert patient. It may be brought about by more or less extensive destruction or disorganization of the cortex, the white matter, or the subcortical (nuclear) structures, either singly or in combination, by one or more pathological processes. The causes of dementia are therefore numerous (Table 18.5) and they have been classified into primary dementia in which the principal damage occurs in the cerebral cortex (in some cases there is associated extrapyramidal and spinal tract degeneration), and secondary dementia resulting from some other primary abnormality in the brain, e.g. infarction, tumour, general paralysis of the insane, toxic and metabolic disturbances, various infections and hydrocephalus.

Table 18.5 Causes of dementia

Causes of dementia
Primary dementias
Alzheimer's disease
Pick's disease
Huntington's disease
Parkinson's disease
Secondary dementias
Vascular
multi-infarct
systemic lupus erythematosus
Traumatic
post-traumatic encephalopathy
subdural haematoma
Post-infective
neurosyphilis – general paralysis of the insane
post-encephalitic syndromes
Creutzfeldt–Jakob disease
acquired immunodeficiency syndrome (AIDS)
Normal pressure hydrocephalus

Primary Dementia

Alzheimer's disease. This is by far the most common of the primary dementias. Females are more commonly affected than males. The aetiology of Alzheimer's disease remains obscure. Some have likened it to an acceleration of the normal ageing process, whilst others have considered it to be a separate entity. At autopsy the brain is atrophied, usually weighing 1000 g or less. The atrophy is accentuated in the frontal and temporal lobes. There is almost always compensatory enlargement of the ventricular system. Microscopy reveals a generalized loss of neurons, gliosis and a large number of **senile (neuritic) plaques** composed of masses of small argyrophilic granules and filaments often with a core of amyloid material in the cortical grey matter (Fig. 18.39). In addition, there are tangles of coarse neurofibrils (**Alzheimer's neurofibrillary degeneration**) in many of the large neurons of the cerebral cortex. It has been established recently that the levels of many biochemical cell markers are reduced in the brain in Alzheimer's disease. There is, however, relatively severe loss of choline acetyltransferase, suggesting a selective loss or dysfunction of cholinergic neurons. An important role for chromosome 21 in the neuropathology of Alzheimer's disease has long been assumed because of the development of senile plaques and neurofibrillary tangles in the brains of patients with Down's syndrome (trisomy 21) who survive to middle age.

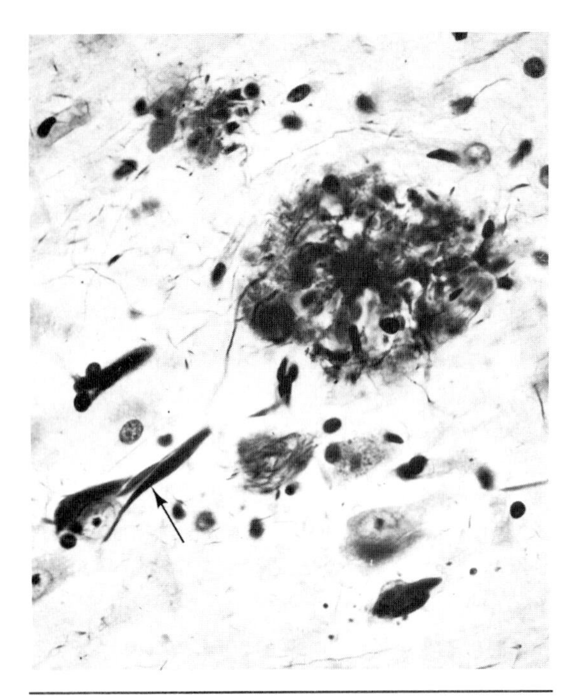

Fig. 18.39 Alzheimer's disease. There is a typical senile plaque composed of filamentous and granular material. A neurofibrillary tangle is seen in a neuron (arrow). (King's amyloid stain.) ×250.

Pick's disease. This is classified as a presenile dementia due to cortical atrophy from loss of neurons, particularly in the frontal and temporal lobes. Some of the surviving neurons are greatly enlarged by a globular argyrophilic material.

Huntington's disease. This is an autosomal dominant disorder in which a progressive dementia is accompanied by involuntary choreiform movements. It usually begins in the third or fourth decades. The incidence is about 4–7 per 100 000 population, and recent studies have linked the disease to the short arm of chromosome 4. At autopsy the brain is usually small, but the most striking feature is selective atrophy of the caudate nucleus. Several neurotransmitter systems are affected, but probably the most important is a reduction in gamma-aminobutyric acid (GABA), together with enzymes associated with it such as glutamic acid decarboxylase.

Secondary Dementias

The pathological basis for some of these has been discussed earlier.

Multi-infarct dementia. Most patients are usually elderly and hypertensive, and the dementia has a step-wise course. Widespread atheroma of the major cerebral arteries results in repeated cerebral infarction. The distribution of the infarcts does not appear to correlate with the development of dementia, and it seems likely that the dementia occurs after a certain volume of the brain – perhaps about 100 ml – has been destroyed. The ventricles are usually enlarged, symmetrically if there are multiple small infarcts in each hemisphere, and asymmetrically if the infarcts involve mainly one hemisphere.

Dementia of normal pressure hydrocephalus is of a disinhibited frontal lobe type, together with urgency of micturition and a widely ataxic gait.

Dementia due to 'slow viruses'. The archetype of this rare cause is Creutzfeldt–Jakob disease, which is linked to a variety of other forms of spongiform encephalopathy (see p. 833).

System Disorders

This is a diverse group of disorders, many of which are familial, have a hereditary basis and are characterized by a progressive degeneration of neurons and their processes within anatomically and functionally defined regions or systems. Patients may present therefore with the clinical features of disease of the sensory or motor systems, cerebellar ataxia with involuntary movements or with dementia, alone or in combination with other neurological abnormalities.

Parkinson's Syndrome (Parkinsonism)

This is a disturbance of motor function characterized by slowing of emotional and voluntary movement, akinesia, muscular rigidity and tremor, and, in some cases, dementia. The syndrome is brought about by damage to, or malfunction of, the nigral system. The majority of cases are idiopathic but types of Parkinsonism with known aetiologies include the post-encephalitic and drug-induced types (phenothiazines). Other causes are vascular, traumatic, and various toxins and poisons such as manganese, carbon monoxide, mercury and more recently, *N*-methyl-4-phenyltetrahydropyridine (MPTP) a byproduct in the synthesis of a meperidine-related opiate, marketed illegally as synthetic heroin.

The condition is brought about by selective and progressive destruction of the pigmented dopaminergic neurons in the substantia nigra and the locus ceruleus of the brain stem. There is destruction of neurons, accompanied by granules of pigment lying free in the parenchyma and within macrophages, and also some astrocytosis. Frequently some of the residual pigmented neurons contain large intracytoplasmic inclusions known as **Lewy bodies**. In advanced cases, **depigmentation of the substantia nigra** is readily apparent macroscopically (Fig. 18.40).

Lesions of the Motor and Sensory Neurons

The main acute disease of lower motor neurons, acute anterior poliomyelitis, has already been described. Chronic progressive degenerative disease of the motor neuron is usually referred to as motor neuron disease. In Friedreich's ataxia there is atrophy in both motor and sensory tracts.

Motor Neuron Disease

In this disease there is a relentless and progressive degeneration of motor neurons. It tends to occur in middle and late adult life and is more common in males than in females. The disease is usually fatal in 2–3 years. Motor neuron disease occurs world wide and has an incidence of approximately 1 per 1000 deaths. There is a particularly high incidence among the native Chamorro population of Guam, accompanied, however, by clinical features of Parkinsonism and dementia. The aetiology is unknown although suspected causes include genetic disorders, viral infection possibly related to poliomyelitis and intoxication with heavy metals.

Three variants are recognized depending on the distribution of the disease process. The commonest is **progressive muscular atrophy** when there is selective involvement of the cervical

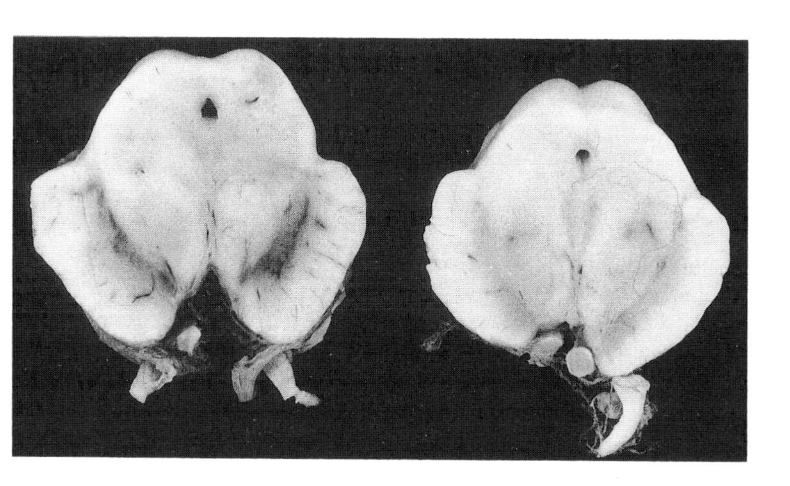

Fig. 18.40 Parkinson's disease. In comparison with the normally pigmented substantia nigra on the left, there is depigmentation of the substantia nigra on the right. (From Adams and Graham, 1988.)

region of the spinal cord, as a result of which there is fibrillation and then atrophy of the small muscles of the hand which soon assumes a characteristic claw-like form. The involvement then spreads to the muscles of the arm and shoulder girdle. Involvement of the cranial nerve nuclei in the brain stem results in **progressive bulbar palsy** with wasting and paralysis of the muscles of the tongue, lips, jaw, larynx and pharynx. The term **amyotrophic lateral sclerosis** is used when upper motor neurons are also affected, leading to degeneration of the corticospinal tracts and a spastic paraparesis. No sharply dividing line can be drawn, however, between these variants. Their names merely emphasize that in any one case the early stages of the disease may have a particular distribution. In the terminal stages there is often widespread involvement of motor neurons in the brain stem and in the spinal cord.

The most conspicuous macrosopic abnormality in the CNS is atrophy of the ventral spinal nerve roots: this is most obvious in the cervical region and in the cauda equina. The ventral horns of the spinal cord appear smaller than normal and there is atrophy of the lateral and anterior columns of the spinal cord in contrast to the striking preservation of the white matter of the posterior columns. The most important microscopic changes are loss of motor neurons and an astrocytosis, features that are particularly easily seen in the ventral horns of the cervical and lumber segments of the spinal cord and in the hypoglossal nuclei of the lower brain stem. Changes in the white matter of the spinal cord are variable, the most common being degeneration of the pyramidal tracts (Fig 18.41). There is severe neurogenic atrophy of affected muscles (see p. 871).

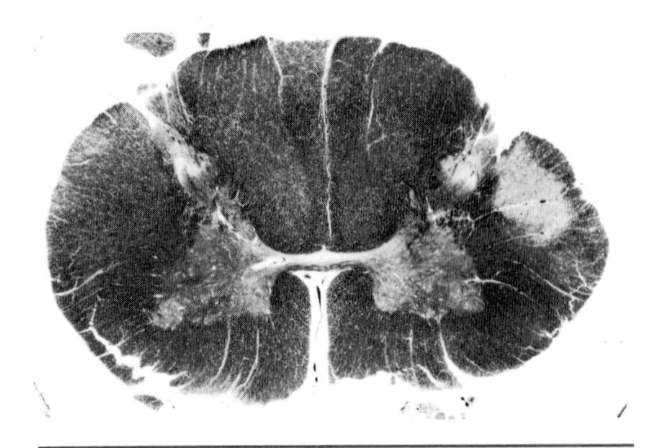

Fig. 18.41 Motor neuron disease. The ventral horns of the grey matter are small. There is some degeneration in the lateral and anterior columns, and preservation of the posterior columns. (Weigert–Pal method).

Friedreich's Ataxia

This condition is inherited as an autosomal recessive and may affect more than one member of a family. Rarely it occurs in successive generations. It usually begins in childhood and the chief symptoms are ataxia with muscular weakness. Lateral curvature of the spine and talipes equinus often develop, and nystagamus and disturbance of speech are also common. In such cases the spinal cord is found to be relatively thin, and there is degeneration of the posterior and lateral columns (Fig. 18.42). The aetiology is unknown. The condition is frequently associated with a chronic progressive myocarditis in which focal coagulative necrosis of the muscle fibres is followed by replacement fibrosis.

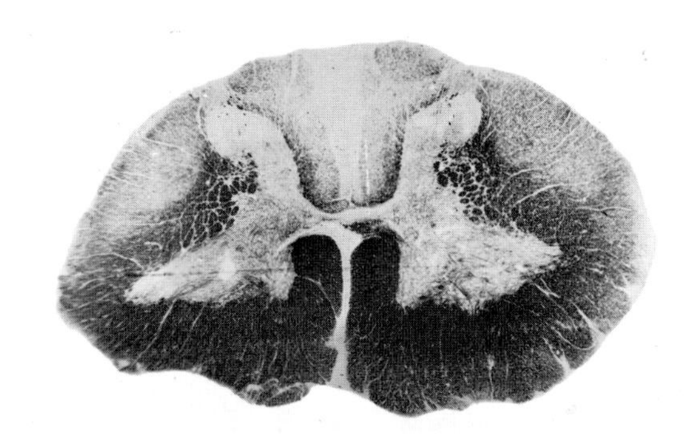

Fig. 18.42 Friedreich's ataxia. There is degeneration in the posterior and lateral columns. (Weigert–Pal method).

Developmental Abnormalities

There are serious developmental abnormalities in between 2 and 3% of all infants at birth, and of these approximately one-third are malformations of the CNS. In over 50% of cases the aetiology of congenital malformations remains undetermined. Important considerations, however, include either singly or in combination genetic factors (e.g. microcephaly), chromosomal abnormalities (such as trisomy 21), and various environmental factors including maternal infections such as rubella and cytomegalovirus, irradiation to the pelvis during the first 4 months of pregnancy, the fetal-alcohol syndrome, pharmaceutical drugs, tobacco and possibly vitamin deficiencies. The CNS is susceptible throughout its various phases of development. The teratogenic effects of an agent depend on its nature, the gestational stage at which it acts and the genetic background of the individual.

Chromosomal Abnormalities

The clinically important disorders in which there is extra chromosomal material and which are characterized by mental retardation include trisomy 21, 18 and 13. Abnormalities of sex chromosomes include the Kleinfelter (XXY) and Turner syndromes (XO), and many are associated with mental retardation.

Down's Syndrome

This has an incidence of 1.4 per 1000 live births: 95% are due to trisomy of chromosome 21 as a result of non-dysjunction at meiosis, 4% to translocation between chromosome 21 and one of the D or G chromosomes, and 1% are mosaics. The incidence in babies born to women over the age of 40 is about 1% and increases with age. The brain is usually small and the characteristic feature in cases more than 30 years of age is the presence of a large number of Alzheimer neurofibrillary tangles and plaques. Quantitative comparison of the tangles and plaques in the hippocampi of patients with Down's syndrome with normal ageing and familial forms of Alzheimer's disease have revealed marked similarity in the regional topography, and have served to highlight the importance of chromosome 21 in these processes.

Defects in the Neural Tube

The incidence in the UK varies from 0.1 to 1% of live births: there is a familial tendency and the risk of recurrence after one affected child is about 5%. Defects of the neural tube may be diagnosed prenatally by the presence of raised alphafetoprotein levels in blood and amniotic fluid and by ultrasonography. Defects of the neural tube are induced by damage occurring during the fourth week of fetal development and are thought to result from a combination of genetic and environmental factors.

Anencephaly

Three-quarters of affected infants are female. The head is retroflexed and appears to sit on the shoulders. The cranial vault is missing, and the base of the skull is flattened. The brain is represented by a small disc-shaped disorganized mass of glia, malformed brain and choroid plexus, the **area cerebrovasculosa**, which sits on the base of the skull and is usually covered by a thin smooth membrane.

Defects of the Spinal Neural Tube

Defects limited to the spine with failure of fusion of the neural arches are called spina bifida (Fig. 18.43). The majority occur in the lumbosacral region.

Spina bifida cystica. In some 80–90% of these the lesion is a myelomeningocele in which the abnormal cord is exposed by a defect in skin, the vertebral arches and meninges: there are often

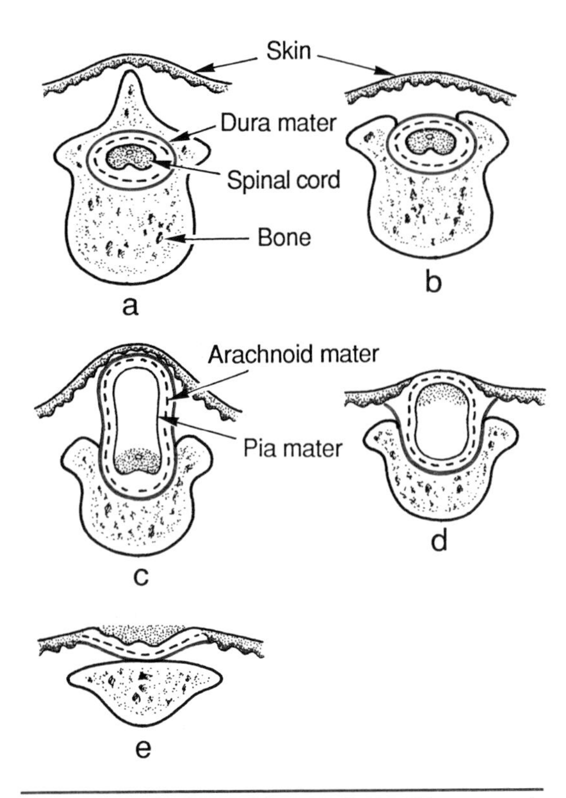

Fig. 18.43 Defects of the neural tube. Diagrammatic representation of spina bifida. **a**, Normal; **b**, spina bifida occulta; **c**, meningocele; **d**, myelomeningocele; **e**, myelocele. (From Adams and Graham, 1988.)

associated abnormalities such as syringomyelia or diastematomyelia. In the remaining 10–20% of cases, the lesion is a meningocele which involves only meninges, vertebral arches and skin and the cord is virtually normal. The quality of life in most of those patients who survive with myelomeningocele is poor, the sequelae including incontinence of urine and faeces, flaccid areflexic weakness of the legs and lumbar kyphosis. Many suffer from moderate or severe mental retardation.

Spina bifida occulta is said to occur in 17% of normal adults as determined by the absence of one or more spinous processes radiologically. Limited to the lumbosacral region, the dysraphic abnormality is covered by skin which may show abnormal pigmentation, a hairy patch or a dermal sinus. In many instances this condition is asymptomatic but neurological disturbances may, however, develop in adult life.

Encephalocele

This condition is a hernia of brain tissue and meninges through a midline defect in the cranial cavity. Females are more commonly affected than males, and in western Europe some 80% occur in the occipital region where an encephalocele protrudes through either the foramen magnum or the squamous occipital bone. Large encephaloceles are usually incompatible with life.

Malformations of the Cerebellum

Chiari Malformations

Chiari originally described three types of malformation affecting the cerebellum, the brain stem and the base of the skull. The type II lesion is also known as the Arnold–Chiari malformation and is, next to anencephaly, the most common severe malformation of the CNS. In the type II malformation there is an abnormality of the hindbrain and cerebellum associated with a lumbar myelomeningocele and with hydrocephalus. There are two main components of the hindbrain abnormality. First, there is displacement of the vermis of the cerebellum through the foramen magnum into the upper portion of the spinal canal, and secondly, there is caudal displacement of the medulla which appears narrow, S-shaped and elongated, much of it lying below the level of the foramen magnum. As a result of the downward displacement of the brain stem into the cervical canal, the lower cranial nerves and cervical nerve roots run a cephalad course from their point of origin. Additional features include a shallow malformed posterior fossa, low insertion of the tentorium, and thickened and fibrotic meninges in relation to both the herniated tissue and the exit foramina of the fourth ventricle. Hydrocephalus is almost invariably present since the exit foramina of the fourth ventricle lie within the spinal canal.

Dandy Walker Malformation

This disorder is associated with a malformation of the cerebellar vermis. The posterior fossa is enlarged with elevations of the torcula, the tentorium and the lateral and straight sinuses. In some two-thirds of cases there are associated anomalies. Its aetiology is uncertain but it may be due to failure of the foramen of Magendie to perforate, leading to dilatation of the fourth ventricle, which subsequently becomes a large cyst in the posterior fossa.

Malformations Involving the Whole Brain

These conditions are commonly the end result of many disease processes related to genetic, chromosomal and environmental factors.

Microcephaly

This denotes a brain that weighs less than 1000 g in adults or less than two standard deviations below the mean normal weight for the age and sex of the patient. It may result from diverse disorders that include degenerative, destructive, or congenital conditions. For example, it may result from congenital infections such as rubella, toxoplasmosis and cytomegalic inclusion body disease, or may be the result of toxins, irradiation and metabolic disorders. It is also common in chromosomal abnormalities. In contrast to the secondary forms of microcephaly, there is a form of primary formative microcephaly in which the frontal and temporal lobes are particularly small and the gyral pattern may be either simplified or more complex than usual.

Megalencephaly

This generally refers to a brain that in the adult weighs more than 1700 g or more than 2.5 standard deviations from the mean normal for the age and sex of the patient. Primary megalencephaly may be an isolated finding, or associated with achondroplasia and endocrine disorders or it may be familial. Secondary megalencephaly may be due to metabolic disorders such as Tay–Sachs disease and certain leucodystrophies. There is also an association with tuberous sclerosis.

Destructive Lesions often Resembling Primary Malformations

This group of disorders is due to the destructive action of agents that act on the brain after its initial period of organogenesis. They therefore resemble developmental abnormalities but in fact are acquired *in utero*. Causal agents include drugs or their metabolites, ionizing radiation and infections such as cytomegalovirus, toxoplasmosis and rubella. Some of the lesions appear to be due to the failure of cerebral perfusion, either from disease of the placenta or hypotension in the mother. The term, **porencephaly**, is applied when part of the brain is replaced by a collection of fluid, covered by meninges, and sometimes in communication with the ventricles. A more severe form of porencephaly is **hydranencephaly** in which there is virtual absence of the cerebral hemisphere except for the basal ganglia and thalami, and the temporal and occipital lobes. This condition is thought to be due to fetal hypoxia.

Phacomatoses

This group of mainly familial disorders is characterized by malformations of the neuraxis together with multiple small tumours which involve neuroectodermal structures. The skin, the eyes and some internal organs such as the kidneys are also commonly involved.

Neurofibromatosis (von Recklinghausen's Disease)

This autosomal dominant disease is relatively common (1 in 3000). In its mildest form the condition may be limited to cutaneous *café au lait* pigmentation and cutaneous neurofibromas. Visceral lesions and elephantiasis may be present. In the central form of the disease there may be various developmental abnormalities. Tumours are common, the most characteristic being bilateral schwannomas of the eighth cranial nerve, and tumours of spinal nerve roots (see p. 866).

Tuberous Sclerosis (Bourneville's Disease)

Tuberous sclerosis, an autosomal dominant, affects 1 per 100 000 subjects. It is characterized clinically by seizures and mental retardation usually presenting in infancy. Other manifestations include adenoma sebaceum of the skin, rhabdomyomas of the heart, angiomyolipomas of the kidney and pancreatic cysts. The brain may be small, normal or of increased size, the most characteristic feature being the presence of pale, firm tubers in the cerebral cortex. These lesions show loss of cortical architecture and contain large bizarre multinucleate neurons and astrocytes. Nodular protuberances are also present in the walls of the ventricles.

The Spinal Cord

The tissue of the spinal cord is similar to that of the brain, but the relative frequencies of various lesions are very different. Specific diseases of the spinal cord are described elsewhere: **subacute combined degeneration** due to vitamin B_{12} deficiency (see p. 842); **syringomyelia** and the system disorders of **motor neuron disease** (see p. 845) and **Friedreich's ataxia** (see p. 846). Lesions of the spinal cord are one of the most serious features of **acute decompression sickness** (p. 99) and related non-thrombotic embolic phenomena including **air embolism** and **fat embolism**. So-called transverse lesions, various types of spinal injury and the consequent ascending and descending Wallerian degeneration within the cord, and vascular lesions will be dealt with here.

The spinal cord in transverse section is shown diagrammatically in Fig. 18.44. The **ascending posterior columns** convey impulses concerned with joint sensation, vibration, pressure discrimination and touch. The columns receive axons from sensory neurons in posterior root ganglia and are added to the posterior columns in a clockwise direction so that the axons from the lumbar and sacral regions are closer to the midline than those from the thoracic and cervical regions. The **spinothalamic tracts** convey the modalities of pain, temperature, touch and deep pressure. The system receives sensory fibres which participate in a complex synaptic network in the dorsal grey horn. The **spinocerebellar tracts** carry afferent (mainly proprioceptive) information.

At the junction of the medulla and the spinal cord the descending corticospinal system that subserves motor function undergoes incomplete decussation, giving rise to two main tracts – a large **lateral corticospinal tract (crossed)** and a **smaller anterior corticospinal tract (uncrossed)**. The latter does not extend further than the upper thoracic region. Within the lateral corticospinal tract the fibres supplying motor nerves that innervate the muscles of the arm are sited medially, whereas those that descend to the lower segments of the cord are placed more laterally.

The descending fibres associated with higher control of sphincter function are also in the lateral white matter of the cord just in front of the lateral corticospinal tracts. Ascending fibres associated with bladder function are in the more superficial part of the lateral white columns.

Transverse Lesions

These occur when partial or complete interruption of the cord is produced by local disease or trauma.

Slowly progressive effects may be produced by **extrinsic tumours** in the extradural space, e.g. metastatic carcinoma (Fig. 18.45) or lym-

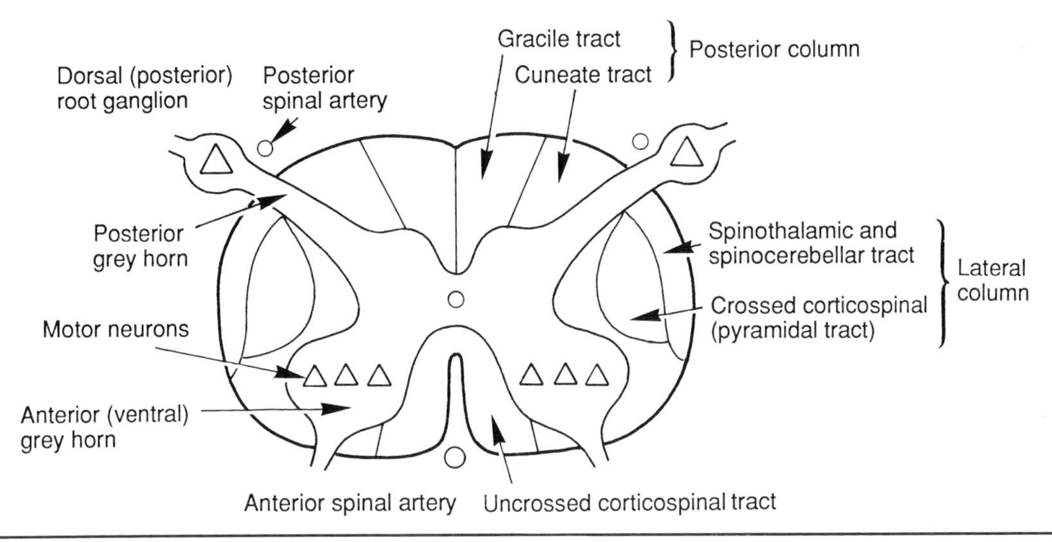

Fig. 18.44 Diagrammatic representation of the main structures within the spinal cord.

phoma, or in the subdural space, e.g. meningioma or schwannoma. **Intrinsic tumours**, e.g. astrocytoma or ependymoma, are rare causes. **Tuberculosis** is still a common cause in various parts of the world. It leads to angular curvature of the spine, 'cold' abscesses and granulomatous masses, any of which can cause pressure on the cord: this may be so severe that infarction of the cord may occur at this level.

The term **Froins' syndrome** refers to changes in CSF that occur when the spinal cord is compressed by a gross lesion which also blocks the subarachnoid space. There is a great increase in protein concentration and the fluid coagulates rapidly after withdrawal; it is often yellow (xanthochromia). There may also be a slight increase in lymphocytes.

Acute transverse lesions may be due to **trauma**, usually a fracture dislocation of the vertebra, **infarction** when the circulation of the anterior spinal artery is impaired, **haemorrhage** usually from a vascular malformation or **acute demyelination**. The term **transverse myelitis** is a clinical rather than a pathological one and is applied when there is an acute transverse lesion of the spinal cord in the absence of a compressive lesion, e.g. due to infarction, demyelination, caisson disease, infection or haemorrhage.

The inevitable consequence of a total or partial transverse lesion of the cord, besides the local damage, is the development of ascending and descending Wallerian degeneration (see p. 807) in the interrupted tracts of the spinal cord. Degeneration occurs in those fibres that are separated from their cell bodies by the lesion and is best demonstrated by the Marchi technique. The degenerating fibres appear black from about a week after onset. The method is applicable until the degenerated myelin has disappeared – that is, for 3 months or so. In older lesions stains for normal myelin should be used since, when the degenerate myelin has become absorbed, the affected tract appears as a pale area.

Ascending Degeneration

If we take as an example a comparatively recent lesion in the lower thoracic spinal cord, the ascending degeneration found in a section taken a few segments above the lesion will involve the posterior columns and the spinothalamic and spinocerebellar tracts (Fig. 18.46). In the cervical region, however, the degeneration in the posterior columns is practically confined to the gracile tracts (Fig. 18.47) because the cuneate tract is composed of ascending fibres that have joined the cord above the level of the lesion. Degeneration of affected axons ascends up to the cuneate and

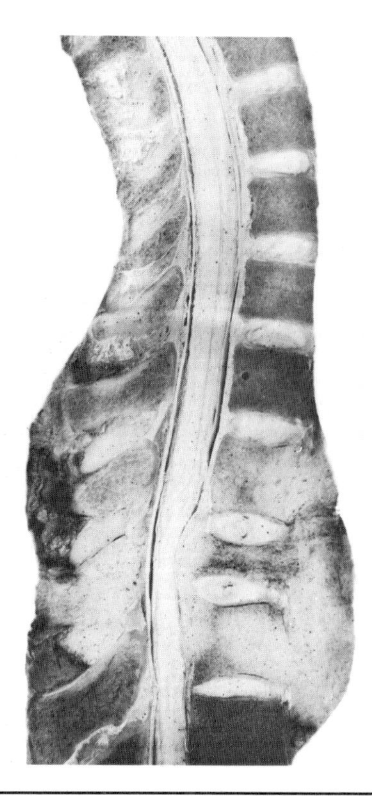

Fig. 18.45 Compression of the spinal cord. Metastatic carcinoma in the vertebral bodies is compressing the spinal cord.

gracile nuclei in the medulla. Ascending degeneration in the posterior spinocerebellar tract extends up to the inferior cerebellar peduncle and into the

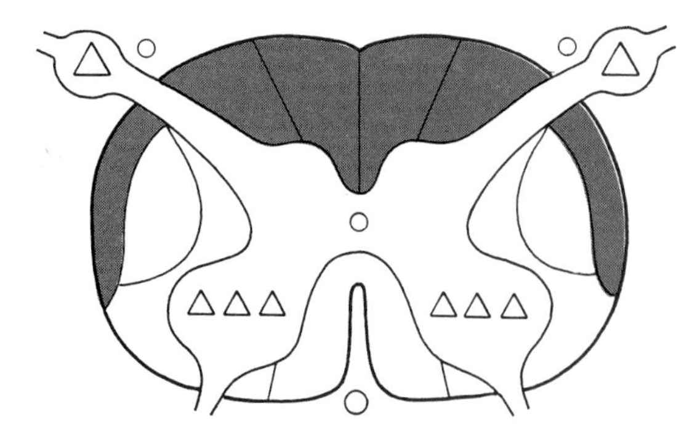

Fig. 18.46 Diagram of spinal cord immediately above a transverse lesion. There is degeneration of the posterior columns and the spinothalamic and spinocerebellar tracts.

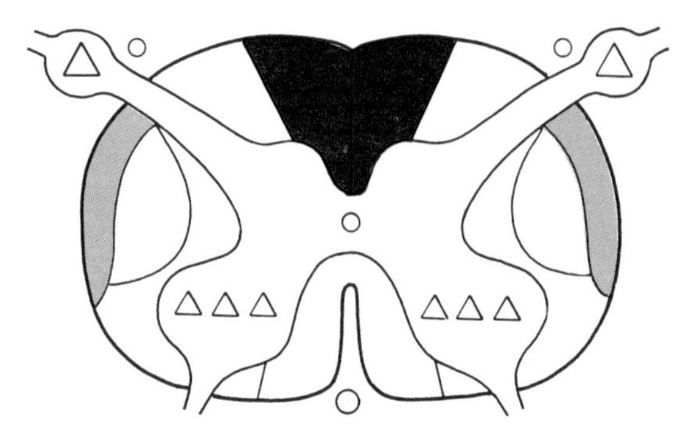

Fig. 18.47 Diagram of spinal cord well above a transverse lesion. There is preservation of the cuneate tracts and there is less severe degeneration in the spinothalamic and spinocerebellar tracts.

cerebellum, and in the anterior spinocerebellar tract to the middle lobe of the cerebellum. In all lesions, loss of myelin and gliosis are most conspicuous in the posterior columns because the inflow of normal myelinated fibres above the lesion masks the loss of myelinated fibres in the spinocerebellar and spinothalamic tracts.

Descending Degeneration

This occurs below a transverse lesion in the cord, and as a result of lesions in certain parts of the brain. With a transverse lesion of the cord, the most marked degeneration is in the crossed (lateral) and uncrossed (anterior) pyramidal tracts (Fig. 18.48). The commonest example due to a

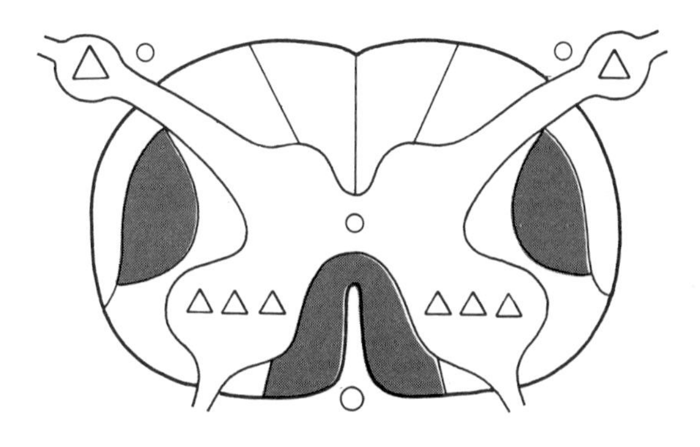

Fig. 18.48 Diagram of spinal cord below a transverse lesion. There is degeneration in the corticospinal tracts.

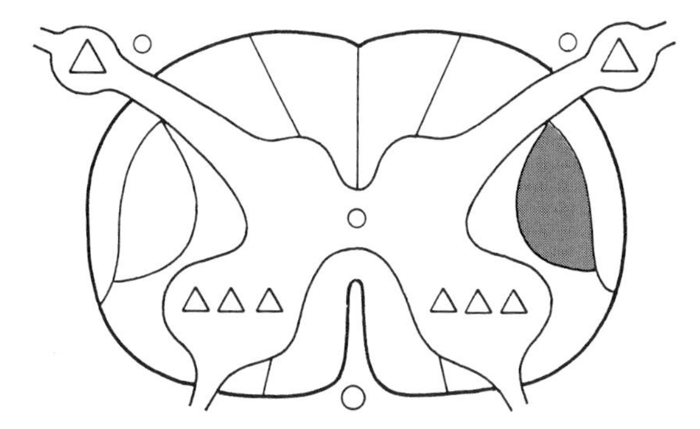

Fig. 18.49 Diagram of spinal cord resulting from an old infarct in the internal capsule. There is degeneration in one corticospinal tract.

lesion of the brain is destruction of the motor fibres in the internal capsule by cerebrovascular disease. There is degeneration of the crossed pyramidal tract on the opposite and of the uncrossed pyramidal tract on the same side (Fig. 18.49). As the uncrossed pyramidal tract does not usually extend below the upper thoracic segments, its degeneration will not be seen in sections below this.

Spinal Injury

These may be non-missile or missile injuries. The former result from subluxations and fracture/dislocations of the vertebral column, and are usually brought about by acute flexion or extension. Missile injuries are caused by such objects as bullets or may be caused by a stab wound. The clinical outcome depends on the extent of irreversible damage at the level of injury where there are varying degrees of haemorrhagic necrosis. The affected cord is soft and swollen and there is often a traumatic **haematomyelia** which is a collection of blood within the cord. This often extends as a fusiform mass for some distance above and below the level of injury. Eventually the dead tissue is removed and the cord becomes greatly narrowed. A delayed – often many years after the accident – result of trauma is the development of **post-traumatic syringomyelia**.

Prolapsed Intervertebral Disc

This is a common cause of compression of the nerve roots and more rarely causes compression of the cord. The intervertebral disc consists of a central nodule of semi-fluid matrix, the nucleus pulposus, surrounded by a ring of fibrous tissue and fibrocartilage, the annulus fibrosus. The posterior segment of the annulus is thinner and less firmly attached to bone and, following unusual stress, part of the matrix of the nucleus pulposus may herniate through it. This lesion, often termed 'slipped disc', usually tracks posterolaterally around the expansion of the posterior longitudinal ligament, appearing at one side and compressing the nerve root in the intervertebral foramen (Fig. 18.50).

Disc protrusions almost always occur in the lumbar spine and L5/S1, L4/L5 and L3/L4 discs are affected in that order of frequency: they also occur occasionally in the cervical spine. If the protrusion is small, localized pain is produced by irritation of the posterior longitudinal ligament: if larger there may also be root pain due to pressure on nerves leaving the spinal column, producing the clinical signs and symptoms of sciatica. The rarer central protrusions are of greater importance since they compress the cauda equina, as a result of which there may be paraparesis and sphincter dysfunction.

Cervical Spondylosis

This results from degeneration of intervertebral discs in the cervical region. The disc spaces are

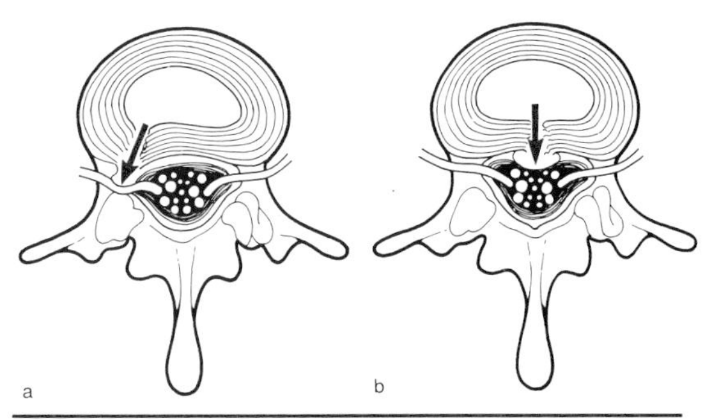

Fig. 18.50 Prolapsed intervertebral disc. **a** Posterolateral protrusion compressing a nerve; **b** central protrusion compressing the cauda equina. (From Adams and Graham, 1988.)

narrowed and transverse bars develop in the vertebral canal as a result of posterior protrusion of the annulus. Osteophytes form and as the spondylosis progresses there may, in addition to compression of nerve roots, be interference with the blood supply to the spinal cord where the vertebral canal is narrowest. The importance of cervical spondylosis is uncertain as it can be demonstrated radiologically in some 50% of adults over the age of 50 and in some 75% over 65. It may be therefore that secondary ischaemic damage in the spinal cord – **cervical myelopathy** – occurs only in individuals where antecedent congenital narrowing of the vertebral canal is aggravated by the development of cervical spondylosis.

Vascular Lesions of the Spinal Cord

Infarction of the spinal cord is usually due to disease of the anterior spinal artery. The blood supply to the ventral portion of the cord may be affected in neurosyphilis, collagen disorders, compression of the segmental artery by tumour, dissecting aneurysm of the aorta and surgery upon the aorta.

Arteriovenous malformations are congenital abnormalities of blood vessels and may present clinically at any age in either sex but are most common in males in the sixth or seventh decade. The commonest site is in the thoracolumbar region and the lesion may be extra- or intradural or within both compartments. The majority of patients present with progressive deterioration of all spinal modalities, simulating cord compression. Only some 10–15% present with a sudden onset of acute cord compression due to haemorrhage.

Malformations of the Spinal Cord

Spina bifida has already been described.

Syringomyelia

This is a cyst-like space (syrinx) or spaces that develop within the cervical cord (syringomyelia) or lower brain stem (syringobulbia). The cavity usually extends through several segments of the cervical cord and as it enlarges the cord becomes swollen and feels somewhat soft. Histologically the tissue around the cavity is seen to consist of large astrocytes. Occasionally, syringomyelia occurs in association with tumours affecting the spinal cord. The effects are due principally to destruction of the cord by the enlarging cavity (Fig. 18.51). The first fibres to be affected are the decussating sensory fibres conveying the sensations of heat and pain: the resulting defect, known as **dissociated anaesthesia**, is a selective insensitivity to heat and pain in the region corresponding to the involved segments of the spinal cord. A neuropathic arthritis occurs, closely similar to that in tabes, but as syringomyelia is usually in the cervical region, the joints of the upper limbs are chiefly involved. Trophic lesions also occur in the skin.

Diastematomyelia

This is the term applied when the cord is split into two by a fibrous or bony spur projecting into the vertebral canal. It occurs predominantly in the

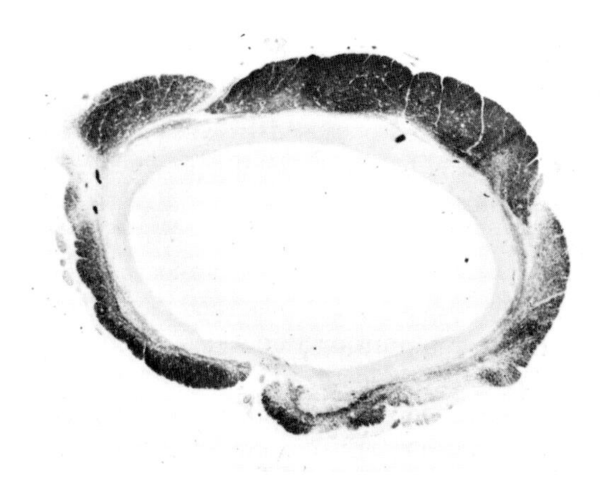

Fig. 18.51 Syringomyelia. There is a large central cavity in the spinal cord in the lower cervical region. (Weigert–Pal method).

thoracolumbar spine and is often associated with other anomalies such as spina bifida occulta and the Arnold–Chiari malformation. There is usually a localized kyphoscoliosis at the site of the lesion.

Tumours of the Nervous System

An abbreviated classification of tumours of the nervous system is given in Table 18.6. Tumours of neuroepithelial tissue have an average annual incidence of between 3 and 4 per 100 000 of the population. Up to the age of 15 years they are the second commonest form of cancer, being exceeded only by leukaemia. Metastatic tumours have a similar incidence. Intracranial tumours may produce local effects which will depend upon their site, e.g. focal epilepsy, hemiparesis or hemianopia, and they also behave as expanding intracranial lesions leading to a raised intracranial pressure. The effective size of the tumour is frequently contributed to by oedema in the adjacent brain; this usually responds dramatically to steroid therapy.

Tumours of nerve sheath cells are discussed on p. 866.

Table 18.6 Classification of tumours of the nervous system

- Tumours of neuroepithelial tissue
  - Astrocytic tumours
    - Astrocytoma
    - Anaplastic astrocytoma
  - Oligodendroglial tumours
    - Oligodendroglioma
    - Anaplastic oligodendroglioma
  - Ependymal and choroid plexus tumours
    - Ependymoma
    - Myxopapillary ependymoma
    - Anaplastic ependymoma
    - Choroid plexus papilloma
  - Neuronal tumours
    - Ganglioglioma
  - Poorly differentiated and embryonal tumours
    - Glioblastoma
    - Medulloblastoma
    - Gliomatosis cerebri
- Tumours of nerve sheath cells
  - Schwannoma (neurilemmoma)
  - Neurofibroma
  - Malignant variants
- Tumours of meningeal tissue
  - Meningioma
  - Anaplastic meningioma
- Primary malignant lymphomas
- Tumours of blood vessel origin
  - Haemangioblastoma
- Other malformative tumours and tumour-like lesions
  - Craniopharyngioma
  - Epidermoid and dermoid cysts
  - Colloid cyst of the third ventricle
- Extensions from regional tumours
  - Glomus jugulare tumour (chemodectoma, paraganglioma)
  - Chordoma
  - Chondroma
  - Chondrosarcoma
- Metastatic tumours

Of the primary tumours overall 60% are gliomas, 20% meningiomas and the rest comprise 20%. Metastatic tumours are as frequent as gliomas so that they comprise 25–30% of all intracranial tumours.

Tumours of Neuroepithelial Tissue

The great majority of tumours of neuroepithelial tissue are derived from the neuroglia, viz. **astrocytes, oligodendrocytes and ependymal cells**, the corresponding tumours **being astrocytoma, oliogodendroglioma** and **ependymoma**. These tumours are known collectively as the **gliomas**. Some are composed of cells that are very similar to mature neuroglial cells, whilst others are anaplastic. The term anaplasia includes features like cellular pleomorphism, loss of cellular differentiation, the presence of mitotic figures, the occurrence of vascular endothelial hyperplasia (Fig. 18.52) and the presence of necrosis (Fig. 18.53).

As in other tissues, the general rule usually applies that the more primitive or undifferentiated the cells are, the more rapid is their growth. The

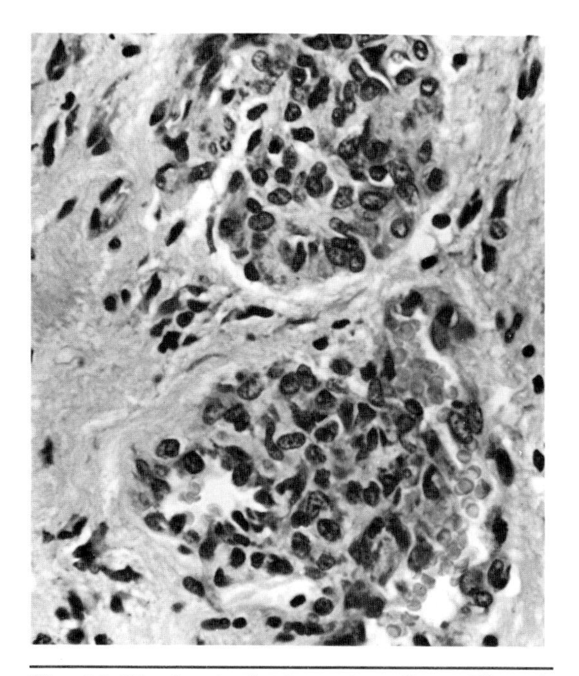

Fig. 18.52 Anaplastic change in a glioma. There is intense capillary endothelial hyperplasia. ×390.

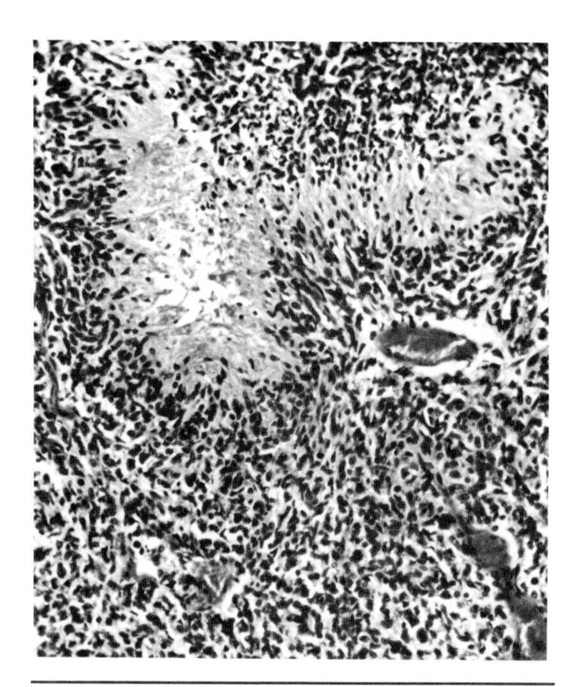

Fig. 18.53 Anaplastic change in a glioma. There are areas of necrosis within the tumour around which there is palisading of tumour cells. ×130.

terms 'benign' and 'malignant' have different connotations than they have with most tumours in other systems of the body: no matter how well differentiated or benign a glioma appears, it almost invariably infiltrates into the adjacent brain; and no matter how poorly differentiated the glioma appears, they very rarely metastasize. Any type of glioma, however, may occasionally spread diffusely throughout the subarachnoid space, this being termed **meningeal gliomatosis**.

Astrocytoma

This is by far the commonest type of glioma. It is a slowly growing, greyish white tumour, usually poorly defined where it merges with the surrounding tissue. Some contain abundant glial fibrils and are tough, almost rubbery: others have scanty glial fibrils and are soft. Cystic change is common (Fig. 18.54), particularly in the cerebellar astrocytoma of childhood. Various types are described, depending on the predominant type of astrocyte, e.g. *fibrillary*, *protoplasmic*, *gemistocytic* or *pilocytic*. On histological examination there is often also microcystic change.

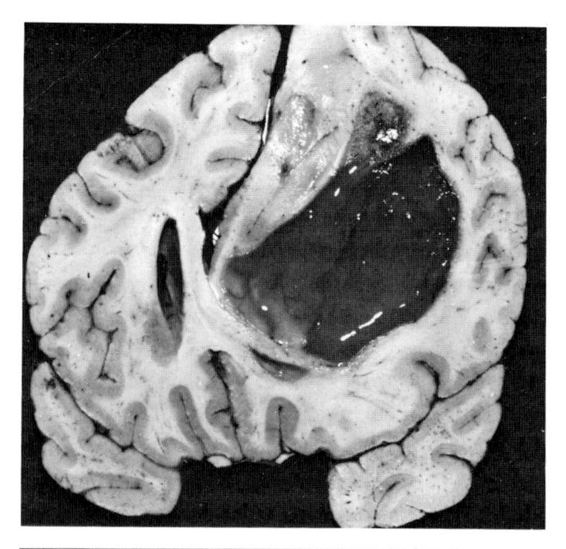

Fig. 18.54 Astrocytoma. There is a cystic tumour in the right frontal lobe. Tumour tissue is identifiable adjacent to the upper pole of the cyst.

Astrocytomas display a marked tendency to become anaplastic: this may be restricted to one part of the tumour or it may be multifocal. The anaplastic areas are haemorrhagic and necrotic and often appear to have a relatively well defined edge. The histological features of anaplasia are as described above.

Oligodendroglioma

They are slowly growing, often rather gelatinous and commonly calcified tumours. The cells are uniformly small and round like normal oligodendroglial cells with clear cytoplasm and distinct cell membranes (Fig. 18.55). Anaplastic change is less common than in astrocytomas.

Ependymoma

Ependymoma tends to be an intraventricular tumour. It occurs most frequently in children, usually in the fourth ventricle. It may also occur within the spinal cord. The tumour cells often have a distinctly epithelial appearance and they are characteristically orientated around small blood vessels but are separated from them by an eosinophilic fibrillary band (Fig. 18.56). Less frequently, columnar cells form small canaliculi. Ependymomas may also become anaplastic.

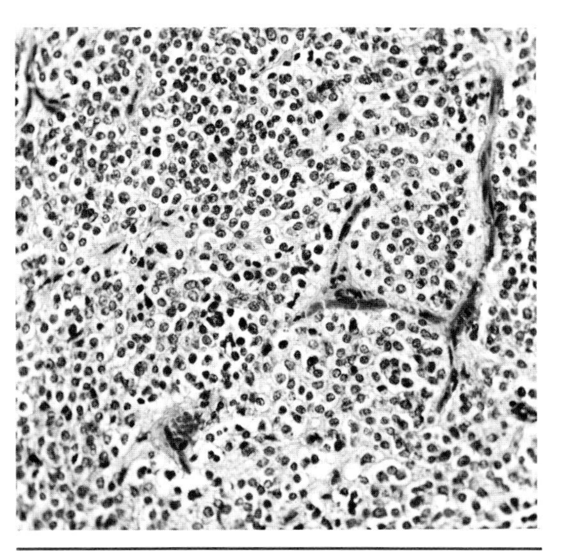

Fig. 18.55 Oligodendroglioma. The tumour is composed of round or oval cells with distinct cell boundaries. ×125.

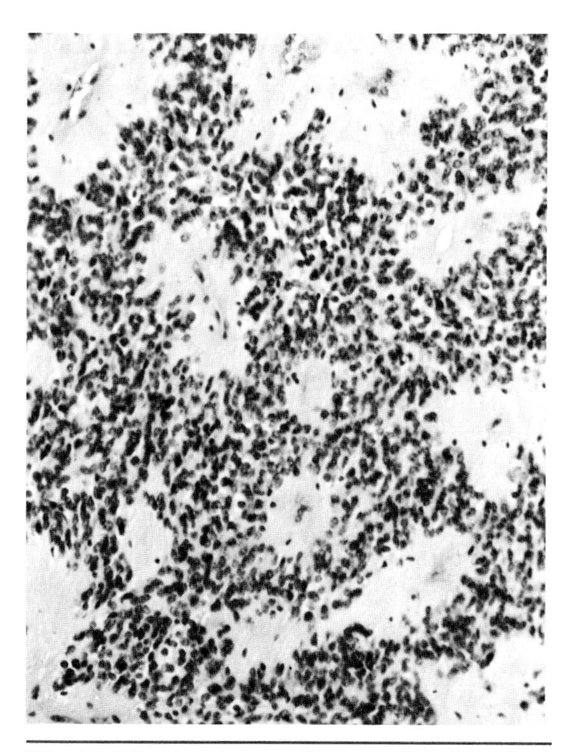

Fig. 18.56 Ependymoma. Perivascular pale fibrillary haloes are characteristic of this type of tumour.

The **myxopapillary ependymoma** arises from the filum terminale. It is a slowly growing, markedly gelatinous tumour that gradually ensheaths the nerve roots of the cauda equina and the caudal part of the spinal cord. The stroma consists of a central vascular core surrounded by mucoid connective tissue and covered in places by cuboidal epithelium.

Closely related to the ependymomas is the **choroid plexus papilloma**. This is also most often seen in children, forming a rounded bulky tumour within a ventricle. The papillae have a vascular connective tissue core covered by columnar epithelium, very similiar in appearance to normal choroid plexus.

Ganglioglioma

This type of tumour is very similar to the non-cystic astrocytomas. In addition to the astrocyomatous element, however, the tumour is interspersed with large bizarre, binucleate, and often multinucleate ganglion cells containing Nissl granules. The tumour may become anaplastic, the anaplastic change usually occurring in the astrocytic element.

Glioblastoma

This is a neuroepithelial tumour that is highly anaplastic throughout. They occur mainly in adults in the cerebral hemispheres and present as rapidly growing, sometimes relatively well-defined masses, with extensive necrosis and haemorrhage (Fig. 18.57). They produce considerable distortion of the brain and often a rapid increase of intracranial pressure. They are highly cellular in the areas that are not necrotic, and there are great variations of cell type ranging from closely packed masses of small anaplastic cells to pleomorphic giant cells (Fig. 18.58). Mitoses are frequent and glial fibrils extremely scanty. Vascular endothelial hyperplasia is usually conspicuous.

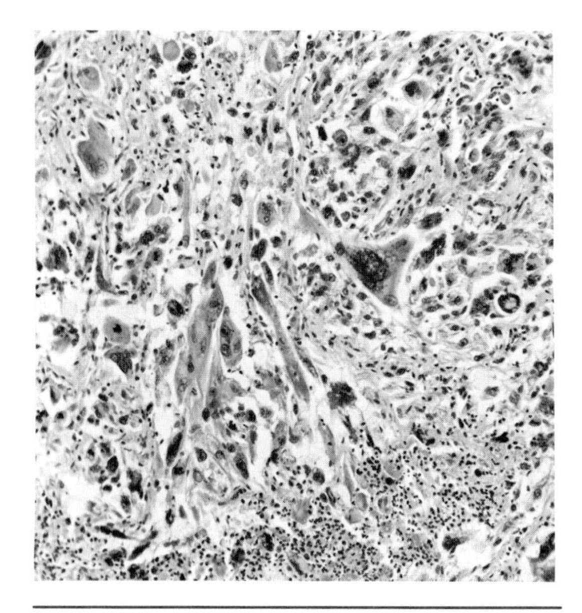

Fig. 18.58 Glioblastoma. There are many aberrant giant cells. ×110.

Medulloblastoma

Medulloblastoma, a tumour of the posterior fossa occurring most often in childhood, may sometimes also occur in young adults. It is a poorly differentiated, rapidly growing tumour that originates in the cerebellum. It usually presents as a soft, greyish white mass protruding into the fourth ventricle. It has a particular predilection for spread throughout the subarachnoid space and it frequently 'seeds' rostrally into the ventricular system and caudally into the spinal subarachnoid space. On histological examination it is composed of closely packed, slightly elongated cells with, not infrequently, rosette formations without a central cavity (Fig. 18.59). Tumours of similar morphology occasion-

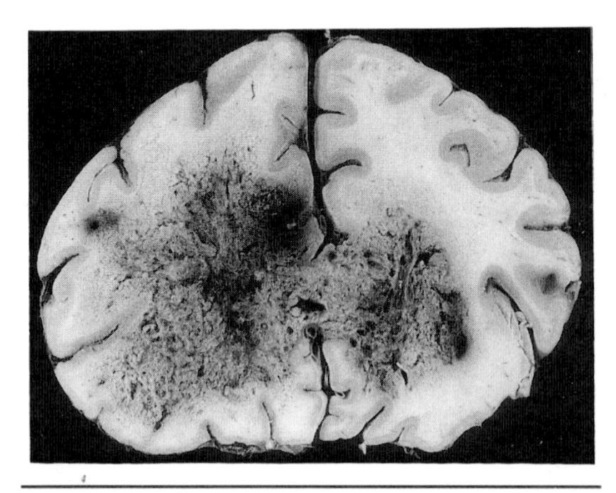

Fig. 18.57 Glioblastoma. Necrotic and haemorrhagic tumour is seen in the corpus callosum and in both frontal lobes.

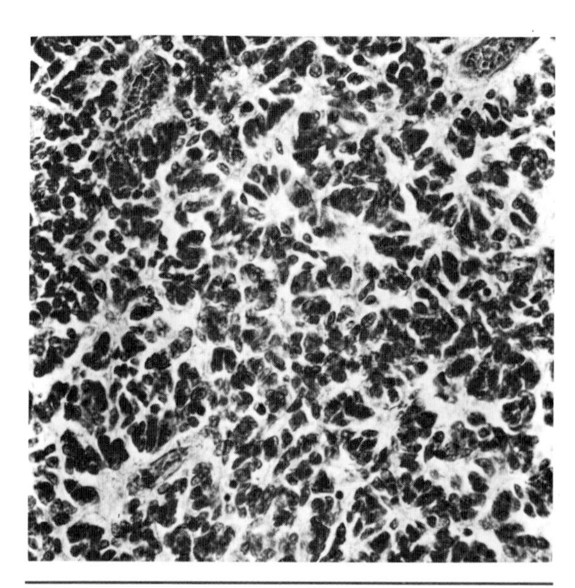

Fig. 18.59 Medulloblastoma. The cells are small, slightly elongated and closely packed. There are some poorly defined rosettes. ×285.

ally occur in the cerebral hemispheres in children when they are referred to as **primitive neuroectodermal tumours**.

Gliomatosis Cerebri

Known previously as diffuse astrocytoma, the brain tissue is diffusely permeated by tumour astrocytes, there usually being remarkable preservation of neurons and their fibres within the tumour. It is a rare tumour but occurs principally in the brain stem and in the spinal cord.

Tumours of Meningeal Tissue

Meningioma

This is a tumour of the arachnoid and many probably originate from arachnoidal granulations. They account for between 15 and 20% of primary intracranial tumours. They are solid, lobulated tumours, well demarcated from the brain tissue into which they project, forming a depression (Fig. 18.60): they are usually firmly attached by a broad base to the dura. They tend to arise adjacent to the major venous sinuses, commonly parasagittally or from the base of the skull, often in the region of the olfactory groove or the sphenoidal ridge. Rarely a meningioma may arise from the tela choroidea and appear as an intraventricular tumour. Spinal meningiomas have similar general features: they are intradural tumours and are a cause of cord compression. Most meningiomas are benign and can often be successfully removed. Some, however, infiltrate the overlying bone which may be greatly thickened.

There are various histological types, the most common being composed of fibrocellular tissue with a somewhat whorled appearance owing to the concentric arrangement of the cells. The whorls may undergo hyaline change and become calcified, resulting in a gritty tumour containing numerous spherical calcified particles – psammoma bodies (Fig. 18.61). Only rarely do meningiomas become anaplastic. Very occasionally meningiomas metastasize, usually to the lungs; this may follow craniotomy with spread into the soft tissues or may result from invasion of a venous sinus.

Primary Malignant Lymphomas

Intrinsic cerebral lymphomas vary greatly in appearance. Some are well defined while others are

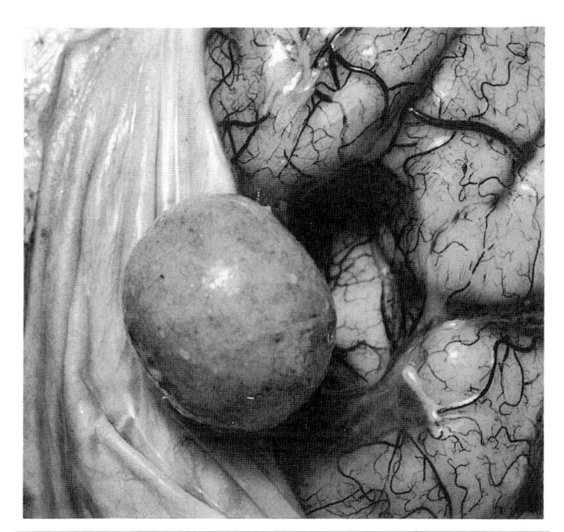

Fig. 18.60 Meningioma. The tumour has produced a depression in the cerebral cortex from which it can readily be withdrawn.

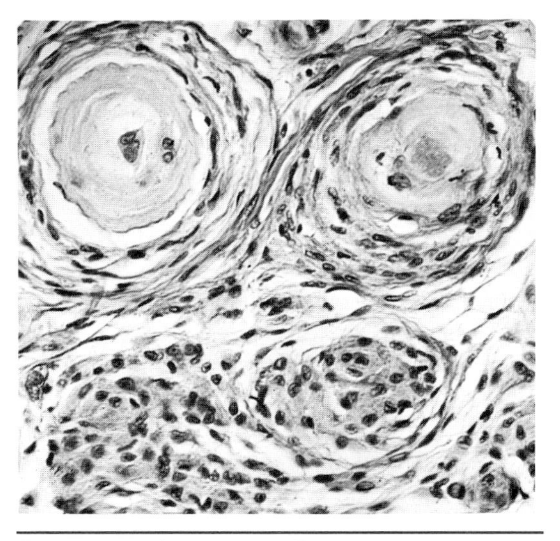

Fig. 18.61 Meningioma. There are whorls of cells, some of which are calcified (psammoma bodies). ×350.

less so, often having a slightly granular appearance. Multicentric deposits are not uncommon. Deposits of lymphoma often seem to replace brain tissue rather than act as expanding lesions: there is therefore often little evidence of the intracranial pressure having been high. A considerable proportion of cerebral lymphomas occur in the absence of any evidence of lymphoma elsewhere in the body. There is an increased incidence of cerebral lymphomas in immunocompromised individuals and in patients with AIDS.

These tumours are basically diffuse, non-Hodgkin lymphomas with structural features similar to those seen elsewhere in the body (see Chapter 15). The majority are of B-cell origin and are high-grade lymphomas.

Tumours of Blood Vessel Origin

Haemangioblastoma

This occurs almost exclusively within the cerebellum in adult life. Occasionally, they arise in relation to the caudal brain stem or the cervical spinal cord. The classic type consists of a large cyst containing xanthochromic fluid and a mural nodule of tumour. Sometimes, however, the tumour is solid. The solid areas usually have a distinctly yellow colour. They are basically benign tumours but recurrence is common, and some recurrent tumours become more aggressive and infiltrate through a craniectomy into the tissues of the scalp. Some patients with a haemangioblastoma also have polycythaemia.

The tumour consists of a closely packed network of vascular channels of varying size and a stroma composed of large polygonal cells that are usually distended with lipid (Fig. 18.62). There is a dense reticulin network throughout the tumour.

Cerebellar haemangioblastomas may exist as solitary or multiple lesions (Lindau's syndrome) but they may also be a component of von Hippel–Lindau's syndrome when there may be similar tumours in the retinae, congenital cysts in the pancreas and the kidneys, and clear cell tumours in the kidney.

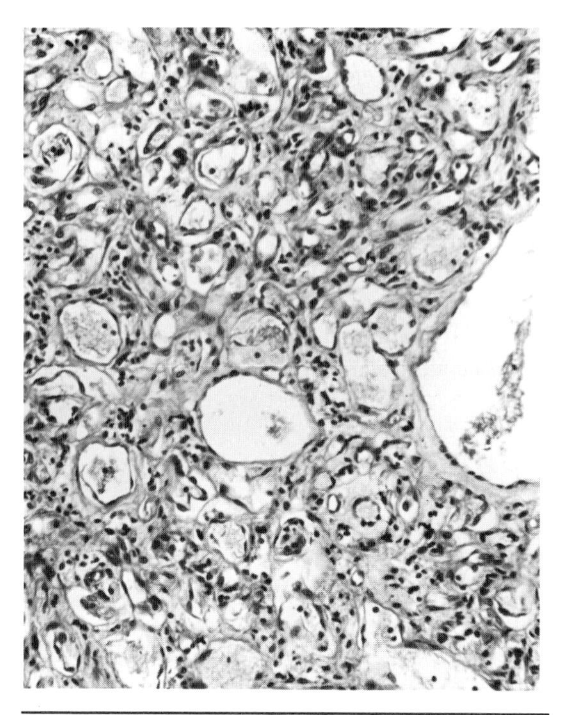

Fig. 18.62 Haemangioblastoma. There is a closely packed network of small blood vessels. ×130.

Malformative Tumours and Tumour-like Lesions

These are very uncommon and are briefly summarized.

Craniopharyngiomas arise in the region of the pituitary stalk from ectopic nests of squamous epithelial cells. They characteristically occur as a suprasellar mass projecting upwards into the hypothalamus and the third ventricle, and downwards into the pituitary fossa. It is an encapsulated, sharply circumscribed tumour, much of which is often cystic, the fluid having the colour and consistency of dark engine oil. The solid areas are rather greyish white and there is usually considerable calcification, usually seen in plain X-rays of the skull.

The solid parts of the tumour are composed of keratinizing stratified squamous epithelium which tends to undergo a peculiar change when the individual cells become separated by clear spaces (Fig. 18.63), thus producing appearances similar to an adamantinoma (ameloblastoma, p. 681). Throughout the tumour there are deposits of keratin, with numerous multinucleate giant cells adjacent to collections of cholesterol, so-called cholesteatomas.

Epidermoid and dermoid cysts are the same as similar cysts that occur elsewhere in the body. They occur particularly in the posterior fossa and in the vertebral canal, when there may be a fistula connecting the cyst with the overlying skin. They also occur within the diploe of the skull.

Colloid cysts of the third ventricle. There is some doubt as to the precise cell of origin of this type of cyst but they develop within the third ventricle, usually contain green, rather gelatinous fluid, and are lined by a flat cuboidal or pseudostratified epithelium that may or may not be ciliated. A colloid cyst may have an intermittent ball-valve effect on the interventricular foramina leading to episodes of high intracranial pressure. Not infrequently, however, a patient with a colloid cyst may die within hours because of acute hydrocephalus.

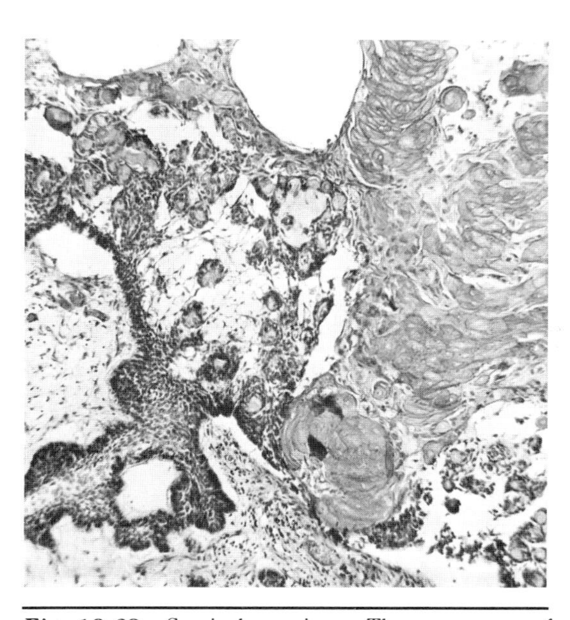

Fig. 18.63 Craniopharyngioma. There are areas of squamous epithelium with a partly adamantinomatous appearance that is produced by the stellate reticulin among the epithelial cells.

Metastatic Tumours

These are common and probably have a prevalence similar to that of the gliomas, i.e. 25–30% of all intracranial tumours. The primary tumour may be of any type but there is a particular predilection for small cell carcinoma of the bronchus to metastasize to the CNS. Other primary sites include breast, kidney, gastrointestinal tract and skin (melanoma). Metastases occur most frequently in the posterior frontal and parietal regions, and in the cerebellum. They are characteristically multiple but not infrequently a patient presents with what appears to be a large, solitary metastasis.

Deposits of metastatic carcinoma are characteristically sharply demarcated from the adjacent brain tissue (Fig. 18.64). They vary greatly in appearance, some being granular, others gelatinous, and others – particularly malignant melanomas – being haemorrhagic. Oedema in the adjacent brain tissue is often marked. Metastatic tumour also occurs quite frequently in the spinal

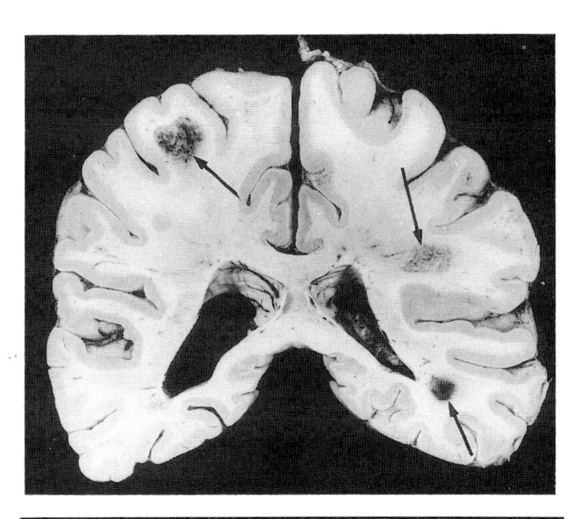

Fig. 18.64 Metastatic carcinoma. There are three metastases (arrows) in this brain slice.

extradural space leading to compression of the cord.

Non-metastatic effects of carcinoma on the nervous system are described on p. 841.

Meningeal carcinomatosis is the commonest type of diffuse meningeal tumour and, in the majority of cases, there is no other evidence of metastatic carcinoma in the brain. The tumour cells may reach the subarachnoid space by spreading centripetally along cranial or spinal nerve roots, but carcinoma cells usually reach the subarachnoid space by haematogenous spread. There may be some slight opacity of the leptomeninges but in other cases there are no macroscopic abnormalities, the diagnosis depending on histological examination. There are, however, sometimes small nodules of tumour on the nerve roots of the cauda equina which tend to be rather matted together and difficult to separate. On histological examination, carcinoma cells are seen diffusely throughout the subarachnoid space. They are particularly conspicuous on the surface of the cerebellum where they often show a tendency to extend into the adjacent cortex along perivascular spaces. The CSF protein is usually elevated and the glucose reduced. Thus, the features of this disease are often very similar to tuberculous meningitis but malignant cells can usually be identified in the CSF.

The leptomeninges may also be seeded with deposits of various leukaemias and this is important in the management of affected patients. Radiation of the CNS is carried out prior to bone marrow transplantation to ensure eradication of these deposits.

Local extension from regional tumours directly into the cranial cavity and spinal cord may occur (Table 18.6).

The Peripheral Nervous System

The peripheral nervous system consists of the dorsal and ventral nerve roots and their endings, the autonomic ganglia and their fibres.

Most peripheral nerves are mixed, carrying somatic motor and sensory, visceral sensory and autonomic fibres. The fibres themselves are of two types, myelinated (1–15 μm in diameter) and unmyelinated (0.4–3 μm in diameter), in each case covered by the supporting cell of the peripheral nervous system, the Schwann cell. Unmyelinated fibres lie in bundles of 5–20 in grooves within the cytoplasm of the Schwann cell, the latter being arranged end to end in series along the axon to form the sheath of Schwann. Each Schwann cell covers a segment about 0.3–1.5 mm long, as is easily seen in myelinated fibres; in these, a flattened sheet of cell membrane is wrapped concentrically round and round an individual axon, like a 'Swiss' or a 'jelly' roll, to form the myelin (Fig. 18.65a). Where the Schwann cells interdigitate, the myelin is interrupted by constrictions called nodes of Ranvier. They play a role in the fast, saltatory conduction which occurs in myelinated as compared to unmyelinated fibres.

Within the peripheral nerve, individual fibres are enclosed in a tube of connective tissue called the **endoneurium**. Mixed bundles of myelinated and unmyelinated fibres are bound together in fascicles by the thick, strong **perineurium**. Finally, the fascicles are surrounded by **epineurium**, the tube which encloses the whole nerve.

Degenerative Changes in Peripheral Nerves

Peripheral nerves show two main types of reaction to injury: (1) axonal degeneration, including Wallerian degeneration, as previously described and resulting from transection of the axon and (2) segmental demyelination. The two often occur together in the individual case but one tends to predominate. The chief clinical reason for distinguishing between the two is in regard to prognosis: if the axon is intact when the pathological process stops, the return of conductive function is much quicker because the Schwann cells can remyelinate a fibre rapidly, whilst if the axon is transected then Wallerian degeneration occurs, and in these cases the axon can only grow at approximately 1 mm per day, from the central stump.

Axonal degeneration follows severe injury or death of a neuron or its axon. Degeneration of the axon is followed rapidly by breakdown of its myelin. Invading macrophages clear the debris, while Schwann cells proliferate ready to form a new myelin sheath. The usual cause of this type of injury is trauma to a peripheral nerve and these changes are seen distal to the site of damage [Wallerian degeneration – Fig. 18.65(2)]. Proximal to the damage the nerve cell body undergoes transient swelling and breakdown of the endoplasmic reticulum (chromatolysis), but recovers to support regeneration of the damaged axon. If the continuity of the endoneurial tubes is preserved, the prognosis for recovery is good although axons regenerate only at the rate of about 1 mm per day. Many axonal sprouts [Fig. 18.65(5)] may not reach the distal stump, however, and will proliferate in the dense scar tissue to form a painful swelling called an *amputation or traumatic neuroma.*

In some peripheral nerve diseases there is a tendency for the injury to axons to occur first and most severely at the distal ends. Axonal degeneration then proceeds backwards toward the neuron. This is called 'dying-back' [Fig. 18.65(3)] and these are the dying back neuropathies or distal axonopathies which present typically with glove and stocking anaesthesia. Finally, axonal degeneration can also be secondary to degeneration of the cell body, as in anterior poliomyelitis or motor neuron disease.

Segmental demyelination occurs when the Schwann cell and myelin sheath are damaged, leaving the axon intact [Fig. 18.65(4)]. The process is usually patchy. Schwann cells are capable of division so that remyelination occurs, provided the cause of the Schwann cell injury is removed. The demyelinated internode is usually replaced by two or more Schwann cells [Fig. 18.65(6)], leading to a decrease in internodal length in this segment. If the damage is repeated, as in certain hereditary neuropathies for example, then the frustrated attempts at healing result in hyperplasia of the Schwann cells with concentric wrapping of their cell processes and the formation of 'onion bulbs' along the nerve fibres [Fig. 18.65(7)].

Peripheral Neuropathies

Neuropathies cause muscle weakness and atrophy, loss or changes in sensation and autonomic effects. With axonal degeneration, muscle fasciculation and wasting will occur but if demyelination occurs these features are absent because there is conduction failure but no denervation.

The diseases which cause peripheral neuropathy can be acute (developing within days), subacute (developing over weeks) or chronic (developing within months to years). One nerve alone may be involved – a **mononeuropathy**, or several individual nerves – **mononeuritis multiplex**, or several in a symmetrical distribution – **polyneuropathy**. In addition, either or both of the two types of degeneration can be present. In addition to the clinical features, the specialized techniques of electrical nerve conduction and nerve biopsy can be helpful in establishing the cause.

Classification of these neuropathies can be very complex but a simplified one is given in Table 18.7 with an indication of the distribution, the clinical features and the type of degeneration. In many clinical cases an aetiological diagnosis cannot be established. The principal types are now discussed briefly.

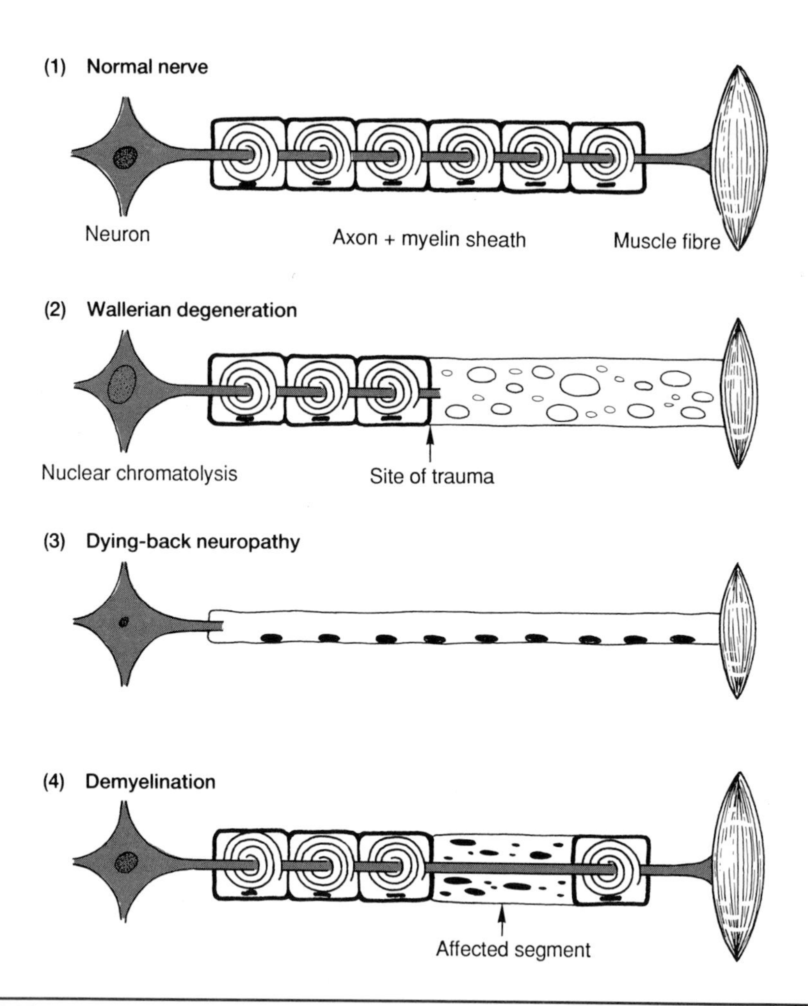

Fig. 18.65 (1) The normal nerve with its myelinated axon and the muscle fibre it supplies. (2) Distal to trauma, both axon and myelin layer degenerate while proximally the motor neuron nucleus swells. (3) In a dying back neuropathy, the axon degenerates, starting distally. The myelin also disappears. (4) In demyelination, the axon remains intact while segments of myelin degenerate. (5) Both axon and Schwann cells show proliferation but repair depends on continuity being established. (6) Remyelination is accompanied by shortening of myelin segments. (7) Continual damage results in hyperplastic Schwann cell proliferation and larger, nodular myelin segments.

Acute Idiopathic Inflammatory Polyneuropathy (Guillain–Barré Syndrome)

This is the commonest demyelinating peripheral neuropathy seen in clinical practice. It usually starts within 1–2 weeks of an acute febrile illness. It may also follow immunization, surgery or mycoplasma infections at approximately the same interval, or be associated with cancer or HIV infection. It presents with the rapid onset of numbness, paraesthesiae and an ascending paralysis, and the patient may need urgent assisted ventilation because of respiratory failure. Cranial nerves can also be affected, especially the oculomotor, while sphincter disturbances and cardiac arrhythmias may follow involvement of the autonomic nervous system. The CSF changes are typical: a greatly increased protein concentration, with very

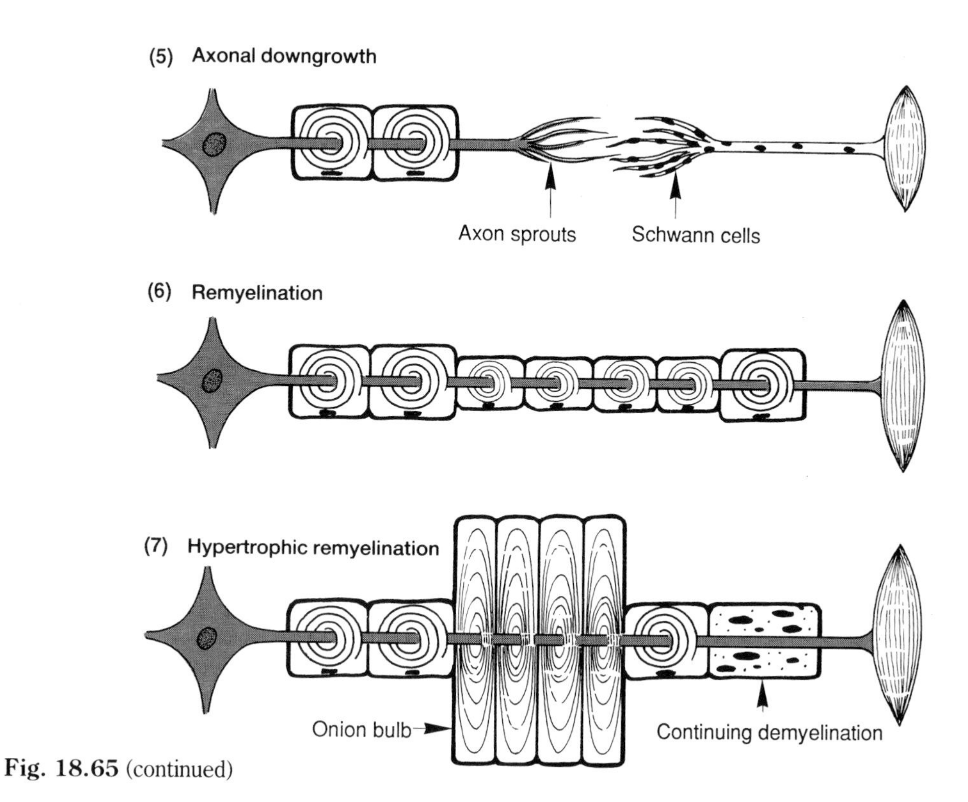

Fig. 18.65 (continued)

few, or no lymphocytes. The high protein content is due to leakage from inflamed blood vessels around the spinal roots.

Any part of the peripheral nervous system involved will show segmental demyelination, with relative sparing of the axons and endoneurial infiltrates of lymphocytes and macrophages. The latter strip off and phagocytose the superficial myelin lamellae. Recovery starts after one to several weeks and may be complete, but a small number of cases go on to develop a chronic, relapsing/remitting disease. In these cases, 'onion bulbs' can be found on the involved nerves. The aetiology of the Guillain–Barré syndrome is considered to be immunological and this is supported by the highly beneficial effect of plasmapheresis if carried out early in the disease.

Other Neuropathies

Diabetes mellitus. This can produce one of several clinical pictures as indicated in Table 18.7. It involves all sizes of fibres, including unmyelinated. The perineurial and endoneurial capillaries show severe luminal narrowing with thickened, reduplicated basal lamina indicating that chronic ischaemia probably plays a major role.

Uraemia. This resolves with a return to normal renal function.

Paraneoplastic. This is one of the many remote effects of carcinoma on the nervous system and is of interest in that its onset often precedes and draws attention to the tumour.

Paraproteinaemias. Neuropathy is relatively common with these disorders. Recently, specific IgM antibody to myelin-associated glycoprotein has been demonstrated in affected nerves, and its presence is associated with the demyelination.

Toxins. Many drugs and environmental agents produce peripheral neuropathies and the numbers are continually increasing. Among those incrimi-

Table 18.7 Classification of peripheral neuropathies

Idiopathic (possibly immunological)	Acute idiopathic inflammatory polyneuropathy: (Guillain–Barré syndrome)	See text
Ischaemia	Diabetes mellitus	Variable clinical picture: focal or multiple: sensory, sensorimotor, autonomic
	Vasculitis	
	Peripheral vascular disease	All ischaemic types show axonal degeneration and some demyelination
	Entrapment neuropathies	
Nutritional	Alcohol abuse Vitamin B deficiency – B_{12} and B_3	Distal sensorimotor; axonal degeneration and demyelination
Infection	Herpes zoster	Single cranial or spinal nerve; sensory neuron loss
	Leprosy	Focal or multiple, axonal degeneration and demyelination
	HIV	Demyelination
Drugs	Isoniazid, vincristine	Distal sensorimotor; axonal degeneration
	cis-Platinum	Distal sensorimotor: demyelination
Metabolic	Uraemia Porphyria	Mainly motor: axonal degeneration
Hereditary	HSN types I–III Werdnig-Hoffmann's disease	See text
Miscellaneous		
Amyloidosis	Hereditary forms more frequently but also in secondary types	Distal sensorimotor; demyelination
Paraproteinaemia	Multiple myeloma Waldenström's macroglobulinaemia	
Paraneoplastic	Carcinoma of bronchus	Variable: sensory or motor; axonal degeneration and demyelination: neuronal loss

nated are nitrofurantoin, diphenylhydantoin, perhexiline maleate and dapsone. Alcohol abuse is a common cause (Fig. 18.66). Chemical agents include lead, arsenic and hexacarbons.

Hereditary motor and sensory neuropathies (HMSN). These are very rare disorders in which a highly selective involvement of lower motor neurons (Werdnig–Hoffmann disease or acute infantile spinal muscular atrophy), primary sensory neurons (hereditary sensory neuropathies) or both, is seen. In peroneal muscular atrophy or Charcot–Marie-Tooth disease (HMSN I) demyelination with 'onion bulbs' occurs, whereas in Déjérine–Sottas disease (HMSN II) the abnormality is thought to be in the neuron and axonal degeneration occurs.

Nerve Sheath Tumours

These tumours may also occur within the cranial cavity and spinal canal. The two major benign peripheral nerve sheath tumours are the schwannoma (neurilemmoma) and the neurofibroma. They are closely related lesions but there are sufficient differences to justify their separation.

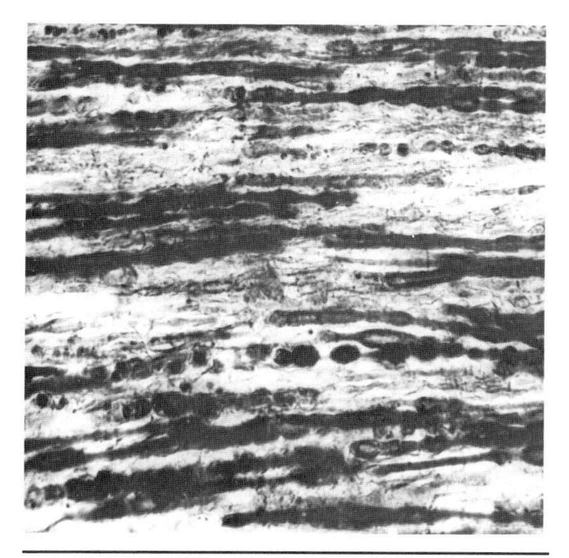

Fig. 18.66 Longitudinal section of peripheral nerve in alcoholic neuropathy showing degeneration of myelin sheaths (Marchi method). × about 400.

Neurofibromatosis is characterized by multiple neurofibromas (and other lesions). Malignant nerve sheath tumours are uncommon. Granular cell tumour (p. 1001) is now regarded as of neural origin.

Schwannoma

This is usually a solitary well circumscribed and encapsulated tumour, typically situated at the periphery of the nerve so that the nerve fibres are stretched over it. Thus, the tumour can often be carefully excised without destroying the nerve. The tumour is derived from Schwann cells. Histologically (Fig. 18.67), there is a variable mixture of appearances. Compact areas in which spindle-shaped cells are arranged in a whorled pattern and with nuclear palisading (Antoni type A tissue) form structures known as Verocay bodies. Elsewhere the tumour cells are stellate and loosely arranged in a myxoid stroma (Antoni type B tissue).

Intracranially, the most common site is the vestibular portion of the eighth cranial nerve, which takes its origin just within the internal auditory meatus, and enlargement of which is usually visible radiologically. Clinically it is often referred to as an 'acoustic neuroma'. The tumour fills the cerebellopontine angle (Fig. 18.68), and eventually produces distortion and displacement of the

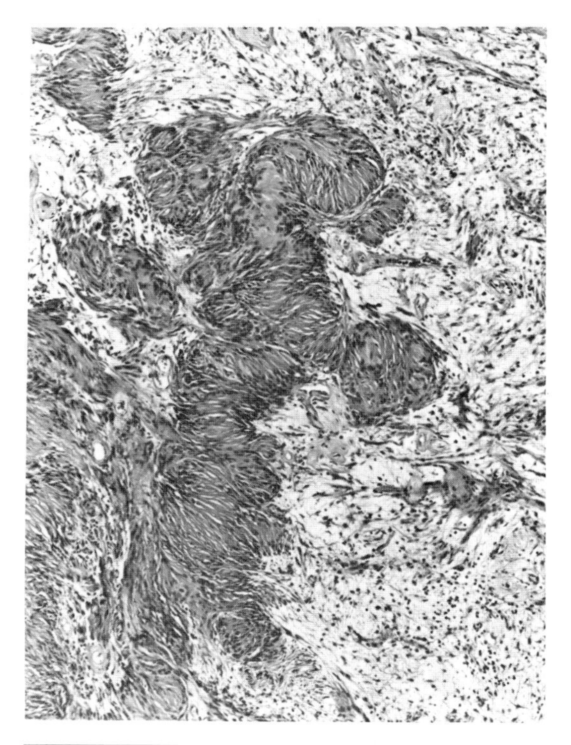

Fig. 18.67 Schwannoma of eighth cranial nerve (acoustic neuroma) showing cellular Antoni type A tissue with whorling and nuclear palisading forming Verocay bodies; surrounding these there is loosely arranged myxoid Antoni type B tissue. ×65.

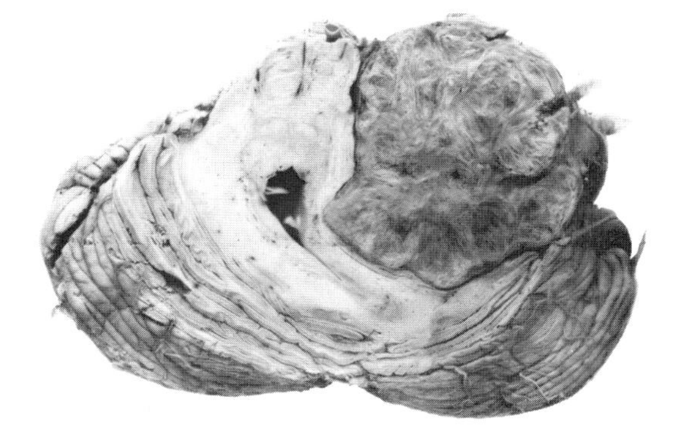

Fig. 18.68 Large schwannoma of the auditory nerve in the cerebellopontine angle, which has caused great displacement of the adjacent structures.

adjacent brain stem and some degree of hydrocephalus. In the spinal canal, schwannomas occur as intradural tumours, almost invariably on dorsal nerve roots, where their main effect is compression of the spinal cord. They may, however, extend through an intervertebral foramen with the production of a 'dumb-bell' tumour.

Neurofibroma

This usually presents as a fusiform swelling on a single nerve resulting from the neoplastic proliferation of fibroblasts and Schwann cells. Sometimes a group of nerves are affected by numerous oval and irregular swellings, this being referred to as a plexiform neurofibroma. Such lesions tend to occur on the scalp and the neck, when the overlying skin becomes firm and nodular. Unlike schwannoma, the nerve fibres run through the tumour; excision of the tumour results in loss of integrity of the nerve.

Histologically, the tumour cells are a mixture of Schwann cells, perineurial cells and fibroblasts, loosely arranged in a myxoid stroma with variable amounts of collagen. Malignant change is rare in solitary lesions but more common in the multiple lesions of neurofibromatosis.

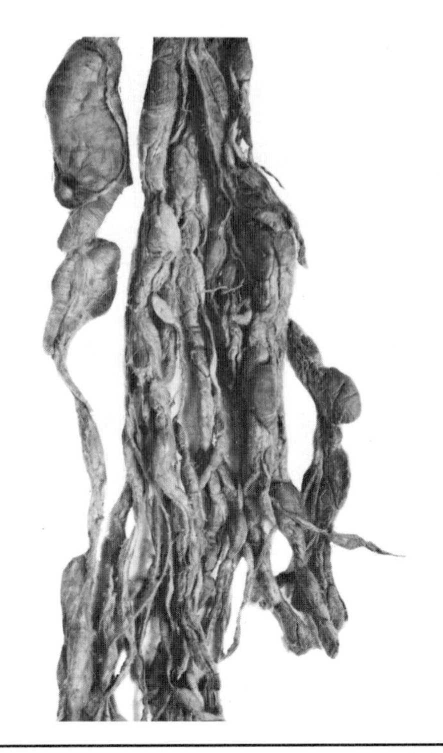

Fig. 18.69 Plexiform neurofibroma of the sciatic nerve and its branches. Note the numerous nodules of various sizes and forms.

Neurofibromatosis

This condition exists in two forms, peripheral and central. In the **peripheral form, neurofibromatosis type-1 (Nf-1 or von Recklinghausen's disease)**, multiple neurofibromas are widely distributed on motor, sensory and autonomic nerves, sometimes forming plexiform neurofibromas (Fig. 18.69), where a major nerve is converted into a 'bag of worms' by widespread overgrowth of Schwann cells. Associated lesions include pigmented skin areas (*café au lait* spots), hamartomas of the iris, skeletal deformities and numerous other abnormalities. Malignant transformation of neurofibromas occurs in about 1% of patients.

This is an uncommon disorder with a frequency of 1 in 30 000 births. It is inherited as an autosomal dominant with a high degree of penetration. Only about 50% of patients have a family history, implying a high rate of mutations. The responsible gene has been localized to chromosome 17 and recently cloned. Preliminary data suggest it may be an anti-oncogene probably involved in the control of the *ras* oncogene. Failure of this control mechanism may account for the excess cellular proliferation seen in neurofibromatosis and the increased risk of neurofibrosarcomas and other neoplasias, e.g. optic nerve glioma and phaeochromocytoma.

In the **central form**, bilateral acoustic neuromas, optic glioma, astrocytoma, meningioma and 'dumb-bell' tumours of the spinal nerve roots are present. In this form few, if any, peripheral neurofibromas are seen and *café au lait* spots are less common.

Malignant Peripheral Nerve Sheath Tumours (Malignant Schwannoma, Neurofibrosarcoma)

Sarcomas of nerve origin are uncommon; typically they form a large mass within a major nerve although sometimes no direct origin from a nerve can be demonstrated. Patients with neurofibromatosis are at increased risk. However, sporadic cases may arise from a normal nerve or a single neurofibroma and only very rarely from a schwannoma. The prognosis is poor, particularly in patients with neurofibromatosis.

Voluntary Muscles

Normal Structure

An individual muscle (Fig. 18.70) consists of bundles of fibres – fascicles – within a connective tissue framework which can be divided into three components, the **endomysium** which separates the individual muscle fibres, the **perimysium** which envelops bundles of fibres, and the **epimysium** which ensheaths the whole muscle. Individual muscle fibres are elongated, multinucleate syncytia up to 10 cm long and 10–100 μm in diameter. The muscle nuclei lie at the periphery of the fibre, under the plasma membrane (**sarcolemma**), which is enclosed in a basal lamina. Each muscle fibre contains sarcoplasm within which are mitochondria together with several hundred to several thousand myofibres, these in turn containing the contractile myofilaments. The latter are made up of overlapping thick filaments of myosin and thin filaments, predominantly of actin, but also containing tropomyosin and troponin. The myofilaments are arranged in parallel (Fig. 18.70) and the cross-striations seen in longitudinal sections result from this parallel arrangement, which is maintained by the cytoskeletal intermediate filaments, desmin, vimentin and synemin.

The functional unit within the myofibril is the sarcomere, which is bounded on either side by a Z-line. Within each sarcomere there are A (anisotropic) bands, mostly of myosin and I (isotropic) bands mostly of actin. The intermediate filaments link the individual myofibrils at the Z-line and also link the myofibrils to the sarcolemma. A tubular network is arranged transversely across the muscle fibre and is thus wrapped round individual myofibrils. The muscle fibre contracts in response to stimulation of the electrically excitable sarcolemma. This envelopes the fibre and extends into it by way of the transverse tubular system. The electrical stimulus releases calcium ions and they activate the chemical processes which produce contraction. During contraction the actin and myosin filaments slide between each other producing shortening of the myofibril. Tension in the muscle is maintained by cross-linkages between the filaments.

The individual motor unit comprises the anterior horn cell and its peripheral nerve fibre, the neuromuscular junction and the myofibres supplied by it. Disease states occur from lesions at any level of the motor unit. The number of myofibres receiving their nerve supply from a single anterior horn cell determines the size of the motor unit: in general, the more delicate the function to be performed, the smaller the size of the unit. Myofibres are divided into types 1 and 2: all the muscle fibres in a motor unit are of the same type, determined by the 'parent' anterior horn cell. **Type 1 (slow-twitch or red) fibres** are highly resistant to fatigue: they are rich in mitochondria and contain a relatively high ratio of lipid to glycogen. These fibres are adapted for long, sustained contractions, such as for posture. In contrast, **type 2 (fast-twitch or white) fibres** are rich in myofibrillar ATPase activity, have fewer mitochondria and contain a high ratio of glycogen to lipid. They are specialized for fine, rapid, powerful movement. Both fibre

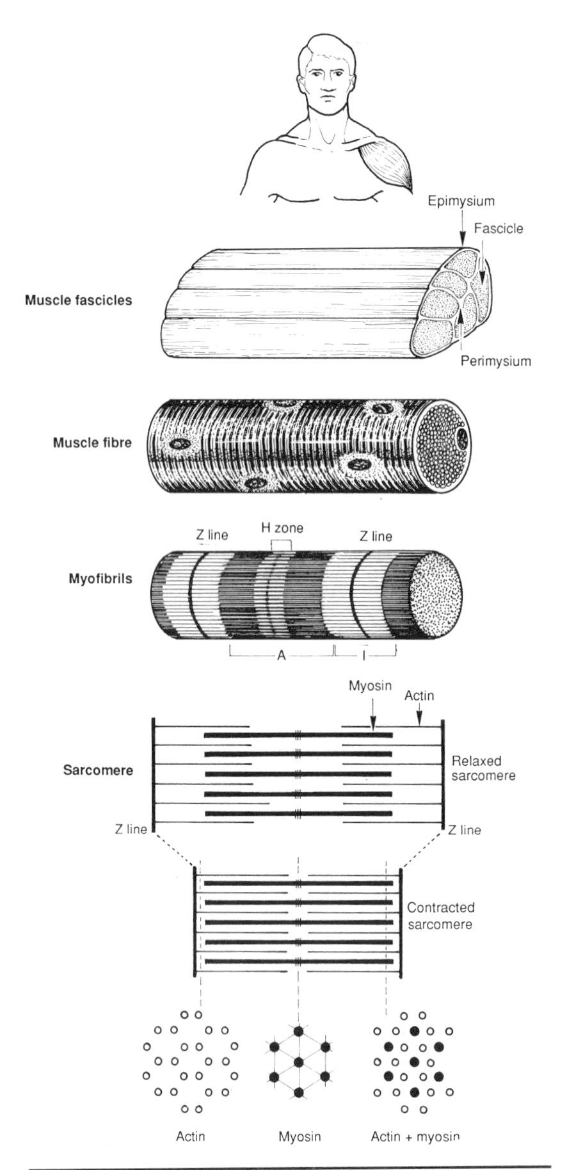

Fig. 18.70 Normal structure of muscle seen at gradually increasing magnification. The fascicles are separated by perimysial connective tissue and bound together by epimysial connective tissue. The muscle fibre is a syncytium and numerous peripheral sarcolemmal nuclei can be seen, together with the strongly contrasting A (dark) and I (light) bands. The A band includes a lighter zone, the H zone and the I band contains the Z line, as shown in the myofibril. The sarcomere, the unit of contraction, extends from Z line to Z line. The explanation for the light and dark zones is seen when the sarcomere is examined at high magnification. Both actin and myosin filaments are present in the A zone, while only actin is found in the I zone.

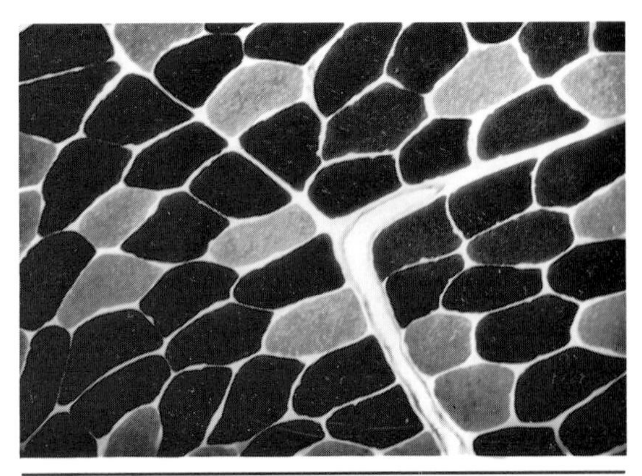

Fig. 18.71 Section of normal muscle showing intermingling of types 1 and 2 fibres. (Frozen section stained for myofibrillar ATPase: type 2 fibres appear darker than type 1.) ×250. (Courtesy Dr W.J.K. Cumming.)

types are found in all skeletal muscle, but their proportions vary according to the main function of the muscle. The fibres of a motor unit do not form a discrete group, but are intermingled with fibres of adjacent units (Fig. 18.71).

Clinical investigation is based on careful examination to determine the pattern of muscle weakness. Electrophysiological studies are used to test the function of the peripheral nerve and to sample muscle fibre reactions. These tests are subject to sample error and are therefore used mainly as a guide to further investigation. The serum creatinine kinase provides an index of muscle fibre damage, usually being increased when there is necrosis.

Muscle Biopsy

Biopsy is usually performed on large proximal limb muscles (e.g. quadriceps or biceps). A muscle which is severely involved by the disease should usually be avoided because the basic pathological process may not be apparent in end-stage muscle disease. Needle biopsies are most commonly done nowadays because they are much less traumatic and can be repeated during the course of the disease.

Histochemical stains are essential in evaluating muscle diseases and in identifying any biochemical abnormalities. They will distinguish between type 1 and type 2 fibres, demonstrate structural abnormalities which cannot be seen on routine histological stains, e.g. enzyme-deficient 'cores' and 'moth-eaten' fibres, show the distribution of mitochondria and suggest enzyme deficiencies in the glycolytic, fat or other metabolic pathways.

The stains used most commonly are:

(1) the myosin adenosine triphosophatase (myofibrillar ATPase) for myofibrils, which, when the section is preincubated in an alkaline buffer at pH 9.4, stains type 2 fibres dark and type 1 fibres pale, while in an acid buffer it produces exactly the opposite effect:

(2) the reduced nicotinamide adenine dinucleotide (NADH) tetrazolium reductase and succinic dehydrogenase stains, both of which stain mitochondria;

(3) a modified Gomori stain which will detect mitochondria, especially clumps of abnormal ones; these latter are responsible for the 'ragged-red' fibre. The thread-like inclusions called 'nemaline rods' are also identified with this stain. Other stains are used to demonstrate glycogen, phosphorylase, phosphofructokinase and adenylate deaminase, all substances with an abnormal muscle distribution in certain diseases (e.g. McArdle's disease). Finally, recently denervated fibres stain intensely dark with the non-specific esterase reaction.

Reactive Changes

The usual pathological changes are modified in muscle because of the specialized development of the contractile apparatus and the fact that the fibre is a syncytium.

Changes in Fibre Size

The fibres in normal adult muscle show a range of diameters and measurement is often important in diagnosis. Muscle fibres hypertrophy in response to an increased work load and atrophy when this is removed. These are physiological responses. Hypertrophy of scattered individual fibres is seen as a compensatory response in chronic denervation.

Neurogenic atrophy follows loss of the nerve supply to the fibre, due to death of the anterior horn cell (e.g. poliomyelitis), peripheral nerve damage, or lesions at the neuromuscular junction (e.g. myasthenia gravis). Since fibres from different motor units are intermingled, denervation of a single motor unit leads to small, angular atrophic fibres scattered between normal fibres (Fig. 18.72). This is called disseminated neurogenic atrophy. If the denervating process is chronic, then group atrophy affecting large or small groups may be seen. Atrophy of fibres at the periphery of the fascicle, **perifascicular atrophy**, is characteristic of the inflammatory myopathy, dermatomyositis, and is thought to be ischaemic. Sometimes the atrophy affects only one type of fibre, e.g. type 1 atrophy is seen in myotonic dystrophy and some of the congenital myopathies. Type 2 atrophy is not specific, being seen in any condition in which there is muscle disease, but it is typically present in steroid myopathy.

Changes in Fibre Distribution

In a normal muscle fibre, responsiveness to acetylcholine is limited to the end-plate zone but in response to denervation, all of the sarcolemma

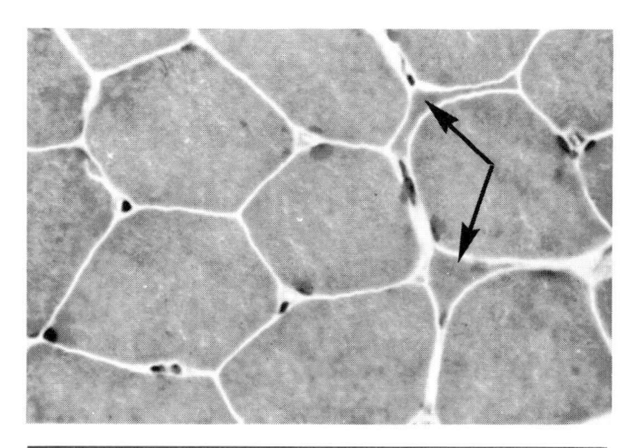

Fig. 18.72 Spinal muscular atrophy, showing two inconspicuous atrophic muscle fibres lying among normal fibres (arrows). ×400. (Courtesy Dr W.J.K. Cumming.)

becomes responsive to acetylcholine. This appears to stimulate the formation of collateral sprouts from intact nerve terminal branches (Fig. 18.73). The fibres then redevelop to normal size and take on the histochemical feature of the fibre type determined by the new nerve. This leads to grouping of fibre types with loss of the normal checkerboard appearance (Fig. 18.74a). When a previously enlarged motor unit is affected, groups of atrophic fibres are seen (Fig. 18.74b).

Nuclear Changes

Less than 3% of fibres in any biopsy usually show central nuclei – more than this number suggests a myopathy. Numerous central or 'internal' nuclei are a feature of myotonic dystrophy and the rare centronuclear myopathy. Nuclear chains probably have the same significance. Clumps of pyknotic nuclei are seen in chronic denervation. Large vesicular nuclei suggest regeneration.

Necrosis

Usually only a segment of the fibre is affected and this appears pale, hyaline or vacuolated and without striations. Sarcolemmal nuclei disappear in any necrotic area, macrophages infiltrate the sarcoplasm and phagocytose the necrotic debris, multinucleate forms sometimes being prominent.

Ischaemia can cause necrosis of large areas of muscle, e.g. in Volkmann's contracture following trauma to the elbow, in polyarteritis nodosa or in the 'anterior compartment syndrome', where strenuous exercise causes swelling of the anterior tibial muscle, compression of its blood supply and necrosis.

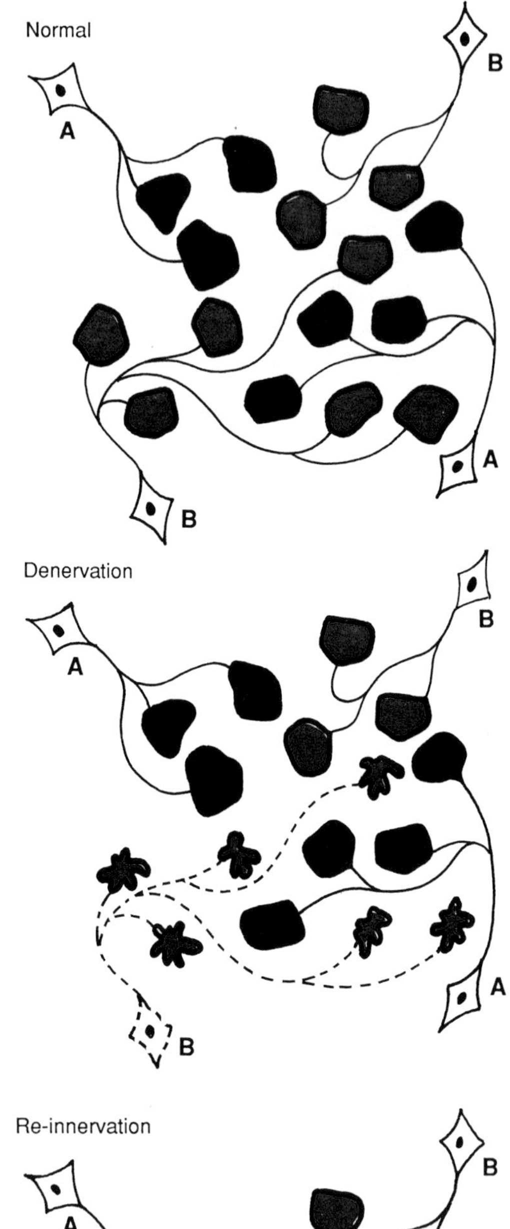

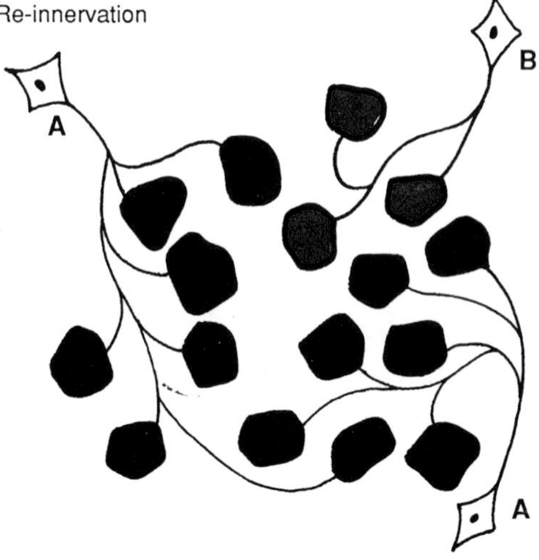

Fig. 18.73 Changes seen in the pattern of type 1 and type 2 fibres in response to denervation and re-innervation. The normal mosaic pattern is seen first with nerves A supplying type 1 (light) and nerves B supplying type 2 (dark) muscle.

Death of a nerve B results in denervation atrophy of the type 1 fibres it supplies. Re-innervation by adjacent twigs from nerves A results in the fibres changing from type 1 to type 2 and the appearance of 'grouping' of dark fibres.

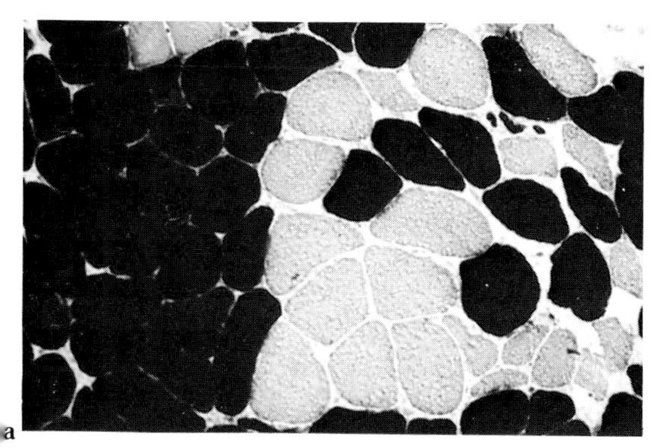

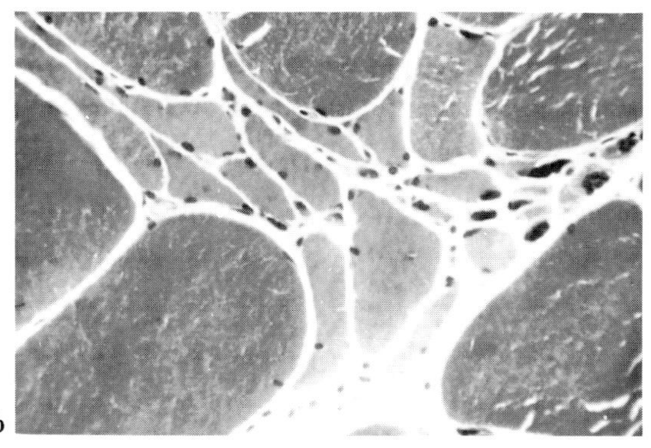

Fig. 18.74 a Spinal muscular atrophy, showing grouping of type 2 fibres resulting from re-innervation and regeneration of denervated fibres. (Frozen section stained for myofibrillar ATPase: type 2 fibres darkly stained.) ×250. **b** Spinal muscular atrophy. Re-innervation has resulted in grouping of fibres of a motor unit. Subsequent denervation has resulted in atrophy of the grouped fibres. ×600. (Courtesy Dr W.J.K. Cumming.)

Changes in Cytochemical Architecture

Sometimes the fibre is granular and stains red with the modified Gomori trichrome stain: this is called a 'ragged-red' fibre. Such a fibre may be found in any myopathy but large numbers are typical of mitochondrial diseases. Structural changes may be seen on the histochemical stains, e.g. central cores, target fibres, 'moth-eaten' fibres, or rod bodies, suggestive of the myopathies.

Regeneration

When voluntary muscle fibres are damaged, their capacity to regenerate depends mainly on whether loss of fibres is accompanied by destruction or loss of their basement membrane and endomysium. When these are lost, little effective regeneration of a fibre occurs, but if they remain intact there may be considerable regeneration. Proliferation of satellite stem cells provides mononuclear myoblasts which fuse to form a new fibre: initially, this has a row of central rounded nuclei and is known as a **myotube**. The nuclei then migrate to the periphery and the fibre assumes its adult form. Fibres which are basophilic on H & E staining are thought to be regenerating, especially if the nuclei are vesicular. This change is common in myopathies, especially in the early stages of Duchenne muscular dystrophy.

Neuromuscular Disorders

This term includes a large group of diseases in which impaired function of motor units presents clinically as weakness. The term myopathy is used for disorders of the muscle fibres; dystrophy is applied to genetically determined myopathies in which there are degenerative changes in the muscle fibres without evidence of a storage disorder. Some of the diseases are neurogenic, i.e. result from lesions of the lower motor neurons and their nerve fibres: others arise from defects of the neuromuscular junction or of the muscle fibres themselves. By convention, the term atrophy is applied to neuromuscular disease when the cause is neurogenic. A simplified classification is given in Table 18.8. Most of the neurogenic disorders listed have been dealt with earlier in this chapter.

As a general rule, when clinical examination shows bilateral symmetry of muscle involvement the patient is likely to have a myopathy, while selective or asymmetric involvement of muscles is likely to be of neurogenic origin.

Table 18.8 Classification of neuromuscular disorders

Myopathic disorders
Genetically determined myopathies
muscular dystrophies
myotonic dystrophies
metabolic myopathies
benign myopathies of childhood
Inflammatory myopathies
idiopathic
viral, bacterial or parasitic infections
Drug-induced and toxic myopathies
Endocrine myopathies
steroid
thyroid
others
Neurogenic disorders
Disorders of neuromuscular transmission (myasthenic syndromes)
myasthenia gravis
Eaton–Lambert syndrome
Disorders of innervation (denervation atrophy)
anterior horn cells: spinal muscular atrophy, motor neuron disease, poliomyelitis
motor nerve roots: vertebral compression, malignant infiltration
peripheral neuropathies:* acquired, genetically determined

This simplifed classification is based on that given by Swash and Schwartz, 1984.
*See Table 18.7.

Genetically Determined Myopathies

Duchenne Muscular Dystrophy

Duchenne muscular dystrophy is the commonest genetic myopathy, with an incidence of approximately 3/10 000 liveborn males. Inheritance is X-linked recessive, the disease being manifest in males and carried by females. Carriers may be detected by serial serum creatine kinase estimations but negative results do not, unfortunately, exclude this state because of random X-chromosome inactivation in females. Carriers may also be detected by tracking the mutant gene within a family using DNA analysis, and this approach has been used successfully for reliable prenatal diagnosis in at-risk pregnancies. Now that the affected gene has been identified, detection should become easier. About 30% of cases arise by mutation and so have no family history.

Duchenne muscular dystrophy is the most severe form of muscular dystrophy and the most rapidly progressive. Affected males present before the age of 5 years with delayed development of motor function, especially a waddling gait and an inability to run. Because of weakness of the pelvic-girdle muscles these children are unable to rise easily from the floor and use their arms to push the trunk into the upright position (Gower's manoeuvre). The majority of boys are confined to a wheelchair by 13 years of age and death, due to respiratory failure or cardiac arrhythmias, occurs usually in the late teens.

Pathological changes in muscle depend on the age of the child at the time of biopsy. Up to 1 year the predominant finding is the presence of frequent hyaline (prenecrotic) and necrotic fibres with adequate regeneration (Fig. 18.75a), but then regenerative capacity declines. There is progressive replacement of the muscle fibres by adipose and fibrous tissue (Fig. 18.75b) and this may, paradoxically, result in apparent hypertrophy (pseudohypertrophy) of affected muscle groups.

The nature of the genetic defect has been established. The gene is present on the short arm of the X chromosome (Xp21) and is a very large genetic locus. Its protein product, dystrophin, is a 400 kDa protein and is a structural component of the sarcolemma and transverse tubules of the muscle fibres. It is present in both skeletal and smooth muscles, and has been highly conserved during evolution. In Duchenne muscular dystrophy deletion of varying lengths or other mutations of the gene occur, and dystrophin production is absent or markedly abnormal (Fig. 18.75c, d). The precise role of dystrophin in muscle function is not clear. It has similarities to spectrin, a component of red cell membranes (p. 601). Absence of dystrophin

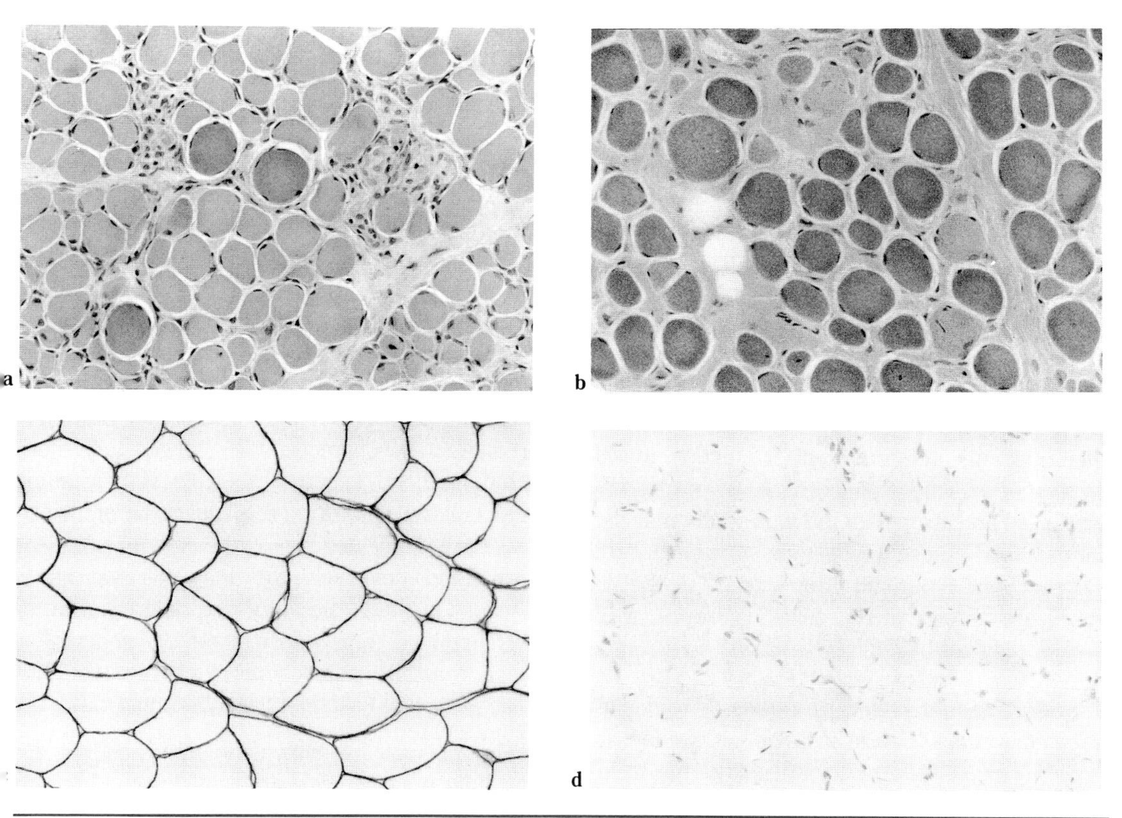

Fig. 18.75 **a** Duchenne muscular dystrophy: note rounded hyaline 'prenecrotic' fibres and necrotic fibres undergoing phagocytosis. **b** Later stage of Duchenne muscular dystrophy showing increase in endomysial and perimysial fibrous connective tissue. ×150. **c** Normal skeletal muscle showing immunolabelling of the protein dystrophin at the surface of the muscle fibres. ×150. **d** Duchenne muscular dystrophy showing absence of dystrophin immunolabelling; nuclei are counterstained with haematoxylin. ×150. (**c** and **d** by courtesy of Dr M. A. Johnson.)

results in dysfunction of the sarcolemmal membrane, allowing ingress of excess calcium ions. Dystrophin testing can now be carried out in muscle biopsies for diagnosis in preclinical cases.

Other Muscular Dystrophies

Becker's muscular dystrophy is also inherited as an X-linked recessive and has an incidence of 0.5/10 000 male births. The age of onset is from 3 to 20 years but it is more benign and death is from 30 to 60 years of age. It is of great interest that this genetic defect occurs at the same locus as for Duchenne muscular dystrophy. Dystrophin is present but it is of an abnormal (increased) molecular size and is quantitatively deficient.

Limb-girdle, facioscapulohumeral and ***oculopharyngeal dystrophy*** are part of a heterogeneous group which present later, have different muscle distributions and progress more slowly. It is likely that molecular analysis will help to characterize these disorders in the future.

Myotonic Dystrophy

This is an autosomal dominant disease due to a mutation on chromosome 19. The clinical presentation is stiffness, which is how the patient describes myotonia, i.e. delayed relaxation of muscle after contraction, and distal weakness, often seen as foot-drop. Involvement of other systems leads to frontal balding, cardiomyopathy, testicular atrophy, cataracts and mental retardation.

Electromyography is helpful in diagnosis because it shows the typical myotonia. The muscle biopsy shows myopathic changes in addition to two unusual features: long chains of central nuclei in the fibres and enlarged muscle spindles with numerous intrafusal fibres. The latter is an interesting change because these are the sensory organs in muscle which are responsive to tension and participate in moderating contraction and in controlling reflexes.

Metabolic Myopathies

In the adult, the clinical symptoms tend to fall into one of two categories: either severe muscle cramps or weakness on exercise, or progressive weakness and atrophy of the limb-girdle muscles. In the child, these myopathies may cause the 'floppy infant syndrome'. Since many of the diseases are autosomal recessive disorders, there may or may not be a family history.

The glycogen storage diseases. Muscles are affected in type II (acid maltase deficiency) and type V (myophosphorylase deficiency – McArdle's disease). Patients with acid maltase deficiency either present in infancy with severe hypotonia and die within one or two years, or late in life with a relentlessly progressive myopathy. Patients with McArdle's disease, however, can lead entirely normal lives provided they avoid strenuous exercise. The fact that they cannot produce lactate during ischaemic exertion is the basis of a serological test for the condition. Excessive glycogen can be seen in the muscle fibres on biopsy.

Periodic paralyses. These syndromes present as episodes of flaccid weakness lasting for hours or days, localized to one group of muscles or with generalized involvement; the respiratory muscles tend to be spared. There is often a family history and the patients tend to be hypo- or hyperkalaemic. The initial attacks are usually followed by complete recovery but later on, irreversible muscle damage occurs. The histological hallmark of all these conditions is a vacuolar myopathy due to dilation of the sarcoplasmic reticulum and the transverse tubules, followed by lysis and the formation of a membrane. The vacuole thus formed communicates with the extracellular space and fills up with extracellular fluid. If it ruptures, damage to the fibre follows.

Mitochondrial myopathies. This is a very mixed group of disorders, of which over 20 are now recognized but which was defined originally on the basis that the mitochondria appeared abnormal. On electron microscopy they may be much larger than normal or more abundant, with bizarre cristae and inclusions. They form subsarcolemmal and intermyofibrillar aggregates which are conspicuous on the Gomori trichrome stain and produce the characteristic 'ragged-red' fibre found in these syndromes. However, in some mitochondrial disorders, e.g. muscle carnitine palmityltransferase deficiency, the organelles appear normal and conversely, they may look abnormal in diseases in which the mitochondria are not primarily involved, e.g. acid maltase deficiency. For these reasons, a biochemical classification has been proposed based on the following groups:

(1) transport or enzymatic mitochondrial defects causing impaired substrate utilization;
(2) defective mitochondrial energy conservation; and
(3) a specific deficiency of one or more mitochondrial respiratory chain components.

Most of these very rare syndromes present with slowly progressive weakness of proximal and distal muscles, exacerbated by exercise, and with or without external ophthalmoplegia. Since the mitochondrial abnormalities may not be confined to muscle there may be other systemic disorders, e.g. affecting the central nervous system causing seizures, dementia and ataxia; short stature; retinopathy; deafness; peripheral neuropathy and cardiac conduction defects.

About 20% of patients have a family history but maternal transmission to offspring is about eight times more frequent than paternal transmissions. This led to the suggestion that mitochondrial DNA might be the site of mutation. During the formation of the zygote, all the mitochondria are contributed by the ovum, thus the mitochondrial genome is transmitted by maternal, non-mendelian inheritance. Mitochondrial DNA encodes 13 peptides which are components of respiratory-chain complexes. Recent work has confirmed that there are mitochondrial DNA deletions in some types.

Benign Myopathies of Childhood

These disorders are characterized clinically as the 'floppy infant syndrome', although sometimes they do not cause symptoms until late in childhood. They are usually inherited, but are very rare. The weakness is usually mild or moderate, muscle wasting is unusual and the course is slowly progressive although some cases may show improvement. They are classified purely on the basis of the muscle biopsy changes and these are related to the development of the muscle fibre. During normal development, fusion of myoblasts is followed by nuclear margination. The nuclei move from the centre to the periphery of the fibre. If nuclear margination fails, myotubes persist – *centronuclear or myotubal myopathy*. Defects in fibre differentiation may lead either to a deficiency or a preponderance of type 1 fibres, i.e. congenital fibre type disproportion. The abnormality may be associated with structural changes in the fibre producing the thread-like or rod-body inclusions of *nemaline myopathy*.

Inflammatory Myopathies

Polymyositis/ Dermatomyositis

Symmetrical progressive limb-girdle weakness is the cardinal presenting clinical feature of polymyositis/dermatomyositis in the child or adult. In childhood, dermatomyositis is seen more commonly than polymyositis, but the similarities in the clinicopathological features, the course of the disease and the response to therapy, suggest that the disease is of the same nature in children and adults.

Patients with this complex present with a proximal weakness which progresses slowly over weeks to months. A heliotrope rash may develop around the eyes, across the bridge of the nose, over the dorsal aspect of the joints of the hands and often on the extensor surface of the thighs. An increased serum creatine kinase concentration, myopathic changes on electromyography, and inflammation, necrosis and phagocytosis on muscle biopsy complete the diagnostic criteria.

About 20% of cases are associated with a connective tissue disorder, SLE, systemic sclerosis or Sjögren's syndrome. An association with carcinoma has also been suggested but it is likely that this is coincidence. Other systems may be affected: the majority of patients have cardiac involvement, usually of the conduction system, producing a risk of sudden death; interstitial pulmonary fibrosis also occurs.

Pathologically, there is widespread patchy necrosis and inflammation, often affecting the peripheral fibres of muscle fascicles (Fig. 18.76). Fibres in various stages of regeneration are seen. The inflammatory infiltrate, which is often perivascular, is composed of lymphocytes, macrophages and occasionally eosinophils.

The aetiology is not known but recent evidence of enteroviral genome in biopsies from patients with dermatomyositis, implicates a persistent coxsackievirus infection. A group of unusual autoantibodies can also be demonstrated in these patients, directed against transfer (t) RNA synthetases, and of which the anti-Jo-1 is directed against histidyl tRNA synthetase. It has been suggested, since viruses are known to bind to

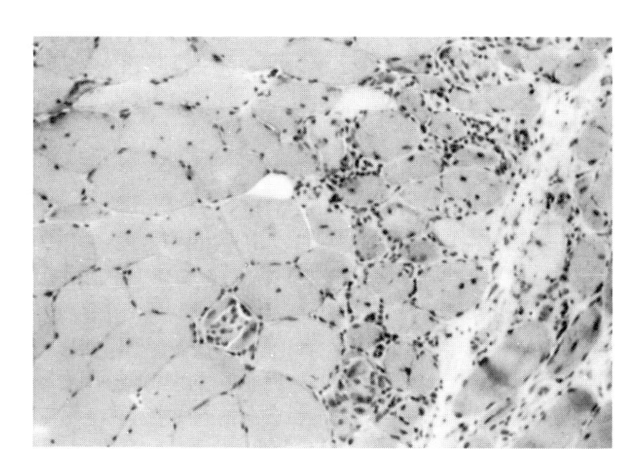

Fig. 18.76 Polymyositis/dermatomyositis, showing an inflammatory infiltrate with necrosis and regeneration affecting muscle fibres. ×200. (Courtesy Dr W.J.K. Cumming.)

active enzyme sites, that in these cases, the antibodies arise as a consequence of molecular mimicry.

Viral, Bacterial or Parasitic Infections

Viral myositis, pyogenic myositis and gas gangrene (p. 299) and parasitic diseases (p. 1188) have been considered elsewhere. Granulomatous inflammation of muscle may occur in sarcoidosis, polyarteritis nodosa and Wegener's granulomatosis.

Drug-induced and Toxic Myopathies

Muscle is very susceptible to the direct effects of toxins and other drugs. Most of these compounds act directly on the muscle fibre, causing necrosis. Clinically, this leads to a limb-girdle syndrome, sometimes associated with myoglobinuria. The serum creatine kinase is usually increased and provides a sensitivie index of muscle involvement. In most cases, removal of the toxin or drug is associated with complete recovery.

Drugs. The commonest drug-induced myopathy is caused by glucocorticoids. It usually affects the proximal lower limb muscles, especially the iliopsoas and quadriceps and its occurrence appears to be related to prolonged treatment and high dosage. Muscle biopsy shows a severe atrophy of type 2 fibres. Recovery of muscle function can be expected after the drug is stopped, but is slow. Other drug reactions include a vacuolar myopathy (chloroquine), necrotizing myopathy (emetine, procainamide and epsilon-aminocaproic acid), and a myasthenic-like disorder caused by penicillamine.

Malignant hyperthermia. This syndrome, occurring in response to anaesthetics such as halothane, consists of a rapid rise in body temperature (up to 1°C every 5 minutes), muscle rigidity, metabolic acidosis and increased serum creatine kinase activity. It is an autosomal dominant disorder with variable penetrance. The sarcolemma becomes abnormally permeable to calcium, and fibre necrosis occurs.

A somewhat similar clinical picture is seen in the **neuroleptic malignant syndrome**. This consists of muscle rigidity, hyperpyrexia, fluctuating coma and increased serum creatine kinase levels. It follows long-term administration of neuroleptic drugs such as the phenothiazines, or the abrupt cessation of dopaminergic therapy in Parkinson's disease.

Toxins. Snake bites may lead to muscle necrosis. Acute alcoholism may lead to hypokalaemia with extensive fibre necrosis and weakness. In the chronic alcoholic, a progressive necrobiotic myopathy develops which often does not improve with alcohol withdrawal.

Endocrine Myopathies

Muscle weakness can be a presenting syndrome in hyperthyroidism or myxoedema and is associated with parathyroid and adrenal disorders. The histological changes are usually mild, consisting of atrophy particularly of type 2 fibres and occasional fibre necrosis.

Disorders of Neuromuscular Transmission

There are two major disorders and each appears to have an immunological basis. The passage of nerve impulses across the synapse at the neuromuscular junction depends on the release of quanta of acetylcholine (ACh) from vesicles in the nerve terminals and their effect on receptors on the adjacent folds of muscle membrane (Fig. 18.77a). In myasthenia gravis, autoantibodies bind to the ACh receptor so that normal stimulation of muscle cannot occur (Fig. 18.77b). Damage is caused to the postsynaptic region. There is some evidence of cross-reactivity between glycoprotein D of herpes simplex and the acetylcholine receptor; this could be important in the pathogenesis of myasthenia gravis. In the Eaton–Lambert syndrome an autoantibody to the voltage-gated Ca^{2+} channels in the nerve causes presynaptic damage. The clinical and electromyographic findings are more useful in diagnosis than muscle biopsy, because ultrastructural analysis of motor end plates is needed to show the specific features.

Myasthenia Gravis

The classical feature of myasthenia gravis is abnormal fatiguability of skeletal muscles, presenting as weakness on exercising muscles and recovery on resting. It occurs predominantly in young women and middle-aged men. In the former, thymic hyperplasia with germinal centres in the medulla is usually found, while in the latter a thymoma may be found, usually of mixed epithelial and lymphocytic type.

The extrinsic ocular and facial muscles are almost always affected early, causing ptosis and diplopia, and there is commonly difficulty in speaking, chewing and swallowing. Symptoms may remain confined to the eyes (ocular form) but more often, generalized muscular weakness develops and respiratory distress may occur, particularly in exacerbations (crises). The disease may progress rapidly, with death in a few months, or slowly over many years, often with fluctuations in severity. Untreated, the commonest cause of death is aspiration pneumonia due to respiratory muscle weakness.

In 90% of patients antibodies to acetylcholine receptors occur (Fig. 18.77), forming the basis of a diagnostic test. However, it has to be remembered that the antibody titre does not correlate with the severity of the disease. Similar antibodies may be present at much lower titres in occasional patients' relatives, individuals with SLE or Down's syndrome, and in the very old. In pregnant women with myasthenia gravis the antibody may cross the placenta and cause **neonatal myasthenia gravis**, a transient disorder in infants which lasts about 6 weeks.

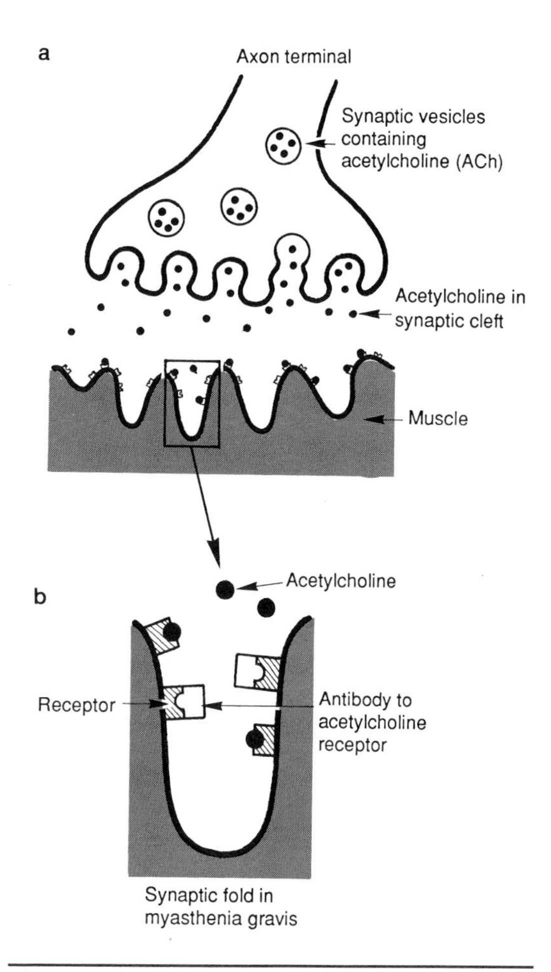

Fig. 18.77 The changes at the neuromuscular junction in myasthenia gravis. **a** Normal neuromuscular junction. Vesicles of acetylcholine are released from the nerve terminal, cross the synaptic cleft and reach their receptors on the junctional fold of sarcolemmal membrane. **b** In myasthenia gravis, specific antibody binds to the acetylcholine receptor and so prevents acetylcholine stimulating the membrane.

Plasmapheresis is useful in myasthenia gravis for treating a severe relapse, preparing the patient for thymectomy or the start of long-term steroid therapy. Its effect lasts for about 6 weeks.

Congenital myasthenia gravis. Congenital myasthenia gravis comprises a heterogeneous group of disorders in which the neuromuscular junction is structurally abnormal but there are no immunological defects.

The Eaton–Lambert Syndrome

In contrast to myasthenia gravis, this syndrome is associated with muscle weakness which improves with repeated exercise. There is usually proximal lower limb weakness and areflexia. In about 50% of cases, there is an associated small cell bronchial carcinoma. The syndrome can also occur with other autoimmune diseases or as an isolated entity.

Neurogenic Disorders with Denervation Atrophy

Spinal Muscular Atrophy

This results from an idiopathic loss of anterior horn cells in infancy. Eventually, re-innervation is no longer possible and the atrophic fibres appear small and rounded with densely stained nuclei (see Fig. 18.72). Secondary 'myopathic' changes may develop with fibre splitting, internal migration of nuclei and fat accumulation.

The clinical symptoms depend on the rate of denervation. When this is rapid the disease runs a short rapidly fatal course – progressive infantile spinal muscular atrophy (Werdnig–Hoffmann disease). When denervation is slower and re-innervation more effective the course is slower – chronic childhood spinal muscular atrophy (Kugelberg–Welander syndrome). The mutant gene responsible for these diseases has been mapped on chromosome 5 (5q12–q14); the nature of the gene product is not known, but presumably it is important in the normal maintenance of anterior horn cells.

The Eye

The pathological changes which occur in the eye and in the orbit are, in many respects, identical to those described in other systems of the body. However, owing to the particular anatomical and functional properties of the eye, there are some important disease processes which lead to blindness and this justifies a separate section.

Applied Anatomy

The structure of the eye is shown diagrammatically in Figs 18.78 and 18.79. Visual acuity depends upon a transparent focusing system (the cornea and lens), transparent media (the aqueous and vitreous) and a normal photoreceptor and neural conducting mechanism. The metabolism of the cornea and lens is maintained by the circulation of the aqueous fluid, which is produced in the ciliary processes and leaves the anterior chamber via the outflow apparatus situated in the inner peripheral cornea adjacent to the root of the iris. The outflow system is a filter which consists of a series of fenestrated collagenous plates (trabeculae) which are covered by phagocytic endothelial cells: this trabecular meshwork is limited externally by the canal of Schlemm. The pressure within the eye is normally 15–20 mmHg (2.0–2.7 kPa) and depends upon aqueous production, the resistance in the outflow system and an intact corneoscleral envelope. Any marked variation in pressure – **ocular hypotension or ocular hypertension** – whether acute or chronic, causes an imbalance in tissue perfusion which leads to metabolic damage, most importantly to the light-sensitive and impulse-conducting neural tissues.

The retina and the pigment epithelium are maintained by blood flow from two separate arterial systems. The inner two-thirds of the thickness of the retinal tissue are supplied by the branches of the central retinal artery, whilst the outer third (the photoreceptor layer) is maintained by the choriocapillaris which is supplied by the posterior ciliary arteries. The photoreceptors detect photons of light in a series of stacked discs (Fig. 18.80). To prevent deterioration in the lipoprotein membranes due to the release of free radicals after photon stimulation, there is constant formation of

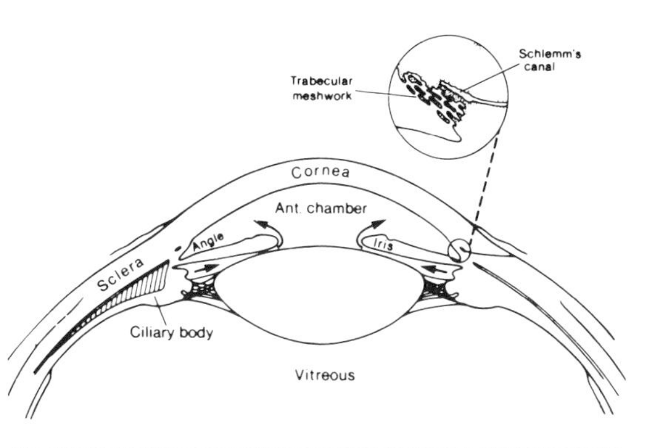

Fig. 18.78 Schematic diagram of the structures of the anterior segment of the eye to show the principal route of aqueous flow.

new discs and phagocytosis of 'spent' discs by the retinal pigment epithelium. Each cell in this monolayer phagocytosis thousands of lipoprotein discs each day and, in addition, supports the photoreceptor cell with the biochemical precursors for disc formation. Abnormalities in the relationship between photoreceptors and the retinal pigment epithelium are the basis for an inherited blinding disease called ***retinitis pigmentosa***, in which there is progressive loss of photoreceptors with proliferation of the retinal pigment epithelium.

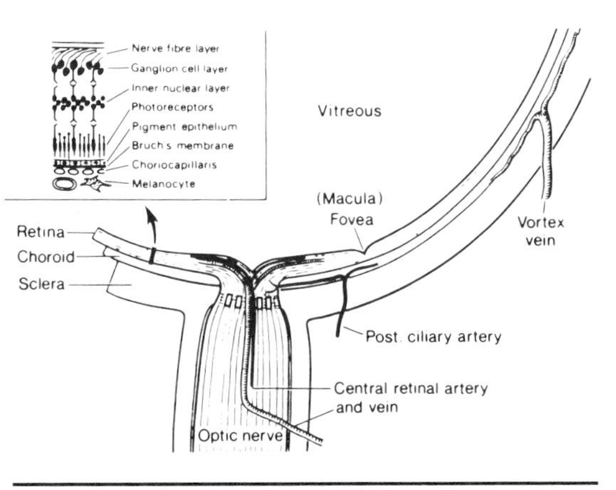

Fig. 18.79 Schematic diagram of the structures of the posterior segment of the eye to show the vascular supply to the choroid, retina and optic disc.

The optic nerve is supplied by the meningeal arteries, and the optic disc or papilla is nourished by blood vessels which are derived from the adjacent (peripapillary) choroid. Because of this vascular arrangement, distinctive patterns of ischaemic damage can occur in the visual sensory system according to the anatomical site of the vascular occlusion or impairment (Fig. 18.81).

Infection in the Eye

Pathogenic micro-organisms of numerous types can invade the eye from the external surface, the adjacent orbital tissues or via the bloodstream. Primary infection by blood-borne bacteria is still important, but is more important as a secondary complication of trauma (accidental or surgical).

The cellular response is, in general, similar to that observed in other tissues, but the eye is particularly vulnerable because the lens and vitreous are avascular, protein-rich structures – ideal media for the proliferation of many pathogenic bacteria. A traumatic ulcer of the cornea complicated by infection may measure only a few millimetres in diameter, but it will seriously impair vision and may necessitate removal of the eye if the ulcer perforates.

Conjunctiva and Cornea

Adenoviruses types 3 and 7 cause a conjunctivitis in which there is hyperplasia of lymphoid tissue in the oedematous and hyperaemic conjunctival stroma – follicular conjunctivitis. **Epidemic conjunctivitis** is due to adenovirus type 8 infection.

The cornea is involved particularly in herpes simplex infection, the epithelium being destroyed in a finger-like or dendritic pattern. ***Herpes simplex* keratitis** is often recurrent, and corneal transparency is destroyed by stromal fibrosis and ingrowth of blood vessels accompanied by inflammatory cells. Dissolution of the corneal stroma is aggravated by the release of collagenases from leucocytes and the damaged corneal cells. When scarring occurs the central cornea can be replaced by a homotransplant.

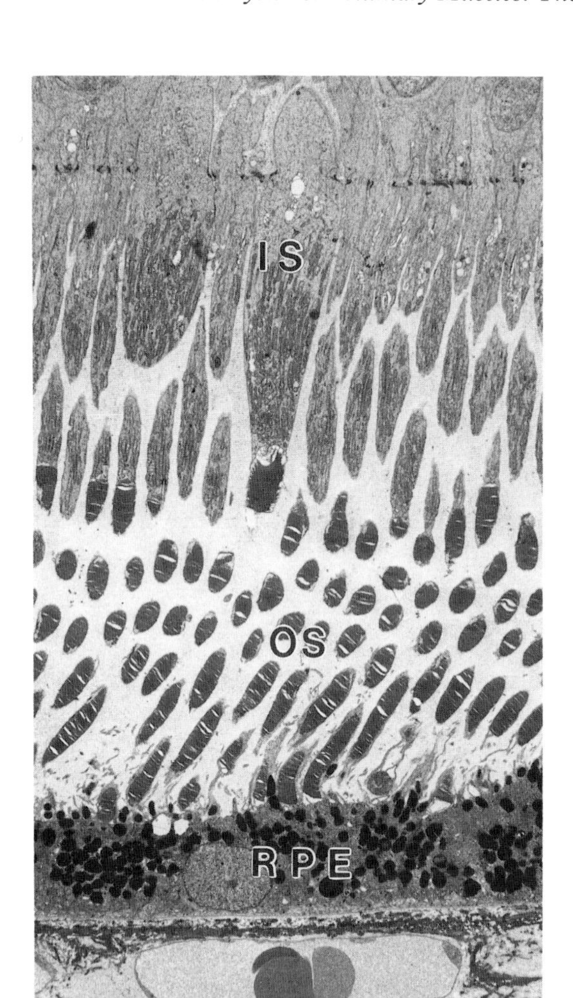

Fig. 18.80 An electron micrograph of the inner segments (IS) and outer segments (OS) of the photoreceptor layer: the tips of the photoreceptors are phagocytosed by the cells in the retinal pigment epithelium (RPE).

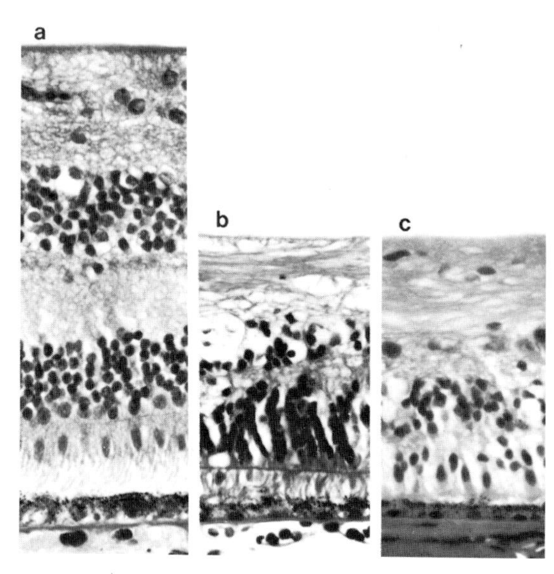

Fig. 18.81 **a** Normal retina. **b** Ischaemic atrophy of the inner retina due to occlusion of the central retinal artery. **c** Ischaemic atrophy of the outer retina due to posterior ciliary artery occlusion. ×240.

Trachoma/Trachoma-inclusion Conjunctivitis or TRIC Infection

Infection caused by *Chlamydia trachomatis* of types A, B and C is common in the tropical zones, and trachoma is responsible for blindness on a massive scale. The organism initially infects the conjunctival epithelium and it can be demonstrated in smears of these cells by the presence of characteristic intracytoplasmic inclusion bodies. The conjunctiva is thickened by a dense lymphocytic infiltrate which commonly extends on to and destroys the superficial peripheral cornea. The healing stage is associated with conjunctival scarring, eyelid distortion and corneal damage by in-turned lashes.

Oculogenital conjunctivitis *Chlamydia trachomatis* (types D–K) commonly infects the genital tract. However, it causes a mild keratoconjunctivitis in individuals living in the temperate zones.

Uvea

In tuberculosis, syphilis and brucellosis the uveal tract (the iris, ciliary body and choroid) is the normal location of the granulomatous reaction – **granulomatous uveitis**. A chronic inflammatory process in the choroid (**choroiditis**) leads to focal destruction of the pigment epithelium and the adjacent retina, which either fuses with the choroid or is detached by leakage of fluid from blood vessels (exudative detachment). In the iris (**iritis**) and ciliary body (**cyclitis**), stromal infiltration by lymphocytes and macrophages leads to exudation of protein into the anterior and posterior chambers: clumps of inflammatory cells adhering to the posterior corneal surface (keratic precipitates) are a classical sign of **iridocyclitis**.

Uveitis of Unknown Aetiology

It should be noted that in many cases the cause of chronic uveitis is unknown, despite intense investigation. The inflammatory infiltrate is predominantly lymphocytic in the uveal tract: involvement of the ciliary body leads to ocular hypotension, which causes choroidal and retinal oedema. Swelling of the nerve fibres in the optic disc – papilloedema (Fig. 18.87c) is also a feature. The release of toxic substances results in degeneration of the lens and inflammation and fibrosis in the vitreous lead to **traction detachment of the retina**. Exudation of proteinaceous material into the subretinal space also contributes to retinal detachment. The end stage of any chronic inflammatory disease is a striking shrinkage of the eye with massive subretinal fibrosis and secondary ossification – phthisis bulbi (Fig. 18.82).

Retina

Retinitis is the most important component of infection due to herpes and cytomegalovirus in AIDS, and the retina is the site of attack in toxoplasmosis and toxocariasis. In drug addicts, fungal infection spreads from the retina into the vitreous.

Autoimmune Disease

Autoimmune reactions occur in the eye in two established disease entities, lens-induced uveitis and sympathetic ophthalmitis. The eye may be involved in all the connective tissue diseases, but the disastrous effects of destruction of collagen in the sclera (scleromalacia) and cornea are noteworthy in rheumatoid arthritis.

Lens-induced Uveitis

Release of degraded lens crystalline protein from a degenerate (cataractous) lens stimulates a T-cell mediated, giant-cell granulomatous reaction around and within the iris and lens.

Sympathetic Ophthalmitis

Trauma to an eye with damage to the iris or the ciliary body may be followed by a T-cell mediated giant-cell granulomatous uveitis in both eyes (Fig. 18.83). This autoimmune inflammatory process can cause bilateral blindness, but is preventable if the injured eye is enucleated within 3 weeks of injury. Current research favours an autoimmune reaction to exposed retinal antigens as the most likely aetiology.

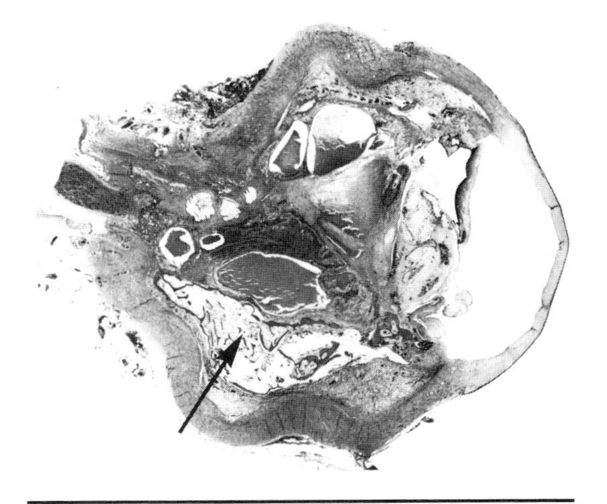

Fig. 18.82 Shrinkage and disorganization of the eye (phthisis bulbi) following inflammation. The retina is detached and the choroid is thickened by oedema and ossification (arrow).

Vascular Disease

Retinal Vascular Disease

Important changes occur when there is focal occlusive disease (diabetes mellitus, malignant hypertension) in the retinal arterioles: the subsequent ischaemia leads to exudation through damaged capillary endothelium. The outer plexiform layer is a zone in which resorption of exudate is undertaken by macrophages: on ophthalmoscopy, the corresponding features are discrete pale yellow areas in the retina and these are described as **hard exudates** (Fig. 18.84). Another clinical feature of focal ischaemia is a **soft exudate** which is a diffuse white thickening resembling a cotton-wool spot in the inner retina. On histological examination, a cotton-wool spot is seen as an interruption of axons in the nerve fibre layer of the retina. The damaged sector is oedematous and contains the bulbous tips of axons (**cytoid bodies**) which have been interrupted and have sealed off (Fig. 18.85). The bulbous swelling is due to continuing axoplasmic flow from the cell body in the parent ganglion cell distal to the interruption.

When small arterioles rupture, the blood tracks within the nerve fibre layer to produce flame-shaped haemorrhages. Conversely, blot or dot haemorrhages are seen when blood accumulates in the outer plexiform layer after rupture of capillaries. Haemorrhages are most prominent when venous outflow is partially impaired by thrombosis in the central retinal vein. The visual consequences of venous occlusion are less serious than those of embolic obliteration of the central artery,

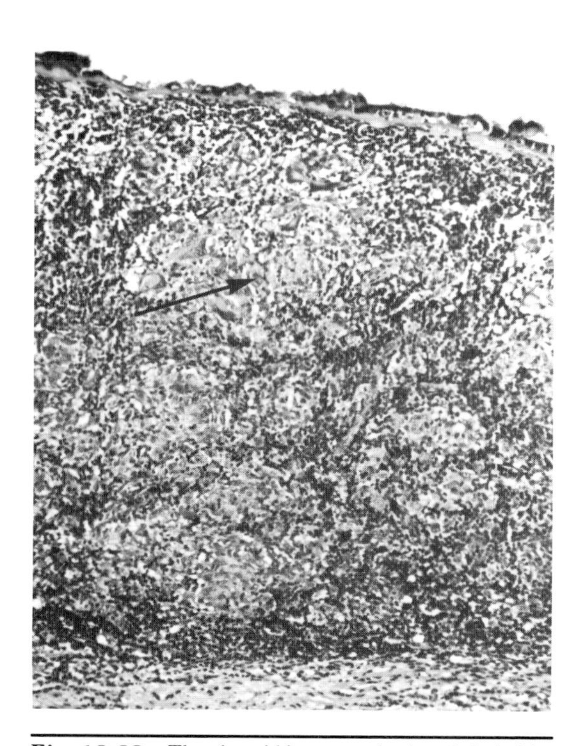

Fig. 18.83 The choroid in sympathetic ophthalmitis; the tissue is infiltrated by a giant-cell granulomatous reaction (arrow). ×370.

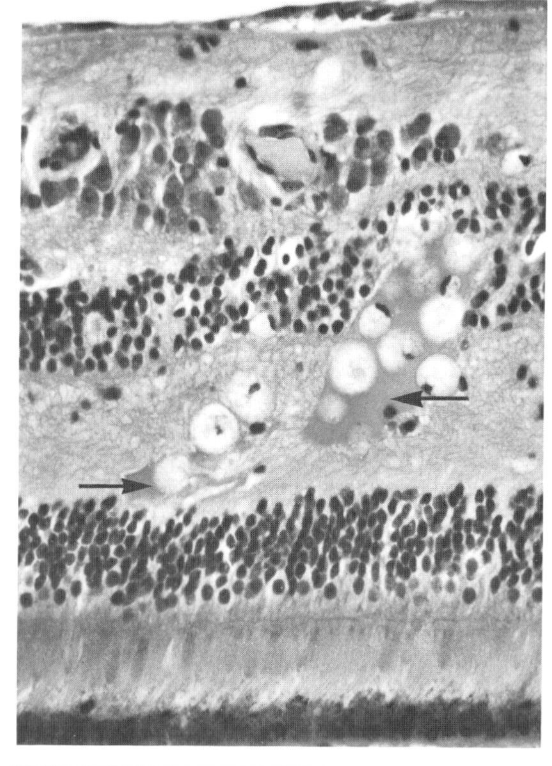

Fig. 18.84 A proteinaceous exudate (arrow) in the inner nuclear and the outer plexiform layers; lipid-laden macrophages are prominent. ×300.

when there is total ischaemic infarction of the retina and immediate loss of vision.

One of the most important responses to focal retinal ischaemia is the release of vasoformative factors from the surviving neural tissue: this causes proliferation of endothelial cells into the ischaemic area. Although this process is potentially beneficial, the delicate newly formed vessels tend to penetrate the vitreous where they stimulate the formation of membranes which cause retinal detachment and blindness. Vasoproliferative retinopathy is a common complication in the later stages of diabetes mellitus, so-called diabetic retinopathy; this can now be controlled by laser treatment.

Age-related Retinal Degeneration

In the elderly, after prolonged irradiation by visible light, the photoreceptors atrophy at the macula and this is accompanied by degenerative changes in the retinal pigment epithelium (age-related macular degeneration). In some patients the degeneration in the retinal pigment epithelium stimulates sub-retinal neovascularization with haemorrhage and fibrosis (senile disciform degeneration of the macula). The overlying photoreceptor tissue is destroyed and loss of central vision is a serious consequence of this common disease.

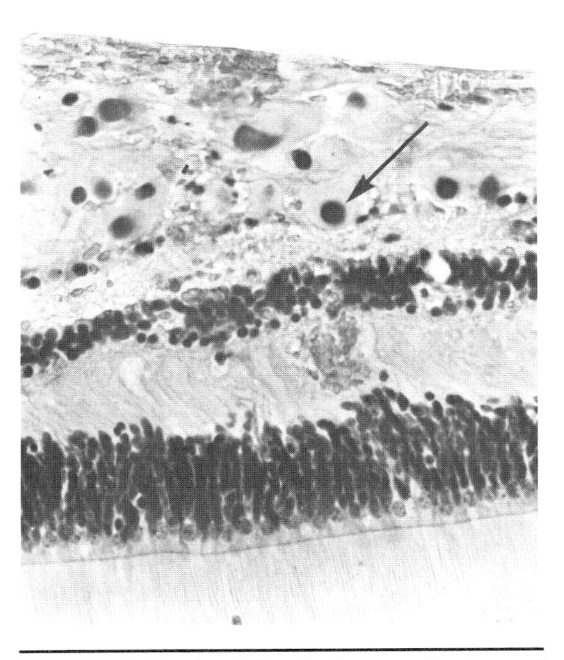

Fig. 18.85 A micro-infarct in the nerve fibre layer of the retina in which the swollen ends of axons (arrow) are seen as large, darkly staining round masses surrounded by paler areas. ×300.

Retinal Detachment

In myopia and in the ageing eye, there are areas of retinal thinning at the equator. Vitreous traction causes tears in the atrophic retina and fluid from the vitreous separates the photoreceptors from the pigment epithelium. This separation deprives the photoreceptors of their metabolic support and there is loss of visual field corresponding to the region of the detachment.

Cataract

The biconvex lens substance is formed by cells which contain crystalline lens proteins. The cells are enclosed in an elastic membrane, the lens capsule. The malleability of the lens permits rapid fine focusing by tension exerted on the lens equator by the ciliary muscle via the zonular fibres. As there is a constant production of new lens fibres at the periphery of the cortex during life, any change in the biochemical composition of the aqueous fluid may result in formation of abnormal (opaque) proteins in the damaged lens cells. Thus, opacities may occur after trauma, in uveitis and in metabolic diseases, e.g. diabetes mellitus and hypocalcaemia. The most common form of cataract, however, is senile cataract which is due to degradation of lens proteins in the oldest central part of the lens: yellow and eventually dark brown proteins are formed. Most cases of cataract are treated successfully by removal of the opaque lens matter and the insertion of a plastic lens implant into the residue of the lens capsule.

Glaucoma

Glaucoma is a generic name for a group of diseases in which, for a variety of reasons, the intraocular pressure increases to a level which impairs the vascular perfusion of the neural tissue and causes blindness. The rise in pressure is due to obstruction to the outflow of aqueous, which occurs either as the result of closure of the chamber angle (iridotrabecular contact) or as the result of an abnormality within the outflow system.

Closed-angle Glaucoma

In the **primary form** the iridocorneal angle is narrow and the anterior chamber is shallow. In such individuals the iris and lens may come into contact when the iris is in mid-dilatation: this prevents the flow of aqueous through the pupil and pressure builds up behind the iris, which becomes further bowed anteriorly and causes further occlusion of the angle (Fig. 18.86). This form of glaucoma is of acute onset, with ocular congestion, corneal oedema and severe pain. Untreated, there is blindness due to ischaemic atrophy of the optic disc.

Secondary closed-angle glaucoma has many causes, but the most common is due to fibrovascular adhesion between iris and cornea following ischaemic retinal disease and uveitis.

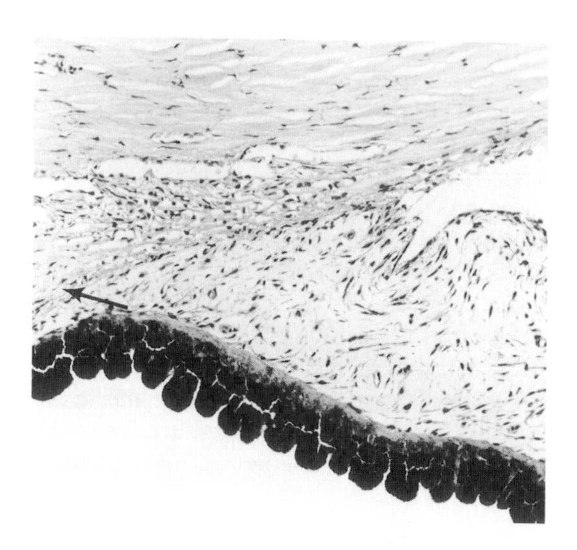

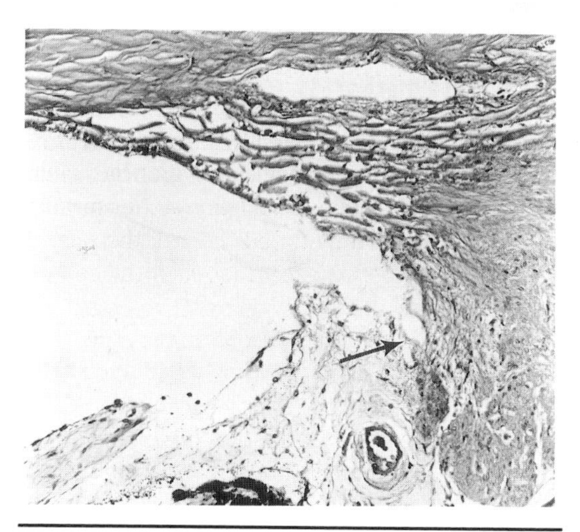

Fig. 18.86 *Upper*: The chamber angle in angle closure glaucoma. The iris is displaced forwards and the stroma has sealed off the outflow system; the iris root is shown by an arrow. *Lower*: The chamber angle in open-angle glaucoma. The trabecular meshwork has thickened and hyalinized trabeculae: note the recess between the trabecular meshwork and the iris root (arrow).

Open-angle Glaucoma

The **primary type** is an insidious disease of the elderly in which a slowly progressive increase in intraocular pressure leads to an interruption of axoplasmic flow in the nerve fibres in sectors of the optic disc: this is often not noticed by the patient, but can be detected clinically by the presence of a field defect (scotoma) which has a characteristic arcuate shape. Modern morphological techniques have not revealed a specific cause for the increased resistance in the outflow system.

In **secondary open-angle glaucoma** the outflow system is obstructed mechanically by cells or particulate matter. In acute or chronic inflammatory disease, inflammatory cells accumulate within the intertrabecular spaces, while obstruction by macrophages occurs after haemorrhage or degenerative liquefaction of the lens cortex. The outflow system can also be obstructed by tumour cell infiltration, e.g. by a malignant melanoma of the iris or ciliary body.

The Effects of Increased Intraocular Pressure

The most serious effects on visual function are due to ischaemic atrophy of the axons in the nerve fibres of the disc, and secondary atrophy in the nerve fibre layer of the retina. Excavation or cupping of the disc may become so advanced that it extends into the optic nerve (Fig. 18.87).

The corneal endothelium maintains dehydration of the stroma and this is necessary for transparency. At high pressure, the endothelial barrier breaks down and the stroma becomes cloudy due to oedema and the epithelium separates (**bullous keratopathy**). At an advanced stage, the uveal tissues become atrophic and fibrosis occurs in ischaemic areas of the iris and choroid; the scleral tissues may stretch to form localized bulges or **staphylomas**.

In infants and children, glaucoma can result from developmental abnormalities in which there is a failure in modelling of the embryonic tissues which are found in the chamber angle in the early stages of intrauterine life. Increasing intraocular pressure causes the malleable infantile eye to expand uniformly and it may become so large that it resembles an ox-eye ('**buphthalmos**').

Tumours

The tumours of the eyelid, conjunctiva and orbital tissues do not differ significantly in morphology and behaviour from those occurring elsewhere. Intraocular tumours are rare, but are important because of the serious effect on vision and their unusual patterns of behaviour.

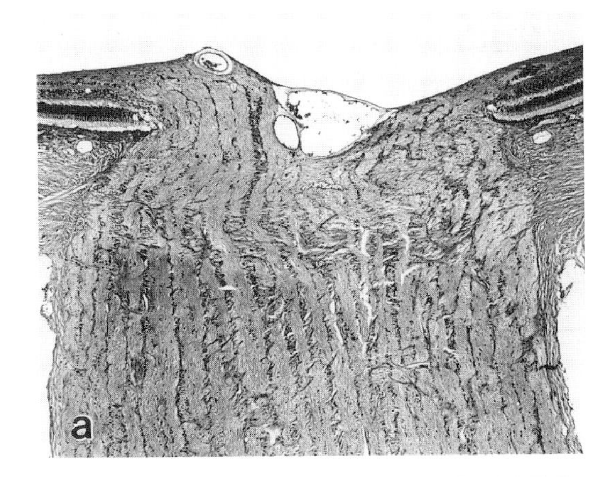

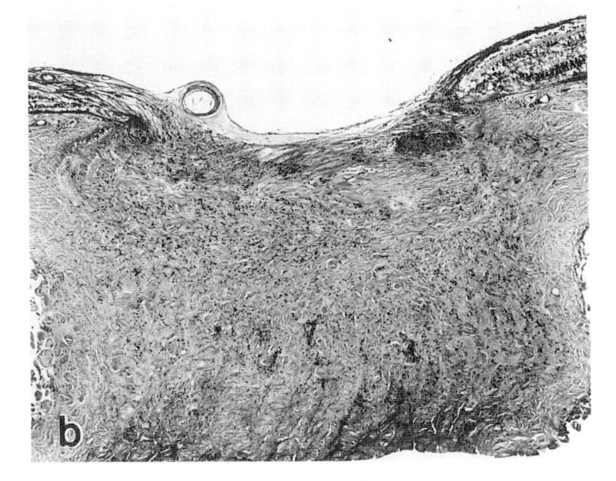

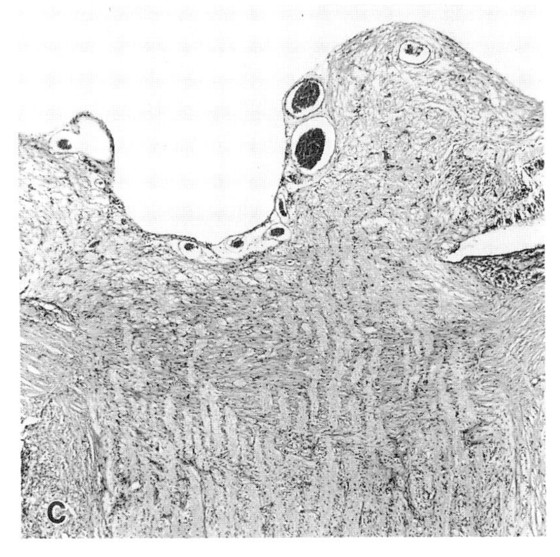

Fig. 18.87 The normal optic disc is shown in **a** for comparison with **b** the atrophic nerve head in glaucoma and **c** the swollen nerve fibre layer in papilloedema.

Benign Naevi and Malignant Melanoma

These are uveal tumours of adult life, derived from the spindle-shaped melanocytes of the uveal tract. **Benign naevi** are common and clinically unimportant, but there is good evidence that some undergo malignant transformation. **Malignant melanomas** are unilateral and solitary and are most commonly situated in the posterior choroid. The tumour expands the choroid, penetrates Bruch's membrane and adopts a characteristic collar-stud shape (Fig. 18.88): alternatively an ovoid mass is formed. Plasma leaks from the tumour into the subretinal space and causes secondary exudative retinal detachment. Microscopically (Fig. 18.88) the tumour cells are either spindle-shaped or round and epithelioid. Predominantly epithelioid tumours have a 10% 15-year survival, considerably worse than mainly spindle-cell tumours, which carry a 60% 15-year survival rate. Growth within the eye leads to disorganization and often to secondary glaucoma, whilst extension usually takes place through intrascleral vascular and neural channels and the choroidal (vortex) veins. This tumour is notorious for producing multiple, rapidly enlarging liver metastases as long as 20 (symptom-free) years after enucleation of the affected eye ('the big liver and glass-eye syndrome'). What happens to the tumour cells seeded in the liver in the latent interval is a matter for speculation, but current theories invoke an immunological suppression of viable metastases.

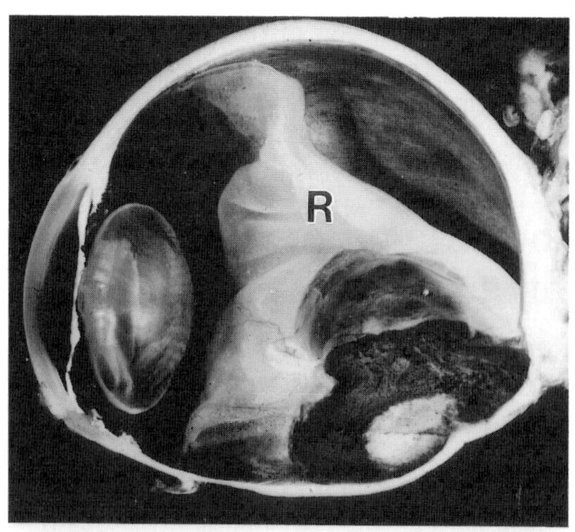

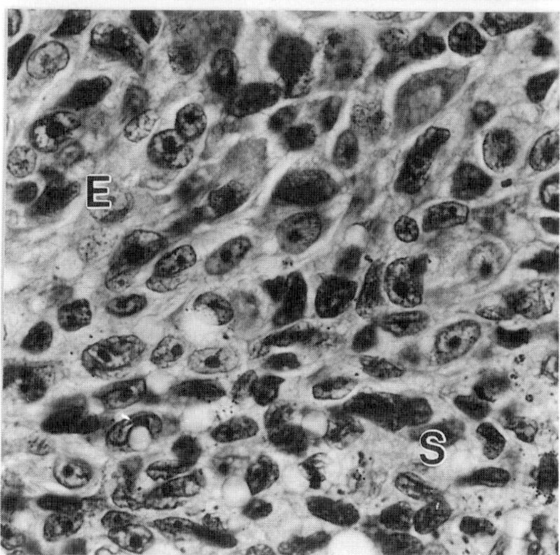

Fig. 18.88 Malignant melanoma of the choroid. *Above,* the tumour has a collar-stud shape and the cut surface is both pigmented and non-pigmented; the retina (R) is detached. *Below,* histology of this tumour reveals large epithelioid cells (E) and smaller spindle cells (S).

Retinoblastoma

This is a malignant tumour of the retina which occurs in infants: the incidence is 1 in 23 000 live births. It affects both sexes equally and in 40% of cases other relatives are affected. These familial cases are inherited as an autosomal dominant and have an additional risk of a second malignancy, especially in soft tissues. Spontaneous non-familial tumours are usually unilateral and present at a later age.

As has been previously described (p. 396) the retinoblastoma gene occurs on the long arm of chromosome 13 (13q14). In order for a tumour to develop, both copies of the retinoblastoma gene must be lost (the 'two-hit' hypothesis), i.e. one copy can act as a suppressor gene or, more appropriately, as an 'anti-retinoblastoma gene'. In familial cases the first hit occurs through inheritance of a mutant allele and the second occurs as a somatic mutation; in non-familial cases two acquired somatic mutations occur, usually in one area of the retina, so that the tumour is unilateral and unifocal.

Blindness in the affected eye causes the child to squint. When the tumour fills the vitreous or detaches the retina, a white mass is seen behind the lens, so that reflected light produces a reflex similar to that seen in a cat's eye in car headlights. On gross examination, a retinoblastoma forms a solid, pale-grey, partially calcified and partially necrotic mass.

The tumour is composed of small, round or oval cells with scanty cytoplasm and a high mitotic rate. A tendency to differentiation is seen in the formation of rosettes, which are circular arrangements of the tumour cells (Fig. 18.89). Extra-ocular extension occurs, either by spread along the optic nerve into the brain or through the sclera into the orbit. Metastases to visceral organs are a late and unusual event. Early enucleation or radiotherapy to the eye achieves a survival rate of the order of 90%.

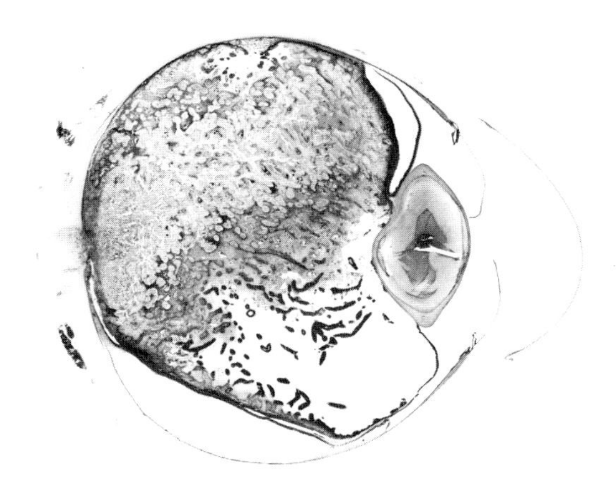

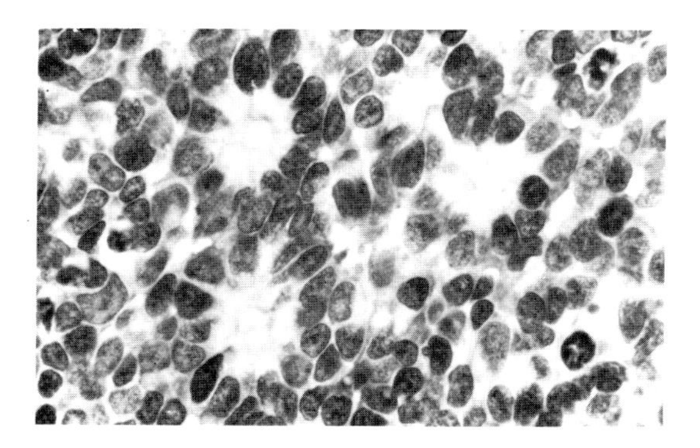

Fig. 18.89 Extensive growth of retinoblastoma within the posterior part of the eye (*above*). ×2.5. The microscopic features includes the typical rosettes (*below*). ×525.

Other Intra-ocular Tumours

Gliomas of the optic nerve are uncommon, but may develop in some 5–10% of patients with neurofibromatosis (p. 868). Nodular hamartomas of the iris are found in 90% of patients with neurofibromatosis. Metastatic tumours (breast, lung, leukaemias) are the most common intra-ocular neoplasms and may be bilateral.

Further Reading

The Nervous Systems

Adams, J. H. and Graham, D. I. (1988). *An Introduction to Neuropathology*. Churchill Livingstone, Edinburgh.

Weller, R. O. (ed.). (1990). *Nervous System, Muscle and Eyes. Systemic Pathology*, 3rd edn, Vol. 4. Churchill Livingstone, Edinburgh.

Voluntary Muscles

Dubowitz, V. (1985). *Muscle Biopsy. A Practical Approach*. Baillière Tindall, London and Philadelphia.

Moraes C. T., diMauro S., Zeviani M., *et al.* (1989). Mitochondrial DNA deletions in progressive external ophthalmoplegia and Kearns–Sayre syndrome. *New England Journal of Medicine* **320**, 1293–9.

Roberts A., Penera S., Lang B., Vincent A., Newson-Davies J. (1985). Paraneoplastic myasthenic syndrome IgG inhibits $^{45}Ca^{2+}$ flux in a human small cell carcinoma line. *Nature* **317**, 737–9.

Swash, M. and Schwarts, M. S. (1984). *Biopsy Pathology of Muscle.* Chapman and Hall Medical, London.

The Eye

Garner, A. and Klintworth, G. (eds). (1982). *Pathobiology of Ocular Disease*, pp. 1732. Marcel Dekker, Inc., New York.

Lee, W. R. (1993). *Ophthalmic histopathology.* Springer-Verlag, London.

Naumann, G. O. H. and Apple, D. (1986). *Pathology of the Eye.* Springer-Verlag, Berlin.

Spencer, W. H. (ed.) (1986). *Ophthalmic Pathology*, Vols 1–3. W. B. Saunders Co., London and Philadelphia.

19

The Kidneys and Urinary Tract

Fine Structure and Function

The kidneys are each composed of about one million nephrons, the major functions of which are to remove from the plasma various waste products of metabolism, and to maintain fluid and acid–base balances and the normal body content of electrolytes. This is achieved by production of a very large volume of glomerular filtrate, which is then subjected to selective reabsorption as it passes down the tubules. The main purpose of this system is to excrete the required quantities of waste products while conserving water and electrolytes. Although only some 0.5% of the total body weight, the kidneys receive 20% of the cardiac output. Nearly all of this passes through the glomeruli, where around 20% of the plasma volume (550 ml/min; 800 litres/day) is filtered off, giving a glomerular filtration rate (GFR) of 120 ml/min (180 litres per day). The process of filtration is aided by the unusually high pressure in the **glomerular capillaries** which is due to their unique position between two arterioles. The capillary walls (Fig. 19.1) consist of the vascular endothelium, which is unusual in having cytoplasmic **fenestrations** allowing direct contact between the contents of the capillary at the site of these fenestrae and the glomerular basement membrane. Outside the basement membrane is a layer of visceral **epithelial cells** or **podocytes**, which make contact with the basement membrane by means of cytoplasmic processes – **foot processes** or **pedicels**. In the spaces (slit pores) between the foot processes there is a thin 'slit membrane' with a central bar. The factors which regulate passage across the glomerular capillary wall include the pressure differences across the wall, the sieving effect of the slit pores and the negative charge of the basement membrane which retards the passage of negatively charged macromolecules, especially proteins.

Each glomerulus is composed of several lobules, the structure of which is shown in Fig. 19.2. The capillary loops lie at the periphery of the lobules, while the core is made up of mesangial

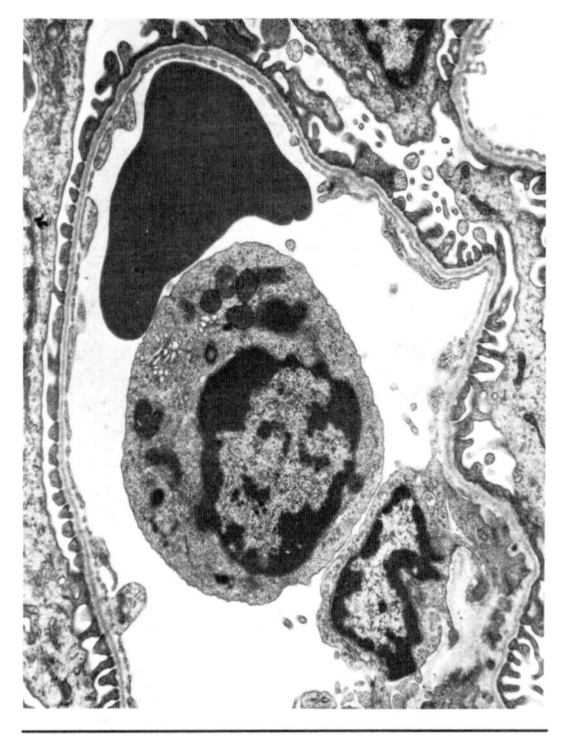

Fig. 19.1 Electron micrograph of glomerular capillary containing a lymphocyte and red cell. Note, from within outwards, the endothelial cytoplasm with fenestrations, the continuous basement membrane, and the foot processes of the epithelium. ×12 000.

cells and basement membrane-like material. The **mesangial cells** have a number of functions, including a structural supportive role; they also contain actomyosin and may regulate blood flow through the glomeruli. They have phagocytic properties and are responsible for maintenance of the basement membrane.

Reabsorption in the **proximal convoluted tubule** is both active and passive. The epithelial cells have a prominent brush border which is seen by electron microscopy to consist of numerous, fine, relatively long microvilli (Fig. 19.3); this increases the cellular absorptive area by a factor of 40. The most important active reabsorption is that of sodium and this function accounts for about 6% of the body's energy needs in the resting state. The driving force of sodium reabsorption leads to passive reabsorption of urea, chloride and water, down concentration, electrical and osmotic gradients, respectively. Most of the filtered glucose

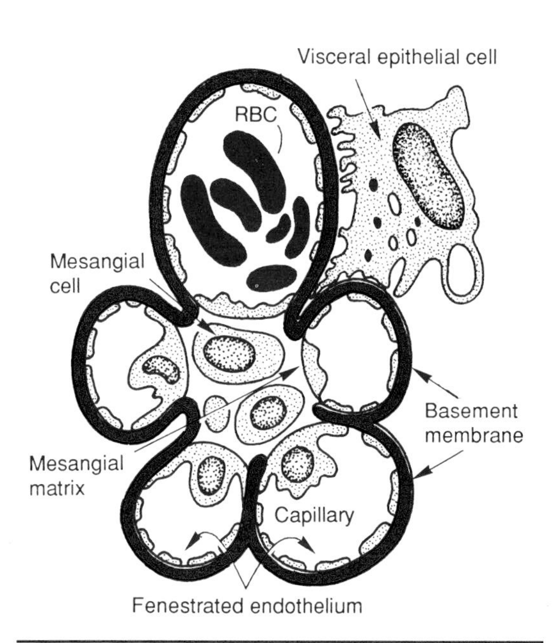

Fig. 19.2 Diagram of a glomerular lobule in cross-section.

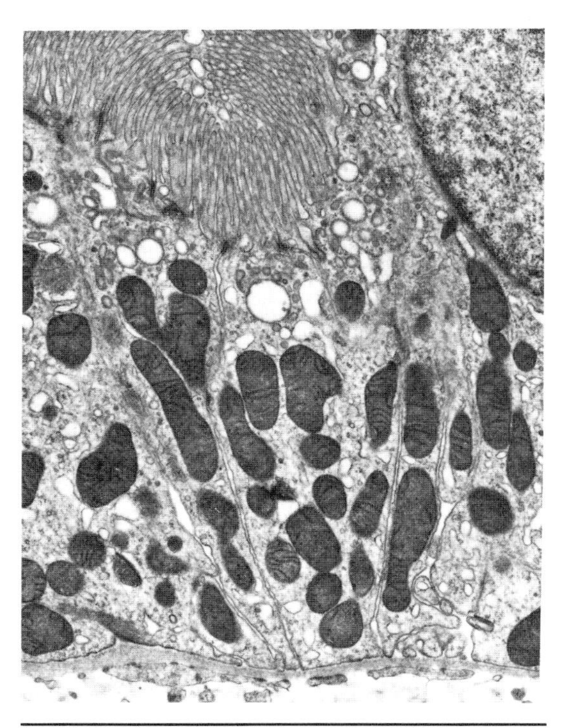

Fig. 19.3 Electron micrograph of parts of two epithelial cells of the proximal convoluted tubule, showing the microvilli (upper left) and numerous mitochondria. The basal part of the epithelium rests on a thin basement membrane. ×11 000.

and amino acids and much of the potassium, bicarbonate and phosphate are also actively reabsorbed.

Thereafter the **thin descending** and **thin ascending limbs of the loop of Henle** allow equilibration between the tubular lumen and interstitium. This maintains the hypertonicity of the interstitium which is essential to the countercurrent multiplier system and thus to the mechanism of urine concentration. The next segment of the nephron is the **thick ascending limb of the loop of Henle** which continues the reabsorptive function of the proximal tubule.

In the **distal convoluted tubule**, active sodium reabsorption again takes place but here it is influenced by aldosterone and in exchange there is secretion of hydrogen ions and potassium. Final adjustment of water balance occurs both in the distal tubule and collecting tubule. In states of water depletion, antidiuretic hormone (ADH) acts on these parts of the tubule to make them permeable to water which is then reabsorbed into the hypertonic interstitium down an osmotic gradient, leading to the production of a low volume, concentrated urine. Thus, tubular function each day reduces the 180 litres of glomerular filtrate to around 1.5 litres of urine which enables waste products such as urea to be excreted in a highly concentrated form.

In addition to their homeostatic and excretory roles, the kidneys also have hormonal and metabolic functions. Specialized cells in the juxtaglomerular apparatus secrete **renin**, an enzyme which proteolytically converts plasma angiotensinogen to angiotensin I. Angiotensin converting enzyme then converts angiotensin I to angiotensin II which raises blood pressure by means of its vasoconstrictor effect and stimulates aldosterone secretion by the adrenal cortex. These phenomena and the fine structure of the **juxtaglomerular apparatus** are described on p. 75.

The kidneys secrete **erythropoietin** which stimulates erythropoiesis (p. 590). Deficiency of erythropoietin is the main cause of the severe anaemia which is characteristic of advanced chronic renal failure.

One of the most important metabolic functions of the kidneys is the hydroxylation of vitamin D. The proximal tubules contain the enzyme 1α hydroxylase which is necessary to convert 25-hydroxyvitamin D_3 [$25(OH)D_3$] to 1,25-dihydroxyvitamin D_3, [$1,25(OH)_2D_3$], the active form of vitamin D_3, whose main effect is to increase calcium absorption from the intestine. The deficiency of $1,25(OH)_2D_3$ which occurs in chronic renal failure has an important role in the production of renal osteodystrophy (p. 949).

Clinical Aspects of Renal Disease

Diseases of the kidney can present in a variety of ways, the six most common of which are outlined here.

(1) The nephrotic syndrome. Heavy proteinuria, which may vary from around 3 grams to more than 10 grams per 24 hours, results in hypoalbuminaemia and generalized oedema: these three features together constitute the nephrotic syndrome. Hyperlipidaemia is an almost invariable feature and hypertension and impaired renal function are frequently present.

The proteinuria is due to increased glomerular permeability and can thus result from a variety of glomerular diseases. The causes are summarized in Table 19.1. In children, minimal change nephrotic syndrome or minimal change disease is the commonest cause, whereas in adults, membranous glomerulonephritis is most commonly found. In addition to glomerulonephritis, the nephrotic syndrome can be caused by systemic disease affecting the glomerulus, e.g. diabetes mellitus. Other aetiological factors include infection, drugs, toxins and neoplastic disease.

In addition to generalized oedema, and sometimes also ascites and pleural effusions, there is a high risk of infections. The kidneys show striking changes. These include generalized enlargement and pallor due to oedema, and frequently a yellow, radial streaking of the cortex due to deposition of lipids (Fig. 19.4). There may be accumulation of 'foamy' lipid-laden macrophages and also giant-cell granulomas around crystals of cholesterol. The proximal tubular cells contain abundant hyaline droplets due to reabsorption of protein and also

Table 19.1 Causes of the nephrotic syndrome

Causes
Primary glomerular diseases
Minimal change disease
Membranous glomerulonephritis
Focal segmental glomerulosclerosis
Mesangiocapillary glomerulonephritis
Diffuse proliferative glomerulonephritis
Focal glomerulonephritis
Systemic disease with secondary glomerular injury
Diabetes mellitus
Amyloidosis
Systemic lupus erythematosus
Henoch–Schönlein purpura
Infections, e.g. quartan malaria, infective endocarditis
Neoplastic diseases, e.g. lymphoma, carcinoma and multiple myeloma
Drugs and toxins
Gold, penicillamine

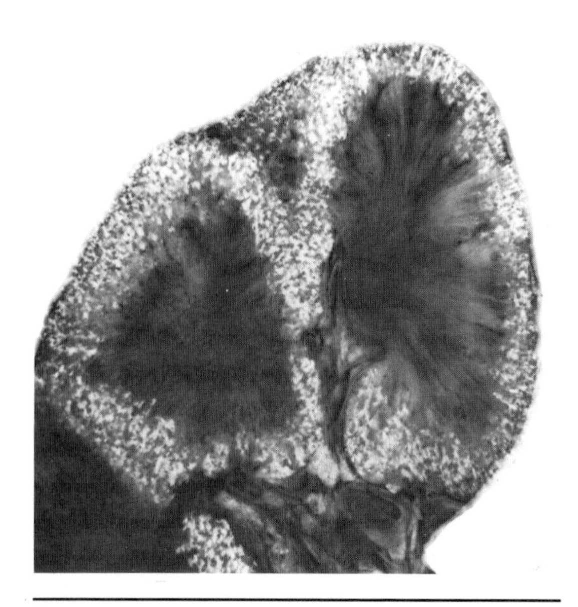

Fig. 19.4 Kidney in nephrotic syndrome, showing abundant cortical deposits of neutral fat and anisotropic lipids. (Photographed using crossed polarizing filters). ×0.8.

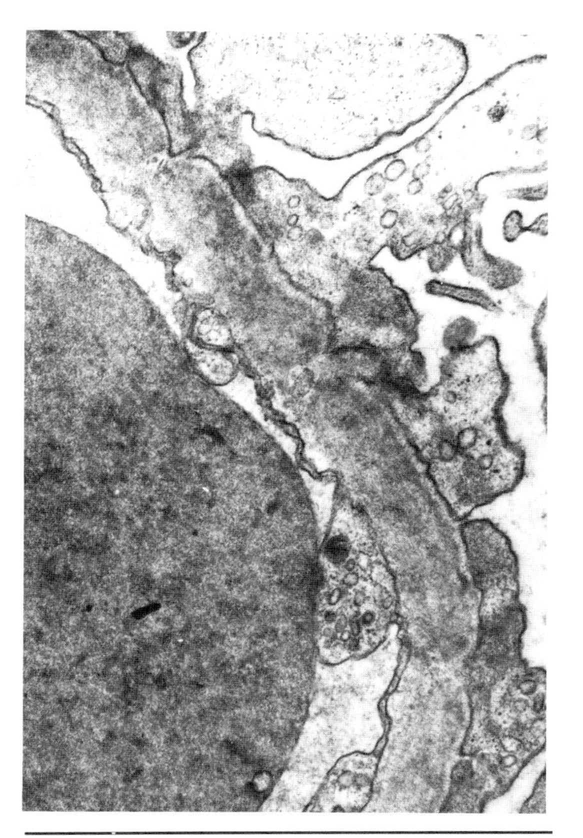

Fig. 19.5 Electron micrograph of glomerular capillary wall in minimal change disease. The only abnormality is fusion of the foot processes. ×18 000.

globules of lipid. Protein casts are present in the distal tubules.

The glomeruli in patients with the nephrotic syndrome show the pathological features of the causal disease. The only feature common to most cases is seen by electron microscopy, and consists of effacement of the foot processes of the epithelial cells, the cytoplasm of which is closely applied to the outer part of the glomerular basement membrane (Fig. 19.5)

(2) The acute nephritic syndrome is virtually synonymous with acute proliferative glomerulonephritis. The clinical features are diffuse oedema, especially in the periorbital region, hypertension with a predisposition to encephalopathy and oliguria. Urine examination reveals proteinuria, haematuria (often giving the urine a smoky appearance) and granular casts.

(3) Asymptomatic proteinuria can result from the same diseases which cause the nephrotic syndrome, the main difference being that the proteinuria is of insufficient degree to cause hypoalbuminaemia and oedema. It will be detected during routine investigation or medical examination.

(4) Painless haematuria is often due to bladder lesions such as a benign or malignant tumour but may also result from renal disease, the commonest example being IgA nephropathy. Microscopic examination of the urine is helpful in localizing the site of blood loss. Red blood cells originating in the lower urinary tract are usually of normal morphology, while those resulting from glomerular disease are dysmorphic, i.e. they are fragmented with a variety of shapes.

(5) Hypertension is usually idiopathic or essential in type but in around 10% of cases is due to underlying parenchymal renal disease. The incidence of hypertension varies among the different types of primary renal disease and the incidence in glomerulonephritis is about 60%. In advanced renal failure the overall incidence is as high as 80%. Another cause of secondary hypertension is renal artery stenosis, usually due to atheroma of the main renal artery or one of its branches. This is uncommon, accounting for less than 5% of all hypertension, but is of importance because of the potential for cure by restoring normal blood flow.

(6) Renal failure is classified as either acute or chronic, each with a lengthy list of causes which are described later. If of long duration, renal failure can lead to a wide variety of complications. Some of these, such as the pruritus, gastrointestinal symptoms, pericarditis and neuropathy result from the uraemia, i.e. accumulation of toxic waste products. Others stem from the various derangements which may accompany progressive renal damage such as the deficiency of erythropoietin, and of $1,25(OH)_2D_3$ and the development of hypertension.

Glomerulonephritis

This term embraces a group of renal diseases in which the lesions are primarily glomerular. Although the name implies inflammation, the typical histological features of inflammation are not present in all types. Glomerulonephritis can be classified on either a clinical or pathological basis but the latter is preferable in view of its greater precision and better correlation with pathogenetic mechanisms, response to therapy and prognosis. Table 19.2 divides glomerulonephritis into the main groups and some of these are then further subdivided in the text. Also some forms of glomerulonephritis consist of diseases confined to the kidney, such as diffuse membranous glomerulonephritis, while with others the disease may be systemic, e.g. SLE. We shall first discuss the aetiology and pathogenesis of glomerulonephritis in general and then deal with each type in turn.

Table 19.2 Classification of glomerulonephritis

Acute diffuse proliferative glomerulonephritis (post-streptococcal glomerulonephritis; post-infectious glomerulonephritis)
Crescentic glomerulonephritis (rapidly progressive glomerulonephritis)
Diffuse membranous glomerulonephritis (idiopathic membranous glomerulonephritis; membranous nephropathy)
Mesangiocapillary glomerulonephritis (membranoproliferative glomerulonephritis)
Type I
Type II
Type III
Focal glomerulonephritis
Primary type: IgA nephropathy
Secondary type
Minimal change nephrotic syndrome (minimal-change disease)
Focal segmental glomerulosclerosis
Chronic glomerulonephritis

Aetiology and Pathogenesis

Immunological Basis

Although no single type of glomerulonephritis is fully understood there is strong evidence that most are due to injury caused by the presence of antigen–antibody complexes in the walls of the glomerular capillaries. Much of this evidence is based on experimental animal work. Immune complexes may localize within the glomeruli in one of three ways:

(1) circulating immune complexes may be filtered out as they pass through the glomerular capillaries;
(2) circulating antibodies may react either with non-basement membrane glomerular antigens or with antigens from the plasma which become trapped in the capillary wall, to form immune complexes *in situ*;
(3) antibodies may form to intrinsic constituents of the glomerular basement membrane.

Deposition of Circulating Immune Complexes Within Glomeruli

Why should immune complexes or antigens circulating in the plasma accumulate preferentially in glomeruli? The kidney receives a relatively large blood supply and the glomeruli are unusual in that their capillaries lie between two arterioles: in consequence, the glomerular capillary pressure is much greater than in other capillary beds. In addition, the normal glomerular capillary wall acts as a progressive sieve: very small molecules and ions pass freely through the endothelial layer, basement membrane and epithelial slit pores to appear in the glomerular filtrate, but cells and very large molecular aggregates are kept within the vascular tree by the pore size of the endothelial cells. Between these two extremes, macromolecules and antigen–antibody complexes can penetrate into the glomerular wall (Fig. 19.6).

It has been suggested that the depth of such penetration depends on a combination of the size, shape and charge of the immune complex. Smaller complexes can penetrate further, as can those that are asymmetrical rather than globular. Furthermore, the basement membrane and the outer membrane of the epithelial cells are negatively charged and will thus repel negatively charged complexes. However, recent studies suggest that circulating complexes usually localize in the mesangium or subendothelial region rather than penetrating into the subepithelial spaces.

In situ *Immune-complex Formation*

Increasing attention has been given recently to the possibility that many forms of immune-complex glomerulonephritis result, not from deposition of circulating immune complexes but from *in situ* complex formation. Animal experiments have suggested that antigens located within glomerular epithelial cells can react with circulating antibodies giving rise to immune complexes localized to the epithelial side of the basement membrane. Further research is required to delineate the relative roles of *in situ* complex formation and deposition of circulating complexes in the pathogenesis of human glomerulonephritis. In both the *in situ* and circulating complex types of disease, immunofluorescence microscopy can be used to demonstrate the complexes which exhibit a typically granular appearance (see Fig. 19.12).

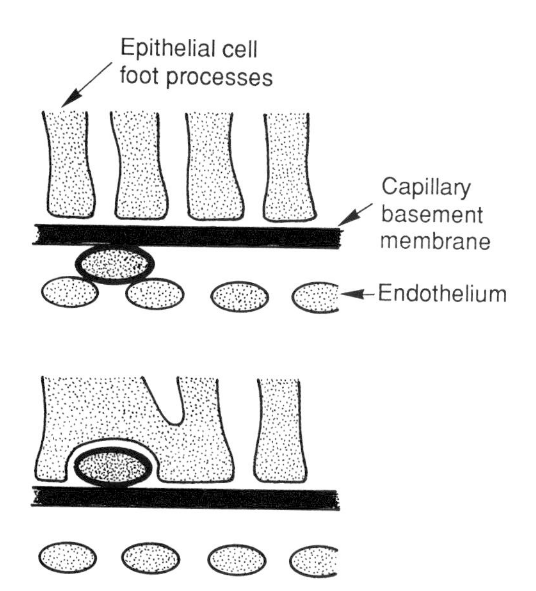

Fig. 19.6 The sites of deposition of immune complexes in the glomerular capillary walls. Larger complexes aggregate on the subendothelial side of the basement membrane (above). Smaller complexes are deposited on the epithelial side of the basement membrane (below).

Antibodies Directed Against the Glomerular Basement Membrane

These can also give rise to experimental and human forms of glomerulonephritis. The classical animal model is nephrotoxic serum nephritis in which glomerular basement membrane antibody raised in another heterologous species and following injection, it binds to antigen in the basement membrane. The injected animal thereafter develops autologous antibodies which are directed against and thus bind to the heterologous antibody along the basement membrane. In this type of glomerulonephritis, fluorescence microscopy shows a characteristic fine linear deposition of antibody (see Fig. 19.13).

Mechanisms of Glomerular Injury

Whether as a result of immune complex formation or deposition of antiglomerular basement membrane antibody, glomerular injury may result in a number of ways. The reaction of antigen and antibody activates the complement system, through either the classical or alternative pathways, with the production of a number of biologically active products including chemotaxins for polymorphonuclear leucocytes and stimulants of monocyte and macrophage function (p. 142). The polymorphs phagocytose the immune complexes and in doing so, secrete numerous lysosomal en-

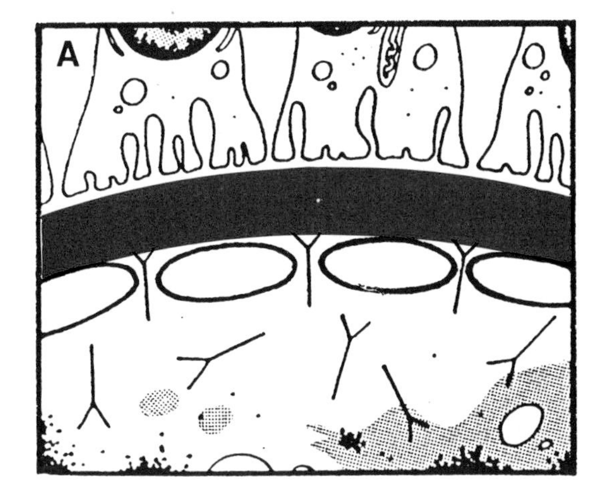

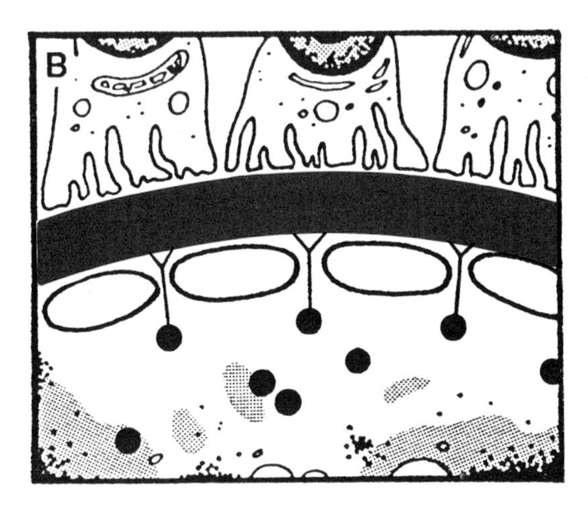

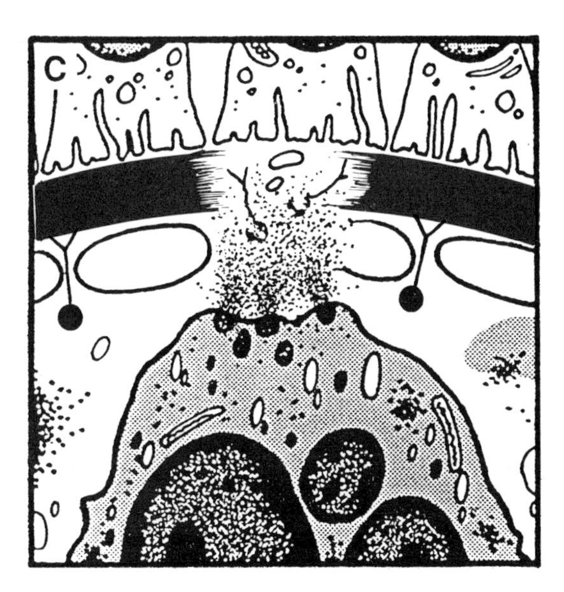

zymes (p. 145) some of which can degrade cell and basement membranes (Fig. 19.7).

There may also be local activation of the coagulation cascade, either secondary to complement activation or to cell damage with the release of various enzymes and protein breakdown products. There is deposition of fibrin in the lumen and walls of the glomerular capillaries, and early administration of anticoagulants in experimental immune-complex nephritis reduces some of the glomerular injury. If the injury to the glomerular capillaries is severe, components of the clotting system may escape into Bowman's space where deposition of fibrin promotes the formation of cellular aggregates or crescents (p. 902), which further impair glomerular function.

In addition to these antibody mediated mechanisms there is increasing evidence for cellular mechanisms in the pathogenesis of glomerulonephritis. Such evidence includes experimental models in which transfer of T lymphocytes can produce lesions in sites where the appropriate antigen is present.

In summary, the pathogenesis of glomerulonephritis involves the formation of immune complexes, mediators such as complement and cellular immune responses which can all combine to produce the end result which we recognize histologically as the various types of glomerulonephritis.

Glomerular Manifestations of Immune-complex Injury

The major histological features of immune-complex glomerular injury can be explained by consideration of the pathogenetic mechanisms.

(1) Hypercellularity is due to an increase in the number of mesangial cells and to emigration and arrest of neutrophil polymorphs and monocytes in response to immune-complex deposition, activation of complement and endothelial injury.

Fig. 19.7 Antibody (—<) fixes to antigen in the basement membrane (A) and the resulting antigen–antibody complex fixes complement (●) (B). As a consequence of complement activation chemotactic factors attract inflammatory cells into the area with the release of lytic enzymes and resultant tissue damage (C).

(2) Thickening of the glomerular capillary basement membrane as seen by light microscopy (the normal basement membrane can only be appreciated by electron microscopy) has a variety of causes. Large subepithelial, intramembranous or subendothelial deposits of immune complexes, swelling of the damaged epithelial or endothelial cells, or prolongation of long mesangial cell processes between the endothelium and basement membrane (see Fig. 19.21) secondary to immune-complex deposition can all give rise to a thickened basement membrane. Production of new basement membrane material may also be stimulated by the presence of immune complexes. The PAS stain or a methenamine silver stain is used to assess basement membrane thickening by light microscopy.

(3) Crescent formation. The escape of fibrin into Bowman's space stimulates the lining epithelial cells to divide and this, together with an admixture of mononuclear phagocytes, produces a crescent-shaped mass of cells which compresses the glomerular tuft, hence the name of the lesion.

These three changes may affect the whole glomerulus but in some instances, the mesangium may be more effective in clearing large subendothelial immune-complex deposits from one lobule of the glomerulus than from another, resulting in a **focal** and **segmental lesion**.

Acute Diffuse Proliferative Glomerulonephritis

Clinical features and course. This type of glomerulonephritis occurs at all ages, although it is more prevalent in children than in adults. It affects males more often than females and usually follows an acute infection with group A haemolytic streptococci – most often pharyngitis (including scarlet fever) in the UK. In developing countries the infection may occur in the skin sores of malnourished children. Only certain (nephritogenic) strains of streptococci give rise to glomerulonephritis. Usually the disease develops 1–2 weeks after the onset of the streptococcal infection; sometimes after a brief latent period of apparent well-being. Acute glomerulonephritis can occasionally result from infection with other bacteria such as *Staphylococcus aureus* and *Streptococcus pneumoniae* and also some viral and protozoal infections, e.g. Epstein–Barr virus and malaria.

Patients usually present with the acute nephritic syndrome (p. 895). The disease can also take a subclinical form, resulting in microscopic haematuria in otherwise well children following a bacterial or viral infection. In childhood the disease usually runs a benign course and some 95% recover completely after an illness lasting a week or two. However, the mortality increases with age and exceeds 50% in patients over the age of 65 years. In these older patients the histological appearances are often those characteristic of crescentic glomerulonephritis. In between these two extremes, the disease may pursue a course characterized by resolution of symptoms but persistence of proteinuria. A number of years later these patients may enter a phase of progressive chronic renal failure. However, the percentage of cases of chronic glomerulonephritis which follow the acute form is small, probably 10% or less.

Laboratory findings. There is moderate proteinuria; microscopy of the urine shows many red blood cells and also granular and red cell casts. Renal function is impaired to a varying degree, with elevation of blood urea and serum creatinine, and depression of glomerular filtration rate as measured by creatinine clearance. In cases of streptococcal origin, the antistreptolysin O titre (ASO titre) will be elevated, and this is one of the types of glomerulonephritis characterized by low serum complement levels.

Pathological features. In acute diffuse proliferative glomerulonephritis the renal cortex is pale due to oedema: in fatal cases it may be up to twice the normal thickness, and glomeruli may be just visible with a hand lens as light grey dots projecting from the cut surface.

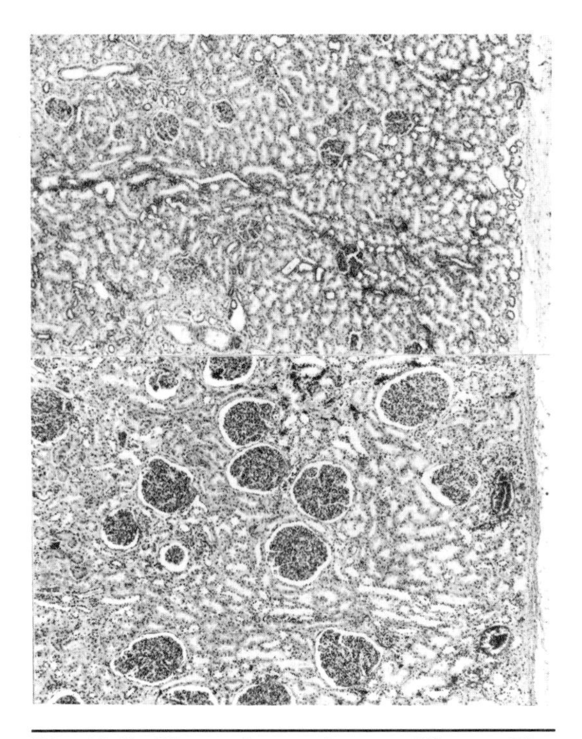

Fig. 19.8 The renal cortex in acute diffuse proliferative glomerulonephritis (below) compared with the cortex of a normal kidney (above). Note the gross enlargement and hypercellularity of the glomeruli. ×30.

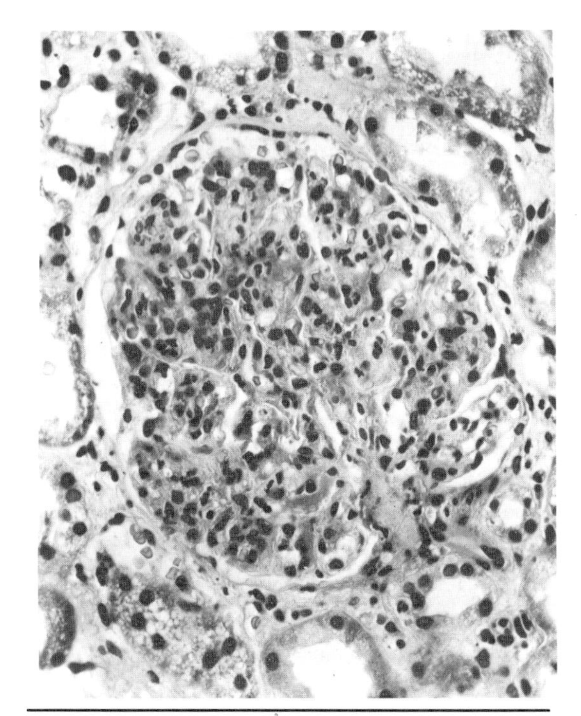

Fig. 19.9 Glomerulus in acute diffuse proliferative glomerulonephritis, showing swelling and increased cellularity of the glomerular tuft. ×200.

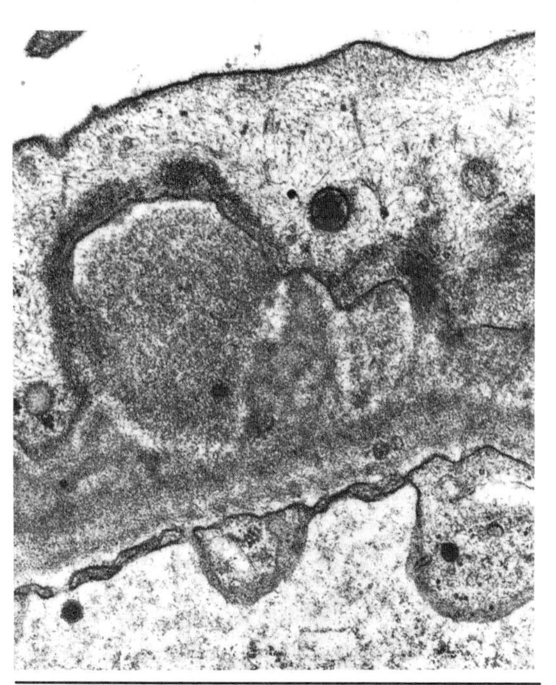

Fig. 19.10 Electron micrograph of part of glomerular capillary wall in acute diffuse glomerulonephritis, showing a large granular subepithelial deposit. Note the fusion of the foot processes (lumen below, urinary space above). ×15 000.

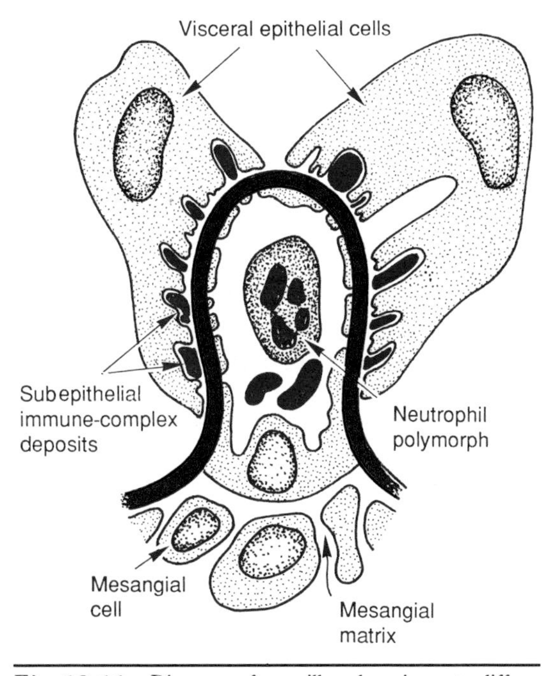

Fig. 19.11 Diagram of a capillary loop in acute diffuse proliferative glomerulonephritis. Note the presence of subepithelial immune-complex deposits, and an excess of mesangial cells. A neutrophil polymorph is present in the capillary lumen.

Microscopically, the appearances are similar in biopsy and autopsy material. The most conspicuous changes are diffuse enlargement and increased cellularity of the glomeruli (Fig. 19.8), the latter being due to an increase in the number of mesangial and endothelial cells and also to the presence of neutrophil polymorphs and macrophages (Fig. 19.9). Crescents are absent or few in typical cases. Electron microscopy shows the presence of subepithelial electron dense dome shaped 'humps' (Figs 19.10 and 19.11) the number of which shows some correlation with the severity of the glomerulonephritis. Smaller deposits may also be seen in the subendothelial space and in the mesangium. Immunofluorescence microscopy shows that the 'humps' correspond to the sites of deposition of IgG and C3 giving a granular pattern to the peripheral capillary loops (Fig. 19.12).

Changes in the remainder of the kidney are secondary to the glomerular damage. Thus, protein and red cell casts may be found in tubular lumina and, in severe cases, ischaemic tubular epithelial damage may be present. The extent and duration of the hypertension is usually insufficient to give rise to vascular damage.

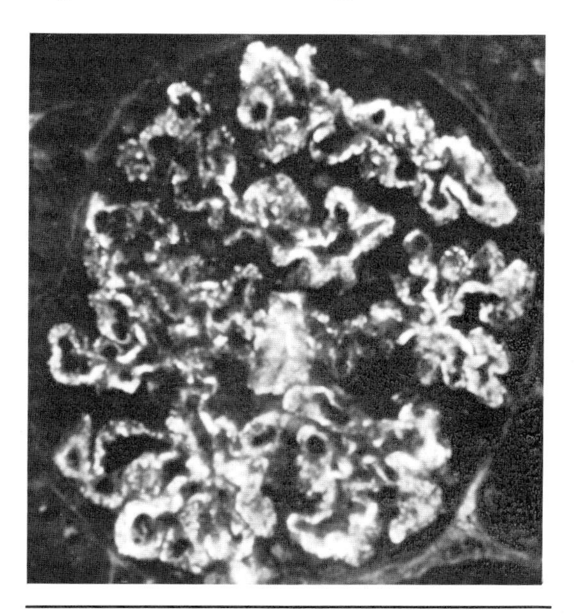

Fig. 19.12 Renal biopsy in acute diffuse glomerulonephritis. Immunofluorescence technique, showing granular and ill-defined deposition of IgG in the glomerular capillary wall. ×350.

With recovery from the disease the glomeruli return to normal, although increased numbers of mesangial cells may persist for many months and their presence may be an indication of a previous episode of acute glomerulonephritis.

Pathogenesis. The demonstration by immunofluorescence microscopy of granular deposits of immunoglobulin (usually mainly IgG) and components of complement in the glomerular capillary walls (Fig. 19.12), together with the detection by electron microscopy of dense subepithelial deposits (Fig. 19.10) are strongly suggestive of the deposition of immune complexes. As acute glomerulonephritis often follows a streptococcal infection it is likely that, in these patients, antibodies to streptococcal products combine with streptococcal antigens in the plasma to produce immune complexes which initially are formed in the presence of antigen excess. In keeping with this, there are low levels of serum complement components, consistent with activation of complement by an antigen–antibody reaction, and an elevated serum ASO titre, indicating previous streptococcal infection. Attempts to demonstrate streptococcal antigen in the glomerular deposits have provided conflicting results: detection of antigen has been reported mostly in biopsy material obtained early in the course of the disease, and it is likely that, later on, the deposited antigen becomes coated by an excess of antibody and thus, obscured. Still later, immunofluorescence microscopy may reveal complement components alone. It is not understood why only certain types of group A streptococci, notably Griffiths types 12, 4, 1, 25 and 49, are nephritogenic, whereas other types are not.

Crescentic (Rapidly Progressive) Glomerulonephritis

This serious form of glomerulonephritis may arise as a primary disease involving only the kidneys or it may be of secondary type, forming part of a multisystem disease (Table 19.3). The primary type may be due to immune-complex deposition but also occurs as an idiopathic form.

Clinical features and course. The onset is usually insidious, with malaise and fluid retention resulting in oedema and dyspnoea. Oliguria and symptoms of uraemia, in particular nausea and vomiting, may follow. This primary form affects both sexes and is commoner in the middle aged and elderly than in children and young adults. As Table 19.3 shows, the secondary type may be associated with a variety of multisystem diseases and the mode of presentation will therefore depend on the associated disease. Goodpasture's syndrome is due to an anti-basement membrane antibody which attaches to both glomerular and pulmonary basement membrane giving rise to acute renal failure and haemoptysis. It is a disease predominantly of young adult males. Confirmation of the diagnosis can be obtained by detection of the antibody in the blood using a radioimmunoassay or enzyme linked immunoabsorbent assay (ELISA), or by the demonstration of linear deposition of immunoglobulin on fluorescence microscopy (Fig. 19.13).

Vasculitis can be of several types but the ones most often associated with crescentic glomerulonephritis are Wegener's granulomatosis and the microscopic form of polyarteritis nodosa. The former is characterized by granulomatous lesions in the upper respiratory tract (p. 527) and the latter by malaise, a purpuric skin rash and (often) joint pains (p. 467). In both types acute renal failure occurs secondarily. The other secondary types of crescentic glomerulonephritis occurring in Henoch–Schönlein syndrome, SLE and infective endocarditis are less common.

Table 19.3 Causes of crescentic (rapidly progressive) glomerulonephritis

Primary
Idiopathic
Post-streptococcal
Secondary
Goodpasture's syndrome
Vasculitic syndromes
Wegener's granulomatosis
polyarteritis nodosa
Henoch–Schönlein syndrome
Systemic lupus erythematosus
Infective endocarditis

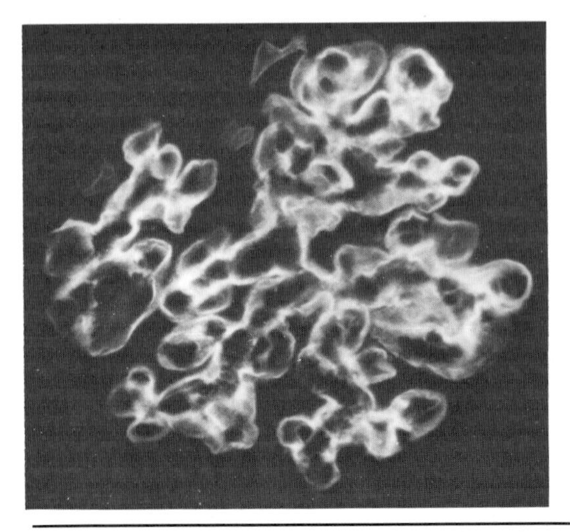

Fig. 19.13 Antibody to glomerular capillary basement membrane in Goodpasture's syndrome, showing the characteristic linear pattern of staining by the immunofluorescence technique.

In all types there will, in the absence of treatment, be progression to irreversible renal failure over a period which may vary from days to months. Immunosuppressive therapy may produce a temporary and/or partial remission but virtually never a complete cure. The most important prognostic factor is the stage at which immunosuppression is introduced. If the patient has become anuric, remission is unusual while if therapy is started earlier, improvement will often follow. The most effective therapy, irrespective of the type of crescentic glomerulonephritis, is a combination of prednisolone and cyclophosphamide.

Pathological changes. The kidneys are normal in size or enlarged due to oedema: on section the cortex is pale, but may show petechial haemorrhages, and the glomeruli stand out conspicuously as grey dots, visible with a lens on the cut surface. In most cases, there is little or no scarring and the surface of the kidneys is smooth.

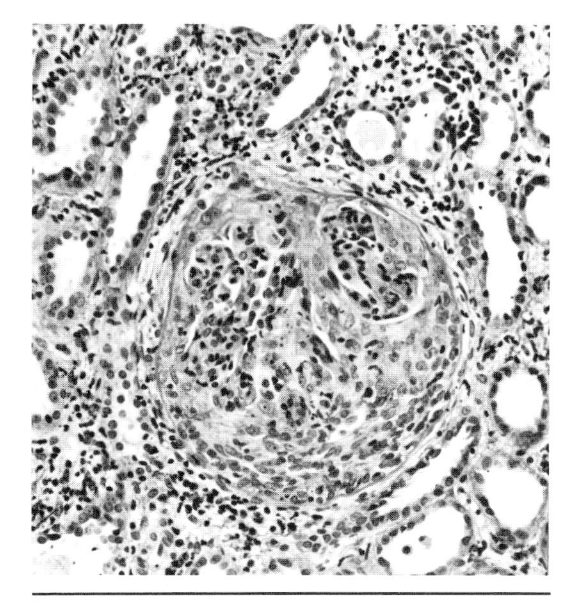

Fig. 19.14 Glomerulus in crescentic glomerulonephritis, showing destruction and fibrosis of parts of the tuft, hypercellularity of the remainder, and formation of a large crescent around the tuft. ×200.

Microscopy shows the most important changes to be glomerular (Fig. 19.14). As in acute diffuse glomerulonephritis, there is proliferation of both endothelial and mesangial cells, with narrowing of the capillary lumina, and variable polymorph infiltration of the tuft. Although all glomeruli are affected, the involvement may be segmental with some lobules more severely affected than others. There may be rupture of the basement membrane, thrombosis and haemorrhagic necrosis of capillaries. The most characteristic histological feature is the formation of crescents. Originally believed to be derived solely from the capsular epithelium, crescents are now known to consist, at least in part, of macrophages derived from emigrated monocytes. They may be segmental or may totally enclose the tuft. Immunofluorescence studies have failed to demonstrate immunoglobulins in crescents, but deposits of fibrin are present. In time the epithelial crescents are usually replaced by connective tissue and severe glomerular scarring occurs. Changes occuring in the tubules are similar to but more severe than those seen in acute diffuse proliferative glomerulonephritis.

Diffuse Membranous Glomerulonephritis

Clinical features and course. The disease is commoner in males, is unusual below the age of 10 years and reaches its peak incidence in middle to old age. It usually presents insidiously as a nephrotic syndrome and may progress to gross oedema also with ascites and pleural effusions. The urinary protein is mainly albumin but consists also of some larger molecular weight globulins and there is often mild microscopic haematuria but never marked haematuria.

Over a 10–15-year period, complete remission will take place in under 30% of patients, proteinuria will persist with stable renal function in about 20% and approximately half the patients will progress to advanced renal failure. Adverse prognostic indicators are deteriorating renal function, increasing proteinuria and hypertension. If remission does occur, subsequent relapse is unusual. The mainstay of treatment is diuretic therapy, while most studies have found that immunosuppressive drugs are not of value. A high protein diet will only increase the proteinuria without raising the serum albumin and is therefore not of value.

Pathological changes. The essential change consists of a diffuse hyaline thickening of the walls of all the glomerular capillaries. In the early stages this is minimal and hard to detect, but it becomes increasingly obvious as the disease progresses. By light microscopy the capillary walls appear thickened, eosinophilic and hyaline (Fig. 19.15) and silver staining techniques give an appearance of spikiness of the basement membrane (Fig. 19.16). The endothelial and mesangial cells appear normal and there is no cellular infiltrate. Electron microscopy shows irregular deposition of dense amorphous material in the outer (i.e. subepithelial) part of the capillary basement membrane (Fig. 19.17) and thickening of the basement membrane between these deposits corresponds to the spikes seen by light microscopic examination of silver preparations. Eventually the 'spikes' of basement membrane thicken still further and envelop the deposits (Fig. 19.18).

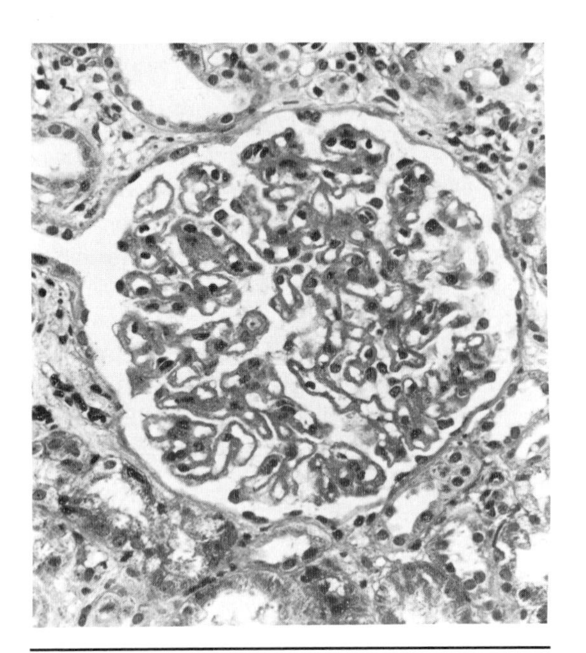

Fig. 19.15 Idiopathic membranous glomerulonephritis. The capillary basement membrane is diffusely and uniformly thickened. ×250.

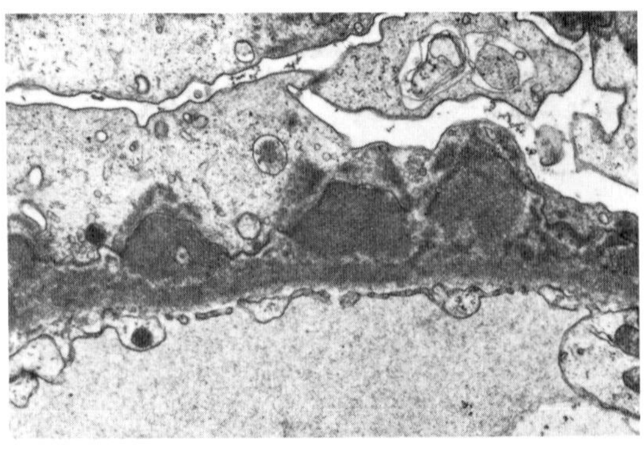

Fig. 19.17 Electron micrograph of segment of glomerular capillary wall in membranous glomerulonephritis (lumen below, urinary space above). The basement membrane is thickened and there are multiple, almost confluent dense deposits on its outer surface. ×16 000.

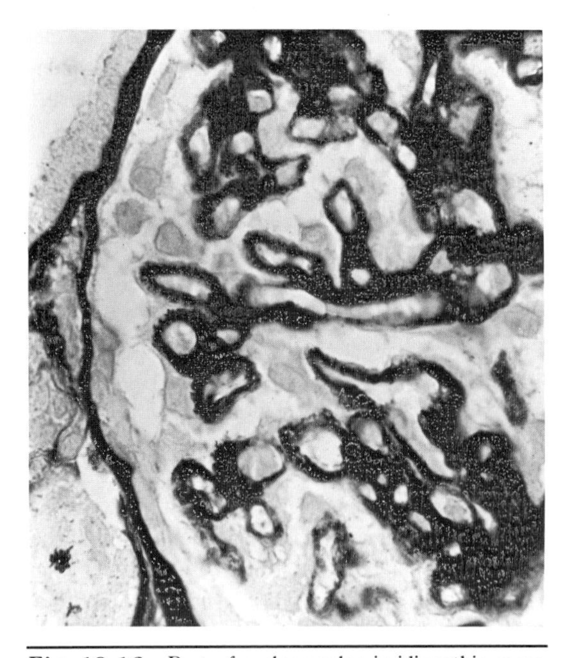

Fig. 19.16 Part of a glomerulus in idiopathic membranous glomerulonephritis, stained by silver impregnation technique and showing the characteristic spiky appearance of the capillary basement membrane. ×475.

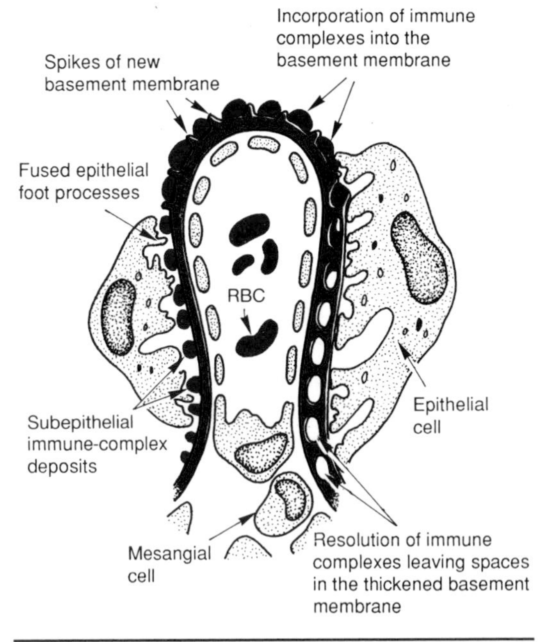

Fig. 19.18 Progression of changes in membranous glomerulonephritis. The subepithelial immune-complex deposits gradually enlarge and the formation of new basement membrane takes place appearing initially as 'spikes' between the immune-complex deposits. The latter are then incorporated into the thickened irregular basement membrane and eventually some complexes may be resolved leaving spaces in the basement membrane.

In the chronic stage of the disease, the thickening of the glomerular capillary walls results in narrowing of the lumina; renal blood flow and GFR are seriously diminished, and uraemia and hypertension develop. Proteinuria diminishes and the oedema tends to subside and may disappear. Microscopy of the kidneys at this stage shows gross diffuse thickening of glomerular capillary walls, some glomeruli being almost solid due to eosinophilic hyaline material. Tubular atrophy from ischaemia accompanies the glomerular hyalinization and interstitial fibrosis occurs, but lipid deposits, indicative of the preceding nephrotic stage, may persist.

Pathogenesis. Immunofluorescence microscopy shows deposition of immunoglobulin, usually mainly IgG, in a granular pattern along the walls of the glomerular capillaries. Deposition of complement is also seen in a similar distribution, but the amounts are often small and this may explain the absence of a cellular inflammatory reaction.

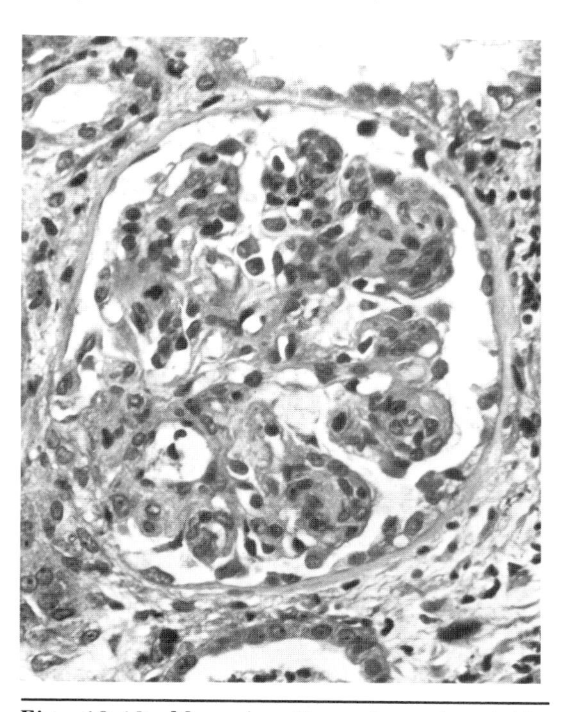

Fig. 19.19 Mesangiocapillary glomerulonephritis. The glomerular lobulation is accentuated, there is increased cellularity, and thickening of capillary walls. ×350.

Attempts to demonstrate circulating immune complexes in cases of membranous glomerulonephritis have been largely unsuccessful, and it is probable that the formation of immune complexes occurs *in situ*. The nature of the antigen is unknown in most cases, but some cases are associated with infections, e.g. malaria, syphilis and hepatitis B virus, with malignant tumours or treatment with certain drugs, notably captopril, penicillamine and gold salts. In all of these associations, the glomerular deposition of IgG suggests an immune-complex basis, the antigens being assumed to be derived from the micro-organisms, tumours or drugs. However, it should be emphasized that, in the vast majority of cases, membranous glomerulonephritis is idiopathic.

Mesangiocapillary (Membrano-proliferative) Glomerulonephritis

The clinical features of mesangiocapillary glomerulonephritis are variable, the commonest being a nephrotic syndrome. Other modes of presentation are asymptomatic proteinuria and an acute nephritic syndrome, the latter being more common in the type II disease. Remission is uncommon with most patients progressing to renal failure. Treatment is symptomatic only, with no benefit from immunosuppressive therapy in any form of the disease.

Pathological changes. At an early stage the glomeruli show diffuse proliferative change with increase in size and number of mesangial and endothelial cells; the mesangium, in particular, shows increased cellularity and the lobular pattern of the glomeruli is accentuated (Fig. 19.19). The capillary lumina are reduced and there is irregular thickening of their walls. Silver stains show, here and there, a double basement membrane (Fig. 19.20).

Two main types are discernible by electron

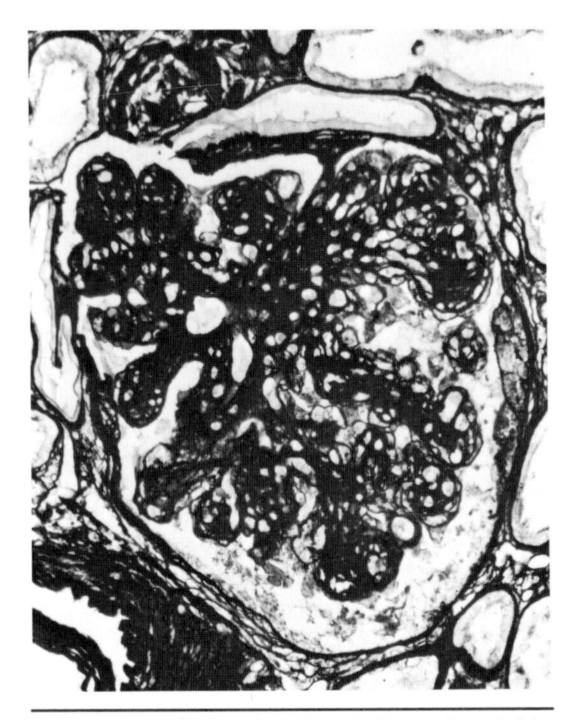

Fig. 19.20 Mesangiocapillary glomerulonephritis. Stained by silver impregnation to show the thickening of the glomerular capillary basement membrane which has a double contour in some peripheral capillary loops. ×350.

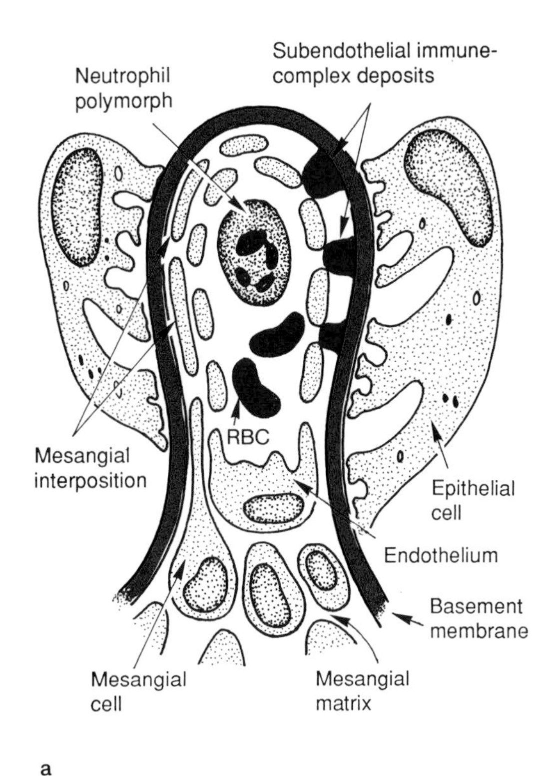

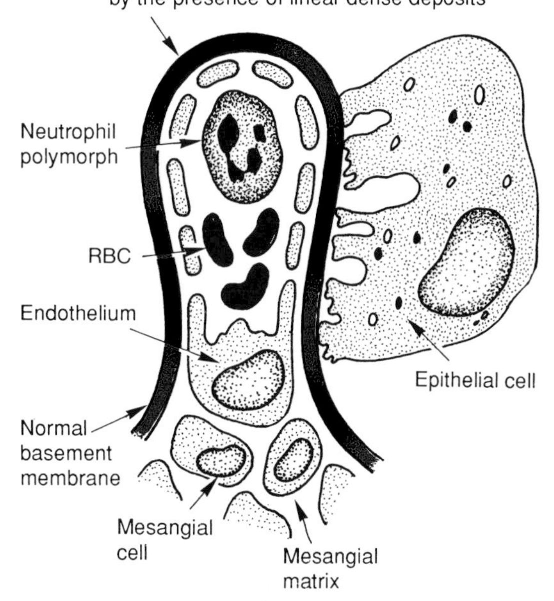

Fig. 19.21 **a** Type I mesangiocapillary glomerulonephritis. The diagram depicts the two main features: mesangial interposition and the presence of subendothelial immune complexes. For the sake of clarity these have been separated in the diagram. In the actual disease process both features would of course be present at the same time. **b** Type II mesangiocapillary glomerulonephritis (dense deposit disease). In this type there is again an excess of mesangial cells and matrix; however, the striking feature is the presence of linear dense deposits within the basement membrane.

microscopy. In type I, discrete irregular deposits are found on the inner (i.e. subendothelial) side of the (original) basement membrane, and there is extension of the cytoplasm of mesangial cells between the endothelium and the basement membrane (mesangial interposition). A second layer of basement membrane is laid down between the endothelium and the mesangial cytoplasmic extension, thus accounting for the double contour seen by some silver stained preparations (Fig. 19.21a). In type II, dense material is deposited within the lamina densa causing a more diffuse thickening of the basement membrane which has led to the use of the term **dense deposit disease** (Fig. 19.21b). A type III with both subendothelial and subepithelial deposits also occurs. In some cases, particularly of the type II, small crescents are formed in the capsule of occasional glomeruli. Type I is approximately ten times more frequent than type II and type III is extremely rare.

As the disease progresses the mesangial cells diminish in number and hyaline material accumulates, while the capillaries become progressively thickened so that glomerulosclerosis and chronic renal failure result.

Pathogenesis. In type I, components of complement and immunoglobulins (IgG and/or IgM) are present in the capillary walls and it is likely that this disease is immune complex in nature. Activation of the complement system by the classical pathway may lead to low serum complement levels. In type II, C3 is deposited along the capillary walls and low serum complement levels are almost invariable. However, in this type the complement system is activated by the alternative pathway due to C3 nephritic factor. This is an autoantibody to the C3 convertase of the alternative pathway (C3bBb). The antibody stabilizes this converting enzyme, thus allowing continuous breakdown of C3. Type II is probably not an immune-complex disease but rather is due to a structural alteration of the glomerular basement membrane. This type may have a familial predisposition and there is a syndrome linking it with partial lipodystrophy. Type III, like type I, is probably immune complex in origin.

In addition to these primary forms of mesangiocapillary glomerulonephritis, a number of conditions can result in a secondary form, probably as a result of immune-complex formation. These include infective endocarditis, infected ventriculoatrial shunts (so-called shunt nephritis) and malaria.

Focal Glomerulonephritis

This may be defined as a glomerulitis affecting only a proportion of the glomeruli. Furthermore, the lesions usually involve only part of the glomerular tuft, and may therefore be described as **focal** and **segmental**. The disease may be primary (IgA nephropathy) or may be secondary to a number of other diseases, notably Henoch–Schönlein syndrome, infective endocarditis and SLE. Also some cases of crescentic glomerulonephritis, in particular those resulting from microscopic polyarteritis or Goodpasture's syndrome, often show the histological picture of focal glomerulonephritis in their early stages.

Pathological changes. The glomerular lesion consists of a cellular proliferation, probably of mesangial cells, affecting the peripheral part of one or more lobules (Fig. 19.22), in some cases accompanied by fibrinoid necrosis of capillary loops: within the lesions, individual capillary lumina may be obliterated by thrombus. Red cells may be present in the capsular space and in the tubules, and small crescents may be formed. The number of glomeruli affected varies considerably. Some patients develop the nephrotic syndrome and the associated renal changes (p. 894) are then seen.

Primary Type: IgA Nephropathy (Berger's Disease)

Now known to be one of the commonest forms of adult glomerulonephritis in the world, the disease

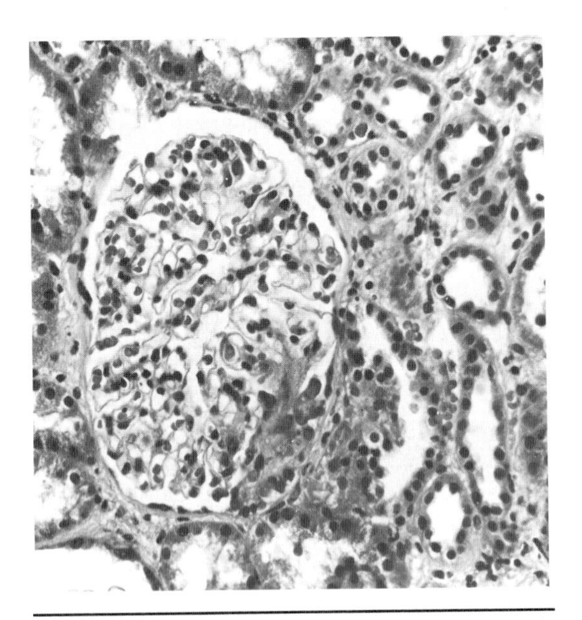

Fig. 19.22 Idiopathic focal glomerulonephritis: early lesion. Note the hypercellularity of the affected part of the tuft on the right. ×200.

presents with a variety of clinical syndromes including recurrent haematuria (often macroscopic), proteinuria and less often, the nephritic or nephrotic syndrome. There is an association with ill defined viral or bacterial inflammation of mucosal surfaces containing IgA and hence, with gluten enteropathy, Crohn's disease and chronic bronchitis. IgA immune-complex formation has been postulated as a causal mechanism and an increased incidence of the disease is found in patients with chronic liver disease (notably alcohol induced) who have an inability to clear such complexes.

Glomerular involvement is variable, mirroring the severity of the clinical symptoms. Immunofluorescence microscopy demonstrates the presence of mesangial IgA deposits, with variable accompanying IgG, IgM and C3. Electron microscopy confirms the presence of electron dense deposits, mainly in the mesangium but also appearing in the subendothelial space in those cases with a more aggressive course. The disease was initially regarded as having a benign course but it is now apparent that at least 25% of patients will progress to chronic renal failure. The disease also may sometimes recur in renal allografts.

Secondary Type

Henoch–Schönlein Syndrome

There is a close relationship between IgA nephropathy and the Henoch–Schönlein syndrome and indeed some workers believe that these are two distinct manifestations of a single disease. The Henoch–Schönlein syndrome occurs mainly in children who present with a purpuric skin rash, joint pains and colic, and there may be a history of streptococcal infection or of hypersensitivity to certain foods. In some cases, there is a fairly mild focal glomerulonephritis associated with the mesangial deposition of IgA and in these patients, renal failure is either mild or transient with complete recovery. A more severe renal lesion may occur, particularly in older patients.

Infective Endocarditis

Renal glomerular lesions are commonly present in infective endocarditis, but often they do not lead to serious impairment of renal function. Focal glomerulonephritis occurs in 10–20% of cases, while in some patients a crescentic glomerulonephritis may occur.

In keeping with an immune-complex mediated lesion, the serum complement levels are depressed, electron microscopy shows the presence of subendothelial and mesangial deposits, and immunofluorescence studies confirm the presence of immunoglobulin. Circulating immune complexes have been demonstrated by some workers.

The clinical presentation may range from asymptomatic proteinuria or microscopic haematuria, which correspond to the milder pathological forms, to renal failure from crescentic glomerulonephritis. In the latter type, immunosuppressive therapy with steroids and cyclophosphamide may produce short- or long-term remission but rarely cure. In association with the renal manifestations, a wide variety of extrarenal features may occur in particular joint symptoms, rash and involvement of various viscera especially the lungs, heart and brain.

Polyarteritis Nodosa

The necrotizing arteritis which is the essential

lesion of this condition usually involves the larger arteries in the kidneys, with aneurysm formation and/or thrombosis, and renal infarcts are commonly present (Fig. 12.20; p. 466). In about one-third of cases, death results from renal failure with hypertension. In the microscopic form of polyarteritis, the vascular lesions show the same features – fibrinoid necrosis and inflammatory changes – but involve mainly the interlobular arteries, afferent glomerular arterioles, and also the glomerular capillaries, giving rise to focal glomerulonephritis. A crescentic glomerulonephritis may also be found, as described on p. 901.

Aetiology and Pathogenesis of Focal Glomerulonephritis

While in focal glomerulonephritis there is evidence of an immunological mechanism, the aetiology is diverse. IgA deposition is obvious in IgA nephropathy and also in the Henoch–Schönlein syndrome, which is probably related. Although glomerular lesions are focal and segmental by light microscopy, the immunoglobulins have a more uniform distribution as shown by immunofluorescence and electron microscopy. It may be that, for some unknown reason, the focal lesions occur in glomerular lobules in which the mesangial cells fail to clear the subendothelial immune-complex deposits.

The available evidence suggests that the diseases which focal glomerulonephritis accompanies are attributable to abnormal immunological reactions. The evidence is strongest in the case of SLE (see below). Lesions resembling those of polyarteritis nodosa occur in serum sickness: fixed immunoglobulins, and in some cases HBsAg, have been observed in the early vascular lesions, although evidence for immune-complex deposition in the glomeruli is not convincing. In infective endocarditis the prolonged infection provides a possible basis for immunological injury from circulating antigen-antibody complexes.

Glomerular Disease in Systemic Lupus Erythematosus (SLE)

An autoimmune disease which affects primarily young women, SLE has a clinically apparent, serious renal component in approximately 60% of patients. The disease is characterized by the production of a variety of autoantibodies to cellular and tissue constituents including nucleic acids and nucleoproteins. Complexes of various sizes are therefore formed and these filter out in mesangial, subendothelial or subepithelial position, in the glomerulus. Immunofluorescence microscopy may therefore demonstrate IgG, IgA, IgM, C3, C4 and C1q in a single glomerulus. As a consequence, so-called **lupus nephritis** may present as a spectrum of glomerulonephritis and, hence, with every possible clinical renal syndrome. It is preferable therefore to discuss this as a separate topic.

The WHO defines five possible classes of lupus nephritis. In class 1 no abnormality is seen by light microscopy and immunofluorescence and electron microscopy are negative. In class 2 mild mesangial abnormalities are seen by light microscopy and mesangial immune-complex deposits are detected by immunofluorescence and electron microscopy. In the other classes immune-complex deposits are, in addition, found in subendothelial positions and light microscopy shows either a focal glomerulonephritis (class 3) or a diffuse proliferative glomerulonephritis (class 4). In some cases massive subendothelial deposits give rise to focal thickening of the glomerular capillary basement membrane with a refractile eosinophilic appearance – the so-called wire loop lesion (Fig. 19.23). In addition hyaline thrombi may be detected in some capillaries. Areas of severe segmental damage show the presence of haematoxyphile bodies – lilac coloured, irregular fragments of damaged nuclei. The latter are pathognomonic for SLE. In class 5 the light and electron microscopic features are those of a membranous glomerulonephritis. Interstitial nephritis (p. 920) is common and in some instances may be the major

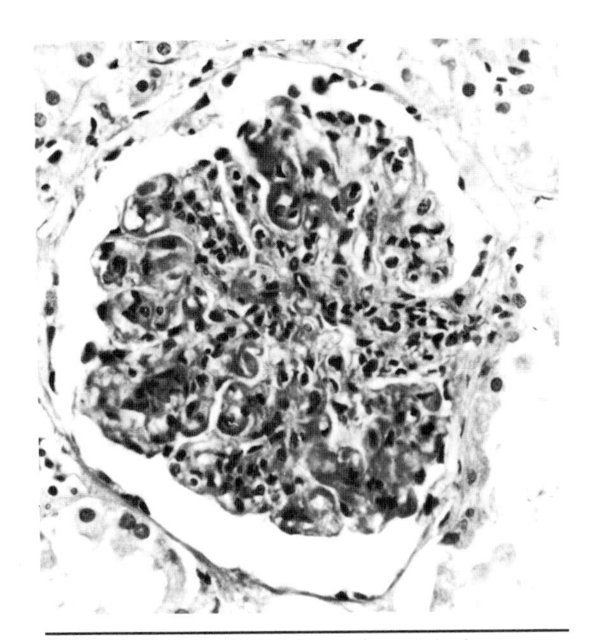

Fig. 19.23 A glomerulus in systemic lupus erythematosus, showing hyaline thickening of some of the capillaries – the 'wire-loop' lesion, and a diffuse increase in cellularity. ×300.

abnormality. Such cases often present with tubular defects. Spontaneous transformation of one class into another may occur and the aim of therapy is to encourage transformation from classes 3 and 4 – the proliferative groups which have a worse prognosis – into groups 1, 2 and 5 which have a more indolent course.

Chronic Glomerulonephritis

It is apparent from the foregoing descriptions of the various types of glomerulonephritis, that an end stage may be reached in which glomerular damage is so extensive that chronic renal failure develops. The time taken to reach this stage, and the rate of progression once it has developed, vary widely. Hypertension, sometimes of the accelerated (malignant) type, may develop and this will, particularly if inadequately treated, aggravate the renal damage. In cases where hypertension is absent or less severe, renal failure will usually progress more slowly.

In many patients with chronic glomerulonephritis there is no history to suggest preceding renal disease, and the renal lesions progress silently until chronic renal failure develops. In such cases, it is often not possible to decide, even by histological examination of the kidneys, what type of glomerulonephritis has led to the chronic stage. Most types of glomerulonephritis can present at this late stage but it is now thought that IgA nephropathy is the commonest type to present in this way.

Pathological changes and pathogenesis. Both kidneys are uniformly and equally reduced in size, sometimes slightly but often to about one-third of normal (Fig. 19.24). The capsule is often firmly adherent and the subcapsular surface uniformly and finely irregular (**'granular contracted kidney'**). There is diffuse thinning of the cortex, while the medullary pyramids are also, although less markedly, shrunken. **In contrast to**

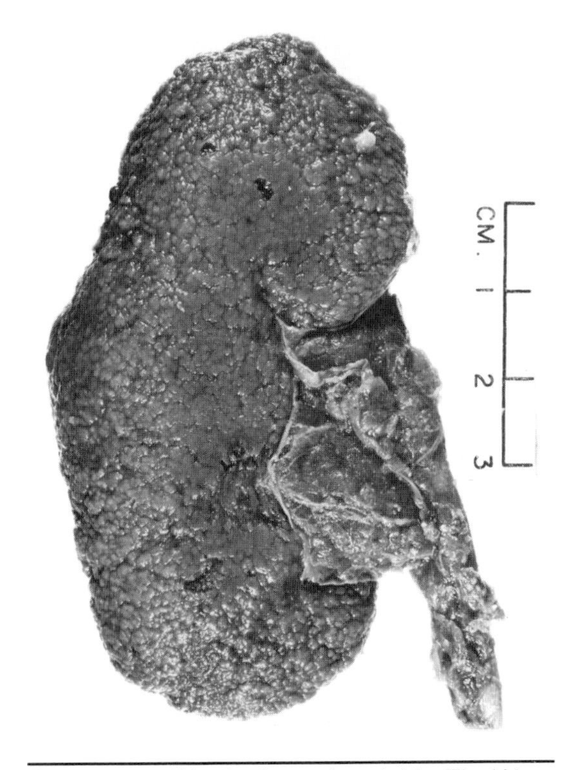

Fig. 19.24 Chronic glomerulonephritis. The kidney is uniformly shrunken, in this case to about half the normal size, and the surface is diffusely granular.

chronic pyelonephritis, the calyces and renal pelvis are not distorted.

Microscopically, it is common to find all degrees of hyalinization of glomeruli. Many are completely hyalinized (Fig. 19.25) and some show partial destruction. The appearances of some glomeruli may still suggest the type of glomerulonephritis responsible, e.g. membranous or crescentic. A few normal glomeruli may remain, and they tend to become hypertrophied. The tubules show extensive atrophy, and there is an increase in the intertubular connective tissue which contains aggregates of lymphocytes and some plasma cells. In cases with some near-normal hypertrophied glomeruli, the corresponding tubules are enlarged and account for the elevations which give the subcapsular surface its granular appearance. They may show hyaline droplets in the epithelial cytoplasm and frequently contain protein casts.

The arcuate and interlobular arteries and the afferent arterioles show hypertensive changes which are likely, by causing ischaemia, to have contributed to the glomerular scarring. When malignant hypertension has supervened the consequent changes (see Fig. 19.42, p. 930) are seen in those glomeruli which have not been destroyed already by the glomerulonephritic process; there may be blood in the capsular spaces and in functioning tubules.

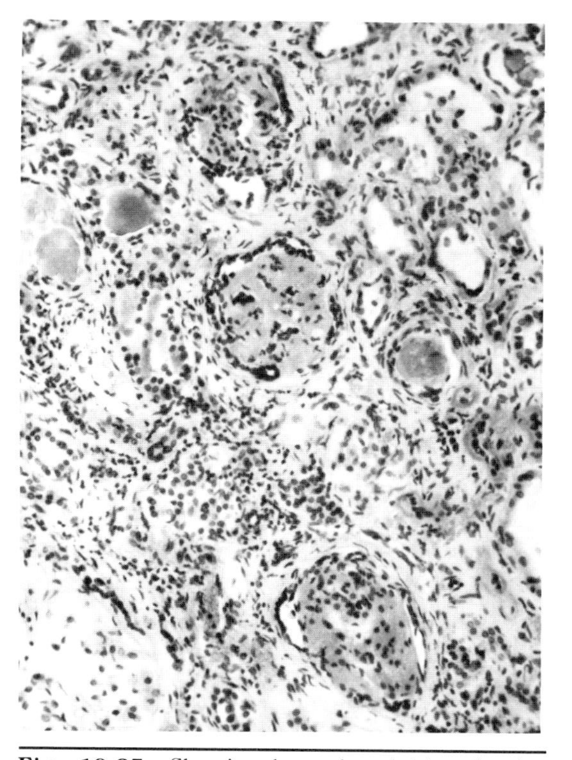

Fig. 19.25 Chronic glomerulonephritis, showing hyalinization of glomeruli; the tubular epithelium is atrophic and there is interstitial fibrosis. ×100.

Miscellaneous Causes of the Nephrotic Syndrome

In addition to the various types of glomerulonephritis, there are two other important intrinsic renal diseases which cause the nephrotic syndrome. These are minimal change nephrotic syndrome and focal glomerulosclerosis. Of the metabolic causes, diabetes mellitus and amyloidosis are the most important.

Minimal-change Nephrotic Syndrome

Clinical features and course. In childhood, the peak incidence occurs between 2 and 6 years, males predominate by 2:1 and the condition accounts for 75% of cases of the nephrotic syndrome. In adults there is an equal sex incidence and it is responsible for up to 25% of cases of the nephrotic syndrome. The hallmarks of this disease are normal blood pressure, normal renal function and absence of red cells on urine microscopy. In the presence of these features, especially in childhood, a renal biopsy is not necessary for confirmation of the diagnosis, unless there is failure to respond to steroid therapy. The proteinuria in this condition is highly selective, i.e. it consists almost exclusively of albumin with negligible quanitities of globulin. However, tests based on this selectivity are not reliable enough for diagnostic purposes. Atopy or allergy are relatively common associated features.

Spontaneous remission may occur, but corticosteroid therapy will usually produce remission within 1–2 weeks and should be given unless there is a strong contraindication. Once proteinuria has disappeared, the corticosteroid is tailed off over 4–8 weeks. In just over 90% of patients a remission will occur with steroid therapy but around 60% will later relapse and two-thirds of these have repeated relapses, although responding on each occasion to a further course of steroids. These frequent relapsers will usually obtain a longer remission following an 8-week course of cyclophosphamide but even this therapy is not curative. However, there is a tendency for long-term remission to occur even in these frequent relapsers after a number of years. Some patients still die from infection supervening on the nephrotic syndrome.

Pathological changes. Microscopically, the glomeruli look normal apart from an appearance of fixed dilatation of the capillaries (Fig. 19.26). The most conspicuous change on electron microscopy is fusion of the foot processes of the epithelial cells, the basement membrane being covered externally by a layer of epithelial cell cytoplasm (see Fig. 19.5): the epithelial cells also show an increase in vacuolation and in some cases the basement membrane is slightly thickened.

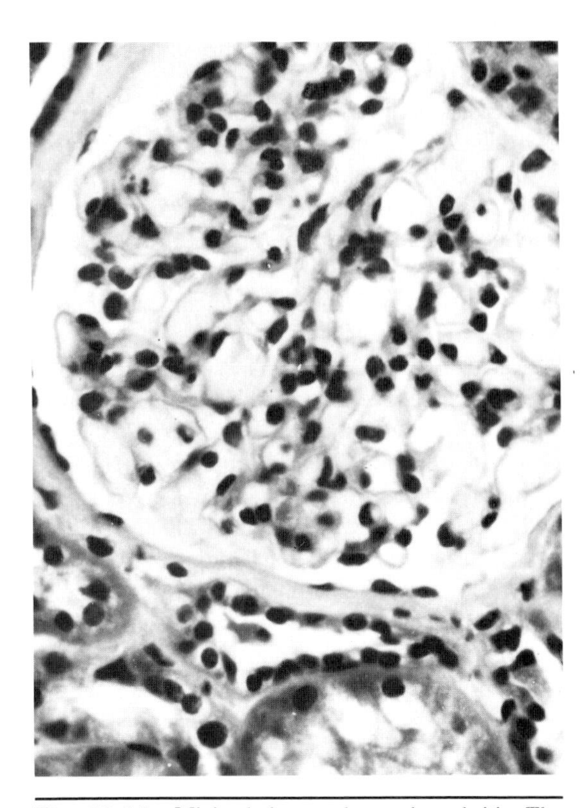

Fig. 19.26 Minimal-change glomerulonephritis. The glomerulus shows no obvious abnormality apart from dilatation of many of the capillaries. ×560.

Pathogenesis. In a high percentage of cases, the condition is idiopathic and with no evidence that immune complexes are involved. However, it can also occur in Hodgkin's disease, non-Hodgkin's lymphoma and occasionally with other tumours. Recent evidence has pointed to loss of the negative electrical charge of the glomerular basement membrane as the central mechanism in allowing filtration of negatively charged protein molecules. The factor(s) responsible for the reduced polyanion content, however, are not known.

Focal Glomerulosclerosis

This accounts for 10–20% of cases of the nephrotic syndrome.

Clinical features and course. The presentation is similar to that of minimal-change nephrotic syndrome. However, proteinuria is less selective and both hypertension and microscopic haematuria are common. The condition is usually resistant to steroid therapy although in some cases there may be an initial response. The prognosis is poor, most cases progressing to renal failure although this may take a number of years. The disease tends to recur in renal transplants. Although most of the glomeruli appear normal, those close to the medulla show sclerosis, consisting of deposition of hyaline material with consequent obliteration of capillaries: this change is at first focal, but gradually destroys whole glomeruli and extends peripherally to involve more glomeruli. There is associated tubular atrophy. Renal biopsy is only diagnostic if it includes some of the deeper, affected glomeruli. It is now thought that patients diagnosed from a superficial renal biopsy as minimal-change nephrotic sydrome, and who eventually develop chronic renal failure, are really missed cases of focal glomerulosclerosis. Immunofluorescence microscopy shows deposition of IgM and complement in an irregular, granular or nodular distribution in association with the focal sclerotic lesions seen on light microscopy.

Diabetes Mellitus

Renal disease is an important complication of diabetes mellitus. It causes chronic renal failure in more than 10% of all diabetics, and in over 40% of those developing diabetes in childhood. The most important pathological lesions are diabetic glomerulosclerosis and hyaline thickening of the afferent glomerular arterioles. The latter is similar to that already described in hypertensives and old people (p. 459), but is more severe in diabetics, both with and without hypertension, and affects also the efferent arterioles to a greater degree than in non-diabetics (Fig. 19.27).

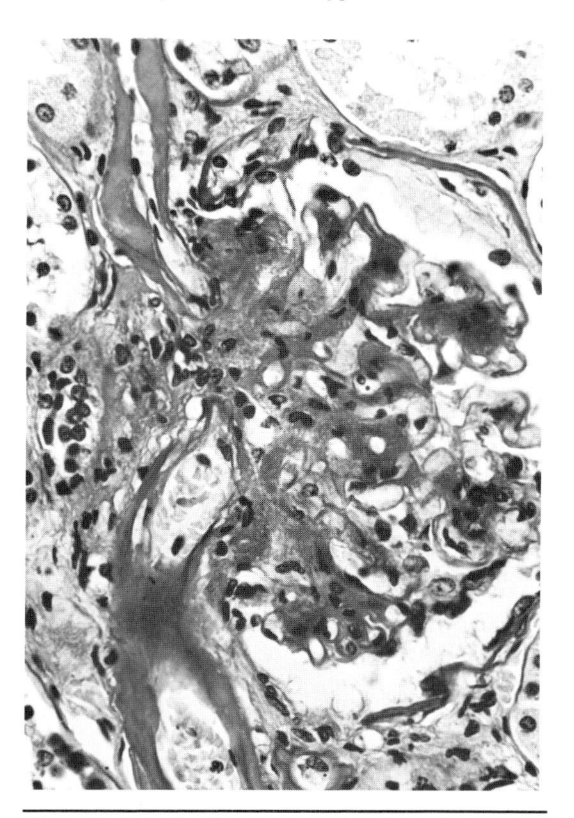

Fig. 19.27 Hyaline change in the afferent and efferent glomerular arterioles in diabetes mellitus. Note also the diffuse glomerulosclerosis. ×250.

Diabetic Glomerulosclerosis

This consists of deposition of eosinophilic, hyaline material in the mesangium of the glomerular lobules. The deposits may be discrete rounded nodules, sometimes laminated, situated near the tip of the lobule and therefore appearing peripheral in the glomerulus (Kimmelstiel–Wilson lesion). Such **nodular glomerulosclerosis** affects lobules and glomeruli unequally, and one or more nodules, of various sizes, may be seen in affected glomeruli (Fig. 19.28). The glomerular capillaries are seen around the margin of the nodules, and may long remain unaffected. Aneurysmal dilatation of some glomerular capillaries and also of some arterioles within the kidney is associated with microaneurysms elsewhere – in particular within the retina. Diabetic nephropathy and retinopathy are almost always associated with one another.

Nodular glomerulosclerosis is usually accom-

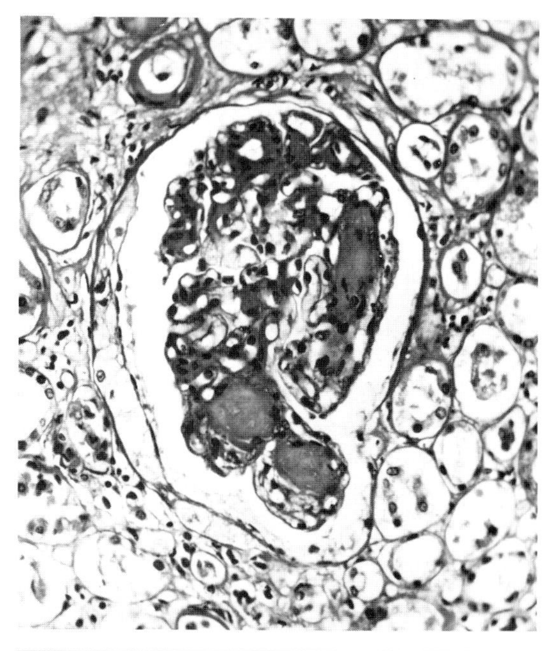

Fig. 19.28 Nodular glomerulosclerosis in diabetes mellitus (Kimmelstiel–Wilson lesion). ×205.

panied by more diffuse deposition of hyaline material in the mesangium of all the glomerular lobules, with associated thickening of the glomerular capillary basement membranes. This **diffuse glomerulosclerosis** may resemble membranous glomerulonephritis, but shows less uniform basement membrane thickening. It may eventually progress to obliteration of most of the capillaries and severe hyalinization of the glomeruli. Ischaemic changes, including obliteration of the capsular space by collagen and glomerular collapse, occur (see Fig. 19.40, p. 929), and are presumably related to hyaline thickening of the afferent arterioles. As a result of glomerulosclerosis, secondary atrophy occurs in the tubules, and the kidneys may be reduced in size with thinning of the cortex and a granular surface.

Diabetic glomerulosclerosis has been reported in 25–50% of diabetics at autopsy. In most instances, the nodular and diffuse forms are combined, but in some the diffuse form occurs alone. It is worth distinguishing between the two forms, for while the nodular lesion is highly characteristic of diabetes, the diffuse lesion is related much more closely to disturbances of renal function.

The pathogenesis of diabetic glomerulosclerosis is not fully understood. It should be regarded as part of the metabolic defect in diabetes mellitus and is closely related to the widespread diabetic microangiopathy which affects many other organs. It is commoner in diabetics with poor blood glucose control but this is probably only one of a number of aetiological factors. In insulin dependent type I diabetics the time interval between diagnosis of the diabetes and renal failure is usually between 15 and 25 years. Although it is shorter in the maturity-onset, non-insulin dependent type II, this is presumably because in these patients the diabetes has often been in existence for a long time before it is diagnosed.

In type I diabetes, the GFR is above normal prior to the onset of renal disease. It is likely that this glomerular hyperfiltration is associated with hypertension within the glomerular blood vessels, and this leads to progressive glomerular damage in the form of nodular glomerulosclerosis. This mechanism of glomerular damage is similar to that described later in the chapter for other types of chronic progressive renal disease. One of the, as yet unexplained, aspects in diabetes is what produces the elevated GFR in the first place. Systemic hypertension is almost invariable in diabetic glomerulosclerosis but, although it accelerates the decline in renal function, it is thought to have a secondary rather than a primary role in that respect. Other possibilities to explain the thickening of the glomerular basement membrane include increased synthesis or decreased removal of various extracellular matrix proteins, or abnormal glycosylation of proteins.

The first detectable abnormality in diabetic glomerulosclerosis is proteinuria and this is followed by the nephrotic syndrome as the protein excretion becomes heavier. Renal function then begins to deteriorate and the patient progresses to advanced renal failure. Hypertension will have become established by the time the patient is nephrotic and is often present earlier during the stage of asymptomatic proteinuria.

Other Renal Changes in Diabetes

The term diabetic nephropathy is applied to the combined renal lesions which occur in the kidney. As already mentioned they are almost always associated with diabetic retinopathy (p. 884). In non-diabetics the renal arteries rarely show severe narrowing from atheroma unless they are involved at their origins by aortic atheromatous plaques. In diabetes, however, severe atheroma does occur in the main renal arteries and their segmental branches and may contribute, in some patients, to the hypertension. **Papillary necrosis** (p. 925) is usually a late complication. Diabetics are susceptible to bacterial infections including urinary tract infections.

Amyloidosis

The kidneys are involved in nearly all cases of secondary amyloidosis and are also commonly affected in primary amyloidosis. The most important site of deposition is around the glomerular capillary basement membrane; this is accompanied by increased permeability, and proteinuria may be sufficiently heavy to cause the nephrotic syndrome. As the deposits increase, capillary narrowing and obliteration ensue, and the glomeruli may be largely replaced by amyloid (Fig. 19.29). Secondary atrophy of the tubules and interstitial fibrosis result from the glomerular lesion, and chronic renal failure gradually supervenes. The kidneys are firm and pale, and tend to be of normal size or slightly enlarged. The glomeruli are usually visible by naked eye after treating a slice of kidney with Lugol's iodine (Fig. 19.30). In cases with the nephrotic syndrome, the usual accompanying features are seen in the kidneys (p. 894).

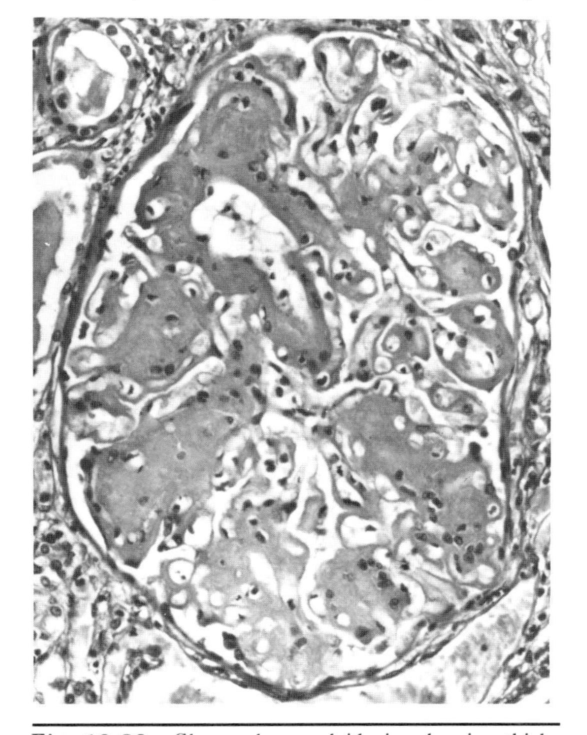

Fig. 19.29 Glomerular amyloidosis, showing thickening and hyaline appearance of capillary walls. ×350.

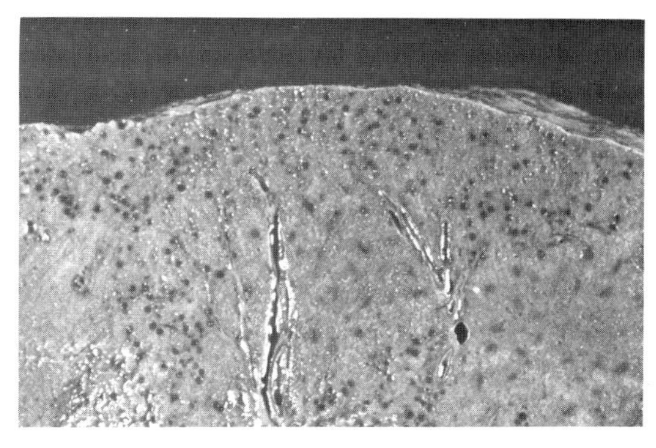

Fig. 19.30 Amyloidosis. A slice of the renal cortex has been treated with Lugol's iodine. The glomeruli contain sufficient amyloid material to be visible as darkly stained spots.

Urinary Tract Infection and Pyelonephritis

Urinary tract infection involves either the bladder (cystitis) or the kidneys and the renal pelves (pyelonephritis) or both. The single most important criterion of urinary tract infection is the presence of bacteria in the urine (bacteriuria). In urine obtained through a bladder catheter the presence of any organisms is significant, while in the commonly used midstream sample there is bound to be some contamination by urethral or perineal organisms. Thus, in such samples a bacterial count of more than 10^5 per ml is the accepted definition of infection. Bacteriuria in the absence of symptoms is termed asymptomatic or covert bacteriuria and it is of importance under two circumstances: first, in infancy, if associated with ureteric reflux, it can lead to ascent of infection to the kidneys; second in pregnancy, where it might be followed by symptomatic infection and can predispose to pre-eclampsia and prematurity.

Urinary tract infection occurring without preceding catheterization or obstruction is usually due to bacteria normally present in the faeces, in most cases *Escherichia coli*, but sometimes *Klebsiella*, *Proteus* spp. or *Pseudomonas* spp. are responsible. Infection complicating obstruction or instrumentation is commonly of mixed bacterial type, *E. coli. Proteus* spp. and staphylococci being most often present. Haematogenous spread may also occur but is much less common; it may arise in the course of acute pyaemia or septicaemia complicating staphylococcal infections or infective endocarditis.

By far the commonest route of infection is along the lumen of the urethra. The incidence of infection is higher in females throughout all age ranges with a sex ratio of 20:1 in children and young adults but this sex ratio falls in old age due to the increasing incidence of prostatic hypertrophy. The female preponderance is due mainly to the ease with which endogenous infections can ascend the short female urethra. Precipitating factors include trauma to the perineum during sexual intercourse or childbirth. Most urinary infections in females occur in anatomically normal urinary tracts and the vast majority of these are confined to the bladder. In a small percentage of females and relatively more often in males, stagnation of urine resulting from urinary tract obstruction is the main aetiological factor. Causes include urethral obstruction by inflammatory scarring or congenital, valve-like mucosal folds, urinary calculi, diverticula and tumours of the bladder, congenital malformations such as double ureters, and neurological disorders, e.g. paraplegia or multiple sclerosis which interfere with emptying of the bladder. In men, prostatic enlargement is the commonest predisposing cause of urinary tract infection.

When confined to the bladder, urinary infection is termed cystitis and is characterized by dysuria, increased frequency of micturition and sometimes haematuria. The ascent of infection to the kidneys is usually due to vesicoureteric reflux, urinary tract obstruction or pregnancy.

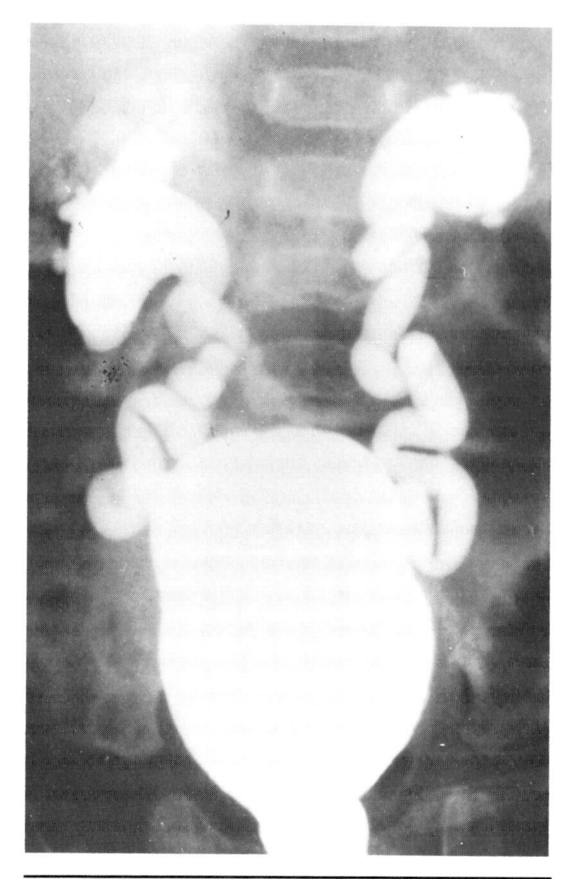

Fig. 19.31 Micturating cystogram in a 1-year-old child. Note the reflux of urine up both ureters as far as the renal pelves. On the right side at the upper pole intra-renal reflux is also evident.

Vesicoureteric reflux consists of the retrograde flow of bladder urine up the ureters during micturition. Reflux is normally prevented by the oblique course of the ureter through the wall of the bladder which effects a valve-like action during contraction of the bladder. However, in infancy the ureters enter the bladder at a less acute angle and reflux is common at this age. In older children and adults, reflux is less common and usually seen in association with pregnancy, urinary tract obstruction or a neurogenic bladder. Reflux is demonstrated by a micturating cystogram in which dye is instilled into the bladder by catheter. Following removal of the catheter, films are taken during micturition when the presence of reflux can be seen. Reflux is graded in severity from I to IV depending on how much of the upper urinary tract is opacified and on the degree of dilatation of the ureters and renal pelves. Grade IV reflux with gross dilatation of the upper urinary tract is illustrated in Fig. 19.31. The main importance of reflux is that it can carry infected urine up to the kidneys. The bladder infection also tends to be perpetuated by the reflux, as the refluxing urine will return to the bladder following micturition and thus there is incomplete bladder emptying. The regular complete 'washing out' of the urinary tract which is an important mechanism in maintaining its sterility is therefore lost. Infection within the renal parenchyma as a consequence of reflux is of particular importance in infancy as it may proceed to chronic pyelonephritis in later childhood or adult life.

In severe reflux, urine may re-enter the renal parenchyma, especially at the upper and lower poles of the kidney where the papillae are compound, i.e. fused. In such papillae the mouths of the collecting ducts are held open and refluxing urine flows readily into them. By contrast, the orifices of the collecting ducts of the simple papillae in the midzone of the kidney have a slit-like opening which collapses on pressure, effectively preventing the entry of refluxing urine. It is of interest that these sites of intra-renal reflux, at the upper and lower poles, are the sites at which scars are most commonly found in chronic pyelonephritis.

Pyelonephritis

Pyelonephritis is a bacteria-induced inflammation of the renal pelvis, calyces and renal parenchyma. It can occur in acute and chronic forms and can affect one or both kidneys. The vast majority of cases are due to ascending infection, often in association with vesicoureteric reflux, while in a very small proportion organisms reach the kidney through the bloodstream. The predominant organisms responsible for ascending infection are faecal flora as has already been mentioned, but virtually any bacteria or fungus can cause renal infection.

Acute Pyelonephritis

Clinical features and course. This condition is uncommon in contrast to acute cystitis. Normal protective mechanisms, however, may break down, predisposing to acute pyelonephritis. Such predisposing conditions include:

(1) urinary tract obstruction, which may be congential or acquired. Structural or functional abnormalities of the urinary tract even without obstruction, such as a neurogenic bladder also predispose to infection.

(2) vesicoureteric reflux.

(3) instrumentation of the urinary tract.

(4) pregnancy.

(5) diabetes mellitus, in which there is a general susceptibility to infection.

(6) immunosuppression.

(7) pre-existing or acquired renal lesions which may cause intra-renal scarring and obstruction, e.g. gout and interstitial nephritis.

The clinical symptoms of acute pyelonephritis are loin pain, with usually a high fever and often rigors. There may also be accompanying symptoms of cystitis. In uncomplicated cases acute episodes resolve within a few days of instituting appropriate antibiotic therapy.

Pathological changes. These comprise acute inflammation of the pelves, calyces and renal parenchyma which, in severe cases, may progress to suppuration. The suppuration may be discrete and focal, involving one or both kidneys. Pale linear streaks of pus may extend radially from the tip of the papillae to the surface of the cortex (Fig. 19.32), where adjacent lesions may fuse to produce extensive abscesses. There may be much destruction of the cortex, although there may be remarkable sparing of glomeruli and blood vessels. The changes tend to be more florid if there is obstruction in the lower urinary tract. When there is virtually total or complete obstruction, pus may accumulate in the pelves and calyces to produce pyonephrosis. Extension through the renal capsule may produce a perinephric abscess.

Chronic Pyelonephritis

The importance of chronic pyelonephritis lies in the various adverse effects of long-standing renal parenchymal scarring rather than the symptoms and signs of infection. It is an important cause of end-stage kidney disease constituting about 15% of patients requiring renal dialysis or transplantation.

Clinical features and course. Two main groups of individuals are predisposed to develop chronic pyelonephritis. First, and the commoner, are those with bacteriuria and ureteric reflux in infancy in whom chronic pyelonephritis manifests itself in late childhood or early adult life. This is sometimes referred to as reflux nephropathy.

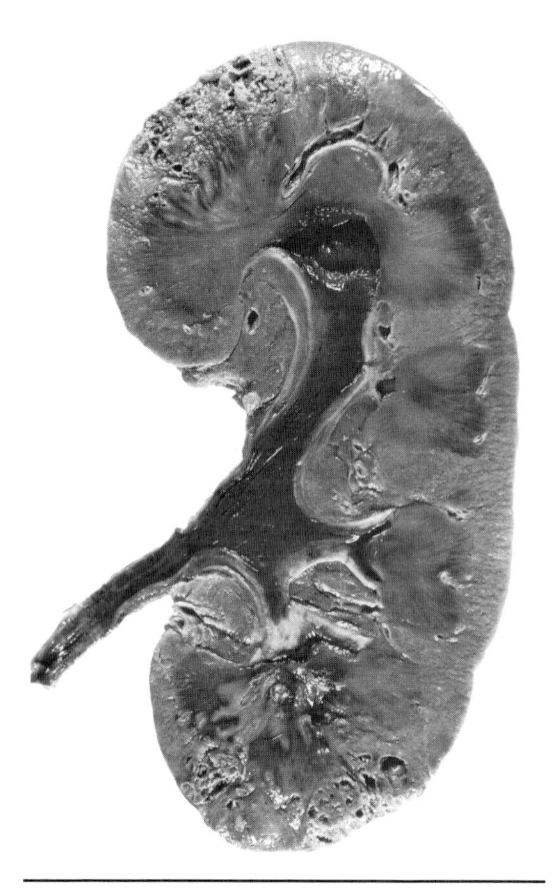

Fig. 19.32 Acute pyelonephritis. In this case the lesions are at the upper and lower poles. Note the cortical abscesses and the streaks of suppuration in the medulla. Note also the acutely inflamed pelvis and ureter.

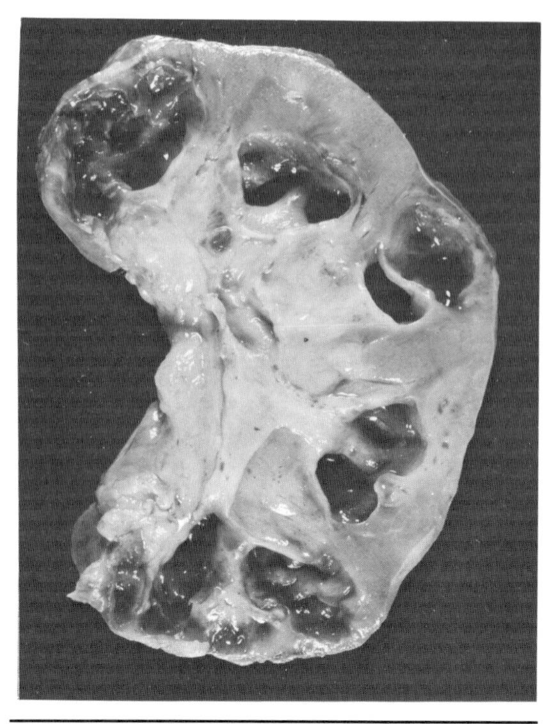

Fig. 19.33 Chronic pyelonephritis, showing dilatation and distortion of the calyces, over some of which the kidney tissue has been largely destroyed and now consists of a thin fibrous layer.

Second are those with anatomical or functional abnormalities of the urinary tract, the former including obstruction and calculi and the latter a neurogenic bladder.

Clinically, there may be a history of recurrent urinary infection but this is by no means invariable. Sometimes there may be a history of failure to thrive in early childhood or of nocturnal enuresis. In bilateral cases the condition usually presents with features of chronic renal failure or hypertension; in 15–20% of those with hypertension it is of the malignant type.

The diagnosis of chronic pyelonephritis is most easily confirmed by intravenous pyelography, in which the typical radiological findings comprise asymmetrical shrinkage of the kidneys, irregularity of renal outline due to cortical scarring and dilatation or disturbance of the calyces opposite the scarred areas. In some patients heavy proteinuria may develop, approaching that seen in the nephrotic syndrome. Such patients show secondary focal segmental glomerulosclerosis and its presence suggests the likelihood of fairly rapid deterioration of renal function.

Pathological changes. The macroscopic appearances of the kidney are important in differentiating chronic pyelonephritic shrinkage from other types of renal scarring. Unlike other forms of chronic tubulointerstitial disease, the pelvic and calyceal walls are thickened and distorted, their mucosa is granular or atrophic, with also scarring of the pyramids and usually calyceal dilatation (Fig. 19.33). In contrast to chronic glomerulonephritis, the renal parenchyma shows irregular asymmetri-

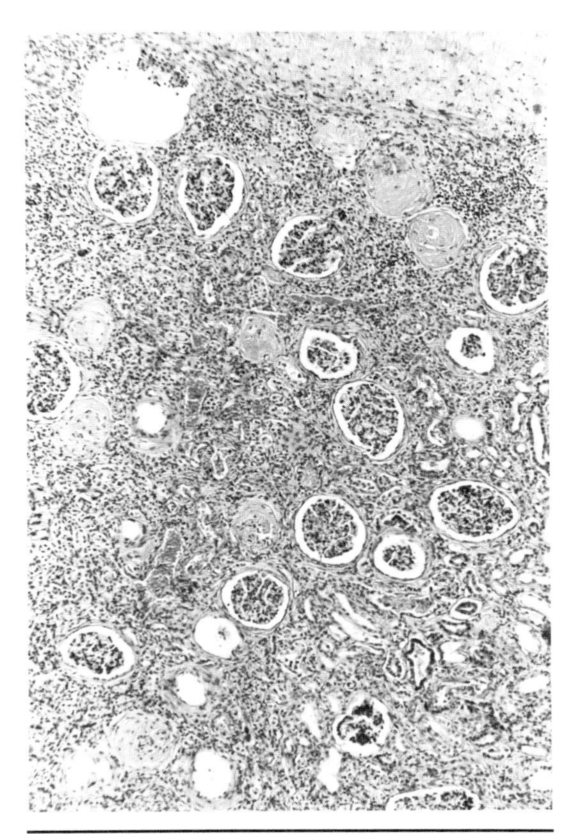

Fig. 19.34 Chronic pyelonephritis. The tubules are greatly atrophied and there is a marked interstitial inflammatory cell infiltrate. Many of the glomeruli still appear normal, but others are completely hyalinized. ×38.

cal scarring and shrinkage, these scars being in close relationship to deformed calyces and being found mainly at the upper and lower poles of the kidney.

Microscopically, the pelvic and calyceal mucosa may be thickened by granulation tissue; there is often submucosal fibrosis and an intense chronic inflammatory cell infiltrate, sometimes with lymphoid follicles. In the parenchymal scars there is tubular atrophy with thickening of their basement membranes and there is an intense inflammatory cell infiltrate of the interstitium (Fig. 19.34) comprising predominantly lymphocytes and plasma cells, but sometimes containing neutrophils and eosinophils. In the late stages of the disease there is dense scar tissue formation and in a 'burnt out' pyelonephritis there may be little active inflammation. Partial destruction of tubules results in survival of isolated segments; these become distended with eosinophilic colloid material, producing a superficial resemblance to thyroid acini, so-called thyroidization. The glomeruli in the scarred areas may appear normal but a spectrum of abnormalities may be seen with concentric periglomerular fibrosis, ischaemic injury, fibrous obliteration and hyalinization of the glomerular tufts. Obliterative endarteritis affects the vessels and arteriolar and glomerular capillary necrosis may occur if there is severe hypertension. In non-scarred areas there may be compensatory glomerular and tubular hypertrophy and vascular change may develop as a result of hypertension.

Xanthogranulomatous pyelonephritis is a distinct but rare form of unilateral chronic pyelonephritis. More common in females, it is associated with chronic infection (*Proteus* spp. in 60% of cases) and obstruction to urinary outflow, often secondary to staghorn calculus. The kidney is enlarged and dilated calyces contain yellowish friable material which histologically contains numerous lipid-laden macrophages. The lesion may resemble a renal cell carcinoma.

Other Forms of Urinary Tract Infection

Tuberculosis. This is becoming increasingly uncommon. The bladder may be affected as a result of direct mucosal infection most often in cases of renal tuberculosis but sometimes in tuberculosis of the genital tract. Tuberculous pyelonephritis results from blood spread, usually from pulmonary lesions. Minute tubercles are seen in acute miliary tuberculosis. Localized lesions of tuberculous pyelonephritis may slowly extend to destroy the kidney(s) (Fig. 19.35). The disease can also involve the ureters, bladder and other pelvic viscera. Renal pelvic involvement often results in haematuria and the renal lesions tend also to suppurate, giving pyuria.

Schistosomiasis (bilharziasis). The bladder is

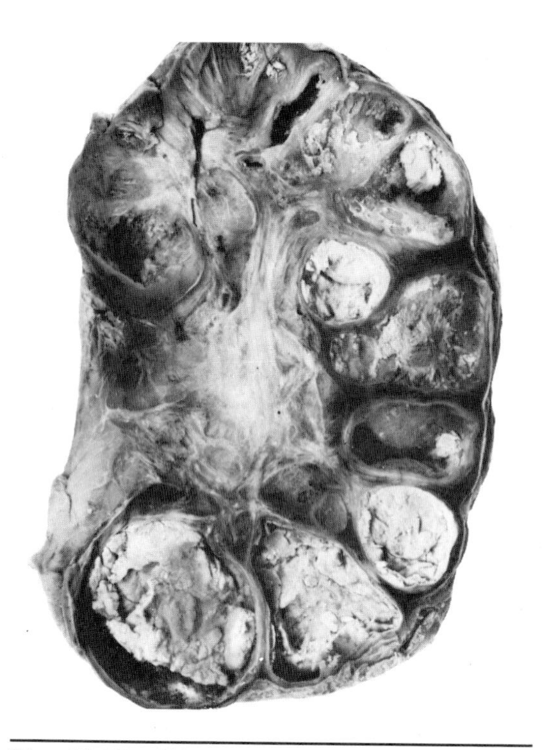

Fig. 19.35 Old tuberculosis of kidney, which has been largely replaced by caseous lesions enclosed by fibrous tissue.

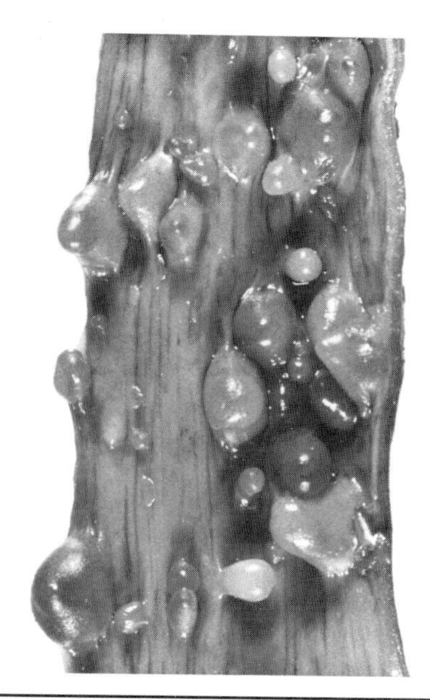

Fig. 19.36 Ureteritis cystica. The thin-walled cysts have formed in sequestered epithelium, but as they enlarged have come to project into the lumen. ×3.

the most frequent site of lesions in infection by *Schistosoma haematobium* (p. 1168). The patients present with haematuria. Microscopy of a bladder biopsy shows a chronic granulomatous cystitis. Bilharzial infection can also predispose to carcinoma of the bladder (p. 943).

Ureteritis cystica. Inflammation of the urinary tract may be followed by formation of multiple small cysts which contain clear fluid and project into the lumen (Fig. 19.36). Apparently, foci of epithelium become sequestrated deep to the surface and form these cysts. The change occurs also in the renal pelves and bladder (**pyelitis** and **cystitis cystica**).

Malakoplakia. This is an uncommon condition found in some cases of chronic cystitis, and is characterized by the formation of soft, rounded, pale, yellowish plaques, up to 2 cm across, on the mucosal surface of the bladder. They consist of cellular granulation tissue and contain macrophages which have large characteristic granules known as Michaelis–Gutmann bodies. Electron microscopy shows them to consist of material probably derived from phagocytosed bacteria. Although uncommon, the condition is important for it may be mistaken clinically for carcinoma.

Tubulointerstitial Diseases

There is a broad category of diseases in which the tubules and interstitium are predominantly affected (Table 19.4). Acute tubular necrosis is also included in this section and is just discussed together with acute renal failure. Some of the conditions, notably pyelonephritis, are discussed elsewhere in this chapter.

Table 19.4 Causes of tubulointerstitial disease of the kidney

Infection
- Acute and chronic pyelonephritis (including renal obstruction and reflux nephropathy)

Drugs and toxins
- Acute interstitial nephritis: sulphonamides, non-steroidal anti-inflammatory drugs
- Chronic interstitial nephritis: analgesic abuse, heavy metals

Metabolic
- Gout: urate nephropathy
- Nephrocalcinosis
- Hypokalaemic nephropathy
- Oxalate nephropathy

Miscellaneous
- Multiple myeloma: myeloma cast nephropathy
- Sjögren's syndrome
- Systemic lupus erythematosus
- Radiation nephritis
- Secondary to glomerulonephritis and/or vascular disease
- Idiopathic interstitial nephritis

Acute Renal Failure and Acute Tubular Necrosis

Acute tubular necrosis is the term applied to the acute renal failure resulting from severe injury to tubular epithelial cells. It is the most important cause of acute renal failure but it should be borne in mind that acute renal failure can arise from a number of causes. **The definition of acute renal failure is very simple – namely, renal failure of sudden onset.** There are three main types, pre-renal, post-renal or obstructive, and renal parenchymal.

Pre-renal. This type occurs in cardiogenic or hypovolaemic shock or peripheral circulatory failure and is characterized by a low volume concentrated urine, only a slightly elevated blood urea and serum creatinine and immediate recovery on effective treatment of the circulatory failure.

Obstructive. Complete obstruction of the urinary outflow tract will produce anuria and acute renal failure. It is usually due to bilateral obstruction at the lower end of ureters resulting from carcinoma of the bladder or uterine cervix. It may also result from a calculus blocking the ureter of a solitary kidney.

Parenchymal. In decreasing order of frequency, it can result from acute tubular necrosis (ATN), crescentic (rapidly progressive) glomerulonephritis, acute interstitial nephritis, hepatorenal syndrome, bilateral renal artery thrombosis, cortical necrosis and papillary necrosis.

Acute Tubular Necrosis

This condition is characterized by the sudden onset of renal failure, usually but not always associated with oliguria. After a period varying from a few days to several weeks, the urine volume rises and normal renal function is restored over the subsequent few weeks. In some milder cases, a normal urine volume is sustained throughout. Although the renal damage is fully reversible the mortality is around 50%, due mainly to death from the illness which precipitated the renal failure. There are two basic mechanisms, ischaemia and nephrotoxicity, accounting for around two-thirds and one-third of cases respectively.

The **ischaemic type** is due to reduced renal perfusion and the classical example is the patient in a state of shock, e.g. following massive haemorrhage. However, particularly in the elderly, much less overt degrees of circulatory failure may produce renal ischaemia sufficient to cause ATN. Patients with ATN due to ischaemia are usually classified under three headings, medical, surgical and obstetric and the commoner causes are shown in Table 19.5. Over the past two decades the obstetric group has shrunk to only a small percentage of the total while the surgical group now constitutes about 75%.

The common **nephrotoxic causes** are also given in Table 19.5. Only the most frequently encountered drugs are listed and the chemical

Table 19.5 Causes of acute tubular necrosis

Ischaemic		
Medical	*Surgical*	*Obstetric*
Septicaemia	Multiple injuries	Ante partum haemorrhage
Gastroenteritis	Peritonitis	Pre-eclampsia
Pneumonia	Pancreatitis	
Leptospirosis	Ruptured abdominal aneurysm	
Myocardial infarction	Burns	
	Cardiac surgery	
Nephrotoxic		
Drugs	*Chemicals*	*Endogenous pigments*
Aminoglycosides	Organic solvents	Haemoglobin (intravascular haemolysis); myoglobin (non-traumatic rhabdomyolysis)
Paracetamol overdose	Glycols	
	Metals, e.g. mercury, arsenic	

causes are diminishing in frequency. One type which is becoming increasingly recognized is non-traumatic rhabdomyolysis; muscle damage due to such causes as status epilepticus and exhaustive exercise can release sufficient myoglobin to exert a nephrotoxic effect.

Pathological Changes

In fatal cases, the kidneys are usually enlarged and the cut surface bulges, due mainly to dilatation of tubules and interstitial oedema. The cortical vessels contain little blood and the cortex appears pale; the medulla is often dark and congested and so the corticomedullary differentiation is accentuated.

Microscopically, the tubular changes are variable and non-specific. The tubular necrosis tends to be focal, involving segments of the proximal and distal convoluted tubules and the ascending limb of the loop of Henle. However, this tubular epithelial necrosis is often not a conspicuous feature and in many cases cannot be seen. Rupture of the basement membrane – tubulorrhexis – may be present with an accompanying inflammatory reaction in the interstitial tissue. An early change seen by electron microscopy is the loss of the normal brush border from the proximal tubular cells. The time at which these cells regain their brush border correlates well with the return of renal function. Proteinaceous, eosinophilic, granular casts are conspicuous in the distal and convoluted tubules. In cases associated with haemoglobinuria, cells containing granules of pigmented material are prominent. There is interstitial oedema. In biopsies taken after the first week, epithelial regeneration with mitotic figures is seen and this regeneration is associated with a return of normal renal function.

Distinctive differences cannot usually be demonstrated between the histological changes in the ischaemic and nephrotoxic types of ATN. An exception is mercuric chloride induced ATN – nowadays a rarity – in which the whole of the proximal tubule may be involved.

Pathogenesis

The pathogenesis of acute renal failure in ATN is not fully understood. Although the main histological abnormalities are seen in the renal tubules, a profound decrease in GFR is probably the main cause of the functional impairment. Four principal mechanisms are thought to be involved:

(1) ***Arteriolar vasoconstriction.*** Reduction in renal blood flow to less than 50% of normal has been demonstrated in acute tubular necrosis and this will result in reduced GFR and oliguria. However, a similar reduction in blood flow may occur in chronic renal failure without oliguria developing. The arteriolar vasoconstriction has been attributed to activation of the renin–angiotensin system as a result of disturbed tubular transport of sodium or chloride.

(2) ***Increased glomerular permeability.*** This could result from ischaemic or toxic effects on glomerular epithelial cells or vascular reactivity. Swelling of glomerular epithelial cells is seen in early ischaemic acute renal failure and again renin–angiotensin mechanisms could modulate glomerular capillary reactivity.

(3) ***Tubular obstruction.*** The presence of necrotic tubular epithelial debris and proteinaceous material results in extensive cast formation, producing a raised intratubular pressure which could contribute to a reduced GFR and also affect afferent arteriolar function.

(4) ***Back leak of tubular fluid*** occurs into the interstitium, due to the tubular damage, producing a further rise in intratubular pressure and thus further aggravating the effects of tubular obstruction.

It seems likely that various combinations of these four and possibly other mechanisms operate in the individual patient and that one or more may predominate, depending on the cause.

Clinicopathological Correlations

Oliguria is common though not invariable in acute tubular necrosis and can last from a few days to several weeks. During the initial phase, both renal blood flow and GFR are markedly reduced. Renal blood flow soon begins to recover but despite this, GFR remains low during the oliguric phase. The low GFR leads to retention of nitrogenous products and this is usually aggravated by increased endogenous protein breakdown resulting from tissue damage. The oliguria itself leads to a tendency to fluid overload unless fluid intake is restricted. In young persons the fluid overload leads mainly to oedema while in the elderly the main risk is cardiac failure. Tubular function is also impaired and this leads to an inability to concentrate the urine; this defect persists through the early recovery phase.

There is acidosis and a very important complication in the oliguric phase is hyperkalaemia, which may be life threatening. This is due to a combination of reduced renal excretion and a shift of potassium from within the cells to the extracellular fluid. In the recovery phase when the urine concentrating power is still reduced, increased electrolyte loss may occur leading to hypokalaemia and/or hyponatraemia.

Tubulointerstitial Injury in Various Systemic Diseases

Gout – Urate Nephropathy

In spite of the high frequency and variety of renal changes in gout, renal failure supervenes in only a small proportion of cases. The main features of gout are described on p. 996. The excretion of an increased amount of urate by the kidneys may result in crystal formation in the medulla. The crystals are deposited mainly in the collecting tubules where they cause local destruction of the tubular wall and become surrounded by a giant-cell reaction and eventually by fibrous tissue. The destructive changes in the collecting tubules result in atrophy of the corresponding nephrons and the kidney may be reduced in size with a granular surface and scarring of the medulla. Urate stones may develop in the renal pelves and may cause renal colic, haematuria and obstruction. A moderate degree of hypertension is common in gout and is accompanied by the usual renal changes.

Multiple Myeloma

Myeloma may affect the kidney in one of two ways. In myeloma cast nephropathy, which may affect more than 50% of patients with the disease, renal dysfunction is the result of light chain (Bence Jones) proteinuria. The light chains are toxic to tubular epithelial cells and in addition, casts comprising light chains and tubular proteins develop in the tubules, and may erode into the interstitium, instigating an inflammatory reaction in which multinucleate giant cells may be conspicuous.

The other way in which myeloma may cause renal disease is by the deposition of paraproteins either in the form of amyloid or kappa light chain fragments in blood vessels, glomeruli and tubules. Both types of renal involvement may present as either acute or chronic renal failure. A similar clinical and pathological picture may occur in light chain disease and Waldenström's macroglobulinaemia.

Nephrocalcinosis

This is the result of calcium deposition in the kidney in idiopathic hypercalciuria or in hypercalciuria secondary to hypercalcaemia from whatever cause, e.g. primary hyperparathyroidism, bone metastases, multiple myeloma and hypervitaminosis D. The calcium first accumulates in and injures tubular epithelial cells; there is deposition on the basement membrane and subsequently, interstitial fibrosis and non-specific chronic inflammation. Chronic renal failure may supervene.

Renal Tubular Acidosis

Deficient tubular function is partly responsible for the acidosis which complicates chronic renal failure (p. 933). The term 'renal tubular acidosis' is, however, restricted to acidosis resulting from a tubular deficiency in the absence of chronic renal failure. It occurs in a number of conditions and traditionally is divided into two types.

In type I, function of the distal part of the tubule is impaired, with a reduced capacity to produce urine of low pH. This may occur as an inherited tubular defect, or as a result of tubular injury from pyelonephritis, hypercalcaemia, urinary tract obstruction or an autoimmune reaction. In type II, there is impaired secretion of hydrogen (H^+) by the proximal tubule. This occurs in association with other tubular defects, e.g. aminoaciduria, renal glycosuria, cystinosis and hypophosphataemia.

In both types of tubular acidosis, there may be hyperchloraemia, osteomalacia or rickets which is resistant to vitamin D, and a danger of deposition of calcium salts in the renal medulla (nephrocalcinosis) which may cause further renal damage. In type I cases, oral administration of alkali is effective, but in type II this is of less value.

The Renal Lesion of Potassium Deficiency

In diseases associated with prolonged potassium depletion, there is an intense hydropic vacuolation of the cells of the proximal tubules (Fig. 19.37), chiefly in the descending straight portion. The lesion is associated with marked loss of concentrating power, but only minimal proteinuria and no urea retention. The commonest causes include: severe and prolonged diarrhoea, e.g. in ulcerative colitis or following purgation; diuretic administration; hyperaldosteronism; Cushing's syndrome; steroid therapy; and diabetic ketoacidosis. The lesion is potentially reversible following potassium administration but permanent functional impairment can occur in long-standing cases.

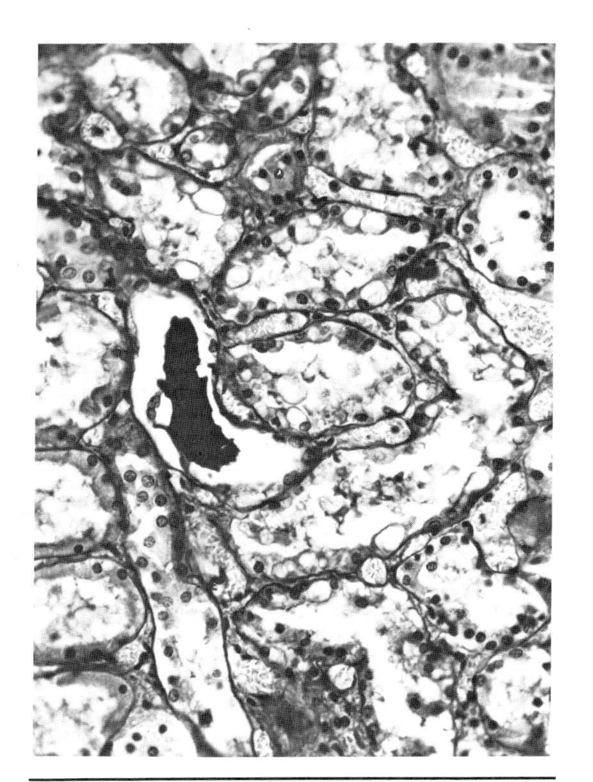

Fig. 19.37 The kidney in severe potassium depletion following prolonged diarrhoea in ulcerative colitis. The cells of the proximal convoluted tubules show gross cytoplasmic vacuolation. ×230.

Interstitial Nephritis due to Drugs and Toxins

The kidney is particularly prone to damage from drugs and chemicals due to a number of factors, notably the very high blood flow in relation to the size of the kidneys and the excretory role of the kidney for these agents and their metabolites. The role of heavy metals in causing membranous glomerulonephritis with a nephrotic syndrome has already been discussed (p. 905) and nephrotoxic acute tubular necrosis is discussed on p. 921. In addition drugs may also cause an acute or chronic interstitial nephritis.

Acute Interstitial Nephritis

First associated with sulphonamides, many drugs are now identified with this form of renal injury. These include non-steroidal anti-inflammatory drugs (NSAIDs), in particular mefenamic acid; diuretics such as frusemide; antibiotics mainly of the synthetic penicillin group; and other agents such as the anticoagulant phenindione.

Clinically, symptoms develop about 2 weeks after commencing the drug. There is fever, haematuria, mild proteinuria, a rising serum creatinine and progression to acute renal failure with oliguria in some patients. Pathologically, there is interstitial oedema, a cellular infiltrate which consists mainly of lymphocytes, plasma cells and sometimes eosinophils and there may be some tubular epithelial necrosis. Granulomas are present in some cases.

Hypersensitivity mechanisms seem likely, the drugs or their metabolites acting as haptens and provoking an immunological reaction following attachment to epithelial or interstitial proteins.

Chronic Interstitial Nephritis

The drugs associated with this are again the NSAIDs and other analgesics of which, in the past, phenacetin was the most important. The changes in the kidney are referred to as **analgesic nephropathy** and comprise interstitial fibrosis and papillary necrosis.

Clinically, there is interference with the ability to concentrate the urine, and pyuria is common. Progressive impairment of renal function often follows and as this develops, a metabolic acidosis and anaemia tend to be prominent features. Sloughing of the necrotic papillae may occur and retrograde or intravenous pyelography may demonstrate the loss of papillae.

The necrosis affects the distal part of some or all of the papillae. The necrotic part may be yellow or white and it is demarcated from the living tissue by a red line of congestion. The necrotic tissue appears structureless and may show patchy calcification. One or more papillae may slough off, leaving an irregular ulcerated surface. Atrophy of the overlying cortex ensues so that the gross appearance of the kidney comes to resemble that of chronic pyelonephritis with intervening patches of more normal and sometimes hypertrophied renal tissue.

Microscopically, the junction between the dead and living papillary tissue is often indistinct and there may be a zone of partial necrosis. The cortex shows tubular loss and atrophy. A distinctive microangiopathy occurs, characterized by the presence of PAS positive material in the vessel wall and this may lead to marked narrowing of the lumen. The resultant ischaemia is an important factor in the pathogenesis of the papillary necrosis although a nephrotoxic effect of the drug may also be important. Papillary necrosis may also be found as a complication of urinary tract obstruction or in diabetes mellitus.

In patients with long-standing analgesic nephropathy, there is an increased incidence of transitional cell carcinoma of the renal pelvis.

Congenital and Hereditary Lesions of the Kidneys and Urinary Tract

Congenital Cystic Kidneys

This occurs in two main forms, one of which does not usually cause illness until beyond the age of 30 years while the other is usually fatal in infancy.

Adult polycystic disease is the commonest form of congenital cystic renal disease. The condition is inherited as an autosomal dominant trait, with a high degree of penetrance. The gene defect is on the short arm of chromosome 16. The kidneys contain a large number of cysts which enlarge throughout life. Death from renal failure does not occur in infancy or childhood, but more than 50% of patients develop symptoms due to hypertension or uraemia in the third or fourth decade.

In adult patients, the kidneys are greatly enlarged and occupied by numerous cysts of various sizes. Functioning renal tissue is gradually compressed by the slowly enlarging cysts and secondary hypertension or chronic renal failure develops. Each kidney may weigh 1 kg or even more (Fig. 19.38) and is easily palpable. The cysts may be of any size up to 4–6 cm in diameter; they usually contain serous fluid, colourless or brownish. The

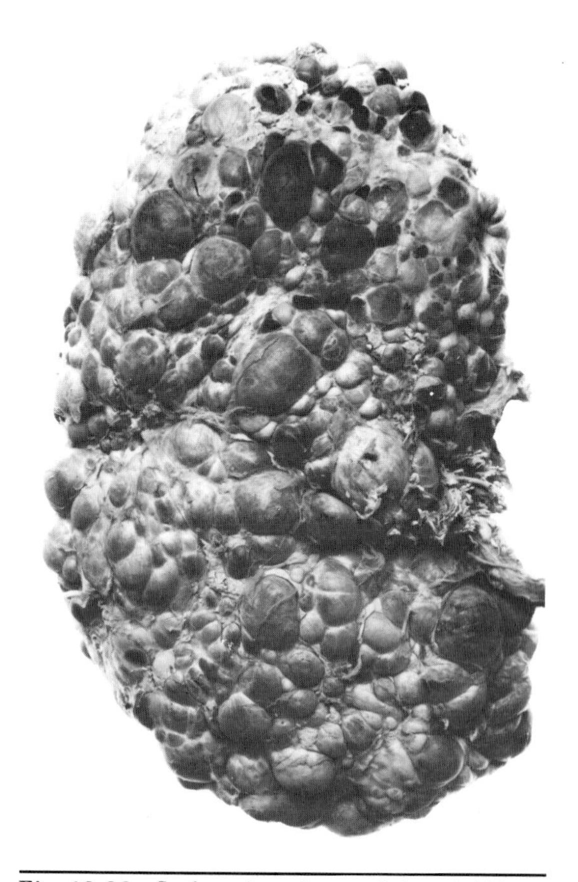

Fig. 19.38 Surface view of congenital cystic kidney, which weighed 1.5 kg.

condition may result from imperfect fusion between the kidney tubules proper and the collecting tubules (which grow up from the extremity of the ureter to meet them) but other embryological explanations have been proposed. There may be accompanying cystic change in the liver, although not sufficient to disturb hepatic function.

Ten per cent of patients with polycystic kidneys die from subarachnoid haemorrhage, this being due to an increased incidence of the congenital vascular abnormality responsible for berry aneurysms. The diagnosis of polycystic kidneys can be made with confidence in early adult life or beyond by ultrasound examination which can visualize cysts greater than 0.5 cm in diameter.

Infantile polycystic disease is rare and usually leads to renal failure in infancy or early childhood. It may be due to an autosomal recessive trait. The kidneys contain multiple elongated radially arranged cysts lined by cuboidal or columnar epithelium. Renal enlargement may be sufficient to interfere with birth or, in liveborn infants, with respiration.

Medullary sponge kidney shows cystic dilatation of the collecting ducts in the papillae. It is usually bilateral and may affect any or all of the papillae in each kidney. Symptoms usually develop after the age of 30, and are due to the formation of calculi within the cysts or to superadded pyelonephritis. The cysts are usually less than 5 mm in diameter and their epithelial lining may be single-layered, squamous or transitional. The diagnosis may be apparent from intravenous pyelograms. Its cause is unknown.

Simple renal cysts are very common and most individuals over the age of 45 have one or more. Occasionally multiple, they show an increasing incidence with age and also in kidneys damaged by pyelonephritis and glomerulonephritis and in end-stage kidneys in patients on chronic dialysis. Such cysts are obviously secondary in nature.

Other Congenital Defects

Renal

These are numerous and some are comparatively common. Occasionally one kidney, usually the left, is absent – agenesis – and in these cases the ureter is also absent. As a result, the surviving kidney undergoes compensatory hypertrophy. This occurs also in hypoplasia of one kidney, which appears usually as an irregular atrophic structure around the upper end of its ureter. If bilateral, hypoplasia will result in renal failure.

Sometimes, the kidneys are fused, most often at the lower pole – 'horseshoe kidney': the two ureters pass in front of the connecting bridge. One kidney, more rarely both, may lie in an ectopic position in front of the sacrum. The kidney is originally composed of five lobules and ordinarily their fusion is complete. If incomplete the term **fetal lobulation** is applied: the condition is of no importance. The arrangement of the renal arteries is very variable and there may be one, two or occasionally multiple arteries.

The Urinary Tract

Renal Pelves and Ureters. The ureter may be double (duplex) in its upper part or in its whole length; in either case, the renal pelvis too is usually duplex. When the duplication is complete, the ureter from the upper part of the kidney opens separately into the bladder, or sometimes into the urethra or a seminal vesicle. Narrowing of a ureter without scarring, possibly of a congenital nature is a common cause of unilateral hydronephrosis. Such abnormalities favour the occurrence of infection.

The bladder. The most important abnormality is a defect of its anterior wall, accompanied by a corresponding median defect of the abdominal wall

– **extroversion** of the bladder. The posterior wall of the bladder is thus exposed and the mucosa undergoes metaplasia in part into squamous epithelium and in part into a columnar mucus-secreting epithelium resembling that of the large intestine. In the male, the urethra remains open on its dorsal aspect, the condition being known as **epispadias**; in the female there is usually a split clitoris. The symphysis pubis is also usually deficient, though this may occur apart from extroversion of the bladder.

In the posterior urethra, valve-like folds of the mucosa may cause obstruction with consequent hypertrophy of the bladder and bilateral hydronephrosis. Other abnormalities of the male urethra include **epispadias** (see above), and **hypospadias** in which it opens on the ventral surface of the penis. Also epispadias may occur as an isolated defect in the presence of a normal bladder.

Hereditary Nephritis

This comprises an uncommon group of syndromes in which there is renal involvement affecting the glomeruli. The pattern of inheritance is complex and may be X-linked or autosomal dominant; in the former the defective gene is on the long arm of the X chromosome.

Alport's syndrome is the commonest, and in this there is high frequency nerve deafness and sometimes an abnormality of the eye in which the lens is more spherical than usual (spherophakia). In females the syndrome is usually characterized by haematuria with well preserved renal function, but in males proteinuria and renal failure may also occur, usually in the first or second decade. Light microscopy of the kidney shows non-specific changes but on electron microscopy there is irregular multilamination and fragmentation of the glomerular and tubular basement membranes. Fluorescence microscopy shows lack of binding of glomerular basement membrane antibodies (such as occur in Goodpasture's syndrome). There is, therefore, some defect of the glomerular basement membrane in these patients.

Vascular Disease of the Kidney

The renal vessels show the usual features of generalized vascular diseases. Atheroma occurs but is much less common than in other arteries of comparable size and, except in patients with diabetes mellitus, it is rarely severe enough to interfere with the renal circulation. Disturbances arise more commonly from involvement and narrowing at the origin of one or rarely both renal arteries by atheromatous plaques. Unilateral renal artery stenosis accounts for less than 5% of cases of hypertension. In addition to atheroma, renal artery stenosis may be the result of fibromuscular dysplasia and this accounts for about a third of cases. Hypertension results from the renal ischaemia (p. 464). It is important to make the diagnosis of unilateral renal artery stenosis as surgical treatment may cure the hypertension.

Renal Changes in Hypertension

The arterial changes in hypertension have already been described and their pathogenesis discussed (p. 458). The arterial tree of the kidney is usually affected more than other organs and this results in varying degrees of renal damage. In benign (essential) hypertension the renal injury is usually slight and there is often minimal functional impairment, whereas in malignant (accelerated) hypertension severe arteriolar damage in the form of arteriolar necrosis gives rise to renal failure.

Benign hypertension. Hypertensive arteriosclerosis of the larger branches of the renal arteries is without any functional effect; the interlobular arteries may be narrowed in severe arteriosclerosis by the fibroelastic intimal thickening, but the most significant lesion, hyaline arteriolosclerosis (p. 459), occurs mainly in the afferent glomerular arterioles (Fig. 19.39) which become tortuous, thick-walled and often severely narrowed. These arterial changes tend to cause ischaemia and individual nephrons are affected. The capillary tuft of the affected glomerulus shrinks, and becomes hyalinized, and Bowman's capsule becomes filled with collagen (Fig. 19.40). The tubules atrophy and are replaced by fibrous tissue often containing some lymphocytes.

In the early stages of hypertension the kidney appears normal, but with prominent arteries visible on the cut surface. As more nephrons are lost there is diffuse thinning of the renal cortex and the kidneys become moderately reduced in size, with an average weight of about 115 g (Fig. 19.41). If enough nephrons are lost there may be hypertrophy of the surviving nephrons. The kidneys are seldom very small and while there may be loss of functional reserve, renal function is not significantly impaired.

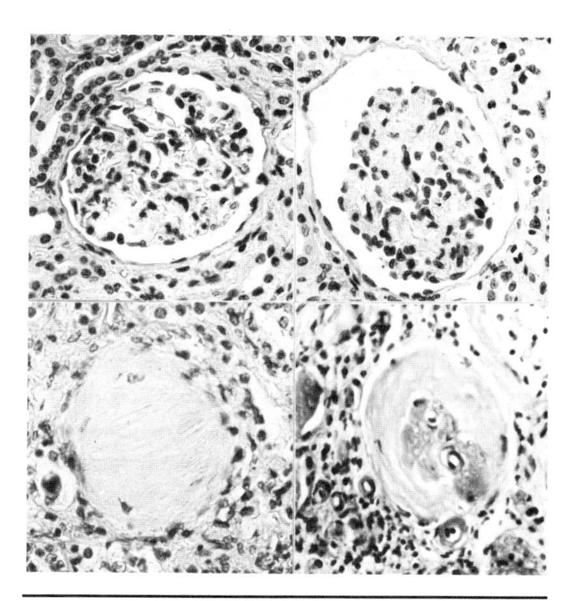

Fig. 19.40 Ischaemic changes in the glomeruli in chronic essential hypertension. The two glomeruli above show partial hyalinization. The lower left is completely hyalinized and the lower right is collapsed, extensively hyalinized, and encased in fibrous tissue which has formed inside Bowman's capsule. Note its hyalinized afferent arteriole (seen below, containing a leucocyte). ×160.

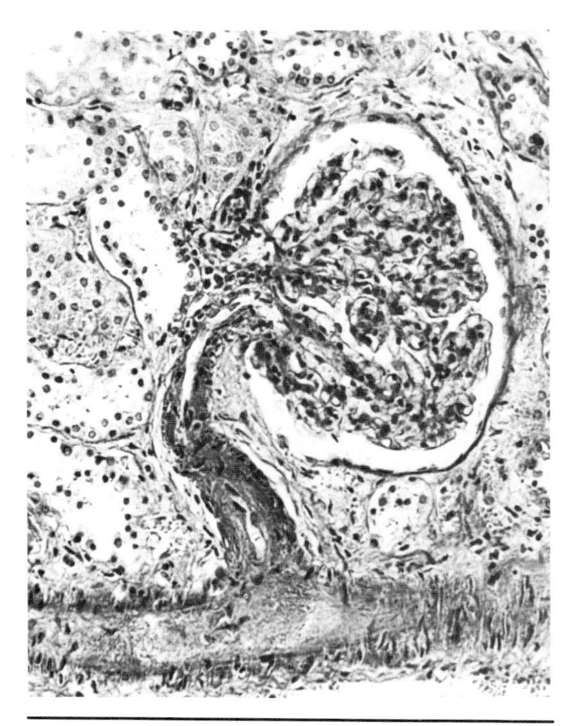

Fig. 19.39 Benign essential hypertension, showing hyaline thickening of an afferent arteriole. ×180.

Malignant (accelerated) hypertension. This may arise acutely, apparently *de novo*, or may supervene after a variable period of benign hypertension (p. 457), and the appearances in the kidney vary accordingly. In the most acute cases the surface of the kidney is smooth and spotted with tiny petechial haemorrhages. The cut surface may show mottling due to multiple tiny infarcts. The interlobular arteries may show intimal thickening. Fibrinoid necrosis affects mainly the distal portions of the interlobular arteries and the afferent arterioles (Fig. 19.42) and may extend into the glomerular tuft. There is often blood or proteinaceous fluid in Bowman's space and sometimes proliferation of the capsular epithelium may give rise to small crescents. A minority of the glomeruli are affected, the severe impairment of

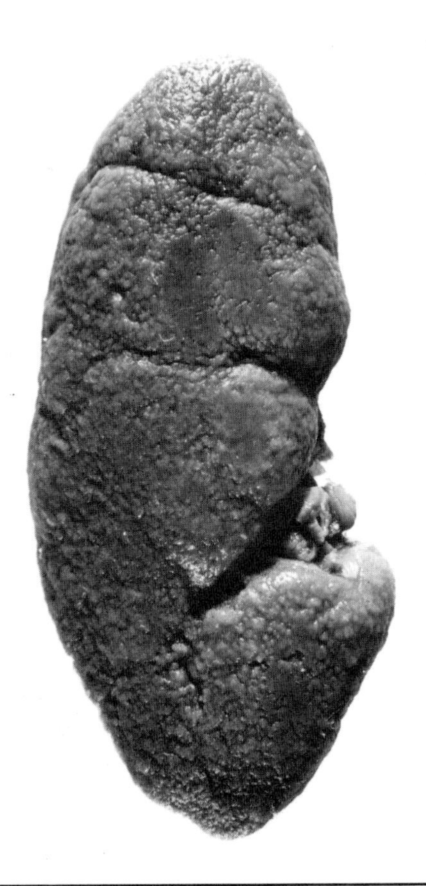

Fig. 19.41 Kidney in long-standing benign essential hypertension, showing slight reduction in size and granularity of the subcapsular surface. ×1.

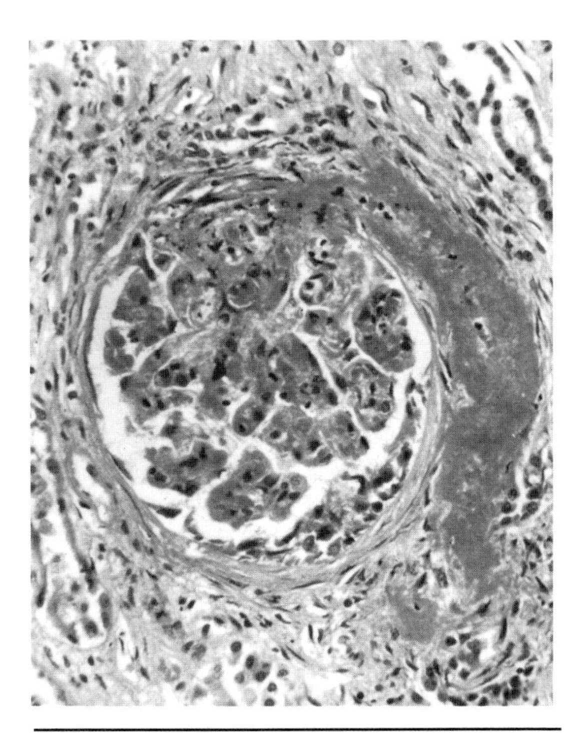

Fig. 19.42 Malignant hypertension. Fibrinoid necrosis of an afferent arteriole and of most of the glomerular tuft. Note also the aggregation of cells in the capsular space (lower right) to form a small crescent. ×180.

renal function being due to ischaemia caused by the severe arterial damage. The tubules may be atrophied or enlarged and usually contain proteinaceous or blood casts.

There is hyperplasia of the renin-secreting cells of the juxtaglomerular apparatus, correlating with the high serum levels of renin and angiotensin II in malignant hypertension. In contrast to benign hypertension, renal failure is common in untreated cases.

Secondary hypertension. Various grades of hypertension may complicate pre-existing renal diseases. Depending on the height and rate of rise of the blood pressure, the renal changes of benign and/or malignant hypertension may be superimposed on those of the primary renal disease.

Renal Changes in the Vasculitic Syndromes

The intrarenal vessels may be involved in polyarteritis nodosa, microscopic polyarteritis and Wegener's granulomatosis. Glomerular involvement may also occur, causing a focal or rapidly progressive crescentic type of glomerulonephritis (p. 901).

The Microangiopathic Disorders

The renal involvement in the microangiopathic complications of diabetes mellitus have been described. There is another group of diseases, however, in which, clinically, there is evidence of red cell haemolysis, microangiopathic haemolytic anaemia, thrombocytopenia, disseminated intravascular coagulation (DIC) and renal failure. The morphological findings favour DIC (see p. 91) as the essential or the most important factor in the pathogenesis of these disorders.

Renal injury in DIC results from obstruction of arterioles and glomerular capillaries by fibrin thrombi (Fig. 19.43). In addition, circulating non-polymerized fibrin and fibrin degradation products pass through the fenestrae of the glomerular capillary endothelium. They may then aggregate on the basement membrane under the endothelium and in the mesangium, in the same fashion as intermediate-sized immune complexes in focal glomerulonephritis. There is mesangial hyperplasia and thickening of the basement membrane. Insudation of the walls of the interlobular arteries with fibrin may also occur, stimulating a proliferative endarteritis resembling that of malignant hypertension. The afferent arterioles may also be permeated by fibrin and undergo fibrinoid necrosis which, as in malignant hypertension, may extend into the glomerular tufts with focal proliferative and necrotic changes. Clinically, the features of renal failure are superimposed on those of the predisposing cause of DIC.

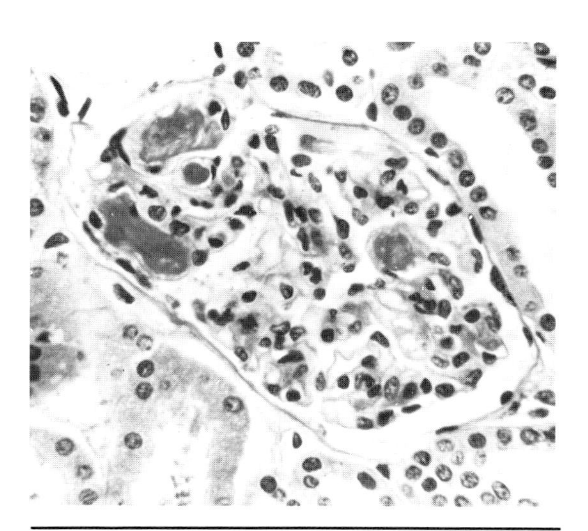

Fig. 19.43 The kidney in disseminated intravascular coagulation. Some of the glomerular capillaries are occluded by fibrin. ×250.

The disorders in which there is an association between microangiopathic haemolytic anaemia and renal disease are the following:

(1) Haemolytic uraemic syndrome which can be of childhood or adult type. In childhood, the onset often follows an upper respiratory or diarrhoeal illness. The main features are acute renal failure, a bleeding tendency, confusion and microangiopathic haemolytic anaemia. In adults too, the illness may follow an episode of diarrhoea but can also occur in late pregnancy, particularly in association with pre-eclampsia and rarely in the post-partum period following an uneventful pregnancy. When preceding diarrhoea occurs in both children and adults a verocytotoxin producing *E. coli* can often be cultured from the stool and it is thought that this verocytotoxin may be the cause of the DIC. Most patients survive but recovery of renal function is often incomplete.

(2) Thrombotic thrombocytopenic purpura, a rare and idiopathic condition which results in fever, variable neurological signs, thrombocytopenic purpura and acute renal failure as well as microangiopathic haemolytic anaemia. There is no effective treatment and the mortality rate is high.

(3) Progressive systemic sclerosis (scleroderma) which is described in more detail on p. 229. The renal manifestations are irreversible renal failure associated with hypertension, often of malignant type. The typical pathological changes are concentric intimal thickening of the interlobular arteries and fibrinoid necrosis of the arterioles, changes very similar to those seen in malignant (accelerated) hypertension.

Renal Cortical Necrosis

Diffuse bilateral cortical necrosis with sparing of the medulla is very uncommon but when present it leads to failure of renal function or to incomplete recovery. It is most frequently associated with pre-eclampsia but may also occur in the haemolytic uraemic syndrome and occasionally in septic shock. It is due mainly to intravascular coagulation.

Chronic Renal Failure, Renal Replacement Therapy and Renal Transplantation

The diseases which can damage the kidneys in a progressive and irreversible way, leading to chronic renal failure are discussed elsewhere in this chapter, and are listed, in descending order of frequency in Table 19.6. Chronic renal failure is the major cause of death from renal disease. The healthy kidney has a large reserve of function and, while the biochemical evidence of renal insufficiency will occur earlier it is only when around 75% of renal function has been lost that the symptoms of chronic renal failure make themselves manifest.

Chronic Renal Failure

Pathophysiology

Animal experiments in which more than 50% of healthy kidney tissue is removed have demonstrated how the kidney adapts to loss of nephrons. In an attempt to maintain a normal internal body environment, hypertrophy of healthy nephrons compensates for the reduction or total loss of function of the diseased ones. Thus, the blood flow to the remaining healthy glomeruli increases and this is accompanied by an increase in their individual GFR. There is, of course, an overall drop in the total GFR. The mechanism of this compensatory process is poorly understood although some studies have suggested a role for prostaglandins. The glomerular hyperfiltration is able to stabilize the amount of nitrogenous waste products in the blood but only at a higher level. For example, with a total GFR of 120 ml/min and a normal blood urea level of 5 mmol/l the amount of urea in the glomerular filtrate will be $(5/1000) \times 120$, i.e. 0.6 mmol/l per minute. A fall in total GFR to 12 ml/min will require a rise in blood urea to 50 mmol/l to restore homeostasis [$(50/1000) \times 12 = 0.6$ mmol/l per min]. Hypertrophy of the tubules also occurs and this is most prominent in the proximal tubule. Functional changes naturally occur also although there is little evidence of this when water and electrolyte intake and non-renal losses are maintained within the usual limits. For example, a reduction in the filtered load of water down to 10% of normal is accompanied by a commensurate decrease in the fraction of water reabsorbed in the tubule from 99% to 92% to maintain a normal urine volume of around 1.5 l/24 h. Similar alterations apply to the handling of electrolytes such as sodium and potassium. Even at this considerably diminished level of renal function, problems only arise when there is a marked change in external water or electrolyte balance. Thus, electrolyte loss from diarrhoea will not be followed in the poorly functioning kidney by the necessary increase in tubular electrolyte reabsorption and so electrolyte depletion will result.

Other tubular functions to be adversely affected by compensatory hypertrophy are the ability to vary urine concentration and to excrete an acid load. The increased volume of glomerular filtrate, combined with a decrease in tubular cell mass, results in a decrease in sodium and chloride re-

Table 19.6 Causes of chronic renal failure in decreasing order of frequency

Glomerulonephritis
Diabetic glomerulosclerosis
Chronic pyelonephritis
Obstructive uropathy
Hypertensive nephrosclerosis
Polycystic kidneys
Drugs and toxins

absorption in the thick ascending limb of the loop of Henle. This in turn results in a reduced hypertonicity in the medulla on which the urine concentrating mechanism depends. Also contributing are an osmotic diuresis due to the high blood urea and possibly decreased responsiveness of the collecting tubule to antidiuretic hormone. The decrease in acidification of the urine is mainly due to reduced ammonia production because of the reduced tubular mass.

A final important aspect is the likelihood that the compensatory process of hyperfiltration has, in the long term, a deleterious effect on the glomerulus, leading eventually to sclerosis. Such an effect can be clearly demonstrated in animal models. The obvious implication of this is that once nephron loss reaches a certain degree, it will become self-perpetuating even if the initial cause of the renal disease becomes inactive.

Clinical Features

The predominant symptom of chronic renal failure is tiredness, due mainly to the accompanying anaemia. Urinary symptoms may include polyuria resulting from the osmotic diuresis. This in turn may cause polydipsia and thirst. Dyspnoea is common, particularly in the older patient, due again to the anaemia and often also to heart failure. Tachypnoea may also be due to the acidosis, in which case it will be unaccompanied by the visible distress of dyspnoea; this type of sighing breathing carries the eponym of Kussmaul's respiration. Hypertension may be a primary cause of chronic renal failure but much more often it is a sequel to the renal disease. Anorexia, nausea, pruritus and vomiting are features of more advanced uraemia while neuromuscular features include myopathy, peripheral neuropathy and encephalopathy with convulsions and intellectual deterioration in the long-term patient.

Biochemical Features

While the blood urea level will reflect the degree of renal failure it is also affected by dietary protein and rate of tissue breakdown, and the serum creatinine is a more accurate guide to renal function. Other nitrogenous products whose blood levels are elevated include uric acid. Serum sodium is often normal but may be low due to decreased tubular capacity to conserve sodium. The same applies to potassium, although in very advanced cases the blood level may become high once the GFR falls to very low levels, or in association with oliguria or severe acidosis. The acidosis is of the metabolic type and is characterized by a lowering of the serum pH, $P\text{CO}_2$ and bicarbonate. The serum phosphate rises due to the decrease in phosphate filtered and this is usually associated with a fall in serum calcium.

Pathological Changes

Cardiopulmonary. Atheroma occurs to a much greater degree in chronic renal failure than in healthy subjects due to a combination of hyperlipidaemia and hypertension, in addition to any risk factors unrelated to the chronic renal failure which the patient may possess. Calcification may also contribute to the vascular disease. Cardiac enlargement, left ventricular hypertrophy and later heart failure are common and the factors causing these include hypertension, anaemia and coronary artery disease.

Fibrinous pericarditis may occur in uraemia and, although often asymptomatic, it may be complicated by a pericardial effusion and sometimes bleeding, leading to pericardial tamponade. A syndrome of 'uraemic lung' used to be described but it is now thought that this is simply pulmonary oedema resulting from left ventricular failure.

Bones/calcium and phosphate metabolism. **Renal osteodystrophy** is a collective term which includes osteomalacia (or in childhood, rickets), osteitis fibrosa cystica and osteosclerosis, One of the two most important primary factors is a deficiency of $1,25(OH)_2D_3$ which results from a lack of the enzyme 25-hydroxyvitamin D_3 1-α-hydroxylase within the kidney. The main consequences are reduced calcium absorption from the intestine and hypocalcaemia which may lead to osteomalacia (or rickets). The hypocalcaemia stimulates the parathyroid glands leading to secondary hyperparathyroidism which manifests itself as osteitis fibrosa cystica. Osteosclerosis is probably a variant of osteitis fibrosa cystica. Patients often have a combination of these different forms of bone disease. Finally, phosphate retention leads to hyperphosphataemia. This contributes to the parathyroid stimulation and to the high Ca × P product in the blood causing metastatic calcification, mainly in blood vessels and around joints.

Haematological. The main haematological consequence is anaemia. It is due mainly to deficiency of the hormone erythropoietin which is synthesized by the kidney. The degree of anaemia is variable but may be severe. Blood transfusion used to be the mainstay of treatment but now synthetic recombinant erythropoietin is available and has a markedly beneficial effect.

Immunological. Uraemia is accompanied by a variable degree of immunodeficiency, both cell mediated and humoral. This predisposes to infection although it does have the compensating advantage of reducing the strength of the rejection reaction following transplantation.

Gastrointestinal. Upper gastrointestinal symptoms are common. Pathological abnormalities are often confined to oesophageal, gastric and duodenal inflammation, so-called uraemic oesophagitis, gastritis and duodenitis.

Neurological. The findings in the central nervous system are non-specific, consisting mainly of degenerative changes, possibly due to parathyroid hormone excess. In the past, aluminium from the tap water resulted in a progressive, fatal dialysis-dependent dementia in haemodialysis patients. Water treatment has eradicated this problem, but the smaller amounts of aluminium absorbed from ingested phosphate binding agents may be a factor in the intellectual deterioration seen in some long-term dialysis patients.

Renal Replacement Therapy

In patients with chronic renal failure, conservative measures maintain a reasonable degree of well-being until the GFR is down to around 5 ml/min, which is equivalent to a serum creatinine of just under 1000 μmol/1. Thereafter symptoms become more severe and the risk of death from complications becomes greater. At this stage a decision has to be made regarding suitability for long-term dialysis. Almost all patients below the age of 70 years are suitable provided they do not have too much damage to other organs – a common example is heart failure – which would result in a very poor life expectancy. Beyond 70 years some patients are suitable but a greater degree of selection is required.

There is a choice between haemodialysis and continuous ambulatory peritoneal dialysis (CAPD). Two groups of patients have fewer complications with CAPD than haemodialysis, namely those with diabetes mellitus or extensive vascular disease, and this therefore is the preferred treatment for them. The main complication of CAPD is peritonitis, resulting from the passage of organisms into the peritoneal cavity. An important systemic complication is obesity due to absorption of glucose from the dialysis fluid.

The main technical complications of haemodialysis are thrombosis or infection of the vessel access site which is usually an arteriovenous fistula but may be a vein loop or prosthetic graft such as goretex. The most important systemic complication is a type of amyloidosis due to the extravascular deposition of β_2 microglobulin, plasma levels of which are markedly elevated in these patients. The main clinical features of the amyloidosis are a carpal tunnel syndrome, joint pain and stiffness. The kidneys from patients who have had prolonged haemodialysis sometimes develop numerous cysts, probably as a result of obstruction by interstitial fibrosis. Adenomas and, much less frequently, adenocarcinomas may be present in the walls of these cysts.

Renal Transplantation

Renal transplantation, first successfully carried out in 1955 between identical twins, is now the preferred treatment modality for chronic renal failure. Improved immunosuppressive therapy now assures a 90% survival of renal allografts at one year post-transplant. The general immunological aspects of allograft rejection are discussed on page 223. Renal allograft rejection remains the commonest cause of graft failure, while other problems include technical difficulties with the vascular and ureteric anastomoses, and acute tubular necrosis resulting from the period of ischaemia between harvesting the donor kidney and its re-anastomosis in the recipient.

Pathology of Rejection

Rejection is classified clinically as hyperacute, acute and chronic.

Hyperacute rejection, within minutes or hours of renal transplantation, occurs when the kidney donor's ABO blood group is incompatible with the recipient, or when, as a result of pregnancy, blood transfusion or a previous transplant, the recipient has developed cytotoxic HLA antibodies reactive with the donor's cells.

In hyperacute rejection, the kidney regains its normal pink colour and starts to produce urine when blood flow is established, but then rapidly becomes soft, cyanotic and anuric. Microscopy shows arrest of polymorphs along the walls of arterioles and venules and in the glomerular and peritubular capillaries. Platelets aggregate in the small vessels and thrombosis and haemorrhage occur. The process is a type 2 or a type 3 (Arthus) hypersensitivity reaction in which circulating antibody reacts with graft antigen. This type of rejection is irreversible and progresses to infarction of the kidney, necessitating its removal. The performance of a cross-match between donor lymphocytes and recipient serum is now standard practice and should prevent this type of rejection.

Acute rejection. Many renal transplant recipients have an episode of acute rejection within a few weeks of transplantation. The graft tends to become enlarged and the patient may develop a fever and fall in urine volume. However, in cyclosporin treated patients, clinical features may be non-existent and the only clue to rejection is a rise in serum creatinine. Microscopically, the changes are predominantly cellular or vascular. **Acute cellular rejection** is a cell mediated or type IV hypersensitivity reaction (p. 219) and the kidney shows interstitial oedema and focal cortical infiltrates of lymphocytes, plasma cells and macrophages. Deposition of immunoglobulin or complement components cannot be detected by immunofluorescence microscopy. This type of rejection usually responds to treatment with high dose steroids or antilymphocyte globulin, and the prognosis is good. **Acute vascular rejection** is a type 2 (cytotoxic antibody) hypersensitivity reaction; lymphocytes are few or absent and immunofluorescence studies show the presence of IgG, IgM and complement components in the walls of blood vessels and of the glomerular capillaries. Platelet thrombi, fibrin and polymorphs are present in the glomerular capillaries and foci of plasmatic vasculosis (p. 459) or fibrinoid necrosis are found in the vessel walls. Interstitial haemorrhage may be present and the intima of some vessels is infiltrated by chronic inflammatory cells. If untreated, the process proceeds to cortical necrosis and may be associated with microangiopathic haemolytic anaemia. Vascular rejection often occurs at an early stage after transplantation, i.e. within the first few weeks , and the response to immunosuppressive therapy is less good than with cellular rejection. Frequently of course, cellular and vascular rejection occur together.

Chronic rejection usually occurs after several

months or years and often in patients who have had acute rejection at an earlier stage. It presents clinically with progressive deterioration in renal function usually with heavy proteinuria and hypertension. Grossly, the kidney is normal in size or enlarged and may appear pale because of ischaemia. Microscopically, the changes are vascular and/or glomerular. The vascular changes represent a continuation of acute vascular rejection; episodic deposition of platelet and fibrin thrombi occurs in the intima of the interlobular and arcuate arteries, which eventually show the circumferential intimal proliferation of endarteritis obliterans, presenting an onion-skin appearance with a marked reduction of the lumen (Fig. 19.44). Lipid-laden macrophages are frequently found in a subintimal position. The consequent ischaemia is reflected in hyperplasia of the juxtaglomerular epithelioid cells (p. 75) and causes atrophy and loss of tubules, and interstitial fibrosis.

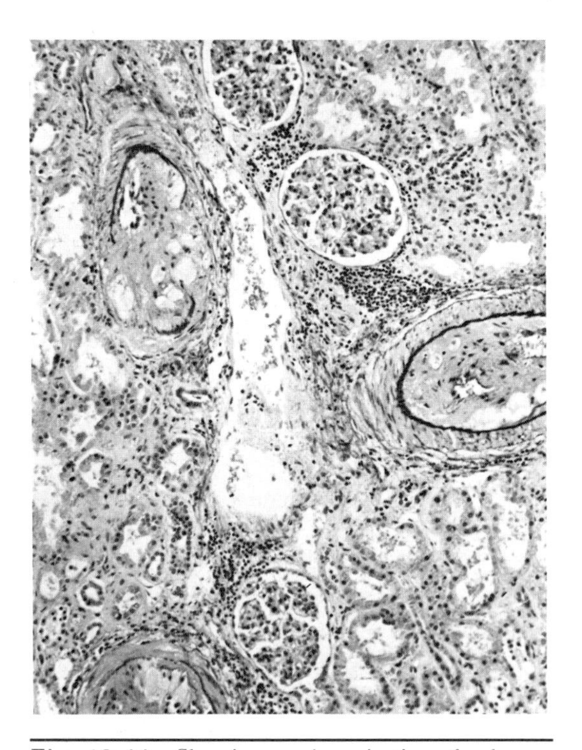

Fig. 19.44 Chronic vascular rejection of a human renal allotransplant. Note the obliterative intimal changes and disruption of the arterial walls. (Professor K. A. Porter.)

The glomerular changes are not specific but mesangial hyperplasia with focal basement membrane thickening is common, giving rise to an appearance resembling mesangiocapillary glomerulonephritis. Various other changes are seen, including focal or segmental glomerular sclerosis and, rarely, the formation of crescents. Chronic rejection leads to progressive deterioration in renal function and sometimes also to a nephrotic syndrome. Graft loss will eventually result and there is no response to anti-rejection therapy.

Other Complications of Renal Transplantation

Opportunistic infections may occur, particularly if large amounts of immunosuppression are required for rejection episodes. Most commonly encountered are those due to cytomegalovirus, **Pneumocystis carinii** and fungi such as *Candida* and *Aspergillus*. However, the bulk of infections are due to the commonly encountered bacteria rather than opportunistic pathogens.

Tumours. There is also a significant increase in malignant tumours in transplant patients, particularly non-Hodgkin's lymphoma and skin tumours.

Recurrence of glomerulonephritis in the allograft may lead to graft failure. IgA nephropathy, type II mesangiocapillary glomerulonephritis and focal glomerulosclerosis are those most liable to recur. Finally, **glomerulonephritis**, usually of the membranous type, may occur **de novo** without any relationship to the recipient's own kidney disease.

Urinary Tract Obstruction

Obstruction in the urinary tract may be of sudden or insidious onset, may be intermittent or complete, may be bilateral or unilateral and may predispose to urinary tract infection and calculus formation.

Aetiology and Effects

A summary of the causes of urinary tract obstruction is given schematically in Fig. 19.45). Serious mechanical obstruction of the urethra is practically confined to the male sex (p. 1065). Neurogenic disturbance of the bladder occurs in spina bifida and following trauma or pressure on the spinal cord. In addition to pressure effects, in pregnancy the effect of high progesterone levels in relaxing smooth muscle may result in functional dilatation of ureters and pelvis with so-called dysfunctional obstruction. In many instances of unilateral hydronephrosis severe narrowing of the ureter occurs at the pelviureteric junction, but without scarring: it may represent a congenital structural abnormality or result from some form of neuromuscular dysfunction. Kinking of the ureter by an aberrant renal artery to the lower pole of the kidney may also cause hydronephrosis (Fig. 19.46).

In urethral obstruction, the chief effect is the

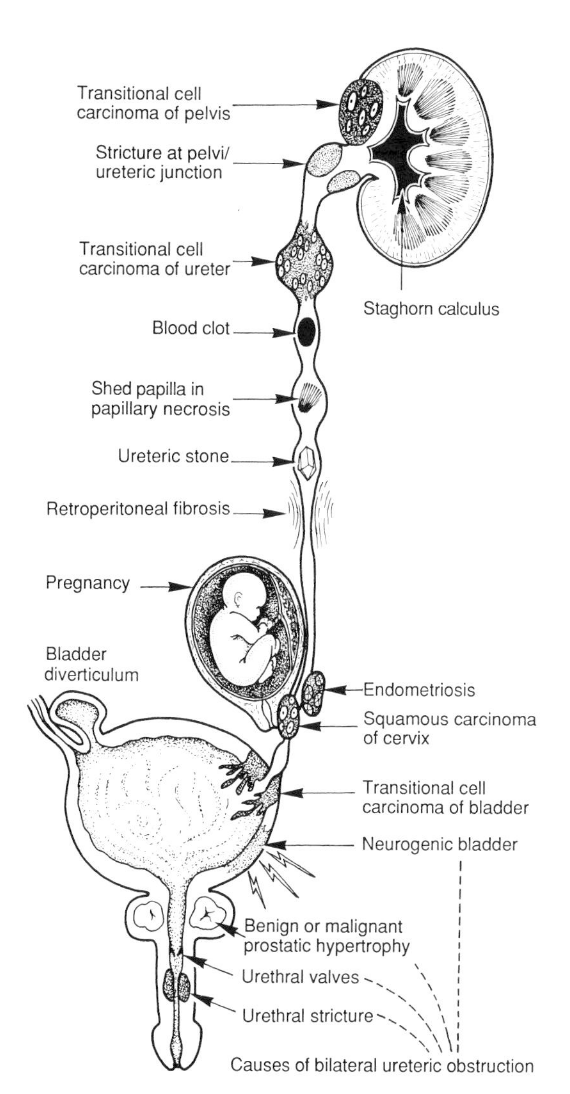

Fig. 19.45 Causes of obstruction to urinary outflow.

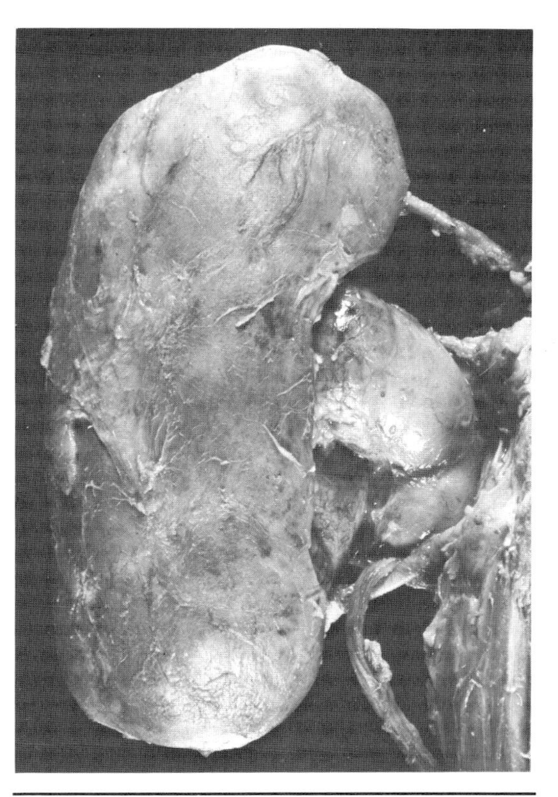

Fig. 19.46 Hydronephrosis with kinking of the ureter around an accessory renal artery to the lower pole of the kidney.

production of variable degrees of hypertrophy and dilatation of the bladder wall. When the outstanding feature is hypertrophy, the muscular part of the wall is thickened and the bands of muscle, which have an interlacing arrangement under the mucosa, enlarge and form prominent ridges or bands with depressions between (Fig. 22.10, p. 1066). Occasionally one of these depressions may become enlarged and form a diverticulum in which infection with suppuration, ulceration and even perforation may follow. Urethral obstruction ultimately leads to dilatation of the ureters and renal pelves – hydroureter and hydronephrosis.

Hydronephrosis

Hydronephrosis is a dilatation of the renal pelvis and calyces due to obstruction of urinary outflow; this can lead to progressive renal atrophy with fibrosis because the pressure in the renal pelvis is transferred back to the collecting tubule and the nephron. Glomerular filtration persists for some time, even with complete obstruction, and so the affected calyces and pelvis may become markedly dilated. Tubular function is affected by the increasing pressure with impaired ability to concentrate the urine.

As the distension progresses the calyces become flattened; the renal parenchyma becomes progressively thinned and may ultimately form a mere rind enclosing a cystic structure in which the normal kidney architecture cannot be defined. Atrophy of the renal parenchyma may be regular or irregular so that some areas may be spared while the rest is severely thinned (Fig. 19.47). Histologically, there is tubular atrophy, glomerular fibrosis and a superimposed chronic inflammatory cell infiltrate.

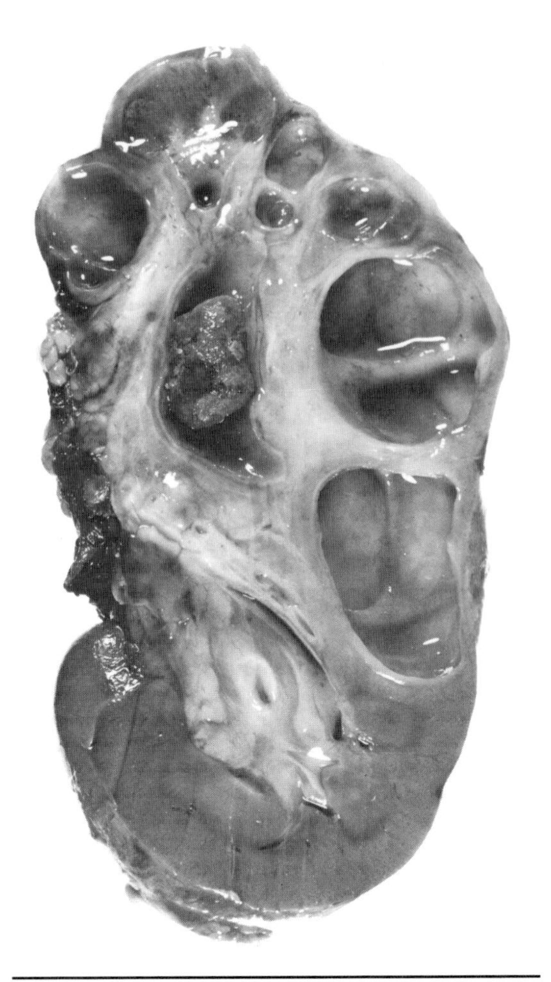

Fig. 19.47 An impacted stone in the renal pelvis, which has caused hydronephrosis and consequent atrophy of the renal tissue. The stone was in such a position that the lower part of the pelvis was not obstructed, and the lower pole of the kidney appears normal.

Clinical features. These depend on the site of obstruction and whether it is sudden and/or complete. Acute obstruction may give rise to pain due to rapid distension; ureteric obstruction due to a renal calculus is exquisitely painful; urethral obstruction due to prostatism will result in bladder distension. Unilateral hydroureter and hydronephrosis may be clinically silent, renal function being maintained by the other kidney. Bilateral complete obstruction will result in rapidly progressive renal failure. Bilateral incomplete obstruction results initially in tubular dysfunction with impairment of urine concentration, producing polyuria and nocturia. Superimposed urinary tract infection will produce additional symptoms, mainly dysuria, fever and loin pain. Renal failure will progress slowly.

Urinary Calculi (Urolithiasis)

Urinary calculi are formed by precipitation of urinary constituents, a small amount of organic material also being incorporated. Deposition is favoured by a highly concentrated urine (and is consequently more common in hot climates), and by secretion of excessive amounts of one or other constituents (oxalate, urate, etc.). Changes in urinary pH and the presence of urinary tract infection also affect calculus formation. Calculi develop in the renal pelvis or ureter, or in the bladder, although some of the latter originate in the kidneys, and subsequently enlarge in the bladder.

Examples of renal stones are shown in Fig. 19.48. The main types are:

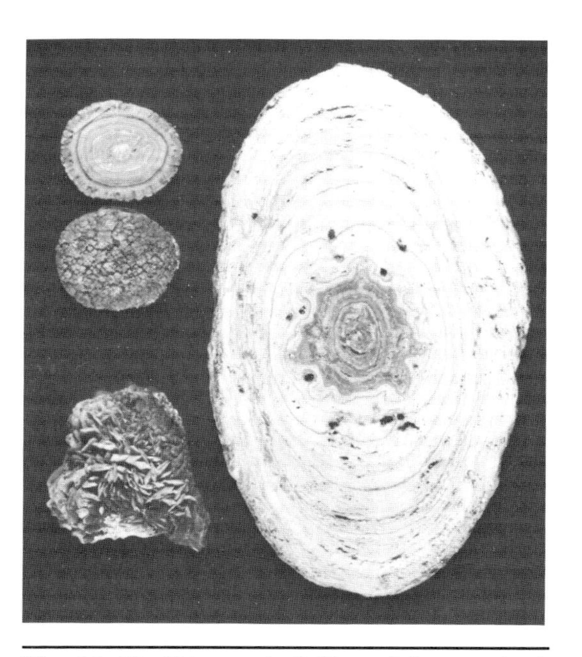

Fig. 19.48 Urinary calculi. Upper left, a renal calculus composed of uric acid and calcium oxalate showing the inner lamellae and rough surface. Lower left, a renal calculus composed mainly of calcium oxalate. Right, a large bladder stone, which started as a urate stone, probably in the renal pelvis, and subsequently gained layers of phosphates while in the bladder. ×1.

(1) calcium containing stones, the calcium salt being either oxalate or phosphate or a mixture of these anions. These are commonest, comprise more than 75% of all urinary calculi, and are laid down in an acid urine.

(2) complex triple phosphate stones including magnesium, ammonium, carbonate and calcium components. These so-called struvite stones comprise 15% of urinary calculi. They are laid down in an alkaline urine. They may form an outer laminated deposit on other stones and are often associated with urinary infection.

(3) a mixture of uric acid and urate–uric acid stones, comprise 5% of urinary calculi and affect 20% of patients with gout. Like calcium containing stones they are laid down in an acid urine. Pure uric acid stones are radiolucent.

(4) cystine stones occur in primary cystinuria and are important in childhood.

The mechanisms of stone formation are complex and ill understood. It requires both **nucleation**, a process whereby the stone deposition is initiated, and **aggregation** whereby the stone grows in size. Some urinary constituents can promote the nucleation of others (e.g. urates can nucleate oxalate precipitates) and this explains why many urinary stones are mixed in composition. An increase in the urinary excretion of a particular substance is usually an important factor, as for example, in hypercalciuria, where the increased excretion of calcium and phosphate very frequently leads to the formation of calculi; hypercalciuria occurs in hyperparathyroidism, chronic resorptive bone disease, prolonged immobilization in bed, sarcoidosis, milk alkali syndrome, but in addition it is sometimes idiopathic.

Renal Calculi

Stones in the renal pelvis may be single or multiple. They are sometimes particularly numerous when there is partial obstruction and dilatation. A single calculus may, however, grow to the size and shape of the dilated pelvis, the so-called staghorn calculus (Fig. 19.49).

A small calculus may pass down the ureter to the bladder, giving rise to renal colic with haematuria. It may be arrested temporarily, usually at the narrow lower end of the ureter. Permanent impaction, usually at the upper or lower ends of the ureter or at the level of the pelvic brim, produces hydronephrosis. When the urine is infected with urea splitting bacteria (e.g. *Proteus* spp.) ammonia is produced and calculi or softer deposits composed of phosphates form in the alkaline urine and are precipitated in the inflamed pelvis. The condition may be accompanied by suppuration (pyonephrosis) and ulceration. The branching staghorn calculi arise in this way and are composed largely of complex hydrated phosphates. A calculus in the renal pelvis, especially when it is movable, may give rise to metaplasia of the lining of the pelvis to stratified squamous epithelium and there is a risk of the development of squamous-cell carcinoma.

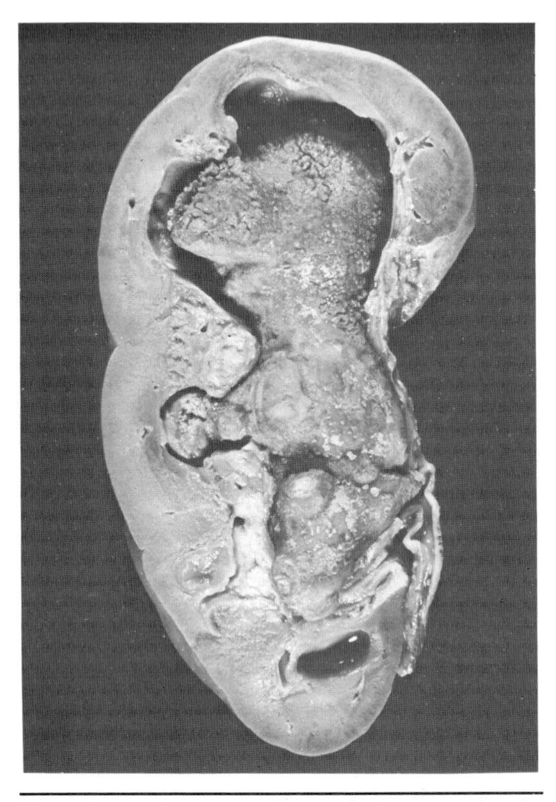

Fig. 19.49 A large 'staghorn' calculus occupying the dilated renal pelvis and calyces.

Bladder Calculi

These may be single or multiple: they are sometimes numerous and like coarse sand. They are now relatively uncommon in developed countries. In many cases calculi form first in the renal pelvis, especially uric acid and oxalate calculi, and pass to the bladder where they increase in size. The larger calculi vary greatly in composition and structure, but as a rule there is a nucleus of primary stone surrounded by concentric laminae.

Bladder stones sometimes grow to measure several centimetres, and may weigh over 300 g in extreme cases. As in the renal pelvis squamous metaplasia may occur. Stones may form without the presence of bacterial infection or inflammation, and lead to mechanical effects – pain and irritation with haematuria, intermittent obstruction, and damage to the bladder mucosa with ulceration. When, however, there is secondary bacterial infection and ammoniacal decomposition of the urine occurs, then triple phosphates and ammonium urate separate out as described above.

Tumours of the Kidney and Urinary Tract

Tumours of the kidney and urinary tract are not uncommon. They tend to bleed and haematuria is the commonest symptom. Infection may also occur and recurrent cystitis is not unusual with ulcerated tumours. Symptoms may also arise from local invasion or distant metastases; metastases, sometimes in unusual sites, may occur with renal cell carcinomas.

Benign Tumours

The commonest benign intra-renal tumour is a small **fibroma** of the medulla derived from the interstitial cells.

Adenomas, which usually develop in the cortex, are more commonly seen in the end-stage kidneys of patients who are on long-term dialysis or have received a renal transplant. Apart from this they are rare. They are usually benign, but occasionally may metastasize. Histologically, they resemble renal cell adenocarcinomas and because of this the size of an adenoma is arbitrarily used as a diagnostic criterion: tumours less than 3 cm in diameter are usually benign and any larger than this may metastasize.

Angiomyolipomas, comprising an admixture of vessels, smooth muscle and adipose tissue, are common in patients with tuberous sclerosis (p. 850). In the renal pelvis **villous papillary tumours** are sometimes seen; they correspond to the papillary tumours of the bladder and they may be concurrent. **Angiomas** are uncommon, occur in the pyramids or just beneath the lining of the pelvis, but even when small, may lead to severe haematuria. **Renin-producing tumours** of the juxtaglomerular apparatus occur but are extremely rare.

Malignant Tumours

Malignant tumours are much less common in the kidneys than in several other organs, but two are of importance – renal cell carcinoma and nephroblastoma. Secondary tumours are not uncommon, although metastases are neither as frequent nor as numerous as might be expected from the large renal blood flow.

Renal Cell Carcinoma (Adenocarcinoma)

Renal cell carcinomas account for 90% of all malignant renal tumours in the adult and they have a peak incidence in the sixth decade. They are often large, and may occur in any part of the kidney. On section, there are usually large areas of dull yellowish tissue, interspersed with vascular, haemorrhagic, cystic and necrotic areas (Fig. 19.50). Although the tumour may often appear to be encapsulated, it is frankly malignant. It commonly grows into the tributaries of the renal vein and may extend along it even into the inferior vena cava. Such venous spread is usually followed by metastases, especially to lungs and bones. Spread also occurs by lymphatics, but often later. Widespread metastases may occur before there are any local signs or symptoms. Invasion and ulceration of the renal pelvis usually causes haematuria.

Microscopically, most of these tumours are

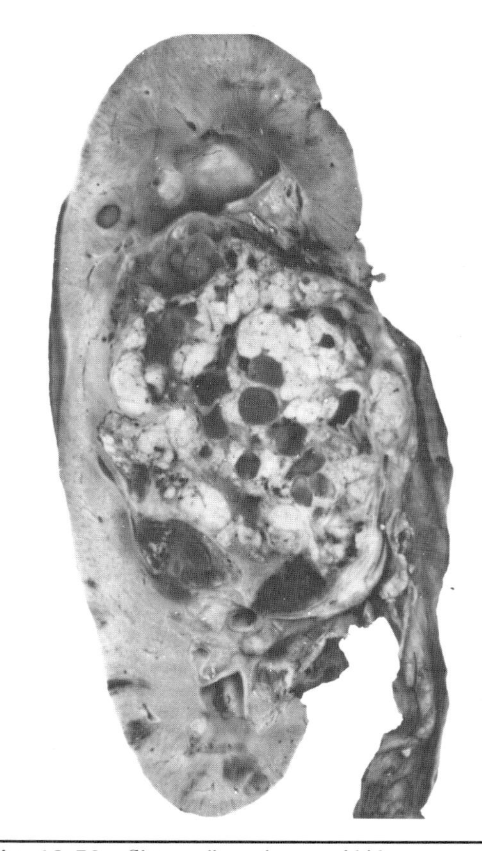

Fig. 19.50 Clear-cell carcinoma of kidney, growing from the central part of the kidney and compressing the renal pelvis. Note the haemorrhagic and gelatinous areas and rounded nodules of whitish tumour.

composed of large, uniform cells with abundant clear cytoplasm (Fig. 19.51) rich in glycogen and lipid. Hence, they are often referred to as clear-cell carcinomas. The cells are arranged in places in solid masses, but often show an acinar arrangement and sometimes papillary processes, or occasionally a papillary cystadenocarcinomatous structure. Some tumours show greater cell pleomorphism and anaplasia, and have a poorer prognosis. Spindle-cell variants of renal carcinoma also occur.

Clinically, haematuria is the most common presenting sign. Loin pain and a palpable mass are other features. Paraneoplastic syndromes are common and related to secretion of hormone-like substances, e.g. hypercalcaemia (parathormone), polycythaemia (erythropoietin), hypertension (renin) and Cushing's syndrome (glucocorticoid).

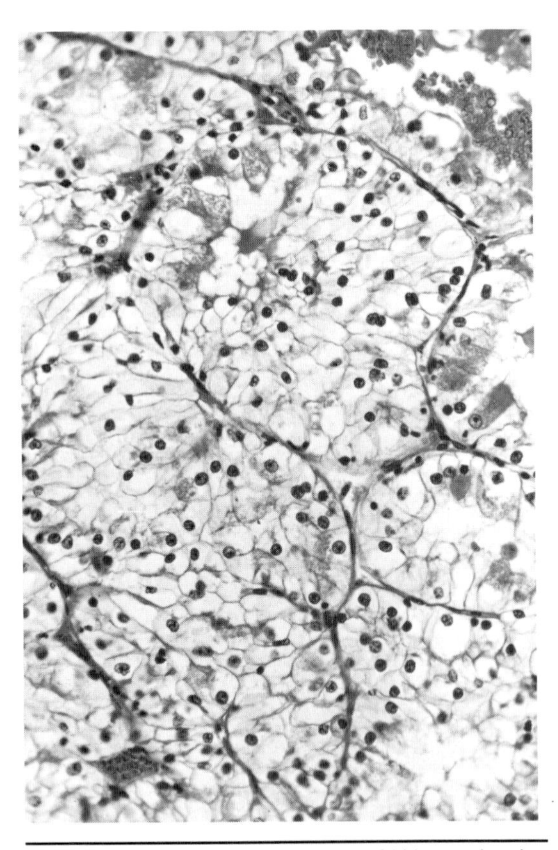

Fig. 19.51 Clear-cell carcinoma of kidney, showing typical empty-looking cells with well defined walls and delicate stroma. ×205.

Nephroblastoma (Wilms' Tumour)

This is an embryonic tumour derived from the renal blastema and with features of a rapidly growing sarcoma. It may reach a large size, and though often remaining enclosed within the renal capsule, rapidly invades blood vessels, producing metastases, chiefly in the lungs. It is most common in the first 3 years of life. Although rare, it is one of the commonest malignant tumours in childhood and sometimes develops in the fetus and may interfere with delivery.

Microscopically, the tumour is composed of spindle-celled tissue, with formation of acini and tubular structures, and apparent transitions may be seen between the spindle cells and those of epithelial type (Fig. 19.52). There may also be imperfect formation of glomeruli. Some tumours may have a more complicated structure, striated or smooth muscle, cartilage, bone or fat being present.

Clinically, the prognosis for patients with Wilms' tumour has dramatically improved in the past 15 years and 90% long-term survival is possible with radiotherapy, combination chemotherapy and surgical resection.

Transitional Cell Tumours

Nearly all tumours of the urinary tract arise from the transitional epithelial lining. Chemical carcinogens are of aetiological importance, and as the whole urothelium is exposed to them, it is not surprising that two or more tumours often occur, either simultaneously or sequentially. Because of its relatively large surface area, the bladder is a commoner site of tumours than the ureters or renal pelves, and the trigone appears to be a particularly common site.

Bladder tumours are a well known industrial

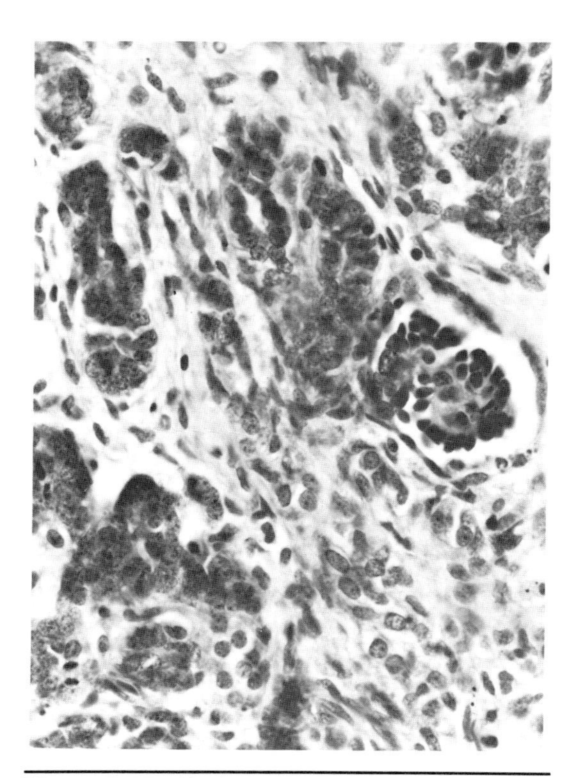

Fig. 19.52 Nephroblastoma, showing spindle-shaped tumour cells and differentiation into imperfect tubules and glomeruli. ×275.

hazard in workers in the aniline dye industry, in which 2-naphthylamine has been incriminated. There is also an increased incidence in workers in the rubber industry, and more recently there is evidence incriminating benzidine and related compounds, and possibly artificial sweeteners such as saccharin. The incidence is also increased in cigarette smokers, and in people who take high doses of analgesics over a long period. A high incidence of bladder tumours complicates infection with *Schistosoma haematobium* (p. 1168).

The grading of transitional cell tumours is prognostically important. We use the following system in which all transitional cell tumours are regarded as carcinomas and are divided into four grades as follows:

Grade I. This is a pedunculated tumour, often less than 1 cm in diameter, which projects into the lumen from a narrow stalk and is composed of fine branching fronds, each of which has a thin central core of vascular connective tissue and a lining which is 3–4 cells thick and resembles very closely the normal transitional epithelium of the urinary tract (Fig. 19.53). Mitoses are rare. Tumours showing this high degree of differentiation behave clinically in a benign fashion and have been referred to as papillomas. They are usually treated by local cauterization and comprise 25–30% of transitional cell tumours of the bladder.

Grade II. They have a structure similar to that of grade I, but differ in having a lining composed of

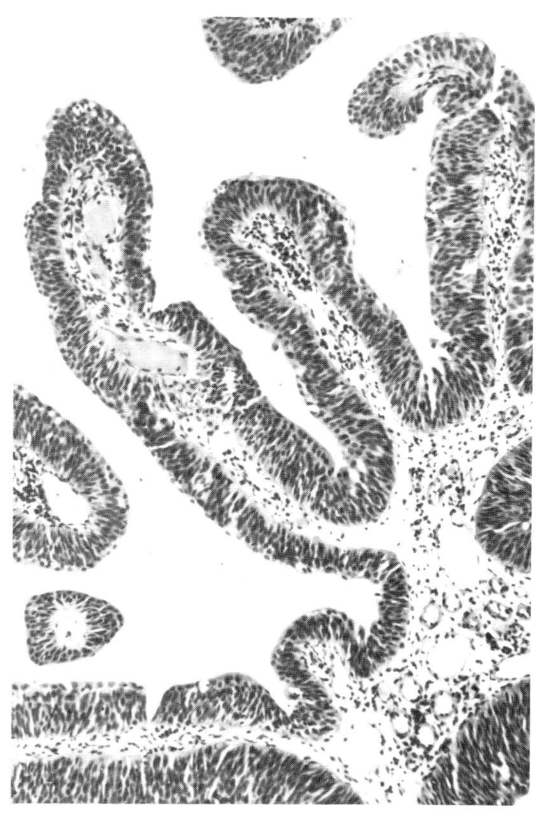

Fig. 19.53 Papilloma of bladder. Part of the tumour, showing the frond-like processes. Where the epithelium has been cut perpendicularly, it is 3–4 cells thick: in other places, oblique section gives a false impression of more cell layers. ×85.

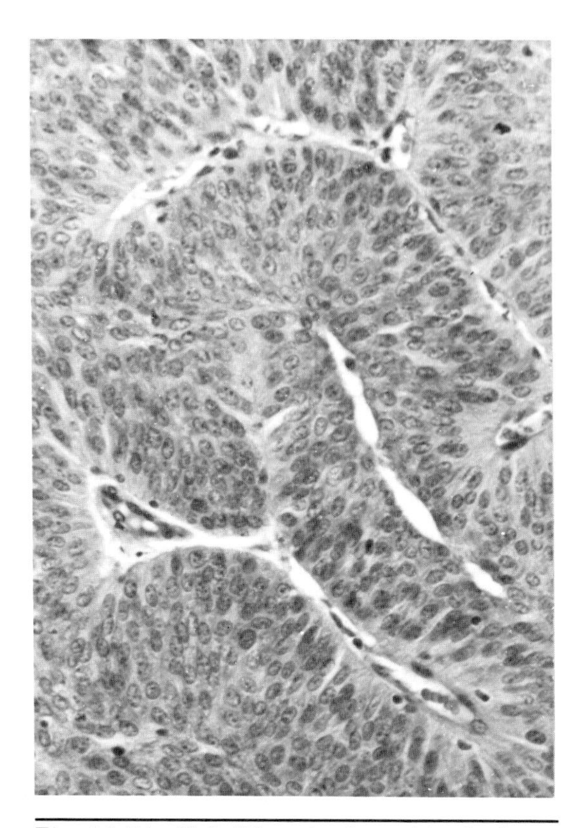

Fig. 19.54 Well differentiated transitional-cell carcinoma of the urinary bladder. ×350.

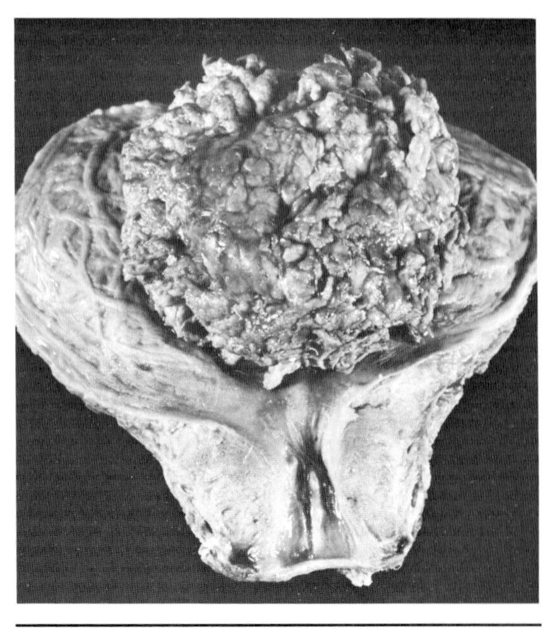

Fig. 19.55 A large papillary carcinoma of the bladder.

more layers of cells (Fig. 19.54) and more than an occasional mitotic figure may be seen. This lesion, as for grade I, tends to be superficial and also has a good prognosis. The larger ones require surgical excision.

Grade III. Here the tumours may have a sessile cauliflower-like appearance (Fig. 19.55) and areas of ulceration and necrosis are frequent. Whilst papillary areas may still be seen microscopically, they are interspersed with more compact areas. Mitotic figures are now easily detected.

Grade IV. In this, the most aggressive type, the tumour has a sessile, often solid appearance with much necrosis and ulceration. Papillary areas are rare and cellular pleomorphism is such that the transitional nature of the tumour is recognized only with difficulty. Mitotic figures are frequent and often atypical and extension of the tumour into the underlying muscle with lymphatic and venous extensions are often apparent: the prognosis is consequently very poor.

While low-grade transitional cell carcinomas of the bladder (grades I and II above) tend to be benign, their behaviour can be unpredictable so that the patients develop recurrent tumours or show progression of their disease. Recurrence may represent the development of new tumours elsewhere in the bladder. *Carcinoma in situ* also occurs in the bladder and is defined as a *flat* epithelial lesion composed of cells which are poorly differentiated and show mitotic activity. The presence of carcinoma *in situ* indicates a greater likelihood of disease progression with invasion. Thus, patients with low-grade tumours and certainly patients with carcinoma *in situ* require careful clinical follow-up.

Other Types of Tumour

Squamous cell carcinoma also occurs in the urinary tract: in some instances it arises from squamous metaplasia attributable to the presence of calculi and chronic inflammation.

Adenocarcinoma is relatively uncommon. It may arise from transitional epithelium and occurs particularly in congenital extroversion of the bladder, when the epithelium undergoes metaplasia to mucus-secreting type. Another possible origin is from remnants of the urachus around the apex of the bladder.

Further Reading

Heptinstall, R. T. (1983). *Pathology of the Kidney*, 3rd edn. Little, Brown & Co., Boston.

Hill, G. S. (ed.) (1989). *Uropathology*. Churchill Livingstone, Edinburgh.

Tisher, C. C. and Brenner, B. M. (1989). *Renal Pathology with Clinical and Functional Correlations*. J. B. Lippincott Co., Philadelphia.

20
Locomotor System

Diseases of Bone

Bone has two main functions. It forms a rigid endoskeleton and has a central role in mineral homoeostasis, principally of calcium and phosphate ions, but also of sodium and magnesium.

Bone is composed of cells, a protein matrix and mineral. There are three cell types. **Osteoblasts** are responsible for bone formation and lie in sheets on the surface of bone trabeculae. During active bone synthesis they are large cells whose cytoplasm contains abundant rough endoplasmic reticulum and Golgi apparatus for protein synthesis and processing, and is rich in alkaline phosphatase for mineralization of the matrix. After completing a cycle of activity osteoblasts become smaller resting cells. **Osteocytes** are mature relatively inactive osteoblasts which lie in lacunae within bone. Long cytoplasmic processes run within canaliculi through bone and connect to other osteocytes and osteoblasts by intercellular junctions. It is speculated that osteocytes are sensitive to electric currents produced by deformation of crystals in bone (piezoelectricity), and so may be involved in control of bone remodelling in response to mechanical stress. **Osteoclasts** are large multinucleated cells: they resorb bone and often lie in the shallow depressions (Howship's lacunae) so formed on the surface of bone. Their plasma membrane is thrown into folds forming a 'ruffled border' adjacent to bone. Lysosomal enzymes including acid phosphatase, collagenase and carbonic anhydrase (generating hydrogen ions) remove mineral and matrix simultaneously. Indeed osteoclasts cannot resorb uncalcified matrix (see rickets and osteomalacia. Osteoclasts are derived from marrow precursors, are closely related to macrophages and are best regarded as belonging to the mononuclear phagocyte system.

The protein matrix of bone consists largely of type I collagen, with small amounts of non-collagenous proteins. Osteoblasts produce both osteonectin, a 32 kDa protein which binds bone collagen and hydroxyapatite crystals, and another hydroxyapatite-binding protein, osteocalcin (mol wt 5.8 kDa) whose synthesis is vitamin K dependent. Serum levels of osteocalcin reflect the level of osteoblastic activity. Hydroxyapatite, a microcrystalline material [$Ca_{10}(PO_4)_6(OH)_2$] forms the mineral matrix. Substantial amounts of sodium, potassium, magnesium, carbonate and citrate are present within the crystalline matrix.

Types of Bone

In man, bone is found in two forms, woven and lamellar. **Woven bone** is formed where bone is laid down rapidly as in fetal growth, during healing of a fracture (Fig. 20.1) and in bone-forming tumours. It contains numerous plump osteocytes and collagen fibres are arranged randomly. **Lamellar bone** is slowly laid down, is structurally strong and forms the adult skeleton. The collagen lies in parallel sheets whose fibres run in different directions, resulting in a laminated structure which is best appreciated when viewed in polarized light (Fig. 20.2). The osteocytes are small and relatively sparse. Adult lamellar bone is arranged in two forms.

Compact bone forms the cortex of bones. Between subperiosteal and endosteal plates of circumferential bone lie Haversian systems (osteons), concentric arrays of bone surrounding a central artery and vein (Fig. 20.3).

Cancellous (spongy) bone, found between the cortices of bones and at the ends of long bones, is composed of plates or trabeculae separated by marrow spaces.

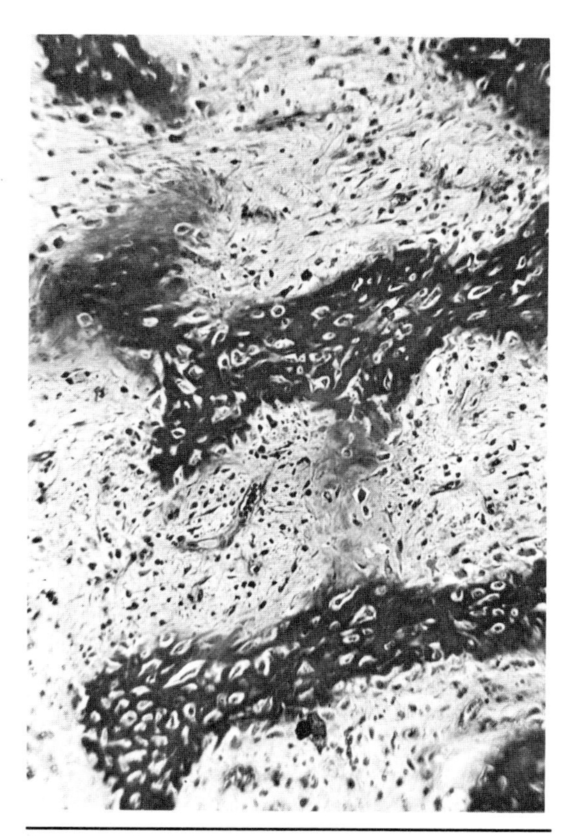

Fig. 20.1 Woven bone, from fracture callus, showing large, closely packed lacunae. ×190.

Turnover of Bone

Bone is constantly being formed and resorbed; approximately 5% of the adult skeleton is replaced annually. Bone remodelling is carried out by osteoclasts and osteoblasts coupled together by chemical mediators in bone remodelling units (BRUs), thus keeping adult bone mass fairly constant. Control of bone turnover is a complex process which remains incompletely understood (Fig. 20.4). Factors which stimulate bone resorption, e.g. parathyroid hormone, vitamin D and interleukin 1, do not act directly on osteoclasts but induce osteoblasts to produce soluble factors which stimulate osteoclastic activity. The osteoblast also secretes collagenase which initiates resorption, and then retracts from the bone surface, allowing osteoclastic activity to proceed. When the phase of resorp-

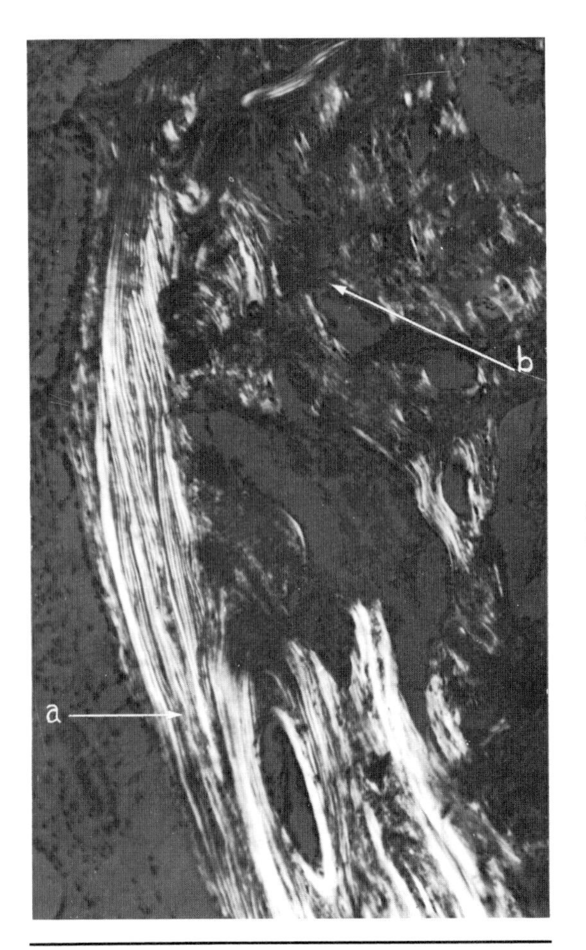

Fig. 20.2 **a** Lamellar bone in polarized light showing the orderly orientation of the bone lamellae. **b** On the surface are some new-formed trabeculae of woven bone; showing lack of lamellar orientation. ×190.

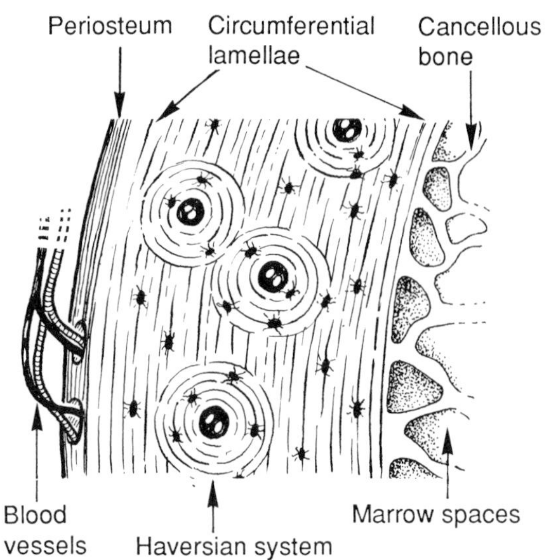

Fig. 20.3 Cortical bone is composed largely of Haversian systems where concentric lamellae are arranged around central blood vessels. Circumferential lamellar bone lies below the periosteum and also forms the endosteal border of the cortex. The marrow spaces lie between trabeculae of cancellous bone. Blood vessels penetrate the periosteum to supply the bone.

tion ceases, osteoblasts synthesize newly formed uncalcified matrix (known as osteoid), which becomes mineralized approximately 10 days later by mechanisms which are poorly understood. A very thin layer of osteoid is therefore a normal finding and may cover up to 20% of the trabecular surface area. A higher proportion is covered by osteoid when there is increased bone formation for any cause. When a section stained by von Kossa's method to demonstrate calcium deposition is viewed in polarized light a lamellar pattern with a maximum of four bright lines can be seen on the bone surface. More than four indicates failure of mineralization. A linear deposit of calcium which can be found along about 60% of the interface between osteoid and bone is known as the calcification front. Because of its abundant surface area and cellularity cancellous bone turns over more rapidly than cortical bone.

Factors Affecting Bone Turnover

Parathyroid hormone (PTH) is a polypeptide of 84 amino acids (mol. wt 9.5 kDa), the N-terminal 34 amino acids of which constitute the biologically active molecule. A fall in serum ionized calcium increases secretion of PTH. This induces bone resorption, increases renal tubular calcium reabsorption, and by promoting synthesis of active metabolites of vitamin D, increases intestinal calcium absorption. These effects combine to return blood calcium towards normal levels. The action of

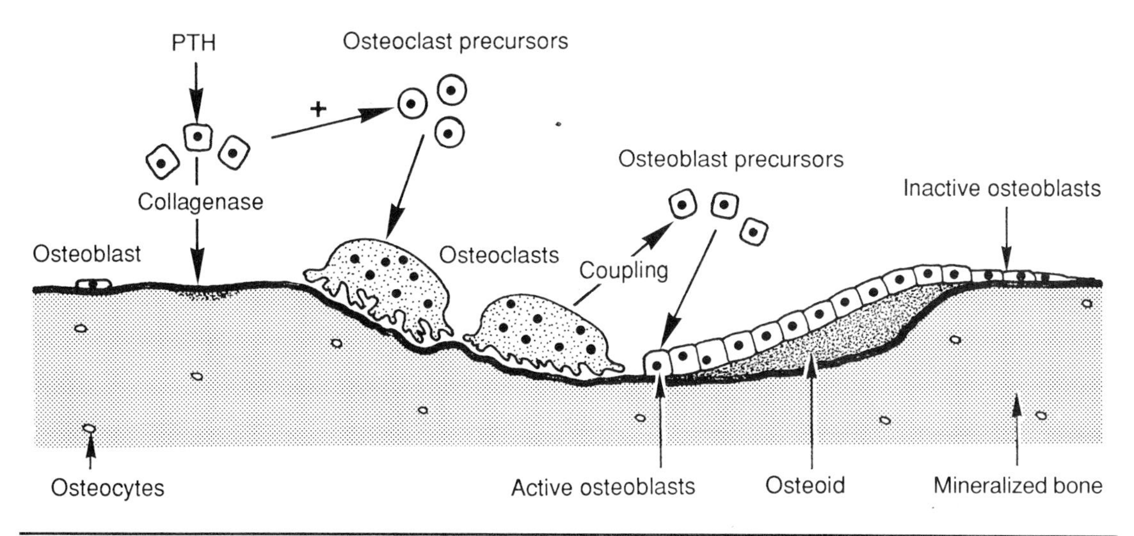

Fig. 20.4 The cycle of bone turnover. Resting osteoblasts are stimulated by agents such as parathyroid hormone to retract from the bone surface and secrete collagenase which initiates bone resorption. Osteoblasts also promote the maturation of osteoclast precursors into osteoclasts which resorb bone forming Howship's lacunae. When resorption ceases coupling signals stimulate osteoblasts to lay down osteoid which is mineralized a few days later. When the original mass of bone is restored osteoblasts become inactive and assume a flattened shape.

PTH on bone is mediated through osteoblasts. Binding of PTH to cell membrane receptors increases intracellular calcium concentration and by increasing adenylate cyclase activity elevates cyclic AMP concentration. The effects of increased levels of PTH on bone are described on pages 955–957.

Vitamin D. The term vitamin D refers to a group of fat-soluble sterols, two of which, 25-hydroxyvitamin D_3 (25(OH)D_3) and 1,25-dihydroxyvitamin D_3 (1,25$(OH)_2D_3$), have major physiological roles. Vitamin D metabolism is summarized in Fig. 20.5. Vitamin D in man is derived from oral intake of ergocalciferol (vitamin D_2) and cholecalciferol (vitamin D_3) and conversion of 7-dehydrocholesterol to vitamin D_3 in the skin by ultraviolet irradiation. Both are converted by a hepatic microsomal 25-hydroxylase enzyme to 25(OH)D_3. This, the major circulating form, is transported to the kidney where mitochondrial hydroxylase systems convert it to 1,25$(OH)_2D_3$, a highly potent substance, or 24,25$(OH)_2D_3$, an apparently inactive substance. Elevated serum PTH levels or low phosphate levels stimulate 1-hydroxylation, while low PTH and high phosphate promote synthesis of 24,25$(OH)_2D_3$. The principal effects of 1,25$(OH)_2D_3$ are to increase intestinal absorption of calcium, and to elevate serum calcium and phosphate levels which promote bone mineralization and suppress PTH activity. In addition, 1,25$(OH)_2D_3$ stimulates bone resorption, promotes the maturation of osteoclast precursors, and stimulates osteocalcin production by osteoblasts.

Calcitonin, a 3.5 kDa polypeptide of 32 amino acids, is produced by the thyroid parafollicular 'C' cells in response to a rise in serum ionized calcium. In pharmacological doses it binds to osteoclasts, increases cAMP levels and diminishes osteoclastic bone resorption. This, and increased renal calcium excretion result in reduced serum calcium levels. The effect of physiological levels of calcitonin is less clear. Nevertheless, its role in the treatment of Paget's disease and hypercalcaemia makes calcitonin an important hormone.

Physical activity. Muscular activity and weight

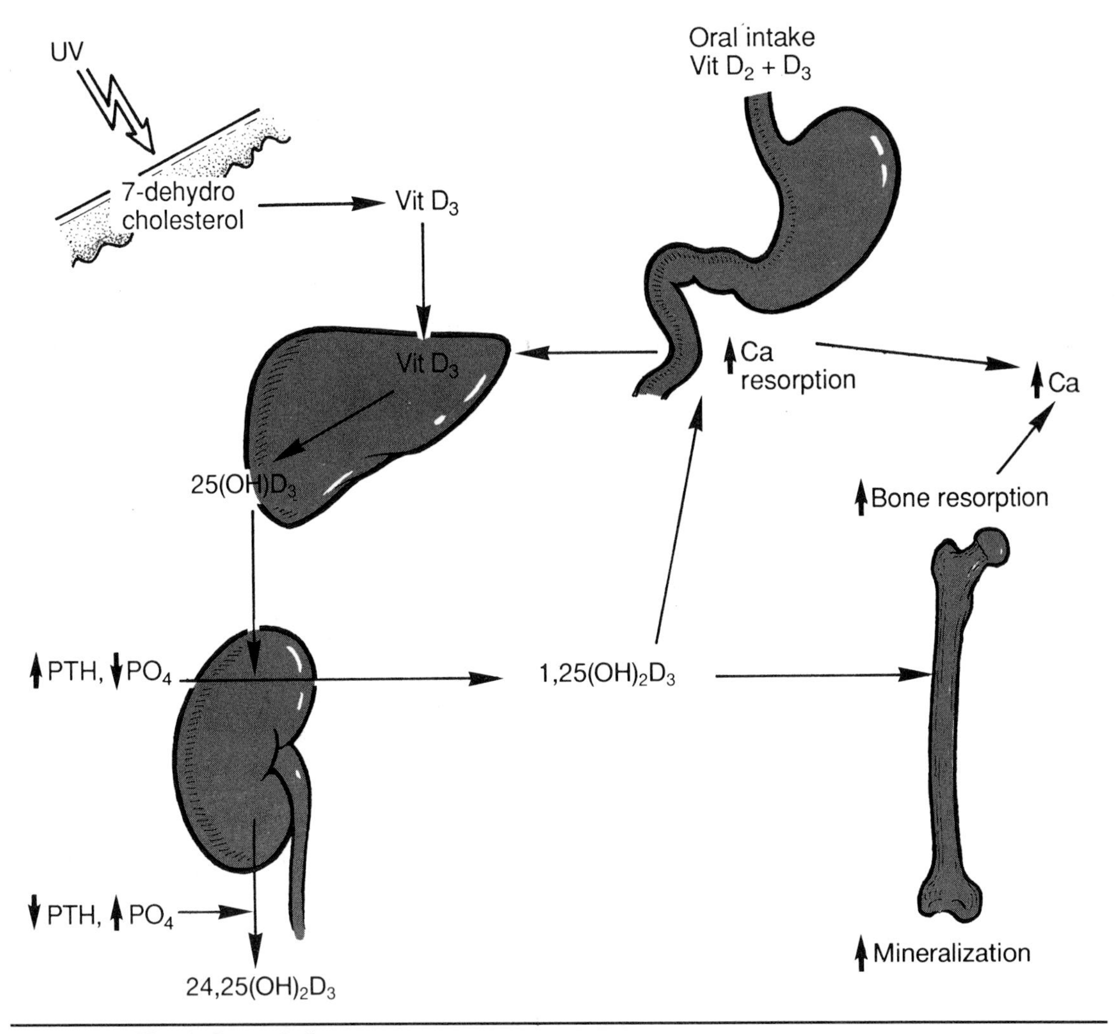

Fig. 20.5 Vitamin D metabolism.

bearing promote osteoblastic activity and increase bone mass, while immobilization leads to a rapid increase in osteoclastic activity, a decrease in osteoblast activity and loss of bone mass (Fig. 20.7).

A number of local factors have been shown to regulate osteoblast and osteoclast function. These include prostaglandins, insulin-like growth factor I, interleukin 1, and tumour necrosis factors α and β.

Metabolic Bone Disease

This term covers a group of generalized skeletal disorders resulting from defective bone formation, resorption or mineralization.

Osteoporosis

The term osteoporosis is used to describe the state where bone mass is reduced below the level

Table 20.1 Causes of osteoporosis

Primary
- Involutional (age related)
- Post-menopausal oestrogen deficiency
- Idiopathic in children and young adults

Secondary
- Immobilization (local or general)
- Endocrine
  - Cushing's syndrome and steroid therapy
  - hypogonadism
  - hyperthyroidism
  - diabetes mellitus
- Malnutrition
  - malabsorption
  - scurvy
- Inflammatory
  - rheumatoid arthritis
- Congenital
  - osteogenesis imperfecta
  - homocystinuria
- Neoplastic
  - multiple myeloma
  - secondary carcinoma
- Liver disease
  - primary biliary cirrhosis

required for its normal structural function. Although reduced in amount, the bone is of normal chemical composition and is fully mineralized. Osteoporosis may occur in a localized form, following immobilization of a limb; this can be regarded simply as a form of disuse atrophy. In generalized osteoporosis the entire skeleton is involved. There are a large number of causes of osteoporosis (Table 20.1). The development of osteoporosis results from an excess of bone resorption over formation, and may be due to increased resorption, decreased formation or both.

It is difficult to make a sharp distinction between the normal decrease in bone mass which accompanies ageing and clinically apparent osteoporosis. Skeletal mass in both sexes diminishes from the fourth decade onwards. Bone loss occurs earlier in women and there is a marked acceleration at the time of the menopause. Loss is most marked at sites of rapid turnover such as the cancellous bone of the vertebrae, ribs, pelvis and ends of long bones. The normal state of decreased bone mass

Table 20.2 Risk factors for post-menopausal osteoporosis

- Premature menopause
- Caucasian ancestry*
- Thin, with small bone structure
- Family history of osteoporosis
- Decreased physical activity
- Cigarette smoking, alcohol abuse
- Low calcium intake

*In general blacks have a heavier bone structure than whites.

in post-menopausal women and elderly men can be described as physiological or involutional osteoporosis. Osteoporosis is described as pathological when bone loss is so severe that there is evidence of mechanical failure of bone. Vertebral crush fractures, often with anterior wedging, lead to severe back pain, kyphosis and loss of height. Fractures after minor injury are common and involve the neck of femur, neck of humerus and distal radius (typically a Colles' fracture); femoral neck fractures in particular are a major cause of morbidity and mortality in the elderly. In the USA, over one million fractures each year are attributable to osteoporosis.

The pathogenesis of osteoporosis is not fully understood. The increased incidence in women with an artificially induced early menopause suggested that oestrogen deficiency was of major importance. Other factors may be implicated. Chronic mild negative calcium balance, increased sensitivity to parathyroid hormone, and reduced mechanical stimulation of osteoblasts due to loss of muscle bulk and a sedentary lifestyle have been suggested. A number of risk factors have been clearly identified for the development of post-menopausal osteoporosis (Table 20.2). Prompt administration of hormone replacement therapy can prevent or at least delay osteoporosis, although treatment must be continued for a long period and may be associated with endometrial hyperplasia and, possibly, endometrial carcinoma.

Once a diagnosis of osteoporosis is made, it is important to investigate the patient for any treatable cause (Table 20.1); although normal bone mass may not be restored, continued loss of bone may be halted or slowed. The patient should be encouraged to keep active; bed rest is best avoided in patients with spinal collapse.

Before a diagnosis of osteoporosis is made, the possibility of multiple myeloma (p. 637) must be excluded as it often gives rise to diffuse bone loss rather than to discrete areas of bone destruction. Less commonly, disseminated carcinoma produces the same pattern of involvement. Rarely, children or young adults develop osteoporosis, usually of uncertain cause.

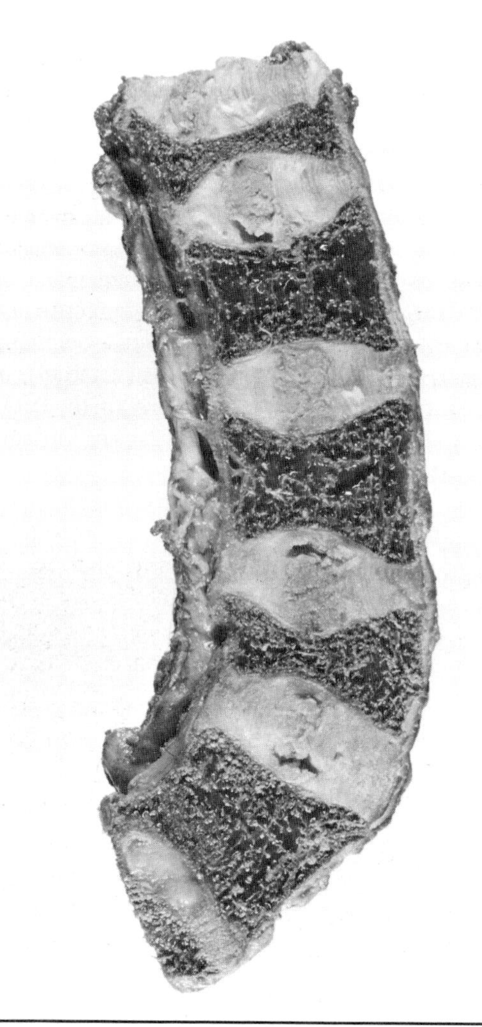

Fig. 20.6 The lumbar spine of this 74-year-old with severe osteoporosis shows bulging of the intervertebral discs and collapse of the vertebral bodies of L1 and L4.

Pathology

Osteoporosis may be recognized radiologically or at autopsy by the appearance of thinned cortices of long bones with loss of cancellous bone. Osteoporosis of the spine leads to vertebral collapse, weakness of the vertebral end plate and bulging of the intervertebral discs – codfish vertebrae (Fig. 20.6). Disc material herniated into the vertebral body is known as a Schmorl's node. On microscopic examination abnormally thin trabeculae of bone are seen, with normal mineralization (Fig. 20.7). There may be evidence of structural failure in the form of healed trabecular microfractures. Thinning of cortical bone is due chiefly to opening up of Haversian systems on the endosteal aspect, so-called cancellization.

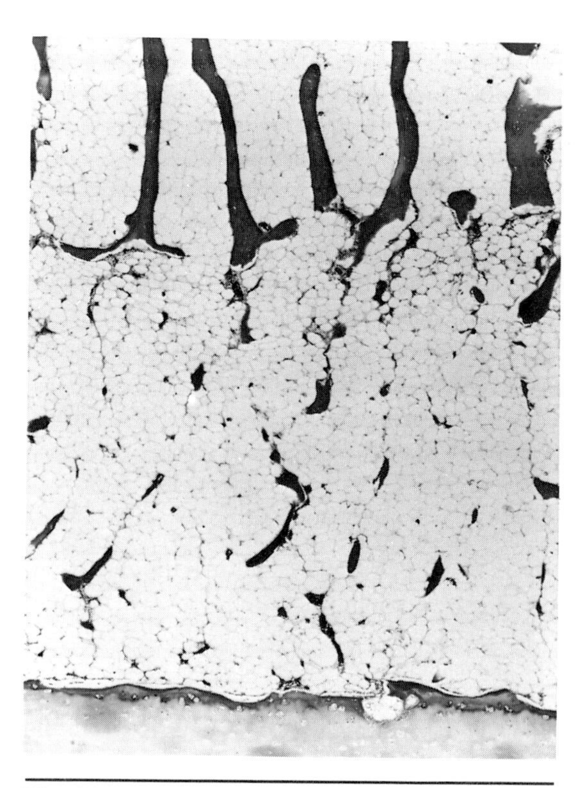

Fig. 20.7 Immobilization osteoporosis. The articular surface is at the bottom of the picture. The subchondral trabeculae have almost completely disappeared and there is active osteoclasis spreading to involve the normal sized trabeculae above them. ×45.

OSTEOMALACIA

Failure of mineralization of bone leads to the accumulation of excessive amounts of osteoid on the surface of bone trabeculae. The bones are abnormally soft, hence the term osteomalacia. In children rickets is characterized by soft bones and, in addition, by defective mineralization of epiphyseal cartilage leading to growth disturbance. The many causes of osteomalacia and rickets are summarized in Table 20.3. The majority of cases are due to vitamin D deficiency (p. 346) or renal failure (p. 894). In the UK vitamin D deficiency is found in the elderly on poor diets, in food faddists and in immigrants from Asian countries, in whom there is reduced exposure to sunlight and diminished cutaneous synthesis of vitamin D_3. The flour used in chapattis may be a factor since it is said to bind calcium and so inhibit its absorption. In many patients osteomalacia is multifactorial.

Table 20.3 Causes of osteomalacia and rickets

Vitamin D deficiency
- Decreased intake or synthesis
  - dietary insufficiency
  - lack of cutaneous exposure to UV light
  - malabsorption, e.g. coeliac disease, pancreatic insufficiency, hepatobiliary disease

Abnormal metabolism
- Drugs, e.g. anticonvulsants (accelerated hepatic degradation of $25(OH)D_3$).
- Deficient renal 1-hydroxylation of $25(OH)D_3$
  - chronic renal failure
  - vitamin D dependent rickets type I
  - tumour associated osteomalacia

Normal levels of vitamin D
- End organ resistance: vitamin D dependent rickets type II
  - chronic hypophosphataemia
  - primary renal phosphate losing syndromes, e.g. familial hypophosphataemic rickets, Fanconi's syndrome
  - chronic phosphate depletion, e.g. aluminium hydroxide antacid abuse
- Defective mineralization with normal calcium, phosphate and vitamin D
  - aluminium toxicity
  - hypophosphatasia (decreased bone alkaline phosphatase)
  - diphosphonate therapy, e.g. for Paget's disease

Patients with osteomalacia usually complain of bone pain and tenderness, with weakness of proximal muscles often resulting in a waddling gait. Pathological fractures may occur (Fig. 20.8). Bowing of long bones and pelvic deformity are rare in adults, but common in children with rickets, in whom there is also retarded growth. The epiphyseal plate is widened and the costochondral junctions swollen giving rise to the so-called 'rickety rosary'. Pelvic deformity produces a narrowed or flattened pelvic outlet which may lead to difficulties in childbirth.

Radiological examination shows a loss of normal bone density (osteopenia) particularly in the long bones. The radiological hallmark of osteomalacia is the Looser's zone (Fig. 20.8), a transverse linear lucency perpendicular to the bone surface, typically of rib, pubic ramus, inner scapular border and long bones. Greenstick fractures are occasionally seen in adults and there may be failure to mineralize fracture callus. In rickets the epiphyseal plate is widened with an irregular cupped metaphysis. The appearance of epiphyseal centres of ossification may be delayed.

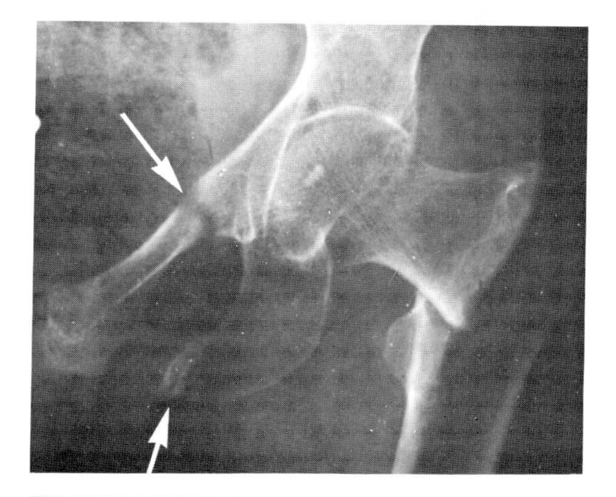

Fig. 20.8 Radiograph of a woman who developed osteomalacia and suffered a pathological fracture of her femur. The radiograph also shows Looser's zones in the pelvic bones (arrowed). (Mr John Chalmers, FRCS.)

Pathology

The delay in mineralization of bone matrix leads to an increase in osteoid which covers more of the trabecular surface and forms thickened seams (Fig. 20.9). When sections stained by von Kossa's method are viewed in polarized light four or more bright laminae are seen. The calcification front is deficient. When hypocalcaemia is present, mild changes of hyperparathyroidism may be found. It is important to realize that an increase in osteoid may occur in many conditions where there is rapid new bone formation such as fracture healing, Paget's disease and hyperparathyroidism. It is the abnormal thickness of osteoid seams and loss of mineralization front which allow the diagnosis of osteomalacia to be made. In rickets, failure to mineralize the matrix of the epiphyseal cartilage prevents osteoclastic resorption of cartilage, and leads to a greatly thickened and irregular hypertrophic zone. There may be extension of cartilage into the metaphysis. The woven bone laid down on the surface of cartilage is also unmineralized and so there is failure to remodel the metaphysis. Treatment of the underlying cause (e.g. oral vitamin D in dietary deficiency) is very rapidly followed by mineralization of matrix and the radiological appearances of the epiphyses revert to normal (Fig. 20.10). Unfortunately bowing of long bones and pelvic deformity usually remain.

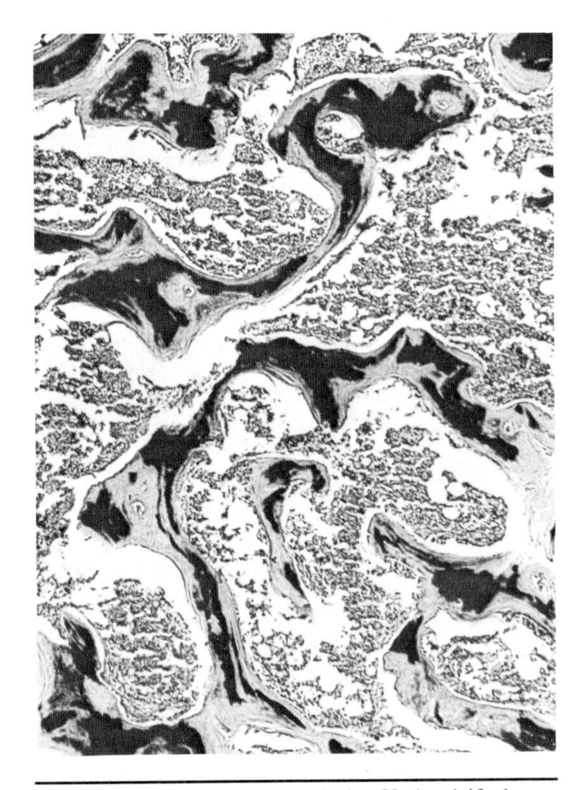

Fig. 20.9 Severe osteomalacia. Undecalcified section stained by von Kossa's method. Only the bone stained black is calcified. There are wide seams of unstained osteoid. ×40.

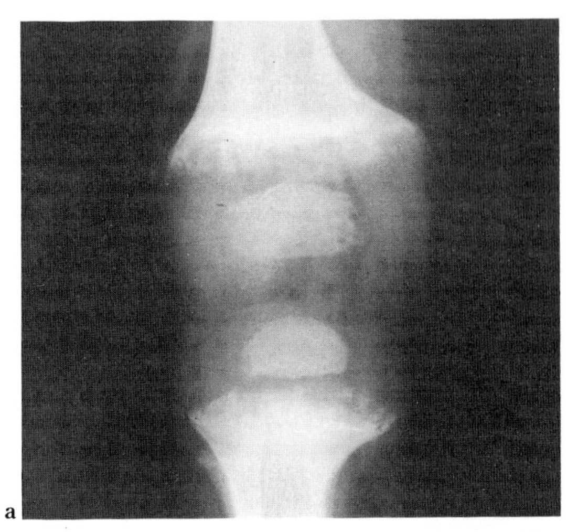

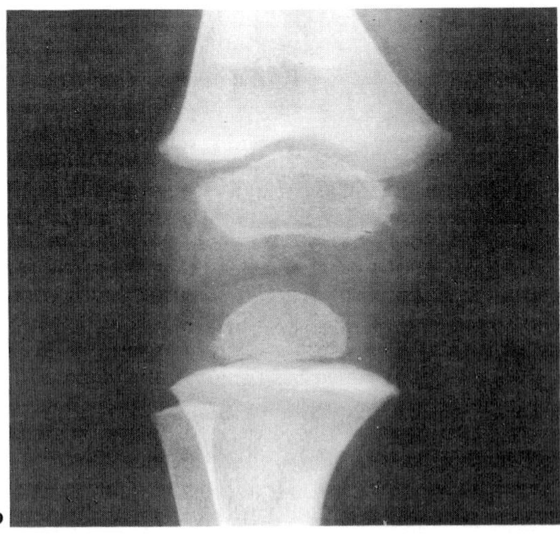

Fig. 20.10 Rickets. **a** Radiograph of the knee of a child with vitamin D deficiency rickets. The epiphyseal plates are widened and irregularly calcified. **b** After 3 months of treatment with oral vitamin D the appearances have returned to normal.

Primary Hyperparathyroidism

Overactivity of the parathyroid glands is classified as primary, secondary or tertiary (p. 1103).

Since the introduction of routine biochemical analysis of serum calcium, hypercalcaemia and primary hyperparathyroidism are much more commonly recognized. Consequently, the majority of patients are asymptomatic with clinically apparent bone disease found in only 5–10% of cases. Some patients complain of bone pain. Radiographs may show generalized osteopenia. A distinctive appearance of subperiosteal cortical resorption, particularly affecting the phalanges and sometimes the outer ends of the clavicles, is highly suggestive of hyperparathyroidism. Occasionally, localized areas of radiolucency, so-called brown tumours, may be seen. Joint disease may also complicate primary hyperparathyroidism with an increased incidence of pseudogout and gout (p. 995).

Pathology

Increased bone resorption is produced by increased numbers of osteoclasts on the surface of, and burrowing within, trabeculae of cancellous bone (Fig. 20.11) and in Haversian systems of cortical bone. Fibrous tissue forms around sites of resorption. Although resorption is accompanied by increased bone formation with prominent osteoblasts lined up on the surface, overall there is loss of bone. As the disease progresses much bone may be resorbed and replaced by small irregular trabeculae of woven bone, with loss of the normal bony architecture. The marrow spaces become filled with fibrous tissue in which cystic degeneration occasionally occurs. These features have led to the descriptive term **osteitis fibrosa cystica**. In some areas bone is replaced by fibrous tissue containing numerous osteoclasts and abundant haemosiderin, forming 'brown tumours' of hyperparathyroidism. These lesions may simulate giant-cell tumour of bone (p. 980); indeed hyperparathyroidism should be excluded before giant-cell tumour is diagnosed in unusual sites such as jaw, skull or phalanges, particularly if multiple lesions are present.

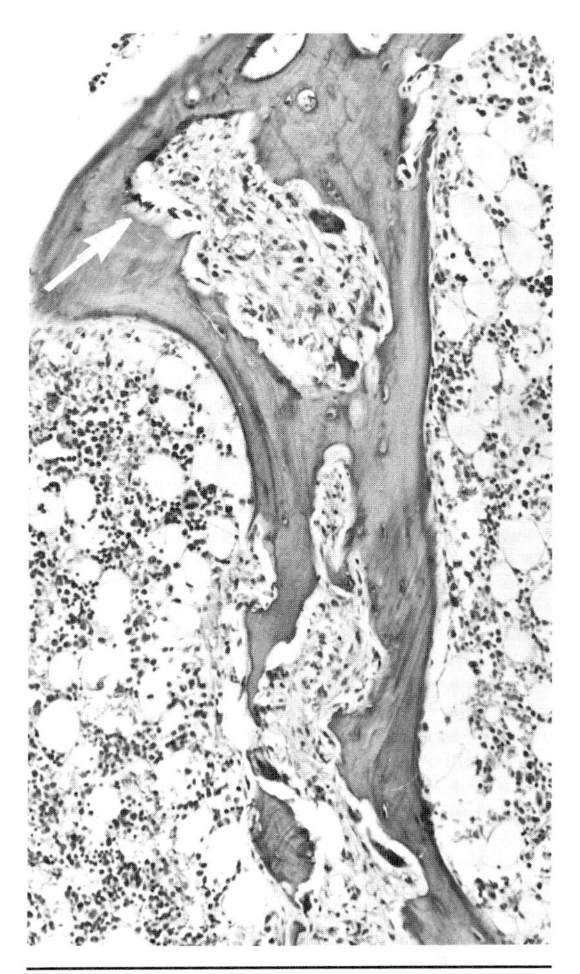

Fig. 20.11 Osteitis fibrosa of hyperparathyroidism. There is osteoclastic resorption of the central part of a bone trabecula with fibrous tissue replacement, so-called dissecting resorption. Some osteoblasts are also seen (arrow). ×100.

Surgical removal of a parathyroid adenoma or of hyperplastic glands is followed by a rapid fall in serum levels of calcium and parathyroid hormone, and diminution of osteoclastic activity. Normal bone structure is usually rapidly restored (Fig. 20.12).

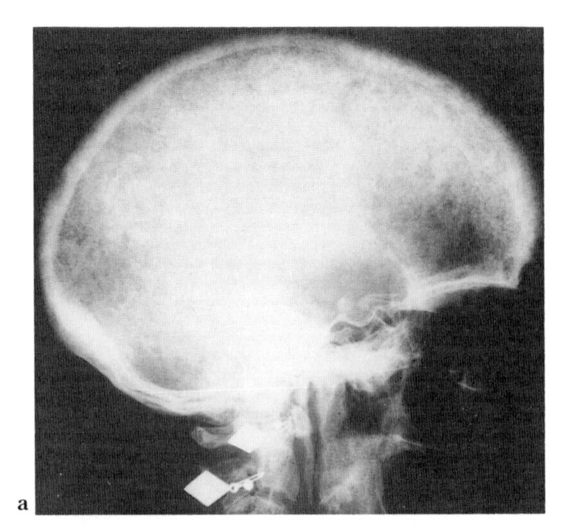

a

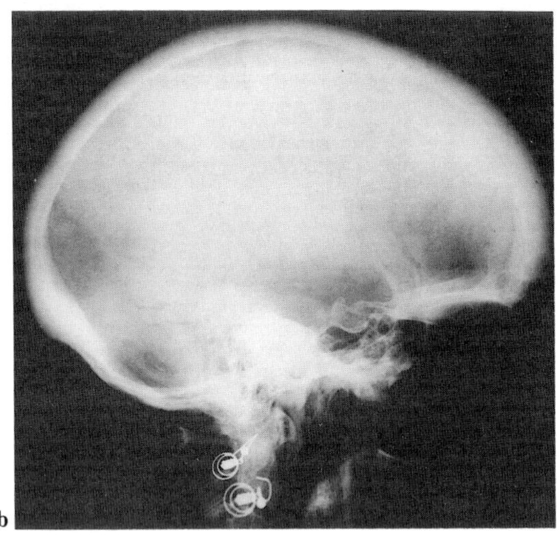

b

Fig. 20.12 Primary hyperparathyroidism. **a** The skull shows a mottled pattern of bone lysis. **b** Six months after removal of a parathyroid adenoma the skull is of normal appearance. The patient has also changed her earrings!

Secondary Hyperparathyroidism

This is a physiological response of hyperplasia and increased PTH secretion to a number of conditions (Table 20.4) whose common factor is hypocalcaemia. Bone changes similar to those described in the primary form may result. The most common cause is chronic renal failure, the bone changes of which are discussed below. In long-standing secondary hyperparathyroidism an autonomous adenoma may develop in a hyperplastic gland, causing **tertiary hyperparathyroidism**.

Table 20.4 Causes of secondary hyperparathyroidism

Chronic renal failure
Vitamin D deficiency – osteomalacia and rickets
Decreased intestinal calcium absorption, e.g. coeliac disease
Increased urinary calcium loss
Renal tubular acidosis
Idiopathic hypercalciuria
Pseudohypoparathyroidism – renal insensitivity to parathyroid hormone

Renal Osteodystrophy

This term is applied to the complex group of bone changes seen in patients with chronic renal failure (p. 932). Features of hyperparathyroidism, osteomalacia and increased bone density (osteosclerosis) may all be seen in varying degree. The pathophysiology of renal osteodystrophy is summarized in Fig. 20.13. Diminished glomerular filtration leads to retention of phosphate and hyperphosphataemia which causes a reciprocal fall in serum calcium. This stimulates parathormone secretion, which effects a return of serum calcium and phosphate levels towards normal. Serum calcium is elevated by increased renal tubular absorption, mobilization of calcium from bone and increased synthesis of $1,25(OH)_2D_3$. Increased urinary excretion of phosphate lowers serum phosphate levels. As renal disease progresses the renal tubule becomes insensitive to PTH, leading to severe hyperphosphataemia, hypocalcaemia and further hyperparathyroidism. Reduced synthesis of $1,25(OH)_2D_3$ results in reduced intestinal calcium absorption and so to osteomalacia. The changes of renal osteodystrophy are often more severe in patients who develop tertiary hyper-

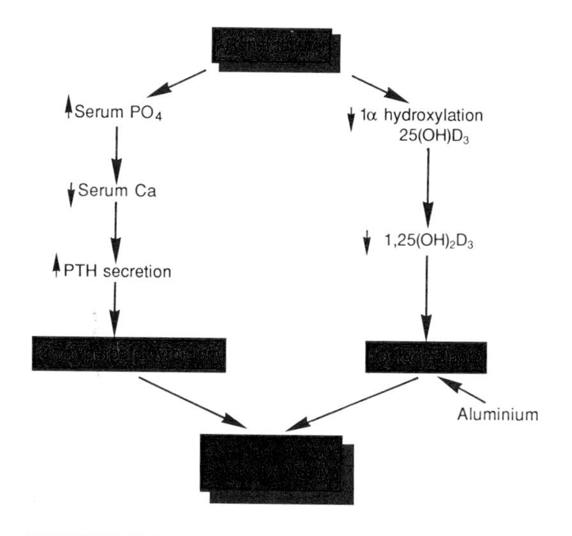

Fig. 20.13 Pathophysiology of renal osteodystrophy (see text).

parathyroidism and in children, who may in addition develop rickets.

Other factors are implicated in the osteomalacia of renal patients. A severe form seen in dialysis patients with bone pain, pathological fracture and muscle weakness was shown to be due to deposition of aluminium at the calcification front, where it completely inhibits normal mineralization. Several sources of aluminium have been identified – dialysis fluid, tap water with high levels, and orally administered aluminium-containing phosphate-binding gels. Increased awareness means that this (like aluminium-induced dementia (p. 934)), is no longer a major clinical problem.

Pathology

Serial bone biopsies of patients with renal failure have shown that the initial abnormality, present in 80–90% of patients, is osteitis fibrosa due to hyperparathyroidism. In keeping with a high turnover state there is frequently an increase in trabecular surface area covered by osteoid, but the seams are of normal thickness and the mineralization front is normal.

Coexistent osteomalacia develops in 20–40% of cases, with thickened osteoid seams and a reduced mineralization front. Osteoclastic resorption of mineralized bone continues deep to the resistant layer of osteoid. Where osteomalacia is due to aluminium this can be demonstrated histologically by staining aluminium at the calcification front.

Osteosclerosis, increased density of bone often due to extensive formation of woven bone, is found in about 30% of patients, usually in the axial skeleton. Areas of sclerosis adjacent to the vertebral end plates give a striped radiological appearance known as a 'rugger jersey spine'.

Effects of Treatment

Hyperparathyroidism may be controlled by oral calcium supplements and phosphate binders. Both osteitis fibrosa and osteomalacia often improve after treatment with $1,25(OH)_2D_3$ or $1\alpha(OH)D_3$, although parathyroidectomy may be necessary in patients who fail to respond to medical management or in those who develop tertiary hyperparathyroidism. Renal osteodystrophy normally responds to renal transplantation. Renal transplant patients are at risk of developing both osteonecrosis, particularly of femoral heads and condyles and osteoporosis. As steroid therapy is implicated in both conditions, the introduction of cyclosporin and consequent reduction of steroid dosage has resulted in a lower incidence of these complications.

Biochemistry of Metabolic Bone Disease

In clinical practice bone biopsy and serum biochemistry are complementary in the assessment of patients with metabolic bone disease. The typical biochemical findings are given in Table 20.5. Serum phosphate and calcium concentrations should be measured in the morning after overnight fasting to avoid variations due to circadian rhythms and dietary intake. Approximately half the serum calcium is ionized and this is the biologically active fraction. The remainder is bound to proteins, especially albumin, and to citrate, phosphate and

Table 20.5 Laboratory results in metabolic bone diseases

	Ca	PO_4	Alk phos	Serum PTH	$25(OH)D_3$
Osteoporosis	N*	N	N	N	N
Osteomalacia (vitamin D deficient)	↓	↓	↑	↑	↓
Primary hyperparathyroidism	↑	↓	N or ↑	↑	N
Renal osteodystrophy	N, ↓ or ↑	N or ↑	N or ↑	↑	N
Paget's disease	N*	N	↑	N	N

*Immobilized patients occasionally develop hypercalcaemia especially if they suffer from extensive Paget's disease.
Typical results are given: N, normal; ↑, increased; ↓ decreased.
PTH, parathyroid hormone; Alk phos, alkaline phosphatase.

bicarbonate. The total serum calcium must therefore be corrected for changes in serum albumin concentration.

Measurement of bone-specific alkaline phosphatase isoenzyme is a more accurate index of osteoblastic activity than serum alkaline phosphatase, as the presence of other isoenzymes, e.g. from liver, may obscure minor changes. Parathyroid hormone is measured by immunoassay using antibodies directed to the initial 34 N-terminal amino acids which confer biological activity.

The most sensitive indicator of vitamin D deficiency is a fall in serum $25(OH)D_3$, as levels of $1,25(OH)_2D_3$ are maintained until deficiency is severe. In renal failure, measurement of $1,25(OH)_2D_3$ indicates the remaining activity of the renal enzyme, $25(OH)D_3$ 1α-hydroxylase.

Paget's Disease of Bone

First described by Sir James Paget in 1877, this is a disorder of excessive turnover of bone resulting in disorganization of bone architecture. Although commonly discussed with metabolic bone diseases it is not a generalized skeletal disorder, but may affect part or all of one, several or many bones. The aetiology is not known, but intranuclear inclusions found in the osteoclasts of patients with Paget's disease resemble those of myxoviruses, while immunohistochemical techniques have supported the theory that Paget's disease is due to viral infection. As yet, nucleic acid hybridization studies have not consistently shown the presence of viral nucleic acid sequences in the osteoclasts of Paget's disease.

The incidence of Paget's disease shows considerable geographical variation. Almost unknown in Japan and Scandinavia and rare in the tropics, it is common in Britain and in people of Anglo-Saxon stock. Occasionally found in young adults, Paget's disease can be detected at autopsy or by radiology in about 3% of patients over 40 years, rising to 10% of those over 80. There is a slight male preponderance. Of this large number of people only about 5% have symptoms, mainly of bone pain. Most frequently vertebrae, pelvis, skull and femur, tibia and humerus are involved.

Radiological Appearances

Paget's disease starts at one site in a bone and gradually extends, the advancing front being lytic. Long bones occasionally show a sharply defined flame shaped area of bone resorption, while localized rarefaction of the skull is known as

osteoporosis circumscripta. As the disease progresses, resorption lessens and bone formation becomes more prominent with patchy sclerosis and coarse trabeculae. The shafts of long bones are thickened on the periosteal and endosteal surfaces so that the bone is enlarged and the marrow cavity narrowed. The weakened bones may be bowed. The skull enlarges and is sometimes three to four times thicker than normal; the distinction between diploë and cancellous bone is gradually lost (Fig. 20.14).

Pathology

In early Paget's disease there is intense activity of osteoclasts which are much larger than normal. Plump osteoblasts rapidly lay down new bone, some of which is woven rather than lamellar, with prominent osteoid seams reflecting increased bone formation. The marrow spaces contain vascular fibrous tissue. Later, as resorption diminishes, trabeculae become thickened and show a 'mosaic' or 'jigsaw' pattern of cement lines indicating previous phases of bone resorption and formation (Fig. 20.15). Normal cortical Haversian systems are replaced by irregularly arranged trabeculae. Eventually the marrow becomes densely fibrosed and the bone surfaces inactive.

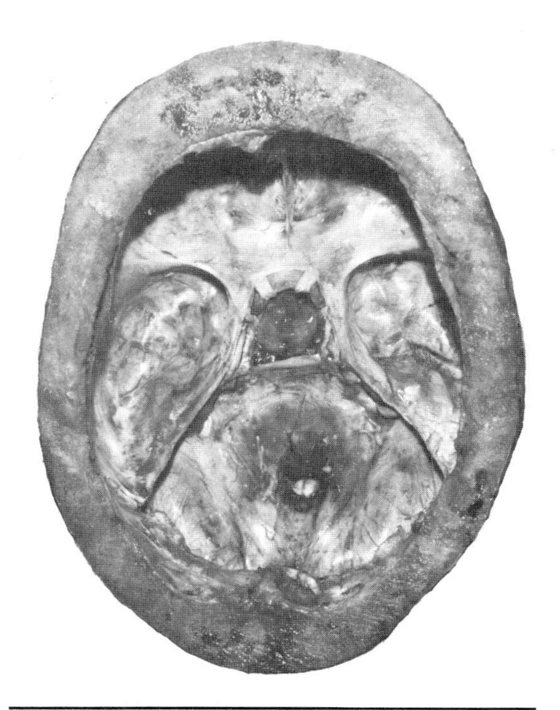

Fig. 20.14 Paget's disease of the skull, showing enormous thickening of the calvarium with loss of distinction of the tables. The sella turcica is much enlarged owing to the fortuitous presence of an adenoma of the pituitary.

Complications

Even when thickened, 'Pagetic' bone is structurally weak due to destruction of cortical Haversian systems; this leads to bowing of long bones and pathological fractures which are often transverse. Bone deformity tends to throw abnormal stresses on joints and predisposes to osteoarthritis. Narrowing of exit foramina of the skull by new bone formation sometimes gives rise to nerve compression, typically of the eighth cranial nerve causing deafness. Similarly, spinal cord compression may follow enlargement, or less commonly, collapse of an involved vertebra. Rarely patients with very extensive Paget's disease have a high cardiac output and compromised

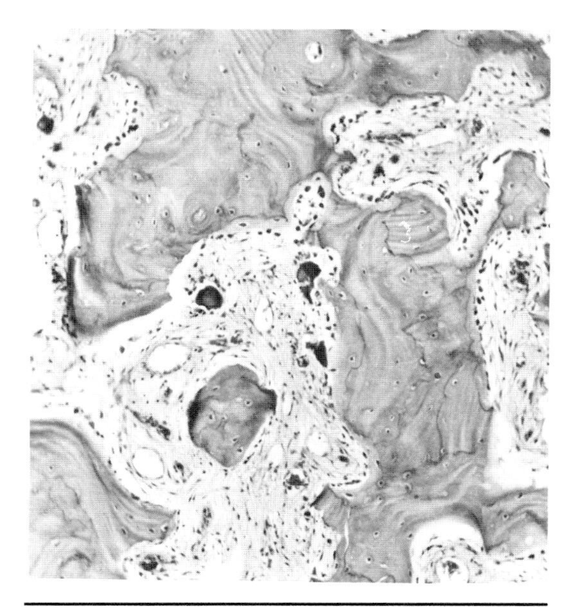

Fig. 20.15 Paget's disease of the femur, showing the typical mosaic structure of the bone, with both active osteoclastic resorption and osteoblastic formation. (Professor J. B. Gibson.) ×90.

cardiac function due to increased blood flow through the affected bones.

Paget's sarcoma. The most serious complication of Paget's disease is the development of sarcoma, but fortunately this is rare, affecting less than 1% of patients. The tumour is usually an osteosarcoma, malignant fibrous histiocytoma, or pleomorphic sarcoma. Although Paget's disease commonly affects vertebrae and skull, sarcoma frequently arises in long bones, especially the femur and humerus. The prognosis in Paget's sarcoma is very poor; most patients develop early pulmonary metastases and die within 2 years.

Generalized Developmental Abnormalities of Bone

Achondroplasia

In this condition, failure of enchondral ossification leads to severe short-limb dwarfism. Achondroplasia is due to a dominant gene with a very high mutation rate; thus, most affected children are born to normal parents. Patients have very distinctive features; the head appears large, the forehead bulging and the root of the nose sunken. The limbs are disproportionately short compared with the trunk and cranium. The hands are broad with fingers of equal length (trident hands). The spinal canal is narrowed and spinal cord compression is common in adults. These changes are a consequence of the failure of normal enchondral ossification. At the epiphyseal line the cartilage cells form short rows or are irregularly arranged, with little or no ossification, resulting in reduced bone growth.

Eighty per cent of affected infants die, usually from neurological complications such as hydrocephalus due to maldevelopment of the skull base. Those less severely affected individuals who survive into adult life have normal intellect.

Osteopetrosis (Marble Bone Disease, Albers-Schönberg Disease)

Defective osteoclastic activity (due, for example, to absence of osteoclast carbonic anhydrase activity, or to an absence of osteoclasts themselves) leads to failure of resorption of the cartilaginous model of bones. The marrow cavities fail to form and anaemia with a peripheral blood leucoerythroblastic reaction (p. 594) develops. In severely affected children anaemia and infections due to leucopenia may be life threatening. The bones are radio-opaque (Fig. 20.16) and show evidence of abnormal remodelling. Although of increased density the bones are structurally abnormal and are subject to pathological fracture. Skull involve-

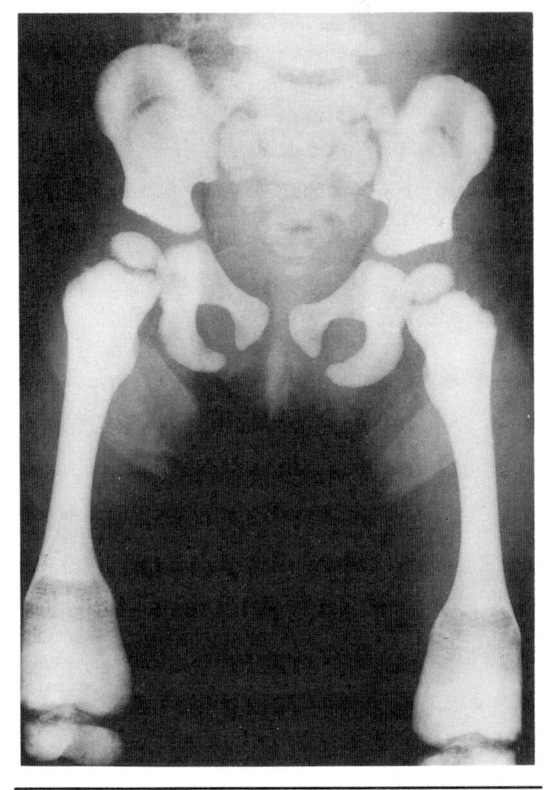

Fig. 20.16 Osteopetrosis. The bones are of increased density and the marrow cavities have not formed. There is defective remodelling of the lower femoral metaphysis which is widened.

ment with narrowing of exit foramina may result in deafness or blindness. The disease is transmitted in a severe form as autosomal recessive, and in a milder autosomal dominant form which is often not recognized until adult life.

Patients with severe disease may be treated by bone marrow transplantation. Donor osteoclasts derived from marrow precursors resorb the cartilaginous matrix and allow remodelling. There may be transient severe hypercalcaemia following this treatment.

Osteogenesis Imperfecta ('Brittle Bone Syndrome')

This term is applied to a group of rare heritable diseases (1 in 20 000–40 000 births) characterized by bone fragility and repeated fractures. The severity of the disease and the age of onset vary widely between patients. Extraskeletal abnormalities, such as abnormal dentine (**dentinogenesis imperfecta**), and cardiac valvular disease and thin sclerae through which the choroid pigment may be seen giving a blue appearance, allow a clinical classification (Table 20.6). It has been established that most cases of osteogenesis imperfecta result from mutations in the structural genes for type I collagen, whose locations are given on p. 44.

The pathological appearances vary in accordance with the severity of the clinical disease. In general, osteoblast activity is defective with a reduction in bone formation. In keeping with reduced matrix formation osteocytes are crowded. The more severely affected the patient the higher the proportion of woven to lamellar bone. The shafts of long bones are thin while the epiphyses are broad and often disorganized. Multiple fractures often result in bowing of limb bones. Hyperplastic fracture callus may simulate the development of a sarcoma.

The radiological appearance of multiple healing fractures of varying ages may be misinterpreted as evidence of 'non-accidental injury', with serious medicolegal implications.

Osteonecrosis

Osteonecrosis (aseptic necrosis, avascular necrosis) refers to death of bone due to interference with its blood supply, unassociated with infection. The most common cause is a fracture that disrupts the major blood supply to an area of bone; the scaphoid and femoral head (Fig. 20.17) are two sites where the distribution of vessels is especially likely to cause clinically important osteonecrosis.

A large number of non-traumatic conditions are associated with osteonecrosis (Table 20.7) and sometimes no clear cause can be found (idiopathic). In some cases the pathogenesis seems clear: in compressed-air workers, nitrogen bubbles form during decompression and block small blood vessels, while in the osteonecrosis complicating steroid therapy and alcohol excess the mechanisms are speculative.

Necrosis may involve the cancellous bone of the shaft of a long bone. The resulting infarct sometimes is seen as an area of increased radiological density due chiefly to calcification of dead marrow.

Table 20.6 Clinical classification of osteogenesis imperfecta

Type I	Autosomal dominant. Osseous fragility, little deformity and normal stature. Blue sclerae, presenile hearing loss, with or without dentinogenesis imperfecta
Type II	New dominant mutations. Severe bone disease, usually lethal in perinatal period, occasional survivors
Type III	Some recessive. Progressive deforming bone disease with dwarfing. Sclerae blue in infancy, normal later
Type IV	Autosomal dominant. More fractures than type I, with deformity and short stature. Normal sclerae, with or without dentinogenesis imperfecta

Modified from Smith (1986).

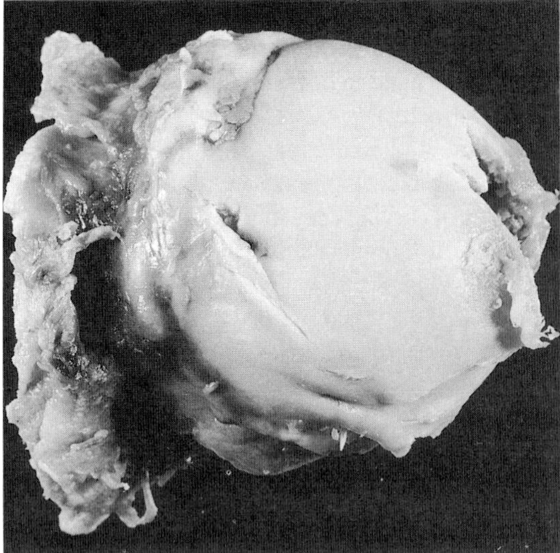

a

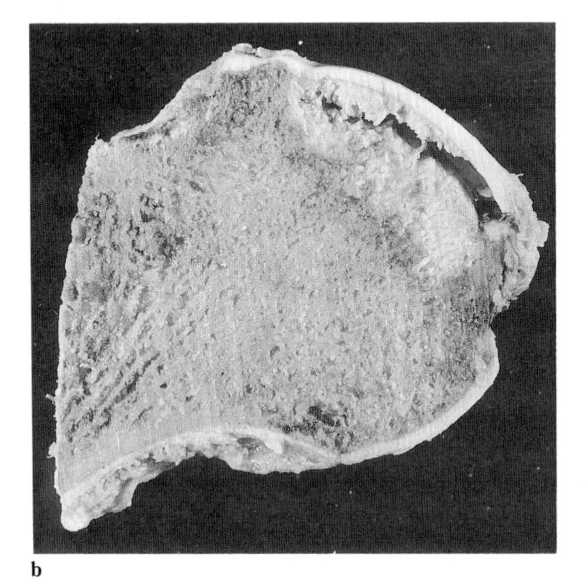

b

Fig. 20.17 Osteonecrosis of the femoral head. **a** The superior surface of the femoral head is depressed with incongruity of the articular cartilage. **b** A subchondral fracture has occurred through a pale wedge shaped area of necrotic bone resulting in a loose flap of articular cartilage and subchondral bone. (Dr M. E. Catto.)

Table 20.7 Causes of osteonecrosis in adults

Trauma
Fracture (especially neck of femur, scaphoid)
Dislocation of hip
Idiopathic
Steroid therapy
Renal transplantation
Alcoholism
Dysbarism (compressed-air workers and divers)
Sickle cell disease
Chronic pancreatitis
Connective tissue diseases, e.g. systemic lupus erythematosus
Gaucher's disease

Such lesions are symptomless, although very rarely a sarcoma may arise in relation to an old bone infarct. In contrast, in juxta-articular sites such as the femoral head or condyles, necrotic trabeculae may eventually collapse with deformity of the joint surface and secondary osteoarthritis.

Whatever the cause or location of osteonecrosis, the histological changes are similar. The earliest sign is necrosis of haemopoietic marrow seen within 2–3 days of removal of its blood supply. Loss of osteocytes from lacunae is a slower process which is not complete for 2–4 weeks, although irreversible changes have occurred much earlier. Initial steps in repair consist of revascularization of dead marrow followed by deposition of live bone on the surface of necrotic trabeculae (appositional new bone). In cancellous bone, removal of dead bone by osteoclastic resorption is often late.

A number of disorders of childhood are known to be due to osteonecrosis, although the aetiology is uncertain. **Perthes' disease** affects the hips of children, particularly boys, who present with pain and a limp. About 10% of cases are bilateral. Pathologically there is osteonecrosis of the femoral epiphysis which may heal without significant deformity or may collapse, often resulting in osteoarthritis in later life. **Osteochondritis dissecans** commonly involves the lateral aspect of the medial femoral condyle, where a wedge shaped area of bone undergoes necrosis. This, with its attached articular cartilage, separates from the articular surface, leaving a well demarcated defect. The loose body (p. 999) may cause locking and damage to the articular cartilage. Many cases follow an episode of trauma. Similar conditions may affect the tarsal navicular (**Köhler's disease**), the lunate (**Kienböck's disease**) and the second metatarsal (**Freiberg's disease**).

Effects of Radiation on Bone

For a general description of the effects of radiation see p. 437. Excessive doses of radiation, whether from external sources or following ingestion of a radionuclide such as radium, may damage bone and cartilage cells directly as well as by obliterating small blood vessels. Bone may become necrotic and is more likely later to become infected. **Osteomyelitis** is particularly likely to follow irradiation of the jaw. **Pathological fracture** of the femoral neck may occur some years after irradiation for pelvic cancer, especially in women. In children inclusion of the epiphyseal cartilage plate in the radiation field may damage the cartilage cells causing **retardation of growth** and sometimes premature closure of the epiphysis.

Neoplasia following Radiation

Leukaemia. External radiation of the skeleton tends to affect most severely the haemopoietic cells of the marrow and is a well established cause of leukaemia. Leukaemia, however, does not seem to have been a common complication of ingested radium which is incorporated into bone.

Bone sarcoma. External radiation of bone carries a relatively small risk of subsequent sarcoma, but due to variation in individual response the 'safe' dosage is uncertain. This small risk is accepted in the treatment of malignancy but, when possible, benign or non-neoplastic lesions, especially in children, are treated by other means. The latent period before development of bone sarcoma is usually from 5 to 20 years. Post-radiation tumours include osteosarcomas, fibrosarcomas or malignant fibrous histiocytomas. In the past, bone sarcoma occurred in as many as 20% of those who ingested doses of radium or its salts.

Infection of Bones and Joints

Acute Osteomyelitis

The incidence of pyogenic infection of bone has declined sharply in developed countries, and the prognosis is greatly improved by antibiotic therapy. Nevertheless, awareness of the disease is important, as delay in diagnosis and treatment may lead to considerable morbidity or even death. Osteomyelitis most commonly occurs in children and adolescents, although the relative incidence in neonates and adults has risen. Any bone may be affected but the metaphyses of long bones (distal femur, proximal tibia and humerus) adjacent to actively growing epiphyses, and the vertebral column are most often involved.

In most cases the organisms are blood borne from a primary focus elsewhere such as a boil, or otitis media. Frequently, no source can be found and it is assumed that there is a minor lesion which is clinically inapparent or has healed. Bone infection may result from contamination of a compound fracture or follow surgery especially when a metallic implant is used. Occasionally it arises by direct spread from an adjacent infection, for example to the jaw from a dental abscess.

The causative organism of most serious infections is coagulase positive staphylococcus, although streptococci and Gram-negative bacilli such as *Escherichia coli*, *Proteus* spp. and *Haemophilus influenzae* are sometimes isolated. Sickle cell anaemia (p. 605) predisposes to infection by salmonellae.

Typically, the patient is unwell with a high fever, and complains of severe pain and tenderness aggravated by any movement. There is often a history of minor trauma to the area. The ESR is almost always elevated, and the white blood count shows an increase in neutrophils, although often this is delayed until more than 24–48 hours after the onset. Radiology is not helpful in early diagnosis since changes frequently do not appear for 7 days or so. If acute osteomyelitis is suspected, blood cultures should be taken and large doses of antibiotics given immediately to avert septicaemia. A high level of suspicion is required to make the diagnosis in immunosuppressed patients who frequently have few symptoms or signs.

Pathology

The following description refers to untreated or antibiotic resistant osteomyelitis. Prompt antibiotic treatment may abort the infection at an early stage before radiological change appears.

The susceptibility of the metaphysis to acute osteomyelitis is, in part, explained by the dilated vascular sinusoids of the marrow spaces where sluggish blood flow provides an ideal site for multiplication of bacteria. This initiates an acute inflammatory response with exudation of protein-rich fluid and neutrophil polymorphs. As intraosseous pressure rises, there is venous and later arterial thrombosis and local bone necrosis. Infection spreads rapidly throughout the marrow spaces so that the medullary cavity is occupied by pus, which penetrates the Haversian systems of the metaphyseal cortex, elevates the periosteum and forms a subperiosteal abscess. The periosteum of the adolescent (unlike that of the adult) is loosely attached and the abscess may surround much of the diaphysis, leading to thrombosis of penetrating arteries. Occlusion of both periosteal and endosteal vessels leads to necrosis of some or all of the diaphysis, the portion of dead bone being known as a **sequestrum**. Small sequestra, particularly in children, tend to be completely absorbed by osteoclastic activity, while larger ones usually persist for months or years, forming a nidus for repeated episodes of infection. As infection becomes less acute, subperiosteal new bone may form a shell around the dead bone (Fig. 20.18). This **involucrum** is irregular and often perforated, allowing pus to track into the surrounding soft tissues, ultimately reaching the skin surface and forming a discharging sinus.

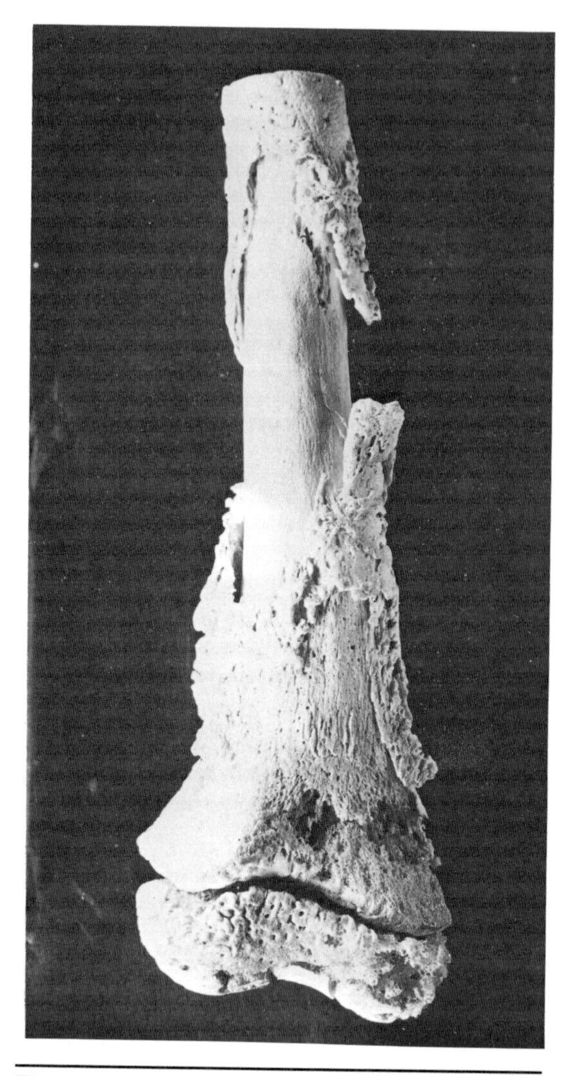

Fig. 20.18 Femur from a case of long-standing suppurative osteomyelitis and periostitis in a child, showing the formation of an irregular involucrum of new bone round the sequestrum.

The epiphysis is usually spared since the epiphyseal plate forms a barrier to direct spread from the metaphysis. In addition, the periosteum is firmly attached to the margin of the plate, preventing spread of the subperiosteal abscess in this direction. In infants, however, metaphyseal blood vessels penetrate the developing epiphyseal plate and anastomose freely with epiphyseal vessels, allowing spread of infection to the epiphysis and also the joint. In adults, after closure of the growth plate, similar extension of infection may result.

Complications

Septicaemia. Spread of infection, particularly when due to staphylococci, may lead to septicaemia with abscesses in lung, kidney or myocardium and acute endocarditis. This accounted for a mortality of 25% before antibiotic therapy was available.

Septic arthritis due to direct spread of infection occurs in those joints, such as the hip and shoulder, where the metaphysis is within the joint capsule. Metastatic blood-borne arthritis may complicate infantile streptococcal or pneumococcal osteomyelitis.

Alteration in growth rate. Damage to the epiphyseal plate, particularly in infants, sometimes leads to growth retardation, while occasionally increased blood flow causes accelerated growth.

Chronic osteomyelitis. Acute osteomyelitis, particularly in adults, may become chronic with recurrent exacerbation of infection with abscesses, discharging sinuses and increasing patchy bone sclerosis. **Secondary amyloidosis** and occasionally **squamous carcinoma** arising in a sinus may complicate very long-standing chronic osteomyelitis.

Subacute Pyogenic Infection

Many patients develop a subacute pyogenic infection with an insidious onset and little fever or malaise. Most cases affect the spine, but other bones may be involved.

Vertebral Osteomyelitis

Infection of the vertebral column is usually haematogenous, either arterial or by retrograde spread through the vertebral venous plexus which communicates directly with pelvic veins and bypasses the vena cava. In about two-thirds of patients the lumbar spine is involved. *Staphylococcus aureus* is the commonest organism; infection with coliforms may follow genitourinary surgery. In most patients the onset is insidious with intermittent attacks of backache and little fever. The initial focus is in or close to the vertebral end plate; infection spreads to involve adjacent disc and cancellous bone of the vertebral body, both of which undergo necrosis. Some collapse of bone occurs with loss of the disc space; reactive new bone formation may cause spontaneous fusion of adjacent vertebrae. As the lesion heals marked bone sclerosis develops.

Brodie's Abscess

This is a form of localized subacute or chronic osteomyelitis which is usually situated in the metaphysis of a long bone, especially the upper end of the tibia. A central cavity containing pus, which may be sterile, is lined by granulation tissue and surrounded by reactive bone sclerosis.

Septic Arthritis

Joint infection may result from haematogenous spread to synovium, from direct extension from acute osteomyelitis, or follow penetrating injury or surgery, especially joint replacement. *Staphylococcus aureus* is the commonest causative organism. Patients with rheumatoid arthritis and those on steroid therapy are at increased risk from joint infection, which often gives rise to few local symptoms.

Neonates, children and adults may all develop septic arthritis. Classically, children and young adults present with high fever and a swollen, hot, extremely painful joint. The patient will not allow any movement of the joint. While an inflamed knee is obvious clinically, inflammation of the hip is readily missed. It is important to be aware that elderly patients, particularly those on steroid therapy, frequently show few signs of systemic upset.

Pathology

The synovium is acutely inflamed with large numbers of neutrophils in the membrane and in the joint fluid. Proteolytic enzymes, released by neutrophils; and plasmin, activated by bacterial enzymes such as staphylokinase, lead to destruction of the articular cartilage (Fig. 20.19). Effective early treatment is likely to preserve joint function, but loss of articular cartilage is followed by functional impairment and sometimes by fibrous or bony ankylosis.

Tuberculosis of Bones and Joints

While the overall incidence of tuberculosis in developed countries has fallen, the relative importance of skeletal infection has increased. Skeletal tuberculosis is almost always due to blood spread from infection elsewhere, usually lung, lymph node or urinary tract; the patient should be investigated to find this source of infection. Direct spread, e.g. from lung to rib or sternum, is rare.

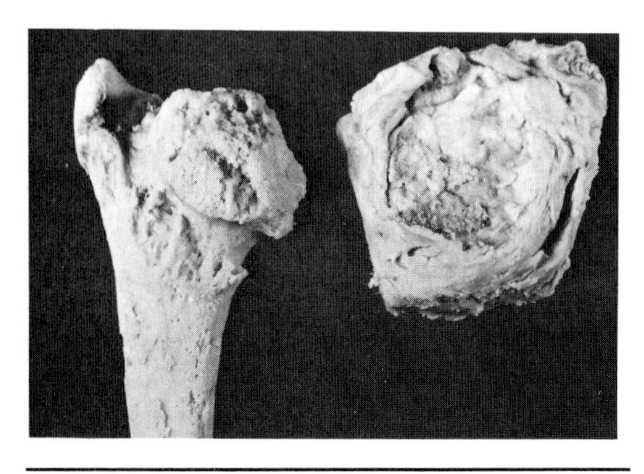

Fig. 20.19 Suppurative arthritis of hip joint. The articular cartilage of both the femoral head and the acetabulum is destroyed and there is erosion of the underlying bone.

With the elimination of bovine tuberculosis, the human strain, *Mycobacterium tuberculosis*, is responsible for most infections in Britain. Early diagnosis and treatment are vital to minimize tissue destruction.

In the third world young children are mainly affected, while in the UK most infections occur in the elderly indigenous population and in adolescent immigrants, usually from the Indian subcontinent. About half of the infections involve the spine (Pott's disease), usually the lower thoracic and lumbar vertebrae. Initially one vertebral body is affected with early involvement of the intervertebral disc. Granulomatous inflammation with caseation destroys bone, causing vertebral collapse. Unlike pyogenic spinal infection, little reactive new bone is formed. A local paraspinal abscess, often visible radiologically, develops and infection may extend along the anterior spinal ligaments to other vertebrae, or track anteriorly along tissue planes. In the lumbar spine infection may spread along the sheath of the psoas muscle to point in the groin as a 'cold' or 'psoas' abscess (Fig. 20.20). Angulation of the spine may occur with a severe kyphus (tuberculous gibbus). About a quarter of patients with vertebral tuberculosis develop spinal cord compression. This may occur either early in the disease due to pressure from an extradural abscess, small sequestra, or disc material, or late if the cord is stretched over the apex of a severe kyphosis. In the latter case the prognosis is poorer.

Healing is by fibrosis with some new bone formation. Tubercle bacilli tend to survive for long periods in walled off caseous material; later, if the patient becomes immunosuppressed, reactivation of the infection may occur.

Tuberculous arthritis results from haematogenous spread of infection to synovium or by extension from an affected intracapsular portion of bone. Granulomatous inflamed synovium invades the subchondral bone and causes its resorption. Dissection of articular cartilage from the underlying bone is characteristic, leading to destruction of the joint surface.

Less commonly, bone involvement occurs in the absence of joint disease, typically with destructive lesions in the metaphysis of long bones, for example at the knee, femoral neck and

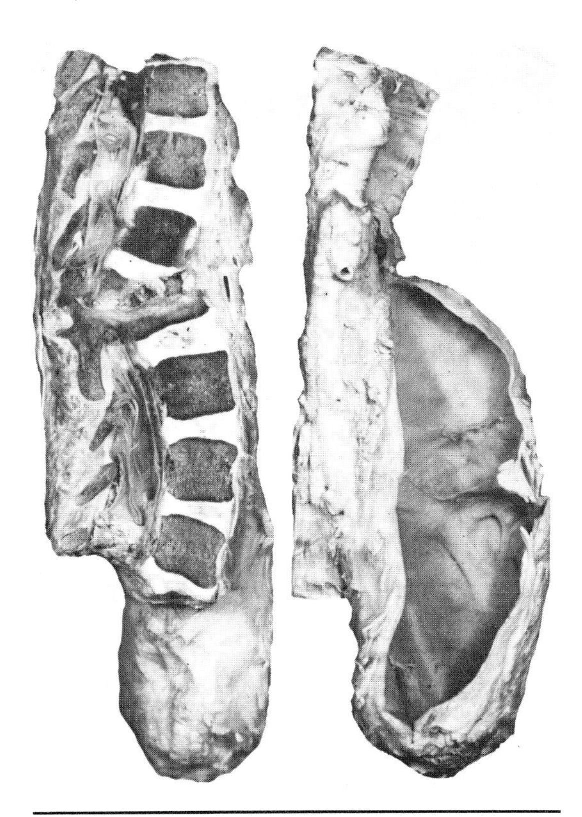

Fig. 20.20 Tuberculosis of spine (Pott's disease). Loss of intervertebral disc and collapse of T12 and L1 with paraplegia and formation of psoas abscess.

greater trochanter. The tubular bones of the hands may be affected (dactylitis). The histological appearances are typical; acid- and alcohol-fast bacilli can often be identified in histological sections; synovium should also be submitted for bacteriological examination.

Other Infections of Bones and Joints

Infections of bones and joints in syphilis and actinomycosis are discussed in Chapter 9.

Gonococcal arthritis. Infection by *Neisseria gonorrhoeae* is now a major cause of bacterial arthritis. Most patients complain of flitting pain in many joints, particularly the knees, ankles, wrists and elbows. Tenosynovitis and a skin rash are often present. It is thought that joint involvement follows a bacteraemic phase after genital infection. However, culture of *N. gonorrhoeae* from inflamed joints is often difficult, and it has been suggested that immune complexes rather than true infection may be the cause of arthritis in some cases. In most patients little permanent joint damage results.

Brucellosis. Infection by the small Gram-negative bacilli of the genus *Brucella* is transmitted to man from infected animals or animal products. Infection of bone and joints is common in patients with chronic brucellosis, and less so in the acute form. Typically one or a few peripheral joints are involved; sacroiliitis is also seen. The organism is difficult to culture, and often the diagnosis can only be supported by the clinical history and positive serological tests. Histologically the synovium or bone contains non-caseating granulomas.

Lyme disease. This is a multisystem infection caused by the spirochete *Borrelia burgdorferi*, which is transmitted by ticks of the genus *Ixodes*, particularly in areas with large deer populations. (The name derives from Lyme, Connecticut where a cluster of children with arthritis led in 1975 to recognition of the disease.) A skin rash (*erythema chronicum migrans*, p. 1110), cardiac, nervous system and osteoarticular involvement have all been described.

Joint manifestations include migratory joint pains, intermittent attacks of acute arthritis and chronic erosive arthritis which, in about 10% of patients causes permanent disability. Large joints, particularly the knee, are affected. Lyme arthritis responds to treatment with high dose penicillin, although irreversible damage may have already occurred.

Viral arthritis. Many common viral infections, e.g. hepatitis B, rubella and its vaccine and parvovirus, are associated with transient arthritis or arthralgia. In all instances the arthritis is nondestructive and does not lead to chronic joint disease.

Infections related to prosthetic joint replacements are discussed on p. 998.

Tumours in Bone

Metastatic Tumours

Metastatic tumours far exceed primary bone tumours in frequency, and may be found at autopsy in 70% of patients dying with disseminated tumour. Almost all are carcinomas, particularly those arising from bronchus, breast, prostate, kidney and thyroid, while in children neuroblastoma often spreads to bone. Metastases occur most commonly in areas where haemopoietic marrow is present, such as the vertebral column, ribs (Fig. 20.21), proximal femur and humerus. Retrograde spread to the spine occurs along the prevertebral venous plexus. Metastases distal to the knee and elbow are rare.

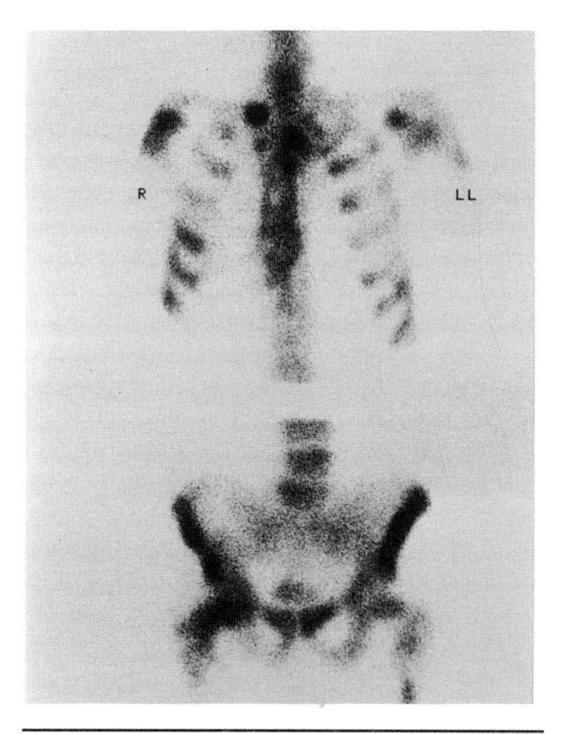

Fig. 20.21 Isotope bone scan. Increased uptake is seen in many bones including the ribs, pelvis, proximal femur and humerus in a patient with disseminated prostatic carcinoma. (Dr Richard Jones.)

Bone metastases usually destroy bone (osteolysis) and may cause vertebral collapse or pathological fracture. Bone is removed by osteoclasts rather than directly by tumour cells. The exact mechanisms are unclear, but many factors produced by tumour cells, such as transforming growth factors α and β and prostaglandins, can stimulate osteoclastic activity. Tumour necrosis factor β appears to be the major osteoclast stimulating factor in multiple myeloma (p. 637). Rarely carcinomas, typically of prostate and sometimes of breast, may induce reactive new bone formation giving rise to osteosclerotic metastases (Fig. 20.22). In these patients serum alkaline phosphatase is often elevated, reflecting increased osteoblastic activity. In patients with disseminated prostatic carcinoma, acid phosphatase of prostatic origin is also elevated (p. 1068). If marrow replacement is very extensive, anaemia with a peripheral blood leucoerythroblastic reaction results (p. 594). Extensive bone destruction may cause hypercalcaemia but, in the absence of bony metastases, 'humoral hypercalcaemia of malignancy' is often due to the production by tumour

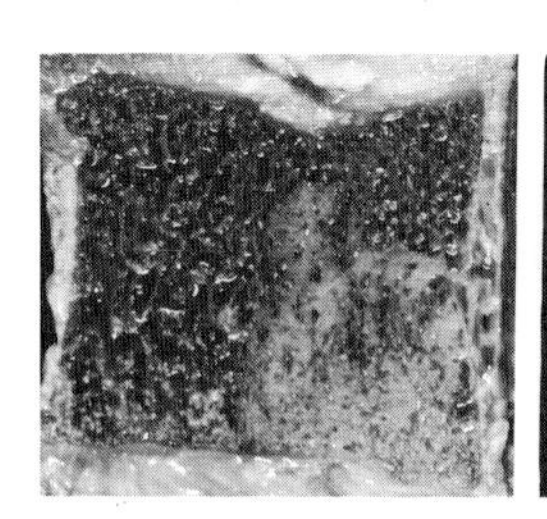

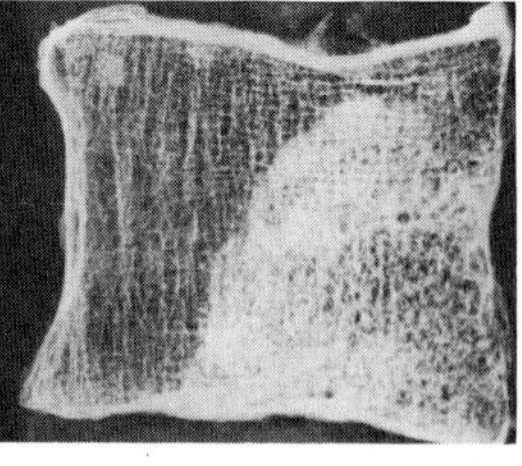

Fig. 20.22 The body of the lumbar vertebra is partially replaced by secondary prostatic carcinoma. The radiograph of a thin slice shows that this has provoked reactive bone sclerosis.

cells of parathyroid hormone related peptide (PTHrP), which has sequence analogies and functional similarity to PTH.

Metastatic tumours in bone occasionally present as solitary lesions, but usually multiple further metastases rapidly develop. Rarely, surgical removal of a primary renal or thyroid carcinoma and a solitary metastasis results in worthwhile remission or cure.

Primary Bone Tumours

Although much less common than metastases, primary tumours are an important cause of disability and death, particularly in the young. As a result of their rarity, expertise in diagnosis and management is increasingly concentrated in regional centres. A simplified classification together with a summary of the typical anatomical location, age range and clinical features is given in Table 20.8.

Benign Bone-forming Tumours

Osteoid osteoma. This benign lesion commonly occurs in the shafts of long bones of adolescents and young adults, particularly males. Patients complain of persistent pain, worse at night and often relieved by aspirin. Radiographs show a small lucent or lightly mineralized **nidus** usually less than 1 cm in diameter (Fig. 20.23). Lesions in the cortex are often surrounded by a mass of sclerotic bone which may obscure the central nidus on plain radiographs. Tomography or radioisotope scans using isotopes such as technetium (^{99}Tc), may be useful in demonstrating the site of lesions embedded in dense cortical bone.

Histologically, the lesion consists of a well defined and highly vascular nidus of irregular trabeculae of woven bone or osteoid formed by cytologically benign osteoblasts. The nidus is surrounded by a variable amount of reactive bone (Fig. 20.24). Symptoms may recur if the lesion is incompletely removed.

Benign osteoblastoma closely resembles osteoid osteoma histologically but it is larger (up to 10 cm diameter) and there is usually little surrounding bone sclerosis. Patients rarely complain of intense pain. Osteoblastoma is frequently situated in the vertebral column where it may cause spinal cord or nerve compression. Occasional osteoblastomas show cytological atypia and a tendency to local recurrence. Distinction of these 'aggressive osteoblastomas' from low grade osteosarcomas is sometimes difficult.

Osteosarcoma

With the exception of multiple myeloma (p. 637), this is the commonest primary malignant tumour arising in bone, with approximately 150 new patients (three cases per million population) diagnosed in Britain each year. Three-quarters of patients are between 10 and 25 years old with males more frequently affected. In more than half the patients over 40 years the tumour complicates Paget's disease. Some tumours arise in previously irradiated bone. Patients typically present with increasing pain and swelling. Pathological fracture is relatively unusual. Most osteosarcomas arise in the medullary cavity of the metaphysis of long bones, with over half around the knee. The proximal humerus and femur and distal radius are other common sites.

Pathology

By definition, osteosarcoma is a malignant tumour where osteoid or bone is formed directly by the tumour cells (Fig. 20.25). The gross appearances vary greatly. Some tumours are densely sclerotic, while others are fleshy; telangiectatic osteosarcomas contain large blood-filled spaces. The naked eye appearances are modified by the response to preoperative chemotherapy which gives rise to large areas of necrosis, haemorrhage and fibrous replacement.

The histological appearances are also very vari-

Table 20.8 Primary bone tumours and tumour-like lesions – clinical and pathological features

	Peak age (years)	Principal site	Radiology/Pathology	Comments
Tumour-like lesions				
Solitary bone cyst	10–20	Humerus, femur (metaphysis)	Well defined lucency, slightly expanding bone. Frequently crack or pathological fracture	Non-neoplastic. Migrates away from growth plate. Frequently recurs after curettage if near plate. Injections of steroids may promote healing
Aneurysmal bone cyst	10–20	Vertebrae, flat bones, long bones (metaphysis)	Eccentric, expanding lytic 'blow out'. Blood-filled spaces, trabeculae of fibrous tissue containing giant cells and woven bone	May heal after biopsy or spontaneously. ABC-like areas in many other lesions
Metaphyseal fibrous defect (non-ossifying fibroma)	5–20	Long bones (metaphysis)	Eccentric, well defined, with scalloped border. Fibroblasts, lipid and haemosiderin laden macrophages. Scattering of osteoclast-like cells	Common, self-healing lesions, often incidental radiological finding. May fracture. Cured by curettage
Fibrous dysplasia	10–30	Ribs, long bones (diaphysis or metaphysis), skull	Lytic lesion (ground glass on X-ray). 'Lobster-claw' woven bone trabeculae form by metaplasia from fibrous stroma	Non-neoplastic. May recur after curettage. May affect multiple bones.
Eosinophil granuloma	5–15	Skull, ribs, vertebrae, long bones (diaphysis or metaphysis)	Punched out lytic lesion; may be ill-defined with periosteal reaction Langerhans' cells with eosinophils	May be multiple. Rarely extraskeletal manifestations which carry worse prognosis
Benign tumours				
Osteoma	40–50	Skull, facial bones, sinuses	Well defined radio-opaque protuberance of dense mainly lamellar bone	
Osteoid osteoma	10–30	Any bone, mainly long bones (often cortex)	Lucent nidus of osteoblastic tissue (<1 cm); usually surrounding reactive sclerosis. Localize by isotope scan	Pain, worse at night, relieved by aspirin. Usually cured by curettage
Osteoblastoma	10–30	Vertebrae (posterior arch), long bones (metaphysis or diaphysis)	Well defined lytic or calcified mass of osteoblastic tissue (>1 cm)	Occasionally recurs after curettage
Enchondroma	10–40	Hands and feet in 60%, long bones (medulla of metaphysis, diaphysis), ribs	Well defined lytic defect, partially calcified. Expands narrow bones. Lobules of cartilage.	Usually cured by curettage. May be multiple, often unilateral (Ollier's disease). Risk of malignancy in axial skeleton

Table 20.8 *Continued*

	Peak age (years)	Principal site	Radiology/Pathology	Comments
Osteochondroma	10–30	Long bones (metaphysis)	Protruding mass of bone with cartilage cap	Developmental abnormality. Cure by excision. Multiple (hereditary) in 10% (diaphyseal aclasis)
Chondroblastoma	10–25	Long bones especially femur, humerus (epiphysis)	Well defined, seldom expanding, lytic area with sclerotic border. Chondroblasts with plaques of chondroid matrix	Occasionally recurs after curettage
Chondromyxoid fibroma	10–30	Long bones, especially tibia, metatarsals (metaphysis)	Well defined eccentric lucency. Myxoid tissue arranged in pseudolobules. May be mistaken for chondrosarcoma	Occasionally recurs after curettage
Haemangioma	20–50	Skull, vertebrae	Multiple lucent areas. May have marked periosteal reaction in skull lesions. Cavernous or capillary vascular spaces	May bleed profusely at biopsy
Tumours of intermediate malignancy				
Desmoplastic fibroma	20–30	Long bones (metaphysis, diaphysis)	Lytic, quite well circumscribed lesion. Cytologically bland fibroblastic tissue	Locally aggressive, non-metastasizing. Rare
Giant-cell tumour	20–40	Long bones (epiphysis, extending into metaphysis)	Eccentrically expanding, ill-defined lytic lesion. Often subperiosteal extension. Mononuclear cells and numerous large osteoclasts	30% recur after curettage. 10% metastasize usually after radiation
Malignant tumours				
Osteosarcoma	10–25	Long bones, 50% around knee (metaphysis)	Lytic or sclerotic destructive lesions with periosteal reaction and soft tissue extension. Variable histology – malignant cells forming osteoid or bone	Early pulmonary metastases. Previous 5-year survival of 20% increasing with multi-agent chemotherapy and surgery
Parosteal osteosarcoma	30–60	Femur, humerus, tibia (bone surface of metaphysis)	Lobulated ossified mass, on surface of bone. Often encircles shaft. Trabeculae of bone and malignant fibrous stroma	Much better prognosis than conventional osteosarcoma. 5-year survival 80%

Table 20.8 *Continued*

	Peak age (years)	Principal site	Radiology/Pathology	Comments
Chondrosarcoma	30–60	Pelvis, ribs, femur, humerus. Central – medulla of metaphysis. Peripheral – surface of metaphysis (in relation to exostosis)	Central – bone expansion, cortical thickening. Often calcified. Peripheral – large irregularly calcified cartilaginous mass with ill-defined margin	Mainly low grade – local recurrence and extension. Cure may require very radical surgery. Rarely high grade with pulmonary metastases. Not responsive to radiotherapy or chemotherapy. 10% 'dedifferentiate' with poor prognosis
Mesenchymal chondrosarcoma	20–60	Any bone; one-third in soft tissue	Lytic destructive lesion. Primitive malignant cells, islands of cartilage	Rare. Very poor prognosis with metastases, sometimes after many years
Ewing's sarcoma	5–20	Long bones (diaphysis or metaphysis), pelvis, ribs, scapulae	Ill-defined lysis. Periosteal reaction (sometimes multilayered) Malignant round cell tumour, glycogen rich, reticulin poor	Highly malignant; 5-year survival improving with chemotherapy
Fibrosarcoma	20–60	Long bones (metaphysis)	Lytic with cortical destruction. Low or high grade	Prognosis depends on grade. High grade, metastasize early to lung
Malignant fibrous histiocytoma (MFH)	20–60	Long bones (metaphysis)	Lytic destructive lesion	Often associated with precursor lesion (see text). Poor prognosis
Paget's sarcoma	50–70	Long bones (diaphysis or metaphysis) pelvis, spine, ribs	Destructive lesion with soft tissue extension, Osteosarcoma, MFH, fibrosarcoma	Rarely multifocal. Most patients die in 18 months with lung metastases
Chordoma	40–60	Sacrococcygeal, base of skull, vertebrae	Large destructive lesions. Lobulated gelatinous tissue, 'physaliphorous' cells	Slow progressive growth; metastases in 10%. Arise from notochord remnants
Adamantinoma		Tibia – usually anterior cortex. Rarely other bones	Single or multiple lytic areas. Poorly defined with soft tissue extension. Fibrous stroma and epithelial elements	Locally aggressive. Metastases in up to 20%
Malignant lymphoma	20–60	Any bone, femur (diaphysis or metaphysis), pelvis	Lytic, destructive. Mainly B-cell non-Hodgkin's lymphoma	If confined to bone over 50% survive 5 years. If generalized have poor prognosis
Multiple myeloma	40–70	Vertebrae, pelvis, ribs, sternum, skull, spine	Punched out lytic lesions or diffuse osteoporosis. Sheets of abnormal plasma cells	Paraproteins, Bence Jones protein, anaemia, renal failure, amyloidosis. Lengthen survival by chemotherapy but rarely 'cure'

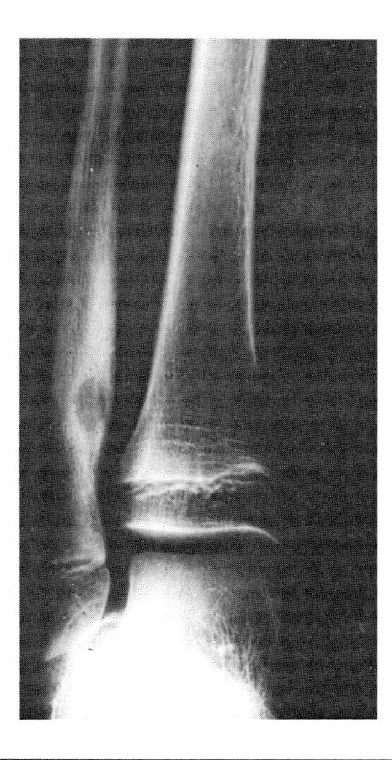

Fig. 20.23 An osteoid osteoma has given rise to an ovoid translucency in the lower end of the fibula. There is a little surrounding reactive bone sclerosis.

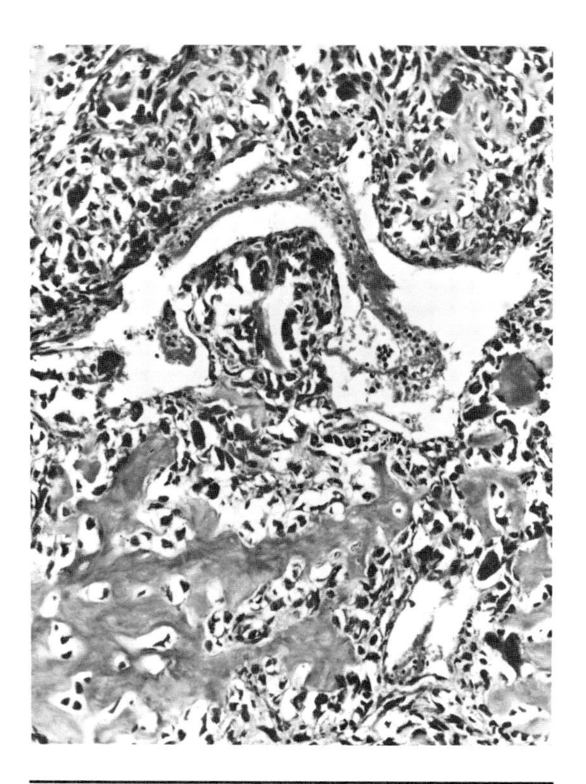

Fig. 20.25 Osteosarcoma. A highly vascular, cellular tumour with osteoid formation well seen in the lower part of the field. ×200.

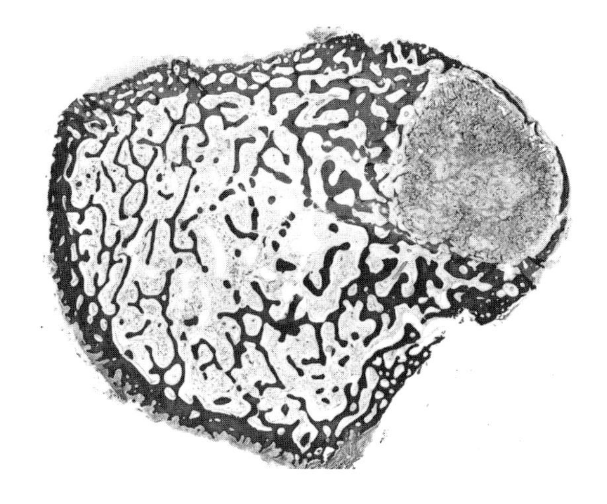

Fig. 20.24 A transverse section of the fibula shows that the small bone trabeculae of the osteoid osteoma have replaced cortical and medullary bone and stimulated slight surrounding reactive sclerosis. ×6.

able. Some tumours contain abundant 'tumour bone'; in others, only small foci of bone or osteoid are present and much of the tumour consists of malignant cartilage or sheets of malignant spindle-shaped cells.

Osteosarcoma spreads within the marrow spaces, occasionally with separate 'skip lesions'. The tumour penetrates and partially destroys the cortex to extend beneath the periosteum and sometimes later into soft tissue (Fig. 20.26). In rapidly growing tumours, when the periosteum is raised, spicules of new bone are laid down perpendicular to the cortex ('sunray spiculation'), while at the junction between raised and normal periosteum Codman's triangle of reactive bone may develop. Although characteristic of osteosarcoma, Codman's triangle is by no means specific for this diagnosis, and occurs in any condition where the periosteum is raised including other bone tu-

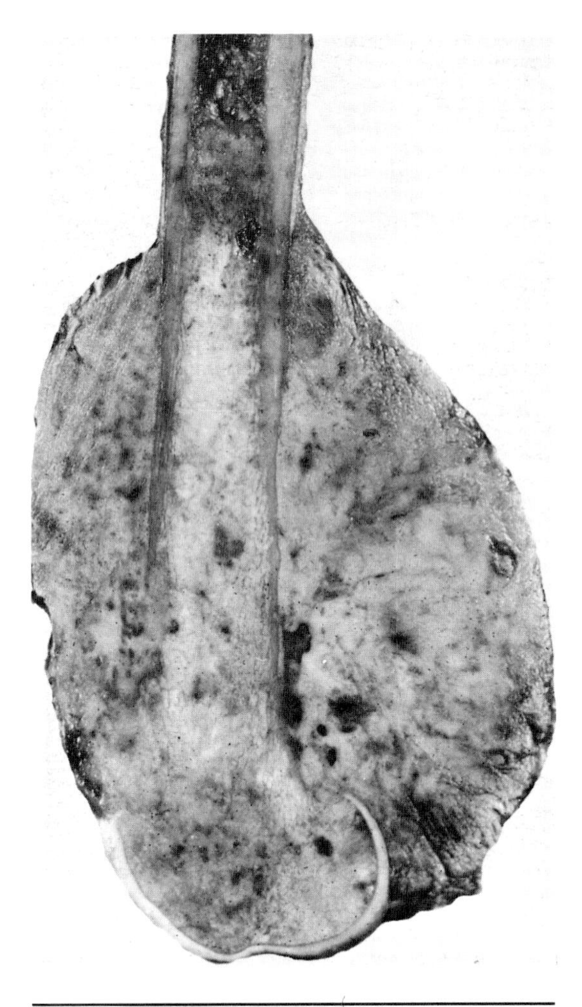

Fig. 20.26 Osteosarcoma of lower end of femur. The medullary tumour has penetrated and partly destroyed the cortex, spreading outwards to form a large subperiosteal mass.

mours, bone infection and early in fracture healing. The epiphyseal cartilage plate acts for a time as a barrier to the spread of tumour, but in many cases microscopic extension into the epiphysis is seen.

Prognosis and Treatment

Osteosarcoma is an aggressive tumour with early blood-borne pulmonary metastases, which may be evident at presentation. It is generally accepted that in most patients undetectable pulmonary micrometastases are already present when the primary tumour is discovered. In an attempt to deal with these silent metastases modern therapy combines preoperative and postoperative chemotherapy with surgery. The development of new techniques allows many patients to be treated by local resection and endoprosthetic replacement, rather than by amputation.

Of patients treated by surgery alone only 20% or so survive 5 years. Recent advances in combination chemotherapy, particularly with adriamycin and cisplatin, have significantly improved survival; approximately 60% of patients survive for 5 years. A better prognosis is seen in young adults compared with children, and when tumours are located in the distal skeleton and jaws. Multifocal osteosarcomas and those arising in Paget's disease have a worse prognosis.

Osteosarcoma on the Surface of Bones

Parosteal osteosarcoma forms a well defined lobulated mass, partly encircling the bone and attached to the cortex by a broad base often on the posterior aspect of the distal femur or on the proximal humerus (Fig. 20.27). Although local recurrence is common, metatastic spread is less frequent and the prognosis better than that of conventional osteosarcoma.

Periosteal osteosarcoma usually contains abundant malignant cartilage and has a prognosis intermediate between that of parosteal and conventional osteosarcoma.

High grade surface osteosarcoma is a rare tumour with a poor prognosis.

Benign Cartilage Tumours

Enchondroma is a benign intramedullary tumour of cartilage. Over half of the cases occur within the tubular bones of the hands and feet, although long bones such as the humerus and femur may be affected. Most enchondromas are symptomless

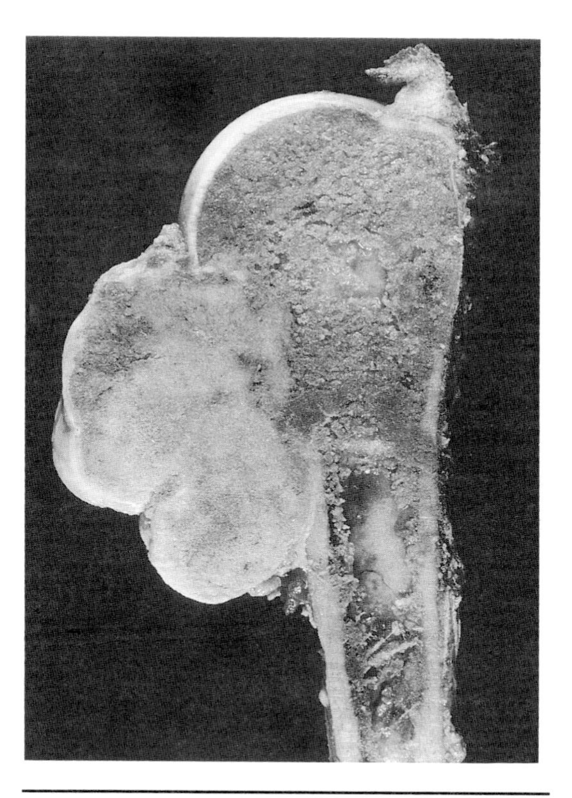

Fig. 20.27 Parosteal osteosarcoma. A well defined lobulated mass lies on the surface of the proximal humerus. The underlying cortex has been eroded and there is early invasion of the medullary cavity.

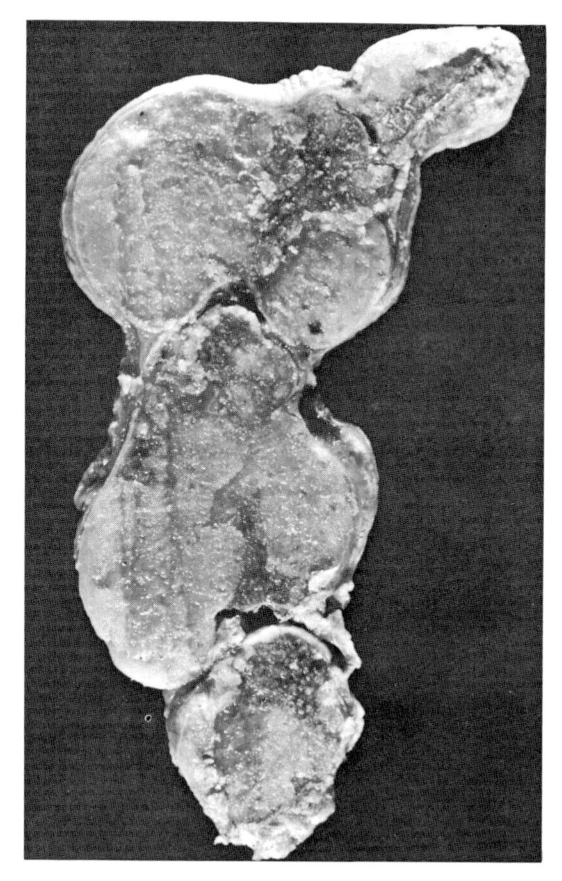

Fig. 20.28 Benign enchondromas of finger. The finger has been amputated just proximal to the metacarpal head. While the joint spaces remain intact each phalanx is replaced by a mass of hyaline cartilage. The cortices have disappeared but periosteum still surrounds the cartilage.

and are incidental radiological findings appearing as radiolucent lytic lesions often with spotty calcification. Patients with a tumour in the hand may complain of swelling or pain following injury, sometimes with a pathological fracture.

In **multiple enchondromatosis** (Fig. 20.28) few or many enchondromas may be present. The hands are almost invariably affected, but there may be involvement of long bones with shortening or deformity. When predominantly unilateral the condition is referred to as **Ollier's disease**. The combination of multiple enchondromatosis and soft tissue haemangiomas is known as **Maffucci's syndrome**. Neither Ollier's disease nor Maffucci's syndrome is an inherited condition.

Chondromas are composed of lobules of blue-grey cartilage, often rather gelatinous. The histological distinction of chondroma of long bones from low-grade chondrosarcoma can be difficult. Chondromas contain small uniform cells with small darkly staining nuclei. The presence of cells with plump nuclei and more than an occasional cell with two such nuclei is suspicious of malignancy if the clinical history and radiological appearances are also worrying. Chondrosarcoma of the tubular bones of the hands and feet is rare. In this site chondromas, especially in multiple enchondromatosis, may be very cellular and show mild cytological atypia without indicating malignancy.

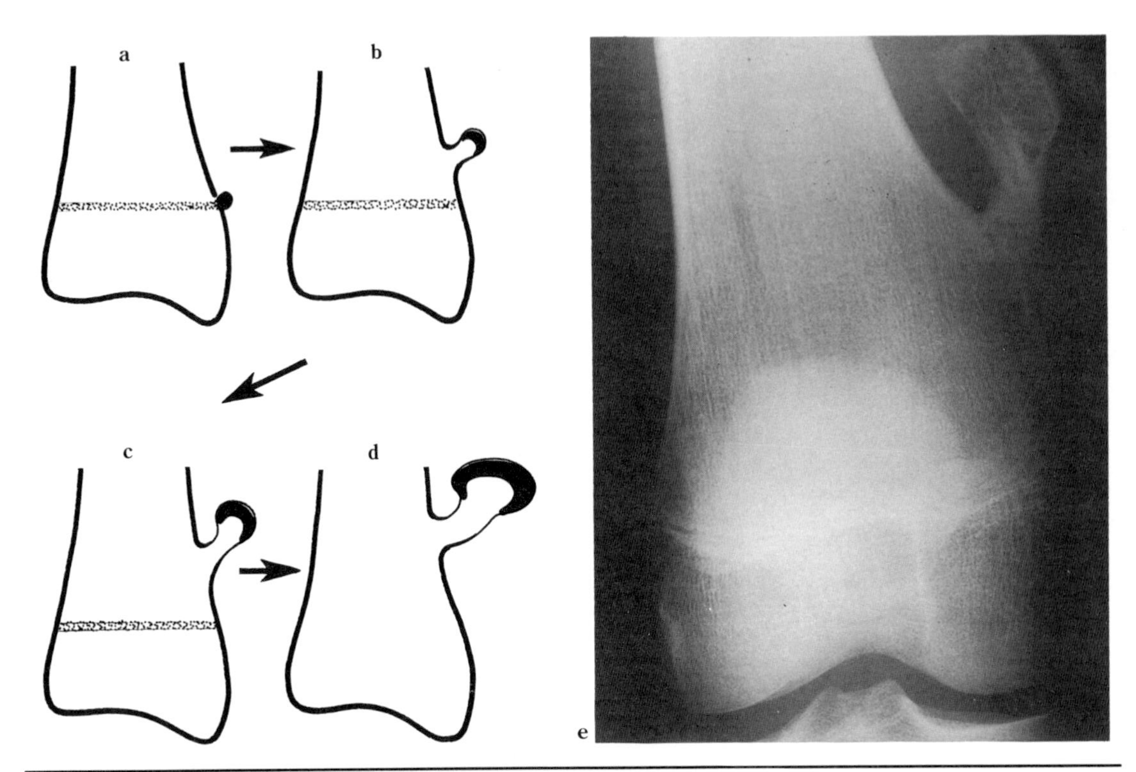

Fig. 20.29 Development of osteocartilaginous exostosis from an outgrowth of the epiphyseal plate **a**. The lesion becomes a cartilage capped lesion on a bony stalk **b**. With bone growth, the epiphyseal plate migrates away from the base of the lesion **c**. Growth of the exostosis usually ceases after skeletal maturity is attained **d**. A radiograph **e** shows an exostosis arising from the distal femoral metaphysis. The cartilaginous cap, being poorly mineralized, is not visualized.

Malignant transformation of solitary enchondromas is rare. In contrast, 25–30% of patients with multiple enchondromatosis develop chondrosarcoma, while the risk is higher in those with Maffucci's syndrome. In addition these patients appear to be at increased risk of non-skeletal malignancies, for example primary brain tumours and pancreatic carcinomas.

Periosteal chondromas usually arise on the metaphyseal surface of tubular bones, and cause scalloping of the underlying cortex. As in chondromas of the hands and feet mild cytological atypia does not imply malignancy.

Osteocartilaginous exostosis (osteochondroma) is the most common benign tumour of bone. It arises as a developmental anomaly at the epiphyseal growth plate (Fig. 20.29). It consists of a bony excrescence whose outer shell and medulla are continuous with that of the bone from which it grows. It is covered by a proliferating cartilage cap which undergoes enchondral ossification. Exostoses may be single or multiple; when multiple the condition is inherited as an autosomal dominant trait and may be associated with some failure of bone remodelling (**hereditary multiple exostoses, diaphyseal aclasis**). Exostoses may arise in any bone formed by enchondral ossification but the metaphyses of long bones, especially the femur, humerus and tibia, are the commonest sites. The lesions are usually first noticed in childhood and adolescence; growth commonly ceases in adult life, and sometimes the cartilaginous cap is completely replaced by bone. Malignant change is rare in solitary exostoses but probably about 10%

of patients attending hospital with multiple lesions develop chondrosarcoma which is almost always of low grade. Population studies suggest that the true incidence of malignant change is even lower. Exostoses of the axial skeleton or proximal limb bones are more likely to become malignant than those in the peripheral skeleton. A growth spurt, resumption of growth or pain which is not associated with fracture of the stalk of the exostosis or with bursitis should raise suspicion of malignancy.

Subungual exostosis, which usually involves the distal phalanx of the great toe and is often painful, is a reactive condition rather than a developmental abnormality or tumour. It commonly arises following infection or trauma as a result of cartilaginous and osseous metaplasia of the fibrous tissue around the terminal part of the distal phalanx. It never becomes malignant.

Chondrosarcoma

Chondrosarcoma usually arises *de novo*, though about 10% of cases are due to malignant change in a pre-existing benign cartilage tumour. The tumour may occur within the medullary cavity (central) (Fig. 20.30) or on the surface of bone (peripheral) usually in relation to an exostosis, but rarely in a subperiosteal location.

Chondrosarcoma usually affects the middle aged and elderly, particularly males. Most tumours arise in the axial skeleton, especially the pelvis, shoulder girdle and ribs, or in the proximal femur and humerus. Unlike enchondroma, chondrosarcoma is very rare in the tubular bones of the hands and feet. Most patients complain of swelling or pain. Indeed, pain associated with a cartilage tumour in the absence of pathological fracture or other mechanical cause is highly suggestive of malignancy.

Pathology

Central tumours consist of lobules or of sheets of cartilage which may permeate throughout the marrow spaces and cause endosteal erosion.

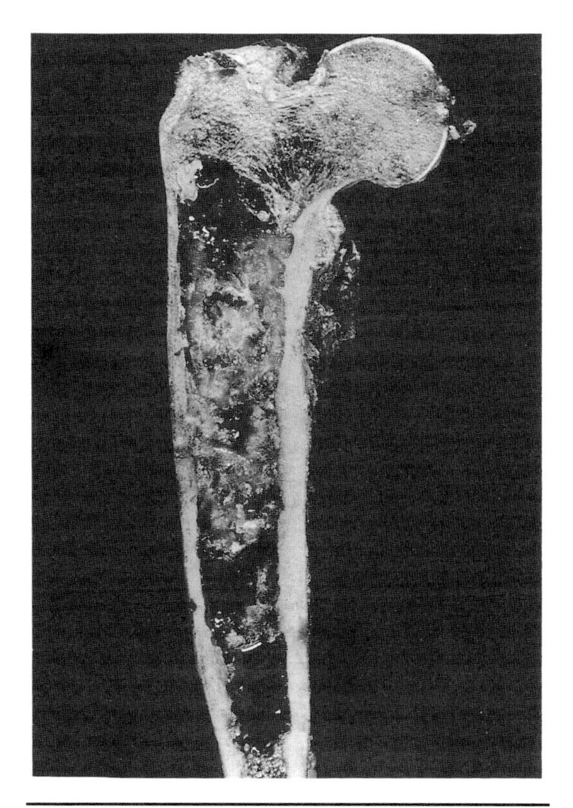

Fig. 20.30 Central chondrosarcoma of the femur. A mass of cartilage is present within the medullary canal. There is mild thickening of the medial femoral cortex, with a little endosteal erosion.

Frequently low-grade tumours produce buttressing of the outer aspect of the cortex, while more aggressive ones tend to destroy the cortex and form a subperiosteal mass. Focal calcification is a distinctive radiological finding. A greatly thickened cartilaginous cap with nodules of proliferating cartilage on the surface suggests that malignant change in an exostosis has occurred.

The histological diagnosis of low-grade chondrosarcoma is difficult, in that most chondrosarcomas do not show the classical features of malignancy such as the marked nuclear pleomorphism and abundant mitoses seen in other types of tumour. The finding, even focally, of many chondrocytes with plump nuclei and moderate numbers of binucleate cells in a cartilage tumour of the axial skeleton is consistent with a diagnosis of malignancy if the clinical and radiological features are also compatible (Fig. 20.31a). These cytological features may be discounted in tumours of the tubular bones of the hands and feet, in multiple enchondromatosis, subperiosteal or soft tissue cartilage tumours, and those in young growing children. The identification of a permeative growth pattern, with sheets of tumour filling marrow spaces between pre-existing bony trabeculae and eroding the cortex, is often helpful in making the diagnosis. Only rare cartilage tumours contain pleomorphic cells and moderate numbers of mitoses; these are of high-grade malignancy (Fig. 20.31b).

Approximately 10% of chondrosarcomas of low or middle grade, typically those arising in the medullary cavity, are accompanied by a high grade component of osteosarcoma or malignant fibrous histiocytoma, which frequently extends to form a large soft tissue mass (Fig. 20.32). The term dedifferentiated chondrosarcoma is applied to these tumours. Both low- and high-grade components are thought to arise from primitive stem cells which differentiate along different pathways. The term dedifferentiation, implying that differentiated cartilage cells revert to less mature forms, is inaccurate, but the term is familiar to orthopaedic surgeons and pathologists and remains in use.

Prognosis and Treatment

Most chondrosarcomas are slow growing tumours; they often run a prolonged course with repeated local recurrences. Tumours of the axial skeleton, especially on recurrence, may be sur-

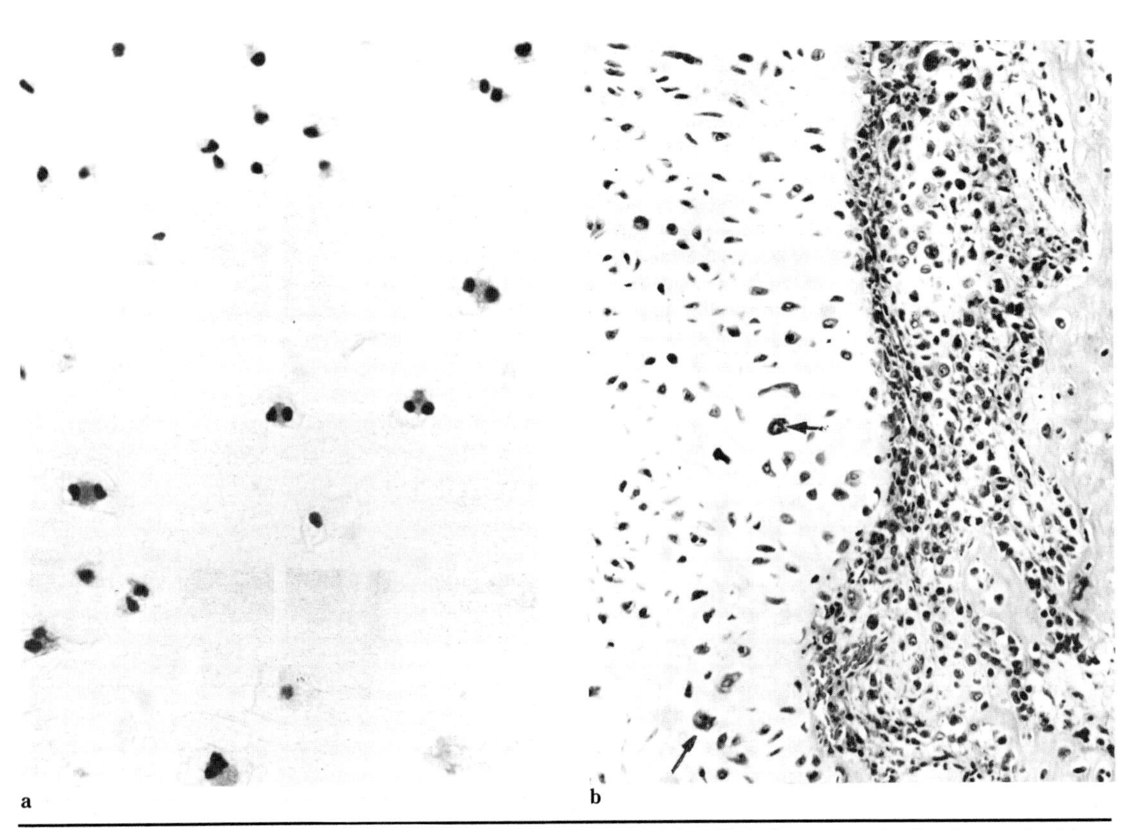

Fig. 20.31 **a** This recurrent low-grade chondrosarcoma of pelvis killed the patient by local spread without metastases. The cartilage matrix is well formed and the tumour is not very cellular but there are numerous foci of chondrocytes with plump double nuclei. ×250. **b** Metastasizing chondrosarcoma of ilium. The cartilage cells vary greatly in size and there are several mitoses, two of which are arrowed. ×100.

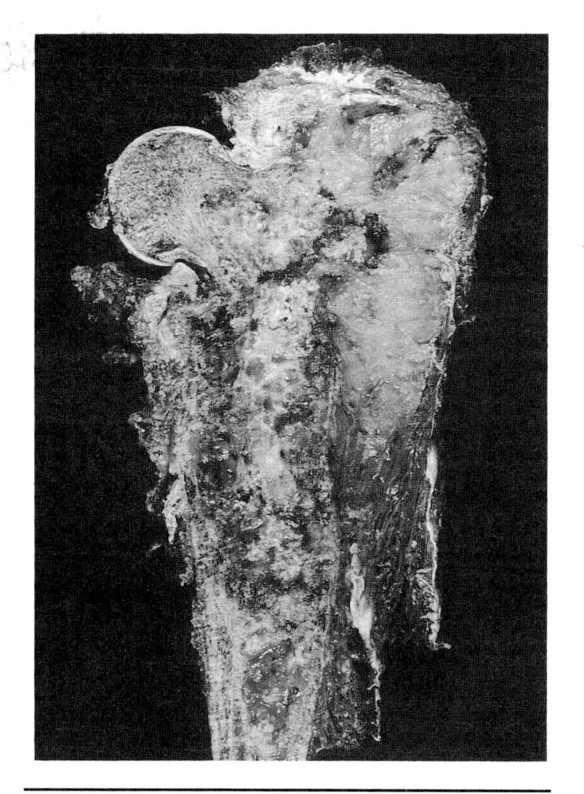

Fig. 20.32 Dedifferentiated chondrosarcoma of femur. A low-grade central chondrosarcoma occupies the medullary canal of the femur. There is a pathological fracture, and the greater trochanter has been destroyed by a fleshy tumour mass which extends widely into overlying skeletal muscle.

gically unresectable and eventually lead to death by involvement of vital structures. Chondrosarcoma has a tendency to implant and grow in soft tissues following biopsy or if tumour is exposed at the time of surgery. This is probably due to the low nutritional requirements of cartilage. Chondrosarcomas rarely metastasize; this occurs mainly in the 15% or so high-grade tumours where vascular permeation and pulmonary metastases are seen and in dedifferentiated chondrosarcomas in which the metastases are composed of the high-grade sarcomatous component. Successful management of chondrosarcoma is best achieved by adequate wide surgical excision at the first operation; this tumour is rarely sensitive to chemotherapy or radiotherapy.

Ewing's Sarcoma

This highly malignant tumour typically affects the diaphysis and metaphysis of long bones of children and adolescents, although pelvis, scapulae and ribs are also common sites. The tumour originates within the medullary cavity but early cortical penetration with periosteal elevation and formation of a soft tissue mass is usual. Radiographs show a moth-eaten pattern of bone destruction, often with parallel layers of reactive periosteal new bone (so-called onion-skin appearance) (Fig. 20.33).

The clinical presentation is usually of pain and swelling, but some patients are unwell with fever and elevation of white cell count and ESR, a picture simulating osteomyelitis. Grossly, the tumour may be very soft; in some cases the appearance at operation resembles pus, supporting the erroneous clinical diagnosis of infection.

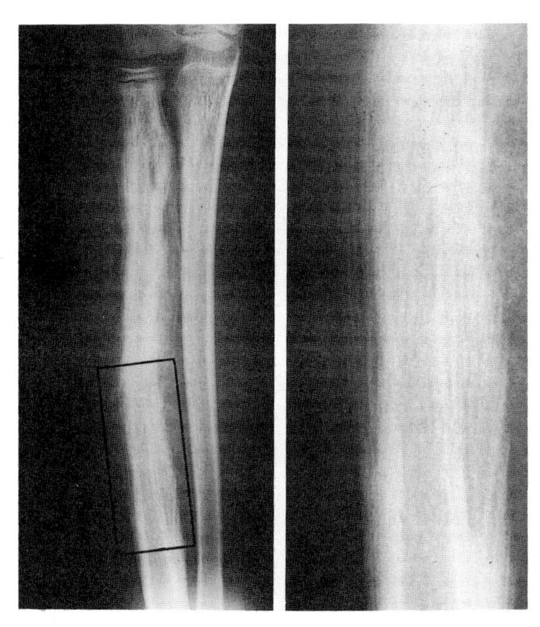

Fig. 20.33 Ewing's sarcoma of the radius. The shaft of the radius shows patchy lysis and sclerosis. The tumour has extended into soft tissue, and there is a layered periosteal reaction, shown at a higher power (right).

Pathology

Histologically, Ewing's sarcoma consists of sheets of uniform small round cells with pale oval nuclei and surprisingly little nuclear pleomorphism or mitotic activity. The cytoplasm is bubbly, and the cell boundaries are indistinct, giving the tumour a syncytial appearance (Fig. 20.34). The presence of intracellular glycogen and minimal intercellular reticulin together with lack of immunohistochemical staining for leucocyte common antigen assists in the distinction from lymphoma of bone. Metastatic neuroblastoma in young children may resemble Ewing's tumour but is associated with raised urinary catecholamine levels.

Prognosis and Treatment

Ewing's tumour is highly aggressive with early metastases to lung and other bones. The prognosis is especially poor in those patients with systemic symptoms, pelvic tumours or large soft tissue masses. Treatment with combination chemotherapy has significantly improved the prognosis. The histogenesis of Ewing's sarcoma is not known, although recent evidence suggests that it is a primitive tumour of neuroectodermal origin. Cytogenetic analysis has shown a reciprocal translocation [t(11;22)(q24;q12)] in many cases.

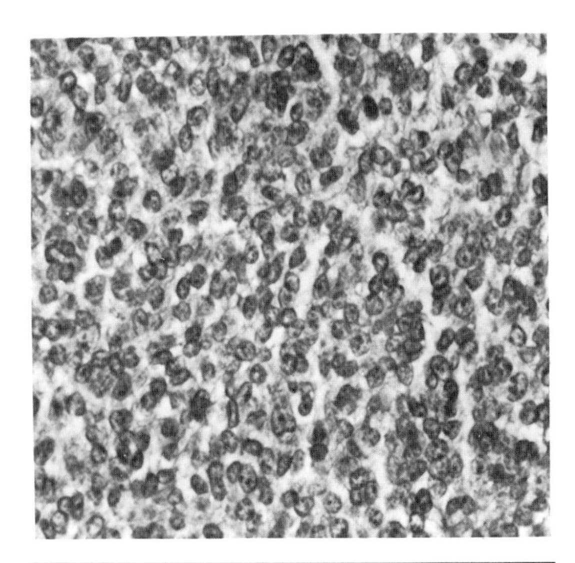

Fig. 20.34 Ewing's tumour of femur showing syncytial structure and uniform cell type. ×450.

Other Tumours in Bone

Giant-cell tumour (osteoclastoma). Giant-cell tumour principally affects patients between 20 and 40 years of age. Although flat bones may be involved, most tumours occur in long bones with half in the distal femur and proximal tibia. Almost all lesions arise in the bone end, although extension into the metaphysis is often seen. Giant-cell tumours are very rarely seen at the site of an open epiphyseal plate.

Giant-cell tumour is a lytic lesion which often causes marked eccentric expansion of the bone end (Fig. 20.35). It is covered initially by a thin shell of subperiosteal bone but after surgery this may later be breached as tumour extends into the soft tissue. Crack fracture of the bone shell or pathological fracture often occurs. Grossly the

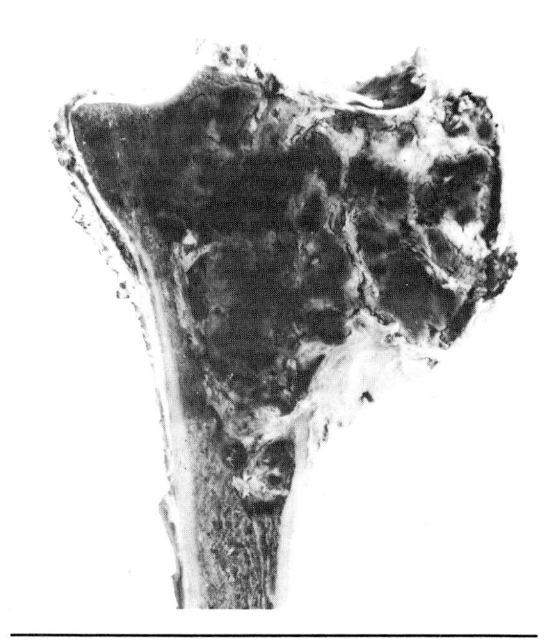

Fig. 20.35 Section of giant-cell tumour of upper end of tibia showing eccentric expansion of the bone end and much haemorrhage within the tumour.

tumour is soft, reddish-grey with areas of haemorrhage and necrosis. Microscopically, plump ovoid or spindle-shaped mononuclear cells are abundantly interspersed with very large osteoclasts (Fig. 20.36). Areas of fibrosis and reactive bone may be found, particularly after fracture or treatment.

Giant-cell tumour is a benign but locally aggressive tumour. The incidence of local recurrence depends on the extent of surgery. About 30% of the cases treated by curettage recur locally, often with soft tissue involvement. About 10% become malignant, usually after radiotherapy treatment, and metastasize to the lungs. These tumours contain areas of fibrosarcoma, malignant fibrous histiocytoma or osteosarcoma. Rarely, giant-cell tumours which appear histologically benign metastasize. These metastases often also lack the histological features of malignancy; in some cases they appear to have limited growth potential, while in others they progress rapidly.

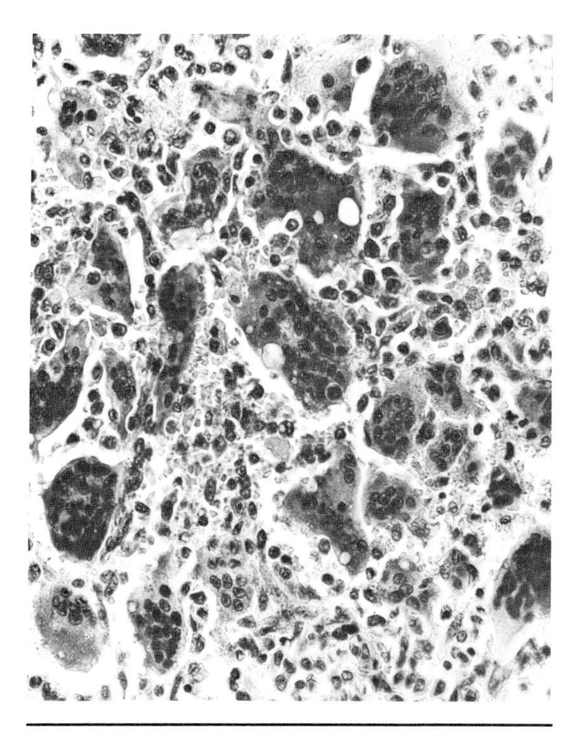

Fig. 20.36 Giant-cell tumour. The nuclei of the mononuclear tumour cells closely resemble those of the multinucleated osteoclasts.

Malignant fibrous histiocytoma (MFH). This group of tumours includes many lesions formerly regarded as fibrosarcomas. A wide age range of patients usually present with pain, swelling or pathological fracture. Typically a destructive lesion is seen in the metaphysis of a long bone. About a third of cases arise in association with pre-existing lesions such as Paget's disease, previous irradiation, long-standing bone infarcts or benign or low-grade malignant cartilage tumours. MFH is an aggressive tumour, early blood-borne metastases being common. The cells of malignant fibrous histiocytoma are typically arranged in short bundles radiating from a central point – a 'storiform' pattern like rush matting or the spokes of a wheel. Large multinucleate tumour cells, osteoclast-like giant cells and foci of lipid-laden macrophages are common, and the tumour is often heavily collagenized. Although histiocytes are present, evidence suggests that these are not neoplastic, and the tumour is probably best regarded as a primitive sarcoma of fibroblast origin.

Fibrosarcoma. The clinical features are very similar to those of MFH. Histologically, fibrosarcoma consists of more uniform spindle-shaped cells arranged in fascicles with a 'herring-bone' pattern. Like MFH the prognosis is poor; 40–50% of patients survive 5 years. Metastatic carcinoma, especially of bronchus and kidney, may have a spindle-cell appearance which can be confused with a fibrosarcoma or MFH.

Non-Hodgkin's lymphoma of bone. Although disseminated non-Hodgkin's lymphoma commonly involves bone, primary malignant lymphoma is relatively rare. Most tumours are diffuse non-Hodgkin's lymphomas of B-cell type, centroblastic or centrocytic/centroblastic (p. 663). In contrast to disseminated lymphoma involving bone, primary bone lymphoma has a relatively good prognosis; over 50% of patients survive 5 years.

Chordoma. This tumour, which is thought to arise from notochordal remnants, affects the sacrum, base of skull and less commonly the vertebrae. Most patients are middle aged or elderly and two-thirds are male. Chordomas are slow growing tumours with symptoms due to pressure on adjacent organs. Sacrococcygeal tumours give rise to pain, symptoms from sacral nerve compression and a palpable mass on rectal examination. Spheno-occipital tumours compress cranial nerves and rarely the pituitary. Chordomas are lobulated gelatinous tumours infiltrating bone and with an extraosseous mass covered by periosteum. Microscopy shows cords of cells in a sea of mucin. Many of the cells are vacuolated, the so-called physaliphorous (bubble-bearing) cells (Fig. 20.37). Chordomas tend to kill by local invasion. About 10% are said to have metastasized at the time of presentation, with up to 30% at autopsy. Chordomas express epithelial antigens such as cytokeratins and epithelial membrane antigen, and also S-100 protein. These features help in the distinction of chordomas from secondary carcinomas which express epithelial antigens but are usually negative for S-100 protein and from chondrosarcomas which are positive for S-100 but negative for epithelial markers.

Tumour-like Lesions of Bone

Fibrous dysplasia. Fibrous dysplasia is a benign fibro-osseous abnormality of bone of unknown aetiology, which may affect one or several bones. Rib, jaw, femur and tibia are common sites. Most patients present in childhood, with mild pain or swelling though sometimes repeated fractures lead to bone deformity. While most lesions stop growing after puberty, occasionally new ones appear. Malignant change is very rare in the absence of radiation therapy.

Fibrous dysplasia often expands the bone, has a well circumscribed border and consists of white gritty fibrous tissue, occasionally with cysts and nodules of cartilage. Histologically, loose spindle-celled fibrous stroma contains scattered curving 'lobster-claw' trabeculae of woven bone (Fig. 20.38). These are not arranged along stress lines

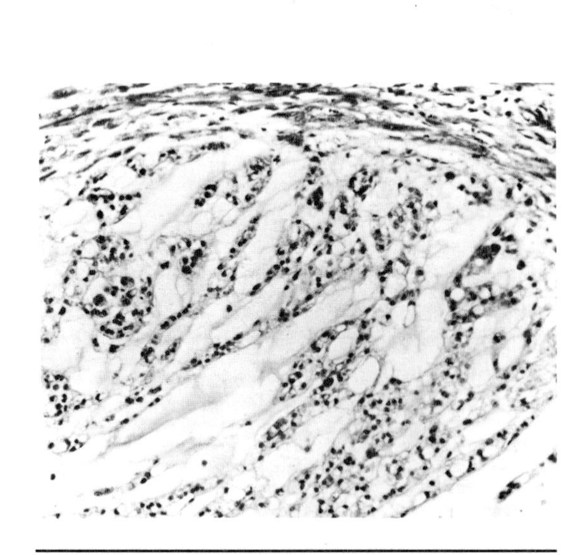

Fig. 20.37 Chordoma from sacrum. Strands of cells, many of them vacuolated, are seen lying in a background of mucinous material. ×140.

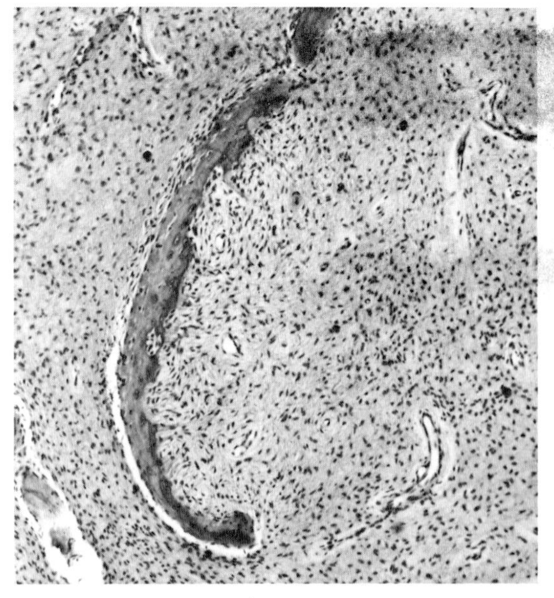

Fig. 20.38 Fibrous dysplasia of bone. The delicately cellular fibrous tissue contains a thin trabecula of woven bone. ×75.

and sometimes give rise to a 'ground-glass' appearance on radiology. Osteoblasts are not present on the surfaces of trabeculae which are formed by metaplasia from the fibrous stroma. The triad of polyostotic fibrous dysplasia (multiple bone involvement), patchy skin pigmentation and precocious puberty is referred to as **Albright's syndrome**. This condition is commoner in girls who may be of short stature due to premature epiphyseal fusion.

Metaphyseal fibrous defect. This is a common developmental abnormality with a distinctive radiological appearance; a radiolucent area with a scalloped sclerotic margin is seen in the metaphyseal cortex of long bones of children. These lesions may disappear spontaneously or enlarge to involve the medullary cavity, when they are known as **non-ossifying fibromas** and sometimes cause pathological fracture. Macroscopically, the lesion has a tan or orange colour due to the presence of some haemosiderin and many lipid-laden macrophages which lie in whorled fibrous tissue containing scattered small osteoclasts.

Eosinophil granuloma. This rare lesion, a localized form of histiocytosis X (p. 655), may occur at any age or site, but most commonly arises in children and young adults with one or more lesions in skull, long bones, vertebrae and pelvis. Sharply outlined lytic lesions are seen, although in long bones cortical erosion with an associated periosteal reaction may suggest malignancy. Vertebral involvement sometimes leads to bony collapse and a flat dense vertebra (vertebra plana). Histologically, groups of pale staining Langerhans' cells are mixed with numerous eosinophils. Patients with solitary or few lesions may be cured by surgery or low doses of radiotherapy; sometimes eosinophil granulomas heal spontaneously. It is important to ascertain whether there is systemic involvement for this worsens the prognosis.

Cysts of Bone

Aneurysmal bone cyst. This lesion of children and young adults may affect any bone but typically the posterior elements of vertebrae and the metaphysis of long bones. Patients complain of pain and of swelling which often increases rapidly. Radiographs show a well circumscribed area of bone lysis, often with very marked eccentric expansion sometimes described as a 'blow out'. A thin shell of new bone is usually present at the subperiosteal margin. Anastomosing blood-filled spaces are seen, separated by fibrous septa containing a few woven bone trabeculae and osteoclastic giant cells (Fig. 20.39). Although aneurysmal bone cysts may simulate a malignant tumour clinically and radiologically, they are benign. They sometimes heal following biopsy or incomplete removal, and are probably not neoplastic. A variety of benign and malignant tumours contain areas of secondary aneurysmal bone cyst change, so the pathologist must examine the entire specimen for any pre-existing lesion.

Simple (unicameral) bone cysts are common findings in children and adolescents and affect the

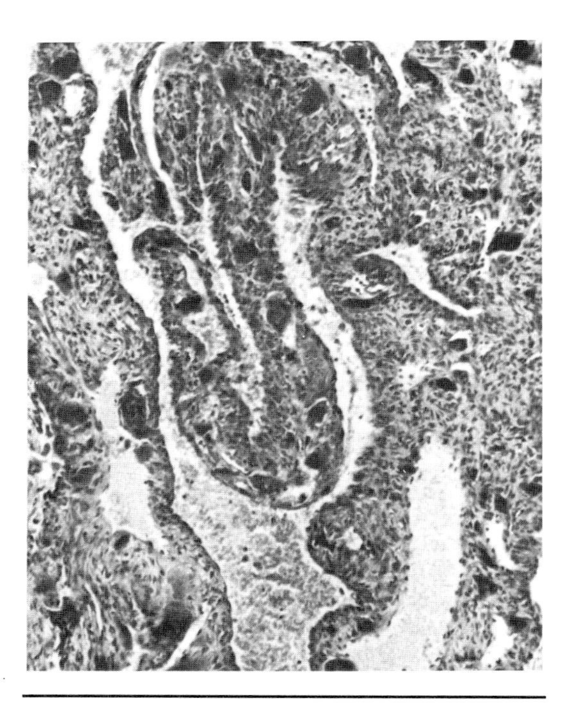

Fig. 20.39 Aneurysmal bone cyst. Vascular spaces lined by strands of fibrous tissue with giant cells. ×45.

metaphyses of the humerus, femur and tibia. The patient typically presents with a crack fracture of the bony shell or a frank pathological fracture. Radiological examination shows a central area of lysis which thins the cortex and slightly expands the bone. Cysts are thought to result from a disturbance of growth at the epiphyseal line and are located in the metaphysis abutting the plate. Serial radiographs often show the epiphysis growing away from the cyst so that the cyst comes to lie in the diaphysis. The cyst is smooth walled and contains clear fluid unless there has been a fracture. The wall of the cyst consists of a layer of fibrous tissue, sometimes containing osteoclasts, haemosiderin and new woven bone. Partially calcified fibrinous deposits are a typical feature. The cysts may be treated by curettage and grafting or by injection of steroids. The cysts adjacent to the epiphyseal plate recur more often than those separated from it.

Subchondral cysts are frequently seen in osteoarthritis. Similar fibrous walled cysts containing mucoid fluid may occur near the bone end in the absence of degenerative joint disease and are referred to as *intraosseous ganglia.*

Hydatid cysts (p. 1174) may occur in bone.

Diseases of Joints

Two types of joint exist. Synovial (diarthrodial) joints have a synovial lining and usually allow large amounts of movement. Synarthroses, joints where movement is very limited, will not be discussed further.

Articular Cartilage

The bone ends are covered by hyaline cartilage, an avascular tissue which provides a smooth, low friction surface allowing joint movement. It is capable of resisting compressive forces by deforming under mechanical loading but recovers its shape on removal of the load. Normal articular cartilage is a smooth bluish translucent material, which is composed of chondrocytes, proteoglycans, collagen and water.

Collagen. Eighty-five to 90% of collagen in articular cartilage is type II, while type V and type IX collagen are also found, chiefly around chondrocytes. Other proteins such as chondronectin and anchorin may link collagen and chondrocytes. In the deep and intermediate zones collagen fibres are orientated perpendicular to the articular surface, while in the superficial zone the fibres lie parallel to the surface, forming the lamina splendens (Fig. 20.40). Articular cartilage adjacent to underlying bone is calcified. A wavy basophilic line indicates the heavily calcified border between calcified and non-calcified cartilage.

Proteoglycans. The intercellular matrix of cartilage contains complexes of proteoglycan core proteins, link proteins, hyaluronic acid and glycosaminoglycans. These macromolecules are capable of binding large amounts of water. The numerous anionic groups on glycosaminoglycan chains cause mutual repulsion. Together these factors endow cartilage with the ability to resist compression. Proteoglycans are not evenly distributed in cartilage, being present in larger amounts in deeper zones and around chondrocytes.

Chondrocytes synthesize matrix components (e.g. collagen and proteoglycans) as well as enzymes (e.g. collagenase) capable of degrading them. As protein synthesizing cells, they contain abundant rough endoplasmic reticulum and prominent Golgi apparatus. They are also capable of

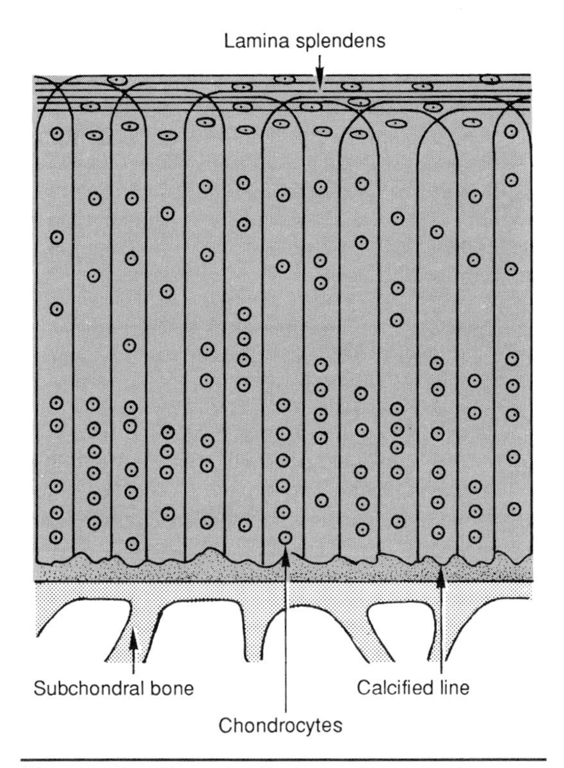

Fig. 20.40 Normal articular cartilage. In the superficial zone collagen fibres are orientated parallel to the surface of the cartilage forming the lamina splendens. Beneath this, the collagen is arranged perpendicular to the surface. A calcified line marks the boundary between articular cartilage and a thin zone of calcified cartilage which abuts on the subchondral bone plate.

phagocytosis, for example of erythrocyte breakdown products in chronic haemarthrosis. The 'lacunae' seen around chondrocytes by light microscopy are an artefact caused by shrinkage of cytoplasm during fixation.

Synovium

The synovial membrane covers all intra-articular structures except articular cartilage and fibrocartilaginous menisci. It consists of a layer of fibrous or adipose tissue supporting a surface of synovial lining cells. These cells are specialized mesenchymal cells, and are not epithelial; they do not have a basement membrane. Electron microscopy and immunostaining have identified subtypes of synovial lining cells. Type I (known to electron microscopists as type A cells) are macrophage-like cells containing lysosomes and expressing macrophage immunophenotype. Type II cells are non-phagocytic cells bearing HLA-DR antigens but no other monocyte markers. Type III cells (type B cells of electron microscopy) are fibroblast-like and contain abundant rough endoplasmic reticulum.

Synovial fluid is an ultrafiltrate of plasma into which hyaluronic acid is secreted by synovial cells. In health this viscous fluid is present in small amounts, acts as a lubricant and especially in adults is of great importance in the nutrition of articular cartilage.

Arthritis

Disorders of the joints are among the most disabling of conditions. They cause serious morbidity to the affected individual, and they are of major economic importance both to the patients, who may have long periods off work, and to society as a whole. Joint replacement is a very common and expensive operation in terms of professional time, bed occupancy and prosthetic materials. About 100 000 total hip replacements are carried out each year in the USA, mostly for osteoarthritis and rheumatoid arthritis.

In this section we will consider osteoarthritis, the most common form of joint disease, and contrast it with rheumatoid arthritis, one of the autoimmune diseases. A number of other inflammatory arthritides will be described, but these are much less common. Infections of joints have already been discussed.

Osteoarthritis

The commonest chronic joint disease, osteoarthritis is largely a disease of the elderly. It is not an inflammatory disorder, but a degenerative disease. Similar degenerative changes are found on radiography or at autopsy in some joints in almost all subjects over 60 years of age. The prevalence of symptomatic disease is much less, but osteoarthritis is a major cause of morbidity. Osteoarthritis principally affects the large weight bearing joints (hip, knee) and the joints of the cervical and lower lumbar spine. Osteoarthritis in the young is usually seen only when there is a predisposing cause (Table 20.9). Primary generalized osteoarthritis, sometimes with a familial incidence and more common in females, affects multiple joints including the interphalangeal joints of the hands. Palpable osteophytes of the distal and proximal interphalangeal joints are known as Heberden's and Bouchard's nodes respectively. Although unsightly, these cause little disability.

Patients complain of pain, relieved by rest, and of stiffness and sometimes crepitus on movement. Osteoarthritis of the hip often results in a characteristic limp (antalgic gait). Spinal involvement, principally of the intervertebral discs and the posterior apophyseal joints is very common, and gives rise to stiffness and pain due to compression of nerve roots, particularly in the cervical spine. Bony spurs may compress the vertebral arteries compromising cerebral blood flow.

Table 20.9 Causes of osteoarthritis

Primary
Secondary
Underlying joint disorders
Intra-articular fracture
Previous infective arthritis
Rheumatoid or other inflammatory arthritis
Osteonecrosis including Perthes' disease
Congenital dislocation of hip
Slipped capital femoral epiphysis
Abnormal stresses
Malaligned fracture
Paget's disease with deformity
? Chronic over-use
Metabolic/endocrine
Ochronosis (alkaptonuria)
Haemochromatosis
Calcium pyrophosphate deposition
Gout
Neuropathic disorders
Peripheral neuropathy in diabetes mellitus
Intra-articular corticosteroids in excess
Tabes dorsalis
Syringomyelia

Pathology

In osteoarthritis changes are seen within the articular cartilage, the underlying bone and, secondarily, within the synovium.

An early change is loss of proteoglycan from the superficial zone of articular cartilage. Disruption of the smooth surface of cartilage follows, initially tangential to the surface (flaking) and then extending vertically into the deeper zones (fibrillation) (Fig. 20.41); this pattern conforms to the arrangement of collagen fibres previously described (p. 984). Proliferation of chondrocytes, forming clusters around fissures, and increased proteoglycan synthesis may be regarded as attempts at healing, but this is unsuccessful and progressive loss of articular cartilage occurs by abrasion, with eventual exposure of the underlying bone.

Along with these changes the subchondral bone trabeculae become greatly thickened particularly in areas of cartilage loss. Here the bone is polished smooth (eburnation) (Fig. 20.41), sometimes with grooves worn in the direction of joint movement (Fig. 20.42). Any marrow spaces exposed tend to become plugged by proliferating fibrocartilage. Cystic spaces containing loose, degenerate fibrous tissue appear in the subchondral marrow spaces and the adjacent trabeculae are thickened.

Marked bone remodelling results in alteration of the contour of the joint surface. This is particularly obvious in osteoarthritis of the femoral head where the superior surface is flattened. At the margin of the articular cartilage outgrowths of proliferating cartilage develop and undergo enchondral ossification to become osteophytes (Fig. 20.43). These may cause deformity and limitation of movement.

The synovium may be normal, but often villous hypertrophy and fibrosis are seen. There is sometimes infiltration by lymphocytes and occasional plasma cells. Abraded fragments of bone and cartilage which become embedded in the synovium

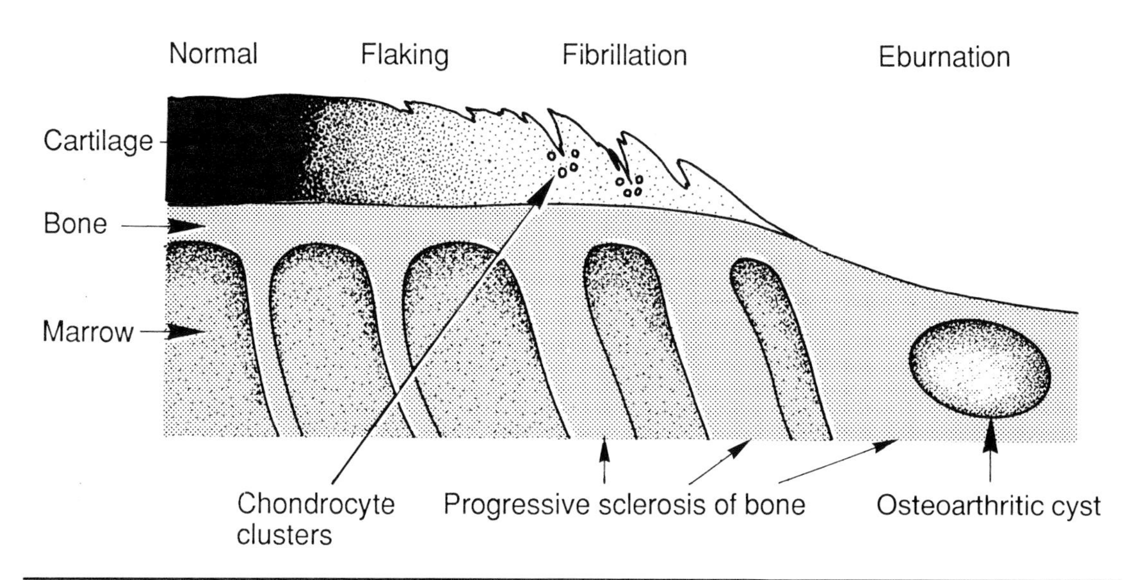

Fig. 20.41 A schematic representation of the sequential changes of osteoarthritis. Loss of proteoglycan from the articular cartilage is followed by superficial flaking and deeper fibrillation. Despite proliferation of chondrocytes loss of articular cartilage occurs with exposure of the underlying bone. These changes are accompanied by progressive sclerosis of the subchondral bone and sometimes by the formation of subchondral cysts.

stimulate mild reactive synovitis (detritus synovitis).

Aetiology and Pathogenesis

Osteoarthritis is not a single disease, but the end result of joint damage from many causes. The reasons for joint destruction in many of the secondary forms of osteoarthritis (Table 20.9) are easy to understand. Thus, loss of articular cartilage due to previous septic or rheumatoid arthritis or an incongruity of the articular surface due to an intra-articular fracture can readily be accepted as leading to further cartilage damage.

The role of chronic overuse as a cause of osteoarthritis, for example in the knees and ankles of footballers and the metatarsophalangeal joints of ballet dancers, is disputed. There is little convincing evidence that chronic loading alone causes osteoarthritis, but little doubt that repeated injuries, to the menisci or ligaments for instance, may be associated with the subsequent development of osteoarthritis.

The pathogenesis of primary osteoarthritis is poorly understood. Alterations in the metabolism of chondrocytes and the biochemistry of the cartilaginous matrix, in particular of proteoglycans, are well defined. The water content of both ageing and osteoarthritic cartilage is increased, and proteoglycan concentration decreased. Some authors believe that the primary change in osteoarthritis is an alteration in the biochemical composition of the articular cartilage and that all other changes are consequences of this. Others have suggested that the primary abnormality is thickening of the subchondral bone plate, which prevents dissipation of compressive forces from cartilage to underlying bone and may lead to cartilage degeneration during repetitive loading.

Recently, much interest has focused on the role of inflammatory mediators such as prostaglandins and interleukin 1, which have been shown to affect chondrocyte metabolism. Interleukin 1, for example, suppresses chondrocyte proteoglycan synthesis. These factors may not initiate osteoarthritis, but are probably involved in progression of cartilage destruction.

The difficulty in interpreting all these findings is in distinguishing those changes which cause

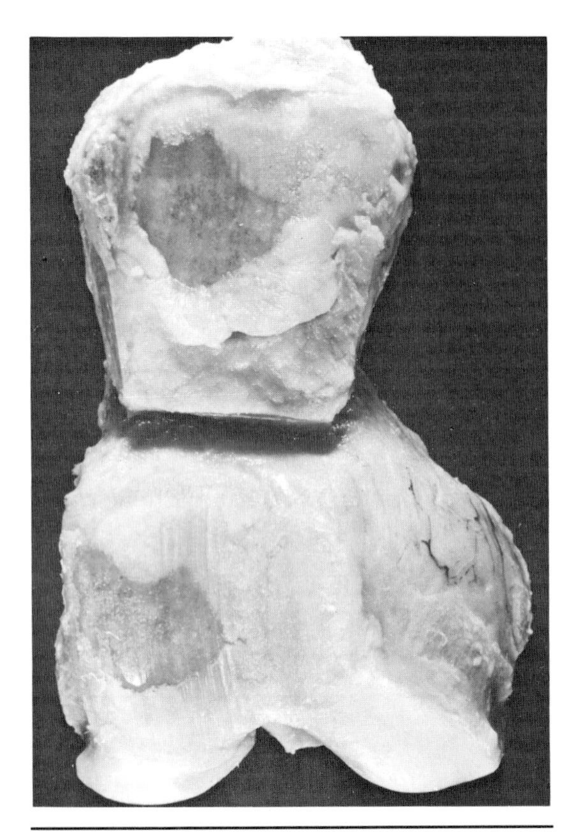

Fig. 20.42 Osteoarthritis of the knee joint has caused complete loss of articular cartilage with exposure of the bone on opposing surfaces of the patella (above) and the femur. There is parallel scoring of the joint surface.

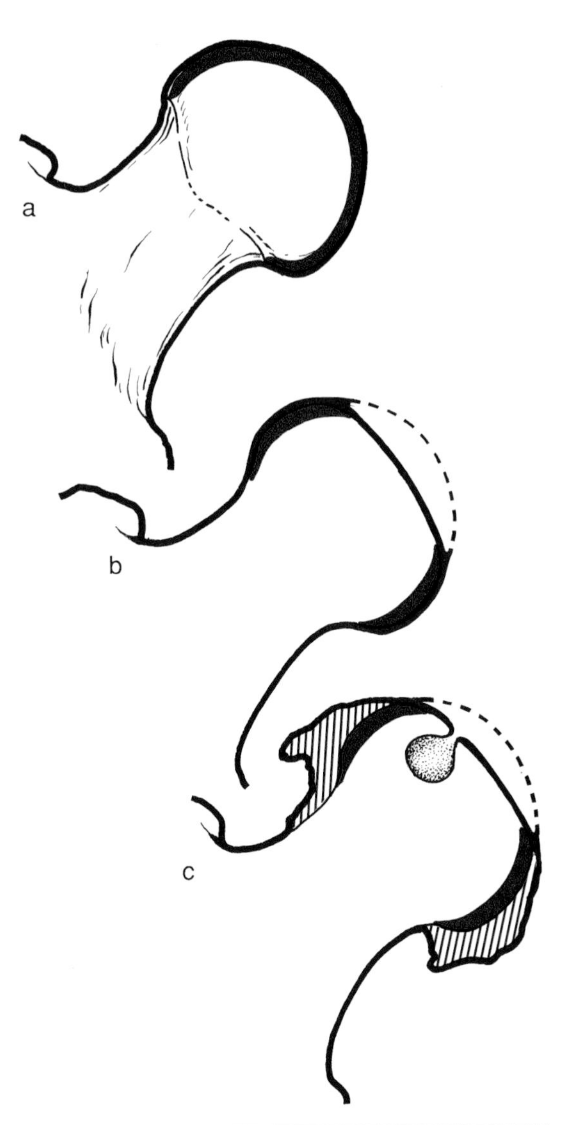

Fig. 20.43 Osteoarthritis of the femoral head. As articular cartilage is lost the femoral head loses its spherical shape **a** and becomes flattened **b**. Osteophytes at the margin are formed **c** by proliferation of cartilage which undergoes enchondral ossification.

osteoarthritis from those which are consequences of the disorder.

Neuropathic Arthropathy (Charcot's Joint)

This accelerated form of osteoarthritis occurs in a joint which has lost proprioceptive and pain sensation (Table 20.9). The cartilage is destroyed and the bone ends become distorted with formation of very large osteophytes. These may fracture, as may the joint surface with hyperplastic callus formation. Progressive disorganization of the joint results, the florid changes contrasting with the relative lack of pain.

Rheumatoid Arthritis (RA)

In contrast to osteoarthritis (Table 20.10), rheumatoid arthritis is a systemic inflammatory disease, the brunt of which usually falls on the joints.

It is common, affecting 1% of the adult population; three-quarters of patients are female. Any age from childhood to old age may be affected, but the onset is typically in the third to fifth decades.

Rheumatoid arthritis may involve any synovial joint, but is usually a symmetrical polyarthritis affecting principally the metacarpophalangeal and proximal interphalangeal joints, the wrist, shoulder and knee. Patients complain of pain and stiffness especially in the morning. The affected joints are warm and swollen due to joint effusion and synovial hyperplasia. The onset is usually insidious over weeks or months, but rarely symptoms may develop acutely in a few days. In most cases the disease follows a course of repeated remissions and relapses, with further loss of function during each relapse. Less commonly, the disease progresses rapidly with joint destruction and severe disability. Some patients have a few attacks of arthritis which resolve without functional loss.

In 85% of patients, **rheumatoid factors** (p. 230) can be identified in the serum and synovial fluid. These are antibodies, usually of IgM, IgG and IgA type, whose antigen binding sites react with the Fc component of IgG forming immune complexes. Patients whose serum contains these antibodies are known as seropositive. This is associated with more aggressive disease than those without rheumatoid factors (seronegative).

Pathology

Joint involvement in RA is characterized by inflammation and hyperplasia of the synovium followed by destruction of articular structures. The synovium is thrown into villous folds often matted together by fibrin (Fig. 20.44); both hypertrophy and hyperplasia of synovial lining cells occur. The synovium is infiltrated by lymphocytes and plasma cells; lymphoid aggregates with germinal centres are often seen (Fig. 20.45). Exudation of fibrin onto the synovial surface occurs, sometimes forming soft loose bodies known as rice bodies. Neutrophil polymorphs are present in synovial fluid from inflamed joints and are seen in the superficial synovium in significant numbers during acute exacerbations.

These changes in the synovium are reversible; however, when granulation tissue grows over the surface of the articular cartilage the **pannus** so

Table 20.10 A comparison of rheumatoid arthritis and osteoarthritis

	Rheumatoid arthritis	Osteoarthritis
Age	Any age, mainly 25–55	Predominantly in elderly
Affected joints	Symmetrical arthritis Metacarpophalangeal, proximal interphalangeal, wrists, shoulders, knees	Often one affected joint – hip, knee, ankle Hereditary form – proximal interphalangeal and distal interphalangeal joints
Synovium	Hyperplastic, dense chronic inflammation	Mild 'secondary' inflammation
Articular cartilage	Eroded by pannus from periphery	Flaking, fibrillation and loss on weight bearing surface
Subchondral bone	Osteoporotic Marginal erosions	Sclerotic Cysts
Osteophytes	Usually absent	Present
Systemic disease	Yes – see text for extra-articular manifestations	No
Pathogenesis	Autoimmune disease	Degenerative

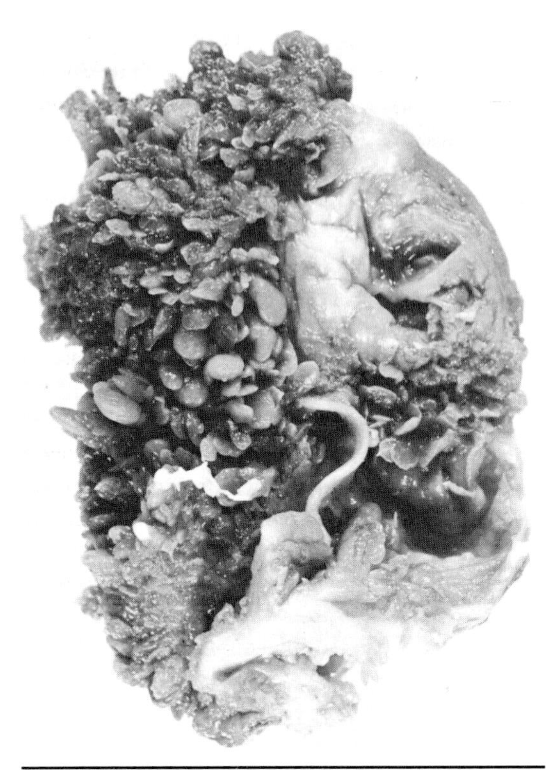

Fig. 20.44 Synovium from a rheumatoid knee joint. The synovial surface is markedly frondose and some of the villi are tipped with white fibrin.

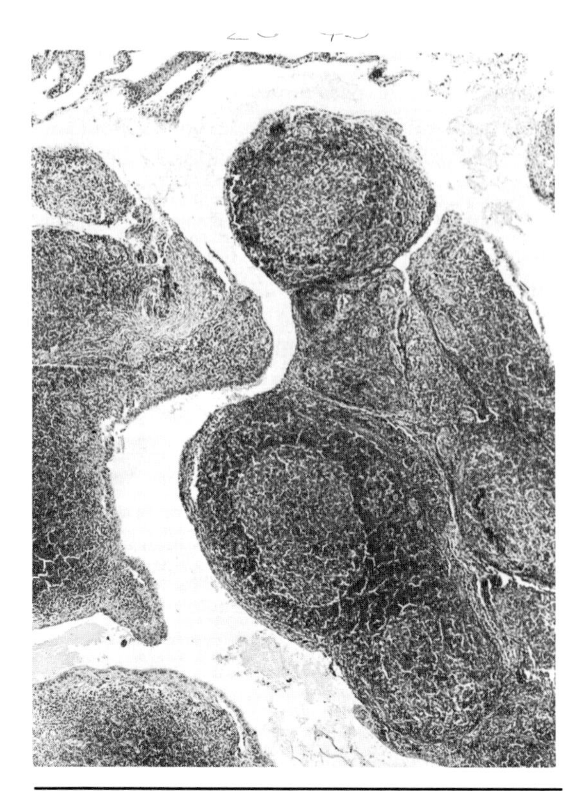

Fig. 20.45 Synovial membrane in chronic rheumatoid arthritis. The synovium shows villous hypertrophy and is extensively infiltrated with lymphocytes, amongst which occur poorly defined germinal centres. Plasma cells also are abundant. ×38.

formed interferes with the nutrition of cartilage and causes enzymatic degradation of its matrix (Fig. 20.46). Permanent joint damage now results. Pannus may spread into the subchondral bone giving rise to radiological 'erosions'. If much articular cartilage is lost, granulation tissue from both sides of the joint forms adhesions, followed sometimes by fibrous union (fibrous ankylosis). Bony ankylosis very occasionally affects the small joints of the hands and feet.

Striking deformities of ulnar deviation of the fingers (Fig. 20.47) with dislocation and subluxation lead to characteristic boutonnière and swan neck deformities. These result from destruction of the joint capsule and also of tendons, which are eroded by inflamed synovium of their sheaths. There is atrophy of muscles surrounding the joints (e.g. interossei in the hand), while a combination of disuse atrophy and local hyperaemia leads to loss of bone close to the bone ends (juxta-articular osteoporosis). Involvement of the cervical spine may cause atlantoaxial subluxation and spinal cord compression. Hyperextension during intubation for general anaesthesia may precipitate neurological damage.

Extra-articular Manifestations of Rheumatoid Arthritis

It must be re-emphasized that RA is a multisystem disease; while its effects on the joints give rise to much morbidity, there are many extra-articular complications which may be severe and life threatening.

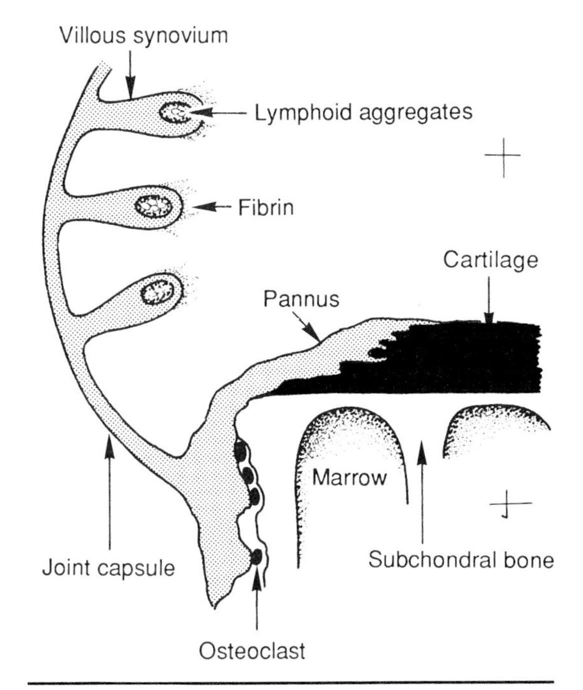

Fig. 20.46 Rheumatoid arthritis. Hyperplastic synovium is thrown up into villous folds containing lymphoid aggregates. A pannus of granulation tissue grows over and erodes the articular cartilage and the subchondral bone undergoes osteoclastic resorption.

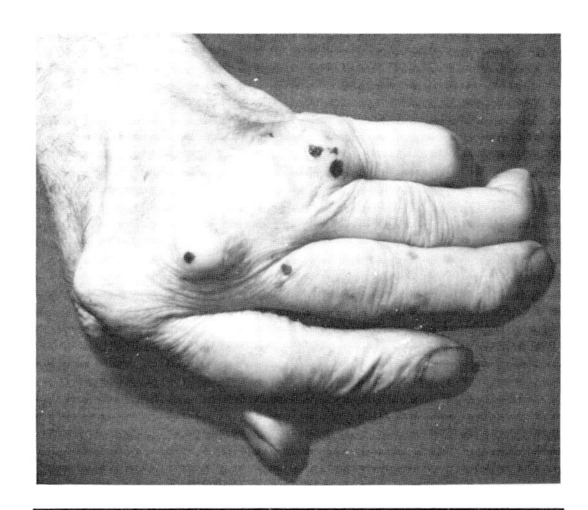

Fig. 20.47 The hand shows the typical severe deformity of rheumatoid arthritis with marked ulnar deviation of the fingers and muscle wasting. Ulcerated rheumatoid nodules are present over the metacarpophalangeal joints.

Rheumatoid nodules. These nodules consist of a central area of fibrinoid necrosis (Fig. 20.48) surrounded by macrophages and fibrous tissue containing chronic inflammatory cells. Rheumatoid nodules are found in 20–35% of patients with RA and are typically located in the subcutaneous tissues over extensor surfaces such as the olecranon process, but may also be seen in the visceral organs. Rheumatoid nodules usually develop in patients who are seropositive; their presence often indicates a more aggressive course.

Vasculitis. Arteritis with fibrinoid necrosis of the vessel wall (p. 464), although rare in RA, usually affects seropositive patients with severe disease. Immune-complex deposition with complement activation is responsible for the damage to the vessel wall. The effects are usually mild with splinter haemorrhages in the nail folds, but gangrene of digits and infarction of viscera occasionally occur. Vasculitis may cause peripheral neuropathy (p. 863).

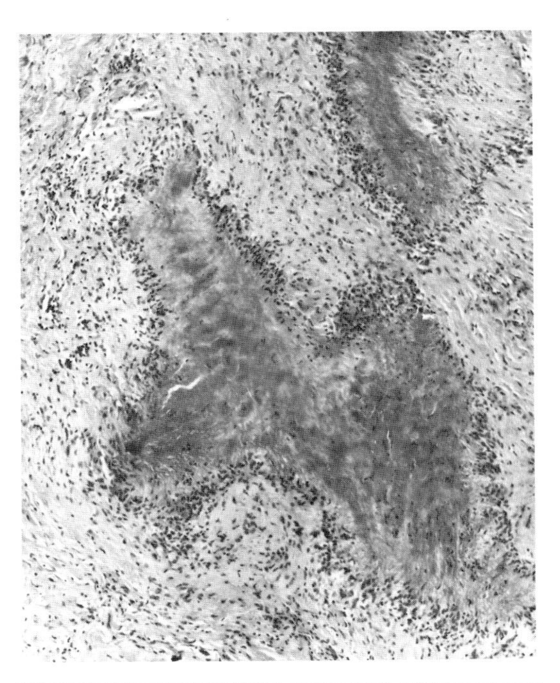

Fig. 20.48 Rheumatoid nodule from the region of the elbow joint. ×90.

Cardiac disease. Rheumatoid nodules in or near the conducting system occasionally lead to heart block, while coronary arteritis is a rare cause of myocardial infarction. It must be emphasized that most myocardial infarction in patients with RA is due to coronary atheroma and thrombosis. Myocarditis and endocarditis are seldom seen.

Pulmonary disease (p. 572). Patients with rheumatoid arthritis sometimes develop diffuse pulmonary fibrosis. Rheumatoid nodules are occasionally found in the lung and very rarely large nodules with central breakdown and widespread fibrosis occur in patients with pneumoconiosis. This is known as Caplan's syndrome. The incidence of this complication has diminished with that of pneumoconiosis.

Serosal inflammation. Pericarditis and pleurisy are often found at autopsy, but, in contrast, are seldom of clinical importance.

Amyloidosis. Rheumatoid arthritis is one of the most common causes of secondary (AA) amyloidosis (p. 246).

Anaemia. Like many chronic diseases, rheumatoid arthritis is often complicated by microcytic hypochromic anaemia (anaemia of chronic disease, p. 619), while non-steroidal anti-inflammatory drugs may produce acute erosive gastritis, with repeated minor episodes of gastrointestinal blood loss and iron deficiency.

Felty's syndrome. Less than 1% of patients with RA, usually those with other extra-articular manifestations, develop splenomegaly with hypersplenism and granulocytopenia which may lead to infections. Nodular regenerative hyperplasia of the liver (p. 750) is seen in some patients with Felty's syndrome, and rarely in others with rheumatoid arthritis.

Eye involvement. Keratoconjunctivitis sicca as part of Sjögren's syndrome (p. 681) is the commonest ocular complication of rheumatoid arthritis. Inflammation of the sclera (scleritis) may lead to perforation of the globe (scleromalacia perforans). Histologically, this is characterized by fibrinoid necrosis of collagen with surrounding histiocytes, a reaction similar to the rheumatoid nodule. Disastrous consequences follow corneal stroma lysis which in contrast is due to release of collagenases; perforation occurs in the absence of a significant inflammatory reaction.

Aetiology and Pathogenesis

Despite much research the cause of rheumatoid arthritis remains unknown. This is a complex problem and only a simplified account can be given. A summary of the mechanisms thought to be responsible is given in Fig. 20.49.

Rheumatoid arthritis is an autoimmune disorder affecting individuals with a genetic predisposition who are exposed to an appropriate antigenic stimulus. Once initiated, the disease appears to be self-perpetuating.

Genetic predisposition. It has long been known that rheumatoid arthritis has a familial tendency, but that not all members of a family are affected. Susceptibility to rheumatoid arthritis is associated with certain alleles of the class II major histo-

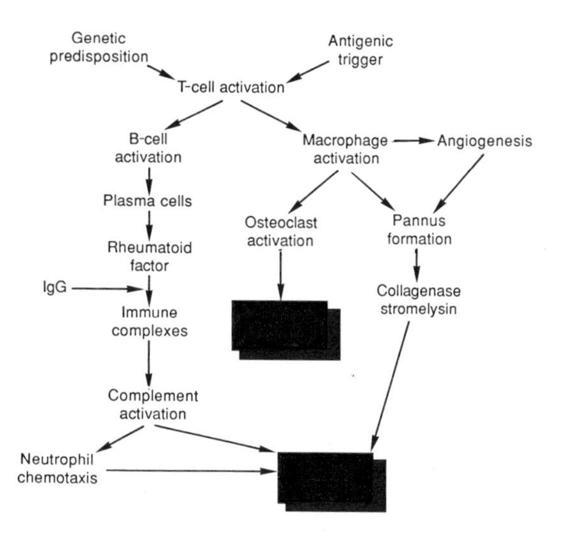

Fig. 20.49 Possible pathogenetic mechanisms of joint destruction in rheumatoid arthritis.

compatibility complex (MHC) particularly HLA-DR4. Class II MHC molecules are expressed on the surface of antigen-presenting cells and are essential for recognition of antigen by T cells. Predisposition to rheumatoid arthritis appears to be conferred by those alleles, such as HLA-DR4, which encode specific amino-acid sequences in the β chain. This results in a particular molecular configuration which may lead to an altered immune response to certain antigens, including auto-antigens (p. 233).

Initiating factors. The trigger for the development of RA has not been identified. It is possible that a variety of different antigenic stimuli may be responsible. The prime suspects have been infective agents, in particular viruses such as Epstein–Barr virus and human parvovirus. Evidence that RA is initiated by an infection is circumstantial; certainly none of the suggested organisms fulfils Koch's postulates.

It has been suggested that endogenous antigens may be responsible for triggering RA. Autoantibodies directed against IgG (rheumatoid factors) and type II collagen are found in the serum and synovial fluid of many patients with RA, but there is no convincing evidence that these have initiated the disease. However, there is little doubt that the immune complexes which form within joints are involved in amplification of the inflammatory process and in tissue destruction.

Development of synovitis. The earliest pathological change found in rheumatoid synovium is a perivascular accumulation of T lymphocytes (principally CD4 positive). It is thought that synovial lining cells and macrophages process antigen and present it to T lymphocytes which then proliferate. Southern blot analysis of T-cell receptor gene rearrangement suggests that relatively few clones of T cells are involved in this process. T cells play an essential role in the activation of B cells and in their differentiation to plasma cells, which produce antibodies including rheumatoid factors. Activated macrophages release many of the proteolytic enzymes involved in cartilage destruction and also stimulate proliferation of endothelial cells (angiogenesis). In this way the synovial membrane mass is greatly increased with an extensive network of new blood vessels, an accumulation of T cells, B cells, plasma cells and macrophages.

Destruction of joint structures. The irreversible destruction of the joint occurs when the proliferating granulation tissue grows over articular cartilage and invades subchondral bone, tendons and joint capsule. Synovial cells and macrophages produce proteolytic enzymes such as collagenase and stromelysin, which are capable of destroying the matrix proteins of cartilage and bone. Cytokines such as interleukin 1 act on chondrocytes to reduce the production of intercellular matrix and also to secrete enzymes such as collagenase which break down existing matrix. Immune complexes formed by rheumatoid factors and IgG activate complement (p. 230) which contributes to tissue damage. Chemotactic factors such as C5a and leukotriene B_4 attract neutrophil polymorphs into the synovial fluid. These cells degranulate with the release of proteinases which participate in the destruction of articular cartilage. Erosion of subchondral bone is largely attributable to activation of osteoclasts by cytokines such as interleukin 1 and by prostaglandins rather than by direct proteolytic action.

Juvenile Rheumatoid Arthritis

This disease differs in several ways from adult rheumatoid arthritis. By definition the disorder starts below the age of 16, most commonly between 1 and 3 years. Patients may present with involvement of many or few joints, or with severe systemic disease which may precede the development of arthritis. These patients have a high spiking fever, often with daily or twice-daily elevations of temperature, accompanied by a distinctive macular rash on the trunk, proximal limbs and over pressure areas. There may be hepatosplenomegaly, lymphadenopathy or serosal inflammation, especially pericarditis.

Juvenile rheumatoid arthritis generally involves the knees, wrists, elbows and ankles and the small joints of the hands and feet. Involvement of the cervical spine and sacroiliac joints is common. Most patients are seronegative. Other features include growth retardation and chronic uveitis which may lead to blindness.

The pathological features resemble those seen in adult rheumatoid arthritis. The disease often persists into adult life but occasionally remits spontaneously.

Seronegative Arthritides

This term is applied to a group of inflammatory polyarthritides in which tests for rheumatoid factor are negative and which tend to involve the sacroiliac joints and the spine (spondylitis) as well as peripheral joints. The group includes ankylosing spondylitis, psoriatic arthropathy, Reiter's syndrome and arthritis associated with Crohn's disease and ulcerative colitis, but excludes cases of seronegative rheumatoid arthritis.

Association with HLA-B27. There is a strong association between seronegative arthritis with sacroiliac involvement and the histocompatibility antigen HLA-B27 (p. 176). About 8% of a general Caucasian population possess this antigen, while over 90% of patients with ankylosing spondylitis, 70–90% with Reiter's syndrome and 50–70% with psoriatic or enteropathic arthropathy with sacroiliitis are positive. It is not known whether HLA-B27 is responsible for ankylosing spondylitis or only a marker for another closely linked gene. Most evidence suggests that the former is true. Patients homozygous for HLA-B27 tend to have more severe disease. Approximately 25% of HLA-B27 positive individuals develop ankylosing spondylitis.

Ankylosing Spondylitis

This is now recognized to be a common disorder with a prevalence of 0.5–1% in Western populations, although in many cases, especially in women, symptoms are mild and recognition depends on radiological changes. Patients, often with a family history and typically in their early twenties, complain of persistent sacroiliac and lumbar pain with limitation of movement. The onset is usually insidious. As many as 20% of patients present with symptoms of pain and swelling relating to asymmetric involvement of the peripheral joints, especially of the lower limbs; during the course of the disease a further 15% develop similar problems. The condition is usually self-limiting but in a minority of patients it progresses until the spine is fused (bamboo spine) (Fig. 20.50). Physiotherapy is important in regulating posture to prevent spinal fusion in a stooped position (Fig. 20.51). When the cervical spine is involved, fracture or atlantoaxial dislocation may occur after minor injury and care must be exercised during anaesthesia.

Ankylosing spondylitis is characterized by inflammation occurring at the bony insertion of ligaments, joint capsule and fibres of the annulus fibrosus of the intervertebral disc. The site of ligamentous insertion is the **enthesis**, and the resultant condition is known as enthesopathy. Inflammation is followed by fibrosis and ossification, particularly at the margins of intervertebral discs, with the formation of bridging spurs of bone (**syndesmophytes**). Similar ossification occurs across the apophyseal and sacroiliac joints, and sometimes the costovertebral joints. The synovitis histologically resembles that seen in rheumatoid arthritis. Bony ankylosis is more common than in rheumatoid arthritis, and may affect large joints, particularly the hips.

Extra-articular manifestations. Patients with ankylosing spondylitis may lose weight and develop a low-grade fever with a high ESR. Uveitis (p. 883) occurs in a quarter of cases, while a similar proportion develop aortitis with aortic incompetence (p. 470). Although chest expansion is often restricted, pulmonary ventilation is usually well maintained. Diffuse bilateral upper lobe fibrosis, of uncertain aetiology, is a well recognized late complication.

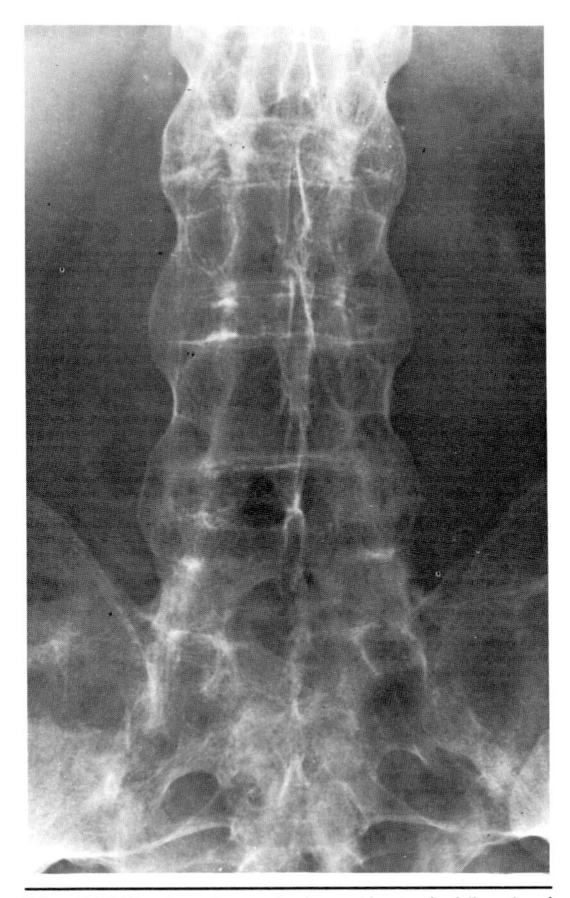

Fig. 20.50 A radiograph shows the typical 'bamboo' spine of late severe ankylosing spondylitis.

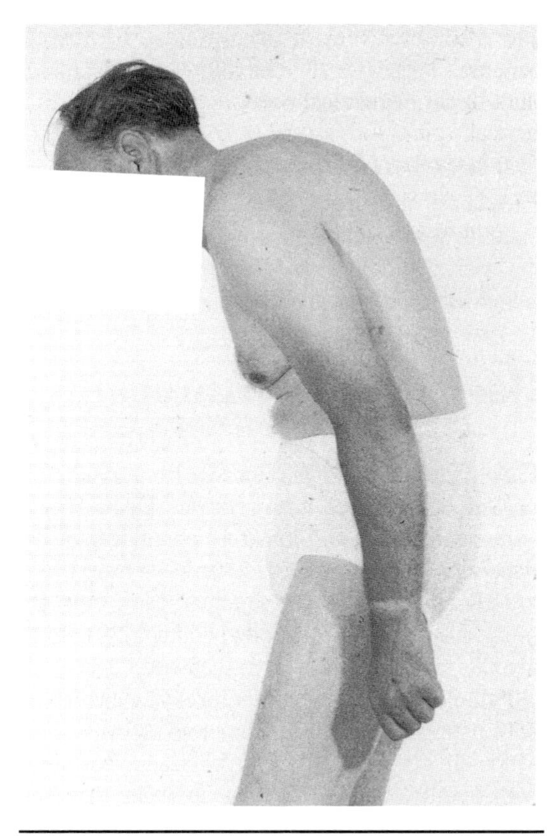

Fig. 20.51 This patient with long-standing ankylosing spondylitis has a characteristic stooped posture due to fusion of the spine.

Reiter's Syndrome

This condition was initially defined as the triad of arthritis, conjunctivitis and urethritis, although some authorities now include patients with other features such as dysentery, balanitis, cervicitis and oral ulceration. Both epidemic (e.g. *Shigella flexneri*) and sporadic cases may occur, some of the latter associated with non-specific urethritis due to chlamydia or mycoplasma. Post-venereal Reiter's syndrome is much more common in males while the epidemic form shows no sexual difference. Most patients are in their twenties. The arthritis typically affects the large weight-bearing joints, the hands, feet and spine, and is often persistent or recurrent. Insertional tendonitis affecting the Achilles tendon and plantar fascia is common.

Psoriatic Arthropathy

Approximately 5% of patients with psoriasis (p. 1115) develop an associated arthritis, typically affecting a few joints with an asymmetrical distribution. The distal interphalangeal joints of the hands and feet, the knees, hips, ankles and wrists are commonly involved. In a small number of patients inflammation is restricted largely to the distal interphalangeal joints, commonly in association with psoriatic pitting of the nails; rarely the arthropathy progresses to osteolysis of the affected phalanges (arthritis mutilans). Sacroiliac and spinal involvement occurs in up to 40% of patients. Pathologically the synovium resembles that of rheumatoid arthritis.

Enteropathic Arthritis

Peripheral and spinal arthritis can be found in patients with Crohn's disease and ulcerative colitis and also following infections with shigella, salmonella, yersinia and campylobacter.

Haemophilic Arthropathy

Patients with haemophilia (p. 90) are at risk of repeated episodes of intra-articular haemorrhage (haemarthrosis) and ultimately about half of the patients develop chronic destructive arthritis. The knees, ankles, elbows, shoulders and hips are most often affected. The joint becomes chronically swollen, with limitation of movement.

Pathologically there are features reminiscent of both osteoarthritis and rheumatoid arthritis. The synovium becomes grossly hyperplastic and laden with haemosiderin. It grows in from the joint margin to cover and erode the articular cartilage. In addition the cartilage becomes fissured and the underlying bone is exposed. Subchondral cysts are found, and there is marked osteophyte formation. Many chondrocytes contain haemosiderin.

Accumulation of iron appears to be of major importance in the pathogenesis of haemophilic arthropathy, both by its effect on chondrocyte metabolism and also by stimulating synovial proliferation. The synovium is capable of producing prostaglandins and degradative enzymes such as collagenase, in quantities similar to those found in rheumatoid arthritis, thus accounting for the erosions.

Arthritis due to Deposition of Crystals

Gout

Gout is associated with hyperuricaemia, defined as an elevated serum urate concentration greater than 7 mg/dl in adult males or 6 mg/dl in adult females. Most hyperuricaemic patients remain asymptomatic; the proportion developing clinical gout increases with the serum urate level.

Hyperuricaemia may be classified as primary or secondary. **Primary gout** refers to those cases where hyperuricaemia is not a consequence of another disorder either acquired or inborn. Primary gout is not a single disease, but a heterogeneous group of disorders. It has long been recognized that gout particularly affects middle-aged males, often those with a family history. Less than 10% of patients are female and the onset usually occurs after the menopause. It appears that multiple genes control the serum urate concentration. In most cases of primary gout the exact mechanism has not been established. Hyperuricaemia is due to increased production, decreased excretion of uric acid, or both. In a minority of cases specific enzyme disorders have been recognized. Increased activity of 5-phosphoribosyl-1-pyrophosphate synthetase (PRPPS) and decreased hypoxanthine guanine phosphoribosyltransferase (HGPRT) activity both result in increased urate production. Both of these rare disorders are X-linked. **Secondary gout** refers to those cases which develop during the course of another disease. Patients with malignancy, particularly leukaemia or myeloproliferative disorders, treated by chemotherapy without uricosuric cover commonly develop gout as a consequence of increased purine catabolism. Many drugs including diuretics interfere with renal excretion of uric acid. Hyperuricaemia may be a consequence of chronic renal failure but gouty arthritis is surprisingly rare. There is a high incidence of gout in patients with hyperparathyroidism.

Acute gout. One or more joints are affected and are exquisitely painful, red and swollen. In over half of the patients the metatarsophalangeal joint of the big toe is the first joint to be affected (*podagra*). Dietary or alcoholic excess, drugs, trauma or surgery often precipitate attacks, usually starting at night and lasting for a few days or weeks. The picture of the port-drinking glutton with an acute attack of podagra is a very familiar one!

Examination of fluid aspirated from an involved joint shows many inflammatory cells, particularly neutrophil polymorphs. Large numbers of needle-shaped crystals are present within and outside cells. Neutrophils phagocytose urate crystals and release lysosomal enzymes and other mediators of inflammation including factors chemotactic for neutrophils.

Chronic 'tophaceous' gout has become less common since the introduction of the uricosuric agent allopurinol. It is associated with the formation of crystalline deposits (**tophi**) of sodium biurate particularly in poorly vascular fibrous tissue, and hyaline and fibro-cartilage. When viewed in plane polarized light the crystals are seen to be strongly negatively birefringent (Fig. 20.52). Tophi are found in the pinna of the ear, in articular cartilage, sometimes with associated degenerative changes, and in periarticular structures (Fig. 20.53). Subchondral and subperiosteal deposition gives rise to punched out lytic lesions in bone. Deposition of urates in the kidney may cause renal failure (p. 923).

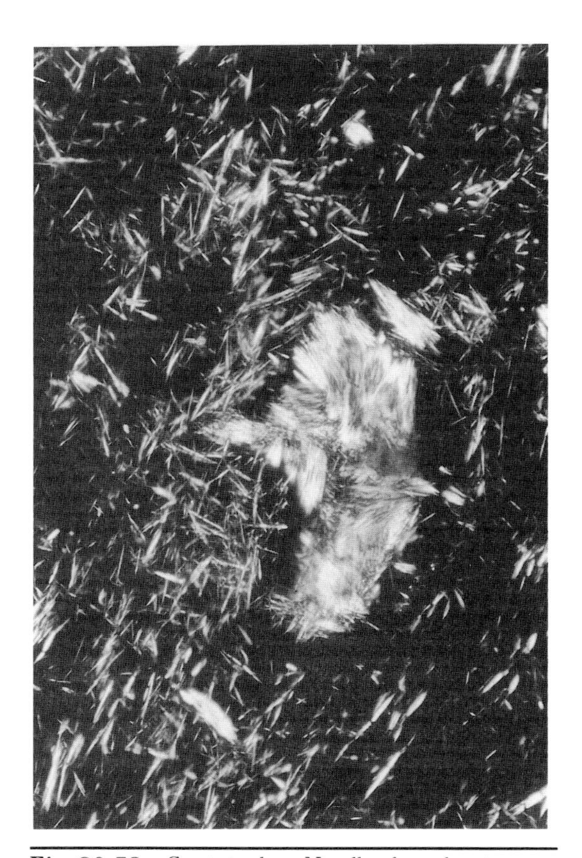

Fig. 20.52 Gouty tophus. Needle-shaped urate crystals are strongly birefringent in polarized light.

Microscopy of tophi shows sheaves of urate crystals surrounded by a florid foreign-body giant-cell and histiocytic reaction. Urate crystals are water soluble; tissue suspected of containing urates should be preserved in alcoholic fixatives for histological examination.

Calcium Pyrophosphate Deposition Disease (CPPD) (Pseudogout)

Calcium pyrophosphate dihydrate crystals are deposited in cartilage and juxta-articular tissues; the large joints, particularly the menisci of the knees of the elderly, are most often affected. Calcium pyrophosphate deposition disease may be familial, secondary to underlying conditions including hyperparathyroidism and haemochromatosis, while associations with gout and diabetes mellitus

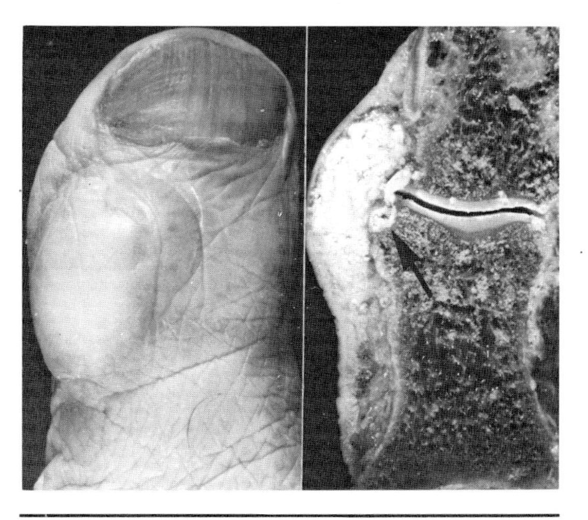

Fig. 20.53 A gouty tophus is seen in the subcutaneous tissue overlying the interphalangeal joint of the great toe. The tophus has produced a little resorption of bone at the joint margin (arrow). The articular cartilage is also flecked with white crystalline material.

have also been noted. When the condition is recognized a cause should be sought.

As in gout, both acute crystal synovitis and chronic deposition may occur. Acute attacks (pseudogout) lasting days to weeks may affect one or several joints, most commonly the knee and often the wrists, elbows, shoulders and ankles. Surgery or illness may precipitate an attack. Synovial fluid contains abundant neutrophils and small rhomboid and rod-shaped crystals (Fig. 20.54), which show weak positive birefringence.

Chronic deposition within the menisci, articular cartilage, ligaments, tendons and joint capsule is detectable on plain radiographs as small calcified foci, an appearance known as **chondrocalcinosis**. This can be detected in 30–60% of subjects over 85 years. Although most are asymptomatic, some patients develop subacute or chronic synovitis with morning stiffness. Others have low-grade chronic symptoms due to degenerative joint disease with or without acute attacks. Rarely, severe destructive arthritis resembling neuropathic arthropathy is seen. On naked eye examination a white chalky 'frosted' precipitate is seen, while microscopy shows clusters of rhomboid and rod-shaped crystals, and a mild foreign-body giant-cell reaction in vascularized sites.

Although a relationship exists between calcium pyrophosphate deposition disease and osteoarthritis, its nature is not clear. Articular deposition of pyrophosphate crystals may predispose to degenerative change, while metabolic abnormalities in osteoarthritic cartilage may favour precipitation of crystals. Finally, since both conditions are very common, their coexistence may be coincidental.

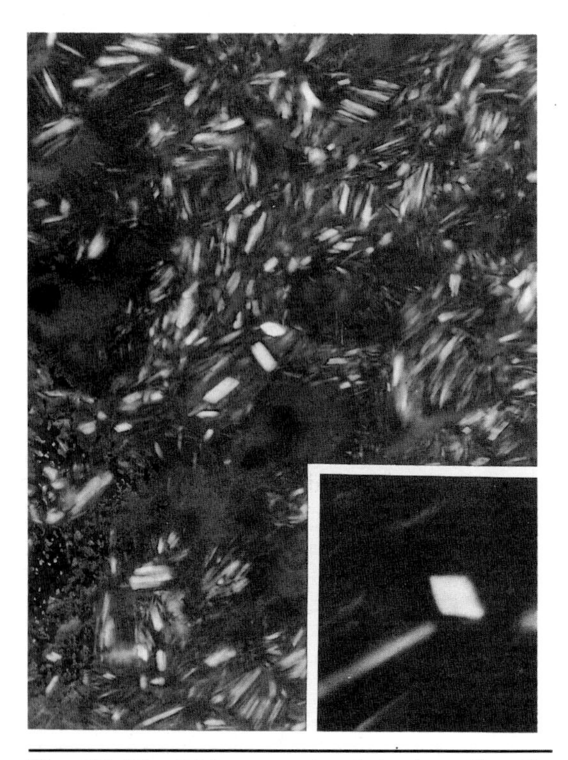

Fig. 20.54 Calcium pyrophosphate deposition disease. The synovial fluid contains numerous birefringent rhomboid and rod-shaped crystals.

Basic Calcium Phosphate (Calcium Apatite) Crystal Deposition Disease

Acute and chronic symptoms such as tendonitis may occur in response to deposition of calcium apatite crystals; recently an association with osteoarthritis has been described, for these crystals may be identified by electron microscopy in the synovial fluid of patients with osteoarthritis. An erosive arthritis has also been described affecting various joints. A rapidly progressive destructive arthritis of the shoulder (so-called 'Milwaukee shoulder') particularly affects elderly females. While it has been suggested that calcium apatite crystals may be responsible for this disorder, it is possible that apatite deposition follows bone destruction. Apatite crystals are not recognizable by light microscopy because of their small size.

Other Disorders of Joints

Pathology of joint replacement. The management of patients with arthritis was revolutionized in the early 1960s by the development of low friction arthroplasties (artificial joints) which can restore mobility and give pain relief. Most prostheses are manufactured from largely inert metallic alloys and high molecular weight polyethylene, and are anchored within the bone by acrylic cement or by ingrowth of bone or fibrous tissue into the prostheses. Implants made from silicone polymers are often used to replace small joints in the hands, usually in rheumatoid arthritis.

Unfortunately, in some patients the prosthesis becomes loose, most often due to mechanical causes. The exact mechanisms are unclear but it is thought that very small movements between the prosthesis and bone, which have different mechanical properties, induce bone resorption. Friction between the components of the prosthesis results in fine wear products of metal or polyethylene which, like fragments of acrylic cement, induce a florid reaction of macrophages and foreign-body giant cells (Fig. 20.55). This also contributes to bone resorption around the prosthetic stem and loosening. It has been suggested that an immune reaction, possibly to the metallic components, is implicated in bone resorption. Patients may experience considerable pain and insertion of a replacement prosthesis is often required.

Although advances in surgical technique, including antibiotic loaded cement and laminar-flow operating theatres, have greatly diminished the incidence of infection of arthroplasties, this remains an important complication especially in the knee. Infection occurs immediately after surgery or appears insidiously months or years later. Superficial wound infections must be treated aggressively to prevent spread to the bone surrounding the prosthesis. Once established, eradication of deep infection is very difficult and it may be necessary to remove the prosthesis. Coagulase positive and negative staphylococci are often responsible, while organisms of low virulence, including anaerobes, may be cultured, sometimes with difficulty.

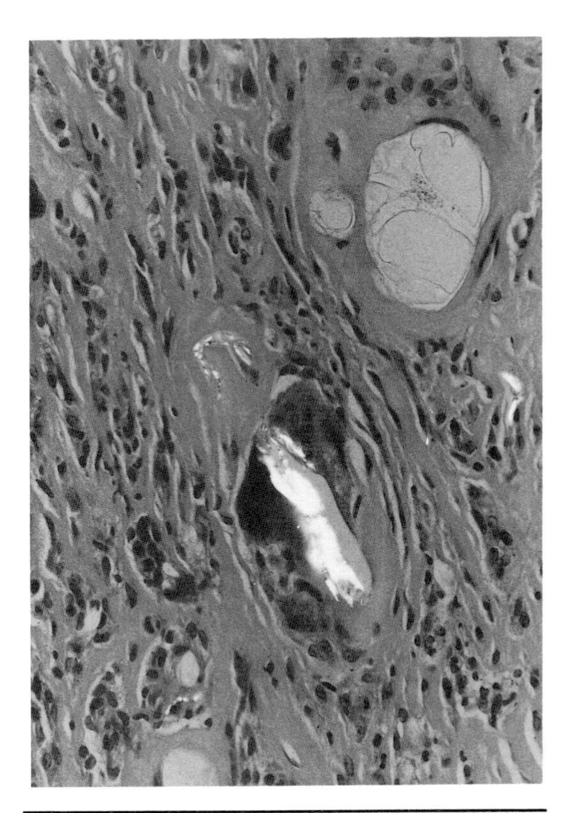

Fig. 20.55 Reaction to a mechanically loosened prosthesis. The section has been photographed through partially crossed polarizing filters. Foreign-body giant cells surround birefringent fragments of high molecular weight polyethylene. Acrylic cement has been removed from the section during processing leaving a little non-birefringent material (top right).

Intra-articular loose bodies. Multiple soft loose bodies (rice or melon-seed bodies) formed from fibrin or necrotic synovium are found in tuberculous or rheumatoid arthritis. Hard loose bodies may cause repeated episodes of locking of the joint, and damage to the articular cartilage resulting in osteoarthritis. There are several varieties. In **synovial chondromatosis** multiple nodules of cartilage form by metaplasia in the synovial membrane and may become ossified (Fig. 20.56). Some nodules become detached and lie free in the synovial fluid. The cartilage may be very cellular and so be mistaken for chondrosarcoma. In **osteochondritis dissecans** (p. 962), the loose body consists of articular cartilage and underlying necrotic bone. The cartilage remains viable and proliferates to cover the bony fragment. Fracture of **marginal osteophytes** in osteoarthritis may occur, particularly in neuropathic

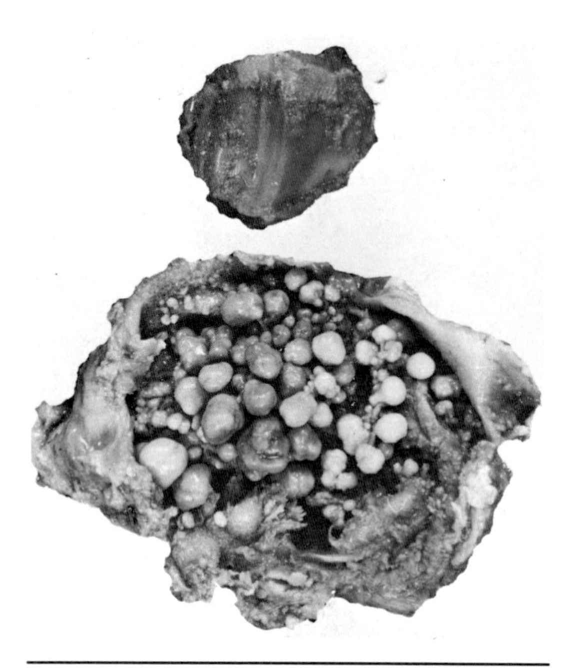

Fig. 20.56 Synovial chondromatosis of the knee joint.

joints. Rarely intra-articular fractures may result in loose bodies.

Pigmented villonodular synovitis (PVNS). This benign proliferative lesion of synovium occurs in two distinct clinical settings. **Localized nodular synovitis** presents as a firm, nodular swelling in the finger, usually in women between 30 and 50 years. It consists of a lobulated nodule arising from tendon sheath or joint and contains giant cells and groups of histiocytes containing abundant haemosiderin and lipid, which impart a tan colour. The lesion occasionally recurs, particularly if there is diffuse involvement of the adjacent synovium, and may also erode bone. Occasionally similar nodules are found in large joints alone or associated with diffuse PVNS.

Diffuse PVNS most often involves the knee or hip joint, causing pain, a blood-stained effusion or locking of the joint. The synovium is thrown up into hyperplastic pigmented villi which become matted together like an orange beard. The enlarged villi are covered by hyperplastic synovial cells and there are numerous macrophages containing haemosiderin and lipid. The diffuse form of PVNS is more difficult to eradicate, and tends to recur. Bone may be eroded especially when the hip joint is involved. Diffuse PVNS may also occur in tendon sheaths and bursae.

Ganglia occur in the soft tissue around joints or tendon sheaths, most commonly on the dorsum of the wrist. They develop by myxoid change in fibrous tissue with formation of thin walled cysts containing clear glairy fluid. Sometimes there is a communication between the ganglion and an adjacent joint and this must be eradicated if recurrence is to be avoided. Similar lesions may occur within the periosteum and also within bone (intraosseous ganglion).

Cyst of semilunar cartilage. Myxoid change may occur in the loose fibrous tissue adjacent to the lateral meniscus or in the meniscus itself, resulting in a lesion histologically identical to a ganglion.

Bursitis. A bursa is a synovial lined sac, and is found chiefly over bony prominences. It may communicate with a joint and is subject to the same disorders. Repeated mild trauma may result in inflammation (as for instance in prepatellar bursitis, 'housemaid's knee').

Amyloidosis. Deposition of amyloid is commonly found in the synovium and degenerate articular cartilage in elderly patients who do not have systemic amyloidosis. Neither its significance nor the exact nature of the amyloid protein is known. Deposition of amyloid of β_2 microglobulin origin within the synovium, articular cartilage and adjacent bone may be found in patients on long-term haemodialysis (p. 934).

Soft Tissue Tumours and Tumour-like Lesions

Skeletal muscle, fat and fibrous tissue, together with the blood vessels and nerves supplying them, are regarded as 'soft tissues'. Tumours of these tissues are classified on the basis of the adult tissue they resemble (Table 20.11). As has been indicated in Chapter 3, differentiation does not necessarily imply histogenesis; thus a rhabdomyosarcoma does not arise from mature skeletal muscle, but rather from primitive cells which differentiate towards skeletal muscle.

The majority of soft tissue tumours, particularly small, superficially situated lesions, are benign. In contrast, large tumours in deep soft tissue are very likely to be malignant even if they appear well encapsulated on naked eye examination. Soft tissue sarcomas are a heterogeneous group of tumours of varying histological type and biological behaviour. Precise histological typing is often difficult. Although uncommon, they cause considerable morbidity and mortality; for this reason a lengthier discussion is given than their frequency alone would warrant. Among tumour-like lesions of soft tissue are the fibromatoses – a group of infiltrative and recurrent lesions which are probably not true tumours – and a small group of benign reactive conditions which tend to grow rapidly and may be confused histologically with sarcomas. Tumours of peripheral nerve are discussed on p. 866, those of blood vessels on p. 478, and fibrous histiocytoma and dermatofibrosarcoma protuberans on p. 1138.

Benign Tumours

Lipoma. This common soft tissue tumour may arise anywhere in the body, but often in the subcutaneous tissues of the back, shoulder and neck, and the proximal parts of the limbs. Patients, mainly women over 40, complain of a slowly growing painless mass. Much less common are lipomas of deep soft tissue; those in retroperitoneum and mediastinum may grow to considerable size and cause symptoms due to pressure. The pathologist must examine these tumours very carefully; some well-differentiated liposarcomas with locally aggressive behaviour closely resemble lipomas histologically. Lipomas are well circumscribed, lobulated, thinly or delicately encapsulated masses of mature adipose tissue. Several variants exist. **Angiolipomas** which contain numerous thin walled capillaries may be painful, especially when microthrombi form within their rich vascular network.

Leiomyomas. Benign smooth muscle tumours are much more common in the uterus and gastrointestinal tract than in soft tissue. Cutaneous leiomyomas arising from erector pili muscles are usually multiple and painful. Those arising from smooth muscle in the genital zones (e.g. dartos muscle in the scrotum) are usually solitary and painless. Vascular leiomyomas, with prominent abnormal thick walled venous channels, typically form painful lumps in the legs of middle-aged patients particularly women. Leiomyomas consist of spindle-shaped cells which closely resemble normal smooth muscle cells.

Chondromas are uncommon lobulated masses of cartilage found in the hands and feet of adults. Many probably arise in synovium. They are sometimes highly cellular and may be mistakenly diagnosed as chondrosarcoma.

Granular cell tumour. This lesion, now thought to be of Schwann cell origin, may occur in many sites but typically in the dermis, the submucosa of, for instance, the larynx, and the muscle of the tongue. The tumour consists of large cells with abundant granular cytoplasm due to the accumulation of numerous secondary lysosomes. The nuclei are small. The tumour cells have an infiltrative

Table 20.11 Soft tissue tumours – clinical and pathological features

	Peak age	Principal site	Pathology	Immuno-cytochemistry Electron microscopy	Comments
Fibrohistiocytic tumours					
DERMATOFIBROMA (cutaneous fibrous histiocytoma)	20–40	Skin, especially extremities	Ill-defined nodule of fibroblasts, blood vessels, haemosiderin and lipid-laden macrophages	Not helpful	Benign. May be multiple. If haemosiderin-laden may simulate melanoma clinically
Atypical fibroxanthoma	Elderly. Young adults	Sun exposed skin. Skin of limbs & trunk	Nodule of highly pleomorphic spindle cells with aberrant mitoses. Small, well defined, confined to dermis	To exclude malignant melanoma and squamous carcinoma	Benign, despite histological appearances
Dermatofibrosarcoma protuberans	25–55	Trunk, proximal limbs	Infiltrating tumour. Spindle cells arranged in storiform pattern (like spokes of a wheel)	Not helpful	Repeated local recurrences unless totally removed
MALIGNANT FIBROUS HISTIOCYTOMA	50–70	Deep soft tissue of limbs, retroperitoneum	Variable, usually pleomorphic cells with storiform pattern	Exclude other forms of differentiation, e.g. peripheral nerve sheath tumour	Pulmonary metastases in 40%
Tumours of adipose tissue					
LIPOMA	40–60	Mainly superficial, trunk, proximal limbs	Encapsulated mature fat	Not required	Benign. Several histological variants, e.g. angiolipoma, spindle-cell lipoma
LIPOSARCOMA	40–70	Retroperitoneum, deep soft tissue of trunk and proximal limbs	Well differentiated, myxoid, round cell and pleomorphic variants	S-100 protein positive. Lipid droplets, basal lamina	All locally recurrent. Round cell and pleomorphic variants metastasize frequently

Table 20.11 *Continued*

	Peak age	Principal site	Pathology	Immuno-cytochemistry Electron microscopy	Comments
Tumours of smooth muscle					
Leiomyoma			Mature smooth muscle cells arising from:	Desmin, smooth muscle actin positive. Thin filaments with focal condensations, basal lamina, micro-pinocytosis.	Benign Often multiple (a) Often painful (a,c)
(a) Cutaneous	15–30	Extensor surfaces	(a) erector pili		
(b) Genital	15–30	Genital area – scrotum, nipples	(b) muscle, e.g. dartos		
(c) Vascular	30–50	Subcutaneous, especially legs	(c) thick walled blood vessels		
LEIOMYOSARCOMA	50–70	(a) Retroperi-toneum, deep soft tissue of limbs (b) Subcutaneous (c) Cutaneous	Smooth muscle of varying differentiation	As above, with variable differentiation	(a) Death by local extension & metastases (b,c) Metastases less common
Tumours of striated muscle					
Rhabdomyoma	>40	Neck, tongue	Large cells with eosinophilic cytoplasm and cross-striations	Desmin and myoglobin positive. Thick and thin filaments; Z band material	Benign Very rare
RHABDOMYOSARCOMA					
Embryonal	Children	Genitourinary tract; head and neck	'Botryoid tumour' (bunch of grapes). Rhabdomyoblasts	As above	Highly malignant. Improved prognosis with chemotherapy, particularly for embryonal variant
Alveolar	Adolescents	Trunk, limbs	Packets of cells with eosinophilic cytoplasm; 'alveolar' pattern	As above	
Pleomorphic (very rare)	Adults	Limbs	Pleomorphic cells, occasional cross-striations	As above	

Table 20.11 *Continued*

	Peak age	Principal site	Pathology	Immuno-cytochemistry Electron microscopy	Comments
Tumours of blood vessels					
HAEMANGIOMA	Children	Head & neck	Capillary or cavernous patterns	Factor VIII related antigen positive, *Ulex europaeus* lectin positive. Weibel–Palade bodies	Benign
Glomus tumour	20–40	Extremities, e.g. subungual	Small nodules comprising small uniform round cells surrounding thin-walled blood vessels	Desmin positive. Thin filaments with focal condensations	Often painful
KAPOSI'S SARCOMA (a) classic (European) (b) endemic (African)	 50–70 30–50	 Skin of distal leg Skin of leg	Histology varies with stage. Spindle cells and proliferating vascular channels	Ultrastructure and immuno-chemistry suggesting endothelial cell origin but it is uncertain whether this is vascular or lymphatic	(a) Prolonged course (b) Variable – more aggressive than classical; some fulminant – visceral involvement
(c) lymphadenopathic (African) (d) transplant-associated (e) HIV associated (particularly male homosexuals)	Children Wide range 20–50	Lymph nodes Skin, sometimes viscera Disseminated – skin and nodes			(c) Rapidly fatal (d) 30% die of visceral involvement (e) Prognosis that of AIDS
ANGIOSARCOMA	40–70	Scalp; limbs (especially lymphoedematous, e.g. post-radiotherapy)	Ill-defined haemorrhagic tumour; well or ill-formed blood vessels	*Ulex europaeus* lectin positive; Factor VIII related antigen often negative	Highly malignant; metastases to lymph node, lung and liver
Peripheral nerve sheath tumours					
SCHWANNOMA	20–50	Head, neck, flexor surfaces of limbs	Encapsulated tumour, cellular (Antoni A) and myxoid areas (Antoni B)	S-100 protein positive. Schwann cells with cytoplasmic processes, basal lamina	Benign. Uncommon in neurofibro-matosis

Table 20.11 *Continued*

	Peak age	Principal site	Pathology	Immuno-cytochemistry Electron microscopy	Comments
NEUROFIBROMA	20–40	Cutaneous nerves	Non-encapsulated. Spindle cells, axons	S-100 protein – variable staining. Mixture of Schwann cells, perineurial cells, fibroblasts	Benign. Multiple tumours in neurofibromatosis. Malignant transformation occurs in 2% of people with neurofibromatosis
Malignant peripheral nerve sheath tumour	20–50	Large nerve trunks	Fusiform mass on nerve trunk	Some S-100 protein positive cells. Schwann cell features	Often associated with neurofibro-matosis. Poor prognosis
GRANULAR CELL TUMOUR	30–50	Tongue, dermis-subcutis of chest wall, arms	Ill-defined yellow nodule. Nests of granular cells. Pseudoepithelio-matous hyperplasia of overlying squamous epithelium	S-100 protein positive. Schwann cell features, numerous lysosomes	Benign
Tumours of cartilage & bone					
Chondroma	30–60	80% fingers	Multinodular lesion of hyaline cartilage	S-100 protein positive	Benign
Mesenchymal chondrosarcoma	15–35	Head and neck, e.g. orbit. Deep soft tissue of limbs	Undifferentiated small cells & islands of cartilage	S-100 protein positive in cartilaginous islands	Highly malignant
Extraskeletal myxoid chondrosarcoma	35–60	Deep soft tissue of limbs	Nodules of myxoid cartilage	Weakly S-100 protein positive. EM – cartilaginous differentiation	Local recurrence. <50% metastasize
Osteosarcoma of soft tissue	40–60	Lower limb, retroperitoneum	Malignant cells form osteoid or bone	Not helpful	Highly malignant. May arise after irradiation. Rare
Tumours of uncertain origin					
Alveolar soft part sarcoma	15–35	Adults – lower limb Children – head & neck	Packets of large rounded cells. Intracellular PAS positive/diastase resistant crystals. Vascular invasion very common	Crystals, 6 nm periodicity	Uncertain histogenesis. Metastases to lungs, brain, skeleton. 10-year survival <50%

Table 20.11 *Continued*

	Peak age	Principal site	Pathology	Immuno-cytochemistry Electron microscopy	Comments
EPITHELIOID SARCOMA	15–35	Hand, forearm, foot	Hard, often ulcerated nodules. Central necrosis. Eosinophilic 'epithelioid' cells	Cytokeratin positive. Epithelial membrane antigen positive. EM – intermediate filaments and cell, junctions	Repeated local recurrences. Metastases to lymph nodes and lung in 45%
Clear-cell sarcoma (malignant melanoma of soft parts)	20–40	Foot, ankle	Nests of clear or eosinophilic cells. Melanin in 50% of cases	S-100 protein positive. Premelano-somes	Local recurrence. Metastases in 45%
Ewing's sarcoma of soft tissue	15–30	Chest wall, paravertebral	As Ewing's sarcoma of bone	Vimentin positive. Glycogen rich	Early pulmonary metastases. Neuroectodermal origin ?
SYNOVIAL SARCOMA	15–40	Limbs, close to large joints	Biphasic pattern of spindle-cell sarcoma with epithelial elements	Cytokeratin, epithelial membrane antigen positive. Epithelial differentiation with desmosomes	Not of synovial origin. Metastases in 50%, often late. Monophasic variants are recognized by cytokeratin expression

Tumours which are common or particularly important are shown in capitals, e.g. HAEMANGIOMA.

growth pattern which may lead to a mistaken diagnosis of malignancy. In addition, the lesion stimulates growth of the overlying epithelium, pseudoepitheliomatous hyperplasia (Fig. 20.57), which may be misinterpreted as infiltrating squamous carcinoma. Malignant granular cell tumours are very rare.

Fibroma. Although fibromas are found in internal organs they are extremely rare in soft tissues. Most benign fibrous lesions are reactive rather than neoplastic, and apart from specific entities such as fibroma of tendon sheath the diagnosis of soft tissue fibroma should virtually never be made.

Malignant Tumours

Most soft tissue sarcomas are well circumscribed masses in deep soft tissue. Although they may appear to be encapsulated, there is microscopic invasion of the surrounding tissues; surgical 'shelling out' of the tumour is almost inevitably followed

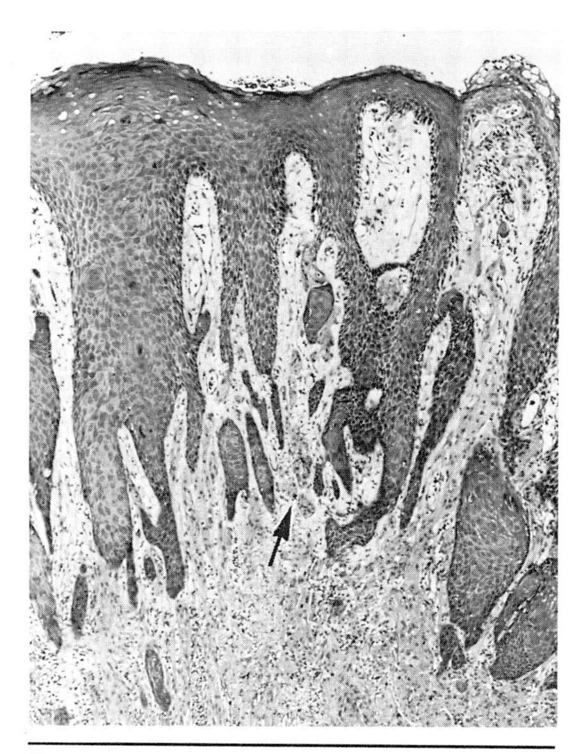

Fig. 20.57 Granular cell myoblastoma of the tongue with marked overlying pseudoepitheliomatous hyperplasia of the squamous mucosa. Small clumps of granular cells are present (arrow).

by local recurrence. The prognosis depends on several factors. The risk of local recurrence is largely related to the adequacy of surgical removal, which itself depends on the anatomical site and the skill of the surgeon. Thus, a tumour confined to a single muscle compartment in the thigh may be completely removed by a 'compartmental excision' while a retroperitoneal tumour or one in the popliteal fossa may be impossible to excise with a covering of normal tissue. Factors influencing the risk of metastases include the histological grade, extent of necrosis of tumour, size and anatomical location. There are a number of histological grading systems, which use different criteria. High-grade tumours tend to metastasize early, while low-grade lesions give problems chiefly from local recurrence or extension. In general the more superficial a tumour and the smaller it is, the better the prognosis. Retroperitoneal tumours tend to have a worse prognosis than those in the limbs.

Histological typing of sarcomas is often difficult. Even using immunocytochemistry and electron microscopy (Table 20.11) 10–20% of tumours can only be reported as '*sarcoma of uncertain histogenesis*'. With few exceptions the grade of a tumour is more important than its histological type in determining prognosis.

Malignant fibrous histiocytoma (MFH). This is the commonest soft tissue sarcoma of adults; it occurs mainly in the deep soft tissue of limbs or in the retroperitoneum in patients over 50. Although several histological subtypes are described, all the tumours contain some areas with cells arranged in a cartwheel or 'storiform' pattern. This is an aggressive pleomorphic sarcoma with a high risk of recurrence and metastasis, and a poor prognosis, particularly when sited in the retroperitoneum. The histogenesis of the tumour is disputed; it is possibly best regarded as a primitive sarcoma of fibroblast origin.

Fibrosarcoma. Many lesions previously diagnosed as fibrosarcoma are now regarded as malignant fibrous histiocytomas, malignant peripheral nerve sheath tumours or monophasic synovial sarcomas. Fibrosarcomas occur in middle-aged adults, especially in the limbs. Histologically, they consist of fascicles of spindle-shaped fibroblastic cells producing variable amounts of collagen and arranged in a 'herring-bone' pattern. Overall mortality rates are around 50%.

Liposarcoma. The age incidence and location are similar to those of MFH. Several histological subtypes are described which show varying degrees of differentiation towards adipose tissue (Fig. 20.58). These all tend to recur locally but have major differences in metastatic potential and survival. Metastases are extremely rare in cases of well differentiated liposarcoma and are unusual in the most common variant, myxoid liposarcoma. In contrast, round cell and pleomorphic liposarcomas are highly malignant tumours with early pulmonary metastases.

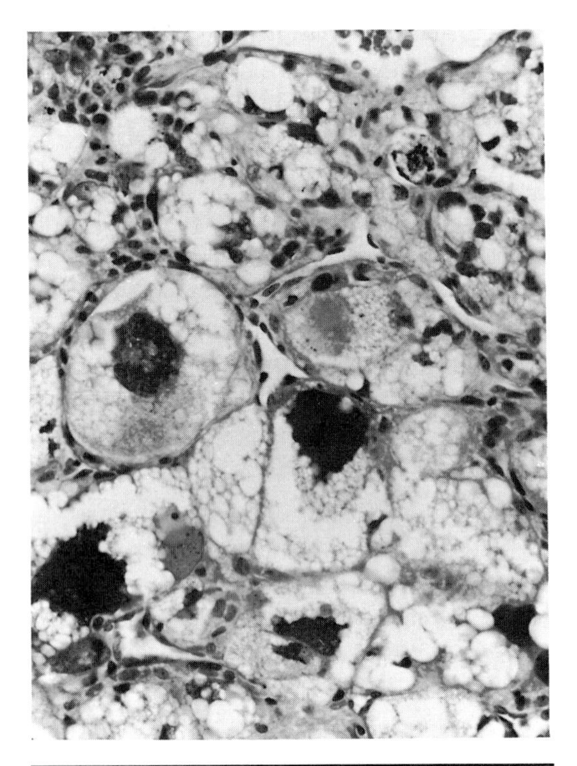

Fig. 20.58 Pleomorphic liposarcoma. Many fatty droplets are present in the cytoplasm of the gigantic lipoblasts with their hyperchromatic nuclei.

Rhabdomyosarcoma is the commonest soft tissue tumour of childhood and adolescence, but is rare in older patients. Three histological types are recognized.

Embryonal rhabdomyosarcoma occurs mainly in children, in the head and neck, genitourinary tract and retroperitoneum. Tumours occurring in the submucosa of, for example, the vagina or bladder, project as grape-like gelatinous masses and are known as 'botryoid' sarcomas. The previously poor prognosis of embryonal rhabdomyosarcoma has improved greatly with the use of chemotherapy, radiotherapy and surgery.

Alveolar rhabdomyosarcomas occur in adolescents, particularly arising in the skeletal muscle of the limbs. Tumour cells adhere to fibrous septa which divide the cells into clumps. Loss of cohesion in the centre of the groups produces an alveolar pattern. The prognosis of this group of tumours has also improved, but less dramatically.

Pleomorphic rhabdomyosarcomas are very rare and occur chiefly in the skeletal muscles of older people. It is often difficult to separate this group from other pleomorphic sarcomas.

In the past the firm diagnosis of rhabdomyosarcoma depended on the identification of cross-striations (Fig. 20.59), similar to those seen in skeletal muscle. Electron microscopy showing thick and thin (myosin and actin) filaments and, more particularly, immunohistochemical staining for desmin and myoglobin have made diagnosis, particularly of the embryonal and alveolar variants, much more reliable.

Leiomyosarcoma. This tumour affects the middle aged and elderly. About half the soft tissue leiomyosarcomas arise in the retroperitoneum and have a poor prognosis; less than 30% of patients survive 5 years. Of the remainder most are found in the dermis or subcutaneous tissue. In keeping with other superficially situated sarcomas the prognosis for these tumours is better; over 90% of patients with dermal tumours and 65% with subcutaneous lesions survive 5 years.

Histologically, leiomyosarcomas consist of spindle-shaped cells arranged in long interlacing fascicles. Many tumours express the intermediate

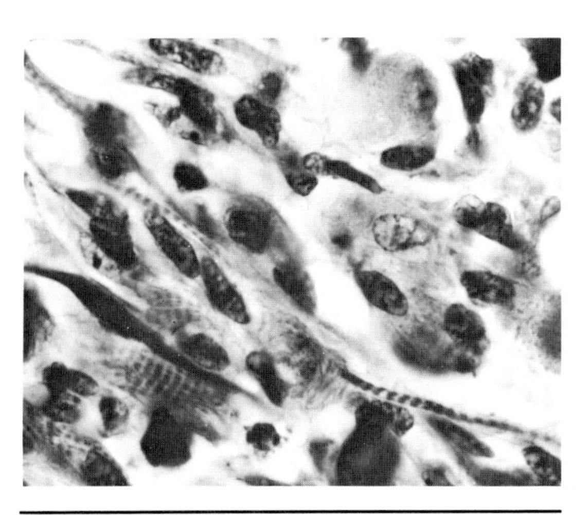

Fig. 20.59 Rhabdomyosarcoma. The myofibrils are best seen in cross-striations of the elongated strap cells but these cells are often hard to find.

filament desmin and smooth muscle actin. The principal criterion in distinguishing malignant and benign smooth muscle tumours is the number of mitotic figures. Nuclear pleomorphism without mitotic activity may be found in leiomyomas.

Synovial sarcoma. Despite its name this tumour is not a tumour of synovium. It is typically found adjacent to, but not within, large joints of adolescents and young adults. Sometimes the lesion has been present for many years and has only recently increased in size. Histologically, a biphasic pattern of a spindle-cell sarcoma with groups of 'epithelial' cells arranged in acini and tubules is usually seen (Fig. 20.60). Some tumours which consist of spindle cells alone are regarded as monophasic synovial sarcomas, and contain individual cells which express epithelial antigens. Synovial sarcoma is an aggressive tumour, with metastases in 50–70% of patients, often many years after diagnosis.

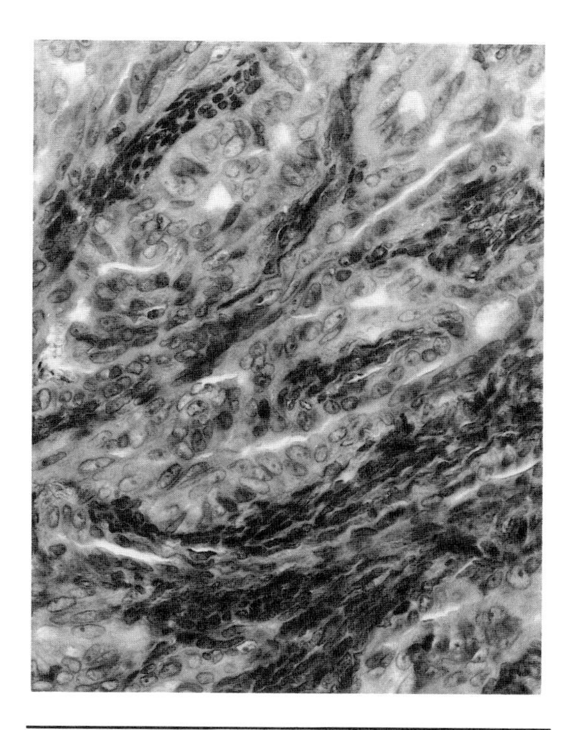

Fig. 20.60 Synovial sarcoma showing a biphasic pattern of spindle-cell sarcoma and epithelial cells arranged in glands.

Tumour-like Lesions of Soft Tissue

Fibromatosis

This term includes several fibrous lesions which have a tendency to infiltrate adjacent tissues and to recur, but not to metastasize.

Palmar fibromatosis (Dupuytren's contracture) begins as a firm nodule in the palm of middle-aged and elderly patients. In time, this extends to form subcutaneous cord-like bands which produce flexion contractures, especially of the fourth and fifth fingers. Histologically, the palmar aponeurosis is expanded by multiple nodules of proliferating, delicate, elongated fibroblasts which, by electron microscopy, are shown to be myofibroblasts, i.e. have contractile filaments. In time these nodules become heavily collagenized and poorly cellular. 'Recurrence' after surgery is common because much of the fascia may be affected by a field change. Similar lesions may occur in the sole of the foot, usually without contracture, (plantar fibromatosis) or in the penis (Peyronie's disease).

Musculo-aponeurotic fibromatosis is seen typically in the muscles of the shoulder and pelvic girdles and in the thigh where it forms a firm white mass which infiltrates widely through muscle (Fig. 20.61), often further than can be identified at surgery. For this reason complete excision is difficult and repeated recurrences are common, sometimes with involvement of major structures such as the brachial plexus. Occasionally there may be difficulty in differential diagnosis from low-grade fibrosarcoma.

Abdominal desmoids are similar lesions seen in the rectus abdominis of women during or after pregnancy but tend to be smaller, less aggressive and less likely to recur following excision.

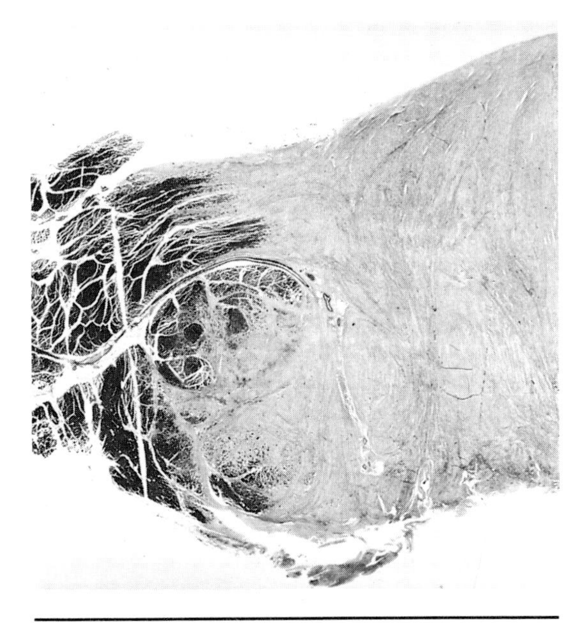

Fig. 20.61 Musculo-aponeurotic fibromatosis. Poorly cellular fibrous tissue has replaced much of the muscle and at its margin is infiltrating amongst the surviving muscle bundles (left). (Reproduced by permission from *Applied Surgical Pathology*, Blackwell Scientific Publications).

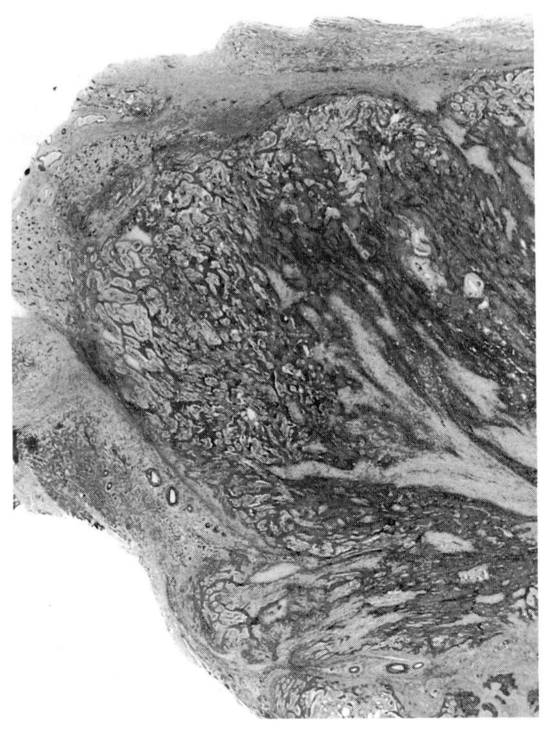

Fig. 20.62 Myositis ossificans. Arcades of woven bone are seen at the periphery of the lesion. Within this shell, less well differentiated trabeculae are seen to the right of the picture.

Reactive Conditions

Nodular fasciitis. The clinical history is usually of a rapidly growing tender nodule in the upper limb, especially the forearm of a young adult. Most often the lesion is subcutaneous, but sometimes muscle or deep fascia are involved. Microscopy shows fibroblasts randomly arranged like cells in tissue culture, with frequent mitotic figures of normal morphology. There is a prominent vascular pattern and small myxoid foci with a scattering of chronic inflammatory cells. The differential diagnosis is from spindle-cell sarcoma. The lesion is entirely benign.

Myositis ossificans occurs mainly in the muscles of the limbs of young people. Patients complain of a rapidly growing soft tissue swelling, sometimes following trauma. Some patients have low-grade fever and an elevated white blood count, sometimes suggesting infection. On microscopy there is a characteristic zoning pattern; a central zone of proliferating fibroblasts merges with areas of primitive bone formation (Fig. 20.62), which usually mature to form a well defined peripheral shell of woven bone in 4–6 weeks. There is a danger that myositis ossificans is misdiagnosed as osteosarcoma particularly in the early stages, before 'zoning' has developed.

Further Reading

Bullough, P. G. and Vigorita, V. J. (1984). *Atlas of Orthopaedic Pathology with Clinical and Radiologic Correlations*. Gower Medical Publishing, New York, London.

Dahlin, D. C. and Unni, K. K. (1986). *Bone Tumors*, 4th edn. Charles C. Thomas, Springfield, Illinois.

Enzinger, F. M. and Weiss, S. W. (1988). *Soft Tissue Tumors*, 2nd edn. The C. V. Mosby Co., St Louis, Missouri.

Fletcher, C. D. M. (1991). Soft tissue tumours: an update. In *Recent Advances in Histopathology*, No. 15, pp. 113–39, eds P. P. Anthony and R. N. M. MacSween. Churchill Livingstone, Edinburgh.

Harris, E. D. Jr. (1990). Rheumatoid arthritis. Pathophysiology and implications for therapy. *New England Journal of Medicine* **322**, 1277–89.

Kelley, W. N., Harris, E. D. Jr., Ruddy, S. and Sledge, C. B. (1989). *Textbook of Rheumatology*, 3rd edn. W. B. Saunders Co., Philadelphia.

Revell, P. A. (1985). *Pathology of Bone*. Springer-Verlag, Berlin.

Smith, R. (1986). Osteogenesis imperfecta. *Clinics in Rheumatic Diseases* **12**, 655–89.

21

The Female Reproductive Tract and the Breast

The Female Reproductive Tract

The Vulva

Dermatological Conditions

The skin of the vulva is part of the body integument and is therefore subject to all the diseases that can afflict the skin elsewhere in the body, such as, for example, psoriasis, pemphigus or lichen planus. Two conditions, namely lichen simplex and lichen sclerosus et atrophicus, do, however, merit special attention, partly because they occur with some frequency in the vulvar skin and partly because these two disorders have, until recently, been regarded, quite illogically, as falling into a separate category of 'vulvar dystrophies'. In the absence of any superimposed intraepithelial neoplasia neither of these two skin lesions is associated with any increased risk of vulvar carcinoma.

Lichen simplex appears as circumscribed areas of thickened, white or red skin, usually on the labia majora. Histologically, the squamous epithelium is thickened and shows acanthosis, elongation of the rete pegs, parakeratosis and hyperkeratosis: there is a chronic inflammatory cell infiltration of the dermis.

Lichen sclerosus et atrophicus (Fig. 21.1) is characterized by thinning of the epidermis, flattening of the dermoepidermal junction, hyalinization of the upper dermis and a chronic inflammatory cell infiltrate of the lower dermis.

Infections

Many vulvar infections, especially those occurring in debilitated women, are of mixed nature but some are due to streptococci or staphylococci, the latter, and also candida infections, occurring with increased frequency in diabetics. The features of the various sexually transmitted diseases which involve the vulva are described in Chapter 8.

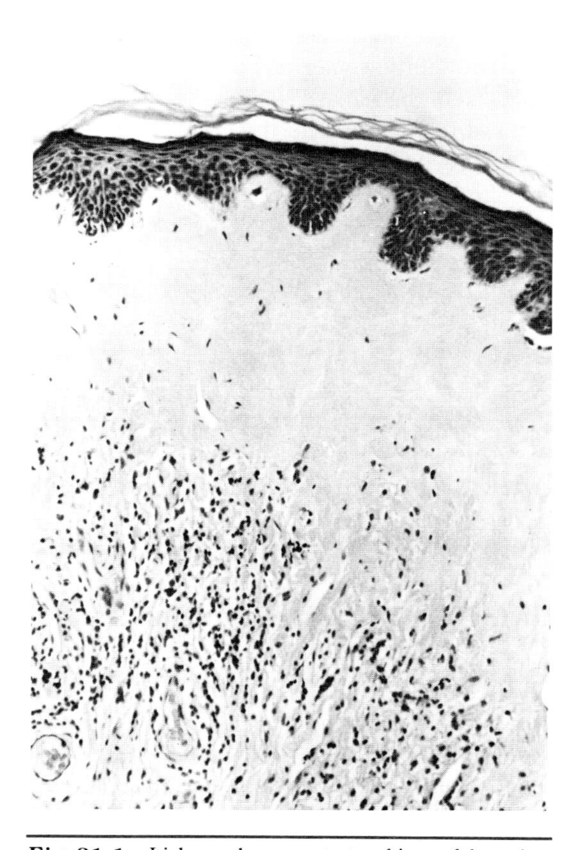

Fig. 21.1 Lichen sclerosus et atrophicus of the vulva. The upper dermis is hyalinized whilst in the deeper part of the dermis there is a non-specific chronic inflammatory cell infiltrate. The epidermis is atrophic. ×150.

Atrophy

Thinning of the vulvar epithelium is common; some degree of atrophy occurs as a physiological response to oestrogen withdrawal in all postmenopausal women and is sometimes sufficiently marked to cause narrowing of the introitus.

Vulvar Intraepithelial Neoplasia

A proportion of vulvar squamous-cell carcinomas arises from abnormal squamous epithelium showing varying degrees of cellular atypia. In the atypical epithelium the cells fail to mature and have an increased nucleocytoplasmic ratio and hyperchromatic nuclei: mitotic figures are often seen above the basal layer and are sometimes of abnormal form. Atypia of this type is now recognized to be an intraepithelial neoplasm, **vulvar intraepithelial neoplasia (VIN)** and is often associated with human papillomavirus infection. If atypical cells occupy less than the full thickness of the epithelium the condition is classed as VIN I or II, whilst if the full thickness of the epithelium is occupied by atypical cells the condition is graded as VIN III and corresponds to carcinoma *in situ*. Relatively few cases of VIN III progress to an invasive cancer and a significant proportion spontaneously regress. Progression to an invasive squamous-cell carcinoma is most likely to occur in elderly women or in immunosuppressed young women.

Tumours

A variety of benign skin neoplasms, such as **papillomas**, **fibromas** and **lipomas**, occur in the vulva and this is a site at which benign sweat gland tumours, **hidradenomas** (p. 1132) are particularly prone to develop.

Malignant vulvar neoplasms are uncommon and most are **squamous-cell carcinomas**. These tumours usually develop in elderly women and can arise from either an epithelium showing the changes of VIN or an otherwise normal squamous epithelium. The tumour may present as an indurated plaque, an ulcer with hard rolled edges or as a warty mass, most commonly on the labia majora; histologically, it is usually, though not invariably, well differentiated. The tumour spreads first to the inguinal lymph nodes: later spread is to femoral, iliac and para-aortic nodes. The overall 5-year survival rate for women treated for a vulvar carcinoma is about 70%: the survival rate is 90% for those without lymph node involvement but falls to between 25 and 60% for those with lymph node metastases.

Rare primary malignant neoplasms of the vulva include **adenocarcinoma of Bartholin's gland, malignant melanoma** and **basal cell carcinoma.**

The Vagina

Infections

Vaginal infections are common but many are non-specific in nature and due to lowered vaginal resistance to bacterial invasion, as occurs, for instance, in vaginal epithelial atrophy resulting from oestrogen deficiency. Specific infections, including those transmitted sexually, may be due to organisms such as *Neisseria gonorrhoeae, Mycoplasma,* herpesvirus, or *Chlamydia,* while candida infection, predisposed to by the high glycogen content of the vaginal epithelium, is common; sexually transmitted infestation with the protozoal parasite *Trichomonas vaginalis* is also very common.

Adenosis

This is characterized by the presence of small glands or cysts in the submocosa of the upper third of the vagina; the epithelium in these may be endocervical, endometrial or tubal in type. This, usually asymptomatic, congenital abnormality is particularly common in girls whose mothers received synthetic oestrogen therapy during pregnancy and, although innocuous in itself, predisposes to the development of an adenocarcinoma.

Tumours

Squamous-cell carcinoma of the vagina is uncommon: it usually occurs in the upper part of the vagina in elderly women and presents as an indurated patch: the tumour is often poorly differentiated and tends to invade the cervix, paravaginal tissues, rectum and bladder, the 5-year survival rate after treatment being only about 30%.

Adenocarcinoma of the vagina was, until recently, of exceptional rarity, but in the last 15 years a considerable number of clear-cell vaginal adenocarcinomas have occurred in girls aged between 15 and 25, mostly in North America. Common to virtually all of these cases has been pre-existing vaginal adenosis and a history of prenatal exposure to synthetic oestrogens, particularly diethylstilboestrol.

The Uterus

The Cervix

Cervicitis

Cervical infection is common, possibly because the complex deep folds of the endocervical crypts offer a relatively protected haven in which micro-organisms can flourish. The inflammatory response to infection may be either acute or chronic, the histological characteristics of the inflammatory process being exactly the same as those seen in comparable infections elsewhere in the body. Many cervical infections are of a non-specific, and probably mixed, bacterial nature, but specific infection with *Neisseria gonorrhoeae*, herpesvirus, *Chlamydia*, mycobacteria, *Trichomonas vaginalis*, and *Treponema pallidum* can occur.

Cervical Ectopy

This term is applied to a red area on the ectocervix which surrounds the external os (Fig. 21.2): this abnormality is often erroneously called an 'erosion'. An ectopy is a physiological change consequent upon an increase in cervical bulk, as occurs at puberty or in pregnancy; this causes an unfolding of the cervix with eversion of the distal endocervix out into what is anatomically the ectocervix. The thin endocervical columnar epithelium is relatively transparent and hence the subepithelial vessels impart to an ectopy its characteristic redness. The exposure of the delicate endocervical epithelium to the acidity of the vagina results in squamous metaplasia, a protective mechanism. This area of squamous metaplasia is often known as the **transformation zone** and is of considerable importance because most cervical carcinomas appear to originate at this site.

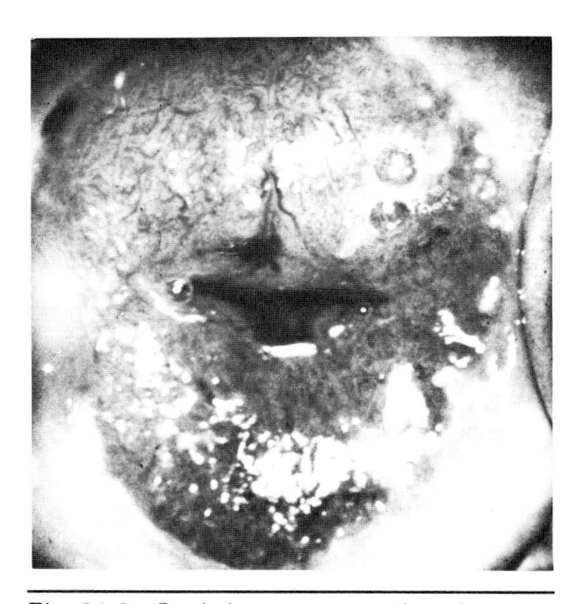

Fig. 21.2 Cervical ectopy as seen through a colposcope. The external os is circumferentially surrounded by thin endocervical epithelium through which the subepithelial vessels are clearly visible.

Premalignant Disease of the Cervix

A squamous-cell carcinoma of the cervix does not usually arise abruptly in otherwise normal cervical squamous epithelium but evolves over a number of years, probably 10–15, from an epithelium which shows progressively severe degrees of abnormality. The early, or premalignant stage of cervical carcinoma is characterized by the presence within the squamous epithelium of cells showing a failure of maturation, loss of polarity, excessive and abnormal mitotic activity, an increased nucleocytoplasmic ratio and both nuclear and cytoplasmic pleomorphism. The term **cervical intraepithelial neoplasia (CIN)** has been introduced to cover the whole spectrum of premalignant change in cervical epithelium. If undifferentiated cells are confined to the lower third of the epithelium the lesion is classed as CIN I whilst if such cells extend into the middle third of the epithelium the term CIN II is applied: if undifferentiated cells extend into the upper third of the epithelium, or occupy its full thickness, the lesion is regarded as CIN III (Fig. 21.3). It should not, however, be assumed that all examples of CIN I or II progress to CIN III or that CIN III will invariably proceed to an invasive carcinoma. Many cases of CIN, at any stage in the evolution of this abnormality, either remain stationary or regress with probably no more than one-third of cases of CIN III advancing to the invasive stage; indeed, it is almost certain that some, probably many, examples of CIN I and II are not truly neoplastic in nature but represent an atypical cellular response to factors such as viral infection. Currently, however, there are no available methods for distinguishing a reactive lesion from one which is truly neoplastic or for the recognition of those cases of CIN which will progress to invasive cancer. Hence, all cases of CIN have to be regarded as potentially invasive: fortunately these epithelial lesions, though asymptomatic, are readily de-

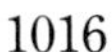

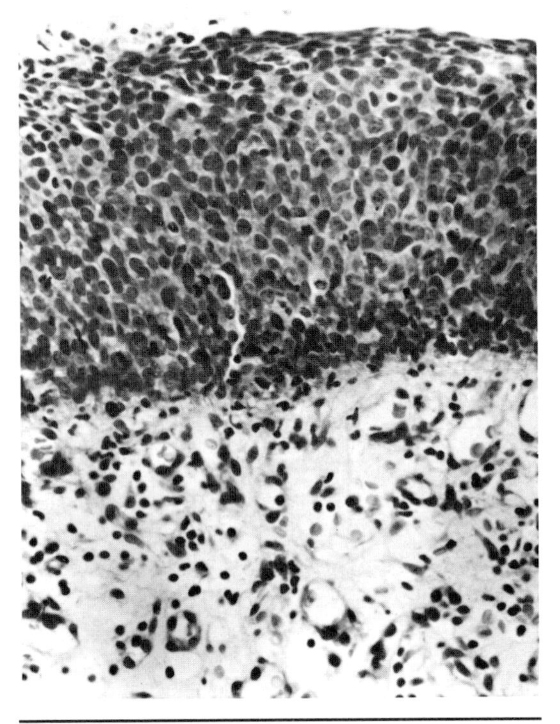

Fig. 21.3 Cervical intraepithelial neoplasia (CIN) grade III of the uterine cervix. The cells in the cervical epithelium show a complete lack of maturation, are pleomorphic and have an increased nucleocytoplasmic ratio. ×275.

tected by cytological examination of cervical smear preparations and their treatment and eradication, by techniques such as cryocautery and laser therapy, are relatively simple. It is hoped that widespread cytological screening and prompt treatment of intraepithelial abnormalities will reduce markedly the incidence of invasive cervical carcinoma.

Malignant Tumours of the Cervix

Seventy per cent of malignant cervical tumours are squamous-cell carcinomas, most of the remainder being either adenocarcinomas or mixed adenosquamous carcinomas.

Squamous-cell Carcinoma

Epidemiological studies have demonstrated an association between squamous-cell carcinoma of the cervix and early marriage, early pregnancy, a high number of pregnancies, sexual promiscuity, divorce, sexually transmitted diseases, prostitution and low socio-economic status. It is virtually certain that the one common link between these various factors is early onset of sexual activity. It is believed that a carcinogen is transmitted sexually by the male at a time when the epithelium of the cervix is in an unstable state, i.e. when the transformation zone is undergoing squamous metaplasia during late adolescence. The nature of this carcinogenic agent remains uncertain but suspicion has fallen on certain strains of human papillomavirus (p. 406). Certainly the role of sexual transmission is indicated by the fact that barrier methods of contraception are associated with a lower incidence of cervical carcinoma and by the apparent proneness of some men to be 'carcinogenic', their sexual partners having an unusually high risk of developing cervical cancer.

Cervical squamous-cell carcinoma may grow out from the surface as a friable, papillary or polypoid mass (Fig. 21.4) or extend deeply into the cervix, converting it into a hard, bulky, nodular mass which eventually ulcerates. The tumour tends to infiltrate as irregular sheets of epithelial cells, sometimes with pointed or spiky margins (Fig. 21.5). Formation of epithelial pearls and keratin is unusual.

The neoplasm invades locally into the uterine body, vagina, parametrial tissues, bladder and rectum; of particular importance is involvement of the ureters, either by direct invasion of their walls or by compression by extrinsic tumour masses. Lymph-node spread occurs at an early stage to pelvic, inguinal, iliac and aortic nodes but spread by the blood, principally to liver, lungs and bone, does not occur until a late stage. Death used to be most commonly due to uraemia consequent upon ureteric obstruction but is now, because of effective pelvic therapy, more usually due to distant metastases. The 5-year cure rate for patients in whom the tumour is confined to the cervix is, with modern therapy, about 85%, falling to between 50

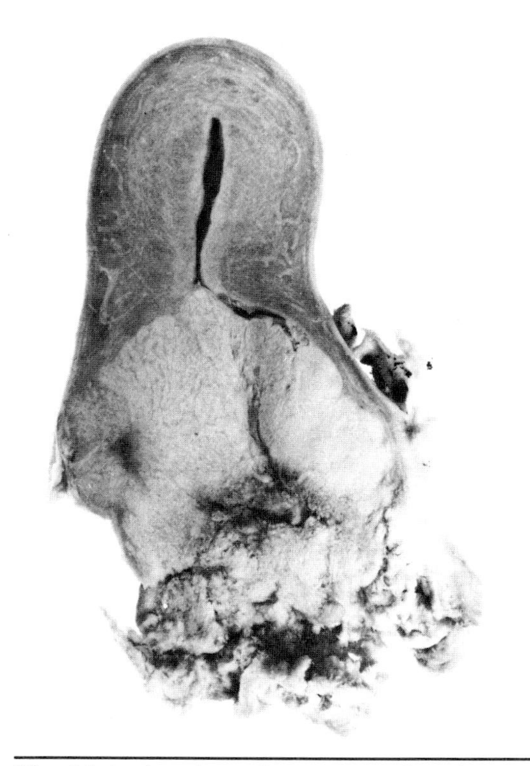

Fig. 21.4 An advanced squamous-cell carcinoma of the uterine cervix.

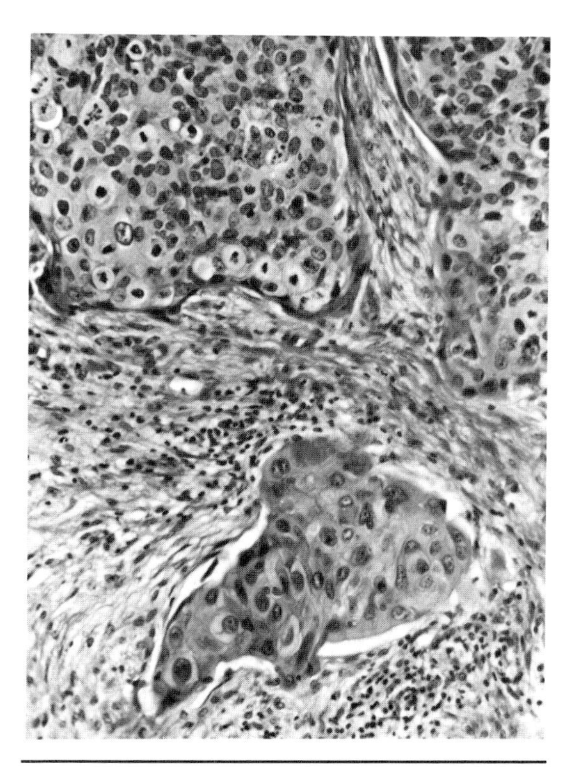

Fig. 21.5 Squamous-cell carcinoma of the uterine cervix showing infiltrating masses of tumour cells. Note the numerous mitotic figures. ×165.

and 75% for those cases with pelvic invasion at the time of treatment.

Adenocarcinoma

The factors listed aetiologically for cervical squamous-cell carcinoma do not apply to cervical adenocarcinoma and indeed the neoplasm is relatively commoner in nullipara. Some adenocarcinomas of clear-cell type occur in young girls exposed prenatally to diethylstilboestrol.

The tumour grows in the endocervix and is commonly well differentiated: it tends to spread upwards into the myometrium and outwards into the pelvis and the 5-year cure rate is relatively poor.

The Endometrium

The endometrium is that part of the uterine lining above the level of the internal os and consists of a basal layer, which is insensitive to hormonal stimulation, and a superficial functional layer which is markedly sensitive to ovarian hormones.

Endometrial Morphology during the Menstrual Cycle

The menstrual cycle is divided into three stages; the **pre-ovulatory**, during which the developing graafian follicle is secreting oestrogens, the **post-ovulatory**, throughout which the corpus luteum is producing both oestrogens and progesterone, and the **menstrual**. During the pre-ovulatory stage the endometrium regenerates and grows under the influence of oestrogen and is said to be in the proliferative phase (Fig. 21.6); the glands are straight and narrow, the stroma is compact and

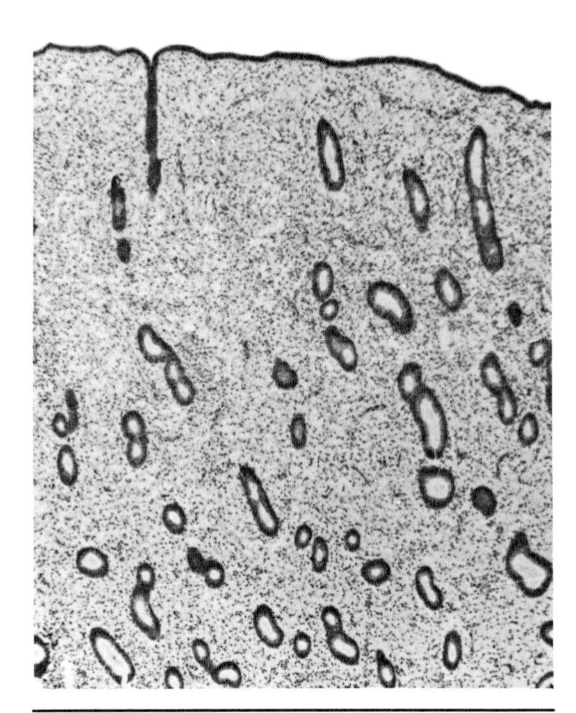

Fig. 21.6 Section of the endometrium on the 10th day of the cycle, showing the appearances of the proliferative phase. The glands are relatively small. ×60.

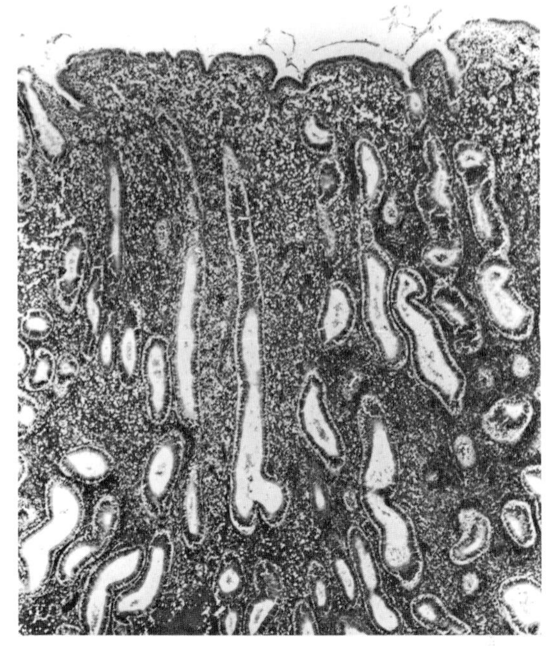

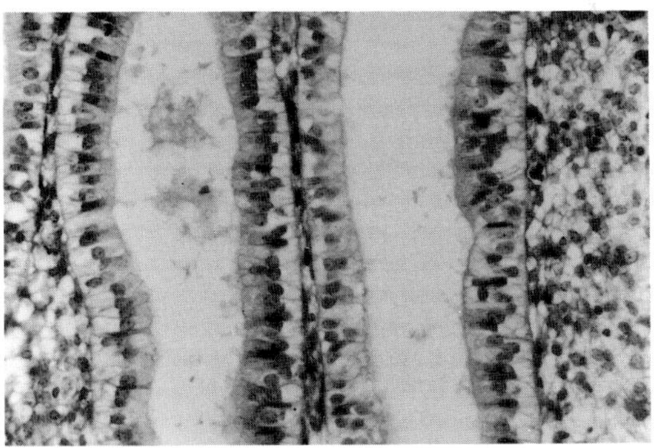

Fig. 21.7 Post-ovulatory endometrium on the 16th day of the cycle. The glands have increased in size and show basal vacuolation. Above, ×30; below, ×245.

cellular and mitotic figures are seen in both the glands and stroma. After ovulation, which usually occurs about the 14th day of the cycle, the endometrium enters the secretory phase, the first morphological evidence of which is the appearance of subnuclear glycogen-containing vacuoles in the glandular epithelial cells (Fig. 21.7); these appear about 36–48 hours after ovulation. As the secretory phase progresses the vacuoles disappear, the epithelial nuclei return to a basal position, the glands become increasingly dilated and tortuous and secretions appear in their lumens (Fig. 21.8); because oestrogens increase endometrial intracapillary hydrostatic pressure the stroma becomes markedly oedematous during the mid-part of the secretory phase. When the corpus luteum begins to degenerate there is a precipitous fall in oestrogen levels, a rapid regression of the stromal oedema and a sudden decrease in thickness of the endometrium with buckling of the spiral vessels, vascular stasis and ischaemic necrosis of the functional layer. As the oedema regresses the stroma becomes compact and the stromal cells take on a decidua-like appearance. Shortly before breakdown of the endometrium the stroma becomes infiltrated by polymorphonuclear leucocytes and these harbingers of overt necrosis are soon followed by disintegration and haemorrhage, the menstrual phase of the cycle now having been reached. Most of the functional layer is lost during menstruation but the basal layer persists to give rise to the regenerative phase of the next cycle.

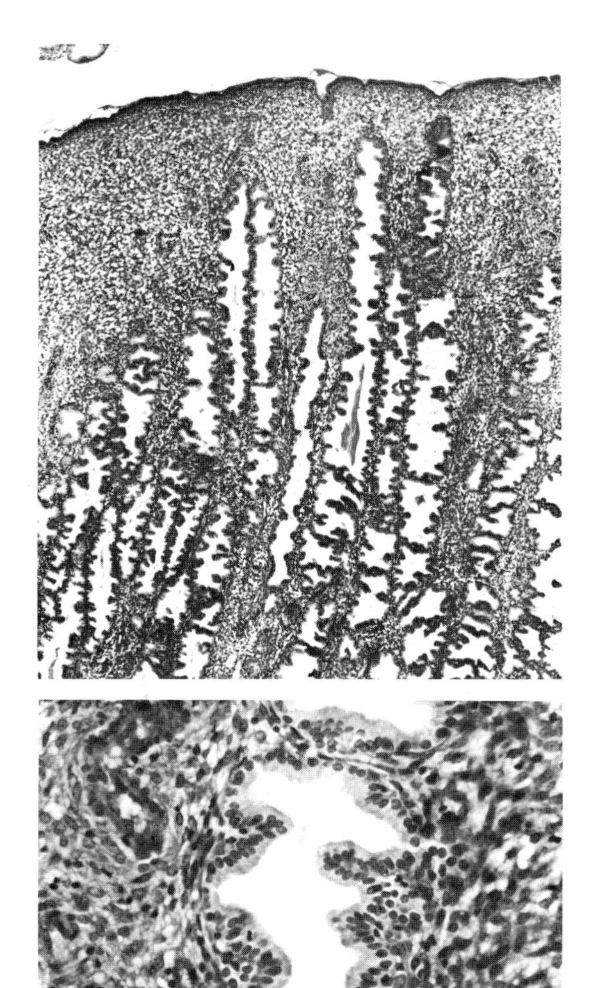

Fig. 21.8 Secretory-stage endometrium on the 25th day of the cycle. The glands contain secretion and are convoluted, presenting a 'saw-tooth' appearance. Above, ×30; below, ×245.

Factors Altering Endometrial Morphology

Pregnancy. The normal cycle will be interrupted if a fertilized ovum implants in the endometrium; when this occurs the corpus luteum persists, the stromal oedema fails to subside completely, the stromal cells become large, plump and polygonal with abundant cytoplasm, the glands enlarge and glandular secretion increases.

Oral contraception. The use of oral steroid contraceptives markedly alters endometrial morphology. The type of pattern seen depends upon the dosage and the type of preparation used, but a very characteristic pattern with the combined type of regime is one of endometrial atrophy in which the glands are small, relatively few and largely inactive, with a compact stroma showing a variable degree of decidua-like change (Fig. 21.9). The endometrium rapidly reverts to normal after stopping oral contraceptives.

Intrauterine contraceptive devices. The effects on the endometrium vary with the type of device used but focal atrophy and fibrosis are commonly seen; foci of haemorrhage and squamous metaplasia may be present whilst there is frequently a mononuclear cell infiltration of the stroma. Cyclical changes continue in the endometrium but the secretory phase tends to be accelerated.

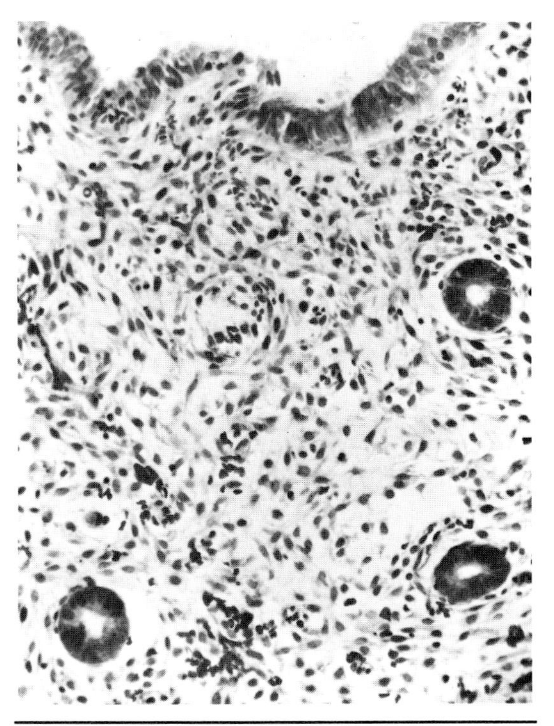

Fig. 21.9 Endometrium from a woman taking a hormonal contraceptive pill. The stroma is abundant while the glands are reduced in number, small and inactive. ×200.

The menopause. Some slight proliferative activity may occur in the endometrium for a year or two after the menopause, but the postmenopausal endometrium undergoes a progressive atrophy and the glands eventually become inactive. Stromal fibrosis is not uncommon and this often leads to obstruction of the necks of many of the glands, which tend to become cystically dilated; the cystic glands are lined by a thin, inactive epithelium.

Endometritis

The endometrium is relatively resistant to infection, partly because of its excellent natural drainage and partly because it is difficult for an infection to become established during reproductive life in a tissue which is regularly shed.

Acute endometritis occurs most commonly after an abortion or parturition, especially if fragments of placenta or membranes are retained in the uterus; a variety of organisms, including streptococci, staphylococci, *Escherichia coli* and pseudomonas, may be implicated. An acute sterile inflammation can also occur with certain types of intrauterine contraceptive device and may also complicate irradiation of the uterus.

The inflamed endometrium is oedematous and congested; with a varying degree of ulceration and tissue destruction and a polymorphonuclear leucocytic infiltration. The cellular infiltrate differs from that which occurs as a physiological event during the late stage of the menstrual cycle by being present, not only in the stroma, but also in the glands, where small intraluminal abscesses are commonly seen.

Non-specific chronic endometritis. A chronic inflammation of the endometrium may follow an acute endometritis but is more commonly chronic from the outset. Macroscopically the endometrium may be somewhat thickened but often appears normal. Chronic inflammation in this site is characterized by the same features as elsewhere in the body and the diagnosis rests upon the finding of a chronic inflammatory cell infiltration of the stroma; the infiltrate must be of more than trivial degree and although occasionally purely lymphocytic in type there is usually an admixture with, and sometimes a predominance of, plasma cells. Some degree of fibroblastic and vascular proliferation may be present, whilst the normal cyclical changes may continue undisturbed, be accentuated or absent.

Chronic endometritis may follow abortion or childbirth and can occur in association with an intrauterine contraceptive device, chronic salpingitis or endometrial adenocarcinoma; furthermore, endometrial tuberculosis can masquerade as a non-specific inflammation.

Tuberculous endometritis is nearly always secondary to tuberculous salpingitis and is now uncommon in Western countries. The disease is often accompanied by infertility but this may well be because of the accompanying tubal lesions rather than a result of endometrial damage, for the normal cyclical changes are not usually interrupted by a tuberculous endometritis. Continued menstrual shedding of the endometrium prevents the disease proceeding to the stage of caseation, and in premenopausal women the characteristic histological finding is a few small scattered tubercles with little or no central caseation. The tubercles are maximally developed, and so most obvious, in the later stages of the menstrual cycle and diagnostic biopsy in suspected cases should always be undertaken at this time. Occasionally, tubercles are absent and the findings are of a non-specific chronic endometritis.

Endometrial tuberculosis is rare in postmenopausal women but when it does occur there is no obstacle to its progression to caseation. In such cases the endometrium may appear as a thickened whitish-yellow, shaggy lining to the uterine cavity and sometimes the latter is itself filled with caseous material; histologically, the endometrium will show confluent caseating tuberculosis.

Endometrial Polyps

The term polyp is a purely descriptive one and does not denote any specific pathological process;

it is, however, usually applied to a focal overgrowth of the endometrium which protrudes into the uterine cavity. Such polyps are common; they may be pedunculated or sessile and are characteristically pink and fleshy with a smooth surface. Histologically, a polyp is covered by columnar epithelium and contains endometrial stroma and glands; the latter are commonly either inactive or show patchy irregular cyclical changes but are, in some cases, responsive to oestrogen but not to progesterone and thus show simple hyperplasia (see below). A pedunculated polyp may undergo torsion, and ulceration of the tip of the polyp may cause bleeding. Malignant change is extremely uncommon.

Endometrial Hyperplasia

Two quite separate conditions are included together under the general term endometrial hyperplasia and a diagnosis of hyperplasia without specification of the type is of no value.

Simple hyperplasia. In this condition the uterus is moderately enlarged whilst the endometrial lining is thickened, often appearing polypoidal. Histologically, the endometrium is diffusely involved and the distinction between functional and basal zones is lost. The endometrial glands are straight and cylindrical but of very variable calibre, some being unusually small, but invariably a number are considerably larger than normal (Fig. 21.10). The glands are lined by narrow columnar cells with basophilic cytoplasm; some multilayering may be present but there is no pleomorphism or cellular atypia. The stromal cells are plump and closely packed, giving a hypercellular appearance. As both stroma and glands share in the hyperplastic process the ratio of glands to stroma is approximately normal.

Simple hyperplasia is due to prolonged, unopposed oestrogenic stimulation of the endometrium, the commonest cause of which is a succession of anovulatory cycles. These occur most frequently in the perimenopausal years but are not uncommon during the menarche and are characterized by the development of a succession of graafian follicles which mature, fail to release their ova, persist for weeks or months and then degenerate; the consequent fluctuations in plasma oestrogen levels lead to intermittent breaking down of the hyperplastic endometrium and irregular heavy bleeding. Simple hyperplasia can also be produced by prolonged oestrogen therapy and by oestrogen-secreting ovarian tumours. Simple hyperplasia is not associated with subsequent adenocarcinoma and should not be regarded as a premalignant condition.

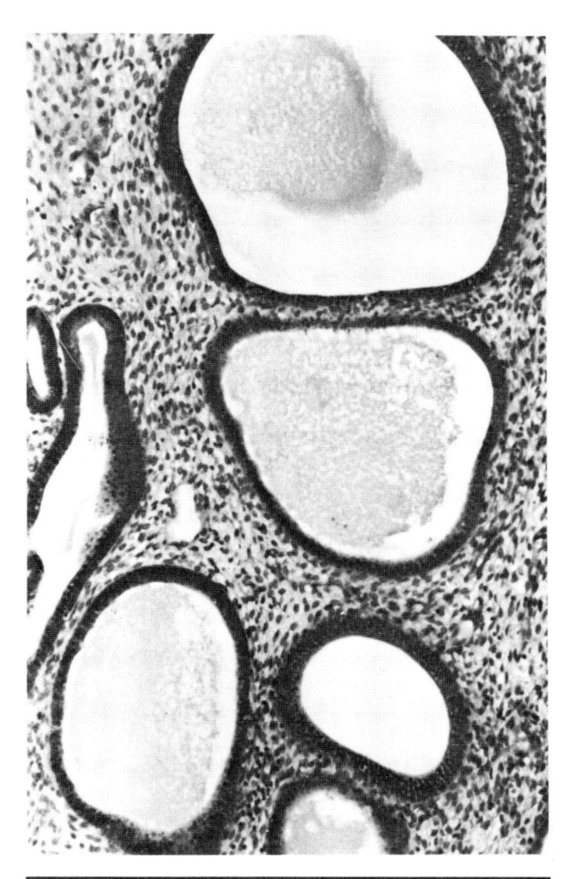

Fig. 21.10 Simple hyperplasia of the endometrium. The glands, many of which are greatly enlarged, are lined by tall darkly staining cells. ×100.

Atypical endometrial hyperplasia may be combined with, or occur independently of, simple hyperplasia; this form of hyperplasia is, however, invariably focal rather than diffuse and is not simply a late stage of simple hyperplasia. Atypical hyperplasia is characterized by irregular glandular proliferation without any accompanying stromal proliferation (Fig. 21.11). The glands are increased in number and crowded together, in severe cases being in direct apposition with each other to give a 'back-to-back' appearance: they are irregular in outline and are lined by tall cells with eosinophilic cytoplasm, the epithelium often being multilayered and forming intraluminal buds. Varying degrees of cellular and nuclear atypia are present and mitotic figures are common and occasionally of abnormal form. In the most extreme cases of typical hyperplasia the distinction from a well differentiated adenocarcinoma may be almost impossible.

Atypical hyperplasia tends to occur under the same circumstances as does simple hyperplasia and is most common around the time of the menopause; the focal nature of the abnormality suggests that while simple hyperplasia is the normal response to prolonged oestrogenic stimulation, atypical hyperplasia represents an abnormal tissue response to this hormonal stimulus. Indeed, it is possible that this lesion is a form of intra-endometrial neoplasia rather than a true hyperplasia. Unlike simple hyperplasia, atypical hyperplasia is associated with a high risk of progression to an endometrial adenocarcinoma; the degree of risk is related to the severity of the atypia and in severe cases is in the region of 50%.

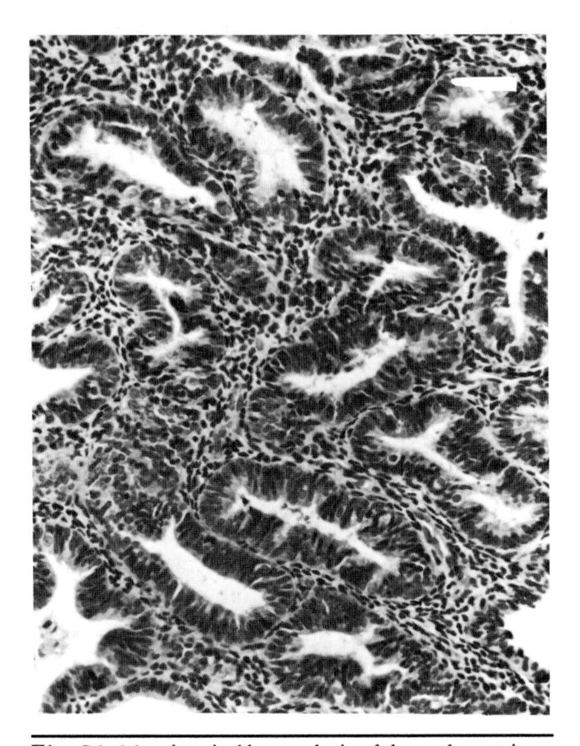

Fig. 21.11 Atypical hyperplasia of the endometrium. Note the crowding of the glands which are of irregular shapes and show evidence of multilayering. ×190.

Malignant Tumours of the Endometrium

Adenocarcinoma

The vast majority of malignant tumours of the endometrium are adenocarcinomas; these occur most commonly between the ages of 50 and 60. Nulliparous women are particularly prone to develop an endometrial adenocarcinoma. There is convincing evidence of a link with obesity, but not with hypertension or diabetes.

The aetiological role of oestrogens has been much debated but there is now little doubt that such hormones can contribute to the development of endometrial adenocarcinomas, as shown by the frequent occurrence of such neoplasms in women with oestrogenic ovarian tumours and their greatly increased incidence in women receiving long-term oestrogen therapy. Most women who develop an endometrial adenocarcinoma do so, however, in the absence of such factors: many of these patients have, however, an increased capacity for converting androstenedione, of adrenal origin, into oestrone in the body fat (hence the association with obesity). Although adenocarcinoma may evolve from an atypical hyperplasia, many such tumours arise from an atrophic endometrium.

The tumour may appear as a localized nodule, plaque or polyp, usually in the upper part of the uterus, but more commonly it presents either as a diffuse nodular or polypoid thickening of the uterine lining (Fig. 21.12), often with superficial ulceration and bleeding, or as a bulky, friable, partially necrotic mass which may fill, or even

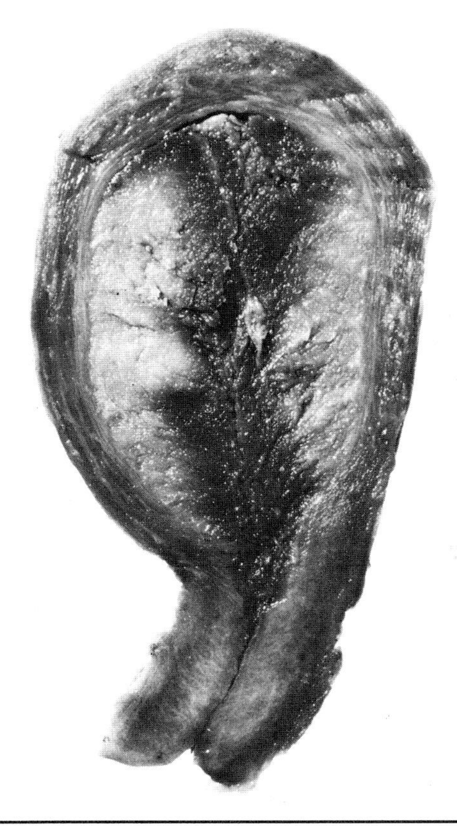

Fig. 21.12 Adenocarcinoma of the endometrium. The tumour has filled and distended the uterine cavity.

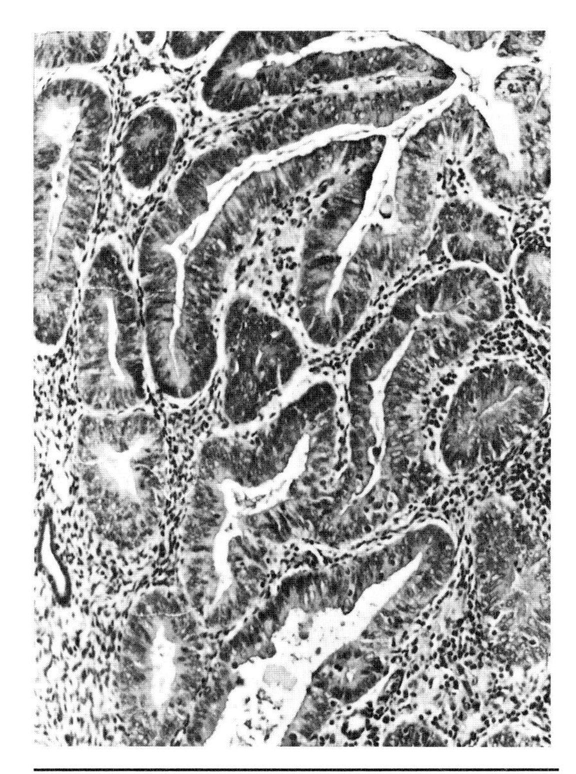

Fig. 21.13 A well differentiated endometrial adenocarcinoma. ×150.

expand, the uterine cavity. The uterus may be slightly or moderately enlarged, and the myometrium, although usually focally thinned by invading tumour, is occasionally diffusely thickened by widely infiltrating neoplastic cells.

The neoplasm is commonly a well differentiated adenocarcinoma (Fig. 21.13) but solid areas, a cribriform pattern and papillary formations are common and sometimes dominant. Foci of intraglandular squamous metaplasia are frequent, but some endometrial adenocarcinomas are admixed with malignant squamous tissue: such tumours, known as **adenosquamous carcinomas**, merit specific identification for they have an unusually poor prognosis.

Endometrial adenocarcinoma invades the myometrium at an early stage but, because of the thickness of this muscular barrier, tends to be confined to the uterus until late in the course of the disease. Eventual penetration of the myometrium leads to parametrial infiltration and tumour deposits in the pelvic peritoneum and pouch of Douglas. Extension along the lumen of the fallopian tube, a particular feature of growths arising in the cornu of the uterus, can result in implants in the ovaries and broad ligament. Vaginal metastases occur by venous or lymphatic dissemination. Lymphatic spread to the para-aortic nodes occurs at an early stage, but involvement of hypogastric and obturator nodes is a late event. Distant metastases to liver and lung are uncommon and death is usually due to the effects of neoplastic infiltration of the pelvis.

The prognosis is related to the degree of differentiation of the tumour and to the clinical stage at the time of diagnosis. The overall 5-year survival rate is in the region of 66%.

Sarcomas

Endometrial sarcomas arise from undifferentiated cells, which not only retain their embryonic potential to develop into endometrial stromal and glandular cells, but also have a capacity to differentiate into connective tissue cells of a type foreign to the uterus, e.g. cartilage, fat, striated muscle. Sarcomas containing only endometrial-type tissue are known as 'homologous' whilst those in which extra-uterine cell types occur are called 'heterologous'. Further, the neoplastic cells may differentiate along only one cellular pathway to give a 'pure' sarcoma or into a variety of cell types to form a 'mixed' sarcoma.

Thus, a sarcoma formed solely of malignant endometrial stromal cells is a **pure homologous sarcoma** whilst a uterine rhabdomyosarcoma is a **pure heterologous sarcoma**. A neoplasm containing both endometrial stromal sarcoma and endometrial adenocarcinoma is a **mixed homologous sarcoma** and is usually known as a **carcinosarcoma** while the presence, in such a tumour, of malignant foci of cartilage or striated muscle indicates a **mixed heterologous sarcoma**, commonly known as a **mixed Müllerian tumour**.

All endometrial sarcomas are rare but the carcinosarcoma and the mixed Müllerian tumour are the least uncommon: both usually develop in elderly women and form large polypoid tumour masses which expand the uterine cavity and extend through the endocervical canal to present in the vagina. The prognosis is very poor.

Endometriosis

Endometriosis is a condition in which tissue identical in all respects to the endometrium is found in sites distant from the uterus (Fig. 21.14). The ectopic tissue occurs most commonly in the ovaries, fallopian tubes, pouch of Douglas, uterine ligaments, rectovaginal septum and the bowel: occasionally, foci of endometriosis are encountered in laparotomy scars, at the umbilicus or in the skin, while exceptional instances of lesions occurring in lymph nodes, limbs, pleura and lung have been recorded.

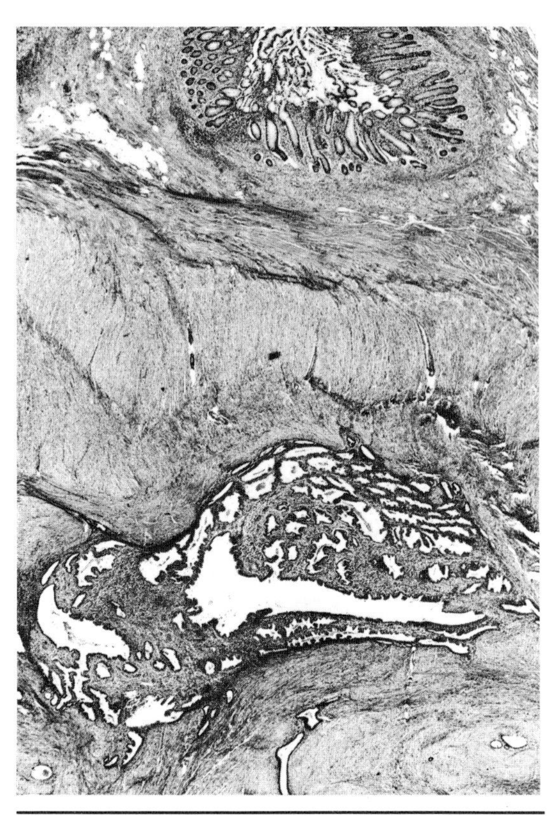

Fig. 21.14 Endometriosis of the appendix and caecum. A focus of endometrial glands and stroma, showing cystic change, is present in the muscular coat of the caecum close to the appendix (seen at top of picture). ×12.

The pathogenesis of this disorder is still far from clear but one possible mechanism is the reflux of viable fragments of endometrial tissue through the tubes during menstruation with subsequent implantation on, and growth in, the ovaries and pelvic peritoneum: certainly, endometriosis in scars appears to be due to implantation of endometrial tissue during uterine surgery. A further possibility is that endometriosis arises ectopically as a result of endometrial metaplasia of the peritoneal serosa; this is a feasible hypothesis and it may be that, in fact, such metaplasia is induced by regurgitated fragments of endometrial tissue which, after initiating the process, subsequently die. The occurrence of endometriosis in distant sites cannot, however, be explained except by invoking haematogenous or lymphatic dissemination and it is probable that there is no single pathogenic mechanism which applies to all cases of this condition.

Macroscopically, pelvic endometriosis is seen as small bluish nodules, often with surrounding fibrosis. In the ovaries the lesions are commonly cystic and contain altered blood; these may reach a considerable size and, because of the dark colour of their contents, are often referred to as 'chocolate cysts'. Ovarian endometriosis is frequently associated with dense adhesions, the ovaries being bound down to the broad ligament or bowel.

Histologically, the lesions of endometriosis consist of both endometrial glands and stroma. The endometrium is, however, usually functional and hence menstrual type bleeding occurs and often obscures and distorts the original histological appearances; indeed, the epithelial component is frequently destroyed and a presumption that the lesion was originally one of endometriosis is then only made possible by the presence of stroma containing many haemosiderin-laden macrophages.

It is the hormonal sensitivity of the endometriotic lesions that is responsible for their role in producing symptoms; recurrent swelling causes pain and repeated bleeding leads to fibrosis. Hence the commonest complaints are of pelvic pain just before and during the menstrual period, deep pain on sexual intercourse and rectal discomfort. Infertility is often noted but the basis of this is obscure as it is not due to tubal occlusion. Malignant change may occasionally occur in both ovarian and extra-ovarian foci of endometriosis.

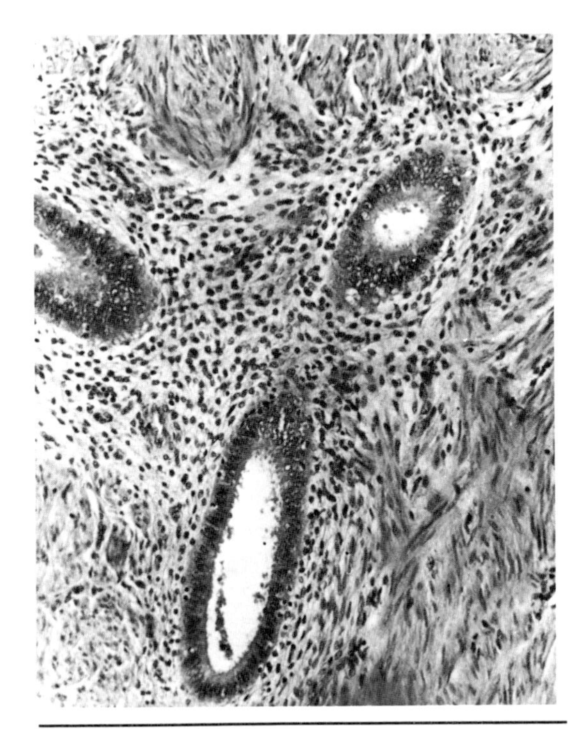

Fig. 21.15 Adenomyosis. A focus of well formed endometrial glands and stroma lying deep within the myometrium. ×150.

The Myometrium

The myometrium is the thick muscular wall of the uterus and is capable of marked alterations in size, capacity and contractility during pregnancy and labour.

Adenomyosis

This common condition is characterized by the presence of endometrial tissue within the myometrium, well below the base of the endometrium (Fig. 21.15). The nodules of ectopic tissue may be distributed diffusely, in which case the uterus shows a roughly symmetrical enlargement, or they may be focal, causing a poorly delineated, tumour-like, asymmetrical thickening of the myometrium. Histologically, foci of adenomyosis are not encapsulated and consist of typical endometrial glands and stroma; the glands are commonly of basal type and hence inactive, but cyclical changes and menstrual bleeding sometimes occur. The myometrial lesions can cause dysmenorrhoea and irregular, excessive bleeding with symptoms usually starting during the fourth decade and persisting until the menopause.

Adenomyosis is due to a downgrowth of basal endometrium into the myometrium and continuity of the ectopic tissue with the endometrium can be demonstrated by serial sectioning.

Benign Tumours

Leiomyomas

These originate from the smooth muscle cells of the myometrium: there is commonly an intermingling with fibrous tissue and these neoplasms are often called **fibroids**. Myometrial leiomyomas are extremely common, usually multiple (Fig. 21.16) and vary in size from tiny 'seedlings' less than 1 cm in diameter to huge masses which fill the abdomen. They may be within the wall, i.e. intramural, in a submucosal site immediately below the endometrium, or lie just beneath the peritoneum to form a subserosal tumour. The submucosal leiomyomas bulge into and distort the uterine cavity and the overlying endometrium is stretched and thinned; these neoplasms may become pedunculated and form a polypoid mass within the uterine cavity which can extend through the cervix into the vagina. The subserosal tumours grow out from the uterine surface, occasionally into the broad ligament, and may also become pedunculated; very rarely such a tumour becomes attached to the omentum or pelvic peritoneum and loses its stalk to become a 'parasitic leiomyoma'.

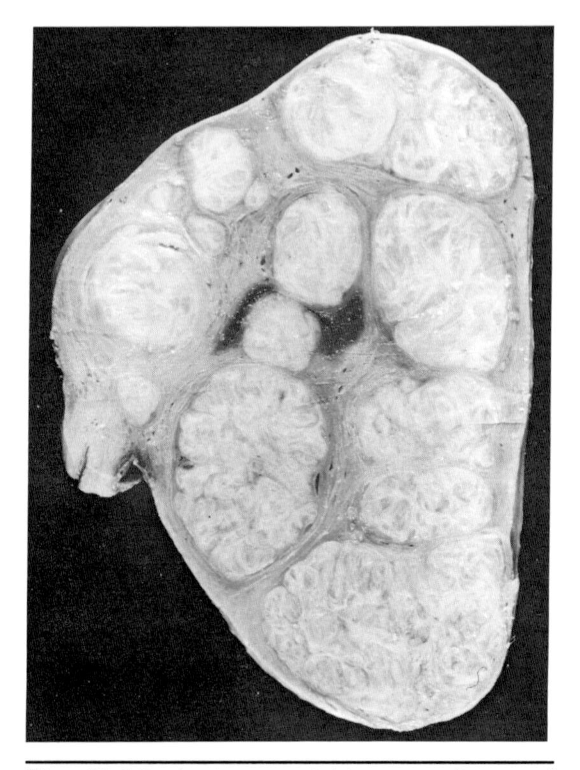

Fig. 21.16 A uterus containing many intramural leiomyomas. The cervix is seen on the left.

Leiomyomas have a well defined, regular outline and a surrounding layer of compressed uterine muscle fibres, giving the appearance of encapsulation; they are firm and their cut surface has a white whorled appearance. Histologically, the neoplasms are formed of interlacing bundles of smooth muscle fibres arranged in twists or whorls; some, known as cellular leiomyomas, contain densely packed spindle cells with elongated nuclei: rarely the smooth muscle fibres are rounded with central nuclei and clear cytoplasm, tumours containing such cells being called epithelioid leiomyomas. In all except the smallest tumours the appearances are altered to a variable degree by degenerative changes which are due to the neoplasm outgrowing its blood supply and thus fibrosis, hyaline change, calcification, patchy necrosis or fatty change are common. Infarction of a leiomyoma is uncommon but a pedunculated tumour may undergo torsion, whilst a specific form of necrosis, known as red degeneration, occurs particularly, but not only, in pregnancy and is characterized by a dull beefy red appearance of the whole tumour; this change may be accompanied by pain and fever and the presence of thrombosed vessels indicates that it is probably due to haemorrhagic infarction of an extremely hyalinized neoplasm.

Uterine leiomyomas appear to be at least partially under hormonal control, for they occur almost entirely during the reproductive years, enlarge during pregnancy and in women on oral contraceptives, and tend to regress after the menopause; nevertheless, attempts to relate them to a hormonal disturbance have been unsuccessful.

Many small leiomyomas are asymptomatic but large tumours can cause pressure effects with pelvic discomfort and frequency of micturition, and complaints of heavy prolonged menstrual bleeding, dysmenorrhoea and reduced fertility are common. Malignant change is rare (see below).

Adenomatoid Tumours

These appear as small subserosal nodules, usually in the cornual region, and consist of numerous small channels lined by endothelial-like cells and set in a connective tissue stroma: they are always benign and are probably derived from the serosa, resembling in their fine structure a benign mesothelioma.

Malignant Tumours

Myometrial **leiomyosarcomas** are rare and may arise either in a pre-existing leiomyoma or directly from the myometrium. They are less well demarcated in appearance than leiomyomas, often show areas of haemorrhage or necrosis, and are characterized histologically by their cellularity, pleomorphism and mitotic activity. Leiomyosarcomas occur most commonly during the sixth decade and have a poor prognosis.

The Fallopian Tubes

The fallopian tubes play a vital role in sperm and ovum transport and damage to them often results in infertility and sometimes in tubal pregnancy (p. 1036).

Salpingitis

Acute salpingitis is virtually always due to an infection which ascends via the uterine cavity and hence takes the form of endosalpingitis. The disease may occur after abortion, parturition or uterine instrumentation and has rather a high incidence in patients with an intrauterine contraceptive device; nevertheless most cases occur in the absence of such factors and are commonly due to a mixture of aerobic and anaerobic organisms of enteric type. *Neisseria gonorrhoeae* is now an uncommon cause of acute salpingitis and indeed the ability of this organism to cause an acute tubal inflammation is doubted by many, who consider that gonococcal salpingitis is usually only transient but inflicts sufficient minor damage to pave the way for subsequent establishment of secondary, mixed infection. *Mycoplasma* and *Chlamydia* are now emerging as important causes of acute salpingitis. In acute salpingitis both tubes are usually involved; they are congested, perhaps slightly swollen, and pus may be seen oozing from the fimbrial ostia, the fimbriae themselves being often swollen, congested and matted. Histologically, there is swelling and congestion of the mucosal folds (plicae) which are infiltrated with polymorphonuclear leucocytes; the lumen often contains pus.

Many cases of acute salpingitis resolve but a proportion pass into a chronic stage with polymorphonuclear, lymphocytic and plasma-cell infiltration (Fig. 21.17) and fibrosis; adhesions between the plicae become established and a complex cribriform pattern often results (Fig. 21.18), this being known as follicular salpingitis. The

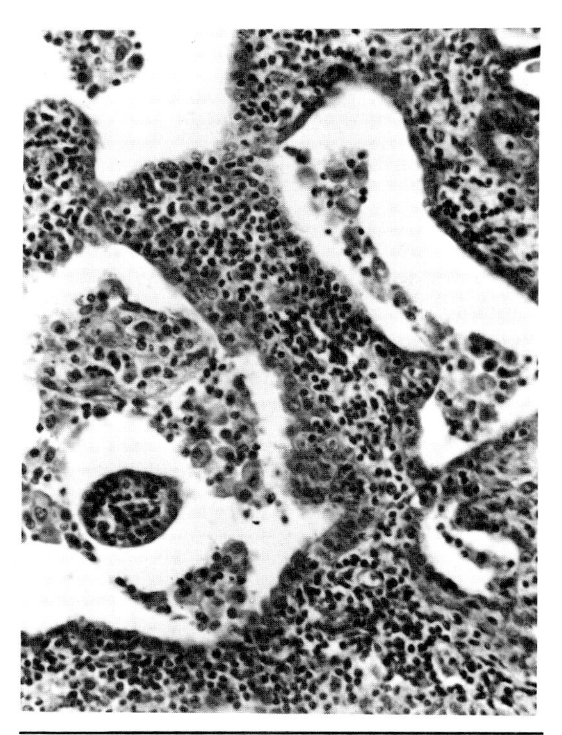

Fig. 21.17 Chronic salpingitis. The plicae are fused, thickened and infiltrated with inflammatory cells. Purulent exudate, containing polymorphs and macrophages is present in the lumen. ×200.

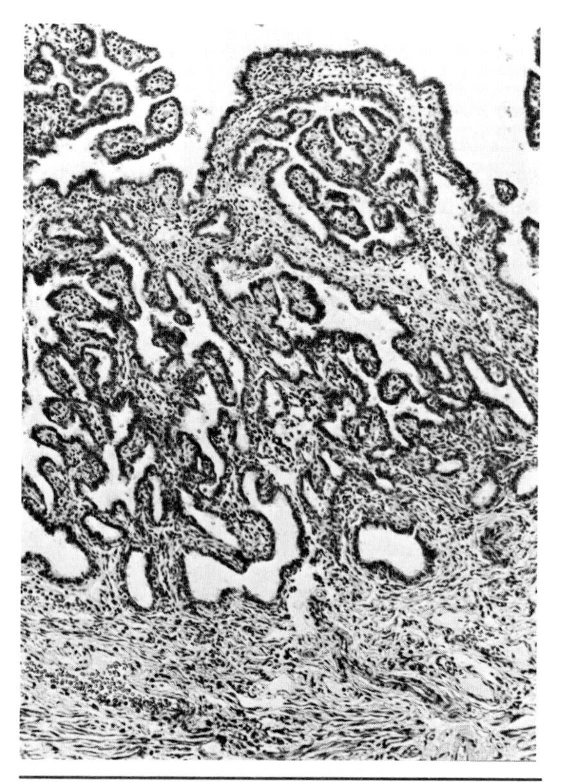

Fig. 21.18 Chronic follicular salpingitis. There is extensive fusion of the plicae, producing blind-ending crypts in the mucosa. ×130.

chronic inflammatory cell infiltrate may persist but often subsides leaving a legacy of residual scarring and deformity.

An acute salpingitis may also result in a pyosalpinx in which the fimbrial ostia become occluded and the tube distended by pus; such a condition may persist but more commonly infection is eliminated and a hydrosalpinx results in which the tube is thin-walled, greatly distended and contains clear watery fluid. The pathogenesis of a hydrosalpinx is not fully understood, for the isthmic end of the tube remains patent and there seems no good reason why the fluid should not drain into the uterus.

Tuberculous salpingitis. The fallopian tubes are usually the first part of the female genital tract to be involved in tuberculosis, tubal infection being almost invariably secondary to extragenital disease and reaching the tube via the blood. The infected tubes are usually moderately or markedly thickened and the tube deformed and bound down to the ovary by dense adhesions: in the less common exudative form of the disease the tube becomes grossly distended and resembles an ordinary pyosalpinx. Histologically, there is a diffuse non-specific chronic inflammatory cell infiltration of the mucosa and tubercles, usually few in number, are found scattered in the mucosa and submucosa; central caseation is usually apparent in the tubercules and foci of caseation often become confluent and rupture through the mucosa into the lumen.

Tumours of the Fallopian Tubes

Benign tumours such as **fibroma, adenoma, haemangioma** and **leiomyoma** are sometimes encountered. **Adenocarcinoma** is rare, bilateral in many cases, sometimes associated clinically with a characteristic watery vaginal discharge, and has a poor prognosis.

The Ovaries

Inflammation

Acute inflammation of the ovary occasionally complicates acute salpingitis and this combination may progress to a tubo-ovarian abscess.

Non-neoplastic Cysts

Cystic change occurs with some frequency in graafian follicles and corpora lutea. Corpus luteum cysts are usually solitary, contain either altered blood or clear amber fluid, are lined by luteinized granulosa and theca cells and, although usually asymptomatic, can rupture and bleed into the peritoneal cavity. Follicular cysts are found in the cortex and are small and unilocular. Their smooth lining is formed of flattened granulosa cells which may secrete sufficient oestrogen to inhibit pituitary FSH secretion and lead to anovulatory cycles with consequent endometrial hyperplasia. Multiple follicular cysts occur in a variety of conditions to give the picture of a polycystic ovary; when multiple cysts are associated with thickening of the ovarian capsule, hyperplasia and luteinization of theca cells and anovulation, there is often an accompanying clinical triad (expressed either partially or fully) of infertility, obesity and hirsutism which is known as the Stein–Leventhal syndrome. The exact pathophysiology of this condition is obscure but it appears that this particular type of polycystic ovary secretes, possibly because of an enzyme defect, an excess of androstenedione.

If the ovaries are subjected to excessive gonadotrophic stimulation, as occurs in patients with a hydatidiform mole and in some women receiving gonadotrophin therapy, cysts, known as theca-lutein cysts, may develop in the luteinized granulosa cells of atretic follicles.

Tumours of the Ovaries

The many different ovarian tumours are classified on the basis of their cell or tissue of origin. A simplified form of the complex classification of ovarian tumours defines five main groups:

(1) tumours derived from the surface epithelium;
(2) tumours of sex cord and stromal origin;
(3) tumours derived from germ cells;
(4) miscellaneous tumours;
(5) metastatic tumours.

Tumours Derived from the Surface Epithelium

Approximately 60% of all ovarian tumours, and 90% of those which are malignant, are derived from the surface epithelium: they are collectively known as the common epithelial tumours. The ovarian surface epithelium is derived from, and is the mature equivalent of, the coelomic epithelium which in embryonic life overlies the gonadal ridge and from which are derived the Müllerian ducts and the tissues to which these give rise, i.e. the tubal and endocervical epithelia and the endometrium. Neoplasms arising from indifferent cells in the surface epithelium retain this embryonic potential for Müllerian differentiation. In some, the tumour epithelium differentiates along an endocervical pathway, producing the mucinous neoplasms; others differentiate into a tubal type of epithelium, forming the serous group of tumours, while a third group differentiates along endometrial lines to produce the endometrioid neoplasms. Surface epithelial tumours also have a potential for differentiating along Wolffian lines to form urothelium, neoplasms containing such epithelium being eponymously called Brenner tumours. The clear cell tumours are probably a morphological variant of the endometrioid group of neoplasms.

All these epithelial neoplasms can exist in benign and malignant forms and those which are malignant are often grouped together as ovarian adenocarcinomas. These are the commonest fatal tumours of the female reproductive system. They form bulky masses which tend to infiltrate locally into the pelvic tissue and seed tumour implants on to the omentum, but they rarely metastasize to extra-abdominal sites.

Patients with ovarian adenocarcinoma have a 5-year survival rate of only 30% and little is known of the aetiology of this form of neoplasia; it is thought that recurrent ovulation, which repeatedly inflicts minor trauma on the surface epithelium, and exposure to exogenous ascending material, such as talc or asbestos, may possibly be of aetiological significance.

In addition to the benign and malignant forms, a third category of tumours of borderline malignancy or tumours of low malignant potential is recognized for epithelial neoplasms. These resemble macroscopically the benign forms but are characterized histologically by changes in their epithelium which suggest malignancy, i.e. multilayering, irregular budding, cellular atypia and mitotic activity, without, however, any evidence of stromal invasion. Most such neoplasms behave in a benign fashion but a few pursue an indolently malignant course over 10 years or more.

Benign mucinous tumours (mucinous cystadenomas) are common and form large cysts with a smooth outer surface; they are usually multilocular and contain clear mucous material. Microscopically, the cyst epithelium is formed of tall mucin-secreting columnar cells which, in most cases, are identical to those lining the endocervix (Fig. 21.19). In a minority, however, the epithelium is of gastrointestinal type and contains argyrophil and Paneth cells; neoplasms containing this enteric type of epithelium may be derived from the surface epithelium from a focus of intestinal metaplasia, but some are thought to be teratomas which have developed along only one tissue line. Benign mucinous cysts may attain a huge size and distend the abdomen; torsion may occur, and occasionally the cyst ruptures and the contents escape into the peritoneal cavity, where tumour cells may become attached and form seedling growths which continue to secrete mucin (pseudomyxoma peritonei). This condition is likely to cause death from matting together and obstruction of the intestine by masses of mucin undergoing organization.

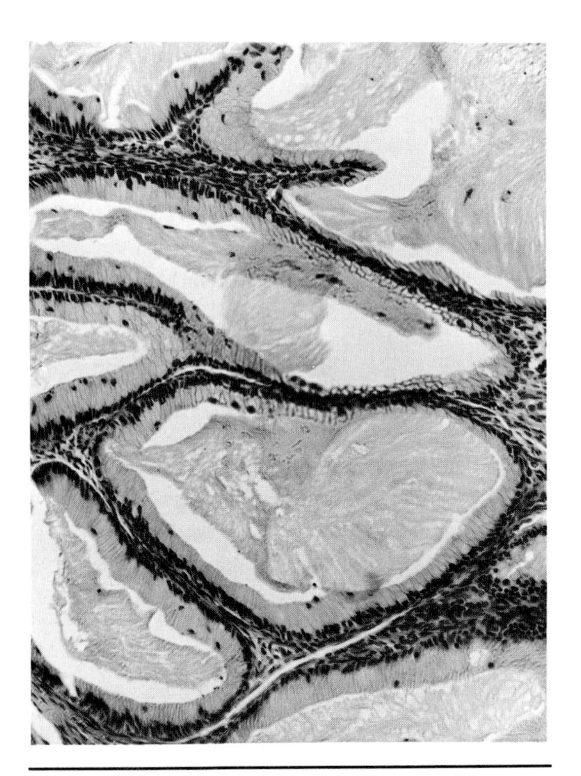

Fig. 21.19 Mucinous cystadenoma of the ovary, showing acini lined by tall columnar epithelium and containing mucous secretion. ×130.

Malignant mucinous tumours (mucinous adenocarcinomas) are often partially solid, and show the usual features of malignancy.

Benign serous tumours (serous cystadenomas) commonly occur as thin-walled unilocular cysts though in some the inner surface shows papillary projections into the lumen. Histologically, the epithelium of these cysts is identical to that of the fallopian tube (Fig. 21.20). Serous tumours may also grow as a papillary warty outgrowth on the surface of the ovary.

Malignant serous tumours (serous cystadenocarcinomas) are usually cystic but contain numerous soft papillary ingrowths and are frequently solid in some areas.

Endometrioid tumours are usually malignant, benign and borderline forms being rare. The tumours, usually solid with areas of haemorrhage, are commonly histologically identical with endometrial adenocarcinomas but any type of endometrial neoplasm can occur in the ovary as a form of endometrioid tumour, e.g. mixed Müllerian tumours. Although most endometrioid neoplasms originate from the surface epithelium, a minority arises from foci of pre-existing ovarian endometriosis.

Brenner tumours are usually small, solid and benign; microscopically, they consist of rounded islands of transitional-type epithelium embedded in

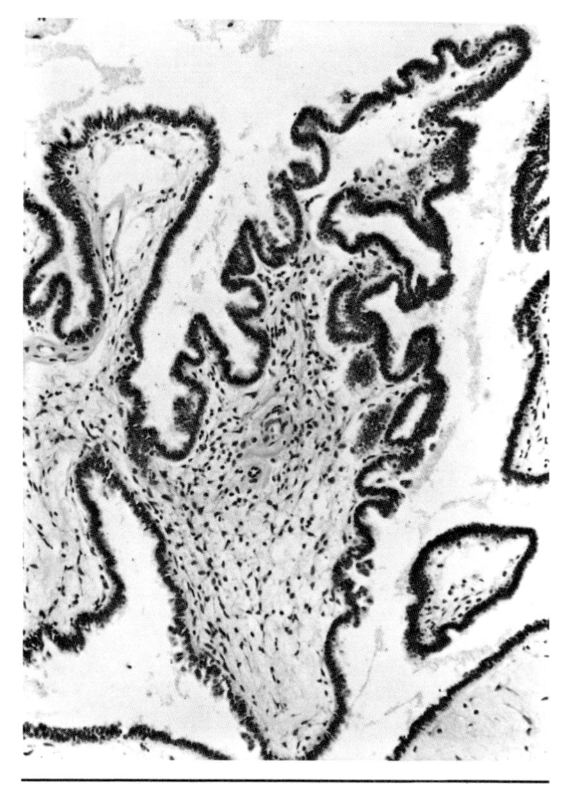

Fig. 21.20 Serous cystadenoma of the ovary, showing papillary processes which are lined by tubal-type epithelium and project into the lumen. ×100.

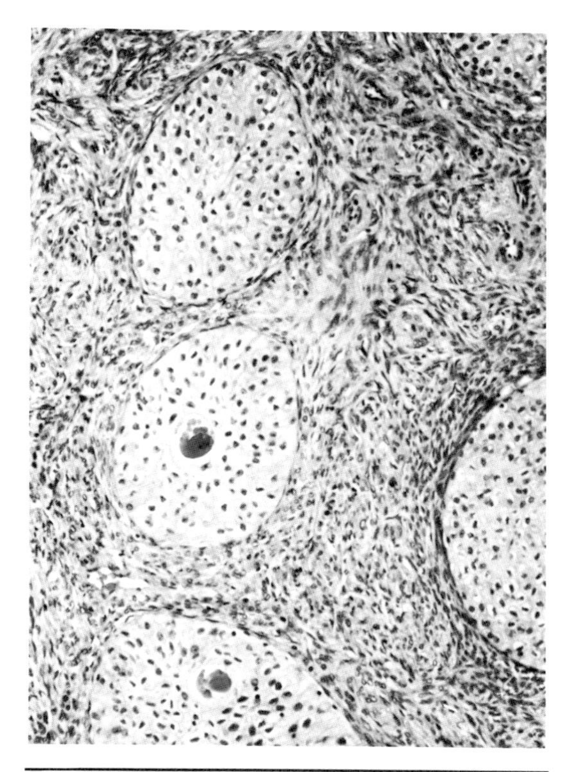

Fig. 21.21 Brenner tumour of the ovary. ×150.

a dense fibrous stroma (Fig. 21.21). Malignant forms are rare.

Clear-cell carcinomas show a complex papillary and tubular pattern intermingled with sheets of clear cells.

Tumours of Sex Cord and Stromal Origin

During the early embryonic stages of gonadal development, cords of cells, possibly derived from the surface epithelium and known as sex cords, envelop the germ cells: at this stage the primitive gonad is capable of developing into either an ovary or a testis and the cells derived from the sex cords can differentiate into either the granulosa cells of the graafian follicle or the Sertoli cells of the seminiferous tubules. There is an interaction between the sex cords and the adjacent primitive gonadal stroma, cells from the latter differentiating into either thecal cells or Leydig cells. Tumours derived from tissues of sex cord or stromal origin retain this bisexual embryonic potential and can differentiate into any of these various cell types either singly or in any combination.

Granulosa-cell tumour is the commonest representative of this group of neoplasms. It is usually small, solid and formed of cells of granulosa type arranged in follicles, trabeculae, islands or sheets; the solid groups of cells often contain tiny cystic spaces filled with eosinophilic fluid and nuclear debris, known as Call–Exner bodies (Fig. 21.22). Granulosa-cell tumours frequently secrete oestrogens and can be responsible for signs of precocious puberty in young girls; in older patients the effects of prolonged oestrogenic stimulation of the endometrium, i.e. hyperplasia and sometimes adenocarcinoma, lead to complications of menor-

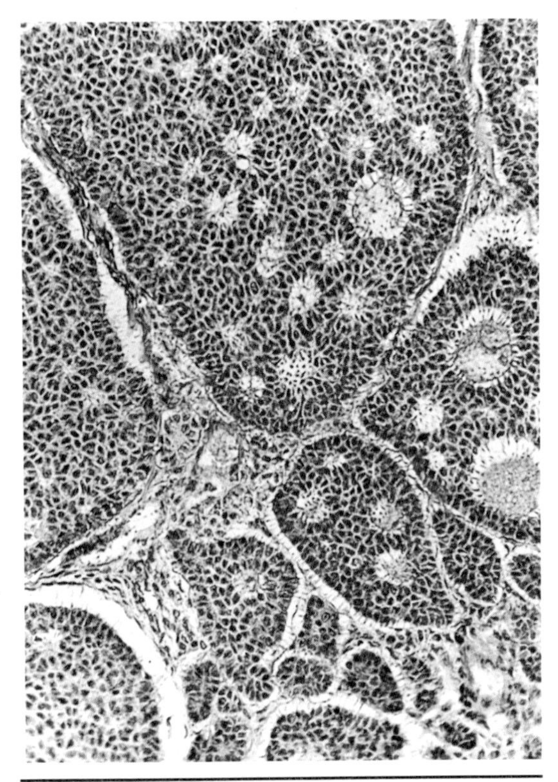

Fig. 21.22 Granulosa-cell tumour of the ovary, showing the characteristic masses of cells with Call–Exner bodies. ×225.

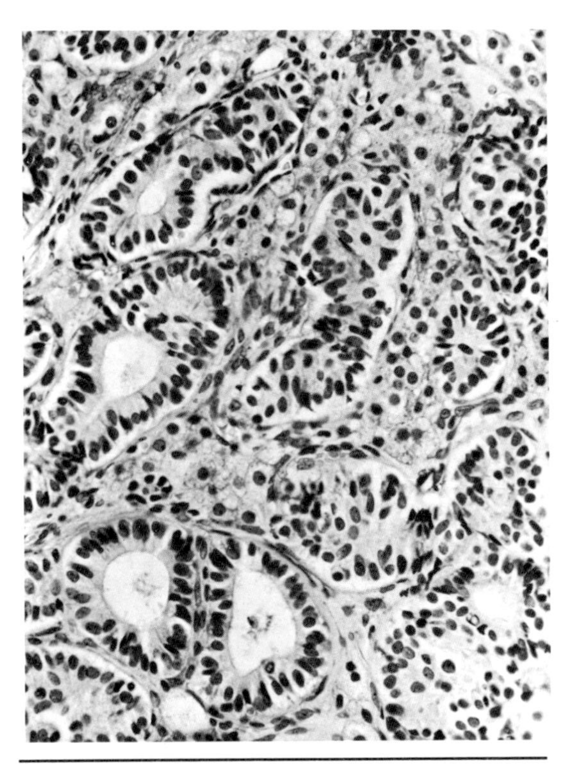

Fig. 21.23 Androblastoma of the ovary showing tubules lined by Sertoli cells and with Leydig cells in the stroma. ×220.

rhagia or postmenopausal bleeding. Granulosa-cell tumours are of low-grade malignancy and may recur after many years; the histological features offer no guide to prognosis but the larger the neoplasm the greater the risk of recurrence.

Many granulosa-cell tumours are pure but some contain an admixture of thecal cells and **pure theca-cell neoplasms** are sometimes encountered: these present as solid, yellowish masses and are formed of plump, lipid-containing spindle-shaped cells. Theca-cell tumours are often oestrogenic and thus produce symptoms similar to those of granulosa-cell tumours; they are, however, almost invariably benign.

Androblastomas are neoplasms composed of Sertoli cells, Leydig cells, or any combination of these cells. Pure Sertoli-cell tumours, which are formed of well differentiated tubules, and pure Leydig cell neoplasms formed of acidophilic Leydig cells, derived either from the stroma or from pre-existing hilar cells, are rare and nearly always benign. Mixed Sertoli–Leydig-cell tumours (Fig. 21.23) are slightly more common and show a very wide range of differentiation, most behaving in a benign fashion but a minority pursuing a malignant course; the histological features are of little prognostic value. Pure Sertoli-cell tumours are sometimes oestrogenic but all other types of androblastomas often secrete androgens and produce some degree of virilization.

Tumours Derived from Germ Cells

Tumours derived from germ cells may show no evidence of either embryonic or extra-embryonic differentiation: such undifferentiated germ-cell neoplasms are known as **dysgerminomas** and are microscopically identical to the seminoma of the testis, sharing with this neoplasm also the attributes of early dissemination to the para-aortic lymph nodes and a marked degree of radiosensitivity.

A germ-cell tumour may, however, differentiate along extra-embryonic pathways into either placental tissue, resulting in the rare and highly malignant ovarian choriocarcinoma, or into yolk-sac tissue to produce the equally uncommon malignant yolk-sac tumour. The latter occurs in young girls, and like the yolk-sac tumour of the testis, has a complex histological structure with elements resembling primitive yolk sac, a similarity further accentuated by the ability of these neoplasms to secrete alpha-fetoprotein. These tumours were, until recently, invariably fatal but many respond well to modern chemotherapy.

Teratomas result from differentiation of a germ-cell tumour into embryonic tissues. The embryonic tissues within a teratoma may be fully mature, i.e. resemble microscopically those seen in adult tissues, and the neoplasm is then benign, or may resemble immature embryonic tissue in which case the tumour tends to behave in a malignant fasion. Most ovarian teratomas are of the mature variety and most of these are cystic. The mature cystic teratoma (Fig. 21.24), often misleadingly called a **dermoid cyst**, accounts for 15–20% of all ovarian neoplasms. It usually takes the form of a large thick-walled cyst containing hairs and pultaceous matter; the cyst is lined by a stratified squamous epithelium and skin adnexae, such as hair follicles, abound; within the wall of the cyst a variety of tissues may be found, amongst which cartilage, bone, teeth, thyroid tissue, gastro-intestinal and respiratory epithelium and neural tissue are the most common. Malignant change supervenes in about 1% of mature cystic teratomas, and usually takes the form of a squamous-cell carcinoma.

Although teratomas classically contain a mixture of tissues, some appear to develop along only one tissue line; thus a few, known as struma ovarii, contain only thyroid tissue while others form a pure carcinoid tumour. Teratomas containing immature tissues are usually solid and occur in children and young adults; although these tumours are malignant, many patients are now being treated successfully by chemotherapy.

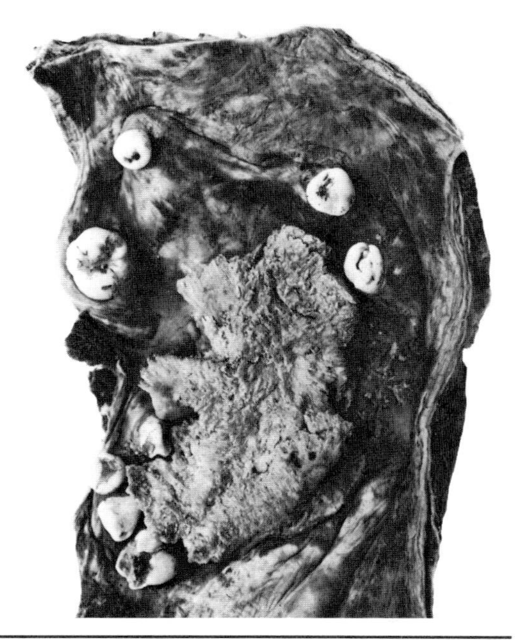

Fig. 21.24 Part of the wall of a mature cystic teratoma ('dermoid cyst') of the ovary, showing irregular growth of teeth from the inner surface of the cyst wall.

Miscellaneous Tumours

Placed in this group are a number of extremely rare tumours of unknown histogenesis, **primary malignant lymphomas** of the ovary and tumours derived from the non-specialized tissues of the ovary. Amongst the latter group the **fibroma** merits special attention partly because it is common and partly because this neoplasm can be associated with ascites and hydrothorax (Meigs' syndrome) which resolve after removal of the ovarian neoplasm.

Metastatic Tumours

The ovary is a common site for metastatic tumour, especially from the uterus, breast and gastrointestinal tract. A particular type of metastatic lesion is the Krukenberg tumour: this is due to transcoelomic spread of a gastric or colonic adenocarcinoma and is characterized by the presence of mucin-containing 'signet-ring' cells scattered in a fibrous stroma which is extremely cellular. This florid stromal reaction is seen before the menopause.

Miscellaneous Conditions of the Female Reproductive Tract

Abnormalities Related to Pregnancy

Hydatidiform Mole

This is an abnormal conceptus in which an embryo is absent and the placental villi are so distended by fluid that they resemble a bunch of grapes. The placental mass is often unduly large and distends the uterine cavity: the villi appear as clusters of tense, translucent, fluid-filled vesicles which commonly measure up to 1 cm and exceptionally as much as 2 cm, in diameter (Fig. 21.25). No trace of an embryo, amniotic sac or umbilical cord is apparent. Microscopically the stroma of the villi is markedly oedematous (Fig. 21.26), often to a degree of complete liquefaction, and no fetal vessels are present. A constant feature is the presence of a variable degree of atypical villous trophoblastic hyperplasia.

Hydatidiform mole occurs most commonly in women aged less than 18 or more than 40 years; it also shows a striking geographical variation in incidence, being uncommon in Europe and North America, rather more common in Australia and of frequent occurrence in the Far East and parts of Africa, India and Latin America. Attempts to explain this regional variation in terms of socioeconomic status or ethnic group have met with little success. There is also a clear-cut relationship between hydatidiform mole and choriocarcinoma, 50% of choriocarcinomas occurring in women who have previously had a hydatidiform mole.

Some light on the cause of this abnormality has been shed by the discovery that 85% of true moles have an XX chromosomal constitution, both X chromosomes being of paternal origin; accordingly, it is postulated that moles arise from the formation and replication of a diploid cell derived from a single sperm that has penetrated a dead or dying ovum. Fifteen per cent of moles have an XY chromosomal constitution, though again both chromosomes are of paternal origin: it is thought that this form of mole is due to the entry of two

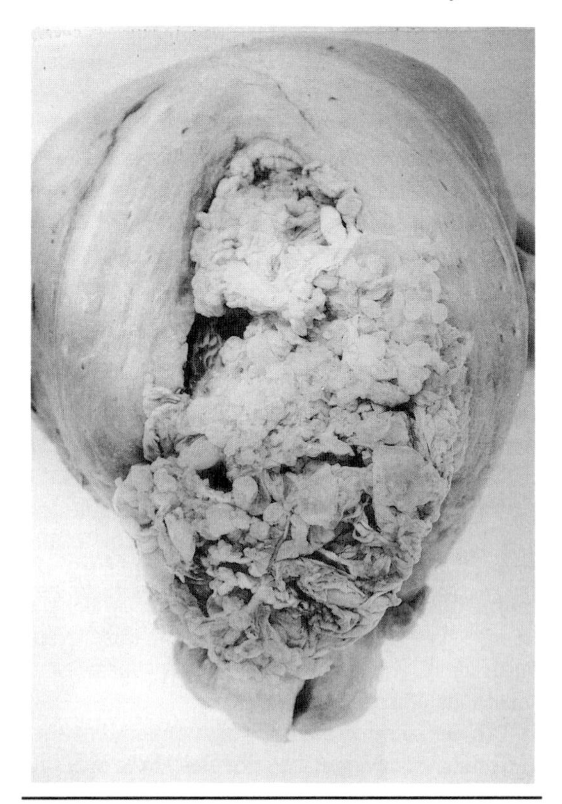

Fig. 21.25 An opened uterus containing a hydatidiform mole.

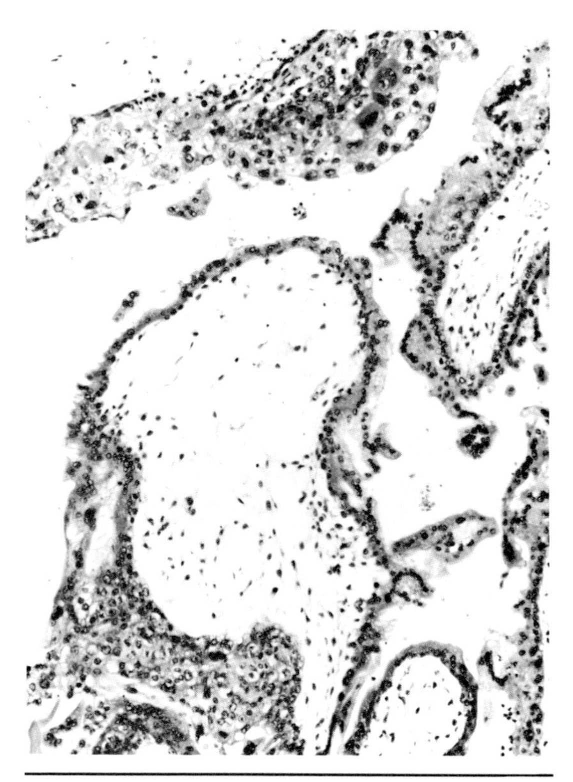

Fig. 21.26 A hydatidiform mole; the placental villi are avascular and markedly oedematous. There is a moderate degree of trophoblastic hyperplasia. ×100. (Dr C. W. Elston.)

sperms into an abnormal ovum, with subsequent fusion and replication.

A mole leads inevitably to abortion, often preceded by unduly rapid uterine enlargement and haemorrhage. After the uterus has been emptied a woman with a mole has a 2–3% risk of eventually developing a choriocarcinoma but, unfortunately, the histological features of any individual mole offer no guide to eventual prognosis, no relationship existing between degree of trophoblastic hyperplasia and the later occurrence of a choriocarcinoma.

Invasive Mole

In most hydatidiform moles the abnormal villi do not invade the myometrium but in 5–10%, the villi will not only invade but may even penetrate through the uterine wall; in such cases the myometrial vessels may be breached and emboli of hydatidiform mole transported to distant sites as 'metastases'. Despite this local invasion and distant spread, this form of mole is not malignant; after removal of the mole the 'metastases' will often regress spontaneously and there is no increased risk of eventual choriocarcinoma.

Partial Mole

This term is applied to placentas in which only a minority of villi show hydatidiform change and atypical trophoblastic proliferation, the distended vesicular villi being scattered amidst otherwise normal placental tissue; a partial mole is often accompanied by a fetus, albeit one that is usually grossly abnormal. A partial mole is not simply a variant of a true mole but is associated with a chromosomal abnormality in the fetus, usually a triploidy.

Choriocarcinoma

This is a malignant tumour of trophoblast and is formed of both cytotrophoblast and syncytiotrophoblast; it is a unique neoplasm in that, being of purely fetal origin, it is a neoplastic allograft in the mother. The aetiology is unknown but the tumour has a geographic pattern of distribution similar to that of hydatidiform mole, being rare in western Europe where it occurs no more than once in 40 000 deliveries. The tumour follows a hydatidiform mole in 50% of cases and an unremarkable abortion in a further 25%: the remainder develop, often after a period of months or years, as a sequel to an apparently normal pregnancy. Choriocarcinomas (and hydatidiform moles) secrete placental human chorionic gonadotrophin (HCG) and assay of serum and urinary levels of this 'tumour marker' are used in patient management.

Because trophoblast has an inherent capacity for invading and eroding blood vessels, the neoplasm is seen within the uterus as a soft, largely haemorrhagic mass (Fig. 21.27). Microscopically, a choriocarcinoma mimics the appearances of an early implanting blastocyst with central cores of mononuclear cytotrophoblast surrounded by a rim of multinucleated syncytiotrophoblast; the trophoblast shows a variable degree of pleomorphism and mitotic activity but no villi are present (Fig. 21.28).

Choriocarcinoma invades rapidly and deeply into the uterine wall but penetration is principally by infiltration into venous sinuses rather than by destruction of the myometrium. Because of this extensive vascular permeation, blood spread occurs at an early stage, principally to the lungs, liver, brain and vagina; metastasis via the lymphatics is uncommon. Despite this pattern of early spread there have been few neoplasms for which the prognosis has been altered so dramatically by the advent of chemotherapy; until recently it was always rapidly fatal, but at least 80% of patients are now permanently cured by treatment with cytotoxic drugs.

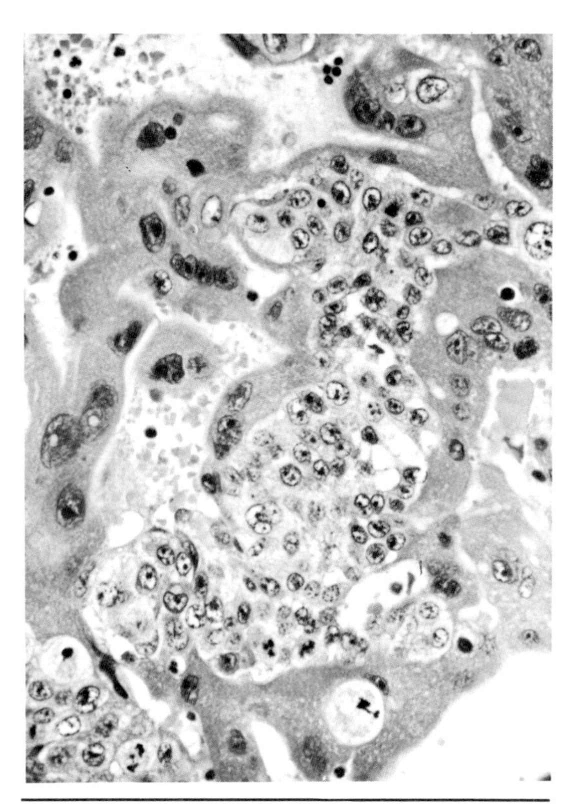

Fig. 21.28 A choriocarcinoma containing both cytotrophoblastic cells and multinucleated clumps of syncytiotrophoblast. ×300. (Dr C. W. Elston.)

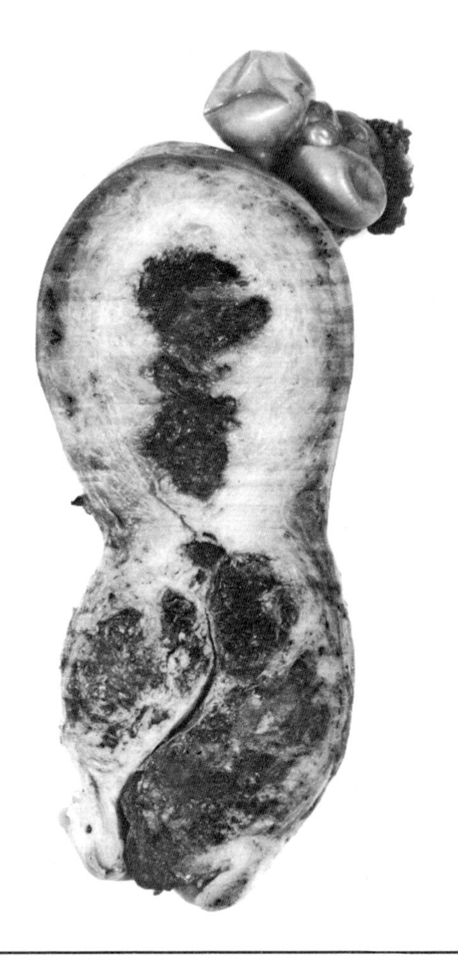

Fig. 21.27 A bisected uterus containing multiple dark haemorrhagic nodules of choriocarcinoma. (Dr C. W. Elston.)

Ectopic Pregnancy

An ectopic pregnancy is one in which a fertilized ovum implants and begins to develop before it reaches its natural site in the uterus. An extra-uterine gestation can develop in the ovary or in the peritoneal cavity, but 97% of ectopic pregnancies occur in the fallopian tubes, most commonly in the ampullary portion. Within the tube, the developing placental tissue evokes an inadequate decidual response and not only invades the muscular wall but also erodes the intramural vessels. Erosion of a large vessel may lead to a haematosalpinx and separation of the conceptus from the tubal wall by haemorrhage; furthermore, the invading trophoblast weakens the tubal wall which may rupture, often with considerable intraperitoneal bleeding. Clinically, these complications are usually accompanied by severe pain and other symptoms of an 'acute abdomen', demanding surgical treatment. Following tubal rupture, the conceptus may implant on to the peritoneum and continue to grow as an intra-abdominal pregnancy, but this is distinctly unusual.

Many cases of tubal pregnancy are clearly due to partial tubal obstruction, usually as a consequence of infection, while some result from the ovum lodging in a tubal diverticulum. Nevertheless, tubal pregnancies can occur in the absence of these lesions and suggested aetiological factors in such cases include delayed ovulation with washing back of the fertilized ovum by menstrual reflux, and transmigration of the ovum, i.e. an ovum released from the ovary traversing the peritoneal cavity to enter the contralateral tube. The incidence of ectopic pregnancy, particularly ovarian, is increased in women who become pregnant in spite of the presence of an intrauterine contraceptive device.

Congenital Abnormalities

During normal female embryogenesis the internal genitalia develop from the two Müllerian ducts which fuse distally to form the uterus and remain separate proximally to form the fallopian tubes. The vagina develops from the urogenital sinus. The Wolffian ducts make no contribution to the female genital tract and undergo atrophy.

The female type of development will occur in neuter embryos and is independent of the presence of functioning ovarian tissue; it is, however, radically altered by the presence of a testis which secretes a substance (not testosterone) that inhibits development of the Müllerian ducts and promotes that of Wolffian ducts; this substance has a purely local action and thus a left-sided testis will only influence development of the reproductive tract on the left side of the body. The external genitalia will always develop along female lines unless virilization is induced during embryonic life by their exposure to testosterone. Congenital abnormalities of the female genital tract thus fall into two broad groups, depending on whether the gonads are normal or abnormal.

Malformations in Women with Normal Ovaries

These patients have normal ovaries and external genitalia and usually a normal chromosomal constitution.

Müllerian duct fusion defects. A total failure of Müllerian duct fusion will result in a reduplication of the uterus and vagina (**uterus didelphys**) while lesser degrees of failure can result in a single vagina with double uterus (**uterus bicollis bicornis**) or a single vagina and cervix with two uterine bodies (**uterus unicollis bicornis**). The lesser forms of fusion defect are compatible with a normal capacity to become pregnant but are associated with a high incidence of abortion, premature delivery and abnormal labour.

Genetic factors contribute to fusion defects which probably result from a very slight physical separation of the two Müllerian ducts at a critical stage of embryogenesis, possibly because of an altered shape of the embryonic pelvis.

Müllerian duct aplasia. Total aplasia is very rare and found only in infants that are also otherwise grossly malformed.

Failure of fusion of Müllerian ducts with urogenital sinus. A failure of fusion between the two structures that make up the vagina leads to vaginal atresia; the uterus may be normal but is more commonly hypoplastic or absent (the Rokitansky–Küster–Hauser syndrome).

Malformations in Women with Abnormal Gonads

Women of this type, though phenotypically female, often, though not invariably, have an abnormal chromosomal karyotype: if any testosterone-secreting tissue is present the external genitalia will show some degree of virilization and are often classed as being 'ambiguous'.

Patients with Turner's syndrome have bilateral **streak gonads** (a strand of undifferentiated stroma on the back of the broad ligament); both the external and internal genitalia develop along normal female lines but remain infantile throughout life. Patients with Turner's syndrome have a 45XO karotype and additional features include short stature and often webbing of the neck. Individuals with mixed gonadal dysgenesis have a streak gonad on one side and a testis on the other; Müllerian development occurs normally on the side with a streak gonad but is inhibited on the other, the external genitalia being ambiguous. True hermaphrodites (p. 1072) may have an ovary on one side and a testis on the other, or bilateral ovotestes, and show a variable pattern of genital development.

Some phenotypic females are, in fact, males with a normal karyotype and normally developed internal male genitalia; their external genitalia are, however, female. These patients have bilateral testes which are capable of producing the factor inhibiting Müllerian development; these individuals suffer, however, either from a defect in testosterone biosynthesis, an inability to convert testosterone to dihydrotestosterone in target tissues, or a complete organ insensitivity to androgen effect, this latter syndrome being known as '**testicular feminization**' or, preferably, as '**androgen insensitivity syndrome**' (p. 1073).

The Breast

The female breast is in the unique position of being a gland which is non-functional except during lactation. It is, nevertheless, subject to hormonal influences, particularly throughout reproductive life, and this probably accounts for most of its pathological changes, which rarely affect the male. By far the most important disease is carcinoma, which usually presents as a palpable lump. Other lesions are mostly of importance because some of them also produce a lump or lumpiness of the breast, or other symptoms which raise the suspicion of carcinoma and must therefore be investigated. The commonest of these are the fibroadenoma, most frequent in the third decade, and fibrocystic change which presents particularly in the pre-menopausal decade. Because of the liability of the breast to injury, traumatic fat necrosis is another cause of a firm lump. Duct ectasia (dilatation of ducts) and duct papilloma may each (like carcinoma) cause a discharge from the nipple. Infection of the breast is rare except during lactation and most congenital abnormalities are of minor importance.

The Normal Breast

The breasts consist of a group of modified apocrine sweat glands which develop from 15 to 25 downgrowths of the epidermis. At first solid cords, they develop a lumen and become the major (segmental) ducts each of which opens separately at the nipple. Each segmental duct gives rise to the branching duct system of a segment of breast tissue. Before puberty the structure of male and female breast tissue is identical. In the female, under the hormonal stimulation of puberty the duct system proliferates and lobules composed of acini and intralobular stroma bud from subsegmental ducts to form physiologically functional terminal

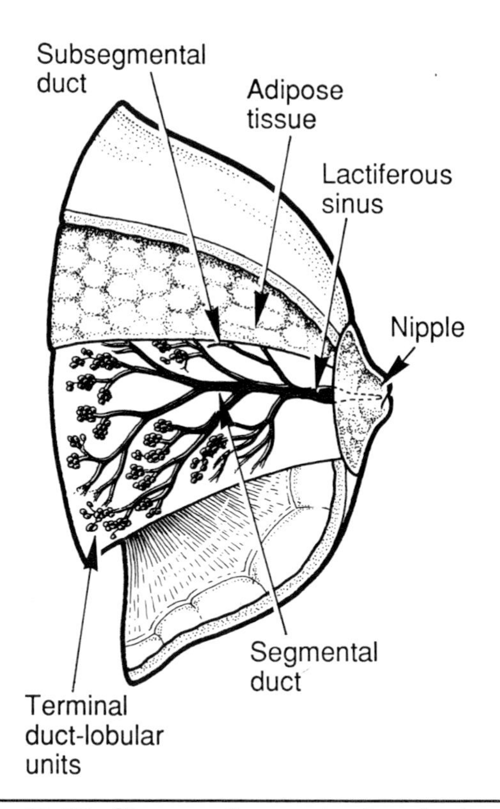

Fig. 21.29 Diagrammatic reconstruction of mature female breast to show the main anatomical structures.

duct lobular units (Fig. 21.29). The interlobular and segmental connective tissue is less cellular and more densely collagenous and during puberty becomes infiltrated with fatty tissue; this accounts for most of the enlargement of the female breast at this time.

Apart from a stratified squamous lining close to the nipple, the ducts and ductules are lined by a two-layered epithelium, an inner layer of cuboidal or columnar cells and an outer discontinuous layer of smaller, contractile myoepithelial cells (Fig. 21.30 and 21.31). The epithelium is invested in a continuous basement membrane and the duct system is ensheathed in a layer of loose connective tissue which is rich in lymphatics. There is little or no elastic tissue in the lobules, but an elastic layer surrounds the extralobular ducts.

The ductal epithelium of the mature female breast has some secretory activity, but the secretion is normally reabsorbed. During pregnancy, proliferation increases and secretory acini develop from the terminal ductular alveoli. After the menopause the breast epithelium atrophies and the lobular connective tissue changes to acellular hyaline collagen; the terminal ductules may virtually disappear, but sometimes become dilated, forming microcysts lined by flattened, attentuated epithelium. Apart from duct ectasia and duct papilloma, most lesions in the breast are believed to arise from the terminal duct lobular unit.

Developmental Abnormalities

Congenital abnormalities of the breast are rare and unimportant, with the exception of **polymastia** and **polythelia** – accessory nipples. These may occur anywhere along the 'milk line' and are sub-

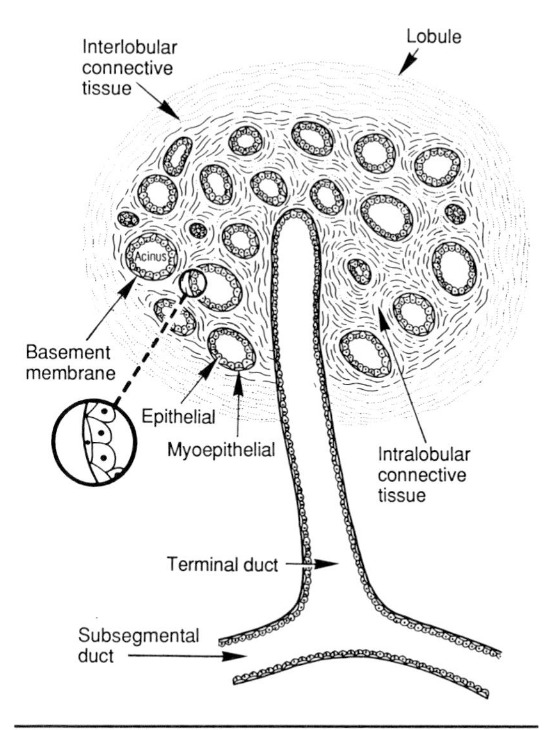

Fig. 21.30 Diagram of a single terminal duct lobular unit showing the relationship between the epithelial and stromal components.

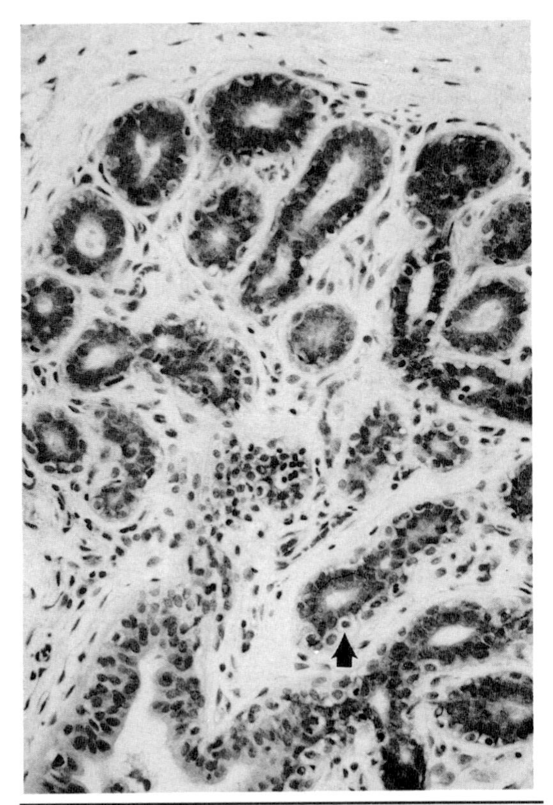

Fig. 21.31 Part of a terminal duct lobular unit. The terminal duct is at the bottom; a two layered epithelium is visible in the acini, the myoepithelial cells (arrow) having a clear cytoplasm.

ject to the same disorders as normally situated breasts.

Failure of development of the breasts at puberty is very uncommon and usually associated with ovarian agenesis, as in Turner's syndrome. Precocious development may also occur, occasionally related to the presence of an ovarian granulosa-cell tumour, but usually for unexplained reasons.

Adolescent or **juvenile hypertrophy** is the commonest developmental abnormality found. At the onset of puberty the breasts grow rapidly and out of proportion, so that they become a severe physical and psychological burden. Rarely, the hypertrophy is unilateral. The cause is unknown and the only effective treatment is surgical reduction. Microscopically, no specific abnormality is seen and the enlargement appears to be due to an overgrowth of adipose and connective tissue.

Benign Breast Lesions

The term benign breast disease is often used clinically to imply a specific pathological entity. This is clearly an oversimplification and there are a number of distinct lesions which merit discussion.

Infections

Acute pyogenic mastitis occurs mainly during lactation and is the result of infection via the ducts or through an abrasion of the nipple. It is most often caused by staphylococci acquired in hospital from the mouth of the suckling infant which has been colonized by the prevalent strain of *Staphylococcus aureus*. Unless effectively treated, staphylococcal mastitis may cause a loculated breast abcess; abscess formation may also occur superficial to or deep to the mammary gland. Acute pyogenic mastitis may become chronic if not treated adequately, and infection with pyogenic bacteria may also start insidiously and persist, but these events are rare. Recurrent or chronic low-grade infection of the subareolar tissue occurs in some women, with scarring, distortion and sometimes fistula formation.

Tuberculosis of the breast is now rare. It may arise by haematogenous, lymphatic or direct spread, usually from the lungs or pleura. It may remain localized as a single caseating lesion, which sometimes discharges through the skin, or it may spread extensively through the breast. In view of its rarity and the occurrence of other lesions with similar histological appearances, tuberculosis of the breast should not be diagnosed unless *Mycobacterium tuberculosis* has been detected in the lesion.

Non-Infective Inflammatory Lesions

Mammary duct ectasia consists of progressive dilatation of large or intermediate ducts with surrounding chronic inflammatory change. It affects one or more segments of the breast and rarely is palpable, like a 'bag of worms'. The dilated ducts contain inspissated fatty material and their walls are thickened (Fig. 21.32). Microscopically, the duct epithelium appears thin and the thickened fibrous wall is usually infiltrated with plasma cells and lymphocytes. Foamy macrophages may be present in the lumen and in the nipple discharge. The periductal elastic tissue is usually increased but may show patchy destruction.

Duct ectasia is often symptomless, but there may be a nipple discharge and contraction of periductal fibrous tissue may cause retraction of the nipple and raise the suspicion of carcinoma. Occasionally a dilated duct ruptures into the surrounding stroma, where its lipid contents promote a persistent inflammatory reaction with accumulation of foamy macrophages and giant cells and fibrosis; the microscopic appearances resemble those of traumatic fat necrosis and the lesion may become palpable as a firm lump. The term plasma cell mastitis is sometimes applied to duct ectasia with an unusually heavy plasma cell infiltration.

The aetiology is uncertain; it tends to occur most often in multipara who have not breast-fed their babies, but occurs also in nullipara. There is increasing evidence that the underlying mechanism for the duct dilatation is periductal inflammation leading to destruction of the elastic network with fibrosis.

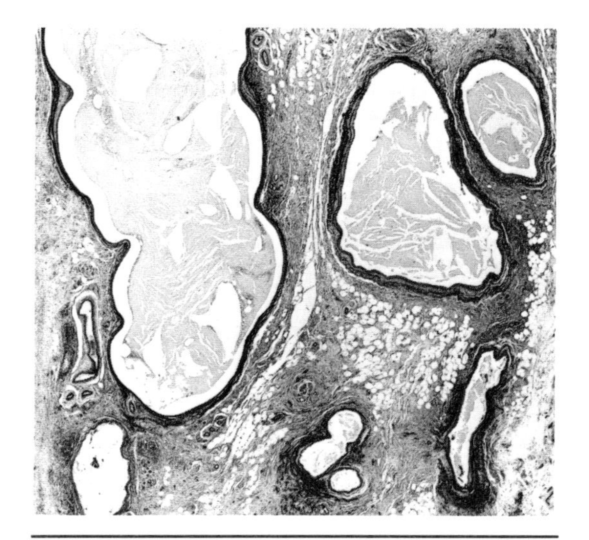

Fig. 21.32 Mammary duct ectasia. The ducts are dilated and filled with fatty material. Their walls are thickened and fibrotic.

Granulomatous mastitis is an uncommon condition in which terminal duct lobular units are the site of an intense chronic inflammatory process with conspicuous giant cells. Terminal duct dilatation may be present, with associated foamy macrophages and, on occasion, actual abscess formation. The condition is often associated with a recent pregnancy but has also been described in nulliparous women. It should properly be termed 'idiopathic' granulomatous mastitis as the aetiology is unknown. No infectious cause has been identified but tuberculosis should always be excluded. Sarcoidosis may also be associated with granulomas in the breast, but these are not confined to lobular structures.

Traumatic fat necrosis. This lesion in the fatty tissue of an obese and pendulous breast is caused by injury, although in many instances it presents as a hard lump in the breast, often without a history of trauma. The initial necrosis is accompanied by haemorrhage and followed by an acute inflammatory reaction. The lesion becomes heavily infiltrated by foamy macrophages containing lipid and often haemosiderin, and crystals of lipid may be deposited and stimulate a foreign-body giant-cell reaction. Granulation tissue forms around the lesion and gradually matures into a thick layer of fibrous tissue which, often together with calcification, accounts for the presentation as a firm or hard lump. The fibrous reaction may result in retraction of the nipple or fixation to the skin, features which increase the clinical resemblance to carcinoma.

Reaction to foreign material. Injection of silicone or paraffin wax to increase the size of the breast is usually without harmful effect but can introduce infection, and occasionally induces a granulomatous giant-cell reaction, causing tenderness and nodularity. Microscopically, fragments of the 'inert' material are seen, surrounded by multinucleated giant cells.

Galactocele

This is a cystic swelling of a lactiferous duct which develops during lactation, apparently due to obstruction of the duct. Initially it contains creamy fluid which gradually becomes watery, and it may induce a granulomatous reaction or become infected.

Fibroadenoma

Although it has previously been the convention to regard fibroadenomas as benign tumours there is considerable evidence to support the view that they are focal areas of lobular hyperplasia rather than true neoplasms. They may present at any age after puberty but are most common in the third decade. Clinically they present as small, firm, well defined mobile lumps, which may occasionally be multiple and bilateral.

Microscopically, the dominant element is a proliferation of loose, cellular, intralobular stroma which is associated with a variable number of tubular structures (Fig. 21.33). The latter appear either as elongated clefts or tubules cut in cross-section. The previous designation of 'intracanalicular' and 'pericanalicular' types, based on these patterns of stroma and epithelium, has no practical or prognostic significance, and can safely be abandoned. Fibroadenomas are usually well circumscribed lesions, but although they are easily enucleated at surgery they are not truly encapsulated. Occasionally, small foci of fibroadenomatous hyperplasia are found in conjunction with fibrocystic change.

The great majority of fibroadenomas are entirely benign lesions which do not predispose to subsequent carcinoma. Indeed, many surgeons avoid surgical excision once the diagnosis has been established on clinical and cytological grounds. Very rarely *in situ* carcinoma, mainly of lobular type, may develop within a fibroadenoma, but this probably means that its epithelium, like that of normal breast, is not immune to carcinogenic agents.

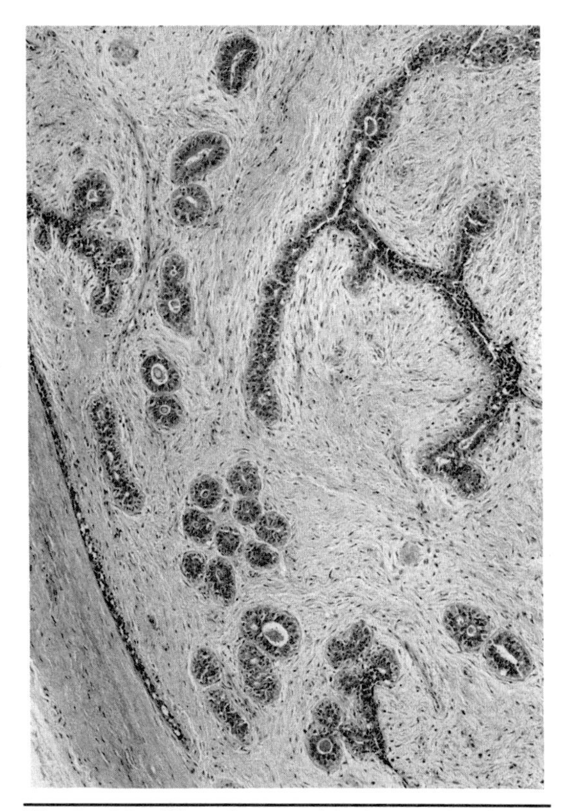

Fig. 21.33 Fibroadenoma of the breast, showing the characteristic loose, cellular stroma and the epithelial clefts and acini.

Fibrocystic Change

A large number of terms has been used as synonyms for a group of changes which present clinically as a lump or lumpiness in the breast during the reproductive decades. They include fibroadenosis, cystic hyperplasia, cystic mastopathy and mammary dysplasia. None is entirely satisfactory but fibrocystic change has become the most widely accepted. The condition is the commonest of all breast lesions, and produces clinical symptoms in at least 10% of women. The peak incidence is in the premenopausal decade. After the menopause there is a sharp decline in symptomatic cases. Microscopically, a range of appearances is seen and the components described below are present in variable amounts from case to case.

Cyst formation results from localized dilatation of lobular and terminal ductules, and is presumably due to obstruction. Cysts are usually multiple (Fig. 21.34) and mostly less than 1 cm in diameter, although occasional larger ones are not unusual. They are thin-walled and appear blue when seen close to the cut surface of biopsy material. The lining epithelium often becomes flattened and may be lost in larger cysts. It may also undergo apocrine metaplasia, the cells becoming larger and columnar with a convex free margin and abundant strongly eosinophilic cytoplasm, like those in apocrine glandular epithelium. An incomplete layer of myoepithelium can usually be detected, at least in places, in the cysts. Like the ductules from which they develop, the cysts are not ensheathed in elastic tissue. Unless haemorrhage has occurred, the cysts contain clear watery or mucinous fluid. Occasionally a cyst ruptures and causes an inflammatory reaction in the adjacent stroma, which may be tender or painful.

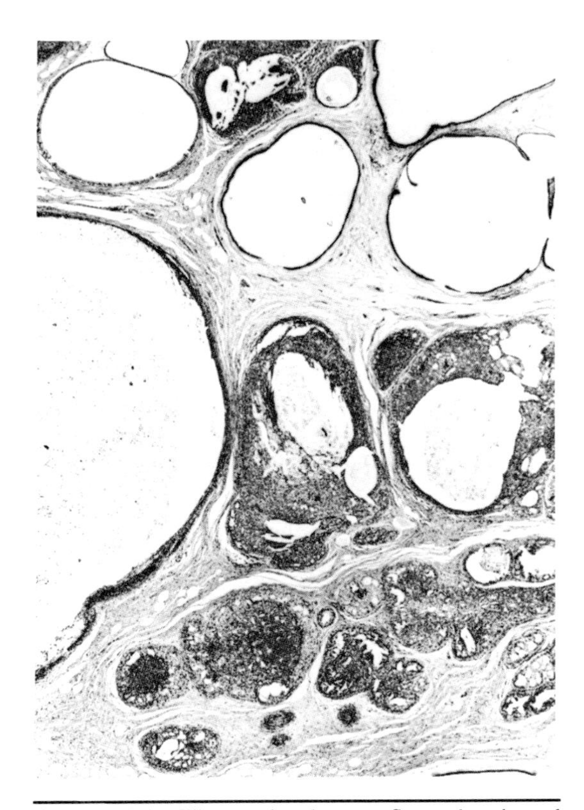

Fig. 21.34 Fibrocystic change. Several enlarged cystic structures are present and there are also ductules exhibiting epithelial hyperplasia.

Adenosis. The broad terms adenosis and fibroadenosis, implying disorders of glandular tissue, are so non-specific and so frequently applied to breast tissue having no discernible abnormality that their use should be abandoned. Even the term 'blunt duct adenosis' is questionable, since it is used by some to describe an organoid hypertrophy of the lobular acini and by others to indicate a minor hyperplasia of acinar cells.

Sclerosing adenosis denotes a more specific proliferation of the terminal duct lobular unit. The changes may be present as tiny microscopic foci in otherwise normal breast tissue, as an integral component of fibrocystic change, or, particularly in younger women, as palpable nodules mimicking tumour masses. Histologically, the normal configuration of a lobule or group of lobules is distorted by a disorderly proliferation of acini and intralobular stromal cells (Fig. 21.35). A whorled pattern of microtubules may be seen but luminal structures are often indistinct. It is usually possible to distinguish, at least focally, a normal two-layered epithelium, but epithelial and myoepithelial cells may appear to proliferate separately. Nuclei are regular, without atypia, and mitoses are infrequent. Sclerosing adenosis is regarded as a benign condition which carries no increased risk of subsequent carcinoma. Its main importance diagnostically stems from the fact that it may be mistaken both radiologically and pathologically for carcinoma. Fine speckled calcification is frequently found in the glandular spaces (Fig. 21.35b) and this may mimic the calcification of *in situ* carcinoma mammographically. Microscopically, the tubular structures may be misinterpreted by inexperienced pathologists as invasive carcinoma, especially in poorly prepared paraffin sections or in frozen sections. Extension of sclerosing adenosis into perineural spaces also occurs in rare cases, and care must be taken not to mistake this for evidence of malignancy.

Epithelial hyperplasia of significant degree occurs in approximately a quarter of cases of

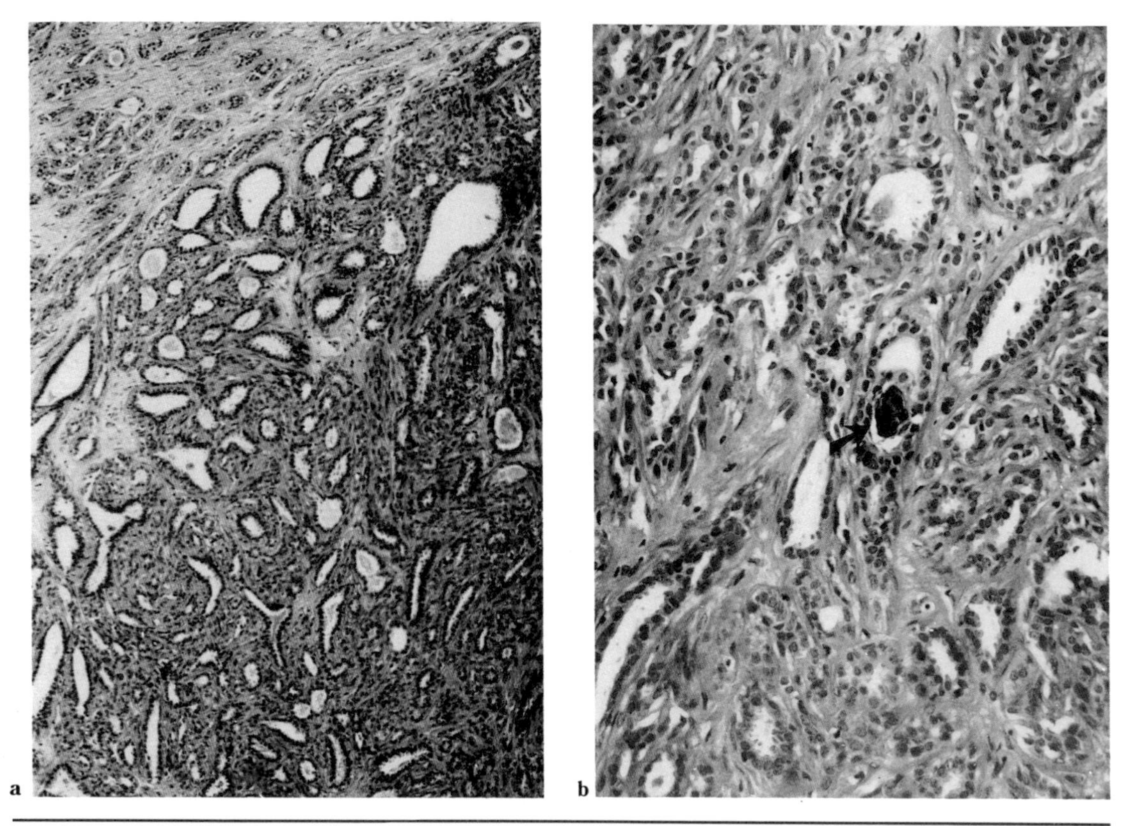

Fig. 21.35 Sclerosing adenosis, showing a nodule **a** composed of a disorderly proliferation of lobular structures. In **b** microtubules are seen with microcalcification (arrow), and there is also a proliferation of stromal cells.

fibrocystic change. In the past, nomenclature has been confusing; European pathologists used the term **epitheliosis** whilst in the United States **papillomatosis** was preferred. For this reason epithelial hyperplasia is now classified as being of usual type or atypical. In **epithelial hyperplasia of usual type** the ductules are lined by several layers of large epithelial cells and the lumen may be obliterated by a solid proliferation (Fig. 21.36). Nuclei are regular, and although occasional mitoses may be present, they are of normal configuration. In a small minority of cases abnormal features are present and diagnostic difficulty may be experienced in distinguishing the changes from carcinoma *in situ*. In **atypical ductal hyperplasia** the commonest pattern is that of an irregular lacy network resembling cribriform ductal carcinoma *in situ*, but lacking the necessary geometric configuration (compare Fig. 21.37 with Fig. 21.41). A micropapillary pattern may also be seen. In **atypical lobular hyperplasia** the appearances resemble those seen in lobular carcinoma *in situ* (compare Fig. 21.38 with Fig. 21.43). Definite hyperplasia is present within lobular acini, but there is no increase in the overall size of lobules and only minimal expansion of acini. There may be partial involvement of some lobules and most acinar lumina are preserved.

Fibrosis. Increase of fibrous stroma occurs in most cases of fibrocystic change, but is difficult to assess. In thin women, the normally fibrous breast stroma of young adult life persists with little change even after the menopause, but in obese women there is a progressive replacement of fibrous by fatty tissue, particularly after the meno-

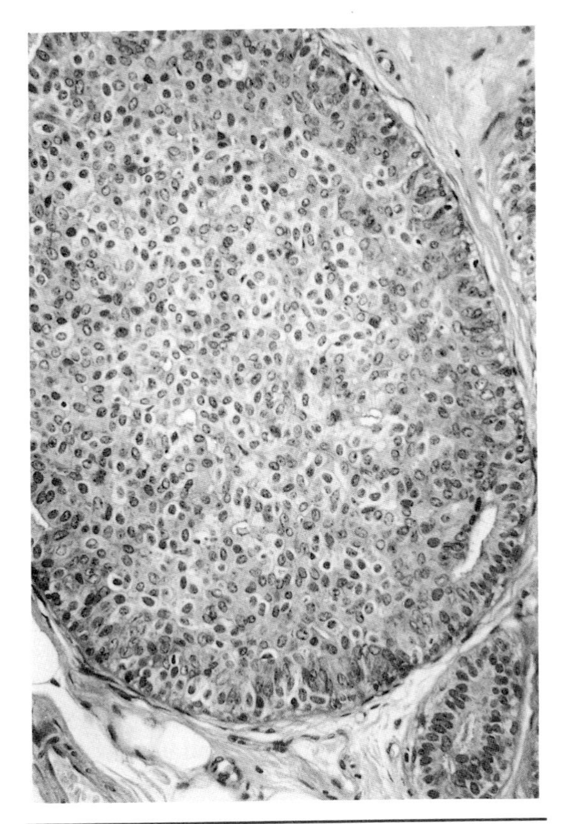

Fig. 21.36 Epithelial hyperplasia of usual type. A ductule is filled with epithelial and myoepithelial cells which exhibit a 'streaming' pattern.

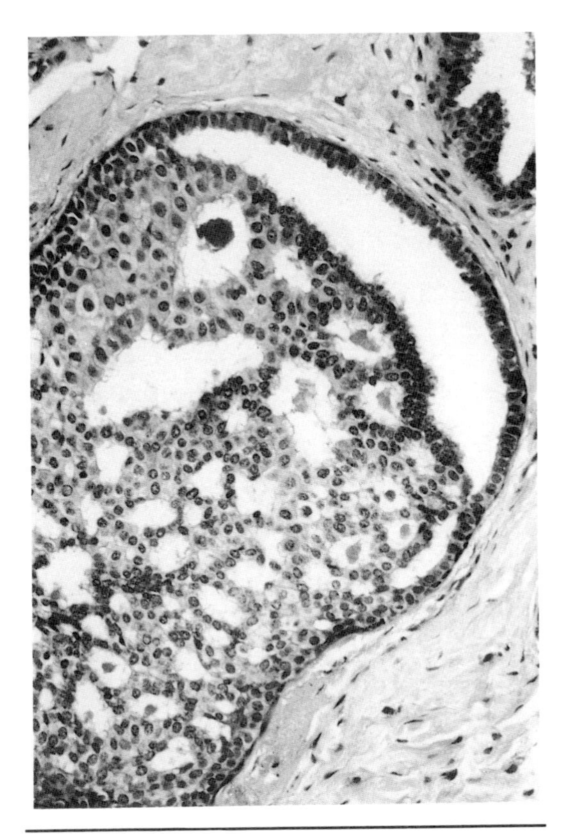

Fig. 21.37 Atypical ductal hyperplasia. The epithelial proliferation forms an irregular network lacking a geometric pattern. There is no nuclear atypia.

pause. As age advances, the fibrous stroma becomes hyaline and relatively acellular, while the epithelial elements atrophy. It is this collagenization of pre-existing stroma without obvious fibroblastic proliferation that is responsible for fibrosis of the breast.

Aetiology

It is widely assumed that fibrocystic change is caused by the influence of hormones on the female breast throughout reproductive life, but this does not explain why the changes are so patchy. An association with menstrual irregularities has been noted, but only in some patients, and there is also a relatively higher incidence in nullipara. Cystic changes in the breast can be produced in animals by administration of oestrogen, but it must be admitted that most patients have no evidence of hormonal imbalance. Furthermore, autopsy studies have shown that asymptomatic fibrocystic change is present in a large percentage of pre- and perimenopausal women, so that its status as a disease entity has been questioned.

Radial Scar and Complex Sclerosing Lesion

A varied and confusing nomenclature has been applied to these distinctive sclerosing lesions of the breast, including 'sclerosing papillary proliferation', 'benign sclerosing ductal proliferation' and 'infiltrating epitheliosis', but the above terms are preferred. Morphologically, they are composed of radiating stellate connective tissue with a dense fibroelastic core. Radial scars vary between 1 and

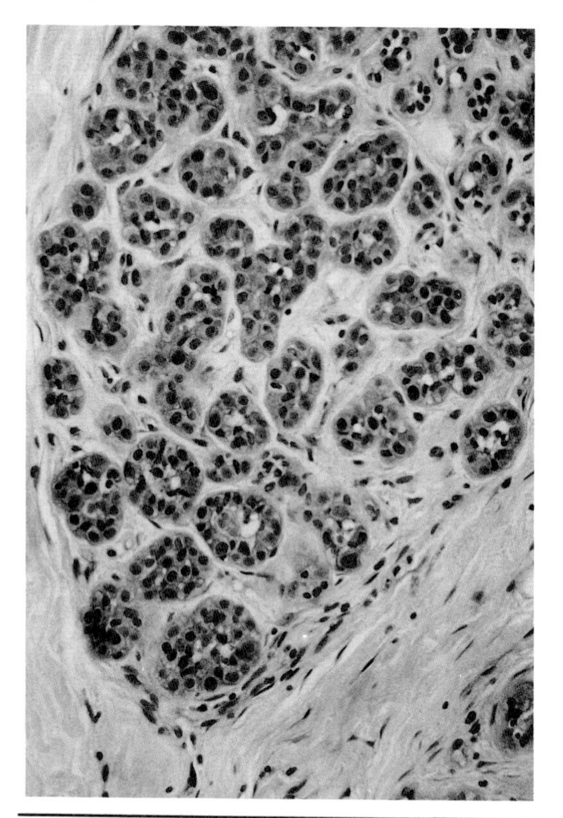

Fig. 21.38 Atypical lobular hyperplasia. Part of a lobule showing a proliferation of epithelial cells within acini which are not expanded and have clear lumina.

10 mm in diameter and complex sclerosing lesions are greater than 10 mm. Within the arms of the stellate configuration, ductules appear drawn in to the centre. A variable degree of epithelial proliferation is present. In complex sclerosing lesions foci of sclerosing adenosis may also be found.

These lesions were initially thought to be uncommon, but as mammography has become more widely used, especially in population screening, they are now known to occur relatively frequently. The precise pathogenesis is unclear, but most evidence suggests that they have a close association with fibrocystic change. Although very rare, cases of both *in situ* and invasive carcinoma arising in radial scars have been described. However, the great majority of radial scars are benign. The risk of subsequent malignancy appears to be related to the degree of epithelial hyperplasia.

Benign Breast Lesions and Risk of Malignancy

The relationship between benign breast lesions and subsequent breast carcinoma has been the subject of great controversy. Many studies have been seriously flawed, and it is only recently, in studies employing careful histopathological review, that a degree of clarity has been achieved. Patients whose biopsies show no epithelial hyperplasia have no increased risk; since this category accounts for approximately 70% of benign biopsies the great majority of women can be reassured, and do not require follow-up. Hyperplasia of usual type gives an increased risk of carcinoma of about double that in women whose breasts are 'normal'; biopsies with usual hyperplasia comprise about 25% of the total. The most significant risk, up to fourfold, occurs with patients whose biopsies show atypical hyperplasia, and this is doubled to eightfold if there is also a family history of breast cancer. However, atypia is found in only 4% of biopsies and atypia with a family history in only 1%. Long-term follow-up is advisable for this very small group; they should be taught breast self-examination and offered regular mammography.

Benign Tumours of the Breast

Adenoma

It is only recently that the existence of a true mammary adenoma has been established. Most previous lesions termed adenoma were really examples of cellular fibroadenoma. Tubular adenomas are sharply circumscribed nodules measuring between 5 and 40 mm. Microscopically they are composed of closely packed ductular structures with little intervening stroma. They are entirely benign.

The status of the so-called lactating adenoma is questionable. Whilst it is possible that some are true tubular adenomas, in the great majority of cases they are in reality areas of lobular proliferation which become prominent and palpable as part of the physiological hyperplasia of the breast during pregnancy.

Adenoma of the nipple is a rare lesion which presents as a reddened rounded nodule, sometimes mimicking Paget's disease. It is composed of proliferating ductal type epithelium which often has a papillary structure. The presence of two layers of epithelium distinguishes the lesion from a carcinoma.

Papilloma

Papillomas are uncommon benign neoplasms, occurring predominantly in middle-aged patients. In the majority of cases the presenting symptom is single duct discharge from the nipple; the discharge may be blood-stained. Microscopically, they consist of a fronded fibrovascular core covered by two-layered duct type epithelium (Fig. 21.39). Duct papillomas can be separated into two main groups, central and peripheral. Central papillomas are usually single and occur in the main nipple ducts. They appear to carry no risk of subsequent carcinoma. Peripheral papillomas are more usually multiple and are associated with other proliferative epithelial changes, including atypical hyperplasia. In such cases there appears to be an increased risk of subsequent carcinoma. Carcinoma may also supervene rarely in cases of intracystic papilloma.

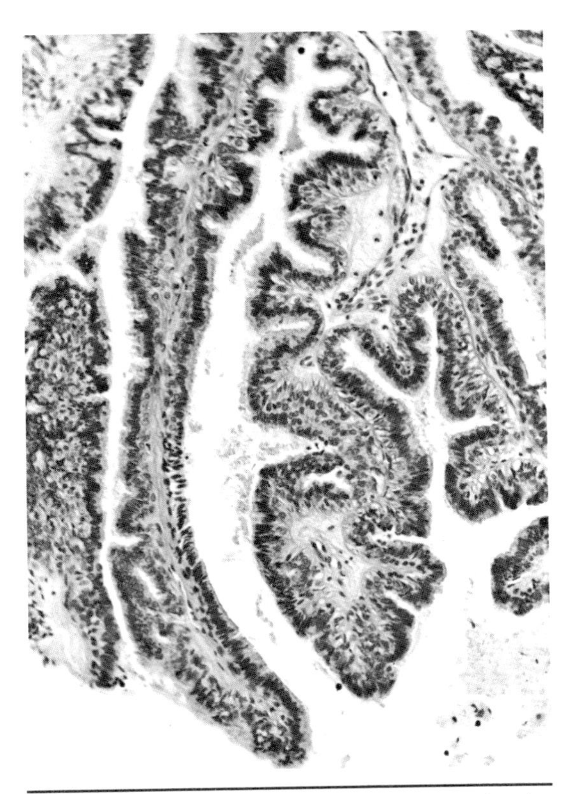

Fig. 21.39 Duct papilloma of breast, showing branching fibrovascular cores covered by epithelium mainly of columnar type.

Malignant Tumours of the Breast

Carcinoma

With the possible exception of skin, breast cancer is the commonest of human female cancers throughout the world. During the mid-1980s mortality from cancer of the breast overtook that of every other female cancer to become the commonest cause of cancer death. Nearly twice as many develop breast cancer as die of it. The incidence and mortality of breast cancer are high and remarkably constant in most developed countries; the frequency is increasing, especially in younger women, and this is not entirely due to an increase in the 'at risk' population. It is more than 200 times commoner in women than in men. Carcinoma of the breast may occur at any age, but is rare before 25 years and most frequent between 40 and 70 years.

About 50% of invasive carcinomas occur in the upper outer quadrant of the breast, the remainder being distributed equally throughout the rest of the breast. A cancer arising in the axillary tail may be mistaken clinically for an enlarged lymph node. The main presenting symptom is a palpable mass and for this reason all lumps in the breast, whatever the age of the patient, must be regarded clinically as possibly malignant until proved otherwise. In practice this usually requires a tissue diagnosis and excellent preoperative methods are available. A core-cutting needle such as the Tru-Cut provides a histological specimen, but increasing use is being made of fine needle aspiration which gives a cytological preparation. Frozen section should only be required if these other methods have proved unsuccessful, and then only if there is a strong suspicion of malignancy. Following the introduction of a national breast screening programme for women aged 50–64 years it is anticipated that improved mammographic technique will enhance the early detection of impalpable lesions.

Types of Breast Carcinoma

Carcinoma of the breast arises from the lining epithelium of the duct system. Previously it was thought that in some cases the origin was ductular and in others it was lobular, but it is now accepted that virtually all cancers are related to the terminal duct lobular unit. For a variable length of time the tumour cells remain confined within the duct system before breaching the basement membrane and invading the breast stroma. As elsewhere, the distinction between *in situ* and infiltrating carcinoma is extremely important and is the main pathological subdivision used.

In Situ Carcinoma

By definition the cytological changes of malignancy are present in the epithelial cells of an *in situ* carcinoma, but the basement membrane remains intact and no invasion is seen. It has become conventional to recognize two types of *in situ* carcinoma of the breast, ductal and lobular. Although both types are now known to arise from the same site, the terminal duct lobular unit, there are morphological and prognostic differences between the two which justify this subdivision.

***Ductal carcinoma* in situ.** In symptomatic series of breast cancer the frequency is approximately 2–5%. In the majority of these cases it presents as a palpable mass. Increasingly, ductal carcinoma *in situ* is being detected by mammography, in screening programmes in asymptomatic women and in such series the frequency may be as high as 15–20%.

Microscopically, a variable number of ducts or ductular structures may be involved. Four morphological patterns are recognized. In the **solid** type the ductules are completely filled by a disorderly proliferation of large epithelial cells with abundant cytoplasm, variable nuclear pleomorphism and increased mitoses. A similar appearance is present in the **comedo** type but in addition there is central necrosis in the lumen (Fig. 21.40) so that lipid-rich yellow debris may be expressed from the cut surface like toothpaste from a tube. **Cribriform** ductal carcinoma *in situ* is characterized by a proliferation of relatively

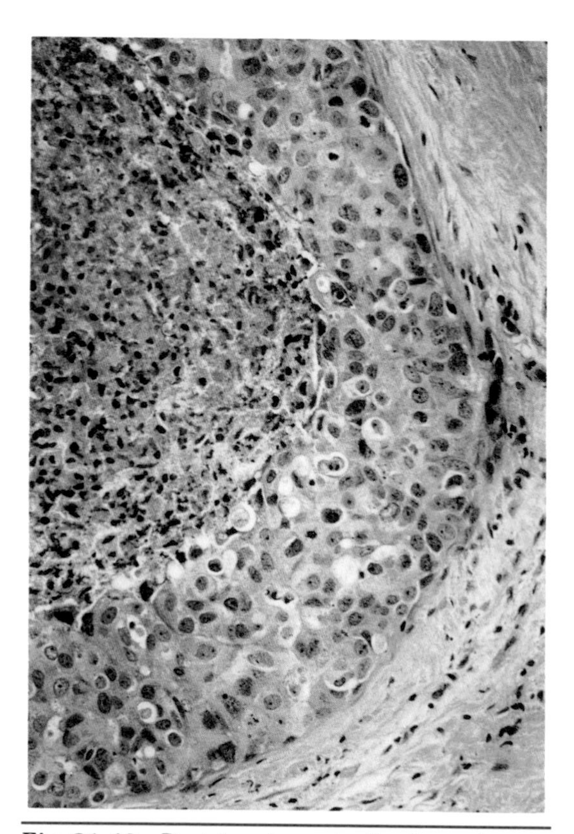

Fig. 21.40 Ductal carcinoma *in situ* of comedo type. The ductule is lined by an irregular proliferation of neoplastic epithelial cells. Note the necrotic debris in the lumen.

small and regular cells which form a geometric 'lacy' network of bridges and trabeculae (Fig. 21.41). The **micropapillary** type also consists of a proliferation of small epithelial cells, which form small papillary projections into the lumen. In some cases a mixture of one or more patterns may be present. Coarse microcalcification in the necrotic luminal debris, or fine clustered calcification in the interstices of the epithelial proliferation form useful diagnostic features for mammographic detection of ductal carcinoma *in situ*.

When ductal carcinoma *in situ* extends along major ducts as far as the nipple, groups of carcinoma cells may enter the deeper layer of the epidermis and spread within it through the nipple and areola. The affected skin shows reactive inflammatory changes in the dermis. These changes produce a characteristic eczematous appearance named **Paget's disease of the breast** after Sir James Paget who described it in 1874. The carcinoma cells usually form clusters within the epidermis (Fig. 21.42) and can be distinguished by their large nuclei, prominent nucleoli and abundant cytoplasm. Paget's disease is always accompanied by an underlying ductal carcinoma *in situ* which may be confined to the nipple ducts or situated deep in the breast. At present the treatment of choice is mastectomy.

In symptomatic cases ductal carcinoma *in situ* is usually confined to one quadrant of the breast, but in a minority of cases multiple separate foci may occur. Examples of the latter are more frequent in cases detected by breast screening. Because of the risk of multifocality many surgeons favour mastectomy as potentially curative therapy, although there is an increasing trend towards con-

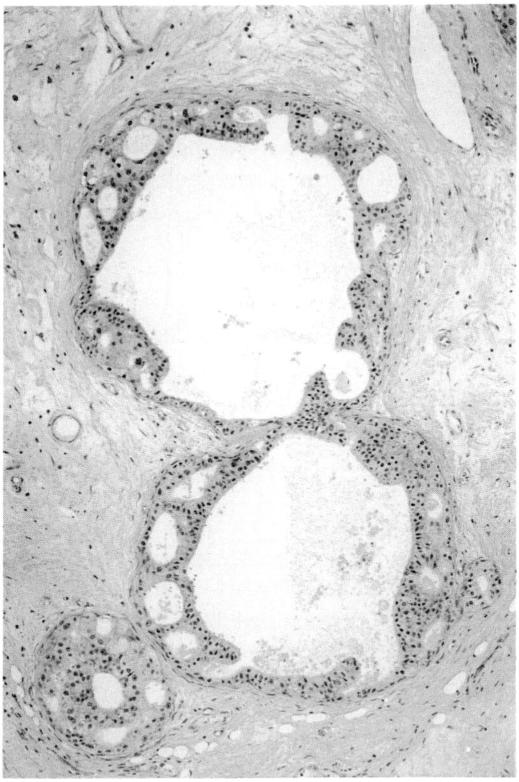

Fig. 21.41 Ductal carcinoma *in situ* of cribriform type. Note the lacy pattern, with rigid geometric epithelial bridges.

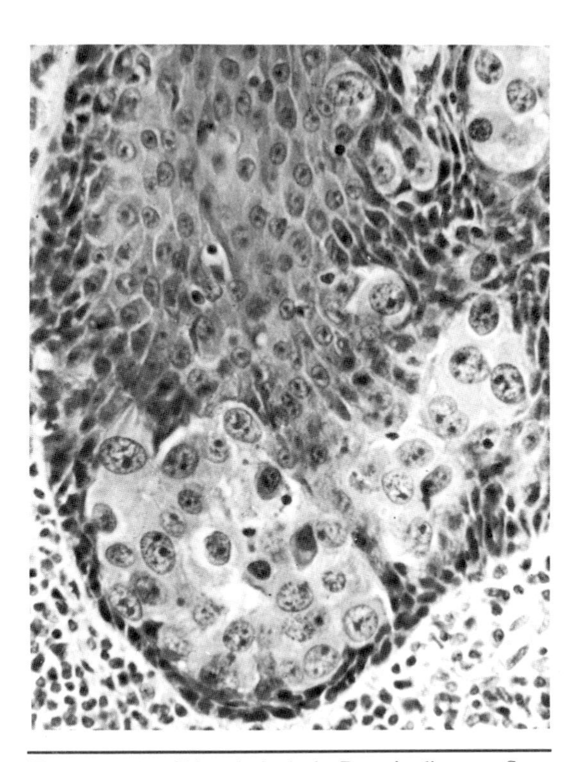

Fig. 21.42 Skin of nipple in Paget's disease. Scattered clumps of carcinoma cells are present in the lower epidermis. There is a marked lymphocytic infiltrate in the dermis.

servation (local excision, with or without postoperative radiotherapy). If primary therapy is adequate the long-term prognosis of ductal carcinoma *in situ* is excellent, with a 10-year survival of greater than 95%.

***Lobular carcinoma* in situ** is much less common than ductal carcinoma *in situ* and is usually an incidental finding in breast tissue removed for fibrocystic change. Microscopically, small, regular, epithelial cells fill and distend the acini of one or more complete lobules (Fig. 21.43). Mitoses are few but the nuclear/cytoplasmic ratio is increased. Basement membranes remain intact. The epithelial proliferation frequently extends into terminal and subsegmental ducts by infiltrating between the duct epithelium and basement membrane, the so-called 'Pagetoid' spread. These changes, however, do not reach the nipple and lobular carcinoma *in situ* is not associated with Paget's disease of the nipple.

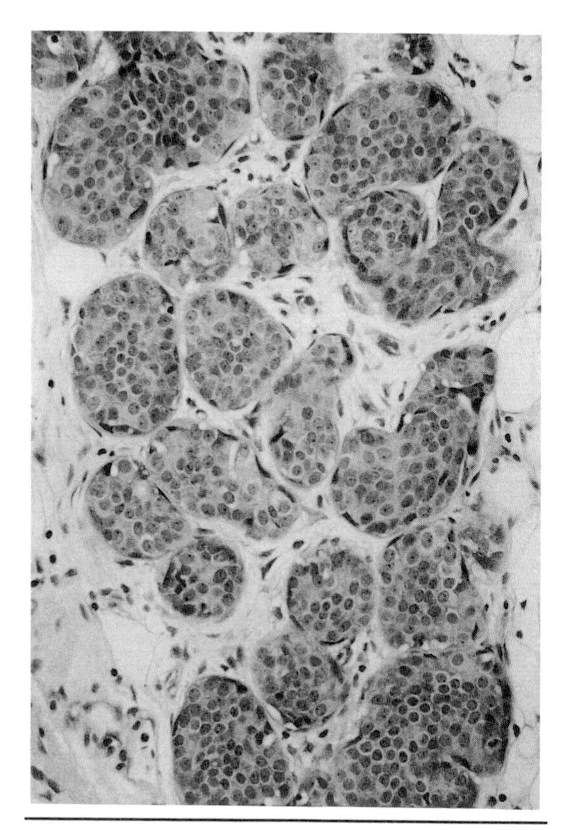

Fig. 21.43 Lobular carcinoma *in situ*. Part of a lobule is shown in which acini are expanded by an epithelial proliferation filling the lumen.

In contrast with ductal carcinoma *in situ*, lobular carcinoma *in situ* is often multifocal and bilateral involvement is reported to occur in up to 30% of cases. Recent follow-up studies have shown that lobular carcinoma *in situ* is best regarded as a risk factor for subsequent invasive carcinoma, and in this respect some authorities link it with atypical lobular hyperplasia under the umbrella term lobular neoplasia. The risk for atypical lobular hyperplasia is approximately fourfold whilst that for lobular carcinoma *in situ* is about tenfold. It is important to note that half the subsequent carcinomas occur in the opposite breast. Careful follow-up is therefore required; the patient should be taught breast self-examination and undergo regular mammography.

Invasive Carcinoma

Invasive carcinoma of the breast arises from a pre-existing *in situ* carcinoma, although by the time the tumour has presented clinically, the *in situ* element may no longer be discernible histologically. A number of different morphological types of invasive breast carcinoma are recognized.

Infiltrating ductal carcinoma – no special type. Over 50% of invasive breast carcinomas fall into this category. Grossly, they form a firm, often hard, moderately defined lump measuring 10–40 mm in diameter. They cut like an unripe pear and it is this type which was traditionally referred to as scirrhous carcinoma (Fig. 21.44). Microscopically, the tumour is composed of cords and sheets of large epithelial cells which infiltrate in a disorganized fashion between dense bands of collagen (Fig. 21.45). The cells vary in size and shape, some tubule formation may be seen and mitoses are usually present, but there are no special morphological features.

Infiltrating lobular carcinoma accounts for approximately 10% of all invasive carcinomas. Although these tumours may have a scirrhous macroscopic appearance similar to ductal carcinoma, more frequently they are softer with an ill-defined

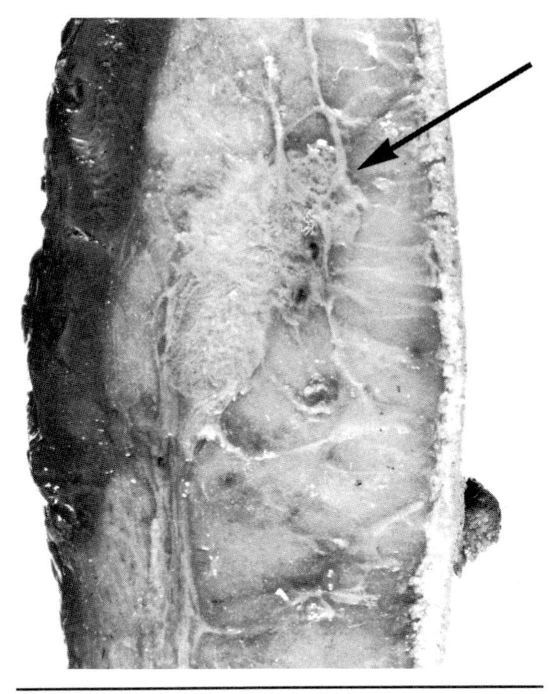

Fig. 21.44 Invasive carcinoma of the breast. The skin of the breast, including the nipple, is seen to the right and the pectoral muscles on the left. The cancer is seen on the cut surface (arrow) as an ill-defined paler area lying in fatty breast tissue.

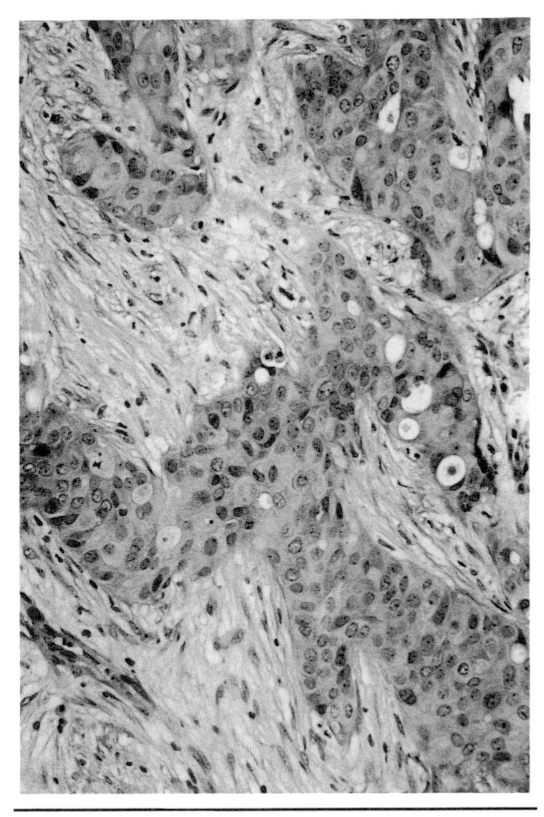

Fig. 21.45 Infiltrating ductal carcinoma. Cords of tumour cells are seen invading into surrounding fibrous stroma.

outline. Microscopically, they are composed of small, regular epithelial cells with infrequent mitoses. Classically, linear cords of cells infiltrate diffusely as discrete or single cells within fine collagen bands giving a so-called targetoid or 'Indian file' pattern (Fig. 21.46).

Tubular carcinomas are uncommon in symptomatic series amounting to about 2% of invasive carcinomas; this frequency increases in screened populations to approximately 15% because impalpable lesions are detected mammographically. Grossly they are small (usually less than 1 cm in diameter), firm and have an irregular stellate outline. Microscopically, there is central elastosis and elongated tubular structures radiate through a cellular fibroblastic stroma (Fig. 21.47). The tubules are lined by a single layer of regular epithelial cells, and lumina are patent. Mitoses are infrequent. Whilst this pure tubular type is uncommon, in about 20% of invasive carcinomas a mixed pattern is seen, where a tubular structure is preserved centrally, but infiltrating ductal or lobular carcinoma is present at the periphery.

Medullary carcinomas account for approximately 3% of invasive carcinomas. Macroscopically, they are well defined and soft, measuring between 10 and 40 mm in diameter. Microscopically, they are composed of syncytial masses of large epithelial cells with a conspicuous lymphoplasmacytoid infiltrate in the stroma and at the periphery. The cells vary markedly in size and shape, and mitoses are frequent.

Mucoid carcinomas are rare (less than 1% of invasive carcinomas). Characteristically they have a well defined gelatinous gross appearance. Histo-

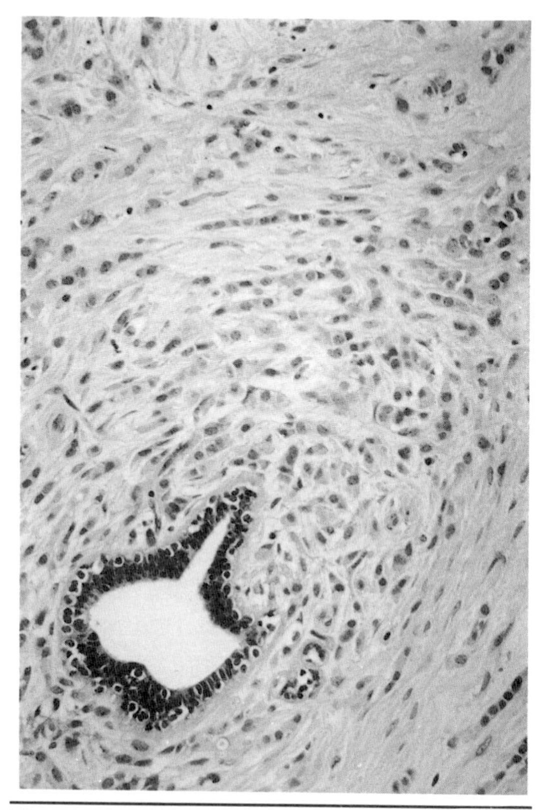

Fig. 21.46 Infiltrating lobular carcinoma. Single files of uniform tumour cells infiltrate the stroma, in a 'targetoid' fashion around a normal ductule.

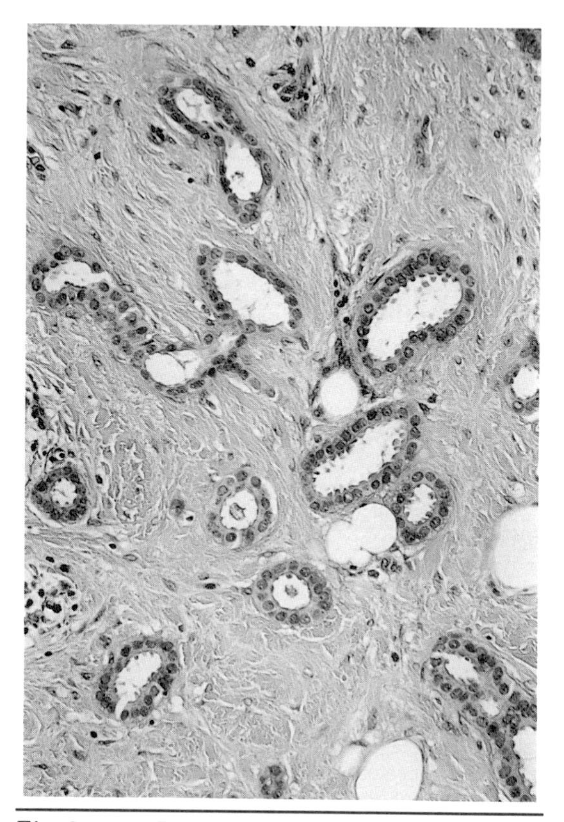

Fig. 21.47 Tubular carcinoma. Note the well formed open tubules composed of a single layer of epithelial cells.

logically, the tumour is composed of clumps of small, regular epithelial cells lying within lakes of mucin.

Papillary carcinomas are also very rare. There may occasionally be evidence of an origin in a pre-existing duct or cyst papilloma but in most cases this is not so. Microscopically, they are composed of papillary structures with fibrovascular cores lined by epithelial cells. Nuclear differentiation is variable.

Other types of invasive breast carcinoma, such as **spindle cell, squamous and secretory** are exceedingly rare. Combinations of the types listed above may also occur.

Routes of Spread

Unfortunately, at the time of diagnosis in symptomatic patients breast cancer is often already widely disseminated. This explains the observation that age-adjusted death rates have remained remarkably constant, and that radical local therapy such as extended radical mastectomy gives no better survival than complete local excision. There are three main ways in which breast cancer may spread from the primary site: local, lymphatic and blood.

Locally, if a tumour remains undetected and continues to grow it will eventually invade the overlying skin and the deep fascia and chest wall. This is termed a 'locally advanced primary'. Careful histological studies have shown that lymphatic permeation can be observed at the periphery of many breast carcinomas. Axillary lymph nodes are involved by metastatic carcinoma in up to 50% of patients with apparently 'operable' tumours. Metastatic carcinoma may also be found in internal mammary lymph nodes, especially if the primary tumour is located in the inner quadrants. Distant metastasis occurs via the bloodstream. Many organs may be involved but the commonest are lung, bone and liver.

Prognosis of Invasive Carcinoma

Few accurate long-term follow-up studies have been carried out and the best is that of Brinkley and Haybittle (1984). They showed that the crude mortality for primary operable breast carcinoma was 40% after 5 years, over 60% at 10 years and approximately 75% at 35 years. Thus, after prolonged follow-up, only a quarter of patients with breast cancer can be considered to be clinically 'cured' whilst three-quarters of an age-matched control population are still alive.

Several pathological factors are known to have an influence on the prognosis of an individual patient. The **size** at diagnosis is important; not surprisingly the smaller the tumour the better the survival. This is the logical basis for breast cancer screening using mammography to detect tumours at a stage before they are palpable. Although the main route for metastasis to other organs is via the bloodstream, **lymphatic invasion** occurs simultaneously and gives a good indication of such spread. Both the number and level of loco-regional lymph nodes involved correlate well with survival; the more nodes involved and the higher the level in the axilla the worse the prognosis. Overall, the 10-year survival is reduced from 75% in patients with histologically uninvolved nodes to 30% in those with metastatic carcinoma in nodes. Size and stage of lymph node involvement are time dependent factors; the longer the tumour has been growing the more advanced they will be.

An important biological factor, which probably remains relatively constant is the degree of **tumour differentiation**. Both tumour type and grade of differentiation correlate well with prognosis. The special tumour types such as tubular, tubular mixed and mucoid carry an excellent long-term survival, infiltrating lobular carcinoma has an intermediate prognosis and infiltrating ductal has a relatively poor prognosis. Histological grade is determined by assessing three histological features, the amount of tubule formation, the degree of nuclear pleomorphism and the mitotic count. Three grades are used ranging from well differentiated (grade 1) with good tubule formation, little pleomorphism and low mitotic counts through moderately differentiated (grade 2) to poorly differentiated tumours (grade 3) with little or no tubule formation, marked pleomorphism and high mitotic counts. Eighty-five per cent of patients with grade 1 tumours are alive 10 years after the diagnosis compared with 35% of patients with grade 3 tumours. Even in the relatively small group of patients who survive 25 years or more death may still occur from breast cancer, indicating that complete cure is a rarity.

Aetiology of Breast Carcinoma

No single causal agent has been found, but a number of predisposing factors have been identified. The incidence of breast cancer, like carcinomas in general, increases with age, but the increase occurs earlier than for most cancers, being most rapid between the ages of 30 and 50 years, after which it rises more slowly to a maximum in old age. The strongest aetiological factor is a positive family history; there is a definite increased risk if a female relative, i.e. mother, maternal grandmother or sister, has had breast cancer. Occasional families exist in which there is a very high incidence of breast cancer, and such evidence points to the possibility of a genetic predisposition. Although differences in racial susceptibility have been established (the incidence is lower in China and Japan) this is almost certainly due to environmental factors, since the incidence rises in 'westernized' Japanese women. There is good evidence that exposure to female sex hormones, and oestrogen in particular, is an important factor in the development of breast cancer, but it is not certain whether there is a systemic effect or an increase in target organ sensitivity. Some risk factors have been identified; apart from the obvious difference in the incidence in men and women, the risk in women is increased by early menarche and late menopause, whilst early first pregnancy and oophorectomy before the age of 35 years have a protective effect. There is still no agreement concerning the role of oral contraceptive therapy in the aetiology of breast cancer. The balance of epidemiological evidence is that users of the pill are at an increased risk. These data, however, are particularly difficult to interpret because of the large number of variable factors involved.

Hormone Dependence

In up to 30% of women with breast cancer the course of the disease may be influenced by alterations in the hormonal background of the patient. This was first demonstrated by Beatson in Glasgow in 1896 when he carried out bilateral oophorectomy in patients with advanced breast cancer. More recently the oestrogen receptor competitor tamoxifen has been used successfully in the treatment of metastatic disease to obtain average remissions of approximately 2–3 years. Measurement of oestrogen receptor protein in tumour samples provides a good prediction of likely response to endocrine therapy; a favourable response is unlikely if oestrogen receptor cannot be detected. Oestrogen receptors can now be identified in tissue sections using immunochemistry.

Miscellaneous Tumours of the Breast

Phyllodes Tumour

These uncommon and unusual tumours are still referred to erroneously as 'giant fibroadenoma' or 'cystosarcoma phyllodes'. They occur predominantly in middle-aged or elderly women and are only rarely seen below the age of 40. They form large, lobulated, circumscribed masses which may grow rapidly to cause unilateral breast enlargement or even skin ulceration. Grossly, they have a whorled cut surface which resembles a compressed leaf bud (Greek phyllon=leaf) with visible clefts and cystic spaces (Fig. 21.48). Microscopically, the elongated cleft-like spaces are lined with epithelial cells and the intervening stroma is cellular (Fig. 21.49). The epithelial cells are regular and entirely benign, although focal hyperplasia may occasionally be present. The stromal cells are plump and may be densely packed; nuclear abnormalities are rare and mitoses variable in number. The great majority of phyllodes tumours are benign and complete excision is curative. Approximately 10% will recur locally after enucleation, due to incomplete excision. True malignant change occurs in less than 5% of cases. The stroma becomes **sarcomatous** and both lymph node and blood-borne metastases may develop, especially if local excision is incomplete.

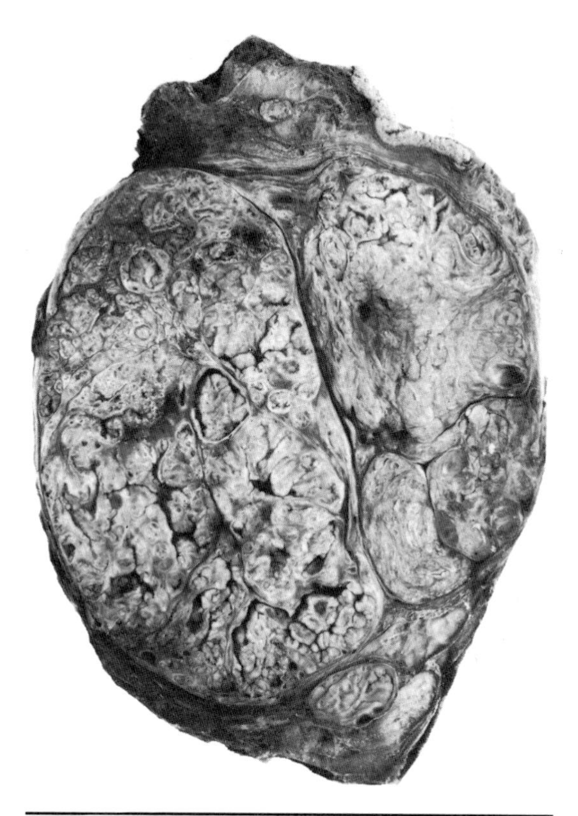

Fig. 21.48 Phyllodes tumour. The resemblance of the cleft-like spaces to a compressed leaf bud is well shown.

Sarcomas

Most types of malignant connective tissue tumour have been described in the breast, but all are exceedingly rare. The prognosis of angiosarcoma, once thought to be invariably fatal, is now known to depend on the degree of differentiation of the vascular endothelium. The behaviour of liposarcoma and malignant fibrous histiocytoma appears to be the same as in other sites in the body.

Lymphomas

The breast is an unusual primary site of lymphomas, diffuse centrocytic/centroblastic being least rare. Its distinction from carcinoma at operation is important in order to avoid unnecessary mutilation. Involvement of the breast in disseminated lymphomas and in granulocytic leukaemia is commoner and occasionally provides the presenting symptoms.

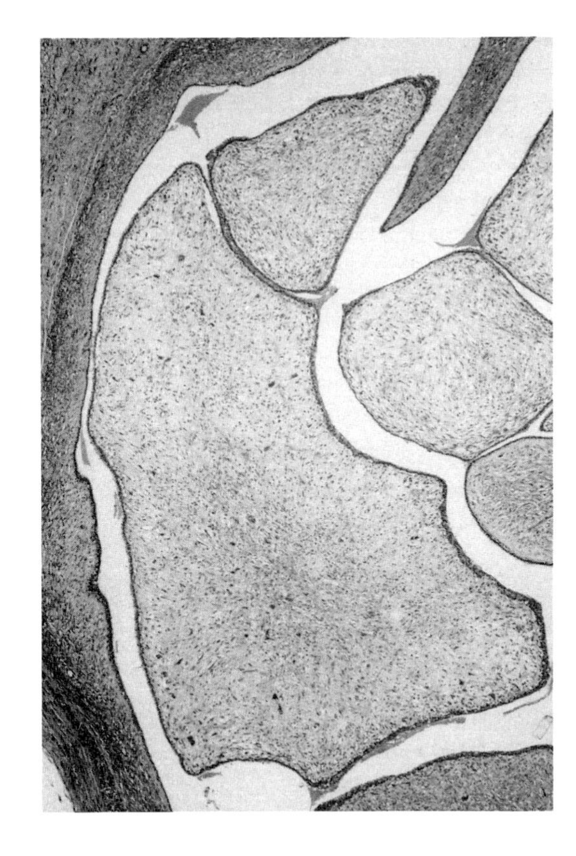

Fig. 21.49 Phyllodes tumour, composed of clefts lined by epithelial cells, with a cellular stroma.

The Male Breast

Hypertrophy (Gynaecomastia)

The male and female breasts are essentially similar until the onset of the secondary sex characters at puberty; in some adolescent males one or both breasts may then enlarge. This is known as pubertal hypertrophy and is rarely marked, but may cause pain or discomfort. It is due mainly to increase of stroma and enlargement of ducts, but without lobule formation; the hyperplastic duct epithelium may be surrounded by a zone of oedematous, fibrillary stroma. It tends to regress and operative removal is rarely necessary. Similar changes may occur in old age. Both pubertal and senile hypertrophy are due to changes in levels of sex hormones.

Gynaecomastia occurs in response to high oestrogen levels, for example in chronic liver disease, in prolonged hormonal therapy for prostatic cancer, and reportedly in workers involved in the manufacture of oestrogens. Less commonly, it is induced by digitalis and some other drugs. Occasionally hypertrophy results from an underlying endocrine disease such as feminizing tumour of the adrenal cortex. Less often testicular injury is causal. In chromatin-positive Klinefelter's syndrome the enlarged breasts show lobules comparable with those of the normal female breast.

Tumours

Tumours are rare. Carcinomas are usually of infiltrating ductal type. Prognosis is often poor because of early spread to lymph nodes and to the chest wall. Paget's disease of the male breast is very rare. Metastatic tumour, e.g. from a bronchial carcinoma, occasionally occurs and the male breast, like that of the female, may be involved in generalized lymphoid neoplasms and the leukaemias.

Further Reading

The Female Reproductive Tract

Anderson, M. C. (ed.) (1991). Female Reproductive System. *Systemic Pathology*, 3rd edn. Vol. 6, pp. 480. Churchill Livingstone, Edinburgh.

Buckley, C. H. and Fox, H. I. (1989). *Biopsy Pathology of the Endometrium*, pp. 278. Chapman and Hall, London.

Coleman, D. V. and Evans, D. M. D. (1989). *Biopsy Pathology and Cytology of the Cervix*, pp. 386. Chapman and Hall, London.

Fox, H. (ed.) (1987). *Haines and Taylor's Obstetrical and Gynaecological Pathology*, 3rd edn, pp. 1331. Churchill Livingstone, Edinburgh.

Fox, H. and Buckley, C. H. (1991). *Pathology for Gynaecologists*, 2nd edn, pp. 304. Edward Arnold, London.

Hendrickson, M. R. and Kempson, R. I. (1980). *Surgical Pathology of the Uterine Corpus*, pp. 589. W. B. Saunders, Philadelphia.

Kurman, R. J. (ed.) (1987). *Blaustein's Pathology of the Female Genital Tract*, 3rd edn. pp. 959. Springer Verlag, New York.

Ridley, C. M. (ed.) (1989). *The Vulva*, pp. 363. Churchill Livingstone, Edinburgh.

Rollason, T. P. (1991). Aspects of ovarian pathology. In *Recent Advances in Histopathology*, No. 15, pp. 195–218, eds P. P. Anthony and R. N. M. MacSween. Churchill Livingstone, Edinburgh.

Roth, L. M. and Czernobilsky, B. (1985). *Tumors and Tumor-like Conditions of the Ovary*, pp. 296. Churchill Livingstone, New York.

Wilkinson, E. J. (ed.) (1987). *Pathology of the Vulva and Vagina*, pp. 340. Churchill Livingstone, New York.

The Breast

Brinkley, D. and Haybittle, J. L. (1984). Long-term survival of women with breast cancer. *Lancet*, **1**, 1118.

Page, D. L. and Anderson, T. J. (1987). *Diagnostic Histopathology of the Breast*, pp. 362. Churchill Livingstone, Edinburgh.

Sloane, J. P. (1985). *Biopsy Pathology of the Breast*, pp. 284. Chapman and Hall Medical, London.

22 The Male Reproductive System

Testis and Epididymis

It is convenient to consider together these two organs which, along with the tunica vaginalis and lower end of the spermatic cord, make up the testicle (i.e. the contents of the scrotal sac).

Inflammatory Lesions

Acute epididymitis is usually a complication of either gonococcal or 'non-specific' urethritis or of urinary tract infections. It results from spread of the infection along the vas deferens and may be bilateral. Persistent or inadequately treated lesions may suppurate and cause destruction of epididymal tubules with consequent sterility. Spread to involve the testis, **epididymo-orchitis**, is less common but may result in much tissue destruction and scarring.

Tuberculosis of the male genital tract is now uncommon in developed countries. It usually results from haematogenous spread from a distant primary site, most commonly in the lungs, and the epididymis is the part most often affected (compare tuberculous salpingitis), although subsequent spread to the prostate gland and bladder may occur. The epididymis becomes enlarged and firm due to caseation and fibrosis (Fig. 22.1) and if untreated, the process may involve the scrotal skin with the formation of chronic discharging sinuses. Curiously, the testis itself is not affected

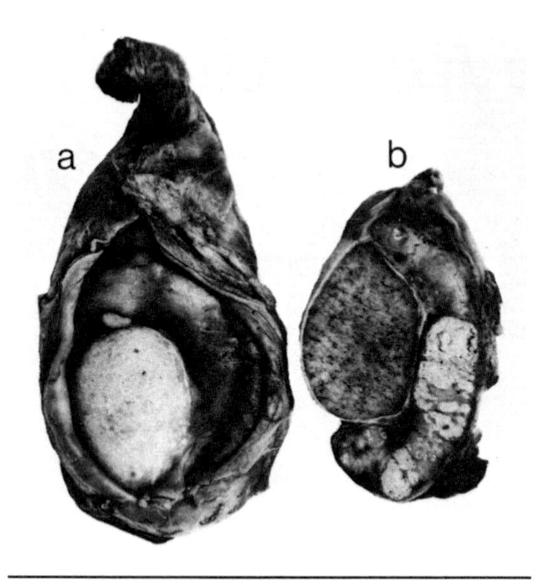

Fig. 22.1 Bilateral epididymal tuberculosis: in **a** the irregularly swollen epididymis is seen above and to the right of the testis: in **b** caseation in the other epididymis is shown on section. × 0.7.

until late on and even then lesions are usually limited to tissue immediately adjacent to the epididymis.

Acute orchitis occurs most commonly as a complication of mumps in post-pubertal males. Infection occurs during the viraemic phase, usually about 6 days after the parotids are involved, although in some patients the orchitis may be the first or only symptom. The testis becomes acutely painful and swollen. The inflammation subsides within a few days but, in a minority of cases, secondary ischaemic damage may result in the testis becoming atrophic. Fortunately, mumps orchitis is bilateral in less than 20% of patients and sterility rarely occurs. Other viruses such as herpes, coxsackie and echo may occasionally cause acute orchitis, and a suppurating orchitis may complicate acute bacterial epididymitis.

Syphilitic orchitis. The testis is very commonly involved in tertiary syphilis, indeed more frequently than any other organ except the aorta. The lesion is usually a classic gumma. A more diffuse chronic interstitial orchitis without necrosis can also develop, especially in inadequately treated patients.

Granulomatous orchitis, of unknown aetiology, causes unilateral painful swelling of the testis, usually in middle-aged men. After a few weeks this subsides leaving an indurated organ with reduced sensitivity to pressure. Histologically, the appearances superficially resemble tuberculosis, with a granulomatous inflammatory infiltrate, including giant cells, surrounding and destroying seminiferous tubules, thus imparting a follicular pattern to the process. An autoimmune pathogenesis has been suspected but with little supporting evidence.

A quite similar histological appearance is seen in the epididymis following extravasation of sperm. These **sperm granulomas** are usually due to distal duct obstruction and are common following vasectomy operations. This suggests that granulomatous orchitis may also be due to a reaction to sperm or tubular epithelium.

Tumours of the Testicle

Approximately 90% of testicular tumours are of germ-cell origin and almost all are malignant. They are all uncommon, accounting for less than 1% of cancer deaths (ovarian tumours account for over 10%). However, the peak incidence of testicular tumours is in early adult life and this makes them one of the most important forms of cancer in young men.

Germ-cell Tumours

Classification. The classification of germ-cell tumours used here is outlined in Fig. 22.2. It is a simplification of the UK Testicular Tumour Panel's recommendations (Pugh, 1976), since their classification is the most widely used in this country and, in terms of current concepts regarding the origin of teratomas, it is histogenetically sound. The other

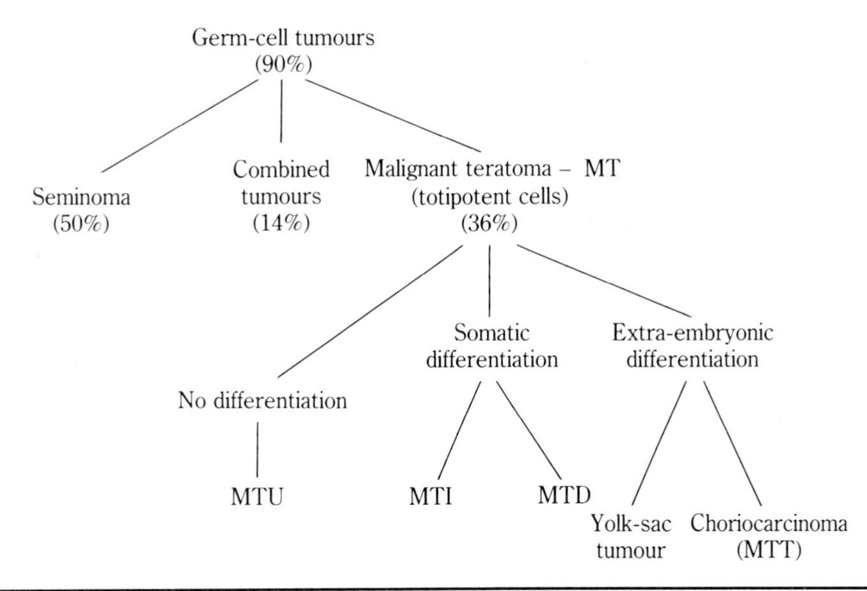

Fig. 22.2 Diagram outlining the classification of germ cell tumours of the testis: the figures in parenthesis indicate the approximate relative frequency of each type as a proportion of all testicular tumours. MTU, malignant teratoma undifferentiated. MTI, MTD, malignant teratoma with differentiation into mature tissue elements, of intermediate degree (I) or well developed (D). MTT, malignant teratoma trophoblastic.

major classification is that of the World Health Organisation (Sobin *et al.*, 1978). These classifications do not correspond exactly and, in particular, in the WHO classification the concept of undifferentiated teratoma is not accepted and the term embryonal carcinoma is used in its place.

Seminoma

This is the commonest malignant tumour of the testis (the ovarian homologue, dysgerminoma, is much less common). Seminoma is almost unknown before puberty, becomes commoner in the 20s, has a peak in the 30s and falls sharply in the 50s. This is in striking contrast to the rise in incidence of most other carcinomas in men after 50 years of age. Like all testicular tumours, it usually presents as a painless enlargement of the testis.

Macroscopically, seminoma typically appears as a well defined, firm, often large, rounded mass within the substance of the testis and only rarely involving the tunica albuginea, epididymis or scrotum. The cut surface is soft but otherwise resembles that of a potato, being uniformly grey-white, solid and opaque (Fig. 22.3a). Haemorrhage and necrosis are unusual (compare teratoma). Microscopically, it is composed of large cells bearing a distinct resemblance to spermatogonia, with abundant pale cytoplasm and large central vesicular nuclei (Fig. 22.4). The cells are arranged in compact aggregates separated by irregular thin strands of stroma. The latter is usually infiltrated, sometimes very heavily, by lymphocytes, and sarcoid-like granulomas are frequently also present; the latter features probably represent a host immune reaction to the tumour and, when pronounced, may signify an improved prognosis.

Two uncommon variants of seminoma are worth mentioning. In **anaplastic seminoma** the tumour cells are larger and more pleomorphic with giant-cell formation and show increased mitotic activity. It may carry a worse prognosis. By contrast, **spermatocytic seminoma**, despite being histologically pleomorphic, carries a better prognosis. Some of the tumour cells resemble spermatocytes, hence the name. It tends to occur in older men, usually over 65, and is never associated with teratomatous elements.

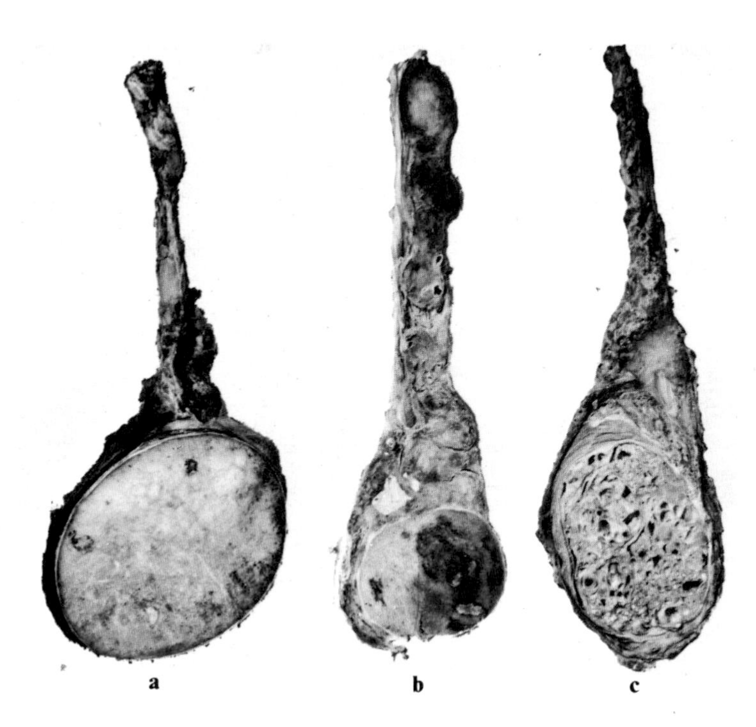

Fig. 22.3 Tumours of the testis. **a** Seminoma: typical solid 'potato' appearance. **b** Undifferentiated teratoma (MTU), mainly solid and haemorrhagic. **c** Unusually well differentiated teratoma (MTD) with multiple cysts.

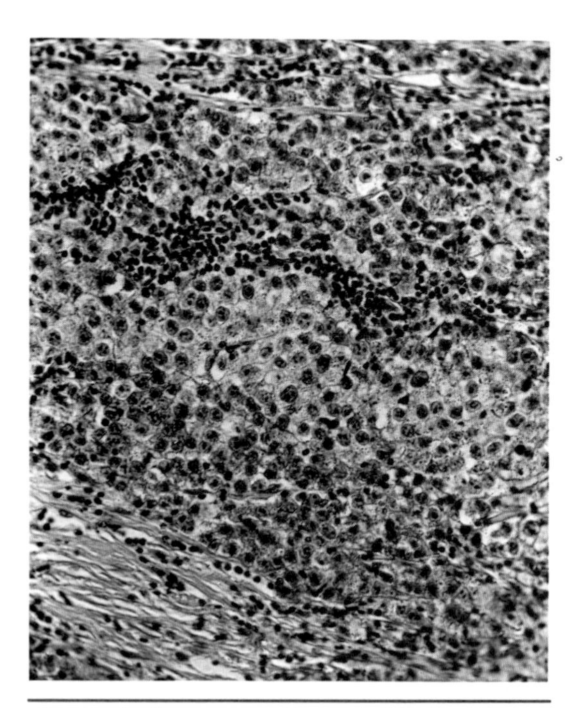

Fig. 22.4 Seminoma of the testis. The tumour consists of masses of large, round, pale staining cells with vesicular nuclei. Note the marked lymphocytic infiltrate. ×210.

Teratoma

A general account of these tumours has been given on p. 370. Testicular teratoma occurs in younger patients than seminoma, the peak incidence being in the 20s and with some cases occurring in childhood. In contrast to ovarian teratoma, testicular teratomas are usually solid and almost invariably malignant. Their gross appearance differs from seminoma in that areas of haemorrhage and necrosis are usually prominent (see Fig. 22.3b). Multiple small cysts may be seen in the better differentiated tumours (see Fig. 22.3c).

Malignant Teratoma Differentiated – MTD (WHO – mature teratoma). These tumours are relatively uncommon and are made up of haphazardly arranged well differentiated tissues (Fig. 22.5) and are similar in appearance to the much commoner benign ovarian teratoma ('dermoid' cyst). However, unlike the ovarian dermoid cyst, MTDs are mainly solid, although they may contain small cysts. They may metastasize even though all the various elements seen are mature and cytologically benign. This is probably because small

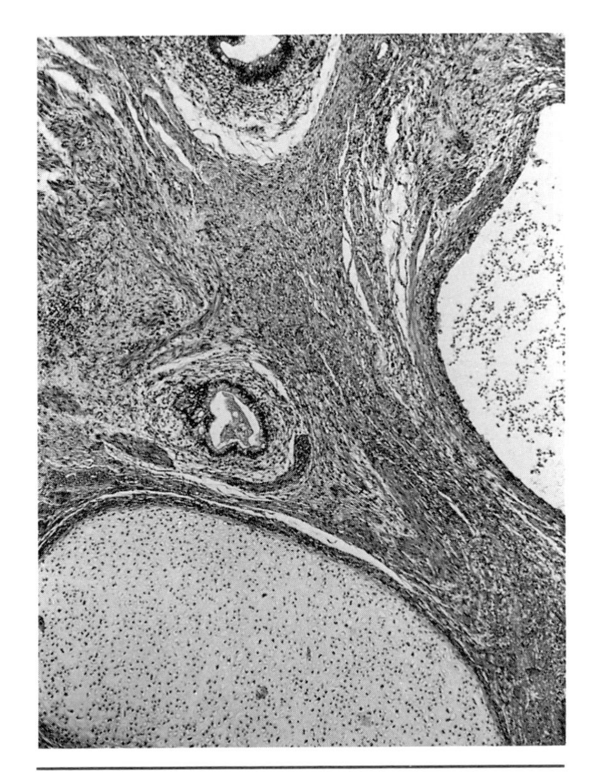

Fig. 22.5 Part of a well differentiated teratoma of the testis (MTD), showing a nodule of cartilage, glandular tissue and cystic spaces, lying in a mature connective tissue stroma containing strands of smooth muscle. ×15.

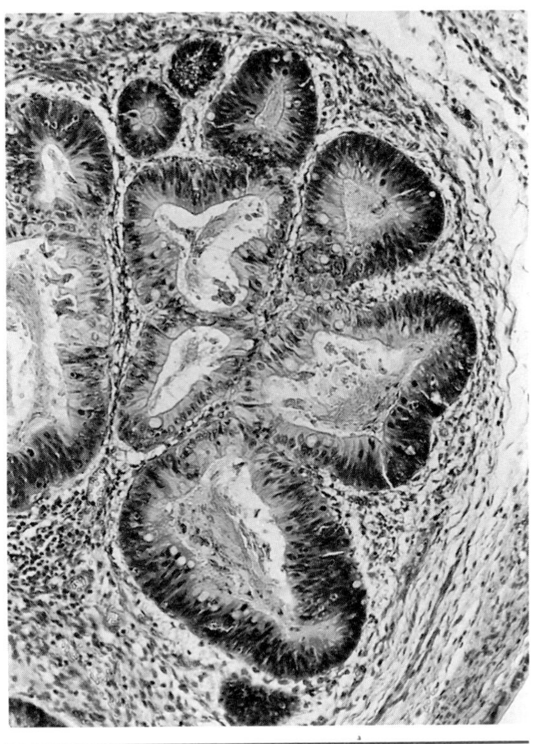

Fig. 22.6 Mucin-secreting glandular tissue in an intermediate teratoma (MTI) showing marked atypia of the glandular epithelium with crowding of nuclei and numerous mitoses. ×45.

foci of less well differentiated tissue are present and remain undetected despite extensive histological sampling. For this reason all MTDs should be regarded as malignant tumours.

Malignant Teratoma Intermediate – MTI (WHO – immature teratoma; teratocarcinoma), is the commonest form of testicular teratoma. These tumours consist of a mixture of tissues showing variable degrees of differentiation (Fig. 22.6) and in addition many contain clearly malignant elements which may be carcinomatous, sarcomatous or anaplastic in appearance (Fig. 22.7).

Malignant Teratoma Undifferentiated – MTU (WHO – embryonal carcinoma). These tumours consist entirely of malignant tissue resembling the malignant elements of MTI (Fig. 22.7). The commonest pattern is masses of large, pleomorphic malignant cells which, in areas, may show attempts at adenocarcinomatous or papillary differentiation.

Tumours with extra embryonic elements. Germ-cell neoplasms may differentiate along placental or yolk-sac lines. Pure **choriocarcinoma** (Fig. 22.8) of the testis (designated malignant teratoma trophoblastic – MTT) is rare, but carries a very poor prognosis even with modern therapy. The primary tumour is often small and the initial presentation may be haemoptysis from haemorrhagic pulmonary metastases.

Pure *yolk-sac tumours* are also very rare; they occur in infants and young boys and histologically consist of poorly differentiated epithelial tissue often organized into papillary formations and mi-

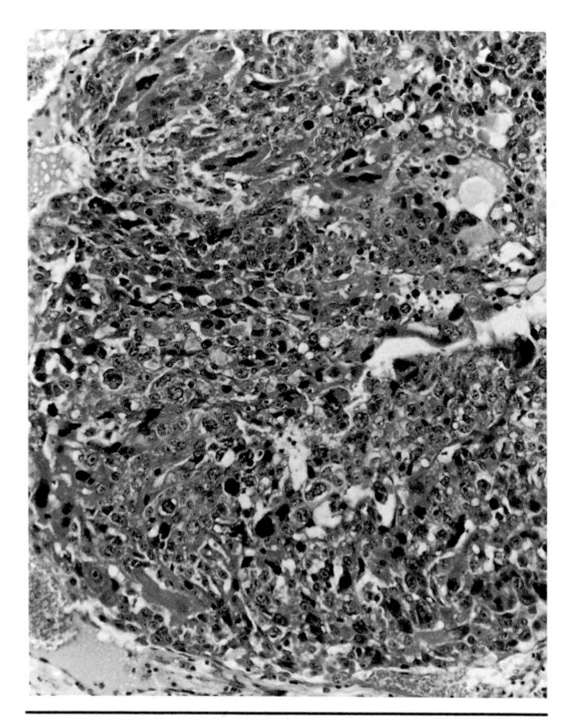

Fig. 22.7 A focus of anaplastic malignant tissue in an intermediate teratoma (MTI). The tumour cells show marked pleomorphism and mitotic activity. Undifferentiated testicular teratomas (MTU) are composed entirely of tissue like this. ×145.

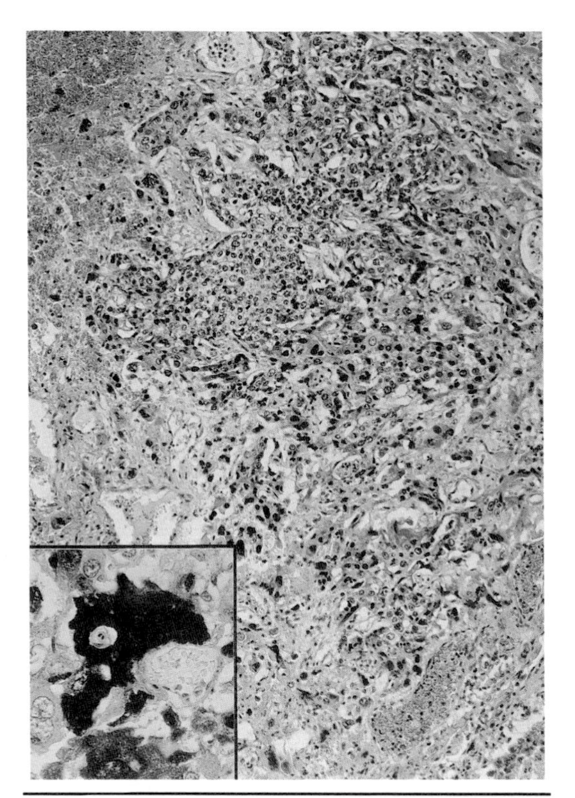

Fig. 22.8 A metastatic pulmonary deposit of choriocarcinoma. The tumour is biphasic, consisting of masses of uniform cytotrophoblastic cells together with syncytiotrophoblastic giant cells. There are areas of necrosis and extensive haemorrhage into the adjacent lung parenchyma (top left). ×120. Inset: syncytiotrophoblastic giant cell stained for HCG. Indirect peroxidase technique. ×200.

crocysts. A form of glomeruloid structure known as a *Schiller–Duval body* is highly characteristic. These tumours, if pure, are less aggressive than MTU or MTI.

Trophoblastic tissue produces human chorionic gonadotrophin (HCG) and yolk-sac tissue produces alpha-fetoprotein (AFP). Each of these substances may be demonstrated in the tumour tissue as well as in the serum. Their detection in the serum is of value in diagnosis, in monitoring the response to treatment, and in detecting the development of metastases.

The use of immunohistochemical methods has demonstrated that extraembryonic tissues occur more frequently in testicular tumours than had been previously suspected using conventional microscopy. Thus, about 75% of MTUs contain foci of either or both types of tissue, while 10% of seminomas contain HCG positive syncytiotrophoblast giant cells, and a smaller proportion contain AFP-positive cells.

Combined germ-cell tumours. In 14% of testicular germ-cell tumours there is a combination of seminomatous and teratomatous elements either mixed together (mixed tumour) or as separate nodules (combined tumour). Extraembryonal elements may also be present and the resulting histological picture may be very complex. In general, the behaviour of these tumours depends on the most malignant element present. Thus, if trophoblastic elements are present these may overgrow the other elements or metastases may consist of pure choriocarcinoma.

Clinical Behaviour and Treatment

Both seminomas and teratomas invade the lymphatics and venules of the spermatic cord which may be palpably thickened (see Fig. 22.3b). Metastases occur to the para-iliac and para-aortic lymph nodes, sometimes extending to those in the thorax. Spread may occur also by the bloodstream, to involve the lungs and, less commonly, the liver. Both tumour types are capable of both patterns of spread but lymphatic spread is more characteristic of seminoma and blood spread of teratoma. All testicular germ-cell tumours, but particularly teratoma, may present with metastatic disease, usually pulmonary lesions or a retroperitoneal tumour mass. The primary tumour may on occasion be microscopical in size and indeed may not be found.

If untreated the prognosis of both seminoma and teratoma is poor but modern therapy has revolutionized the outcome. Seminoma is one of the most radiosensitive of all tumours and orchidectomy coupled with abdominal radiotherapy achieves a 95% cure rate. Even patients with lung metastases have a relatively good prognosis. Treatment of teratoma by combination chemotherapy, including particularly cisplatin, combined with debulking surgery (including the removal of pulmonary metastases) has achieved remarkable results, the cure rate now approaching that of seminoma. If the patient shows no progression for 2 years after therapy then recurrence is unlikely.

Aetiology and Pathogenesis of Testicular Germ-cell Tumours

The incidence of this group of tumours is undoubtedly increasing but the causal factors are not understood. Genetic factors are apparent in only rare cases affecting twins or fathers and sons. Geographical differences exist, much higher rates being observed in the UK and USA than in the Far East. Racial differences also seem to be important – Caucasians have a higher incidence than Negroes and a lower incidence than Jews in any given community. This, however, may in part be due to, as yet unidentified, environmental factors.

The major risk factor so far identified is cryptorchidism. Up to 10% of germ-cell tumours (usually seminoma) arise in maldescended gonads and the increased risk has been variously calculated as being between 10 and 40 times that in descended organs. There is also an increased risk of tumour in the contralateral, normally-descended testis, suggesting there are common factors, possibly hormonal, which predispose to cryptorchidism and to tumour development. Ectopic and abdominal testes seem to carry a higher risk than organs which have descended to the inquinal canal and this perhaps also reflects that, in these cases, the gonads are likely to be more abnormal. This risk is sufficient to justify surgical abdominal exploration

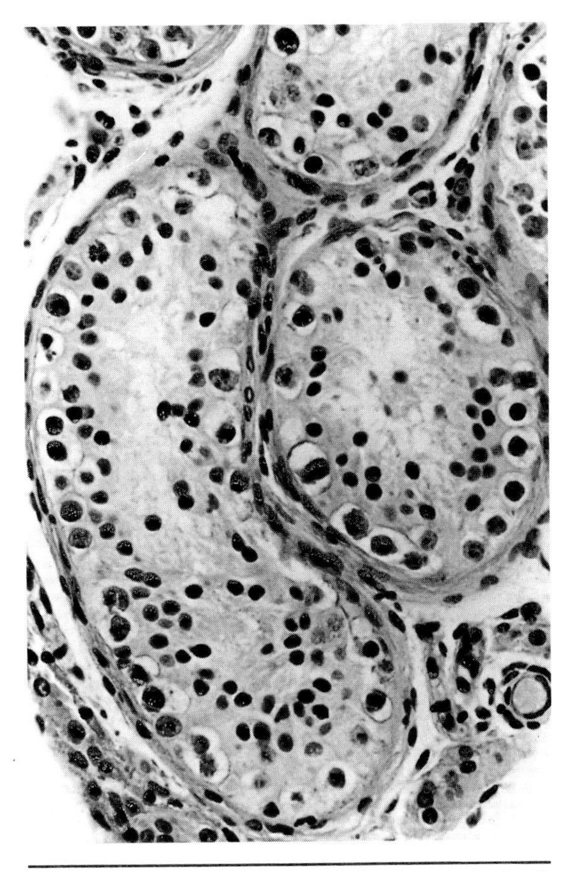

Fig. 22.9 Premalignant change in the germinal epithelium in an undescended testis. Note the abnormally large spermatogonia with vacuolated cytoplasm and large hyperchromatic nuclei. (By courtesy of Dr R. A. Risdon and the *Journal of Pathology*.)

and removal of such organs. Testes present in the inquinal canal should be resited in the scrotum (orchidopexy) and this operation both reduces the increased risk of subsequent neoplasia and increases the chances of fertility, if carried out when the child is less than 3–4 years old. Maldescended testes removed in later life may show focal cytological abnormalities in the seminiferous epithelium and this is regarded as premalignant change, or *in situ* carcinoma (Fig. 22.9).

Other Tumours of the Testicle

Gonadal Stromal/Sex Cord Tumours

These are not as common as their homologues in the ovary and together comprise 2–3% of testicular tumours.

Leydig-cell tumours form a well circumscribed, often lobulated, brown coloured mass which consists microscopically of sheets of uniform eosinophilic cells. Characteristic elongated intracellular Reinke crystalloids are present in half of the cases. Leydig-cell tumours are often hormonally active, producing either testosterone or oestrogens, and endocrine effects such as gynaecomastia or sexual precocity may be the presenting feature. Almost all of these tumours are benign.

Sertoli-cell tumours are less common than Leydig-cell tumours but 20% are malignant. They may produce hormones, usually oestrogens. One-third of Sertoli-cell tumours have small admixed foci of Leydig cells.

Lymphoma. Secondary malignant lymphomas and leukaemias may occur in the testis in the context of systemic disease. This is particularly important in the treatment of childhood leukaemia where the testes may act as a reservoir for the disease, leading to relapse after drug-induced remission. Primary lymphoma of the testis is of diffuse, non-Hodgkin's type, usually B cell. It becomes the commonest primary testicular neoplasm in men over 60 years and accounts for about 7% of primary testicular tumours.

Adenomatoid tumour. This is an uncommon benign tumour which usually presents as a small mass in the epididymis. It is of mesothelial origin.

Mesenchymal tumours such as leiomyoma are occasionally found in relation to the testis or epididymis; malignant mesenchymal tumours are very rare.

Metastatic tumours of the testicle are uncommon.

Male Infertility

Approximately 15% of married couples are infertile. Though the figures are not very reliable, the responsible partner is generally held to be the male or female in roughly equal numbers, with a third group in which both partners are subfertile. This suggests that at least 5% of males are infertile and while some cases are psychological, endocrine or drug induced, the majority are due to lesions of the genital organs, particularly the testes. The causes of male infertility may be conveniently divided into pretesticular, testicular and post-testicular groups and the principal ones are listed in Table 22.1.

Miscellaneous Lesions

Hydrocele. This is a collection of clear, usually straw-coloured, fluid within the tunica vaginalis. It can usually be distinguished from testicular enlargement by transillumination. Hydroceles may be part of a generalized oedema but the majority are idiopathic. However, it is most important to exclude inflammatory or neoplastic disease of the testicle which may be both causing the accumulation of fluid and being concealed by it. Purulent fluid within the tunica vaginalis is usually due to

Table 22.1 The main causes of male infertility

Pretesticular causes
Hypopituitarism
Oestrogen excess
endogenous: hepatic cirrhosis; adrenal or gonadal tumours
exogenous: treatment for prostatic cancer
Testicular causes
Cryptorchidism
Klinefelter's syndrome
Germ-cell aplasia
Hypospermatogenesis/maturation arrest
idiopathic
severe systemic illness, e.g. uraemia
toxic chemicals, e.g. lead
elevated temperature: varicocele; pyrexial illnesses; occupational, e.g. blast furnance workers
Irradiation
Post-inflammatory, e.g. mumps
Post-testicular causes
Blockage of efferent ducts
congenital
acquired: post-inflammatory; post-vasectomy; iatrogenic, e.g. post-herniorrhaphy
Abnormal seminal fluid or sperm maturation – idiopathic
Impotence; many causes

underlying epididymitis. A haematocele may result from trauma or testicular tumours.

Torsion of the testicle may follow violent exercise but also occurs, paradoxically, during sleep. It is most common in pubescent and adolescent boys. It presents with acute pain and swelling of the organ. Torsion is sometimes mistaken clinically for acute epididymo-orchitis with disastrous consequences. It may occur in infancy, when it is difficult to diagnose and missed cases may be the basis for infertility in adulthood. The torsion usually affects the intravaginal portion of the spermatic cord and a particularly long intravaginal segment predisposes (the so-called bell-clapper anomaly). Torsion causes venous obstruction with acute congestion which progresses to venous infarction, necessitating orchidectomy if unrelieved. The treatment is immediate surgery, with untwisting of the cord and, to prevent recurrence, both testes should be fixed in position by suturing to the dartos musculature.

Varicocele. This refers to varicosity of the veins of the pampiniform plexus which surrounds the spermatic cord. It is produced by venous obstruction and the same factors that cause varicose veins elsewhere. Varicocele is almost invariably more pronounced on the left side because of the longer course of the left testicular vein and its right angled junction with the left renal vein. Minor degrees of varicocele are extremely common and subfertility may be caused because the increased scrotal temperature reduces spermatogenesis. The testis may be smaller than normal, suggesting that ischaemic atrophy due to the chronic venous congestion may also contribute to the infertility.

Cysts in relation to the epididymis are quite common. Some arise from embryological remnants. A **spermatocele** is an epididymal cyst in which spermatozoa can be found; it results from obstruction of an epididymal tubule.

Prostate Gland, Vas Deferens and Seminal Vesicles

Inflammatory Lesions

Apart from infection, the vas deferens and seminal vesicles are seldom the site of pathological changes. In gonorrhoea and urinary tract infections, the organisms may cause suppuration in the seminal vesicles or prostate and spread along the vas to involve the epididymis. Acute prostatitis may also follow surgical instrumentation of the urethra or of the prostate itself. Chlamydial infections are also common but usually milder.

Chronic prostatitis may result from acute infections and a number of other causes. The prostate is initially enlarged and tender but may eventually become fibrosed and shrunken. Urethral obstruction may occur and the lesion may be mistaken clinically for prostatic carcinoma. **Tuberculosis** of the prostate shows characteristic granulomatous caseating lesions and may involve the whole gland. Tuberculosis may extend in either direction along the vas, depending on whether the initial site of infection of the genital tract was by haematogenous involvement of the epididymis, or by extension from the kidney to the urinary bladder and then to the prostate and vas.

Granulomatous prostatitis is a rare condition in which an inflammatory infiltrate, including giant cells, is present in relation to prostatic ducts and glands. It may be a reaction to retained secretion (compare granulomatous orchitis). Histologically, it may mimic tuberculosis. A characteristic type of palisading granuloma which mimics a rheumatoid nodule may be seen in the prostate following surgery and is caused by a reaction to damaged collagen.

Allergic (eosinophilic) prostatitis with focal necrosis and heavy infiltration with eosinophils has been associated with allergic conditions, particularly asthma. Eosinophilic prostatitis may also occur because of parasitic infestation, e.g. *Schistosoma haematobium* (p. 1168).

Benign Nodular Hyperplasia (BNH) of the Prostate Gland

This is not a neoplastic process but represents an overgrowth of prostatic glandular tissue and smooth muscle and is comparable to conditions such as nodular goitre and cystic hyperplasia of the breast. It is very common and the incidence increases with age. By the age of 80 over 75% of males are affected to some degree although only some 5% have significant symptoms. The cause is obscure but hormonal factors must be important: BNH does not occur in eunuchs or castrated men. BNH is not regarded as premalignant.

The process starts in the periurethral prostatic glands (Fig. 22.10) and the growth occurs mainly on each side of the urethra (in the so-called lateral lobes), although often there is a localized hyperplasia of the tissue just behind the urethra to form a rounded mass which projects into the bladder (the so-called median lobe). The hyperplastic tissue is

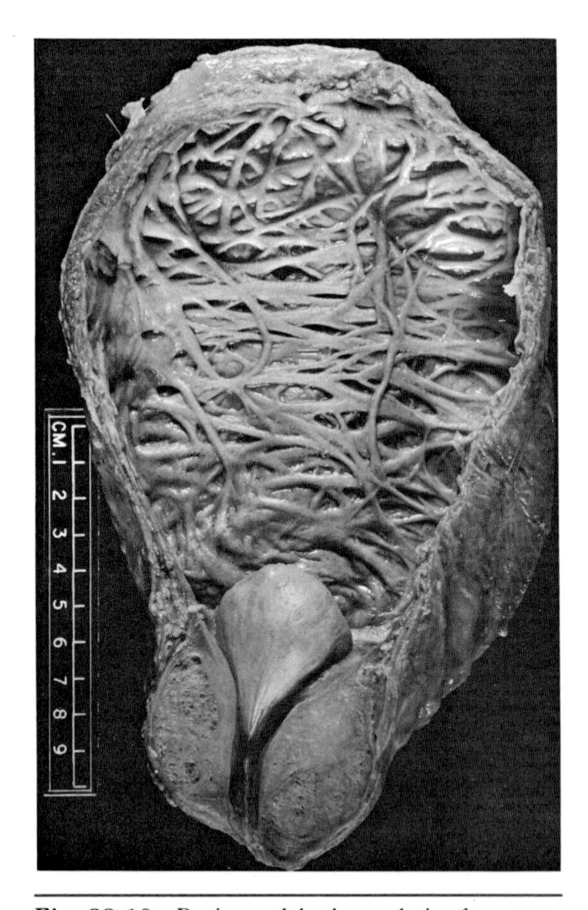

Fig. 22.10 Benign nodular hyperplasia of prostate. The 'middle lobe' is prominent, but the main bulk is on each side of the urethra ('lateral lobes'). The compressed peripheral part of the prostate can be seen as a rim round the outside of the 'lateral lobes'. Though the prostatic urethra is not obviously narrowed, the hypertrophied and dilated bladder with prominent muscle bundles (trabeculation) provides clear evidence of obstruction. ×0.5.

usually firm, white and nodular but it may sometimes show areas of inflammation, abscess formation or infarction. Microscopically, there is an increase in both the glandular elements and the stroma (Fig. 22.11). The glands are usually arranged in well defined lobules and the acini are lined by tall columnar cells beneath which there is a basal cell layer. The hyperplastic epithelium may extend into the lumina of the acini forming small papilliform projections. Some of the acini may be dilated and small retention cysts can form. Tiny concentric concretions known as *corpora amylacea,* formed from inspissated secretion, are commonly found, and deposition of oxalates and phosphates may produce prostatic calculi. The connective tissue stroma usually contains a substantial proportion of smooth muscle fibres. Fibromuscular hyperplasia is most prominent in the earlier stages of the process but in some cases it may be predominant, forming nodules in which glandular elements are scant.

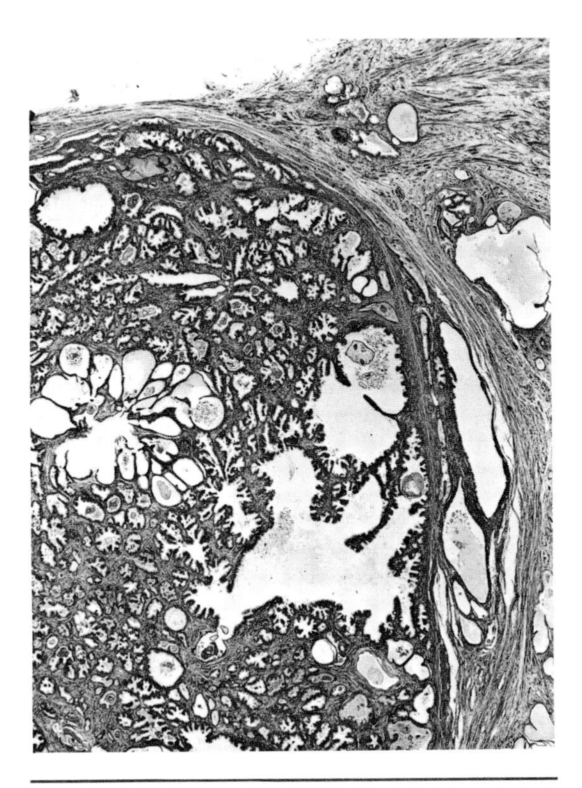

Fig. 22.11 Benign nodular hyperplasia of the prostate. The large adenoma-like nodule that fills most of the field shows predominantly glandular overgrowth, with small cysts. In the actively growing area at top right, the stroma, with numerous smooth muscle fibres, is much more prominent. ×10.

Clinical Features

Prostatic hyperplasia is the most important cause of urinary obstruction and infection in older men (p. 937). Although the prostatic urethra is distorted by BNH it is rarely significantly stenosed, and the effects on bladder function result from a complex disturbance of the bladder sphincter mechanism by the obtruding prostate rather than by simple obstruction. Accordingly, the symptoms of 'prostatism' are more diverse than those of simple obstruction and the severity of the symptoms does not correlate closely with prostatic size. There may be acute retention of urine or chronic partial obstruction, sometimes with 'overflow incontinence'. Acute obstruction may be precipitated by infection or acute congestion of the gland caused by ingestion of alcohol or as part of the venous congestion of cardiac failure. Chronic obstruction leads to hypertrophy and dilatation of the bladder (Fig. 22.10), followed in time by hydroureter and hydronephrosis. If unrelieved, chronic renal failure may result. Urinary tract infection due to *Escherichia coli* or mixed bacterial flora is frequently superadded; ascending spread of infection resulting in pyelonephritis.

Treatment is surgical. In the older operation of abdominal (retropubic or transvesical) prostatectomy the hyperplastic tissue was enucleated, leaving behind a rim of compressed peripheral prostatic tissue. The mass so removed could vary from 50 to 150 g (normal weight of prostate 20 g) but was sometimes much larger. In the modern operation of transurethral resection (TUR) the periurethral prostatic tissue is removed piecemeal in the form of 'chips'.

Carcinoma of the Prostate

This is now one of the commonest cancers of an internal organ in males in the developed countries, its mortality rate being exceeded only by carcinomas of the bronchus, stomach and large intestine. Carcinoma of the prostate has its principal incidence later in life than most other cancers, and its increasing incidence over the last 20 years is mainly attributable to the increased number of elderly men in the population. There are marked racial and geographical variations in incidence, however. American Negroes have the highest incidence in the world, considerably greater than white Americans and greater than black Africans. There is a very low incidence in Chinese and Japanese.

The tumour usually arises on the posterior aspect and at the periphery of the gland, outwith the area chiefly affected by BNH. Since both are common lesions prostatic carcinoma and BNH frequently coexist but, as already stated, there is virtually no evidence that BNH is causally related to the development of malignancy.

The large majority of prostatic carcinomas are adenocarcinomas. The degree of differentiation of the tumour is an important prognostic indicator. In the Gleeson classification (Gleeson, 1977) the tumours are graded on a scale of 1–5. Grade I tumours are very well differentiated, may indeed be difficult to distinguish from BNH and consist of uniform tumour cells arranged in small acini (so-called microacinar pattern) and mitoses are scanty. Grade 5 tumours are anaplastic, and usually show marked cellular pleomorphism and a high mitotic rate.

The tumour spreads within the gland and may cause urethral obstruction. However, because it often arises from the periphery of the gland it soon spreads to adjacent tissues and may have metastasized widely and silently before urinary symptoms appear. Spread may be: (1) lymphatic, initially to presacral, iliac and para-aortic lymph nodes but often extending widely; (2) retrograde venous, to the lumbar spine; (3) by the bloodstream causing widespread metastases, with a marked predilection for the skeleton. Bony metastases due to prostatic carcinoma are typically *osteosclerotic*, i.e. they cause new bone formation, in contrast with the osteolytic lesions seen with most other metastatic carcinomas. They appear dense on X-rays and such a finding is highly suggestive of prostatic carcinoma.

Two highly specific markers for prostatic carcinoma are available. Prostatic epithelium produces prostatic acid phosphatase and an immunohistochemically characterized prostatic specific antigen. Increased serum levels of prostatic acid phosphatase occur with metastatic disease and are of value in establishing the clinical diagnosis and in monitoring a response to treatment. Both prostatic acid phosphatase and prostatic specific antigen can be demonstrated by immunohistochemical techniques, and this is helpful in establishing that metastatic adenocarcinoma is of prostatic origin and therefore that hormonal therapy may be beneficial.

'Latent Carcinoma'

Microscopic foci of carcinoma are often found incidentally in prostatectomy specimens or in the prostate at autopsy. The microscopical appearances are indistinguishable from those of clinically overt, well differentiated prostatic carcinoma. The incidence of these 'latent' carcinomas depends largely on the age of the patient and the thoroughness of the search. They may be found in about half of prostates in men in their 50s and in practically 100% in those over 75 years. The biological significance of 'latent carcinoma' is uncertain but the incidence of subsequent overt prostatic carcinoma, in men in whom this lesion is discovered accidentally in prostatectomy specimens, is little or no more than in the general population as a whole (Byar, 1972). The incidental finding of a 'latent carcinoma' is therefore not an indication for anticancer therapy or more extensive surgery.

Clinical Course and Treatment

The poor prognosis of prostatic carcinoma relates chiefly to the large proportion of tumours which have spread beyond the gland at the time of diagnosis and are therefore not amenable to complete surgical removal. When lymph node metastases and bony metastases are present the prognosis is extremely poor, with a 5–10-year survival rate of less than 35%, whereas patients in whom the tumour is confined to the gland may expect a 75% survival.

Clinical management comprises surgery, radiotherapy and endocrine treatment. Carcinoma of the prostate is a good example of a hormone-dependent tumour, testosterone promoting cell growth. The response to orchidectomy is often dramatic, the pain of bone metastases being relieved within hours of the operation. Tumour growth is slowed down or arrested, and metastases may even regress. Microscopy shows degenerative changes with cytoplasmic vacuolation and nuclear pyknosis in many of the tumour cells. Similar benefit may be obtained from the administration of oestrogens which, by suppressing pituitary luteinizing hormone (LH), reduces testosterone secretion by Leydig cells. Oestrogens also act directly on the tumour cells themselves, and a histological feature characteristic of oestrogen administration is the development of squamous metaplasia in both benign and malignant prostatic glands. However, in elderly men, oestrogen administration may aggravate ischaemic heart disease and may precipitate cardiac failure. Long-term use of analogues of luteinizing hormone releasing hormone (LHRH) (e.g. buserelin) also suppresses LH secretion and in turn testosterone secretion. (The analogues suppress or exhaust hypothalamic LHRH but do not themselves stimulate LH secretion.) Unfortunately, even patients who respond initially to hormonal manipulation usually relapse within a few years, the tumour appearing to 'escape' from hormonal control.

Urethra, Penis and Scrotum

Urethra

Urethritis. Gonococcal urethritis may be acute or chronic, and in the chronic form may produce a urethral stricture. Repeated reinfection, inadequate treatment and persistent suppuration in the periurethral glads are the major factors. *E. coli* and other faecal organisms, chlamydia and mycoplasma are other causal agents. In non-specific urethritis no organism can be isolated. This can occur in isolation or may be accompanied by arthritis and conjunctivitis in **Reiter's syndrome**.

Urethral stricture may be due to gonorrhoea and may also follow traumatic injury to the membranous part of the urethra, the result of surgical instrumentation and falls onto the perineum or pelvic fractures.

Tumours. By far the commonest tumour is involvement by genital or venereal warts (condyloma acuminatum, which may be multiple due to infection with human papillomaviruses (HPV). Squamous-cell carcinomas are very uncommon.

Penis

Balanoposthitis is an inflammation of the inner surface of the prepuce (balanitis) and adjacent surface of the glans penis (posthitis) and is usually caused by pyogenic bacteria, including occasionally the gonococcus. A tight foreskin (phimosis) and lack of personal hygiene predispose. Ulcerated lesions on the penis may be due to a variety of venereal infections including syphilis (primary chancre), chancroid, lymphogranuloma venereum, granuloma inguinale and genital herpes, usually HSV type 2.

Peyronie's disease is a circumscribed fibrous thickening of the connective tissue around the corpora cavernosa. It causes pain and curvature of the erect penis (phallocampsis). It appears to be related to the fibromatoses (p. 1009).

Priapism is persistent painful erection of the penis. It is caused by thrombosis in the prostatic venous plexus and the corpora cavernosa. This may be idiopathic but sometimes blood dyscrasias such as leukaemia or polycythaemia are responsible. Rarely, priapism may be due to infiltration of the penile venous sinuses by metastatic carcinoma.

Tumours

Condyloma acuminatum is the commonest tumour of the penis. It is venereally contracted and caused by the human papillomavirus (HPV) types 6 and 11. It forms a reddish papillary growth, often large, which usually involves the glans, prepuce or urinary meatus. Condyloma acuminatum must not be confused with **condyloma latum**; the latter is not neoplastic and represents the highly infective, penile lesion of secondary syphilis. Pigmented naevi may occur on the penis.

Squamous-cell carcinoma of the penis, seen usually after the age of 50, is an uncommon tumour in Europe and North America but the incidence varies greatly. It is very common in some regions of Africa, Asia and Latin America. If circumcision is done shortly after birth, penile carcinoma practically never develops: circumcision round puberty, as practised by Moslems, only partly reduces the incidence. It seems likely that the development of carcinoma is related to poor personal hygiene and the carcinogenic effect of retained inspissated smegma, factors that are enhanced by failure to circumcise. Patients with penile carcinoma frequently have phimosis. In addition, carcinoma of the penis has been associated with infection by human papillomaviruses (particularly HPV 16 and HPV 18), implying a venereal element in the aetiology (compare carcinoma of the uterine cervix). Like carcinoma of the cervix, carcinoma of the penis has two main gross forms: a solitary papillary exophytic mass and an indolent infiltrating ulcer. Treatment is surgical resection. Distant spread is by the lymphatics, initially to the inguinal nodes, and occurs relatively late. **Bowen's disease** (p. 1130) may affect the penis, as also may an uncommon lesion known as **erythroplasia of Queyrat**, and which is histologically very similar to Bowen's disease. Both of these lesions are regarded as forms of squamous-cell carcinoma *in situ*.

Malignant melanoma may arise in penile skin, either *de novo*, or from a pre-existing naevus.

Scrotum

Fournier's gangrene is an acute necrotizing inflammatory process involving the skin and subcutaneous tissue of the scrotum and penis. It occurs in healthy young men and in most cases the cause is obscure. A minority of cases follow minor injuries or surgical procedures to the perineum, and cases have been described in patients undergoing chemotherapy for malignant disease.

Idiopathic calcinosis of the scrotum is the presence in the scrotal skin of numerous, painless, dermal nodules composed of chalky material. There is usually a prominent foreign-body giant-cell reaction to this material and occasionally squamous epithelium is included in the lesions, suggesting that they may represent massive calcification of the contents of epidermoid cysts.

Scrotal pseudotumour is the name given to prominent peritesticular fibrosis, involving the tunica albuginea and tunica vaginalis testis. This produces diffuse or nodular thickening, thus mimicking a tumour. The lesion is probably the result of a low-grade non-specific inflammatory process ('nodular periorchitis').

Tumours

Most of the many varieties of skin tumours can occur in the scrotal skin but apart from condyloma acuminatum all are uncommon. **Squamous-cell**

carcinoma of the scrotum (Fig. 22.12), although very rare now in this country, is of interest because, not only was it the first occupational cancer to be recognized, but it was the first time that chemical carcinogenesis was appreciated in the causation of tumours. In 1775 Sir Percival Pott described carcinoma of the scrotum in London chimney sweeps. The localization appears to depend on the ability of the rugose scrotal skin to retain dirt and the tumour is produced by chemical carcinogens within the retained soot. The effect is a specific one, since other workers with carbon, e.g. coal-miners, do not run this risk. Precautions to prevent soiling of the scrotal skin and improved personal hygiene have virtually eliminated scrotal cancer.

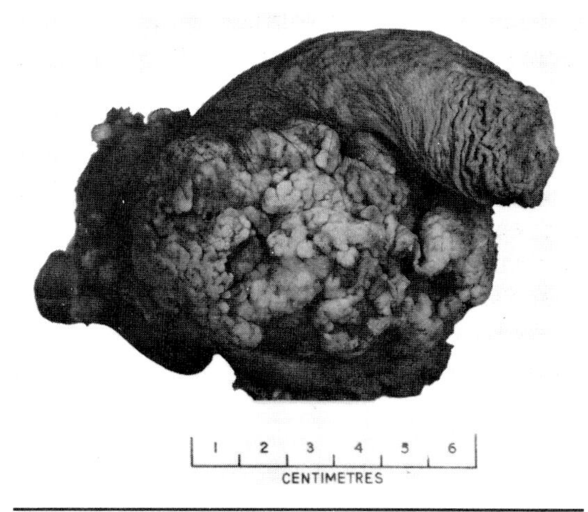

Fig. 22.12 Advanced squamous-cell carcinoma of the scrotum showing an ulcerated papillary tumour mass.

Congenital Abnormalities of the Male Genital Tract

Sex Chromosome Disorders and Intersexes

The cytogenetic aspects of these have been outlined in Chapter 2 and the malformations which can occur in the female are discussed in the preceding chapter. Essentially, one is dealing with (1) disorders of genetic sex, determined by the presence or absence of a Y chromosome and which results in gonodal dysgenesis and true hermaphroditism: and (2) disorders of phenotypic sex, in which the gonads are consistent with the genotype but in which there are physical ambiguities producing pseudohermaphroditism. The pathological effects of this are extremely variable and show considerable overlap. The important aspects, in the context of this chapter, are the occurrence of germ-cell defects and of intersexes and the topic is discussed under these headings.

Germ-cell Defects

Absence or near absence of germ cells can be subdivided into two main types, chromosomal and non-chromosomal (in which, as yet, no genetic mechanism has been demonstrated).

Chromosomal: Klinefelter's Syndrome and its Variants

This is one of the commonest of chromosomal disorders affecting approximately 1 in 1000 male births. In 85% of cases the karyotype is 47,XXY: in the others there are a number of variants – mosaics 46,XY/47,XXXY and also 48,XXXY, 48,XXYY and 49,XXXXY, so that more than two X chromosomes and more than one Y chromosome may occur. The presence of a Y chromosome, whose sex determining region is on the short arm, ensures the formation of testes and a male phenotype, but the presence of two or more X chromosomes prevents normal gonadal development at puberty. Hypogonadism is therefore, a constant feature of this syndrome. In addition, individuals with Klinefelter's syndrome are often eunuchoid in appearance and have variable degrees of feminization with lack of facial hair, a female hair distribution and gynaecomastia. Some degree of mental defect is also common but not invariable. The testes are small, usually under 5 g each in weight (normal testicular weight is over 20 g) and the penis is small. The seminiferous tubules are very small and hyalinized ('ghost' tubules) and only a small proportion are lined by Sertoli cells: surviving germ cells are inconspicuous. Most of the testicular volume is made up of masses of Leydig cells. This, however, is not a true hyperplasia of Leydig cells and is a consequence of the marked reduction in testicular volume due to atrophy of the seminiferous tubules. True Leydig cell hyperplasia is thought to be very rare in man.

The mechanisms responsible for the failure of gonadal development are not known. Serum FSH levels are high and the testosterone/oestrogen ratio is abnormal, the extent of this probably determining the degree of feminization which occurs. The diagnosis is confirmed on karyotype analysis. However, the presence of Barr bodies, representing the additional and inactive X chromosome(s) (Fig. 22.13) affords a rapid means of diagnosis which can be carried out on a buccal smear.

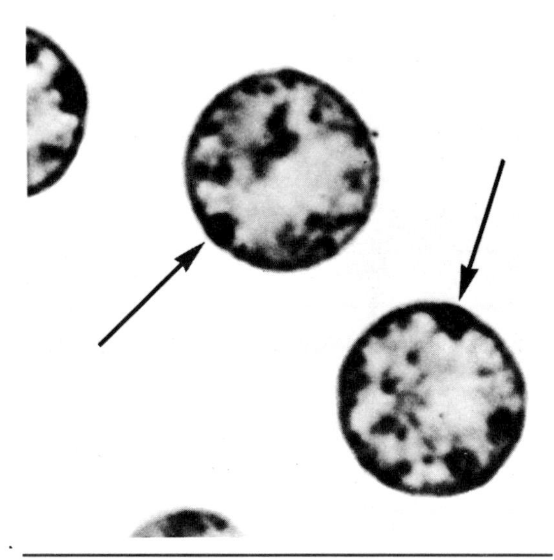

Fig. 22.13 Nuclear sex chromatin (Barr bodies), identical to that of normal females, in the Leydig cells of a testicular biopsy from a case of 47,XXY Klinefelter's syndrome. ×1500.

Non-chromosomal: Germ-cell Aplasia

This condition has also been called chromatin negative Klinefelter's syndrome or the del Castillo syndrome. There is absence or near absence of germ cells and, although the exact cause is unknown, most cases are thought to be congenital in origin. The phenotypic effects are similar to those of 47,XXY cases but less pronounced, except for infertility which is nearly invariable. Thus, a eunuchoid body type is less common and there is no associated mental defect. The testes are not so small and the histological abnormalities less severe. The tubules are generally well preserved but are lined entirely by tall, pale-staining, Sertoli cells. Between the tubules there is an apparent excess of Leydig cells but this 'pseudohyperplasia' is not as marked as in 47,XXY cases. Some cases are partial and foci of spermatogenesis may be seen producing oligospermia rather than azoospermia.

Intersexes

Affected individuals present some of the physical characteristics of both sexes. The principal varieties are the following.

Chromosomal Intersexes

Klinefelter's syndrome and its variants and Turner's syndrome – 45,XO – are the commonest types. In these, and in contrast to the next group, the phenotypic abnormalities are far less intersexual than the chromosomal picture.

Hermaphroditism

True hermaphrodites are extremely rare. They possess both testicular and ovarian tissue. There may be an ovary on one side and a testis on the other or various mixtures of the two may be combined in so-called **ovotestes**. The genitalia are often a mixture of male and female organs or indeterminate between the two, although the dominant effect of a testis often results in the external genitalia being predominantly male at birth. Breast development and other signs of feminization appear at puberty. The mechanisms of this aberrant development are obscure. Some cases are true mosaics, mixtures of 46,XX and 46,XY cells derived from a single zygote: others are apparently 46,XX karyotypes in which the sex determining region of the short arm of the Y chromosome has been translocated to the top of the short arm of the X.

Male pseudohermaphroditism. The gonads are testes and these individuals are 46,XY. The external genitalia, however, are imperfectly developed and phenotypically more closely resemble that of the female. Minor abnormalities such as bifid scrotum and hypospadias probably represent lesser degrees of this condition.

In some cases there is thought to be inadequate androgen production by the testes *in utero* producing defective virilization of the embryo. In the majority of cases, however, there is a genetically determined defect of androgen receptors which renders the target cells insensitive – **androgen insensitivity syndrome**. There is thus, unopposed oestrogen activity leading to so-called testicular feminization. The affected gene is on the X chromosome and transmission is sex-linked recessive. Offspring of carriers have an equal chance of being normal males, normal females, carriers (but otherwise normal females) and affected, sterile phenotypic females.

Female pseudohermaphroditism. This is more easily understood. All cases are genetically 46,XX; the gonads are ovaries, but there is virilization of the external genitalia due to excessive or inappropriate adrenal androgen production by the fetus, so-called adrenal virilism (p. 110). It is worth remembering that a child of doubtful phenotypic sex at birth is usually, either a genetic female with adrenal virilism or a male pseudohermaphrodite. Examination of a buccal smear for Barr bodies will reliably differentiate between them.

Cryptorchidism (undescended testis). During fetal life the testes migrate from their site of development in the genital ridge down through the abdominal cavity and then through the inguinal canal into the scrotum, the track of this migration being marked by the course of the testicular arteries and veins. Although in most cases both testes are present in the scrotum at birth, a smaller proportion (around 10%) will complete their descent normally by the age of 3 years. In about 1% of males, however, one or both testes become arrested at some point in their descent, the most common site being around the internal inguinal ring. This is usually an isolated abnormality but is also seen as part of the syndrome associated with trisomy 13. The consequence of this, namely an increased risk (between 10- and 40-fold) of developing germ-cell tumours and infertility (if bilateral, and this occurs in 15% of cases) have already been discussed. A distinction is sometimes made between undescended and **ectopic testes**. In the latter the testis has strayed from the normal path of descent and is found in an abnormal location within the abdominal cavity.

Miscellaneous Abnormalities

Congenital inguinal hernia. In this relatively common condition the fetal connection between the peritoneal sac and the tunica vaginalis remains patent, allowing abdominal contents to pass through the inguinal canal into the scrotum (**persistent processus vaginalis**), thus producing an inguinal hernia of indirect type.

Hypospadias is the commonest malformation of the urethra occurring in one of every 350 males. The external urinary meatus fails to reach the end of the penis and opens at some point along its undersurface or even in the perineum. By contrast **epispadias**, in which the urethra opens on the dorsal surface, is rare.

Congenital valves of the posterior urethra (Young's valves) are often symmetrical and usually occur below the verumontanum. They allow the passage of a catheter but obstruct the outflow of urine. They are a rare but important cause of urinary obstruction in neonates; if incomplete they may not present until adolescence or adult life by which time the prostatic urethra may be markedly dilated and bladder hypertrophy with diverticula may be present.

Congenital bladder neck obstruction (Marion's disease) is analogous to hypertrophic pyloric stenosis and gives rise to symptoms identical to those of congenital valves.

Rare congenital defects include bifid scrotum; absence or duplication or fusion of the testes (synorchism); and a variety of congenital strictures or atresias which cause blockage of the outflow tract in the epididymis and vas.

Further Reading

Byar, D. P. (1972). Survival of patients with incidentally found microscopic cancer of the prostate: results of a clinical trial of conservative treatment. *Journal of Urology* **108**, 908–13.

Gleeson, D. F. (1977). The Veterans Administration Cooperative Urological Research Group: Histological grading and clinical staging of prostatic carcinoma. In *Urological Pathology, The Prostate,* Chapter 9, pp. 171–98, ed. M. Tannenbam, Lea and Febiger, Philadelphia.

Grigor, K. M. (1991). Germ-cell tumours of the testis. In *Recent Advances in Histopathology,* No. 15, pp. 177–94, eds P. P. Anthony and R. N. M. MacSween. Churchill Livingstone, Edinburgh.

Lennox, B. (1981). The infertile testis. In *Recent Advances in Histopathology,* No. 11, pp. 135–48, eds P. P. Anthony and R. N. M. MacSween. Churchill Livingstone, Edinburgh.

Pugh, R. C. B. (ed.) (1976). *Pathology of the Testis,* pp. 487. Blackwell Scientific, Oxford and London.

Sobin, L. H. Thomas, L. B., Percy, C. and Henson, D. E. (eds) (1978). *A Coded Compendium of the International Histological Classification of Tumours,* pp. 116. World Health Organisation, Geneva.

23

Endocrine Pathology

The endocrine system comprises two main components. The classical endocrine organs include the pituitary, thyroid, adrenal, parathyroid glands, the islets of Langerhans in the pancreas, the ovary and testis and the pineal. The diffuse endocrine system consists of cells dispersed singly or in small groups throughout various non-endocrine organs, including the gastrointestinal tract, lung and skin.

The cells of the diffuse system may be identified by their affinity for silver (argyrophilia). This is demonstrated by impregnation techniques, when an exogenous silver-reducing agent is included in the incubation. These will identify all the diffuse endocrine cells. In addition, some of these cells, particularly in the small intestine, have the capacity to reduce silver without the addition of an exogenous agent. These are known as argentaffin cells. They share a variety of other cytochemical features including a capacity for amine precursor uptake and decarboxylation, hence the term APUD cells. Pearse formulated a unifying theory proposing that the cells of the diffuse endocrine system had a common origin from the neural crest, constituting a neuroendocrine system. It is now clear, however, that cells of the diffuse endocrine system have a variety of embryological origins and that many of them differentiate from local multipotent stem cells. Their common features reflect the similarity of their neuroendocrine functions.

The endocrine system plays its putative role in regulating physiological functions by secreting hormones which affect specific target cells bearing the appropriate hormone receptor. In addition to classical endocrine action, paracrine or autocrine pathways may also operate. Endocrine glands in turn are under complex regulatory control with a variety of stimulatory and inhibitory signals. This includes negative feedback by hormones secreted by target glands. In addition, there is evidence of significant cyclical activity of secretion and the circulating levels of many hormones show a marked circadian variation.

The symptoms and signs of many endocrine diseases are the result either of hyperfunction or hypofunction of the appropriate gland with resulting perturbations in physiological signalling pathways. Thus, endocrine tumours may release excessive amounts of a hormone in an autonomous fashion, leading to hyperstimulation of the target cells. In contrast, destruction of an endocrine gland will result in deficiency of the hormone normally produced. In addition, however, two other mechanisms may be involved in producing endocrine disease: (1) when hormone/hormone interactions occur, e.g. in the endometrium, there may be dysfunction so that hormone activities get out of phase and this results in clinical effects; (2) the target cell may be unable to respond to a hormone messenger, either due to deficiency of a functional receptor, or to abnormalities in post-receptor pathways.

An understanding of endocrine pathology requires a basic knowledge of the normal pathways regulating the function of the gland involved, and of the general signal transduction mechanisms by which chemical messengers, including hormones, induce their effects in the target cell. These have been discussed in detail in Chapter 1.

This chapter will deal mainly with the pathology of the classical endocrine organs. Diseases of the diffuse endocrine system are not fully characterized as yet but, where appropriate, these have been dealt with in the relevant systemic chapters. The pathology of the islets of Langerhans is discussed on p. 798 *et seq.*

Investigative Techniques

With standard histological staining techniques, little information can be obtained on the specific functional aspects of endocrine pathology. The application of the following methods is essential in many cases for a full diagnosis.

Immunohistochemistry

The development of antibodies to a wide variety of hormonal peptides has permitted a fuller characterization of normal endocrine cells and of hormone production in various diseases (Fig. 23.1). In addition, various non-hormonal proteins are present in a wide variety of endocrine cells. These include the chromogranins, which are constituents of neurosecretory granules, and synaptophysin, a granule membrane protein. Antibodies to these proteins can be used to identify tumours as endocrine, even when it is uncertain what hormone is present. Some neuroendocrine tumours show very little granule storage and antibodies to cytoplasmic proteins such as PGP 9.5 and the enzyme neuron-specific enolase may be useful in these cases. It is usual to apply a range of such antibodies when investigating a difficult tumour.

Electron microscopy. This has been a powerful tool in the investigation of the endocrine system, particularly when coupled with immunocytochemistry. Very precise classification of individual cell types is possible. In the peptide/amine producing cells, this is based on the size and shape of the neurosecretory granules and on the general morphology and distribution of organelles. In some cells these features are highly specific as in the crystalline granule of insulin secreting cells, Fig. 23.2.

In situ hybridization (p. 58). It is possible to detect specific messenger RNAs (mRNAs) in

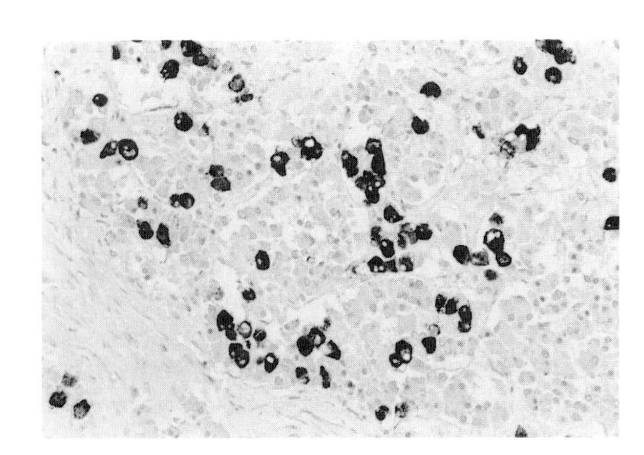

Fig. 23.1 Section of adenohypophysis stained by the immunoperoxidase technique with antibody to ACTH. ACTH cells are scattered among immunonegative cells, which are producing other pituitary hormones.

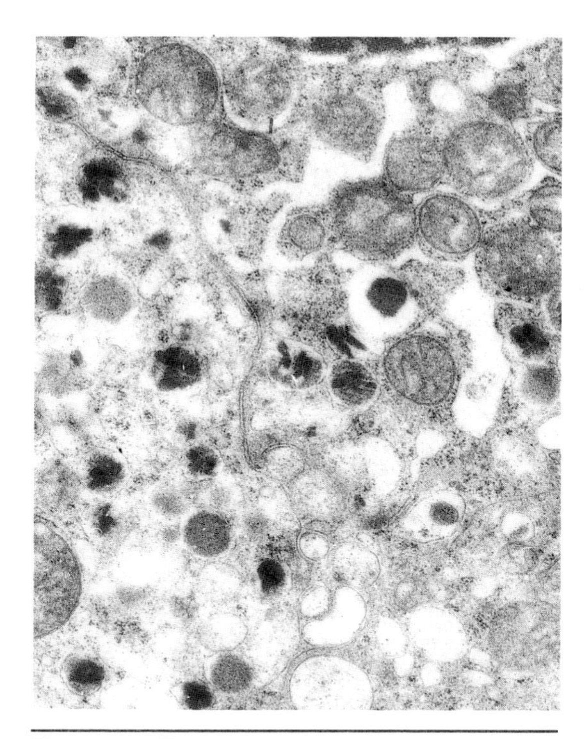

Fig. 23.2 Electron micrograph of cells from an insulinoma. The neurosecretory granules contain crystalline material, which is known to be characteristic in shape and size for insulin.

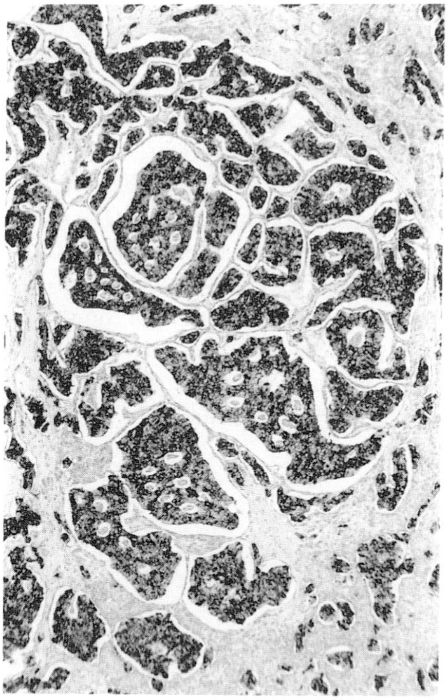

Fig. 23.3 *In situ* hybridization reaction on a somatostatin-secreting tumour of pancreas, using an oligodeoxynucleotide probe directly linked to alkaline phosphatase. Somatostatin mRNA (black staining) is detected in variable quantities in individual tumour cells.

tissue sections, by applying probes consisting of sequences of nucleotides complementary to part of the specific mRNA. These are labelled using radioisotopes or non-isotopic chemicals. The site of binding can then be detected using autoradiography or standard histochemical or immunohistochemical techniques (Fig. 23.3). In conjunction with immunocytochemistry, this gives us a more accurate and dynamic assessment of the function of endocrine cells in tissue sections in health and disease.

The Pituitary Gland and the Hypothalamus

The anterior pituitary (adenohypophysis) develops from an upgrowth of the primitive oral cavity known as Rathke's pouch. As this extends upwards it is met by a downgrowth from the floor of the third ventricle which becomes the posterior pituitary (neurohypophysis). The gland comes to lie in a bony cavity, the **sella turcica**. This is covered by a layer of dura, the diaphragma sellae, which is perforated by the pituitary stalk. In the adult male the gland weighs about 600 mg, in the parous female up to 800 mg.

The blood supply is mainly by the hypothalamic–

pituitary portal system. The primary capillary plexus lies in the median eminence of the hypothalamus and blood passes down venous channels on the pituitary stalk to the secondary capillary plexus within the anterior lobe. Thus, hypothalamic hormones pass directly to the anterior pituitary. There is evidence that arterial blood supply may reach areas of the anterior lobe directly via branches of the trabecular arteries situated in the fibrous core in the lateral parts of the gland. The posterior pituitary has a direct arterial supply. Since the anatomy, blood supply and functions of the two lobes differ, they will be dealt with separately.

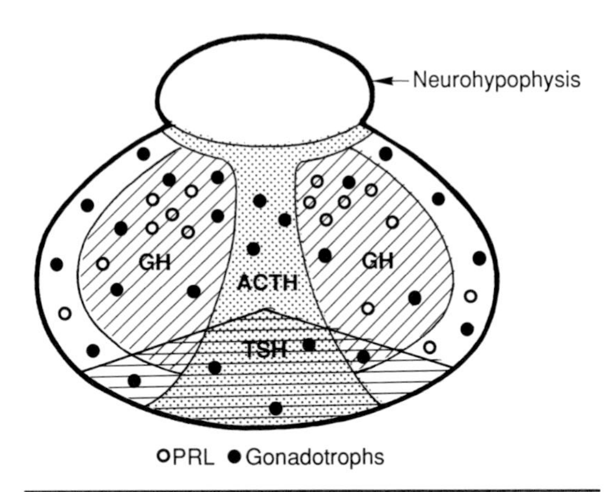

Fig. 23.4 Schematic representation of the distribution of the various hormone-producing cell types in a transverse section of human pituitary gland. ACTH cells (corticotrophs) are situated mainly in the median wedge, along the junction with, and extending into the posterior lobe in variable numbers. GH cells (somatotrophs) are mainly in the lateral wings; TSH cells (thyrotrophs) are in a wedge shaped area anteriorly. PRL cells, lactotrophs, are present in higher numbers in the posterolateral parts of the gland and gonadotrophs (producing both FSH and LH) are randomly distributed.

Adenohypophysis

The anterior pituitary comprises 75% of the whole gland and produces a variety of hormones – growth hormone (GH), prolactin (PRL), thyroid stimulating hormone (TSH), adrenocorticotrophic hormone (ACTH), and the gonadotrophic hormones, follicle stimulating hormone (FSH) and luteinizing hormone (LH). Historically, the cells have been divided into three categories, based on standard histochemical techniques – eosinophil, basophil and chromophobe. GH and PRL were thought to be produced by eosinophils and ACTH and glycoprotein hormones by basophils. It was proposed that chromophobes might represent either precursors for hormone-producing cells or effete cells. Such a classification is no longer acceptable, since immunohistochemistry and ultrastructural analysis now permit the identification of each specific hormone-producing cell type. The distribution of the various hormone-producing cell types is non-random within the human pituitary, an important point when assessing some aspects of pituitary pathology (e.g. hyperplasia). Their general distribution in transverse section is shown in Fig. 23.4. A group of non-hormone-producing cells is also randomly distributed. These **folliculostellate cells** extend processes between other cells and may either have a macrophage-like role or exert paracrine effects on hormone-producing cells. A number of novel peptides including galanin have been shown to be co-localized and co-secreted with classical hormones in the pituitary. Their functions are unknown and whether they have paracrine actions or are secreted as hormones is as yet unclear.

Control of Anterior Pituitary Function

The hypothalamus secretes a variety of releasing and inhibitory factors into the portal blood to control the function of the anterior pituitary gland. There is also negative feedback by hormones produced by the peripheral target glands on both pituitary and hypothalamus and also by pituitary hormones themselves in the hypothalamus. Basal levels of many anterior pituitary hormones show a marked circadian rhythm and may also be altered by external stimuli.

Growth hormone synthesis and secretion are

regulated in an integrated manner by two main hypothalamic factors. Growth hormone releasing factor (GRF) stimulates while somatostatin inhibits release. Growth hormone has multiple direct actions on metabolism while others are mediated indirectly by the somatomedins, or insulin-like growth factors (IGF), particularly IGF_1 produced by the liver in response to growth hormone. Direct effects include stimulation of RNA and protein synthesis in the liver and muscle and lipolysis of fat stores. Skeletal growth is effected by IGF, which also exerts negative feedback on GH release in the pituitary.

Adrenocorticotrophic hormone is a 39 amino-acid peptide derived from a large precursor molecule, pro-opiomelanocortin (POMC). Its release is stimulated by corticotrophin releasing factor (CRF) and vasopressin. It regulates the secretion of glucocorticoids by the adrenal cortex; these exert negative feedback on both CRF and ACTH production.

Glycoprotein hormones. FSH, LH and TSH are glycoproteins consisting of two subunits. The α-subunit is common to all three, but each has a specific β-subunit. The gonadotrophins FSH and LH are produced in the same cells (gonadotrophs). In men, FSH stimulates spermatogenesis and LH regulates Leydig cell function. In women, FSH is involved in regulation of follicle growth, while LH is related to ovulation and the development of the corpus luteum. Both the absolute and relative levels of the two hormones vary with the menstrual cycle. The hypothalamic peptide gonadotrophin releasing hormone (GnRH) is important in the stimulation of FSH and LH secretion while androgens and oestrogens exert negative feedback.

TSH stimulates the thyroid follicular cells. Its secretion is regulated by a hypothalamic tripeptide, thyrotrophin releasing hormone (TRH) and there is negative feedback by thyroid hormones.

Prolactin is a polypeptide hormone which has stimulatory effects on the breast during lactation. Circulating basal levels of PRL are similar in men and women, but no specific function has yet been identified in the male. In contrast to the other pituitary hormones, the dominant regulatory influence of the hypothalamus is in inhibiting PRL release, effected mainly by dopamine. Thyrotrophin releasing hormone stimulates PRL release.

Pathology of the Adenohypophysis

Pituitary Adenomas

Pituitary adenomas are the most common lesion of the anterior pituitary gland and may be found in over 20% of unselected autopsy cases. However, only a small proportion of adenomas are clinically apparent, patients often presenting with syndromes related to hypersecretion of specific hormones. They may occur as part of the inherited multiple endocrine neoplasia type I (MEN I) syndrome (p. 1105). Adenomas are divided into microadenomas (<10 mm diameter) and macroadenomas (>10 mm). In patients with larger tumours, symptoms may be related to compression of surrounding structures: visual disturbances such as homonymous hemianopia due to pressure on the optic chiasma or optic nerves (Fig. 23.5) and headache due to raised intracranial pressure are common. Pressure atrophy of the adjacent

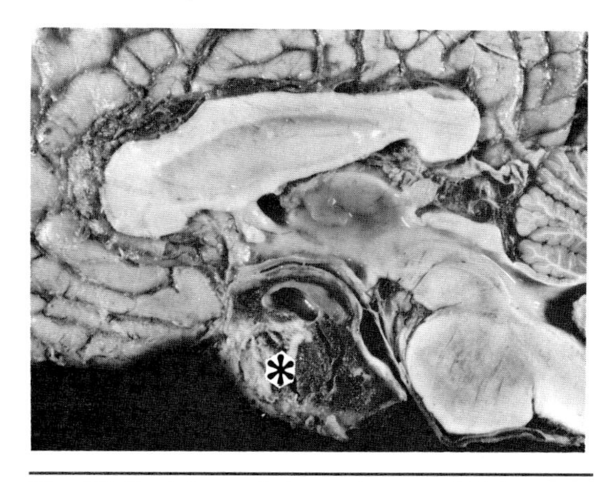

Fig. 23.5 A large pituitary adenoma which has compressed the optic chiasma. The tumour is haemorrhagic and shows cystic change.

normal gland may cause hypopituitarism. Lateral extension into the cavernous sinus may prevent complete surgical removal and allow postoperative persistence of symptoms with hormonally active tumours. Occasional tumours show extremely aggressive behaviour, with extension into the hypothalamus and brain, and this may eventually result in raised intracranial pressure. Such local invasion does not indicate malignancy; pituitary carcinomas with proven metastases are extremely rare.

Classification is based primarily on hormonal immunoreactivity. Many tumours contain more than one cell type, even when clinical symptoms are attributable to only one hormone, and all cell populations should be documented. Further detailed subclassification requires ultrastructural analysis without which some specific diagnoses cannot be made (Kovacs and Horvath, 1987). This approach is now leading to the recognition of behavioural differences among subtypes of tumours associated with the same clinical syndrome. An outline of their classification with the relative distribution of the various types of tumour found in surgical practice is shown in Table 23.1.

Table 23.1 Classification of pituitary adenomas and incidence in surgical practice

Tumour type	Incidence (%)
Immunoreactive for GH	14
Immunoreactive for PRL	27.5
Immunoreactive for ACTH	14
TSH cell adenoma	1
Gonadotroph adenoma	6
Mixed GH cell – PRL cell adenoma	5
Acidophil stem cell adenoma	2.5
Mammosomatotroph adenoma	1.5
Other plurihormonal adenomas	4
Non-immunoreactive adenomas	
Null cell adenoma	16
Oncocytoma	8.5

The data are abstracted from several publications by Kovacs and Horvath. Classification is based primarily on immunocytochemistry and further on ultrastructural analysis.

Aetiology. The causes of pituitary tumours are not yet fully understood. Hyperstimulation by hypothalamic releasing factors may play a role in some cases. ACTH producing tumours can occur in Addison's disease and TSH producing tumours in primary hypothyroidism, where levels of releasing factors are increased due to lack of negative feedback from target gland hormones. GRF stimulation causes proliferation of GH cells in the normal pituitary. There is recent evidence that, in a subgroup of GH cell adenomas, mutations are present in the gene for the G_s α-subunit that inhibit GTPase activity, thus producing a permanently activated G_s, continued elevation of cAMP and therefore uncontrolled stimulus to secretion of GH and to GH cell proliferation. The putative oncogene produced by these mutations is termed *gsp* (for G_s protein).

In addition, alterations in the local microenvironment have been implicated in the pathogenesis of adenomas. The presence of direct arterial blood supply in localized areas of the anterior lobe might expose the cells to growth factors which are not present in high concentration in portal blood. In addition, hypothalamic peptides might not gain access and the imbalance produced could result in abnormal proliferation and tumorigenesis. The latter might be of relevance in the genesis of PRL cell adenomas, by preventing local access of dopamine to lactotrophs.

Other Tumours and Cysts

In many pituitaries small cysts occur along the junction of the anterior and posterior lobes. They represent remnants of Rathke's cleft, and occasionally, one may enlarge causing atrophy of the rest of the gland. Craniopharyngiomas (p. 860) arise from remnants of Rathke's pouch. They are usually suprasellar, occasionally intrasellar. They may produce hypopituitarism by pressure atrophy of the pituitary or of the area of the hypothalamus which secretes pituitary releasing factors. They also interfere with the blood supply to the anterior lobe by pressure on the pituitary stalk. Rarely, tumours may arise from the connective tissue elements in the pituitary – fibroma, angioma, etc. It is extremely unusual to find metastatic tumour in the anterior lobe.

Inflammatory Conditions

Acute inflammation is extremely rare but may occur as a direct extension of infection from neighbouring areas. Autoimmune hypophysitis is much less common than any autoimmune disease of the other endocrine glands. It usually follows pregnancy and may resolve spontaneously. Granulomatous inflammation may involve the pituitary, e.g. tuberculosis or sarcoidosis, and can lead to hypopituitarism directly or as a result of extension to the hypothalamus. In AIDS, the pituitary appears to be relatively frequently involved by cytomegalovirus, but other opportunistic infections are rare.

Circulatory Disturbances

Small pituitary infarcts are common at autopsy, but three-quarters of the gland must be destroyed before there is evidence of endocrine deficiency. In areas where obstetric care is poor, the commonest cause of hypopituitarism is Sheehan's syndrome, in which necrosis of the anterior lobe occurs in patients suffering severe postpartum haemorrhage. The exact pathogenesis is unclear, but predisposing factors are the low pressure portal vascular supply, general hypotension and the enlargement of the pituitary which occurs during pregnancy. Infarcts may also occur in patients on long-term ventilation, in disseminated intravascular coagulation, sickle cell disease, diabetes mellitus or raised intracranial pressure.

In a small proportion of pituitary adenomas, haemorrhage into the tumour (pituitary apoplexy) may present as an emergency due to raised intracranial pressure. The haemorrhage causes destruction of the tumour, with regression of symptoms of hormonal excess.

Hyperfunction of the Adenohypophysis

This is usually due to hypersecretion of hormone by a pituitary adenoma. Less commonly, central or hypothalamic abnormalities may result in hyperstimulation of the gland. Rarely, non-pituitary tumours (e.g. carcinoids and islet cell tumours of pancreas) may produce hypothalamic releasing hormones in an 'ectopic' manner, resulting in pituitary hyperstimulation. The most important clinical syndromes are acromegaly and gigantism due to excess GH, the effects of hyperprolactinaemia, and Cushing's disease caused by excess ACTH.

Acromegaly and Gigantism

Acromegaly means enlargement of the extremities. It occurs when excess GH secretion occurs after fusion of the epiphyses. There is marked overgrowth of soft tissues and bone; the hands and feet enlarge and there is a characteristic facial appearance, with widening of the nose and prognathism (Fig. 23.6). The irregular bone growth often leads to osteoarthritis. Entrapment of nerves results in pain and paraesthesia. There is enlargement of internal organs, often with cardiomegaly and hypertension. Patients with untreated acromegaly have approximately twice the expected mortality rate, mainly from cardiovascular disease. The general effects of GH on metabolism are reflected in abnormal glucose tolerance, with frank diabetes mellitus in a minority of cases. Failure to suppress plasma GH in response to oral glucose administration is used as a diagnostic test. In some patients, the changes in appearance may stop progressing after a few years, although GH levels remain high. The other metabolic effects often continue.

When hypersecretion of GH occurs before the epiphyses close, it results in gigantism, with proportionate increase in length and thickness of bones; epiphyseal fusion is delayed. If GH hypersecretion persists after the epiphyses close the features of acromegaly are then superimposed.

Most patients with acromegaly have a pituitary adenoma. In 30–40% of cases, there is also PRL

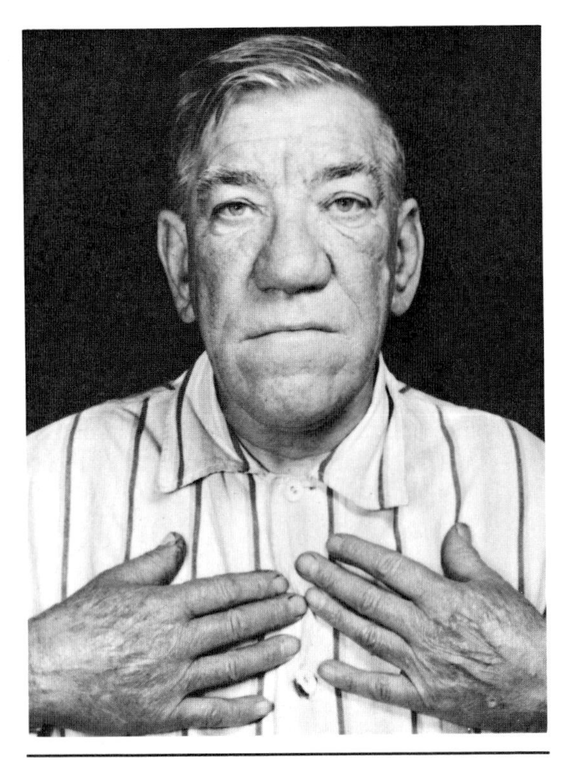

Fig. 23.6 Acromegaly, illustrating the thickening of the nose and enlargement of the lower jaw.

secretion, which gives rise to galactorrhoea in some patients. In addition, 40% of GH secreting adenomas are immunoreactive for the α-subunit of the glycoprotein hormones but this is not associated with any obvious endocrine symptoms. Rarely, the disease is associated with production of GRF by a pancreatic islet cell tumour or a hypothalamic gangliocytoma (p. 1084).

Hyperprolactinaemia

PRL is the hormone most commonly secreted by pituitary adenomas. In women, excessive PRL secretion is often associated with amenorrhoea and infertility and, in a proportion of cases, galactorrhoea. In men, excessive secretion is usually asymptomatic, but occasionally causes loss of libido or infertility. In premenopausal women, amenorrhoea and galactorrhoea are obvious and dramatic symptoms meriting prompt investigation so that the tumours are diagnosed early and are often microadenomas. However, in men and in postmenopausal women the absence of obvious hormonal effects means that the tumour will usually present clinically only if large enough to cause local pressure effects.

Other causes of hyperprolactinaemia include destructive lesions of the hypothalamus, and pressure on the pituitary stalk by other types of pituitary adenoma, which will interfere with the normal transport of dopamine to the anterior pituitary. Treatment with drugs which alter endogenous dopamine turnover or with dopamine receptor antagonists (e.g. methyldopa, reserpine, metoclopramide, phenothiazines) will also raise serum PRL concentrations. Finally, it should be remembered that physiological hyperprolactinaemia occurs in pregnancy.

Cushing's Disease

Cushing's syndrome (p. 1098) is the result of excessive glucocorticoid secretion by the adrenal glands. In about two-thirds of cases, this is due to excessive stimulation of the adrenals secondary to hypersecretion of ACTH by the pituitary. The majority of these patients have an ACTH cell adenoma, and surgical removal results in cure. A minority have ACTH cell hyperplasia, which is presumed to be secondary to a central or hypothalamic abnormality. Rarely, ectopic secretion of CRF may result in hyperstimulation of ACTH secretion. In all variants of Cushing's syndrome, non-tumourous pituitary corticotrophs show a characteristic appearance, known as Crooke's hyaline change (Fig. 23.7). This results from aggregation of cytokeratin intermediate filaments, a change similar to that which results in Mallory body formation in liver cells (p. 763). It is thought to be the effect of high levels of glucocorticoids, since exogenous administration for therapeutic purposes may also induce Crooke's hyaline change.

Hypersecretion of Other Hormones

Rarely, TSH secreting tumours may result in thyrotoxicosis. Gonadotrophin secreting tumours account for about 6% of tumours (Table 23.1) but rarely give rise to clinical symptoms. Isolated

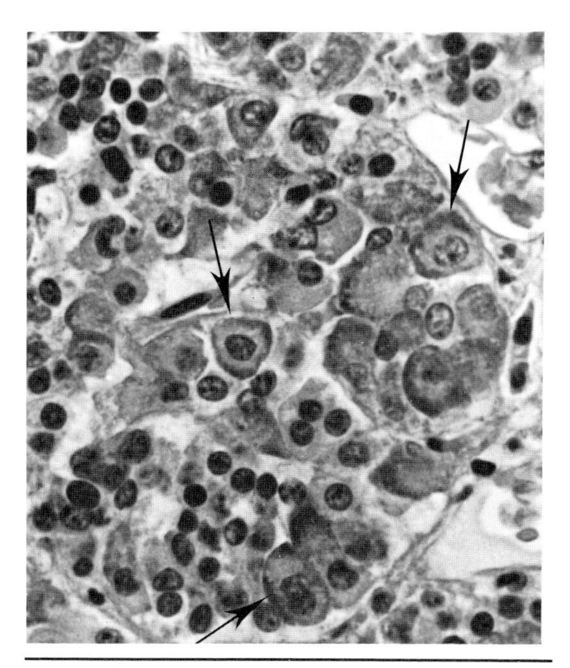

Fig. 23.7 Adenohypophysis in Cushing's syndrome showing Crooke's hyaline change in the ACTH cells (arrows).

hypersecretion of glycoprotein α-subunit is also reported, but again this is clinically undetectable and is usually identified on the basis of biochemical analysis in patients with clinically nonfunctioning tumours, or on follow-up of a patient with a tumour shown to be immunoreactive for α-subunit.

Hypopituitarism

Multiple hormone deficiencies are usually the result of a destructive process involving the gland itself, the pituitary stalk or the hypothalamus. The most common cause is pressure from an expanding pituitary tumour. Sheehan's syndrome (postpartum pituitary necrosis) is now relatively uncommon in the Western world, but is still the major cause of hypopituitarism in developing countries, where obstetric care is less advanced. Pituitary surgery and irradiation of the pituitary or adjacent structures may also result in hypopituitarism, the latter several years after treatment. Occasional cases are the result of trauma, inflammation, including autoimmune hypophysitis, or intrasellar tumours other than pituitary adenomas. Suprasellar tumours (e.g. craniopharyngioma) may affect the stalk, the hypothalamus or the pituitary. Granulomatous diseases and histiocytosis X (p. 655) may infiltrate the hypothalamus affecting the production of releasing hormones.

The clinical manifestations of hypopituitarism are variable, and may depend on the underlying cause. For example, the patient with an enlarging pituitary tumour may complain primarily of symptoms relating to local pressure. The effects of gonadotrophin deficiency are usually the first to present clinically; in women, there may be amenorrhoea, loss of secondary sex characteristics and loss of libido and in men, impotence. Circulating levels of GH are also low at the time of presentation, but this does not give rise to clinical signs. Deficiency of TSH and ACTH follows, with hypothyroidism and hypoadrenalism. This may eventually lead to hypotension, nausea, vomiting and, occasionally, fatal collapse.

Isolated hormonal deficiencies are usually manifest in children and the underlying cause is unknown. GH deficiency results in growth retardation, usually noticed after one year of age. In contrast to many other forms of dwarfism e.g. achondroplasia (p. 960), these children are of normal proportion. In Kallman's syndrome isolated gonadotrophin hyposecretion occurs, resulting in failure to undergo puberty. This is associated with anosmia and is due to the lack of development of the area of the hypothalamus giving rise to the cell bodies of both GnRH neurons and the olfactory nerves. Patients may respond to GnRH therapy.

Neurohypophysis

The posterior pituitary consists of nerve fibres, blood vessels and supportive tissues. It secretes two hormones, **oxytocin** and **vasopressin** (antidiuretic hormone). These are synthesized in cell bodies within the supraoptic and paraventricular nuclei of the hypothalamus and pass down the nerve fibres to the posterior lobe bound to carrier proteins, the **neurophysins**. Oxytocin causes contraction of uterine smooth muscle and ejection of milk in lactation. It has no known effects in males, and no syndromes have been identified in association with hormonal excess or deficiency. Vasopressin regulates water balance by stimulating reabsorption of water in the distal tubules and collecting ducts of the kidney.

Diabetes Insipidus

This is the result of lack of vasopressin. Patients have polyuria (often over 10 l/24 h) and polydipsia. The urine is dilute even when the patient is deprived of fluid. This latter feature distinguishes the disease from **psychogenic polydipsia**. In some cases, there is no obvious cause, the idiopathic variant; this may be sporadic or familial. Other causes are destructive lesions of the hypothalamus including tumours, granulomatous disease and histiocytosis X. It may also follow head injury or neurosurgical procedures.

Inappropriate Secretion of Vasopressin

Absolute or relative excess secretion of vasopressin results in hyponatraemia and hypo-osmolality due to water retention. Vomiting, muscle cramps and weakness result, sometimes leading to coma and death. It is most commonly caused by ectopic secretion of vasopressin by an oat cell carcinoma of lung. It may also occur in cases of meningitis, subarachnoid haemorrhage, following head injury or in patients with pneumonia, or on mechanical ventilation, although in these cases the mechanism of hypersecretion is unclear.

Tumours

Metastases may be identified in 1–3% of cancer patients particularly from breast and lung, but rarely cause clinical symptoms. Gangliocytomas, which also occur in the hypothalamus, may sometimes involve the neuro- and the adeno-hypophysis.

Hypothalamus

The hypothalamus is bounded on its lower surface by the optic chiasm anteriorly, laterally by the optic tracts and posteriorly by the mamillary bodies. It comprises several nuclei of neuronal cell bodies and nerve tracts. It controls many of the endocrine functions of the body by secreting/releasing and inhibiting factors which regulate anterior pituitary secretion. It is in direct continuity with the neurohypophysis via the pituitary stalk. In addition, it regulates many of the basic bodily functions such as eating, drinking, body temperature and emotional responses. Granulomatous inflammation including **sarcoidosis** or involvement in **histiocytosis X** may result in hypopituitarism and diabetes insipidus. Tumours are most commonly **gliomas** or **germinomas** (similar to seminomas). Again, these may cause destruction of nuclei and tracts. The extremely rare **gangliocytoma** (consisting of ganglion cells and glial cells) may secrete hypothalamic releasing hormones, causing hypersecretion of one of the pituitary hormones (e.g. growth hormone causing acromegaly). At the same time, it may result in hyposecretion of other hormones due to hypothalamic destruction.

The Thyroid Gland

The thyroid is normally situated just below the cricoid cartilage and consists of two lateral lobes joined by the isthmus. In 50% of people, a pyramidal lobe is present above the isthmus. The gland weighs 15–25 g in the normal adult. Histologically, it consists mainly of follicles, lined by cuboidal epithelium, which contain varying amounts of colloid, the storage form of thyroglobulin. Among the follicular cells in the middle and upper portions of the lateral lobes are scattered C cells, which produce calcitonin. The follicular elements are endodermal in origin, derived from a downgrowth of the primitive pharynx. The C cells are neuroectodermal, arising from the ultimobranchial bodies which develop from the ventral portions of the fourth pharyngeal pouches.

The thyroid follicles produce the hormones thyroxine – tetraiodothyronine, T4 and tri-iodothyronine, T3 (Fig. 23.8). Inorganic iodide is actively trapped and concentrated by the gland. It is then oxidized by a thyroid peroxidase present at the apical cell membrane of the follicular cells, and binds to tyrosine residues on thyroglobulin to form mono- and di-iodotyrosine. Coupling of the iodotyrosines produces T4 or T3. These hormones are then stored in thyroglobulin in the colloid of the thyroid follicles. TSH stimulation results in endocytosis of thyroglobulin into the follicular cells. There is fusion with lysosomes and thyroglobulin is broken down with release of T4 and T3, which then pass into the bloodstream. The iodotyrosines released are deiodinated by a dehalogenase enzyme and the iodine recycled.

The circulating thyroid hormones are largely bound to thyroxine binding globulin (TBG) and thyroxine binding prealbumin (TBPA) and only a small proportion circulate in the active free form. In peripheral tissues T4 is deiodinated to produce T3 or reverse T3, of which only T3 is active and predominantly responsible for the metabolic effects of the thyroid. These effects involve modulation of fat, protein and carbohydrate metabolism. The hormone acts mainly by binding to specific nuclear receptors and regulating expression of specific genes including growth hormone and various enzymes involved in key metabolic path-

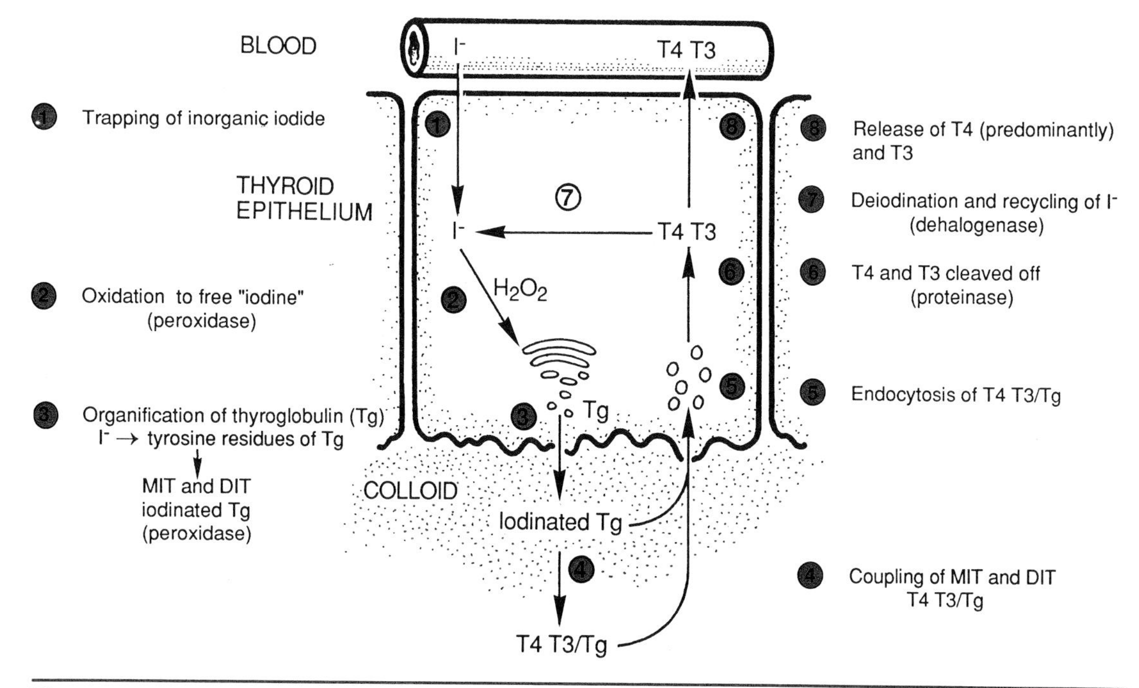

Fig. 23.8 Figure to illustrate the steps involved in the biosynthesis of the thyroid hormones. Inherited abnormalities in the biosynthesis resulting in dyshormogenetic goitre may involve: 1, 3, 4 and 7. Those associated with 3 comprise a heterogeneous group in some of which an abnormal thyroglobulin is synthesized; in Pendred's syndrome there is a partial organification defect plus sensorineural deafness.

ways. These hormones, therefore, have very significant regulatory effects on general cell metabolism.

Patients with thyroid disease usually present either as the result of thyroid swelling – **goitre** – or because of the effects of excess or deficiency of thyroid hormones. It is appropriate to outline the clinical features of hyperthyroidism and hypothyroidism before discussing the various thyroid lesions with which they may be associated.

Hyperthyroidism

This is known clinically as thyrotoxicosis and is due to hypersecretion of thyroid hormone. There is weight loss but increased appetite; the patient is weak but hyperkinetic, nervous, irritable and emotionally labile. There is heat intolerance, excessive sweating, a fine tremor, tachycardia and an increased cardiac output; palpitation and breathlessness may occur. In older patients atrial fibrillation is often present, and cardiac failure may be the presenting feature. A staring appearance with lid retraction and infrequent blinking is due to contraction of levator palpebrae superioris which has a sympathetic innervation. This clinical sign, and indeed many of the clinical features of thyrotoxicosis are due to increased sensitivity to circulating adrenaline as a result of enhanced β-adrenergic responsiveness, an example of hormone/hormone interaction.

The most common cause is Graves' disease, accounting for up to 80% of cases. Toxic nodular goitre is implicated in around 10%, particularly in middle-aged and elderly patients and a toxic nodule (adenoma) accounts for another 5–10%. It may be seen in early Hashimoto's thyroiditis, so called hashitoxicosis. Other causes are rare and include TSH secretion from a pituitary adenoma; ingestion of thyroid hormone; and the sudden hyperthyroidism which may occur if large doses of iodine are given to a patient with a large non-toxic nodular goitre which can then synthesize excessive quantities of thyroid hormones (the Jod–Basedow phenomenon).

Hypothyroidism

In the adult, this is known as **myxoedema**. The symptoms will depend on the severity of the hormone deficiency. The patient is lethargic, and may have impaired intellectual function which, in untreated patients, can lead to frank psychosis (myxoedema madness). The skin and hair are dry and accumulation of mucopolysaccharides in the dermis causes coarsening of the features (Fig. 23.9). Similar deposits around nerves may cause pain and paraesthesia, while involvement of the larynx and tongue results in the voice becoming gruff. The patient gains weight, feels cold and may develop hypothermia. Blood cholesterol levels are increased, and the raised levels of TRH may cause hyperprolactinaemia.

The commonest cause is autoimmune thyroiditis, either primary myxoedema or Hashimoto's disease. It may also occur with severe iodine deficiency or in patients with dyshormonogenesis; following thyroid surgery or radioiodine therapy; and as a result of the ingestion of antithyroid drugs or goitrogenic chemicals. Finally, hypopituitarism will result in hypothyroidism secondary to decreased TSH secretion.

Cretinism is due to severe hypothyroidism in infancy. The baby often appears normal at birth, but soon shows signs of mental retardation, neuromuscular abnormalities, deaf-mutism and retarded growth. There is a typical facial appearance, with coarse features and an enlarged tongue (Fig. 23.10). Cretinism may occasionally be due to thyroid agenesis or hypoplasia and a goitre is absent. In areas of endemic goitre, maternal iodine deficiency may give rise to cretinism associated with nodular goitre in the child. *Sporadic goitrous cretinism* is usually caused by congenital absence of one of the enzymes involved in the biosynthesis of thyroxine (Fig. 23.8), or to defective peripheral responses to the hormone. This leads to decreased negative feedback on the pituitary and increased TSH secretion with stimulation of thyroid growth. The goitre is usually diffuse with severe hyperplasia and little evidence of colloid storage. It is extremely important to

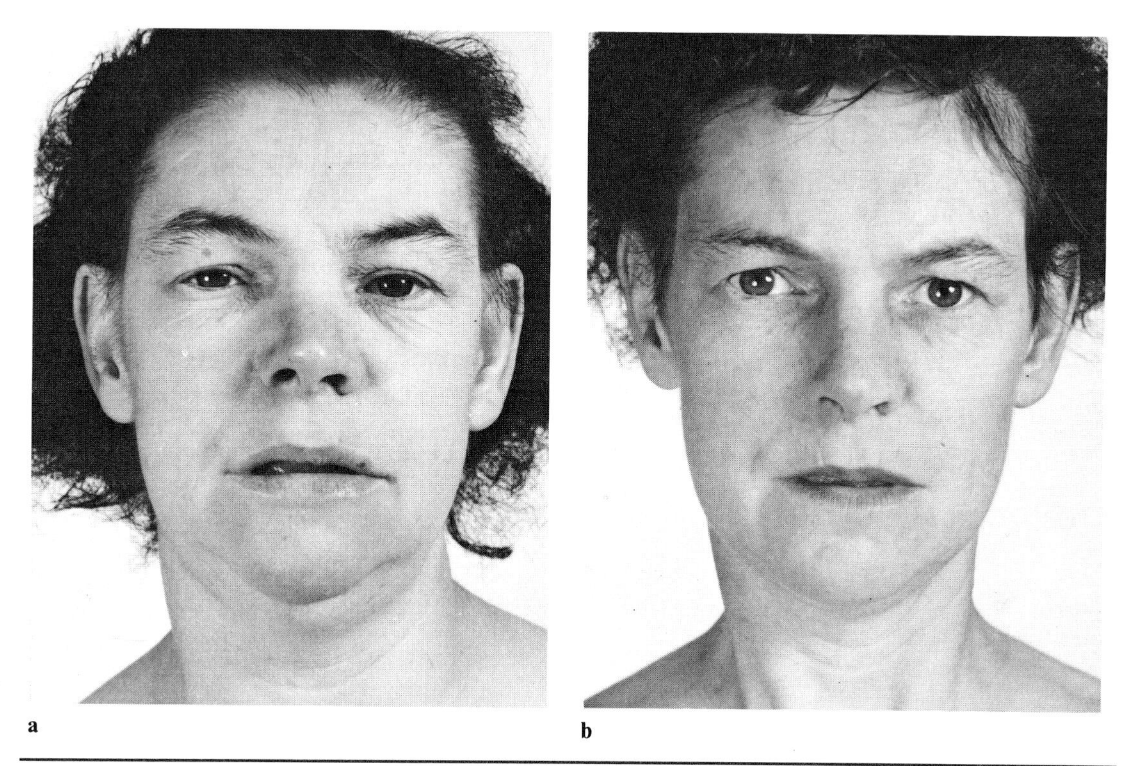

Fig. 23.9 Myxoedema. **a** Before treatment: note the coarsening of the features. **b** After treatment with thyroxine.

make the diagnosis of cretinism at an early stage and to institute hormone replacement therapy in order to prevent mental retardation.

Functional Disorders of the Thyroid Gland

Non-toxic Nodular Goitre

This is the commonest lesion in thyroid pathology and reflects compensatory thyroid hyperplasia in the context of absolute or relative iodine deficiency. On epidemiological grounds, two forms can be defined – endemic and sporadic.

Endemic goitre is defined as the occurrence of non-toxic goitre in more than 10% of a population. Since the main natural dietary source of iodine is seafood, this usually occurs in mountainous areas or in areas far from the sea, e.g. the Alps, the Himalayas, and the Andes. In Western society, the incidence has decreased in these areas since the introduction of iodized salt. The goitre often presents in childhood and there is a less marked female predominance than in the sporadic type.

Sporadic non-toxic goitre is due to a relative lack of iodine in individual patients. This may result: (1) from poor dietary intake; (2) from inherited deficiency of the various enzymes involved in the biosynthesis of thyroxine as shown in Fig. 23.8; (3) from ingestion of specific chemicals which interfere with thyroid hormone synthesis – goitrogens. These include vegetables of the *Bras-*

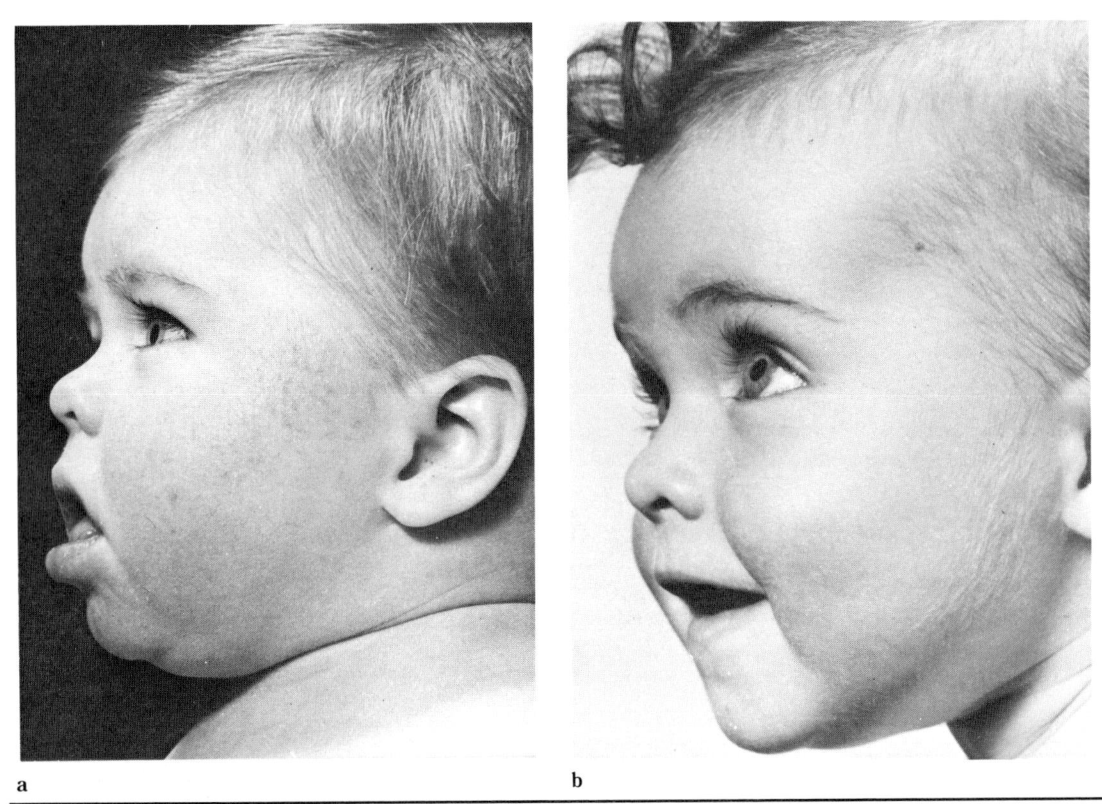

Fig. 23.10 A cretin aged 17 months. **a** Note the enlarged protruding tongue, coarse dry skin and dull expression. **b** This shows the effects of thyroxine treatment for 2 months.

sica family, e.g. cabbage and Brussel sprouts, and excessive fluoride in water. Drugs may also be involved, such as para-amino salicylic acid, sulphonylureas and, in some individuals, iodides in expectorants; and finally (4) possibly as part of the spectrum of autoimmune thyroid disease with the production of growth stimulating immunoglobulins. This mechanism at present remains unproven.

Sporadic goitre is ten times more common in women. It often presents around puberty or in relation to pregnancy and lactation when iodine requirements are increased. Most patients are clinically euthyroid, although TSH levels may be slightly increased.

In the early stages, diffuse hypertrophy and hyperplasia of follicular cells occur with depletion of colloid (**parenchymatous goitre**) which is followed by involution of the epithelium and accumulation of colloid (**colloid goitre**). Subsequent episodes of stimulation appear to result in more focal hyperplasia with variable involution. There is often vascular damage with haemorrhage and scarring. This eventually leads to the classical picture of **multinodular goitre** which comprises nodules consisting of follicles of varying size and colloid content, some cystic, separated by fibrous tissue containing haemosiderin laden macrophages and variable numbers of other inflammatory cells. The gland may weigh up to 500 g and occasionally several hundred grams and there is usually marked asymmetry (Fig. 23.11). In rare cases, it may cause compression of the recurrent laryngeal nerve, the trachea or oesophagus.

In some cases, one nodule may be much larger than the others (dominant nodule) giving rise to suspicion of tumour. Fine needle aspiration cytology may be useful in the differential diagnosis but

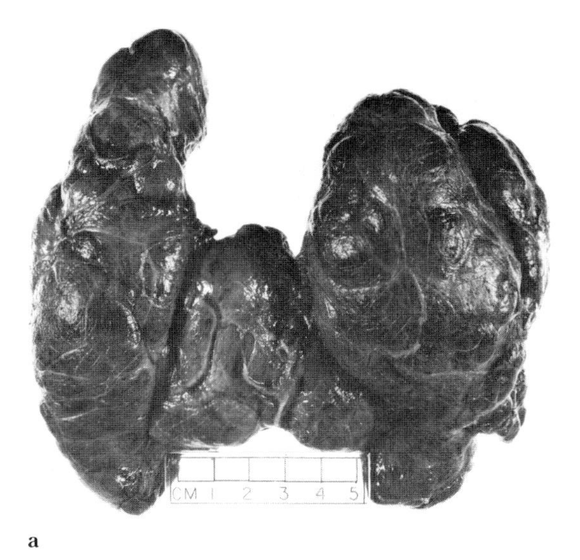

a

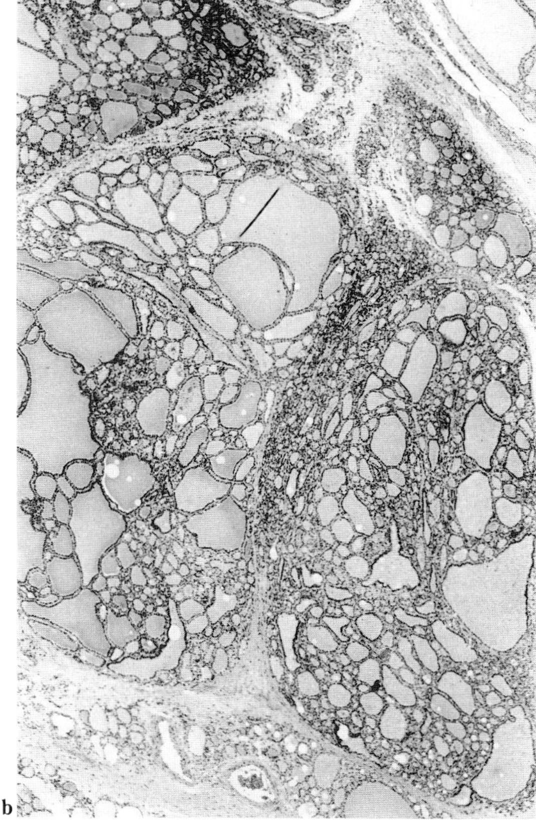

b

Fig. 23.11 Multinodular goitre. **a** There is general thyroid enlargement, with an obvious nodular configuration, and marked asymmetry. **b** Nodularity is confirmed on histological examination.

partial thyroidectomy may be required to make this distinction. In occasional patients, particularly in an older age group, secondary hyperplasia may occur in multinodular goitre, **toxic nodular goitre**, resulting in hyperthyroidism. The underlying mechanisms are unclear.

Autoimmune Thyroid Disease

This group of diseases, Hashimoto's thyroiditis, primary myxoedema and Graves' disease, are characterized by lymphoid infiltration of the gland and by the presence of circulating autoantibodies to various components of thyroid follicular cells (Table 23.2). Many of these play an active role in the pathogenesis of the diseases. Thyroid stimulating immunoglobulins (TSI) are TSH-receptor antibodies which activate the receptor and stimulate secretion of thyroid hormones with resultant hyperthyroidism. Others are thought to promote thyroid growth (TGI), and may be important in causing the goitre of Hashimoto's disease. The presence of blocking antibodies reacting with the TSH receptor may contribute to hypothyroidism.

There is a familial association between the thyroid autoimmune diseases and other organ-specific autoimmune disease (p. 227), including Addison's disease, type I diabetes mellitus and pernicious anaemia.

Although the role of autoimmunity in chronic focal thyroiditis and lymphocytic thyroiditis is less clear, they will also be considered under this heading.

Table 23.2 Autoantibodies in thyroid diseases

	Comment
Antimicrosomal Antithyroglobulin Anti-C2 (second colloid antigen)	May be present in 10% of normal adults, particularly women, and in 80% or more of patients with autoimmune thyroid disease. Of limited diagnostic value
Anti-TSH receptor	
Thyroid stimulating immunoglobulin (TSI)	See text
Thyroid growth immunoglobulin (TGI)	See text
'Blocking' antibody	May induce hypothyroidism and may be goitrogenic

Hashimoto's Thyroiditis

This is a disease mainly of middle-aged women, female to male ratio 20:1. There is a familial occurrence and an increased prevalence of HLA-DR5, suggesting a role for genetic factors. The patient presents with a painless goitre and in the early stages is usually euthyroid. However, hypothyroidism develops in around 80% of cases. The thyroid is widely infiltrated and replaced by lymphoid cells, plasma cells and macrophages and there is germinal centre formation (Fig. 23.12a). The thyroid follicular cells are enlarged, with eosinophilic granular cytoplasm (Fig. 23.12b) due to the accumulation of mitochondria. This is known as Askanazy or Hürthle cell change. In some cases fibrosis is very prominent and in men this variant is more commonly seen. High titre microsomal antibodies are present in most cases, and 50% of patients have antibodies to thyroglobulin. Occasionally, patients present with hyperthyroidism and this may be due to the presence of thyroid stimulating immunoglobulins (TSI).

Graves' Disease

This form of autoimmune thyroiditis is characterized by diffuse thyroid hyperplasia with hyperthyroidism. It is five times more common in females than in males, occurring mainly between 20 and 40 years and there is an increased prevalence of HLA-DR3. Some patients also have exophthalmos – protrusion of the globe (Fig. 23.13) – probably due to the presence of autoantibodies to the extraocular muscles; in advanced cases there is also inflammation of other tissues in the orbit. Pretibial myxoedema, an infiltrate of the dermis and of unknown aetiology, is present in 10–15% of patients.

The thyroid gland is uniformly enlarged, up to about three times its normal size. In the untreated case, the thyroid epithelium is hyperplastic, sometimes with papillary infolding, and there is little colloid storage (Fig. 23.14a). Lymphocytic infiltration is present, but is usually less than in the other autoimmune diseases. Germinal centres may be present.

Because of the significant metabolic abnormalities, surgery in a hyperthyroid patient poses considerable risks and before thyroidectomy patients are usually treated with antithyroid drugs with or without iodine. This induces changes in the morphology of the gland. Iodine causes reduction in vascularity and colloid accumulation (Fig. 23.14b) while antithyroid drugs cause more marked hyperplasia, and the resultant picture may be extremely complex.

Primary Myxoedema

In this condition, mainly of elderly women, there is very severe atrophy of the thyroid. The gland is replaced by fibrous tissue and a lymphoid infiltrate (Fig. 23.15) and what follicular tissue remains usually shows squamous metaplasia. Such patients are severely hypothyroid.

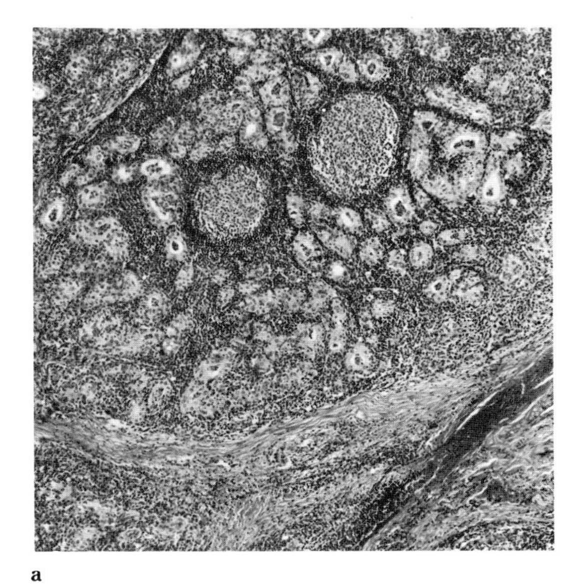

a

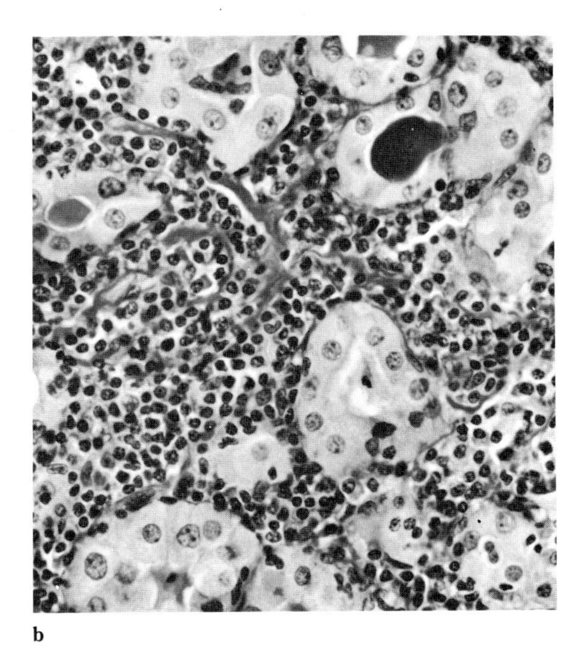

b

Fig. 23.12 Hashimoto's thyroiditis. **a** There is a diffuse lymphoid infiltrate, germinal centres, fibrosis and small acini. **b** At higher power, the lymphoplasmacytic infiltrate is seen, and the follicular cells show typical Askanazy cell change.

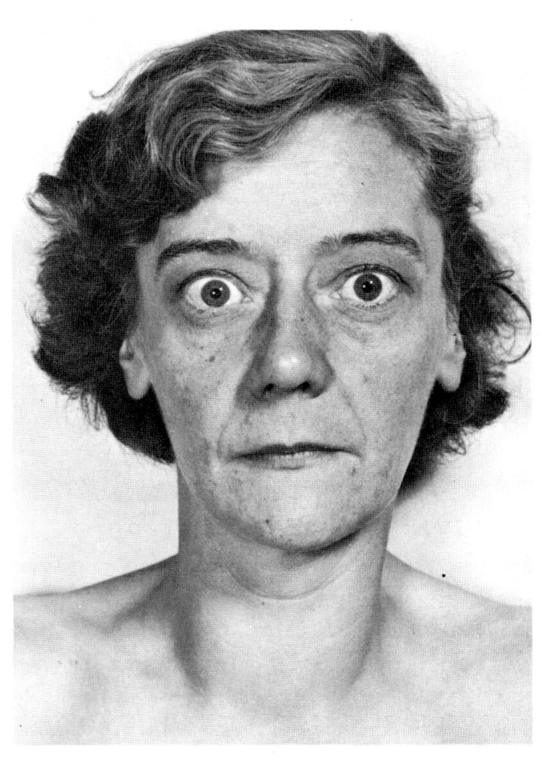

Fig. 23.13 Thyrotoxicosis due to Graves' disease. There is diffuse thyroid enlargement and the patient has prominent eyes (exophthalmos).

Lymphocytic Thyroiditis

This disease of children and young adults usually presents with goitre, sometimes associated with hyperthyroidism. There is a diffuse lymphoplasmacytic infiltrate with moderate germinal centre formation, but Hürthle cell change is not seen. Thyroid autoantibodies may be present but in low titre. It has been suggested that it is an early precursor form of Hashimoto's disease.

Focal Chronic Thyroiditis

In autopsy series, focal lymphoid infiltration is seen in about 15–20% of thyroid glands from patients who had no clinical evidence of thyroid disease. However, since the incidence correlates well with the overall occurrence of thyroid autoantibodies in the general population, it is thought to reflect some form of autoimmune response. Its

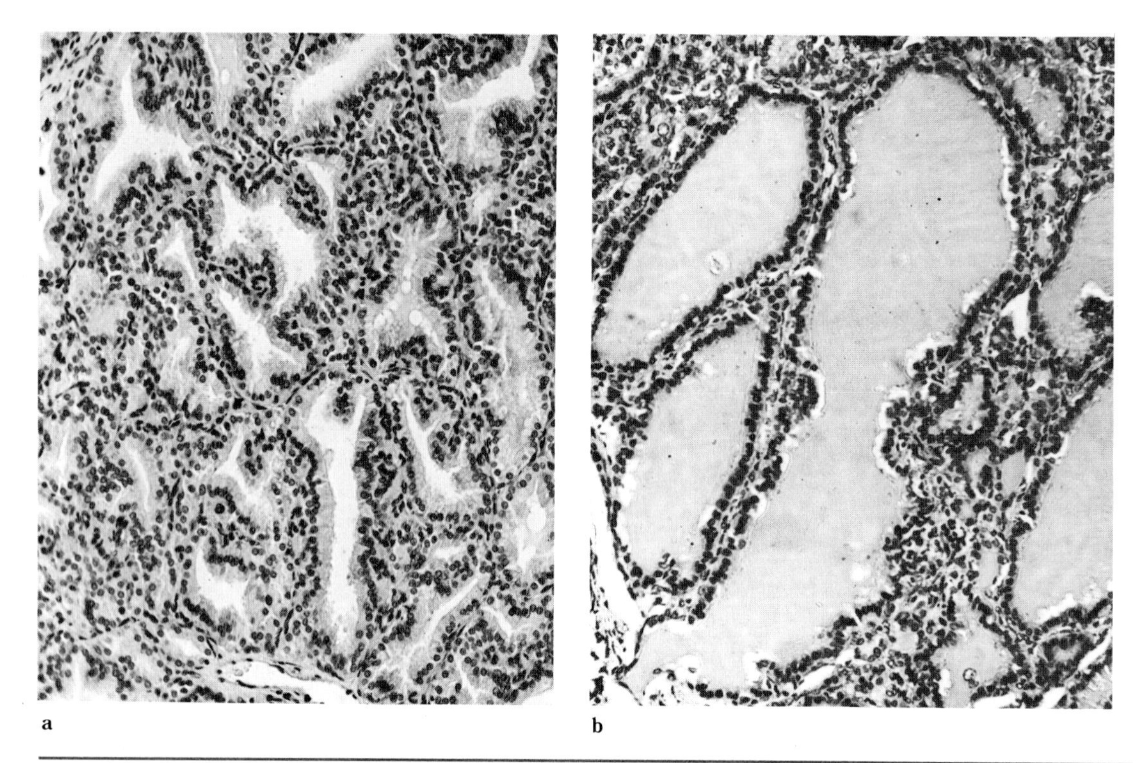

Fig. 23.14 The thyroid in Graves' disease. **a** Untreated: the epithelial cells are columnar and there is virtually no colloid. **b** After treatment with iodine for 10 days: the epithelium is cuboidal and some colloid has accumulated.

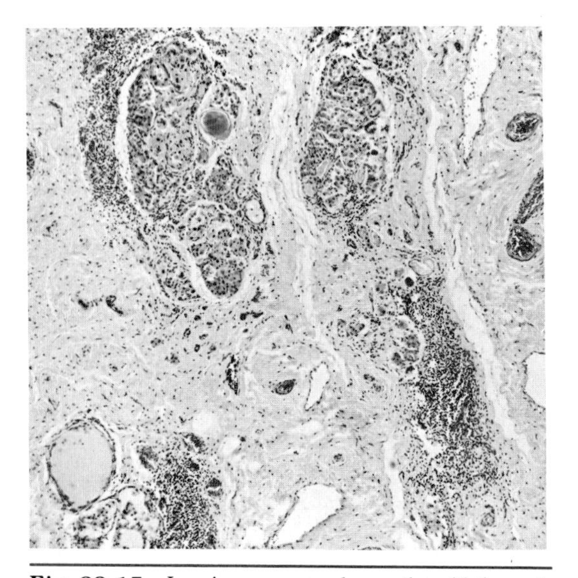

Fig. 23.15 In primary myxoedema, thyroid tissue is largely destroyed and replaced by fibrous tissue. The small islands of thyroid epithelium remaining show changes of chronic thyroiditis.

exact relationship to the other diseases is unclear, and it may represent a reaction to a variety of insults.

Other Forms of Thyroiditis

Acute thyroiditis may occasionally develop in bacteraemic states, with localized abscess formation. In immunosuppressed patients, fungal thyroiditis may occur.

Giant-cell (de Quervain's) thyroiditis, is a subacute thyroiditis which presents as a painful goitre. It is thought to be viral in origin, and is often associated with a prodromal illness and fever or preceded by an upper respiratory infection. Three-quarters of cases are in women mainly in the 20–50 age group. In some, there is initial hyperthyroidism, but the condition is self-limiting. Antithyroid antibodies may be transiently detected in some patients. The thyroid initially shows acute inflammation with neutrophil polymorphs followed by a local lymphohistiocytic granulomatous reaction with giant-cell formation, and varying degrees of fibrosis may be present.

Riedel's thyroiditis. This very rare disease is characterized by replacement of thyroid tissue by dense fibrous tissue. It may present as a goitre, but there may be tracheal symptoms or damage to the recurrent laryngeal nerve, due to extension of the fibrosis beyond the thyroid gland, mimicking malignancy. The cause is unknown, but some patients also have retroperitoneal or mediastinal fibrosis (p. 739).

Thyroid Tumours

Benign and malignant thyroid tumours usually present clinically as solitary nodules and the majority of these are 'cold' on thyroid scan (i.e. they concentrate less radioiodine than the surrounding gland). Of clinically apparent solitary nodules about 70% represent a dominant nodule in a multinodular goitre. The remainder are tumours, the majority of which are benign. In men and in young people, however, cold nodules should be regarded with more suspicion than in middle-aged women. Thyroid cancer is rare, accounting for less than 1.0% of all cancers and less than 0.5% of all deaths from cancer.

Tumours can arise from both follicular epithelium and C cells. The majority are follicular adenomas. Malignant tumours of follicular cell origin fall into two main groups – papillary and follicular carcinomas – which behave differently. Medullary carcinomas arise from C cells.

Follicular Adenoma

These are the commonest thyroid neoplasms, presenting most frequently in women over 30 years. Infrequently, an adenoma may be the cause of hyperthyroidism (toxic adenoma) and will show as a 'hot' nodule on a thyroid scan. Adenomas are usually encapsulated and compress the surrounding normal gland. Haemorrhage, degenerative changes and fibrosis may occur.

Histologically, most show a microfollicular pattern, with little colloid storage (fetal adenoma) but a variety of other subtypes may be identified, e.g. colloid adenoma, with marked colloid storage. Some are composed of Hürthle cells. These differences in appearance, however, have no bearing on tumour behaviour. As in other areas of endocrine pathology, it is sometimes difficult for the histopathologist to make the distinction between a true adenoma and a circumscribed hyperplastic nodule in a non-toxic goitre. In clinical terms, however, this should not alter patient management.

Papillary Carcinoma

In practice, all papillary neoplasms of the thyroid are regarded as malignant. They account for 60–70% of all thyroid cancers, occurring in young adults (peak 30–40 years) and are three times more common in women. They are not well encapsulated and many appear multifocal within the gland, most probably due to intraglandular lymphatic metastases. This propensity for lymphatic spread is also manifest by the presence of lymph node metastases in the neck in 40% of cases at the time of diagnosis. This finding does not, however, alter prognosis and the 5-year survival rate approaches 90%. Distant metastases to lung or bone are uncommon with this tumour but, if present in the lung at the time of diagnosis, reduce the 5-year survival to around 75%. Papillary carcinomas may be very small and sometimes a patient will present with a lymph node metastasis in the neck and very careful sectioning of the thyroid is required to find a minute primary tumour.

These tumours have a characteristic cytological appearance with optically clear or grooved nuclei (so-called Orphan Annie nuclei). Many tumours show sclerosis, and calcispherites (psammoma bodies) are present in about half the cases. As the name suggests, most have an overall papillary structure (Fig. 23.16). Some show a mixed papillary and follicular pattern and rarely, a tumour with

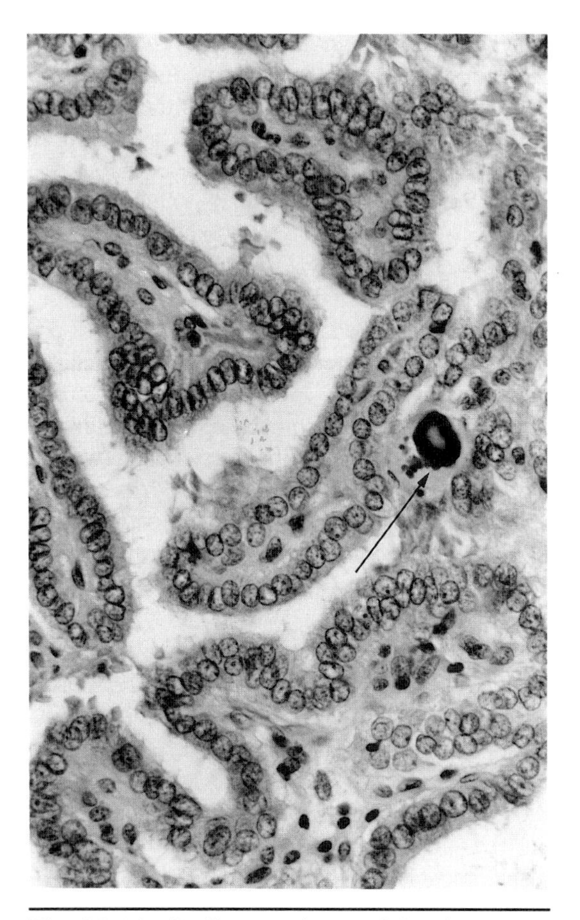

Fig. 23.16 Papillary carcinoma of thyroid showing papillae with fibrovascular cores, and optically clear nuclei and a psammoma body (arrow).

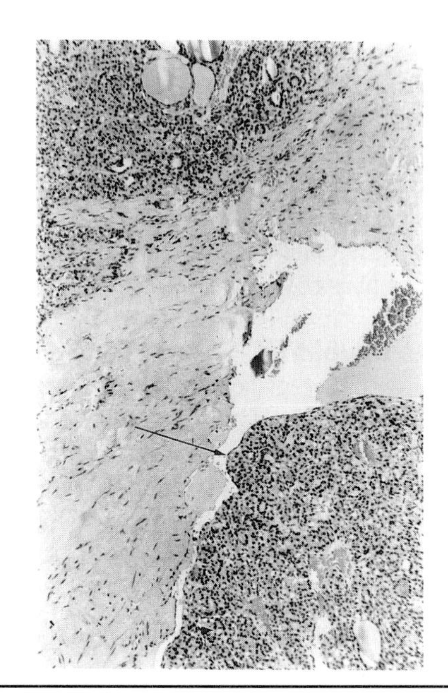

Fig. 23.17 Follicular carcinoma of thyroid showing vascular invasion with a tongue of tumour cells within a vessel lumen (arrow).

the cytological features of papillary carcinoma may have an overall follicular structure (the follicular variant of papillary carcinoma). These, however, behave in the same fashion as the classical papillary tumour.

Follicular Carcinoma

These comprise 15–20% of all thyroid cancers, but in areas of endemic goitre, account for a higher proportion of cases. They are also more common in women and the peak incidence is in the fifth decade, one-third of cases occurring over the age of 50 years. Distant blood-borne metastases occur, particularly to bone and lung. The prognosis is worse than in papillary carcinoma, with an overall survival rate of 50%. Follicular carcinomas can be divided into two groups: first, widely invasive tumours which spread throughout the normal glandular tissue and are dispersed in blood vessels: and secondly, encapsulated 'microinvasive' tumours where malignancy is identified by microscopic invasion of the fibrous capsule and of blood vessels (Fig. 23.17). The most important prognostic factor is the extent of invasion, patients with an encapsulated tumour faring better than those in whom it is widely invasive.

Medullary Carcinoma

These account for 5–10% of thyroid cancers, and 10–20% are familial, forming part of the MEN 2 (multiple endocrine neoplasia) syndrome (p. 1105). They are slightly more common in women. The sporadic type is usually unilateral and the majority present in the fifth or sixth decade. In contrast, the familial variant is usually bilateral and multifocal, arising on a background of C-cell hyperplasia, and often presenting before the age of 25 years. If medullary carcinoma and C-cell hyperplasia are identified in a gland, it is important to screen family members for raised calcitonin levels or other features of MEN 2. Prophylactic thyroidectomy should be performed in affected family members at the stage of C-cell hyperplasia to prevent the development of tumour.

Histologically, medullary carcinoma consists of solid irregular groups and cords of cells. Calcitonin immunoreactivity can be demonstrated in the tumour cells in all cases (Fig. 23.18). The tumours may produce other hormones, including bombesin, serotonin and ACTH and give rise to ectopic hormone syndromes. Amyloid, thought to be derived from the calcitonin precursor, is identified in about 50% of cases. Medullary carcinoma spreads by both vascular and lymphatic channels, resulting in lymph node and distant metastases. Although very long survival times have been reported when no metastases are identified at the time of diagnosis, the overall 10-year survival rate is about 50%. However, tumours associated with MEN 2b are extremely aggressive and usually fatal.

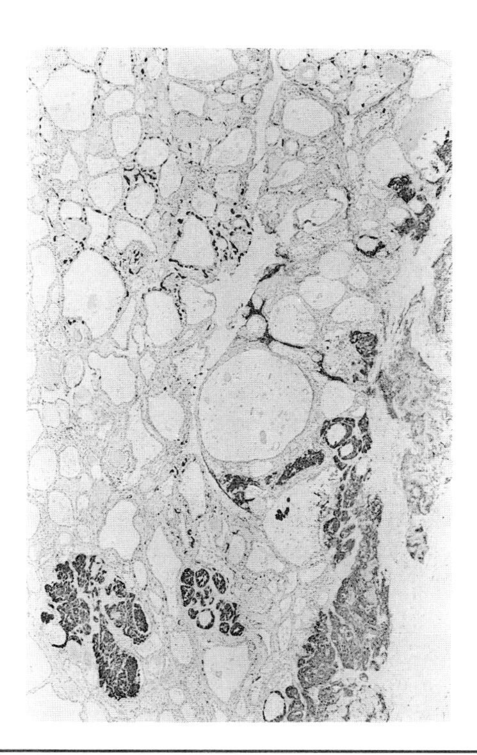

Fig. 23.18 Medullary carcinoma of thyroid stained by immunoperoxidase technique with an antibody to calcitonin. Tumour cells arranged in small groups or lobules are immunopositive. The dense hyaline material between the cells is amyloid. The adjacent gland shows an increase in the number of C cells.

Anaplastic Tumours

Around 5–10% of thyroid carcinomas are anaplastic. They occur mainly in women between 60 and 70 years old. They grow rapidly and are highly malignant, often showing signs of both local invasion and distant metastases at the time of presentation. Microscopically, as the name suggests, they are very poorly differentiated, often with bizarre giant cells. They probably arise from follicular or papillary carcinomas, areas of which may sometimes be identified. There is often a history of a long-standing thyroid mass with recent expansion.

Aetiology of Thyroid Carcinoma

The differences in differentiation and behavioural patterns between papillary and follicular carcinomas would suggest that different mechanisms might be involved in their genesis. It is unclear whether iodine deficiency has any significant effect on the overall incidence of thyroid tumours. Nevertheless, it may play some role in determining the type of tumour, in that follicular carcinomas comprise a greater proportion of tumours in iodine deficient areas. This is supported by the fact that where iodine has been added to the diet in areas of endemic goitre, the ratio of papillary to follicular tumours then approaches that of populations with a normal iodine intake. External radiation may play a role in the induction of some tumours of papillary type, and an increased incidence of such tumours followed the use of the atomic bomb in Hiroshima and was also reported following therapeutic irradiation of the head and neck in early childhood.

Recent studies have investigated molecular

genetic aspects of thyroid tumours. Interestingly, it has been shown that while 80% of follicular tumours express activated *ras* oncogenes, this occurs in only 20% of papillary tumours (Lemoine *et al.*, 1988). These activated oncogenes are present in follicular adenomas as well as carcinomas, suggesting that *ras* mutation represents an early event in the development of follicular tumours.

A DNA sequence has recently been isolated from papillary carcinomas which will transform cells on transfection. It appears to have resulted from the rearrangement of an unknown amino-terminal sequence to the tyrosine kinase domain of the *ret* proto-oncogene and has been designated the *PTC* oncogene (for papillary thyroid carcinoma).

The genetic abnormalities in medullary carcinoma as part of MEN 2 are now being clarified, but little is known of the molecular basis for the sporadic variant.

Other Tumours

Benign and malignant tumours may rarely arise from the connective tissue and vascular components of the thyroid (e.g. haemangioma). Occasionally, metastatic tumour may be present, most usually from lung, breast and gastrointestinal tract.

Lymphomas

B-cell lymphomas of follicle centre cell type may arise in the thyroid, and in 80% of cases are associated with Hashimoto's disease. The prevalence of lymphoma in Hashimoto's disease is about 1–2%. Since the thyroid is derived from the primitive gut, thyroid lymphocytes are regarded as forming part of the mucosa-associated lymphoid tissue (MALT) (p. 172). Many thyroid lymphomas show lymphoepithelial lesions, a feature commonly seen in MALT lymphomas (p. 731). Initially, the tumour is confined to the thyroid, but may disseminate to local and distant lymph nodes, and to Peyer's patches of the gastrointestinal tract, thus reflecting the normal circulation of gut-associated lymphocytes. Plasmacytoma, which may produce thyroid autoantibodies, is an even rarer complication of Hashimoto's disease.

Miscellaneous Thyroid Disorders

Congenital abnormalities. Congenital absence of the thyroid and hypoplasia have already been discussed as causes of cretinism. Occasionally, abnormalities of descent occur, the commonest being **lingual thyroid**. **Thyroglossal duct cysts** develop from persistence of the lower part of the tubal downgrowth which gives rise to the thyroid. They are situated in the midline of the neck and may rupture. They are usually lined by respiratory epithelium often surrounded by lymphoid tissue and thyroid remnants may be seen.

Amyloid deposition may cause a goitre (amyloid goitre), either as an isolated finding or as part of systemic amyloidosis. This is not to be confused with the calcitonin derived amyloid in medullary carcinoma.

The Adrenal Glands

The adrenal glands lie above the kidneys and comprise the cortex, derived from the mesoderm of the urogenital ridge, and the medulla, which is of neuroectodermal origin. The adrenal is divided into head, body and tail, and in the normal gland, medulla is present only in the head and body. The normal adrenal in the adult weighs 4–4.5 g at surgery or in cases of sudden death. However, at hospital autopsy, the average weight is 6 g. This is due to the stress of the terminal illness causing excessive stimulation by ACTH and cortical growth. The pathology of the cortex and medulla differs and will be dealt with separately.

Adrenal Cortex

The adrenal cortex is responsible for the synthesis of a number of steroid hormones. It consists of three zones: the **zona glomerulosa**, dispersed focally in the subcapsular region; the **zona fasciculata**, forming the major part with lipid laden cells arranged in parallel cords; and the inner **zona reticularis**, with anastomosing clusters of compact or eosinophilic cells. The major pathways of adrenal steroidogenesis are shown in Fig. 23.19.

The **zona glomerulosa** synthesizes mineralocorticoids, mainly aldosterone. Its function is regulated by the renin–angiotensin system (p. 75). The zona reticularis and fasciculata act as a single unit and produce glucocorticoids, the most important of which is cortisol. Androgens and oestrogens are also produced but in the normal adult the amounts secreted are not functionally significant. The **zona reticularis** acts as the functional zone, the **zona fasiculata** as a reserve zone. Stimulation by ACTH results in broadening of the reticularis and a reduction in the width of fasciculata.

Aldosterone plays a major role in the regulation of plasma volume and of potassium homeostasis. It increases the renal tubular reabsorption of sodium and chloride. Aldosterone also increases renal tubular secretion of potassium. Glucocorticoids have wide ranging effects on general metabolism. They promote gluconeogenesis and oppose the action of insulin, inhibit protein synthesis and increase protein catabolism. They act on vascular smooth muscle, thus raising blood pressure. They have anti-inflammatory properties, and inhibit the phagocytic and bactericidal activities of polymorphs and macrophages. They are immunosuppressive, by a cytotoxic effect on lymphocytes, particularly T cells (p. 224). Healing is inhibited, due to suppression of the formation of granulation tissue and abnormal collagen maturation (p. 161). Effects on bone formation and calcium absorption lead to osteoporosis (p. 950).

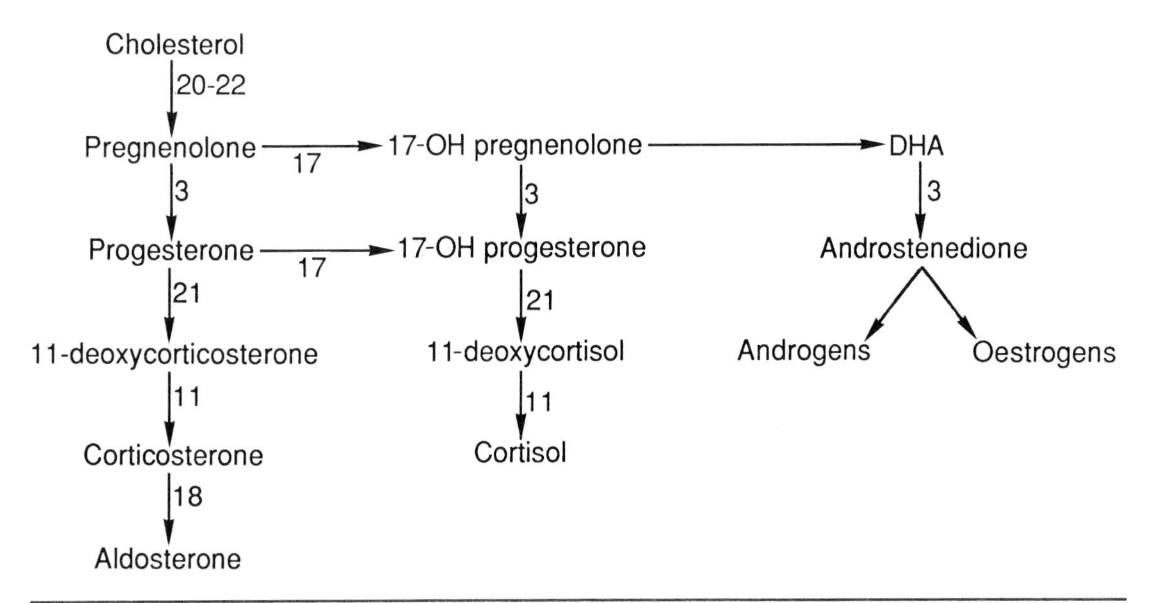

Fig. 23.19 Pathways of adrenal steroidogenesis. Enzymes involved: 20-22 – 20,22-desmolase; 3 – 3β-hydroxysteroid dehydrogenase; 21–21-hydroxylase; 11–11β-hydroxylase; 18–18-hydroxylase (only present in zona glomerulosa); 17–17α-hydroxylase; DHA–dehydroepiandrosterone.

Adrenal Tumours

The true incidence of both benign and malignant adrenocortical tumours is unknown. Nodules, apparent to the naked eye and sometimes measuring several centimetres in diameter, may be identified in up to 5% of unselected autopsies but it has not yet been established whether these are neoplastic or hyperplastic. They occur more commonly in patients with vascular disease, in whom it is suggested that focal ischaemic necrosis of areas of the cortex is followed by regenerative activity. This would suggest that the majority are hyperplastic. However, the resolution of the question will require the application of techniques to establish clonality: a true neoplasm would be expected to be clonal in origin (i.e. derived from a single cell) while hyperplastic nodules would be polyclonal. With increasing use of CT scans for the investigation of intra-abdominal pathology, a significant number of adrenal nodules are now identified in life. This raises the problem of whether to remove them or not. At present, if the nodule is less than 3 cm in diameter and there is no evidence of abnormal hormonal secretion, surgical intervention is deemed unnecessary.

Adenoma

Functional adrenal adenomas may be associated with excessive secretion of cortisol, aldosterone or sex steroids. The tumours resemble normal adrenocortical cells histologically with varying proportions of clear (fasciculata-like) and compact (reticularis-like) cells. Aldosterone-secreting tumours may also contain glomerulosa-like cells and hybrid cells, sharing features of both glomerulosa and fasciculata.

Carcinoma

Some adrenocortical tumours are frankly malignant, with metastases present at the time of first clinical presentation. The prognosis is extremely poor. If metastases are not present, the distinction between benign and potentially malignant tumours is extremely difficult. Larger tumours (>100 g) are more likely to be malignant but carcinomas of less than 50 g have been reported. Adrenocortical tumours which secrete androgens or large tumours which are non-functional are more likely to be malignant. Histologically, there is no single criterion of malignancy and prognosis has to be based on a multifactorial anlaysis including mitotic rate, distribution of cell type, the presence of necrosis, fibrosis and vascular invasion. Virilism or the absence of hormonal secretion from a larger tumour also suggest malignancy.

Aetiology

The causes of adrenocortical tumours are unclear. Recent studies have identified mutations in the gene for the α chain of the inhibitory G protein G_{i2} in some cases. The amino-acid substitutions generated would inhibit GTPase activity and thus activate α_{i2}. Although the physiological role of the G_{i2} gene in the adrenal is unknown, the presence of an activated α chain would obviously disrupt whatever basic physiological pathway is involved. The authors have therefore proposed that these mutations convert the α_{i2} gene into a putative oncogene, *gip 2* (for G inhibitory protein 2).

Adrenocortical Hyperfunction

There are three main syndromes within this spectrum. Cushing's syndrome results from the prolonged hypersecretion of cortisol; Conn's syndrome from primary hyperaldosteronism and the adrenogenital syndrome from excessive secretion of androgens or, less commonly, oestrogens.

Cushing's Syndrome

Cushing's syndrome comprises a well recognized group of clinical signs and symptoms due to excessive circulating glucocorticoids. Because of the wide ranging effects of cortisol on metabolism, there is a high morbidity and mortality in untreated patients. The syndrome occurs most commonly in women, but may present in men, and rarely, in children.

Increased protein breakdown leads to loss of muscle bulk, particularly on the limbs; centripetal deposition of fat results in moon face, buffalo hump and truncal obesity; inhibition of protein synthesis and abnormal collagen maturation cause abdominal striae (Fig. 23.20). There is hypertension. Osteoporosis may lead to vertebral collapse. Proximal myopathy is common. Diminished glucose tolerance is present, with hyperglycaemia and glycosuria in up to 20% of cases. Wound healing may be delayed. Mental symptoms are common with depression and sometimes psychosis. In some cases, there is also excess secretion of androgens, with hirsutism, amenorrhoea and virilization.

While there are three main causes as discussed below, it must be remembered that the **long-term therapeutic administration of glucocorticoids** may produce the features of Cushing's syndrome and such patients are referred to as 'Cushingoid'.

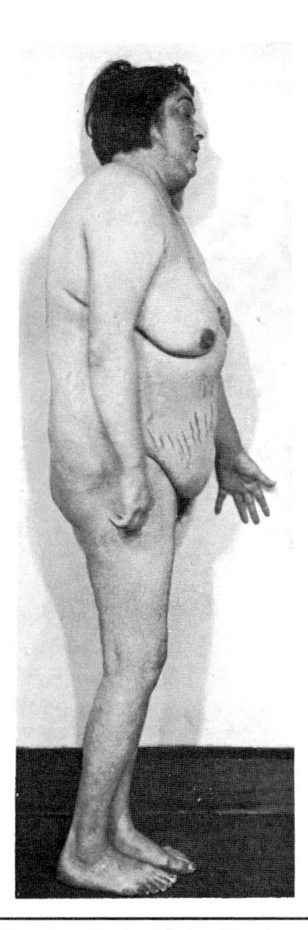

Fig. 23.20 A patient with Cushing's syndrome. Note the characteristic obesity of face, neck and trunk, dusky cyanosis, and facial hair and striae of the abdominal skin.

Cushing's disease (pituitary-driven Cushing's syndrome). This accounts for about 70% of cases of Cushing's syndrome. Excess ACTH secretion from the pituitary gland results in hyperstimulation of the adrenals and bilateral adrenal hyperplasia which may be diffuse or nodular. In diffuse hyperplasia the cortex is broadened; most glands weigh between 6 and 12 g (Fig. 23.21). Nodular hyperplasia is less common; obvious nodules up to 2.5 cm in diameter are present and the glands are markedly enlarged. Whether this develops from diffuse hyperplasia in long-standing disease is unclear. There are raised plasma glucocorticoid levels which can, however, be suppressed by high doses of dexamethasone. ACTH

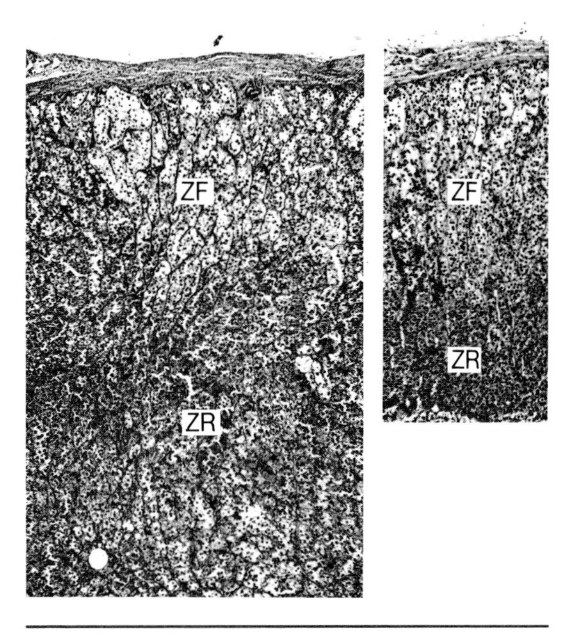

Fig. 23.21 Hyperplasia of the adrenal cortex in pituitary-dependent Cushing's syndrome **a** compared with a normal adrenal **b**. There is a general increase in width of the cortex with a relative increase in the width of the zona reticularis (ZR) and reduction in the zona fasciculata (ZF).

levels are usually just above the normal reference range, with loss of normal circadian rhythm.

Adrenal tumours. Adrenal tumours with autonomous secretion of cortisol account for about 20% of cases in adults, 80% of tumours occurring in women. Approximately half of these adrenal tumours are malignant, although the problems of making this distinction have already been discussed. Adrenal tumours account for 50% of Cushing's syndrome in children and carcinoma is more common. Cushing's syndrome with features of virilization (so-called 'mixed' Cushing's syndrome) is often seen in association with large, especially malignant tumours.

Because of increased glucocorticoid feedback, ACTH secretion is suppressed. This results in atrophy of the contralateral adrenal and of the adrenal remnant adjacent to the tumour. When the tumour is surgically removed, it is necessary, therefore, to administer glucocorticoids to the patient until ACTH secretion is re-established and regeneration of the remaining adrenal tissue occurs.

Biochemically, there are raised plasma glucocorticoid levels, which cannot be suppressed by high doses of dexamethasone. Plasma ACTH levels are low or undetectable due to the increased negative feedback by the high levels of cortisol.

Ectopic ACTH syndrome. In the remaining cases of Cushing's syndrome, there is secretion of ACTH from a non-pituitary tumour. These include small cell carcinoma of lung, thymic carcinoids and islet cell tumours of pancreas. With small cell carcinomas of lung, the full blown clinical picture of Cushing's syndrome may not develop because of the concomitant effects of a rapidly progressive cancer.

The large amounts of ACTH and related peptides secreted by the tumour produce bilateral adrenal hyperplasia. The adrenal weights are usually much heavier than in pituitary dependent Cushing's syndrome, ranging from 12 to over 20 g for a single gland.

Biochemical analysis shows high levels of plasma glucocorticoids which are not suppressed by high dose dexamethasone. There are raised ACTH levels, usually higher than in Cushing's disease. CT scans of appropriate sites may often localize the tumour.

Other causes. A rare cause of Cushing's syndrome, usually in young people, is primary adrenocortical nodular dysplasia in which the cortex is of normal weight, but consists of heavily pigmented lipofuscin containing nodules interspersed with atrophic cortex. The aetiology is unknown.

Hyperaldosteronism

Primary hyperaldosteronism – Conn's syndrome. This is characterized by hypertension, periodic muscle weakness or paralysis, muscle cramps and tetany, nocturia and polyuria. The biochemical features are hypokalaemia, metabolic alkalosis (high serum bicarbonate), high plasma aldosterone and low plasma renin levels, indicating autonomous secretion of aldosterone. In 80% of cases, it is due to an adrenal adenoma, three-quarters of these occurring in women. Carcinomas have been reported only rarely. In the remainder, there is bilateral hyperplasia of the zona glomerulosa of unknown aetiology. In cases with an adenoma, surgical removal is curative if performed before the vascular changes of hypertension become established.

Secondary hyperaldosteronism. Increased activity of the renin–angiotensin system will stimulate aldosterone secretion. This may occur in a wide variety of kidney diseases in which there is renal ischaemia (p. 464), in oedema (p. 76) and occasionally with a renin-secreting tumour (p. 941) or as a result of oestrogen administration. In contrast to Conn's syndrome, plasma aldosterone and renin levels are both high.

Adrenogenital Syndrome

Tumour associated. Androgens are more commonly secreted in excess than oestrogens and, in females, cause virilism (hirsutism and enlargement of the clitoris). This may occur in association with both benign and malignant tumours, sometimes as an isolated finding, sometimes in association with Cushing's syndrome ('mixed syndrome'). Very rarely, tumours, mostly carcinomas, may secrete oestrogens; in males, there is feminization with gynaecomastia, and testicular and penile atrophy and in female children there may be precocious puberty.

Congenital adrenal hyperplasia. This is a group of diseases due to congenital deficiency of one of the enzymes involved in the synthesis of cortisol (see Fig. 23.19). They are autosomal recessive and most present in infancy or early childhood. Although they are rare conditions, it is important to be aware of their existence because steroid replacement therapy at an early stage is important for normal life. Reduction in cortisol secretion results in decreased negative feedback. Hypersecretion of ACTH follows in an attempt to produce normal amounts of cortisol. In most cases this also results in the excess production of androgens. In some instances, there is also excessive secretion of intermediate steroids with mineralocorticoid effects. The clinical syndromes depend on the particular steroids secreted in each case.

In all cases, hyperstimulation results in adrenocortical hyperplasia. Each adrenal weighs an average of 15 g (normal range 1.5–3 g) and has a characteristic cerebriform appearance. Histologically, in most variants, the cortex is composed entirely of reticularis-like cells, with no lipid storage. Only in the rare 20,22-desmolase deficiency is there excessive cholesterol accumulation, because cholesterol cannot be converted to pregnenolone.

The commonest form is **21-hydroxylase deficiency** which occurs with a mean incidence of 1 in 14 000. Female infants are born with an enlarged clitoris and may have fusion of the labia (Fig. 23.22). The internal reproductive organs are normal. Males present with precocious puberty usually in early childhood. In two-thirds of cases, aldosterone synthesis is also impaired. Virilism is then accompanied by features of salt loss with dehydration, vomiting and hypotensive collapse. Deficiency of **11β-hydroxylase** is one-fifth as common. Deoxycorticosterone accumulates along with androgens, causing hypertension in addition to virilism.

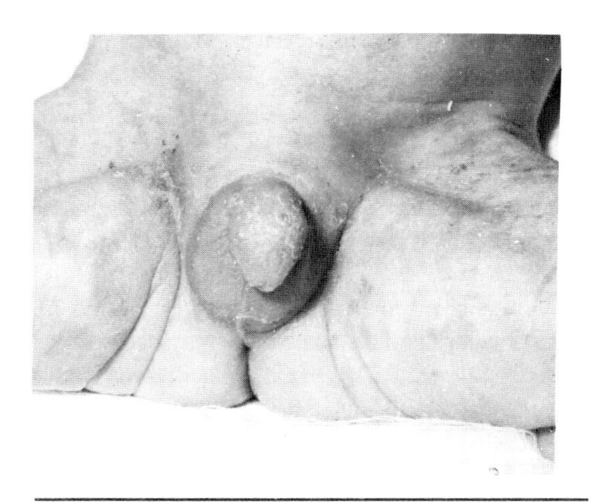

Fig. 23.22 Abnormal external genitalia of female child due to the action of androgens in a case of androgenital syndrome with 21-hydroxylase deficiency.

Adrenocortical Hypofunction

In both acute and chronic hypofunction around 90% of the cortex must be destroyed before clinical symptoms are present. Adrenocortical failure may be the result of primary disease of the adrenal gland, or it may be secondary to lack of ACTH release from the pituitary, most commonly as one aspect of panhypopituitarism.

Acute Adrenocortical Insufficiency

This may occur in septicaemic states, particularly due to meningococcal infection and is known as the **Waterhouse–Friedrichsen syndrome**. It is associated less frequently with other bacteraemic infections, including pneumococcus, staphylococcus or *Haemophilus influenzae*. The clinical presentation is of vomiting, salt loss with hyponatraemia, hyperkalaemia, hypoglycaemia and dehydration causing collapse, hypotension and sometimes death. Patients often have high fever, and a purpuric rash. There is haemorrhage into the adrenal glands, with extensive cortical necrosis. Although in the past it was thought that the adrenocortical failure played a major role in the vascular collapse in this disease, it is now realized that it is only one of several contributory factors, the major one being the massive bacteraemia and endotoxaemia.

Acute adrenocortical failure superimposed on chronic failure (Addisonian crisis) may occur when increased demands are made on a chronically failing adrenal cortex by, for example, infection or trauma. In addition, lack of corticosteroid cover in adrenalectomized patients may precipitate adrenal failure, as may the sudden withdrawal of glucocorticoids from patients on long-term treatment. It is critically important therefore that patients receiving glucocorticoids should be made fully aware of the risk of discontinuing these drugs. Acute adrenocortical failure may also be part of the acute presentation of congenital adrenal hyperplasia.

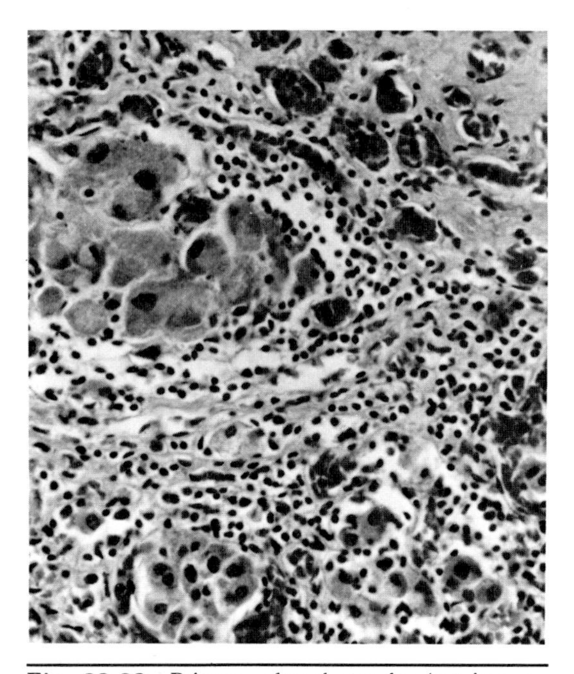

Fig. 23.23 Primary adrenal atrophy (autoimmune adrenalitis) in Addison's disease. Most of the cortical cells have been destroyed and the cortex consists mainly of vascular fibrous tissue. In places there are residual foci of enlarged cortical cells with associated lymphocytic and plasma cell infiltration.

Chronic Adrenocortical Insufficiency – Addison's Disease

In chronic adrenal insufficiency, there is general lethargy, muscle weakness, hypotension, anorexia and pigmentation of skin and mucous membranes. The commonest cause of chronic insufficiency is now **autoimmune adrenalitis**, which accounts for 75% of cases. The adrenals are atrophic with an infiltrate of lymphocytes and plasma cells (Fig. 23.23). The medulla is not affected. There is an association with other organ-specific autoimmune diseases, such as autoimmune thyroid disease, pernicious anaemia (p. 615), vitiligo and insulin-dependent diabetes mellitus (p. 799).

The second most common cause is **tuberculosis**, in which the medulla is also destroyed. The adrenals are enlarged (Fig. 23.24), and consist of masses of caseous material often with calcification which may be seen on X-ray. Occasionally amyloidosis, fungal infection or secondary tumour may result in adrenal failure.

Chronic adrenal insufficiency results in ACTH-cell hyperplasia with increased ACTH secretion by the pituitary. Occasionally an adenoma may form.

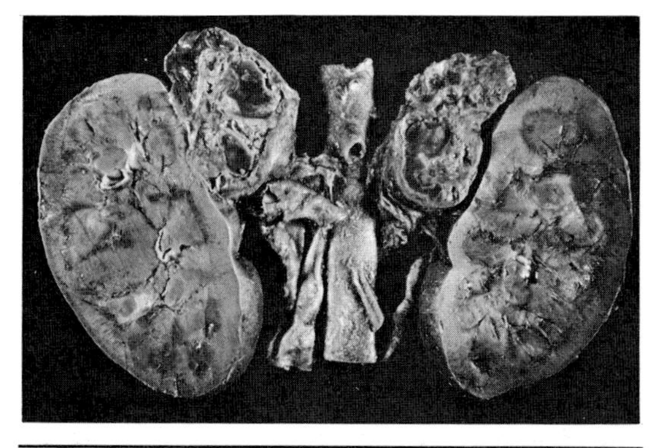

Fig. 23.24 Adrenal glands in tuberculous Addison's disease, showing extensive caseation and enlargement.

Adrenal Medulla

The adrenal medulla consists mainly of phaeochromocytes, or chromaffin cells, the latter name referring to their ability to reduce chrome salts to metallic chromium producing a brown colour reaction. In addition, there are scattered ganglion cells, autonomic nerve fibres and a population of dendritic sustenacular cells. The phaeochromocytes produce adrenaline and noradrenaline from tyrosine, with dopa and dopamine as intermediates. These catecholamines are secreted rapidly following stress, and they exert a wide range of adaptive effects.

Tumours

These are uncommon but may produce well-recognized clinical syndromes.

Phaeochromocytoma

These arise from the chromaffin cells, and produce symptoms as a result of secretion of catecholamines. They include hypertension, palpitation, sweating and sometimes collapse. There is hyperglycaemia and glycosuria. They occur in both sexes across a wide age range, but are uncommon in children: 10% are bilateral; 10% are familial, often found as part of the MEN 2 syndrome and arising on a background of medullary hyperplasia; 10% are malignant. They usually consist of cells arranged in an alveolar or trabecular pattern and, as with many other endocrine tumours, it is impossible to predict tumour behaviour in individual cases, metastasis being the only absolute criterion of malignancy. Occasionally they may secrete various peptides, giving rise to ectopic ACTH syndrome, and the watery diarrhoea, hypokalaemia, achlorhydria (WDHA) syndrome due to secretion of vasoactive intestinal polypeptide (VIP).

Morphologically similar tumours may arise in extra-adrenal paraganglia, where they are known as paragangliomas. The most common site for paraganglioma associated with hypertension is the organ of Zuckerkandl. These are more often malignant than are intra-adrenal tumours.

Other Tumours

Neuroblastoma is a tumour arising in children from the primitive cells of the medulla. Benign tumours may arise from the other components of the medulla and include **neurofibroma** and **ganglioneuroma**, fibroma and angioma.

Occasionally pseudocysts may develop, due to haemorrhage into adrenal tumours. Haemopoietic tissue is frequently seen as an incidental finding in the adrenal at autopsy. Rarely, this may coexist with adipose tissue, the so-called myelolipoma. Metastases are common, particularly from bronchial carcinoma.

The Parathyroid Glands

The parathyroids develop from the third and fourth branchial pouches. There are usually four, lying posterior to the thyroid gland, two at the upper and two at the lower poles. However, one or more may be intrathyroidal, or lie in the lower neck or upper mediastinum in close relationship to the thymus, which also develops from the third branchial pouch. The total weight is 120 mg in adult males and 140 mg in females, the upper limit of normal for an individual gland being 50 mg. They consist of two main cell types: (1) **chief cells**, the main functional group are usually eosinophilic, but may have a clear cell appearance, depending on the intracellular glycogen content; and (2) **oxyphil cells**, which are slightly larger, with a strongly eosinophilic rather granular cytoplasm, due to the presence of large numbers of mitochondria. The number of these cells increases with age. Stromal fat is present after puberty, and constitutes up to 30% of the normal adult gland.

The parathyroids secrete **parathormone**, an 84 amino-acid peptide, cleaved to a hormonally active N-terminal peptide of 34 amino acids which has a major role in regulating calcium metabolism and raising blood calcium levels. This is achieved by several mechanisms: mobilization of calcium from bone (p. 948), increased reabsorption by the kidney and indirectly by stimulation of synthesis of 1,25-dihydroxyvitamin D_3 (1,25$(OH)_2D_3$) in the kidney (p. 950), which increases calcium absorption from the gut. The secretion of parathormone appears to be controlled directly by calcium levels.

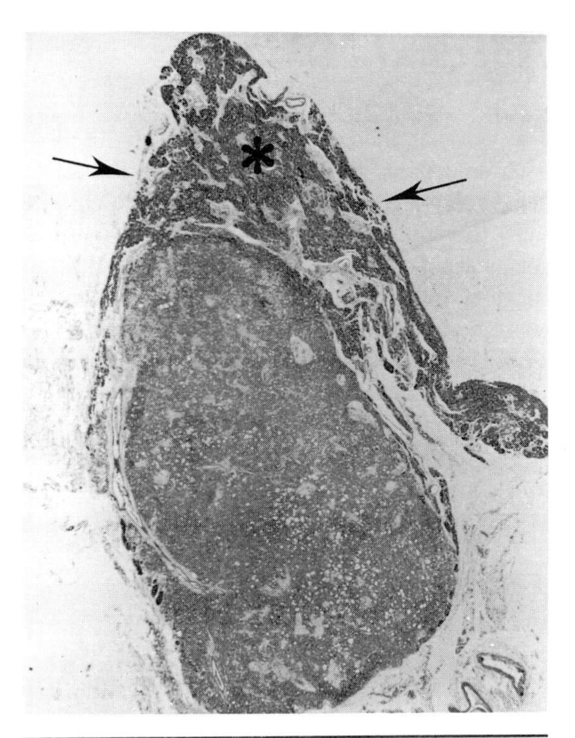

Fig. 23.25 Parathyroid adenoma. The fairly uniform adenoma is surrounded by a rim of normal parathyroid (stained darker) in which the parathyroid cells are interspersed with adipose tissue.

Hyperparathyroidism

This may be classified as primary or secondary. In primary hyperparathyroidism there is excessive secretion of parathormone without any apparent physiological stimulus. Secondary hyperparathyroidism occurs when the glands are exposed to increased physiological stimulation, most often in chronic renal failure.

Primary Hyperparathyroidism

Excessive secretion of parathormone results in hypercalcaemia, hypophosphataemia and increased excretion of calcium in the urine. The disease occurs most often in middle age, with a slight preponderance of women. Patients may present with general tiredness and muscular weakness. In the past, more than 50% of patients presented with symptoms of renal calculi. Nowadays, with earlier, more detailed biochemical investigation of patients with these general symptoms, primary hyperparathyroidism is often diagnosed before renal calculi and severe bone disease, with osteitis fibrosa cystica (p. 955) have developed. Other complications include duodenal ulceration and acute pancreatitis. Metastatic calcification may occur in the kidney, causing nephrocalcinosis and renal failure and in the soft tissues, heart and other organs.

In 80% of patients, the disease is due to a single **parathyroid adenoma** (Fig. 23.25). This is usually tan coloured and consists histologically of chief cells with a variable content of clear and oxyphil cells. Occasional adenomas are of oxyphil cell type. There is often a compressed rim of normal gland. In 15–20% of cases there is enlargement of more than one gland which is thought to be **primary hyperplasia**. Histologically, there is an admixture of chief, oxyphil and transitional oxyphil cells. It is therefore important for the surgeon to examine all parathyroids in order to exclude this diagnosis. In 2–3% of cases the disease is caused by a **parathyroid carcinoma**. As with other endocrine tumours, this is a difficult histological diagnosis to make. The presence of broad fibrous bands, mitotic activity and invasion of capsule and blood vessels are indicative of malignancy.

Primary hyperparathyroidism may occur as part of the MEN 1 and 2 syndromes, and in these cases hyperplasia is the more common diagnosis.

Secondary Hyperparathyroidism

Persistent low serum levels of ionized calcium will result in increased stimulation of parathormone release from the parathyroid glands, and result in hyperplasia indistinguishable on morphological grounds from primary hyperplasia. This occurs most commonly in chronic renal failure but may also be seen in malabsorption syndromes and with vitamin D deficiency.

Occasionally a patient with secondary hyperparathyroidism becomes hypercalcaemic. This is referred to as **tertiary hyperparathyroidism**. It is thought that some cells in a parathyroid gland become autonomous, i.e. insensitive to the controlling effects of Ca^{2+}, and an inappropriately high level of parathormone results. In some cases an adenomatous nodule may develop.

Hypoparathyroidism

Deficiency of parathormone results in hypocalcaemia and hyperphosphataemia. The low calcium levels cause increased muscular tone and if severe, characteristic muscle spasms, known as tetany. There may also be mental changes and convulsions, and patients often develop cataracts.

The most common cause is surgical removal of the parathyroids, sometimes inadvertently during thyroidectomy or head and neck surgery. The condition also forms part of the diGeorge syndrome (p. 239) in which there is failure of development of the third and fourth branchial pouches, and thus aplasia or hypoplasia of both thymus and parathyroid glands. This variant presents more commonly in infants or children than in adults. Finally, the parathyroid gland may very occasionally be involved by autoimmune disease. In such cases, there may be a familial association with autoimmune diseases of other endocrine glands.

Pseudohypoparathyroidism. In this condition, circulating parathormone levels are normal or elevated, but the patient is hypocalcaemic and hyperphosphataemic, indicating a lack of response to the hormone. Many of these patients have been shown to have low levels of the α-subunit of G_s protein, and it is suggested that this may be the mechanism for the reduced response. Multiple somatic abnormalities occur in this disease including short stature, soft tissue calcification and mental retardation. Although the serum Ca^{2+} is low the calcium phosphate product is elevated. It may be that these somatic effects are also related to reduced intracellular responses to ligands acting via a G_s protein.

Multiple Endocrine Neoplasia (MEN) Syndromes

In these uncommon syndromes, tumours or hyperplasia occur in more than one endocrine gland either in the same individual or in members of a family. There are two main types, which are inherited as autosomal dominants. Although rare, it is important to recognize their existence because, once an index case is diagnosed, screening of family members is important to detect other affected individuals. Most of these tumours develop on a basis of hyperplasia, and by detecting biochemical abnormalities at this stage, it is possible to undertake prophylactic surgery and prevent progression to tumour.

MEN Type 1 (Wermer's Syndrome)

This syndrome is now thought to be linked to genetic abnormalities on the long arm of chromosome 11. Parathyroid tumours occur in 95% of patients; these are accompanied by pancreatic islet cell tumours producing gastrin, insulin, pancreatic polypeptide or occasionally glucagon. Pituitary tumours also occur, the majority secreting prolactin or growth hormone.

MEN Type 2

This has two main variants. The gene for MEN 2a has been mapped to an area near the centromere on chromosome 10. MEN 2b has not been so accurately mapped as yet, but it is thought that it may be the result of different mutations at the same locus.

MEN 2a (Sipple's syndrome). Medullary carcinoma of thyroid is the main tumour, and it is accompanied by phaeochromocytoma in about 50% of cases and by parathyroid adenoma or hyperplasia in up to 40%. The thyroid and adrenal tumours are preceded by hyperplasia.

MEN 2b. Medullary carcinoma of thyroid and phaeochromocytoma are associated with neuromas in the mucosa of the lips, tongue, eyelids and cornea. Ganglioneuromas develop in the gut. Medullary carcinoma of thyroid is extremely aggressive in this form of the disease and invariably fatal.

The Pineal Gland

This tiny gland is situated above the posterior part of the third ventricle. Its functions are unclear, but it secretes melatonin, which may play some role in the regulation of body rhythms. The commonest lesions are tumours occurring mainly in childhood, and include gliomas, teratomas and tumours morphologically indistinguishable from seminomas (p. 1059). These cause local pressure effects with hydrocephalus and ocular paralyses. They may also be associated with precocious puberty, although the mechanism of induction is unclear.

Further Reading

Kovacs, K. and Asa, S. (eds) (1990). *Functional Endocrine Pathology*. Blackwell Scientific Publications, Boston.

Kovacs, K. and Horvath, E. (1986). Tumours of the pituitary gland. *Atlas of Tumour Pathology, Fascicle 21*, Second Series, Hartmann, W. H. and Sobin, L. H. (eds). Armed Forces Institute of Pathology, Washington.

Thakker, R. V. and Ponder, B. A. J. (1988). Multiple endocrine neoplasia. *Baillière's Clinical Endocrinology and Metabolism* **2**, 1031–67.

24
The Skin

The skin is a highly complex organ which performs numerous functions including protection against ultraviolet irradiation, infection and mechanical trauma; temperature regulation; absorption and excretion of fluid; metabolism of vitamin D; immunological surveillance; sensory perception and cosmesis.

Epidermis

The light microscopic appearances of the skin are shown in diagrammatic form in Fig. 24.1. The thickness of the epidermis and its overlying corneal layer and the number and types of adnexal structures vary considerably between different body sites. The epidermis is a keratinizing stratified squamous epithelium from which arises the adnexal skin structures – the sebaceous glands, sweat glands, nails and hair. It comprises four clearly defined layers in which there is progressive maturation from the basal germinative layer to the outermost acellular protective corneal layer.

Ultrastructurally the epidermal cells, **keratinocytes**, are seen to contain abundant filamentous material consisting of cytokeratins. These are a class of intermediate filament (p. 8) which form part of the cytoskeleton of the keratinocyte. The germinative **basal layer** cells contain only low molecular weight cytokeratins but the more specialized differentiated cells of the upper layers contain both low and high molecular weight cytokeratins. The keratinocytes are anchored together by intercellular junctions termed desmosomes. These may be seen on light microscopy as tiny 'spines' around the cell boundaries, particularly in the **stratum spinosum** which derives its name from this feature. Within the cytoplasm of the cells of the stratum spinosum and **stratum granulosum** there are granules termed Odland bodies. These are discharged by the granular layer cells into the intercellular space where they act as a water barrier and they are also important in cell cohesion within the lower stratum corneum. The cells of the stratum granulosum also contain large, easily visible basophilic granules termed keratohyaline granules, one of the constituents of which is a precursor of the protein filaggrin. This protein is present in the **stratum corneum** which forms the major physical barrier of the skin and consists of a complex network of keratin filaments

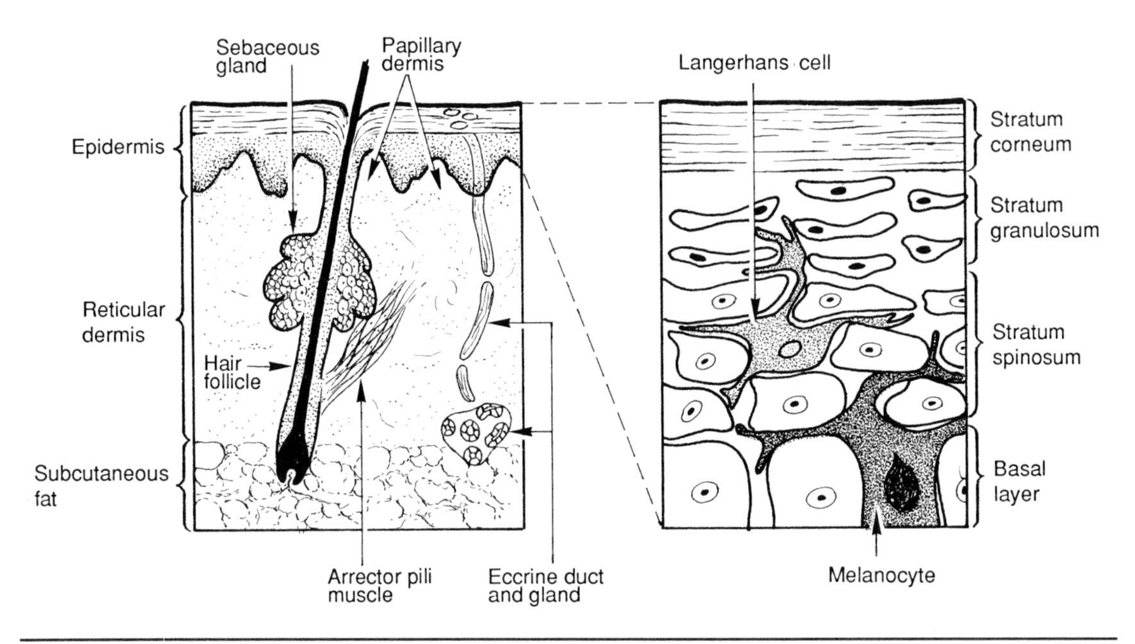

Fig. 24.1 The microanatomy of the skin (left) and the layers of the epidermis (right).

'glued' together by filaggrin. The keratinocytes in the stratum corneum are non-viable and cell nuclei are not present under normal circumstances.

The **basement membrane zone** is a complex area between the epidermis and the dermis (Fig. 24.2). A basic understanding of its structure is helpful as it may be altered or damaged in some inherited disorders, e.g. epidermolysis bullosa, and is a site of deposition of immune complexes, e.g. in bullous pemphigoid. The basal cells of the epidermis are attached to the basement membrane zone by hemidesmosomes. Immediately under the basal cell there is a clear area, the lamina lucida, and beneath this there is the lamina densa which is composed primarily of type IV collagen and has a barrier function, restricting the passage of high molecular weight molecules. It is connected to the dermis by anchoring fibrils composed predominantly of type VII collagen.

Although the most numerous cells in the epidermis are the keratinocytes, several other cell types are present. These include melanocytes, Langerhans cells and neuroendocrine cells.

Melanocytes migrate during fetal life from the neural crest to the basal layer of the epidermis. They are dendritic cells but appear as rounded cells with clear cytoplasm in routine fixed tissue sections. They contain membrane-bound organelles termed melanosomes in which melanin pigment is synthesized. This pigment protects the

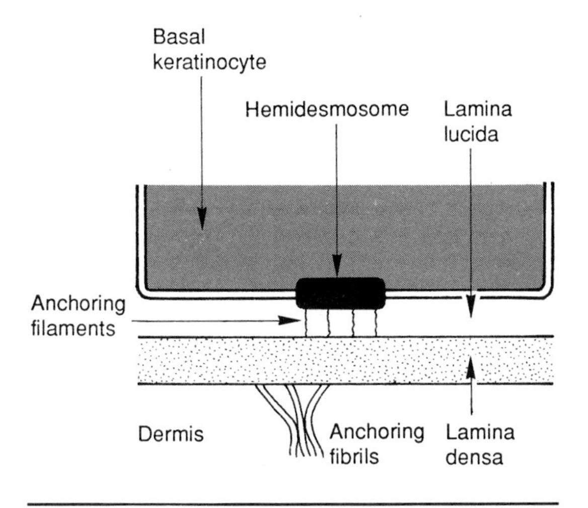

Fig. 24.2 Basement membrane zone of human skin.

skin from the harmful effects of ultraviolet irradiation and is transferred to keratinocytes of the basal and spinous layers of the epidermis from the dendritic processes of the melanocytes.

Langerhans cells are also dendritic cells and are present in the suprabasal layers of the epidermis and in smaller numbers in the dermis. They are difficult to identify in routine fixed tissue sections but they can be demonstrated by immunohistochemical techniques as they bear the CD1 antigen on their surface. They possess surface receptors for the Fc component of IgG and for C3 and they express HLA-DR on their surface. Ultrastructurally, they contain characteristic granules in their cytoplasm termed Birbeck granules. These bone marrow derived cells belong to the mononuclear phagocyte series and are important in the processing and presentation of antigen. They are thought to play an important role in delayed hypersensitivity reactions such as contact dermatitis.

Neuroendocrine cells (Merkel cells) of the skin cannot be demonstrated reliably by conventional microscopy. They are found in association with intraepidermal peripheral nerve endings and ultrastructurally, possess cytoplasmic membrane-bound dense-core granules similar to those found in other cells of the diffuse endocrine system. They contain neuron-specific enolase (NSE) which allows them to be demonstrated by immunostaining. Merkel cells are thought to function as mechanoreceptors. They are irregularly distributed but are found predominantly on the lips, in the oral cavity, in relation to hair follicles and on the finger tips.

Dermis

The epidermis is supported by the dermis which is divided into two areas, the superficial or **papillary dermis** and the deep or **reticular dermis**. Both areas are composed of collagen, elastic tissue and ground substance and are richly supplied by blood vessels and nerves. The collagen in the reticular dermis is predominantly type I whilst the papillary dermis consists mainly of the finer type III collagen. The dermis also contains the skin adnexae such as hair follicles and their associated sebaceous glands, eccrine sweat glands and, in some sites, apocrine sweat glands.

Terminology in Skin Pathology

Certain terms are used commonly in dermatopathology and are defined here.

Acantholysis: a disturbance of the intercellular connections between keratinocytes with a resultant loss of cell-to-cell cohesion. Individual keratinocytes detach from one another and the acantholytic cells take on a more rounded appearance than usual. One of the diseases in which this process occurs is pemphigus vulgaris where the damage to the intercellular connections is immunologically mediated (p. 1118).

Acanthosis: thickening of the epidermis due mainly to increase of the stratum spinosum.

Bulla: a large (greater than 5 mm diameter) fluid filled blister.

Vesicle: a small (less than 5 mm diameter) fluid filled blister.

Dyskeratosis: premature keratinization of single cells or groups of cells within the epidermis.

Hyperkeratosis: thickening of the corneal layer of the epidermis.

Parakeratosis: the presence of nuclei within the stratum corneum as a result of abnormal maturation of the epidermis.

Spongiosis: the presence of intercellular oedema fluid within the epidermis.

Non-neoplastic Disorders of the Skin

Infections of the Skin

Bacterial Infection

Infective Folliculitis

Superficial infection of the hair follicle by *Staphylococcus aureus* is a common disorder leading to formation of small red pustules which resolve following discharge of pus. If, however, the follicle fails to discharge its contents the infection spreads into the adjacent dermis resulting in a furuncle or 'boil' (p. 294).

Impetigo

This is a superficial skin infection caused by *Staphylococcus aureus* or less commonly by haemolytic streptococci. It occurs in children and immunosuppressed patients and causes crusted superficial vesicles around the nose and mouth.

Staphylococcal Scalded Skin Syndrome

This condition occurs mainly in children and neonates and is due to the effects of a toxin produced by *Staphylococcus aureus* usually of phage type 71. The original infection may be occult or in the upper respiratory tract or middle ear. The child develops a spreading erythematous rash with superficial peeling of the skin. Histological examination shows a split in the granular layer of the epidermis with little inflammation. The prognosis is relatively good in infants but the rare cases described in adults carry a considerable mortality.

Mycobacterial Infection

The most common form of tuberculosis of the skin is referred to as **lupus vulgaris**. It is usually the result of haematogenous spread from a distant tuberculous focus. One or more reddish patches are present on the face particularly around the nose and, on close inspection, small yellow-brown gelatinous nodules, 'apple-jelly nodules', may be seen. The lesions show typical tuberculous granulomas, often with little or no caseation. These are present in the superficial dermis and may extend up to the epidermis and ulcerate. The condition progresses slowly and results in scarring and disfigurement.

Atypical mycobacteria such as *Mycobacterium marinum* may infect the skin. This organism can infect minor skin abrasions and injuries and may cause lesions on the hands of individuals who keep tropical fish tanks or may be contracted from swimming pools ('swimming pool granuloma').

Leprosy is discussed on p. 308.

Spirochaetal Infection

Lyme Disease (Erythema Chronicum Migrans)

This infection occurs in Europe and in North America where it has recently generated considerable publicity. It takes its name from the town in Connecticut where the first major outbreak was reported. It is caused by the spirochaete *Borrelia burgdorferi* and is transmitted by tick bites. Patients develop an erythematous skin rash which starts around a tick bite. There may be neurological, cardiac and joint complications and residual arthritis may be a long-term sequela (p. 967).

The cutaneous manifestations of **syphilis** are discussed on p. 317.

Viral Infection

Human Papillomavirus Infection

The human papillomavirus (HPV) is a DNA virus. Over 40 subtypes have now been identified. The **common wart (verruca vulgaris)** is caused by HPV types 2, 4 and 7. It is seen particularly in children and occurs most often on the hands and fingers. Florid crops of viral warts may be seen in immunosuppressed patients, e.g. following renal transplantation. Histologically, there is a thickened epidermis which is thrown into papillary folds; the rete ridges are elongated and those at the periphery curve inwards (Fig. 24.3). There is hyperkeratosis which, in young lesions, alternates with parakeratosis. The cells in the upper layers of the epidermis have a vacuolated cytoplasm with eosinophilic inclusions and some contain large clumped keratohyaline granules. Basophilic nuclear inclusions may be identifiable.

The **plantar wart** caused by HPV 1, 2 and 4 occurs on the sole of the foot and may be deep and painful when caused by HPV 1.

The **plane wart (verruca plana)** is most common on the face and hands and is caused by HPV 3. It shows less papillomatosis than the common wart and diffuse vacuolation of the cells in the granular layer.

Other examples of HPV infection include the **condyloma acuminatum** or genital wart (p. 1069) and **Bowenoid papulosis** of the genitalia.

Molluscum Contagiosum

This common lesion is caused by a pox virus which measures 300 × 240 × 230 nm and is shaped like a brick with a dumb-bell shaped DNA core. It occurs on the face, trunk and limbs of children and in adults may occur on the genitalia following sexual transmission. The lesions are often multiple and consist of small firm umbilicated papules. Microscopically, there is a downgrowth of epidermis into the dermis (Fig. 24.4). The keratinocytes contain

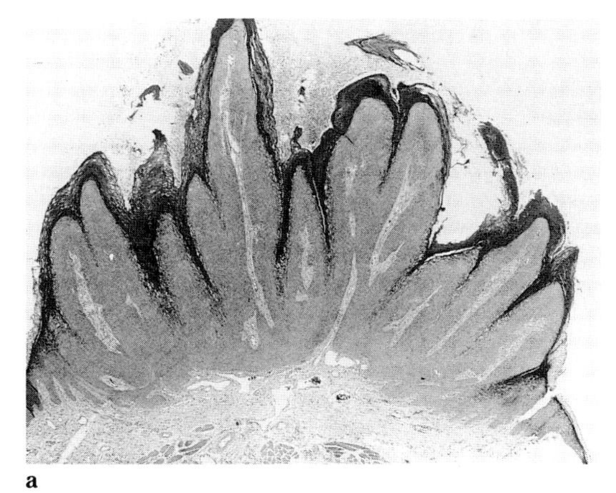

a

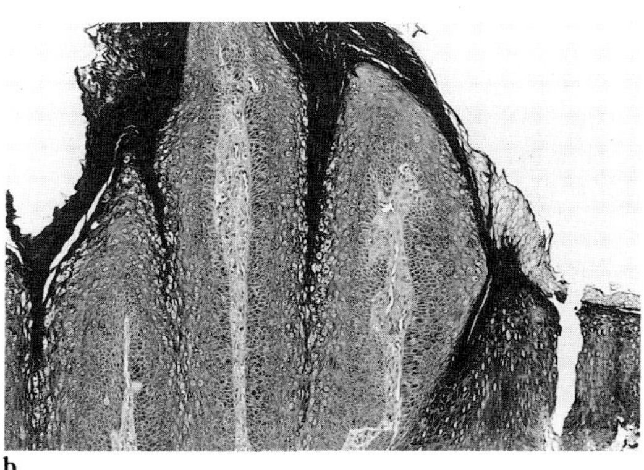

b

Fig. 24.3 **a** Verruca vulgaris. Note hyperkeratosis, papillomatosis and inward curving of peripheral rete ridges. ×28. **b** Verruca vulgaris. Marked vacuolation of cytoplasm of keratinocytes in upper epidermis. ×110.

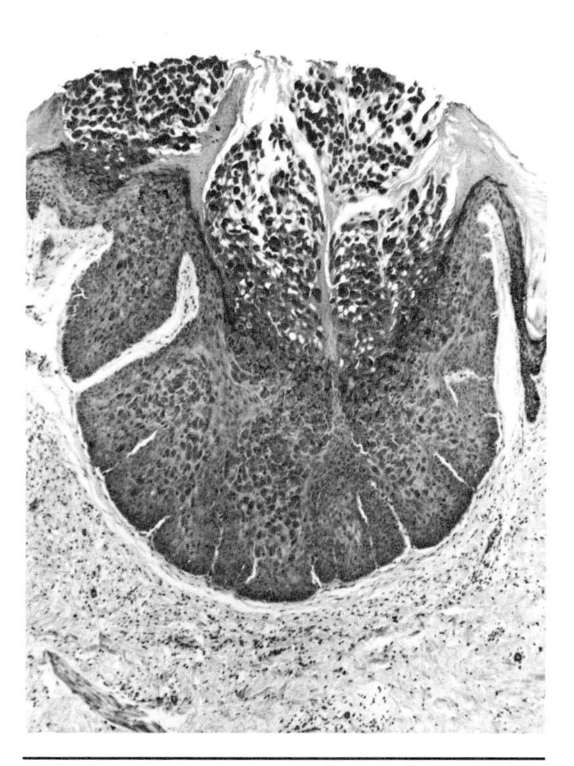

Fig. 24.4 Molluscum contagiosum. The lesion is a sharply localized epithelial proliferation with enlargement of the keratinocytes by cytoplasmic inclusion bodies. ×70.

a large intracytoplasmic inclusion body, composed of many virions, which compresses the nucleus to one side and becomes more basophilic, forming the Henderson–Paterson body as the cell reaches the surface.

Herpes Simplex Virus

Herpes simplex virus (HSV) type 1 is responsible for recurrent 'cold sores' around the mouth. Most people acquire the infection asymptomatically in childhood and thereafter the virus remains latent, but it may reactivate due to sunburn, a febrile illness or stress, producing the typical lesions around the lips. The virus may colonize the skin of children with atopic dermatitis causing a severe condition known as Kaposi's varicelliform eruption. HSV type 2 causes genital herpes and is transmitted by sexual contact. The histological features of herpes simplex infection are virtually identical to those of herpes zoster.

Varicella and Herpes Zoster

Varicella virus infection is the cause of chickenpox which is most commonly seen in childhood. The virus can persist for years in the posterior root ganglia and herpes zoster ('shingles') occurs usually in adults as a result of reactivation of this latent infection (p. 327). The virus reaches the skin, presumably via the sensory nerves, and produces a crop of painful lesions in the area supplied by a nerve – most commonly on the trunk, face or arm. Histologically there is intracellular oedema of the keratinocytes (balloon degeneration) progressing to rupture of the cells to produce an intraepidermal vesicle. Some cell walls persist as strands within the vesicle (reticular degeneration). Multinucleated epidermal cells and intranuclear inclusion bodies are often seen (Fig. 24.5).

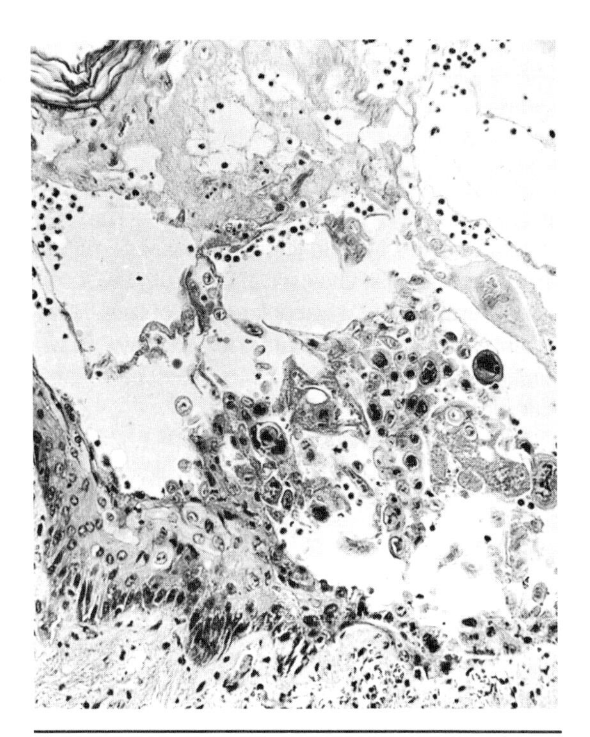

Fig. 24.5 Zoster. Multilocular intra-epidermal bulla, showing large swollen cells (balloon degeneration) and strands of cell walls traversing the bulla (reticular degeneration). ×350.

Fungal Infection

Superficial fungal infection of the skin caused by a variety of dermatophytes is not uncommon. They infect the keratin layer but do not extend into the deeper layers. Dermatophyte infections include *Tinea capitis* (ringworm of the scalp), *Tinea pedis* (athlete's foot) and *Tinea versicolor* which causes widespread areas of hypo- and hyperpigmentation on the trunk in coloured and white skins respectively.

Infection by *Candida albicans* can take a number of forms. Acute mucocutaneous candidiasis occurs as a complication of antibiotic or corticosteroid treatment or in the warm moist environment of the skin folds in obese individuals and infants. Vulvovaginal candida infection is common in pregnancy when the lowered vaginal pH promotes growth of the fungus. Chronic mucocutaneous candida infection occurs in patients with impaired cell mediated immunity and is one of the infections associated with the acquired immunodeficiency syndrome (AIDS).

Arthropod Infestation

The most common infestation is by the itch mite *Acarus scabiei* which causes scabies. The female mite burrows into the epidermis where it deposits its eggs. The lesions may be widespread but are particularly seen around the wrists and hands and in the genital region. They are intensely itchy, especially at night.

Non-infective Inflammatory Skin Diseases

Numerous conditions fall into this category, some rare and some extremely common. Three diseases – dermatitis, psoriasis and acne vulgaris – together comprise the vast majority of referrals to dermatology clinics for non-neoplastic disease and are discussed below. Other disorders discussed in this section include lichen planus, the bullous diseases, vascular and connective tissue diseases and granulomatous disorders.

Dermatitis (Eczema)

The term 'dermatitis' (often used synonymously with 'eczema') strictly speaking should refer to any inflammation of the skin; however, it is applied in a restricted sense in dermatology to a particular reaction of the skin which causes a set of recognizable clinical and histological features. Both the epidermis and dermis are involved in dermatitis and it may be seen in one of three stages which sometimes, but by no means always, show a progression from one to the next:

Acute dermatitis. The skin is red and there is weeping of a serous exudate. Sometimes small vesicles are present. The epidermis shows spongiosis which separates the keratinocytes. The spongiosis may become confluent with the formation of intraepidermal vesicles (Fig. 24.6). The dermis is oedematous and contains a mild inflammatory infiltrate consisting predominantly of lymphocytes and histiocytes.

Subacute dermatitis. The skin is again red but there is less exudation. There is often a severe itch with excoriation and crusting. Microscopically, there is less spongiosis and vesiculation, the epidermis is acanthotic and there is surface parakeratosis.

Chronic dermatitis. The skin becomes thickened and leathery due to long-standing scratching

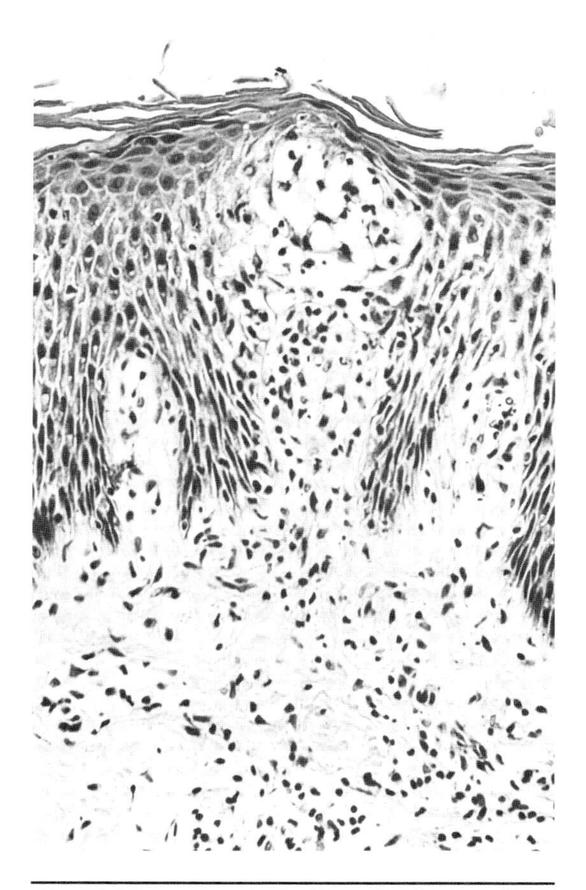

Fig. 24.6 Acute dermatitis, showing an intraepidermal vesicle containing leucocytes and degenerate epithelial cells. ×200.

and rubbing. There is marked acanthosis of the epidermis with hyperkeratosis and often parakeratosis. The upper dermis may be scarred and there is a chronic inflammatory cell infiltrate in the dermis (Fig. 24.7).

Despite the clinical and histological similarities there are wide differences in the aetiology and pathogenesis of the various types of dermatitis. These distinctions form the basis of a simplified method of classification into atopic and contact dermatitis and dermatitis of unknown aetiology.

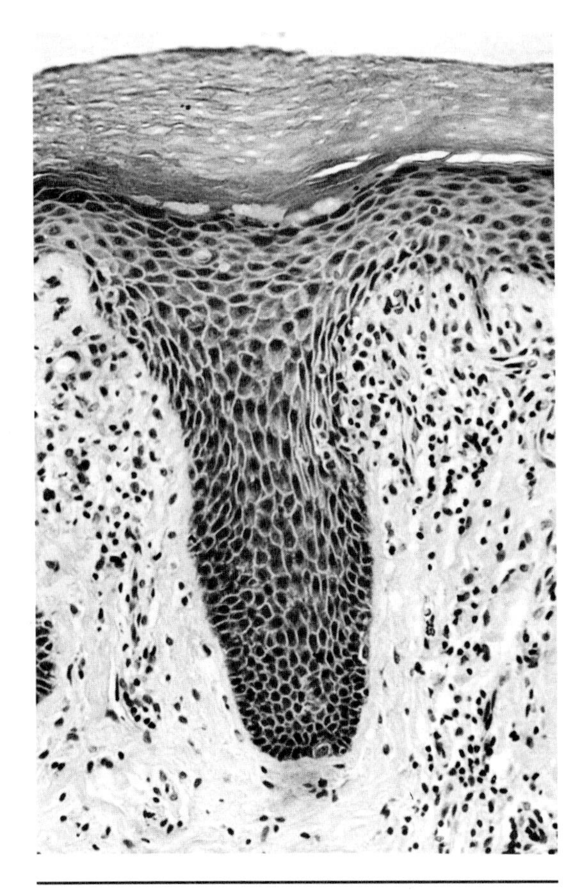

Fig. 24.7 Chronic dermatitis. There is hyperkeratosis, elongation of the rete ridges and a perivascular inflammatory infiltrate in the upper dermis. ×300.

Atopic Dermatitis

This is most common in infants and children and causes an intensely itchy rash which the child may constantly scratch, resulting in secondary infection. The disease may improve after adolescence and often completely clears, although some cases persist into adulthood. Atopic dermatitis is associated with excessive production of IgE to a variety of common allergens (p. 208). There is also a reduction in circulating CD8 positive suppressor T lymphocytes. Affected individuals may have a positive family history and may also suffer from asthma or hay fever.

Contact Dermatitis

This can be divided into two groups.

Contact irritant dermatitis is caused by direct damage to the skin by a number of potent irritants such as strong acid or alkali, detergent, phenol, etc.

Contact allergic dermatitis is caused by a type 4 delayed hypersensitivity reaction. Common allergens include nickel, chromate, dyes and synthetic rubber. Many compounds which cause contact allergic dermatitis are low molecular weight haptens which require to combine with an epidermal protein to become immunogenic. This conjugation probably occurs on the surface of a Langerhans cell. The subsequent cellular immune response is dependent on the hapten–protein complex being processed by the HLA-DR positive Langerhans cell and then presented to a specifically sensitized CD4 positive T-helper lymphocyte which is then stimulated to release a variety of lymphokines.

Dermatitis of Unknown Aetiology

This includes such clinically distinct disorders as seborrhoeic dermatitis and nummular dermatitis. **Seborrhoeic dermatitis** may show some resemblance to psoriasis. It affects areas rich in sebaceous glands such as the scalp and forehead, the eyelids and the upper chest. It is very common and often severe in patients with AIDS. **Nummular dermatitis** is a form of chronic dermatitis which causes characteristic coin shaped 'discoid' lesions.

Psoriasis

Psoriasis affects at least 1–2% of the population and in its classical form presents as well defined, red, oval plaques on the extensor surfaces of the knees and elbows, and on the sacrum and scalp. The lesions are covered by a fine silvery scale which, when gently scraped off, reveals fine bleeding points underneath (Auspitz sign). Some patients with chronic psoriasis show pitting of the finger and toe nails, and a small percentage develop a chronic seronegative arthritis (p. 995) which in some cases can closely resemble rheumatoid arthritis.

Microscopically, psoriatic plaques show acanthosis of the epidermis with regular elongation of club-shaped rete ridges. There is a parakeratotic scale on the surface which contains small collections of neutrophil polymorphs (Munro microabscesses) which have migrated through the epidermis from capillaries in the upper dermis. There is thinning of the epidermis over the broadened dermal papillae (Fig. 24.8).

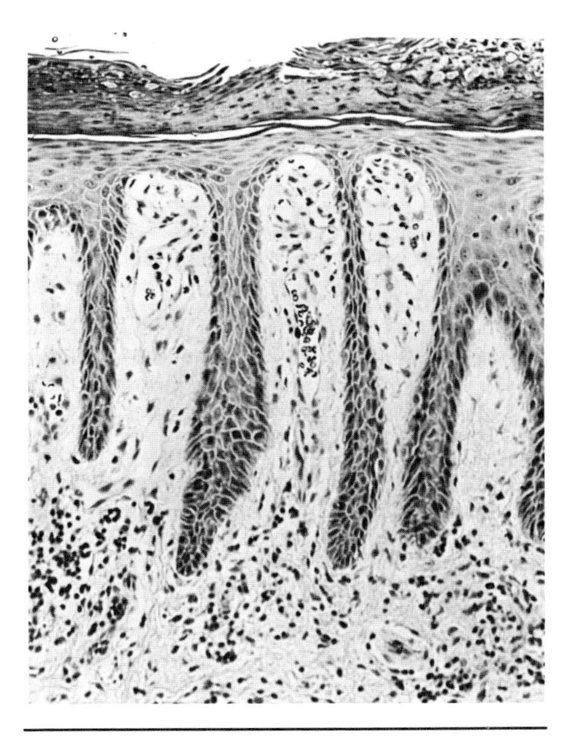

Fig. 24.8 Psoriasis. The surface is covered by a parakeratotic scale containing numerous polymorphonuclear leucocytes. The rete ridges are elongated and the suprapapillary epidermis is thinned. ×150.

Aetiology and Pathogenesis

Approximately one-third of affected individuals have a family history of the disease, and there is an association with the class I MHC antigens HLA-B13, HLA-B17, HLA-Bw16 and HLA-Cw6. A variety of stimuli, including trauma, infection and sunburn can precipitate psoriasis.

Although the aetiology is unknown, a number of abnormalities have been detected in psoriatic skin. One of these is a marked increase in the epidermal cell proliferation rate with a corresponding reduction in the transit time of keratinocytes through the epidermis. The germinative layer of the epidermis may be up to three layers thick compared to a single basal layer in normal skin. The acceleration of cell proliferation may be related to a disturbance in the normal ratio of the cyclic nucleotides adenosine 3,5-monophosphate (cAMP) and guanosine 3,5-monophosphate (cGMP) which are closely involved in cell proliferation. In psoriasis there is a reduction in cAMP and an increase in cGMP in the epidermal cells.

Acne Vulgaris

Acne vulgaris, a very common disorder, usually begins around puberty and particularly affects the face, chest and upper back. There is plugging of the pilosebaceous follicle by keratin and sebum, resulting in an expanded follicle termed a 'comedo'. If the comedo is connected to the surface of the epidermis it is visible as a 'blackhead' but if the canal is blocked a 'whitehead' forms. The whitehead is liable to rupture into the surrounding dermis, provoking an intense inflammatory reaction and causing the familiar pustules and nodules of acne. In severe cases there may be marked cyst formation and residual scarring.

The cause of acne is unknown; however, circulating androgens may be elevated, especially in severe cases. The onset of acne at puberty coincides with a rise in circulating androgens. Sebum production is also important in the development of the disorder. Acne occurs in sites which are rich in sebaceous glands and in some severe cases the administration of 13-*cis*-retinoic acid, which reduces sebum production, has a beneficial effect. The skin commensal *Propionibacterium acnes* may also contribute to the development of acne and the therapeutic effect of oral tetracycline may be due to suppression of this organism although this is not proven.

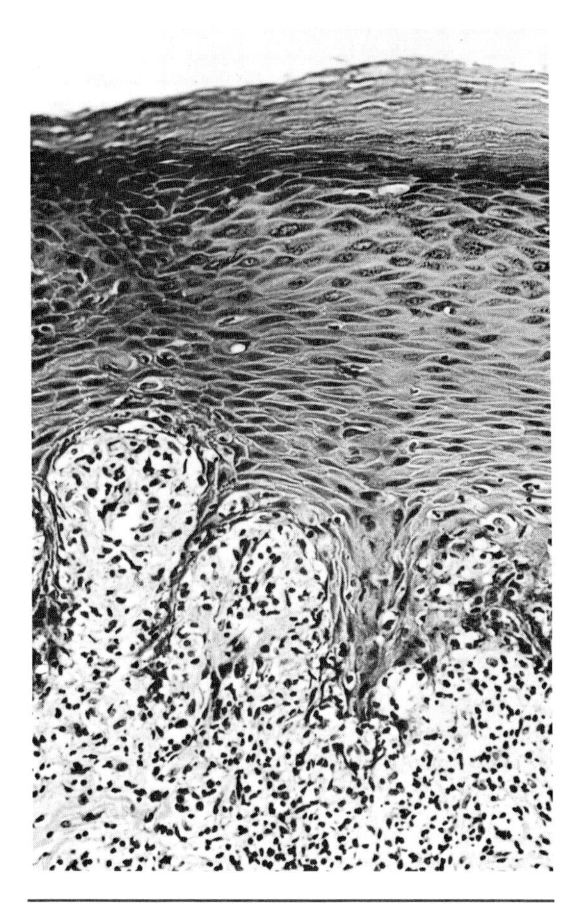

Fig. 24.9 Lichen planus. Note the hypertrophy of the granular layer and the saw-tooth appearance of the rete ridges. ×200.

Lichen Planus

Small itchy violaceous papules affecting the forearms, legs and genitalia, together with white narrow streaks on the buccal mucosa (see Fig. 16.5), characterize this disorder. Delicate networks of white lines (Wickham's striae) may be seen on the surface of the lesions.

Microscopically (Fig. 24.9) there is acanthosis of the epidermis, the base of which has a characteristic jagged, 'saw-toothed' appearance. There is liquefaction degeneration of the basal layer, a destructive process in which there is necrosis of basal keratinocytes the remains of which can be identified as anuclear, eosinophilic colloid bodies at the dermoepidermal junction. A dense band of lymphocytes is present in the upper dermis. The aetiology of lichen planus is unknown but it may involve a delayed hypersensitivity reaction to an epidermal antigen. Epidermal Langerhans cells are present in increased numbers in the early stages of the disease and the lymphocytic infiltrate is predominantly of the CD4 positive T-helper/inducer subset. Certain drugs such as gold (used in severe rheumatoid arthritis) can cause skin rashes similar to lichen planus.

Bullous Diseases

The major bullous diseases are summarized in Table 24.1. A number are immunologically mediated and immunofluorescence (IF) tests play an important role in their investigation. In the indirect IF test, a fresh tissue substrate such as baboon oesophagus is treated successively with the patient's serum and fluorescein-labelled anti-immunoglobulin in order to detect the presence of antibodies to a constituent of squamous epithelium. In the direct IF test, unfixed cryostat sections of the patient's skin are treated with fluorescein-labelled anti-immunoglobulins and

Table 24.1 The major bullous diseases

	Clinical presentation	Site of blister	Additional histological features	Immunopathology
Pemphigus vulgaris	Fragile blisters and erosions on skin and mucosae	Intraepidermal	Acantholytic keratinocytes float in the bulla cavity	Intercellular IgG deposits in epidermis and circulating IgG antibodies to intercellular material (titre correlates with disease severity)
Bullous pemphigoid	Tense bullae; elderly patients; may involve oral mucosa	Subepidermal	Often numerous eosinophils in the dermis and bulla	Linear deposits of IgG and C3 along basement membrane (lamina lucida). Circulating anti-basement membrane IgG
Epidermolysis bullosa (congenital)	Blisters during infancy or childhood	Subepidermal	No associated inflammation	None
Epidermis bullosa acquisita	Blistering after trauma in adults	Subepidermal	No associated inflammation	Linear subepidermal deposits of IgG and C3 (under lamina densa); circulating anti-basement membrane IgG
Herpes gestationis	Itchy vesicles in pregnancy and puerperium	Subepidermal	Numerous eosinophils, dermal oedema and basal cell necrosis	Linear C3 deposits along basement membrane (lamina lucida); circulating herpes gestationis factor, a complement-fixing anti-basement membrane IgG
Dermatitis herpetiformis	Itchy vesicles in young adults; associated with gluten sensitive enteropathy (coeliac disease)	Subepidermal	Neutrophils in upper dermis, 'papillary, microabscesses'	Granular IgA deposits in dermal papillae under lamina densa; no similar circulating antibody demonstrable
Porphyria cutanea tarda	Blistering and scarring in sun-exposed skin in adults	Subepidermal	PAS positive material around dermal blood vessels	IgG 'trapped' by fibrillar material in blood vessel walls
Erythema multiforme	Acute eruption – may follow viral infection, drugs, etc.	Subepidermal	Keratinocyte necrosis; roof of bulla formed by necrotic epidermis	Immunoglobulin and complement deposits in walls of vessels

antibodies to complement components in order to detect *in vivo* deposition of antibody and complement in the skin.

Pemphigus

The pemphigus group of diseases is characterized by loss of cohesion between the epidermal keratinocytes (acantholysis) resulting in an intraepidermal blister. The loss of cellular cohesion is caused by autoantibodies directed against a glycoprotein on the surface of the keratinocytes. Direct IF tests show IgG and often complement deposited in the intercellular region of the epidermis. Indirect IF tests show circulating antibody to a constituent of the intercellular substance of squamous epithelium (Fig. 24.10). The titre of the circulating antibody tends to reflect the severity of the disease and may be used to monitor therapy.

There are four main types of pemphigus. The most important form of the disease is **pemphigus vulgaris**, an uncommon disease of the middle-aged and elderly. It may begin with blisters and erosions in the mouth or genitalia. The skin lesions consist of bullae which because they are intraepidermal are very fragile and easily rupture, leaving raw erosions which can be extensive and lead to a high mortality rate in the absence of treatment with systemic corticosteroids and immunosuppressants. Histologically, the acantholysis occurs just above the basal layer of the epidermis (Fig. 24.11) and individual rounded keratinocytes may be seen floating in the cavity of the intraepidermal bulla. The basal cells remain attached to the dermis, an appearance which has been likened to a row of tombstones. **Pemphigus vegetans** is a variant of pemphigus vulgaris but the blisters tend to heal with verrucous vegetations. A characteristic histological feature is the presence of numerous eosinophils in the dermis and in epidermal 'abscesses'. **Pemphigus foliaceus** has a better prognosis than pemphigus vulgaris and may affect younger adults. The site of the intraepidermal split is much higher in the epidermis, usually in the granular layer. A mild form of pemphigus foliaceus is **pemphigus erythematosus** (Senear–Usher syndrome) which may remain localized to the head and neck. It may show a clinical resemblance to lupus erythematosus and indeed, direct IF tests show both intercellular positivity and a 'lupus band' (p. 1121) in many cases. This type of pemphigus may be associated with myasthenia gravis and thymoma.

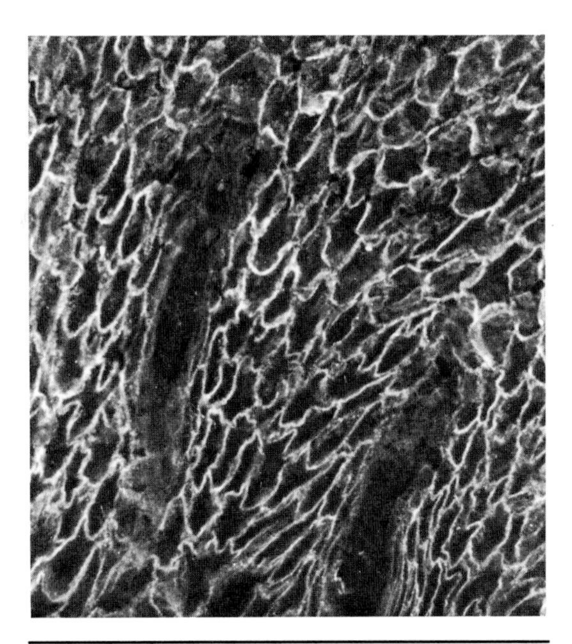

Fig. 24.10 Pemphigus vulgaris. Intercellular immunofluorescence staining in squamous epithelium. Indirect immunofluorescence technique. ×300.

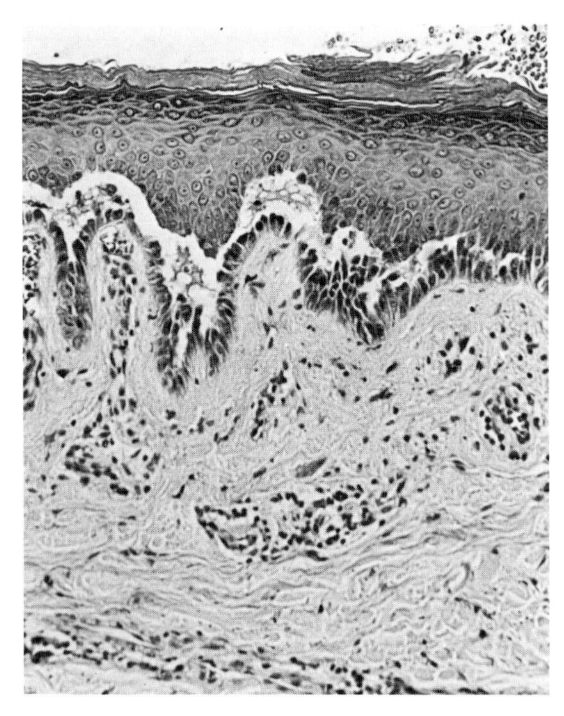

Fig. 24.11 Pemphigus vulgaris. Intraepidermal bulla containing acantholytic cells, best seen just above the basal layer of the epidermis. ×150.

Bullous Pemphigoid

This disease most commonly affects the elderly causing large tense bullae which can be extensive or may be localized to the lower limbs. Involvement of the oral mucosa is common. The condition can be life-threatening but it is usually controlled by corticosteroids. The blisters are subepidermal and the blister cavities and adjacent dermis often contain an infiltrate of eosinophil polymorphs. Circulating antibody, usually IgG class, to a component of the basement membrane zone of squamous epithelium is demonstrable in approximately 70% of cases and in almost 100% of cases there is linear deposition of antibody and complement in the basement membrane region of the patient's skin (Fig. 24.12). There is no correlation between the titre of circulating antibody and the severity of the disease. The bullous pemphigoid antigen has been identified as a normal component of the basement membrane zone and is a glycoprotein located both extracellularly within the lamina lucida and within the basal keratinocytes closely associated with the hemidesmosomes.

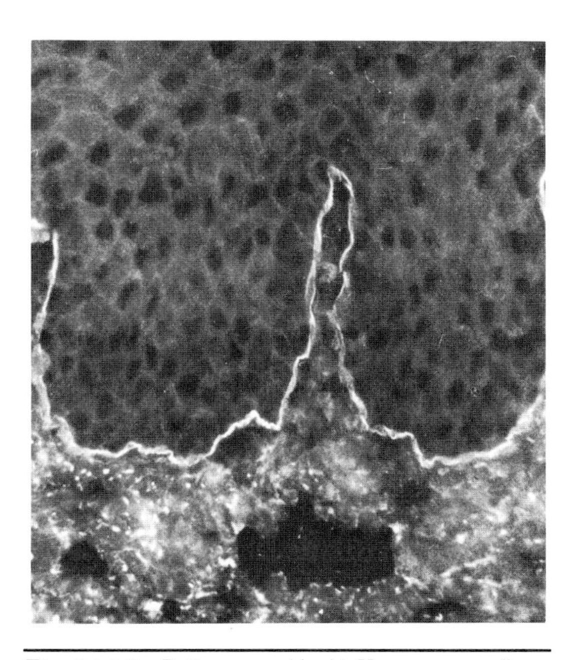

Fig. 24.12 Bullous pemphigoid. Homogeneous linear immunofluorescence of basement membrane. Direct immunofluorescence technique. ×300.

Cicatricial pemphigoid is a chronic scarring disease which affects the mucosae, particularly the oral mucosa. The conjunctivae may be involved, leading to visual impairment. Bullae are sometimes present on the skin. In most cases direct IF is positive for linear antibody deposition along the basement membrane of the mucosal squamous epithelium but circulating antibodies are only rarely detected by conventional indirect IF studies.

Epidermolysis Bullosa Acquisita

This is the only form of epidermolysis bullosa (Table 24.1) which is not inherited. The disease starts in adult life with blistering on trauma and subsequent scarring. Affected sites include the wrists, fingers and feet. It may be associated with autoimmune diseases, chronic inflammatory bowel disease and internal malignancies. The bulla is subepidermal and immunofluorescence findings are similar to those in bullous pemphigoid. However, immunoelectron microscopy shows that the immunoglobulin deposits are just beneath the lamina densa in contrast to their location within the lamina lucida in bullous pemphigoid.

Herpes Gestationis (Pemphigoid Gestationis)

Presenting as a rare itchy vesicular eruption during pregnancy or the puerperium, this disease usually recurs with subsequent pregnancies and may carry an increased risk of abortion. The bullous lesions are caused by basal cell necrosis leading to a subepidermal bulla. Numerous eosinophils are associated with the lesions. In almost 100% of cases direct IF tests show complement (C3) deposited in a linear distribution along the basement membrane zone and this has been shown to be within the lamina lucida. The patient may have circulating IgG antibody, so-called herpes gestationis factor, which, *in vitro*, can be shown to be capable of fixing complement on the basement membrane zone of normal human skin.

Dermatitis Herpetiformis

This chronic condition is most common in early adult life and causes a widespread eruption of groups of intensely itchy papules and vesicles which respond well to the drug dapsone. Affected patients have a high incidence of HLA-B8 and HLA-Dw3. The vast majority show histological evidence of jejunal villous atrophy associated with a gluten sensitive enteropathy (p. 723); however, only a small proportion show clinical signs of malabsorption. The vesicles of dermatitis herpetiformis are subepidermal in location (Fig. 24.13) and adjacent to the vesicle there is a characteristic accumulation of neutrophil polymorphs in the dermal papillae. Granular deposits of IgA, demonstrable by direct IF tests, are present in the dermal papillae of uninvolved skin but are not found (presumably because they are destroyed) in involved and even sometimes in perilesional skin. No similar circulating antibody is detectable in the serum. The IgA deposited in the skin contains J chains, implying that it is dimeric and suggesting an origin in the gut mucosa. Immunoelectron microscopy has shown the IgA to be deposited in the area of the anchoring fibrils beneath the lamina densa.

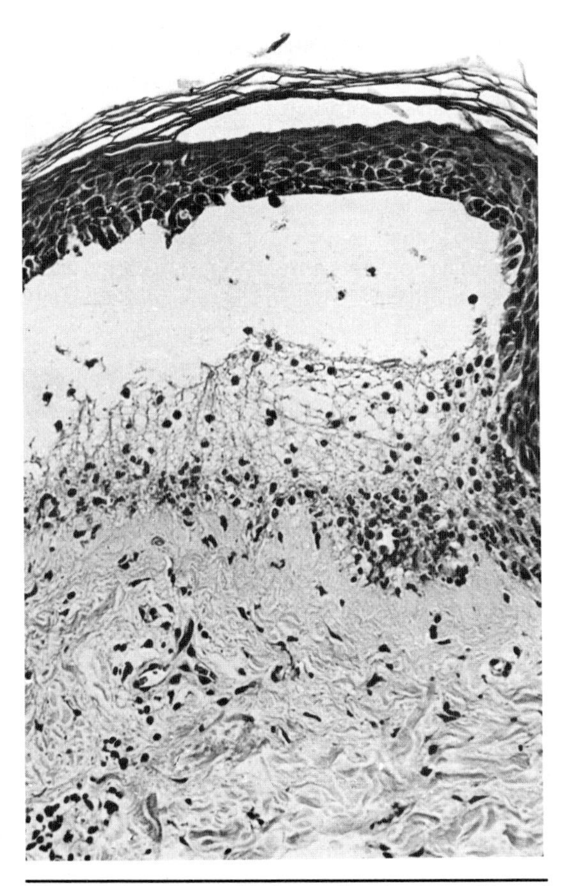

Fig. 24.13 Dermatitis herpetiformis. Subepidermal bulla containing fibrin and neutrophil polymorphs. ×200.

Linear IgA dermatosis. A small number of patients show linear rather than granular deposition of IgA by direct immunofluorescence. These patients have a low incidence of HLA-B8 and of gluten sensitive enteropathy in contrast to classical dermatitis herpetiformis. Their rash may resemble that of bullous pemphigoid.

Chronic bullous dermatosis of childhood. Classical dermatitis herpetiformis is rare in childhood. Chronic bullous dermatosis is a self-limiting disorder in which linear deposits of IgA are found along the basement membrane zone. Like dermatitis herpetiformis the incidence of HLA-B8 is high but there is no gluten sensitive enteropathy and circulating anti-basement membrane IgA antibodies are common.

Porphyria

All the forms of porphyria except the acute intermittent type show cutaneous photosensitive manifestations. These vary clinically, but the histological features are always similar. PAS positive material consisting of reduplicated type IV basement membrane collagen is present in the walls of small dermal blood vessels and sometimes along the dermoepidermal junction. The disease is not immunologically mediated although IF tests may show IgG which has been trapped by the excessive fibrillar material in blood vessel walls.

Erythema Multiforme

The mechanisms underlying erythema multiforme are not fully understood. It is likely, however, to be an immune complex mediated disease. The aetiology is usually unknown but it may follow viral infections such as herpes simplex or the ingestion of certain drugs. It has a variable clinical appearance and may be macular, papular or bullous. Typical 'target lesions' may be seen, consisting of a circular erythematous area with a central vesicle. A severe, sometimes fatal form is the **Stevens–Johnson syndrome**, in which there are extensive haemorrhagic erosions involving the mucous membranes. The term **toxic epidermal necrolysis** is used to describe extensive blistering with detachment of the epidermis and widespread denuding of skin. This is sometimes related to an adverse drug reaction and is probably a severe variant of erythema multiforme.

The histological features of erythema multiforme comprise a mixed inflammatory cell infiltrate in the dermis with necrosis of individual keratinocytes within the epidermis. This necrosis may become confluent and necrosis of the basal cell layer may result in formation of a subepidermal bulla, the roof of which consists of epidermis showing coagulative necrosis (Fig. 24.14).

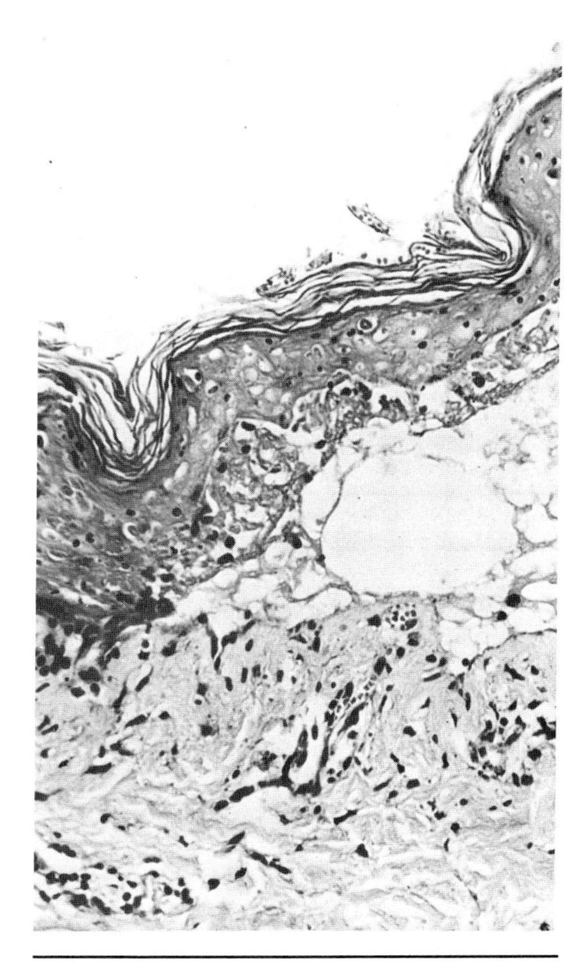

Fig. 24.14 Erythema multiforme. Subepidermal bulla roofed by necrotic epidermis. ×200.

Connective Tissue Diseases

Lupus Erythematosus

This disorder encompasses a clinical spectrum ranging from chronic discoid lupus erythematosus (CDLE), which is confined to the skin and shows no systemic involvement, to systemic lupus erythematosus (SLE) in which visceral lesions predominate and in which cutaneous lesions may or may not be present. In CDLE the lesions usually arise in sun-exposed sites and consist of red scaly patches which often heal with scarring. In the scalp this scarring may lead to permanent hair loss. Autoantibodies to a variety of nuclear constituents are present in the serum of most patients with SLE (p. 229) but are much rarer in CDLE. The histological features of SLE and CDLE overlap to a considerable extent. The epidermis is atrophic and hyperkeratotic and there is keratin plugging of the hair follicles. The basal layer shows liquefaction degeneration similar to that seen in lichen planus. There is a patchy lymphocytic infiltrate in the dermis, particularly around adnexal structures, and there is oedema of the upper dermis (Figs 24.15 and 24.16).

Direct immunofluorescence testing shows, in most cases, a coarse band of IgG in the vicinity of the basement membrane of the epidermis in both types of lupus erythematosus. This 'lupus band' is seen only in clinically affected skin in CDLE but in SLE it is present not only in affected skin but also in normal skin from sun-exposed sites. A lupus band may be seen in some cases of SLE in clinically normal, non-sun-exposed sites: this tends to reflect a high degree of disease activity with a higher risk of renal involvement. Immunoelectron micro-

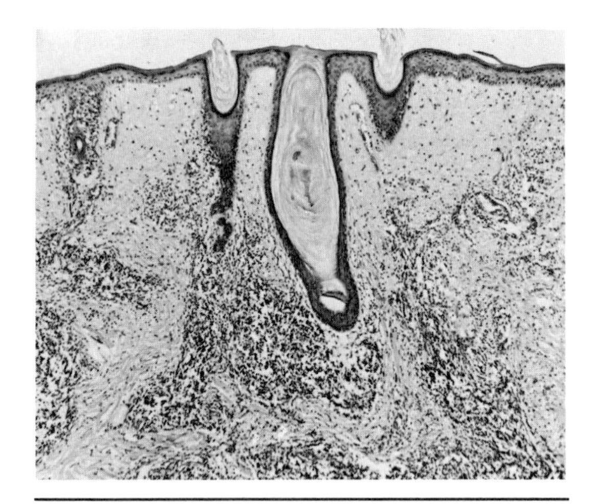

Fig. 24.15 Chronic discoid lupus erythematosus. Flattening of rete ridges, follicular plugging and focal lymphocytic infiltration of the dermis are seen. ×40.

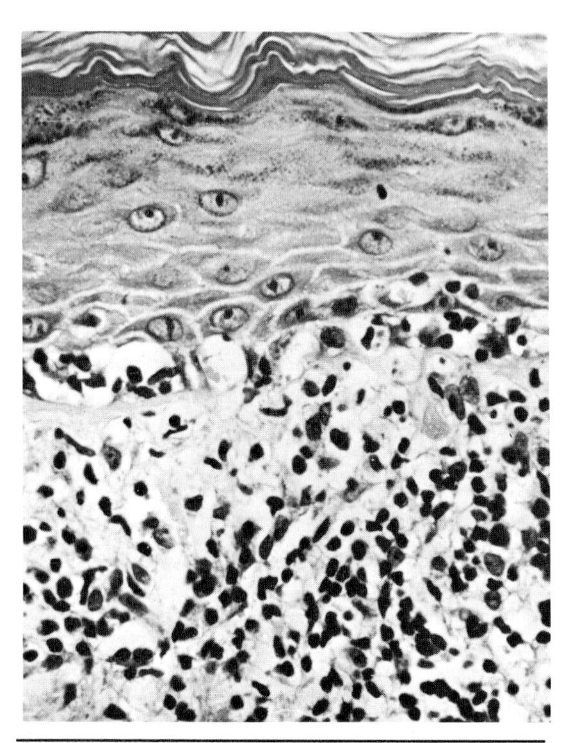

Fig. 24.16 Chronic discoid lupus erythematosus. Liquefaction degeneration of the basal layer of the epidermis. ×300.

scopy shows the site of immune complex deposition to be just beneath the lamina densa.

Progressive Systemic sclerosis

Progressive systemic sclerosis involves both the skin and internal organs (p. 231). The cutaneous lesions (scleroderma) consist of oedema and thickening of the skin which becomes tight, shiny and tethered down to the subcutaneous fat. In addition the fingertips often show ischaemic changes.

Morphoea is a localized skin disease which is clinically and histologically similar to the cutaneous lesions of progressive systemic sclerosis. The skin shows areas of ivory coloured hardening and in the early stages an erythematous halo is seen at the margin of the lesion. It is not associated with internal organ involvement. Some recent studies have suggested a possible relationship between morphoea and the spirochaete *Borrelia burgdorferi*, the organism responsible for Lyme disease (p. 867). This requires further evaluation but raises the possibility of antibiotic treatment in active disease.

In both progressive systemic sclerosis and morphoea the dermal collagen bundles show marked swelling and thickening and this sclerosis extends deep into the subcutaneous fat (Fig. 24.17). There is often accompanying atrophy of dermal adnexal structures. Prominent thickening of the intima of dermal blood vessels may be seen.

Another localized skin disease, **lichen sclerosus et atrophicus**, may closely resemble morphoea both clinically and microscopically. Any area of skin may be affected but it is most common in the vulva (Fig. 21.1, p. 1013). The upper dermis has a glassy homogeneous appearance and there is an absence of elastic fibres in this area. In the mid-dermis there is a band of chronic inflammatory cells.

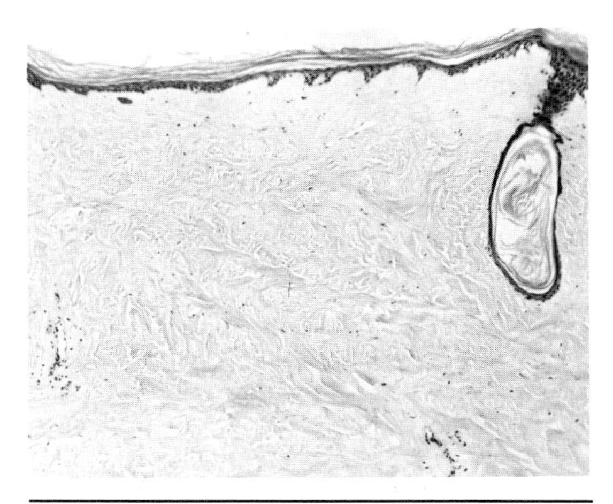

Fig. 24.17 Morphoea. Note the flattening of the rete ridges and the increase in thickness of the dermal collagen. Dermal appendages are absent. ×40.

Disorders of the Blood Vessels and Subcutaneous Fat

Purpura

In **senile purpura** large ecchymoses are present on the arms and hands of the elderly due to deficient collagen formation around dermal blood vessels. Purpuric skin lesions are also present in the vitamin C deficiency disease of **scurvy** where there may also be bleeding into muscles and joints and from the gums. The deficiency of ascorbic acid results in defective collagen synthesis due to an inability to hydroxylate proline.

'Small vessel' (Leucocytoclastic) Vasculitis

Acute vasculitis affecting small dermal blood vessels of venular size is not uncommon in the skin. It is immune complex mediated and has a number of different associations including infections, drugs, autoimmune diseases and internal malignancies. The skin lesions are purpuric and are most numerous in dependent sites such as the lower legs or, in bed-bound patients, the lumbosacral region. There is usually no associated systemic vasculitis but in Henoch–Schönlein purpura (p. 471), a disease most common in children, there is associated joint pain, gastrointestinal bleeding and glomerulonephritis.

Immunofluorescence studies show deposition of immunoglobulin and complement in small blood vessel walls. The presence of immune complexes is thought to activate the complement cascade and trigger an acute inflammatory reaction. Neutrophil polymorphs are present within and around venular walls and often show varying degrees of karyorrhexis leading to large amounts of 'nuclear dust' in the vicinity of blood vessels (Fig. 24.18), hence the term leucocytoclastic vasculitis. There may also be fibrinoid necrosis of vessel walls and thrombosis of some inflamed blood vessels.

The blood vessels of the skin may also be involved in systemic vasculitides such as polyarteritis nodosa and Wegener's granulomatosis

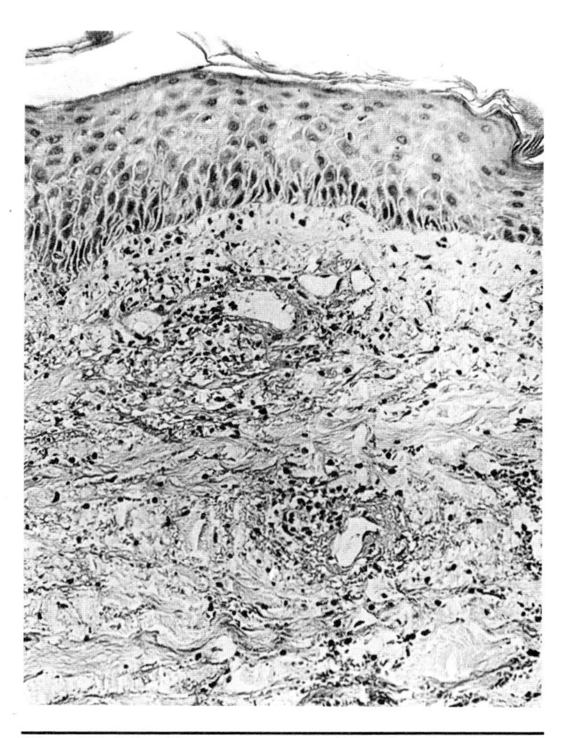

Fig. 24.18 Cutaneous vasculitis showing fibrinoid necrosis of dermal vessels. There is haemorrhage under the epidermis and a marked perivascular inflammatory infiltrate. ×200.

where there is involvement not only of small but also of medium sized vessels in the dermis and subcutis. Necrotizing granulomas are sometimes seen in the skin in Wegener's granulomatosis.

Erythema Nodosum

Erythema nodosum is associated with a variety of diseases including sarcoidosis, streptococcal throat infections, chronic inflammatory bowel disease, gastrointestinal infection with *Yersinia enterocolitica* and drug reactions. It usually occurs in young people and produces red, tender nodules in the lower legs. Histologically, the lesions consist of chronic inflammation in the subcutaneous fat, particularly in the fibrous septa which divide the fat into lobules. The subcutaneous blood vessels do not usually show acute vasculitic changes but there is intimal thickening with oedema and chronic inflammation of vessel walls. The pathogenesis is unknown and there is no evidence that it is an immune complex mediated disease.

Erythema Induratum (Nodular Vasculitis)

Red, tender subcutaneous nodules develop on the calves in erythema induratum, a disease which affects women more commonly than men. Ulceration and subsequent scarring are common. In some cases the disease develops as an immunological reaction to tuberculosis elsewhere in the body but the lesions themselves are sterile. The histological features vary from severe necrotizing granulomatous inflammation of the subcutaneous fat with vasculitis to a vasculitis with only minimal granulomatous inflammation in the fat, when the disease is termed nodular vasculitis.

Panniculitis in Alpha-1-antitrypsin Deficiency

In addition to pulmonary emphysema (p. 551) and hepatic cirrhosis (p. 772), severe inflammation and necrosis of subcutaneous fat may occur in alpha-1-antitrypsin deficiency, usually in homozygotes with the PiZZ phenotype. Patients develop recurrent nodules which tend to break down and discharge a yellowish fluid. Lesions usually appear after trauma and are found most often on the trunk.

Granulomatous Inflammation in the Skin

There are numerous causes of granulomas in the skin. These include tuberculosis, leprosy, syphilis, deep fungal infections and sarcoidosis. Foreign body responses may be seen to keratin and hair, paraffin and greases, plant materials such as thorns, suture material and minerals including beryllium, zirconium and silica.

Granuloma Annulare and Necrobiosis Lipoidica

Granuloma annulare is a relatively common condition seen mainly in children and young adults as groups of raised papules forming an annular pattern on the fingers or backs of the hands. Necrobiosis lipoidica is associated in many but not all cases with diabetes mellitus and occurs most often on the legs as reddish patches with a yellow centre.

Both conditions show a similar histological appearance with a central area of collagen degeneration surrounded by macrophages in a palisaded arrangement (Fig. 24.19). In general, the granuloma formation in necrobiosis lipoidica extends more deeply into the dermis and subcutis than in granuloma annulare.

Hereditary and Congenital Diseases

There is a large number of congenital skin diseases almost all of which are very rare. Only a small selection are described below.

Epidermolysis bullosa comprises a group of blistering diseases which, apart from one variant, epidermolysis bullosa acquisita, are all inherited,

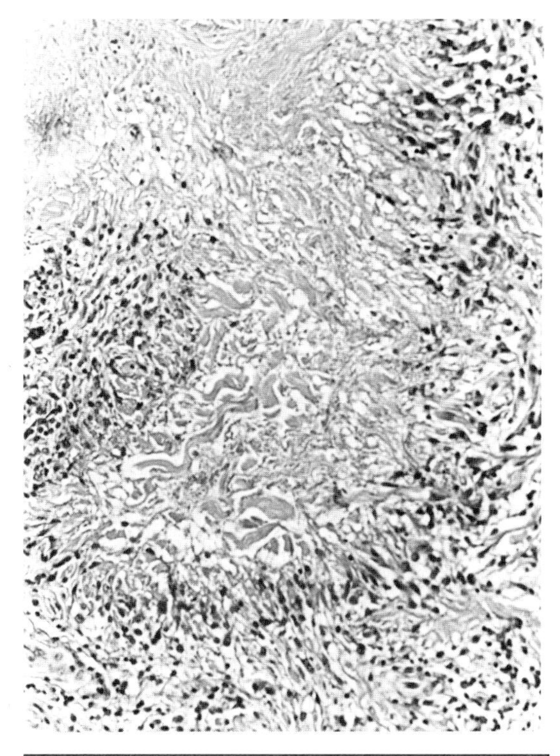

Fig. 24.19 Granuloma annulare. The lesion consists of a central acellular area of necrosis which is surrounded by a palisade of macrophages and, more peripherally, a mixture of chronic inflammatory cells. ×150.

the mode of inheritance varying with different subtypes. Blisters are present at birth or develop in childhood, and death may occur in infancy in some of the more severe forms. Histologically, blisters are subepidermal and are associated with minimal inflammation. The different subtypes cannot be distinguished by light microscopy but by electron microscopy it is possible to divide epidermolysis bullosa into three broad categories: **epidermal** in which the split is a result of cytolytic changes within the basal cells of the epidermis; **junctional** in which the split is within the lamina lucida and where there is an abnormality of the hemidesmosomes; **dermal** in which the split is below the basal lamina and where the anchoring fibrils are abnormal. Prenatal diagnosis is now possible on fetal skin biopsy at 18–20 weeks of gestation and may be offered where there is a known risk of a child having one of the severe, potentially fatal forms.

Ichthyosis comprises a number of conditions in which the skin is dry and covered by scales. The autosomal dominant form, **ichthyosis vulgaris**, is one of the more common congenital skin diseases and in some cases it is associated with atopic dermatitis. The characteristic feature of ichthyosis vulgaris is hyperkeratosis with thinning or absence of the granular layer: this is an exception to the general rule that hyperkeratosis is associated with thickening of the granular layer. The abnormality of the keratohyaline granules is due to a defect in the synthesis of the protein filaggrin. There is a rare X-linked recessive form of ichthyosis which is associated with a deficiency of the enzyme steroid sulphatase. This enzyme acts on cholesteryl sulphate, a product of the Odland bodies (p. 1107) which promote cellular adhesion in the lower corneal layer. Absence of the enzyme results in increased adhesion and disturbance of desquamation.

Pseudoxanthoma elasticum is an inherited disorder of elastic tissue in which there is a tendency for elastic fibres to undergo calcification. There are both autosomal dominant and autosomal recessive forms of the disease. Skin lesions are patchy in distribution and consist of yellow papules involving the sides of the neck, the groins and the axillae. The skin is loose and wrinkled. In the eye, the abnormal elastic fibres in Bruch's membrane cause the formation of angioid streaks in the fundi and vision may be impaired. Involvement of vascular elastica leads to gastrointestinal bleeding, angina and intermittent claudication.

Urticaria pigmentosa. This group of disorders is associated with an increased number of mast cells in the dermis. The disease may present at birth or in early childhood or it may develop in adult life. In children the disease tends to regress spontaneously but this is not the case in adults. The most common presentation is of multiple, itchy, brown pigmented macules and papules on the trunk. Very rarely potentially fatal **systemic**

mastocytosis, with widespread infiltration of internal organs, may occur.

Xeroderma pigmentosum is an autosomal recessive disease in which there is a defect in the ability to excise and repair segments of DNA damaged by ultraviolet irradiation. Affected children show atrophy, severe freckling and premature ageing changes in the skin. In addition, and at an early age they develop multiple cutaneous tumours including basal and squamous-cell carcinomas and malignant melanomas.

Tumours of the Skin

Benign Epidermal Tumours

Basal cell Papilloma (Seborrhoeic Keratosis)

This is a common benign warty growth, seen most often in the elderly. Almost any site may be affected but it occurs most frequently on the face, chest and back. Microscopically, the tumour has an exophytic growth pattern and is raised above the surface of the epidermis. The tumour cells are small and basophilic, resembling the basal cells of the epidermis. Keratin is characteristically formed in spherical masses termed **horn cysts** within the tumour (Fig. 24.20). There may be abundant melanin pigment within the lesion which may result in clinical confusion with malignant melanoma and excision is usually performed either for this reason or for cosmesis. Malignant change very rarely, if ever, occurs.

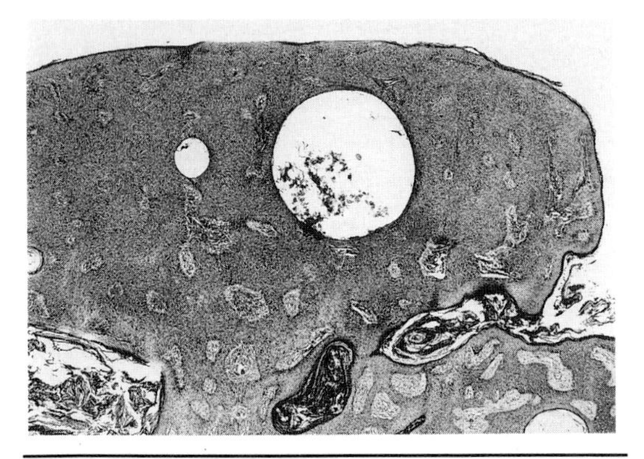

Fig. 24.20 Basal-cell papilloma. Exophytic tumour consisting of small basal-like cells and horn cysts. ×35.

Squamous Papilloma

The great majority of squamous papillomas of the skin are simple viral warts. Two less common squamous papillomas which are clinically distinctive but histologically resemble a viral wart are the linear epidermal naevus and acanthosis nigricans.

Linear epidermal naevus. Multiple hyperkeratotic warty lesions, presenting at birth or in childhood, occur in a linear distribution on the trunk or extremities. They may be localized to one area or may be widespread and disfiguring. The latter form is associated with abnormalities of the skeleton and central nervous system.

Acanthosis nigricans. In this disorder hyperkeratotic, pigmented patches are present on the neck, axillae and genitalia. Some forms of acanthosis nigricans occur in association with internal malignancies especially carcinoma of the stomach. In other cases the lesions may be inherited or associated with endocrine diseases such as Cushing's syndrome, diabetes mellitus and polycystic ovaries.

Keratoacanthoma

This tumour-like lesion deserves special mention because it is a benign self-healing lesion which can, however, be mistaken both clinically and microscopically for invasive squamous-cell carcinoma. It occurs on the face and other sun-exposed sites of adults. A nodule appears in the skin and grows

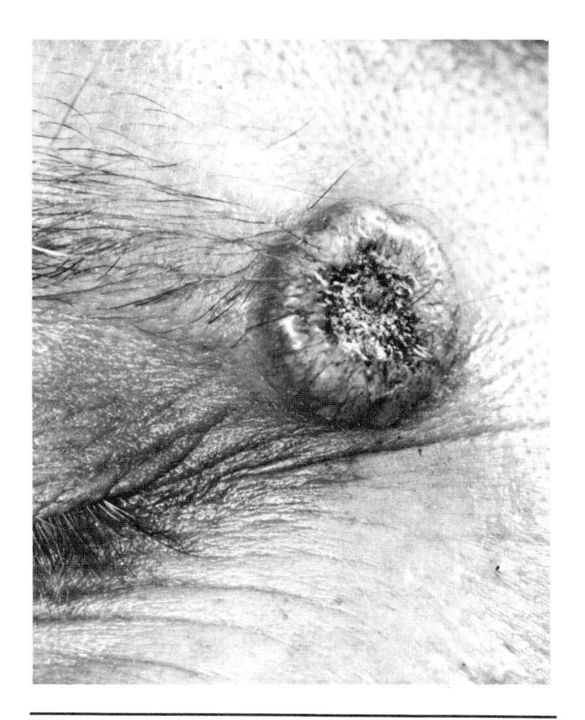

Fig. 24.21 Keratoacanthoma. Clinical photograph of an 8-week-old lesion near the eye. A firm rounded nodule with epidermis stretched over the edge, and a central crater where the keratin core is exposed. ×1.5.

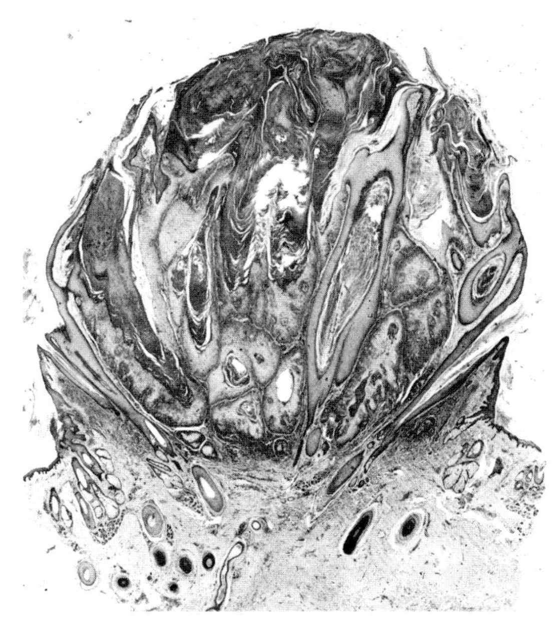

Fig. 24.22 Keratoacanthoma. A lesion about the same age as Fig. 24.21. Note the resemblance to squamous-cell carcinoma. ×10.

rapidly for about 8 weeks, producing a mass of 10–20 mm diameter with a central keratin filled dimple (Fig. 24.21). It usually spontaneously involutes within 6 months. Microscopically, there is marked proliferation of keratinizing squamous epithelium with downgrowths into the dermis resembling invasive tumour. On closer inspection, however, the lesion is superficial with the apparently invasive component lying at or above the level of the sweat glands. A characteristic feature is seen at the edge of the lesion where the epidermis is thrown up into peripheral shoulders (Fig. 24.22).

Malignant Epithelial Tumours ('Non-melanoma Skin Cancer')

The most important aetiological factor for all types of skin cancer is excessive exposure to ultraviolet B (UVB) light (wavelength 290–320 nm) in the form of natural sunlight. The greater the cumulative lifetime exposure the higher is the risk of developing non-melanoma skin cancer – basal- and squamous-cell carcinomas. These tumours are therefore most common on sun-exposed sites of the body. Their incidence is greater in outdoor than in indoor workers, rises with increasing age and they are much more common in light skinned than in dark skinned races. In addition their incidence directly increases with proximity to the equator. There is current concern about what effect depletion of the ozone layer, which acts as a protective barrier to UV radiation, will have on the incidence of skin cancer. The recent rise in the use of sunbeds which utilize long-wave UVA light has stimulated investigation into the possible harmful effects of UVA radiation. Animal experiments have shown an increase in non-melanoma skin cancer with long-term UVA exposure and there may be a similar risk to humans.

Basal-cell Carcinoma

Basal-cell carcinoma is the most frequent malignant skin tumour. It occurs most commonly in the elderly and can present almost anywhere on the skin except palms and soles. Over 70% of cases occur on the face, especially in sites such as the naso-labial fold which are particularly rich in sebaceous glands.

The typical basal-cell carcinoma (rodent ulcer) begins as a small nodule the centre of which breaks down, forming an ulcer which, as the tumour grows, develops a characteristic raised, rolled translucent or pearly border. Small dilated blood vessels are visible over the surface of the tumour. **Extrafacial** basal-cell carcinomas are flat plaque-like lesions which resemble Bowen's disease but which, on close inspection, still retain a raised edge. Another variant is the infiltrative **morphoeic** basal-cell carcinoma which presents as a firm indurated scar-like area often in the nasolabial fold. The margins are ill-defined and the lesion may therefore be incompletely excised. Basal-cell carcinoma is a locally malignant tumour and metastases are excessively rare. If neglected, however, or incompletely excised, it may erode deeply and show extensive destruction of facial structures such as the orbit and nose.

Histologically, a basal-cell carcinoma consists of islands of small, dark cells resembling the basal cells of the epidermis. In most cases the tumour appears to arise from the epidermal basal layer and invades the underlying dermis (Fig. 24.23). Eventually there is ulceration of the epidermis over the central portion of the tumour and the characteristic rolled border is due to lateral invasion of the tumour under the intact epidermis at the periphery. Each island of tumour cells is surrounded by a well defined columnar layer which forms a peripheral palisade (Fig. 24.24). The tumour may show heavy melanin pigmentation and can occasionally be confused clinically with a malignant melanoma. In the extrafacial form of basal-cell carcinoma the tumour islands have a more superficial location and tend to bud downwards from the epidermis with a typical, apparently multifocal appearance (Fig. 24.25). The morphoeic basal-cell carcinoma shows thin cords of infiltrative tumour within a dense fibrous stroma resulting in the ill-defined edge of these tumours.

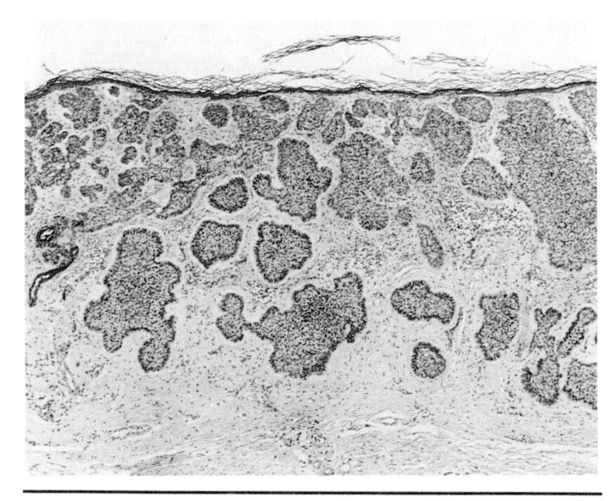

Fig. 24.23 Basal-cell carcinoma. Islands of small basal-like cells invade the dermis. ×35.

Squamous-cell Carcinoma

Squamous-cell carcinoma is the next most common malignant skin tumour after basal-cell carcinoma. It may arise anywhere on the body surface but is most common on sun-exposed sites, particularly the face, dorsum of the hand, pinna of the ear and lower lip. Like basal-cell carcinoma, the most important aetiological factor is prolonged exposure to excessive sunlight, but some cases are due to exposure to carcinogens such as tars and creosote or to previous ingestion of arsenic which was once a component of medicinal tonics. A small number arise in old scars or at the edges of chronic ulcers and sinuses (the so-called Marjolin's

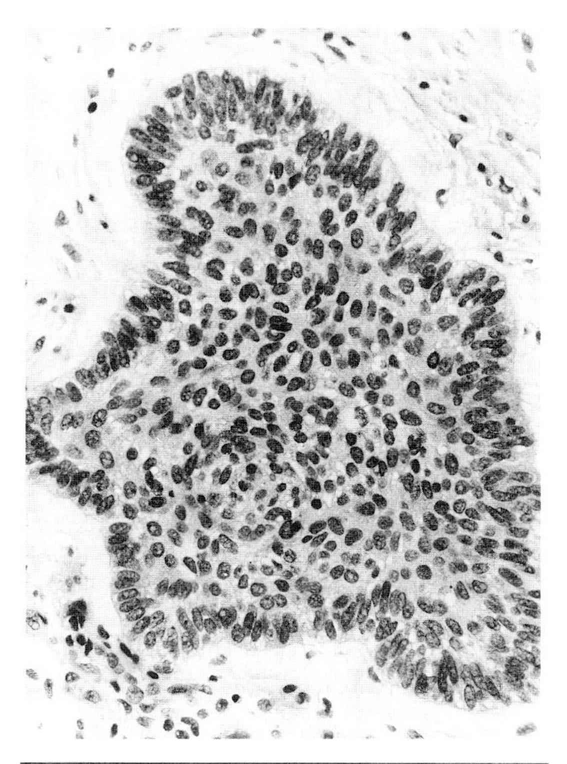

Fig. 24.24 Basal-cell carcinoma. Note palisaded arrangement of nuclei at the periphery of the lobule. ×250.

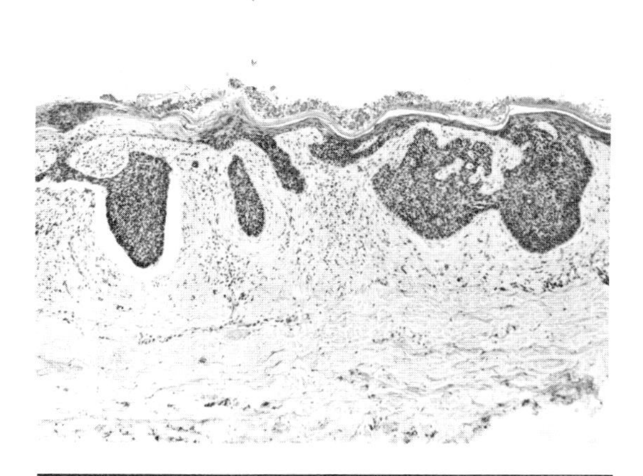

Fig. 24.25 Basal-cell carcinoma, showing the apparently multicentric origin from the base of the epidermis. ×20.

ulcer). There is a higher than expected incidence of cutaneous squamous carcinoma in immunosuppressed individuals such as renal transplant patients and the tumour may behave more aggressively in this group.

Microscopically, squamous carcinomas of the skin are usually well differentiated with abundant keratin formation. In general the prognosis is good with an overall metastatic rate of 3%. Tumours arising in scars and chronic ulcers metastasize more often than those due to sun damage and metastases are also more frequent from tumours of the lower lip than from other sites.

Premalignant Squamous Lesions

Two disorders, actinic keratosis and Bowen's disease, show premalignant changes of the epidermis ranging from mild dysplasia to carcinoma *in situ*.

Actinic (solar, senile) keratosis. Lesions of actinic keratosis arise in skin which shows evidence of sun damage such as loss of elasticity, atrophy and irregular pigmentation. Commonly affected sites include the face and back of hands and there are often multiple lesions consisting of dry, roughened areas of skin thickening.

The epidermis shows varying degrees of dysplasia, ranging from mild disorganization and cellular atypia involving only the lowermost layers of the epidermis to severe dysplasia affecting the full thickness of the epidermis. Overlying the dysplastic epidermis there is usually parakeratosis reflecting abnormal epidermal maturation. The epithelium of the mouths of the hair follicles and sweat glands is not usually dysplastic and therefore there is no parakeratosis overlying these structures although the keratin layer is usually thickened. This gives rise to the classical histological feature of alternating columns of hyperkeratosis and parakeratosis (Fig. 24.26).

The incidence of development of invasive squamous carcinoma from these lesions is difficult to determine. Estimates of the proportion of patients with actinic keratoses who develop squamous carcinoma vary widely from 1 to 20% in different studies.

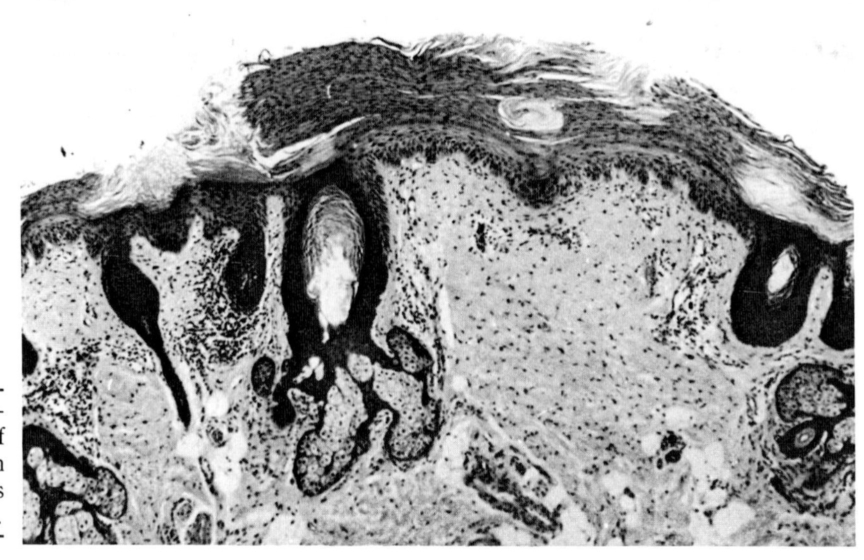

Fig. 24.26 Actinic keratosis, showing a patch of epithelial atrophy with dysplasia, hyperkeratosis and parakeratosis. ×25.

Bowen's disease. Bowen's disease presents as a sharply defined, red, scaly patch which may occur on exposed or covered sites. Clinically it may be mistaken for a patch of psoriasis or dermatitis. On exposed sites chronic exposure to sunlight is a factor. Some elderly patients give a history of previous ingestion of arsenic-containing medicinal tonics.

The epidermis shows full thickness dysplasia which also involves the epithelium of intraepidermal adnexal structures. There is marked cellular atypia and abnormal mitotic figures and multinucleated cells may be frequent (Fig. 24.27). Although the histological appearances are of carcinoma *in situ*, invasive squamous carcinoma rarely supervenes and only then after a long time interval.

Adnexal Tumours

As a group adnexal tumours are far less common than tumours arising from the epidermis. They can occur on virtually any site but are most common in the head and neck region. Eccrine sweat gland tumours may arise from the intraepidermal or the dermal portion of the sweat duct or from the secretory coils. Tumours also arise from the apocrine sweat glands and from the pilosebaceous follicles. Their subclassification is complex and may be found in specialized textbooks of dermatopathology. A simplified list is found in Table 24.2. The majority of adnexal tumours are benign or occasionally locally aggressive; however, eccrine sweat gland and sebaceous gland carcinomas, although rare, have the potential for systemic metastases.

Melanocytic Tumours

Melanocytic Naevi

Early in fetal life melanocytes migrate from the neural crest and settle in the skin, the uveal tract of the eye and the leptomeninges. Those that migrate to the skin come to lie among the basal cells of the epidermis. The ratio of melanocytes to basal cells varies from approximately 1:10 to 1:5, de-

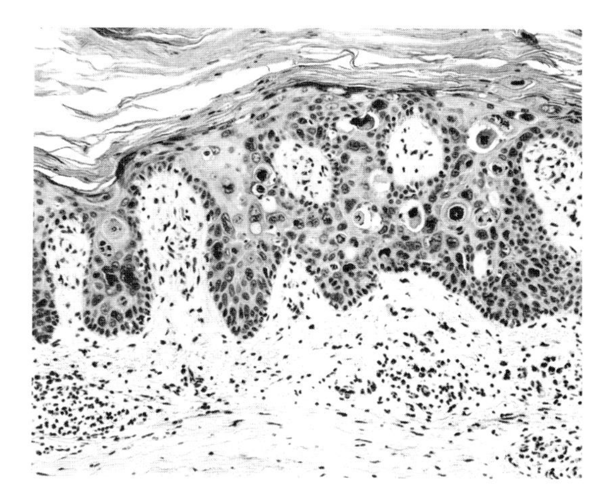

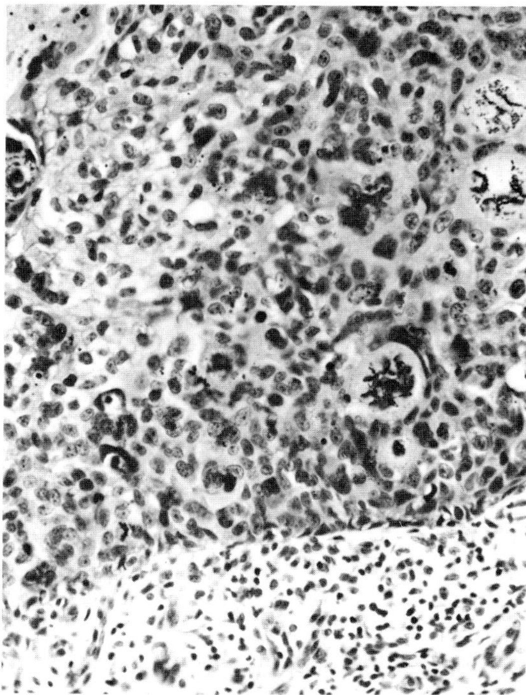

Fig. 24.27 Bowen's disease of the skin. Above, showing the large, abnormal cells in the epidermis. ×60. Below, showing more cellular detail, including enlarged and clumped nuclei and aberrant mitoses. ×160.

pending on the anatomical site. The number of melanocytes per unit area of skin is constant irrespective of race or skin colour, but melanin pigment synthesis is greater in dark skinned than in light skinned races.

The term melanocytic naevus will be used in this chapter and is synonymous with the widely used term 'pigmented mole'. Common melanocytic naevi are derived from epidermal melanocytes and most young adults have approximately 20–25 such lesions, the numbers decreasing with advancing age. These naevi are classified as acquired, i.e. they appear after birth, most often between the ages of 12 and 30 years. The risk of malignant change occurring in acquired naevi is extremely small. Melanocytic naevi should not be confused with freckles in which there is an increase in melanin pigmentation of the basal layer without an increase in the numbers of melanocytes.

The probable evolution of melanocytic naevi is shown in diagrammatic form in Fig. 24.28. It is thought that during childhood or adolescence the normal ratio of melanocytes to epidermal basal cells is disturbed at some sites and the melanocytes become too numerous to be accommodated in their normal position. The initial lesion in their development is a **junctional naevus** which presents as a flat blemish varying in colour from pale to dark brown and is seen most often in children and teenagers. The melanocytes in the basal layer undergo focal proliferation and enlargement and lose their dendritic processes. They are now termed naevus cells and are present in small nests which bulge down into the dermis but which remain attached to the epidermis (Fig. 24.29). This appearance is termed junctional activity.

As the patient ages, some of the naevus cells in the epidermis in a junctional pigmented naevus eventually 'drop off' and come to lie in small nests within the dermis while there is still some overlying junctional activity. The lesion is then termed a **compound naevus** and is the most common melanocytic naevus seen in young adults. Clinically, the compound naevus is usually raised above the surface, is sometimes papillomatous and varies in colour from pale brown to black.

In older adults the junctional activity ceases and only the intradermal component of the lesion remains and constitutes an **intradermal naevus** (Fig. 24.30). Clinically, an intradermal naevus is often flesh coloured. It may be a dome-shaped, raised, sessile lesion or can be pedunculated. As the lesion ages the naevus cells become smaller

Table 24.2 Skin appendage tumours

Differentiation	
Eccrine sweat glands	Eccrine hidrocystoma: solitary or multiple – face, especially periorbital
	Syringoma: multiple lesions – face, especially lower eyelids
	Eccrine poroma: usually solitary, often sole of foot
	Eccrine spiradenoma: solitary, any site, often tender
	Eccrine hidradenoma: usually solitary. Any site
	Chondroid syringoma: solitary, head and neck
	Eccrine carcinoma: head and neck, metastases common
Apocrine sweat gland	Apocrine hidrocystoma: solitary, bluish cyst on face.
	Syringocystadenoma papilliferum: presents at birth or in childhood on scalp
	Hidradenoma papilliferum: solitary nodule in genital or perianal region of female
	Cylindroma: head and neck; multiple lesions may occur on scalp (turban tumour)
	Apocrine carcinoma: very rare; axilla or genital; local or widespread metastases
Hair follicle	Proliferating tricholemmal cyst: scalp, may develop from simple pilar cyst
	Tricholemmoma: solitary, on face; multiple lesions associated with breast cancer (Cowden's syndrome)
	Pilomatricoma: solitary lesion on head and neck; often in children
	Trichofolliculoma: solitary on face; central pore with tuft of white hair
	Trichoepithelioma: solitary or multiple; head and neck
Sebaceous gland	Sebaceous adenoma: very rare; head and neck
	Sebaceous carcinoma: eyelid; aggressive course with metastases

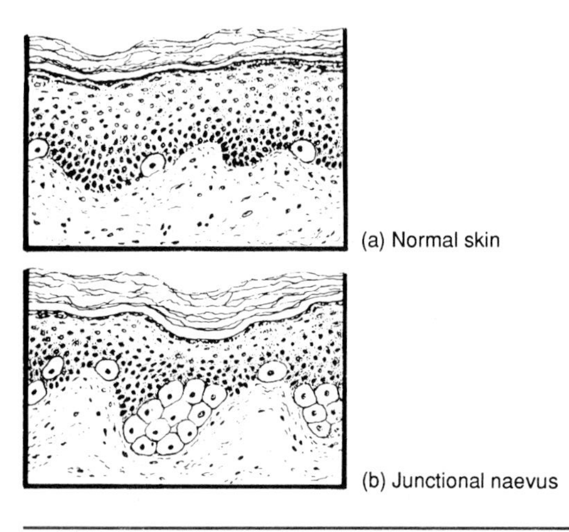

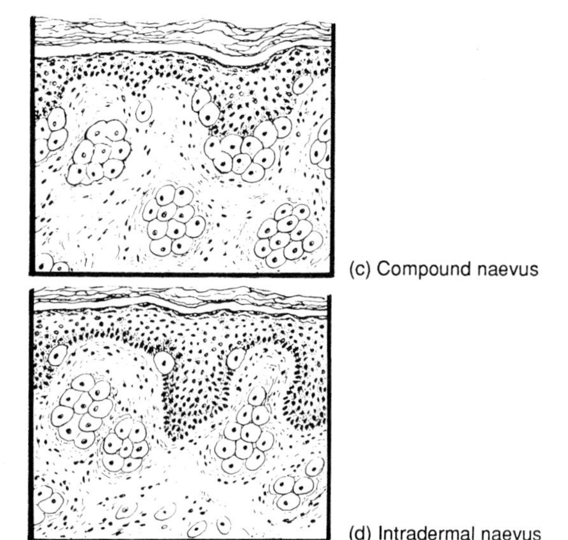

Fig. 24.28 Diagram of the evolution of a melanocytic naevus (see text).

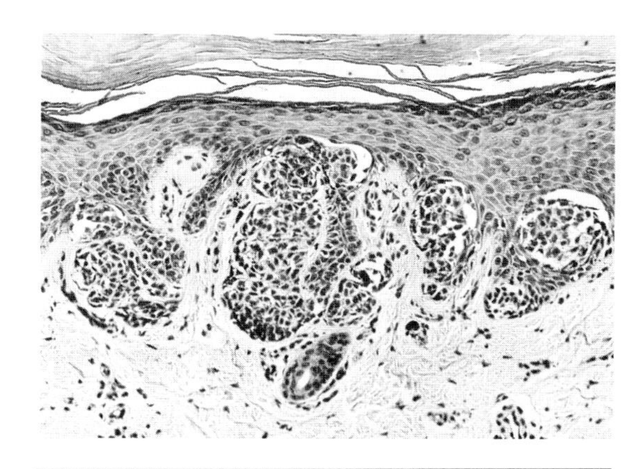

Fig. 24.29 Junctional melanocytic naevus. Nests of naevus cells bulge into the dermis from the basal layer of the epidermis. ×100.

and more spindle shaped and there is increasing fibrosis in its deep aspect.

Variants of Melanocytic Naevi

Spitz naevus is a benign compound naevus which can occur at any age but is particularly common in children and young adults. It is a dome-shaped, reddish lesion which may clinically resemble a vascular lesion, particularly a pyogenic granuloma (p. 1139). Histologically, the margins of the Spitz naevus are well defined but the cells are larger than ordinary naevus cells, there may be mitotic activity and there is a considerable degree of cellular pleomorphism (Fig. 24.31). Melanin pigment is usually sparse. There may be acanthosis of the overlying epidermis and two oft-quoted features, seen most often in Spitz naevi in young

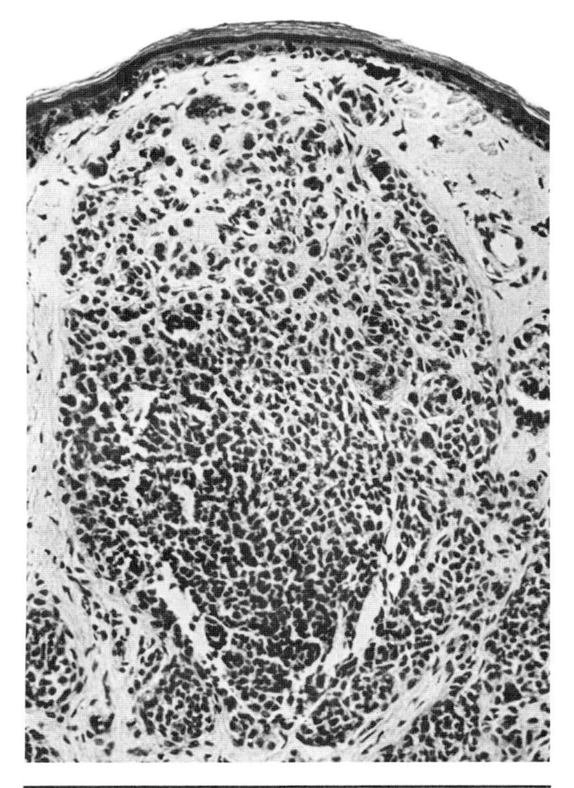

Fig. 24.30 Intradermal naevus. Collections of small naevus cells in the dermis with no junctional activity. ×220.

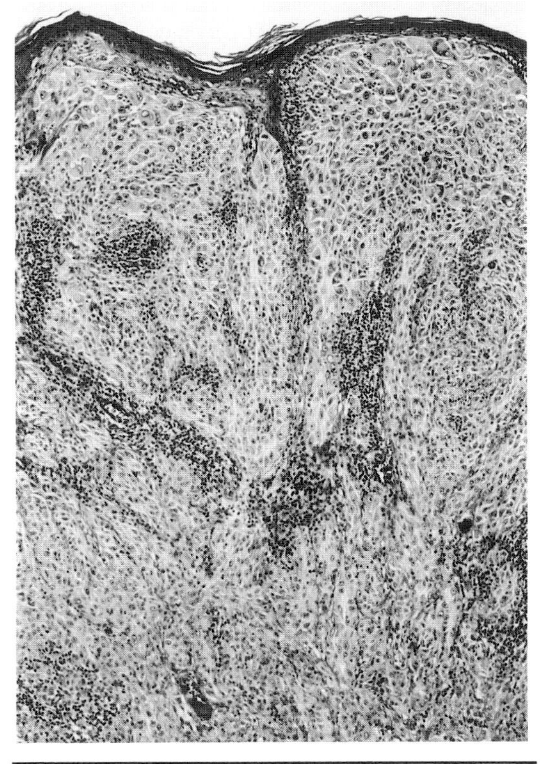

Fig. 24.31 Spitz naevus. Large pleomorphic naevus cells some of which are multinucleated. Cells vary from rounded to more spindle shaped deeper in the dermis. ×220.

children, are the presence of upper dermal oedema and telangiectatic blood vessels. Differentiation from malignant melanoma can be very difficult but features favouring a Spitz naevus include a lack of abnormal mitotic figures, a decrease in size of the naevus cells in the deep part of the lesion and well defined margins to the lesion.

Congenital naevi. Unlike the common acquired naevi, which they resemble but are not identical with histologically, congenital naevi are present at birth. They can be divided broadly into two groups, giant and small. Giant congenital naevi are extensive pigmented lesions which may cover a large area of the body surface and are often hairy. They may be associated with diffuse pigmentation of the leptomeninges. They carry a definite risk of developing malignant melanoma, estimates of the risk varying from 6 to 12% of cases. Recent interest has been shown in small (less than 1.5 cm diameter) congenital naevi as possible precursors of malignant melanoma but this has not yet been definitely proven.

Blue naevus. Occasionally some melanocytes are halted in their migration to the epidermis from the neural crest during fetal life and are arrested in the dermis where they retain their dendritic morphology and are usually deeply pigmented. Clinically, these lesions are blue in colour as a result of an optical effect due to their depth beneath the surface and they are seen most frequently in children and young adults often on the dorsa of the hands or feet.

Dysplastic Naevus Syndrome

This disorder occurs in a familial form, probably autosomal dominant, although apparently sporadic cases also occur. Affected patients develop large numbers of melanocytic naevi which have clinically atypical features such as a larger than average size, irregular edges and variable pigmentation. These naevi occur most often on the trunk, especially the back, and there may a history of atypical naevi and sometimes of malignant melanoma in the family. Histologically, they are junctional or compound naevi which have ill-defined margins and show mild pleomorphism of the naevus cells. The risk for the patient of developing malignant melanoma depends on whether there is a family or personal history of melanoma. As an extreme example it has been calculated that a patient with dysplastic naevi and a previous melanoma and who has two relatives with a history of melanoma has virtually a 100% chance of developing a second melanoma. Patients with the dysplastic naevus syndrome should be regularly followed up and examined for any change in their lesions, preferably using serial clinical photographs for comparison. In addition, the relatives of affected individuals should be examined.

Malignant Melanoma

Malignant melanoma is important because of its increasing incidence, as shown in figures from Europe, Australia and the USA, and because it is a life-threatening tumour which in many cases affects young and middle-aged adults. As with non-melanoma skin cancer, the most important aetiological factor is excessive sun exposure but, unlike basal- and squamous-cell carcinomas, cumulative lifetime exposure is not as important as short sharp bursts of intense exposure accompanied by severe sunburn. An exception to this is lentigo maligna melanoma which occurs in an older age group and, like non-melanoma skin cancers, appears to be more related to long-term sun exposure. Individuals at greatest risk are fair skinned with blue eyes and blonde or red hair who do not tan but have a tendency to freckle and who have a large number of common acquired naevi. An increased risk is also found in patients with dysplastic naevus syndrome or giant congenital naevi. Clinical features which suggest the possibility of a pigmented lesion being a malignant melanoma include development of itch or inflammation in the lesion, increase in size, irregular colour and shape, and ulceration or bleeding. If there is any suspicion the lesion should be excised and examined microscopically.

The vast majority of melanomas begin in the basal layer of the epidermis. The malignant cells may spread in all directions within the epidermis (radial growth phase) and the tumour at this stage is incapable of metastasizing. Subsequently the tumour spreads downwards into the dermis (vertical growth phase) and now it has the potential to metastasize. Clinically the radial growth phase appears as a flat irregular area of pigmentation and the vertical growth phase as a pigmented nodule within this area. The tumour has four clinicopathological subtypes; lentigo maligna melanoma, superficial spreading melanoma, nodular melanoma and acral lentiginous melanoma.

Lentigo Maligna and Lentigo Maligna Melanoma

Lentigo maligna is a slowly growing, flat pigmented lesion arising on sun-exposed skin, principally of the head and neck, of the elderly. The basal layer of the epidermis is replaced by pleomorphic melanocytes which have a high nuclear/cytoplasmic ratio and which extend down the basal layer of hair follicles (Fig. 24.32). The epidermis is usually atrophic and there is degeneration and matting of elastic tissue in the dermis, so-called solar elastosis. There is no invasion of the dermis by malignant melanocytes and so there is no potential to metastasize. Eventually, however, sometimes after many years, a proportion of lesions show dermal invasion. The tumour is now termed lentigo maligna melanoma and may metastasize.

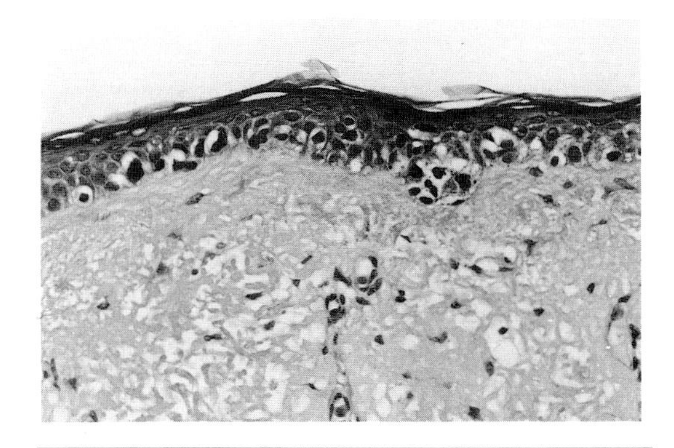

Fig. 24.32 Lentigo maligna. Replacement of the epidermal basal layer by atypical melanocytes. The dermis shows solar elastosis. ×250.

Superficial Spreading Melanoma

Although some cases of superficial spreading melanoma are diagnosed and treated at the early preinvasive stage of radial growth, the vast majority have invaded the dermis at the time of presentation. This is the most common form of invasive melanoma. Females are affected more often than males and the most common sites are the lower leg for women and the trunk, especially the back, for men. There is widespread invasion of the epidermis by large malignant melanocytes with pale cytoplasm and dermal invasion by nests of similar cells (Fig. 24.33).

Nodular Melanoma

Nodular melanoma has no clinically or histologically evident radial growth phase and consists of a pigmented nodule with no surrounding flat area of pigmentation. Ulceration is common. Presumably a short radial growth phase does exist but dermal invasion occurs so rapidly that a preinvasive stage is not apparent. Microscopically, invasive melanoma cells are present in the dermis with abnormal junctional activity in the epidermis immediately overlying the tumour but no radial spread of tumour into the adjacent epidermis.

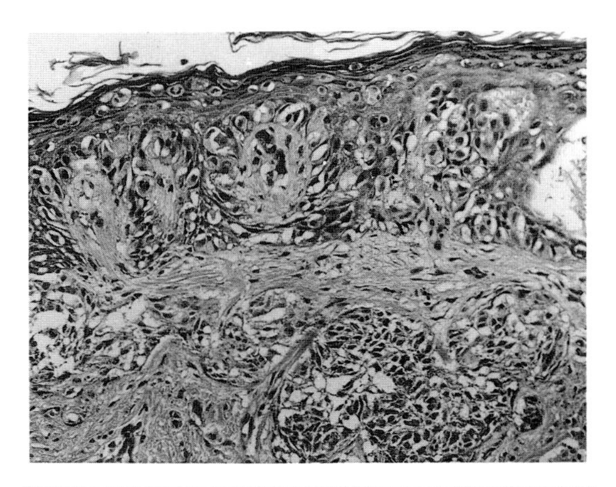

Fig. 24.33 Superficial spreading melanoma. Malignant melanocytic cells invade the dermis and spread through the upper layers of the epidermis. ×110.

Acral/Mucosal Lentiginous Melanomas

These are variants arising on the palms and soles and on the mucosal surfaces respectively. Microscopically they are similar to lentigo maligna melanoma except that solar elastosis is not present and the epithelium is not atrophic.

Prognostic Features in Malignant Melanoma

By far the most important prognostic factor is the thickness of the melanoma measured microscopically from the top of the granular layer of the epidermis to the deepest point of invasive tumour in the dermis and expressed in millimetres. This is termed the Breslow thickness (Fig. 24.34). The thicker the tumour the worse the prognosis, e.g. in the UK the 5-year disease-free survival of patients with a melanoma less than 1.5 mm in thickness is 90% compared to 40% for patients with a melanoma over 3.5 mm thick. Measurement of the level of invasion of the dermis (Clark level) is also used but is not as accurate a guide as the Breslow thickness; the outlook is best when the tumour is confined to the superficial dermis and worst when it extends into the subcutaneous fat. Other poor prognostic features are the presence of vascular invasion by tumour cells, ulceration and a high mitotic rate. Males have a poorer prognosis than females and the site of the tumour appears to be important, trunk melanomas behaving more aggressively than those at other sites.

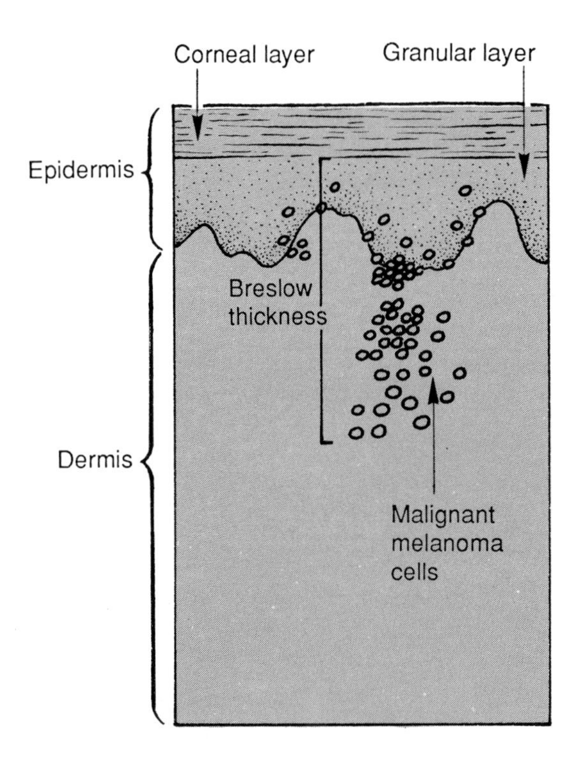

Fig. 24.34 Breslow thickness of malignant melanoma is measured in millimetres from the top of the stratum granulosum to the deepest invasive tumour cell.

The disease may occur in three stages: stage I in which there are no metastases, stage II in which there are metastases to regional lymph nodes, and stage III in which there is disseminated disease. Distant metastases occur to the liver, brain and lungs and to unusual sites such as bowel and heart. Widespread metastases may also appear in the skin and subcutaneous tissue.

Cutaneous Lymphomas

The skin may be involved in advanced systemic non-Hodgkin's lymphomas and rarely in advanced Hodgkin's disease but the most common cutaneous lymphoma is mycosis fungoides.

Mycosis Fungoides

This is a cutaneous T-cell lymphoma which may remain confined to the skin but in a proportion of cases shows systemic and lymph node involvement. Some patients develop the 'Sézary syndrome' – a generalized erythematous skin rash with lymphadenopathy and large atypical T lymphocytes circulating in the bloodstream. Mycosis fungoides is clinically classified into three stages, the earliest patch stage, the plaque stage and the advanced tumour stage. By no means all patients progress from the early stages to more advanced disease and it has been proposed that the disease is initially a chronic T-cell reaction to persistent antigenic stimulation, in some cases the T-cell proliferation becoming neoplastic. In support of this hypothesis are studies which have demonstrated clonal rearrangement of the T-cell receptor β-chain gene in advanced mycosis fungoides but not in the early stages of the disease. There is some evidence to suggest that the antigen may be a retrovirus infection and HTLV-1 antibodies have been found in the serum of some patients.

In established cases the upper dermis is infiltrated by atypical lymphocytes with hyperchromatic, convoluted nuclei. These tend to invade the epidermis and form small aggregates termed Pautrier microabscesses (Fig. 24.35). The infiltrate consists predominantly of CD4 positive T lymphocytes. Epidermal Langerhans cells are increased in number in early mycosis fungoides and may be seen in contact with clusters of the atypical T cells; Langerhans cells are also present within the dermal infiltrate.

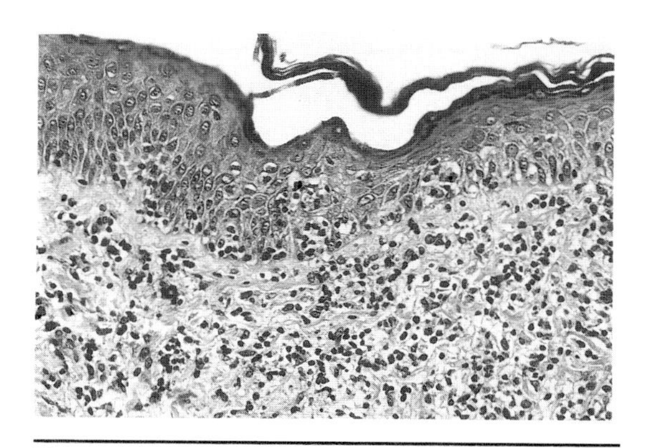

Fig. 24.35 Mycosis fungoides. Pautrier microabscesses are present in the epidermis. There is an infiltrate of atypical lymphoid cells in the dermis. ×180.

Tumours of the Dermis

Merkel Cell Carcinoma (Neuroendocrine Carcinoma)

This is an aggressive tumour which usually occurs on sun-exposed skin, particularly of the head and neck, in the elderly. It is most commonly a solitary firm nodule and usually does not ulcerate. There is a high rate of local recurrence and of regional lymph node metastases, and death due to systemic metastases occurs in approximately 25% of cases.

Histologically, the tumour consists of aggregates, cords or trabeculae of basophilic, round cells with scanty cytoplasm within the dermis and subcutaneous fat. Invasion of the epidermis is rare. Numerous mitotic figures are present. Ultrastructurally the cells contain cytoplasmic membrane-bound dense core granules as seen in cells of the APUD series and they show positive immunostaining for neuron-specific enolase. The differential diagnosis includes metastatic small cell carcinoma of lung, which is also of APUD cell origin, and a chest X-ray should be performed to exclude this diagnosis. The exact cell of origin of this predominantly dermal tumour is unknown as the normal location of the Merkel cell is the epidermis. It may, however, arise from Merkel cells arrested in the dermis in transit from the neural crest to the epidermis.

Mesenchymal Dermal Tumours

Benign mesenchymal tumours such as neurofibromas, lipomas and leiomyomas are not uncommon in the dermis and subcutaneous fat. Certain tumours merit special consideration and are discussed below.

Fibrohistiocytic Tumours

Dermatofibroma (benign fibrous histiocytoma, sclerosing haemangioma). This common benign lesion occurs most often on the limbs of adults and presents as a smooth, firm, red-brown nodule. The histological features are variable but it is usually a poorly circumscribed dermal nodule composed of interlacing bundles of spindle cells, lipid-laden macrophages and giant cells (Fig. 24.36). The lesion often contains small capillary blood vessels and haemosiderin pigment is often scattered through the lesion. There is a variable amount of collagen production.

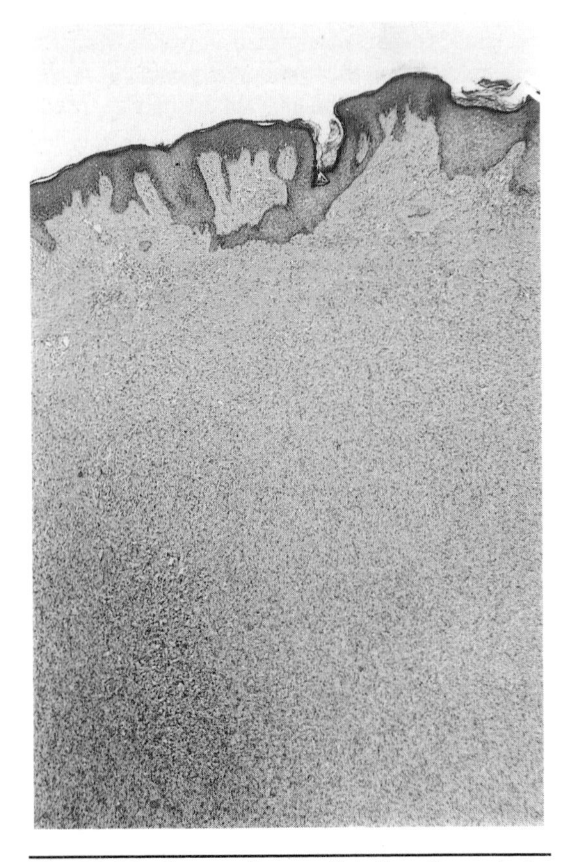

Fig. 24.36 Dermatofibroma. Spindle-cell vascular lesion in the dermis with acanthosis of the overlying epidermis. ×55.

Dermatofibrosarcoma protuberans. This slowly growing dermal tumour occurs on the trunk and lower limbs of adults. It may extend from the dermis into subcutaneous fat and is composed of uniform spindle cells which show a 'cartwheel' or 'storiform' arrangement and scattered mitotic figures (Fig. 24.37). It rarely metastasizes but often locally recurs unless widely excised.

Atypical fibroxanthoma. This tumour occurs most commonly on the sun-exposed skin of the head and neck of the elderly, but is occasionally also found on the extremities of younger adults. It presents as a firm nodule which may be ulcerated. It is a dermal tumour with little extension into subcutaneous fat and is composed of a mixture of spindle cells, plump histiocytic-type cells and bizarre giant cells which are cytologically malignant and display numerous atypical mitotic figures. Despite this histological appearance these lesions are subject only to local recurrence and metastases are rare. The histological features are very similar to the malignant fibrous histiocytoma (MFH) of soft tissue and it is thought that atypical fibroxanthoma represents a superficial variant of MFH which has a good prognosis due to its superficial location.

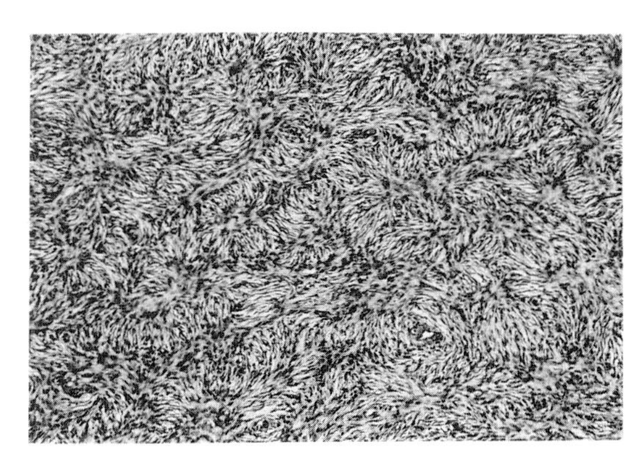

Fig. 24.37 Dermatofibrosarcoma. Tumour shows characteristic storiform pattern. ×110.

Vascular Tumours

Pyogenic Granuloma

This is a common lesion which is thought by some to be reactive rather than truly neoplastic. It occurs at any age and presents as a rapidly growing, red, pedunculated nodule which is often ulcerated. It is seen most commonly on the head and neck and on the gingivae of pregnant women. The nodule is composed of numerous capillary blood vessels set in an oedematous stroma which is often heavily inflamed.

Haemangioma

There are two main types of benign haemangioma of the skin, the capillary and the cavernous haemangioma. The **capillary haemangioma** presents in the neonatal period as a bright red strawberry birthmark which may arise at any site. Most cases spontaneously involute during childhood. Microscopic examination shows large lobular aggregates of capillary sized blood vessels lined by prominent endothelial cells (Fig. 24.38). The **cavernous haemangioma** also appears in infancy but shows little tendency to spontaneous involution. Large dilated thin walled blood vessels are seen histologically in the dermis and subcutaneous fat.

Glomus Tumour

The glomus tumour is usually a solitary tumour arising from the glomus body, a specialized vascular structure concerned with temperature regulation which is most often found in the fingers. The tumour also occurs most frequently on the fingers, especially in a subungual position. It is usually a small reddish nodule and is characteristically exquisitely tender or painful. Histologically, it is a well circumscribed lesion consisting of blood vessels surrounded by small uniform glomus cells with eosinophilic cytoplasm (Fig. 24.39). These cells have ultrastructural features of modified smooth muscle cells.

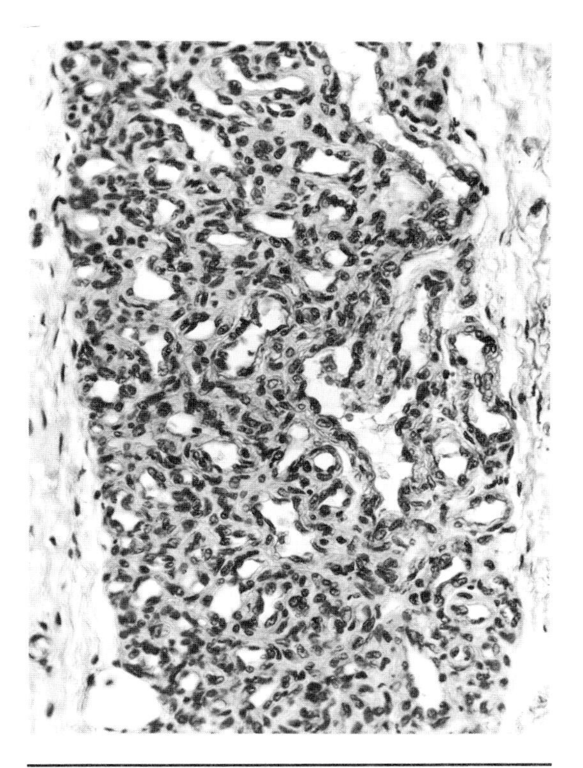

Fig. 24.38 Capillary haemangioma showing well formed capillaries with prominent endothelial cells. The solid areas between capillaries include many cells which appear to be endothelial cells not related to a lumen. ×200.

Angiosarcoma

Angiosarcoma of the skin is a rare malignant tumour which occurs in two clinical settings, either in a chronically lymphoedematous limb, especially the arm after a radical mastectomy and radiotherapy for breast carcinoma (Stewart–Treves syndrome), or on the head and neck, particularly the scalp, of elderly individuals. The tumour presents as red plaques and nodules which may be very extensive and tend to ulcerate. The prognosis is very poor and regional lymph node and blood-borne metastases occur but death may occur before this in head and neck tumours as a result of extensive local destructive effects. Microscopically, the tumour consists of an anastomosing network of vascular channels, lined by atypical endothelial cells, dissecting through the dermal

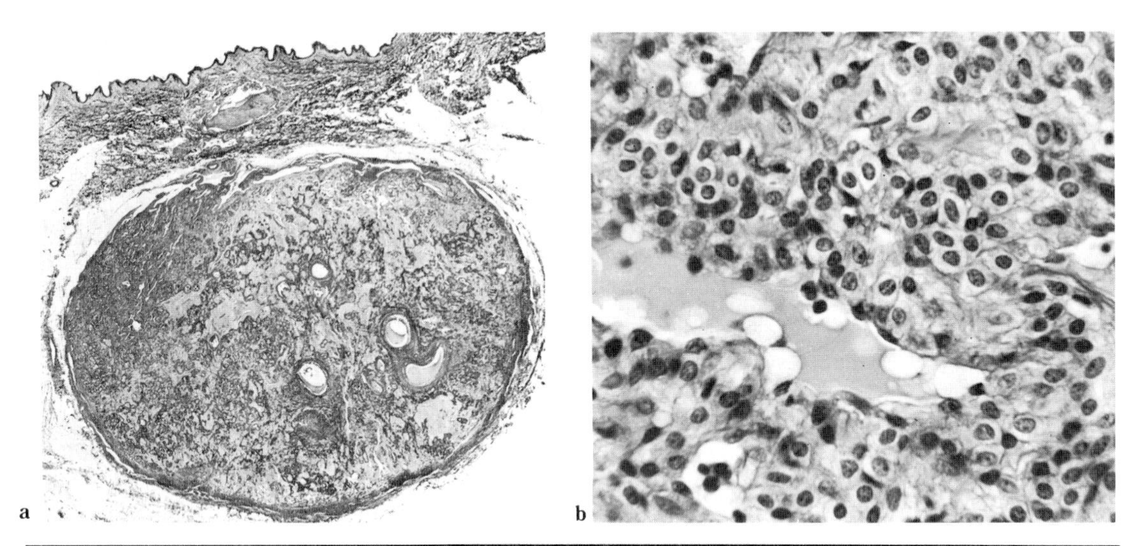

Fig. 24.39 **a** Glomus tumour. Small subcutaneous encapsulated growth showing the coiled arteriole. ×8. **b** Glomus cells surrounding a vascular space. ×350.

collagen. Areas of poorly differentiated solid spindle-cell tumour may be present.

Kaposi's Sarcoma

Although traditionally regarded as a malignant tumour there is current controversy over whether Kaposi's sarcoma is indeed a true neoplasm or a multifocal vascular proliferation.

There are five main forms of Kaposi's sarcoma.

(1) The **classical** sporadic form as described by Kaposi in 1872 is seen in the Western world and occurs as red-blue plaques or nodules on the distal lower extremities of elderly males. It is particularly associated with individuals of Mediterranean extraction and with Eastern European Jews. It has an indolent course and death is often due to an unrelated cause. Patients have a higher than normal incidence of other malignant tumours, especially malignant lymphoma.

(2) In parts of sub-Saharan Africa the disease is **endemic** in the black population and affects predominantly males usually of 30–50 years of age. The clinical course is very variable, some cases behaving like sporadic Kaposi's sarcoma, some with aggressive local disease with florid fungating skin lesions and local lymph node involvement and some with widespread systemic disease.

(3) A rapidly fatal **lymphadenopathic** variant occurs in African children in whom there is widespread lymph node involvement, often without cutaneous lesions.

(4) Transplant-associated Kaposi's sarcoma occurs in a small proportion (less than 1%) of patients on prolonged immunosuppressive therapy following organ transplants. Lesions occur in the skin and systemically. The course is usually more aggressive than in sporadic Kaposi's sarcoma and is fatal in 30% of patients.

(5) In recent years Kaposi's sarcoma has been recognized as an **AIDS-associated** disease. It occurs far more frequently in homosexual males with AIDS than in other at-risk groups and the reasons for this are uncertain. Skin lesions are usually small, pink or purple patches and are often multiple, involving the head and neck, trunk, arms and hard palate. Multiple lesions in extracutaneous sites such as lymph nodes, gastrointestinal tract and liver are also found. These patients die of the other complications of AIDS (p. 243).

All forms of Kaposi's sarcoma may be seen in three stages, an early patch stage, a plaque stage and a nodular stage. In AIDS-related Kaposi's sarcoma the lesions are often seen at the early patch stage, which is the most difficult to diagnose histologically as lesions may resemble granulation tissue (Fig. 24.40). There is an increased number of small blood vessels in the dermis and these have a rather jagged outline and show a tendency to dissect through the dermal collagen. They are often surrounded by extravasated erythrocytes, and mild infiltrate of plasma cells. At later stages in the disease there are two components, a proliferation of vascular channels lined by endothelial cells, and a fibrosarcoma-like spindle-cell component in which small sieve-like spaces are present which contain red blood cells (Fig. 24.41). There may be scattered haemosiderin pigment and plasma cells may be numerous. There is still debate over whether Kaposi's sarcoma is of lymphatic or vascular endothelial cell origin.

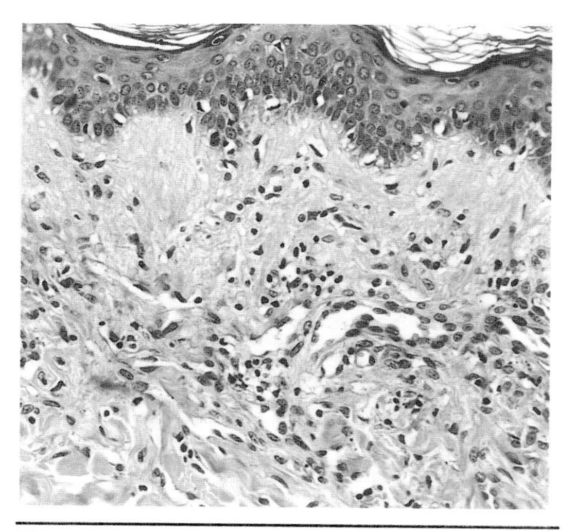

Fig. 24.40 Kaposi's sarcoma in AIDS patient – patch stage. Note proliferation of small blood vessels in the upper dermis. The vessels have an irregular jagged outline and are surrounded by chronic inflammation. ×180.

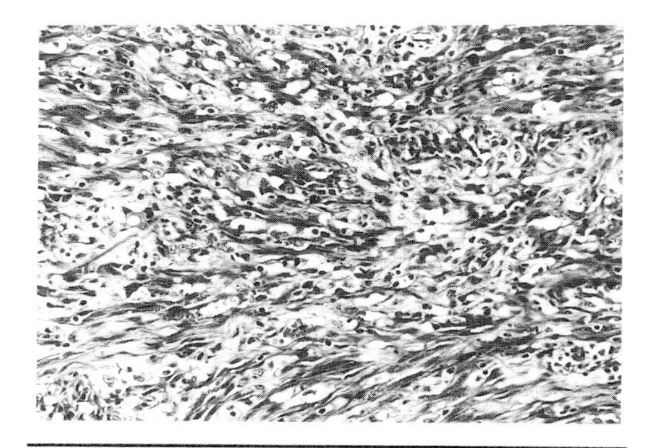

Fig. 24.41 Tumour stage Kaposi's sarcoma. Spindle-cells with sieve-like spaces containing erythrocytes. ×110.

Further Reading

Enzinger, F. M. and Weiss, S. W. (1988). *Soft Tissue Tumours*, 2nd edn. C. V. Mosby, St Louis.

Fitzpatrick, T. B., Eisen, A. Z., Wolff, K., Freedberg, I. M. and Austen, K. F. (1987). *Dermatology in General Medicine*, 3rd. edn (2 vols). McGraw-Hill, New York.

Harawi, S. J. and O'Hara, C. J. (1989). *Pathology and Pathophysiology of AIDS and HIV-related Diseases*, Chapters 6 and 9. Chapman and Hall, London.

Lever, W. F. and Schaumburg-Lever, G. (1990). *Histopathology of the Skin*. J. B. Lippincott, Philadelphia.

McKee, P. H. (1989). *Pathology of the Skin*. J. B. Lippincott, Philadelphia.

MacKie, R. M. (1989). *Skin Cancer*. Martin Dunitz, London.

Rook, A., Wilkinson, D. S., Ebling, F. J. G., Champion, R. H. and Burton, J. L. (1986). *Textbook of Dermatology*, 4th edn (3 vols). Blackwell Scientific, Oxford.

25

Diseases Caused by Parasitic Protozoa and Metazoa

Parasitic diseases result from infection by protozoa, helminths (worms) and some arthropods. They have an immense influence on the lives of man and all lower vertebrates, producing a great variety of illnesses with effects ranging from the rapidly fatal through the chronically morbid to the incidental and asymptomatic. About 30 000 species of protozoa and a similar number of helminths are known, most of them free-living, the minority parasitic. Of these, only 20 or so genera of protozoa and about 100 species of worms afflict man. Yet the genus *Plasmodium* alone – the cause of the malarias – is a major, sometimes the major public health problem in 70 countries with one-third of the world's population at risk from infection. In Africa alone, it is estimated that malaria kills directly or indirectly one million children each year. Similarly, the two species of hookworm may be found in one-quarter of all people on earth and are a significant cause of chronic anaemia and consequent debility and loss of work output.

Parasitic diseases are not synonymous with tropical diseases. Although parasitic infections are more common in warm climates, 'tropical diseases' are also the natural results of poverty, overcrowding, malnutrition, lack of clean water and of adequate disposal of excreta. The interactions of these factors with the prevailing parasites constitute medicine in the tropics. In developed countries, many parasites are endemic at a low level, e.g. amoebae and hydatid cysts, and several at a high level, such as threadworms, *Toxoplasma* and scabetic mites. New diseases have emerged, for example the acquired immune deficiency syndrome (AIDS, p. 243) with its frequent opportunistic infections by ubiquitous but normally non-pathogenic parasites such as *Pneumocystis*. Also over one billion passengers travel by air each year around the world; visitors to endemic zones can bring back their newly acquired parasites to developed countries before the incubation periods are over, and present clinically at home. These considerations emphasize the significance of parasitic illnesses in all nations and the necessity of recognizing them.

This chapter gives a synoptic account of the pathological changes induced by the major parasites, along with brief clinical descriptions. Life cycles, usually considered an unnecessary burden on the memory, are kept to the minimum needed for understanding the disease processes. The importance of immunopathology is emphasized and the outlines of diagnostic tests are stated. For further details of the life cycles of parasites and accounts of their intermediate hosts, the student is referred to standard texts on parasitology and medical entomology.

Parasite pathophysiology. Some general features are worth introducing at this point:

(1) The intensity of infection, i.e. the number of parasites present in a host, often determines whether an infection is asymptomatic, mild or debilitating. A few hookworms or *Strongyloides* are of slight clinical consequence; hundreds may be fatal.

(2) In the absence of effective host resistance, protozoa can replicate within the host and may build up fatal intensities, e.g. in cerebral malaria and toxoplasmosis. At the other extreme, as with *Entamoeba histolytica*, the host may pass cysts chronically and suffer no ill effects. By contrast, most helminths do not multiply in the host, but increase in number by repeated infections.

(3) Resistance to parasites is a vast and complex subject. Man is resistant to some protozoa which nevertheless can cause opportunistic infection: an example is *Pneumocystis carinii*, a cause of severe, often fatal pneumonia in subjects with depressed immunity. Other protozoa multiply readily in man and cause disease in most of those infected, but they stimulate an immune response with consequently increasing resistance. Such acquired immunity helps to explain the varying features of infection by a parasite in different age groups in endemic zones, and also the different patterns of disease seen in non-immune visitors, as compared with inhabitants who have been exposed to infection all their lives and have acquired a degree of protective immunity. Thus, unprotected visitors to malarial zones acquiring *Plasmodium falciparum* infection may die of cerebral malaria, but this is uncommon in local inhabitants. In the latter, acute malaria is mainly seen in childhood and during pregnancy.

(4) The mechanisms by which parasites cause disease in the host vary enormously. In the schistosomiases, the damage is wrought by a hypersensitivity reaction to the eggs laid by the worm's host, i.e. immunopathology. At the other end of the scale, the lesions of amoebiasis are due almost entirely to tissue necrosis caused directly by the amoebae.

(5) In the highly endemic zones multiple parasitism is the rule. A typical African peasant may harbour hookworms, schistosomes, ascarid worms and a filarial worm, in addition to a chronic low level of malarial parasitaemia.

(6) The pathophysiology of parasitic infections is complicated by the close interdependence, in susceptible populations, of infection, nutrition and immunity. This is particularly important where malnutrition is common. Infections such as malaria and hookworms reduce nutrition by causing chronic ill health; malnutrition increases the severity of many protozoal, bacterial and viral illnesses; and heavy parasite loads impair non-specific and immune cellular defence mechanisms. Yet, as an illustration of our lack of full understanding of the complexities involved, there is the paradoxical observation that severe oedematous malnutrition in children (kwashiorkor) appears to protect them against the cerebral form of malaria.

(7) Finally, a few parasites are known to be associated aetiologically with cancer: *Schistosoma haematobium* with bladder cancer, opisthorchiasis with cholangiocarcinoma and malaria with Burkitt's

lymphoma. In none of these is the parasite known to produce any carcinogenic agent; rather, they appear to act as promoters or by causing immunosuppression.

Diseases Caused by Protozoa

Protozoa are small unicellular eukaryotic cells which range in size from 1 to 150 μm, although most parasitic species are at the smaller end of the scale. They have short generation times, high reproductive rates and variable means of evading the host immune response. The major human protozoal diseases are malaria, the leishmaniases, the trypanosomiases and amoebiasis. In developed countries, the commonest is toxoplasmosis.

Malaria

This ancient disease is still the scourge of the tropics and subtropics. Africa, the Middle East, Asia and China, and Central and South America are all endemic zones, with tens of millions of cases annually. Non-endemic countries see malaria frequently as an imported but uninvited guest in travellers. Temperate areas in the USA and Europe have been cleared but elsewhere attempts to obliterate the disease have been hindered by lack of finance, wars and political upheavals, acquisition of resistance to insecticides by the mosquito and to drugs by the parasite. Consequently, in most endemic areas the aim is now control rather than elimination.

Four species of *Plasmodium* affect man, *P. falciparum*, *P. vivax*, *P. malariae* and *P. ovale*, of which *P. falciparum* is the most important. Malaria is a complex multisystem disease. Erythrocytes, the brain, lungs, kidney and placenta are the main sites of pathology. The case fatality rate for *P. falciparum* is approximately 2%.

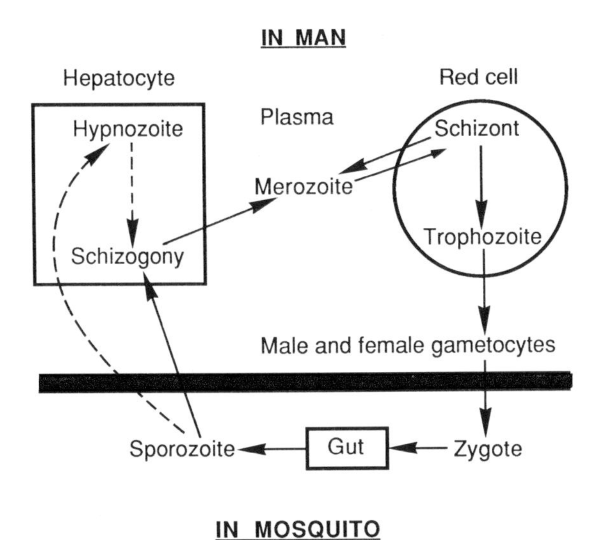

Fig. 25.1 Life cycle of malaria parasites. The hypnozoite pathway (interrupted lines) applies only to *Plasmodium vivax* and *Plasmodium ovale*.

Life Cycle (Fig. 25.1)

Females of *Anopheles* species of mosquito are the vectors of malaria. They bite man to obtain a blood meal necessary for the development of their own progeny. When man is bitten by an infected mosquito, **sporozoites** (10 μm long) are injected. These rapidly leave the circulation and enter hepatocytes, where asexual multiplication occurs and the progeny, called **merozoites** (1 μm diameter) are released into the circulation when the infected liver cells rupture (Fig. 25.2). This exo-erythrocytic schizogony (literally: multiplication outside the blood) takes from 5 to 15 days, depending on the *Plasmodium* species, and determines the incubation period of malaria.

The merozoites enter red cells and become **trophozoites**; at first, they have a ring form (Fig. 25.3), but then enlarge to fill the cell. Further asexual division occurs, forming a **schizont** composed of many merozoites (Fig. 25.4). The developing parasite feeds on the haemoglobin and brown breakdown pigment called haemozoin is

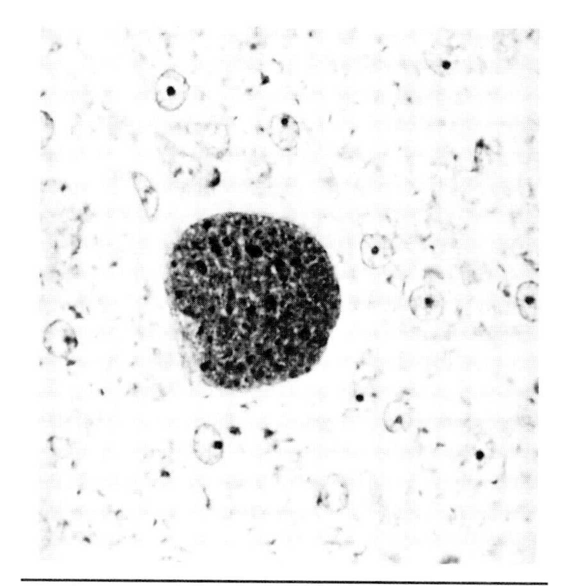

Fig. 25.2 A liver cell distended by numerous merozoites in the early stage of malarial infection. ×1000.

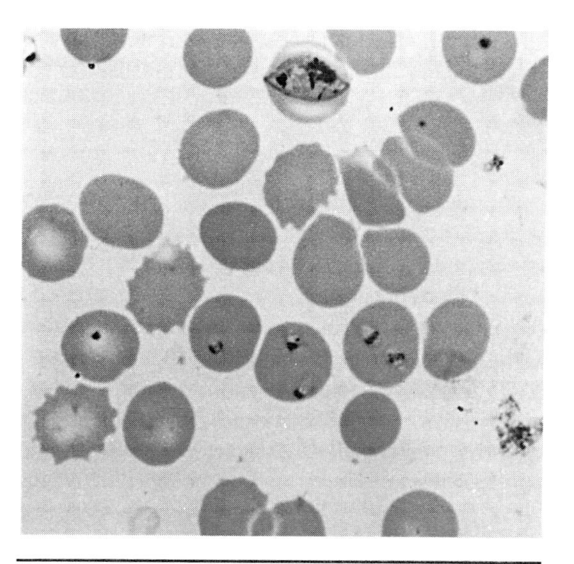

Fig. 25.3 Blood smear showing ring forms of *Plasmodium falciparum* in red cells. Some cells contain two parasites. The large crescentic form also present is a gametocyte. ×1000.

seen in the red cells. The erythrocytes rupture, releasing the merozoites which then invade other red cells. This erythrocytic cycle is characteristically synchronous; it takes 48 hours in *P. vivax*, *P. ovale* and *P. falciparum* and 72 hours in *P. malariae* infections and this determines the periodicity of the clinical paroxysms of fever and chills in acute malaria.

Some merozoites do not develop asexually but differentiate into male and female **gametocytes**. The mosquito takes these up in a blood meal from an infected individual; they fuse in the mosquito gut to form a zygote which multiplies to produce thousands of sporozoites. These enter the mosquito's salivary gland and are injected into man when it bites.

In *P. vivax* and *P. ovale* infections, relapses are now known to be the result of persistent liver parasites called **hypnozoites** (literally: sleeping animals) which develop directly from the sporozoites. They lie dormant as 1 μm bodies in hepatocytes, emerging months or years later to release merozoites into the blood.

Malaria may also be contracted from infected blood by blood transfusion and by syringes shared among intravenous drug abusers. Transplacental

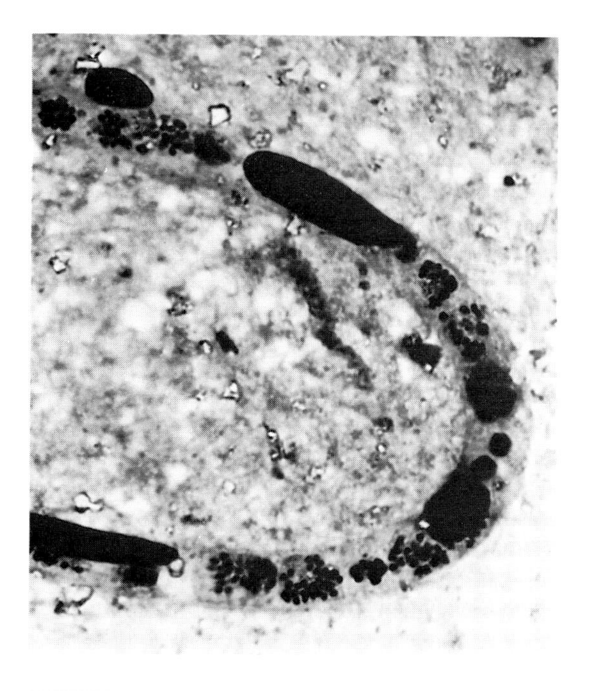

Fig. 25.4 *Plasmodium falciparum* schizonts inside a cerebral capillary in a fatal case of cerebral malaria. The numerous merozoites which fill the red cell schizonts are seen as tiny black dots. The large nuclei belong to endothelial cells. ×1250.

infection is uncommon; it presents as anaemia and splenomegaly in early infancy. The morphology of the various parasite forms in the erythrocytic cycle are characteristic for each species and serve to differentiate them diagnostically.

P. falciparum infections are potentially fatal, while the others are not. This is due to several factors: (1) *P. falciparum* produces more merozoites from the schizogony cycles in the liver and red cells than the other species, and so causes higher levels of parasitaemia; (2) red cells harbouring *P. falciparum* adhere to endothelium. They are sequestered in the capillaries of the viscera where they impede blood flow and cause ischaemic damage.

Clinical Features

Malaria presents with sudden onset of fever, headache, myalgia and a haemolytic anaemia. In the first attack, the bouts occur at regular intervals, coinciding with the release of merozoites from burst red cells: every 2 days with *P. vivax* ('benign tertian' malaria), *P. ovale* ('ovale tertian') and *P. falciparum* ('malignant tertian') and every 3 days with *P. malariae* ('quartan malaria'). Elimination of parasites in the blood is curative for *P. falciparum* and *P. malariae*, but *P. vivax* and *P. ovale* malarias may, as described above, relapse months or years later in the absence of re-infection. In endemic zones with constant re-infections, an acquired immunity is built up in survivors. Passive immunity from maternal antibodies lasts about 6 months from birth, then waves of severe infection ensue but become less severe after a decade or so. Thereafter, attacks of acute malaria occur most often in pregnant women because the maternal sinuses of the placenta provide a particularly favourable site for intra-erythrocytic schizogony. Low fetal weight is a result.

Overwhelming infection with parasitaemias around 10^{12}/l of blood is responsible for hyperpyrexia and anaemia and for the **algid malaria shock syndrome** with peripheral vascular collapse: disseminated intravascular coagulation also occurs but is not common. Severe pulmonary oedema may be seen after treatment has commenced and is due to both shock and overenthusiastic intravenous infusions in patients with impaired renal function.

The malarias of *P. vivax, P. ovale* and *P. malariae* cause much chronic ill health through fever and anaemia but, apart from the quartan malaria nephrotic syndrome, are seldom fatal. *P. falciparum* infection has a fatality rate that is highest in children in endemic areas and in non-immune visitors who are not taking effective antimalarial prophylaxis.

The malarias are diagnosed by finding the parasite in the blood. Serodiagnosis is still being developed but is aimed more at epidemiology than at individuals. A light parasitaemia is most readily detected by examining thick films, but the thin film is usually needed to recognize the infecting species.

Pathological Changes

Haematological. The anaemia of malaria is multifactorial, and in endemic zones is commonly complicated by iron and folate deficiency. The most important factor is destruction of parasitized red cells, producing the general features of a haemolytic anaemia (p. 599): haemolysis occurs both intravascularly and by extravascular destruction in the spleen, but splenectomy makes malaria worse by impairing parasite clearance. Blood films show a variable parasitaemia, usually affecting 2% or less of the red cells except in falciparum infections when, in spite of sequestration of infected cells, up to 30% parasitaemias may be seen in non-immunes; levels over 25% are commonly fatal. The anaemia is normochromic; there may be a reticulocytosis, and a leucopenia with relative monocytosis is common. Dyserythropoiesis (p. 611) is uncommon. A variably positive Coombs' test does not correlate with the haemoglobin level, and immune haemolysis of parasitized and non-parasitized cells by bound antibody or immune complexes (which appear in the blood in malaria) is therefore apparently of minor importance. An exception to this is **blackwater fever**, an acute intravascular haemolysis during falciparum malaria in non-immunes, often following quinine therapy: the effects are those of massive haemolysis, notably prostration, fever, acute anaemia, shock and acute renal failure. The renal tubules are filled with debris and haemoglobin products, and show acute tubular necrosis due to the state of shock.

The lymphoreticular system. Malaria causes hyperplasia of the lymphoreticular system and the prevalence of malaria in a community may be gauged by the proportion of children with palpable spleens. In the acute attack, spleen and liver enlarge and become dark browny-grey as does the bone marrow. The sinusoids are congested with parasitized red cells and haemozoin pigment is plentiful in splenic macrophages and Kupffer cells (Fig. 25.5). Sinus histocytosis is seen in the lymph nodes and spleen. Following clearance of parasites from the blood, the pigment in the liver is carried in macrophages from the sinusoids to the portal tracts. The haemopoietic marrow is hyperplastic and contains abundant haemozoin pigment.

Tropical splenomegaly syndrome – hyper-reactive malarial splenomegaly. The latter term is better in that the syndrome is an idiosyncratic immunological response to malaria. Affected adults in areas endemic for falciparum malaria develop massive splenomegaly without obvious cause, i.e. not due to schistosomiasis, cirrhosis or portal vein thrombosis. The splenomegaly is likely to be related aetiologically to malaria because: (1) it is restricted to endemic zones; (2) patients with the syndrome have higher mean levels of antimalarial antibodies in the serum than controls, and also a very high serum IgM level; (3) it is rare in people with sickle-cell trait, who are partially protected against malaria; and (4) the splenomegaly regresses with long-term antimalarial treatment. The main clinical effects are those of hypersplenism and a dragging pain in the left flank. Parasitaemia is very scanty or absent. The spleen may weigh 3 kg or more and on section is firm and dark red. Histologically, there is hyperplasia of both the red and white pulp, but minimal or no pigment. The most characteristic histological change is hepatic sinusoidal lymphocytosis (Fig. 25.6).

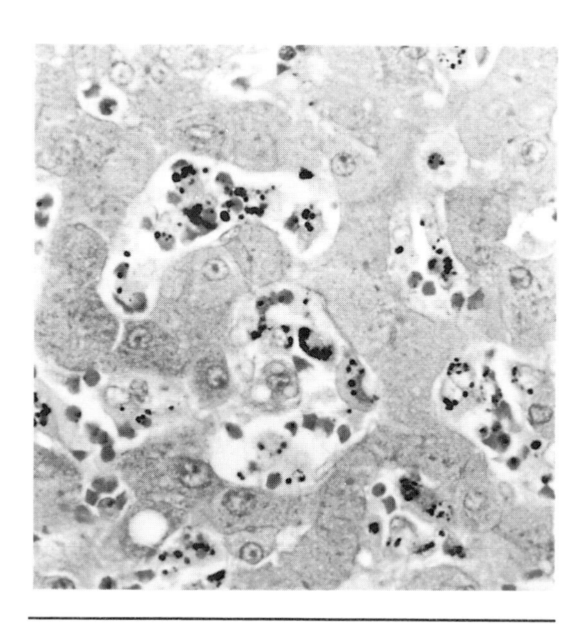

Fig. 25.5 The liver in falciparum malaria: parasitized red cells are just visible and there are plentiful dark granules of haemozoin within the Kupffer cells. ×1000.

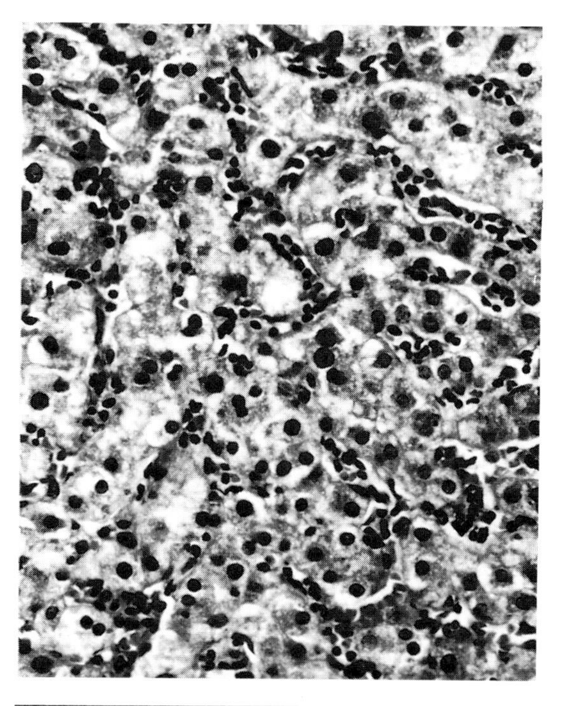

Fig. 25.6 The liver in tropical splenomegaly syndrome: the sinusoids contain numerous mature lymphocytes – hepatic sinusoidal lymphocytosis. ×400.

Burkitt's lymphoma (p. 408) is limited geographically to highly endemic malaria zones, where it forms the commonest malignancy in childhood. In these zones, virtually all children are infected with both the Epstein–Barr virus and malaria parasites; in a small proportion of them, repeated attacks of malaria apparently permit the oncogenic potential of EBV in B cells to be expressed as a B-cell lymphoma.

The kidneys. The renal tubules are damaged during blackwater fever and in the algid malaria syndrome. Circulating immune complexes are commonly present in malaria, and two types of immune-complex glomerulonephritis occur. The first is a reversible acute proliferative glomerulonephritis seen in some non-immune patients with acute *P. falciparum* infection. The second, **quartan malaria nephrotic syndrome**, occurs in a small percentage of children with chronic *P. malariae* infection. Biopsy shows focal or diffuse membranous glomerulonephritis and, later on, chronic glomerulonephritis. Deposits of *P. malariae* antigen, immunoglobulin and complement can sometimes be detected in the glomerular capillary walls. The condition has a poor prognosis; it does not respond to antimalarials, and progresses to chronic renal failure.

Cerebral malaria is the cause of death in falciparum malaria in non-immunes. Clinically, there is clouding of consciousness, fits and sometimes focal neurological signs. Intensive therapy saves many patients, and residual neurological deficits are uncommon. In fatal cases the brain is congested, often with petechial haemorrhages in the subcortical white matter (Fig. 25.7). Gross haemozoin pigmentation is not a feature, nor is infarction, unless the patient has been maintained on a ventilator after brain death. Microscopy shows microvascular congestion and large numbers of parasitized red cells sticking to the vascular endothelium (Fig. 25.4). Changes sometimes present include pericapillary demyelination and pericapillary ring haemorrhages (Fig. 25.8). The pathogenesis of the condition is not yet certain. The demyelination and ring haemorrhages appear to be related to vascular disruption (a similar picture is seen in systemic fat embolism). Erythrocytes parasitized by *P. falciparum* demonstrate electron dense deposits ('knobs') under the surface membrane, at which site there is adhesion to the surface of endothelium, i.e. the red cells become 'sticky' (Fig. 25.9).

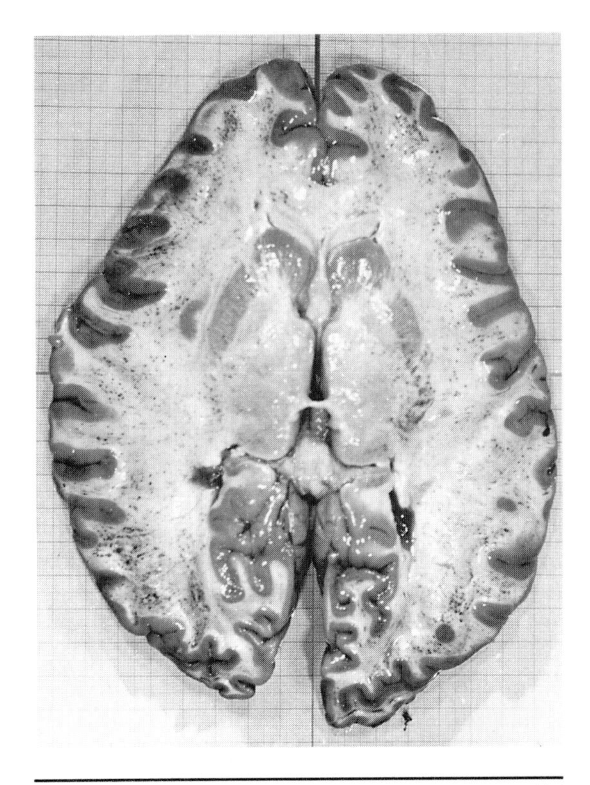

Fig. 25.7 The brain in cerebral malaria. Petechial haemorrhages are widespread throughout the white matter.

The Leishmaniases

These diseases are caused by flagellate protozoa of the genus *Leishmania*. With few exceptions they are zoonoses, i.e. infections primarily of animals with man as an incidental victim. Transmission is by the bite of sandflies. Some 500 000 new cases occur world wide per annum, and these include visitors to endemic zones. Three broad clinicopathological groups of diseases result (Table 25.1). The taxonomy of the leishmanias is com-

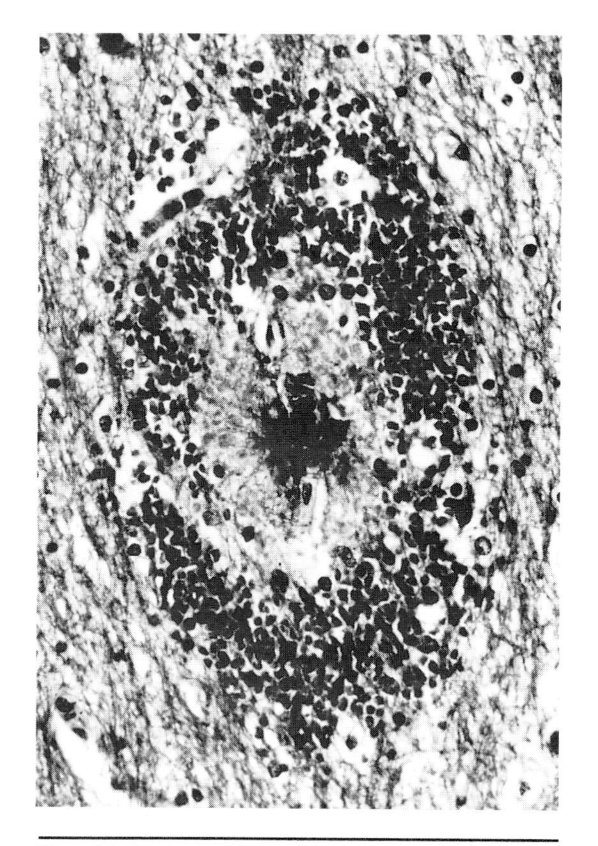

Fig. 25.8 A ring haemorrhage in cerebral malaria. The central vessel is plugged with fibrin and the immediate surrounding white matter is necrotic. Peripheral to that is a ring of red cells (stained black). ×400.

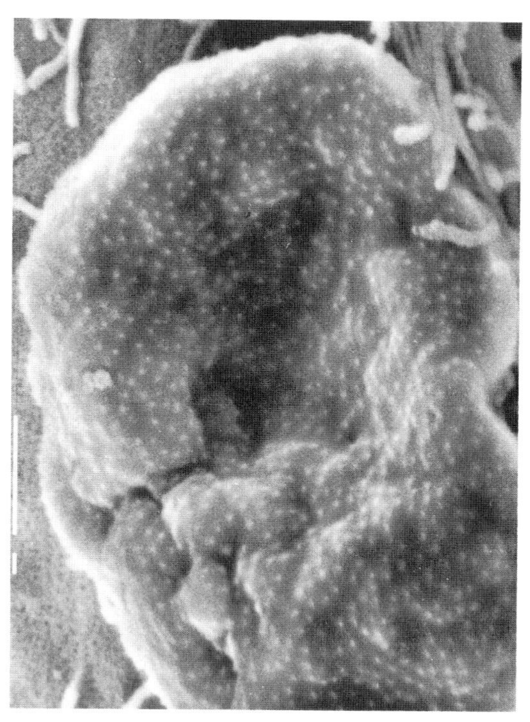

Fig. 25.9 Scanning electron photomicrograph of an erythrocyte infected by *Plasmodium falciparum*. Uninfected red cells have a smooth surface. Parasitized cells are covered in small, protruberant 'knobs', composed of parasite molecules and rearranged erythrocyte membrane skeletal components. The 'knobs' are the sites of adhesion of these cells to endothelial cells. (Photo by courtesy of Prof. M. Hommel, Liverpool School of Tropical Medicine.)

Table 25.1 The types and geographical distribution of leishmaniasis

Disease	Parasite	Distribution
Cutaneous leishmaniasis ('oriental sore')	*L. tropica* *L. major*	Africa, Asia, Middle East
	L. infantum	Southern Europe
	L. mexicana	South and Central America
Mucocutaneous leishmaniasis ('espundia')	*L. brasiliensis*	South and Central America
Visceral leishmaniasis ('kala-azar')	*L. donovani*	Asia, Africa, S. America
	L. infantum	Southern Europe

plex: DNA and isoenzyme analyses of the parasites are used to distinguish the various species.

The leishmanias are intracellular parasites, and cell mediated immunity is therefore involved in resistance and in their elimination. After an infective bite, injected leishmanias are taken up by macrophages, transform into non-flagellate **amastigotes** (literally: no whip) and multiply by binary fission. The amastigotes of all species are morphologically similar: they are round or ovoid bodies of 1.5–3 μm diameter with a thin cell membrane, a dense nucleus and a rod-shaped kinetoplast in the cytoplasm. They are also known as Leishman–Donovan (L–D) bodies (Fig. 25.10).

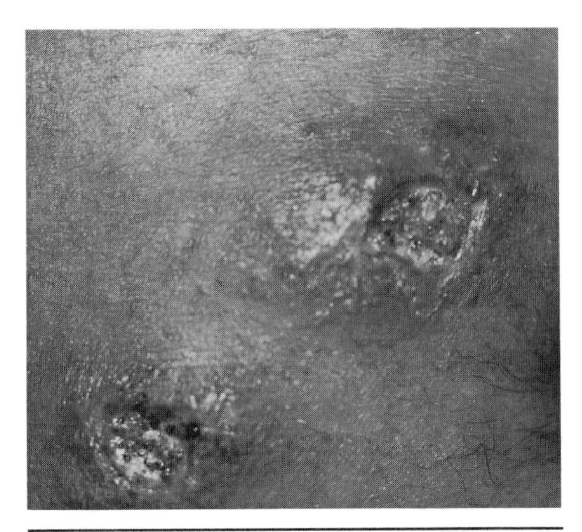

Fig. 25.11 Two lesions of cutaneous leishmaniasis near the umbilicus. The erythematous papules have broken down to form crateriform ulcers. (Slide kindly supplied by Dr D. Evans, London School of Hygiene and Tropical Medicine.)

Cutaneous Leishmaniasis

This is generally a localized self-healing condition. At the site of a bite, a papule develops and breaks down to form a crateriform ulcer (Fig. 25.11). Secondary bacterial infection often supervenes, but healing takes place over weeks or months, leaving a scar. Microscopically, the early lesion consists of dermal macrophages filled with amastigotes (Fig. 25.12); later there is an intense infiltration of lymphocytes and plasma cells followed by necrosis, granulomas and gradual elimination of the parasites. L–D bodies can usually be

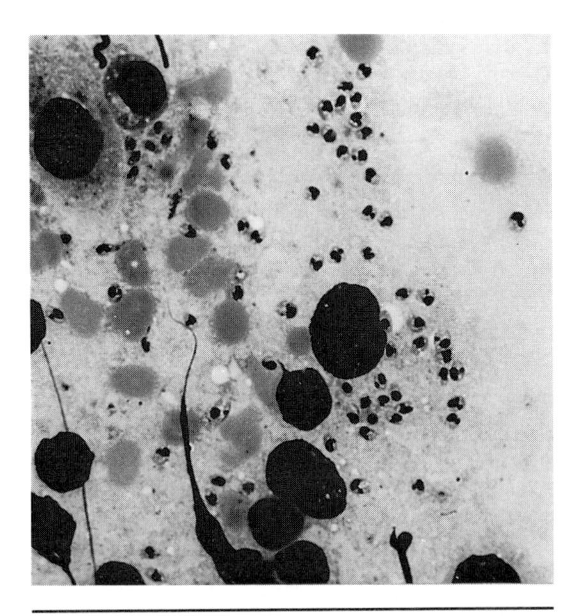

Fig. 25.10 Numerous Leishman–Donovan bodies in a splenic aspirate from a case of visceral leishmaniasis. The comma-shaped bodies next to the nuclei are the kinetoplasts. ×1000.

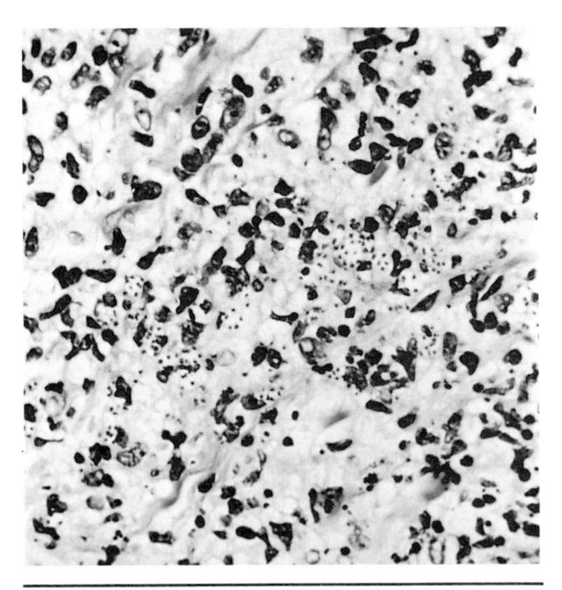

Fig. 25.12 Early lesion of cutaneous leishmaniasis. Amastigotes are seen as abundant small dark bodies within dermal macrophages. ×250.

detected microscopically in an aspirate or biopsy of the lesion, or if necessary by culture. Occasionally the host response in cutaneous leishmaniasis is inadequate and large areas of the skin become and remain filled with heavily parasitized macrophages. This condition of **diffuse cutaneous leishmaniasis** is analogous to lepromatous leprosy, and indeed there is evidence of a similar immunopathological spectrum of host–parasite relationships in both conditions.

Mucocutaneous Leishmaniasis

L. brasiliensis infection starts like ordinary cutaneous leishmaniasis, with lesions on the head, limbs or trunk. These heal, but metastatic lesions appear at mucocutaneous junctions, commonly in the nose and the upper lip. These secondary lesions do not heal, but progress destructively, eroding skin, mucosa and cartilage and often causing gross disfigurement. Secondary bacterial infection complicates the picture. There is necrosis and a mixed inflammatory infiltrate including macrophage granulomas, in which the parasites are scanty or undetectable.

Visceral Leishmaniasis

This is the classical *L. donovani* disease to which is applied the term **kala-azar** (Hindi for 'black fever', so named because fair skinned patients become hyperpigmented). The disease is the result of anergic failure to react to the intracellular parasites, which disseminate throughout the lymphoreticular system. There is hepatosplenomegaly, lymphadenopathy, cachexia, fever and pancytopenia. The incubation period is several months, and without treatment the disease is usually fatal from intercurrent bacterial infection such as pneumonia. In the form of the disease caused by *L. infantum*, subclinical illness and recovery from infection are common, unless, as is increasingly seen, the patient is immunocompromised by HIV infection.

The pancytopenia results from hypersplenism and marrow replacement by parasitized macrophages. The susceptibility to secondary infection is multifactorial; leucopenia, T-cell suppression and deficient antigen handling by parasitized macrophages all contribute. There is also a polyclonal B-cell proliferation in the tissues, producing a characteristic high level of IgG and IgM in the serum, only part of which is anti-leishmanial antibody.

The liver in visceral leishmaniasis is large and pale; the spleen is massively enlarged, commonly weighing 3 kg or more, and on section is firm and red. The red marrow is hyperplastic. Histologically, amastigotes are abundant in the macrophages of the liver, spleen, marrow, lymph nodes and lamina propria of the gut, but necrosis is rare. Liver sinusoids are distended by hypertrophied parasitized Kupffer cells (Fig. 25.13); sinus histiocytosis and paracortical cell depletion are seen in the lymph nodes, and there is gross hyperplasia of the splenic red pulp. Plasma cells are also increased in these organs. An analogy of

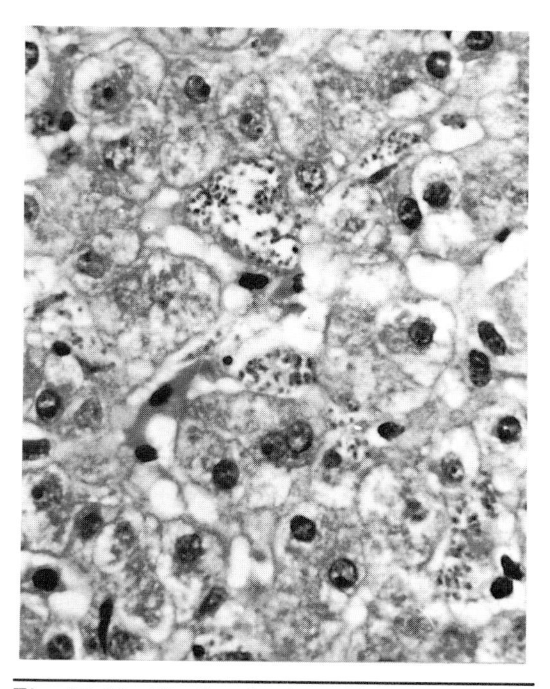

Fig. 25.13 The liver in visceral leishmaniasis. Hypertrophied Kupffer cells are filled with small L–D bodies. ×400.

this disease is *Mycobacterium avium-intracellulare* infection in immunosuppressed patients, where macrophages of the lymphoreticular system become filled with acid-fast bacilli, yet without necrosis or formation of tubercules.

Visceral leishmaniasis is diagnosed by finding L-D bodies in smears from spleen or marrow aspirates (see Fig. 25.10), and by liver biopsy.

The Trypanosomiases

Insect-transmitted flagellates of the genus *Trypanosoma* cause two entirely distinct diseases in man – the African trypanosomiasis (sleeping sickness) and South American trypanosomiasis (Chagas' disease). The trypanosomes in the blood (**trypomastigotes**) in both diseases are undulating elongated slender cells, 15–30 μm long, with a nucleus and a posterior kinetoplast with a flagellum arising from it (Fig. 25.14). In fresh preparations they wriggle rapidly and continuously and can be detected at low magnification by the disturbance they create among the adjacent red cells. In African trypanosomiasis the parasite remains extracellular in location, but in Chagas' disease it enters tissue cells and assumes a small **amastigote** form (like a *Leishmania*) and transforms back to the trypomastigote form during subsequent episodes of parasitaemia.

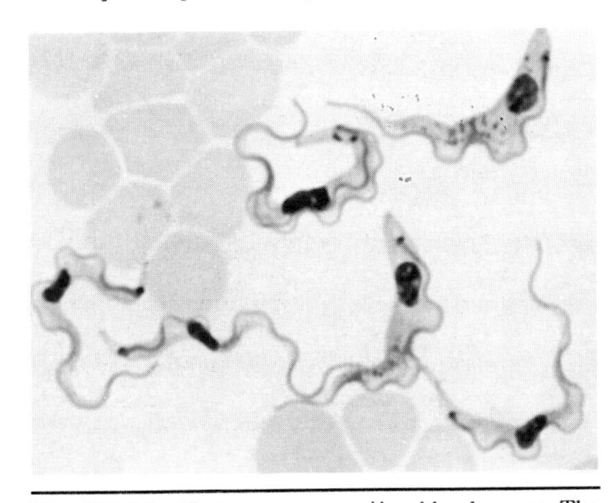

Fig. 25.14 *Trypanosoma cruzi* in a blood smear. The flagellum is seen arising from the kinetoplast body. ×1200.

African Trypanosomiases

About 45 million people in West, Central and East Africa are at risk from sleeping sickness, which is fatal without treatment. Related trypanosomes are an even more important cause of disease in cattle so that much of the African savannah is uninhabitable by livestock. The human disease may occur in epidemics and depopulate large areas. Two forms of the disease are seen: that caused by *Trypanosoma brucei (T. b.) gambiense* in West and Central Africa is restricted to man, whilst that caused by *Trypanosoma brucei (T. b.) rhodesiense* in Central and East Africa has a reservoir in game animals, and is the more fulminant form. All trypanosomiases in Africa are transmitted by tsetse flies. Transplacental transmission is very uncommon.

The parasites multiply by binary fission at the site of the tsetse fly bite. The ensuing oedema and inflammation result in a trypanosomal chancre. Invasion of the blood follows and various grades of parasitaemia persist until terminated by death or treatment. The trypanosomes may divide in the blood to peak numbers exceeding 1.5×10^9/l.

Clinical Features and Course

There is fever, anaemia, mild splenomegaly, lymphadenopathy, a puffy face and skin rashes. Sooner or later after blood invasion has occurred, the trypanosomes enter the central nervous system. Headache, behavioural changes, neurological signs and altered sleep rhythm gradually lead to semi-coma. Death follows from inanition and secondary infection, within months in the florid *T. b. rhodesiense* form and within months to years in the *T. b. gambiense* infection. In *T. b. rhodesiense* infection, there are heavier parasitaemias, often pancarditis, and in some cases an immune-complex glomerulonephritis or disseminated intravascular coagulation.

The diagnosis of African trypanosomiasis depends on finding the parasites in the blood, lymph node aspirate or CSF. In late *T.b. gambiense* infection, blood trypanosomes may be exceedingly scanty, and haemoconcentration techniques may be needed. A raised CSF IgM concentration is almost pathognomonic of cerebral trypanosomiasis.

Immunological factors. The parasitaemia of both forms of African trypanosomiasis is periodic. Antibodies are produced to trypanosomal antigens and opsonize the parasites, which are cleared from the blood by phagocytes in the liver, spleen, etc. However, a few parasites with different surface antigenic determinants survive and they multiply to produce a new wave of parasitaemia. Further antibody production follows, but the same phenomenon occurs, and the results are repeated episodes of parasitaemia at roughly weekly intervals and increasingly high levels of IgM in the blood. This phenomenon of **antigenic variation** by the parasite and subsequent multiplication of new clones of parasites non-reactive with the 'old' antibodies thus allows the trypanosome to evade the host immune response. A B-cell mitogen may also be produced by the parasite, since only a fraction of the IgM is antitrypanosomal antibody. There is a general depression of immune responses which contributes to the development of intercurrent infection. One cause of the anaemia in trypanosomiasis is immune adherence of antibodies and immune complexes to erythrocytes, which may undergo 'bystander lysis' in the spleen.

Pathological Changes

The spleen and lymph nodes show sinus histiocytosis and plasma cell proliferation, with depletion of the T-cell zones. A chronic valvulitis and myocarditis with involvement of the cardiac conducting system in seen in some East African cases.

When the central nervous system is involved, the CSF protein and IgM levels rise and lymphocytes, morular cells (see below) and also trypanosomes are found in the CSF. The neural lesion is a **meningoencephalitis**. Grossly, the meninges are congested. In acute cases, there is narrowing of the ventricles due to brain swelling, but in long-standing *T. b. gambiense* infections there may be some cerebral atrophy and secondary hydrocephalus. Microscopy shows the features of a chronic meningitis and focal encephalitis, particularly in the brainstem. Lymphocytes and plasma cells infiltrate the meninges and the perivascular spaces to produce perivascular cuffing. There is reactive gliosis, and near vessels the characteristic morular cells of Mott can be seen (Fig. 25.15). These are plasma cells containing large refractile vesicles stuffed with IgM (Russell bodies).

The cause of cerebral injury in trypanosomal encephalitis is one of the mysteries of tropical pathology, and trypanosomes are not seen in brain tissues. Probably there is an interaction between activitated lymphocytes and astrocytes (which enclose cerebral vessels). Various cytokines are secreted which increase the inflammation and also affect cerebral function.

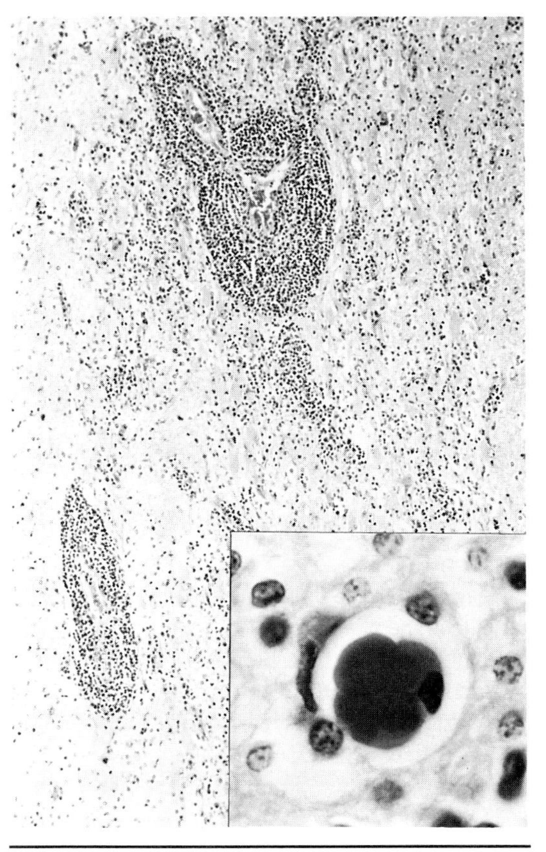

Fig. 25.15 Pons in a case of *Trypanosoma rhodesiense* infection. There is encephalitis with marked perivascular cuffing by lymphocytes. ×100. Inset: a morular cell of Mott – a plasma cell distended by large Russell bodies containing IgM. ×1000.

South American Trypanosomiasis (Chagas' Disease)

At least 10 million people in South and Central America are infected with *Trypanosoma cruzi*, the causal agent of Chagas' disease, though not all show clinical disease. The clinical syndromes are acute Chagas' disease with a mortality of 5–10% followed by a latent asymptomatic period of 10–20 years, after which chronic Chagas' disease becomes manifest in about 30% of infected people. It frequently presents with congestive cardiac failure, and this is the commonest single cause of admission to adult medical wards in many South American hospitals.

Initial infection is usually acquired in childhood when an infective reduviid bug takes a blood meal and deposits flagellate forms of *T. cruzi* in its faeces on the skin. The victim rubs the parasites into the skin when scratching the bite. Transmission may also occur transplacentally or by transfusion of infected blood. The local inflammation and oedema produce a trypanosomal chancre or chagoma. If the parasite enters near the eye, the resulting eyelid oedema and conjunctivitis are known as Romana's sign. After about 2 weeks, the amastigote parasites transform back into trypomastigotes and spread by the blood to infect many types of cell, including myocardium, glial cells of the central nervous system, cells of the myenteric plexus in the gut and cells of the lymphoreticular system.

Chagas' disease is diagnosed by finding the parasite in the blood or by specific serology. In the latent or chronic phases, parasitaemia is often very low and sometimes the diagnosis can be confirmed only by allowing an uninfected reduviid bug to feed on the patient and examining it later for vector stages of the parasite (xenodiagnosis).

Acute Chagas' Disease

The main clinical features are due to myocarditis and encephalitis. The heart is dilated, and the muscle soft and focally haemorrhagic, and microscopy shows clusters of amastigotes in the myocardial cells (Fig. 25.16): rupture of these cells induces a lymphocytic, plasma cell and macrophage reaction with phagocytosis of the parasites. Antibodies to *T. cruzi* persist in the latent phase, and although chemotherapy may abolish this transient phase of parasitaemia, the tissue amastigotes persist.

Chronic Chagas' Disease

This has two main aspects: cardiac failure and the megasyndromes.

There is cardiomegaly, heart block, arrhythmias, increasing congestive failure and embolic phenomena from mural thrombosis in the left ventricle. The heart may weigh up to 1 kg. All the chambers are dilated and there is often an apical aneurysm. Histologically, there is chronic inflammation, fibrosis of the myocardium and scattered

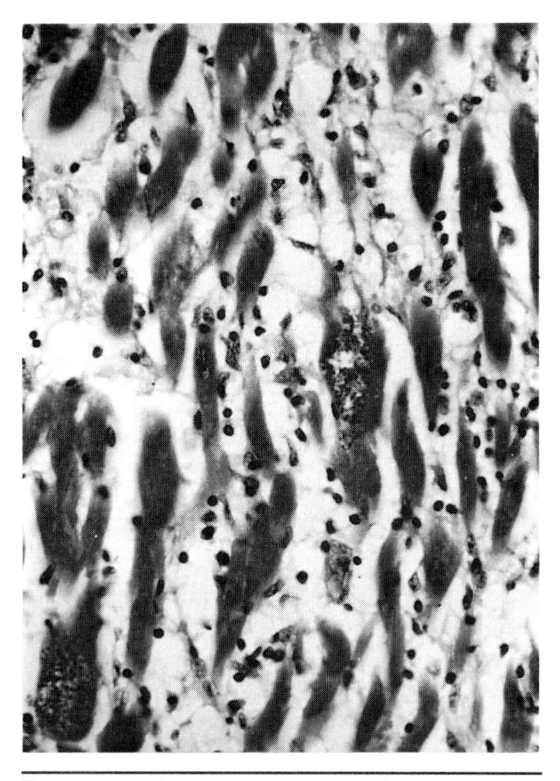

Fig. 25.16 Acute chagasic myocarditis. The myocardium is oedematous and inflamed, and clusters of tiny black dots (amastigotes of *Trypanosoma cruzi*) are seen in two myocytes. ×400.

hypertrophied muscle fibres, but at this stage parasitized myofibres are few and are found in less than 50% of cases. Inflammation and fibrosis also affect the conducting system with reduction of nodal ganglion cells.

The megasyndromes are caused by gross dilatation of the alimentary canal, principally the oesophagus and colon, with the symptoms of stasis. The dilated alimentary tract shows thinning of the wall with variable mural inflammation and scarring. Myenteric plexus ganglion cells are greatly reduced in number.

These chronic lesions are probably caused by delayed hypersensitivity reactions to parasitized muscle and neurons, and possibly also by cytotoxic antibody. During the acute phase of the disease, trypanosomal antigens are released from disrupted infected cells. These antigens bind to other cells and render them susceptible to later attack by the host's anti-*T. cruzi* response. In the majority of those affected, low levels of the cell mediated immunity result in a balanced state in which both host and parasite survive.

The Amoebiases

Two groups of amoebae are pathogenic for man, the most important being the intestinal amoeba, *Entamoeba histolytica*. Many other intestinal amoebae are described, such as *Entamoeba coli* and *Iodamoeba bütschlii*, but these are harmless commensals and are important only because they may be mistaken for *E. histolytica* or vice versa. The second type of pathogenic amoebae are the free-living *Naegleria* and *Acanthamoeba* species.

Entamoeba histolytica

Infection with this parasite can cause amoebic dysentry and amoebic 'abscesses' in the liver and other viscera. Some 10% of the world's population carry *E. histolytica* in their bowel. The proportion is highest in the cities of the tropics and subtropics, but no country is free of infection. Man acquires amoebae by ingesting food or water contaminated by cysts derived from human faeces, there being no animal reservoir. The cysts are hardy and resist drying: following ingestion, they excyst in the small intestine and release four motile **trophozoites**, which are 20–30 μm in diameter and have a single nucleus (see Fig. 25.18). They are anaerobic, feed on gut bacteria and multiply by binary fission. Most people who are infected are asymptomatic healthy carriers; the amoebae reside in the lumen of the proximal colon and do not damage the mucosa but encyst to form quadrinucleate cysts that are excreted in the faeces.

It is now evident that the occurrence of invasive symptomatic disease, to which the term amoebiasis should be properly restricted, depends on both parasite and host factors. By enzyme chromatographic studies, many different strains (or zymodemes) of *E. histolytica* have now been identified, only a few of which have caused invasive disease in man. The other strains, though morphologically identical, are non-pathogenic. The luminal enterobacteria are also probably involved in the expression of pathogenicity by some synergistic action with the amoebae. Certain immunosuppressive states such as pregnancy and steroid therapy predispose to invasive disease, but the mechanisms of natural resistance are unknown.

Pathogenic amoebae lyse cells and tissues; direct contact between amoeba and target cell is necessary; the amoeba secretes an ionophore. The target cell membrane is made leaky so that cytoplasmic ions escape and the cell dies. The host inflammatory reaction is variable and induced by cell injury rather than directly by the amoebae. Healing of the lesions is usually accompanied by minimal scarring and, in contrast to many other parasitic infections, no recognizable hypersensitivity reactions contribute to the pathology of amoebiasis.

Intestinal Amoebiasis

Invasion usually occurs in the caecum and sigmoid colon, rarely in the ileum and appendix. There is early superficial necrosis of the mucosa with adjacent oedema and the amoebae then invade the submucosa (Fig. 25.17) where they tend to spread

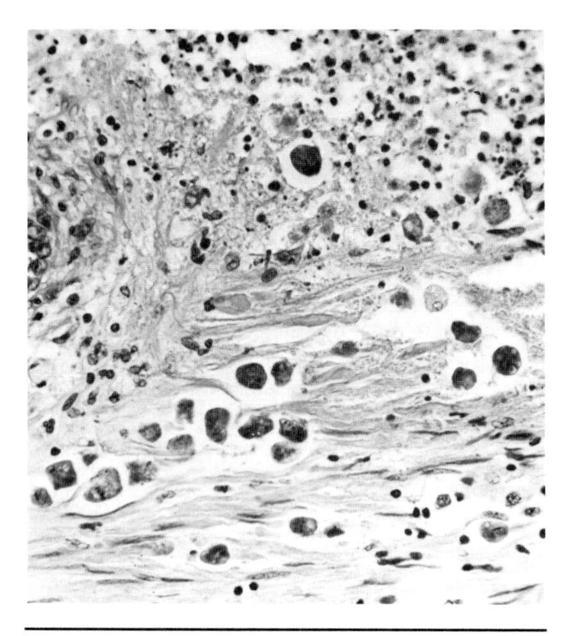

Fig. 25.17 Amoebic ulcer of the colon. The upper part of the field consists of necrotic mucosa and exudate. Below this, the amoebae are seen digesting the submucosa, but with remarkably little cellular reaction. ×200.

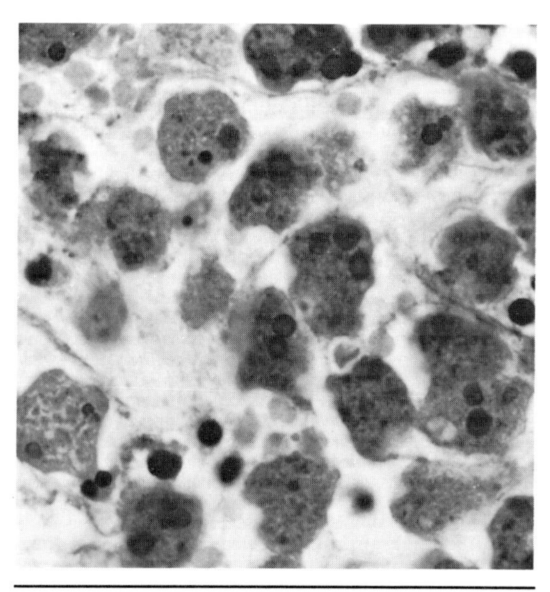

Fig. 25.18 *Entamoeba histolytica* trophozoites near a colonic ulcer. In addition to the nucleus, they also contain phagocytosed red cells (stained dark). ×100.

laterally. This undermines the mucosa and produces the characteristic flask-shaped ulcer. The ulcers may stay discrete or become confluent with sloughing of large areas of mucosa. The stools are foul-smelling, loose, mucoid and tinged with blood.

The early invasive lesion may heal spontaneously or progress to pan-colonic ulceration and dilatation and sometimes perforation, with consequent peritonitis, which has a high mortality and is more likely to occur in patients misdiagnosed as ulcerative colitis and treated with glucocorticoids.

Histologically, the mucosal cells degenerate and the amoebae are often best seen in the adjacent mucous exudate. They appear rounded in form, or amoeboid with pseudopodia, and when invasive they contain phagocytosed red cells (Fig. 25.18). The lesions are infiltrated by plasma cells, macrophages and polymorphs. As the trophozoites invade deeper, they are concentrated at the advancing edge of the lesion, and the overlying mucosa shows ischaemic necrosis.

Proctosigmoidoscopy often shows scattered foci of ulceration surrounded by oedematous mucosa, appearances which differ from those of ulcerative colitis and Crohn's disease and may suggest the correct diagnosis. Confirmation of the active disease can usually be made by identifying the mobile amoebae in a fresh specimen of stool; healthy carriers and patients with chronic indolent disease excrete only cysts. The amoebae can also usually be detected by biopsy of an ulcer. The indirect immunofluorescence test for antibody to *E. histolytica* is usually positive in amoebiasis and negative in healthy carriers.

Amoeboma or *amoebic pseudotumour of the colon* is an uncommon complication of intestinal amoebiasis. After invasion of the submucosa, the infection may remain localized and form a large mass of granulation and fibrous tissue, which may obstruct the lumen. The differential diagnosis is with carcinoma of the colon.

Extra-intestinal Amoebiasis

Amoebiasis of the skin is an uncommon complication of colorectal disease. It usually results from direct spread to the anus or vulval area or to the skin around a colostomy site. Penile amoebiasis is the result of anal intercourse with an infected person. All the skin lesions ulcerate with a foul slough. There is marked epidermal hyperplasia at the edges, which may easily be mistaken histologically for squamous-cell carcinoma, but numerous amoebae can usually be seen at the ulcer margin.

Hepatic amoebiasis arises as a sequel to colonic invasion. Trophozoites are carried in the portal venous system to the liver where they multiply and produce small zones of necrosis of liver cells: these enlarge and become confluent, producing one or more cavities (**amoebic 'abscesses'**), which may grow to more than 10 cm in diameter and are usually in the right lobe. Clinically, they present as fever, polymorphonuclear leucocytosis, hepatomegaly and right hypochondrial pain. Jaundice is uncommon.

Grossly, an abscess has a shaggy pale peripheral necrotic rim and contains thick reddish-brown fluid (often likened to anchovy sauce) composed of necrotic liver-cell debris, fibrin and blood. Histologically, trophozoites may be numerous or scanty in the wall of the cavity. Surrounding the zone of necrotic cells, the liver is oedematous and chronically inflamed (Fig. 25.19); polymorphs are not present in or around the cavity, which is therefore not a true abscess.

Without treatment, hepatic amoebiasis is usually fatal. Clinical dignosis is supported by a characteristic pattern on ultrasonography and a high titre of antibody to *E. histolytica*. Concurrent intestinal amoebiasis is found in less than 50% of cases, and the stool may be negative even for cysts. Aspiration is generally reserved for very large 'abscesses' and those about to rupture, as indicated by a local friction rub. Modern chemotherapy is very effective for this condition.

Complications include rupture and spread beyond the liver. Rupture into the pleural, peritoneal or pericardial cavities has a considerable mortality. From the pleural cavity, the infection can spread to the **lungs** with the formation of a pulmonary 'abscess' and a bronchopleural fistula; necrotic material may then be coughed up. Haematogenous dissemination to other organs including the **brain**, occasionally also results in amoebic 'abscesses'.

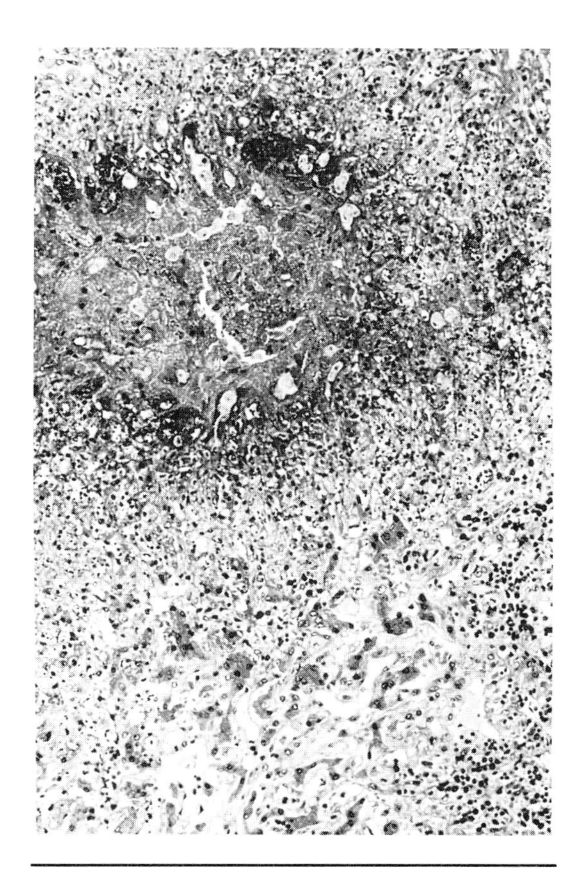

Fig. 25.19 Early amoebic 'abscess' of liver. The liver is inflamed and oedematous, and there is a central zone of necrosis. The amoebae are seen as pale bodies toward the periphery of the necrosis. ×125.

Naegleria fowleri

Naegleria fowleri occurs in warm water such as natural hot springs. The amoebae may enter the nasal passages and invade the central nervous system along the olfactory neuroepithelium. Children are usually affected and the clinical course is of a rapid and fatal meningoencephalitis unless it is treated aggressively.

Giardiasis

Infection with *Giardia lamblia* is world wide. It is acquired by ingesting cysts contaminating food or water. The life cycle is similar to that of *Entamoeba histolytica* except that it colonizes the small bowel and infections are not so chronic.

After ingestion, the cysts break open in the duodenum, releasing trophozoites which then multiply by binary fission so that, within a few days, millions of parasites cover the surface of the villi of the small intenstine. The trophozoites are pear-shaped, 15 μm long and adhere to the enterocytes by their sucker discs. They do not invade the mucosa. Usually giardiasis is a self-limiting condition, although the immunological means of eliminating the parasite are not well understood. About 70% of infections are asymptomatic; the minority cause a diarrhoea lasting some weeks. Fewer than 10% of patients suffer chronic diarrhoea and malabsorption.

The histology of the symptomatic cases shows jejunal villi varying in architecture from normal to subtotal atrophy; malabsorption is usually associated with atrophy. Trophozoites are seen near the surface of the mucosa (Fig. 25.20). Plasma cells are plentiful in the lamina propria and increased intraepithelial lymphocytes are usual, but the villi are less atrophic than is usual in coeliac disease. In patients with defective IgA production who may suffer severe giardiasis, plasma cells are scanty but submucosal nodular lymphoid hyperplasia may be present. Pathophysiological mechanisms proposed for symptomatic giardiasis include the physical covering up of the villi by the parasites, direct damage to the enterocytes, bacterial co-infection and immunopathological reactions involving antibody.

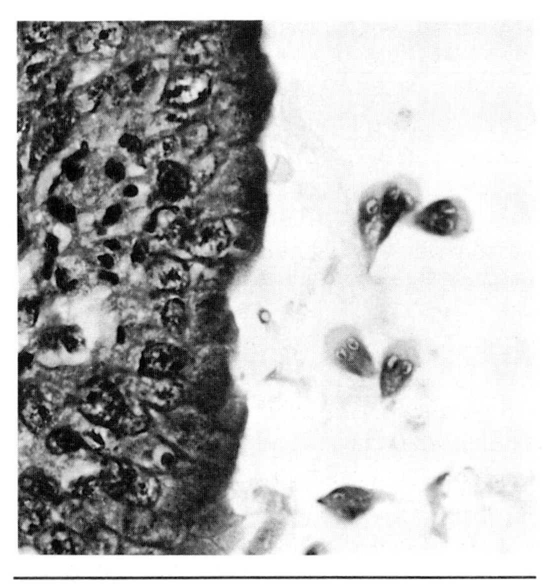

Fig. 25.20 The binucleate trophozoites of *Giardia lamblia* adjacent to jejunal epithelium. ×1000.

Giardiasis is diagnosed by finding cysts in the faeces or trophozoites in jejunal aspirate and biopsy material. The indirect immunofluorscence test for circulating antibodies is positive in 90% of patients with chronic infection and malabsorption.

Coccidiosis

The term coccidiosis indicates disease caused by coccidian protozoa. They include *Toxoplasma gondii, Cryptosporidium* and *Isospora belli.* They all have complex life cycles inside gut enterocytes of the definitive host; infective oocysts are shed in the faeces.

Toxoplasmosis

Toxoplasmosis is a very common worldwide infection caused by the protozoon *Toxoplasma gondii.* From serological studies in many populations, it is evident that about 20% of people have acquired the infection by the age of 20 years, and up to 50% by the age of 70. The infection is usually asymptomatic, but a small minority develop one of the following clinical syndromes: (1) acute acquired toxoplasmosis; (2) congenital toxoplasmosis; (3) ocular toxoplasmosis; and (4) toxoplasmosis in the immunocompromised host.

Life Cycle

The definitive host for *T. gondii* is the cat, in whose intestinal epithelium there is a sexual reproductive cycle via schizogony and gametogony to produce oocysts. A wide variety of other mammals (including man) may act as intermediate host, and in these, two forms of the parasite exist: proliferating trophozoites (or **tachyzoites**) and **bradyzoites** in tissue cysts. The trophozoite is a crescentic cell about 4 × 2 μm without a kinetoplast. It is an intracellular parasite which proliferates by binary fission, causing disruption and death of the host cell. In the early phase of infection, it avoids destruction by phagocyte lysosomes. The tissue cysts are found in many host cells and contain hundreds of bradyzoites (Fig. 25.21), which are smaller than the tachyzoites.

Man acquires toxoplasmosis by ingesting either oocysts from cat faeces or tissue cysts in the undercooked meat of other intermediate hosts, such as sheep, cow and pig. The cysts rupture in the intestine, releasing parasites which rapidly penetrate the intestinal cells and enter macrophages. These intracellular tachyzoites are then disseminated via lymphatics and the bloodstream throughout the body and enter many host-cell types, particularly those of heart muscle and the central nervous system. Inside these cells the tachyzoites replicate. In time, the host mounts a combined humoral and cell mediated immune response to the parasite. The latter is the more important in inhibiting the spread and multiplication of the tachyzoites. Finally, in the uncomplicated case, the parasites persist as bradyzoites in tissue cysts – **the latent infection phase**. The cysts remain in various parts of the body for many years and probably for the duration of the host's life.

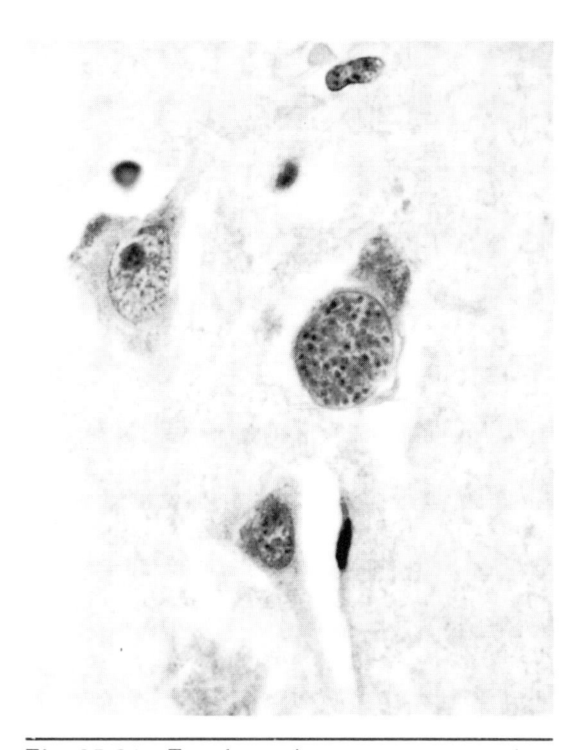

Fig. 25.21 *Toxoplasma* tissue cyst: numerous bradyzoites are seen as small dots inside a cyst in a cerebral neuron. ×1000.

Clinical and Pathological Features

Acute acquired toxoplasmosis. This presents clinically as malaise and fever; if severe, there may be myocarditis and encephalitis. Moderate splenomegaly is usual and in the later stage there may be lymph node enlargment. The disease thus mimics infectious mononucleosis or lymphoma. It may last from weeks to a few months but nearly always there is complete recovery. In the affected tissues, multiplication of the tachyzoites is associated with focal inflammation. The lymphadenopathy, which usually involves the posterior cervical nodes, has characteristic though not pathognomonic histological features. There is follicular hyperplasia and sinus histocytosis. The most suggestive diagnostic feature is focal aggregation of epithelioid macrophages in the paracortex and within the follicles themselves. Although the nodes are involved in the acute phase of infection, parasites are rarely seen in them.

Congenital toxoplasmosis. About 30% of women who acquire toxoplasmosis in pregnancy (usually asymptomatically) transmit the infection to the fetus via the placenta. A woman who already has toxoplasmosis antibodies cannot transmit infection. If the infection occurs in the first trimester, the result may be abortion or severe congenital morbidity: the risk of severe fetal disability decreases progressively the later the infection, and most fetuses infected during mid or late pregnancy are born free of disease.

The classic tetrad of congenital toxoplasmosis is hydrocephalus or microencephaly, chorioretinitis and cerebral calcification. Widespread intracerebral dissemination of tachyzoites results in much cerebral necrosis and inflammation. This damage is caused partly by the destructive effect of tachyzoites, but hypersensitivity reactions are probably also involved. The ensuing tissue swelling and vascular thrombosis produce hydrocephalus (Fig. 25.22). Periventricular dystrophic calcification is characteristic. Milder sequelae of congenital infection can take months or years to appear and include chorioretinitis, squints, deafness, mental retardation and epilepsy.

Ocular toxoplasmosis. Infection of the uveal tract of the eye is usually secondary to congenital rather than acquired infection. The retina and choroid in the posterior part of the eye are mainly involved, and the condition presents with blurred vision and pain. After the acute necrosis and inflammation have resolved, the tissue cysts persist and the infection may become active again at any time.

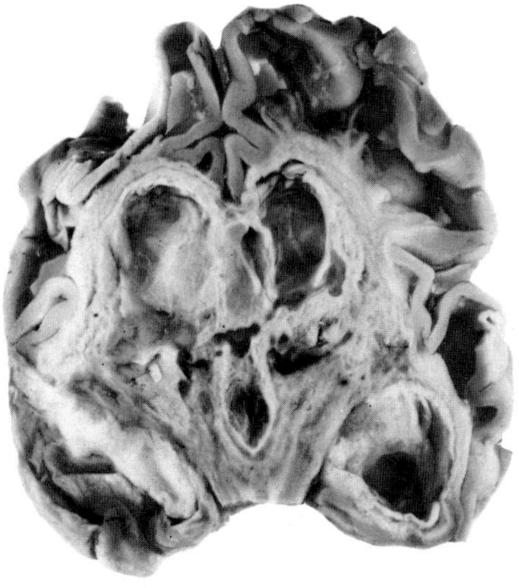

Fig. 25.22 Congenital toxoplasmosis. Coronal section of the brain of a 2-month-old infant. There is extensive cystic and gelatinous degeneration of the cerebral hemispheres and hydrocephalus.

Toxoplasmosis in the immunocompromised host. People who have previously acquired *T. gondii*, with or without manifestations of disease, may suffer a devastating relapse if their immune defences, particularly cell mediated immunity, are impaired. The tissue cysts rupture and release the bradyzoites. These enter adjacent cells, become active tachyzoites and cause necrosis. The organs most commonly damaged are the brain and the heart. Toxoplasma encephalitis is a common feature of AIDS.

The diagnosis of toxoplasmosis is made either by finding parasites in the tissues, or by serology. Infected tissue may also be injected into mice which are examined for toxoplasmosis 6 weeks later. Serological tests include the Sabin–Feldman dye test which utilizes live tachyzoites, and a variety of immunofluorescence tests and complement fixation tests using soluble antigens. A rising titre of IgM antibody indicates recent infection.

Cryptosporidiosis

Cryptosporidium was long assumed to affect only animals, but is now increasingly recognized as a cause of diarrhoea in man. It is acquired faeco-orally, from calves and probably from infected people.

In immunocompetent people *Cryptosporidium* induces an acute, self-limiting watery diarrhoea lasting about one week. Global surveys of childhood diarrhoea find *Cryptosporidium* in up to 15% of episodes. The 2–3 μm parasite infects enterocytes in the small and large bowel. It resides just inside the luminal surface microvilli or membrane (Fig. 25.23), in large numbers. There is a variable inflammation of the lamina propria. The pathogenesis of the diarrhoea is uncertain, but may be a toxic secretory process analogous to cholera.

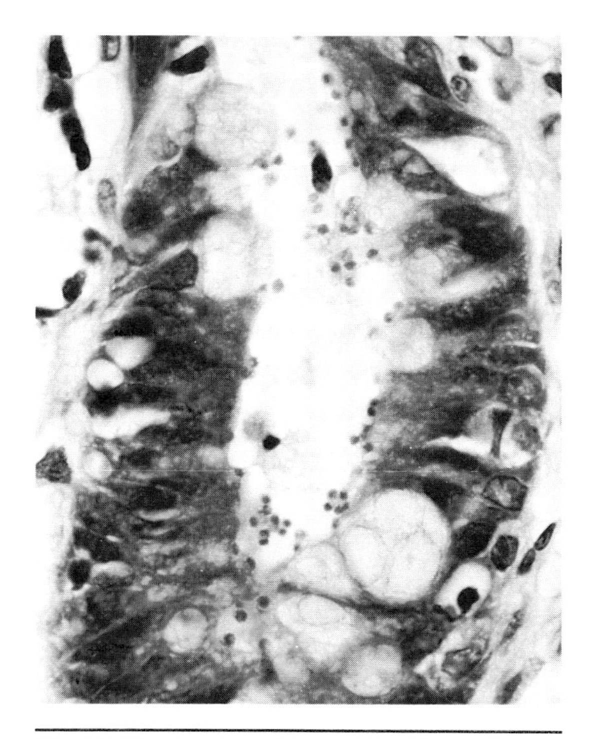

Fig. 25.23 *Cryptosporidium* colitis. The small round parasites are seen on the surface of the epithelium of the intestinal crypts. ×1000.

In immunocompromised patients, *Cryptosporidium* is associated with a persistent watery diarrhoea which is often fatal (chemotherapy is of no avail). In developed countries, this infection is found in up to 15% of AIDS patients with diarrhoea; but in Africa, over 50% of such patients may have cryptosporidiosis, reflecting a higher environmental prevalence. The infection may be diagnosed by biopsy, but usually is detected by staining oocytes in a smear of faeces using the Ziehl–Neelsen method.

Isosporiasis

Infection with *Isospora belli* is less frequent than with *Cryptosporidium*, but it has a similar association with HIV infection and diarrhoea. It is an intra-enterocyte infection of small bowel, and is diagnosed by finding the oocysts in the faeces.

Pneumocystosis

The life cycle of *Pneumocystis carinii* is not yet delineated. From recent DNA studies, it is probably a fungus rather than a protozoon. It probably exists in the atmosphere and is constantly inhaled into the lung alveoli. Only in immunocompromised people does disease result, producing *Pneumocystis carinii* pneumonia.

Until recently, the infection was most often seen in neonates and in adults with malignant disease. However, in developed countries, up to 80% of HIV-infected people suffer and die from *Pneumocystis* pneumonia. It is less common in AIDS patients in the tropics.

The parasite multiplies, filling the alveolar spaces. Gas transfer is impeded and there is dyspnoea. Chest radiography shows a characteristic reticulonodular shadowing (Fig. 25.24). In fatal

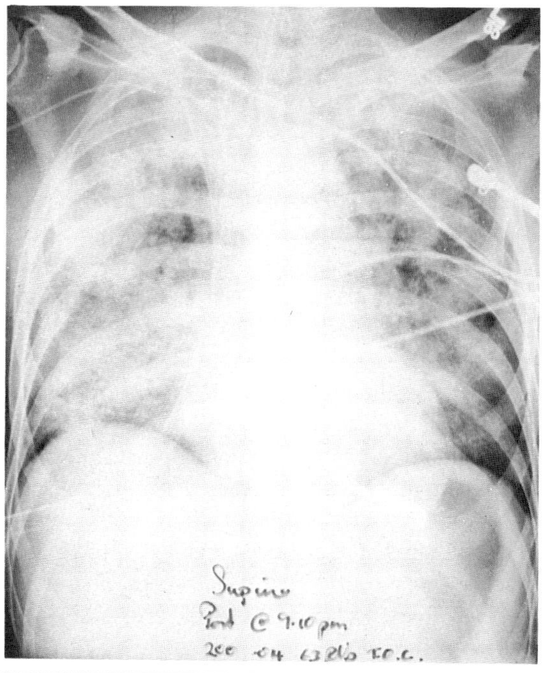

Fig. 25.24 Chest X-ray of patient with severe *Pneumocystis carinii* pneumonia showing bilateral upper and lower zone fluffy infiltrate. The patient was immunocompromised because of a T-cell lymphoma. At autopsy the combined weight of the consolidated lungs was 2.5 kg.

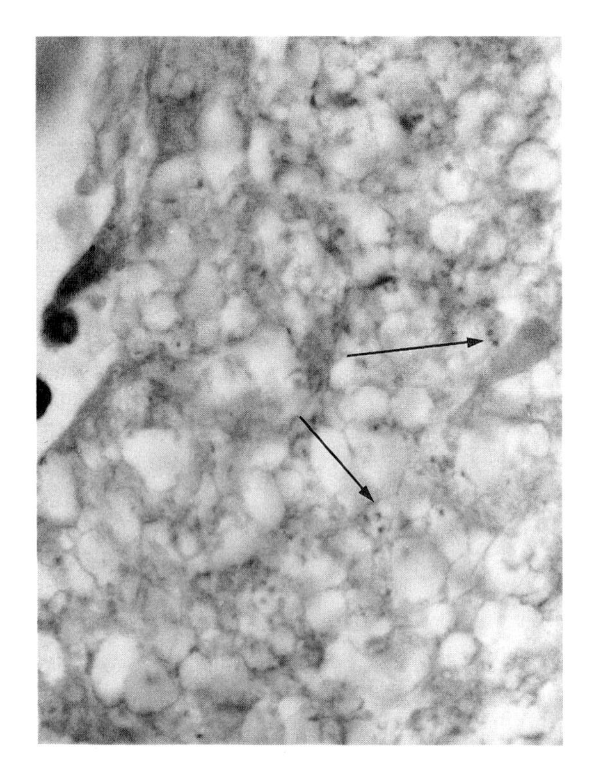

cases, the lungs are dry, consolidated and grey in colour. Histologically, there is a variable lymphocytic and plasma cell infiltrate in the alveolar walls, hence the older term 'plasma cell pneumonia'. The alveoli and terminal bronchioles contain foamy material in which there are round and oval cysts about 5 μm in diameter (Fig. 25.25). The diagnosis is made by microscopy of bronchial washings or a lung biopsy. Serology is unhelpful since most people are seropositive for *Pneumocystis* through asymptomatic exposure.

Fig. 25.25 *Pneumocystis carinii* in lung alveolus. The cysts are round and tightly packed, giving a foamy appearance. In some, trophozoites are seen (arrows). ×1000.

Diseases Caused by Helminths

Helminths (worms) comprise two main phyla, the platyhelminths (flatworms) and the nematodes (roundworms). Flatworms are divided into cestodes (tapeworms) and trematodes (flukes). The size range of parasitic worms is enormous: at one end of the scale are some nematode larvae 0.1 mm long, and at the other are some tapeworms which can reach 10 m in length.

Man may be infected by adult tapeworms in the gut lumen or by larval stages in many viscera; one tapeworm (*Taenia solium*) can have both effects. The trematode flukes reside in blood vessels, bile ducts, lungs or the gut. The more numerous species of nematodes are even more diverse, between them parasitizing virtually every tissue.

Broadly speaking, helminth-induced disease relates to the intensity of infection. A plot of the numbers of parasites per host against numbers of people infected by that parasite usually follows a Poisson distribution: most people have relatively few worms and suffer mildly or not at all, whilst a minority with a heavy infection have considerable morbidity and mortality. Only in a few of the helminthiases is a single worm able to induce significant disease: examples of this are an *Ascaris* worm obstructing the bile duct, and a hydatid cyst blocking the flow of CSF in the brain.

In some infections, the sheer number of worms and their products appear sufficient to account for disease (e.g. the hookworms and ascarid infections). In others, such as some filariases, the more severe disease states may be associated paradoxically with a reduced parasite load but a high degree of hypersensitivity to worm antigens. In schistosomiasis, to take an intermediate example, the severity of disease depends on both the intensity of infection and the host immune reaction.

Immunity to helminth infections is variable and reflects both the intensity of exposure and individual resistance. Even in the most heavily endemic areas where, for example, 95% of the population may have ascarid intestinal worms, a few people with presumably similar exposure to infection do not acquire, or do not keep, the worms. This probably represents a high innate or rapidly acquired immune resistance. Among those with demonstrable parasites, there is a spectrum of clinical, parasitological, pathological and immunological phenomena which indicate not only a wide range of resulting infection intensities, but also a very complex set of host–parasite relationships. Their crucial interaction is well exemplified by *Strongyloides stercoralis* infection, where immunocompetent people may have a few worms in the gut for years with no ill effects, and yet can suffer an overwhelming disseminated infection if their host defences become defective. This implies that, for this parasite at least, the immunity system is constantly operating in the bowel to contain the infection, even though it cannot eliminate it.

Eosinophil leucocytosis is a common feature of nearly all helminth infections (in contrast to its virtual absence in protozoal diseases). The cause is generally assumed to be immunological, with eosinophil chemotactic factors produced by type 1 and type 4 hypersensitivity reactions, both of which are common in worm infections. The function of the eosinophil is obscure, although there is evidence that in one disease, schistosomiasis, it is associated with resistance to infection. The finding of a raised eosinophil count often starts a search for faecal and urinary ova, or larvae in the blood. The relevance of any positive parasitological findings to a patient's problems should always be considered carefully. For example, a middle-aged expatriate working in Africa who presents with blood in the stool, has a mild eosinophilia and is excreting ova of *Schistosoma mansoni*, may still have a carcinoma of the caecum as the cause of his symptoms.

As with all parasitic infections, diagnosis of helminthic diseases should be made by finding the worm. Serological techniques of antibody and antigen detection may eventually prove easier, more reliable and perhaps cheaper, but current methods of worm antibody detection are plagued by cross-reactions between species (particularly with the nematodes) and by a lack of distinction between previous and new, active infections. The specificity, sensitivity and availability of such tests will undoubtedly increase in the future.

Trematode Infections

Trematode worms (also known as flukes) cause chronic infection in many tissues of man, including the bowel lumen, the blood vessels, the lungs and the bile ducts. Apart from the species causing schistosomiasis, they are hermaphrodite and they all utilize specific freshwater snails as intermediate hosts. By far the most important trematodes are the blood vessel flukes – the schistosomes – which cause cystitis, intestinal ulceration, hepatic fibrosis, portal hypertension and splenomegaly. These parasites, and the two liver flukes (*Fasciola* and *Opisthorchis*), which live in the bile ducts, will be described in this section.

Adult trematodes do not multiply in the human host. The presence of the few worms in the majority of those infected is tolerated with little inconvenience; overt clinical disease follows when the number of parasites is large or when the adults and/or eggs are in an ectopic site in the body.

Schistosomiasis (Bilharzia)

The three main *Schistosoma* species, *S. haematobium*, *S. mansoni* and *S. japonicum*, between them infect 10% of the world's population. The resulting disease, schistosomiasis, is the most important parasitic disease after malaria. *S. haematobium* causes urinary schistosomiasis; *S. mansoni* and *S. japonicum* both cause hepatosplenic and intestinal schistosomiasis. Table 25.2 gives further geographical, pathological and parasitological details. *S. japonicum* infection is a zoonosis; the other two species affect only man.

The simplistic equation: 'Man + Snails + Water = Schistosomiasis' is valid because of the high reproductive potential of the life cycle. The peak

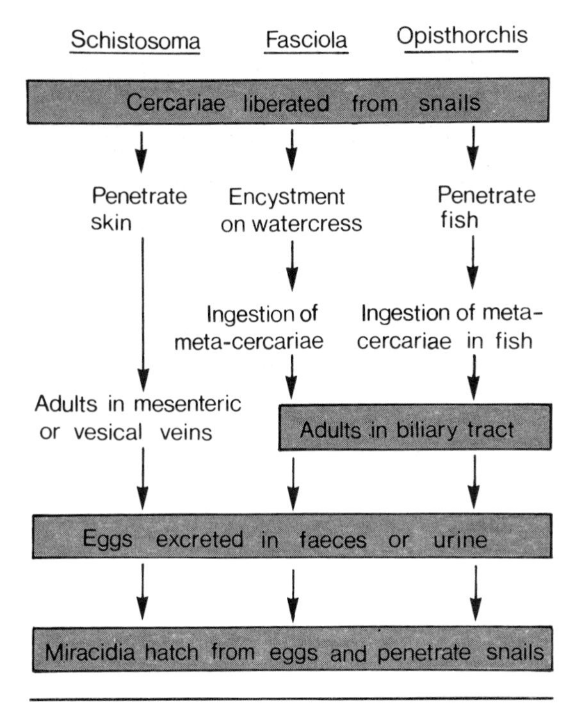

Fig. 25.26 Life cycle of the parasitic trematode worms.

age of infection is in the first two decades of life, and in many areas the prevalence at this age approaches 100%. Thereafter the prevalence and intensity of infection decline, but in those with moderate to heavy infections, schistosomiasis causes chronic morbidity, with a mortality estimated at 2–10%. It is a predominantly rural disease, a scourge of peasant farmers, and is acquired through contact with water. Children in particular, with their high infection levels, indiscriminate habits of excretion, and predilection for playing in water, are very important in propagating the disease.

Life Cycle (Fig. 25.26)

Schistosome eggs in urine or faeces hatch in fresh water and the emerging larva (*miracidium*) penetrates a snail of the appropriate species. After further development in the snail, vast numbers of *cercariae* are released into the water. These are elongated, actively motile larvae, of 360 × 60 μm with a forked tail (Fig. 25.27) and head glands that secrete cytolytic substances. They can penetrate

Table 25.2 Summary of the major features of the schistosomiases

Schistosome	Distribution	Habitat of adult worms	Features of ova	Pathology of chronic phase
S. mansoni	Africa, South America, the Caribbean	Mesenteric and portal veins	Lateral spine	1. Hepatic fibrosis, portal hypertension, splenomegaly 2. Intestinal erosions and polyps 3. Pulmonary hypertension and right ventricular failure
S. japonicum	China, South East Asia, the Phillipines	Mesenteric and portal veins	Rudimentary lateral spine	As for *S. mansoni*
S. haematobium	Africa, the Middle East	Perivesical and rectal veins	Terminal spine	1. Chronic cystitis, hydronephrosis, bladder carcinoma 2. Rectal lesions 3. Pulmonary hypertension and right ventricular failure

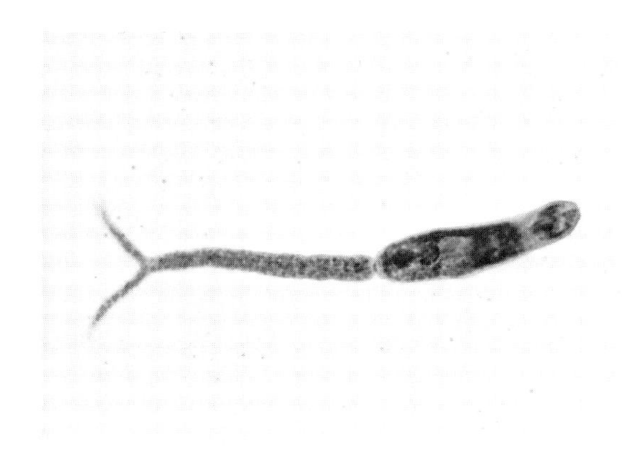

Fig. 25.27 Schistosome cercaria. Note the constriction where the head detaches from the forked tail on skin penetration. ×220.

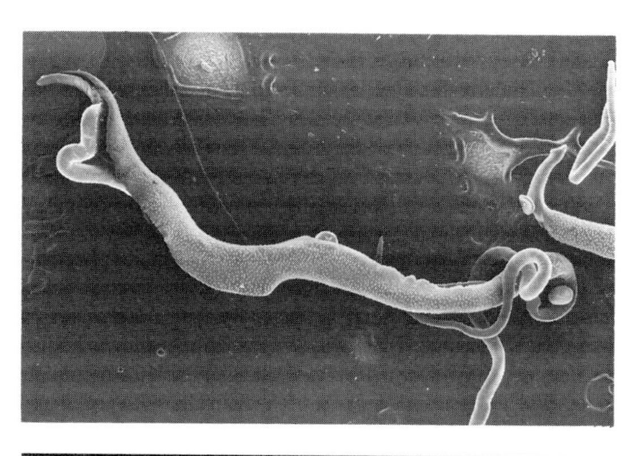

Fig. 25.28 Scanning electron micrograph of a pair of *Schistosoma japonicum* worms. The female is longer, thinner and smooth, and lies in the gynaecophoric canal of the male, whose surface appears speckled. ×15.

human epidermis in less than 5 minutes, during which the tail is lost and the larva is then termed a *schistosomulum*. After a few days in the dermis, it enters a venule and is arrested in the lung, where it grows. It then migrates via the systemic circulation to the liver and enters portal veins where final maturation takes place. Thereafter, the adult schistosomes migrate by the bloodstream to their definitive locations: *S. mansoni* and *S. japonicum* to the mesenteric and portal veins and *S. haematobium* to the perivesical venous plexus and rectal veins. Attached to the endothelium of the veins by their suckers, male and female worms pair up and live in connubial bliss, the female lying in the gynaecophoric canal of the male (Fig. 25.28). They feed on red cells and excrete a dark haemozoin pigment very similar to that produced by malarial parasites. A month after skin penetration, *S. mansoni* and *S. japonicum* worms start laying eggs; this commences after about 8 weeks with *S. haematobium*.

The adult males are about 10 mm long and the females are about 15 mm, depending on the species. Each worm pair of *S. japonicum* lays about 3000 eggs daily, and *S. haematobium* and *S. mansoni* about 300. Schistosome worms can live for over 20 years, although the mean life-span is usually 3–5 years. Infection usually increases steadily as new larvae are acquired. Data on *S. mansoni* infections in Brazil indicate that those people with 10 or fewer pairs of worms in the body have little significant clinical disease. Individuals with severe liver fibrosis have 150–300 worm pairs. The highest number of worm pairs recorded at autopsy is 1608 in a case of schistosomal colitis. The presence of adult worms in the veins induces no direct host reaction, for during their maturation the schistosomula become non-antigenic by acquiring a coat of host molecules, especially A, B, H and Lewis blood group glycolipids, and this acts as a protective disguise.

The eggs are characteristic in shape and size for each species: those of *S. mansoni* (Fig. 25.29) and *S. haematobium* are about 140 × 60 μm and those of *S. japonicum* are 85 × 60 μm. The position of the spine on the eggshell is a distinguishing feature (see Table 25.2). The larval miracidium inside the egg is viable for about 3 weeks. After this it degenerates if the egg has not hatched in water. Roughly half of the eggs are excreted in the faeces or urine, the rest being retained. It is the host reaction to the eggs that causes the significant pathology in schistosomiasis.

Clinical and Pathological Features

The various phases of infection have their distinct features. The host develops an immune response to the antigenic secretion of the head glands of

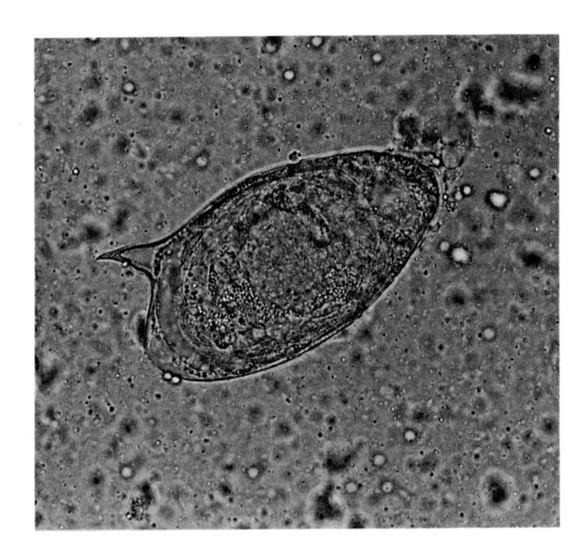

Fig. 25.29 Egg of *Schistosoma mansoni* with characteristic lateral spine containing the granular-appearing miracidium. ×400.

schistosomolum and to surface antigens of the schistosomolum and ova. Penetration of the skin by cercariae causes a transient local inflammatory reaction. In many cases this is clinically evident as a rash – 'swimmers' itch' or **cercarial dermatitis**. It is probably a hypersensitivity reaction and may account for the modest resistance to reinfection that develops in schistosomiasis. Type 1 and type 4 hypersensitivity reactions with IgG antibody-dependent eosinophil reactions are thought to be involved.

Before or shortly after the onset of egg-laying by the worms, there may be a constitutional reaction to a heavy synchronous infection, particularly if this is the first exposure. Fever, cough, diarrhoea, urticaria, hepatosplenomegaly, and a marked eosinophil leucocytosis characterize this phase, known as the **Katayama syndrome**, which may last for days or weeks. The types of hypersensitivity involved are unclear: it has some features of a type 3 (immune-complex) reaction but other types of reaction, kinin activation and even endotoxic shock, may also be involved.

However, neither cercarial dermatitis nor the Katayama syndrome constitute the major problems in schistosomiasis. The reaction to the eggs is the important feature. Wherever the eggs are found, in the liver, bowel or bladder, or in other sites such as the skin, the venule they are in is disrupted and a cellular reaction occurs around the egg. This involves polymorphs initially, then macrophages, lymphocytes and eosinophils, and the evolution of an epithelioid cell granuloma (see Fig. 25.30a) with giant cells and sometimes central necrosis. Plasma cells accumulate around the granuloma. Like granulomas due to other agents, schistosomal granulomas heal with fibrosis. The eggshell and miracidium are phagocytosed, although many eggs resist full degradation and remain as calcified shells. The characteristic fibrosis and scarring of organs in schistosomiasis are the result of coalescence of fibrosis around thousands or millions of eggs. The cause of the florid reaction to schistosome eggs is immunological, a classic example of a type 4 hypersensitivity. Excretion of eggs is accompanied by inflammation of the mucosae with the focal erosions at the sites of escape of eggs; this causes the acute cystitis, colitis and ileitis seen in schistosomiasis.

Diagnosis

Schistosomiasis is diagnosed by finding the eggs. All three species excrete eggs in the faeces, and they may be seen microscopically in faecal suspensions. Alternatively, a biopsy of rectal mucosa can be pressed between two slides and examined for eggs. Histological examination of rectal and liver biopsies is overall a less sensitive method, but biopsy is necessary to diagnose the grosser lesions such as bilharziomas. Similarly, in urinary schistosomiasis, examination of urine sediment for eggs is straightforward; cystoscopy and biopsy is used for complex lesions. The schistosome species is identified by the shape of the egg and the position of the spine (Table 25.2). Serology for schistosomiasis, using egg antigens and the enzyme-linked immunosorbent assay technique, is very sensitive. However, most of the available tests do not discriminate old from new infections, and they are used mainly for epidemiological purposes.

S. mansoni and *S. japonicum* Infections

These parasites affect predominantly the bowel and liver. Roughly half the eggs laid in the portal and mesenteric veins are carried to the liver, the rest remaining in the bowel wall or passing into the lumen.

The Liver

The eggs lodge in the portal venules and induce granulomas (Fig. 25.30a). Over months and years, the granulomas heal with fibrosis, and gradually the portal tracts become linked by fibrous tissue. In heavy infections, e.g. with over 100 worm pairs, there is often massive fibrosis around major portal tracts. This scarring may be up to 2 cm across and is known as **Symmers' clay pipestem fibrosis** – the pictorial analogy is with the white stems of clay pipes being thrust into the liver substance (Fig. 25.30b). Such fibrosis is not a true cirrhosis because the basic architecture is maintained beyond the portal fibrosis. Blood vessels proliferate with the formation of shunts between hepatic arterioles and portal venules. Dark brown haemozoin pigment granules are found in portal macrophages and Kupffer cells.

The effects of schistosomal liver disease depend on the intensity of infection and the infected individual's fibrogenic response – which varies widely between individuals. If this is mild, there is little clinical upset, but when fibrosis is marked there are several secondary phenomena. The most important is **portal hypertension**, due to the fibrosis and the intrahepatic arteriovenous shunting. Oesophageal varices, ascites and splenomegaly with hypersplenism follow; the splenomegaly which may be up to 1.5 kg is in part a consequence of reactive lymphoid hyperplasia. Because the architecture is preserved, liver function is relatively unaffected by schistosomiasis and hepatic encephalopathy is uncommon. There is no

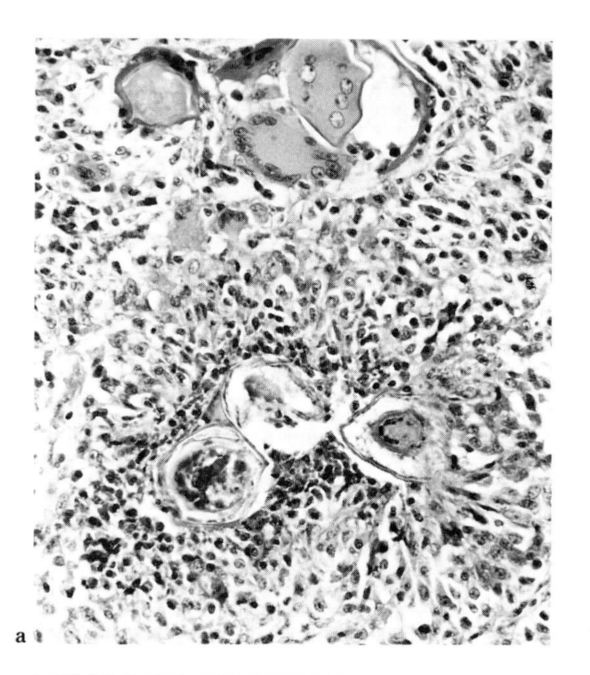

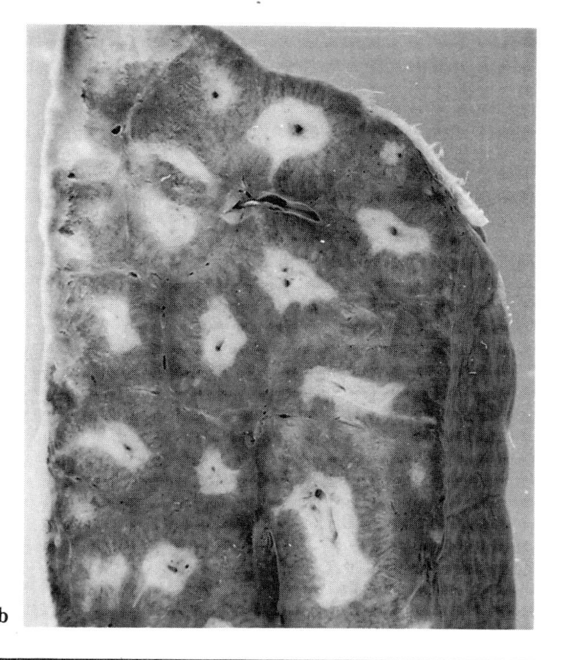

Fig. 25.30 Liver in *S. mansoni* infection. **a** Schistosomal granuloma; three eggs are seen inside an epithelioid-cell granuloma with eosinophils and plasma cells. At the top, part of an older granuloma is seen with giant cells phagocytosing fragments of eggshell. ×235. **b** Macroscopic features showing Symmers' clay pipestem fibrosis. (Picture kindly supplied by the Wellcome Museum of Medical Science.)

predisposition to hepatocellular carcinoma. Because schistosomiasis is such a prevalent disease, it is the commonest single cause of portal hypertension in the world. *S. haematobium* does not significantly affect the liver.

The Intestine

All three schistosome species affect the bowel. *S. mansoni* and *S. japonicum* eggs affect the whole bowel from duodenum to rectum; *S. haematobium* eggs are usually confined to the appendix and large bowel. The acute inflammatory lesions around eggs in the gut wall and the mucosa cause bleeding and diarrhoea: grossly they appear as small raised granular foci with haemorrhagic points. **Schistosomal polyps**, consisting of masses of eggs in the submucosa and inflamed hyperplastic mucosa may develop in the large bowel (Fig. 25.31). They are usually due to a pair of worms blocking a draining venule and pouring eggs continuously into it. The polyps can obstruct the lumen and can form the apex of an intussusception. Elsewhere, there may be focal fibrosis of the bowel. In the serosa and mesentery, nodules composed of eggs, granulomas and fibrosis are occasionally found – so-called **bilharziomas**. Despite the widespread intestinal disease, schistosomiasis does not cause malabsorption. Nor does it predispose to colorectal carcinoma. Specimens of acute appendicitis in endemic areas often contain schistosome eggs in the submucosa, but there is no aetiological relationship between the two diseases.

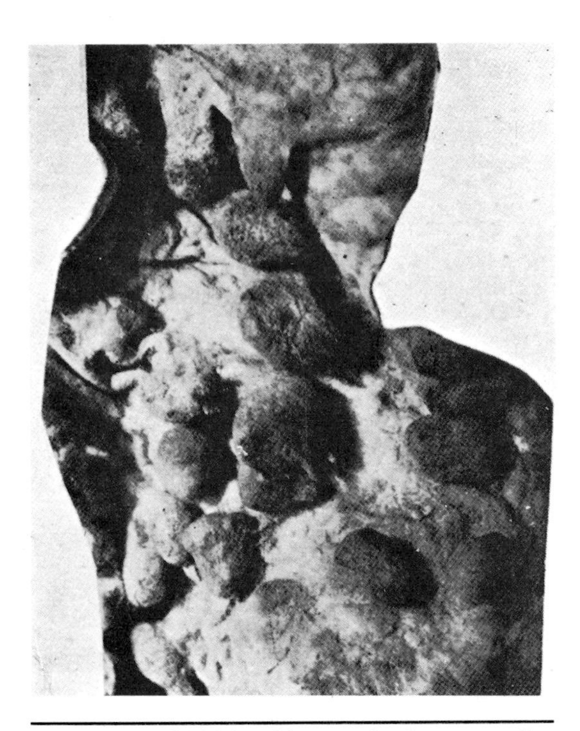

Fig. 25.31 Multiple schistosomal polyps protruding from colonic mucosa. (Picture kindly donated by the Wellcome Museum of Medical Science.)

S. haematobium Infection

The Urinary Bladder and Ureters

Eggs laid by worms in the veins of the bladder induce an intense inflammatory reaction in the mucosa and underlying connective tissue. Eggs passing through the mucosa cause focal erosion of the epithelium. The clinical effects are a painful cystitis and haematuria (characteristically at the end of micturition), which can lead to chronic iron deficiency. Historically, Egypt, where *S. haematobium* is highly prevalent, was known as the 'land of menstruating males'.

Cystoscopically, the mucosa appears granular. The inflammation causes a reactive hyperplasia of the urothelium, and in a very heavy infection gross polyps (Fig. 25.32) result from the hyperplasia and the underlying inflammation (Fig. 25.33). Thus, in the acute stage the mucosa appears hyperaemic and thickened. Histologically, eggs are seen in the venules, in and under the mucosa, surrounded by a heavy diffuse eosinophil infiltrate and by granulomas. The hyperplastic epithelium is often metaplastic, with a glandular or squamous appearance. Adult worms are commonly seen in veins in the outer part of the bladder wall.

As the infection becomes chronic, there are several additional features. Retained eggs tend to calcify and remain in the bladder wall: eventually they are so numerous that a plain X-ray of the

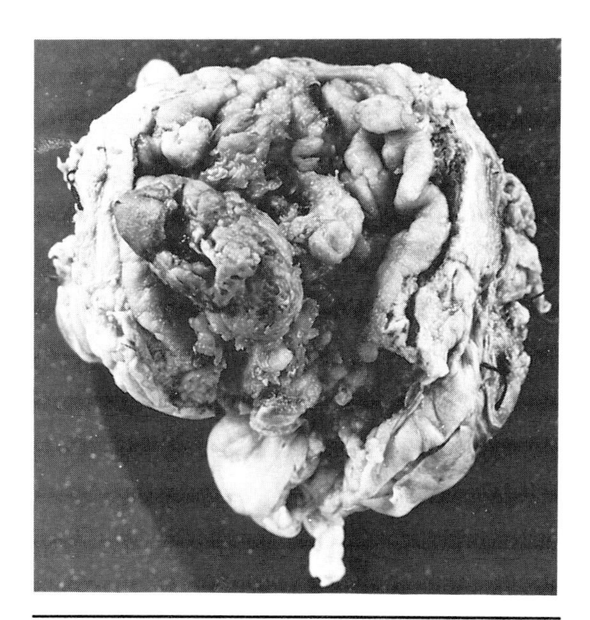

Fig. 25.32 Large polyps in the urinary bladder in severe *Schistosoma haematobium* infection.

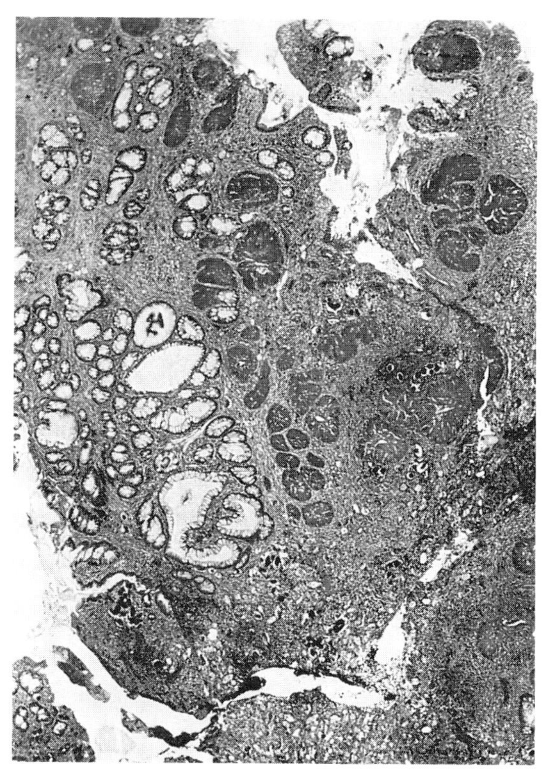

Fig. 25.33 Schistosomiasis of the urinary bladder, showing glandular metaplasia of the surface epithelium, chronic inflammation and fibrosis. ×80.

pelvis will show the viscus as a thick calcified ring. The muscular coat and submucosa become rigid as a result of scarring, and this may affect bladder contraction, so that emptying is incomplete. Secondary bacterial cystitis with coliforms and salmonellae follows in a proportion of cases. Microscopically, vast numbers of calcified eggs are seen embedded in a fibrous stroma, beneath an attenuated epithelium often of stratified squamous type.

The ureters are commonly affected and the pathology is similar to that in the bladder. Inflammation and fibrosis at the lower end of the ureter cause obstruction, and hydronephrosis develops in up to a quarter of infected children in some parts of Africa. However, treatment by anti-schistosomal drugs results in relief of the obstructive uropathy in most early cases.

Carcinoma of the bladder. Heavy *S. haematobium* infection predisposes to bladder cancer, which accounts for about one-quarter of deaths from this infection and has a peak incidence between 40 and 60 years. Unlike the usual bladder cancer, the schistosomiasis-associated tumour is usually a well differentiated squamous-cell carcinoma. It grows from the posterior or lateral wall and projects into the bladder lumen, forming a keratinizing mass, but also invades through the wall and later metastasizes. Its aetiology is uncertain: neither the worms nor the eggs have been shown to produce any carcinogenic agent. The best explanation is as follows: (1) chronic urinary schistosomiasis causes squamous metaplasia of the urothelium and predisposes to Gram-negative bacterial cystitis; (2) the bacteria (e.g. *Escherichia coli*) produce nitrosamines by breakdown of dietary nitrites and nitrates excreted in the urine; (3) the carcinogenic nitrosamines act on the squamous epithelium as initiating agents; and (4) the persistent inflammation and epithelial irritation induced by the schistosomal infection act as promoting factors.

Other genitourinary involvement. *S. haematobium* in the pelvis can lay eggs in other organs of the genitourinary tract. Thus, schistosomal granulomas are commonly found in the epididymis, testis, prostate and seminal vesicles. In women, the ovaries, fallopian tubes and cervix are affected; in the cervix, the inflammation and epithelial proliferation may be so marked as to simulate carcinoma. Schistosomiasis has, however, no aetiological relationship to cervical carcinoma although that tumour is particularly common in developing countries. In both sexes, itchy nodules in the groin areas can result from ectopic egg deposition in the dermis.

Other Lesions in Schistosomiasis

Schistosome worms do not always follow the classical migration pathways, and adults may end up anywhere in the body. If they pair and lay eggs, typical granulomatous inflammation results. The most severe 'ectopic' schistosomal lesions are found in the **central nervous system.** *S. japonicum* worms can inhabit the veins inside the skull, and *S. mansoni* and *S. haematobium* worms can live within vertebral veins. In the neural tissue, the eggs and inflammation produce space occupying lesions, resulting in focal neurological signs and sometimes paraplegia. Definite diagnosis can be made only by biopsy of a lesion. It is notable that visitors to the tropics who acquire schistosomiasis often demonstrate atypical clinical patterns compared with local inhabitants infected from an early age.

When portosystemic venous anastosomes are established in schistosomal portal hypertension, eggs can pass from the abdominal veins to the **lungs**. This also occurs in *S. haematobium* infections, because the pelvic veins drain into the inferior vena cava. The eggs impact in the pulmonary arterioles and induce a granulomatous reaction with arteritis and fibrosis (Fig. 25.34). If the infection is heavy, arterial plexiform lesions associated with pulmonary hypertension are formed throughout the lungs, and right ventricular failure develops in a small proportion of cases.

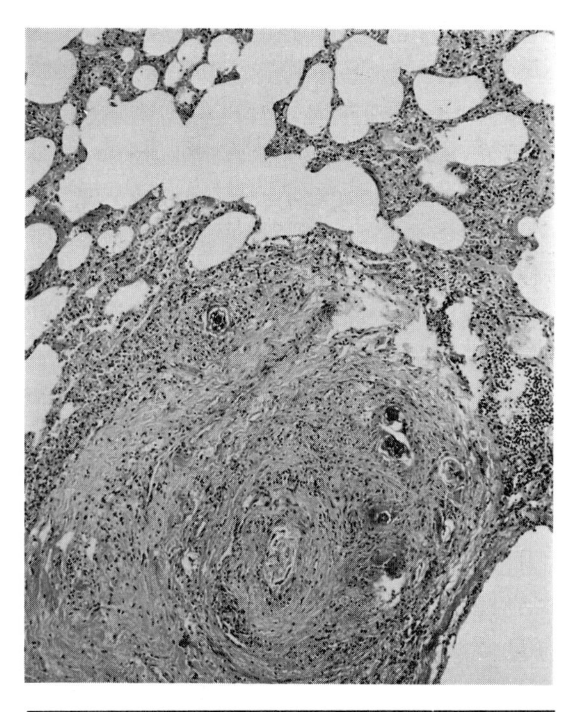

Fig. 25.34 Schistosomal pulmonary hypertension. Small pulmonary artery with eggs and fibrosis. ×80.

Circulating immune complexes are present in schistosomiasis, and in the **kidneys** an immune complex glomerulonephritis of mesangiocapillary type (p. 905) has been described in *S. mansoni* infections (but not with other species). This lesion is, however, much less common than obstructive uropathy resulting from *S. haematobium* infection.

Fascioliasis

Sheep and cattle are the main definitive hosts of *Fasciola hepatica*; sheep liver-rot is a veterinary problem in most sheep-raising areas of the world. Man is only occasionally infected from contaminated watercress (see trematode life cycle, Fig. 25.26). The worms burrow directly into the liver parenchyma, leaving a trail of necrosis and inflammation (Fig. 25.35). In the acute phase, the patient has a tender enlarged liver, fever and eosinophil leucocytosis. The worms gain access to the bile ducts where they mature into leaf-life

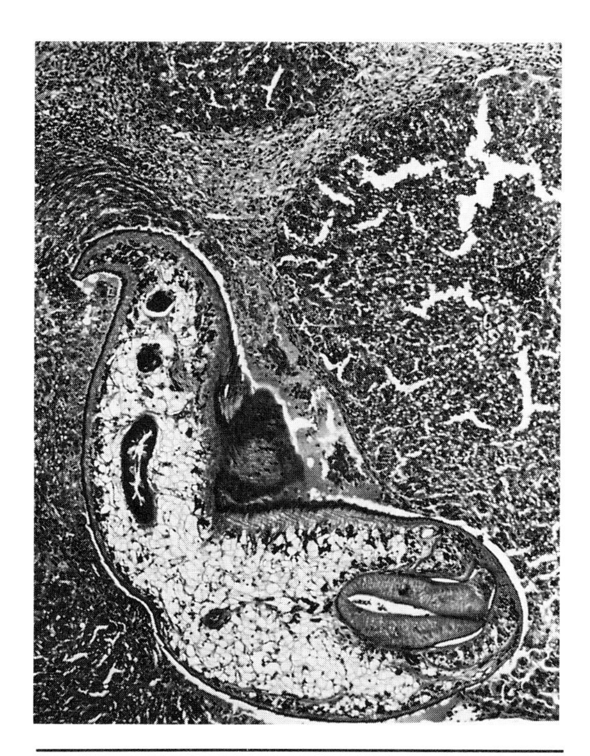

Fig. 25.35 Young *Fasciola hepatica* worm burrowing through the liver. ×80.

adults (about 30 × 10 mm) and remain attached to the biliary mucosa, laying their eggs in the bile.

The adult worms induce hyperplasia of the biliary epithelium, periductal inflammation and some fibrosis. Most patients have only a few worms; the hepatic symptoms subside and there is spontaneous recovery after a year or so. Heavier infections may cause obstructive jaundice. Unlike opisthorchiasis, fascioliasis does not predispose to the development of cholangiocarcinoma.

The diagnosis of fascioliasis can be difficult because eggs are usually scanty in the faeces; serology is helpful when they cannot be found.

Opisthorchiasis

The most important of the three *Opisthorchis* species affecting man is *O. sinensis* (formerly *Clonorchis sinensis*). Up to 75% of people in the endemic zones in the Far East may be infected, but as with most helminthiases, only those with heavy infections – in this case, hundreds to thousands of worms in the liver – suffer symptoms of permanent organ damage.

The metacercariae ingested during consumption of raw fish excyst in the duodenum and pass through the ampulla of Vater into the biliary system. The adults do not invade but attach to the biliary tract epithelium, mainly in the intrahepatic bile ducts but also in the common bile and cystic ducts and the gallbladder. The worms live for up to 20 years, each releasing a thousand or so eggs daily into the bile. Opisthorchiasis is diagnosed by finding the eggs in the faeces. The worms are flat in shape, measure about 16 × 4 mm and feed on the epithelium (Fig. 25.36). Reactive hyperplasia

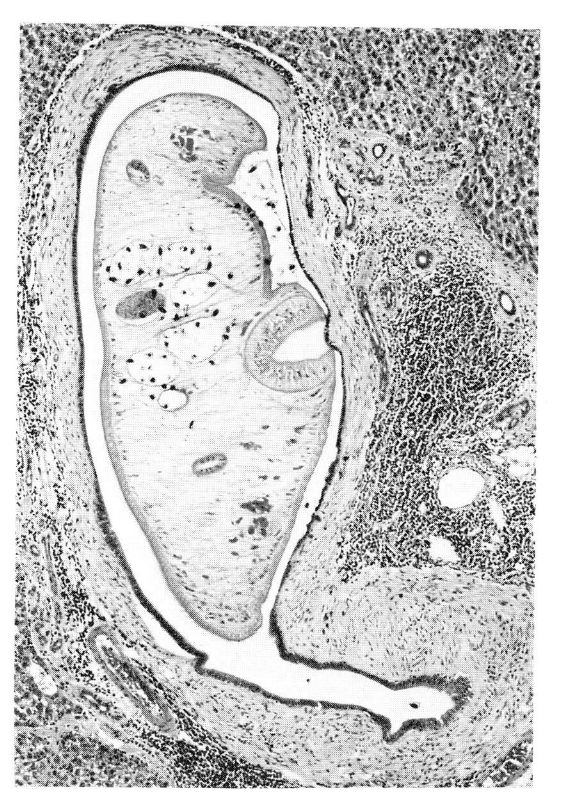

Fig. 25.36 *Opisthorchis* adult attached to the biliary epithelium by its sucker. There is marked periductal fibrosis. Several small dark ova are seen in the coiled uterus of the worm. ×65.

of the biliary epithelium, periductal inflammation and fibrosis follow.

Pathology results from worms obstructing bile ducts with consequent secondary infection and suppurative cholangitis, fibrosis, bile retention cysts, biliary stones (often containing a dead worm), and cholecystitis if worms or stones obstruct the cystic duct. Intrahepatic cholangiocarcinoma is relatively common in patients with a heavy infection. The worms probably act as promoters by their irritant action on the biliary epithelium. Biliary cirrhosis and pancreatitis are rare complications. Damage to the bile duct can also lead to a chronic carrier state with *Salmonella* species.

Cestode Infections

Adult cestodes or tapeworms are flat, ribbon-shaped, segmented worms of sometimes vast length which reside in the intestinal lumen of a definitive host. Their life cycle requires an intermediate host, in which the larvae often take the form of cysts in the tissues. Man can be infected with both adult and larval stages although it is the larval forms which are most harmful. The important human cestode infections are the taeniases, cysticerosis, and hydatid disease. All cestodes have a common life cycle (Fig. 25.37): the adult in the intestine sheds gravid segments containing numerous eggs into the faeces. The eggs contaminate the soil, are ingested by an intermediate host, and hatch into **oncospheres** or larvae, which invade through the intestinal mucosa and disseminate to various viscera. In the infections to be considered in detail here, this spread is haematogenous and the larvae develop into cysts that contain one or more tiny rounded bodies termed **scolices**, which are the heads of future adult worms. When tissues containing the cysts are eaten by carnivores, including man, a scolex attaches to the gut mucosa by means of suckers or hooks and grows into the worm as a chain of segments (**proglottids**). Self- or cross-fertilization of segments occurs and the distal gravid segments are shed.

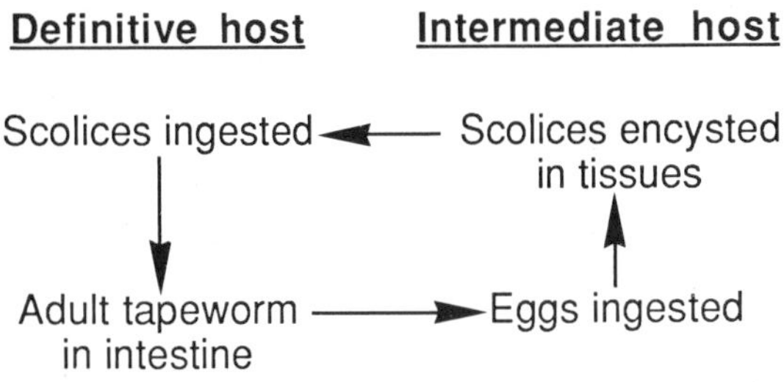

Fig. 25.37 Life cycle of *Taenia* and *Echinococcus* tapeworms.

Taeniases

Man is the only definitive host for *Taenia solium* (the pork tapeworm) and *Taenia saginata* (the beef tapeworm). The worms are cosmopolitan and about 100 million people are infected. Like all cestodiases, their epidemiology depends less on climate than on the distribution of the intermediate hosts. The worms are acquired by eating undercooked or raw measly (i.e. cyst-containing) meat from domestic pigs and bovines.

The final length of an adult *T. solium* is about 6 metres, whilst *T. saginata* can reach 10 metres. They consist of hundreds of 1 cm square, flat segments (Fig. 25.38), and their lifespan is several years. Usually only one worm is present in the intestine and it generally has little effect on the host. Symptoms of mild dyspepsia and fullness are common but there is no malabsorption or weight loss. Psychological upset on seeing moving segments in the faeces or occasionally the unpleasant sensation of a segment wriggling through the anus are more relevant consequences.

These infections are diagnosed by finding either segments or eggs in the faeces; although the eggs of the two species are identical, their segments may be differentiated by the pattern of the uterus.

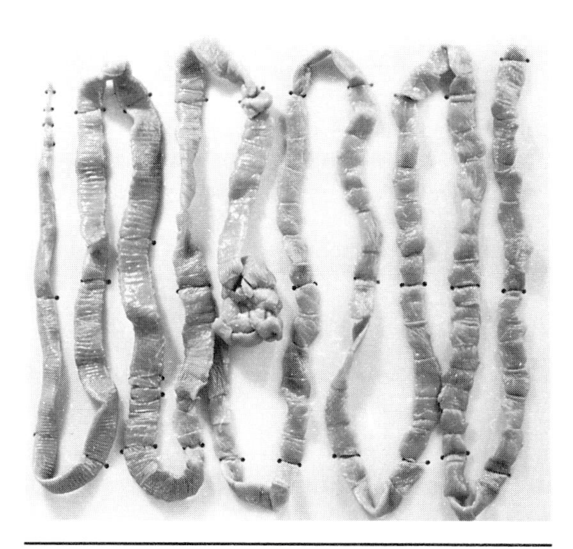

Fig. 25.38 An adult *Taenia* tapeworm. The head (scolex) is the small section at the top left. The mature gravid square segments are evident in the distal half. (St Thomas's Hospital Medical School Pathology Museum.)

Parasitologically and clinically, the significant difference is that while eggs of *T. saginata* cannot develop further in man, those of *T. solium* can do so, resulting in cysticercosis.

Diphyllobothriasis

Diphyllobothrium latum is a relatively uncommon intestinal parasite of temperate zones. A larva is eaten in infected fresh-water fish, and grows into the longest of all helminths, measuring up to 10 metres. Like the taenias usually only one tapeworm develops and it lives for many years attached to the ileal mucosa.

Pathologically, the only serious (but rare) effect of infection arises from the worm's consumption of dietary vitamin B_{12} in competition with the host (p. 614). In Finland, 10% of people with diphyllobothriasis have some degree of megaloblastic erythropoiesis, but only 2% are actually anaemic as a result. In other parts of the world, diphyllobothriasis is asymptomatic.

Cysticercosis

The relationship betwen man and *Taenia solium* is most unusual in that man can be host to both the adult and the larval form; the latter results in cysticercosis.

The larvae form 5 × 10 mm cysts which act as space-occupying lesions in many viscera and cause particular damage if located in the brain or eye. Less than 25% of people with cysticercosis also harbour an adult *T. solium* in the bowel, the majority of cyst infections being acquired by ingesting eggs from the environment rather than by regurgitating back into the stomach a gravid segment of the host's own tapeworm. The cysts grow slowly and the incubation period may be several years.

The disease is common in many tropical and subtropical regions where, like tuberculosis, it is a far more frequent cause of cerebral lesions than primary brain tumours. A patient may have hundreds of cysts distributed in skeletal muscle (Fig. 25.39), subcutis, heart, the central nervous system and the eye. The cyst is a fluid-filled bladder containing one scolex (Fig. 25.40). While it is alive, it elicits little inflammatory reaction. After some years, it dies and stimulates the formation of florid granulation tissue with foreign-body giant cells but little tissue eosinophilia. Finally, the degenerate shrunken cyst becomes calcified and enclosed in a fibrous capsule.

Cysts are most frequent in skeletal muscle where they are usually asymptomatic and often discovered by chance when an X-ray reveals calcified nodules. They may present as soft nodules under the skin. In the brain, the cysts act as space-occupying lesions in the meninges, parenchyma and ventricles. Because the nervous tissue is compressible, the cysts may grow to 2 cm in diameter: focal neurological signs and epilepsy are frequent, and hydrocephalus can result from a blockage of the third ventricle or aqueduct by a cyst. As the cysts die, the host reaction can aggravate the clinical effects, and may cause symptoms in previously silent infections. The mortality from neurocysticercosis may exceed 10%. In the eye, cysts are found in the retina, vitreous or anterior

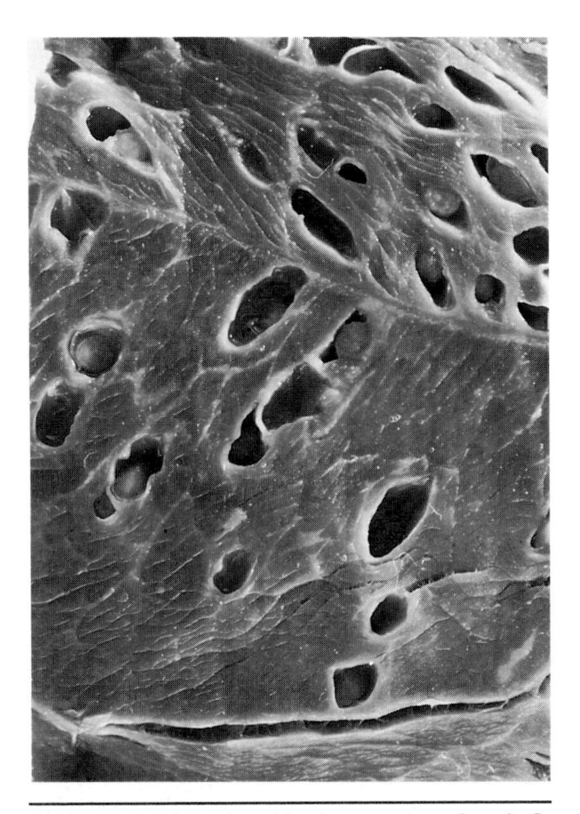

Fig. 25.39 Muscle with numerous cysticerci. In many of them, the scolex can be seen as a solid ball within the bladder-like cyst. ×2. (St Thomas's Hospital Medical School Pathology Museum.)

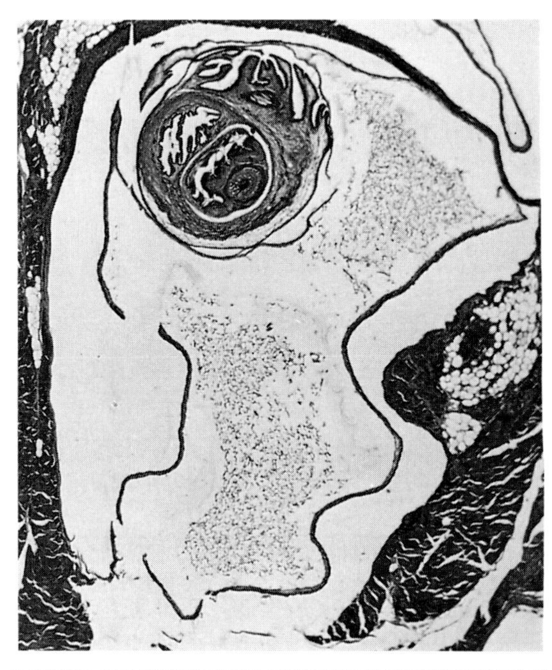

Fig. 25.40 Cysticercus in muscle. Inside the cyst is the scolex, which is inverted. The central targetoid structure is a sucker. ×20.

chamber; optical defects and blindness may follow, with secondary reactions such as conjunctivitis, uveitis, retinitis and finally optic atrophy.

Diagnosis of cysticercosis may be difficult. Biopsy of a subcutaneous lump will give a ready answer, but confirmation of neurocysticercosis is not always possible. Computerized axial tomography shows up most cysts, and can monitor their disappearance with medical therapy. Serological diagnostic techniques are improving, but cases with only central nervous system involvement may be seronegative.

Hydatid Disease (Echinococcosis)

Hydatid disease, caused by the larvae of *Echinococcus granulosus*, is the most serious tapeworm infection in man. One or more large cysts in the viscera behave as chronic space-occupying lesions. Medical therapy is uncertain and surgery is difficult with the risk of dissemination of cyst material: this is a metastasizing parasite.

Life Cycle

The adult tapeworms are 5–9 mm long and live in the small bowel of dogs. Eggs eaten by sheep and cattle, which are the main intermediate hosts, develop into hyatid cysts in their viscera. Offal containing cysts is consumed by the dogs. Man acquires cysts by eating eggs from dogs coats or faeces. Man is probably not always a dead end for the parasite, since some African tribes in endemic areas lay out the bodies of their dead to be eaten by canine carnivores. Hyatid disease is prevalent in sheep-raising countries in all latitudes: early this century, up to a third of the population of Iceland had cysts, and in Southern Australia half the dogs are infected with adult *E. granulosus*. The disease is a major problem in the Middle East, North and sub-Saharan Africa, and South America.

Clinical and Pathological Features

When eggs are ingested by man, the oncospheres hatch out, pass through the duodenal mucosa, and then by the portal vein to the liver, where cysts may develop or the embryos may disseminate by the bloodstream to other organs. The cyst grows slowly, reaching 1–5 cm in diameter by 6 months, and a final size of 5 to over 20 cm. Whatever the tissue, a hydatid cyst has a similar structure (Fig. 25.41). There is a surrounding host fibrous capsule enclosing the cyst wall, which is 1 mm thick, white, acellular, soft, chitinous and laminated. Inside is a thin cellular lining, the germinal membrane, from which develop the scolices. Smaller cysts (daughter cysts or brood capsules) develop from the germinal membrane inside the main cyst and these also generate scolices (Fig. 25.42). Thus, fertile cysts contain myriads of scolices, which are visible as grains of 'hydatid sand' in the otherwise clear or slightly yellowish cyst fluid. The cyst may rupture, spilling fragments of germinal membrane and scolices, which can form new hydatid cysts nearby.

An infected person may have one or several hydatid cysts: 50% of them are in the liver, usually in the right lobe, where they produce hepatomegaly and occasionally obstruct the portal vein and bile duct. Cysts in the lung are rather less common, causing pressure collapse of the affected lobe, haemoptysis and pleural effusion. Any other organ of the body can be involved, notably the spleen (hydatids are the commonest form of splenic cyst) and even the breast. In the peritoneal cavity, where the host reaction is slight, multiple cysts expand to produce great abdominal swelling. Bone hydatids occur in about 2% of cases and are very difficult to remove: in the vertebrae, they

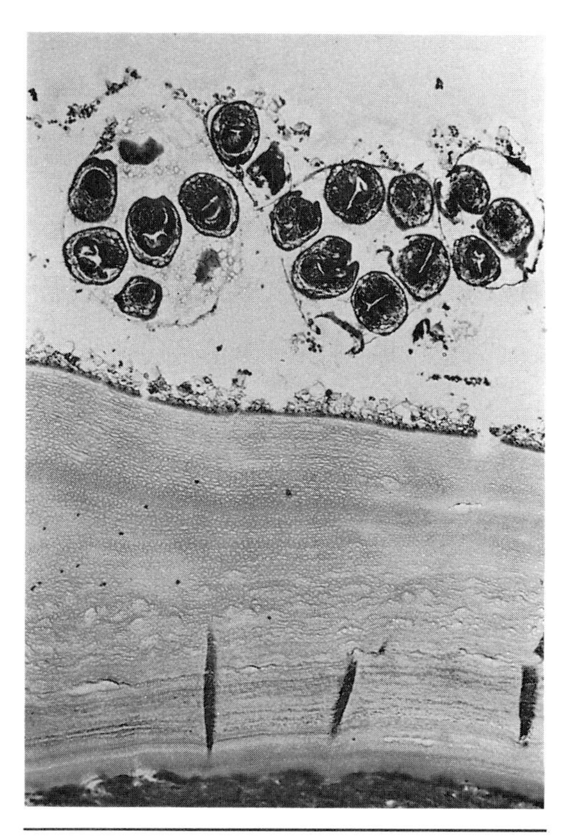

Fig. 25.41 The lining of a hydatid cyst. From the bottom upwards are the host fibrous capsule (stained dark), the pale laminated cyst wall, the thin cellular germinal membrane and, lying in the cyst cavity, three brood capsules containing round scolices. ×95.

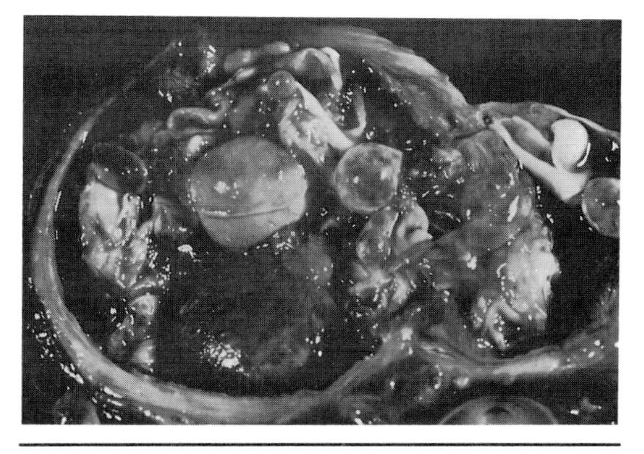

Fig. 25.42 Hydatid cyst of liver. Several daughter cysts, some collapsed, are lying in the main cyst. Note the fibrous capsule around the cyst.

produce relentless spinal cord compression and vertebral collapse. Similarly, cysts in the brain cause focal signs and obstruct the flow of CSF with resulting hydrocephalus. In addition to causing pain, cysts in the kidneys are in uncommon cause of renal failure. *In areas of the world where hydatid disease is highly prevalent, all tumours in any organ should be suspected of being hydatids until proved otherwise.*

In addition to the pathological effects of organ compression, allergic reactions occur if a cyst ruptures spontaneously or through trauma. The spillage of hydatid antigens results in a type 1 reaction with dyspnoea, cyanosis and circulatory collapse; in suspected cases of a cyst in the liver, needle biopsy should not be attempted for this reason. The treatment of a hydatid cyst is problematic. Surgery is still the choice for accessible cysts causing clinically important compression, but care is needed not to spill any of the contents. To prevent metastasis of fertile germinal membrane, hepatic cysts are instilled with formaldehyde after exposure, before proceeding with their removal. Recurrent peritoneal cysts are a common complication of surgery on the liver. Lung cysts may be removed intact, using positive pressure ventilation. Overall the mortality of diagnosed hydatid disease is about 10%. Although there is evidence of an immune host response to hydatid antigens, there is no effective resistance to infection.

Diagnosis

Serology is reasonably specific, and the Casoni skin test is obsolete. Radiology and ultrasound examination are useful to locate hydatid cysts. Occasionally a lung hydatid ruptures into a bronchus, and hooklets from dead scolices may be seen microscopically in the sputum.

Nematode Infections

Nematodes are cylindrical smooth worms which grow to adult size by several moults. They are dioecious, i.e. of separate sexes, and they tend to be long-lived. With the exception of *Strongyloides stercoralis*, their life cycles include an obligatory phase outside the human host. Some of the species require also an intermediate host. The most important nematode infections are the intestinal worms and the filariases. Also considered in this section are trichinosis and the larva migrans syndromes.

Intestinal Nematodes

Intestinal nematodes are ubiquitous, and even if man avoids infection by those adapted to him alone, he may be parasitized by the larvae of roundworms living in the gut of lower animals.

The most important intestinal nematodes are *Enterobius vermicularis, Trichuris trichiura*, the two hookworms (*Necator americanus* and *Ancylostoma duodenale*), *Strongyloides stercoralis* and *Ascaris lumbricoides*. Their life cycles are of varying complexity (Fig. 25.43) and they are acquired either by ingesting ova or by active penetration of the skin by larvae living in the soil. None of them has an intermediate host, but one of them, *Strongyloides stercoralis*, is unique in that it can maintain its cycle entirely within the human body. The other species have a finite lifespan and the infections die out unless new worms are acquired. Further details of these parasites are given in Table 25.3.

Enterobiasis (Oxyuriasis)

This condition is world wide and possibly the commonest human infection after the common cold. It is caused by *Enterobius vermicularis*, and has many synonyms including **oxyuriasis**, **pinworm** and **threadworm** infection. The highest prevalence is in children.

The worms are acquired by ingesting eggs, either one's own or from the environment (Fig. 25.43). The larvae in the eggs hatch in the ileum

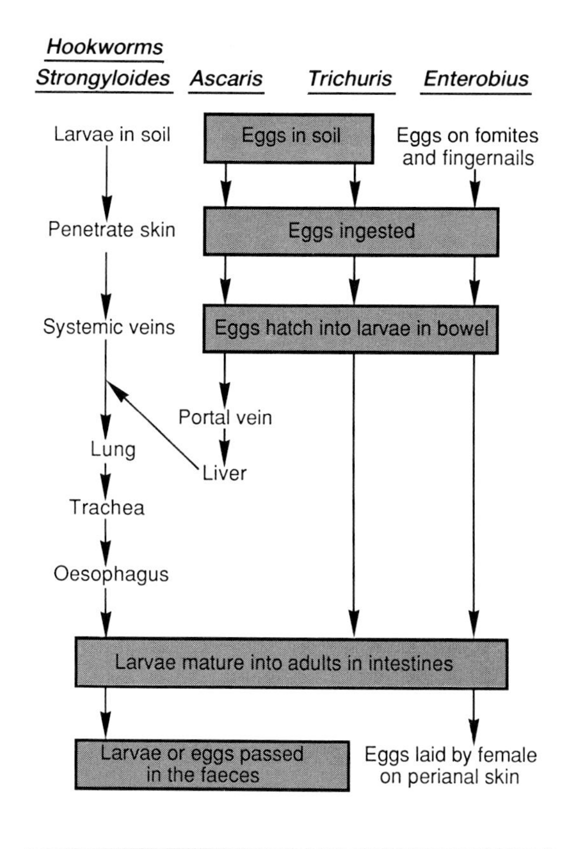

Fig. 25.43 Life cycles of the intestinal nematode worms.

and the mature worms move to the appendix (Fig. 25.44) and large intestine where the males and females mate. The gravid females migrate out of the anus at night and each lays about 10 000 eggs on the perianal skin and then dies. The eggs are dispersed on bed clothes, personal clothes, the floor and the walls, and some are picked up under the fingernails to autoinfect the subject later on. This cycle of infection lasts 4–6 weeks; the ubiquity of the eggs accounts for the ease of re-infection.

The clinical phenomena are primarily itching of the perianal skin (*pruritus ani*) and, in women, the vulval skin. This is a reaction to the worm proteins and the eggs. The adult worms in the bowel lumen have no significant local effect; as initiators of acute appendicitis they are probably unimportant.

An uncommon complication of enterobiasis is seen if a gravid female worm migrates up the female genital tract or invades through a bowel mucosal defect, by which routes a worm can reach the peritoneal cavity. When it dies it provokes an intense eosinophil and granulomatous reaction with central necrosis and abscess formation. Thus endometritis, salpingitis, serosal and liver nodules can occur. The lesions are bacteriologically sterile but in the liver they can masquerade as metastatic tumour deposits.

Table 25.3 Features and effects of the common intestinal nematodes of man

Parasite	Adult female: length in mm	Location	Lifespan	Clinical effects
Enterobius	10–12	Colon, appendix	4 weeks	Pruritus ani; rarely intra-abdominal abscesses
Trichuris	30–50	Colon	1–2 years	Diarrhoea, rectal prolapse
Hookworms	10–12	Jejunum	5 years	Blood loss, iron-deficiency anaemia, pneumonitis, dermatitis
Strongyloides	2	Ileum	Unknown (persists by autoinfection)	Diarrhoea, malabsorption, pneumonitis, dermatitis: hyperinfection, visceral dissemination
Ascaris	200–400	Ileum	1–2 years	Bowel and bile duct obstruction, pneumonitis

Adult worms may be seen in the stools or around the anus at night. Examination of faeces for ova is unrewarding, and the easiest method of diagnosing enterobiasis is by applying clear sticky tape to the anal skin of the subject after sleeping. The eggs adhere to the tape and can be identified by examining it microscopically.

Trichuriasis (Whipworm Infection)

Trichuris trichiura is also widespread and about 500 million people are affected throughout the world. Like ascariasis, trichuriasis is particularly common where human faeces are used as fertilizer ('night soil'). Eggs are ingested with soil or vegetables and hatch in the ileum. The mature adults are about 50 mm long and live in the colon and rectum with their thin anterior end attached to the mucosa and the long, wider, coiled posterior part (the 'whip') hanging in the lumen (Fig. 25.45). The female lays about 5000 eggs per day into the faeces.

Mild infections are symptomless. Heavy infections with hundreds of worms are associated with diarrhoea, and occasionally rectal prolapse in children. The mucosal damage from the physical attachment can also lead to significant blood loss and iron-deficiency anaemia if more than 1000 worms are present. Diagnosis is made by finding eggs in the faeces or by seeing the worms on sigmoidoscopy.

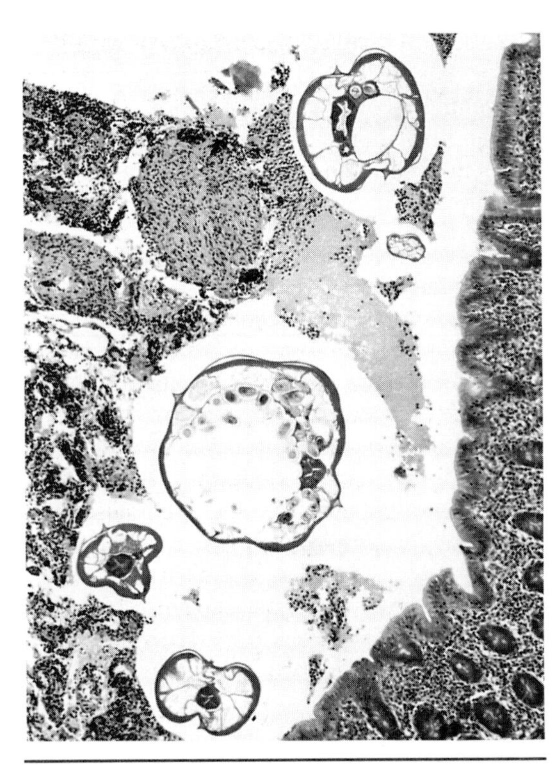

Fig. 25.44 Lumen of the appendix, showing cross-sections of *Enterobius vermicularis* adults. The paired lateral spines on the outer cuticle of the worms are characteristic. ×80.

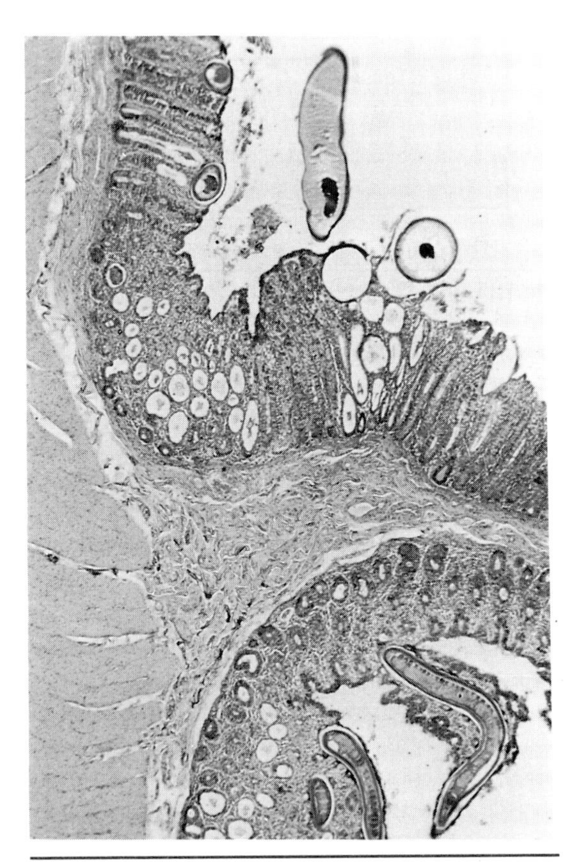

Fig. 25.45 Colonic mucosa, showing several *Trichuris* worms. The narrower anterior ends are buried in the mucosa whilst the broader posterior ends lie in the lumen. ×28.

Ancylostomiasis (Hookworm Infection)

Hookworm infection of the bowel is one of the most important human afflictions. At least 700 million people are infected and a proportion suffer debilitating chronic anaemia as a consequence. The two species of human hookworm, *Necator americanus* and *Ancylostoma duodenale*, have similar morphology and life cycles (Fig. 25.43). They are both found in the tropics and subtropics and *A. duodenale* also extends into temperate regions. (In 1909 the forerunner of the Rockefeller Foundation was instituted for the sole purpose of eliminating hookworm infection from the USA and Puerto Rico: it has yet to succeed.)

Life Cycle

The parasite has an obligate phase in the soil, where eggs deposited in faeces hatch into larvae. The larvae actively penetrate human skin, usually bare feet, and are carried in the venous blood to the lungs. Whilst developing, larvae break into the alveoli, crawl up the airways to the pharynx, and are swallowed. The mature adults reside in the jejunum, attached to the villi. *N. americanus* females lay about 5000 eggs per day, and *A. duodenale* up to 20 000 eggs per day.

Clinical and Pathological Features

These depend on the intensity of infection and on previous exposure. Repeated infection sensitizes the host so that penetrating larvae cause an intensely itchy dermatitis – '**ground itch**'. This inflammation may be a manifestation of resistance, because partial immunity does develop to the infection. During the phase of migration through the lungs, a heavy infection can induce an eosinophil leucocytosis and a pneumonitis, **Loeffler's pneumonitis**, although this is not as severe as the syndrome seen in ascariasis.

The most important clinical effects arise from the attachment of the worms to the jejunal mucosa (Fig. 25.46). The worm is 10 mm long: it attaches to the mucosa by grasping a villus in its mouth, wriggles continuously and sucks blood from the villus. It also secretes an anticoagulant, and even when a hookworm detaches and moves to another part of the mucosa, bleeding continues for a while. Each *N. americanus* worm causes the loss of 0.03 ml of blood daily, and *A. duodenale* a loss of 0.1 ml per day. An individual may harbour up to 2000 worms, but even a few hundred cause **iron-deficiency anaemia**, which is often aggravated by a diet low in iron. The worms live for about 5 years and are a very important cause of debility from anaemia. Infection is diagnosed by finding the eggs (identical in the two species) in the faeces.

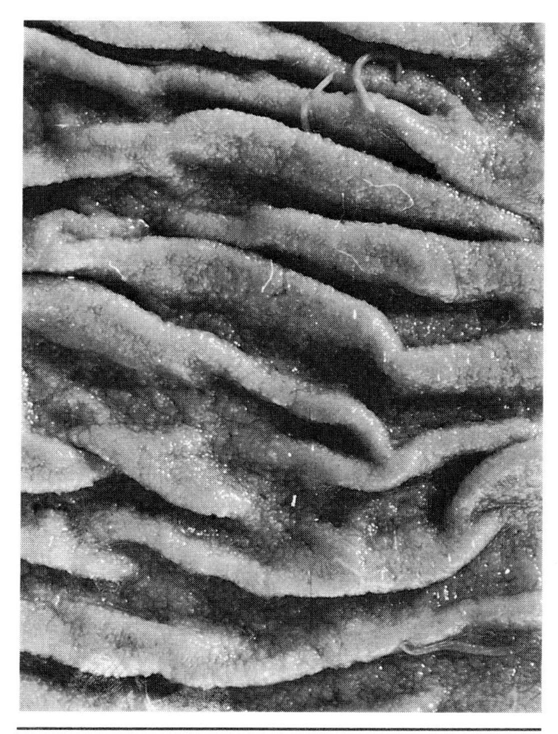

Fig. 25.46 Mucosa of ileum with three hookworms attached (two towards the top, one near the bottom of the picture. (St Thomas' Hospital Medical School Pathology Museum.)

Strongyloidiasis

Infection with *Strongyloides stercoralis* is endemic in the tropics and subtropics with an estimated

100–200 million cases. An unusual feature affecting the life cycle of this worm is the ability of its eggs to hatch and invade without being excreted by the host. By this means, the parasite can persist for decades after a person has left an area of infection. Recent surveys of British ex-servicemen who were prisoners of war in Burma between 1941 and 1945 have shown that up to 20% of them still carry *Strongyloides stercoralis* in their bowel.

Life Cycle

The life cycle of *S. stercoralis* (Fig. 25.43) is similar to that of the hookworms but only female worms are found. They lay eggs parthenogenetically. The eggs hatch in the lumen of the intestine, and most of the larvae are passed with the faeces. Some larvae mature into infective forms by the time they reach the anus and can penetrate the perianal skin directly, then pass via the lungs to the bowel and maintain the infection even in the absence of fresh invasion from parasites in the soil. Migrating larvae may cause wheals in the skin. This autoinfective cycle is, however, usually prevented by protective immune mechanisms in the bowel; massive autoinfection, however, occurs in subjects with defective cell mediated immunity. Not only do larvae penetrate the skin to recycle and increase the parasite load, but they can also invade the bowel mucosa and disseminate via the bloodstream and lymph throughout the body – the 'hyperinfection syndrome'.

Clinical and Pathological Features

In the normal light infection, the small bowel mucosa is hardly disturbed. The **hyperinfection syndrome** of strongyloidiasis is life-threatening. The typical cases are people with chronic infection (usually asymptomatic) who are treated by immunosuppressive drugs, e.g. following organ transplantation, or who are grossly malnourished or develop a lymphoma or some other neoplasm which depresses immunity. There is severe diarrhoea, malabsorption, hepatomegaly and prostration. In addition to the effects of widespread visceral spread of larvae, *Escherichia coli* septicaemia is common, the bacilli entering the blood through breaches in the bowel mucosa. The entire gut is dilated, oedematous and haemorrhagic. Microscopically, the mucosa is grossly inflamed and distorted by innumerable adult worms and larvae (Fig. 25.47). Larvae are seen also in the liver, lungs, brain and meninges, and are surrounded by an acute inflammatory reaction. The syndrome is fatal unless treated, and it is a diagnosis to be considered in immunocompromised patients with unexplained multi-organ damage.

Strongyloidiasis is diagnosed by detecting larvae in the faeces. In the hyperinfection syndrome, larvae can be found in large numbers in a gastric aspirate and sputum, as well as in the stools. Serology may be useful.

Ascariasis

Ascaris lumbricoides is by far the largest intestinal nematode, measuring 20–40 cm in length and 5–6 mm in diameter. Much of the pathology of ascariasis is due to worms obstructing viscera.

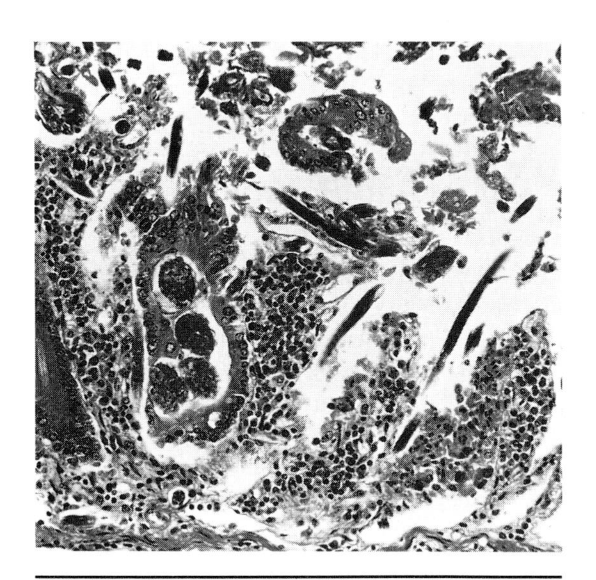

Fig. 25.47 Ileal mucosa in *Strongyloides* hyperinfection. Inside the crypt on the left are four cross-sections of the adult female worm. Above and to the right, several thinner elongated larvae are seen. ×200.

The condition is world wide and about 800 million people are infected. The reproductive effects of *Ascaris* are remarkable, each female laying about 200 000 eggs per day into the faeces. Consequently, infection is prevalent where hygienic standards are low, especially if human faeces are used as an agricultural fertilizer.

The **life cycle** is complicated (Fig. 25.43) because the larvae hatching from ingested eggs have to pass through the lungs during their maturation. They invade the ileal mucosa, travel by the portal vein to the liver and then via the bloodstream to the lungs. There they moult twice and enter the alveoli: after this, their passage is as for the hookworms.

Clinical and Pathological Features

Light infections are symptomless. The overt clinical and pathological effects of ascariasis occur in two phases. During the **larval migration phase**, a heavy synchronous infection (from ingesting a hundred or more eggs) results in a transient hepatitis and pneumonitis as a reaction to the migrating larvae. The pulmonary symptoms include cough, dyspnoea, fever and sometimes haemoptysis. Chest X-ray shows widespread dense pulmonary infiltrates and there is an eosinophil leucocytosis. This condition, known as **Loeffler's syndrome**, comes on 5 days after ingesting the eggs and lasts about 10 days. The lungs are focally consolidated and microscopy shows interstitial pneumonia and eosinophils and fibrin in the alveoli around the small *Ascaris* larvae. The pneumonitis is more severe than that seen in hookworm infection because a heavy synchronous infection is commoner in ascariasis and also because the larvae moult in the lungs, releasing more antigenic material.

Once the worms have matured in the ileum, the **adult worm phase** of the disease ensues. Generally 50 or more worms are needed to produce symptoms although ascariasis is one of the few helminth diseases where a single worm, by blocking at a critical site, can cause morbidity and even death. Tangled masses of worms can produce intermittent or complete intestinal obstruction, commonly at the ileocaecal valve (Fig. 25.48). They may also form the centre of a volvulus, and rarely, by obstructing the lumen of the appendix, may cause acute appendicitis. Serious complications arise if an ascarid enters and blocks the bile duct; biliary colic and sometimes ascending cholangitis and liver abscesses may follow. Should the adult female ascend into the liver and deposit eggs there, a granulomatous abscess may form around the degenerating worm and eggs. Blocking of the pancreatic duct is an unusual cause of pancreatitis. Rarely, the worms also perforate the intestine, with resulting peritonitis. The wanderlust of *Ascaris* is dramatically shown when adults occasionally appear from the nose, mouth, urethra or vagina. In addition to their physical effects, these large worms can compromise the nutrition of the host; it is estimated that a child with 26 ascarids

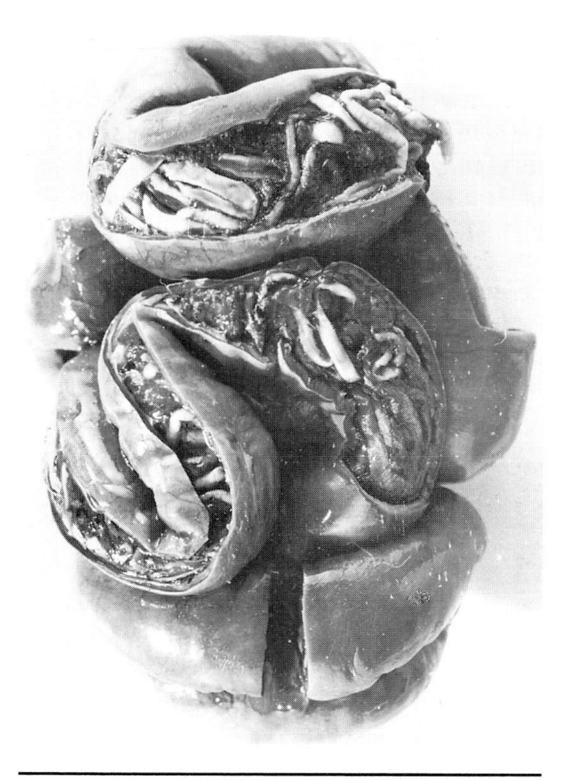

Fig. 25.48 *Ascaris lumbricoides* causing small bowel obstruction. A long bolus of worms fills the lumen. (St Thomas's Hospital Medical School of Pathology Museum.)

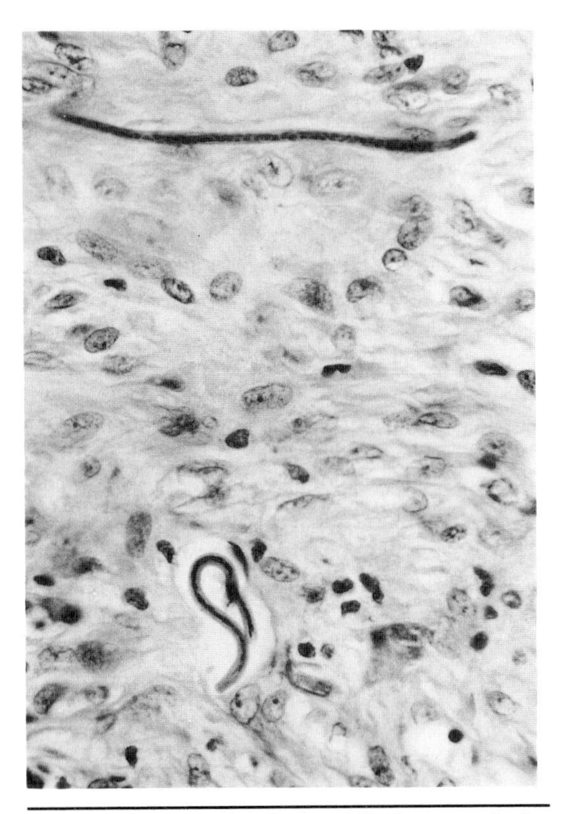

Fig. 25.49 Two microfilariae of *Onchocerca volvulus* in skin with accompanying fibrosing reaction.

loses one-tenth of the total dietary protein intake to the worms.

There is some evidence of a partial acquired immunity to *Ascaris* in older people. The worms live for 1–2 years, and transmission is often seasonal. The infection is diagnosed by finding the eggs in the faeces. In Loeffler's syndrome, larvae may also be seen in the sputum.

Filariasis

This group of diseases is caused by several genera of tissue-dwelling, long thin filarial worms. All are transmitted by biting insects, the adult worms live as paired couples in man, and the females produce embryos called **microfilariae**. These are worm-like motile larvae ranging in length from 250 to 300 μm (Fig. 25.49). In onchocerciasis, the microfilariae wander in the dermis and ocular tissues, but in the lymphatic filariases they live in the blood. When a suitable insect bites an infected person, the microfilariae are ingested and develop into larval forms infective for man. Morphologically, the adults and microfilariae are characteristic for each species of filaria. Some of the major features of the filariases are shown in Table 25.4.

Table 25.4 Types and features of filariasis

	Female parasite (size in mm)	Intermediate host	Numbers affected (× 10^6	Geographical distribution	Effects
Lymphatic filariasis	*Wuchereria bancrofti* (100 × 0.25) *Brugia malayi* (100 × 0.25)	*Culex* mosquito *Mansonia* mosquito	90	Sub-Saharan Africa, India, S.E. Asia, Pacific islands, central and S. America S.E. Asia (*Brugia*)	Lymphadenitis, elephantiasis, tropical pulmonary eosinophilia
Onchocerciasis	*Onchocerca volvulus* (500 × 0.3)	*Simulium* blackfly	17	Sub-Saharan Africa, Central America	Subcutaneous nodules, dermatitis, blindness
Loiasis	*Loa loa* (70 × 0.5)	*Chrysops* fly	20	West and Central Africa	Migratory subcutaneous swellings

Lymphatic Filariasis

The clinical, parasitological and pathological features of infection with *Wuchereria bancrofti* and *Brugia malayi* are similar and are considered together.

Life Cycle

The larvae are injected into the skin by a mosquito and migrate by lymphatics to the draining lymph nodes. During the next year, they develop into adults and reside in the afferent lymphatics and the cortical sinuses of the nodes. The females release **microfilariae** into the lymph from where they pass into the blood. Microfilariae do not circulate in the blood constantly, but stay in the lung capillaries during the day and emerge into the peripheral circulation at night. This nocturnal periodicity is thought to depend on the oxygen tension of the blood during sleep and corresponds with the nocturnal biting habits of the vector mosquitoes. In the endemic zones, filarial worms are acquired progressively from infancy onwards, with peak prevalence in early adulthood. The adult worms live for 10–18 years and there is some degree of concomitant immunity against infection. In many places, infection rates are 50% or more but, as with most helminth infections, the majority of those infected (i.e. those with detectable microfilaraemia) remain free of symptoms.

Clinical and Pathological Features

The adult worms are located predominantly in the lymph nodes of the groin and axilla. The essential clinicopathological features arise from the host reaction to the adult worms, particularly degenerating ones. No toxic factor is secreted by these forms and, with the exception of the syndrome of tropical pulmonary eosinophilia, the microfilariae do not cause lesions.

Living worms in the lymphatics cause a perilymphatic inflammation and fibrosis, but they do not occlude the lumens. However, their physical presence has a dilating effect with subsequent lymphatic incompetence and lymphoedema. Degenerating worms elicit a predominantly cell-mediated immune response with a granulomatous reaction, eosinophilia and fibrosis (Fig. 25.50), and this blocks the afferent lymphatics. Eventually the dead worms calcify.

In the early years of infection, there may be recurrent episodes of **acute filariasis** with fever, lymphadenitis and retrograde lymphangitis. The pathogenesis is not clear, but there is thought to be a transient Arthus-type reaction to worm antigens or secondary bacterial infections in the dependent limb. After many years, signs of overt **chronic filariasis** develop in a small proportion of those infected. Interestingly, visitors who acquire lymphatic filariasis, e.g. military personnel, never develop chronic infections and elephantiasis. The permanent lymphatic dilatation and obstruction caused by the adult worms results in transudation of protein-rich lymph into the dependent tissues. The regions commonly affected are the legs and arms, the scrotum, and

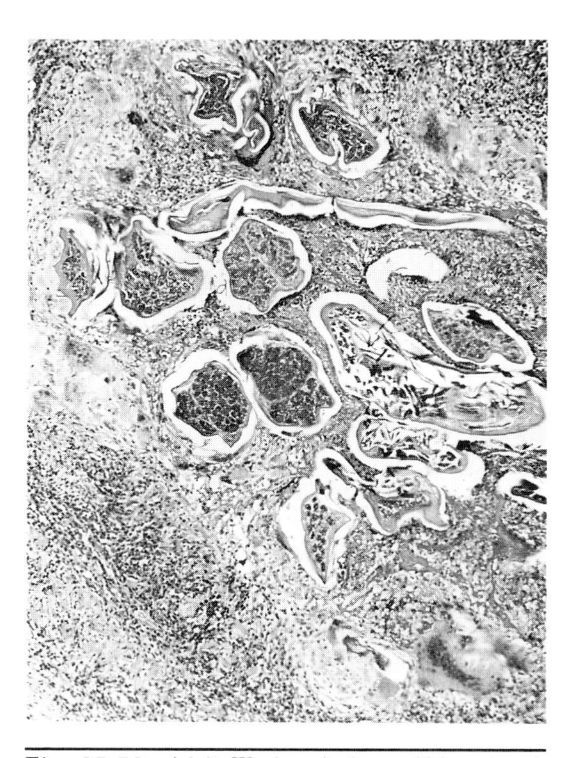

Fig. 25.50 Adult *Wuchereria bancrofti* in a lymph node. Fragments of the coiled worm with a giant-cell granulomatous reaction. ×70.

sometimes the breasts and vulva. The lymphoedema induces a chronic inflammatory and fibroblastic reaction in the dermis and subcutis, with ensuing hardening and gross enlargement of the soft tissues – **elephantiasis** (Fig. 25.51).

Histologically, there is dilatation of dermal lymphatics and the epidermis is often so hyperplastic that the skin of the foot takes on a verrucose appearance – '**mossy foot**'. At this late stage, chemotherapy for filariasis does not reverse the elephantiasis. Within the scrotum, lymph may accumulate in a hydrocele in which microfilariae are sometimes found. If intra-abdominal lymph nodes are infected and obstructed, the lymph can leak back into the peritoneum and produce ascites. Similar leakage from the bladder wall into its lumen, results in chyluria.

Tropical pulmonary eosinophilia. A small percentage of people with either *W. bancrofti* or *B. malayi* infections suffer from nocturnal attacks of fever, asthma and eosinophil leucocytosis. They have very high serum levels of IgE (some of which is antifilarial antibody) but microfilariae are not found in the blood. Chest radiography reveals widespread pulmonary infiltrates, and lung biopsy shows microfilariae surrounded by a granulomatous reaction. It appears that these individuals develop a type 1 hypersensitivity reaction to microfilarial antigens, and that this syndrome is a form of 'occult filariasis' in which microfilariae are effectively cleared from the blood by the host immune reaction. A parallel hypersensitivity probably underlines the production of elephantiasis and the other sequelae of chronic lymphatic filariasis: the affected victims react more strongly than usual to degenerating adult worms, and thus incur more lymphatic damage.

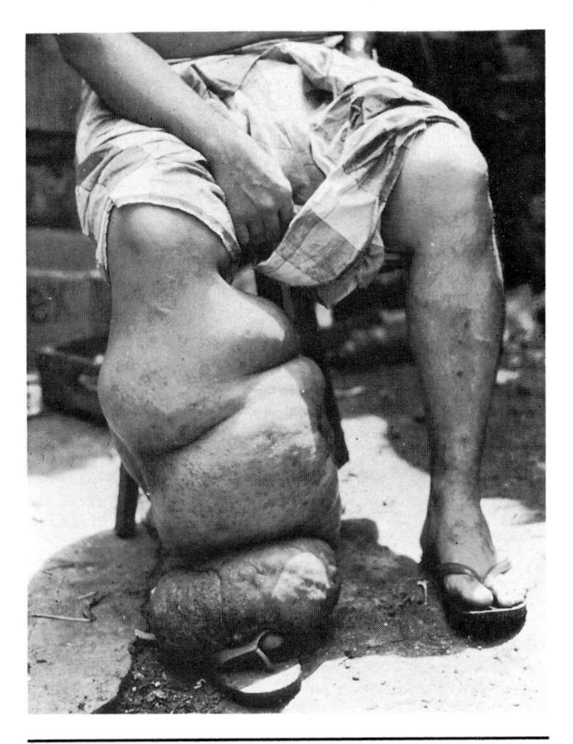

Fig. 25.51 Gross elephantiasis of the right leg due to *Brugia malayi* infection. (Photograph kindly supplied by Dr R. Muller, Commonwealth Institute of Parasitology.)

Diagnosis

The microfilariae are found in the blood (by nocturnal sampling) only in the early stages of lymphatic filariasis, and it may be difficult to distinguish the chronic disease from other environmental causes of lymphoedema such as silica lymphadenopathy. The diagnostic value of serology is limited by the wide antigenic overlap with many other nematodes, and also by the disappearance of antibodies in chronic infection. Although of little use in endemic areas, serology is of diagnostic value in visitors to endemic areas. Eosinophil leucocytosis is characteristic only in the early stages of filariasis.

Onchocerciasis

Onchocerciasis is a chronic disease caused by *Onchocerca volvulus* (Table 25.4). Infection begins in infancy and in many endemic zones everyone is affected by the age of 20. It is a rural disease and the vectors breed by swift streams and rivers; as with schistosomiasis, dams and hydroelectric schemes provide new breeding sites for the vector. Depending on the local prevalence and intensity of infection, up to one-tenth of people in some villages may be partially sighted or blind because of onchocerciasis, which is also known as '**river blindness**'. Consequently, many fertile areas in tropical Africa are abandoned by the population to avoid the disease.

Life Cycle

The larvae, transmitted by an infected *Simulium* fly, migrate via lymphatics to subcutaneous sites over bony prominences, particularly over the iliac crests, ribs, shoulders and cranium. There they mature into pairing adults, the males and females lying coiled around each other. During a lifespan of some 10–15 years, female worms liberate hundreds of thousands of microfilariae, which can live up to 24 months. They do not enter the blood, but wander through the adjacent dermis where only a small proportion will be taken up by a biting vector.

Clinical and Pathological Features

The presence of the adults in non-critical body sites is of no great direct significance. The microfilariae are responsible for the more serious effects. Microfilariae of *O. volvulus* do not secrete any known toxin, and apart from fibrosis they induce no reaction until they degenerate and cease to be motile, when they elicit an eosinophil, mast-cell and histiocytic reaction. Blood eosinophilia is usually marked in onchocerciasis except in advanced and burnt-out cases. Degeneration of microfilariae may occur through natural ageing or from the administration of microfilaricidal drugs.

It is an important feature of onchocerciasis that the main form of current treatment is with diethylcarbamazine, a microfilaricidal drug that has little or no effect on the adult filariae; it does not kill microfilariae *in vitro*, but induces an acute inflammatory response to them, probably by unmasking antigens on their surface. As a result, there is fever, and inflammation develops wherever microfilariae are present in the body, with an acute aggravation of symptoms and signs of the disease. This is known as the **Mazzotti reaction**, and is distinctive enough to be used as a diagnostic test for onchocerciasis. In the presence of a heavy infection, however, such rapid induction of a widespread reaction may be dangerous.

Subcutaneous nodules. The coiled male and female adults induce a fibrous reaction and become palpable nodules or **onchocercomas** (Fig. 25.52). Histologically, the worms are surrounded by a variable chronic inflammatory cell infiltrate and eosinophil reaction with much fibrosis (Fig. 25.53). When they degenerate, they are phagocytosed by giant cells.

Skin lesions. Clinically, the majority of people with untreated onchocerciasis have relatively mild dermatitis. There is pruritus, and in the early stages a rash of small discrete papules. As a result of chronic microfilaria-induced inflammation and scratching, the skin eventually becomes hyperplastic and lichenified. Finally it loses its elasticity, becomes atrophic, focally depigmented and hangs in folds.

The intensity of the lesions caused by the presence of microfilariae in the dermis depends on the

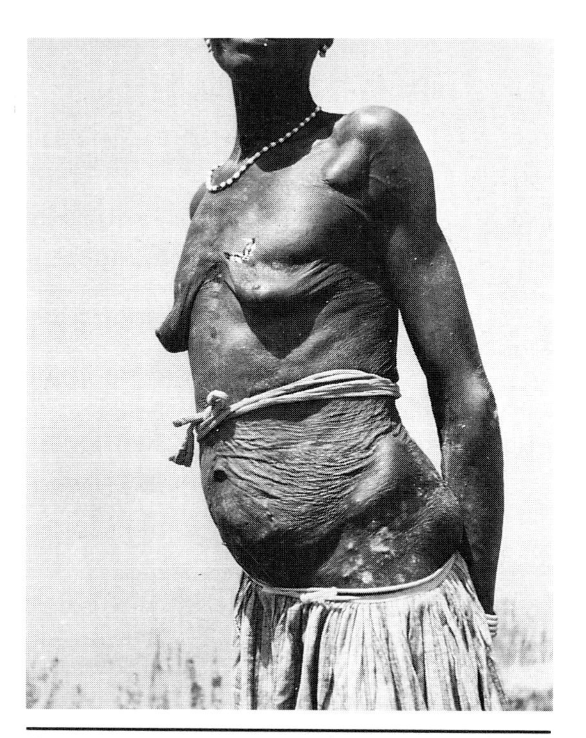

Fig. 25.52 Chronic onchocerciasis. Subcutaneous nodules containing adult worms (onchocercomas) are visible on the shoulder and the iliac crest. Also present are the depigmented areas (above the skirt) and hanging folds of skin due to chronic dermatitis.

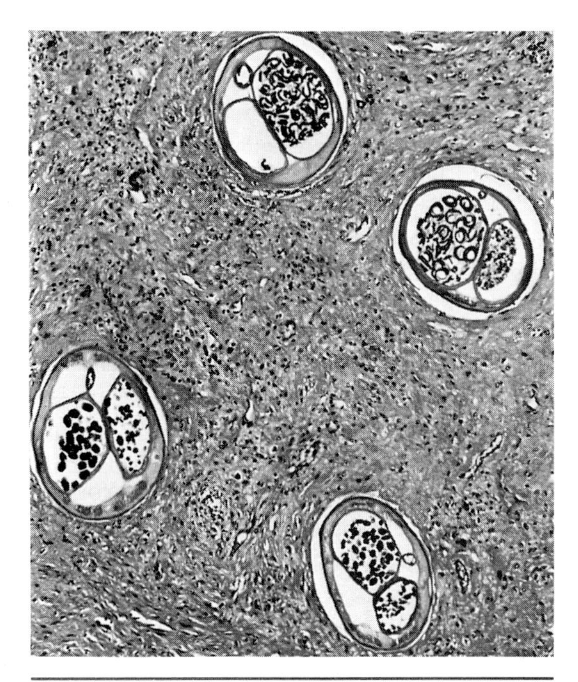

Fig. 25.53 Section through an adult female *Onchocerca volvulus* in the subcutaneous tissues. Several cross-sections of the coiled worm are seen with the uterus containing many microfilariae. ×75.

intensity of infection and on the strength of the host reaction. Skin testing with onchocercal antigens has shown that those with the strongest delayed hypersensitivity reaction have the most active dermatitis and the least number of microfilariae in the skin. Conversely, those with many microfilariae may have little reaction. This is reminiscent of lymphatic filariasis where those reacting more strongly to worm antigens have the more severe disease. The reaction around degenerating microfilariae depends also on antibody-dependent eosinophil cytotoxicity: IgG antibody binds to the microfilarial surface and mediates degranulation of eosinophils, with injury to the microfilariae. A similar phenomenon occurs in the skin in schistosomiasis, when schistosomula are damaged by antibody-dependent eosinophil cytotoxicity.

Histologically, variable numbers of microfilariae are seen in the upper dermis. There is an inflammatory reaction with infiltration of eosinophils, lymphocytes, plasma cells and macrophages, both perivascularly and focally around microfilariae.

Diagnosis is made by demonstrating microfilariae in skin snips; small fragments of skin are snipped off with a razor blade, immersed in saline, and examined later for emerging microfilariae. This also provides a guide to the intensity of infection.

Eye lesions. Although the skin lesions are distressing to the patient, the ocular damage in onchocerciasis is more disabling. Eye lesions are a consequence of heavy and chronic infection with a high density of microfilariae in the dermis of the periocular skin. Microfilariae reach the anterior parts of the eye via the ciliary vessels and the bulbar conjunctiva; they may reach the posterior parts – the retina and the vitreous – via the optic nerve.

The clinicopathological sequelae in the eye are as follows: (1) punctate keratitis, seen as transient fluffy white spots on the cornea, results from an oedematous inflammatory reaction to degenerating microfilariae; (2) sclerosing keratitis, which is an extension of granulation tissue coming in from the limbus and permanently scarring the cornea, a significant cause of blindness; (3) microfilariae may also float free in the fluid of the anterior chamber, cause iritis and the formation of anterior synechiae with secondary glaucoma; and (4) in the posterior chamber, foci of microfilaria-induced retinitis and depigmentation occur. Damage to the optic nerve may cause optic atrophy.

Lymph nodes. The groin and axillary nodes usually show perifollicular fibrosis. In those people with very severe, ulcerating dermatitis, the nodes may have marked follicular hyperplasia and be enlarged. Lymphoedema and elephantiasis are rarely found in this disease.

Loiasis (Eye Worm Infection)

Infection with the filarial worm *Loa Loa* (Table 25.4) is characterized by fleeting areas of subcutaneous oedema although many infections are asymptomatic.

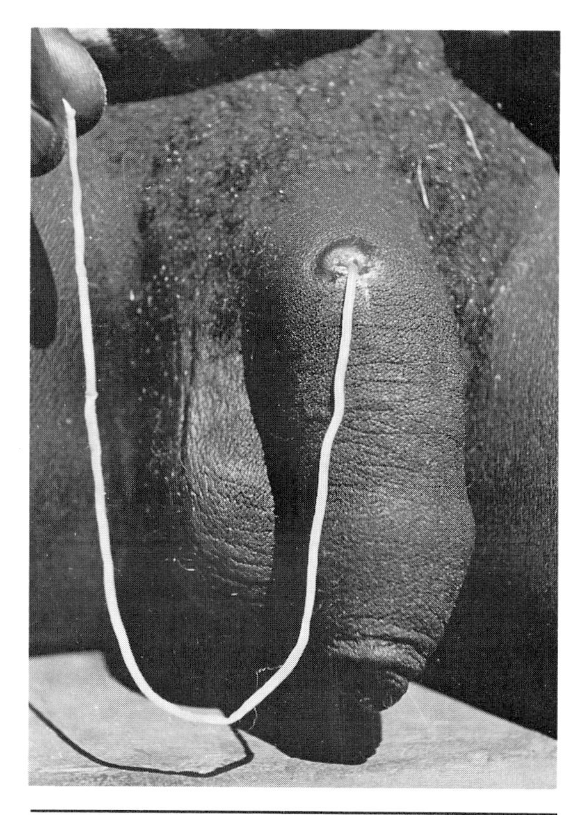

Fig. 25.54 A guinea-worm, *Dracunculus medinensis*, being withdrawn from a blister on the shaft of the penis. (Picture kindly supplied by Dr R. Muller, Commonwealth Institute of Parasitology.)

Life Cycle

The *Chrysops* fly ingests the microfilariae from an infected host and injects infective larvae when it takes a blood meal. The worms mature and mate in the subcutaneous tissues and the females deposit microfilariae which enter the capillaries and circulate in the blood. The female adults live for up to 17 years.

Clinical and Pathological Features

Neither adult nor microfilariae elicit any significant direct injury. The adults move continuously in the superficial tissues, and induce local allergic erythematosus and oedematous swellings ('**Calabar swellings**') which last a few days. These may occur anywhere on the body but are found particularly around the orbit and in the extremities: they are hot, itchy, and may be painful, so that joint movement is impaired. The worm may also cross the eye in the subconjunctival tissues – moving at about 1 cm per minute – where it causes allergic irritation. A rare but serious phenomenon is meningoencephalitis. *Loa loa* is the most frequent filarial invader of the central nervous system, and microfilariae may be found in the CSF.

Histologically, granulomatous reactions are seen around degenerating adults. The diagnosis is made by seeing the migrating worm in the eye, and by finding the microfilariae in the blood, where they appear during the day (like their vector fly).

Other Nematode Infections

Dracunculiasis (Dracontiasis)

Infection with the 'guinea-worm', *Dracunculus medinensis*, is a classic example of a rural, water-borne, seasonal disease arising from the contamination of water used for drinking and washing. Its effects are a blistering and cellulitis of the limbs which, by making movement painful, reduces the productive activity of farmers, often during the harvesting period. Over 1 million people are infected annually throughout Africa, the Middle East and India.

Life Cycle

The infection occurs where people immerse their limbs in wells or cisterns used also for drinking water and which becomes colonized by small crustacean *Cyclops*. When infected individuals immerse their limbs, *Dracunculus* larvae escape into the water and are ingested by *Cyclops*, in which they develop into a form infective for man in about 2 weeks. When infected *Cyclops* are swallowed in the water, they are digested and larvae are released into the gut. They burrow through the gut wall, and migrate through the abdomen to the subcutaneous tissues where they mature and mate; the males then die and are absorbed. The gravid females exhibit geotropism and migrate to the extremities, in most cases the lower limbs. The female is now a cylindrical white worm of about 60 cm × 1.5 mm with some 3 million larvae in its uterus. The worm's head glands secrete irritant (and antigenic) substances which induce a blister in the overlying skin. This is itchy and painful. The blister bursts, and on contact with water, the female extrudes larvae, gradually emerging further out of the skin, until without intervention, it is completely expelled by 4 weeks (Fig. 25.54). Not all gravid worms emerge onto the skin; some degenerate in the deep tissues and calcify, and may be detected by radiography. The complete life cycle from ingestion of larvae in *Cyclops* to expulsion of larvae from the body takes a year, and coincides with the annual dry season when water levels are low and hence densities of *Cyclops* and of expelled larvae in the water are high.

Clinical and Pathological Features

There is no protective immunity to guinea-worm and repeated infections occur. The clinical features are: (1) awareness of a moving subcutaneous worm; (2) allergic phenomena such as urticaria, fever, nausea, diarrhoea and vomiting just before the blister formation; and (3) the local skin reactions to the female worm. If the worm bursts in the tissues during larval expulsion, there is a severe reaction due to the worm antigens and larvae, with cellulitis, myositis and abscess formation. Secondary bacterial infection often supervenes, and acute arthritis can result if the lesion is near a joint. The skin lesions are also a focus for infection with tetanus spores. During infection, blood eosinophilia is usual.

The diagnosis of the guinea-worm infection is usually obvious. The time-honoured treatment is to accelerate the emergence of the adult female (Fig. 25.54) by daily immersion of the site of exit and gradually winding the worm out onto a stick. Antibiotics may also be required.

Trichinosis (Trichinellosis)

Trichinella spiralis is a parasitic nematode worm with many hosts, including the pig, boar and rat. The parasite is acquired by eating the flesh of an infected animal and is thus found only in carnivores. Man is infected by eating undercooked pork, usually in sausage, and is a dead-end for the parasite, because, although a suitable host, his flesh is now seldom eaten.

Larvae are released from cysts in ingested muscle and mature into adult worms in the ileum. About a week later the fecund females release numerous larvae which invade the mucosa and spread by the blood. The adult worms are later expelled from the gut by an immune reaction. Larvae in the blood invade many tissues. Those entering skeletal muscle fibres become encysted and remain alive, while in other organs they are destroyed by a granulomatous and eosinophil reaction.

The human disease often occurs in epidemics originating from a single source of infected meat. In 90%, infections are light, but symptoms usually develop when there are more than 10 larvae per gram of skeletal muscle: they include the classical picture of diffuse myalgia, facial oedema and fever, with an eosinophil leucocytosis. Very heavy infections (up to 5000 larvae per gram of tongue muscle have been observed) result in a myocarditis, pneumonitis and encephalitis, and are sometimes fatal. In one autopsy, James Paget noted more 'creatures (worms) than the whole population of the earth'!

During the invasive stage, biopsy shows a marked myositis, but the infected muscle cell becomes a 'nurse cell' in which the larva (100 × 6 μm) lies coiled up in a hyaline cyst wall (Fig. 25.55) and remains alive for some years before it eventually dies and becomes calcified.

Larva Migrans

Many helminths whose definitive host are lower animals can nevertheless infect man. Their larvae enter the body (see below) and wander locally or systemically, but are unable to mature to adult forms in the wrong host and soon die, causing inflammatory lesions in their wake. Two types of disease result, cutaneous and visceral larva migrans.

Cutaneous larva migrans. The commonest cause is infection with dog hookworm larvae, which penetrate the skin and move in the deep dermis in a serpiginous fashion at a rate of a few centimetres a day, provoking an itchy erythematosus raised reaction – **creeping eruption**. Another parasite group causing cutaneous larva migrans is the bird schistosomes; their cercariae can penetrate human skin and induce an itchy cercarial dermatitis. Outbreaks of this condition have occurred in the UK from swimming in snail-infested gravel pits.

Visceral larva migrans is caused by ingestion of eggs of several species of zoophilic worms, the commonest being *Toxocara*. Adult *Toxocara canis* ascarid worms live in the intestine of dogs in all parts of the world and their eggs are deposited in the faeces. Children acquire visceral larva migrans by ingesting eggs in contaminated soil or food. The larvae are released from the eggs in the gut, penetrate the gut wall, and disseminate by the blood to many organs.

The clinicopathological features depend on the location of the larvae. Pulmonary infection causes cough and dyspnoea, while liver and CNS involvement result respectively in hepatomegaly and focal neurological signs. Fever is common and a marked eosinophil leucocytosis (over 20×10^9/l) is usual. In the tissues, small larvae measuring about 400×20 μm are surrounded by a giant-cell granulomatous reaction with aggregation of eosinophils (Fig. 25.56). The most important manifestation of

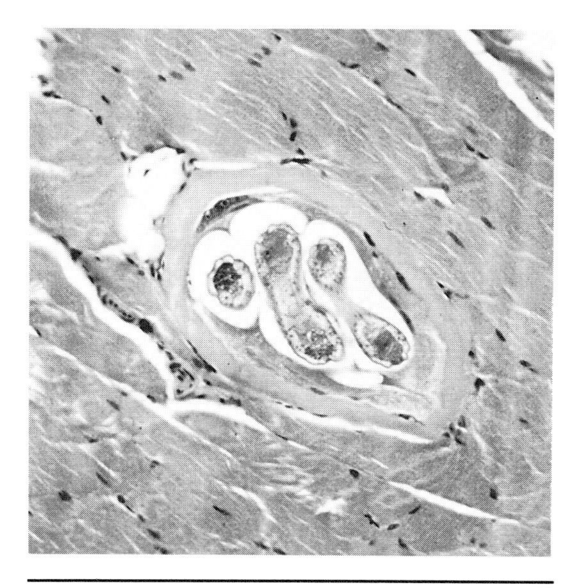

Fig. 25.55 Larva of *Trichinella spiralis* within a skeletal muscle cell ('nurse cell'). A hyaline layer has formed round the coiled parasite. ×200.

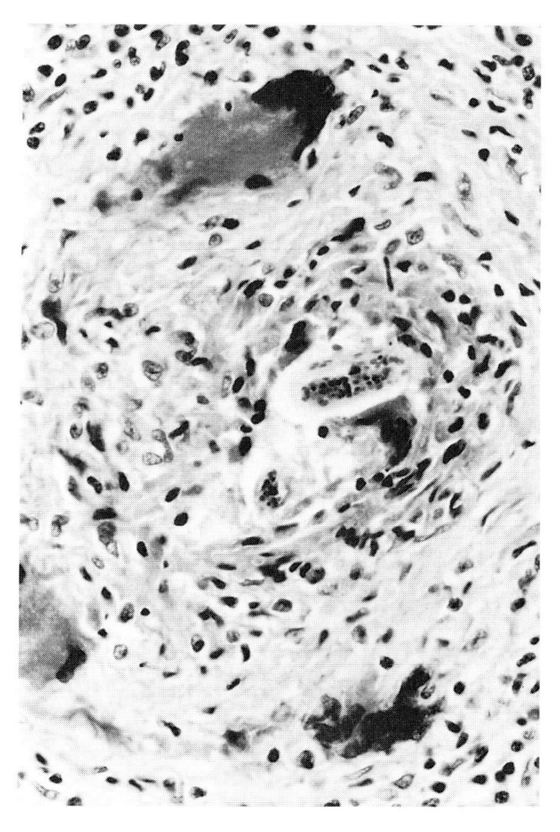

Fig. 25.56 Larva of *Toxocara canis* in a giant-cell granuloma. The fragments of the larva are recognizable by their multiple small nuclei. The lesion was in the pons of a 2-year-old child. ×230. (Section kindly supplied by Dr C. Scholtz, London Hospital Medical College.)

toxocariasis is involvement of the eye, resulting in a granulomatous endophthalmitis which clinically may resemble a retinoblastoma and lead to unnecessary removal of the eye.

Further Reading

Beaver, P. C., Jung, R. C. and Cupp, E. W. (1984). *Clinical Parasitology*. Lea and Febiger, Philadelphia.

Weatherall, D. J., Ledingham, J. G. G. and Warrell, D. A. (1987). Protozoal and helminth infection sections. In *Oxford Textbook of Medicine*, 2nd Edition, pp. 5.446–5.591. Oxford University Press, Oxford.

Index

Note:

Entries in bold, refer to major index key words, though not specifically those key terms in bold in the text. The index is in a letter-by-letter order.

Abbreviations used in sub-entries without clarification:

ADH	antidiuretic hormone
EBV	Epstein–Barr virus
HIV	human immunodeficiency virus
LDL	low density lipoprotein
HTLV-1	human T-cell leukaemia virus